TIETZ FUNDAMENTALS OF

# CLINICAL CHEMISTRY and
# MOLECULAR DIAGNOSTICS

# NINTH EDITION

## TIETZ FUNDAMENTALS OF
# CLINICAL CHEMISTRY and
# MOLECULAR DIAGNOSTICS

**Nader Rifai, PhD**
Professor of Pathology
Harvard Medical School
The Orah S. Platt Chair in Laboratory Medicine
Director of Clinical Chemistry
Boston Children's Hospital
Boston, MA, United States

**Rossa W.K. Chiu, MBBS, PhD, FHKAM, FRCPA**
Professor of Chemical Pathology
Department of Chemical Pathology
The Chinese University of Hong Kong
Hong Kong, China

**Ian Young, MD, FRCP, FRCPath**
Professor of Medicine
Centre for Public Health
Queen's University Belfast
Belfast, United Kingdom

**Carl T. Wittwer, MD, PhD**
Professor Emeritus, Pathology
University of Utah
Salt Lake City, UT, United States

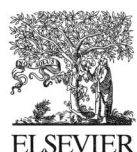

ELSEVIER

Elsevier
3251 Riverport Lane
St. Louis, Missouri 63043

*Content Development Specialist:* Kristen Helm
*Senior Content Strategist:* Kelly Skelton
*Senior Project Manager:* Joanna Souch
*Design Direction:* Ryan Cook

Printed in India

Last digit is the print number:  9  8  7  6  5  4  3  2

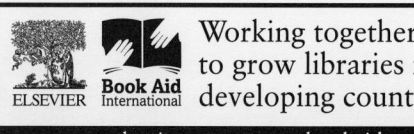

# CONTRIBUTORS

**Aasne K. Aarsand, MD, PhD**
Director
Norwegian Porphyria Centre (NAPOS)
Department of Medical Biochemistry and
Pharmacology
Haukeland University Hospital
Bergen, Norway;
Consultant Medical Biochemist
Norwegian Organization for Quality
Improvement of Laboratory
Examinations
Haraldplass Deaconess Hospital
Bergen, Norway

**Khosrow Adeli, PhD, FCACB, DABCC**
Director
Department of Clinical Biochemistry
The Hospital for Sick Children
Toronto, ON, Canada;
Professor
Department of Clinical Biochemistry
University of Toronto
Toronto, ON, Canada

**David N. Alter, MD MPH**
Associate Professor of Pathology
Department of Pathology and Laboratory
Medicine
Emory University School of Medicine
Atlanta, GA, United States

**Fred S. Apple, PhD**
Medical Staff
Department of Laboratory Medicine and
Pathology
Hennepin Healthcare/Hennepin County
Medical Center
Minneapolis, MN, United States;
Professor
Department of Laboratory Medicine and
Pathology
University of Minnesota
Minneapolis, MN, United States;
Principal Investigator Cardiac Biomarkers
Trials Laboratory (CBTL)
Hennepin Healthcare Research Institute
Minneapolis, MN, United States

**Michael N. Badminton, BSc, MBChB,
PhD, FRCPath**
Professor
Institute for Medical Education
School of Medicine, Cardiff University
Cardiff, Wales, United Kingdom;
Professor
Department of Medical Biochemistry
University Hospital of Wales
Cardiff, Wales, United Kingdom

**Tony Badrick, BAppSc, BSc, BA,
MLitSt, MBA, PhD, PhD, FAACB,
FAIMS, FRCPA (Hon), FACB,
FFScRCPA**
Associate Professor
Faculty of Health Sciences and Medicine
Bond University
Robina, QLD, Australia;
CEO
RCPA Quality Assurance Programs
Sydney, NSW, Australia

**Lindsay A.L. Bazydlo, PhD, DABCC**
Associate Professor
Department of Pathology
University of Virginia
Charlottesville, VA, United States

**Laura K. Bechtel, PhD, DABCC**
Director of Chemistry and Toxicology
Lab Admin
Kaiser Permanente Colorado
Denver, CO, United States

**Marc Berg, MD**
Clinical Professor
Department of Pediatrics
Stanford University
Palo Alto, CA, United States

**Roger L. Bertholf, PhD, DABCC,
FAACC, MASCP**
Medical Director of Clinical Chemistry
Department of Pathology and Genomic
Medicine
Houston Methodist Hospital
Houston, TX, United States;
Professor of Clinical Pathology and
Laboratory Medicine
Weill Cornell Medicine
New York, NY, United States

**Lee M. Blum, PhD, F-ABFT**
Assistant Laboratory Director/Toxicologist
Quality Assurance
NMS Labs, Inc.
Horsham, PA, United States

**Mary Kathryn Bohn, PhD**
Clinical Chemistry Fellow
Department of Laboratory Medicine and
Pathobiology
University of Toronto
Toronto, ON, Canada

**James C. Boyd, MD**
Associate Professor Emeritus
Department of Pathology
University of Virginia Health System
Charlottesville, VA, United States

**Julie A. Braga, MD**
Assistant Professor
Obstetrics and Gynecology
Dartmouth Hitchcock Medical Center
Lebanon, NH, United States

**Jing Cao, PhD, DABCC**
Associate Professor
Department of Pathology
University of Texas Southwestern Medical
Center
Dallas, TX, United States

**Mark A. Cervinski, PhD**
Associate Professor
Department of Pathology and Laboratory
Medicine
The Geisel School of Medicine at
Dartmouth
Hanover, NH, United States;
Director of Clinical Chemistry
Department of Pathology and Laboratory
Medicine
Dartmouth-Hitchcock Medical Center
Lebanon, NH, United States

**Rossa W.K. Chiu, MBBS, PhD,
FHKAM, FRCPA**
Professor of Chemical Pathology
Department of Chemical Pathology
The Chinese University of Hong Kong
Hong Kong, China

**Nigel J. Clarke, BSc (Hons), PhD**
Chief Laboratory Officer and VP R&D
Quest Diagnostics Nichols Institute
San Juan Capistrano, CA, United States

**Timothy J. Cole, BSc(Hons), PhD**
Professor
Department of Biochemistry and
Molecular Biology
Monash University
Melbourne, VIC, Australia

**Andrew R. Crawford, MD**
Assistant Professor of Medicine
Department of Medicine, Endocrinology
Section
Dartmouth-Hitchcock Medical Center
Lebanon, NH, United States

**Michael P. Delaney, BSc, MD, FRCP, LLM**
Department of Renal Medicine
East Kent Hospitals University NHS
    Foundation Trust
Kent, United Kingdom

**Dennis J. Dietzen, PhD, DABCC, FAACC**
Professor
Department of Pathology and
    Immunology
Washington University School of Medicine
St. Louis, MO, United States;
Medical Director
Laboratory Services
St. Louis Children's Hospital
St. Louis, MO, United States

**Leslie Donato, PhD**
Lab Director
Department of Laboratory Medicine and
    Pathology
Mayo Clinic
Rochester, MN, United States

**Graeme Eisenhofer, PhD**
Professor & Chief, Division of Clinical
    Neurochemistry
Institute of Clinical Chemistry &
    Laboratory Medicine
Department of Medicine III
Faculty of Medicine Technische
Universität Dresden
Dresden, Germany

**Christina Ellervik, MD, PhD, DMSci**
Associate Medical Director
Department of Laboratory Medicine
Boston Children's Hospital
Boston, MA, United States;
Professor
Department of Clinical Medicine
Faculty of Health and Medical Sciences
University of Copenhagen
Copenhagen, Denmark;
Assistant Professor
Department of Pathology
Harvard Medical School
Boston, MA, United States

**Jonathan R. Genzen, MD, PhD**
Associate Professor
Department of Pathology
University of Utah
Salt Lake City, UT, United States;
Chief Operating Officer
ARUP Laboratories
Salt Lake City, UT, United States

**David S. Hage, PhD**
Hewett University Professor
Chemistry Department
University of Nebraska
Lincoln, NE, United States

**David John Halsall, PhD**
Department of Blood Sciences
Cambridge University Hospitals NHS Trust
Cambridge, United Kingdom

**Victoria Higgins, PhD**
Clinical Chemist
Medical Affairs
DynaLIFE Medical Labs
Edmonton, AB, Canada;
Clinical Lecturer
Department of Laboratory Medicine and
    Pathobiology
University of Alberta
Edmonton, AB, Canada

**Daniel T. Holmes, BSc, MD, FRCPC**
Clinical Professor
Department of Pathology and Laboratory
    Medicine
University of British Columbia
Vancouver, BC, Canada;
Department Head and Medical Director
Department of Pathology and Laboratory
    Medicine
St. Paul's Hospital
Vancouver, BC, Canada

**Christopher P. Holstege, MD**
Professor
Department of Emergency Medicine &
    Pediatrics
University of Virginia School of Medicine
Charlottesville, VA, United States;
Chief
Division of Medical Toxicology
University of Virginia School of Medicine
Charlottesville, VA, United States;
Director
Blue Ridge Poison Center
University of Virginia Health
Charlottesville, VA, United States

**John Greg Howe, PhD, FABMG, DABCC**
Professor
Department of Laboratory Medicine
Yale University School of Medicine
New Haven, CT, United States

**Ilenia Infusino, MD**
Research Centre for Metrological
    Traceability in Laboratory Medicine
    (CIRME)
University of Milan
Milan, Italy

**Allan S. Jaffe, MD**
Professor
Department of Medicine/Cardiology
Mayo Clinic
Rochester, MN, United States;
Professor
Department of Laboratory Medicine and
    Pathology
Mayo Clinic
Rochester, MN, United States;
Wayne and Kathryn Preisel Professor of
    Cardiovascular Disease Research
Department of Medicine/Cardiology
Mayo Clinic
Rochester, MN, United States

**Graham R.D. Jones, MBBS, BSc(med), DPhil**
Chemical Pathology, Sydpath
St Vincent's Hospital
Darlinghurst, NSW, Australia;
Conjoint Associate Professor
Faculty of Medicine
University of New South Wales
Kensington, NSW, Australia

**Patricia M. Jones, PhD, DABCC, FAACC**
Professor
Department of Pathology
UT Southwestern Medical Center
Dallas, TX, United States;
Clinical Director, Chemistry
Department of Pathology
Children's Medical Center
Dallas, TX, United States

**Peter A. Kavsak, PhD**
Professor
Department of Pathology and Molecular
    Medicine
McMaster University
Hamilton, ON, Canada;
Clinical Chemist
Department of Laboratory Medicine
Hamilton Health Sciences
Hamilton, ON, Canada

**Mark D. Kellogg, PhD**
Director of Quality Programs
Department of Laboratory Medicine
Boston Children's Hospital
Boston, MA, United States;
Assistant Professor of Pathology
Harvard Medical School
Boston, MA, United States

**Mark M. Kushnir, PhD**
Scientific Director, Mass Spectrometry R&D
ARUP Institute for Clinical &
    Experimental Pathology
ARUP Laboratories
Salt Lake City, UT, United States;
Adjunct Professor
Department of Pathology
University of Utah
Salt Lake City, UT, United States

**Edmund J. Lamb, BSc, MSc, PhD, FRCPath**
Clinical Director of Pathology and
    Consultant Clinical Scientist
Department of Pathology
East Kent Hospitals University NHS
    Foundation Trust
Kent, United Kingdom

**James P. Landers, BS, PhD**
Professor
Department of Chemistry
University of Virginia
Charlottesville, VA, United States

**Loralie Langman, PhD**
Professor
Department of Laboratory Medicine and
    Pathology
Mayo Clinic College of Medicine
Rochester, MN, United States

**Kristian Linnet, MD, DMSc**
Professor
Department of Forensic Chemistry
University of Copenhagen
Copenhagen, Denmark

**Dennis Lo, DM, DPhil**
Li Ka Shing Professor of Medicine
Department of Chemical Pathology
The Chinese University of Hong Kong
Shatin, New Territories
Hong Kong, China

**Stanley Lo, PhD**
Professor of Pathology
Department of Pathology
Medical College of Wisconsin
Milwaukee, WI, United States;
Associate Director Clinical Laboratories
Department of Pathology and Laboratory
    Medicine
Children's Wisconsin
Milwaukee, WI, United States

**Nicola Longo, MD, PhD**
Professor
Department of Pediatrics, Pathology,
    Nutrition and Integrative Physiology
University of Utah
Salt Lake City, UT, United States

**Christopher McCudden, PhD**
Associate Professor
Department of Pathology and Laboratory
    Medicine
University of Ottawa
Ottawa, ON, Canada

**Gwendolyn A. McMillin, PhD**
Professor
Department of Pathology
University of Utah
Salt Lake City, UT, United States;
Medical Director
Department of Clinical Toxicology and
    Pharmacogenomics
ARUP Laboratories
Salt Lake City, UT, United States

**Jeffery W. Meeusen, PhD**
Cardiovascular Laboratory Medicine,
    Co-Director
Department of Laboratory Medicine and
    Pathology
Mayo Clinic
Rochester, MN, United States

**Melissa B. Miller, PhD, D(ABMM), F(AAM)**
Professor
Department of Pathology and Laboratory
    Medicine
UNC School of Medicine
Chapel Hill, NC, United States;
Director
Clinical Microbiology and Molecular
    Microbiology Laboratories
UNC Medical Center
Chapel Hill, NC, United States

**W. Greg Miller, PhD**
Professor
Department of Pathology
Virginia Commonwealth University
Richmond, VA, United States;
Co-Director of Clinical Chemistry
Director of Pathology Information
    Systems
Virginia Commonwealth University
    Medical Center
Richmond, VA, United States

**Michael C. Milone, MD, PhD**
Associate Professor
Department of Pathology and Laboratory
    Medicine
Hospital of the University of Pennsylvania
Philadelphia, PA, United States

**Karel G.M. Moons, MD**
Julius Centre for Health Sciences and
    Primary Care
University Medical Center Utrecht
Utrecht University
Utrecht, The Netherlands

**Heba H. Mostafa, MD, PhD, D(ABMM)**
Associate Professor of Pathology, Director
    of Molecular Virology
Department of Pathology
Johns Hopkins School of Medicine
Baltimore, MD, United States

**Robert D. Nerenz, PhD, DABCC**
Associate Professor
Department of Pathology and Laboratory
    Medicine
Medical College of Wisconsin
Milwaukee, WI, United States;
Co-Director of Clinical Chemistry
Department of Pathology and Laboratory
    Medicine
Medical College of Wisconsin
Milwaukee, WI, United States

**Birte Nygaard, MD, PhD**
Associated Professor
Herlev Gentofte Hospital
Department of Internal Medicine
University of Copenhagen
Herlev, Denmark

**Prasad V.A. Pamidi, PhD**
Senior Director of Sensor and Reagent
    Development
Acute Care Dx R&D
Werfen
Bedford, MA, United States

**Mauro Panteghini, MD**
Full Professor of Clinical Biochemistry
    and Clinical Molecular Biology
Department of Biomedical and Clinical
    Sciences
University of Milan
Milan, Italy

**Jason Y. Park, MD, PhD**
Professor
Department of Pathology
University of Texas Southwestern Medical
    Center
Dallas, TX, United States

**Marzia Pasquali, PhD, FACMG**
Professor
Department of Pathology
University of Utah/ARUP Laboratories
Salt Lake City, UT, United States

**Khushbu Patel, PhD, DABCC**
Assistant Professor
Department of Pathology and Laboratory
    Medicine
University of Pennsylvania
Philadelphia, PA, United States;
Clinical Director, Chemistry and Point-
    of-Care
Department of Pathology and Laboratory
    Medicine
Children's Hospital of Philadelphia
Philadelphia, PA, United States

**Tahir Pillay, MBChB, PhD (Cantab), FRCPath(Lon)**
Professor of Chemical Pathology
Department of Chemical Pathology
University of Pretoria
Pretoria, Gauteng, South Africa;
Chief Specialist
Department of Chemical Pathology
National Health Laboratory Service
Pretoria, Gauteng, South Africa

**Victoria M. Pratt, PhD, FACMG**
Director, Scientific Affairs for
    Pharmacogenetics
Agena Bioscience
San Diego, CA, United States

**Alan T. Remaley, MD, PhD**
Senior Investigator
National Institutes of Health
National Heart, Lung, and Blood Institute
Bethesda, MD, United States

**Nader Rifai, PhD**
Professor of Pathology
Department of Pathology
Harvard Medical School
Boston, MA, United States;
The Orah S. Platt Chair in Laboratory
    Medicine
Boston Children's Hospital
Boston, MA, United States;
Director of Clinical Chemistry
Department of Laboratory Medicine
Boston Children's Hospital
Boston, MA, United States

**Alan L. Rockwood, PhD, DABCC**
President
Rockwood Scientific Consulting
Salt Lake City, UT, United States;
Professor (Clinical) Emeritus
Department of Pathology
University of Utah School of Medicine
Salt Lake City, UT, United States

**Thomas G. Rosano, PhD**
Division Head of Laboratory Medicine
Director of Clinical Chemistry
Professor of Pathology and Laboratory
    Medicine
Albany Medical Center
Albany, NY, United States

**William Rosenberg, MA, MB, BS, DPhil, FRCP**
Peter Scheuer Chair of Liver Diseases
Institute for Liver and Digestive Health
Division of Medicine
University College London
London, United Kingdom

**David B. Sacks, MB, ChB, FRCPath**
Adjunct Professor
Department of Medicine
Georgetown University
Washington, DC, United States;
Clinical Professor
Department of Pathology
George Washington University
Washington, DC, United States;
Senior Investigator
Department of Laboratory Medicine
National Institutes of Health
Bethesda, MD, United States;
Honorary Professor
Department of Clinical Laboratory Sciences
University of Cape Town
Cape Town, South Africa

**Sverre Sandberg, MD, PhD**
Director
Norwegian Organisation for Quality
    Improvement of Laboratory
    Examinations, Noklus
Haraldsplass Deaconess Hospital
Bergen, Norway;
Professor
Institute of Public Health and Primary
    Health Care
University of Bergen
Bergen, Norway;
Director
Norwegian Porphyria Centre
Haukeland University Hospital
Bergen, Norway

**Caroline Schmitt, PharmD, PhD**
Associate Professor
Department of Biochemistry and
    Molecular Biology
Université de Paris
Paris, France;
French Centre of Porphyrias
Louis Mourier Hospital
Assistance Publique-Hôpitaux de Paris
Colombes, France

**Leslie M. Shaw, BS, PhD**
Professor
Department of Pathology and Laboratory
    Medicine
Perelman School of Medicine
University of Pennsylvania
Philadelphia, PA, United States;
Director Toxicology Laboratory
Department of Pathology and Laboratory
    Medicine
Perelman School of Medicine
University of Pennsylvania
Philadelphia, PA, United States;
Director, Biomarker Research Laboratory
Department of Pathology and Laboratory
    Medicine
Perelman School of Medicine
University of Pennsylvania
Philadelphia, PA, United States

**Roy A. Sherwood, BSc, MSc, DPhil**
Professor of Clinical Biochemistry
Department of Clinical Biochemistry
King's College London
London, United Kingdom

**Ana-Maria Simundic, PhD**
Head of Department
Department of Medical Laboratory
    Diagnostics
University Hospital Sveti Duh
Zagreb, Croatia;
Professor
Department of Medical Biochemistry and
    Hematology
Faculty of Pharmacy and Biochemistry
University of Zagreb
Zagreb, Croatia

**Ravinder Sodi, PhD, DIC, FRCPath, CSci, EUSpLM**
Department of Biochemistry
Broomfield Hospital
Mid & South Essex NHS Trust
Chelmsford, United Kingdom

**Frederick G. Strathmann, PhD, MBA, DABCC (CC, TC)**
SVP US Business
MOBILion Systems
Chadds Ford, PA, United States

**Catharine Sturgeon, BSc, PhD**
Department of Laboratory Medicine
Royal Infirmary of Edinburgh
Edinburgh, United Kingdom

**Dorine W. Swinkels, MD, PhD**
Professor of Experimental Clinical
    Chemistry
Department of Laboratory Medicine
Radboud University Medical Center
Nijmegen, The Netherlands;
Sanquin Blood Bank
Amsterdam, The Netherlands

**Sudeep Tanwar, MBBS, MRCP, PhD**
Department of Gastroenterology
Barts Health NHS Trust
London, United Kingdom

**Mia Wadelius, MD, PhD**
Professor
Department of Medical Sciences, Clinical
    Pharmacogenomics
Uppsala University
Uppsala, Sweden;
Senior Physician
Department of Clinical Pharmacology
Uppsala University Hospital
Uppsala, Sweden

**Natalie E. Walsham, MBiochem, MSc,
DipRCPath**
Consultant Clinical Scientist
Department of Biochemistry
Dartford and Gravesham NHS Trust
Kent, United Kingdom

**Ping Wang, PhD**
Professor of Pathology and Laboratory
    Medicine
Department of Pathology and Laboratory
    Medicine
University of Pennsylvania
Philadelphia, PA, United States;
Director of Clinical Chemistry and Core
    Laboratory
Hospital of the University of Pennsylvania
Philadelphia, PA, United States

**Maria Alice V. Willrich, PhD, DABCC,
FAACC**
Associate Professor of Laboratory
    Medicine and Pathology
Department of Laboratory Medicine and
    Pathology
Mayo Clinic
Rochester, MN, United States

**Carl T. Wittwer, MD, PhD**
Professor Emeritus
Department of Pathology
University of Utah
Salt Lake City, UT, United States

**Ian Young, MD, FRCP, FRCPath**
Professor of Medicine
Centre for Public Health
Queen's University Belfast
Belfast, United Kingdom

**Stefan Zimmerman, MD**
Head of Division Bacteriology
Department of Infectious Diseases
University Hospital Heidelberg
Heidelberg, Germany

We are pleased to introduce the ninth edition of *Tietz Fundamentals of Clinical Chemistry and Molecular Diagnostics*. We built on the earlier edition to produce a state-of-the-art product for students, trainees, and practicing clinical laboratory scientists.

Chapters were updated to present the most current and relevant information. We aimed to harmonize the presentation of information among chapters while retaining the personality and unique style of each author, hoping for a readable, educational text.

Unlike most other textbooks, all chapters in this edition were reviewed by two individuals: an associate editor and a senior editor. We believe that these efforts have led to a better product. In addition, we made a concerted effort to create an *international* rather than an *American* product to reflect different practices from around the world; for example, all measurements are presented both in traditional and SI units.

In addition to the print format of *Fundamentals*, a wealth of supplementary educational materials including clinical case studies, biochemical calculations, multiple-choice questions, and references are available on the Elsevier Evolve platform for an enhanced learning experience. In addition, we are pleased to have included over 50 adaptive learning courses to complement the chapters; adaptive learning is the closest to personalized education. A simple registration is required to have access to the courses; readers are strongly encouraged to take advantage of this added resource.

This project has been a true group effort and represents the collective intellect, knowledge, and experience of over 100 international leaders in laboratory medicine. We are in debt not only to the authors and editors of the chapters but also to the contributors of the supplementary materials that greatly enrich the product. We are grateful to Elsevier, and particularly to Kristen Helm, for supporting us throughout this project.

We sincerely hope that this product will be a valuable educational and reference resource for the clinical laboratory scientists' community worldwide.

**Nader Rifai**
**Rossa W.K. Chiu**
**Ian Young**
**Carl T. Wittwer**

# CONTENTS

1

# Clinical Chemistry and Molecular Diagnostics

*Nader Rifai, Rossa W.K. Chiu, Ian Young, and Carl T. Wittwer\**

## OBJECTIVES

1. Define the following terms:
   - Ethics
   - Laboratory medicine
   - Molecular diagnostics
2. List and explain the reasons for performing a laboratory test.
3. Describe the field of laboratory medicine, including subdisciplines, information handling, and ethical issues.
4. Describe the role of the clinical chemist.
5. Describe the possible career paths for the clinical chemist.

6. State the applications of molecular diagnostics in laboratory medicine.
7. List and explain five ethical issues that confront laboratorians; describe the critical importance of maintaining confidentiality in the laboratory.
8. Evaluate a possible confidentiality or conflict of interest issue and determine whether it is an ethics violation.
9. State the roles of authors, editors, reviewers, and publishers in providing high-quality scientific publications.

## KEY WORDS AND DEFINITIONS

**Ethics**  Culturally acceptable and expected attitudes and behavior governing the conduct of an individual or the members of a profession.

**Laboratory medicine**  A component of laboratory science that is involved in the selection, provision, and interpretation of testing of individual specimens for purposes of clinical and health assessments.

**Laboratory testing**  A process conducted in a clinical laboratory to rule in or rule out a diagnosis, to select and monitor disease treatment, to provide a prognosis, to screen for a disease, or to determine the severity of and monitor a physiological disturbance.

**Molecular diagnostics**  Use of molecular biology techniques to predict, prevent, diagnose, and monitor disease, including the selection and optimization of therapies.

According to the definition of the International Federation of Clinical Chemistry and Laboratory Medicine (IFCC), "Clinical Chemistry is the largest subdiscipline of **Laboratory Medicine** which is a multidisciplinary medical and scientific specialty with several interacting subdisciplines, such as hematology, immunology, clinical biochemistry, and others. Through these activities clinical chemists influence the practice of medicine for the benefit of the public."

Clinical laboratories provide in vitro testing of chemical, biochemical, and genetic markers in various fluids or tissues of the human body to screen for a disease, confirm or exclude a diagnosis, help to select or monitor a treatment, or assess prognosis. **Laboratory testing** impacts health care delivery to virtually every patient.

The disciplines of *clinical chemistry* and *molecular diagnostics* elicit different images. For clinical chemistry, one thinks of pH measurements or large chemistry analyzers, whereas molecular diagnostics conjures up the human genome project, companion diagnostics, and personalized and precision medicine. Although clinical chemistry is at the core of laboratory medicine, molecular diagnostics is a more recent but explosive upstart. Clinical chemistry excels in random access testing, but molecular diagnostics has evolved massively parallel methods. On the surface, these disciplines appear clearly different.

However, consider the meaning behind the words that compose "clinical chemistry" and "molecular diagnostics." Chemistry by its very nature is molecular, and the study of molecules is chemistry. There is no difference here. Perhaps the "molecular" in "molecular diagnostics" suggests complex polymers with meaningful sequence, excluding simpler chemicals. DNA and RNA sequences largely define life, and

*The authors gratefully acknowledge the contributions by David E. Bruns, François A. Rousseau, Andrea Rita Horvath, and Carl A. Burtis on which portions of this chapter are based.

powerful technologies for nucleic acids now eclipse those for other complex polymers such as proteins and carbohydrates. In common parlance, molecular diagnostics is dominated by nucleic acids. The words "clinical" and "diagnostics" are also similar, connecting both fields to human disease. "Clinical" is more generic than "diagnostics," but again in common use, "molecular diagnostics" includes not only diagnostics but prognosis and genetic predisposition as well. In each two-word combination, the sum is greater than its parts, with combined meanings evolving to fit needs and interest. We believe that molecular diagnostics is best viewed as a subset of clinical chemistry.

## LOOKING BACK

The examination of body fluids for the diagnosis of disease is certainly not a modern concept. The Greeks noticed before 400 BCE that ants are attracted to "sweet urine." However, laboratory testing was not always appreciated by clinicians; the famous Dublin physician Robert James Graves (1796–1853) once remarked, "Few and scanty, indeed, are the rays of light which chemistry has flung on the vital mysteries," and the pioneer Max Josef von Pettenkofer (1818–1901) stated that clinicians use their chemistry laboratory services only when needed for "luxurious embellishment for a clinical lecture." Such views have changed throughout the years, and laboratory testing has proven to be a useful tool to clinicians who have grown to depend and rely on laboratory testing in the routine management of their patients (Box 1.1).

Although it may be difficult to pinpoint the exact date when the concept of the clinical laboratory was born, an article titled "Hospital Construction" by Francis H. Brown was published in 1861 in the *Boston Medical and Surgical Journal*, the precursor of the *New England Journal of Medicine*. Dr. Brown stated, "[Every hospital should have] a small room at the end of the ward to serve as a general laboratory … necessary small cooking might be accomplished here; dishes and other articles washed, etc.; and it would serve as a general storeroom for brooms, pails, and other articles." Although Baron Justus von Liebig (1803–1873) boasted that his clinical laboratory performed more than 400 tests per annum, the average mid- to large-sized laboratory nowadays performs several million tests yearly: the images presented in Fig. 1.1

depict this striking contrast between the legendary Otto Folin in his biochemistry laboratory at McLean Hospital in Boston in 1905 and the University of Utah Clinical Laboratory/ARUP Laboratories more than a century later.

The term *clinical chemistry* was purportedly coined by Charles Henry Ralfe (1842–1896) of London Hospital when he used it as the title of his 1883 treatise. The first laboratory attached to a hospital was established in 1886 in Munich, Germany, by Hugo Wilhelm von Ziemssen. In the United States the first clinical laboratory was The William Pepper Laboratory of Clinical Medicine, established in 1895 at the University of Pennsylvania in Philadelphia. While there may be some uncertainty about the first hospital laboratory, the concept had become sufficiently well established by the late 1880s to enter popular culture. Arthur Conan Doyle, writing in 1887, set the first meeting of Sherlock Holmes and Dr. Watson in 1881 in the chemical laboratory in St. Bartholomew's Hospital, London, where Holmes had just discovered a reagent which "is precipitated by haemoglobin, and by nothing else" (A Study in Scarlet). Hopefully, the excitement experienced by Holmes at this discovery is still felt by laboratory specialists today.

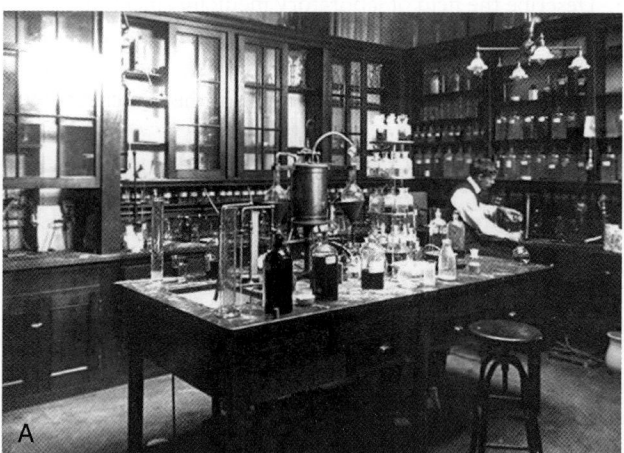

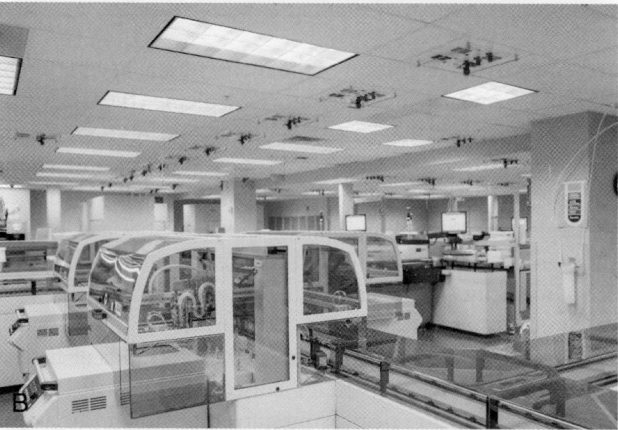

**Fig. 1.1** Early and modern clinical laboratories. (A) The legendary Otto Folin in his biochemistry laboratory at McLean Hospital in Boston in 1905 and (B) the University of Utah Clinical Laboratory/ARUP Laboratories, Salt Lake City, UT, more than a century later. (A, from http://en.wikipedia.org/wiki/File:1905_Otto_Folin_in_biochemistry_lab_at_McLean_Hospital_byAHFolsom_Harvard.png; B, courtesy of ARUP Laboratories.)

---

**BOX 1.1   Uses of Testing in the Clinical Laboratory**

- Confirming a clinical suspicion (which could include making a diagnosis)
- Excluding a diagnosis
- Assisting in selection, optimization, and monitoring of treatment
- Providing a prognosis
- Screening for disease in the absence of clinical signs or symptoms
- Establishing and monitoring the severity of a physiological disturbance

Molecular diagnostics has more recent origins. "Molecular diagnosis" was first mentioned in 1968 as the title of a *New England Journal of Medicine* editorial, commenting on a new inborn error of metabolism that overproduced oxalic acid, resulting in kidney stones. "Molecular" referred to an enzymatic pathway and the substrates, not nucleic acid variants. Twenty years later, additional articles describing "molecular diagnostics" began to appear. In 1986, molecular diagnostics was defined as, "… the detection and quantification of specific genes by nucleic acid hybridization procedures," exemplified by speciation of plant nematodes. In 1987, molecular diagnostics was used to describe mapping of antigenic substances by affinity chromatography using immobilized antibodies. In 1988 the term was used to describe methods for detecting gene amplification and rearrangement using Southern blotting. With the advent of polymerase chain reaction (PCR), the term "molecular diagnostics" became more common, its use doubling in the medical literature every 6 to 7 years. By 1997, commercial real-time PCR instruments solidified "molecular diagnostics" as a branch of clinical chemistry and laboratory medicine. Today, everyone knows about PCR testing for SARS-CoV-2 because of the COVID-19 pandemic.

## EXPANDING BOUNDARIES DEFINED BY TECHNOLOGY

Unlike other specialties in laboratory medicine, clinical chemistry is very much influenced and shaped by technology. No discipline in laboratory medicine uses more technologies than clinical chemistry. Technologies that evolved over time not only changed practice but also remodeled the boundaries of the traditional clinical chemistry laboratory. For example, with the emergence of immunochemical techniques in the 1970s, the US Food and Drug Administration approved many tests for the measurement of proteins, small molecule hormones, and drugs, a development that profoundly changed clinical chemistry and its armamentarium of testing. Integrated automated platforms later enabled the measurement of hormones and therapeutic drugs by immunoassays simultaneously with electrolytes, glucose, and other general chemistry tests, thus subsuming the "endocrine lab" and the "drug lab."

Serologic tests for hepatitis and human immunodeficiency virus (HIV) and tests for autoimmune diseases also moved from their traditional home in microbiology and immunology to chemistry analyzers. Immunoglobulin analysis followed a similar path. The typical clinical chemistry laboratory includes testing for general chemistries, specific proteins and immunoglobulins, therapeutic and abused drugs, blood gases, hormones, biogenic amines, porphyrins, vitamins, and trace elements. Testing for inborn errors of metabolism (such as the measurements of amino acids and organic acids), measurements of coagulation factors, general hematologic testing, and serologic assays can belong either to the clinical chemistry laboratory or to another subspecialty, depending on the institution.

Clinical chemists have embraced technology over the years and used it effectively to derive answers to clinical questions. In modern clinical chemistry laboratories, technologies include spectrophotometry, atomic absorption, flame emission photometry, nephelometry, electrochemical and optical sensor technologies, electrophoresis, and chromatography. The influence of automation, information technology, and miniaturization is evident in current clinical chemistry laboratories. Mass spectrometry, once thought of as a research tool, is playing an ever-growing role in clinical chemistry for the measurement of both small molecules and peptides, and more recently proteins. Point-of-care testing is a disruptive innovation that decentralizes laboratory testing and presents the clinical chemist with many challenges and opportunities.

Molecular diagnostics has forever changed virology and microbiology, introducing faster and more sensitive methods based on nucleic acid amplification rather than microbial replication. Nanotechnology, microfluidics, electrical impedance, reflectance spectroscopy, and time-resolved fluorescence are only a few of the technologies used in point-of-care testing for proteins, drugs, DNA, and analysis of metabolites in small samples of whole blood. Molecular diagnostics in particular impacts diverse specialties, including infectious disease, genetics, and oncology, providing new tools for study at a molecular detail never before considered. In summary, the boundaries of clinical chemistry expand with technology, making the profession vibrant, interesting, and ever evolving.

The scope of the profession is constantly changing for the very same reasons. Scientific and technological developments, medical needs, patient demands, and economic pressures bring various disciplines of medicine closer together, and this integration results in more effective health care. For example, companion diagnostics, which help predict therapeutic responses and individualize patient treatment options, bring together pharmacy and medical laboratories. Point-of-care testing in real time with medical intervention breaks the walls of laboratories to bring the profession closer to clinicians and patients. New disruptive technologies (e.g., "lab on a chip," nanotechnology, home monitoring) as well as movement toward patient empowerment and direct-to-consumer testing bring laboratory testing closer to patients. All of these developments present special challenges to the future generations of laboratory professionals both in terms of how they should be trained and how they will practice.

Technology alone is not the answer to more effective and cost-effective clinical practice. The laboratory data obtained must be meaningful and support clinical management decisions. The generation of more data does not necessarily lead to better patient management and outcomes. In the 1960s and 1970s, with the advent of automated clinical analyzers, laboratories reported chemistry panels of 10 to 20 results. More recently, dense data from expression arrays, genome-wide association studies, epigenomics, and microRNA analyses excel in discovery research, but translation to clinical practice has been slower than anticipated. The promise of greater clinical significance with larger data sets seems intuitive, but history suggests caution. Clinical chemists in this world of "big data" translate high-quality measurement *data* into clinically relevant *information*. This information—when integrated with clinical history and presentation, clinical signs, and an understanding of pathophysiology—becomes *knowledge*. As the data to be integrated become more complex and voluminous, computational algorithms and even artificial intelligence are beginning to add value to this knowledge generation process. Knowledge, in the context of the experience and judgment of the clinician, is converted to *wisdom* that translates to clinical action for improved patient outcomes.

## HOW IS CLINICAL CHEMISTRY PRACTICED?

Although the majority of clinical chemists choose a career in a clinical laboratory environment, many work in the in vitro diagnostics (IVD), pharmaceutical, and most recently biotechnology industries. Clinical chemists, by virtue of their training, are translational researchers who are capable of developing, evaluating, and validating biochemical and genetic assays for clinical use; they develop skills that are essential for new biomarker assays, reagent kits, and companion diagnostics. Clinical chemists also provide interfaces between researchers, clinicians, the clinical laboratory, and the IVD industry to help translate biomarker research into clinically meaningful decisions and actions.

Clinical chemists practicing in the IVD, the biotechnology, or the pharmaceutical industry may not need to routinely interact with clinicians or interpret laboratory results, but they understand and appreciate the clinical utility and relevance of the assays and companion diagnostics they are developing and thus contribute more effectively to the development of diagnostics that improve health. The daily practice of the profession has changed over time. In the 1960s and 1970s, clinical chemists developed laboratory tests. At present, de novo assay development is still active only in certain areas such as chromatography, mass spectrometry, and molecular diagnostics.

However, as the profession matured and the instrumentation changed from open systems to "black boxes," the traditional analytical focus of the profession has significantly diminished. Clinical chemists are now more active in the preanalytical and postanalytical phases of testing and in establishing processes such as how best to select the right test for the right patient and to communicate test results to clinicians and patients in a medically meaningful way, how to build laboratory processes that reduce error, and how to continuously improve the quality of laboratory practices (Box 1.2).

In the current health care environment, there is increasing emphasis on clinical impact and cost effectiveness. Laboratories are expected to demonstrate evidence of improved measurable clinical outcomes and the usefulness and added value of tests to clinical decision making. Proving the fact that laboratory testing contributes to improved patient outcomes is challenging because the relationship between testing and clinical outcomes is mostly indirect. Nevertheless, clinical chemists should move away from being just providers of high-quality data. Transforming laboratory data to information and knowledge

> ### BOX 1.2   Functions of the Laboratory Professional
> - Develop and validate de novo laboratory tests to meet clinical needs.
> - Evaluate and characterize the analytical and clinical performance of laboratory tests.
> - Present laboratory results to clinicians in an effective manner.
> - Provide education and advice on the selection and interpretation of laboratory tests as part of the clinical team.
> - Determine the cost effectiveness and intrinsic value of laboratory tests.
> - Participate in the development of clinical testing algorithms and clinical practice guidelines.
> - Ensure compliance with regulatory requirements.
> - Participate in quality assurance and improvement of the laboratory service.
> - Teach and train future generations of laboratory specialists.
> - Participate in basic or clinical research.

> ### BOX 1.3   Ethical Issues in Clinical Chemistry and Molecular Diagnostics
> - Confidentiality of patient medical information
> - Allocation of resources
> - Codes of conduct
> - Publishing issues
> - Conflicts of interest

requires more skills in information and information management technology, evidence-based medicine, epidemiology, data mining, and translational research. It also requires a shift of thinking from essentialism to consequentialism and from technology-driven to customer-focused and patient-centered laboratory medicine.

To summarize, today's clinical chemists are laboratory professionals who are trained in pathophysiology and technology. The execution of their daily duties, which are more clinically or technology oriented, is influenced by their training (such as MD vs. PhD), interests, institutional needs, and the country where they practice. Clearly the practice of our profession has evolved over the past half a century, and there are even more challenges on the horizon that will expand and change its scope and role and enhance its diversity.

## GUIDING PRINCIPLES OF PRACTICING THE PROFESSION

As in other branches of medicine, practitioners in the clinical laboratory are faced with ethical issues, often on a daily basis; examples are listed in Box 1.3.

## CONFIDENTIALITY OF PATIENT INFORMATION

Safeguarding the confidentiality of patient's personal and medical information is one of the fundamental ethical principles of the practice of medicine. Upholding of these principles prescribes how some laboratory activities are practiced.

The laboratory holds vast amounts of data covering patient's identifiers, demographics as well as health and disease status. The patient's morbid state and future risks for illnesses and death may be described or defined by such information. While laboratory information systems are built to facilitate timely access to the data, the data must be stored in a secure format with measures in place to prevent unwarranted access.

On the other hand, development of new tests requires the use of patient samples and access to patient medical information by the laboratory. Ethical judgments are required regarding the type of informed consent that is needed from patients for use of their samples and clinical information.

Broad coverage genetic testing is becoming more of a routine affair. Prominent in the news in the first and second decades of this millennium has been the issue of confidentiality of genetic information. Legislation was considered necessary to prevent denial of health insurance or employment to people found by DNA testing to be at risk of disease. The power of DNA information lies in its heritability. Predictions can be made on the phenotypes and traits of a person's parents, relatives, and offspring based on an individual's DNA profile. In the event of having identified a clinically significant incidental finding, the right to personal confidentiality against the potential duty to disclose the information to at-risk family members is a current subject of debate among stakeholders. Clinical laboratory professionals are actively participating in the development of such disclosure and clinical management guidelines that will need to adapt to the changing standards of information disclosure or non-disclosure.

## ALLOCATION OF RESOURCES

Because resources are finite, laboratory professionals must make ethically responsible decisions about allocation of resources. There is often a trade-off between cost and quality. What is best for patients generally? How can the most good be done with the available resources? For laboratorians in business, creative accounting may tarnish the profession if patient care is not kept paramount.

## CODES OF CONDUCT

Most professional organizations publish a code of conduct that requires adherence by their members. For example, the American Association for Clinical Chemistry (AACC) has published ethical guidelines that require AACC members to endorse principles of ethical conduct in their professional activities, including (1) selection and performance of clinical procedures, (2) research and development, (3) teaching, (4) management, (5) administration, and (6) other forms of professional service.

## PUBLISHING ISSUES

Publication of documents having high scientific integrity depends on editors, authors, and reviewers all working in concert in an environment governed by high ethical standards.

Editors are responsible for the overall process, including identifying reviewers, evaluating the reviews and the authors' response to them, and making the final decision of whether to accept or reject a manuscript. Editors are also responsible for establishing policies and procedures to ensure consistency in the editorial process as well as a conflict-of-interest policy for all involved.

Authors are responsible for honest and complete reporting of original data produced in ethically conducted research studies. Practices such as fraud, plagiarism (verbatim, mosaic), and falsification or fabrication of data are unacceptable. Other practices to be avoided include duplicate publication, redundant publication, and inappropriate authorship credit. In addition, ethical policies require that factors that might influence the interpretation of study findings must be revealed, such as the role of the commercial sponsor in the (1) design and conduct of the study, (2) interpretation of results, and (3) preparation of the manuscript.

Reviewers must provide a timely, fair, and impartial assessment of manuscripts. They must maintain confidentiality and never contact the authors until after the publication of the report. Finally, reviewers must excuse themselves from the review process if they perceive a conflict of interest. Most journals now require authors to complete conflict of interest forms and delineate each author's contribution.

## CONFLICTS OF INTEREST

The interrelationships between practitioners in the medical field and commercial suppliers of drugs, devices, and equipment can be positive or negative. Concerns led the National Institutes of Health in 1995 to require official institutional review of financial disclosure by researchers and management in situations when disclosure indicates potential or actual conflicts of interest. In 2009, the Institute of Medicine issued a report that questioned inappropriate relationships between pharmaceutical and device companies and physicians and other health care professionals. Similarly, the relationship between clinical laboratory professionals and manufacturers and providers of diagnostic equipment and supplies can be scrutinized.

As a consequence of these concerns and as a result of the enactment of various laws designed to prevent fraud, abuse, and waste in Medicare, Medicaid, and other health care reimbursement programs, professional organizations that represent manufacturers of IVD and other device and health care companies have published codes of ethics that include gifts and entertainment, consulting arrangements and royalties, reimbursement for testing, education, and donations for charitable and philanthropic purposes.

## WHAT IS IN THIS TEXTBOOK?

In this textbook, we have assembled what is essential to effectively practice clinical chemistry and molecular diagnostics. We begin with introductory chapters that describe the basics of laboratory medicine, including statistics, sample handling, preanalytical processes, reference intervals, and quality control. This is followed by a section on analytical techniques and applications, describing the main methods used in clinical chemistry, including immunoassays, mass spectrometry, and point-of-care testing. Next, all the major analytes are discussed, including enzymes, tumor markers, therapeutic drugs, and toxicology, among many others. This is followed by a section on pathophysiology that covers disease states and malfunction of different organ systems that correlate with abnormal laboratory findings. Finally, our last section is dedicated to molecular diagnostics, perhaps the fastest growing field in clinical chemistry. An appendix tabulates reference intervals for the clinical laboratory. The online version includes clinical cases, podcasts, and biochemical calculations. Our aim is to provide current scientific and practical knowledge to support laboratory professionals with knowledge resources that interface between science and technology on the one hand and the clinician and the patient on the other.

## POINTS TO REMEMBER

- Clinical chemistry is the largest subdiscipline of laboratory medicine, and molecular diagnostics is a subset of clinical chemistry.
- Clinical chemistry is a profession that has been shaped and defined by technology.
- The role of clinical chemists evolved over time from analytically and technology focused to customer and patient centered.
- Clinical chemists are translational researchers who convert laboratory data to clinical knowledge.
- Career paths of clinical chemists are heterogeneous and include work in clinical laboratories and in vitro diagnostics, biotechnology, and pharmaceutical industries.
- Clinical chemists must adhere to guiding principles of practicing the profession, which include maintaining confidentiality of genetic and medical information, using resources appropriately, abiding by codes of conduct, following ethical publishing rules, and managing and disclosing conflict of interest.

## REVIEW QUESTIONS

1. The clinical laboratory discipline that is used most often to assess inherited disease through study of the genome is:
   a. Transfusion services
   b. Clinical chemistry
   c. Molecular diagnostics
   d. Hematology
   e. Clinical microbiology

2. When a practitioner in clinical chemistry has an inappropriate personal relationship with a commercial supplier of chemistry analyzers, there may be a potential issue with:
   a. Publication ethics
   b. Confidentiality
   c. Selection of treatment
   d. Conflict of interest
   e. Lack of transparency

3. "Molecular testing" involves the clinical analysis of:
   a. Atoms and molecules
   b. Nucleic acids
   c. Cellular components of blood
   d. The physical structure of compounds
   e. Posttranslational modification of proteins

4. Which one of the following is not considered an ethical issue facing a clinical laboratorian?
   a. Allocation of resources
   b. Conflicts of interest
   c. Discussion of one's salary
   d. Maintenance of confidentiality
   e. Discussing manuscripts under review

5. With respect to handling of patient information, it is inappropriate to:
   a. Store and keep record of patient identifiers
   b. Publicly disclose without obtaining the patient's consent
   c. Store securely in the laboratory laformation system
   d. Monitor data access by laboratory personnel
   e. Include genetic information

6. Which of the following is not considered part of the role of a journal editor?
   a. Establishing conflict-of-interest policy for editors
   b. Determining the direction of the journal
   c. Being responsible for the integrity of the overall review process
   d. Establishing the subscription price
   e. Developing journal policies

7. Molecular diagnostics
   a. Is as old as clinical chemistry
   b. Focuses on long polymers of carbohydrates
   c. Has a long history of providing multiplex assays that translate to clinical practice
   d. Studies the quantity or sequence of nucleic acids
   e. Is none of the above

8. Manuscript reviewers should do all of the following except:
   a. Excuse themselves if they have a conflict of interest regarding the manuscript
   b. Complete the review in a timely fashion
   c. Contact the author if they have a question
   d. Provide a thorough examination of the manuscript
   e. Provide useful comments to the authors

9. Which of the following statements is not part of the professional role of the clinical laboratory specialist?
   a. Develop and validate de novo laboratory tests to meet clinical needs
   b. Evaluate and characterize the analytical and clinical performance of laboratory tests
   c. Decide the pricing of the test and market laboratory services
   d. Present laboratory results to clinicians in an effective manner
   e. Determine cost-effectiveness and intrinsic value of laboratory tests

## SUGGESTED READINGS

Annesley TM, Boyd JC, Rifai N. Publication ethics: clinical chemistry editorial standards. *Clin Chem.* 2009;55:1–4.

Hallworth MJ, Epner PL, Ebert C, et al. Current evidence and future perspectives on the effective practice of patient-centered laboratory medicine. *Clin Chem.* 2015;61:589–599.

Jassam N, Lake J, Dabrowska M, et al. The European Federation of Clinical Chemistry and Laboratory Medicine syllabus for postgraduate education and training for specialists in laboratory medicine: version 5-2018. *Clin Chem Lab Med.* 2018;56:1846–1863.

McMurray J, Zérah S, Hallworth M, et al. The European Register of Specialists in Clinical Chemistry and Laboratory Medicine: guide to the Register, version 3-2010. *Clin Chem Lab Med.* 2010;48:999–1008.

Rifai N, Annesley T, Boyd J. International year of chemistry 2011: clinical chemistry celebrates. *Clin Chem.* 2010;56(12):1783–1785.

# 2

# Analytical and Clinical Evaluation of Methods

*Kristian Linnet, Karel G.M. Moons, and James C. Boyd*

## OBJECTIVES

1. Define the following:
   - Analytical measurement range
   - Analytical specificity
   - Bias
   - Coefficient of variation
   - Correlation coefficient
   - Difference curve
   - Error model
   - Frequency distribution
   - Gaussian probability distribution
   - Limit of detection
   - Linearity
   - Mean
   - Median
   - Population
   - Precision
   - Random error
   - Random sample
   - Regression analysis
   - Sample
   - Standard deviation
   - Systematic error
   - Student *t* distribution
   - Trueness
   - Uncertainty
2. List and describe three criteria that must be considerations in laboratory method selection, including the specific parameters involved in each criterion.
3. Compare population and sample mean, population parameter and sample statistic, and population standard deviation and sample standard deviation, including a description of each, symbols used to express these, how they are calculated, and the information they provide.
4. State the connection of the following concepts to analytical methods:
   - Accuracy
   - Analytical sensitivity
   - Analytical specificity
   - Calibration
   - Limit of detection
   - Linearity
   - Precision
   - Repeatability
   - Reproducibility
5. List two common approaches used to objectively analyze data in a methods comparison study.
6. Describe the components of a difference plot, including the plot's use in method comparison and how the plot is interpreted.
7. Discuss assessment of error in an objective analysis of data in method comparison, including how error occurrence relates to an assay's performance characteristics, the difference between random and systematic error, what causes error, and how error is evaluated in a difference plot.
8. For the following types of analyses, list the components of the analysis, its application in method comparison, how it is computed, how outliers affect it, and how the results are interpreted:
   - Deming regression
   - Nonparametric regression
   - Ordinary least-squares regression
   - Regression
9. Describe the calibration hierarchy, including the tracing of values of routine clinical chemistry measurements to a primary reference, how the values are obtained, and the methods involved; draw a calibration hierarchy given a specific analyte.
10. Discuss the concept of uncertainty in relation to clinical laboratory results, including the components of the standard uncertainty formula and two ways in which uncertainty is assessed.
11. Given appropriate values, state the formula and calculate the following:
    - Coefficient of variation
    - Coefficient of variation percent
    - Deming regression
    - Linear regression
    - Population mean
    - Precision analyses
    - Standard deviation
    - Standard uncertainty
    - Likelihood ratio
    - Odds ratio
    - Predictive value
    - Prevalence
    - Receiver operating characteristic curve
    - Sensitivity
    - Specificity
    - True/false positive
    - True/false negative

12. State the formulas for and calculate, given appropriate information, the following: sensitivity, specificity, predictive value for positive/negative tests (posterior probabilities), odds ratio, and positive/negative likelihood ratio.
13. State the relationship between high sensitivity and false negatives; state the relationship between high specificity and false positives.
14. Compare dichotomous and continuous tests; include definition, sensitivity/specificity, and a clinical example of each type of test.
15. State how the predictive value of a laboratory test (posterior probability) is affected by prevalence.
16. Construct and interpret a receiver operating characteristic curve using data from a diagnostic test study.
17. Describe the added value of combination testing as it is used in the clinical laboratory; include examples, diagnostic usefulness, and associated problems.

## KEY WORDS AND DEFINITIONS

**Accuracy**  Closeness of agreement of a single measurement with "true value."

**Analyte**  The substance being analyzed in an analytical procedure.

**Analytical measurement range**  The analyte concentration range over which measurements are within the declared tolerances for imprecision and bias; also referred to as *reportable range*.

**Analytical sensitivity**  The ability of an analytical method to assess small variations in the concentration of analyte.

**Analytical specificity**  The ability of an assay procedure to determine specifically the concentration of the target analyte in the presence of potentially interfering substances or factors in the sample matrix.

**Assay comparison**  Comparison of measurements by two methods that is carried out objectively using statistical procedures and graphics displays.

**Bias**  In an analytical method, the difference between the average value and the true value that is expressed numerically and is inversely related to the trueness.

**Calibration**  In relation to analytical methods, a function that describes the relationship between instrument signal and concentration of analyte.

**Coefficient of variation**  Relative standard deviation.

**Commutability**  The equivalence of the mathematical relationships between the results of different measurement procedures for a reference material and for representative samples from healthy and diseased individuals.

**Correlation coefficient**  Measure of association between two variables.

**Deming regression**  Least-squares regression analysis taking measurement errors in both variables into account.

**Difference plot**  A bias plot that shows the dispersion of observed differences between the measurements of two methods as a function of the average concentration of the measurements; also referred to as *Bland-Altman plot*.

**Error model**  A model of the error structure.

**Frequency distribution**  A distribution of the frequency (ordinate) as a function of the variable value (abscissa), that is, a histogram of absolute or relative frequencies.

**Gaussian probability distribution**  Bell-shaped relative frequency distribution described under basic statistics.

**Likelihood ratio**  The probability of occurrence of a specific test value given that the disease is present divided by the probability of the same test value given that the disease was absent.

**Linearity**  Range of values for which there is a linear relationship between concentration and signal.

**Limit of detection**  An assay characteristic defined as the lowest value that significantly exceeds the measurements of a blank sample.

**Matrix**  In relation to analytical methods, the material (human serum, urine, etc.) that contains analytes.

**Mean**  Arithmetic average of variables. See Basic Statistics.

**Median**  Equal to the 50th percentile of a set of variables. See Basic Statistics.

**Negative predictive value**  The proportion of subjects with a negative test who do not have the disease.

**Odds ratio**  The probability of the presence of a specific disease divided by the probability of its absence.

**Ordinary least-squares regression (OLR) analysis**  A method used to estimate the unknown parameters in a linear regression assessment performed to minimize the sum of squared vertical distances between observed responses and responses predicted by linear approximation.

**Population**  In relation to analytical methods, the complete set of all observations that might occur as the result of performing a particular procedure according to specified conditions.

**Positive predictive value**  The proportion of subjects with a positive test who have the disease.

**Precision**  The closeness of agreement between independent results of measurements obtained under stipulated conditions. Usually expressed as the standard deviation.

**Prevalence**  The frequency of disease in the study population examined.

**Random error**  Error that arises from imprecision of measurement of the type that is described by a Gaussian distribution (e.g., caused by pipetting variability, signal variability).

**Random sample**  A random sample from a population is one in which each member has an equal chance of being selected.

**Receiver operating characteristic curve**  A graph of sensitivity versus 1 − specificity for all possible cutoff values of a diagnostic test.

**Reference measurement procedure**  A procedure of highest analytical quality that has been shown to yield values having an uncertainty of measurement commensurate with its intended use, especially in assessing the trueness of other measurement procedures for the same quantity and in characterizing reference materials.

**Regression analysis**  A statistical analysis that compares measurement relations between two analytical methods.

**Repeatability**  Closeness of agreement between results of successive measurements carried out under the same conditions (i.e., corresponding to within-run precision).

**Reproducibility**  Closeness of agreement between results of successive measurements carried out under changed conditions (e.g., corresponding to between-runs precision).

**Sample**  A finite set of variables drawn from an infinite population of variables.

**Sensitivity**  The proportion of subjects with disease who have a positive test result.

**Specificity**  The proportion of subjects without disease who have a negative test result.

**Standard deviation**  Square root of the sum of squared deviations from the mean divided by the number of variables minus one. See under Basic Statistics.

**Student *t* distribution**  Distribution related to the Gaussian distribution given a limited sample size. See under Basic Statistics.

**Systematic error**  Error in measurement that arises from calibration bias or nonspecificity of an assay and, in the course of a number of analyses of the same analyte, remains constant (y-intercept deviation from zero) or varies in a proportional way (slope deviation from unity) based on the analyte concentration.

**Traceability**  In relation to analytical methods, a concept based on a chain of comparisons of measurements that lead to a known reference value done to ensure reasonable agreement between measurements of routine methods.

**Trueness**  A qualitative term that describes the closeness of agreement between the average value obtained from a large series of results of measurements and a true value.

**Uncertainty**  A parameter associated with the result of a measurement that characterizes the dispersion of the values that could reasonably be attributed to the measure; more briefly, uncertainty is a parameter characterizing the range of values within which the value of the quantity being measured is expected to lie.

## ASSAY SELECTION OVERVIEW

The introduction of new or revised laboratory tests, markers, or assays is a common occurrence in the clinical laboratory. Test selection and evaluation are key steps in the process of implementing new measurement procedures (Fig. 2.1).

Evaluation of tests, markers, or assays in the clinical laboratory is influenced strongly by guidelines and accreditation or other regulatory standards. The Clinical and Laboratory Standards Institute (CLSI) has published a series of consensus protocols for clinical chemistry laboratories and manufacturers to follow when evaluating methods (http://www.clsi.org). The International Organization for Standardization (ISO) has also developed several documents related to method evaluation (ISOs). In addition, meeting laboratory accreditation requirements has become an important aspect in most countries. Abbreviations are listed in Box 2.1.

### Analytical Performance Criteria

In evaluation of a laboratory test, (1) trueness (formerly termed accuracy), (2) precision, (3) analytical range, (4) detection limit, and (5) analytical specificity are of prime importance. The sections in this chapter on laboratory test evaluation and comparison contain detailed outlines of these concepts. Estimated test performance parameters should be related to analytical performance specifications that ensure acceptable clinical use of the test and its results. For more details related to the recommended models for setting

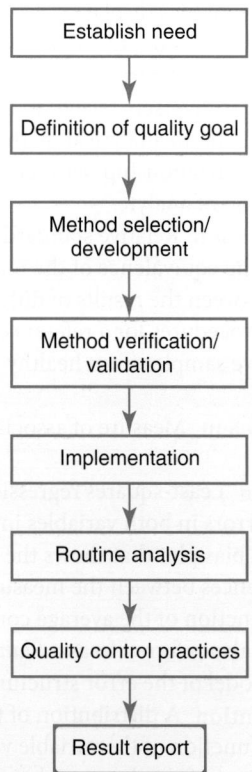

Fig. 2.1 A flow diagram that illustrates the process of introducing a new assay into routine use.

| CI | Confidence interval |
|---|---|
| CV | Coefficient of variation (= SD/$x$, where $x$ is the concentration) |
| CV% | = CV × 100% |
| $CV_A$ | Analytical coefficient of variation |
| $CV_{RB}$ | Sample-related random bias coefficient of variation |
| ISO | International Organization for Standardization |
| OLR | Ordinary least-squares regression analysis |
| SD | Standard deviation |
| SEM | Standard error of the mean $\left(= SD / \sqrt{N}\right)$ |
| $SD_A$ | Analytical standard deviation |
| $SD_{RB}$ | Sample-related random bias standard deviation |
| $x_m$ | Mean |
| $x_{mw}$ | Weighted mean |

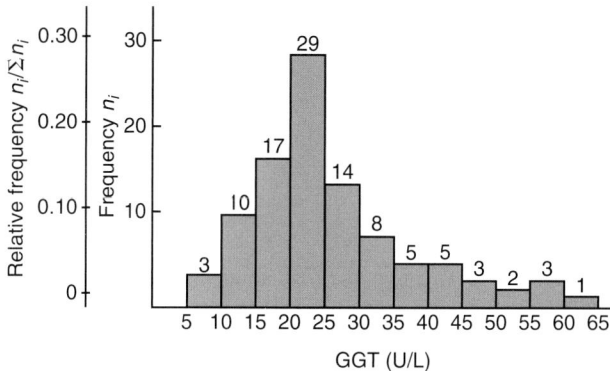

**Fig. 2.2** Frequency distribution of 100 gamma-glutamyltransferase (*GGT*) values.

analytical performance specifications, readers are referred to Chapters 4 and 7. From a practical point of view, the reliable performance of a test in routine use is of importance when used by different operators and with different batches of reagents over long time periods.

## BASIC STATISTICS

In this section, fundamental statistical concepts and techniques are introduced in the context of typical analytical investigations. The basic concepts of (1) populations, (2) samples, (3) parameters, (4) statistics, and (5) probability distributions are defined and illustrated. Two important probability distributions—Gaussian and Student *t*—are introduced and discussed.

### Frequency Distribution

A graphical device for displaying a large set of laboratory test results is the **frequency distribution**, also called a *histogram*. Fig. 2.2 shows a frequency distribution displaying the results of serum gamma-glutamyltransferase (GGT) measurements of 100 apparently healthy 20- to 29-year-old men. The frequency distribution is constructed by dividing the measurement scale into cells of equal width; counting the number, $n_i$, of values that fall within each cell; and drawing a rectangle above each cell whose area (and height because the cell widths are all equal) is proportional to $n_i$. In this example, the selected cells were 5 to 9, 10 to 14, 15 to 19, 20 to 24, 25 to 29, and so on, with 60 to 64 being the last cell (range of values, 5 to 64 U/L). The ordinate axis of the frequency distribution gives the number of values falling within each cell. When this number is divided by the total number of values in the data set, the relative frequency in each cell is obtained.

Often, the position of the value for an individual within a distribution of values is useful medically. The *nonparametric* approach can be used to determine directly the *percentile* of a given subject. Having ranked $N$ subjects according to their values, the *n*-percentile, $Perc_n$, may be estimated as the value of the $[N(n/100) + 0.5]$ ordered observation. In the case of a

non-integer value, interpolation is carried out between neighbor values. The 50th percentile is the median of the distribution.

### Population and Sample

It is useful to obtain information and draw conclusions about the characteristics of the test results for one or more target populations. In the GGT example, interest is focused on the location and spread of the population of GGT values for 20- to 29-year-old healthy men. Thus, a working definition of a **population** is the complete set of all observations that might occur as a result of performing a particular procedure according to specified conditions.

Most target populations of interest in clinical chemistry are in principle very large (millions of individuals) and so are impossible to study in their entirety. Usually, a subgroup of observations is taken from the population as a basis for forming conclusions about population characteristics. The group of observations that has been selected from the population is called a **sample**. For example, the 100 GGT values make up a sample from a respective target population. However, a sample is used to study the characteristics of a population only if it has been properly selected. For instance, if the analyst is interested in the population of GGT values over various lots of materials and some time period, the sample must be selected to be representative of these factors, as well as of age, sex, and health factors of the individuals in the targeted population. Consequently, an exact specification of the target population(s) is necessary before a plan for obtaining the sample(s) can be designed. In this chapter, a sample is also used as a specimen, depending on the context.

### Probability and Probability Distributions

Consider again the frequency distribution in Fig. 2.2. In addition to the general location and spread of the GGT determinations, other useful information can be easily extracted from this frequency distribution. For instance, 96% (96 of 100) of the determinations are less than 55 U/L, and 91% (91 of 100) are greater than or equal to 10 but less than 50 U/L. Because the cell interval is 5 U/L in this example, statements such as these can be made only to the nearest 5 U/L. A larger sample

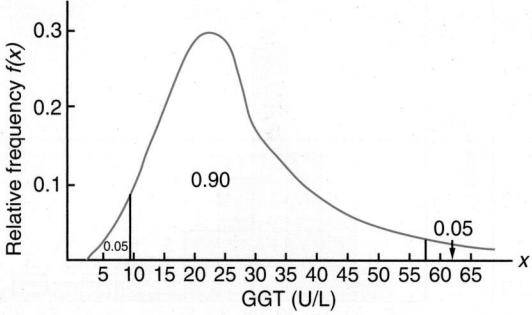

Fig. 2.3 Population frequency distribution of gamma-glutamyltransferase (GGT) values.

would allow a smaller cell interval and more refined statements. For a sufficiently large sample, the cell interval can be made so small that the frequency distribution can be approximated by a continuous, smooth curve, similar to that shown in Fig. 2.3. In fact, if the sample is large enough, this can be considered a close representation of the "true" target *population frequency distribution*. In general, the functional form of the population frequency distribution curve of a variable $x$ is denoted by $f(x)$.

The population frequency distribution allows us to make probability statements about the GGT of a randomly selected member of the population of healthy 20- to 29-year-old men. For example, the probability $\Pr(x_a < x < x_b)$ that the GGT value $x$ is greater than $x_a$ but less than $x_b$ is equal to the area under the population frequency distribution between $x_a$ and $x_b$. For example, if $x_a = 9$ and $x_b = 58$, then from Fig. 2.3, $\Pr(9 < x < 58) = 0.90$. Because the population frequency distribution provides all information related to probabilities of a randomly selected member of the population, it is called the probability distribution of the population. Although the true probability distribution is never exactly known in practice, it can be approximated with a large sample of observations (test results).

## Parameters: Descriptive Measures of a Population

Any population of values can be described by measures of its characteristics. A *parameter* is a constant that describes some particular characteristic of a population. Although most populations of interest in analytical work are infinite in size, for the following definitions, the population will be considered to be of finite size $N$, where $N$ is very large.

One important characteristic of a population is its *central location*. The parameter most commonly used to describe the central location of a population of $N$ values is the *population mean* ($\mu$):

$$\mu = \frac{\sum x_i}{N}$$

An alternative parameter that indicates the central tendency of a population is the median, which is defined as the 50th percentile, $\mathrm{Perc}_{50}$.

Another important characteristic is the *dispersion* of values about the population mean. A parameter very useful in

describing this dispersion of a population of $N$ values is the *population variance* $\sigma^2$ (sigma squared):

$$\sigma^2 = \frac{\sum (x_i - \mu)^2}{N}$$

The *population standard deviation (SD)* $\sigma$, the positive square root of the population variance, is a parameter frequently used to describe the population dispersion in the same units (e.g., mg/dL) as the population values. For a Gaussian distribution, 95% of the population of values are located within the mean $\pm 1.96\ \sigma$. If a distribution is non-Gaussian (e.g., asymmetric), an alternative measure of dispersion based on the percentiles may be more appropriate, such as the distance between the 25th and 75th percentiles (the interquartile interval).

## Statistics: Descriptive Measures of the Sample

As noted earlier, clinical chemists usually have at hand only a sample of observations (i.e., test results) from the overarching targeted population. A *statistic* is a value calculated from the observations in a sample to estimate a particular characteristic of the target population. As introduced earlier, the sample mean $x_m$ is the arithmetical average of a sample, which is an estimate of $\mu$. Likewise, the sample **standard deviation** (SD) is an estimate of $\sigma$, and the **coefficient of variation** (CV) is the ratio of the SD to the mean multiplied by 100%. The equations used to calculate $x_m$, SD, and CV, respectively, are as follows:

$$x_m = \frac{\sum x_i}{N}$$

$$SD = \frac{\sqrt{\sum (x_i - x_m)^2}}{N-1} = \frac{\sqrt{\sum x_i^2 - \frac{\left(\sum x_i\right)^2}{N}}}{N-1}$$

$$CV = \frac{SD}{x_m} \times 100\,\%$$

where $x_i$ is an individual measurement and $N$ is the number of sample measurements.

The SD is an estimate of the dispersion of the distribution. In addition, from the SD, an estimate of the uncertainty of $x_m$ can be derived as an estimate of $\mu$ (see later discussion).

## Random Sampling

A random sample of individuals from a target population is one in which each member of the population has an equal chance of being selected. A **random sample** is one in which each member of the sample can be considered to be a random selection from the target population. Although much of statistical analysis and interpretation depends on the assumption of a random sample from some population, actual data collection often does not satisfy this assumption. In particular, for sequentially generated data, it is often true that observations adjacent to each other tend to be more alike than observations separated in time.

## Gaussian Probability Distribution

The **Gaussian probability distribution**, illustrated in Fig. 2.4, is of fundamental importance in statistics for several reasons. As mentioned earlier, a particular test result $x$ will not usually be equal to the true value $\mu$ of the specimen being measured. Rather, associated with this particular test result $x$ will be a particular measurement error $\varepsilon = x - \mu$, which is the result of many contributing sources of error. Pure measurement errors tend to follow a probability distribution similar to that shown in Fig. 2.4, where the errors are symmetrically distributed, with smaller errors occurring more frequently than larger ones, and with an expected value of 0. This important fact is known as the central limit effect for distribution of errors: if a measurement error $\varepsilon$ is the sum of many independent sources of error, such as $\varepsilon_1$, $\varepsilon_2$, ..., $\varepsilon_k$, several of which are major contributors, the probability distribution of the measurement error $\varepsilon$ will tend to be Gaussian as the number of sources of error becomes large.

Another reason for the importance of the Gaussian probability distribution is that many statistical procedures are based on the assumption of a Gaussian distribution of values; this approach is commonly referred to as *parametric*. Furthermore, these procedures usually are not seriously invalidated by departures from this assumption. Finally, the magnitude of the uncertainty associated with sample statistics can be ascertained based on the fact that many sample statistics computed from large samples have a Gaussian probability distribution.

The Gaussian probability distribution is completely characterized by its mean $\mu$ and its variance $\sigma^2$. The notation $N(\mu, \sigma^2)$ is often used for the distribution of a variable that is Gaussian with mean $\mu$ and variance $\sigma^2$. Probability statements about a variable $x$ that follows an $N(\mu, \sigma^2)$ distribution are usually made by considering the variable $z$,

$$z = \frac{x - \mu}{\sigma}$$

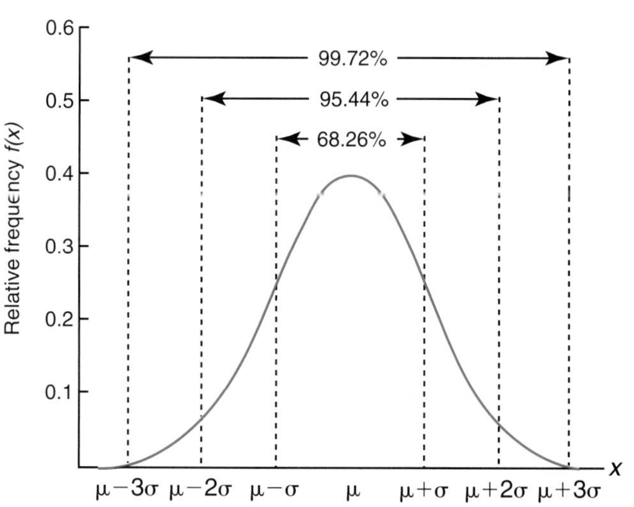

which is called the *standard Gaussian variable*. The variable $z$ has a Gaussian probability distribution with $\mu = 0$ and $\sigma^2 = 1$, that is, $z$ is $N(0, 1)$. The probablility that $x$ is within $2\sigma$ of $\mu$ (i.e., $\Pr(|x - \mu| < 2\sigma) =$) is 0.9544. Most computer spreadsheet programs can calculate probabilities for all values of $z$.

## Student $t$ Probability Distribution

To determine probabilities associated with a Gaussian distribution, it is necessary to know the population SD $\sigma$. In actual practice, $\sigma$ is often unknown, so $z$ cannot be calculated. However, if a random sample can be taken from the Gaussian population, the sample SD can be calculated, by substituting SD for $\sigma$, and computing the value $t$:

$$t = \frac{x - \mu}{\text{SD}}$$

Under these conditions, the variable $t$ has a probability distribution called the **Student t distribution**. The $t$ distribution is a family of distributions depending on the degrees of freedom $v (= N - 1)$ for the sample SD. Several $t$ distributions from this family are shown in Fig. 2.5. When the size of the sample and the degrees of freedom for SD are infinite, there is no uncertainty in SD, so the $t$ distribution is identical to the standard Gaussian distribution. However, when the sample size is small, the uncertainty in SD causes the $t$ distribution to have greater dispersion and heavier tails than the standard Gaussian distribution, as illustrated in Fig. 2.5. At sample sizes above 30, the difference between the $t$ distribution and the Gaussian distribution becomes relatively small and can usually be neglected. Most computer spreadsheet programs can calculate probabilities for all values of $t$, given the degrees of freedom for SD.

The Student $t$ distribution is commonly used in significance tests, such as comparison of sample means, or in testing conducted if a regression slope differs significantly from 1. Descriptions of these tests can be found in statistics textbooks. Another important application is the estimation of confidence intervals (CIs). CIs are intervals that indicate the uncertainty of a given sample estimate. For example, it can be proved that $X_m \pm t_{\text{alpha}}(\text{SD}/N^{0.5})$ provides an approximate 2*alpha*-CI for the mean. A common value for *alpha* is 0.025 or 2.5%, which thus results in a 0.95% or 95% CI. Given sample sizes of 30 or higher, $t_{\text{alpha}}$ is about 2. $(\text{SD}/N^{0.5})$ is called the

Fig. 2.4 The Gaussian probability distribution.

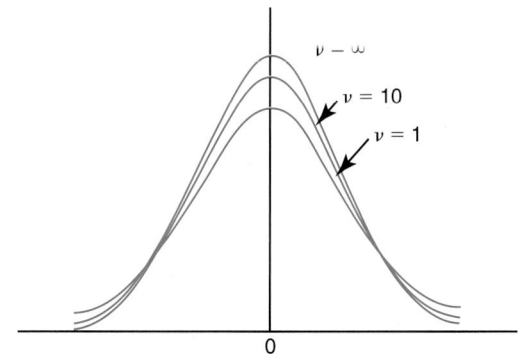

Fig. 2.5 The $t$ distribution for $v = 1$, 10, and $\infty$.

standard error (SE) of the mean. A CI should be interpreted as follows. Suppose a sampling experiment of drawing 30 observations from a Gaussian population of values is repeated 100 times, and in each case, the 95% CI of the mean is calculated as described. Then, in 95% of the drawings, the true mean $\mu$ is included in the 95% CI. According to the central limit theorem, distributions of mean values converge toward the Gaussian distribution irrespective of the primary type of distribution of $x$. This means that the 95% CI is a robust estimate only minimally influenced by deviations from the Gaussian distribution. In the same way, the $t$-test is robust toward deviations from normality.

## Nonparametric Statistics

Distribution-free statistics, often called nonparametric statistics, provide an alternative to parametric statistical procedures that assume data to have Gaussian distributions. For example, distributions of reference values are often skewed and so do not conform to the Gaussian distribution (see Chapter 5 on reference intervals). Formally, to judge whether a distribution is Gaussian or not, a goodness of fit test should be conducted. A commonly used test is the Kolmogorov-Smirnov test, in which the shape of the sample distribution is compared with the shape presumed for a Gaussian distribution. If the difference exceeds a given critical value, the hypothesis of a Gaussian distribution is rejected, and it is then appropriate to apply nonparametric statistics. A special problem is the occurrence of outliers (i.e., single measurements highly deviating from the remaining measurements). Outliers may rely on biological factors and so be of real significance (e.g., in the context of estimating reference intervals) or they may be related to clerical errors. Special tests exist for handling outliers.

Given that a distribution is non-Gaussian, it is appropriate to apply nonparametric descriptive statistics based on the percentile or quantile concept. The $n$-percentile, $Perc_n$, of a sample of $N$ values may be estimated as the value of the $[N (n/100) + 0.5]$ ordered observation. In the case of a noninteger value, interpolation is carried out between neighbor values. The median is the 50th percentile, which is used as a measure of the center of the distribution. For the GGT example, we would order the $N = 100$ values according to size. The median or 50th percentile is then the value of the $[100 (50/100) + 0.5 = 50.5]$ ordered observation (the interpolated value between the 50th and 51st ordered values). The 2.5th and 97.5th percentiles are values of the $[100 (2.5/100) + 0.5 = 3]$ and $[100 (97.5/100) + 0.5 = 98]$ ordered observations, respectively. When a 95% reference interval is estimated, a nonparametric approach is often preferable because many distributions of reference values are asymmetric. Generally, distributions based on the many biological sources of variation are often non-Gaussian compared with distributions of pure measurement errors that usually are Gaussian.

The nonparametric counterpart to the $t$-test is the Mann-Whitney test, which provides a significance test for the difference between median values of the two groups to be compared, given the same shape of the distributions. When there are more than two groups, the Kruskal-Wallis test can be applied.

## Categorical Variables

When dealing with qualitative tests and in the context of evaluating diagnostic testing, categorical variables that only take the value positive or negative come into play. The performance is here given as proportions or percentages, which are proportions multiplied by 100. For example, the **diagnostic sensitivity** of a test is the proportion of diseased subjects who have a positive result. Having tested, for example, 100 patients, 80 might have had a positive test result. The sensitivity then is 0.8% or 80%. Exact estimates of the uncertainty can be derived from the so-called binomial distribution, but for practical purposes, an approximate expression for the 95% CI is usually applied as the estimated proportion $P \pm 2SE$, where the SE in this context is derived as:

$$SE = [P(1 - P) / N]^{0.5}$$

where $P$ is here a proportion and not a percentage. In the example, the SE equals 0.0016 and so the 95% CI is 0.77 to 0.83 or 77% to 83%. The applied approximate formula for the SE is regarded as reasonably valid when $NP$ and $N(1 - P)$ both are equal to or higher than 5.

## TECHNICAL VALIDITY OF ANALYTICAL ASSAYS

This section defines the basic concepts used in this chapter: (1) **calibration**, (2) **trueness** and **accuracy**, (3) precision, (4) linearity, (5) **limit of detection** (LOD), (6) limit of quantification, (7) **specificity**, and (8) others.

### Calibration

The calibration function is the relation between instrument signal $(y)$ and concentration of **analyte** $(x)$, that is,

$$y = f(x)$$

The inverse of this function, also called the measuring function, yields the concentration from response:

$$x = f^{-1}(y)$$

This relationship is established by measurement of samples with known quantities of analyte (calibrators). Solutions of pure chemical standards should be distinguished from samples with known quantities of analyte present in the typical **matrix** that is to be measured (e.g., human serum). The first situation applies typically to a **reference measurement procedure** that is not influenced by matrix effects; the second case corresponds typically to a routine method that often is influenced by matrix components and so preferably is calibrated using the relevant matrix. Calibration functions may be linear or curved and, in the case of immunoassays, may often take a special form (e.g., modeled by the four-parameter logistic curve). An alternative, model-free approach is to

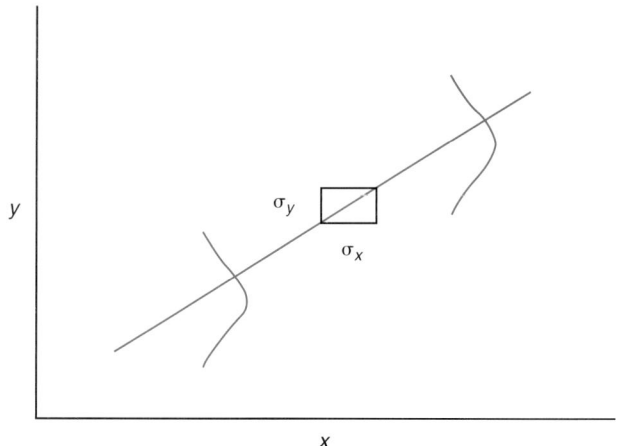

**Fig. 2.6** Relation between concentration (*x*) and signal response (*y*) for a linear calibration function. The dispersion in signal response ($\sigma_y$) is projected onto the *x*-axis and is called assay imprecision [$\sigma_x$ ($=\sigma_A$)].

estimate a smoothed spline curve, which often is performed for immunoassays. If the assumed calibration function does not correctly reflect the true relationship between instrument response and analyte concentration, a **systematic error** or **bias** is likely to be associated with the analytical method.

The precision of the analytical method depends on the stability of the instrument response for a given quantity of analyte. In principle, a random dispersion of instrument signal (vertical direction) at a given true concentration transforms into dispersion on the measurement scale (horizontal direction), as is shown schematically (Fig. 2.6). If the calibration function is linear and the imprecision of the signal response is the same over the analytical measurement range, the analytical SD ($SD_A$) of the method tends to be constant over the analytical measurement range (see Fig. 2.6). If the imprecision increases proportionally to the signal response, the analytical SD of the method tends to increase proportionally to the concentration *(x)*, which means that the *relative* imprecision (CV = SD/*x*) may be constant over the analytical measurement range assuming that the intercept of the calibration line is zero.

## Trueness and Accuracy

Trueness of measurements is defined as closeness of agreement between the average value obtained from a large series of results of measurements and the true value.

The difference between the average value (strictly, the mathematical expectation) and the true value is the *bias*, which is expressed numerically and so is inversely related to the trueness. *Trueness* is a qualitative term that can be expressed, for example, as low, medium, or high. From a theoretical point of view, the exact true value for a clinical sample is not available; instead, an "accepted reference value" is used, which is the "true" value that can be determined in practice. Trueness can be evaluated by comparison of measurements by the new test and by some preselected reference measurement procedure, both on the same sample or individuals.

The ISO has introduced the trueness expression as a replacement for the term *accuracy*, which now has gained a

slightly different meaning. Accuracy is the closeness of agreement between the result of a measurement and a true concentration of the analyte. Accuracy thus is influenced by both bias and imprecision and in this way reflects the total error. Accuracy, which is also a qualitative term, is inversely related to the "uncertainty" of measurement, which can be quantified as described later (Table 2.1).

In relation to trueness, the concepts *recovery*, *drift*, and *carryover* may also be considered. *Recovery* is the fraction or percentage increase in concentration that is measured in relation to the amount added. Recovery experiments are typically carried out in the field of drug analysis. It is useful to distinguish between *extraction recovery*, which often is interpreted as the fraction of compound that is carried through an extraction process, and the recovery measured by the entire analytical procedure, in which the addition of an internal standard compensates for losses in the extraction procedure. A recovery close to 100% is a prerequisite for a high degree of trueness, but it does not ensure unbiased results because possible nonspecificity against matrix components (e.g., an interfering substance) is not detected in a recovery experiment. *Drift* is caused by instrument or reagent instability over time, so that calibration becomes gradually biased. Assay *carryover* also must be close to zero to ensure unbiased results.

## Precision

**Precision** has been defined as the closeness of agreement between independent results of measurements obtained under stipulated conditions. The degree of precision is usually derived from statistical measures of imprecision, such as SD or CV (CV = SD/*x*, where *x* is the measurement concentration), which is inversely related to precision. Imprecision of measurements is solely related to the **random error** of measurements and has no relation to the trueness of measurements.

Precision is specified as follows:

*Repeatability*: **Repeatability** is the closeness of agreement between results of successive measurements carried out under the same conditions (i.e., corresponding to within-run precision).

*Reproducibility*: **Reproducibility** is the closeness of agreement between results of measurements performed under changed conditions of measurements (e.g., time, operators, calibrators, reagent lots). Two specifications of reproducibility are often used: total or between-run precision in the laboratory, often termed *intermediate precision*, and inter-laboratory precision (e.g., as observed in external quality assessment schemes [EQAS]) (see Table 2.1).

The total SD ($\sigma_T$) may be divided into within-run and between-run components using the principle of analysis of variance of components (variance is the squared SD):

$$\sigma_T^2 = \sigma_{\text{Within-run}}^2 + \sigma_{\text{Between-run}}^2$$

In laboratory studies of analytical variation, estimates of imprecision are obtained. It is important to have an adequate number so that analytical variation is not underestimated.

**TABLE 2.1    Overview of Qualitative Terms and Quantitative Measures Related to Method Performance**

| Qualitative Concept | Quantitative Measure |
|---|---|
| **Trueness** | **Bias** |
| Closeness of agreement of mean value with "true value" | A measure of the systematic error |
| **Precision** | **Imprecision (SD)** |
| Repeatability (within run) | A measure of the dispersion of random errors |
| Intermediate precision (long term) | |
| Reproducibility (interlaboratory) | |
| **Accuracy** | **Error of Measurement** |
| Closeness of agreement of a single measurement with "true value" | Comprises both random and systematic influences |

*SD*, Standard deviation.

Commonly, the number 20 is given as a reasonable number of observations (e.g., suggested in the CLSI guideline for manufacturers). To verify method precision by users, it has been recommended to run internal QC samples for 5 consecutive days in five replicates.

To estimate both the within-run imprecision and the total imprecision, a common approach is to measure duplicate control samples in a series of runs. Suppose, for example, that a control is measured in duplicate for 20 runs, in which case 20 observations are present with respect to both components. The dispersion of the means ($x_m$) of the duplicates is given as follows:

$$\sigma 2 = \frac{\sigma_{\text{Within-run}}^2}{2} + \sigma_{\text{Between-run}}^2$$

From the 20 sets of duplicates, the within-run SD can be derived using the following formula:

$$SD_{\text{Within-run}} = \left[ \Sigma \frac{d_i^2}{(2 \times 20)} \right]^{0.5}$$

where $d_i$ refers to the difference between the $i$th set of duplicates. When SDs are estimated, the concept degrees of freedom *(df)* is used. In a simple situation, the number of degrees of freedom equals $N - 1$. For $N$ duplicates, the number of degrees of freedom is $N (2 - 1) = N$. Thus both variance components are derived in this way. The advantage of this approach is that the within-run estimate is based on several runs so that an average estimate is obtained rather than only an estimate for one particular run if all 20 observations had been obtained in the same run.

Generally, the estimate of the imprecision improves as more observations become available. Exact confidence limits for the SD can be derived from the $\chi^2$ distribution. A graphical display of 95% CIs at various sample sizes is shown in Fig. 2.7. For example, suppose we have estimated the imprecision as an SD of 5.0 on the basis of $N = 20$ observations. From the figure, the 95% CI extends from about $0.75 \times 5.0$ to about $1.45 \times 5.0$, that is, from 3.8 to 7.3.

Precision often depends on the concentration of analyte being considered. A presentation of precision as a function of

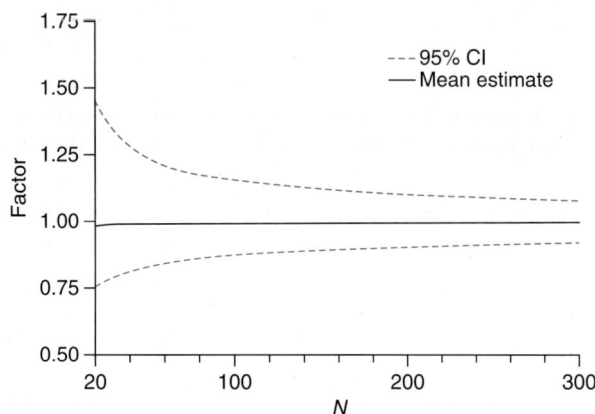

**Fig. 2.7** Relation between factors indicating the 95% confidence intervals *(CIs)* of standard deviations (SDs) and the sample size. The true SD is 1, and the solid line indicates the mean estimate, which is slightly downward biased at small sample sizes.

analyte concentration is the precision profile, which usually is plotted in terms of the SD or the CV as a function of analyte concentration (Fig. 2.8).

## Linearity

Linearity refers to the relationship between measured and expected values over the analytical measurement range. Linearity may be considered in relation to actual or relative analyte concentrations. In the latter case, a dilution series of a sample may be examined. This dilution series examines whether the measured concentration changes as expected according to the proportional relationship between samples introduced by the dilution factor. Dilution is usually carried out with an appropriate sample matrix (e.g., human serum [individual or pooled serum] or a verified sample diluent).

Evaluation of linearity can be performed visually or by statistical tests. When repeated measurements are available at each concentration, the random variation between measurements and the variation around an estimated regression line may be evaluated by an *F*-test. When significant nonlinearity is found, it may be useful to explore nonlinear alternatives to the linear regression line (i.e., polynomials of higher degrees). Another approach is to assess the residuals of an estimated regression line. An additional consideration for evaluating

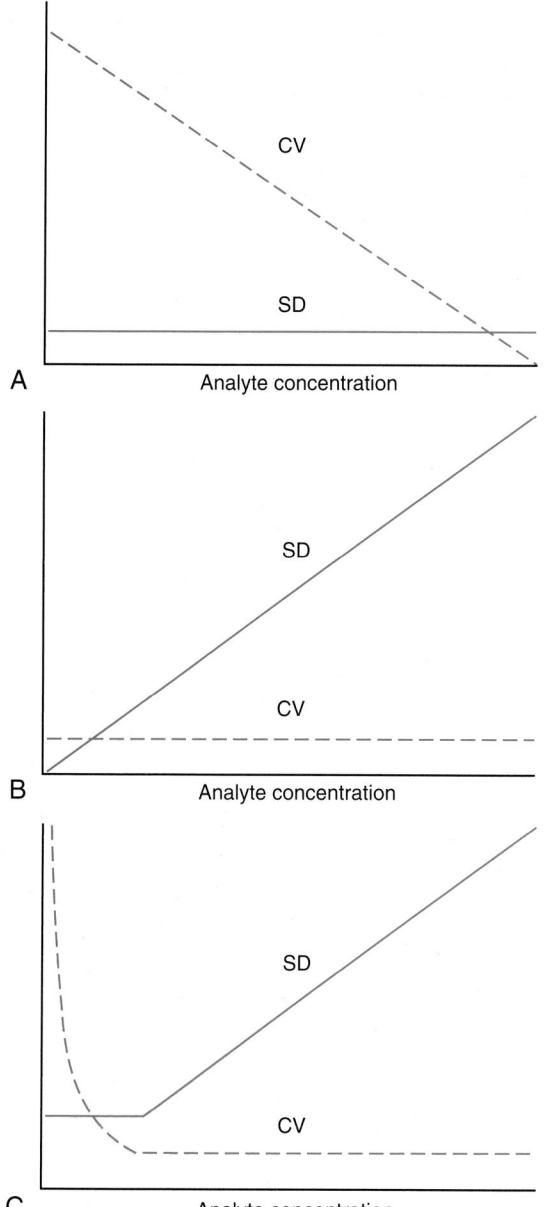

**Fig. 2.8** Relations between analyte concentration and standard deviation *(SD)*/coefficient of variation *(CV)*. (A) The SD is constant, so that the CV varies inversely with the analyte concentration. (B) The CV is constant because of a proportional relationship between concentration and SD. (C) A mixed situation with constant SD in the low range and a proportional relationship in the rest of the analytical measurement range.

proportional concentration relationships is whether an estimated regression line passes through zero or not.

## Analytical Measurement Range and Limits of Quantification

The **analytical measurement range** (measuring interval, reportable range) is the analyte concentration range over which measurements are within the declared tolerances for imprecision and bias of the method. Taking drug assays as an example, there exist (arbitrary) requirements of a CV% of less than 15% and a bias of less than 15%. The measurement range

then extends from the lowest concentration (lower limit of quantification [LLOQ]) to the highest concentration (upper limit of quantification [ULOQ]) for which these performance specifications are fulfilled. The LLOQ is medically important for many analytes, for example, thyroid-stimulating hormone (TSH), where low TSH results are useful for the diagnosis of hyperthyroidism.

The LOD may be defined as the lowest value that significantly exceeds the measurements of a blank sample. Thus the limit has been estimated on the basis of repeated measurements of a blank sample and has been *reported* as the mean plus 2 or 3 SDs of the blank measurements. In the interval from LOD up to LLOQ, a result should be reported as "detected" but not provided as a quantitative result.

The LLOQ of an assay should not be confused with analytical sensitivity. The **analytical sensitivity** is defined as ability of an analytical method to assess small differences in the concentration of analyte. The analytical sensitivity depends on the precision of the method. The smallest difference that will be statistically significant equals $2 \times \sqrt{2} \times SD_A$ at a 5% significance level.

## Analytical Specificity and Interference

**Analytical specificity** is the ability of an assay procedure to determine the concentration of the target analyte without influence from potentially interfering substances or factors in the sample matrix (e.g., hyperlipemia, hemolysis, bilirubin, antibodies, other metabolic molecules, degradation products of the analyte, exogenous substances, anticoagulants).

---

### POINTS TO REMEMBER

- Technical validation of analytical methods focuses on (1) calibration, (2) trueness and accuracy, (3) precision, (4) linearity, (5) LOD, (6) limit of quantification, (7) specificity, and (8) others.
- The difference between the average measured value and the true value is the *bias*, which can be evaluated by comparison of measurements by the new test and by some preselected reference measurement procedure, both on the same sample or individuals.
- The degree of precision is usually expressed on the basis of statistical measures of imprecision, such as SD or CV (CV = SD/*x*, where *x* is the measurement concentration).
- The measurement range extends from the lowest concentration (LLOQ) to the highest concentration (ULOQ) for which the analytical performance specifications (imprecision, bias) are fulfilled.
- Analytical specificity is the ability of an assay procedure to determine the concentration of the target analyte without influence from potentially interfering substances or factors in the sample matrix.

---

## ASSAY COMPARISON

Comparison of measurements by two assays can be carried out by parallel measurements of a set of patient samples. To prevent artificial matrix-induced differences, fresh patient samples are the optimal material. A nearly even distribution of values over the analytical measurement range is also preferable. In an ordinary laboratory, comparison of two routine assays is the most frequently occurring situation. Less commonly, comparison of a routine assay with a reference measurement procedure is undertaken. When two routine assays are compared, it is not possible to establish that one set of measurements is the correct one. Rather, the question is whether the new assay can replace the existing one without a systematic change in result values. To address this question, a statistical procedure with graphics display should be applied. A difference (bias) plot, which shows differences as a function of the average concentration of measurements (Bland-Altman plot), or a **regression analysis.**

## Basic Error Model

The occurrence of measurement errors is related to the performance characteristics of the assay. It is important to distinguish between pure, random measurement errors, which are present in all measurement procedures, and errors related to incorrect calibration and nonspecificity of the assay. Whereas a reference measurement procedure is associated only with pure random error, a routine method, additionally, is likely to have some bias related to errors in calibration and limitations with regard to specificity. Whereas an erroneous calibration function gives rise to a systematic error, nonspecificity gives an error that typically varies from sample to sample. The error related to nonspecificity thus has a random character, but in contrast to the pure measurement error, it cannot be reduced by repeated measurements of a sample. Although errors related to nonspecificity for a group of samples look like random errors, for the individual sample, this type of error is a bias. Because this bias varies from sample to sample, it has been called a *sample-related random bias*. In the following section, the various error components are incorporated into a formal **error model**.

### Measured Value, Target Value, Modified Target Value, and True Value

Taking into account that an analytical method measures analyte concentrations with some random measurement error, it is necessary to distinguish between the actual, measured value and the average result obtained if the given sample was measured an infinite number of times. If the assay is a reference assay without bias and nonspecificity, the following simple relationship holds:

$$x_i = X_{\text{True}i} + \varepsilon_i$$

where $x_i$ represents the measured value, $X_{\text{True}i}$ is the average value for an infinite number of measurements, and $\varepsilon_i$ is the deviation of the measured value from the average value. If the sample was measured repeatedly, the average of $\varepsilon_i$ would be zero and the SD would equal the analytical SD ($\sigma_A$) of the reference measurement procedure. Pure, random measurement error will usually be Gaussian distributed.

In the case of a routine assay, the relationship between the measured value for a sample and the true value becomes more complicated:

$$x_i = X_{\text{True}i} + \text{Cal-Bias} + \text{Random-Bias}_i + \varepsilon_i$$

The *Cal-Bias* term (calibration bias) is a systematic error related to the calibration of the method. This systematic error may be a constant for all measurements corresponding to an offset error, or it may be a function of the analyte concentration (e.g., corresponding to a slope deviation in the case of a linear calibration function). The *Random-Bias*$_i$ term is a bias that is specific for a given sample related to nonspecificity of the method. It may arise because of codetermination of substances that vary in concentration from sample to sample. For example, a chromogenic creatinine method codetermines some other components with creatinine in serum.

The final term in the equation above is the random measurement error term, $\varepsilon_i$. If an infinite number of measurements of a specific sample is performed by the routine method, the random measurement error term $\varepsilon_i$ would be zero. The cal-bias and the random-bias$_i$, however, would be unchanged. Thus the average value of an infinite number of measurements would equal the sum of the true value and these bias terms. This average value may be regarded as the target value ($X_{\text{Target}i}$) of the given sample for the routine method:

$$X_{\text{Target}i} = X_{\text{True}i} + \text{Cal-Bias} + \text{Random-Bias}_i$$

As mentioned, the calibration bias represents a systematic error component in relation to the true values measured by a reference measurement procedure. In the context of regression analysis, this systematic error corresponds to the intercept and the slope deviation from unity when a routine method is compared with a reference measurement procedure (outlined in detail later). It is convenient to introduce a modified target value expression ($X_{\text{Target}i}$) for the routine method to delineate this systematic calibration bias, so that:

$$X_{\text{Target}i} = X_{\text{True}i} + \text{Cal-Bias}$$

Thus, for a set of samples measured by a routine method, the $X_{\text{Target}i}$ values are distributed around the respective $X_{\text{Target}i}$ values with an SD, which is called $\sigma_{\text{RB}}$.

If the assay is a reference method without bias and nonspecificity, the target value and the modified target value equal the true value, that is,

$$X_{\text{Target}i} = X_{\text{Target}i} = X_{\text{True}i}$$

The error model is outlined in Fig. 2.9.

### Calibration Bias and Random Bias

For an individual measurement, the total error is the deviation of $x_i$ from the true value, that is,

$$\text{Total error of } x_i = \text{Cal-Bias} + \text{Random-Bias}_i + \varepsilon_i$$

Estimation of the bias terms requires parallel measurements between the method in question and a reference method. With regard to calibration bias, the possibility of lot-to-lot variation in analytical kit sets should be recognized. Lot-to-lot variation shows up as a calibration bias that changes from lot to lot.

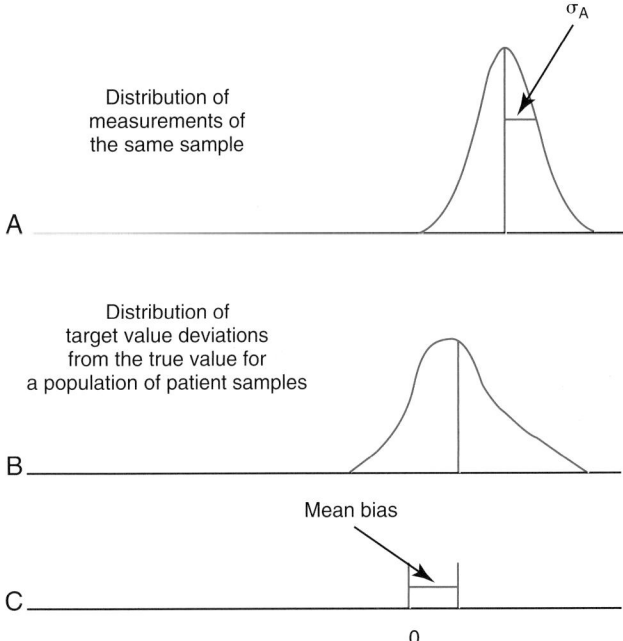

A

B

C

0

**Fig. 2.9** Outline of basic error model for measurements by a routine assay. (A) The distribution of repeated measurements of the *same* sample, representing a normal distribution around the target value ($X_{Target_i}$) *(vertical line)* of the sample with a dispersion corresponding to the analytical standard deviation, $\sigma_A$. (B) Schematic outline of the dispersion of target value deviations from the respective true values for a population of patient samples. A distribution of an arbitrary form is displayed. The standard deviation equals $\sigma_{RB}$. The vertical line indicates the mean of the distribution. (C) The distance from zero to the mean of the target value deviations from the true values represents the calibration bias (mean bias = cal-bias) of the assay.

The previous exposition defines the total error in broader terms than is often seen. A traditional total error expression is:

$$\text{Total error} = \text{Bias} + 2\,\text{SD}_A$$

This is often interpreted as the calibration bias plus 2 $SD_A$. If a one-sided statistical perspective is taken, the expression is modified to Bias + 1.65 $SD_A$, indicating that 5% of results are located outside the limit. Interpreting the bias as identical to the calibration bias may lead to an underestimation of the total error.

Random bias related to sample-specific interferences may take several forms. It may be a regularly occurring additional random error component, perhaps of the same order of magnitude as the analytical error. In this context, it is natural to quantify the error in the form of an SD or CV. The most straightforward procedure is to carry out a method comparison study based on a set of patient samples in which one of the methods is a reference method, as outlined later. Another form of sample-related random interference is more rarely occurring gross errors, which typically are seen in the context of immunoassays and are related to unexpected antibody interactions. Such an error usually shows up as an outlier in method comparison studies. Outliers should be investigated to identify their cause, which may be an important limitation in using a given assay.

## Assay Comparison Data Model

Here we consider the error model described earlier in relation to the method comparison situation. For a given sample measured by two analytical methods, 1 and 2, the following equations apply:

$$x1_i = X1_{Target_i} + \varepsilon1_i = X_{True_i} + \text{Cal-Bias1}$$
$$+ \text{Random-Bias1}_i + \varepsilon1_i$$

$$x2_i = X2_{Target_i} + \varepsilon2_i = X_{True_i} + \text{Cal-Bias2}$$
$$+ \text{Random-Bias2}_i + \varepsilon2_i$$

In the following, some typical situations using this general model are described. First, comparison of a routine assay with a reference measurement procedure will be treated. Second, comparison of two routine assays is considered.

Assuming method 1 is a reference method, the bias components disappear by definition, and the following situation can be described:

$$x1_i = X1_{Target_i} + \varepsilon1_i = X_{True_i} + \varepsilon1_i$$

$$x2_i = X2_{Target_i} + \varepsilon2_i = X_{True_i} + \text{Cal-Bias2}$$
$$+ \text{Random-Bias2}_i + \varepsilon2_i$$

The paired differences become

$$\left(x2_i - x1_i\right) = \text{Cal-Bias2} + \text{Random-Bias2}_i + \left(\varepsilon2_i - \varepsilon1_i\right)$$

We thus have an expression consisting of a systematic error term (calibration bias of method 2) and two random terms. The Random-Bias2 term is distributed around Cal-Bias2 according to an undefined distribution. ($\varepsilon2_i - \varepsilon1_i$) is a difference between two random measurement errors that are independent and, commonly, Gaussian distributed. However, we remind readers that the SD for analytical methods often depends on the concentration, as mentioned earlier. For analytes with a wide analytical measurement range (e.g., some hormones), both sample-related random interferences and analytical SDs are likely to depend on the measurement concentration, often in a roughly proportional manner. It may then be more useful to evaluate the *relative* differences—$(x2_i - x1_i)/[(x2_i + x1_i)/2]$—and accordingly express mean and random bias and analytical error as proportions.

In the comparison of two routine methods, the paired differences become

$$\left(x2_i - x1_i\right) = \left(\text{Cal-Bias2} - \text{Cal-Bias1}\right)$$
$$+ \left(\text{Random-Bias2}_i - \text{Random-Bias1}_i\right)$$
$$+ \left(\varepsilon2_i - \varepsilon1_i\right)$$

The expression again consists of a constant term, the difference between the two calibration biases, and two random terms. The first random term is a difference between two random-bias components that may or may not be independent. If the two field methods are based on the same measurement principle, the random-bias terms are likely to be correlated. For example, two chromogenic methods for creatinine are likely to be subject to interference from the same chromogenic compounds present in a given serum sample. On the other hand, a chromogenic method and an enzymatic creatinine method are subject to different types of interfering compounds, and the random-bias terms may be relatively independent. In the $\varepsilon 2_i - \varepsilon 1_i$ term, the same relationships as described previously are likely to apply. The general form of the expressed differences is the same in the two situations and the same statistical principles apply.

## Planning a Method Comparison Study

Several points require attention, including the (1) number of samples necessary, (2) distribution of analyte concentrations (preferably uniform over the analytical measurement range), and (3) representativeness of the samples. To address the latter point, samples from relevant patient categories should be included, so that possible interference phenomena can be discovered. Practical aspects related to storage and treatment of samples (e.g., container) and possible artifacts induced by storage (e.g., freezing of samples) and addition of anticoagulants should be considered. Comparison of measurements should preferably be undertaken over several days (e.g., at least 5 days) so that the comparison of methods does not become dependent on the performance of the methods in one particular analytical run. The CLSI guideline EP-09-A3, "Method Comparison and Bias Estimation Using Patient Samples," suggests measurement of 40 samples in duplicate by each method when a new method is introduced in the laboratory as a substitute for an established one. Additionally, 100 samples in duplicate is proposed for a vendor of an analytical test system. The EP15 guideline "User Verification of Manufacturer's Claims" suggests a more condensed approach based on a bias or difference plot for 20 samples.

## Difference (Bland-Altman) Plot

The Bland-Altman plot is usually understood as a plot of the differences against the average results of the methods. Thus the **difference plot** in this version provides information on the relation between differences and concentration, which is useful in evaluating whether problems exist at certain ranges (e.g., in the high range) caused by nonlinearity of one of the methods. It may also be of interest to observe whether differences tend to increase proportionally with the concentration or whether they are independent of concentration.

The basic version of the difference plot requires plotting of the differences against the average of the measurements. Fig. 2.10 shows the plot for the drug assay comparison data. The interval ±2 SD of the differences is often delineated around the mean difference. To assess whether the bias is significantly different from zero, the SE of the mean difference is estimated as the SD divided by the square root of the number of paired measurements ($SE = SD/N^{0.5}$) and tested against zero by a $t$-test ($t = [Mean − 0]/SE$).

Nonparametric limits may also be considered. A constant bias over the analytical measurement range changes the average concentration away from zero. The presence of sample-related random interferences increases the width of

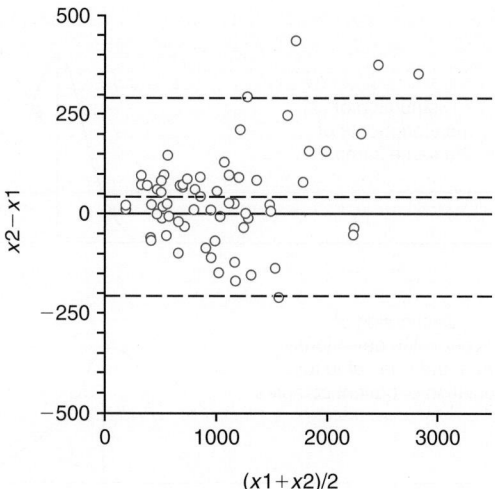

**Fig. 2.10** Bland-Altman plot of differences for the drug comparison example. The differences are plotted against the average concentration. The mean difference (42 nmol/L) with ±2 standard deviation of differences is shown *(dashed lines)*.

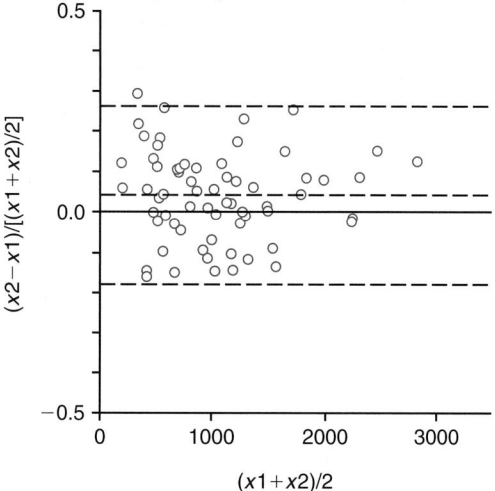

**Fig. 2.11** Bland-Altman plot of *relative* differences for the drug comparison example. The differences are plotted against the average concentration. The mean relative difference (0.042) with ±2 standard deviation of relative differences is shown *(dashed lines)*.

the distribution. If the calibration bias depends on the concentration, if the dispersion varies with the concentration, or if both occur, the relations become more complex, and the interval mean ±2 SD of the differences may not fit very well as a 95% interval throughout the analytical measurement range.

The displayed Bland-Altman plot for the drug assay comparison data (see Fig. 2.10) shows a tendency toward increasing scatter with increasing concentration, which is a reflection of increasing random error with concentration. Thus a plot of the relative differences against the average concentration is of relevance (Fig. 2.11).

## Regression Analysis

Regression analysis has the advantage that it allows the relation between the target values for the two compared methods to be studied over the full analytical measurement range. In linear regression analysis, it is assumed that the systematic difference between target values can be modeled as a constant systematic difference (intercept deviation from zero) combined with a proportional systematic difference (slope deviation from unity), usually related to a discrepancy with regard to calibration of the methods. In situations when random errors have a constant SD, unweighted regression procedures are used (e.g., **Deming regression** analysis). For cases with SDs that are proportional to the concentration, the weighted Deming regression procedure is preferred.

As outlined previously, we distinguish between the measured value ($x_i$) and the target value ($X_{Targeti}$) of a sample subjected to analysis by a given method. In linear regression analysis, we assume a linear relationship between values devoid of random error of any kind. Thus, to operate with a linear relationship between values without random measurement error and sample-related random bias, we have to introduce modified target values:

$$X1'_{Targeti} = X1_{Targeti} + \text{Random-Bias1}_i >$$

$$X2'_{Targeti} = X2_{Targeti} + \text{Random-Bias2}_i$$

where we now assume a linear relationship between these modified target values:

$$X2'_{Targeti} = \alpha_0 + \beta X1'_{Targeti}$$

In this model, $\alpha_0$ corresponds to a constant difference with regard to calibration, and ($\beta - 1$) is a proportional deviation. Thus the systematic error or calibration difference between the measurements corresponds to

$$X2'_{Targeti} - X1'_{Targeti} = \alpha_0 + (\beta - 1) X1'_{Targeti}$$

Because of sample-related random interferences and measurement imprecision (of the type that can be described by a Gaussian distribution, e.g., caused by pipetting variability, signal variability), individually measured pairs of values ($x1_i$, $x2_i$) will be scattered around the line expressing the relationship between $X1'_{Targeti}$ and $X2'_{Targeti}$. Fig. 2.12 outlines schematically how the random distribution of $x1$ and $x2$ values occurs around the regression line. We have

$$x1_i = X1'_{Targeti} + \varepsilon1_i = X1_{Targeti} + \text{Random-Bias1}_i + \varepsilon1_i$$

$$x2_i = X2'_{Targeti} + \varepsilon2_i = X2_{Targeti} + \text{Random-Bias2}_i + \varepsilon2_i$$

The random error components may be expressed as SDs, and generally, we can assume that sample-related random bias (SD $\sigma_{RB}$) and analytical imprecision (SD $\sigma_A$) are independent for each analyte, yielding the relations

$$\sigma_{ex1}^2 = \sigma_{RB1}^2 + \sigma_{A1}^2$$

$$\sigma_{ex2}^2 = \sigma_{RB2}^2 + \sigma_{A2}^2$$

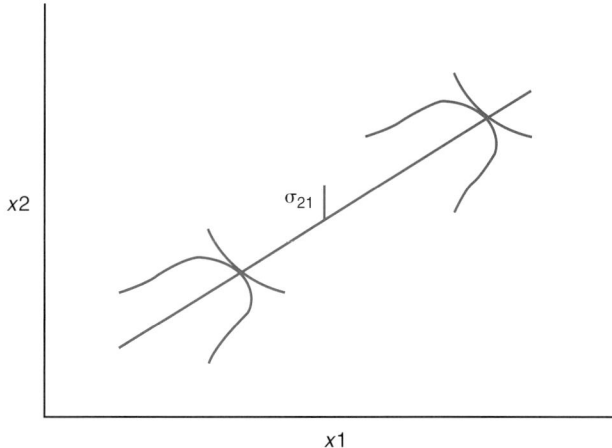

**Fig. 2.12** Outline of the relation between $x1$ and $x2$ values measured by two assays subject to random errors with constant standard deviations over the analytical measurement range. A linear relationship between the modified target values ($X1'_{Targeti}$, $X2'_{Targeti}$) is presumed. The $x1_i$ and $x2_i$ values are Gaussian distributed around $X1'_{Targeti}$ and $X2'_{Targeti}$, respectively, as schematically shown. $\sigma_{21}$ ($\sigma_{yx}$) is demarcated.

$\sigma_{ex1}$ and $\sigma_{ex2}$ are the total SDs of the distributions of $x1_i$ and $x2_i$ around their respective modified target values, $X1'_{Targeti}$ and $X2'_{Targeti}$. The sample-related random-bias components for methods 1 and 2 may not necessarily be independent. They also may not be Gaussian distributed, contrary to the analytical components. Thus, when a regression procedure is applied, the explicit assumptions to take into account should be considered. In situations without random-bias components of any significance, the relationships simplify to

$$\sigma_{ex1}^2 = \sigma_{A1}^2$$

$$\sigma_{ex2}^2 = \sigma_{A2}^2$$

In this situation, it usually can be assumed that the error distributions are Gaussian, and estimates of the analytical SDs may be available from QC data.

Another methodologic problem concerns the question of whether the dispersion of sample-related random bias and the analytical imprecision are constant or change with the analyte concentration. In cases with a considerable range (i.e., a decade or longer), this phenomenon should also be taken into account when a regression analysis is applied. Fig. 2.13 schematically shows how dispersions may increase proportionally with concentration.

## Deming Regression Analysis and Ordinary Least-Squares Regression Analysis (Constant Standard Deviations)

To reliably estimate the relationship between modified target values (i.e., $a_0$ for $\alpha_0$ and $b$ for $\beta$), a regression procedure taking into account errors in both $x1$ and $x2$ is preferable (i.e., Deming approach) (see Fig. 2.12). Although the **ordinary least-squares regression** (OLR) procedure is commonly used in method comparison studies, it does not take errors

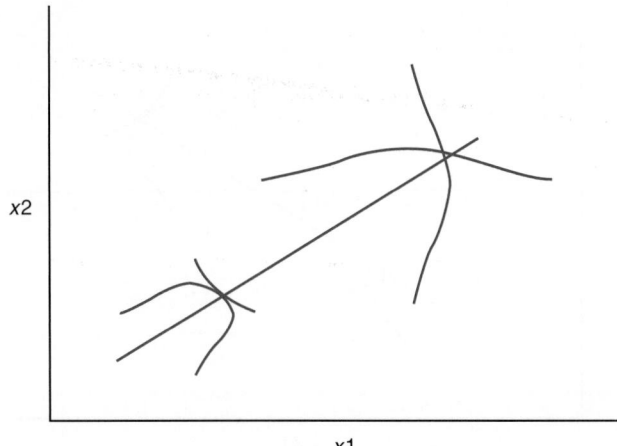

$x2$

$x1$

**Fig. 2.13** Outline of the relation between $x1$ and $x2$ values measured by two assays subject to proportional random errors. A linear relationship between the modified target values is assumed. The $x1_i$ and $x2_i$ values are Gaussian distributed around $X1'_{Target i}$ and $X2'_{Target i}$, respectively, with increasing scatter at higher concentrations, as is shown schematically.

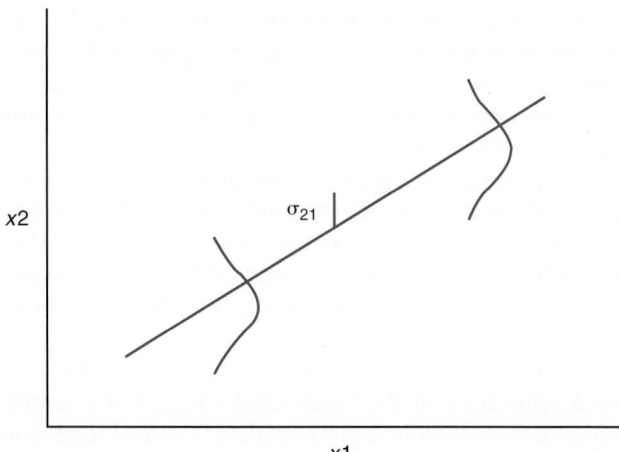

$x2$

$\sigma_{21}$

$x1$

**Fig. 2.14** The model assumed in ordinary least-squares regression. The $x2$ values are Gaussian distributed around the line with constant standard deviation over the analytical measurement range. The $x1$ values are assumed to be without random error. $\sigma_{21}$ ($\sigma_{yx}$) is shown.

in $x1$ into account but is based on the assumption that only the $x2$ measurements are subject to random errors (Fig. 2.14). In the Deming procedure, the sum of squared distances from measured sets of values ($x1_i$, $x2_i$) to the regression line is minimized at an angle determined by the ratio between SDs for the random variations of $x1$ and $x2$. It can be proven theoretically that, given Gaussian *error* distributions, this estimation procedure is optimal. It should here be noted that it is the *error* distributions that should be Gaussian, not the dispersion of values over the measurement range. In Fig. 2.15, the symmetric case is illustrated with a regression slope of 1 and equal SDs for the random variations of $x1$ and $x2$, in which case the sum of squared distances is minimized orthogonally in relation to the line.

OLR regression is not recommended except in special situations. In OLR, the sum of squared distances is minimized in the vertical direction to the line (see Fig. 2.15). The neglect of the random error in $x1$ induces a downward biased slope estimate, which depends on the ratio between the SD for the random error in $x1$ and the SD of the $X1'$ target values. Fig. 2.16 shows the bias as a function of the ratio of the random error SD to the SD of the $X1'$ target value dispersion. For a ratio up to 0.1, the bias is less than 1%. At a ratio of 0.33, the bias amounts to 10%. In a given case, the analytical SD (e.g., from QC data) can be divided by the SD of the measured $x1$ values, which approximately equals the SD of $X1'$ target values. As an example, a typical comparison study for two serum sodium methods may be associated with a downward-directed slope bias of about 10% (Fig. 2.17).

## Computation Procedures for Ordinary Least-Squares Regression and Deming Regression

Assuming no errors in $x1$ and a Gaussian error distribution of $x2$ with constant SD throughout the analytical measurement range, OLR is the optimal estimation procedure.

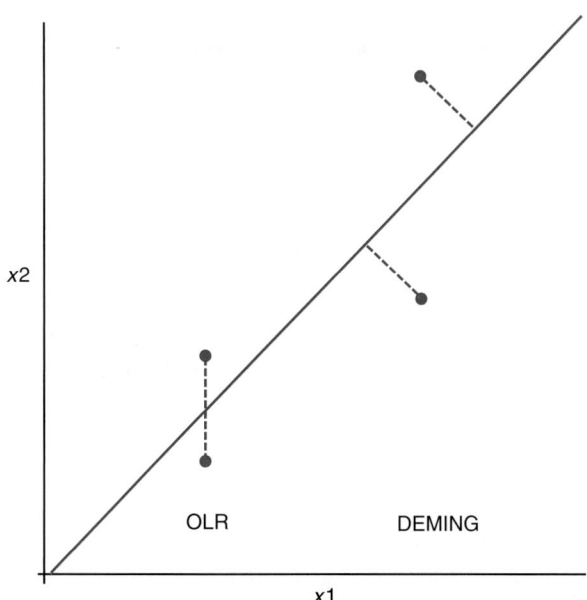

$x2$

OLR          DEMING

$x1$

**Fig. 2.15** In ordinary least-squares regression *(OLR)*, the sum of squared deviations from the line is minimized in the vertical direction. In Deming regression analysis, the sum of squared deviations is minimized at an angle to the line, depending on the random error ratio. Here the symmetric case is displayed with orthogonal deviations. (From Linnet K. The performance of Deming regression analysis in case of a misspecified analytical error ratio. *Clin Chem.* 1998;44:1024–1031.)

Given errors in both $x1$ and $x2$, the Deming approach is the method of choice. It should be noted for these parametric procedures that only the *error* distributions must be Gaussian or normal to ensure the nominal type I errors for associated statistical tests for slope and intercept hold true. The procedures are generally robust toward deviations from normality, but they are sensitive to outliers because of the squaring principle. Finally, the distribution of the $x1$ and $x2$ values over the measurement range does not have to be normal. A uniform distribution over the analytical

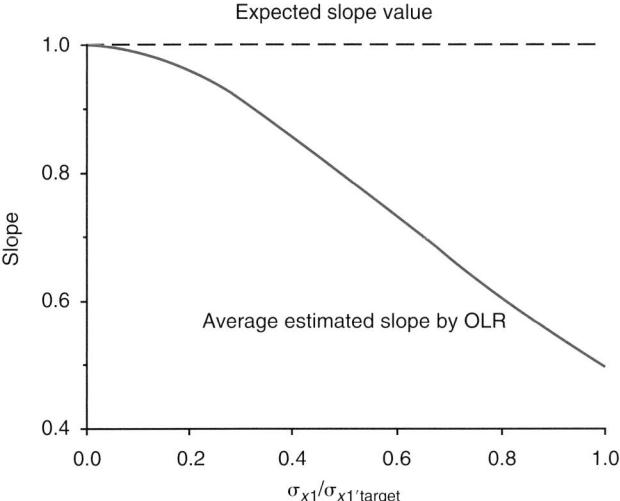

**Fig. 2.16** Relations between the true (expected) slope value and the average estimated slope by ordinary least-squares regression *(OLR)*. The bias of the OLR slope estimate increases negatively for increasing ratios of the standard deviation (SD) random error in $x1$ to the SD of the $X1$ target value distribution.

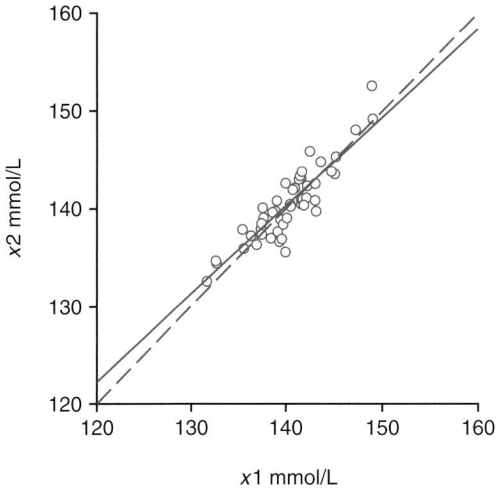

**Fig. 2.17** Simulated comparison of two sodium methods. The *solid line* indicates the average estimated ordinary least-squares regression (OLR) line, and the *dotted line* is the identity line. Even though no systematic difference is evident between the two methods, the average OLR line deviates from the identity line corresponding to a downward slope bias of about 10%.

measurement range is generally of advantage, but the distribution in principle may take any form. For both procedures, we may evaluate the SD of the dispersion in the *vertical* direction around the line (commonly denoted $SD_{y \cdot x}$ and here given as $SD_{21}$). We have

$$SD_{21} = \left[ \Sigma (x2_i - X2 \,'_{\text{Targetest}i})^2 \,/\, (N-2) \right]^{0.5}$$

Further discussion regarding the interpretation of $SD_{21}$ will be given later.

To compute the slope in Deming regression analysis, the ratio between the SDs of the random errors of $x1$ and $x2$ is necessary, that is,

$$\lambda = \left( \sigma_{RB1}^2 + \sigma_{A1}^2 \right) / \left( \sigma_{RB2}^2 + \sigma_{A2}^2 \right)$$

$SD_A$s can be estimated from duplicate sets of measurements as

$$SD_{A1}^2 = (1/2N) \left[ \Sigma (x1_{2i} - x1_{1i})^2 \right]$$

$$SD_{A2}^2 = (1/2N) \left[ \Sigma (x2_{2i} - x2_{1i})^2 \right]$$

If a specific value for $\lambda$ is not available and the two routine methods that are compared are likely to be associated with random errors of the same order of magnitude, $\lambda$ can be set to 1. The Deming procedure is generally relatively insensitive to a misspecification of the $\lambda$ value.

Formulas for computing slope $(\beta)$, intercept $(\alpha_0)$, and their SEs are available from other sources and are not provided here.

## Evaluation of the Random Error Around an Estimated Regression *Line*

The estimated slope and intercept provide an estimate of the systematic difference or calibration bias between two methods over the analytical measurement range. An estimate of the random error is the dispersion around the line in the vertical direction, which is quantified as $SD_{y \cdot x}$ (here denoted $SD_{21}$). We have here without sample-related random interferences

$$\sigma_{21}^2 = \beta^2 \sigma_{A1}^2 + \sigma_{A2}^2$$

Thus $\sigma_{21}$ reflects the random error both in $x1$ (with a rescaling) and in $x2$. Often $\beta$ is close to unity, and in this case, $\sigma_{21}^2$ becomes approximately the sum of the individual squared SDs. This relation holds true for both Deming and OLR analyses. Frequently, OLR is applied in situations associated with random measurement error in both $x1$ and $x2$, and in these situations, $\sigma_{21}$ reflects the errors in both.

The presence of sample-related random interferences in both $x1$ and $x2$ gives the following expression:

$$\sigma_{21}^2 = \left( \beta^2 \sigma_{A1}^2 + \sigma_{A2}^2 \right) + \left( \beta^2 \sigma_{RB1}^2 + \sigma_{RB2}^2 \right)$$

Thus the $\sigma_{21}$ value is influenced by the slope value and the analytical error components $\sigma_{A1}$ and $\sigma_{A2}$ (grouped in the first bracket) and $\sigma_{RB1}$ and $\sigma_{RB2}$ (grouped in the second bracket). In many cases, the slope is close to unity, in which case we have simple addition of the components. Information on the analytical components is usually available from duplicate sets of measurements or from QC data. On this basis, the combined random bias term in the second bracket can be derived by subtracting the analytical components from $\sigma_{21}$. Overall, it can be judged whether the total random error is acceptable or not. The systematic difference can be adjusted for relatively easily by rescaling one of the sets of measurements. However, if the random error term is very large, such a rescaling does not ensure equivalency of measurements with regard to individual samples.

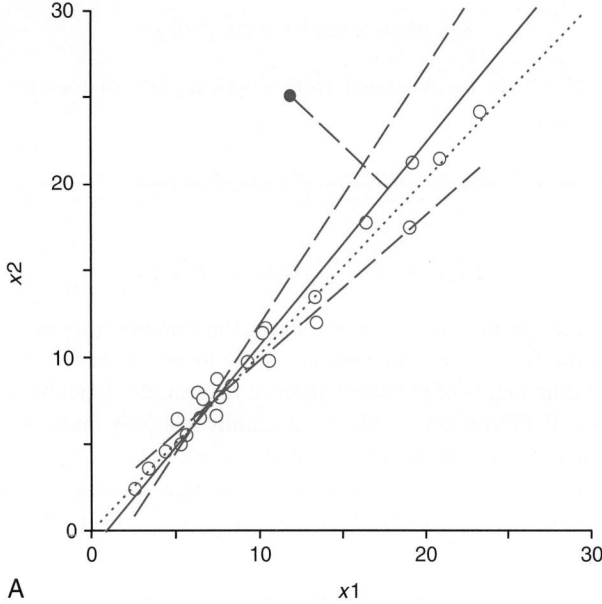

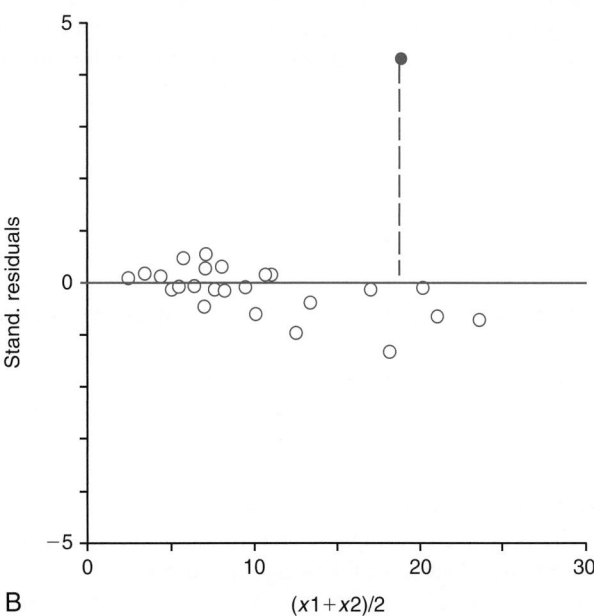

**Fig. 2.18** (A) A scatter plot with the Deming regression line *(solid line)* with an outlier *(filled point)*. The *dotted straight line* is the diagonal, and the *curved dashed lines* demarcate the 95% confidence region. (B) Standardized residuals plot with indication of the outlier.

### Assessment of Outliers

The distance from a suspected outlier to the line is recorded in SD units, and the outlier is rejected if the distance exceeds a predetermined limit (e.g., 3 or 4 SD units). In the case of OLR, the SD unit equals $SD_{21}$, and the vertical distance is considered. For Deming regression analysis, the unit is the SD of the deviation of the points from the line at an angle determined by the error variance ratio $\lambda$. A plot of these deviations, a so-called residuals plot, conveniently illustrates the occurrence of outliers. Fig. 2.18A illustrates an example of Deming regression analysis with occurrence of an outlier and the associated residuals plot (see Fig. 2.18B), which clearly shows the outlier

pattern. In this example, the residuals plot was standardized to unit SD. Use of an outlier limit of 4 SD units in this example led to rejection of the outlier, and a reanalysis was undertaken. In this example, rejection of the outlier changed the slope from 1.14 to 1.03. With regard to outliers, the reason for their presence should be investigated as a method limitation (e.g., possibly a nonspecificity for the analyte).

### Correlation Coefficient

The ordinary **correlation coefficient**, $\varrho$, also called the Pearson product moment correlation coefficient, is estimated as $r$ from sums of squared deviations for $x1$ and $x2$ values as follows:

$$r = p / (uq)^{0.5}$$

where

$$p = \Sigma \left( x1_i - x1_m \right) \left( x2_i - x2_m \right)$$

$$u = \Sigma (x1_i - x1_m)^2 \text{ and } q = \Sigma (x2_i - x2_m)^2$$

and

$$x1_m = \frac{\Sigma x1_i}{N} \text{ and } x2_m = \Sigma x2_i / N$$

The correlation coefficient $r$ is a *relative* indicator of the amount of dispersion around the regression line. If the numeric interval of values is short, $r$ tends to be low, and vice versa for a long range of values. For example, consider simulated examples, where the random errors of $x1$ and $x2$ are the same but the width of the distributions of measured values differs (Fig. 2.19A and B). In A, the target values are uniformly distributed over the range of 1 to 3, and in B, the range is 1 to 6. The random error SD is presumed constant, and it is set to 0.15 for both $x1$ and $x2$, corresponding to a CV of 5% at the value 3. Given sets of 50 paired measurements, the correlation coefficient is 0.93 in case A and 0.99 in case B. Furthermore, a single point located outside the range of the rest of the observations exerts a strong influence, resulting in a value of 0.97 (see Fig. 2.19C).

Although $\sigma_{21}$ is the relevant measure for random error in method comparison studies, $\varrho$ is still incorrectly used as a supposed measure of agreement between two methods. A systematic difference due to a difference regarding calibration is not expressed through $\varrho$ but solely in the form of an intercept ($\alpha_0$) deviation from zero or a slope ($\beta$) deviation from unity.

### Regression Analysis in Cases of Proportional Random Error

For analytes with extended ranges (e.g., 1 or several decades), the $SD_A$ is seldom constant. Rather, a proportional relationship may apply. This may also be true for the random bias components. In this situation, the regression procedures described previously may still be used, but they are not optimal because the SEs of slope and intercept become larger than is the case when a weighted form of regression analysis is applied. Given a proportional

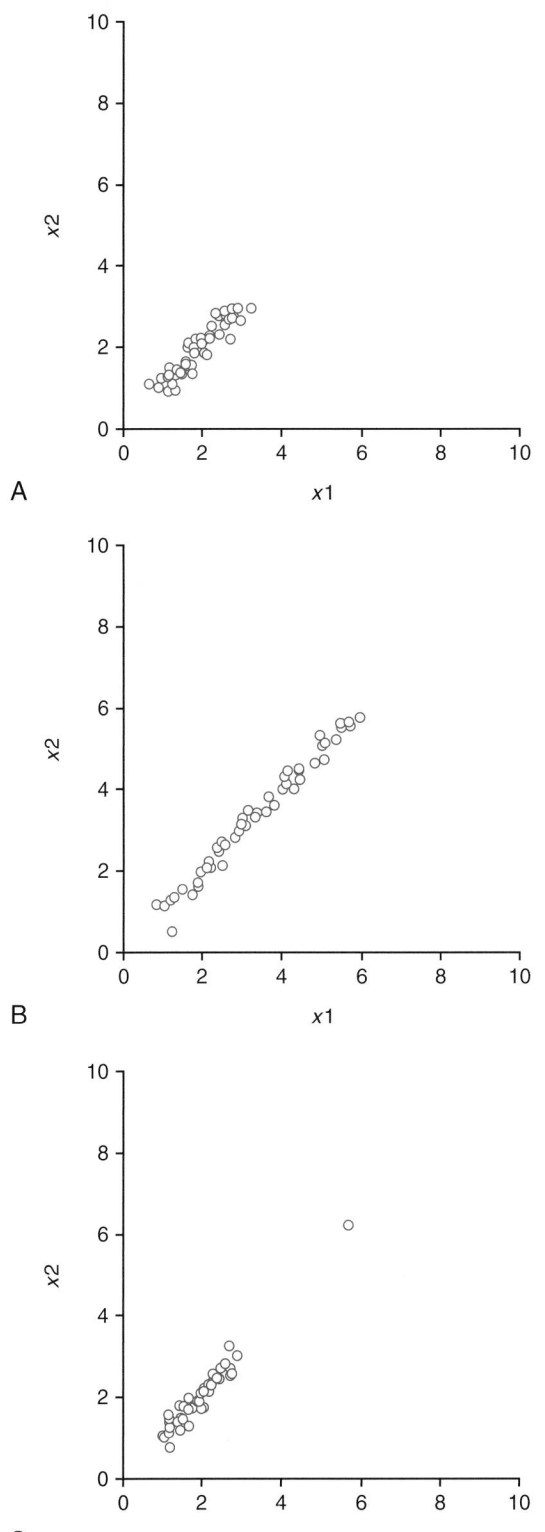

A

B

C

**Fig. 2.19** Scatter plots illustrating the effect of the range on the value of the correlation coefficient $\varrho$. (A) Target values are uniformly distributed over the range 1 to 3 with random errors of both $x1$ and $x2$ corresponding to a standard deviation (SD) of 5% of the target value at 3 (constant error SDs). (B) The range is extended to 1 to 6 with the same random error levels. The correlation coefficient equals 0.93 in A and 0.99 in B. (C) The effect of a single aberrant point is shown. Forty-nine of the target values are distributed over the range 1 to 3, with a single point at 6. The correlation coefficient is 0.97.

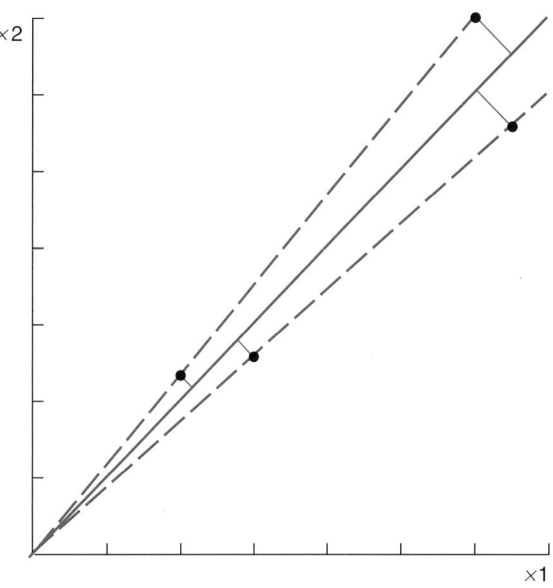

**Fig. 2.20** Distances from data points to the line in weighted Deming regression assuming proportional random errors in $x1$ and $x2$. The symmetric case is illustrated with equal random errors and a slope of unity yielding orthogonal projections onto the line. (Modified from Linnet K. Necessary sample size for method comparison studies based on regression analysis. *Clin Chem.* 1999;45:882–894. Used with permission.)

relationship, a weighted procedure assigns larger weights to observations in the low range; low-range observations are more precise than measurements at higher concentrations that are subject to larger random errors. More specifically, weights are applied in the computations that are inversely proportional to the squared SDs (variances) that express the random error. In the weighted modification of the Deming procedure, distances from $(x1_i, x2_i)$ to the line are inversely weighted according to the squared SDs at a given concentration (Fig. 2.20).

## Testing for Linearity

Splitting of the systematic error into a constant and a proportional component depends on the assumption of linearity. A convenient test is a runs test, which in principle assesses whether negative and positive deviations from the points to the line are randomly distributed. The term *run* here relates to a sequence of deviations with the same sign. Consider, for example, the situation with a downward trend of $x2$ values at the upper end of the analytical measurement range (Fig. 2.21A). The SDs from the line (i.e., the residuals) will tend to be negative in this area instead of being randomly distributed above and below the line (see Fig. 2.21B).

## Nonparametric Regression Analysis (Passing-Bablok Procedure)

The slope and the intercept may be estimated by a nonparametric procedure, which is robust to outliers and requires no assumptions of Gaussian error distributions. The method takes measurement errors for both $x1$ and $x2$ into account, but it presumes that the ratio between random errors is related to the slope in a fixed manner:

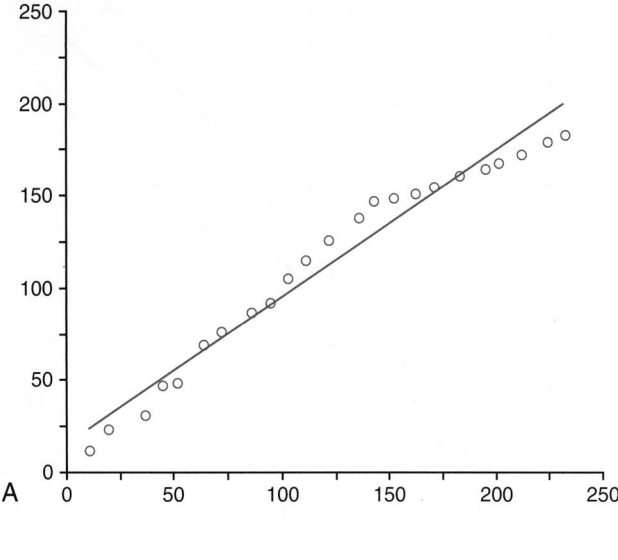

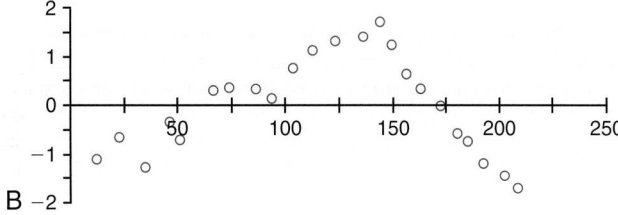

**Fig. 2.21** (A) Scatter plot showing an example of nonlinearity in the form of downward-deviating $x2$ values at the upper part of the range. (B) Plot of residuals showing the effects of nonlinearity. At the upper end of the analytical measurement range, a sequence (run) of negative residuals is present.

$$\lambda = \left(SD^2_{RB1} + SD^2_{A1}\right) / \left(SD^2_{RB2} + SD^2_{A2}\right) = 1/\beta^2$$

Otherwise, a biased slope estimate is obtained. The procedure may be applied both in situations with random errors with constant SDs and in cases with proportional SDs. The method is not as efficient as the corresponding parametric procedures. Slope and intercept with CIs are provided, together with Spearman's rank correlation coefficient.

### Interpretation of Systematic Differences Between Methods Obtained on the Basis of Regression Analysis

A systematic difference between two methods is identified if the estimated intercept differs significantly from zero or if the slope deviates significantly from 1. This is decided on the basis of $t$-tests:

$$t = (a_0 - 0) / SE(a_0)$$

$$t = (b - 1) / SE(b)$$

The $t$-tests can be supplemented with 95% CIs.

$SE(a_0)$ and $SE(b)$ are the SEs of the estimated intercept $a_0$ and the slope $b$, respectively. SEs can be derived by a computerized resampling principle called *the jackknife procedure*, which in practice can be carried out using appropriate software. Having estimated $a_0$ and $b$, we have the estimate of the

systematic difference between the methods, $D_c$, at a selected concentration, $X1'_{Targetc}$:

$$D_c = X2'_{Targetestc} - X1'_{Targetc} = a_0 + (b-1) X1'_{Targetc}$$

$X2'_{Targetc}$ is the estimated $X2'$ target value at $X1'_c$. Note that $D_c$ refers to the *systematic difference* (i.e., the difference between modified target values corresponding to a calibration difference). The SE of $D_c$ can be derived by the jackknife procedure using a software program. By evaluating the SE throughout the analytical measurement range, a confidence region for the estimated line can be displayed. If method comparison is performed to assess the calibration to a reference measurement procedure, correction of a significant systematic difference $Delta_c$ will often be performed by recalibration $[x2_{rec} = (x1 - a_0)/b]$. The associated standard uncertainty is the SE of $Delta_c$.

### Example of Application of Regression Analysis (Weighted Deming Analysis)

Application of weighted Deming regression analysis may be illustrated by the comparison of drug assays example ($N = 65$ ($x1, x2$) single measurements). As outlined in the section on the Bland-Altman plot (see Fig. 2.10), in this example the random error of the differences increases with the concentration, suggesting that the weighted form of Deming regression analysis is appropriate. Fig. 2.22 shows (A) the estimated regression line with 95% confidence bands and (B) a plot of normalized residuals. The nearly homogeneous scatter in the residuals plot supports the assumed proportional random error model and the assumption of linearity. The slope estimate (1.014) is not significantly different from 1 (95% CI: 0.97 to 1.06), and the intercept is not significantly different from zero (95% CI: −6.7 to 47.4) (Table 2.2). A runs test for linearity does not contradict the assumption of linearity. The amount of random error is quantified in the form of the $SD_{21}$ proportionality factor equal to 0.11, or 11%. In the present example, with a slope close to unity and two routine methods with assumed random errors of about the same magnitude, we divide the random error by the square root of 2 and get $CV_{x1} = CV_{x2} = 7.8\%$. QC data in the laboratory have provided $CV_{AS}$ of 6.1% and 7.2% for methods 1 and 2, respectively. Thus, in this example, the random error may be attributed largely to analytical error. The assay principle for both methods is high performance liquid chromatography (HPLC), which generally is a rather specific measurement principle; considerable random bias effects are not expected in this case.

In Table 2.2, estimated systematic differences at the limits of the therapeutic interval (300 and 2000 nmol/L) are displayed (24.6 and 48.9 nmol/L, respectively). This corresponds to percentage values of 8.2% and 2.4%, respectively. Estimated SEs by the jackknife procedure yield the 95% CIs, as shown in the table. At the low concentration, the difference is significant (95% CI: 5.7 to 44 nmol/L; does not include zero), which is not the case at the high level (95% CI: −19 to 117 nmol/L). Even though the intercept

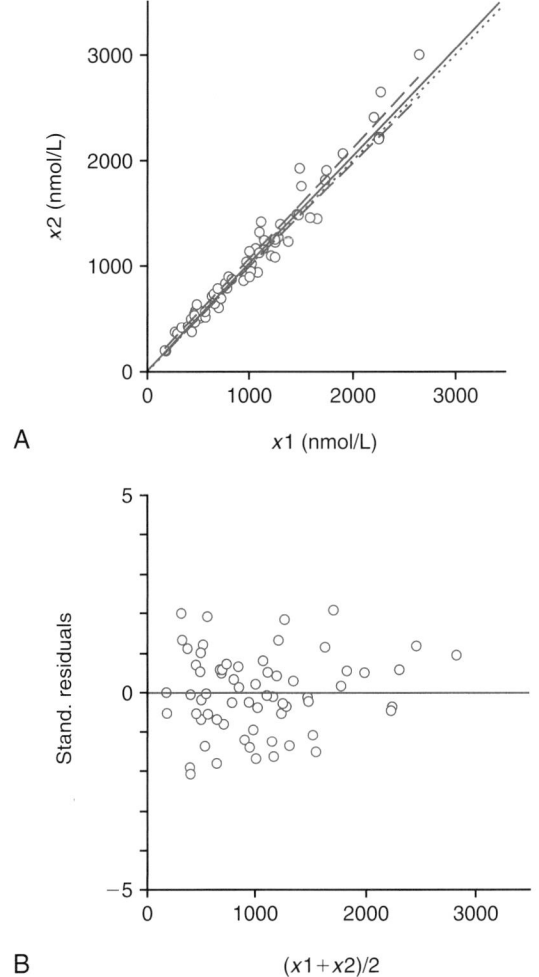

**Fig. 2.22** An example of weighted Deming regression analysis for the comparison of drug assays. (A) The *solid line* is the estimated weighted Deming regression line, the *dashed curves* indicate the 95% confidence region, and the *dotted line* is the line of identity. (B) A plot of residuals standardized to unit standard deviation. The homogeneous scatter supports the assumed proportional error model and the assumption of linearity.

**TABLE 2.2 Results of Weighted Deming Regression Analysis for the Comparison of Drug Assays Example, *n* = 65 Single (*x*1, *x*2) Measurements**

| | Estimate | SE | 95% CI |
|---|---|---|---|
| Slope *(b)* | 1.014 | 0.022 | 0.97–1.06 |
| Intercept *(a₀)* | 20.3 | 13.5 | −6.7 to 47.4 |
| Weighted correlation coefficient | 0.98 | | |
| SD₂₁ proportionality factor | 0.11 | | |
| Runs test for linearity | NS | | |
| $Delta_c = X_2 - X_1$ at $X_c = 300$ | 24.6 | 9.5 | 5.72–43.6 |
| $Delta_c = X_2 - X_1$ at $X_c = 2000$ | 48.9 | 34.2 | −19.3 to 117 |

*CI,* Confidence interval; *NS,* not significant; *SD,* standard deviation; *SE,* standard error.

and slope estimates separately are not significantly different from the null hypothesis values of 0 and 1, respectively, the combined difference *Delta_c* is significant at low

concentrations in this example. If the difference is considered of medical importance and both methods are to be used simultaneously in the laboratory, recalibration of one of the methods might be considered.

## MONITORING SERIAL RESULTS

An important aspect of clinical chemistry is monitoring of disease or treatment (e.g., tumor markers in cases of cancer, drug concentrations in cases of therapeutic drug monitoring). To assess changes in a rational way, various imprecision components have to be taken into account. Biologic within-subject variation ($SD_I$) and preanalytical ($SD_{PA}$) and analytical variation ($SD_A$) all have to be recognized. Assuming that preanalytical variation is already included in the estimated within-subject variation SD, a total SD ($SD_T$) can be estimated as follows:

$$SD_T^2 = SD_{WithinB}^2 + SD_A^2$$

The limit for statistically significant changes then is [*fx2*], where *k* depends on the desired probability level. Considering a two-sided 5% level, *k* is 1.96. The corresponding one-sided factor is 1.65. If a higher probability level is desired, *k* should be increased.

## TRACEABILITY

To ensure reasonable agreement between measurements of routine methods, the concept of **traceability** comes into focus. (See also Chapter 7 for further detail.) Traceability is based on an unbroken chain of comparisons of measurements leading to a known reference value (Fig. 2.23). For well-established analytes, a hierarchy of methods exists with *a reference measurement procedure* at the top, *selected measurement procedures* at an intermediate level, and finally *routine measurement procedures* at the bottom. A reference measurement procedure is a fully understood procedure of highest analytical quality containing a complete uncertainty budget given in Système Internationale (SI) units. Reference procedures are used to measure the analyte concentration in *secondary reference materials,* which typically have the same matrix as samples that are to be measured by routine procedures (e.g., human serum). Secondary reference materials are usually of high analytical quality, and certified secondary reference materials must be validated for **commutability** with clinical samples if they are intended for use as trueness controls for routine methods. Otherwise, their use is restricted to selected measurement procedures for which they are intended. The certificate of analysis should state the methods for which the secondary reference materials have been validated to be commutable with clinical samples. When no information is given for commutability, it must be assumed that the reference material is not commutable with clinical samples, and the user has the responsibility to validate commutability for the methods of interest.

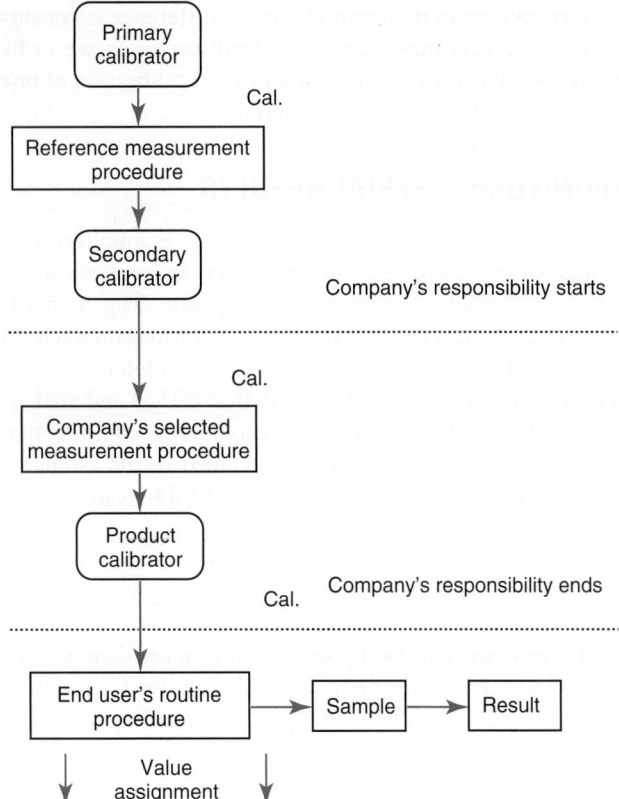

**Fig. 2.23** The calibration hierarchy from a reference measurement procedure to a routine assay. The uncertainty increases from top to bottom. *Cal.*, Calibration.

## Uncertainty Concept

According to the ISO's "Guide to the Expression of Uncertainty in Measurement" (GUM), **uncertainty** is formally defined as "a parameter associated with the result of a measurement that characterizes the dispersion of the values that could reasonably be attributed to the measurand." In practice, this means that the uncertainty is given as an interval around a reported laboratory result that specifies the location of the true value with a given probability (e.g., 95%). In general, the uncertainty of a result, which is traceable to a particular reference, is the uncertainty of that reference together with the overall uncertainty of the traceability chain.

In the outline of the uncertainty concept, it is assumed that any known systematic error components of a measurement method have been corrected, and the specified uncertainty includes uncertainty associated with correction of the systematic error(s). A distinction between type A and B uncertainties is made. Type A uncertainties are frequency-based estimates of SDs (e.g., an SD of the imprecision). Type B uncertainties are uncertainty components for which frequency-based SDs are not available. Instead, uncertainty is estimated by other approaches or by the opinion of experts. Finally, the total uncertainty is derived from a combination of all sources of launcertainty and can be expressed as a *standard uncertainty* ($u_{st}$), which is equivalent

to an SD. By multiplication of a standard uncertainty with a *coverage factor (k)*, the uncertainty corresponding to a specified probability level is derived, for example, multiplication with a coverage factor of 2 yields a probability level of $\approx$95%, given a Gaussian distribution. When the total uncertainty of an analytical result obtained by a routine method is considered ($u_{st}$), preanalytical variation ($u_{PAst}$), method imprecision ($u_{Ast}$), sample-related random interferences ($u_{RBst}$), and uncertainty related to calibration and bias corrections (traceability) ($u_{Tracst}$) should be taken into account. In expressing the uncertainty components as standard uncertainties, we have:

$$u_{st} = \left[ u_{PAst}^2 + u_{Ast}^2 + u_{RBst}^2 + u_{Tracst}^2 \right]^{0.5}$$

In principle, uncertainty can be judged *directly* from measurement comparisons ("top down") or *indirectly* from an analysis of individual error sources according to the law of error propagation ("error budget," "bottom up").

### Example of Direct Assessment of Uncertainty on the Basis of Measurements of a Commutable Certified Reference Material

Suppose a CRM is available that was validated to be *commutable* with patient samples for a given routine method with a specified value of 10.0 mmol/L and a standard uncertainty of 0.2 mmol/L. Ten repeated measurements in independent runs give a mean value of 10.3 mmol/L with SD 0.5 mmol/L. The SE of the mean is then [*fx3*]. The mean is not significantly different from the assigned value [$t = (10.3 - 10.0)/(0.2^2 + 0.16^2)^{0.5} = 1.17$]. The total standard uncertainty with regard to traceability is then $u_{Tracst} = (0.16^2 + 0.2^2)^{0.5} = 0.26$ mmol/L. If the bias had been significant, a correction to the method could have been carried out, and the standard uncertainty would then be the same at the given concentration. Thus, measurements of the CRM provide an estimate of the uncertainty related to traceability, *given the assumption of commutability with patient samples*. The other components have to be estimated separately. Concerning method imprecision, long-term imprecision (e.g., observed from QC measurements) should be used rather than the short-term SD observed for CRM material. Here we suppose that the long-term $SD_A$ is 0.8 mmol/L. Data on preanalytical variation can be obtained by sampling in duplicates from a series of patients or can be a matter of judgment (type B uncertainty) based on literature data or data on similar analytes. We here suppose that $SD_{PA}$ equals half the analytical SD (i.e., 0.4 mmol/L). Finally, we lack data on a possible sample-related random bias component, which we may choose to ignore in the present example. The standard uncertainty of the results then becomes

$$\begin{aligned} u_{st} &= \left[ u_{PAst}^2 + u_{Ast}^2 + u_{RBst}^2 + u_{Tracst}^2 \right]^{0.5} \\ &= \left( 0.4^2 + 0.8^2 + 0.26^2 \right)^{0.5} \\ &= 0.93 \, (mmol/L) \end{aligned}$$

In this case, the major uncertainty component is the long-term imprecision in the laboratory. To attain a reasonably precise uncertainty estimate, estimated SDs should be based on an appropriate number of repetitions. In the subsection on method precision, it can be seen that $N = 30$ repetitions provides SD estimates with 95% CIs extending from about 20% below to 35% above an estimated value (see Fig. 2.7), which may be regarded as reasonable.

### Indirect Evaluation of Uncertainty by Quantification of Individual Error Source Components

On the basis of a detailed quantitative model of the analytical procedure, the standard approach is to assess the standard uncertainties associated with individual input parameters and combine them according to the law of propagation of uncertainties. The relationship between the combined standard uncertainty $u_c(y)$ of a value $y$ and the uncertainty of the *independent* parameters $x_1, x_2, \ldots, x_n$, on which it depends, is

$$u_c\left[y\left(x_1, x_2, \ldots\right)\right] = \left[\Sigma c_i^2 u(x_1)^2\right]^{0.5}$$

where $c_i$ is a sensitivity coefficient (the partial differential of $y$ with respect to $x_i$). These sensitivity coefficients indicate how the value of $y$ varies with changes in the input parameter $x_i$. If the variables are not independent, the relationship becomes

$$u_c\left[y\left(x_1, x_2, \ldots\right)\right] = \left[\Sigma c_i^2 u(x_1)^2 + \Sigma c_i c_k u(x_i, x_k)^2\right]^{0.5}$$

where $u(x_i, x_k)$ is the covariance between $x_i$ and $x_k$, and $c_i$ and $c_k$ are the sensitivity coefficients. The covariance is related to the correlation coefficient $\varrho_{ik}$ by

$$u(x_i, x_k) = u(x_i)\, u(x_k)\, \rho_{ik}$$

This is a complex relationship that usually will be difficult to evaluate in practice. In many situations, however, the contributing factors are independent, thus simplifying the picture. Below, some simple examples of combined expressions are shown. The rules are presented in the form of combining SDs or CVs given *independent* input components.

$$q = x + y \quad SD(q) = \left[SD(x)^2 + SD(y)^2\right]^{0.5}$$

$$q = x - y \quad SD(q) = \left[SD(x)^2 + SD(y)^2\right]^{0.5}$$

$$q = ax \quad SD(q) = a\,SD(x) \text{ and } CV(q) = CV(x)$$

$$q = x^p \quad CV(q) = pCV(x)$$

$$q = xy \quad CV(q) = \left[CV(x)^2 + CV(y)^2\right]^{0.5}$$

$$q = \frac{x}{y} \quad CV(q) = \left[CV(x)^2 + CV(y)^2\right]^{0.5}$$

The formulas shown may be used, for example, to calculate the combined uncertainty of a calibrator solution from the uncertainties of the reference compound, the weighting, and dilution steps. In some situations, a Monte Carlo simulation model of a complex analytical method may be established to estimate the combined uncertainty of the method on the basis of input uncertainties.

> **POINTS TO REMEMBER**
> - For well-established analytes, a hierarchy of methods exists with *a reference measurement procedure* at the top, *selected measurement procedures* at an intermediate level, and finally *routine measurement procedures* at the bottom.
> - The uncertainty is given as an interval around a reported laboratory result that specifies the location of the true value with a given probability (e.g., 95%).
> - The uncertainty of a result, which is traceable to a particular reference, is the uncertainty of that reference together with the overall uncertainty of the traceability chain.
> - The uncertainty can be judged *directly* from measurement comparisons ("top down") or *indirectly* from an analysis of individual error sources according to the law of error propagation ("error budget," "bottom up").

## DIAGNOSTIC ACCURACY OF LABORATORY TESTS

We here consider the basic steps for evaluation of the clinical accuracy of laboratory tests. In diagnostic accuracy studies, the measurements or results of one (or more) laboratory test under evaluation (i.e., the so-called index test) are compared with the results of a reference standard or method. This reference is the best prevailing test or strategy that is used to establish the presence or absence of the disease of interest. This reference standard is conducted and its results interpreted as blindly for and independently from the index test(s) results as possible. Test accuracy studies show the concordance in results of the index test(s) with the presence or absence of disease as defined by the reference standard results. These studies provide information regarding the frequency of types of errors (i.e., false positive and negative test results) by the index test in relation to the reference standard.

### Diagnostic Accuracy, Sensitivity, and Specificity of a Test in Isolation

In a diagnostic accuracy study, the results of the index test are compared with those of a reference test in the same individuals, all of whom are suspected to have the target disease (the suspected disease cohort design). The simplest situation is a comparison of a single index test, with only two result categories (i.e., a dichotomous or binary index test) to a reference standard (i.e., a single-test accuracy study). The ideal dichotomous index test correctly identifies all individuals as diseased or non-diseased with an error rate of zero. A zero error rate is only possible when there is no overlap between index test results in the diseased and non-diseased individuals. However, when there is overlap in index test results, some individuals are classified wrongly as shown below in an example concerning the diagnosis of deep venous thrombosis (DVT) using a D-dimer index test. When using a quantitative (continuous) index test to classify individuals as diseased or nondiseased, a cutoff value needs to be chosen to estimate these error rates. This results in a so-called dichotomized index test.

Values of the dichotomous or dichotomized index test that exceed the cutoff in individuals having the target disease are classified as true positives (TP) (Fig. 2.24). Similarly, index test results lower than the cutoff in nondiseased individuals are true negatives (TN). Accordingly, index test results below the cutoff in truly diseased subjects are false negative (FN), and index test results exceeding the cutoff in truly nondiseased subjects are false positive (FP). Based on the frequencies of FN and FP results, an overall error rate or non-error rate can be derived. The overall diagnostic accuracy of an index test is then defined as the fraction of true classifications out of all classifications:

$$\text{Diagnostic accuracy} = (TN + TP) / (TN + TP + FP + FN)$$

This is an overall non-error rate that can be subdivided into the non-error rate of the nondiseased individuals, which is the specificity of the test, and the non-error rate of diseased individuals, which is the sensitivity of the test:

$$\text{Specificity} = TN / (TN + FP)$$

$$\text{Sensitivity} = TP / (TP + FN)$$

Whereas a very specific test provides negative results for all or almost all subjects who are free of the target disease, a very sensitive test detects all or almost all diseased subjects. To assess the (im)precision of these estimates, CIs should be specified as described under *Categorical Variables*. Table 2.3 displays the widths of the 95% CIs at various sample sizes of 20 to 1000 for two selected proportions. The specificity and sensitivity of two tests applied in the same study subjects can be statistically compared using the McNemar's test.

| Test result | Disease status | |
|---|---|---|
| | **Diseased** | **Nondiseased** |
| **Positive** | TP | FP |
| **Negative** | FN | TN |

**Fig. 2.24** The basic 2-by-2 table for estimating the diagnostic accuracy of a dichotomized quantitative test result. Positive test results are divided into true positives *(TPs)* and false positives *(FPs)* and negative results into true negatives *(TNs)* and false negatives *(FNs)*. (From Linnet K, Bossuyt PM, Moons KG, et al. Quantifying the accuracy of a diagnostic test or marker. *Clin Chem.* 2012;58:1292–1301.)

## Clinical Example: Accuracy of D-Dimer Test in Diagnosis of Deep Venous Thrombosis

We illustrate the concepts using some of the empirical data of a previously published study in primary care patients suspected of having DVT, the target disease (Fig. 2.25).

The study consisted of 2086 patients suspected of DVT, where DVT was defined as present in patients manifesting at least one of the following symptoms or signs: presence of swelling, redness, or pain in the leg. All patients were given a standardized diagnostic workup, including medical history; clinical examination; and testing for D-dimer, the (quantitative) index test. The reference procedure consisted of repeated compression ultrasonography tests and was performed in all patients, blinded to and independent of the index test results. A total of 416 (20%) of the 2086 included patients had DVT.

Applying a commonly used cutoff of 500 µg/L or greater for the (originally) quantitative D-dimer assay (dashed line in Fig. 2.25), the sensitivity was 0.97 (i.e., 3% of the subjects with DVT had a value <500 µg/L). The specificity was only 0.37. The resulting overall diagnostic accuracy was 0.50. Whereas the test displayed good sensitivity at this threshold, detecting all but 3% of those having DVT, its specificity at this test threshold was relatively low, resulting in many FP results. The SEs were 0.012 for the specificity and 0.008 for the sensitivity, resulting in CIs of 0.356 to 0.402 and 0.955 to 0.987, respectively.

## Receiver Operating Characteristic Curves

For a quantitative index test, the specificity and sensitivity depend on the selected cutoff point. A plot of the sensitivity and specificity pairs for all possible cutoff values over the measurement range provides the so-called **receiver operating characteristic (ROC) curve** (Fig. 2.26) Usually, sensitivity ($y$) is plotted against ($1 - $ specificity) ($x$) at each possible cutoff value. The better the performance of the test, the higher

**TABLE 2.3   Relationship Between Sample Size and 95% Confidence Intervals of a Proportion (e.g., a Sensitivity or Specificity): Selected Examples of Proportions of 0.05 and 0.80**

| Sample Size | 95% CI of a Proportion of 0.05 | 95% CI of a Proportion of 0.80 |
|---|---|---|
| 20 | 0.00–0.25 | 0.56–0.94 |
| 60 | 0.01–0.14 | 0.68–0.90 |
| 100 | 0.02–0.11 | 0.71–0.87 |
| 500 | 0.03–0.07 | 0.76–0.83 |
| 1000 | 0.04–0.07 | 0.77–0.82 |

*CI,* Confidence interval.

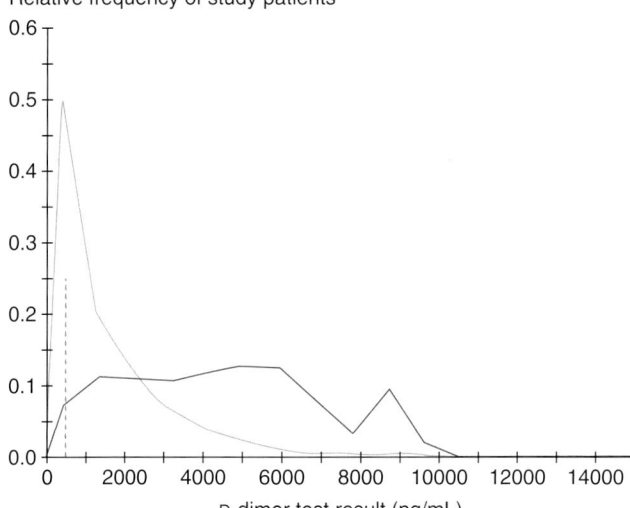

**Fig. 2.25** Distribution of the quantitative D-dimer values for deep venous thrombosis (DVT) and non-DVT subjects in the example study. *Light blue line,* non-DVT; *blue line,* DVT. The *dashed line* indicates the commonly used cutoff value of 500 µg/L. (From Linnet K, Bossuyt PM, Moons KG, et al. Quantifying the accuracy of a diagnostic test or marker. *Clin Chem.* 2012;58:1292–1301.)

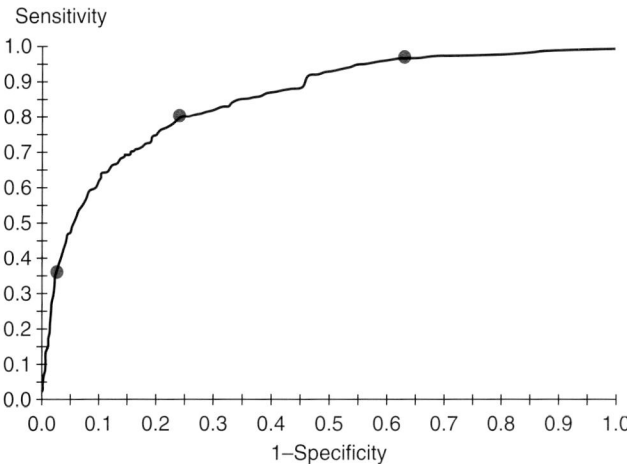

**Fig. 2.26** Receiver operating characteristic curve of the D-dimer assay result for diagnosis of deep venous thrombosis in our example study. The *blue markers* correspond to various cutoff choices (from left to right, 5435, 2133, and 500 µg/L). (From Linnet K, Bossuyt PM, Moons KG, et al. Quantifying the accuracy of a diagnostic test or marker. *Clin Chem.* 2012;58:1292–1301.)

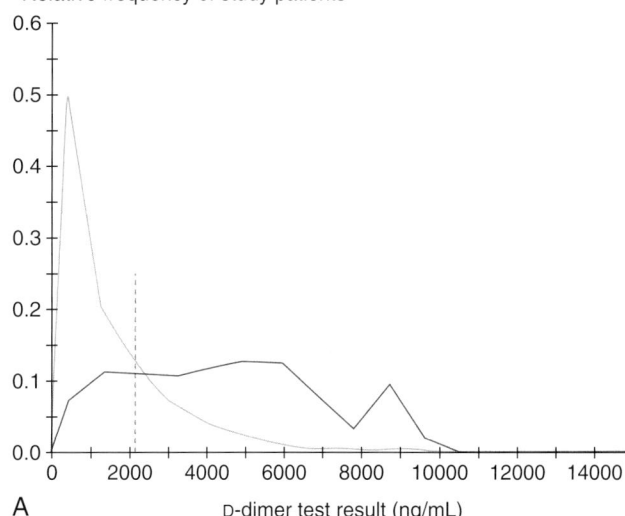

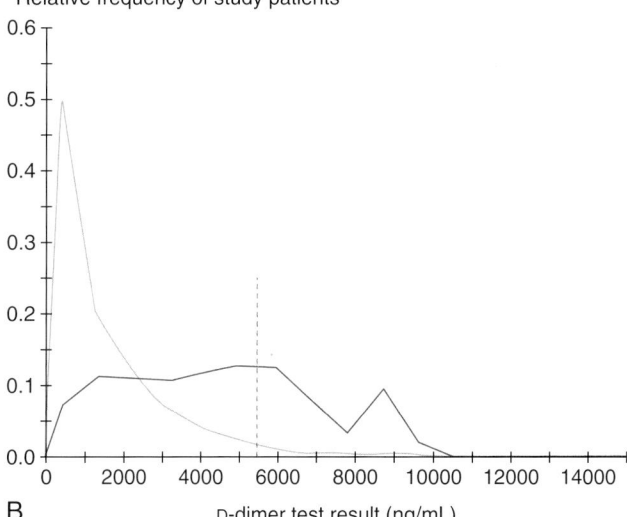

**Fig. 2.27** Alternative cutoffs to 500 µg/L in the D-dimer example. (A) Cutoff (2133 µg/L) giving maximum value of the sum of the specificity and sensitivity. (B) Cutoff (5435 µg/L) providing a high specificity (0.975). *Light blue line,* non–deep venous thrombosis (DVT); *blue line,* DVT. The *dashed line* indicates the cutoff value. (From Linnet K, Bossuyt PM, Moons KG, et al. Quantifying the accuracy of a diagnostic test or marker. *Clin Chem.* 2012;58:1292–1301.)

the ROC curve is located in the left, upper region of the plot. With use of the ROC curve, an appropriate combination of specificity and sensitivity may be chosen, and the corresponding cutoff then selected.

An area under the ROC curve (i.e., the ROC area or so-called concordance or c-index) can be assessed by either parametric or nonparametric statistics. Given an SE of the ROC area or c-index, it is possible to test whether the area significantly exceeds 0.5, which would demonstrate that the index test performs better than chance. A worthless test has an area of 0.5. Furthermore, using the SE, also a 95% CI can be derived for the ROC area or c-index. For the D-dimer test

example, the area under the ROC curve was 0.86 (SE, 0.011), with a 95% CI of 0.84 to 0.88.

## Selection of Cutoff Value in Case of Quantitative Index Tests

The specificity and sensitivity determined for an index test almost always vary inversely over the range of possible cut-offs. The cutoff point that provides the maximum of the sum of the specificity and sensitivity *could* be selected. In the D-dimer example, this cutoff would be close to 2000 µg/L, yielding a specificity of 0.76 and a sensitivity of 0.80 (Fig. 2.27A). However, this method of cutoff selection is commonly not recommended. The selection should rather be based on the intended purpose of the index test. If an index test is applied primarily to rule out the presence of disease (e.g., in the case of the D-dimer assay for exclusion of DVT), the cutoff point should be at the lower end of the distribution of values of diseased individuals (see Fig. 2.25) (e.g., a cutoff of 500 μg/L). At this cutoff, the sensitivity approaches 1.0. But attaining such a high sensitivity is at the cost of a loss of specificity because of overlap of test values in the diseased and nondiseased individuals. Conversely, when FP results are judged unacceptable, the cutoff should be toward the upper limit of the distribution of values for the nondiseased group. For the D-dimer test example, a cutoff value corresponding to the 97.5 percentile of the distribution of values for those not having DVT (5435 μg/L) resulted in a specificity of 0.975, but now the sensitivity was only 0.36 (i.e., nearly the opposite of the situation with a cutoff of 500 μg/L) (see Fig. 2.27B).

## Posterior Probabilities (Predictive Values)

Unlike sensitivity and specificity, the **positive predictive value** assesses the probability of having the disease given a positive test result, $P(D|Tpos)$, whereas the **negative predictive value** assesses the probability of not having the disease given a negative test result $P(Non\text{-}D|Tneg)$. The probability of the presence of the target disease given the index test result is an example of a so-called posterior disease probability, where the prior probability corresponds to the **prevalence** of the disease in the given situation. The prevalence of disease ($P[D]$) in the study sample is the a priori (pretest) probability of disease.

Given a positive test result (Tpos), the posterior disease probability is estimated as the fraction of TP out of all test result positives:

$$P(D|Tpos) = TP / (TP + FP)$$

Analogously for a negative result (Tneg), the probability that the given disease is absent is

$$P(Non\text{-}D|Tneg) = TN / (TN + FN)$$

Just as with sensitivity and specificity values, these posterior disease probabilities depend on the selected cutoff point for a quantitative test. In case of a dichotomous or dichotomized index test, these posterior probabilities are also called predictive values. They are highly dependent on the disease prevalence.

From the Bayes rule, the following relations exist:

$$P(D|Tpos) =$$
$$[\text{Sensitivity} \times P(D)] / [\text{Sensitivity} \times P(D)$$
$$+ (1 - \text{Specificity})(1 - P(D))]$$

$$P(Non\text{-}D|Tneg) =$$
$$[\text{Sensitivity} \times (1 - P(D))] / [\text{Specificity} \times (1 - P(D))$$
$$+ P(D) \times (1 - \text{Specificity})]$$

## Likelihood Ratios and Odds Ratios

From relative frequency distributions for results of the index test in the nondiseased and diseased groups, the so-called

diagnostic **likelihood ratio** (LR) of an index test result ($X$) can be calculated as the ratio between the heights of the relative frequency ($f$) distributions at that specific test value. We get:

$$LR(X) = f_D(X) / f_{Non\text{-}D}(X)$$

In case the relative frequency of the distribution of diseased individuals is higher than that of the nondiseased individuals, the ratio exceeds 1. This indicates that disease is more likely than nondisease given this particular index test result. More formally, the ratio can be used to calculate posterior disease probabilities given specific values of the index test ($X$) and the disease prevalence (D):

$$P(D|X) = P(D) \times LR(X) / [P(D) \times LR(X) + (1 - P(D))]$$

or a more simple calculation can be carried out using odds instead of probabilities:

$$Odds(D|X) = Odds(D) \times LR(X)$$

based on the relation:

$$Odds = P / (1 - P)$$

Odds is an alternative way of expressing probabilities commonly used in betting games in Anglo-Saxon countries. For example, a probability of 0.80, or 80%, corresponds to an odds value of 4 according to the formula above. The higher the odds, the closer a probability is to one. From the equation, the posterior odds are equal to the prior odds multiplied by the diagnostic LR for the result X.

For a dichotomous or dichotomized index test, the following relationships apply:

$$LR(pos) = \text{Sensitivity} / (1 - \text{Specificity})$$

$$LR(neg) = (1 - \text{Sensitivity}) / \text{Specificity}$$

A simple way of achieving the posttest probability of disease from the prevalence (pretest probability of disease) and the diagnostic LR is to use the Fagan nomogram. An example is the estimation of the probability of DVT from testing for D-dimer.

## Comparison of Diagnostic Accuracy of Two Tests in Isolation

The diagnostic accuracy—that is, the ability to detect or exclude the target disease as determined by the reference method—of a new diagnostic index test is usually compared with another, established, index test. We here focus on the pure performances of the tests without consideration of other tests (i.e., we consider each test in isolation). When comparing the accuracy of two or more diagnostic index tests, a paired design is generally preferable for reasons of both validity and efficiency. In the target disease-suspected patients, the two index tests under comparison and the reference standard are performed on all subjects, again independently and

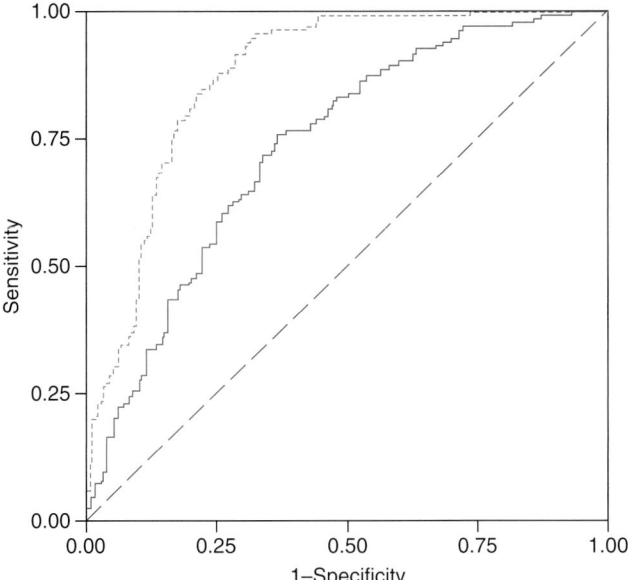

Fig. 2.28 Comparison of the receiver operating characteristic curves of two hypothetical index tests for the same target disease undertaken in the same individuals. The *dotted blue curve* represents a superior diagnostic test, both with regard to sensitivity and specificity over all possible cutoff points. The *dashed diagonal* represents a worthless test, with equal probability of a false-positive (1 − Specificity) and false-negative (1 − Sensitivity) result across all cutoff values (i.e., flipping a coin test). (From Linnet K, Bossuyt PM, Moons KG, et al. Quantifying the accuracy of a diagnostic test or marker. *Clin Chem.* 2012;58:1292–1301.)

blinded with regard to each other's test results. An example of a paired comparison is displayed in Fig. 2.28. Overall, the index test having the largest area under the ROC curve represents the best test. Preferably, CIs of areas and differences of areas should be provided.

The STARD (Standards for Reporting of Diagnostic Accuracy Studies) initiative (Box 2.2) and the so-called QUADAS-2 (Quality Assessment Tool for Diagnostic Accuracy Studies) aim at improving diagnostic accuracy studies (http://www.quadas.org).

## Diagnostic Accuracy of a Test in the Clinical Context

The diagnostic process commonly consists of a series of sequential steps in which much diagnostic information (i.e., diagnostic test results) is acquired. After each step, the physician intuitively judges the probability of the target disease being present. The initial step always consists of patient history and physical signs. If uncertainty about the presence and type of disease remains, subsequent tests are performed, often in another stepwise fashion. These supplementary tests may consist of simple blood or urine tests or be imaging, electrophysiology, or genetic tests, or even later in the process more invasive testing such as biopsy, angiography, or arthroscopy. The supplementary information of each subsequent test is implicitly added to the already collected diagnostic information, and the

target disease probability is constantly updated. This process continues until the target disease can be included or excluded with sufficient certainty.

Diagnostic test studies should reflect the steps in the diagnostic process so that the added value of such tests in excess of the information that is already present can be assessed. Depending on the situation, studies may reveal that the diagnostic information of any subsequent test is already supplied by the simpler previous test results. When regarded in isolation, such subsequent test or marker may indeed show diagnostic accuracy or value, but when assessed in the overall diagnostic workup, it does not. Such a case can arise because different tests may gauge the same underlying pathologic processes to varying degrees and thus provide related diagnostic information.

### Clinical Example: Added Value of d-Dimer Testing in the Diagnosis of Suspected Deep Venous Thrombosis

The same DVT case study described earlier is considered. A total of 2086 patients were suspected of DVT, having at least one of the following symptoms: swelling, redness, or pain in the leg. All patients had a standardized diagnostic workup consisting of index tests from medical history taking, physical examination, and quantitative D-dimer testing. The reference standard was repeated compression ultrasonography, according to current clinical practice, carried out in all patients independent of the results of the index tests and blinded regarding all preceding collected index test results. In total, 416 of the 2068 included patients (20%) had DVT confirmed by ultrasonography. We focus on estimating the added value of D-dimer testing to the information provided by history taking and physical examination.

A multivariable statistical approach is needed to assess the diagnostic accuracy of combined index test results. Logistic regression models express the probability of DVT (on the logit scale) as a linear function of the included index test results. Note that index test results may be included as binary, categorical, or even continuous results. Table 2.4 (model 1) shows the results from history and physical examination test results that were significantly related to DVT in the multivariable analysis, here defined as a multivariable **odds ratio** significantly ($P < .05$) different from 1 (no association).

To quantify whether the quantitative D-dimer assay result has added diagnostic value beyond the history and physical examination results combined, the basic model 1 was simply extended by including the index test D-dimer value, resulting in model 2 (see Table 2.4). After the inclusion of the D-dimer assay result, the regression coefficients of most history and physical tests in model 2 are found to be different from those in model 1: They now express the contribution of the corresponding test results, given a specific D-dimer result. This change reveals that the history and physical and the D-dimer results are indeed correlated and partly provide the same diagnostic information regarding whether DVT is present or not. The trend of lower regression coefficients of

## BOX 2.2 STARD 2015: An Updated List of Essential Items for Reporting Diagnostic Accuracy Studies

**Title or Abstract**

1. Identification as a study of diagnostic accuracy using at least one measure of accuracy (e.g., sensitivity, specificity, predictive values, AUC)

**Abstract**

2. Structured summary of study design, methods, results, and conclusions (for specific guidance, see STARD for Abstracts)

**Introduction**

3. Scientific and clinical background, including the intended use and clinical role of the index test
4. Study objectives and hypotheses

**Methods**

*Study Design*

5. Whether data collection was planned before the index test and reference standard were performed (prospective study) or after (retrospective study)

*Participants*

6. Eligibility criteria
7. On what basis potentially eligible participants were identified (e.g., symptoms, results from previous tests, inclusion in registry)
8. Where and when potentially eligible participants were identified (setting, location, and dates)
9. Whether participants formed a consecutive, random, or convenience series

*Test Methods*

10a. Index test, in sufficient detail to allow replication
10b. Reference standard, in sufficient detail to allow replication
11. Rationale for choosing the reference standard (if alternatives exist)
12a. Definition of and rationale for test positivity cutoffs or result categories of the index test, distinguishing prespecified from exploratory
12b. Definition of and rationale for test positivity cutoffs or result categories of the reference standard, distinguishing prespecified from exploratory
13a. Whether clinical information and reference standard results were available to the performers or readers of the index test

13b. Whether clinical information and index test results were available to the assessors of the reference standard

*Analysis*

14. Methods for estimating or comparing measures of diagnostic accuracy
15. How indeterminate index test or reference standard results were handled
16. How missing data on the index test and reference standard were handled
17. Any analyses of variability in diagnostic accuracy, distinguishing prespecified from exploratory
18. Intended sample size and how it was determined

**Results**

*Participants*

19. Flow of participants, using a diagram
20. Baseline demographic and clinical characteristics of participants
21. Distribution of severity of disease in those with the target condition
22. Distribution of alternative diagnoses in those without the target condition
23. Time interval and any clinical interventions between index test and reference standard

*Test Results*

23. Cross-tabulation of the index test results (or their distribution) by the results of the reference standard
24. Estimates of diagnostic accuracy and their precision (e.g., 95% CIs)
25. Any adverse events from performing the index test or the reference standard

**Discussion**

26. Study limitations, including sources of potential bias, statistical uncertainty, and generalizability
27. Implications for practice, including the intended use and clinical role of the index test

**Other Information**

28. Registration number and name of registry
29. Where the full study protocol can be accessed
30. Sources of funding and other support; role of funders

*AUC,* Area under the curve; *CI,* confidence interval; *STARD,* Standards for Reporting of Diagnostic Accuracy Studies.
From Bossuyt PM, Reitsma JB, Bruns DE, et al. STARD 2015: an updated list of essential items for reporting diagnostic accuracy studies. *Clin Chem.* 2015;61(12):1446–1452.

most findings can be interpreted as follows: A portion of the information supplied by the history and physical items is now replaced by the D-dimer assay result.

### Diagnostic Accuracy of Combinations of Diagnostic Tests: Receiver Operating Characteristic Area

The multivariable diagnostic model, which is based on a combination of diagnostic index tests, as exemplified in models

1 and 2 in Table 2.4, can be considered as a single (overall or combined) quantitative index test, consisting of a composite of individual index tests. The test result of this "combined index test model" for each study patient is simply the calculated posterior probability of DVT presence given the observed pattern of the individual index test results in that patient. (See the footnote to Table 2.4 on how to calculate this probability of disease presence.)

## TABLE 2.4   Basic and Extended Multivariable Diagnostic Model to Discriminate Between Deep Venous Thrombosis Presence Versus Absence[a]

| | MODEL 1 (BASIC MODEL) | | | MODEL 2 (BASIC MODEL + D-DIMER) | | |
|---|---|---|---|---|---|---|
| | Regression Coefficient (SE) | OR (95% CI) | P value | Regression Coefficient (SE) | OR (95% CI) | P value |
| (Intercept) | −3.70 (0.26) | — | <.01 | −4.94 (0.32) | — | <.01 |
| Presence of malignancy | 0.62 (0.22) | 1.9 (1.2–2.9) | <.01 | 0.22 (0.26) | 1.2 (0.7–2.1) | 0.41 |
| Recent surgery | 0.44 (0.16) | 1.6 (1.1–2.1) | <.01 | 0.003 (0.19) | 1.0 (0.7–1.5) | 0.99 |
| Absence of leg trauma | 0.75 (0.18) | 2.1 (1.5–3.0) | <.01 | 0.67 (0.20) | 2.0 (1.3–2.9) | <.01 |
| Vein distension | 0.48 (0.13) | 1.6 (1.1—2.1) | <.01 | 0.25 (0.16) | 1.3 (0.9–1.8) | 0.12 |
| Pain on walking | 0.41 (0.15) | 1.5 (1.1–2.0) | <.01 | 0.46 (0.18) | 1.6 (1.1–2.3) | 0.01 |
| Swelling whole leg | 0.36 (0.12) | 1.4 (1.1–1.8) | <.01 | 0.47 (0.14) | 1.6 (1.2–2.1) | <.01 |
| Difference in calf circumference (per cm) | 0.36 (0.04) | 1.4 (1.3–1.5) | <.01 | 0.29 (0.04) | 1.3 (1.2–1.4) | <.01 |
| D-Dimer (per 500 ng/mL) | NA | NA | NA | 0.29 (0.02) | 1.3 (1.3–1.4) | <.01 |

[a]Exp (regression coefficient) is the odds ratio (OR) of a diagnostic test result. For example, an odds ratio of 2 for absence of leg trauma (model 2) means that a suspected patient without a recent leg trauma has a two times higher chance of having deep venous thrombosis (DVT) than a patient with a recent leg trauma (because in the latter the leg trauma would more likely be the cause of the presenting symptoms and signs). Similarly, an odds ratio of 1.3 for calf difference in cm (model 2) means that for every centimeter increase in calf circumference difference, a patient has a 1.3 times (or 30%) higher chance of having DVT.

A diagnostic model can be considered as a single overall or combined test consisting of different test results, with the probability of DVT presence as its test result. For example, for a male subject without malignancy, recent surgery, or leg trauma but with vein distension and a painful, not swollen leg when walking with a calf difference of 6 cm the formula is (model 1):

$$Z = -3.70 + 0.62*0 + 0.44*0 + 0.75*0 + 0.48*1 + 0.41*1 + 0.36*0 + 0.36*6 = -0.65$$

The probability for this patient of the presence of DVT based on the basic model then is exp (−0.65)/(1 + exp[−0.65]) = 34%.

*CI,* Confidence interval; *NA,* not applicable; *SE,* standard error.

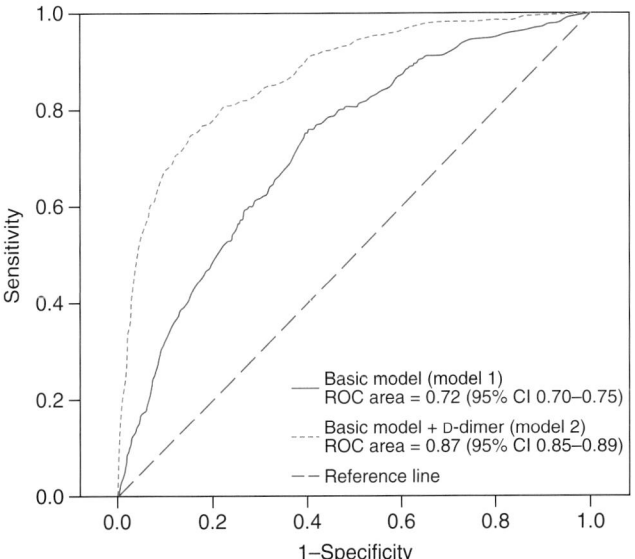

**Fig. 2.29** Receiver operating characteristic *(ROC)* curves for the combination of history and physical examination tests before and after addition of the D-dimer assay result. (From Moonc KG, de Groot JA, Linnet K, et al. Quantifying the added value of a diagnostic test or marker. *Clin Chem.* 2012;58:1408–1417.)

As for single continuous index tests described earlier, also for "test combinations" combined into a single multivariable model, the ROC area (*c*-statistic) can be calculated to indicate the ability of this "test combination" to discriminate between the presence versus absence of the target disease (here DVT). Fig. 2.29 shows the ROC curves and areas for models 1 and 2.

Adding the quantitative D-dimer assay to model 1 mediated an increase in the ROC area from 0.72 to 0.87, a considerable and statistically significant gain (*P* < .01).

## Impact of Diagnostic Tests

When thinking about approaches to evaluate the impact of diagnostic tests on medical decision making, patient outcomes, and health care at large, it is useful to describe the pathways through which benefits (and risks) of using the test are likely to occur. This so-called *working pathway* provides a framework (Fig. 2.30) to explain how a given test leads to benefits or risks for patients' health or health care. Such working pathways include:

1. The anticipated technical or analytical capabilities of the test
2. The unintended and intended results and effects of the test (e.g., benefits of diagnosis and treatment) when applied in the targeted context
3. Those individuals in whom these effects are likely to occur (e.g., in the targeted patients or in the care providers)
4. The anticipated mechanisms through which these potential effects will occur
5. Existing care in the targeted context and individuals
6. The expected time frame in which potential risks and benefits might occur

A clear description of the working pathway of a new test can determine the current benefits (and risks) of prevailing care in the intended medical context. It also helps determine

## POINTS TO REMEMBER

- The diagnostic accuracy of a test indicates the frequency and type of errors that a test will produce when differentiating between patients with and without the target disease.
- The cohort design based on patients suspected of the diseases targeted by the index test is generally preferable for evaluating diagnostic accuracy.
- It is not meaningful to regard estimates of diagnostic performance as properties of the test itself but rather to interpret them as depending on the setting in which the index test was applied and dependent on other tests that are commonly used in that setting.
- Focus has been on approaches and measures for quantification of the diagnostic accuracy of combinations of index tests and of the added value of a new diagnostic test beyond existing diagnostic tests.

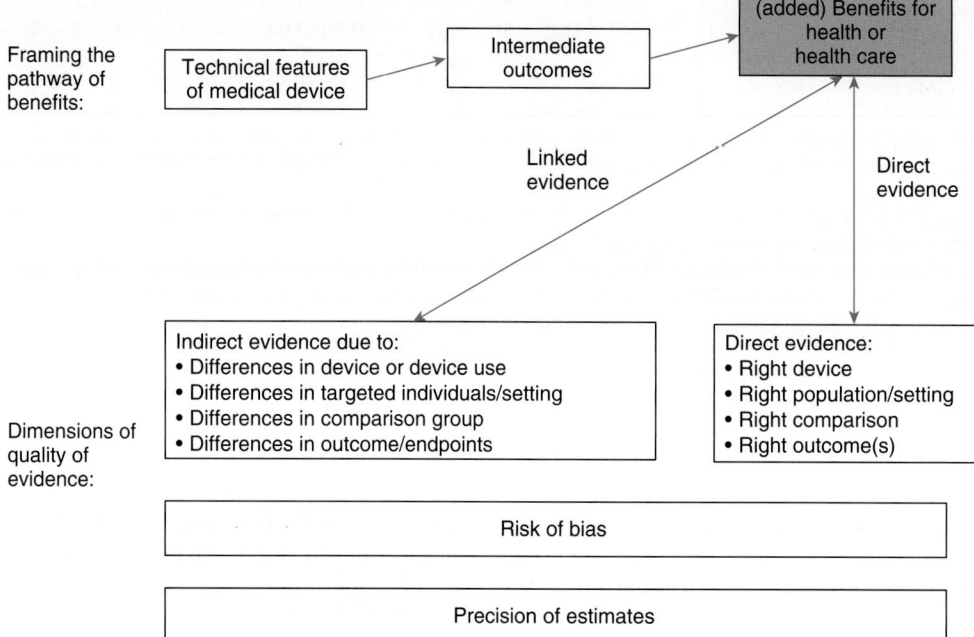

**Fig. 2.30** Relationship between the pathway through which devices may lead to benefits or added benefits for health or health care and the three dimensions of quality for evidence (indirectness of evidence, risk of bias, precision of estimates). (From KNAW. *Evaluation of New Technology in Health Care. In Need of Guidance for Relevant Evidence.* Amsterdam: KNAW; 2014.)

what added value or benefits the new test must provide to improve existing care and what evidence is necessary to quantify whether these (added) benefits are indeed achieved at what risks or costs.

## REVIEW QUESTIONS

1. Which statement applies to a sample of values drawn from a Gaussian distribution?
   a. The central location is best described by the median.
   b. The dispersion is best described by the interquartile range.
   c. The distribution of the values is likely to be asymmetric.
   d. The $t$ distribution is useful for estimation of the 95% CI for the mean value.

2. The analytical specificity of an assay is:
   a. the ability of an assay procedure to determine the concentration of a target analyte in the presence of interfering substances in the sample matrix.
   b. the detection limit of a method.
   c. the ability of an analytical method to assess small variations in the concentration of analyte.
   d. the analyte concentration range over which measurements are within the declared tolerances for imprecision and bias of the method.

3. Two analytical methods are to be compared by analysis in parallel of a suitable number of patient samples. Which of the following is correct?
   a. Ordinary least-squares regression analysis is the most appropriate data analysis approach.
   b. It is generally recommended that the manufacturer use 40 samples for comparison and the user laboratory 100 samples.
   c. A calibration difference is most typically disclosed by an intercept estimate significantly different from zero obtained by regression analysis.
   d. In case of constant CV%s, the Bland-Altman difference plot shows an increasing scatter of the measured differences at increasing measurement values.

4. In a regression analysis comparing results of two methods, the $y$-intercept is calculated to be 2.0 and the slope is 3. This indicates a(n):
   a. calibration error.
   b. uncertainty.
   c. systematic difference.
   d. interference in one method.

5. Which one of the following, when stated as an interval around a reported laboratory result, will specify the location of the true value with a given probability?
   a. Traceability
   b. Coefficient of variation
   c. Trueness
   d. Uncertainty

6. The traceability chain extends downwards from the reference measurement procedure to the routine analytical method. Which of the following is correct?
   a. A reference measurement procedure is sensitive to matrix effects.
   b. The standard uncertainty indicates a 95% uncertainty interval.
   c. Harmonization of laboratory measurements do not presuppose traceability to a reference measurement procedure.
   d. The reference measurement procedure is always more precise than the routine analytical method.

7. The diagnostic accuracy of a test is assessed on a number of subjects suspected of having a given target disease. Which of the following is correct?
   a. The diagnostic accuracy is characteristic for the test and is not influenced by the actual setting in which it is evaluated.
   b. The ROC area provides a measure of the diagnostic accuracy, which is not dependent on a selected cut-off value.
   c. When the cut-off value of a quantitative test is increased, the specificity declines and the sensitivity increases.
   d. In order to rule out the presence of disease, it is important that the specificity is high.

8. The probability of the presence of a specific disease divided by the probability of its absence is the:
   a. likelihood ratio.
   b. odds ratio.
   c. prevalence.
   d. predictive value.

9. When a receiver operating characteristic curve is plotted, the $x$-axis represents the:
   a. false-positive rate.
   b. true-positive rate.
   c. false-negative rate.
   d. true-negative rate.

10. A new test is added to an existing set of diagnostic procedures. Which of the following is correct?
    a. The diagnostic accuracy of the new test is the most important point to consider.
    b. A multivariate data treatment based on logistic regression analysis presupposes quantitative test results.
    c. It is unlikely that results from several tests are correlated.
    d. The difference between the ROC curve area after addition of the new test and the area of the ROC curve of the original diagnostic procedure expresses the added value of the new test.

## SUGGESTED READINGS

Bland JM, Altman DG. Statistical methods for assessing agreement between two methods of clinical measurement. *Lancet*. 1986;1(8476):307–310.

Bossuyt PM, Reitsma JB, Bruns DE, et al. An updated list of essential items for reporting diagnostic accuracy studies. *Clin Chem*. 2015;61:1446–1452.

Bossuyt PMM, Reitsma JB, Linnet K, et al. Beyond diagnostic accuracy: the clinical utility of diagnostic tests. *Clin Chem*. 2012;58:1636–1643.

Dybkær R. Vocabulary for use in measurement procedures and description of reference materials in laboratory medicine. *Eur J Clin Chem Clin Biochem*. 1997;35:141–173.

Hendriksen JMT, Geersing GJ, van Voorthuizen SC, et al. The cost-effectiveness of point-of-care D-dimer tests compared with a laboratory test to rule out deep venous thrombosis in primary care. *Expert Rev Mol Diagnost*. 2015;15:125–136.

Horvath AR, Lord SJ, StJohn A, et al. From biomarkers to medical tests: the changing landscape of test evaluation. *Clin Chem Acta*. 2014;427:49–57.

Krouwer JS. Setting performance goals and evaluating total analytical error for diagnostic assays. *Clin Chem*. 2002;48:919–927.

Linnet K, Bossuyt PM, Moons KG, et al. Quantifying the accuracy of a diagnostic test or marker. *Clin Chem*. 2012;58:1292–1301.

Linnet K. Estimation of the linear relationship between the measurements of two methods with proportional errors. *Statist Med*. 1990;9:1463–1473.

Linnet K. Evaluation of regression procedures for methods comparison studies. *Clin Chem*. 31993;9:424–432.

Linnet K. Limitations of the paired *t*-test for evaluation of method comparison data. *Clin Chem*. 1999;45:314–315.

Linnet K. Nonparametric estimation of reference intervals by simple and bootstrap-based procedures. *Clin Chem*. 2000;46:867–869.

Moons KG. Criteria for scientific evaluation of novel markers: a perspective. *Clin Chem*. 2010;56:537–541.

Moons KG, Altman DG, Reitsma JB, et al. Transparent Reporting of a multivariable prediction model for Individual Prognosis or Diagnosis (TRIPOD): explanation and elaboration. *Ann Intern Med*. 2015;162(1):W1–W73.

Moons KG, Biesheuvel CJ, Grobbee DE. Test research versus diagnostic research. *Clin Chem*. 2004;50(3):473–476.

Moons KG, de Groot JA, Linnet K, et al. Quantifying the added value of a diagnostic test or marker. *Clin. Chem*. 2012;58:1408–1417.

Moons KG, Grobbee DE. Diagnostic studies as multivariable, prediction research. *J Epidemiol Commun Health*. 2002;56(5):337–338.

Moons KG, van Es GA, Deckers JW, et al. Limitations of sensitivity, specificity, likelihood ratio, and Bayes' theorem in assessing diagnostic probabilities: a clinical example. *Epidemiology*. 1997;8(1):12–17.

Obuchowski NA, Lieber ML, Wians Jr FH. ROC curves in clinical chemistry: uses, misuses, and possible solutions. *Clin Chem*. 2004;50:1118–1125.

Oudega R, Moons KG, Hoes AW. Ruling out deep venous thrombosis in primary care. A simple diagnostic algorithm including D-dimer testing. *Thromb Haemost*. 2005;94:200–205.

Passing H, Bablok W. Comparison of several regression procedures for method comparison studies and determination of sample sizes. *J Clin Chem Clin Biochem*. 1984;22:431–445.

Pencina MJ, D'Agostino RB, Vasan RS. Statistical methods for assessment of added usefulness of new biomarkers. *Clin Chem Lab Med*. 2010;48:1703–1711.

Snedecor GW, Cochran WG. *Statistical Methods*. 8th ed. Ames, IA: Iowa State University Press; 1989; 75: 121, 140–142, 170–4, 177, 237–8, 279.

Vesper HW, Thienpont LM. Traceability in laboratory medicine. *Clin Chem*. 2009;55:1067–1075.

# Preanalytical Variation

*Ana-Maria Simundic*

## OBJECTIVES

1. List major sources of variability in preanalytical phase.
2. Define the following terms:
   - Modifiable and unmodifiable influencing factors
   - Endogenous and exogenous interference factors
   - In vivo and in vitro hemolysis
   - Lipemia
   - Icterus
   - First morning urine
   - Timed urine specimen
   - First void urine
   - Midstream urine
   - Suprapubic urine aspiration
   - Unstimulated whole saliva
   - Stimulated saliva
3. State how to deal with modifiable and nonmodifiable influencing factors.
4. Summarize the requirements for a proper definition of the fasting state.
5. Describe mechanisms through which hemolysis, icterus, and lipemia affect various assays and parameters.
6. Describe ways of removal of lipids from the sample.
7. Identify major preanalytical issues related to some specific laboratory tests or sample types.
8. Define optimal sample type for blood gas analysis.
9. Describe proper procedure for saliva collection.
10. Explain the difference between stimulated and unstimulated saliva collection.
11. List advantages and challenges of using saliva as a diagnostic specimen.
12. Describe how cold agglutinins, cryoglobulins, and ethylenediaminetetraacetic acid "(EDTA)-dependent antibodies" interfere with hematologic analytes.

## KEY WORDS AND DEFINITIONS

**Cold agglutinins** Antibodies specific for erythrocyte surface carbohydrate antigens, which bind to the erythrocyte surface at 0°C to 4°C.

**Cryoglobulins** Immunoglobulins with temperature-dependent solubility that precipitate at temperatures below 37°C.

**Endogenous interferences** Interferences that originate from the substances present in the patient sample.

**Exogenous interferences** The effect of various substances added to the patient sample (anticoagulants, gel particles, infusions, etc.).

**First morning urine** A urine specimen that is collected immediately after arising from bed after an overnight sleep (also called overnight or early morning urine).

**First void urine** The first portion of the urine (usually the first 15 to 50 mL) passed at any time of the day.

**Hemolysis** A process of membrane disruption of erythrocytes and other blood cells, accompanied by the subsequent release of cell components into the plasma and red coloration of the serum or plasma after centrifugation.

**Icterus** A clinical condition that is associated with a change of the color of the serum due to the increase of bilirubin concentration above 5.9 mg/dL or 100 μmol/L.

**In vitro hemolysis** Hemolysis that occurs outside of the patient at various steps of the preanalytical phase (during blood sampling, sample handling, delivery to the laboratory, and sample storage).

**In vivo hemolysis** Hemolysis that occurs within the body, before the blood has been drawn and is a result of a pathologic condition.

**Influencing factors** In vivo and in vitro effects on laboratory results of biological origin that modify the concentration of the affected analyte in a method-independent way.

**Interference factors** Compounds and mechanisms in a biological specimen that alter the result of an analyte thus leading to falsely increased or decreased laboratory test results for that analyte.

**Laboratory error** Any error that occurs throughout the total testing process (i.e., preanalytical phase, analytical phase, and postanalytical phase).

**Lipemia** Turbidity of the sample visible to the naked eye, which is caused by light scattering due to the presence of large lipoprotein particles.

**Midstream urine** A urine specimen collected during the middle of a urine flow after the urinary opening has been carefully cleaned (also called clean catch urine specimen).

**Modifiable influencing factors** Influencing factors that can be controlled by patient action.

**Preanalytical phase** Part of the total testing process that encompasses test requesting, patient preparation, sampling, sample transport, delivery to the laboratory, and sample handling before analysis.

**Stimulated saliva** A saliva sample obtained by the stimulation of salivation with citric acid or by oral movements (yawning, chewing paraffin or gum) and collected through adsorbing saliva with cotton rolls, cotton swabs, or filter paper.

**Suprapubic aspiration** A specific way of urine collection performed by aspirating urine from the distended bladder through the abdominal wall.

**Timed urine specimen** A urine specimen that is collected at a specified time or in relation to some activity (e.g., before a meal, after a meal, before therapy, exercise) during a 24-hour period.

**Unmodifiable influencing factors** Factors that lead to unavoidable changes in analyte concentration and cannot be controlled by patient action.

**Unstimulated whole saliva** A saliva sample collected either passively or by spitting into a collector vial.

# PREANALYTICAL PHASE

The annual incidence of premature patient deaths associated with some form of preventable medical error in the United States has been estimated to be 98,000 per year. More recent data indicate that the actual mortality caused by preventable medical errors might even be fourfold higher. Laboratory errors significantly contribute to the overall error frequency in health care. They can lead to diagnostic errors (i.e., missed diagnosis, misdiagnosis, and delayed diagnosis) and consequent patient harm, and increased health care expenditure. The preanalytical phase is recognized as the most vulnerable part of the total testing process and it accounts for two-thirds of all laboratory errors and may be attributed to various causes. Many preanalytical steps are performed outside the laboratory and are not under the direct supervision of laboratory staff. Furthermore, many individuals are involved in various preanalytical steps and those individuals have different levels of education and professional background. Finally, safe practice standards for many activities and procedures (1) are either not available, or (2) available but are not evidence based, or (3) there is a low level of compliance with those standards.

The ISO 15189 accreditation standard clearly defines that medical laboratories are responsible for the management and quality of the preexamination phase. It is the role of the laboratorian to ensure that the right sample is taken from the right patient, at the right time, and that correct test results are provided to the requesting physician in a timely manner. If the quality of the specimen is compromised to a degree where the expected effect is larger than the allowable error, causing clinically significant bias, the sample should be rejected for analysis. The guiding principle should be: "No result is always better than a bad result."

## Influencing and Interference Factors

### Influencing Factors

Influencing factors are effects on laboratory results of biological origin which can occur in vivo (most common) and in vitro (during sample transport and storage). Biological factors modify the concentration of the analyte in a method-independent way.

These factors are either present in the healthy individual, like circadian rhythms, or appear as an effect of a disease and its treatment. Examples of modifiable influencing factors are diet, time of the day, or time of the year (season), whereas unmodifiable influencing factors are gender, ethnicity, genetic background, etc.

*Modifiable influencing factors.* Changes occurring due to the time of sampling may affect the concentrations of various analytes. These changes can be linear (in a chronological order) and cyclic (of a repetitive nature, such as seasonal changes, or changes due to the menstrual cycle).

Several analytes tend to fluctuate in terms of their plasma concentration over the course of a day (i.e., circadian rhythm). For example, the concentration of cortisol is highest in the morning and lowest at night. To avoid the potential effect of analyte changes during the day, reference intervals are defined for blood sampling between 7 and 9 a.m.

Besides the circadian rhythm, some analytes can exhibit significant changes due to the biological changes that occur in hormone patterns during menstruation. For example, aldosterone concentration in plasma is twice as high before ovulation as in the follicular phase.

Diet also may substantially affect the composition of plasma. Differences in serum composition may occur respective to the source of nutrients, the number of meals, and the proportion of nutrients in a diet. Effects from diet can be either long-term or acute. Long-term effects of diet may occur over a couple of days or longer. For example, a diet rich in fat leads to increased serum triglyceride concentration, whereas a diet rich in carbohydrates decreases serum protein and lipid concentrations. Vegetarians tend to have lower concentrations of plasma cholesterol, triglycerides, and creatinine with reduced urinary excretion of creatinine, and a higher urinary pH, as a result of reduced intake of precursors of acid metabolites. Most of the changes described are corrected following the restoration of good nutrition.

Acute effects of diet and other influencing factors occur immediately or shortly after ingestion of food or fluid intake. For example, the decrease of plasma glucose and increase of lactate are the acute effects of ethanol consumption, which occur as early as 2 to 4 hours after the ingestion. Tobacco smoking leads to a number of acute changes in the concentration of fatty acids, epinephrine, free glycerol, aldosterone,

## TABLE 3.1 Unavoidable Influences on Laboratory Results

| Influence | Examples of Analyte Concentrations Changed | Remarks |
|---|---|---|
| Age | Alkaline phosphatase, LDL-cholesterol, hormones, creatinine | Provide age-dependent reference intervals |
| Race | Creatine kinase higher in black than in white males | Provide race-specific reference intervals |
| | Granulocytes higher in white than in black | |
| | Creatinine higher in black than in white | |
| Gender | Alanine aminotransferase, γ-glutamyltransferase, creatinine | Provide gender-specific reference intervals |
| Pregnancy | Triglycerides ↑, homocysteine ↓ during pregnancy | Document months of pregnancy with laboratory results |
| Altitude | CRP, hemoglobin ↑, transferrin ↓ | Consider weeks of adaptation, when coming from or going to high altitude |

*CRP,* C-reactive protein; *LDL,* low-density lipoprotein.

and cortisol. These changes occur within 1 hour of smoking one to five cigarettes. Moreover, within only 10 minutes of smoking a single cigarette, there is an increase in glucose concentration by up to 10 mg/dL (0.56 mmol/L). This increase may persist for 1 hour.

Physical activity of varying duration and intensity may lead to substantial changes in the plasma composition, and the extent of this change depends on several factors, such as training status, fluid intake, electrolytes, carbohydrates, and even the ambient temperature, etc. For example, even a mild physical effort, like clenching a fist during venous blood sampling, can increase the concentration of potassium and should therefore be avoided. Intensive exercise is associated with transient elevations of cardiac biomarkers, markers of muscle damage, enhanced platelet aggregation, leukocytosis, elevation of tissue-plasminogen activator levels, and activation of the fibrinolytic system.

Some modifiable biological influence factors, such as diet, can be controlled by patient action, whereas some others (e.g., age) are noncontrollable. Proper standardization of controllable preanalytical variables will lead to the significant reduction of preanalytical variability.

To ensure standardization of patient preparation for blood sampling, the following general requirements should be applied to all blood tests in the fasting state:
1. Blood should be drawn preferably in the morning from 7 to 9 a.m.
2. Fasting should last for 12 hours, during which water consumption is permitted.
3. Alcohol should be avoided for 24 hours before blood sampling.
4. In the morning before blood sampling, patients should refrain from cigarette smoking and caffeine-containing drinks (tea, coffee, etc.).

*Unmodifiable influencing factors.* Various biological factors, known as **unmodifiable influencing factors**, lead to changes in analyte concentration, which are unavoidable (Table 3.1). These factors should be considered when interpreting laboratory results because their influence cannot be prevented by preanalytical standardization. Possible ways to address these factors are to partition reference intervals for age, race, gender, month of pregnancy, and so on (see Chapter 5).

## Interference Factors

**Interference factors** have the ability to alter the result of any analyte after the specimen has been collected, thus leading to falsely increased or decreased laboratory test results for that analyte. Their effect is assay dependent.

Interferences can be endogenous and exogenous. **Endogenous interferences** are biological constituents of the sample. They originate from the substances present in the patient sample whereas exogenous interferences are either present in the sample (drugs, herbal components, etc.) or are added to the sample during or after sampling. **Exogenous interferences** relate to the effect of various substances added to the patient sample, such as separator gels, anticoagulants, surfactants, etc., all of which may cause significant interference.

Possible endogenous interference factors include:
1. Glucose
2. Paraproteins
3. Free hemoglobin (i.e., hemolysis)
4. Lipids (i.e., lipemia)
5. Bilirubin (i.e., **icterus**)

Possible exogenous interference factors include:
1. Drugs
2. Herbal components
3. Anticoagulants
4. Tube additives
5. Tube gels
6. Intravenous infusions

## POINTS TO REMEMBER

**Influencing and Interference Factors**
- Influencing factors lead to changes in the quantity of the analyte in a method-independent way
- Influencing factors may be changeable (e.g., diet, time of the day) or unchangeable (e.g., gender, ethnicity, genetic background)
- The effect of influencing factors may be reduced through the standardization of preanalytical conditions
- Interferences are mechanisms and factors that lead to falsely increased or decreased results of laboratory tests
- Interference factors and their mechanisms differ with respect to the intended analyte and analytical method, and may be reduced or eliminated by selecting a more specific method

# ENDOGENOUS INTERFERENCE FACTORS

## Hemolysis

### Definition and Background

**Hemolysis** is a process of membrane disruption of erythrocytes and other blood cells, accompanied by the subsequent release of cell components into the plasma and red coloration of the serum (or plasma) to various degrees, after centrifugation. Though hemoglobin is the most abundant protein in red blood cells, hemolysis is not necessarily always associated with the release of hemoglobin into the surrounding extracellular fluid. For example, if a blood sample is stored at a low temperature, low molecular intracellular components (e.g., electrolytes) diffuse from the cells, but hemoglobin will not. Furthermore, the efflux of cell components due to cell lysis affects all blood cells (i.e., platelets and white blood cells) and not only erythrocytes. Therefore it is important to remember that red coloration of the serum or plasma can never accurately predict the concentration of analytes released from blood cell components.

Hemolysis is the most common preanalytical error and cause of sample rejection. Its frequency is up to 30% and accounts for almost 60% of unsuitable specimens. The frequency of hemolysis largely depends on the collection facility, the phlebotomy personnel, and the characteristics of the patient population. The highest frequency of hemolysis has been observed in samples from emergency departments, pediatric departments, and intensive care units, whereas hemolysis has proven to be the least frequent in outpatient phlebotomy centers where blood sampling is done by specialized laboratory staff. These differences are due to the level of knowledge and skills of the staff performing blood collection procedures.

There are two major sources of hemolysis: (1) in vivo and (2) in vitro hemolysis. **In vivo hemolysis** occurs within the body, before the blood has been drawn and is a result of a pathologic condition. Hemolysis in vivo may occur as a result of numerous biochemical (enzyme deficiencies, erythrocyte membrane defects, hemoglobinopathies), physical (prolonged marching, drumming, prosthetic heart valves), chemical (ethanol, drug overdose, toxins, snake venom), immunologic (autoantibodies) mechanisms, and infections (babesiosis, malaria). The most common causes of in vivo hemolysis are a reaction to incompatible transfusion and autoimmune hemolytic anemia.

In vivo hemolysis is not very common and accounts for only 3% of all hemolyzed samples. Laboratories should have a procedure in place for distinguishing in vivo and in vitro hemolysis. In vivo hemolysis should always be suspected when patient blood is hemolyzed over a longer period of time, after repeated blood sampling, even after special care has been taken to avoid hemolysis. Decreased concentration of haptoglobin in serum and free hemoglobin in urine are the most pronounced and specific laboratory signs of in vivo hemolysis. Haptoglobin is a protein that binds free hemoglobin in the circulation to prevent oxidative damage induced by hemoglobin. Once released from the erythrocyte into the plasma, hemoglobin forms complexes with haptoglobin, and those complexes are removed from the circulation by macrophages.

In more pronounced cases of in vivo hemolysis, haptoglobin in serum can be undetectable (i.e., below the limit of detection), whereas its concentration in cases of in vitro hemolysis remains unchanged. When in vivo hemolysis is confirmed, the laboratory should not reject hemolyzed samples for analysis, since parameters in hemolyzed samples reflect the actual patient condition and are relevant for adequate patient care (diagnosis, therapy management, monitoring).

**In vitro hemolysis** occurs outside of the patient at various steps of the preanalytical phase (e.g., blood sampling, sample handling, delivery to the laboratory, and sample storage).

### Mechanisms of Hemolysis Interference

Hemolysis is an endogenous interference that causes clinically relevant bias of patient results through several distinct mechanisms.

*Spectrophotometric interference.* Spectrophotometric interference of hemolysis occurs due to the ability of hemoglobin to absorb light at the following wavelengths: 415, 540, and 570 nm. This characteristic of hemoglobin causes optical interference, which can lead to either falsely increased or decreased concentrations of the measured parameters. The direction and degree of the interference largely depend on the analyte and the method.

*Release of cell components into the sample.* Some components are present in blood cells in concentrations that are several times higher than those in the extracellular space (i.e., plasma or serum). Table 3.2 shows some of the most pronounced differences between intracellular and extracellular concentrations in red cells.

From this, it follows that there is a dramatic increase in the concentration of the listed analytes measured in hemolyzed plasma (or serum) due to the efflux of those substances from erythrocytes.

Since intracellular components may also escape from platelets during clotting, there is a marked difference in the potassium concentration between serum and plasma. The mean estimated difference in the concentration of potassium in serum and plasma is 0.36 ± 0.18 mmol/L and this difference is positively associated with the platelet count. Plasma

### TABLE 3.2 Ratio Between Intracellular and Extracellular Concentration of Various Parameters in Red Cells

| Analyte | Intracellular Concentration (Compared to Extracellular) |
|---|---|
| LDH (lactate dehydrogenase) | ↑160× |
| Inorganic phosphate | ↑100× |
| Potassium | ↑40× |
| AST (aspartate aminotransferase) | ↑40× |
| Folic acid | ↑30× |
| ALT (alanine aminotransferase) | ↑7× |
| Magnesium | ↑3× |

Note: The most pronounced effect of hemolysis is seen for LDH. LDH activity may be increased by >20% in mildly hemolyzed samples and as much as >350% in grossly hemolyzed samples.

is therefore the recommended sample type for the accurate measurement of potassium.

*Sample dilution.* Some analytes, such as albumin, bilirubin, glucose, and sodium, are present in much higher concentrations in plasma than in blood cells. For those parameters, hemolysis will cause a dilution effect and their concentrations will be lower in hemolyzed samples. The effect of sample dilution causes clinically significant bias only at a higher degree of hemolysis. For example, glucose is negatively affected by severe hemolysis (−8.3%) only when the concentration of free hemoglobin is greater than 3 g/L.

*Chemical interference.* Various blood cell components may affect the analyte measurement procedure by directly or indirectly competing for molecules in the reagents, inhibiting indicator reactions or modifying the analyte by complexation, proteolysis, or precipitation. One such effect is caused by the enzyme, adenylate kinase, present in erythrocytes, as well as in platelets. When released from the cells during hemolysis, adenylate kinase may compete for adenosine diphosphate (ADP) with creatine kinase in a creatine kinase assay if inhibitors are not supplied in the reaction mixture. Furthermore, hemoglobin released from erythrocytes during hemolysis may interfere with various assays through its pseudo-peroxidase activity. Pseudo-peroxidase activity of free hemoglobin released from erythrocytes interferes in the assay for measurement of bilirubin concentration through the inhibition of the formation of diazonium salt.

Hemolysis may cause a clinically significant interference on a wide range of analytes in immunochemistry assays. This interference is caused by modifying the reaction analytes (antigens and antibodies) by the proteolytic action of cathepsin E, the major proteolytic enzyme in mature erythrocytes. Proteolytic enzymes released from erythrocytes may mask or potentially enhance epitope recognition in various immunoassays. Interference caused by proteolytic activity may cause measurement bias of various degrees and directions, depending on the assay.

## Lipemia

Lipemia is defined as turbidity of the sample visible to the naked eye. This turbidity is caused by light scattering due to the presence of large lipoprotein particles. The increase in concentration of lipoproteins in blood most commonly occurs due to postprandial triglyceride increase, parenteral lipid infusions, or some lipid disorders. Not all lipoproteins have equal contribution to the sample turbidity. The effect of lipoprotein particles on sample turbidity depends on the size of the particles. Chylomicrons and very-low-density lipoproteins (VLDLs), the largest lipoprotein particles in the circulation, have the greatest contribution to sample turbidity. To avoid postprandial lipemia, patients are requested to fast for 12 hours before blood sampling.

### Mechanisms of Interference Caused by Lipemia

Lipemia is an important endogenous interference that may cause clinically relevant bias of patient results through the following mechanisms:

*Spectrophotometric interference.* Lipemia causes interference by light absorbance and light scattering. A lipemic sample absorbs light, decreasing the intensity of the light passing through the sample. This absorption occurs in the 300 to 700 nm wavelengths. Sample absorbance rises with the decreasing wavelengths and is maximal in the ultraviolet range. That is why many enzymatic methods in which the end product is measured at 340 nm are strongly affected by lipemia.

Lipemic samples also cause light scattering. Light scattering occurs in all directions and its intensity depends on the number and size of lipoprotein particles and the wavelength of measurement. For this reason, light scattering of lipoprotein particles causes significant interference with turbidimetry and nephelometry. In methods where the transmittance of light is inversely proportional to the concentration of the analyte, in the absence of the sample blank, sample turbidity causes positive bias. However, in some competitive assays where the transmittance of light is directly proportional to the concentration of the analyte, sample turbidity will cause negative bias.

*Interference caused by the volume depletion effect.* Plasma in healthy individuals in the fasting state consists of only a minor portion of lipids (<10% of the total plasma volume). The rest of the plasma is water. The increase in the concentration of lipoprotein particles leads to an increase in the plasma volume occupied by lipids. Particles that are not lipid soluble are displaced by the lipids to the water part of the plasma. Through this mechanism, lipemia may lead to the false decrease of the concentration of the measured analyte, in all methods in which the concentration of respective analyte is measured in the total plasma volume (e.g., pseudo-hyponatremia if sodium is measured by flame photometry and indirect measurement using ion-selective electrodes, but not in direct potentiometry).

*Interference caused by partitioning of the sample.* Upon centrifugation of a lipemic sample, lipoproteins are not homogeneously distributed in the serum or plasma due to the lipid gradient. Water-soluble analytes are more concentrated in the lower layer of the plasma or serum, whereas lipids and lipid-soluble analytes, such as drugs and some lipid-soluble hormones, are more concentrated in the top lipid-rich layer. This is especially important in automated chemistry analyzers with a fixed path length of the sample probe. Test results may differ for those analytes that are not evenly distributed between the lipid and water portions of the sample, depending on the part of the specimen from which the probe takes the sample for analysis.

*Interference caused by physicochemical mechanisms.* Excess lipoproteins in blood may interfere with electrophoretic and chromatographic methods by causing abnormal peaks. Elevated levels of triglycerides and lipoprotein particles may disturb the electrophoretic pattern as well as falsely increase the relative percentage of the prealbumin, albumin, and α1- and α2-globulin regions. Moreover, lipemia may affect some immunochemistry assays by masking the binding sites on antigens and antibodies, and thus physically interfere with antigen–antibody binding.

### Removal of Lipids From the Sample

Unlike hemolysis, the interference caused by lipemia can be fully eliminated or at least reduced, by removing the excess lipids from the sample. Methods for lipid removal include ultracentrifugation, high-speed centrifugation, and some lipid-clearing agents.

Ultracentrifugation is the recommended method for the removal of the excess of lipids in the sample. Ultracentrifuges use the centrifugation force of almost 200,000 g and are very effective in clearing lipemic sera by separating lipids, especially chylomicrons (top layer), from the aqueous part (lower layer) of the sample. After centrifugation, the infranatant (lower part of the sample) can be analyzed. It should be kept in mind that by removing the upper lipid layer one also removes lipid-soluble analytes such as drugs and hormones. Results reported from ultracentrifuged samples or samples from which lipids have been removed in any other way should be appropriately annotated to ensure clinicians are aware that the sample has been manipulated to obtain the reported results.

In laboratories where ultracentrifuge is not available, high-speed centrifugation using the microcentrifuge with a maximum centrifugation speed of up to 20,000 g for 15 minutes at room temperature may serve as an acceptable alternative.

Lipid-clearing agents are widely used in many laboratories due to their low cost, convenience, and ease of use. Those agents (cyclodextrin, polyethylene glycol, dextran sulfate, hexane, and others) may vary in their ability to extract lipids from a lipemic sample and may lead to reduction of a significant amount of protein from the sample. It is therefore very important for laboratories to verify the performance of such reagents before their routine use.

## Icterus

The normal concentration of bilirubin in human plasma (or serum) is up to 20 $\mu$mol/L. A change in the color of the serum (or plasma) becomes detectable when bilirubin concentration exceeds 34 $\mu$mol/L. Bilirubin concentrations above 100 $\mu$mol/L are clinically defined as icterus. Bilirubin interferes with numerous chemistry tests, such as enzymes (alanine aminotransferase, alkaline phosphatase, creatine kinase, lipase), electrolytes, metabolites (urea, creatinine, glucose), lipids (cholesterol, triglycerides), proteins (albumin, total proteins, immunoglobulin [Ig]-G), hormones (estradiol, beta-human chorionic gonadotropin [$\beta$-hCG], free T3), and even some drugs (gentamicin, phenobarbital, theophylline, tobramycin). As is the case for hemolysis and lipemia, interference caused by bilirubin differs between instruments and assays.

Unfortunately, there is not much that can be done by the laboratory to remove or minimize the effect of icteric interference. Possible options are diluting the sample (possible only for analytes present at high enough concentrations in the blood) and testing the requested analytes with a different method or on a different instrument for which icterus does not cause clinically significant interference.

### Mechanisms of Interference Caused by Icterus

Icterus interferes through two mechanisms: spectrophotometric interference and by interfering with chemical reactions. It is important to recognize that both mechanisms may occur simultaneously in one sample.

Bilirubin causes spectrophotometric interference due to its ability to absorb light in the wide range of wavelengths between 400 and 540 nm.

Chemical interference of bilirubin is exerted through its interaction with various components in the blood. For example, bilirubin produces negative bias on assays that involve $H_2O_2$ as an intermediate reaction (e.g., cholesterol, glucose, uric acid, triglycerides).

## Detection of Hemolysis, Lipemia, and Icterus

Hemolysis becomes visible at the concentration of 0.3 to 0.5 g/L of free hemoglobin and the intensity of the red color of the serum or plasma further increases with the increase in concentration of free serum hemoglobin (Fig. 3.1A). Lipemia causes sample turbidity, which approximately corresponds to the concentration of serum triglycerides (see Fig. 3.1B). Increased concentrations of serum bilirubin lead to yellow-to-orange coloration of the serum, and the change of the color correlates with the increasing concentration of the bilirubin in serum (see Fig. 3.1C).

Detection of the degree of hemolysis, icterus, and lipemia by visual inspection is highly unreliable and should be replaced with automated detection. Most high-throughput chemistry analyzers currently available on the market have the ability to detect serum indices by the use of semi-quantitative, spectrophotometric measurement, and grading the interfering substances into categories. The serum index is automatically reported for every sample and can be used to determine the degree of interference and its effect on the requested parameters. Such systems are highly reproducible and provide an objective and standardized way to screen for common interferences and manage specimen rejection via built-in rules in analyzer software.

Although the information about serum indices and their cut-offs for tested analytes are provided by the manufacturers of in vitro diagnostic systems and reagents, their claims are often not complete, accurate, and reproducible. It is therefore good practice for a laboratory to perform its own verification of serum indices. Alternatively, laboratories may rely on the evidence from the literature, if available and of adequate quality.

As for all other laboratory methods, analytical quality of serum indices should be continuously monitored by using appropriate internal quality control (IQC) and through participation in an external quality assessment (EQA) program. IQC material for serum indices has been recently made available on the market by several manufacturers.

## EXOGENOUS INTERFERENCE FACTORS

The effects of exogenous interfering substances are difficult to identify. They are introduced into the sample in different ways; for example, through therapy (drugs, natural preparations for self-medication, or supportive therapy), diagnostic procedures (contrast media), by accidental exposures and poisonings (with drugs, herbs, household chemicals, etc.), and through contamination of the sample during sample handling (from rubber tube stoppers, lubricants, anticoagulants, or surfactants) or sample analysis (antibiotics used for reagent and buffer stability).

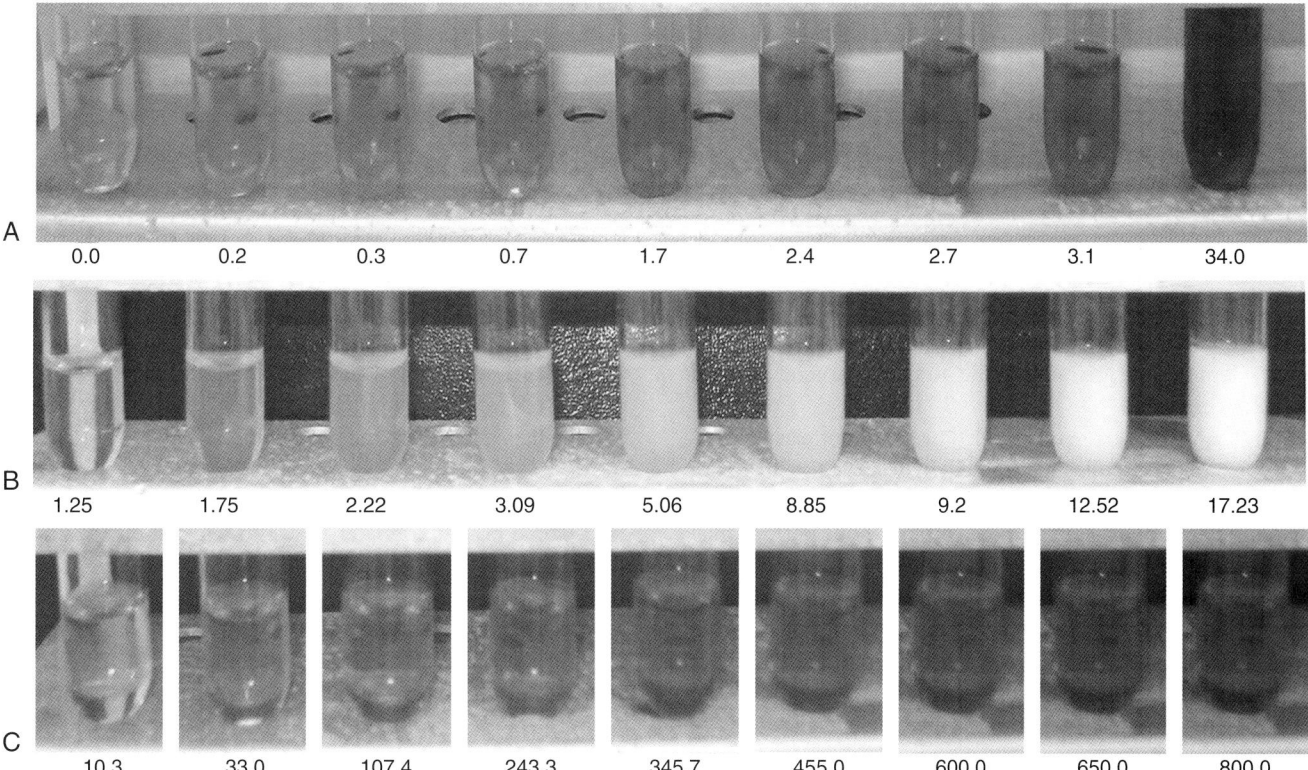

**Fig. 3.1** (A) Hemolysis—the intensity of the red color of the serum and corresponding concentrations of free serum hemoglobin. (B) Lipemia—the degree of turbidity and corresponding concentrations of triglycerides. (C) Icterus—the intensity of the yellow color of the serum and corresponding concentrations of bilirubin. (Courtesy Clinical Institute of Chemistry, University Hospital Center "Sestre Milosrdnice," Zagreb, Croatia.)

---

**POINTS TO REMEMBER**

**Hemolysis, Lipemia, Icterus**
- Visual assessment of the degree of hemolysis, lipemia, and icterus is not reliable and leads to errors.
- Hemolysis is the most common preanalytical error and most common cause of sample rejection.
- Hemolysis may cause clinically relevant bias through spectrophotometric and chemical interference, sample dilution, and the release of cell components into the sample.
- Lipemia causes interference by spectrophotometric interference (light absorbance and light scattering), by the volume depletion effect, by partitioning of the sample, and by physicochemical mechanisms (e.g., disturbance of the electrophoretic pattern).
- Laboratories should verify the performance of lipid removal reagents before their routine use, since they may not be appropriate for a wide range of analytes due to their low recovery.
- Different forms of bilirubin cause varying degrees of interference with different laboratory methods, and the same forms of bilirubin act differently with the same assays on different instruments.

## SPECIFIC CONSIDERATIONS

Besides the general aspects of preanalytical quality (i.e., patient and sample identification, controllable and noncontrollable variables), some specific aspects related to urine,

saliva, and blood gas testing are of particular relevance to laboratory medicine. The following sections deal with the preanalytical aspects of sample types other than serum or plasma, and other types of testing that deserve special preanalytical considerations.

### Influences and Interferences in Urine Testing

Some of the most important preanalytical issues in the analysis of urine are patient preparation, choice of urine type, type of collection vessel, sample stability during transport and storage, sample homogeneity, and sample contamination. These aspects are covered below.

### Types of Urine

Not every urine sample is fit for the purpose of every type of laboratory testing. The possible types of urine samples and their intended use are described in Table 3.3.

When collecting urine specimens, in order to prevent contamination with bacteria that normally reside on the skin, hygiene of the hands and genitalia is essential. Hands should be washed with soap, thoroughly rinsed with water, and dried. Not only proper washing with soap but also thorough rinsing is extremely important, as baby soaps are known to cause significant interference with tetrahydrocannabinol (THC) immunoassays. To prevent sample contamination by skin microorganisms, it is very important not to touch the inner surface of the cap and the container during collection.

## TABLE 3.3  Urine Specimens and Their Diagnostic Use

| Urine Type | Use |
| --- | --- |
| First morning urine | Urine sediment, test strip |
| Second morning urine | Proteins, urinalysis |
| Timed urine (6–24 h) | Hormones, drugs, electrolytes |
| First void urine | Chlamydia |
| Midstream urine | Urinalysis, microbiologic examination |
| Urine obtained through a catheter or sterile suprapubic aspiration | Exclusion and confirmation of urinary tract infection |

Urine should be collected while holding the skin folds (labia) apart (females) or retracting the foreskin (uncircumcised men) during voiding.

**First morning urine** (also called overnight or early morning specimen) is collected immediately after arising from an overnight sleep. Exceptionally, in patients suffering from insomnia or in night-shift workers, other 8-hour periods may also be used for the purpose of first morning urine collection. It is important that the patient's bladder is emptied immediately before going to sleep and that any amount of urine voided during the night is also collected and pooled together with the first voided morning specimen.

**Timed urine specimens** are collected at a specified time or in relation to some activity (e.g., before a meal, after a meal, before therapy, before exercise, and so on) during a 24-hour period. The exact time of the collection should always be reported with a test report.

**First void urine** comprises the first portion of the urine (usually the first 15 to 50 mL) passed at any time of the day. It is collected after a patient has not urinated for at least 1 to 2 hours. The exact time depends on the sensitivity of the actual test method and is usually designated on the method insert sheet.

**Midstream urine** (also called clean catch specimen) is a specimen collected during the middle of a urine flow after the urinary opening has been carefully cleaned. The first amount of urine should be passed into the toilet instead of the container. This will prevent contamination with skin, vaginal or urethral cells, and bacteria. The mid-portion of the urine is collected and once the container is filled, the rest of urine is voided into the toilet until the bladder is empty.

**Suprapubic aspiration** and catheterization are procedures usually applied for bacteriologic studies to obtain uncontaminated urine. A suprapubic specimen is collected by aspirating urine from the distended bladder through the abdominal wall, while catheterization enters the bladder through the urethra. Both collection methods use the sterile technique.

The ideal container for any urine specimen is a wide-mouthed bottle of appropriate size. Containers should be clean, leakproof, particle-free, and preferably made of a clear, disposable material that is inert with regard to urinary constituents. If urine is to be transported, the container used during transportation should have a secure closure to prevent leakage of the contents during transportation. If the urine is to be analyzed bacteriologically, containers have to be sterile.

For pediatric and newborn patients, urine specimen collection bags with hypoallergenic skin adhesive should be used. First, the pubic and perineal areas should be cleaned with soap and water. Then, the adhesive strip should be pressed all around the vulva or the bag fixed over the penis and the flaps pressed to the perineum.

### Transport and Storage of Sample

Since some urine parameters have limited stability in unpreserved urine, temperature and time conditions during transport and storage of urine are very important to ensure adequate sample quality. Urine samples may be stored for up to 1 hour at room temperature and up to 4 hours if refrigerated without significant variation in the results of the physical, chemical, and morphologic analysis of particles. Chemical constituents in urine (for test strip analysis) are stable for 24 hours if urine has been kept at +4°C.

> **POINTS TO REMEMBER**
>
> **Urine**
> - The contamination rate is much lower in urine specimens collected after proper hand and genital hygiene.
> - Laboratories should provide instructions to patients about reasons for urine collection, how to prepare for urine sampling (e.g., effects of diet and fluid intake, diuresis, exercise, and other interferents), and how to properly collect urine.
> - Stability of different analytes in urine is limited and decreases during prolonged storage and at higher temperatures.
> - Preservatives like ethanol, polyethylene glycol, sodium fluoride, mercuric chloride, boric acid, and formaldehyde- and formate-based solutions may enhance the stability of urine particles.
> - The addition of urine stabilizers inhibits the bacterial growth, metabolic processes, and degradation of urine analytes and particles.

### Saliva

Saliva is produced by *major* salivary glands (parotid, submandibular, and sublingual glands) and by oral secretion of the mucus by hundreds of *minor* salivary glands. The primary function of saliva is to provide oral protection by lubrication, digestion, and an immune response. Saliva is an attractive alternative to blood because it is collected noninvasively. As a diagnostic sample, saliva offers many advantages as well as some challenges (Box 3.1).

## BOX 3.1  Advantages and Challenges of Using Saliva as a Diagnostic Specimen

| Advantages | Challenges |
| --- | --- |
| • Rapid and easy collection by minimally trained individuals<br>• Sampling can be done by patients, at home, out of hospital<br>• Multiple sample collection is possible<br>• Procedure safe and painless for the patient<br>• Convenient for children, psychiatric patients, and stress research<br>• Availability<br>• Low cost associated with sampling (skilled staff not required)<br>• Convenient method for population screening programs<br>• Low risk of infections associated with sampling | • Low analyte concentration<br>• Some analytes may be affected by circadian cycle<br>• Questionable recovery for some analytes<br>• Risk of contamination during collection<br>• Difficult sampling and low patient compliance (in small children) |

## Types of Saliva Samples

The easiest way to collect saliva is to collect whole oral fluid (whole saliva). Whole saliva is representative of the oral milieu. However, depending on the intended aim of the sample collection and analyte to be tested, some other sample types are also possible. Various sampling techniques and devices are available. Whereas collection of whole oral fluid is an easy procedure, other sampling methods are more complicated; they require trained staff and are not commonly used.

Whole saliva may be collected as unstimulated (mostly produced by the submandibular glands) and stimulated (originating predominantly from the parotid glands) samples. Stimulation of saliva is obtained by oral movements (yawning, chewing paraffin or gum), or using a cotton roll soaked with citric acid. It has to be noted that stimulated and unstimulated saliva are of different origins (produced by different salivary glands) and composition (concentration of some analytes may vary), and thus are not equally suitable for all assays.

Several commercially available devices may be used for collection of saliva. Unstimulated whole saliva can be collected by:
- Passive drooling into the plastic vial
- Spitting into the collector vial

Passive drooling is considered by many to be the gold standard collection method for many analytes, as it enables collection of a representative portion of saliva present in the oral cavity. Moreover, passive drooling is preferred over spitting, since saliva collected by spitting is more likely to be contaminated with bacteria.

Stimulated saliva may be obtained by adsorbing saliva with cotton rolls, cotton swabs, or filter paper. Cotton is not an ideal collection material, not only due to its unpleasant texture but also because it may induce some variations in salivary immunoassays (some analytes are difficult to elute from cotton). To address this problem, some synthetic materials have been made available, such as inert polymers, polystyrene, rayon, and polyester. It must be emphasized that the composition of saliva collected by the use of various adsorbent devices may differ from the whole saliva, as adsorbent devices mostly collect localized saliva.

## Patient Preparation for Saliva Sampling

The laboratory is responsible for providing information to the patient about the purpose of saliva collection, as well as how to prepare for collection, and how to collect saliva. To avoid sample contamination, it is recommended to wear gloves during saliva collection. Below are some important measures aimed to minimize errors and ensure high-quality saliva samples:
- If not otherwise decided by the requesting physician, saliva should be collected in the morning, preferably in the fasting state (the exact time of collection is important, as some analytes may have diurnal variations)
- The patient should wash his/her face with water and soap and rinse it thoroughly to avoid contamination with facial creams and lotions
- The patient should not consume alcohol 12 hours before the collection
- The patient should not brush or floss his or her teeth at least 30 minutes before the collection
- The patient should not have any dental work done 2 days before the collection (dental bleeding may affect the test results)
- The patient should not ingest any food and drinks (except water) within 30 minutes before the collection
- The patient should not chew gum for at least 30 minutes before the collection
- Before collection, the patient should rinse his or her mouth with water to remove some food remnants. To avoid sample dilution with water, the sample should be collected 10 to 15 minutes after rinsing the mouth.

Any sample visibly contaminated with blood or food remnants should be rejected for analysis, and sample re-collection should be requested.

## Preanalytical Aspects of Arterial Blood Gas Testing

Blood sampling for assessing the oxygenation status of the patient or acid–base balance should be done when a patient is in a stable, resting state, to ensure that test results reflect the actual condition of the patient. Furthermore, the exact time of the blood collection should always be recorded and reported with a test result. Any deviation from the steady state should be noted as a comment and accompany the test report in order to allow proper interpretation of the results and appropriate patient management.

Relevant patient condition determinants (at the time of blood collection) are:

- Patient status (resting, exercising, crying, anxious)
- Ventilatory setting (spontaneous breathing or assisted mechanical ventilation)
- Mode of oxygen delivery (fraction of inspired oxygen [$FiO_2$] through nasal cannula or Venturi mask)
- Respiratory rate (hyperventilation, hypoventilation)
- Body temperature

If a patient's condition is changing, sufficient time should be allowed for the patient to stabilize. If there has been any change in the patient ventilatory setting or the mode of oxygen delivery, the patient should also be left in the resting state to stabilize. For patients without pulmonary disease, a period of 3 to 5 minutes is usually enough to stabilize. However, in patients with pulmonary disease, this period is significantly longer. For most patients, 20 to 30 minutes is adequate time to reach a stable state following ventilatory changes.

Arterial blood collected under anaerobic conditions and anticoagulated with lyophilized balanced Li-heparin is the ideal sample type for an accurate evaluation of the gas exchange function of the lungs ($PO_2$ and $PCO_2$). If arterial blood is not available (e.g., neonates, small children, patients with burns), and during medical transport and prehospital critical care, a capillary sample is an acceptable alternative. Capillary blood sampling is not recommended in patients with circulatory shock, poorly perfused (cyanotic), infected, inflamed, swollen, or edematous tissues. For more details on blood gas analysis and sample collection and processing, see Chapters 6 and 24.

## Hemostasis Testing

Some specific considerations related to hemostasis testing are associated with the type of anticoagulant, sampling technique (fasting state, length of the venous stasis, order of draw, sampling from a catheter), sample handling (centrifugation), transport, and storage prior to analysis.

Samples for hemostasis testing should be anticoagulated with 3.2% sodium citrate, although 3.8% may also be acceptable. It is important that the same concentration of sodium citrate is used within the laboratory, since clotting times may be longer in 3.8% than in 3.2% sodium citrate.

The mixing of samples is extremely important for adequate sample coagulation. Samples must be promptly mixed to avoid in vitro clot formation. Tubes should be mixed by gentle inversion (at 180 degrees) several times. For proper mixing, instructions from the tube manufacturer should be followed. Vigorous mixing and shaking the tubes is discouraged, as it may lead to sample hemolysis, plus the activation of platelets and coagulation factors, resulting in false shortening of clotting times and even the possible false increasing of clotting factor activity. The transport of samples by pneumatic tubes is still under discussion. While some claim that pneumatic tube transport is acceptable for routine hematology and coagulation testing, others argue that it is not appropriate for platelet aggregation studies. It is therefore recommended that each institution verifies the acceptability of their tube transport systems by comparing paired samples for differences.

Samples with visible clots should not be accepted for hemostasis testing. To prevent clot formation during blood sampling, handling, and transport, the following situations should be avoided:

- Blood flow (during blood sampling) too slow
- Collecting the sample into a syringe and then transferring it into a citrated tube
- Tubes underfilled
- Prolonged use of tourniquet (longer than 1 minute)
- Considerable manipulation of the vein by the needle
- Incomplete mixing

Clot formation induces the activation of platelets and clotting factors and the release of granules from the platelets, and it may cause false results in coagulation assays. It is very important to point out that even small clots that are invisible to the human eye may significantly impact coagulation assays.

The required blood-to-anticoagulant ratio is 9:1 and it is therefore very important that tubes for coagulation assays are filled to the mark noted on the tube. Acceptable deviation is a maximum 10% of the total volume; overfilling or underfilling the designated volume is strictly discouraged as this can introduce bias in test results. Laboratories should have preanalytical procedures in place for the rejection of over- or underfilled tubes. Other anticoagulants (e.g., ethylenediaminetetraacetic acid [EDTA] or heparin) are not acceptable for hemostasis testing, since they lead to erroneous results and cause clinically significant errors.

A standardized order of draw has been recommended, with the coagulation tube as the first tube. Although a "discard" tube before the coagulation tube has long been recommended, more recent evidence suggests that it may not be necessary. If intravenous catheter systems are used for blood sampling, five to six times the dead space (priming) volume of the catheter should be discarded prior to blood sampling.

Following collection, citrated samples should ideally be transported to the laboratory immediately and at room temperature, but no later than within 1 hour of blood draw. All coagulation assays should be performed in fresh samples. Blood samples for coagulation testing must be kept at room temperature (20°C to 25°C) until analysis. Storage at a lower temperature, or on ice, and sample freezing are discouraged as some coagulation factors are activated by cold.

Whole blood coagulation assays should be performed within 4 hours after blood sampling. For platelet function assays, samples should rest (at room temperature) for 30 minutes before analysis. Platelet function assays require the careful preparation of platelet-rich plasma by centrifugation of the blood at 200 to 250 g for 10 minutes without application of a centrifuge brake. To generate platelet-poor plasma, centrifugation is normally performed at 1500 g at room temperature for 10 to 15 minutes. Higher speed with a shorter centrifugation time is not recommended, as this may induce hemolysis and activation of platelets.

## Hematology

EDTA is the anticoagulant of choice for hematology testing given its efficacy in preserving cellular morphology. Due to its higher solubility, lower osmotic effect, and best overall performance, the International Council for Standardization in Haematology (ICSH) recommends dipotassium EDTA salt as the anticoagulant of choice for hematology testing.

Blood tubes should be filled to ±10% of the stated draw volume. In underfilled EDTA tubes, cell count and hematocrit might be falsely decreased due to the excess EDTA. In overfilled tubes, clot formation and platelet clumping is likely to occur, due to difficulty of appropriate mixing.

In some individuals, EDTA may cause pseudothrombocytopenia (i.e., platelet clumping or platelet satellitism [platelet adhering to neutrophils]) and subsequently inaccurate platelet results. Since most cell counters are not able to identify this preanalytical problem, platelets are thus counted as white blood cells, resulting in spurious leukocytosis and false thrombocytopenia. EDTA-induced pseudothrombocytopenia has so far been observed in healthy and diseased individuals and is not related to gender and age. The hypothesized mechanism in pseudothrombocytopenia involves IgM autoantibodies, directed against platelet IIb/IIIa fibrinogen receptors. This is further supported by the fact that platelets from patients with Glanzmann thrombasthenia (in which platelets have either defective or low levels of glycoprotein IIb/IIIa) do not react with autoantibodies from pseudothrombocytopenic patients.

EDTA anticoagulated blood should be stored at room temperature and analyzed within 6 hours of collection. Stability of hematologic parameters may differ depending on the parameter that is being measured, the instrument type, the transport, and the storage conditions. Therefore, on some occasions, a shorter time is necessary to ensure accurate and reliable results, whereas some parameters show excellent stability even over much longer time intervals. Some parameters are very stable (hemoglobin and red blood cells), while some others are not (reticulocytes, mean cell volume, and hematocrit). The stability of hematologic parameters is improved if samples are kept at 4°C. The following are the data provided by the ICSH on the stability of some hematology parameters:

- Hemoglobin concentration and red blood cell count are stable up to 72 hours, if blood is kept at 4°C
- Platelet and reticulocyte count are stable for 24 to 72 hours if blood is stored at 4°C
- White blood cell count with automated differential count is stable for at least 24 hours, if blood is kept at 4°C, and up to 6 hours if stored at room temperature
- Peripheral blood smear should be made from blood stored no longer than 1 hour at room temperature (18°C to 25°C)

Since stability may vary depending on the instrument, it is the responsibility of the individual laboratory to verify the stability of hematologic parameters on the instruments used in their laboratory.

Antibodies may affect the cell count of erythrocytes, leukocytes, and platelets. The following antibodies are known to interfere with hematologic analytes:
- Cold agglutinins (erythrocyte specific)
- Cryoglobulins
- EDTA-dependent antibodies with thrombocyte and leukocyte specificity

### Cold Agglutinins

Cold agglutinins are monoclonal or polyclonal antibodies specific for erythrocyte surface carbohydrate antigens, which bind to the erythrocyte surface at 0°C to 4°C. Binding of these antibodies causes agglutination of erythrocytes, induces complement activation and hemolysis, and impairs peripheral circulation. Some rare cases of cold agglutinins toward platelets have also been described, causing pseudothrombocytopenia independent of EDTA.

Cold agglutinins, if undetected, may cause diagnostic confusion and lead to subsequent extensive diagnostic workup as well as wrong and unnecessary therapy, risking patient safety and increasing health care costs. It is therefore very important to recognize cold agglutinins promptly.

Cold agglutinins should be suspected if the following anomalies are observed:
- Red blood cell count too low (in the presence of normal hemoglobin concentration)
- Significantly increased mean corpuscular volume (MCV) values
- Significantly low values of calculated hematocrit in samples with too high mean corpuscular hemoglobin (MCH) and MCH concentration (MCHC) values without any obvious explanation
- Falsely elevated white blood cell and platelet count

White blood cell and platelet counts may be falsely elevated because agglutinates, depending on their size, are either counted in the leukocyte or platelet channel. The blood smear may also show agglutination of erythrocytes. For adequate analysis of samples in which cold agglutinins are suspected, it is essential to warm up the EDTA blood sample at 37°C and analyze it immediately afterwards. This anomaly will appear again if a sample is kept at 4°C and analyzed cold.

### Cryoglobulins

Cryoglobulins are immunoglobulins with temperature-dependent solubility that precipitate at temperatures below 37°C. Cryoglobulins are often associated with infections, autoimmune disorders, and malignancies, and cause organ damage through immune-mediated mechanisms and vascular damage due to increased viscosity of the blood. The precipitation of cryoglobulins depends on the immunoglobulin class to which they belong. Also, precipitation is absent at pH less than 5.0 or more than 8.0.

In samples kept at room temperature, cryoglobulins tend to form globular or cylindrical precipitates, which are then counted by automated hematologic analyzers as cells, thus affecting hematologic laboratory tests and leading to false leukocytosis (pseudoleukocytosis), or false thrombocytosis

(pseudothrombocytosis). The degree of pseudoleukocytosis and pseudothrombocytosis depends on the time of exposure, temperature, cryoglobulin concentration, and the interaction of cryoglobulins with other plasma proteins. The following indices may point to the presence of cryoglobulins:
- Very different cell counts in different investigations
- Blue sediments in differential count samples

- In a sample warmed up to 37°C, significantly lower cell counts are measured

As is the case with cold agglutinins, for adequate analysis of samples in which cryoglobulins are suspected, blood sample should be kept warm at 37°C and analyzed immediately afterward.

## REVIEW QUESTIONS

1. Which of the following statements best describes the way interference factors may be reduced or eliminated?
   a. By standardizing the preanalytical conditions
   b. By providing proper instructions to the patients on how to prepare for blood sampling
   c. By selecting a more specific method
   d. By selecting the appropriate sampling procedure
   e. By maintaining the analytical variability (method $CV_A$) to a minimum
2. Spectrophotometric interference of hemolysis occurs due to the ability of hemoglobin to absorb light at which wavelengths?
   a. 400, 500, and 600 nm
   b. 550 and 570 nm
   c. 540 and 600 nm
   d. 415 and 540 nm
   e. 415, 540, and 570 nm
3. Recommended sample for the accurate measurement of potassium is which of the following?
   a. Plasma
   b. Serum
   c. Whole blood
   d. Capillary blood
   e. Arterial blood
4. Which of the following statements is true for lipid testing and testing for lipid-soluble drugs and hormones?

   a. Testing should always be done in a delipidated sample.
   b. Testing should always be done on the native sample before delipidation.
   c. Delipidation does not affect the concentration of lipids and lipid-soluble drugs.
   d. The most suitable delipidation method is ultracentrifugation.
   e. The most suitable delipidation method is lipid removal using the lipid clearing agents.
5. Major sources of exogenous interferences are described below, *except* which one?
   a. Prescribed medications
   b. Supportive medical therapy like parenteral emulsions, contrast media agents, or infusion solutions
   c. Dietary supplements
   d. Accidental exposure and poisoning
   e. In vivo hemolysis
6. According to the International Council for Standardization in Haematology, the anticoagulant of choice for hematology testing is:
   a. dipotassium EDTA.
   b. tripotassium EDTA.
   c. disodium EDTA.
   d. 3.8% sodium citrate.
   e. 3.2% sodium citrate.

## SUGGESTED READINGS

Baird G. Preanalytical considerations in blood gas analysis. *Biochemia Medica.* 2013;23(1):19–27.

Banfi G, Germagnoli L. Preanalytical phase in haematology. *J Med Biochem.* 2008;27:348–353.

Bonar R, Favaloro EJ, Adcock DM. Quality in coagulation and haemostasis testing. *Biochemia Medica.* 2010;20:184–199.

Chiappin S, Antonelli G, Gatti R, et al. Saliva specimen: a new laboratory tool for diagnostic and basic investigation. *Clinica Chimica Acta.* 2007;383(1–2):30–40.

Delanghe J, Speeckaert M. Preanalytical requirements of urinalysis. *Biochemia Medica.* 2014;24(1):89–104.

Dimeski G. Interference testing. *Clin Biochemist Rev.* 2008;29(suppl. 1):S43–S48.

Dimeski G, Jones BW. Lipaemic samples: effective process for lipid reduction using high speed centrifugation compared with ultracentrifugation. *Biochemia Medica.* 2011;21:86–94.

Favaloro EJ, Adcock Funk DM, Lippi G. Pre-analytical variables in coagulation testing associated with diagnostic errors in hemostasis. *Lab Med.* 2012;43(2):1–10.

Harrison P, Mackie I, Mumford A, et al. Guidelines for the laboratory investigation of heritable disorders of platelet function. *Brit J Haematol.* 2011;155(1):30–44. 2012.

International Council for Standardization in Haematology (ICSH). Recommendations of the ICSH for ethylene diamine tetraacetic acid anticoagulation of blood for blood cell counting and sizing: expert panel on cytometry. *Am J Clin Pathol.* 1993;100:371–372.

Lippi G, Daves M, Mattiuzzi C. Interference of medical contrast media on laboratory testing. *Biochemia Medica.* 2014;24:80–88.

Lippi G, Franchini M, Montagnana M, et al. Quality and reliability of routine coagulation testing: can we trust that sample? *Blood Coagul Fibrinolysis.* 2006;17:513–519.

Narayanan S. The preanalytic phase—an important component of laboratory medicine. *Am J Clin Pathol.* 2000;113:429–452.

Nikolac N. Lipemia: causes, interference mechanisms, detection and management. *Biochemia Medica.* 2014;24(1):57–67.

Nunes LA, Mussavira S, Bindhu OS. Clinical and diagnostic utility of saliva as a non-invasive diagnostic fluid: a systematic review. *Biochemia Medica (Zagreb)*. 2015;25(2):177–192.

Saracevic A, Nikolac N, Simundic AM. The evaluation and comparison of consecutive high speed centrifugation and LipoClear® reagent for lipemia removal. *Clin Biochem*. 2014;47(4–5):309–314.

Simundic AM. Blood gases, ions and electrolytes; Who is doing phlebotomy in Europe? In: Guder WG, Narayanan S, eds. *Pre-Examination Procedures in Laboratory Diagnostics. Preanalytical Aspects and Their Impact on the Quality of Medical Laboratory Results*. De Gruyter; 2015.

Simundic AM, Cornes M, Grankvist K, et al. Standardization of collection requirements for fasting samples: for the Working Group on Preanalytical Phase (WG-PA) of the European Federation of Clinical Chemistry and Laboratory Medicine (EFLM). *Clinica Chimica Acta*. 2014;432:33–37.

Simundic AM, Nikolac N, Guder WG. Preanalytical variation and preexamination processes. In: Rifai N, Horvath R, Wittwer, eds. *Tietz Textbook of Clinical Chemistry and Molecular Diagnostics*. 6th ed. Elsevier; 2017.

Zini G. International Council for Standardization in Haematology (ICSH) stability of complete blood count parameters with storage: toward defined specifications for different diagnostic applications. *Intl J Lab Hematol*. 2014;36(2):111–113.

# Biological Variation and Analytical Performance Specifications

*Sverre Sandberg and Aasne K. Aarsand*

## OBJECTIVES

1. Explain the nature and different types of biological variation.
2. Describe how biological variation studies are performed and how estimates of within- and between-subject biological variation can be generated.
3. Understand how biological variation data are reference data, and where high-quality data can be found.
4. Discuss different applications such as reference change values, index of individuality and personalized reference intervals.
5. Describe the various models for setting analytical performance specifications, and critically assess the advantages and disadvantages of each model.

## KEY WORDS AND DEFINITIONS

**Analytical performance specifications (APS)** The numerical standards of examination performance required to facilitate optimum patient care.

**Analytical variation ($CV_A/SD_A$)** Variation of the concentration of a measurand in a sample measured several times with the same measurement procedure (imprecision).

**Between-subject biological variation ($CV_G$)** The variation in the concentration/activity of a measurand among the homeostatic set points of different individuals.

**Biological variation (BV)** Variation in the concentration/activity of a measurand in the body.

**Critical difference** The change between two results that with a certain probability can be explained by analytical and within-subject biological variation. The preferred synonym is reference change value (RCV; see later).

**Index of individuality (II)** The ratio between the analytical and within-subject biological variation to the between-subject biological variation

$$II = \left( CV_A^2 + CV_I^2 \right)^{1/2} / CV_G$$

**Reference change value** The change between two results that with a certain probability can be explained by analytical and within-subject biological variation.

**Within-subject biological variation ($CV_I/SD_I$)** Variation of the concentration/activity of a measurand around a homeostatic set point within a single individual.

**Within-person biological variation ($CV_P/SD_P$)** This is used to describe the biological variation around the homeostatic set point in an individual, when this is estimated based on the individual's own data.

Many types of variation influence numerical results generated in laboratory medicine. Most measurands are characterized by a random variation of the concentration around a homeostatic set point. In addition, some measurands have biological variations over the span of life and other predictable cyclical variations. Knowledge of the generation and application of biological variation data is essential for the correct interpretation of laboratory test results and are described in detail in this chapter.

## NATURE OF BIOLOGICAL VARIATION AND CENTRAL CONCEPTS

Different sources of variation contribute to the uncertainty of any result generated in laboratory medicine. **Biological variation** is one of the most important and must be taken into account when results are interpreted.

There are various types of biological variation. The concentration or activity of some measurands changes over the span of life—some slowly and some more quickly, particularly at times of physiological change, such as the neonatal period, childhood, puberty, menopause, and old age. To help interpret laboratory data, this variation is taken care of by the creation of age- and/or sex-stratified (partitioned) reference intervals when these are needed. In addition, many measurands have predictable cyclical rhythms in their concentrations. These can be daily, monthly, or seasonal in nature. The major ramifications for interpretation are that reference intervals cannot be generated for every point during these cycles. An important type of biological variation is random

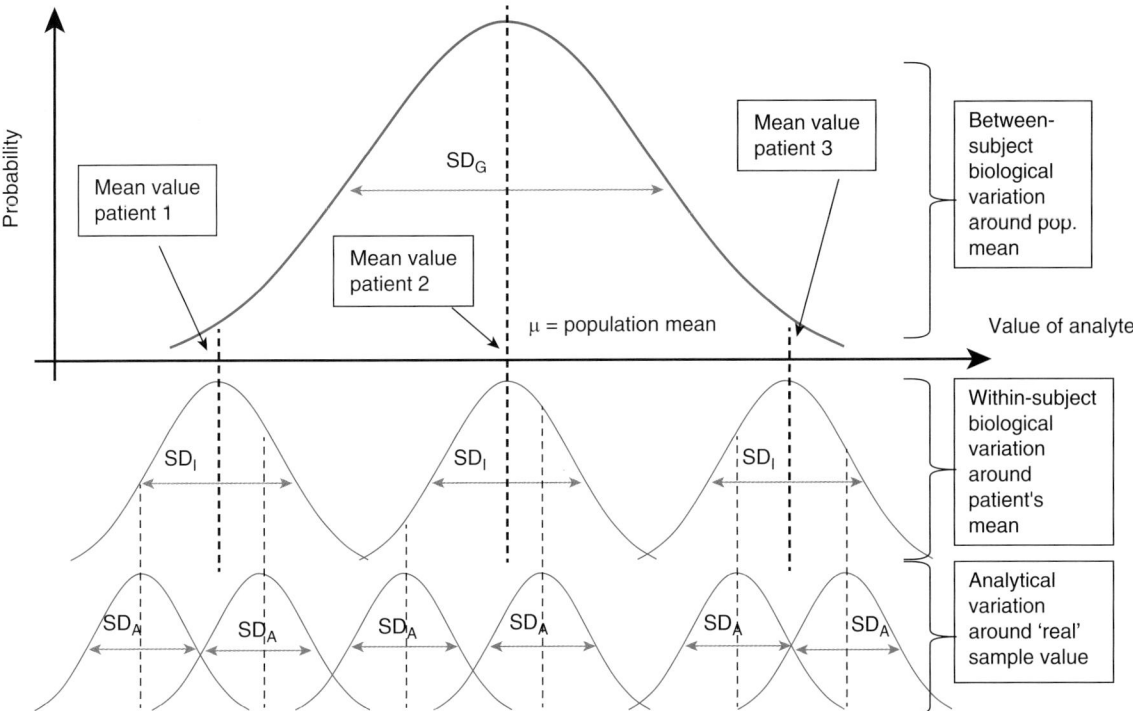

**Fig 4.1** The relationship between the between-subject $(SD_G)$, within-subject $(SD_I)$ and analytical $(SD_A)$ variation. (Adapted from Røraas T, Petersen PH, Sandberg S. Confidence intervals and power calculations for within-person biological variation: effect of analytical imprecision, number of replicates, number of samples, and number of individuals. *Clin Chem.* 2012;58:1306–1313.)

biological variation, which is the variation of the concentration/activity of a measurand around a homeostatic set point within a single individual (i.e., the **within-subject variation** [$CV_I/SD_I$]). The variation among the homeostatic set points of individuals is defined as the **between-subject variation** ($CV_G/SD_G$). The different abbreviations, in the form of CVs and SDs, indicate if the variations are expressed as coefficient of variation (CV) or in the form of standard deviations (SD). The random biological variation of a measurand in a population at a steady state can be separated into three components (Fig. 4.1): (1) the between-subject biological variation around the population mean concentration, (2) the random within-subject biological variation around the mean concentration of the subject, and (3) the **analytical variation** around the measured mean concentration of the measurand. In the figure these variations are displayed as being as normally distributed, which is not always the case.

The individuality of a measurand and the use of conventional population-based reference intervals are determined by comparison of the within-subject and between-subject biological variations. **Personalized reference intervals** (prRI) can be established based on knowledge of the homeostatic set point and estimates of within-subject biological variation derived either for the relevant population or for the individual. Estimates of $CV_I$ and analytical imprecision can be used to create **reference change values (RCVs)**, sometimes called **critical differences**, to assess the probability that the difference between two consecutive results in an individual can be explained by analytical and within-subject biological variation. **Analytical performance specifications**

(APS) for imprecision, bias, total allowable error, measurement uncertainty, and other characteristics can be created using estimates of within- and between-subject biological variation.

## GENERATION OF DATA ON COMPONENTS OF BIOLOGICAL VARIATION

Biological variation studies are usually undertaken as prospective experimental studies that include a higher number of specimens taken from a smaller cohort of reference individuals. Estimates are thereafter derived from a traditional statistical approach such as, for example, analysis of variance (ANOVA) or similar methods, or more recently by alternative approaches such as Bayesian statistics. Additionally, there is a renewed interest in basing estimates on a lower number of specimens, using a larger cohort of data (big data) from, for example, laboratory information systems.

### Prospective Experimental Studies
### Design of Studies

Production of numerical data on biological variation is traditionally obtained by taking specimens from a cohort of healthy individuals, or well-defined patient groups in steady state, using the following approach, as detailed by Fraser and Harris:

- Select a group of reference individuals
- Take a set of specimens from each of the individuals at regular time intervals while minimizing all sources of preanalytical variation

- Transport specimens in a standardized way and store aliquots under controlled conditions until ready for analysis
- Undertake the analyses in duplicate within a single run if possible, while minimizing analytical sources of variation
- Assess data for clinically significant events, trends and statistical outliers and confirm that all results are homogeneously distributed, if to be analyzed by traditional statistical methods
- Dissect out the $CV_A$, $CV_I$, and $CV_G$ components.

This design has been widely used and is very suitable for those measurands that have a low $CV_I$ and are under strict homeostatic control. Historically, many studies have collected (e.g., 10 specimens on a weekly basis from 20 individuals recruited from a smaller cohort of reference individuals) typically healthy individuals, such as hospital workers. However, this small-scale design may be problematic, especially as we often will want to evaluate whether subgroups (e.g., related to sex) are associated with different $CV_I$ estimates. The power of a study and the reliability of the derived biological variation estimates depend on the number of included individuals, samples and replicates and on the ratio between the $CV_A$ and the $CV_I$ estimates. Generally, it is preferable to have a relatively high number of specimens from each individual. However, if the influence of factors such as age and sex on the $CV_I$ is under study, it is important that an adequate number of individuals is included in each sub-group to detect clinically important differences. If the $CV_A$ is high compared to the $CV_I$, either the total number of specimens or the number of replicate analyses should be increased (see recommended references).

Some measurands for which biological variation estimates are sought may be unstable and examinations must therefore be performed soon after the collection of specimens (e.g., for hematologic measurands such as mean cell volume and number of erythrocytes per volume). In this case, to obtain the necessary statistically unconfounded estimate of $CV_I$, the $CV_A$ is estimated by analyzing all specimens taken at each sampling point, in duplicate. However, this only represents the within-run CV. Thus, in addition, quality control materials, preferentially commutable in the relevant concentrations, have to be analyzed between each run to ascertain that variation due to systematic deviations in the examination procedure between each examination is excluded.

### Data Analysis—Traditional Approach

During the study collection period, participants must at regular intervals be assessed clinically and by relevant laboratory analyses to identify (e.g., intercurrent disease) changes in medication or other factors that may influence the measurands the study is aiming to collect biological variation data for. Because of this, either single data points or all the results of a participant may have to be excluded, prior to further data assessment. Thereafter, it is important (1) to verify that all the included individuals are in a steady state; (2) to exclude outliers in the data set; and (3) to assess whether the individuals have a homogeneously distributed individual $CV_I$. The number of data points and subjects excluded following

these analyses, as well as the number of data used to derive the components of biological variation, should always be reported. This provides an indication of the representative nature of the data and underscores its suitability for wide application

***Steady state.*** The calculation of biological variation data assumes that the individuals assessed are in a "steady state," that is, that the homeostatic set points do not change during the time span of the study. If this is not the case, data should be transformed to a "steady state," for example, by correcting for trends using regression analysis or using other methods such as multiple of medians (MoM) and its natural logarithm.

***Data transformation / normal distribution.*** As most biological data are naturally logarithmically distributed, it is usually preferable to perform both the examination and calculations on the logarithms of the observations. This both helps in extracting the CVs and ensuring that the data distribution is closer to normal. If the data are not normally distributed, confidence intervals cannot be calculated using formula-based methods. It is important to specify that the normality relates to the model effects; that is, both the analytical variation around the true sample value and the individuals' variation around their homeostatic set point are normally distributed. It does not relate to the total pooled data. Pooling the standardized residuals for each level, namely, residuals from replicates (difference between replicates and mean of replicates from each sample), residuals from samples (difference between mean of samples and mean for the individual), and residuals from subjects (differences between individual means and total mean) can be used to assess normality.

Example: Assume observations of 2.25, 2.50, and 2.75 are from individual A and 3.50, 4.00, and 4.50 from individual B. Standardized residuals are generated by first dividing by the mean for each individual. Individual A has an average of 2.50, so standardized observations are 0.90, 1.00, and 1.10, and corresponding standardized residuals are −0.10, 0.00, and 0.10. Individual B has an average of 4.00, standardized observations 0.875, 1.00, and 1.125, and corresponding residuals −0.125, 0.00, and 0.125. The pooled standardized residuals are (−0.10, 0.00, 0.10, −0.125, 0.00, 0.125). The standardized residuals can then be examined using Kolmogorov-Smirnov or Anderson-Darling or other techniques for the assessment of normality. If a log-transformation is applied, it is important to transform the estimated SDs back to CVs afterwards. An alternative approach is using the CV-ANOVA as described by Røraas and colleagues (see recommended references).

***Outliers.*** The assessment of outliers is important because extreme values may lead to erroneous estimates of the components of biological variation. It is important that this assessment is done using the same measure of variability that is estimated; that is, if CVs are estimated, the calculations should be performed on data expressed as CVs. Outlier assessments are performed at three levels: (1) between duplicates or replicates, (2) between samples within an individual, and (3) between individuals. Failure to remove outliers in the replicates can result in a falsely high $CV_A$ and an erroneous $CV_I$, while failure to remove outliers from results from each

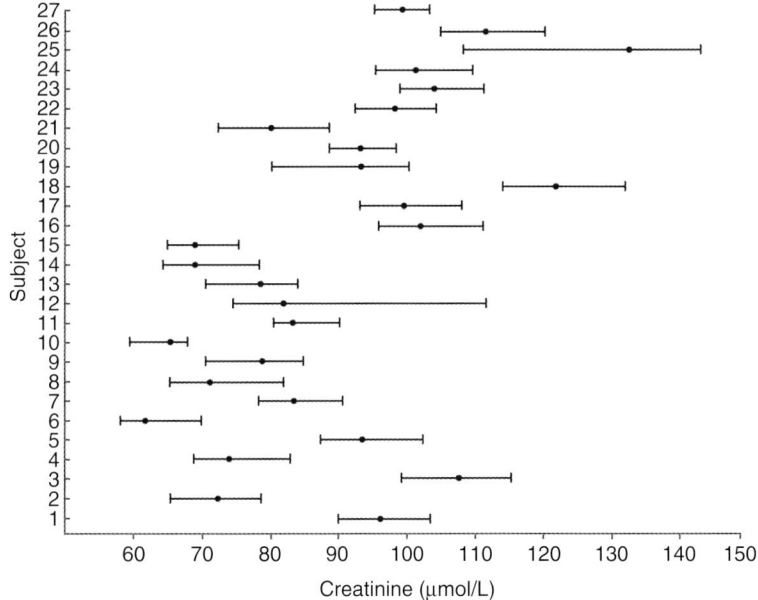

**Fig. 4.2** Means and extreme values for serum creatinine in 27 older adults. Note: 100 µmol/L = 1.13 mg/dL. (From Fraser CG. Inherent biological variation and reference values. *Clin Chem Lab Med.* 2004;42:758–764.)

of the individuals can result in a falsely increased $CV_I$. Finally, outliers among the mean values of the individuals (level 3) are assessed. A simple strategy to perform this process is to use Reed's criterion—that the difference between any mean value and the next value in the series should be less than one-third of the overall range of all values. Another useful approach for the assessment of outliers between individuals is a simple graphical approach in which the mean values and the range of all these values are plotted for each individual (on the *y*-axis) against concentration or activity (on the *x*-axis). An example is provided in Fig. 4.2 and discussed later in this chapter. Failure to exclude outliers of the mean values of the different individuals will result in a falsely large $CV_G$, and because the overall mean value will be different; this may also affect $CV_A$ and $CV_I$ depending on the transformation chosen.

*Homogeneity.* Applications of within-subject biological variation data, for example for estimation of the RCVs, depend on the within-subject variation data being homogeneously distributed. If the specimens have not been obtained from a homogeneous population, the results will not be representative of the population, only an average individual, and stratified analysis by subgroups should be applied if possible. Thus, although estimates of $CV_I$ and RCVs can be calculated, these are not generalizable to the overall population. It is therefore important to know that the ranked cumulative distributions of the variances in specimens drawn from a homogeneous population are distributed around the true variance of the population according to $\chi^2/df$ ($\chi^2$ distribution for degrees of freedom according to the individual sample sizes). This can be illustrated by plotting the cumulated ranked fractions of within-subject variations as a function of the within-subject variation estimates on a Rankit scale (Fig. 4.3). If homogeneous, this curve will fit to the theoretical of the square root of the pooled variance multiplied by $\chi^2/df$. Variance homogeneity can also be tested further by Bartlett's

test. Although Cochrane's test of the variances of the mean values of the specimens is primarily an outlier test, it also can be used as a test for homogeneity.

If some subjects have to be removed in order to achieve variance homogeneity, it is recommended to check if the excluded individuals share common traits that can explain their heterogeneity, which can be valuable information to the applicability of the estimated $CV_I$.

***Calculation of analytical and biological variation.*** There are several estimators available: ANOVA, maximum likelihood (ML), restricted maximum likelihood (REML), minimum variance quadratic unbiased estimator (MIVQUE), and weighted analysis of means (WAM). For balanced designs, the choice of estimator is not important; however, for unbalanced designs, the estimators can yield different results and should be chosen carefully. These estimators are available in most statistical software packages using general linear models or generalized linear models.

In previous publications, many have not used formal ANOVA but instead have simply used subtracted variances. The thesis is that, because preanalytical sources of variation have been minimized and can be considered negligible, the total CV ($CV_T$) of a set of results from each cohort of individuals includes $CV_A$, $CV_I$, and $CV_G$. Then, because:

$$CV_T = \left[(CV_A)^2 + (CV_I)^2 + (CV_G)^2\right]^{1/2}$$

the components can be calculated by simple subtraction. However, this approach will require calculations including degrees of freedom and, therefore, a formal ANOVA is a simpler approach for correct calculations and can take into account unbalanced designs. Additionally, in many of these studies, $CV_A$ has been estimated based on quality control materials, the outliers have not been assessed, and a normal distribution and homogeneity of data are assumed;

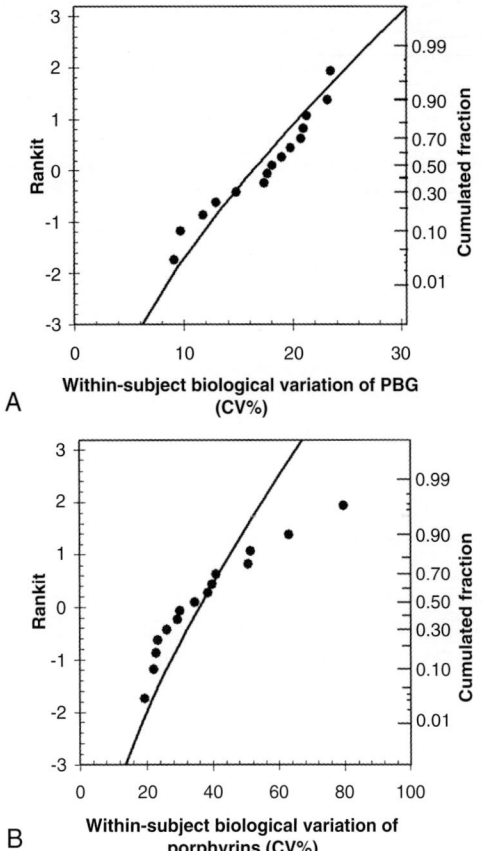

**Fig. 4.3** Variance homogeneity plots. Rankit plots show the accumulated fractions as function of within-subject biological coefficient of variations (CVs). The filled circles represent individual CVs for healthy individuals; the *line* indicates the expected distribution of measured CV for "true" CV values of 17.3% for porphobilinogen *(PBG)* (A) and 28.1% for porphyrins (B). The Cochrane test gives values of 0.11 for PBG and 0.25 for porphyrins, and a value indicating heterogeneity is >0.17. (From Aarsand AK., Petersen PH, Sandberg S. Estimation and application of biological variation of urinary delta-aminolevulinic acid and porphobilinogen in healthy individuals and in patients with acute intermittent porphyria. *Clin Chem.* 2006;52:650–656.)

in consequence, estimates of the components of biological variation are likely to be less precise. Generally, CV-ANOVA methods are recommended.

### Data Analysis—Bayesian Approach

Bayesian statistical models using adaptive Student-*t* distributions instead of the normal distributions can be used to deliver estimates of biological variation.

This model disregards the assumption of normality and makes the model robust to extreme observations which is an advantage over traditional methods such as ANOVA. Thus, laborious statistical operations, associated with possible subjectivity in data trimming to achieve homogeneity and exclusion of outliers, are not required. The Bayesian model delivers individual personal $CV_P$ that can be used to explore heterogeneity, assess relevant sub-groups or to identify individuals not belonging to the group (Fig. 4.4). It is then also possible to assess correlations between the $CV_P$ and (e.g., age or homeostatic set

points) and to calculate prRI. The model also provides the ability to use prior knowledge, which makes precise inference from previous studies of similar analytes possible.

### Retrospective Studies

Results from patient cohorts from hospital data such as pathology laboratory databases may be used to derive biological variation estimates. This is particularly relevant if the measurand in question is not present in matrices from apparently healthy subjects (such as unusual proteins found in myeloma) or if it would be unacceptable or unethical to collect specimens from individuals, for example, children. Assessment of data collected for diagnostic or monitoring purposes also provides the ability to assess sub-groups including different states of health, the effect of time between sampling, or other factors, without the efforts of prospectively collecting large data sets. For many analytes requested for a patient, the levels of the analytes are not impacted by non-relevant pathology and may represent values obtained for the healthy population. A recent study detailing how to use big data derived from pathology databases for estimating $CV_I$ and RCVs for a wide range of routine chemistry and hematology tests reported results equivalent to those delivered by traditional methods. With this approach, cohorts consisting of a large number of individuals, where at least two samples have been collected for routine clinical purposes, are used.

## QUALITY OF BIOLOGICAL VARIATION DATA AND DATABASES

The applications of biological variation data for diagnosis and monitoring of disease and setting APS in the laboratory deliver a requirement that biological variation data must be robust and of high quality. Furthermore, the data must be relevant for the laboratory in which they will be used, both in terms of results being transferable to the examination method in use and relevant for the populations the laboratory serves. Those who use published biological variation data for diagnosis and monitoring must appraise the data similarly to the approach that is usually applied when adopting population-based reference intervals from previously published studies. Many data have been generated over the last 50 years on the components of biological variation for a broad range of measurands. Different databases summarizing available biological variation data have been available, such as the historical online database established by the Analytical Quality Commission of the Spanish Society of Laboratory Medicine (SEQC^ML). However, much of the historic data do not fulfill today's standards or applied outdated analytical methods and are thus no longer fit for purpose. Following the 1st Strategic Conference of the European Federation of Clinical Chemistry and Laboratory Medicine (EFLM) in 2014, the EFLM established a Task Group within the Working Group for Biological Variation, with the objective to appraise available biological variation data and to establish and publish a new Biological Variation Database. As part of this work, the Task Group and the Working Group developed the Biological Variation Data Critical Appraisal Checklist (BIVAC), a standard for

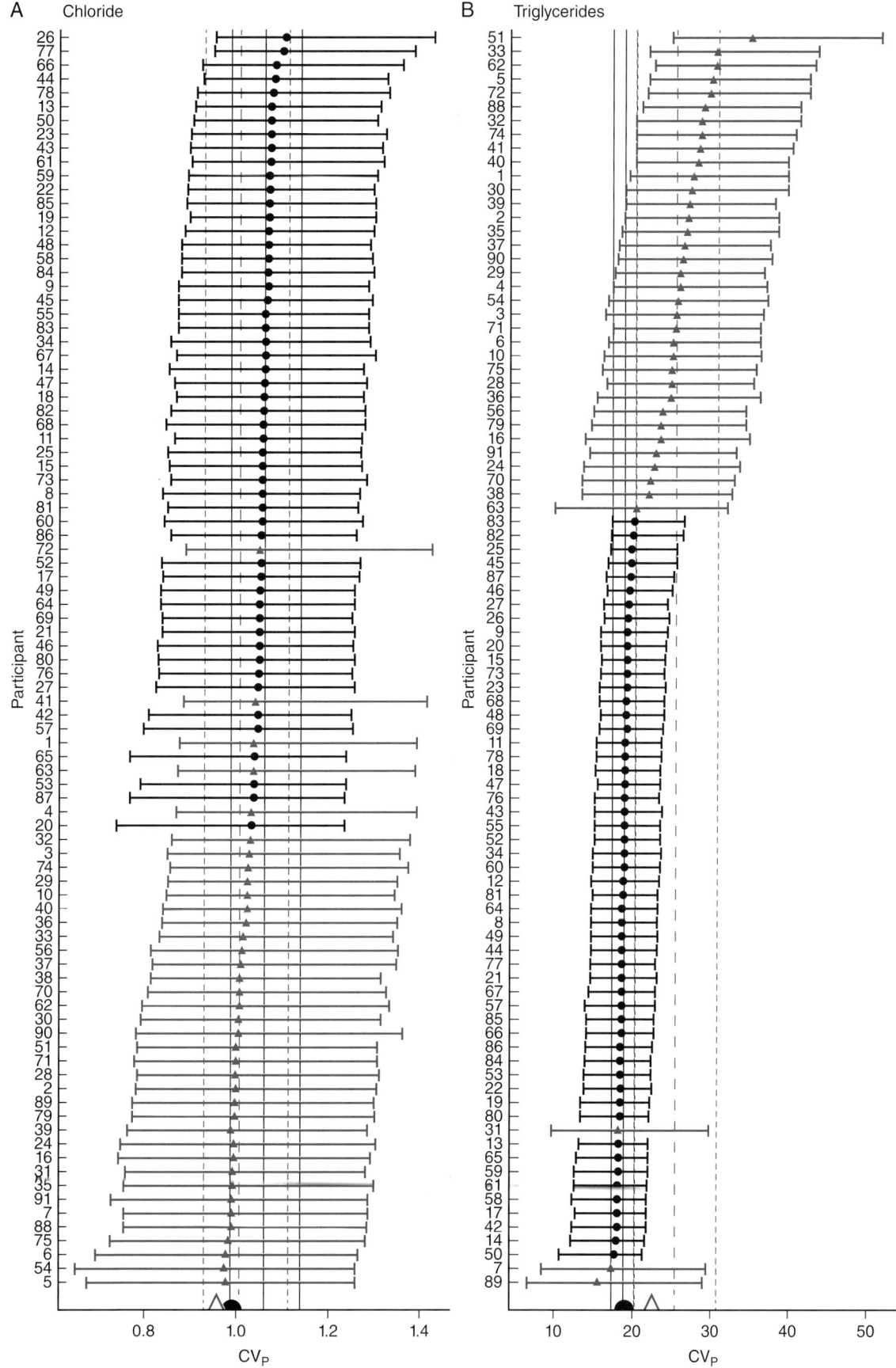

**Fig. 4.4** The within-person biological variation estimates, CV$_P$, with 95% CrI (credible interval) for women (black circles) and men (blue triangles) for chloride (A) and triglycerides (B), derived by a Bayesian model on results from the European Biological Variation Study *(EuBIVAS)*. The participants are sorted by their CV$_P$. The CV$_I$ estimates indicated on the *x* axis by a black circle for women and blue triangle for men are derived by coefficient of variation-analysis of variance *(CV-ANOVA)* on the same data set. The vertical lines show the 20%, 50%, and 80% percentiles for the predicted distributions for CV$_P$. (From Røraas T, Sandberg S, Aarsand AK, et al. A Bayesian approach to biological variation analysis. *Clin Chem.* 2019;65:995–1005.)

**TABLE 4.1    The Quality Items of the Biological Variation Data Critical Appraisal Checklist With Achievable Scores**

| Quality Item Number | Quality Item | ACHIEVABLE SCORES | | | |
|---|---|---|---|---|---|
| 1 | Scale | A | B | - | - |
| 2 | Subjects | A | B | C | D |
| 3 | Samples | A | B | C | D |
| 4 | Measurand | A | B | C | D |
| 5 | Pre-analytical procedures | A | B | C | - |
| 6 | Estimates of analytical variation | A | B | C | - |
| 7 | Steady state | A | B | C | - |
| 8 | Outliers | A | B | C | - |
| 9 | Normally distributed data | A | B | - | - |
| 10 | Variance homogeneity | A | - | C | - |
| 11 | Statistical method | A | B | C | - |
| 12 | Confidence limits | A | - | C | - |
| 13 | Number of included results | A | B | C | - |
| 14 | Concentrations | A | B | - | - |

Adapted from Aarsand AK, Røraas T, Fernandez-Calle P, et al. The Biological Variation Data Critical Appraisal Checklist: a standard for evaluating studies on biological variation. *Clin Chem*. 2018;64:501–514.

evaluating biological variation studies. The BIVAC is designed to assess the quality of biological variation publications by verifying whether all essential elements that may impact upon veracity and utility of the associated biological variation estimates are included in the study. It consists of 14 quality items (Table 4.1) and focuses on the effect of study design, the measurement procedure and statistical handling of data on $CV_I$ estimates. The BIVAC not only allows for appraisal of already published studies, it also, in combination with the Biological Variation Data Reporting Checklist, provides a framework that may help those planning and performing future studies, to ensure that all essential elements are included.

Second, the groups developed a meta-analysis approach to pool estimates from BIVAC-compliant studies with similar study design to provide global biological variation estimates. Finally, the two groups designed and populated a new biological variation database, the EFLM Biological Variation Database (https://biologicalvariation.eu) that provides global biological variation estimates based on systematic reviews and meta-analysis of quality-assessed studies. The database also contains information about reference change values and analytical performance specifications. Here, for all included studies, both the BIVAC scores as well as a biological variation minimum data set, encompassing around 30 descriptive items, are published, thus offering an updated source of quality-assessed data for users worldwide. An overview of many of the recent initiatives in the area of biological variation is published in the 2022 special issue of *Clinical Chemistry and Laboratory Medicine* entitled: Biological variation—8 years after the 1st Strategic Conference of EFLM.

## BIOLOGICAL VARIATION IN DIFFERENT STATES OF HEALTH AND SETTINGS

Some argue that many of the data on the components of biological variation are inappropriate for wide use in laboratory medicine because they have been derived, in general, from studies on healthy individuals, and not on patients with disease who are the source of most requests for examinations. Previous research has indicated that estimates of $CV_I$ are generally independent of the state of health, except when the measurand is one that is pathologically changed, such as tumor markers in patients with cancers. For frequently requested measurands, studies have been published for various conditions such as different sampling intervals (within-day, daily/weekly/monthly), age groups (pediatric, adult, elderly) and states of well-being, but there are generally few high-quality studies and there is a lack of evidence for drawing conclusions on differences in biological variation estimates in these different settings. For less frequently requested measurands, there may be only single studies or studies of low quality available, and no data for different population groups or sampling intervals.

## INTERPRETATION AND USE OF DATA

### Index of Individuality

The results of most examinations in laboratory medicine are compared with conventional population-based reference intervals or sometimes fixed limits for clinical decision-making. Reference intervals typically represent the values found in 95% of the reference population. The $CV_G$ obtained by biological variation studies should not be confused with the population-based reference interval which is calculated by using one specimen from a larger number of individuals and "includes" all three variations $CV_G$, $CV_I$, and $CV_A$. The ramification of biological variation on the use of reference intervals is determined by the individuality of the measurand.

Fig. 4.2 shows the means and extreme values of a cohort of 27 older adults for serum creatinine concentration. Subjects 1 to 13 were women and subjects 14 to 27 were men. The conventional reference intervals for creatinine at the time of study for individuals older than 55 years of age were 60 to 98 μmol/L (0.68 to 1.10 mg/dL) for women and 66 to 128 μmol/L

(0.75 to 1.45 mg/dL) for men. The following conclusions can be drawn when assessing the data in Fig. 4.2:
- No individual has values that span the entire reference interval.
- Most individuals have all values within the reference interval.
- The means of the values of most individuals lie within the reference interval, but they are different from each other.
- A few individuals have values that span the lower or the upper reference limit, and these individuals have values that change from usual to unusual over time.

It is clear that $CV_I$ of creatinine is smaller than the $CV_G$. In numerical terms, current meta-analysis-derived estimates are $CV_I$ of 4.5% and $CV_G$ is 14.1%. Thus, $CV_I$ is less than $CV_G$, meaning that the measurand has marked individuality. This characteristic can be expressed mathematically as an **index of individuality (II)** and is best calculated as: $II = \left(CV_A^2 + CV_I^2\right)^{1/2}/CV_G$. It is common now for II to be simplified as $CV_I/CV_G$. This is satisfactory if $CV_A$ is less than ½ $CV_I$, as is often the case with modern analytical technology and methodology because $CV_A$ will then contribute little to the numerator $CV_A^2 + CV_I^2$. Most common measurands have marked individuality with a low II.

This example provides a biological explanation for the fact that serum creatinine concentration when compared with conventional reference intervals, even if partitioned by age or sex, does not have high sensitivity for the detection of mild renal impairment, and provides a sound rationale for the benefits of the estimated glomerular filtration rate. The estimated glomerular filtration rate uses formulae that take age, sex, and ethnicity into account, as well as the serum creatinine concentration. This example also highlights that most measurands examined in laboratory medicine are not very useful in population screening or in case finding.

### Consequences for Population-Based Reference Intervals

The consequences of individuality were first postulated by Harris, who showed that, when II is high (the criterion usually applied is II >1.4), the distribution of values from any single individual will cover much of the entire dispersion of the reference interval derived from values found in reference individuals. In contrast, if II is low (especially when II is <0.6), the dispersion of values for any individual will span only a small part of the conventional population-based reference interval. By this follows that when II is low, most individuals can have values that are unusual for them, but these will often lie within the reference interval. Thus, taking one specimen

from an individual and comparing, for example, its creatinine result to the population-based reference interval will not be an effective way of picking up the small changes often seen in early pathological processes. However, when only one sample is examined in an individual, the II will have no influence on the percentage of false positives and true positives detected, irrespective of whether the upper reference limit or a clinical decision limit is used. However, if a "confirmatory" measurement is performed, the II is important. For quantities with a very low II, such as creatinine, the new result will be close to the first, and will only provide limited new information. For quantities with a high II, a repeat measurement will decrease the number of true positives and false positives.

If II is defined as $CV_I/CV_G$, this ratio must be made larger to make conventional population-based reference intervals of higher clinical usefulness, especially in diagnosis, case finding, and screening, when no previous results on an individual are available. This is sometimes easily achieved because $CV_G$ can be made smaller by stratifying (or partitioning) the data. An example is shown in Table 4.2 for urine creatinine, where the II for the total cohort is 0.46; therefore, the reference interval is of low usefulness for monitoring individuals. However, for men and women taken separately, the II are 1.83 and 1.42, respectively, and reference intervals will have a higher utility.

### Reference Change Values

Most laboratory results are used for monitoring diseases. Because most measurands have marked individuality and low II, conventional population-based reference intervals provide limited assistance when serial results of an individual need to be interpreted.

Harris first introduced the concept of evaluating consecutive measurements in 1975 and 1976, and the concept was later simplified and introduced by Harris and Yasaka as the RCV, sometimes also referred to as *critical difference*.

The result of one examination will have: dispersion $= Z \times \left(SD_A^2 + SD_I^2\right)^{1/2}$, where $Z$ is the $Z$-score equal to the number of SDs appropriate for the probability desired and the $SD_A$ and the $SD_I$ refer to the analytical and biological variation, in SDs. The result of a second examination will have the same dispersion, so the total dispersion of two results will be $2^{1/2} \times Z \times \left(SD_A^2 + SD_I^2\right)^{1/2}$. Thus, for the difference between two results in the same individual, with a certain probability, to be explained by analytical and within-subject biological variation, this inherent difference due to $SD_A$ and $SD_I$ must be exceeded, and this is the RCV.

This original "classical" RCV formula is in principle only applicable when SDs are used (i.e., changes expressed in units). When using estimates in the form of CVs (i.e., percentages, transformation is required). This is because the sum of normally distributed variables is normally distributed, but the ratio between normally distributed variables is not. The difference between measurements M1 and M2 is defined as (M2−M1)/M1=M2/M1 −1, and if M1 and M2 are normally distributed, M2/M1 is not and the classical RCV formula

| TABLE 4.2 Within-Subject and Between-Subject Biological Variation of Urine Creatinine and Indices of Individuality |||| 
|---|---|---|---|
| Group | CV$_I$ (%) | CV$_G$ (%) | II |
| Men (n = 7) | 11.0 | 6.0 | 1.83 |
| Women (n = 8) | 15.7 | 11.0 | 1.42 |
| Total | 13.0 | 28.2 | 0.46 |

will not provide the correct differences, which in reality are skewed.

A sufficient approximation for RCV using published estimates of $CV_I$ and the laboratory's own estimate of $CV_A$ can be established by the formula:

$$SD_A^2 = \log_e\left(\left(\frac{CV_A}{100}\right)^2 + 1\right)$$

$$SD_I^2 = \log_e\left(\left(\frac{CV_I}{100}\right)^2 + 1\right)$$

$$RCV = \pm 100 \times \left(\exp\left(+Z_\alpha \times \sqrt{2} \times \sqrt{SD_A^2 + SD_I^2}\right) - 1\right)$$

If, as an example, using a published estimate of $CV_I$ of 5.1% for a measurand and the between-run $CV_A$ from a routine laboratory of 1.4%, $SD_I^2 = \log_e\left(0.051_A^2 + 1\right) = 0.00259762$ and $SD_A^2 = \log_e\left(0.014_A^2 + 1\right) = 0.00019598$. The RCV in % can then be calculated as

$$RCV = \pm 100 \times \left(\exp\left(\pm 1.65 \times \sqrt{2} \times \right.\right.$$
$$\left.\left. \sqrt{0.00019598 + 0.00259762}\right) - 1\right)$$
$$= (-11.6\% + 13.1\%).$$

(i.e., the RCVs are skewed), with bigger tolerance for a rise than a fall in values.

If, however, using estimates given as CVs in the $RCV_{SD}$, one would obtain the following result:

$$RCV\% = 100\% \times 1.64 \times \sqrt{2} \times$$
$$\sqrt{0.051 \times 0.051 + 0.014 \times 0.014}$$
$$= \pm 12.5\%$$

Using the log transformation is therefore most important when the included $CV_I$ and/or $CV_A$ estimates are high.

It is usually assumed that preanalytical sources of variation are negligible, and in clinical and laboratory practice this means having well-documented standard operating procedures for patient preparation and specimen collection, transport, and handling before analysis, as well as appropriate training of staff performing these tasks. Moreover, it is important to realize that changes in the bias of the analysis between the collections of the serial specimens can also add to the RCV; as a difference due to bias in percentage terms, $\Delta B$, the formula becomes $RCV = \Delta B + 2^{1/2} \times Z \times \left(SD_A^2 + SD_I^2\right)^{1/2}$. However, in a single laboratory, the main source of $\Delta B$ over time is due to recalibration, and this "random" bias is usually an integral component of the longer-term $CV_A$ as estimated from replicate analyses of internal quality control materials. Thus, it can be assumed that a "systematic" bias of the analysis does not change during the period between the two analyses, and the simpler RCV formula applies when the long-term $CV_A$ is used.

It is often assumed that a Z-score of 1.96 for $P < .05$ (and sometimes also 2.58 for $P < .01$) is appropriate. It is almost ubiquitously stated in studies on biological variation that the RCV is calculated as $2.77 \times \left(SD_A^2 + SD_I^2\right)^{1/2}$. This is incorrect for various reasons. These Z-scores are termed bidirectional (or two-tailed or two-sided), and this infers that the difference between the two serial results can be either an increase or a decrease. However, in most situations, clinical decisions rely on the assessment of a significant decrease (e.g., of $HbA_{1c}$ after treatment for diabetes mellitus or in glucose after adjustment of insulin dosage) or a significant increase in the measurand (e.g., an increase in serum creatinine to assess acute kidney injury, or serum troponin after acute chest pain). Thus, unidirectional (one-tailed or one-sided) Z-scores must be used in most clinical situations to facilitate correct interpretation; these are 1.65 for $P < .05$ and 2.33 for $P < .01$. Precise definition of the real clinical setting and accurate description of what is considered a "change" in terms of "increase" or "decrease" and their many synonyms are required for correct calculation and use of RCVs in clinical decision-making.

It is also important to recognize that clinical decision-making is not always done at $P < .05$, which is the most used probability in analysis of research data. The semantics used are crucial to understanding the probability that is clinically appropriate. The probability used will always be dependent on the consequences of the actions taken if RCV is exceeded; the advantage of an action must always be weighted against the consequences/risk of no action. RCVs should be used in a spectrum of post-analytical processes, including provision of graphs and tables of change versus probability, delta-checking, and flagging of significant changes at different levels of probability on electronic and paper reports of results of examinations.

In addition, the RCV for each laboratory will always depend on the $CV_A$ in that laboratory. Furthermore, it is important that the $CV_I$ estimate is representative for the population for whom it will be used. This means that when RCV is interpreted for diagnostic purposes, exceeding the RCV limits means that the change is unlikely explained by analytical and within-subject biological variation. When RCV is interpreted for monitoring purposes, we assume that the $CV_I$ is similar for healthy and diseased persons and therefore expect changes are of the same order. This depends on the disease not affecting the measurand that is being monitored. This will likely usually be the case, but in some cases, the biological variation for diseased persons will be different from healthy, such as glucose in diabetes mellitus patients. In addition, the time interval used for obtaining both the $CV_A$ and the $CV_I$ must be comparable to the one used in practice. As an example, if HbA1c is controlled every 6 months in a diabetic patient, the applied $CV_I$ should be representative for such a sampling interval and the $CV_A$ should be taken from the internal quality control during this period and should reflect the relevant concentration.

Traditional RCVs are believed by some to be rather simplistic, especially because they only address how likely it is that a certain change can be explained by analytical and within-subject biological variation, but not the probability that a change in the disease state has occurred. A tool for better understanding and interpreting measured differences in monitoring has therefore been suggested. This concept takes into account the distribution of a diseased population. The concepts of sensitivity, specificity, likelihood ratios, and odds used for diagnostic test accuracy evaluations can then be applied to monitoring by substituting measured concentrations with measured differences.

The probability of significance of any difference seen in clinical practice between two results can be calculated using a simple rearrangement of the RCV equation making the $Z$-score (and thus the probability) the unknown, namely:

$$Z = \text{difference} / \left[ 2^{1/2} \times \left( SD_A^2 + SD_I^2 \right)^{1/2} \right]$$

Thus, the formula calculates the probability of significance of the observed change and lets the person interpreting the result decide, in that clinical context, what is good enough a percentage certainty for them.

## Personalized Reference Intervals

The index of individuality gives an idea about the usefulness of a population-based reference intervals for a specific measurand. A low II indicates that most individuals can have values that are unusual for them, but the values will often lie within the population-based reference interval. A reference interval fitted specifically for the person being monitored (i.e., a "personalized" reference interval) would be a better solution. Over time, different models have been developed to assess serial results from an individual, some of them based on the homeostatic model, as the prRI concept described below, and some more complex. For calculating the prRI, you first have to estimate the homeostatic set point; this is achieved by calculating the mean of previous test results obtained in a steady-state situation, and you also need an estimate of the analytical variation ($SD_A$). Thereafter, the prRI can be constructed in two ways: (1) using the person's own within-person biological variation estimate ($SD_P$) or (2) using the within-subject biological variation estimate ($SD_I$) derived from a population similar to the person you are monitoring. The prRI can thereafter be derived as

$$prRI = HSP \pm k \times \sqrt{\frac{(n+1)}{n} \left( SD_A^2 + SD_B^2 \right)}$$

where HSP is the homeostatic set point; $k$ is a constant depending on the type of distribution (normal distribution [z] in case of population-based $SD_I$ and $t$ distribution in case of $SD_P$) and the probability, n is the number of previous test results and the $SD_B$ refers to either the $SD_P$ or the $SD_I$. In principle, using $SD_P$ to calculate the prRI is preferred. However, to get a reliable estimate of the $SD_P$ you need more than five previous test results. This will often be a limitation, and it will therefore be easier to construct the prRI using the $SD_I$, but you still need at least three samples to establish the HSP. The two models will give rather similar prRIs if the presuppositions

for the models are fulfilled. It is possible to estimate prRIs for all measurands where you have repeated measurements from a steady state situation, and prRI has the potential to be useful in diagnosing and follow-up of patients.

## Number of Samples Needed

Examination result variation can be reduced by multiple sampling (or multiple examinations), and the variation is made smaller by the square root of the number of replicates. To estimate the number of specimens needed to determine the homeostatic set point within a certain percentage error with a stated probability, a simple rearrangement of the usual standard error of the mean formula is used, namely:

$$n = \left( \frac{Z \times \sqrt{CV_A^2 + CV_I^2}}{D} \right)^2$$

where $Z$ is the $Z$-score appropriate for the probability, and $D$ is the desired percentage closeness to the homeostatic set point. It is important to note that taking multiple specimens and undertaking replicate analyses does affect the overall variability of the individual analytical result; the dispersion (expressed as 1 CV) can be calculated as:

$$\text{Dispersion} = Z \times \sqrt{\frac{CV_A^2}{nA} + \frac{CV_I^2}{nS}}$$

where $Z$ is the number of standard deviations appropriate to the probability selected, nA is the number of replicate examinations, and nS is the number of specimens. The relative magnitudes of $CV_A$ and $CV_I$ are important in deciding if a lower dispersion is required, whether it is better to undertake replicate analyses on one specimen or singleton analysis on multiple specimens.

## Development of New Measurement Procedures

The introduction of new tests is an ongoing task for the in vitro diagnostic (IVD) industry and also for many medical laboratories. To do this a dynamic cyclic model moving back and forth between different components is used. The components which are essential in the clinical pathway are: analytical performance, clinical performance, clinical effectiveness, and cost-effectiveness. First of all, it is important to define clinical specifications and how the intended application of the biomarker in the clinical pathway should drive each component of test evaluation. It is important to emphasize the interaction of the different components, and that clinical effectiveness data should be fed back to refine analytical and clinical performances to achieve improved outcomes. Desirable clinical performance criteria for a test are the ability to predict a diagnosis or clinically significant event. To be able to do that it is, among other factors, important that the test has a high signal-to-noise ratio, for example, a single test result is likely to detect a clinically significant change and to differentiate it from what can be explained by biological and analytical variation.

Moreover, the data are also necessary for objective analysis of the often somewhat subjective guidelines from professional bodies. The latter provide recommendations on interpretation of the numerical results of examinations and on examination performance specifications; however, these recommendations often do not consider analytical or biological variation.

## ANALYTICAL PERFORMANCE SPECIFICATIONS

Analytical performance specifications (APS) are in principle the numerical standards of examination performance required to facilitate optimum patient care. APS are used for example to set control rules for internal and external quality control and acceptable lot-to-lot variation (see Chapter 7). Over time, many different models to set APS have evolved. Following pioneering studies on the definition of the components of biological variation, a College of American Pathologists conference held in 1976 supported the concept that APS should be best based on biology. The consensus statement, restated in current terms and symbols, was: "For group screening, in which an individual is to be selected from a population, a specification for imprecision ($CV_A$) is defined as: $CV_A = 0.5 \times \left(CV_I^2 + CV_G^2\right)^{1/2}$" and "For individual single and multipoint testing, in which an individual is evaluated on the basis of discrimination values: $CV_A = 0.5 \times CV_I$."

The Stockholm Conference held in 1999 on "Strategies to set global analytical quality specifications in laboratory medicine" advocated the ubiquitous application of a hierarchical structure of approaches, based on a model proposed by Fraser and Petersen.

The hierarchy had five levels, stated as: (1) evaluation of the effect of analytical performance on clinical outcomes in specific clinical settings; (2) evaluation of the effect of analytical performance on clinical decisions in general, using (a) data based on components of biological variation or (b) analysis of clinicians' opinions; (3) published professional recommendations from (a) national and international expert bodies or (b) expert local groups or individuals; (4) performance goals set by (a) regulatory bodies or (b) organizers of external quality assessment (EQA) schemes; and (5) goals based on

the current state of the art as (a) demonstrated by data from EQA or proficiency testing scheme, or (b) found in current publications on methodology. Since the Stockholm conference, there have been further proposals for setting APS, and all of these have included biological variation data in their derivation.

In 2014, the EFLM organized the 1st Strategic Conference on how to define APS. The presentations are available on the EFLM website. The consensus statement and formal papers emanating from the speakers are included in a Special Issue of *Clinical Chemistry and Laboratory Medicine* published in 2015, representing a resource on different aspects of setting APS. In the consensus statement from the Strategic Conference, the hierarchy was simplified and represented by three different models to set APS (Table 4.3):

*Model 1.* Based on the effect of analytical performance on clinical outcomes

This can, in principle, be established using different types of studies:

    a. Direct outcome studies—investigating the impact of analytical performance of the test on clinical outcomes;

    b. Indirect outcome studies—investigating the impact of analytical performance of the test on clinical classifications or decisions and thereby on the probability of patient outcomes, such as by simulation or decision analysis.

The advantage of this approach is that it addresses the influence of analytical performance on clinical outcomes that are relevant to patients and society. The primary disadvantage is that it is only useful for examinations where the links between the test, clinical decision-making, and clinical outcomes are straightforward and strong.

*Model 2.* Based on components of biological variation of the measurand

This attempts to minimize the ratio of "analytical noise" to the biological signal. The advantage is that it can be applied to most measurands for which population-based or subject-specific biological variation data can be established. There are limitations to this approach that has been dealt with earlier in this chapter

*Model 3.* Based on state of the art

This relates to the highest level of analytical performance technically achievable. The advantage of this model is that

## TABLE 4.3 Advantages and Disadvantages of the Three Models Used to Set Analytical Performance Specifications

| Model Based on | Study/Principle | Advantage | Disadvantage |
|---|---|---|---|
| Clinical outcomes | Outcome studies (type 1a and type 1b) | Address the medical needs of patients and society | Difficult to perform studies. Possible for only a limited number of measurands |
| Biological variation | Studies on biological variation Minimize analytical noise to biological signal | Can be applied to most measurands | Reliable data can be difficult to obtain |
| State of the art | Empirical data | Easy to obtain data | Does not relate to what is medically needed (outcome) or to noise/signal minimalization |

state-of-the-art performance data are readily available. An overview of the different models as well as their advantages and disadvantages are provided in Table 4.2. Some measurands can have different performance specifications defined when the test has multiple intended clinical applications.

## Analytical Performance Specifications for Imprecision

In most cases, the APS for $CV_A$ is simply taken as $CV_A = 0.5 \times CV_I$, with the rationale that the noise (analytical imprecision) is then small (12%), compared to the $CV_I$ when using this 0.5 factor. The factor for optimum and minimum performance specifications are arbitrarily set to 0.25 and 0.75, respectively.

## Analytical Performance Specifications for Bias

Analytical bias was not considered in most early works on setting APS, possibly because the thesis was that laboratories all had their own reference intervals to which the results of their analyses were compared. However, as the interest in harmonization of laboratory data across time and geography increased, and the benefits for harmonized reference intervals were appreciated, criteria for bias needed to be developed. Therefore, it was proposed that the APS for bias ($B$), to allow the use of harmonized reference intervals, should be $B < 0.25 \left( CV_I^2 + CV_G^2 \right)^{1/2}$. It must be emphasized, however, that this was not intended as a general formula for a bias specification, but to be used for diagnosis when laboratories wanted to share common reference intervals. Other models combine analytical (state of the art) and biological variation. What formulae to apply should be dependent on the situation in which it is to be used.

## Specifications for Total Allowable Error/ Maximum Allowable Measurement Uncertainty

As the concepts of total laboratory quality management evolved, and the idea that random and systematic sources of variation (imprecision and bias) were both important, it became clear that it was important to have a measure of the total error/maximum measurement uncertainty, since this is the most relevant, from a clinical point of view. Here we present two ways of calculating this.

### Total Allowable Error

It was proposed that a linear model of combining imprecision and bias could be used to set APS for what was termed total allowable error (TAE) as a simple linear addition, $P < .05$:

$$TAE < 1.64 \times 0.5 CV_I + 0.25 \left( CV_I^2 + CV_G^2 \right)^{1/2}$$

where the latter represents the assay bias and the 1.64 $\times$ 0.5 $CV_I$ adds imprecision at the 95% probability level. The disadvantages of this particular model include that there is no theoretical basis for combining imprecision and bias in a

linear way and that it results in overestimation of the allowable total error. For these reasons, this approach should be applied with caution. However, the linear error model is widely used in current practice in laboratory medicine because the formula is simple to use and to calculate, albeit sometimes with a different multiplier for the imprecision term, to deliver different levels of probability.

### Maximum Allowable Measurement Uncertainty

Using the total allowable measurement uncertainty (MAu) model, the basic principles are that the bias should be corrected, and all the remaining sources of variation should be added linearly as variances. In this model, the allowable standard measurement uncertainty can be set as 0.5 $\times$ $CV_I$ and the expanded measurement uncertainty (i.e., the MAU) will then be $k \times 0.5 \times CV_I$), where the factor 0.5 refers to desirable APS. The "$k$" is the coverage factor of for example 2 or 3, to obtain a certain level of confidence. The most used coverage factor is 2. From this follows that for desirable APS,

$$MAU < 2 \times 0.5 * CV_I$$

The factors for optimum and minimum performance specifications are, in line with APS for imprecision, arbitrarily set to 0.25 and 0.75, respectively.

## OVERALL CONCLUSIONS

Most analytes are characterized by random biological variation around a homeostatic set point, where these set points vary between different individuals. Though a vast amount of biological variation data has been published over the past 50 years, some is no longer relevant or fit for purpose and it is important to always assess the quality and relevance of the data prior to applying them for clinical and laboratory applications. Numerical estimates of within-subject and between-subject biological variation are best generated by analysis of a series of specimens taken from a cohort of individuals, analyzed in duplicate, and followed by statistical analysis of the sources of variation, or by analysis of big data. Biological variation data have numerous applications, including establishing APS, the determination of the individuality of a measurand and the usefulness of conventional population-based reference intervals, the statistical significance of changes in serial results from an individual as well as deriving prRI.

The recommended models for establishing APS are
1. To examine the impact of analytical performance on clinical outcome
2. To minimize analytical noise to biological variation and
3. To use state of the art examination methods.

For each of the models there are "sub-models" to set APS for imprecision, bias, total allowable error and total allowable measurement uncertainty. The selection of the model and method to set APS should be decided for the specific measurand, its intended use as well as available data.

## POINTS TO REMEMBER

Most measurands are characterized by random variation around a homeostatic set point: in addition, biological variation may be cyclical and daily, monthly, or seasonal.

The generation of high-quality data on within-subject and between-subject components of biological variation requires adherence to strict experimental and statistical protocols.

Biological variation estimates have been published for many measurands and updated, quality-assessed data can be found in the EFLM Biological Variation Database (https://biologicalvariation.eu), which also contains information about analytical performance specifications and reference change values.

Data on biological variation are used, inter alia, to determine:
- The individuality of a measurand and the usefulness of conventional population-based reference intervals and the calculation of prRI
- The statistical significance of changes in serial results in an individual and the probability that any change documented is larger than analytical and biological variation
- APS for imprecision, bias, total allowable error, and total allowable measurement uncertainty.

## REVIEW QUESTIONS

1. Which of the following usually best describes the variation in the concentration or activity of most measurands in laboratory medicine?
   a. Circadian rhythms
   b. Monthly cycles
   c. Systematic trends
   d. Random variations
   e. Seasonal fluctuations
2. Which of the following strategies is recommended to best set general analytical performance specifications?
   a. Effect of analytical performance on clinical outcomes
   b. Fractions of biological variation component estimates
   c. Professional body recommendations
   d. The limits of acceptance used in external quality assessment or proficiency testing
   e. The state of the art
3. Which of the following is irrelevant to the creation of Reference Change Values?
   a. Within-subject biological variation
   b. Analytical bias
   c. Analytical imprecision
   d. Preanalytical sources of variation
   e. Between-subject biological variation
4. What analytical imprecision should be used when the reference change value is to be created for a measurand that will be used by your own laboratory?
   a. The analytical imprecision obtained from duplicate analyses obtained during the study of the biological variation
   b. The best analytical imprecision you can obtain in your laboratory
   c. The analytical imprecision obtained in your laboratory during the same time period as the time interval between the samples examined
   d. The analytical imprecision as assessed from an external quality assessment scheme
   e. The analytical imprecision documented in the manufacturer's literature
5. Which of the following represents the individuality of most measurands in laboratory medicine?
   a. The index of individuality is high
   b. The index of individuality is low
   c. The measurand has low individuality
   d. The within-subject variation is larger than the between-subject variation
   e. The analytical imprecision is lower than the within-subject variation

## SUGGESTED READINGS

Aarsand AK, Kristoffersen AH, Sandberg S, et al. The European Biological Variation Study (EuBIVAS): biological variation data for coagulation markers estimated by a Bayesian model. Clin Chem. 2021;67:1259–1270.

Aarsand AK, Røraas T, Bartlett WA, et al. Harmonization initiatives in the generation, reporting and application of biological variation data. Clin Chem Lab Med. 2018;60:1629–1636.

Aarsand AK, Røraas T, Fernandez-Calle P, et al. The biological variation data critical appraisal checklist: A standard for evaluating studies on biological variation. Clin Chem. 2018;64:501–514.

Bartlett WA, Braga F, Carobene A, et al. A checklist for critical appraisal of studies of biological variation. Clin Chem Lab Med. 2015;53:879–885.

Carobene A, Aarsand AK, Bartlett WA, et al. The European Biological Variation Study (EuBIVAS): a summary report. Clin Chem Lab Med. 2022;60:505–517.

Ceriotti F, Fernandez-Calle P, Klee GG, et al. Criteria for assigning laboratory measurands to models for analytical performance specifications defined in the 1st EFLM Strategic Conference. Clin Chem Lab Med. 2017;55:189–194.

Fraser CG. Biological Variation: From Principles to Practice. Washington, DC: AACC Press; 2001.

Fraser CG, Harris EK. Generation and application of data on biological variation in clinical chemistry. Crit Rev Clin Lab Sci. 1989;27:409–437.

Fraser CG, Petersen PH. Analytical performance characteristics should be judged against objective quality specifications. Clin Chem. 1999;45:321–323.

Jones GRD. Estimates of within-subject biological variation derived from pathology databases: an approach to allow assessment of the effects of age, sex, time between sample collections, and analyte concentration on reference change values. *Clin Chem.* 2019;65:579–588.

Kenny D, Fraser CG, Petersen HP, et al. Stockholm Consensus Statement 1999. *Scand J Clin Lab Invest.* 1999;59:585.

Klee GG. Establishment of outcome-related analytic performance goals. *Clin Chem.* 2010;56:714–722.

Petersen PH, Sandberg S, Fraser CG, et al. Influence of index of individuality on false positives in repeated sampling from healthy individuals. *Clin Chem Lab Med.* 2001;39:160–165.

Petersen PH, Sandberg S, Iglesias N, et al. 'Likelihood-ratio' and 'odds' applied to monitoring of patients as a supplement to 'Reference Change Value' (RCV). *Clin Chem Lab Med.* 2008;46:157–164.

Ricos C, Iglesias N, García-Lario JV, et al. Within-subject biological variation in disease: collated data and clinical consequences. *Ann Clin Biochem.* 2007;44:343–352.

Røraas T, Petersen PH, Sandberg S. Confidence intervals and power calculations for within-person biological variation: effect of analytical imprecision, number of replicates, number of samples, and number of individuals. *Clin Chem.* 2012;58:1306–1313.

Røraas T, Sandberg S, Aarsand AK, et al. A Bayesian approach to biological variation analysis. *Clin Chem.* 2019;65:995–1005.

Røraas T, Støve B, Petersen PH, et al. Biological variation: the effect of different distributions on estimated within-person variation and reference change values. *Clin Chem.* 2016;62:725–736.

Sandberg S, Carobene A, Aarsand AK. Biological variation—eight years after the 1st Strategic Conference of EFLM. *Clin Chem Lab Med.* 2022;60:465–468.

Sandberg S, Fraser CG, Horvath AR, et al. Defining analytical performance specifications: consensus statement from the 1st strategic conference of the European Federation of Clinical Chemistry and Laboratory Medicine. *Clin Chem Lab Med.* 2015;53:833–835.

# 5

# Establishment and Use of Reference Intervals

*Graham R.D. Jones\**

## OBJECTIVES

1. Define the following:
   - Direct and indirect methods for establishing reference intervals
   - Exclusion criteria
   - Interpercentile interval
   - Outlier
   - Partitioning; partitioning criteria
   - Population-based reference value
   - Predictive value
   - Prevalence
   - Random sample
   - Range
   - Reference individual
   - Reference interval
   - Reference limits
   - Reference population
   - Reference value
   - Selection criteria
   - Subject-based reference value
   - Transferability or transference
2. List three conditions that are essential when a valid comparison of individual laboratory results with reference values is performed; state the need for establishing reference intervals.
3. Give three examples of exclusion criteria used in the production of health-associated reference values; give three examples of partitioning criteria used to subgroup a reference group.
4. State why standardization of specimen collection is important when reference values are established.
5. Compare the terms *reference value* and *reference interval;* list three categories of reference intervals.
6. Briefly state the parametric and nonparametric statistical methods of determining an interpercentile interval; state the important assumption that must be made when parametric statistics are used.
7. State the difference between direct and indirect reference interval studies.
8. State the limitation of using population-based reference intervals instead of subject-based reference intervals, and state a solution to this limitation.
9. Discuss the issue of transferability of reference values with regard to prerequisites and solutions to the issue.
10. Outline the process of selecting a reference interval for use in a laboratory

## KEY WORDS AND DEFINITIONS

**Direct reference interval study** A reference interval study where samples are collected from reference individuals under specified conditions for the purpose of determining a reference interval.

**Indirect reference interval study** A reference interval study using results measured on samples collected for a purpose other than to determine reference intervals.

**Nonparametric analysis** A statistical approach to reference value analysis that requires no assumptions about the nature of the distribution; thus, it can be applied to distributions that are Gaussian or non-Gaussian.

**Parametric analysis** A statistical approach to reference value analysis that describes a population distribution based on parameters that require specific distributional assumptions. For example, it usually requires that the distribution of values be Gaussian (or that the values be mathematically transformed so that they become Gaussian) and is described by the parameters mean and standard deviation.

**Partitioning** The use of specific criteria in the subclassification of reference groups to reduce the variation in each group; the most commonly used criteria are age and sex.

**Reference individual** An individual selected as the basis for comparison with individuals under clinical investigation through the use of defined criteria.

**Reference interval (population based)** A set of values usually defined by an upper reference limit and a lower reference limit, representing a specified proportion of the reference population; this is frequently the central 95% of values from the reference population.

**Reference interval (subject based)** A set of values usually defined by an upper reference limit and a lower reference limit, representing a specified proportion of the values

*The author gratefully acknowledge the original contributions by Helge Eric Solberg and Gary Horowitz on which major portions of this chapter are based.

from a reference individual; this is frequently the central 95% of values from the reference individual.

**Reference population** An undefined number of individuals that represent the demographic for which the reference intervals will be used. Reference individuals are chosen from this larger population, preferably at random, to provide reference samples for the establishment of a reference interval.

**Reference value** A value obtained by observation or measurement of a particular type of quantity on a reference individual; results of a certain type of quantity obtained from a single individual or group of individuals corresponding to a stated description.

**Selection criteria** A set of criteria that define the desired characteristics of a reference individual. The specific criteria chosen will depend on the purpose of the reference interval and the specific population the reference interval is intended to represent.

**Transferability or transference** The adoption by a laboratory of reference intervals that were previously established elsewhere. Procedures for validation of reference intervals must be completed by the adopting laboratory prior to the use of the transferred reference interval to ensure that they are appropriate to the laboratory's patient population and laboratory methods.

---

In medical practice, information collected during (1) patient interviews, (2) clinical examinations, and (3) supplementary investigations are interpreted by comparison with reference information. If the condition of the patient resembles that typical of a particular disease, the clinician or health care provider may base the diagnosis on these observations (positive diagnosis). This diagnosis is also made more likely if observed symptoms and signs do not fit the patterns that characterize a set of alternative diseases (diagnosis by exclusion).

Interpretation of medical laboratory data is an example of decision-making by comparison. We therefore need *reference values* for all tests performed in the clinical laboratory, not only from healthy individuals but also from patients with relevant diseases. Ideally, observed values should be related to several collections of reference values, such as values from (1) healthy people, (2) general ambulant population, (3) undifferentiated hospital inpatient population, and (4) people with relevant diseases, and (5) to previous values from the same subjects. A patient's laboratory result is simply not medically useful if appropriate data for comparison are lacking. Establishment and use of such reference values are the topics of this chapter. In practice, reference values and derived reference limits are usually only formally determined and presented on reports for healthy subjects. Other populations (e.g., people with typical diseases) are more commonly described in textbooks or guidelines or held in clinicians' minds; however, the principles remain the same.

## ESTABLISHMENT OF REFERENCE INTERVALS

Certain conditions are mandatory for making a valid comparison of a patient's laboratory results with reference values:
1. The group(s) of reference individuals should be clearly defined.
2. The patient examined should resemble sufficiently the reference individuals (in all groups selected for comparison) in all respects other than those under investigation (i.e., the presence or absence of the condition under consideration).
3. The conditions under which the samples were obtained and processed for analysis should be known and not affect the comparison, including specimen type where relevant.

4. All quantities compared should be of the same type (i.e., the measurand must be the same).
5. All laboratory results should be produced with the use of adequately standardized methods under sufficient analytical quality control (see Chapter 7).
6. The clinical sensitivity, clinical specificity, and disease prevalence in the populations tested should be known so that laboratory tests can be interpreted intelligently (see Chapter 2).

## Background

The terms *normal values* and *normal ranges* have been used frequently in the past. Confusion arose because the word *normal* has several very different connotations. Consequently, this term is now considered obsolete and should not be used. Instead, the International Federation of Clinical Chemistry and Laboratory Medicine (IFCC) recommends use of the term *reference values* and related terms, such as *reference individual, reference limit, reference interval (RI),* and *observed values.* **Reference values** are results of a certain type of quantity obtained from a single individual or group of individuals corresponding to a stated description, which must be spelled out and made available for use by others.

A short description of qualifiers associated with the term *reference values,* such as *health-associated reference values* (close to what was understood by the obsolete term *normal values*), is convenient. Other examples of such qualifying words are (1) *patient with diabetes,* (2) *patient with diabetes in hospital,* and (3) *ambulatory patient with diabetes.* These short descriptions prevent the common misunderstanding that reference values are associated only with health.

A further distinction is made between subject-based and population-based reference values. *Subject-based reference values* are previous values from the same individual, obtained when the individual was in a defined state of health. *Population-based reference values* are those obtained from a group of systematically defined reference individuals and are usually the values referred to when the term *reference values* is used with no qualifying words. The immediately following sections refer to studies to determine reference intervals which are described as **direct reference interval studies**. These are studies where samples are collected from subjects for the specific purpose of determining a reference interval. This is the preferred method for determining a reference interval. An alternate process, the **indirect reference interval study**, used results on samples measured for other purposes, typically those available in a routine pathology database. Indirect studies will be further explained later in the text.

## Selection of Reference Individuals

A set of explicit criteria should be used to determine which individuals should be included in the group of **reference individuals.** Such criteria include (1) statements describing the source population, (2) specifications of criteria for health, and, if relevant (3) specifications for the disease of interest. The selection of reference individuals is based essentially on the application of these defined criteria to the entire group of examined candidates. The required characteristics of the reference values determine which criteria should be used in the selection process. As examples, the left-hand column of Table 5.1 provides some examples of criteria that should be considered when *excluding* individuals in the production of health-associated reference values.

Ideally the group of reference individuals should be a *random sample* of all individuals in the parent population who meet the **selection criteria**. However, a strictly random sampling scheme is exceedingly difficult to obtain in most situations for a variety of practical reasons. For example, it would imply the examination and application of selection criteria to the entire population (thousands or millions of individuals) and the random selection of a subset of individuals among those accepted. Therefore, using the best reference sample obtained after all practical considerations have been applied

is necessary. Data then should be used and interpreted with due caution because of the possible bias introduced by the non-randomness of the sample selection process. For example, a study recruiting from office workers may introduce a bias by excluding subjects doing manual work or spending more hours outdoors.

Often, separate reference values for sex, age group, and other criteria are necessary. Thus, it is important to define the *partitioning* criteria for the subclassification of the set of selected reference individuals. Some examples are provided in the right-hand column of Table 5.1. It should be noted that some criteria can be used as either exclusion or partitioning criteria, depending on the nature of the study. In practice, each partition could require more than 120 samples; therefore, the number of partitions should usually be kept as small as possible to obtain sufficient sample sizes for the derivation of valid statistical estimates. Current reporting practices with reference limits commonly reported alongside cumulative results over time are also made more complex by frequent age-related changes.

Age and sex are the most frequently used criteria for partitioning because several analytes vary significantly with these variables. Age may be categorized by equal intervals (e.g., by decades) or by intervals that are narrower in the periods of life where greater variation is observed. Partitioning based on age and sex are also easiest to implement for result reporting, as this information is available on the pathology request form and is easily entered into laboratory information systems. In addition, the use of qualitative age groups (e.g., [1] postnatal, [2] infancy, [3] childhood, [4] prepubertal, [5] pubertal, [6] adult, [7] premenopausal, [8] menopausal, and [9] geriatric) often may be appropriate although applying exact definitions becomes difficult. Other clinical criteria such as stages of puberty or of the menstrual cycle are also important for some analytes, but this information is rarely made available to the laboratory. Height and weight also have been used as criteria for the categorization of children, but laboratory information systems or electronic health records may not link these data to laboratory test results, which may complicate accurate determination of using these factors for pediatric reference intervals.

## Specimen Collection

Preanalytical standardization of (1) preparation of individuals before sample collection, (2) the sample collection itself, and (3) handling of the sample before analysis may eliminate or minimize bias or variation from these factors. These steps may reduce "noise" that otherwise may conceal important biological "signals" of disease, risk, or treatment effect.

The magnitudes of preanalytical sources of variation clearly are not equal for different analytes (see Chapter 3). Therefore, one may argue that one should consider only those factors that cause unwanted variation in the biological quantity for which reference value production is intended.

| TABLE 5.1 | Examples of Exclusion and Partitioning Criteria | |
| --- | --- |
| **Exclusion Criteria** | **Partitioning Criteria** |
| Age | Age |
| Alcohol intake | Blood group |
| Blood donation (recent) | Circadian variation |
| Drug abuse | Ethnicity |
| Exercise intensity (recent) | Exercise intensity (recent) |
| Fasting vs. nonfasting | Fasting vs. nonfasting |
| Sex | Sex |
| Hospitalization (recent) | Menstrual cycle (by stage) |
| Hypertension | |
| Illness (recent) | |
| Lactation | |
| Obesity | Obesity |
| Occupation | Posture (when sampled) |
| Oral contraceptives | |
| Pregnancy | Pregnancy (by stage) |
| Prescription drugs | Prescription drugs |
| Recent transfusion | |

Body posture during sample collection is, for instance, highly relevant for the establishment of reference values for nondiffusible analytes, such as albumin or cholesterol in serum, but is irrelevant for diffusible ones, such as serum sodium.

However, performing separate studies to allow for different preanalytical conditions for each constituent is impractical. In addition, several constituents are typically analyzed in the same clinical specimens. For these reasons, standardized procedures are recommended for sample collection, accounting for the requirements that will enable all the constituents under study to be measured accurately.

A special problem is caused by possible effects of therapeutic drug ingestion before sample collection. A distinction may be made between indispensable and dispensable medications. The latter category of drugs should be avoided for at least 2 days before specimen collection. The use of indispensable drugs, such as contraceptive pills or essential medication, may be a criterion for exclusion or partition.

## Analytical Procedures and Quality Control

Essential components of the required definition of a set of reference values are specifications concerning (1) analysis method, including information on equipment, reagents, calibrators, metrological traceability, analytical precision, analytical specificity, types of raw data, and calculation method; (2) quality control (see Chapter 7); and (3) reliability criteria (see Chapter 2). Specifications should be carefully described so that another investigator will be able to reproduce the study and evaluate comparability of the reference values with values obtained by the methods used for production of the patient's values in a routine laboratory. To ensure comparability between reference and observed values, the same analytical method should be used, or more specifically, assays with the same metrological traceability and analytical specificity. Data to ensure valid comparison with reference values can also come from published papers and external quality assurance programs using commutable samples. Alternatively (or in addition), one can establish comparability of methods and populations by analyzing 20 samples from reference individuals and ensuring that no more than two values fall outside the proposed limits, noting that this process does not ensure comparability for results distant from the reference interval.

## Statistical Treatment of Reference Values

After the analysis of the reference specimens is performed, the reference values are subjected to a statistical treatment, which includes (1) partitioning of the reference values into appropriate groups, (2) inspection of the distribution of each group, (3) identification of outliers, and (4) determination of reference limits and their uncertainties.

## Partitioning of Reference Values

The subset of reference individuals and the corresponding reference values may be partitioned according to sex, age, and other characteristics (see Table 5.1). **Partitioning** is also known as *stratification, categorization,* or *subgrouping,* and its results are called *partitions, strata, categories, classes,* or *subgroups.* Such partitioning gives rise to narrower and potentially more appropriate reference intervals. For example, serum creatinine reference intervals for adult males and adult females overlap but are different because of the typical sex-related differences in muscle mass and renal function. Combining them into a single interval would reduce the clinical utility of the reference intervals for each of the sexes. Various statistical criteria for partitioning have been suggested, and all feature the need to collect sufficient data to allow evaluation of the partitions separately and then, if appropriate, to combine them. For example, one may test for differences in means or in standard deviations (SDs) of the separate distributions. However, note that differences in means or differences in variability may be *statistically* significant and still too small *clinically* to justify replacing a single overall reference interval with several class-specific intervals. Harris and Boyd in 1995 and Lahti and coworkers in 2004 have developed other criteria for partitioning and statistical methods for this purpose.

In the following sections a homogeneous reference distribution is assumed to exist—either the complete sample distribution (if partitioning is unnecessary) or a subclass distribution after partitioning.

### Inspection of Distribution

It is advisable to display the reference distribution graphically and subsequently to inspect it. A histogram, as shown in Fig. 5.1, is prepared manually or by a computer program. Examination of the histogram serves as a safeguard against the misapplication or misinterpretation of statistical methods, and it may provide valuable information about the data. The following characteristics should be sought in an examination of the distribution:

1. Highly deviating values (outliers) may represent erroneous values.
2. Bimodal or polymodal distributions have more than one peak and may indicate that the distribution is

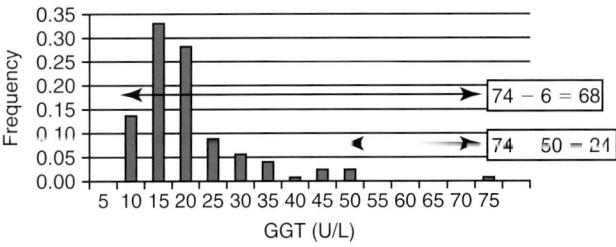

**Fig. 5.1** Observed distribution of 124 γ-glutamyltransferase (GGT) values in serum (U/L). This distribution is clearly not Gaussian; it appears skewed to the right. The *upper arrow* indicates the range of observed values (highest − lowest, or 74 − 6 = 68); the *lower arrow* indicates the difference between the highest value and the next highest value (74 − 50 = 24). Because the quotient (24/68 = 0.35) exceeds 0.33, Dixon's range test indicates that the highest value is an outlier and therefore is omitted from all further analyses.

nonhomogeneous because of the mixing of two or more distributions. If nonhomogeneity is the case, the criteria used to select reference individuals should be reevaluated or partitioning of the values according to age, sex, or other relevant factors attempted.

3. The shape of the distribution may be asymmetrical (skewed) or more or less peaked than the symmetrical and bell-shaped Gaussian distribution (non-Gaussian kurtosis).

4. Visual inspection may provide initial estimates of the location of reference limits that are useful as checks on the validity of later computations.

## Identification and Handling of Outliers

An outlier is an erroneous value that deviates significantly from the proper reference values. Visual inspection of a histogram is a useful initial method for identification of possible outliers. However, the inspector must keep in mind that values near the farthest point on the long tail of a skewed distribution may easily be misinterpreted as outliers. If the distribution is positively skewed, inspection of a histogram displaying the logarithms or other transformation (e.g., Box Cox transformation) of the values may aid in the identification of outliers. Some outliers may be identified by statistical tests, but no single method will detect outliers in every situation that may occur. Two main problems are often encountered:

1. Many tests assume that the type of the true distribution is known before the tests are used. For example, some tests specifically require that the distribution be Gaussian. However, biologic distributions are very often non-Gaussian, and their types seldom are known in advance. The Dixon-Reed range test, described in IFCC's recommendation, is relatively robust and involves identification of the extreme value as an outlier if the difference between the two highest (or lowest) values in the distribution exceeds one-third of the range of all values (see Fig. 5.1).

2. Several tests for outliers assume that the data contain only a single outlier. Thus, the range test may fail in the presence of several outliers. This problem is more relevant with larger data sets.

One approach published in 2005 may provide a solution to both of these problems in some cases. The algorithm involves mathematically transforming the data, if required, so as to approximate a Gaussian distribution, calculating the range of the central 50% of the resulting distribution, and then subtracting 150% of this value from the 25th percentile and adding 150% of this value to the 75th percentile. Any values beyond these limits, sometimes referred to as Tukey fences, are considered outliers.

Deviating values identified as possible outliers should not be discarded automatically. Where possible, values should be included or excluded on a rational basis. The records of the suspect values should be checked and any errors corrected. In some cases, deviating values should be rejected because noncorrectable causes have been found, such as previously unrecognized conditions that qualify individuals for exclusion from the group of reference individuals.

## Determination of Reference Limits

In clinical practice an observed patient's value is compared with the corresponding **reference interval**, which is bounded by a pair of reference limits. This interval, which may be defined in different ways, is a useful condensation of the information carried by the total set of reference values.

The terms *reference limits* and *clinical decision limits* should not be confused. Reference limits describe the reference distribution and provide information about the observed variation of values in the selected set of reference individuals. Thus, comparison of new values with these limits conveys only information about similarity to the given set of reference values. In contrast, clinical decision limits aim to provide optimal separation among clinical categories. Such limits usually are based on analysis of reference values from several groups of individuals (e.g., healthy individuals, patients with relevant diseases) and thus are used for diagnosis. Alternatively, such values are established scientifically on the basis of outcome studies and guide decisions on treatment. For an example of decision limits currently in widespread use, the reader is referred to American College of Cardiology/American Heart Association guidelines for cholesterol or the World Health Organization (WHO) guidelines for the diagnosis of diabetes mellitus.

As discussed earlier, the term *reference range* has been used for the term *reference interval*, but this use should be discouraged because the statistical term *range* denotes the difference (a single value!) between maximum and minimum values in a distribution.

In laboratory medicine the reference interval is generally determined as an interpercentile interval, as it is (1) simple to estimate, (2) very widely used, and (3) recommended by the IFCC. It is defined as an interval bounded by two percentiles of the reference distribution. A percentile denotes a value that divides the reference distribution such that a specified percentage of its values has magnitudes less than or equal to the limiting value. For example, if 47 U/L is the 97.5 percentile of serum $\gamma$-glutamyltransferase (GGT) values, then 97.5% of the values are equal to or less than this value, with 2.5% greater than this value.

The definition of the reference interval as the central 95% interval bounded by the 2.5 and 97.5 percentiles is an arbitrary but common convention (i.e., 2.5% of the values are cut off in both tails of the reference distribution). Another size or an asymmetrical location of the reference interval may be more appropriate in particular cases. As an example, the 99 percentile is recommended as the upper reference limit for serum cardiac troponin testing.

The degree of uncertainty associated with a given percentile is important in the estimation of a population value;

the magnitude of this uncertainty depends on the size of the sample, which increases when the number of observations is low. If the assumption of random sampling is fulfilled, determination of the confidence interval (CI) of the percentile (i.e., the limits within which the true percentile is located with a specified degree of confidence) is possible. The 0.90 confidence interval of the 97.5 percentile (upper reference limit) for serum GGT may, for example, be 39 to 50 U/L. The true percentile would be expected in this interval with a confidence limit of 0.90 if all serum GGT concentrations in the total **reference population** were measured. The minimum sample size required for estimation of the 2.5 and 97.5 percentiles is 40 values, but at least 120 reference values are required to determine the 0.9 CI of the reference limits. Thus 120 sample are required to be able to assess whether the accuracy of the reference limits established will meet clinical need, or whether the results of two reference intervals studies based on the same stated population are actually different. At more extreme percentiles (e.g., 99 percentile) a larger number is required to determine the CI.

The interpercentile interval can be determined by both parametric and nonparametric statistical techniques. The **parametric** method for the determination of percentiles and their confidence intervals assumes a certain type of distribution, and it is based on estimates of population parameters, such as the mean and SD. For example, a parametric method is used if the true distribution is believed to be Gaussian and reference limits (percentiles) are determined as the values located 2 SDs less than and greater than the mean. Most parametric methods in fact are based on the Gaussian distribution. If the reference distribution has another shape, mathematical functions that transform data to approximately Gaussian shape may be used. Any factors used in the transformation are then additional parameters which describe the distribution. In contrast, the **nonparametric** method makes no assumptions concerning the type of distribution and does not use estimates of distribution parameters. The percentiles are determined simply by cutting off the required percentage of values in each tail of the subset reference distribution.

When the results obtained by these two methods are compared, the estimates of the percentiles usually are very similar. In general, the simple and reliable nonparametric method is preferable to the parametric method.

## POINTS TO REMEMBER

The preferred method to establish reference intervals is nonparametric analysis, which:
- Requires a minimum of 120 reference values per partition
- Should include consideration of outlier exclusion
- Can be applied to any distribution of values without transformation; specifically, does not require a Gaussian distribution, as most other methods do
- Involves simple mathematical skills
- Is the method endorsed by CLSI and IFCC
- Must be supported by visual inspection of the distribution

*Nonparametric method.* Several nonparametric methods are available, but those based on ranked data are simple and reliable and allow nonparametric estimation of the confidence intervals of the percentiles.

The steps in a nonparametric procedure are as follows:
1. Sort the $n$ reference values in ascending order of magnitude, and rank the values. The minimum value has rank number 1, the next value number 2, and so on, until the maximum value, rank $n$, is reached. Consecutive rank numbers should be given to two or more values that are equal ("ties"). Spreadsheet software such as EXCEL is often used to sort and rank this type of data.
2. Compute the rank numbers of the 2.5 and 97.5 percentiles as $0.025(n + 1)$ and $0.975(n + 1)$, respectively.
3. Determine the percentiles by finding the original reference values that correspond to the computed rank numbers, provided that the rank numbers are integers. Otherwise, interpolation between the two limiting values is necessary.
4. Finally, determine the confidence interval of each percentile by using the binomial distribution. Table 5.2 facilitates this step for the 0.90 confidence interval of 2.5 and 97.5 percentiles. The bounding rank numbers for each percentile may be located in the table.

Tables 5.3 and 5.4 show an example of the nonparametric determination of percentiles using the serum GGT values shown in Fig. 5.1.

### TABLE 5.2 Nonparametric Confidence Intervals of Reference Limits[a]

| Sample Size | RANK NUMBERS | |
| --- | --- | --- |
| | Lower | Upper |
| 119–132 | 1 | 7 |
| 133–160 | 1 | 8 |
| 161–187 | 1 | 9 |
| 188–189 | 2 | 9 |
| 190–218 | 2 | 10 |
| 219–248 | 2 | 11 |
| 249–249 | 2 | 12 |
| 250–279 | 3 | 12 |
| 280–307 | 3 | 13 |
| 308–309 | 4 | 13 |
| 310–340 | 4 | 14 |
| 341–363 | 4 | 15 |
| 364–372 | 5 | 15 |
| 373–403 | 5 | 16 |
| 404–417 | 5 | 17 |
| 418–435 | 6 | 17 |
| 436–468 | 6 | 18 |
| 469–470 | 6 | 19 |
| 471–500 | 7 | 19 |

[a]The table shows the rank numbers of the 0.90 confidence interval of the 2.5 percentile for samples with 119–500 values. To obtain the corresponding rank numbers of the 97.5 percentile, subtract the rank numbers in the table from ($n$ = 1), where $n$ is the sample size. From International Federation of Clinical Chemistry and Laboratory Medicine (IFCC), Expert Panel on Theory of Reference Values. Approved recommendation on the theory of reference values.

## TABLE 5.3  γ-Glutamyltransferase (GGT) Values Used in the Nonparametric Determination of Reference Intervals

| GGT Value (U/L) | Frequency | Rank Order |
|---|---|---|
| 6 | 1 | 1 |
| 7 | 2 | 2, 3 |
| 8 | 6 | 4–9 |
| 9 | 4 | 10–13 |
| 10 | 4 | 14–17 |
| 11 | 9 | 18–26 |
| 12 | 7 | 27–33 |
| 13 | 7 | 34–40 |
| 14 | 9 | 41–49 |
| 15 | 9 | 50–58 |
| 16 | 8 | 59–66 |
| 17 | 11 | 67–77 |
| 18 | 8 | 78–85 |
| 19 | 5 | 86–90 |
| 20 | 3 | 91–93 |
| 21 | 2 | 94, 95 |
| 22 | 2 | 96, 97 |
| 23 | 2 | 98, 99 |
| 24 | 2 | 100, 101 |
| 25 | 3 | 102–104 |
| 26 | 2 | 105, 106 |
| 27 | 1 | 107 |
| 28 | 1 | 108 |
| 29 | 2 | 109, 110 |
| 30 | 1 | 111 |
| 32 | 2 | 112, 113 |
| 34 | 2 | 114, 115 |
| 35 | 1 | 116 |
| 39 | 1 | 117 |
| 42 | 2 | 118, 119 |
| 45 | 1 | 120 |
| 47 | 1 | 121 |
| 48 | 1 | 122 |
| 50 | 1 | 123 |

## TABLE 5.4  Nonparametric Determination of Reference Interval[a]

**Calculation of Rank Numbers of Percentiles**

| | |
|---|---|
| Lower | 0.025 (123 + 1) = 3.1 (i.e., Rank #3) |
| Upper | 0.975 (123 + 1) = 120.9 (i.e., Rank #121) |

**Original Values Corresponding to These Rank Numbers**

| | |
|---|---|
| Lower limit (2.5 percentile) | 7 U/L |
| Upper limit (97.5 percentile) | 47 U/L |

**Rank Numbers and Values of the 0.90 Confidence Limits**

*Lower Reference Limits*

| | |
|---|---|
| Rank numbers (see Table 5.2) | #1 and #7 |
| Values | 6 and 8 U/L |

*Upper Reference Limits*

| | |
|---|---|
| Rank numbers (see Table 5.2) | (123 + 1) − 7 = #117 and (123 + 1) − 1 = #123 |
| Values | 39 and 50 U/L |

**Summary**

| | |
|---|---|
| Lower reference limit | 7 (6–8) U/L |
| Upper reference limit | 47 (39–50) U/L |

[a]The table shows an example using the γ-glutamyltransferase (GGT) results listed in Table 5.3.

*Parametric method.* The parametric method is more complicated than the nonparametric method and usually requires the use of a computer statistics program when large data sets are processed. Additionally, the parametric method assumes that the true distribution is Gaussian. Therefore, it is critical to test the goodness-of-fit level of the reference distribution to a hypothetical Gaussian distribution. A simple test is examination of the cumulative frequency plotted on Gaussian probability paper (see Fig. 5.2B); the plot should be close to a straight line if the distribution is Gaussian. In addition, many statistical computer programs have goodness-of-fit tests (e.g., tests based on coefficients of skewness and kurtosis, the Kolmogorov-Smirnov test, the Anderson-Darling test).

If the reference distribution does not differ significantly from the Gaussian distribution, the 2.5 and 97.5 percentiles are estimated by values approximately 2 SDs on each side of the mean or more precisely:

$$2.5 \text{ Percentile: } \bar{x} - 1.96 \times SD$$

$$97.5 \text{ Percentile: } \bar{x} + 1.96 \times SD$$

The 0.90 confidence interval of each percentile is estimated by the following two limits:

$$\text{Lower confidence limit} = \text{percentile limit} - 2.81\frac{SD}{\sqrt{n}}$$

$$\text{Upper confidence limit} = \text{percentile limit} + 2.81\frac{SD}{\sqrt{n}}$$

If the reference distribution is non-Gaussian, mathematical transformation of data may adjust the shape to approximate the Gaussian distribution. One frequent observation of interest is that logarithmically transformed values of a distribution with a long right tail (positively skewed) fit the Gaussian distribution rather closely (see Fig. 5.2D). In other cases, a Box-Cox transformation selected to produce the closest Gaussian fit is commonly used. This information provides the basis for the common use of logarithmic and Box-Cox transformations when reference limits are estimated, as described in the following section.

To apply the parametric procedure to transformed data, the process is very similar, as shown in the following steps. In this example a log transformation is used; however, the principle is the same for any transformation:

1. Transform data with the logarithmic function $y = \log_{10}(x)$ (or $y = \ln[x]$). Then test the fit to the Gaussian distribution by using

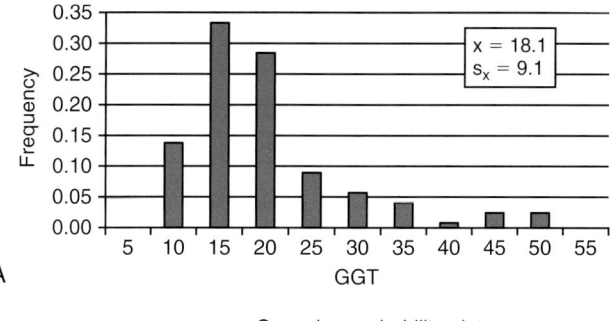

A

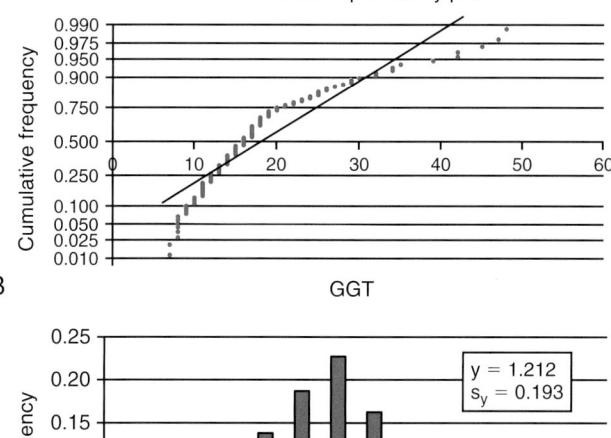

B

C

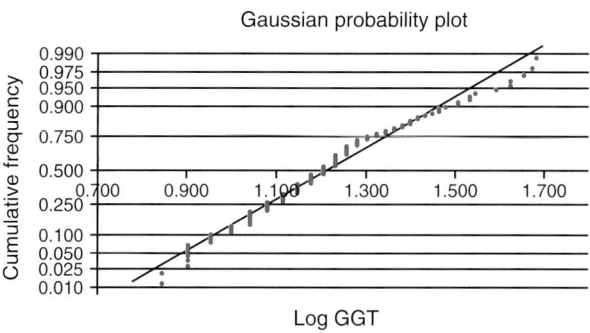

D

**Fig. 5.2** Distribution of 123 remaining γ-glutamyltransferase *(GGT)* values from reference subjects. (A) A histogram of the original, untransformed data. (B) The cumulative frequency of the data from (A) plotted on Gaussian probability paper. (C) A histogram of the logarithmic transformed data. (D) The cumulative frequency of the data from (C), plotted on Gaussian probability paper.

the methods described previously (note for Box-Cox transformations, the degree of transformation can be adjusted to give an optimal fit). [If transformations fail, the simple nonparametric method previously described should be used.]

2. If the transformation is successful, compute the *mean* ($\bar{y}$) and the standard deviation ($SD_y$) of the transformed data.

3. Estimate the percentiles and their confidence intervals in the transformed scale by using the formulas presented previously, substituting $\bar{y}$ for $\bar{x}$ and $SD_y$ for SD.

4. Reconvert the percentiles and their confidence intervals to the original data scale by using inverse functions (e.g., antilogarithms).

As shown in Fig. 5.2D, the mean and the SD of the serum GGT values in Fig. 5.1 after logarithmic ($\log_{10}$) transformation are $\bar{y} = 1.212$ and $SD_y = 0.193$. The 2.5 percentile is:

$$1.212 - 1.96 \times 0.193 = 0.835$$

$$2.5 \text{ percentile} = 10^{0.835} = 6.84$$

The lower reference limit of serum GGT thus is 7 U/L. The 0.90 confidence interval of this percentile is:

$$1.212 - 2.81 \times \left(0.193 / \sqrt{123}\right) = 0.786$$

$$\text{Lower confidence limit} = 10^{0.786} = 6.1$$

$$1.212 + 2.81 \times \left(0.193 / \sqrt{123}\right) = 0.884$$

$$\text{Upper confidence limit} = 10^{0.884} = 7.7$$

that is, 6 to 8 U/L. The 97.5 percentile (and its 0.90 confidence interval) is, using the same method, 40 U/L (35 to 44 U/L).

Table 5.5 demonstrates that the nonparametric method and the parametric method (using the transformed data) result in similar estimates of reference limits (percentiles).

## Other Sources for Reference Limits

Other than locally performed direct reference interval studies, common sources for reference limits include manufacturers' package inserts, peer-reviewed publications, local studies, and multicenter trials. More recently there have been considerable advances in the use of stored laboratory data to develop or validate reference intervals.

One advantage of using manufacturers' package inserts is that there should be no analytical issues, provided the method is stable over time and place. However, comparability of the patient populations, and of other preanalytical issues, must be ensured. Unfortunately, manufacturer's supplied reference intervals commonly do not provide sufficient information about the reference population, or the statistical processes used, to thoroughly assess their suitability, providing another reason that they should not be used uncritically.

As to peer-reviewed publications, when a laboratory considers adopting such reference limits, both method and population comparability must be addressed, but these tasks may be considerably easier for the laboratory than performing its own reference interval study. For example, the CALIPER initiative established, using the techniques described earlier, pediatric reference intervals partitioned by age, sex, and ethnicity, for over 40 different assays. As the authors emphasized, the published reference limits were specific to the methods they used. This type of publication is of tremendous value, as it was well designed with large patient numbers and provided information well beyond the scope of all routine laboratories.

Another source for reference limits is multicenter studies. In contrast to the CALIPER initiative, in which all the analyses were performed by a single laboratory, these studies

**TABLE 5.5    Summary of Glutamyltransferase Reference Interval Determination by Three Methods**

| Method | Lower Limit (Confidence Interval) | Upper Limit (Confidence Interval) | Values Below Lower Limit | Values Above Upper Limit |
|---|---|---|---|---|
| Nonparametric | 7 (6–8) | 47 (39–50) | 1 | 2 |
| Parametric-untransformed data | 0 (–2 to 2) | 36 (34–38) | 0 | 7 |
| Parametric-transformed data | 7 (6–8) | 40 (35–44) | 1 | 6 |

The table summarizes the 95% reference intervals and associated 90% confidence limits generated by each of three methods for the same data set. The numbers of observed values deemed lower and higher than the corresponding interval for each method are given in the last two columns. Because the original data are positively skewed, note that the parametric techniques generate intervals that are biased low. Note too that the parametric technique on untransformed data has a lower confidence interval, which is actually <0.

seek to pool data from many laboratories spread over large regions and potentially among different countries. Although this decreases the number of recruited reference individuals from each laboratory, it also typically increases the number of analytical methods involved for each assay. Despite global efforts at harmonization and standardization, these multi-center studies have repeatedly shown that current methods do not always produce interchangeable results, and therefore methods to ensure method comparability are still needed. When the same method is used at all sites, there is the advantage that the analytical variability is more likely to reflect the variation seen in individual laboratories over time.

### Indirect Reference Values

A growth area for development of reference intervals are the so-called "indirect" methods. In contrast to a formal reference interval study with a reference population selected for the specific purpose (direct studies), indirect studies use data collected for routine purposes. There are now a range of available techniques from the simple graphical methods of Bhattacharya and Hoffman, both dating from the 1960s, to a range of modern computerized methods, including the DGKL method and RefineR. The principles applied are similar, which is to try and identify a central distribution which is taken to represent a population unaffected by disease, condition, or partition. This is typically a Gaussian distribution, either directly or following transformation. These methods have many advantages over direct methods, including time taken, the number of samples available (often in the tens- to hundreds-of-thousands), minimal costs (no sample collections or additional measurements), and the fact that the analytical and pre-analytical factors exactly match those used in routine measurements. However, care must be taken with the selection of the data, and generally a data cleaning process is applied. Commonly used protocols may include limiting samples to general practice samples, only allowing one sample per patient, or only samples from patients with one collection in a time period (more unwell patients are likely to have more testing), and limiting inclusion based on other results, for example assessing TSH only when free T4 results are available and within defined limits.

### Transferability of Reference Values

Determining reliable reference values for each test in the laboratory's repertoire is a major task that is often far beyond the capabilities of the individual laboratory. Therefore, it would be convenient if reference values derived from the other sources described above could be used. A major prerequisite for transfer of reference values is that the populations must be comparable, and no relevant ethnic, social, or environmental differences must be noted between them. If the populations are not comparable, a separate source of reference intervals must found.

Other factors that should not be overlooked include adherence to explicit, standardized protocols for (1) qualifying reference individuals, (2) preparing those individuals for specimen collection, (3) performing specimen collection, and (4) sample handling.

### Analytical Issues

In practice, even if the populations are comparable and preanalytical standards are met, the problem of analytical transferability remains. The optimal, but usually unrealistic, situation assumes that analytical methods, including their calibration and quality assurance, are identical in the laboratories. The starting point for this assumption is that the methods must be traceable to the same reference standards. However, this must be verified, for example by appropriate Quality Assurance data, peer reviewed data, or local sample exchange. If the methods are not equivalent, development and application of a mathematical transfer function is required.

### Verification of Transfer

When a laboratory seeks to adopt reference values from any other source, it is vital that the laboratory verifies the appropriateness of those values for its own use. This verification serves as the final check that both the analytical method and the laboratory's own population are comparable with that used for the original reference value study.

The principle is comparison of local data with the selected reference interval. A simple practical approach has been recommended by the Clinical and Laboratory Standards Institute (CLSI): With a sample size of 20 reference values, one verifies the appropriateness of a proposed reference interval as long as no more than two values are outside the proposed limits.

It is good laboratory practice to support this type of study with assessment against local clinical data. This may include a local indirect study as mentioned above, or assessment of expected flagging rates for high and low values. In addition to identifying possible transferability issues, this process can alert the laboratory to the number of flagged results their clinicians will be seeing in practice.

## Process of Selecting Reference Intervals

Laboratories are responsible for, and usually take the lead in, providing reference limits for their test results. However, there are complicated decisions involved in the process, and the final selection of reference limits will influence the decisions of many physicians about their patients. While laboratory professionals will take the lead in the process, a multidisciplinary group, including relevant clinical specialists, should ideally be involved in making the final decisions. The process starts with understanding the pathophysiology of the analyte, and identifying what pathological and physiological factors affect the results. This assessment allows establishment of the ideal reference population, the likely need for partitioning, relevant exclusions, and controllable sample collection factors (e.g., time of day, fasting or nonfasting). Next is an understanding of the pre-analytical and analytical factors. With this information, data should be sought from all available sources. These should include manufacturer's data, peer reviewed publications, local studies (if performed), any guidance from professional organizations, and analysis of local data. The quality and relevance of the sources used should be assessed and more weight given to the most relevant data. If all sources provide similar values for the reference interval, there can be confidence that the interval is likely correct. If there is wide variation in reference intervals from various sources, then the sources of the variation should be considered. Each reference interval source is based on a process with uncertainties which must be considered in assessing differences between studies. On the basis of all available data, a final interval is selected. Consideration can be given to the number of significant figures for the reference limits with rounded values easier to recall, and too many significant figures suggesting an accuracy which may not be present.

The process should be documented, including all data sources and the reasons for the final decision. This is important when it comes to reviewing the intervals at a later date. Further, reference interval assessment should be revisited periodically; just because an interval has been used for a long time, does not make it correct for the current circumstances or method used. If there is a change in reference intervals, the change must be clearly communicated to users, with the report indicating which interval to apply to reported data.

# USE OF REFERENCE INTERVALS

In practice, interpreting medical laboratory data requires comparison of the patient's values with reference values, which are most commonly expressed as reference intervals.

## Presentation of an Observed Value in Relation to Reference Values

An observed value (patient's value) is interpreted by comparison with reference values. This comparison is often similar to hypothesis testing, but it is seldom statistical testing in the strict sense. Thus, it is advisable to consider the reference values as the yardstick for a less formal assessment than hypothesis testing.

The clinician or health care provider should be supplied with as much information about the reference values as necessary for the interpretation of the patient's test value. Reference intervals for all laboratory tests may be presented to clinicians or health care providers in a booklet, website or APP, together with information about the analysis methods and their imprecision, along with descriptions of the reference values. A convenient presentation of the observed value and the reference interval on the same report, whether electronic or paper, is required for the busy clinician or health care provider. The laboratory computer system can select the appropriate age- and sex-specific reference interval from the database and print it next to the test result. Results relative to reference intervals can also be provided in graphical form. In some countries, there are specific recommendations for the uniform formatting of laboratory reports, an important factor to facilitate ease of reading and interpretation of reports by clinicians and, more commonly, the patient as well.

An observed value may be classified as low, usual, or high, depending on its location in relation to the reference interval. On reports, a convenient practice is to flag unusual results (e.g., through use of the letters L and H for low and high, respectively). Again, this formatting is defined in some locations to make reports from different laboratories similar.

Another method of classification is expressing the observed value by a mathematical distance measure. For example, the well-known SD unit, or normal equivalent deviation, also known as a z-score is such a measure. It is calculated as the difference between the observed value and the mean of the reference values divided by their SD. However, this measure is unreliable if the distribution of values is skewed. Values beyond approximately 2 SD imply that the value is beyond the central 95% of the reference interval. Indeed, by using the SD unit deviation value, one determines the percentile of the observed value (e.g., values greater than 3.0 SD occur in only less than 0.15% of people in the reference distribution).

## Subject-Based Reference Intervals

Fig. 5.3 illustrates the inherent problem associated with **population-based reference intervals**. The figure shows two hypothetical reference distributions. One represents the common reference distribution based on single samples obtained from a group of several different reference individuals. This

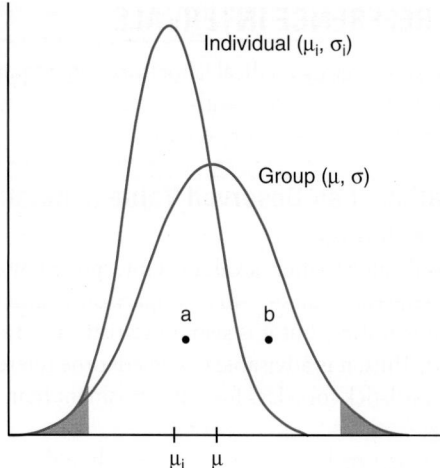

**Fig. 5.3** The relationship between population-based and subject-based reference distributions and reference intervals. The example is hypothetical, and the two distributions are, for simplicity, Gaussian. Hypothetical means and standard deviations are μ and σ (for the population) and $\mu_i$ and $\sigma_i$ (individual, i). (Modified from Harris EK. Effects of intra- and interindividual variation on the appropriate use of normal ranges. *Clin Chem.* 1974;20:1536.)

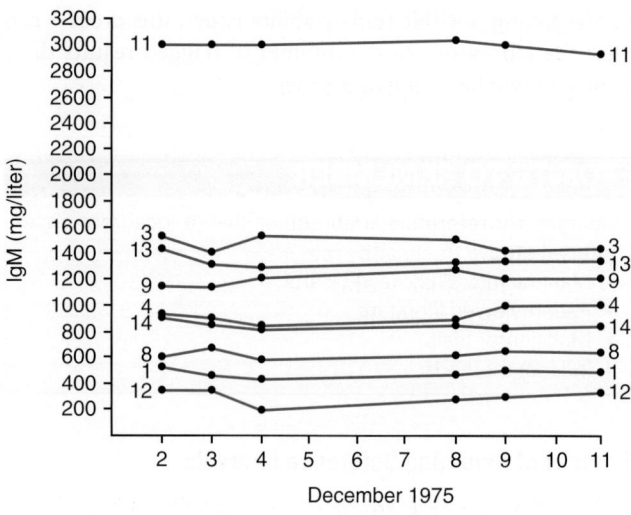

**Fig. 5.4** Serial immunoglobulin M (IgM) values over several days from reference individuals. Note that intraindividual variability is very small compared with interindividual variability. (From Statland BE, Winkel P, Killingsworth LM. Factors contributing to intra-individual variation of serum constituents: 6. Physiological day-to-day variation in concentrations of 10 specific proteins in sera. *Clin Chem.* 1976;22:1635–1636.)

distribution has a true (hypothetical) mean μ and an SD of σ. The other distribution is based on several samples collected over time in a single individual, the *i*th individual. Its hypothetical mean is $\mu_i$ and the SD, $\sigma_i$.

If an observed value is located outside the subject's 2.5 and 97.5 percentiles (i.e., the personal or **subject-based reference interval**), the cause may be a change in biochemical status, suggesting the presence of disease. Fig. 5.3 demonstrates that such an observed value still may be within the population-based reference interval. The sensitivity of the latter interval to changes in a subject's biochemical status depends accordingly on the location of the individual's mean $\mu_i$ relative to the common mean μ and to the relative magnitudes of the corresponding SDs, $\sigma_i$ and σ. A mean $\mu_i$ close to μ and a small $\sigma_i$ relative to σ may conceal the individual's changes entirely within the population-based reference interval.

Two specific examples may help to clarify this concept. Fig. 5.4 depicts immunoglobulin M (IgM) values from several healthy individuals over the course of several days. As illustrated, intraindividual differences are small as compared with interindividual differences. Even though the population-based reference interval might extend from 200 to 1600 mg/L, in practice it would be unusual (abnormal) for any patient's IgM value to change by more than 200 mg/L, even if the value remained within the population-based reference interval. Similarly, it is well known that any given patient's serum creatinine value is reasonably constant, and this is related both to glomerular filtration rate (GFR) and to lean muscle mass. If the latter is constant, changes in GFR are inversely proportional to the serum creatinine (see Chapters 21 and 35); that is, even though a typical (population-based) male reference interval for serum creatinine might extend from 64 to 104 μmol/L (0.7 to 1.2 mg/dL), a change from 65 to 100 μmol/L in a given patient would be distinctly abnormal, representing loss of over one third of the GFR.

At least one solution is known for the problem of the limitations of population-based reference intervals for certain tests. With this solution, the subject's previous values, obtained in a well-defined state of health, are used as the reference for any future value. Application of subject-based reference values becomes more feasible as "health screening" by laboratory tests and computer storage of results become available to large sections of the general population. A common application of this concept is the Reference Change Value; however, this is usually based on the changes relative to a single previous result.

## Limitations to Reference Intervals

As stated above, reference intervals can be determined for any group of subjects, both with and without a specific medical condition. In practice, most laboratory supplied reference intervals are best described as "health associated reference intervals" (i.e., representing values that may be expected in a healthy person). For these reference intervals, important caveats require consideration. They are not established to either define or rule out any medical condition and are usually not assessed for this purpose. Even with regard to health, usual intervals are set up to be "wrong" 5% of the time. Often, patients and caregivers have inflated expectations regarding the use of usual reference intervals, believing that all flagged results indicate disease, and that disease is excluded with results within the reference intervals. It is the role of validated clinical decision points to provide diagnostic information with determined levels of sensitivity and specificity. Having recognized the limitations of usual reference intervals, they have been described as "the most commonly used decision support tool in laboratory medicine" and provide a shorthand, uniform way of identifying test results requiring further consideration.

## When "Normal" May Appear to Be "Abnormal" and Vice Versa

Some, if not many, clinical laboratory test results are related to other clinical laboratory test results. For example, consider the relatively common situation of a patient with a low serum albumin. Because of the relationship between total calcium and albumin in serum (see Chapter 39), a total serum calcium concentration in the healthy reference interval might actually be pathologically high in this patient, and a total serum calcium concentration less than the lower reference limit might be healthy.

As another example, consider prostate-specific antigen (PSA) concentration in a post-prostatectomy patient or thyroglobulin in a post-thyroidectomy patient. In these cases, it would be "healthy" to have undetectable concentrations of these measurands, and it would be distinctly abnormal to have detectable levels. In these cases, the problem is that the traditional reference population used in setting clinical decision points and associated result flags is not appropriate.

In other words, even when reference limit studies are done well, one needs to remember there are dependencies that can render those reference limits misleading.

## REVIEW QUESTIONS

1. A "subject-based" reference value is:
   a. obtained from a group of systematically defined reference individuals.
   b. the equivalent of a *reference value* when no qualifying words are used.
   c. based on several samples collected over time in a single individual.
   d. based on all results from the parent population fulfilling the selection criteria.
2. When reference values are established, the criteria used to determine which individuals should be included in the group of reference individuals are referred to as:
   a. exclusion criteria.
   b. inclusion criteria.
   c. partition criteria.
   d. selection criteria.
3. The advantages of indirect methods for determining or verifying reference intervals include all of the following except:
   a. The pre-analytical factors are the same as are used for patient care.
   b. The analytical factors are the same as used for patient care.
   c. The indirect method is more expensive than the direct methods.
   d. It is possible to include many thousands of results in the procedure.
4. In the selection of reference individuals, subclassifying a set of these individuals into homogeneous groups is referred to as:
   a. partitioning.
   b. excluding.
   c. transferring.
   d. including.
5. When reference limits are determined, the statistical method that assumes that the true distribution of reference values is a Gaussian (normal) distribution is the:
   a. nonparametric method.
   b. parametric method.
   c. interpercentile interval method.
   d. predictive value.

## SUGGESTED READINGS

Ammer T, Schützenmeister A, Prokosch HU, et al. refineR: a novel algorithm for reference interval estimation from real-world data. *Sci Rep.* 2021;11:16023.

Brewster LM, Mairuhu G, Sturk A, et al. Distribution of creatine kinase in the general population: implications for statin therapy. *Am Heart J.* 2007;154:655–661.

Clinical and Laboratory Standards Institute. *Defining, Establishing, and Verifying Reference Intervals in the Clinical Laboratory.* CLSI Document C28-A3c. Wayne, PA: Clinical and Laboratory Standards Institute; 2010.

Colantonio DA, Kyriakopoulou L, Chan MK, et al. Closing the gaps in pediatric laboratory reference intervals: a CALIPER database of 40 biochemical markers in a healthy and multiethnic population of children. *Clin Chem.* 2012;58:854–868.

Ferré-Masferrer M, Fuentes-Arderiu X, Alvarez-Funes V, et al. Multicentric reference values: shared reference limits. *Eur J Clin Chem Clin Biochem.* 1997;35:715–718.

Fraser CG. *Biological Variation: From Principles to Practice.* Washington, DC: AACC Press; 2001:15–17.

Haeckel R, Wosniok W, Streichert T. Members of the Section Guide Limits of the DGKL. Review of potentials and limitations of indirect approaches for estimating reference limits intervals of quantitative procedures in laboratory medicine. *J Lab Med.* 2021;45(2):35–53.

Harris EK, Boyd JC. *Statistical Bases of Reference Values in Laboratory Medicine.* New York: Marcel Dekker; 1995.

Horn PS, Feng L, Li Y, Pesce AJ. Effect of outliers and nonhealthy individuals on reference interval estimation. *Clin Chem.* 2001;47:2137–2145.

Horowitz G, Jones GRD. Establishment and use of reference values. In: Rifai N, Horvath AR, Wittwer CT, eds. *Tietz Textbook of Clinical Chemistry and Molecular Diagnostics.* 6th ed. St Louis: Elsevier; 2017:170–194.

International Federation of Clinical Chemistry and Laboratory Medicine (IFCC), Expert Panel on Theory of Reference Values. Approved recommendation on the theory of reference values. Part 1. The concept of reference values. *J Clin Chem Clin Biochem.* 1987;25:337–342.

Part 2. Selection of individuals for the production of reference values. *J Clin Chem Clin Biochem.* 1987;25:639–644.

Part 3. Preparation of individuals and collection of specimens for the production of reference values. *J Clin Chem Clin Biochem*. 1988;26:593–598.

Part 4. Control of analytical variation in the production, transfer, and application of reference values. *Eur J Clin Chem Clin Biochem*. 1991;29:531–535.

Part 5. Statistical treatment of collected reference values: determination of reference limits. *J Clin Chem Clin Biochem*. 1987;25:645–656.

Part 6. Presentation of observed values related to reference values. *J Clin Chem Clin Biochem*. 1987;25:657–662.

Jones GRD, Haeckel R, Loh TP, et al. Indirect methods for reference interval determination – review and recommendations. *Clin Chem Lab Med*. 2019;57:20–29.

Kearon C, Ginsberg JS, Douketis J, et al. An evaluation of D-dimer in the diagnosis of pulmonary embolism: a randomized trial. *Ann Intern Med*. 2006;144:812–821.

Lahti A, Petersen PH, Boyd JC, et al. Partitioning of nongaussian-distributed biochemical reference data into subgroups. *Clin Chem*. 2004;50:891–900.

Rustad P, Felding P. Transnational biological reference intervals: procedures and examples from the Nordic Reference Interval Project. *Scand J Clin Lab Invest*. 2004;64:265–441.

Rustad P, Felding P, Franzson L, et al. The Nordic Reference Interval Project 2000: recommended reference intervals for 25 common biochemical properties. *Scand J Clin Lab Invest*. 2004;64:271–284.

Solberg HE. The IFCC recommendation on estimation of reference intervals. The RefVal Program. *Clin Chem Lab Med*. 2004;42:710–714.

Solberg HE, Grasbeck R. Reference values. *Advan Clin Chem*. 1989;27:1–79.

Solberg HE, Lahti A. Detection of outliers in reference distributions: performance of Horn's algorithm. *Clin Chem*. 2005;51:2326–2332.

Stone NJ, Robinson JG, Lichtenstein AH, et al. 2013 ACC/AHA guideline on the treatment of blood cholesterol to reduce atherosclerotic cardiovascular risk in adults. *J Am Coll Cardiol*. 2014;63:2889–2934.

Yamamoto Y, Hosogaya S, Osawa S, et al. Nationwide multicenter study aimed at the establishment of common reference intervals for standardized clinical laboratory tests in Japan. *Clin Chem Lab Med*. 2013;51:1663–1672.

# Specimen Collection, Processing, and Other Preanalytical Variables

*Khushbu Patel and Patricia M. Jones*

## OBJECTIVES

1. Define the following terms:
   - Anticoagulant
   - Hemolysis
   - Order of draw
   - Phlebotomy
   - Plasma versus serum
   - Preanalytical error
   - Venipuncture
2. List types of biologic specimens that are analyzed in a clinical laboratory.
3. Summarize the steps that are performed by a phlebotomist in obtaining a blood sample by venipuncture.
4. List the general effects on analytes caused by the following:
   - Pumping a fist before venipuncture
   - Stress
   - Tube collection order of draw
   - Time of collection related to diurnal variation
   - Prolonged venous occlusion with a tourniquet
   - Incomplete tube filling
5. Discuss order of draw for collecting multiple tubes of blood, including color of stopper and associated additive, need for tube filling and inversion, and reason for filling tubes in a specific order.
6. Describe the order of draw for multiple collections from skin puncture and why it is different from venipuncture collections.
7. Describe the skin puncture collection technique, including methods of stimulating blood flow.
8. Explain the difference between serum and plasma.
9. Compare the difference in composition, if any, between serum and plasma specimens for the following analytes:
   - Calcium
   - Cholesterol
   - Albumin
   - Creatinine
   - Total protein
   - Glucose
   - Potassium
10. List the different types of anticoagulants and how each prevents blood from coagulating as well as example analytical uses.
11. Describe how hemolysis affects measurement of certain analytes.
12. List different uses of random versus 24-hour urine collections; list two methods of urine preservation and discuss the use of each.
13. Outline the procedure for collecting a timed urine specimen.
14. List clinical chemistry analyses performed on the following specimen types:
    - Feces
    - Cerebrospinal fluid (CSF)
    - Saliva
    - Buccal cells
    - Hair and nails

## KEY WORDS AND DEFINITIONS

**Additives** Compounds added to biologic specimens to prevent them from clotting or to preserve the constituents of a specimen.

**Anticoagulant** Any substance that prevents blood from clotting.

**Coagulation (clotting)** The sequential process by which the multiple coagulation factors of blood interact in the coagulation cascade, resulting in formation of an insoluble fibrin clot.

**Diurnal variation** Variation that occurs in the amount of a substance during a 24-hour period.

**Hemolysis** Disruption of the red cell membrane causing release of hemoglobin and other components of red blood cells.

**Phlebotomy** The puncture of a blood vessel to collect blood.

**Plasma** The noncellular component of anticoagulated whole blood after centrifugation; plasma contains clotting factors.

**Preanalytical errors** Factors that affect specimens before tests are performed and that can lead to error if not controlled; they are classified as controllable or uncontrollable.

**Preservative**  A substance or preparation added to a specimen to prevent changes in the constituents of a specimen.

**Serum**  The noncellular component of blood obtained after centrifugation from a sample in which coagulation has occurred.

**Skin puncture**  Collection of capillary blood usually from a pediatric patient by making a thin cut in the skin, usually

at the heel of the foot in infants and in fingers in pediatric patients once they are walking.

**Specimen**  A sample or portion of body fluid or tissue collected for examination, study, or analysis.

**Venipuncture**  All of the steps involved in obtaining an appropriate and identified blood specimen from an individual's vein.

Proper collection, processing, storage, and transport of common sample types used for diagnostic testing are critical to the provision of quality test results. Each step involved, as well as factors associated with the patient, can be the source of errors that cause inaccurate results. Minimizing these errors will result in more reliable information for use by health care professionals in providing quality patient care.

This chapter provides a review of the most common specimen types and discusses how they are (1) collected, (2) identified, (3) processed, (4) stored, and (5) transported. Differences between adult and pediatric collection are highlighted.

## PATIENT IDENTIFICATION

Before any specimen is collected, the phlebotomist must confirm the identity of the patient using two or three items of identification (e.g., name, medical record number, date of birth). In specialized situations, such as paternity testing or other tests of medicolegal importance, establishment of a chain of custody for the specimen may require that additional patient identification, such as a photograph, be provided.

Identification must be an active process, with the patient stating his or her name and the phlebotomist verifying information either on the patient's wrist band or on the test requisition form or computer order. In the case of pediatric patients the parent or guardian should be present and be asked to actively provide identification of the child in a manner to prevent a yes or no answer from an often-distracted parent, such as: "Please tell me the name of your child."

## TYPES OF SPECIMENS

Types of biologic **specimens** that are analyzed in clinical laboratories include (1) whole blood; (2) serum; (3) plasma; (4) urine; (5) feces; (6) saliva; (7) other body fluids such as spinal, synovial, amniotic, pleural, pericardial, and ascitic fluids; and (8) cells and various types of solid tissue. The World Health Organization and the Clinical and Laboratory Standards Institute (CLSI) have published several guidelines for collecting many different types of specimens under standardized conditions (Table 6.1).

### Blood

Blood for analysis may be obtained from veins, arteries, or capillaries. Venous blood is usually the specimen of choice. Arterial puncture is used mainly for blood gas analyses. In young children and for many point-of-care tests, skin puncture is frequently used to obtain capillary blood. The process of collecting blood is known as **phlebotomy** (from *phleb*, which means vein, and *tome*, to cut or incise) and should always be performed by a trained **phlebotomist**.

#### Venipuncture

In the clinical laboratory, **venipuncture** is defined as all of the steps involved in obtaining an appropriate and identified blood specimen from a patient's vein (CLSI GP41, see Table 6.1).

*Preliminary steps.* Prior to collection, the patient should be asked about latex allergies, and if necessary the phlebotomist should secure nonlatex equipment. Any signed consent forms or special requisitions should be completed.

Before collection, the phlebotomist should dress in personal protective equipment (PPE), such as an impervious gown and gloves. PPE and adherence to standard precautions limit the spread of infectious disease from one patient to another and promote the safety of the phlebotomist. PPE is often brightly colored in pediatric institutions, where small children may be frightened of anyone in a white coat or gown. When collecting specimens from a patient in isolation in a hospital, the phlebotomist must often dress in specialized PPE. The extent of the precautions required varies with the nature of the patient's illness and the institution's policies and bloodborne pathogen plan.

If appropriate, the phlebotomist should verify that the patient has fasted, identify what medications are being taken or have been discontinued as required, and determine any other relevant information. The patient should be comfortable, seated or supine, and should have been in this position for as long as possible before the specimen is drawn. At no time should venipuncture be performed on a standing patient.

Infants and young children may need to be held to prevent movement. A young child may be held sitting upright in a parent's lap, with the parent helping to support and hold the patient and arm still (Fig. 6.1). An infant's blood is often drawn with the infant in a supine position, and the infant may

## TABLE 6.1   Clinical and Laboratory Standards Institute Documents Related to Specimen Collection, Processing, and Transport

| Document Name | Document Number |
| --- | --- |
| Accuracy in patient and sample identification | GP33 |
| Blood collection on filter paper for newborn screening programs | NBS01-A6 |
| Collection, transport, and processing of blood specimens for testing plasma-based coagulation assays and molecular hemostasis assay | H21-A5 |
| Collection, transport, preparation, and storage of specimens for molecular methods | MM13-A |
| Procedures and devices for the collection of diagnostic capillary blood specimens | GP42-Ed7 |
| Procedures for the handling and processing of blood specimens for common laboratory tests | GP44-A4 |
| Collection of diagnostic venous blood specimens | GP41-Ed7 |
| Blood gas and pH analysis and related measurements | C46-A2 (archived) |
| Protection of laboratory workers from occupationally acquired infections | M29-A3 |
| Urinalysis | GP16-A3 (archived) |
| Qualifying, selecting, and evaluating a referral laboratory | QMS05 |
| Tubes and additives for venous and capillary blood specimen collection | GP39-A6 (archived) |

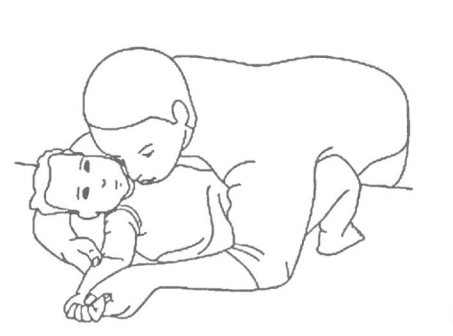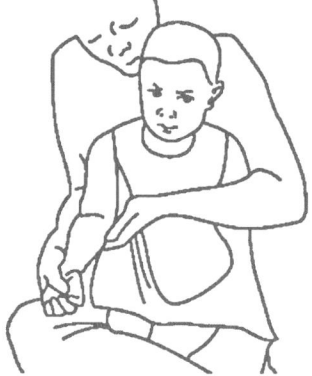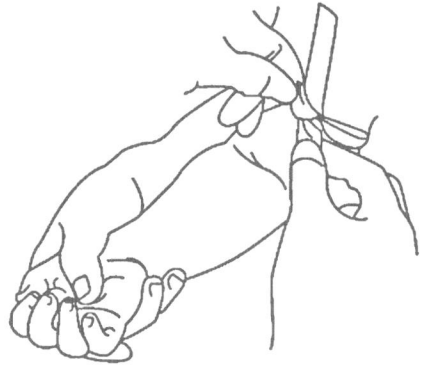

Fig. 6.1 Holding a child for venipuncture. (Modified from World Health Organization. WHO guidelines on drawing blood: best practices in phlebotomy. In *Pediatric and Neonatal Blood Sampling*. Geneva: World Health Organization; 2010. http://www.ncbi.nlm.nih.gov/books/NBK138647.)

be swaddled in a blanket, or a papoose board may be used to restrain movement.

Either of the patient's arms should be extended in a straight line from the shoulder to the wrist. An arm with extensive scarring or a hematoma at the intended collection site should be avoided.

Before performing a venipuncture, the phlebotomist should estimate the volume of blood to be drawn and select the appropriate number and types of tubes for the tests requested. This may be facilitated by computer-generated collection recommendations and should be designed to collect the minimum amount necessary for testing. Estimating volume of blood to be drawn is especially critical in a pediatric setting where the amount of blood available to be collected may be limited. Newborn infants have a total blood volume of approximately 350 mL, thus blood collection in the pediatric population should not exceed 2.5% of the total blood volume present, which can be calculated from the pediatric patient's weight. Iatrogenic blood loss can lead to unnecessary blood transfusions and increased risk of exposure to bloodborne pathogens.

In addition to tubes, an appropriate needle must be selected. The most commonly used sizes for adults are 19- to 22-gauge (the larger the gauge number, the smaller the diameter of the lumen). The usual choice for an adult is 20-gauge. In pediatric patients, 23- to 25-gauge needles are most commonly used, with 23-gauge being the preferred size for very small infant veins. Even for larger volumes of blood, rarely will a needle larger than a 21-gauge be used in pediatrics because it will not fit into the vein easily. A needle is typically 1.5 inches (3.7 cm) long, but 1-inch (2.5-cm) needles, usually attached to a winged or butterfly collection set, are also used in pediatrics and geriatrics. Finally, the phlebotomist should ensure post-draw safety devices are available, including convenient and safe access to disposal devices for contaminated needles and associated devices and appropriate post-draw supplies (gauze and bandage).

***Location.*** The median cubital vein in the antecubital fossa, or crook of the elbow, is the preferred site for collecting venous blood in adults because the vein is large and close to the surface of the skin. Veins on the back of the hand or at the ankle may be used, although these should be avoided in people with diabetes or with poor circulation. However, in infants and children younger than 2 years old, collection from superficial veins is recommended, and dorsal hand veins are preferred over the median cubital vein. A complete listing of sites that must not be used for venipuncture, sites that can be used with physician permission, and sites that should be avoided is given in CLSI GP41 (see Table 6.1).

*Preparation of the site.* The area around the intended puncture site should be cleaned with institutionally approved cleanser. Commonly used materials are a prepackaged alcohol swab, a gauze pad saturated with 70% isopropanol, or a benzalkonium chloride solution. Cleaning of the puncture site should be done with a circular motion from the site outward. The skin should be allowed to dry in the air. No alcohol or cleanser should remain on the skin because traces may increase patient discomfort, cause hemolysis, and invalidate test results.

*Timing.* The time at which a specimen is obtained is important for blood constituents that undergo marked **diurnal variation** (e.g., corticosteroids, iron), those for which a fasting sample has been requested, and those used to monitor drug therapy. In each case the timing should match the conditions under which reference intervals or clinical decision points were determined.

*Venous occlusion.* After the skin is cleaned, a blood pressure cuff or a tourniquet is applied 4 to 6 inches (10 to 15 cm) above the intended puncture site for adults. This obstructs the return of venous blood to the heart and distends the veins (**venous occlusion**). When a blood pressure cuff is used, it is usually inflated to approximately 60 mm Hg (8.0 kPa). If a dorsal hand vein is being accessed in pediatrics, no tourniquet is used. The phlebotomist applies enough pressure with the hand holding the patient's wrist and hand to occlude and distend the vein.

A tourniquet cannot be in place for longer than 1 minute as the composition of blood changes with longer venous occlusion. Although the changes that occur in 1 minute are slight, marked changes have been observed after 1 to 3 minutes for some chemistry analytes. The composition of blood drawn first is most representative of the composition of circulating blood and the least affected by fluid shifts where protein-bound components and other large molecules will be concentrated; water-soluble smaller molecules such as electrolytes may be less affected. The first-drawn specimen should therefore be used for analytes such as calcium and other analytes that are both protein bound and pertinent to critical medical decisions. A uniform procedure for the order of draw for tests is used (see later). If only a small volume of blood is collected, the priority of which tests to perform should be established in consultation with the ordering physician.

Two special notes on the collection process: (1) Pumping of the fist before venipuncture should be avoided. Instruct the patient to make a fist and hold it. Pumping causes an increase in plasma potassium, phosphate, and lactate concentrations. Increased lactate lowers blood pH and causes the plasma ionized calcium concentration to increase. (2) The stress associated with blood collection can have effects on patients at any age. Thus plasma concentrations of analytes affected by stress, such as cortisol, thyroid-stimulating hormone, and growth hormone, may increase. Stress occurs particularly in young children who are frightened, struggling, and held in physical restraint. Collection under these conditions may cause adrenal stimulation, leading to an increased plasma glucose concentration, or may create increases in the serum activities of enzymes that originate in skeletal muscle.

*Order of draw for multiple blood specimens.* In a few patients, backflow from blood tubes into veins occurs owing to a decrease in venous pressure but can be minimized if the arm is held downward. When collecting multiple specimens with an evacuated tube system, one of the primary concerns is to prevent cross-contamination between tubes. To minimize these and other problems, blood should be collected into tubes in the order outlined in Table 6.2.

*Collection with evacuated blood tubes.* Evacuated blood tubes are usually considered to be safer, less expensive, more convenient, and easier to use than syringes. Tubes vary by the type of **additive** and the volume of the tube. The different types of additives are identified by the color of the stopper

| TABLE 6.2 | Recommended Order of Draw for Multiple Specimen Collection | |
| --- | --- | --- |
| **Stopper Color** | **Contents** | **Inversions** |
| Yellow | Sterile media for blood culture | 8 |
| Royal blue | No additive | 0 |
| Clear | Nonadditive; discard tube if no royal blue used | 0 |
| Light blue | Sodium citrate | 3–4 |
| Gold/red | Serum separator tube | 5 |
| Red/red, orange/yellow, royal blue | Serum tube, with or without clot activator, with or without gel | 5 |
| Green | Heparin tube with or without gel | 8 |
| Tan (glass) | Sodium heparin | 8 |
| Royal blue | Sodium heparin, sodium EDTA (trace metal free) | 8 |
| Lavender, pearl white, pink/pink, tan (plastic) | EDTA tubes, with or without gel | 8 |
| Gray | Glycolytic inhibitor | 8 |
| Yellow (glass) | ACD for molecular studies and cell culture | 8 |

*ACD,* Acid citrate dextrose; *EDTA,* ethylenediaminetetraacetic acid.
Note that inversions are specific to manufacturer and should be conducted per instructions for use provided with the collection tubes.
Modified from information in Clinical and Laboratory Standards Institute. *Tubes and Additives for Venous Blood Specimen Collection: CLSI-Approved Standard H1-A5.* 5th ed. Wayne, PA: Clinical and Laboratory Standards Institute; 2003; and Kiechle FL, ed. *So You're Going to Collect a Blood Specimen: An Introduction to Phlebotomy.* 11th ed. Northfield, IL: College of American Pathologists; 2005.

used. Color coding of specimen collection tubes is not yet harmonized and may vary according to manufacturers (CLSI GP39, see Table 6.1 and Table 6.2). Serum or plasma separator tubes are available that contain an inert, polymer gel material that settles like a disk between cells and supernatant when the tube is centrifuged. Release of intracellular components into the supernatant is thus generally prevented. Note that all specimen collection containers, including less commonly used tubes, must be validated by each laboratory before use if not approved by the manufacturer for the specific analysis to be conducted.

Blood collected into a tube containing one additive should never be transferred into other tubes because the first additive may interfere with tests for which a different additive is specified. For example, ethylenediaminetetraacetic acid (EDTA) contamination can cause an erroneously reported hyperkalemia or hypocalcemia when an inappropriate tube type is analyzed.

Collection into the tube occurs until the vacuum is exhausted. It is critically important that the evacuated tube be filled completely. Many additives, particularly for coagulation testing, are provided at concentrations in the tube based on a "full and proper" collection; both short and too-full draws can be a source of **preanalytical error.** They can significantly affect the testing parameters that are based on a properly collected sample. Vacuum tubes should never be opened and filled from a syringe or other source.

***Blood collection with a syringe.*** Syringes are customarily used for patients with difficult veins and for blood gas analysis. The syringe with the needle attached should be aligned with the vein to be entered and the needle pushed into the vein with the bevel up and at an angle to the skin of approximately 15 degrees. When the initial resistance of the vein wall is overcome, forward pressure on the syringe is eased, and the blood is withdrawn by very gently pulling back the plunger of the syringe. Vigorous withdrawal of blood into a syringe during collection or forceful transfer from the syringe to the receiving vessel may cause hemolysis of blood, making the sample invalid for testing.

After filling the syringe and completing the collection, if the sample needs to be transferred to an evacuated tube, a transfer device should be used to puncture the cap of the tube. The tube should be allowed to fill passively using its vacuum.

***Completion of collection.*** When blood collection is complete and the needle withdrawn, a dry gauze pad should be held tightly over the puncture site with the arm raised to stop residual bleeding and promote the clotting process. All used supplies should be discarded in a hazardous waste receptacle.

Tubes should then be labeled per institutional policy. Many institutions recommend showing the labeled tube to the patient to further confirm correct identification.

***Venipuncture in children.*** The techniques for venipuncture in children and adults are similar. However, children are likely to make unexpected movements, and assistance in holding them is often desirable. Although a syringe or an evacuated blood tube system may be used to collect specimens, a syringe with a winged butterfly collection set is commonly used in younger children. The pressure on a syringe can be more easily controlled by the phlebotomist than the vacuum pressure in an evacuated tube, preventing the pressure from pulling small veins closed. In the pediatric population, alternative collection through skin puncture is also used.

## Skin Puncture

**Skin puncture** is an open collection technique in which the skin is punctured by a lancet and a small volume of blood is collected into a microdevice. In practice, skin puncture is used in situations in which (1) sample volume is limited (e.g., pediatric applications), (2) repeated venipunctures have resulted in vein damage, or (3) patients have been burned or bandaged and veins are unavailable. This technique is also commonly used when the sample is to be applied directly to a testing device in a point-of-care testing situation or to filter paper. It is most often performed on the tip of the finger or the heels of infants. In an infant younger than 6 months, the lateral or medial plantar surface of the heel should be used for skin puncture (Fig. 6.2). These areas are the fleshiest part of the foot in an infant, with the most distance between the skin surface and the underlying bone, decreasing the risk of inadvertently hitting bone and causing a bone infection. The back of the heel and the toes should not be used. Blood collection from anywhere on the foot should be avoided on ambulatory patients; thus, when an infant starts walking, a heel stick should no longer be performed. Lancets are made specifically for a heel stick or a finger stick and should not be used interchangeably because they have different tip lengths (Table 6.3). The finger-stick procedure should not be performed on infants younger than 6 months because no commercially available device punctures shallow enough to avoid bones. The complete procedure for collecting blood from infants using skin puncture is described in CLSI GP42-Ed7 (see Table 6.1).

To collect by skin puncture, the phlebotomist first cleans the skin with an approved cleaning solution. Once the skin is dry, it is quickly punctured by a sharp stab with a lancet. To minimize the possibility of infection, a different site should be selected for each puncture. The finger should be held in such a way that gravity assists collection of blood at the fingertip and the lancet held to make the incision as close to perpendicular to the fingernail as possible. Massage of the finger to stimulate

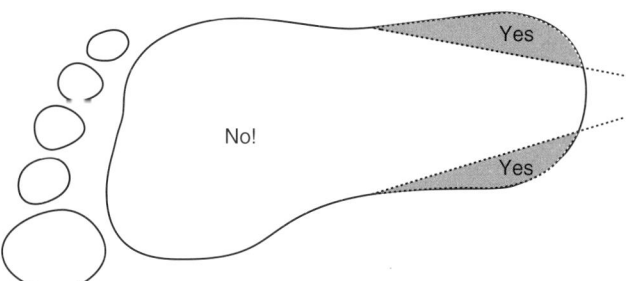

**Fig. 6.2** Acceptable sites for skin puncture to collect blood from an infant's foot. (Modified from Blumenfeld TA, Turi GK, Blanc WA. Recommended site and depth of newborn heel skin punctures based on anatomical measurements and histopathology. *Lancet.* 1979;1:230–233. Reprinted with permission from Elsevier.)

**TABLE 6.3  Tip Lengths in Finger- and Heel-Stick Devices**

| Collection Type and Age of Use | Tip Length (mm) |
|---|---|
| Heel stick: premature infants | 0.85 |
| Heel stick: term infants to 6 months old | 1.25 |
| Heel stick: 6 months to 1 year | 1.25 |
| Finger stick: walking to 8 years | 1.5 |
| Finger stick: >8 years | 1.75–2.2 |

**TABLE 6.4  Order of Draw for Skin Puncture: Capillary Blood**

| Usage or Additive | Tube Top Color |
|---|---|
| Blood gases (heparin) | Microhematocrit tubes |
| Ethylenediaminetetraacetic acid | Lavender |
| Heparin | Green |
| Other additives | Light blue, gray |
| Nonadditives | Red, tiger, yellow |

blood flow should be avoided because it causes the outflow of debris and tissue fluid, which does not have the same composition as plasma. To improve circulation of the blood, the finger or heel may be warmed by application of a warm, wet washcloth or a specialized device, such as a heel warmer, for 3 minutes before cleaning and the lancet is applied. Proper warming will increase capillary blood flow, improving the ability to collect the sample. Analytes in the sample will also approach arterial blood values. In a cold heel, the values more approximate venous blood. The first drop of blood is wiped off, and subsequent drops are transferred to the appropriate collection tube. Filling should be done rapidly to prevent clotting, and introduction of air bubbles should be prevented.

A variety of collection tubes are commercially available for capillary blood collection. Samples should be collected by dripping or capillary action from the puncture site into the small tubes. Scooping along the skin with the edge of the tube should be avoided because it increases hemolysis. The correct order of filling of these devices differs from evacuated blood tubes because tube additive carryover is not a problem and the blood begins clotting as soon as the puncture is made. Anticoagulant tubes, especially the EDTA tube for the complete blood count (CBC), are collected first while blood is flowing well, and the serum tubes are collected last (Table 6.4).

For collection of blood specimens on filter paper for molecular genetic testing and neonatal screening (CLSI MM13-A and NBS01-A6, see Table 6.1), the skin is cleaned and punctured as described previously. The first drop of blood is wiped away and the filter paper is gently touched against a large drop of blood that is allowed to soak into the paper to fill the marked circle. Only a single application per circle should be made. The procedure is repeated to fill all the circles. The filter paper should be properly labeled and then dried following manufacturer instructions before storage in a labeled paper envelope.

### Arterial Puncture

Arterial puncture requires considerable skill and is usually performed only by physicians or trained personnel. Preferred sites of arterial puncture are, in order, the (1) radial artery at the wrist, (2) brachial artery in the elbow, and (3) femoral artery in the groin, with sites in the arm used most often. The proper technique for arterial puncture is described in CLSI C46-A2 (see Table 6.1).

### Anticoagulants and Preservatives for Blood

**Serum** is defined as that portion of blood that remains after **coagulation** has occurred and the cells have been removed

and is the specimen of choice for many analyses. Samples are collected into tubes with no additive or with a clot activator and must be allowed to completely clot before further processing. **Plasma** is defined as the noncellular component of anticoagulated whole blood after the cellular components have been removed. Heparinized plasma is increasingly being used for routine chemistry testing to decrease turnaround time because it is not necessary to wait for the blood to clot. However, considerable differences may be observed between the concentrations of certain analytes (such as total protein) in serum and in plasma. For molecular diagnostics, anticoagulated whole blood or plasma is more likely to be the specimen of choice for either genomic DNA isolation from the white blood cells (WBCs) or viral identification and quantification from plasma.

For any assay provided for clinical use, manufacturers specify the appropriate sample type(s) for which they have validated the assay. Use of different sample types must be validated by laboratory personnel before use.

*Heparin.* Heparin is the most widely used **anticoagulant** for chemistry testing. It is available as sodium, potassium, lithium, and ammonium salts, all of which can adequately prevent coagulation by accelerating the action of antithrombin III, which neutralizes thrombin and prevents the formation of fibrin from fibrinogen. Heparin is naturally occurring and has the disadvantages of high cost and anticoagulation is temporary compared to the anticoagulants discussed later. The use of lithium or ammonium heparin is unacceptable for lithium and ammonia measurements, respectively.

It should be noted that heparin is unacceptable for most tests performed using polymerase chain reaction (PCR) because of inhibition of the polymerase enzyme by this large molecule. DNA can be extracted from heparinized samples, but amplification may be reduced, and the effect of heparin on any molecular diagnostic assay should be assessed as part of a method validation study.

*Ethylenediaminetetraacetic acid.* EDTA is a chelating agent of divalent cations such as $Ca^{2+}$ and $Mg^{2+}$ that is particularly useful for (1) hematologic examinations including transfusion medicine applications, (2) measurement of intracellular drugs such as cyclosporine or tacrolimus, (3) $HbA_{1c}$ analysis, (4) isolation of genomic DNA, and (5) qualitative and quantitative virus determinations by molecular techniques. It is used most commonly as the tri-potassium salt. EDTA prevents coagulation by binding calcium, which is essential for the clotting mechanism.

Because it chelates calcium, magnesium, and iron, EDTA is unsuitable for specimens for these analyses. In addition, EDTA inhibits alkaline phosphatase and creatine kinase activities.

*Sodium fluoride.* Sodium fluoride (NaF) is a weak anticoagulant that is often added as a preservative for blood glucose and lactate. As a preservative, it is often used together with another anticoagulant such as potassium oxalate. It exerts its **preservative** action by inhibiting the enzyme systems involved in glycolysis, although such inhibition is not immediate, and a certain amount of glycolysis occurs during the first hour after collection. Without an antiglycolytic agent, the blood glucose concentration decreases approximately 10 mg/dL (0.56 mmol/L) per hour at 25°C. The rate of decrease is faster in newborns because of the increased metabolic activity of erythrocytes and in leukemic patients because of the high metabolic activity and number of the WBCs. Newer formulations containing both NaF and citrate or EDTA immediately inhibit glycolysis and preserve glucose in the specimen for at least 24 hours.

*Citrate.* Sodium citrate solution, in a ratio of one part to nine parts of blood, is widely used for coagulation studies. The correct ratio of blood to anticoagulant is critical to achieve proper coagulation measurements because the anticoagulant effect is reversed by addition of standard amounts of $Ca^{2+}$ that are based on a proper collection volume. Because citrate chelates calcium, it is unsuitable as an anticoagulant for specimens for measurement of this element. It also inhibits aminotransferases and alkaline phosphatase.

*Acid citrate dextrose.* When both the form and function of the cellular components are required, such as for cytogenetic testing, samples are generally collected into acid citrate dextrose (ACD) anticoagulant. There are two ACD tube designations: ACD A and ACD B. These differ only by the concentrations of the additives. Both enhance the vitality and recovery of WBCs for several days after collection of the specimen.

*Oxalates.* Sodium, potassium, ammonium, and lithium oxalates inhibit blood coagulation by forming rather insoluble complexes with calcium ions.

Oxalate inhibits several enzymes, including acid and alkaline phosphatases, amylase, and lactate dehydrogenase (LDH), and may cause precipitation of calcium as the oxalate salt.

*Iodoacetate.* Sodium iodoacetate is an effective antiglycolytic agent (with the same caveats mentioned earlier) and a substitute for NaF. It inhibits creatine kinase but appears to have no notable effects on other clinical tests.

## Influence of Site of Collection on Blood Composition

Blood obtained from different sites differs in composition. In general, properly collected skin puncture blood is more similar to arterial blood than to venous blood, with no clinically significant differences between freely flowing capillary blood and arterial blood in pH, $PCO_2$, $PO_2$, and oxygen saturation. The $PCO_2$ of venous blood is up to 6 to 7 mm Hg (0.8 to 0.9 kPa) higher. Venous blood glucose is as much as 7 mg/dL (0.39 mmol/L) less than capillary blood glucose.

## Collection of Blood From Intravenous or Arterial Lines

When blood is collected from a central venous catheter or arterial line, it is necessary to ensure that the composition of the specimen is not affected by the fluid being infused into the patient. With clinical approval, fluid may be shut off using the stopcock on the catheter, and blood is aspirated through the stopcock and discarded before the specimen is withdrawn. The goal is to aspirate approximately two times the dead-space volume of the line before collecting the sample for testing for noncoagulation tests. Generally, 5 mL is sufficient for this purpose. Aspirating this blood and clearing the lines is equally important for molecular diagnostics and coagulation testing because the stopcock is often heavily saturated with heparin. Collection of samples for therapeutic drug monitoring should not be done from the line used for the infusion, irrespective of the time since infusion or amount of blood aspirated, because the drug may adhere to the line and leak into the collected sample.

In theory, blood may be collected from the veins of an arm below an IV line without interference from the fluid being infused because retrograde blood flow does not occur in the veins and the fluid being infused must first circulate through the heart and return before it reaches the sampling site. However, collection from the arm without the IV line is strongly recommended.

## Hemolysis

**Hemolysis** is defined as the disruption of the RBC membrane, resulting in the release of hemoglobin, and may be the consequence of intravascular events (in vivo hemolysis) or may occur subsequent to or during blood collection (in vitro hemolysis). Serum and plasma show visual evidence of hemolysis when the hemoglobin concentration exceeds 50 mg/dL (7.7 µmol/L). Slight hemolysis has little effect on most test values. Test interference at this concentration may be observed on those constituents that are present at a higher concentration in erythrocytes than in plasma, such LDH, aspartate transaminase (AST), potassium, magnesium, and phosphate. Most manufacturers provide data on the effects of hemolysis on the analytical performance of individual tests, and this should be evaluated in the selection of individual methods. Laboratory personnel must define at what level of hemolysis results should be held and not reported to prevent poor clinical action on unreliable test results.

In molecular diagnostic testing, hemoglobin may interfere with the amplification reaction. In some situations, the isolation of nucleic acid is sufficiently selective that free hemoglobin from the ruptured cells is removed and will not cause a problem. However, with hemolyzed blood, alternative or additional extraction methods are usually needed to ensure that RNA is fully and accurately transcribed and that the greatest amplification of DNA is achieved.

## Urine

The timing of urine specimen collection is dictated by the tests to be performed. Untimed or random specimens are suitable for some chemical tests, and other tests require urine specimens be collected over a predetermined interval of time, such as 4, 12, or 24 hours. A clean, early morning, fasting specimen is usually the most concentrated specimen and thus is preferred for microscopic examinations and for the detection of abnormal amounts of constituents such as proteins, or of unusual compounds such as chorionic gonadotropin. The clean timed specimen is one obtained at specific times of the day or during certain phases of the act of micturition. Although bacterial examination of the first 10 mL of urine voided is most appropriate to detect urethritis, the midstream specimen is best for investigating bladder disorders. The double-voided specimen is the urine excreted during a timed period after complete emptying of the bladder; it is used, for example, to assess glucose excretion during a glucose tolerance test. Similarly, in some metabolic disorders, urine must be collected during or immediately after symptoms of the disease appear.

When they are to be tested for their alcohol and drugs of abuse content, urine specimens are collected under rigorous conditions, often including enhanced patient identification and special collection facilities where water that could be used for urine dilution is restricted or colored, for example. It is necessary for laboratory personnel to be aware of the relevant legal requirements for this type of testing and plan in advance how these samples and the supporting paperwork will be collected and handled.

Catheter specimens are used for microbiologic examination in critically ill patients and in those with urinary tract obstruction but should not normally be necessary just for examination of chemical constituents. The suprapubic tap specimen is a useful alternative because the tap is unlikely to cause infection. After appropriate cleaning of the skin over the full bladder, a 22-gauge spinal needle is passed through a small wheal made by a local anesthetic. The bladder is penetrated and the urine withdrawn into the syringe.

Even though tests in the clinical laboratory are not usually affected by lack of sterile collection procedures, the patient's genitalia should be cleaned before each voiding to minimize the transfer of surface bacteria to the urine.

Currently, urine is an uncommon specimen type in the molecular diagnostic laboratory for genomic testing, although some laboratories use urine samples for bladder cancer screening and monitoring of therapy for bladder cancer. However, urine is frequently used for molecular testing for infectious agents, such as *Chlamydia,* a common sexually transmitted organism, or BK virus, associated with potential rejection or failure of transplanted kidneys. Because most requests involve a specific organism, an untimed or random urine specimen collected into a sterile container with no preservative is usually acceptable.

### Timed Urine Specimens

The collection period for timed specimens should be long enough to minimize the influence of short-term biologic variations. When specimens are to be collected over a specified period of time, the patient's close adherence to instructions to the collection procedure and restrictions to diet or drug ingestion is critically important and a common source of a preanalytical variable. The bladder must be emptied at the time the collection is to begin and this urine discarded. Thereafter all urine must be collected until the end of the scheduled time, including emptying of the bladder at the end of the collection period. Precautions should be taken to prevent fecal contamination of the urine. When the collection is made over several hours, urine should be passed into a separate container at each voiding and then emptied into a larger container for the complete specimen. This two-step procedure prevents the danger of patients splashing themselves with a preservative, such as acid that may be included in the collection device. The large container generally should be stored at 4°C during the entire collection period.

Urine should not be collected at the same time for two or more tests requiring different preservatives. Removal of aliquots during the collection procedure is not permissible even when the volume removed is measured and corrected because excretion of most compounds varies throughout the day. Appropriate information regarding the collection, including warnings with respect to handling of the specimen, should appear on the container label.

When a timed collection is complete, the specimen should be delivered without delay to the clinical laboratory, where the volume should be measured by using graduated cylinders or by weighing the container and the urine when pre-weighed or uniform containers are used. The mass in grams may be reported as if it were the volume in milliliters.

Before a specimen is transferred into small containers for each of the ordered tests, it must be thoroughly mixed to ensure homogeneity because the specific gravity, volume, and composition of the urine all may vary throughout the collection period and settling may occur.

### Collection of Urine and Feces From Children

Collection of any type of urine specimen from an infant is difficult, with timed collections being the most problematic. The approved method for collecting a random urine specimen from an infant involves a process known as bagging. A plastic bag (e.g., U-Bag, Hollister, Chicago, IL) is placed around the infant's genitalia after cleaning and then is held in place by a mild adhesive (Fig. 6.3). The baby's diaper is reapplied to help hold the bag in place. As soon as voiding has occurred, the bag containing the urine sample is removed and emptied into a regular urine collection cup. A newer technique for clean catch urine collections referred to as the Quick-Wee method involves the cutaneous stimulation of the suprapubic area using gauze soaked in cold liquid. Although in common use, collection of urine in cotton balls or diapers and wringing them out for the urine sample is not an acceptable urine collection method and results in contaminated samples. Invasive collection methods include catheterization or a suprapubic aspiration, which sample urine directly from the bladder. Although these invasive methods are more reliable, they

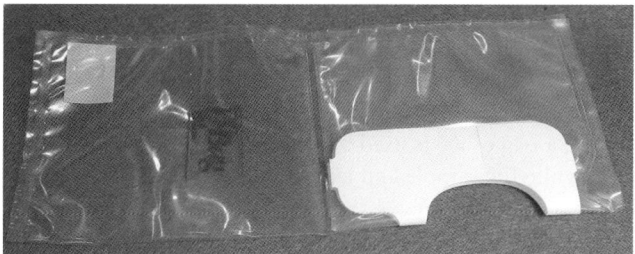

**Fig. 6.3** Urine collection device used in children.

cause pain and distress to the patient and require expertise to perform. In infants and very young children requiring a rare 24-hour urine collection, hospitalization and catheterization are often required to obtain a complete collection.

## Urine Preservatives

Preservatives for urine (CLSI GP16-A3, see Table 6.1) are usually added to reduce bacterial action or chemical decomposition or to solubilize constituents that otherwise might precipitate out of solution. Some specimens should not have *any* preservatives added because of the possibility of interference with analytical methods.

One of the most acceptable forms of preservation of urine specimens is refrigeration immediately after collection; it is even more successful when combined with chemical preservation. Acidification to a pH less than 3 is widely used to preserve 24-hour specimens for determination of calcium, steroids, adrenaline, noradrenaline, and vanillylmandelic acid. However, precipitation of urates will occur, making the sample unsuitable for measurement of uric acid.

A mild base, such as sodium bicarbonate or a small amount of sodium hydroxide, is used to preserve porphyrins, urobilinogen, and uric acid. pH should be adjusted to between 8 and 9.

## Feces

Fecal samples are required for fecal occult blood testing and fecal calprotectin measurement, both used to assess patients having gastrointestinal inflammation. Small aliquots of feces are frequently analyzed to detect the presence of "hidden" or occult blood. Tests for occult blood should be done on aliquots of excreted stools rather than on material obtained on the glove of a physician doing a rectal examination because this procedure may cause enough bleeding to produce a positive result. Fecal calprotectin requires a fresh random fecal specimen that is either frozen or refrigerated prior to analysis within 72 hours post-collection.

In newborns the first specimen from the bowel (meconium) may be used for detection of maternal drug use during the gestational period, which requires specific attention to the details of collection and identification similar to the chain of custody procedure for urine collection discussed earlier. Feces from infants and children may be screened for tryptic activity or for increased fecal fat concentrations, both of which can be indicators of cystic fibrosis. Fecal material is also commonly collected in childhood for the detection of parasites (ova and parasites [O & P]), enteric disease organisms such as *Salmonella* and *Shigella*, and viruses, all of which are useful in sorting out the differential diagnosis of diarrhea. Fecal testing is also used for helping to determine causes of malabsorption.

Usually, no preservative is added to the feces, but the container should be kept refrigerated throughout the collection period, and care should be taken to prevent contamination from urine. When the collection is complete, the container and feces are weighed, and the mass of excreted feces is calculated. Results are generally reported as activity per unit weight.

## Other Body Fluids

Specimens may be collected for analysis from a range of different body fluids. These include cerebrospinal fluid (CSF), pleural fluid, ascitic fluid, pericardial fluid, amniotic fluid, synovial fluid, and others. These fluids are tested for a variety of chemistries, which the laboratory will have validated for the specific tests.

## Buccal Cells

Collection of buccal cells (cells of the oral cavity of epithelial origin) has been identified as providing an excellent source of genomic DNA, as well as being less invasive than collection of blood. It is particularly useful for collecting cells with the patient's genomic DNA when the patient has had blood transfusions and thus another person's DNA or after bone marrow transplantation when the circulating blood cells are derived wholly or partially from the donor of the bone marrow. Two methods are used commonly to collect buccal cells: rinsing with mouthwash and using swabs or cytobrushes.

Rinsing of the oral cavity generally provides a higher yield of cells than can be obtained by using swabs. Mouthwash solutions high in phenol and ethanol are destructive to recovered cells and should be avoided. It is necessary for laboratory staff to validate a list of acceptable solutions.

For swabs, a sterile Dacron or rayon swab with a plastic shaft is preferred because calcium alginate swabs or swabs with wooden sticks may contain substances that inhibit PCR-based testing. After collection, the swab or cytobrush should be stored in an airtight plastic container or immersed in liquid, such as phosphate-buffered saline or viral transport medium.

## Hair and Nails

Currently, the use of hair or nails in molecular diagnostics is limited to forensic analysis (genomic DNA identification). Hair and fingernails or toenails have been used for trace metal and drug analyses, with the potential advantage of timing of exposure if separate segments of longer hair are analyzed, although no standards for such testing currently exist. Use of such samples requires laboratory staff to validate the processes.

## HANDLING OF SPECIMENS FOR ANALYSIS

Steps that are important for ensuring a valid specimen for analysis include (1) identification, (2) preservation, (3) separation and storage, and (4) transport.

# MAINTENANCE OF SPECIMEN IDENTIFICATION

Although the collection of an acceptable specimen is a key aspect of excellent testing, proper identification of the specimen must be maintained at each step of the testing process to ensure that the correct result is reported for the correct patient at all times. The minimum information on any label associated with a specific specimen should include the patient's first and last name and the patient-specific identifier. The collection date and time as well as the health care professional's identity must be available in the LIS. If any of these elements is not available or entered into the LIS, the information must be written on each collection tube at the time of collection so that the information can be entered into the LIS once the specimen is received in the laboratory. All labels should conform to the laboratory's stated requirements. In the United States, there is no specific labeling used for samples from patients with infectious diseases. Standard precautions should always be used, meaning that all specimens should be treated as if they are potentially infectious. Additionally, samples from patients suspected to have known, high-risk pathogens (e.g., hemorrhagic viruses such as Ebola) will have separate, pre-prepared sample handling protocols that may or may not involve the routine laboratory. For these samples proactive procedures must be in place unless the sample can be rendered safe (e.g., by heat treatment), in which case again standard universal precautions should be used.

In practice, every specimen container must be adequately labeled, even if the specimen must be placed in ice or if the container is so small that the label must be folded like a flag around the tube, as might happen with a capillary blood tube. Labels should always be placed on the cup or tube directly and not ever just on the cap.

It is critical that samples be positively identified through all steps of processing and analysis. Aliquoting a sample from the primary collection container to one or more other containers configured for the instrumentation requires close attention to proper labeling and tracking of the sample identifiers to ensure samples are not switched. Good work practice includes "piece work" in which only a single patient's samples are in the work area at one time, the area is clean with no old labels present, and the worker is not disturbed. Because the majority of samples received from pediatric patients are in microtubes, most samples need to be aliquoted, poured into a microsampling device, or hand loaded onto instruments that use whole blood, because these systems are not made to deal with such small tubes. This extra handling of the specimens offers opportunities for error and thus requires more strict attention to detail and analysis of the possible risks during design of the process.

## Preservation of Specimens

Specimens must be properly treated both during transport to the laboratory and from the time the serum, plasma, or cells have been separated until analysis. For some tests, specimens must be kept at 4°C from the time the blood is drawn until the specimens are analyzed or until the serum or plasma is separated from the cells to minimize metabolism and degradation of sample components. Transfer of these specimens to the laboratory must be done by placing the specimen container on ice; a bag of ice is used to surround the sample to keep it cool while the sample and label are not subjected to possible water contamination.

For all test constituents that are thermally labile, serum and plasma should be separated from cells in a refrigerated centrifuge. Some specimens may need to be protected from both daylight and fluorescent light to prevent photodegradation, although the use of plastic, rather than glass, tubes has decreased this preanalytical variable.

For specimens that are collected in a remote facility with infrequent transportation by courier to a central laboratory, proper specimen processing must be done in the remote facility so that appropriately separated and preserved plasma or serum is delivered to the laboratory.

## Add-On Requests

In the interest of preventing additional phlebotomies and to assess a clinical situation from a specimen collected at a specific time, many physicians request an "add-on" test (i.e., for the laboratory staff to perform a test on a sample already in the laboratory and processed). This is especially true in specimens collected from pediatric patients, and samples from an emergency department, where additional testing from the time of presentation may be needed after a clinical diagnosis has been made or narrowed by the clinician. Each laboratory must establish its own guidelines for what will be allowed.

## Separation and Storage of Specimens

Plasma or serum should be separated from cells as soon as possible and certainly within 2 hours for some but not all analytes. Premature separation of serum may permit continued formation of fibrin after centrifugation, which can clog sampling devices in testing equipment. If it is impossible to centrifuge a blood specimen within 2 hours, the specimen should be held at room temperature rather than at 4°C to decrease any effect on potassium measurement caused by leakage from the RBCs by inhibition of the $Na^+,K^+$-ATPase pump. For most plasma samples used for molecular diagnostics, the plasma should be removed from the primary tube promptly after centrifugation and held at −20°C. In all instances of freezing a sample, frost-free freezers should be avoided because they have a wide temperature swing during the freeze-thaw cycle.

Primary specimen tubes should always be centrifuged with the original cap in place. Such containment reduces evaporation, which occurs rapidly in a warm centrifuge with the air currents set up by centrifugation. Caps on the original tube also prevent aerosolization of infectious particles. Specimen tubes with requested testing for volatiles, such as ethanol, *must* have the initial cap in place while they are spun to prevent release of the volatile compound and result in an artificially reduced measurement. Centrifuging specimens with the cap in place also maintains anaerobic conditions, which are important in the measurement of carbon dioxide and ionized calcium.

## Transport of Specimens

Hemolysis may occur in pneumatic tube systems unless the tubes are completely filled and movement of the blood tubes inside the specimen carrier is prevented. The pneumatic tube system should be designed to eliminate sharp curves and sudden stops of specimen carriers. However, with many systems, the plasma hemoglobin concentration may be increased, and the serum activity of RBC enzymes, such as LDH and AST, may also be increased. There are also tests that cannot be transported to the laboratory via a pneumatic tube system such as platelet function testing where samples must be hand delivered to the laboratory.

Although the remaining discussion uses the specific example of referral laboratory testing, many of the issues discussed, such as regulations related to shipping, are also relevant to a laboratory that receives specimens from outlying clinics. This may involve validating specific transport or storage conditions that differ from existing CLSI recommendations. Before a referral laboratory is used for any tests, the quality of its work should be verified by the referring laboratory. Guidelines for selection and evaluation of a referral laboratory have been published (QMS05, see Table 6.1). For laboratories accredited by the College of American Pathologists (CAP), it is a requirement that the referring laboratory validate that the referral laboratory is CLIA'88 certified by obtaining a copy of the Clinical Laboratory Improvement Act (CLIA) certificate before specimens are shipped. For molecular diagnostic testing, this is of particular importance because often the latest genetic test being requested by a physician has not yet been moved from research interest status to patient care status and may not be available in a CLIA-certified laboratory.

Specimen type and quantity and specimen handling requirements of the referral laboratory must be observed, and in laboratories operating under CLIA'88 regulations, test results reported by a referral laboratory must be identified as such when they are filed in a patient's medical record. Most reference laboratories have lower minimum volume requirements for pediatric specimens than for adult specimens, but these lower minimums may preclude being able to retest the sample if there is a problem with the initial analysis. The tube and transport condition for the specimen should be constructed such that the contents do not escape if the container is exposed to extremes of heat, cold, or sunlight. Reduced pressure may be encountered during air transport, together with vibration, and specimens should be protected from these adverse conditions by a suitable container. Variability in temperature is a significant factor causing instability of test constituents.

Polypropylene and polyethylene containers are usually suitable for specimen transport. Containers must be leak-proof and should have a Teflon-lined screw cap that does not loosen under the variety of temperatures to which the container may be exposed. The materials of both stopper and container must be inert and must not have any effect on the concentration of the analyte.

For transport of frozen or refrigerated specimens, a Styrofoam container should be used. The container should be vented to prevent buildup of carbon dioxide under pressure and a possible explosion. Solid carbon dioxide (dry ice) is the most convenient refrigerant material for keeping specimens frozen. The amount of dry ice required in a container depends on the size of the container, the efficiency of its insulation, and the length of time for which the specimens must be kept frozen.

Various laws and regulations apply to the shipment of biologic specimens. Although such regulations theoretically apply only to etiologic agents (known infectious agents), all specimens should be transported as if the same regulations apply. Airlines deem dry ice a hazardous material; therefore the transport of most clinical laboratory specimens is affected and those who package the specimens should be trained in the appropriate regulations, such as those published by the International Air Transport Association.

The various modes of transport of specimens influence the shipping time and cost, and each laboratory staff needs to make its own assessment as to adequate service. The objective is to ensure that the properly collected, processed, and identified specimen arrives at the testing facility in time and under the correct storage conditions so that the analytical phase can proceed.

## CONCLUSION

Accurate test results (the right result for the right patient) begin and end with the integrity of the sample. Integrity can be assured only through proper preparation of the patient; choice of sample container; collection of the sample; and finally transport, processing, and storage of the collected sample, with each step maintaining accurate identification. For these reasons, best laboratory practice demands attention to detail and following appropriate protocols. It is incumbent on laboratory professionals to delineate their processes in complete policies and procedures that not only cover the routine and correct procedures but also cover the unusual. These should include how to handle the process when the system breaks down and steps are not properly performed and may need to be addressed case by case by the laboratory director. Preanalytical variables can be lessened or even avoided if these steps are followed.

---

### POINTS TO REMEMBER

- Proper identification of the patient is essential; samples should be properly labeled at all steps, especially if separated from the primary collection container.
- Collection of all samples must be in the correct tube type; once a sample is in a tube with additives it cannot be transferred to a different tube with additives.
- Attention to the details related to processing of the collected sample (time, temperature, special handling) should always follow validated policies.
- The accurate result for any patient's sample (that will be acted on by the clinician) depends on adherence to all policies and procedures.

## REVIEW QUESTIONS

1. Identify the incorrect specimen collection scenario below.
   a. Ask a parent to name a pediatric patient.
   b. Ask an adult patient to state his or her name and another identifier.
   c. Show the patient or parent the labeled tube after collection is complete.
   d. Check the room and bed number of the patient to be collected and proceed with collection.
   e. Contact a translation service for a patient unable to speak the local language.

2. Identify the correct tube additive and biochemical action below:
   a. A sodium fluoride tube helps to prevent glycolysis and is used for glucose measurement.
   b. A sodium citrate tube with total chelation of calcium allows effective coagulation testing.
   c. A no additive, no gel plasma sample does not need to clot before use.
   d. An EDTA anticoagulated specimen can be used for calcium determination.
   e. Lithium heparin tubes are widely used for chemistry tests and require clotting before use.

3. Patients should not pump their fists after the tourniquet is applied because:
   a. it may cause venous stasis not under the control of the collector.
   b. it will affect the chemical interaction between the tube additive and the patient's blood.
   c. metabolic activity of the blood and muscles will affect analytes such as potassium and calcium through effects on pH.
   d. it will affect the distribution of analytes between plasma and serum.
   e. it will make it more difficult to find the patient's vein.

4. For urine collections, which of the following is true?
   a. Samples should be kept at room temperature for timed collections.
   b. Proper collection technique on an infant utilizes "bagging" with a small plastic collection bag
   c. Preservatives in a 24-hour collection jug do not need to be identified to the patient.
   d. A 24-hour collection includes the first morning urine sample both at the start and the finish of collection.
   e. A "clean catch" is not necessary for urine culture collections.

5. Additional testing (add-ons) performed on a previous sample requires:
   a. any sample that was collected within the appropriate time frame.
   b. a sample that has been sitting at room temperature.
   c. sufficient sample volume left on a sample of the correct type for the add-on assay.
   d. using an unlabeled aliquot of the original sample.
   e. an additional sample be collected for the test.

## SUGGESTED READINGS

Arena J, Emparanza JI, Nogués A, Burls A. Skin to calcaneus distance in the neonate. *Arch Dis Child Fetal Neonatal Ed.* 2005;90(4):F328–F331.

Cornes MP, Ford C, Gama R. Spurious hyperkalaemia due to EDTA contamination: common and not always easy to identify. *Ann Clin Biochem.* 2008;45:601–603.

Farnsworth CW, Webber DM, Krekeler JA, et al. Parameters for validating a hospital pneumatic tube system. *Clin Chem.* 2019;65(5):694–702.

Fokker M. Stability of glucose in plasma with different anticoagulants. *Clin Chem Lab Med.* 2014;52:1057–1060.

Garza D, Becan-McBride K. Capillary or dermal blood specimens. In: Garza D, Becan-McBride K, eds. *Phlebotomy Handbook: Blood Specimen Collection From Basic to Advanced.* 10th ed. Upper Saddle River, NJ: Pearson Prentice Hall; 2019:371–395.

Garza D, Becan-McBride K. Pediatric and geriatric procedures. In: Garza D, Becan-McBride K, eds. *Phlebotomy Handbook: Blood Specimen Collection From Basic to Advanced.* 10th ed. Upper Saddle River, NJ: Pearson Prentice Hall; 2019:423–457.

Green AMI, Gray J. *Neonatology & Laboratory Medicine.* London, UK: ACB Venture Publications; 2003.

Haverstick DM, Brill 2nd LB, Scott MG, et al. Preanalytical variables in measurement of free (ionized) calcium in lithium heparin-containing blood collection tubes. *Clin Chim Acta.* 2009;403:102–104.

Hoeltke LB. The challenge of phlebotomy. In: Hoeltke LB, ed. *The Complete Textbook of Phlebotomy.* 3rd ed. Clifton Park, NJ: Thomas Delmar Learning; 2006:227–248.

Jones PM, Patel K. Pediatric clinical biochemistry: why is it different?. In: Dietzen D, Bennett MJ, Wong E, eds. *Biochemical and Molecular Basis of Pediatric Disease.* 5th ed. Cambridge, MA: Elsevier, Academic Press; 2021. chap 1, 1–13.

Kaufman J, Fitzpatrick P, Tosif S, et al. Faster clean catch urine collection (Quick-Wee method) from infants: randomised controlled trial. *BMJ.* 2017;357:j1341.

Mikesh LM, Bruns DE. Stabilization of glucose in blood specimens: mechanism of delay in fluoride inhibition of glycolysis. *Clin Chem.* 2008;54:930–932.

Mullins GR, Harrison JH, Bruns DE. Smartphone monitoring of pneumatic tube system-induced sample hemolysis. *Clin Chim Acta.* 2016;462:1–5.

Pupek A, Matthewson B, Whitman E, et al. Comparison of pneumatic tube system with manual transport for routine chemistry, hematology, coagulation and blood gas tests. *Clin Chem Lab Med.* 2017;55(10):1537–1544.

Ridefelt P, Åkerfeldt T, Helmersson-Karlqvist J. Increased plasma glucose levels after change of recommendation from NaF to citrate blood collection tubes. *Clin Biochem.* 2014;47:625–628.

WHO guidelines on drawing blood: best practices in phlebotomy. In: *Pediatric and Neonatal Blood Sampling* (Chapter 6). Geneva: World Health Organization; 2010. http://www.ncbi.nlm.nih.gov/books/NBK138647/.

Young DS. *Effects of Preanalytical Variable on Clinical Laboratory Tests.* 3rd ed. Washington, DC: AACC Press; 2007.

Zhang DJ, Elswick RK, Miller WG, Bailey JL. Effect of serum-clot contact time on clinical chemistry laboratory results. *Clin Chem.* 1998;44(6):1325–1333.

# Quality Control of the Analytical Examination Process

*W. Greg Miller and Sverre Sandberg*

## OBJECTIVES

1. Define the following:
   - Coefficient of variation
   - External quality control
   - Internal quality control
   - Levey-Jennings chart
   - Mean
   - Proficiency testing
   - Quality control plan
   - Quality control rules
   - Sigma metric
   - Standard deviation (SD)
   - SD interval
2. Explain how to establish a target value and SD for use with a quality control (QC) material in the following situations: a new lot of QC material replaces an existing lot for an analyte; a new measurement procedure replaces an existing procedure for the same analyte; a new measurement procedure for a new analyte is introduced to the laboratory.
3. Explain how to establish rules for evaluating QC sample results to confirm that results for patient samples from a

measurement procedure are acceptable to make medical decisions.
4. Explain how to verify QC target values following a reagent lot change.
5. Explain the components of a QC plan and how the plan is established.
6. Explain the actions taken when a failed QC result is obtained.
7. Explain how to evaluate results from external quality assessment (EQA) or proficiency testing.
8. Explain why peer group evaluation is used in EQA and what information a laboratory gets about its measurement procedure performance from the data.
9. Explain the limitations in using peer group mean values to assess the relationship of results among different measurement procedures.
10. Explain the value of EQA that uses commutable samples.
11. Explain how QC information is documented and reviewed by laboratory staff.

## KEY WORDS AND DEFINITIONS

**Coefficient of variation** Also called *relative standard deviation*; calculated as the standard deviation (SD) divided by the mean and multiplied by 100 to express in percent.

**External quality assessment** Also called *external quality control or proficiency testing;* an assessment process in which samples that simulate patient specimens are received from an external organization and results compared to those from other laboratories or from a reference method to determine that a measurement procedure's performance meets preestablished criteria to be suitable for use in medical decisions.

**Internal quality control** Frequently referred to as quality control; term used to refer to quality control samples measured to confirm that results from a measurement procedure are suitable for use.

**Levey-Jennings chart** A graphical display with observed control values plotted on the *y*-axis and time (typically in days) shown on the *x*-axis. The *y*-axis shows the target value with plus and minus 1, 2, and 3 SDs indicated. Control limits can be indicated but are not practical to

show on the chart when multiple control rules are used for evaluation of quality control results.

**Mean** The arithmetic average of a series of numbers such as results of repeated measurements of a quality control sample. The mean of a series of replicate results for a quality control material is used as the target value for future measurements of that quality control material.

**Proficiency testing** Another term for external quality assessment.

**Quality assessment** Protocols to confirm that the laboratory service meets the needs of medical providers who use laboratory results for medical decisions. Quality assessment includes preanalytical, analytical, and postanalytical components of quality.

**Quality control** Statistical and/or nonstatistical check protocols, typically using quality control samples that are surrogates for the patient samples being tested, to assess that results from a measurement procedure meet preestablished criteria to be suitable for use in medical decisions.

**Quality control plan** A document that describes the organization and operation of the internal quality control process.

**Quality control rules** A set of rules based on the difference between results for one or more quality control samples and their target values to make a decision that the measurement procedure performance is producing results for patient samples that are suitable for use in medical decisions.

**Sigma metric** A value that expresses the variation in performance of a measurement procedure relative to the allowable variability in results to be suitable for medical decisions expressed in SD units. Six-sigma performance

means that six SDs of measurement procedure variation fit within the allowable limits for acceptable performance.

**Standard deviation** A statistical value that estimates the dispersion of replicate values around a mean value. A SD assumes a Gaussian distribution of values that is typically observed for numeric quality control results.

**Standard deviation interval** The number of SDs an individual result is from a mean value calculated as mean minus individual value divided by SD. The SD interval can be positive or negative relative to the mean value.

The purpose of a clinical laboratory test is to provide information on the pathophysiological condition of an individual patient to assist with diagnosis, therapy, or risk for a disease. **Internal quality control,** frequently referred to as **quality control** (QC), is a statistical sampling approach performed by a laboratory on a regular schedule to assess performance of its measuring systems. External QC, frequently referred to as **external quality assessment** (EQA) or **proficiency testing** (PT), is an approach to assess measuring system performance by comparison of results for samples measured by a group of different laboratories. Both types of QC are addressed in this chapter.

Internal QC evaluates a measurement procedure by periodically measuring a QC sample for which the expected result is known in advance. If the result for a QC sample is within acceptable limits of the known value, the measurement procedure is verified to be performing as expected, and results for patient samples can be reported with high probability that they are suitable for clinical use. If a QC result is not within acceptable limits, the measurement procedure is not performing correctly, there is a high probability that results for patient samples are not suitable for clinical use, and corrective action is necessary. Patient sample measurements could need to be repeated when the measurement procedure has been restored to its stable performance condition. If erroneous patient results have already been reported before an error condition is identified, a corrected report must be issued.

Measurement procedures fall into one of two general categories from a **QC plan** perspective. One type of procedure is a "batch" measurement process in which the results for patient samples and QC samples are completed before the results are reported. The other type of procedure is a "continuous" measurement process in which patient sample results are reported during the interval between measurement of QC samples. For continuous measurement procedures, there is a possibility that erroneous results have already been reported if an error condition is identified by the next QC samples measurements. In either category, QC procedures only identify error conditions present at the point in time when a QC sample is measured.

The design of a QC plan must consider the analytical performance capability of a measurement procedure and the risk of harm to a patient that might occur if an erroneous laboratory test result is used for a clinical care decision.

**POINTS TO REMEMBER**

**Internal Quality Control**
- The primary role of internal QC is to confirm that patient results are correct and to identify possible errors before they will affect patient care decisions.

# MEASUREMENT PROCEDURE PERFORMANCE AS A PREREQUISITE FOR A QUALITY CONTROL PLAN

## Analytical Bias and Imprecision

Fig. 7.1 illustrates the meaning of bias and imprecision for a measurement procedure. The horizontal axis represents the numeric value for an individual result, and the vertical axis represents the number of repeated measurements with the same value made on samples of a QC material. The blue line shows the dispersion of results for repeated measurements of the same QC material, which is the random imprecision of the measurement. The **standard deviation** (SD) is a measure of expected imprecision in a measurement procedure when it is performing within specifications. The mean of repeated measurements of a QC sample becomes the target.

Fig. 7.1B illustrates that if a systematic bias (error) occurs in the measurements, the mean value shifts to another value. Note that the imprecision is the same as before the bias occurred because it is unlikely, although not impossible, that a change in imprecision would occur at the same time as a bias shift. The primary purpose of measuring QC samples is to statistically evaluate the measurement procedure to verify that it continues to perform within the specifications consistent with its acceptable expected stable condition or to identify that a change in performance occurred that needs to be corrected. QC result acceptance criteria are based on the probability for an individual QC result to be different from the variability in results expected when the measurement procedure is performing in a stable condition within its specifications.

Fig. 7.2 shows a **Levey-Jennings chart** that is the most common presentation for evaluating QC results. This format shows each QC result sequentially over time and allows a quick visual assessment of performance. Assuming the measurement procedure is performing in a stable condition, the mean value represents the target (or expected) value for the QC result, and the SD lines represent the expected imprecision. Assuming a Gaussian (normal) distribution

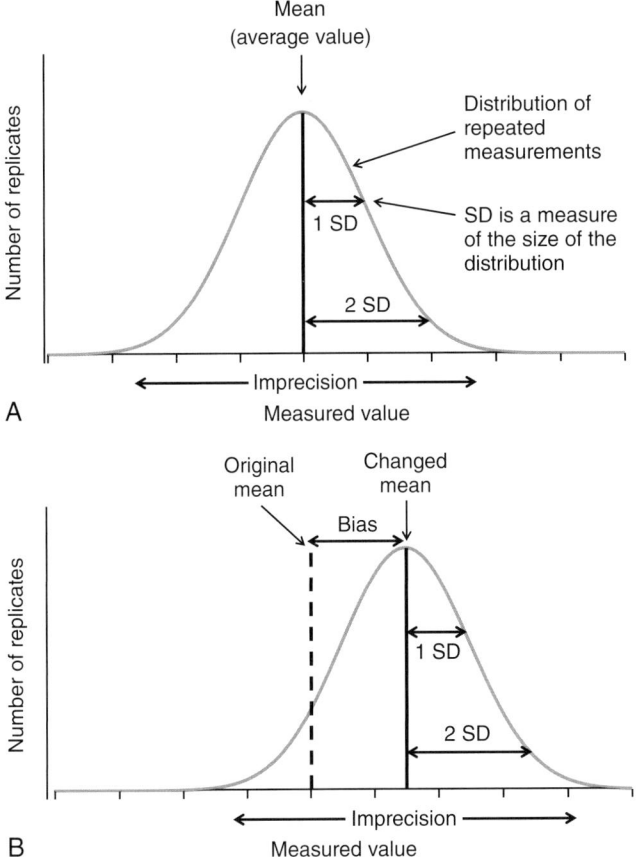

**Fig. 7.1** (A) Distribution of results showing the mean value and expected imprecision for repeated measurements of a quality control sample. (B) Bias when a change in calibration has occurred. *SD*, Standard deviation. (From Miller WG. Quality control. In: *Henry's Clinical Diagnosis and Management by Laboratory Methods*. 23rd ed. Philadelphia: Elsevier; 2016.)

of imprecision, the results should be distributed uniformly around the mean with results observed more frequently closer to the mean than near the extremes of the distribution. The data show fluctuations in performance at different intervals and illustrate the importance of calculating the SD over a long enough time interval to appropriately include all sources of variability in the measurement procedure. Note that a small number of results in Fig. 7.2 exceed 2 SDs, and three results slightly exceed 3 SDs, which is expected for an approximately Gaussian distribution of imprecision. The number of results expected within the **standard deviation intervals** (SDIs) is:

- ±1 SDI = 68.3% of observations
- ±2 SDI = 95.4% of observations
- ±3 SDI = 99.7% of observations

Interpretation of an individual QC result is based on its probability to be part of the expected distribution of results for the measurement procedure when the procedure is performing correctly. Note that evaluation of individual QC results may be performed by computer algorithms without visual examination of a Levey-Jennings chart.

## Performance of a Measurement Procedure for Its Intended Medical Use

It is necessary to determine how the performance of a measurement procedure relates to the medical requirements for interpreting results to determine the frequency to measure QC samples and the criteria to use to evaluate the QC results. The **sigma metric** is commonly used to assess how well a measurement procedure performs relative to the medical requirement. For laboratory measurements, the sigma metric is calculated as:

$$\text{Sigma} = \frac{(TE_a - |\,bias\,|)}{SD}$$

where $TE_a$ is the total error allowed based on medical requirements, and absolute value of bias and SD refer to performance

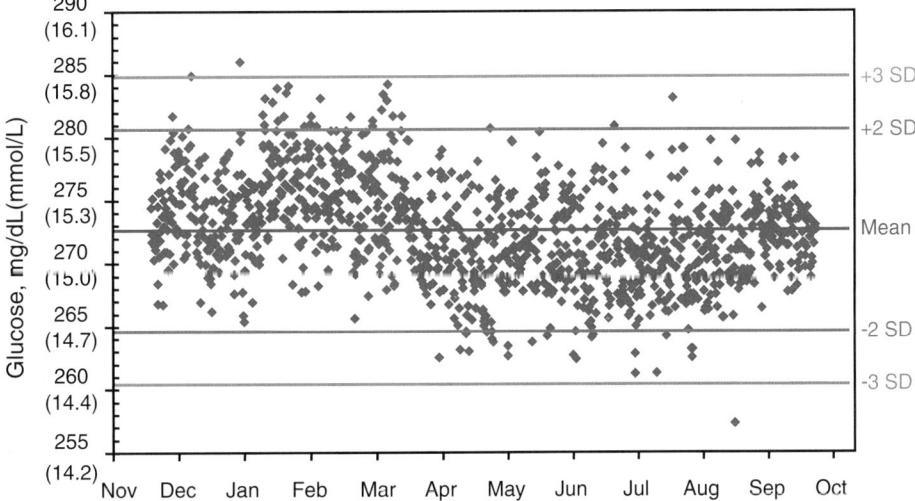

**Fig. 7.2** Levey-Jennings chart of quality control (QC) results (*n* = 1232) for a single lot of QC material used over a 10-month period. *SD*, Standard deviation. (Reprinted with permission from Miller WG, Nichols JH. Quality control. In: Clarke WA, ed. *Contemporary Practice in Clinical Chemistry*. 2nd ed. Washington, DC: AACC Press; 2011.)

characteristics of the measurement procedure. The SD is estimated from the QC data. It is critically important that the estimate of SD be made using QC data that represent all or most components of variability that occur over an extended time period. The bias is difficult for a laboratory to estimate because it is difficult to evaluate if a particular measurement procedure has a bias compared with a reliable estimate of a true value such as a reference measurement procedure. For internal QC, a laboratory is usually interested to determine if a bias has occurred compared with the condition established by calibration of a measurement procedure, and if a bias has occurred it will be corrected. Consequently, the bias is usually assumed to be zero for calculating sigma.

$TE_a$ represents the measurement procedure performance required for medical decisions based on a test result. $TE_a$ can be estimated using three models. The preferred model (model 1) is to set a performance specification based on an outcome study such as the impact of analytical performance on the clinical outcome. Outcome studies are only possible for a small number of analytes and typically indirectly used in clinical practice guidelines.

Model 2 bases the $TE_a$ on a fraction of the within and between individual biological variations of the measurand (the substance or analyte being measured in a clinical sample). (For additional information on biological variation and analytical performance specifications refer to Chapter 4.) This model minimizes the ratio of the "analytical noise" to the "biologic signal," with an assumption that a small ratio will identify measurement procedure performance that relates to the medical requirements. A database of optimal, desirable, and minimal $TE_a$ based on biological variation is available (https://biologicalvariation.eu/ accessed May 5, 2023).

Model 3 bases the performance specifications on the "state of the art," which is the performance capability of a measurement procedure usually derived from QC data. The laboratory should consult with clinical care providers to agree on an appropriate $TE_a$ for the patient population served.

Because sigma assumes a Gaussian or normal distribution for repeated measurements, the probability of a defect (i.e., an erroneous laboratory result) can be predicted. The term *six-sigma* refers to a condition when the variability in the measurement process is sufficiently smaller than the medical requirement that erroneous results are very uncommon. Fig. 7.3A shows a six-sigma test that has the $TE_a$ limits 6 SDs away from the center point of the distribution of variability in measurements when the procedure is performing correctly and there is no bias (black line). A small amount of bias, shown in the blue line, or increased imprecision will have little influence on the number of erroneous results produced, and the risk of producing an erroneous result even with some loss of performance is very low. Consequently, less stringent QC is suitable.

Fig. 7.3B shows a three-sigma measurement procedure that has the $TE_a$ limits 3 SDs away from the center point of the expected distribution of variability in measurements (black line). In the three-sigma situation, a small amount of bias, shown in the blue line, or increased imprecision will cause the number of erroneous results to increase substantially. More frequent QC and more stringent acceptance criteria will allow the laboratory

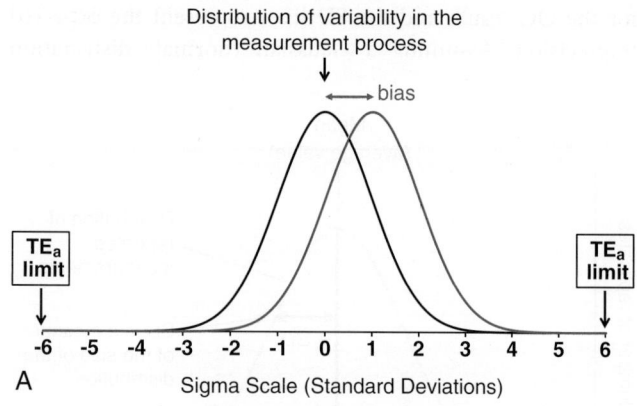

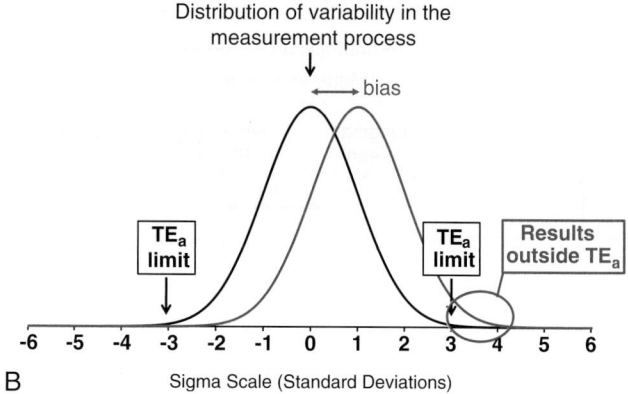

**Fig. 7.3** Test performance relative to the sigma scale to describe how well performance meets medical requirements expressed as the allowable total error *(TE$_a$)*. (A) A six-sigma measurement procedure. (B) A three-sigma measurement procedure. The black line shows zero bias, and the blue line shows a 1 SD shift in bias.

to identify when small changes in performance occur so they can be corrected to minimize the risk of harm to a patient from erroneous results being acted on to make clinical care decisions.

### POINTS TO REMEMBER

- The performance characteristics of a measurement procedure when it is performing in a stable in-control condition must be known.
- The allowable total error for a measurement procedure must be established based on requirements for using a laboratory result in patient care decisions.
- The sigma metric represents the probability that a given number of erroneous results may occur when the test measurement procedure is performing to its specifications.

## DEVELOPING A QUALITY CONTROL PLAN AND IMPLEMENTING INTERNAL QUALITY CONTROL PROCEDURES

### Selection of Quality Control Materials

In general, two different concentrations of QC materials are necessary for adequate statistical QC. For quantitative measurement procedures, QC materials should be selected to provide analyte concentrations that represent clinical decision values over the analytical measuring interval of the measurement procedure. More than two concentrations of QC materials may be needed when there are several important medical decision values. In practice, laboratories are frequently limited by concentrations available in commercial QC products. For procedures with extraction or other pretreatment steps, controls must be used to include any pretreatment steps. For qualitative tests, QC values should assess the performance near a threshold for a classification decision.

The QC materials must be manufactured to provide a stable product that can be used for an extended time period when possible. Use of a single lot for a year or more allows reliable interpretive criteria to be established that will minimize the effort and uncertainty associated with QC lot changes.

## Limitations of Quality Control Materials

An important limitation of most QC materials, which also applies to EQA or PT materials, is called noncommutability with patient samples. Fig. 7.4A shows that a commutable QC material gives a result that closely agrees with results for authentic patient samples with the same amount of analyte when measured by different procedures. Fig. 7.4B shows that results for a noncommutable QC material have a different relationship than observed for patient samples when measured by different procedures. QC and EQA/PT materials are typically noncommutable with patient samples because the serum, blood, or other biologic fluid matrix is usually altered from that of a patient sample during product manufacturing, for example, by use of partially purified human and nonhuman additives to achieve desired concentrations and various stabilization additives and processes. The impact of the matrix alteration on the recovery of an analyte is not predictable and is frequently different for different lots of QC material, for different lots of reagent within a given measurement procedure, and for different measurement procedures. Because of the noncommutability limitation, special procedures are

required when changing lots of reagent or comparing QC results among two or more measurement procedures (see later sections).

A second limitation of QC materials is gradual deterioration of the analyte during storage and after reconstitution, thawing, or vial opening.

## Frequency to Measure Quality Control Samples

The frequency with which to measure QC samples depends on several considerations. Regulatory requirements may specify a minimum frequency for QC measurements. The instructions for use from measurement procedure manufacturers may specify a minimum or recommended QC frequency. The risk of action being taken for a patient before a measurement error of clinical importance is detected is an important consideration for more frequent QC measurements than based on regulatory requirements or manufacturer's recommendations.

### Analytical Stability of the Measurement Procedure

The more stable the measurement procedure, the less frequently a QC evaluation needs to be performed. Some measurement procedures, particularly point-of-care (POC) devices, have been designed with sophisticated built-in control procedures to mitigate the risk that an erroneous result may be produced. These measurement systems may be sufficiently stable and self-monitored to justify reduced frequency of traditional QC sample testing.

### Risk of Harm to a Patient and Number of Patients Who May Be at Risk

More frequent QC sampling is appropriate to avoid the situation of discovering a measurement procedure defect many hours after a physician has made a clinical treatment or nontreatment decision based on an erroneous result. For example, QC sampling performed on a 24-hour cycle might be performed at 9 a.m. If QC results indicate a measurement procedure problem, the erroneous condition could have started at any time during the previous 24 hours. If the problem had

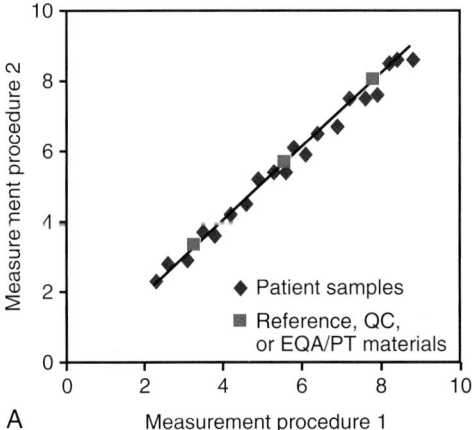
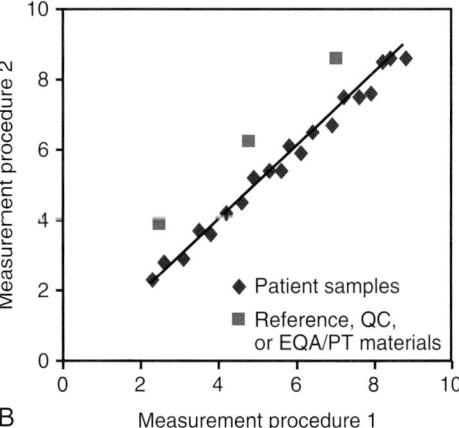

**Fig. 7.4** Illustration of commutable and noncommutable materials. (A) Commutable materials *(blue squares)* have the same relationship between two measurement procedures as observed for patient samples *(black diamonds)*. (B) Noncommutable materials have a different relationship than observed for patient samples. *EQA,* External quality assessment; *PT,* proficiency testing; *QC,* quality control.

occurred at 3 p.m. the previous day, erroneous results could have been reported for 18 hours, likely putting a large number of patients at risk of an inappropriate care decision.

The Clinical and Laboratory Standards Institute (CLSI) has published guideline EP23 addressing risk-based QC procedures. The document provides guidance on how to develop a QC plan based on evaluation of risk of harm to a patient and assessment of the effectiveness of risk mitigation procedures. In general terms, the laboratory director makes a judgment that suitable built-in and laboratory-applied controls are in place and that a result has a high probability to be correct at the time it is reported for clinical use.

### Event-Based Quality Control Sample Measurement

It is necessary when using a continuous measurement system to measure QC samples before and after scheduled events such as recalibration or maintenance that may alter the current performance condition. Each of these operations is intended to restore the measurement conditions to optimal specifications and to correct for any calibration drift or component deterioration that may have occurred. If QC samples are not measured before such scheduled events, a laboratory will not know if an error condition may have occurred since the last time QC samples were measured. It is also necessary to measure QC samples after these events to verify that the operations were performed correctly and that measurement procedure performance meets specifications before restarting to measure patient samples.

### Establishing the Quality Control Target Value and Standard Deviation That Represent a Stable Measurement Operating Condition

QC target values and acceptable performance limits are established to optimize the probability to detect a measurement defect that is large enough to have an impact on clinical care while minimizing the frequency of "false alerts" caused by statistical limitations of the criteria used to evaluate QC results.

### Quality Control Material Target Value

The generally accepted minimum protocol for target value assignment is to use the mean from at least 10 measurements of the QC material on 10 different days when the measurement procedure is correctly calibrated and performing to its specifications. Because all sources of variability cannot be captured in 10 measurements, it is recommended to update the target value after more data have been acquired during use of the QC material. If a 10-day protocol is not possible (e.g., if an emergency replacement of a lot of QC material is necessary), a provisional target value can be established with fewer data but should be updated when additional QC results are available. It is important to emphasize that the target value only represents the mean of the QC results measured under stable conditions and is not the true value.

### Quality Control Material Standard Deviation

The SD must represent the variability expected for a measurement procedure over an extended time interval to include all sources of variability when its performance meets its specifications. Measurement variability has short time interval components (such as pipetting volume), gradual changes (such as pipette seal deterioration or coating of cuvette or electrode surfaces), or variable and sometimes long intervals (such as calibration cycles, reagent replenishment, and maintenance procedures). An SD that represents stable measurement performance can usually be estimated from the cumulative SD over a 6- to 12-month period for a single lot of QC material because most expected sources of variation are likely to be represented. Fig. 7.5 illustrates the fluctuation in SD that occurred when calculated for monthly intervals compared with the relatively stable value observed for the cumulative SD after a period of 6 months. Note that the cumulative SD is not the average of the monthly values but is the SD determined from all individual results obtained over a time interval since the lot of QC material was first used. If the imprecision expected during normal stable operation is underestimated, the acceptable range for QC results will be too small, and the false-alert rate will be unacceptably high.

When a measurement procedure has been established in a laboratory and a new lot of QC material is being introduced, the target value for the new lot of QC material is used along with the well-established SD from the previous lot. This practice is appropriate because in most cases, measurement imprecision is a property of the measurement procedure and equipment used and is unlikely to change with a different lot of QC material.

When a new measurement procedure replaces an existing procedure, the SD for the existing procedure can in many cases be used as the initial SD for the new measurement procedure until the SD for the new measurement procedure has been established. An assumption is made that the new measurement procedure has approximately the same or better performance than the existing procedure, and that the SD for the existing measurement procedure was appropriate to ensure the results were suitable for use in medical decisions.

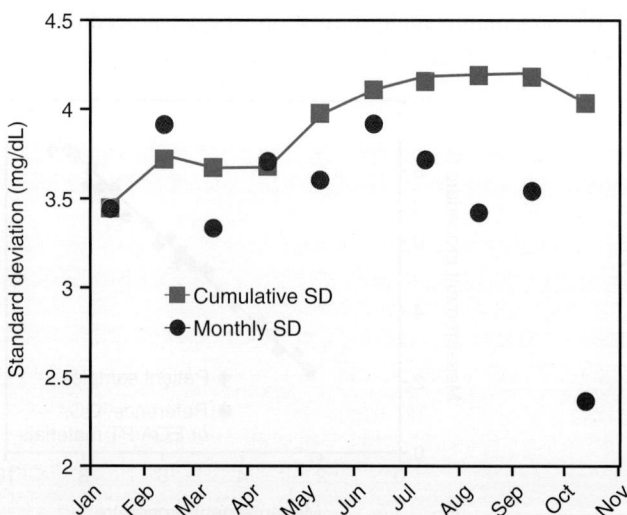

**Fig. 7.5** Cumulative standard deviation (SD) versus single monthly values calculated from the data in Fig. 7.2. (From Miller WG. Quality control. In: *Henry's Clinical Diagnosis and Management by Laboratory Method.* 23rd ed. Philadelphia: Elsevier; 2016.)

Consequently, the SD for the existing measurement procedure is likely to be suitable for QC decisions for the new measurement procedure.

If a measurement procedure for a new analyte is introduced, there will not be any historical performance information. The SD is based on QC data obtained during the measurement procedure validation. A minimum of 20 observations on different days is recommended for the initial estimate of the SD. This initial estimate of SD will likely be an underestimate because it does not include all sources of variability and must be updated when sufficient QC results have been accumulated to include most sources of variability.

### Quality Control Materials With Preassigned Values

Some QC materials are provided by the measurement procedure manufacturer with preassigned target values and acceptable ranges intended to confirm that the measurement procedure meets the manufacturer's specifications. Such assigned values may be used to verify the manufacturer's specifications. However, it is recommended that both the target value and the SD should be reevaluated and assigned by the laboratory after adequate replicate results have been obtained because the QC interpretive **rules** used in a single laboratory should reflect performance for the measurement procedure in that laboratory.

QC materials with assigned target values and SDs are also available from third-party manufacturers (i.e., manufacturers not affiliated with the measurement procedure manufacturer) and typically have values that are applicable to specifically stated measurement procedures and reagent lots to accommodate the influence of noncommutability. However, a laboratory should determine a target value and SD that reflect the operating conditions in that laboratory to ensure optimal assessment of QC results to identify an erroneous measurement condition.

### Establishing Rules to Evaluate Quality Control Results

The acceptable range and rules for interpretation of QC results are based on the probability of detecting an analytical error condition with an acceptably small false-alert rate.

The conventional way to express QC interpretive rules is by using an abbreviation nomenclature popularized among clinical laboratories by Westgard and summarized in Table 7.1. Note that fractional SDIs can be used as in the $2_{2.5S}$ and $8_{1.5S}$ examples and that combinations of numbers of controls and limits can be used as appropriate for QC interpretive rules. Trend detection procedures such as cumulative sum (CUSUM) or exponentially weighted moving average (EWMA) are recommended if supported by an available computer system because they are more powerful for detecting trends than approaches based on counting the number of sequential observations exceeding a specified SDI. A trend rule can be set to give an alert as a warning that may not require discontinuing testing but indicate that a problem is developing that should be investigated.

The efficiency of QC interpretive rules can be improved by combining two or more rules and applying them simultaneously as multirule criteria. For example, the $1_{3S}/2_{2S}$ multirule identifies an error condition if one control exceeds ±3 SD from the target value or if two controls exceed ±2 SDs in the same direction from the target value. The $1_{3S}/2_{2S}$ multirule has a low false-alert rate but improved probability to detect a bias error of a given magnitude.

In practice, empirical judgment is frequently used to establish acceptance criteria (rules) to evaluate QC results based on data acquired over a long enough period of time to adequately estimate the expected variability when a measurement procedure is working correctly. An empirical approach can be used by obtaining a set of QC data that represents stable measurement procedure performance over a time interval expected to include most sources of variability. Using those data, the false-alert rate for a rule can be determined, and bias errors of different magnitudes can be added to estimate the ability of a rule, or a combination of rules, to identify that error. Table 7.2 gives an example of an empirically developed multirule for a 6-sigma measurement procedure. Such control rules should allow the laboratory to detect errors before they are of a magnitude that will affect clinical decisions. A $10_x$ rule was not used because it would have increased the false-alert rate by 10.6%. A $10_x$ rule or other rule that counts the number of sequential QC results on one side of the target value is not recommended because this condition typically does not indicate a problem with clinical interpretation of patient results when the magnitude of the difference from the target value is small. Counting the number of sequential results that exceed a larger SD from the target value, such as $8_{1.5S}$ in this example, is more likely to represent a measurement condition that might need investigation.

For measurement procedures with small sigma values, small deviations from the expected performance need to be identified. Consequently, more stringent QC practices need to be used such as selecting a $1_{2S}$ rule that will give an alert at smaller error conditions, using additional rules in a multirule set, measuring QC more frequently, using more than two QC samples, and not releasing patient results until QC assessment is complete for the time interval during which patient samples were measured. More stringent QC rules will have more false alerts, but this is an unavoidable cost when lower sigma measurement procedures are used.

### Specifying the Quality Control Plan

The preceding subsections describe the considerations for each component in a QC plan. The laboratory director is responsible for considering the components, making judgments regarding the considerations, and approving the final plan for each analyte measured in a laboratory. A plan for internal QC specifies the following components:

- The number of QC samples to be measured and the approximate concentrations of analytes in those controls
- How to set the target value for each QC sample
- How to set the SD for each QC sample to be used in the QC rules
- The rules for evaluating the QC results
- The frequency to test the QC samples

TABLE 7.1 **Abbreviation Nomenclature for Quality Control Evaluation Rules**

| Rule | Meaning | Detects | Levey-Jennings Chart Examples |
|------|---------|---------|-------------------------------|
| $1_{2S}$ | One observation exceeds 2 SDs from the target value. The $1_{2S}$ rule is not recommended except for low sigma measurement procedures because it has a high false-alert rate. | Bias or imprecision | |
| $1_{3S}$ | One observation exceeds 3 SDs from the target value. | Bias or large imprecision | |

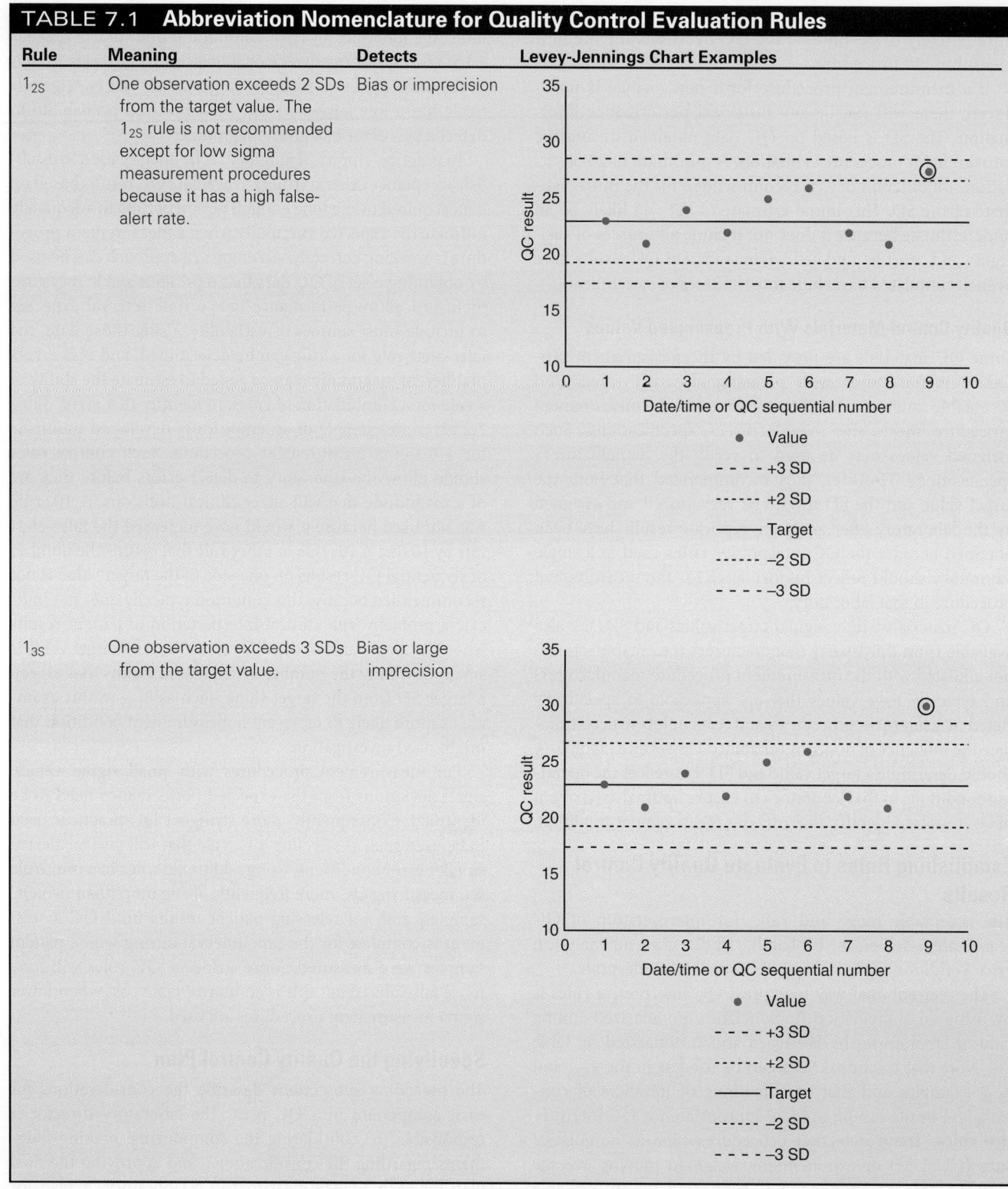

## TABLE 7.1   Abbreviation Nomenclature for Quality Control Evaluation Rules—cont'd

| Rule | Meaning | Detects | Levey-Jennings Chart Examples |
|------|---------|---------|-------------------------------|
| $2_{2S}$ ($2_{2.5S}$) | Observations for two QC samples measured at approximately the same time, or two sequential results for the same QC sample, exceed 2 SDs (or 2.5 SDs) from the target value in the same direction. | Bias | 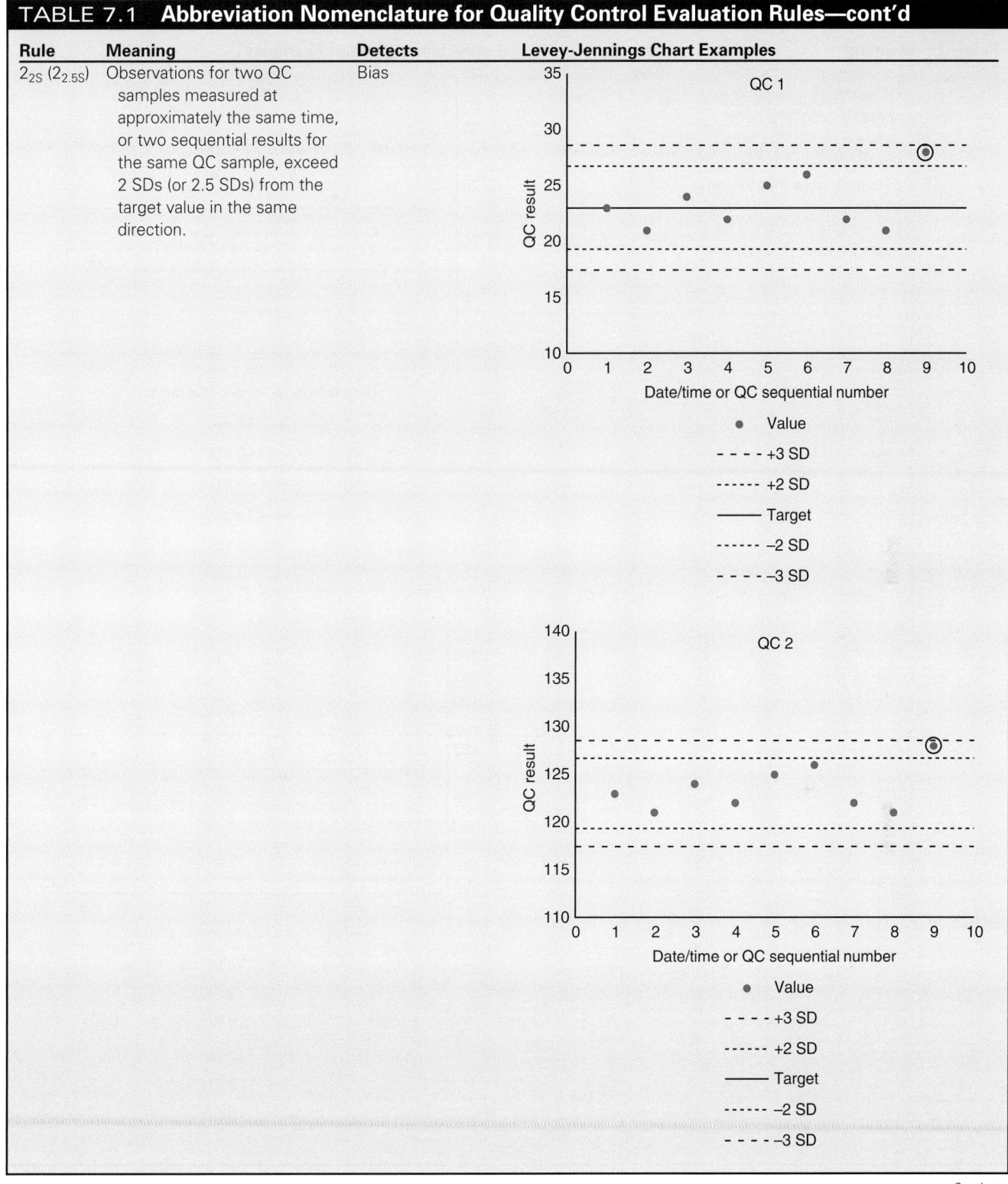 |

*Continued*

## TABLE 7.1    Abbreviation Nomenclature for Quality Control Evaluation Rules—cont'd

| Rule | Meaning | Detects | Levey-Jennings Chart Examples |
|------|---------|---------|-------------------------------|
| 2 of 3$_{2S}$ | Two observations for three QC samples measured at approximately the same time exceed 2 SDs from the target value in the same direction. Note that this type of rule is used when three QC materials are used for a measurement procedure. | Bias | 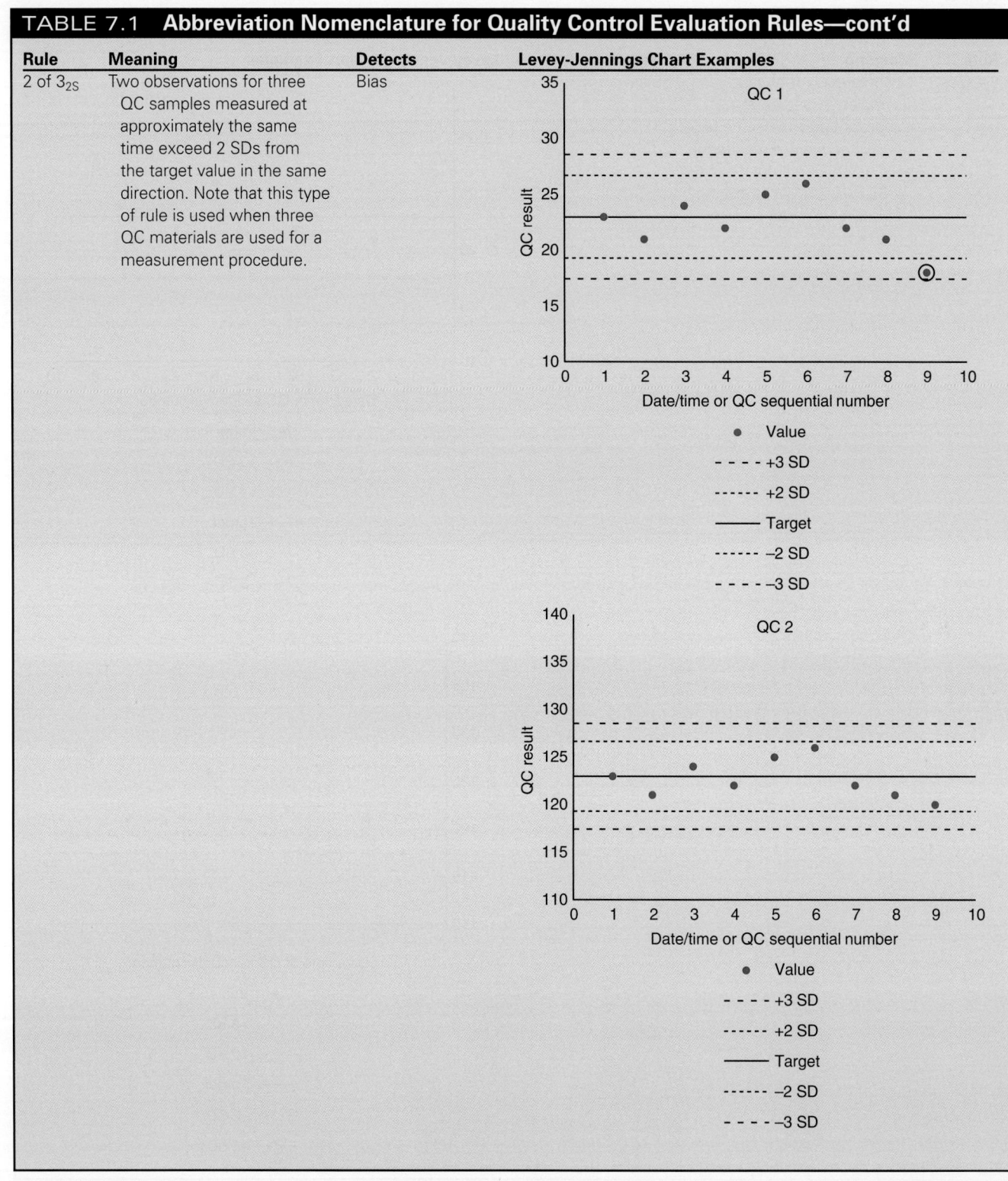 |

## TABLE 7.1 Abbreviation Nomenclature for Quality Control Evaluation Rules—cont'd

| Rule | Meaning | Detects | Levey-Jennings Chart Examples |
|------|---------|---------|-------------------------------|
| | | | 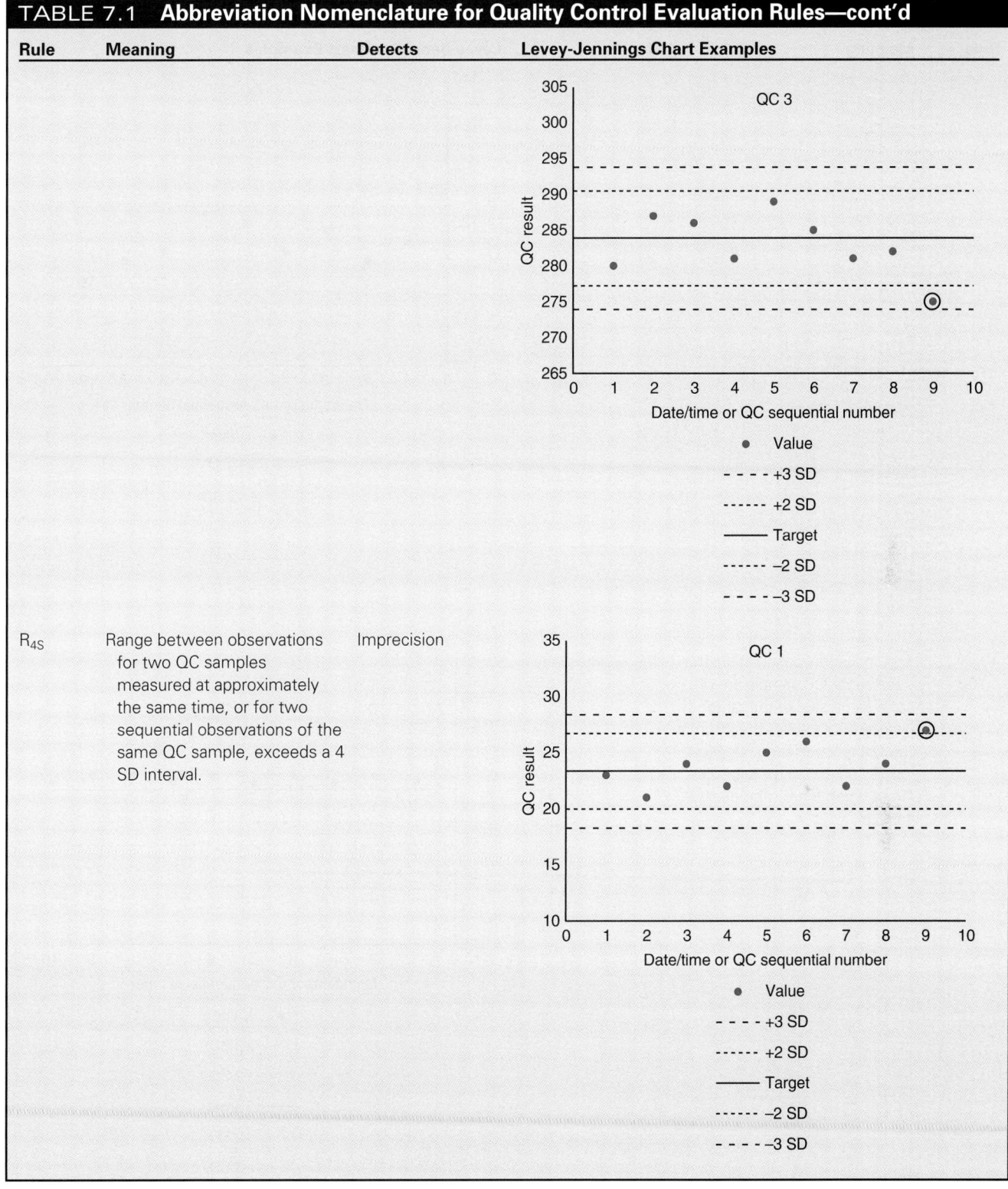 |
| $R_{4S}$ | Range between observations for two QC samples measured at approximately the same time, or for two sequential observations of the same QC sample, exceeds a 4 SD interval. | Imprecision | |

*Continued*

| TABLE 7.1 | Abbreviation Nomenclature for Quality Control Evaluation Rules—cont'd | | |
|---|---|---|---|
| **Rule** | **Meaning** | **Detects** | **Levey-Jennings Chart Examples** |
| | | | 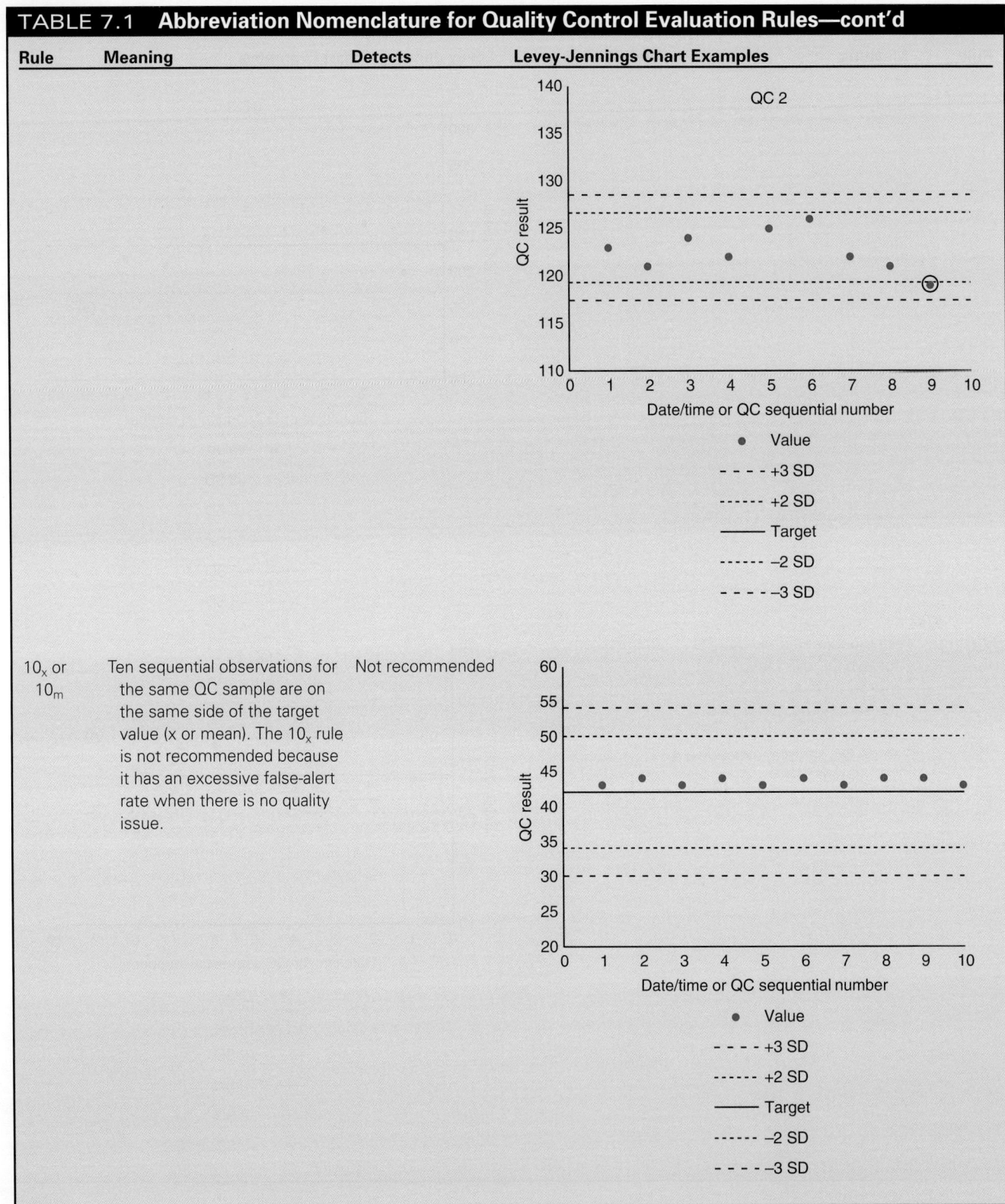 |
| $10_x$ or $10_m$ | Ten sequential observations for the same QC sample are on the same side of the target value (x or mean). The $10_x$ rule is not recommended because it has an excessive false-alert rate when there is no quality issue. | Not recommended | |

## TABLE 7.1  Abbreviation Nomenclature for Quality Control Evaluation Rules—cont'd

| Rule | Meaning | Detects | Levey-Jennings Chart Examples |
|---|---|---|---|
| $8_{1S}$ ($8_{1.5S}$) | Eight sequential observations for the same QC sample exceed 1 SD (or 1.5 SD) in the same direction from the target value. | Bias trend | |
| CUSUM | CUSUM of SDI for the current and previous results. | Bias trend | |

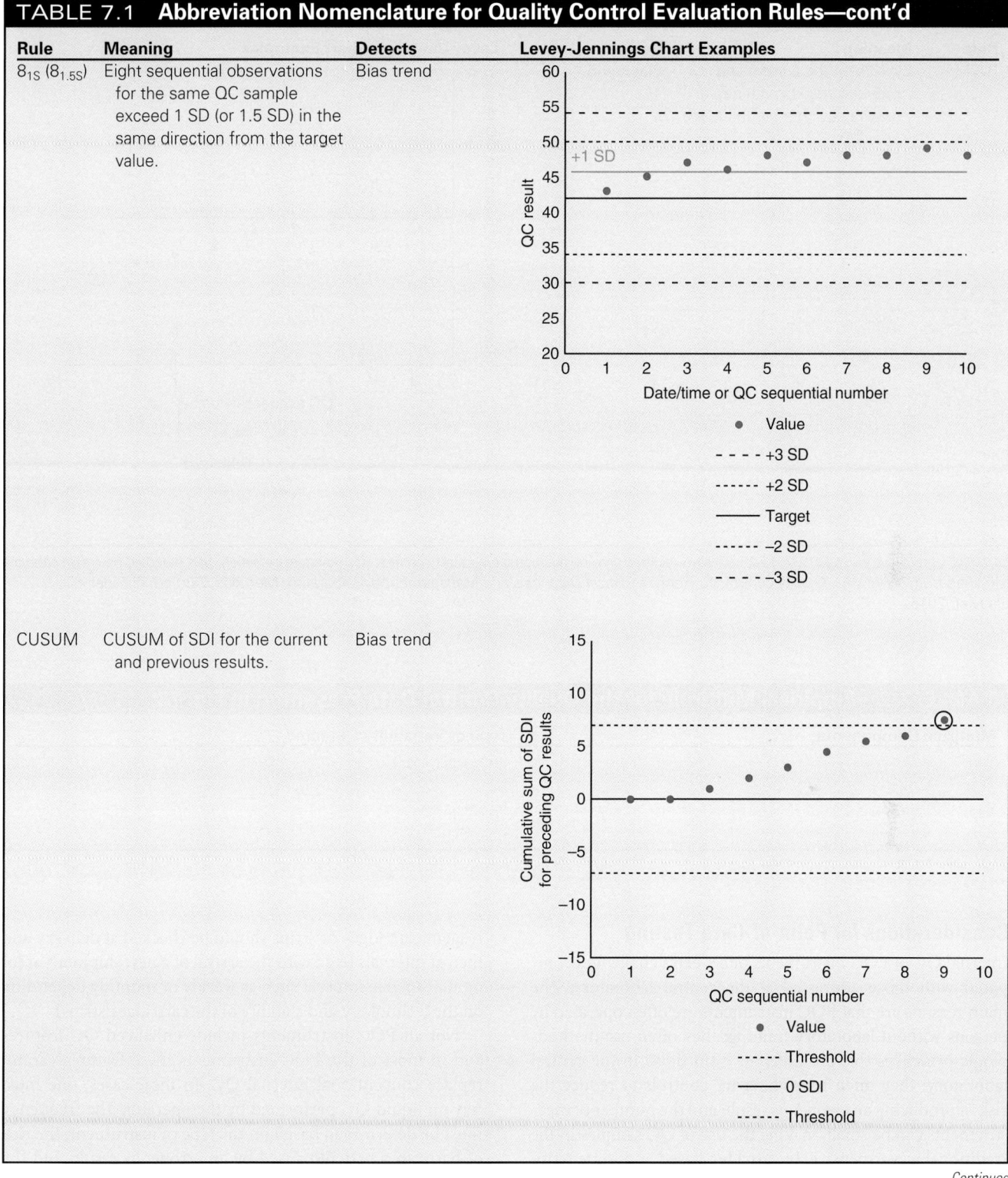

| Rule | Meaning | Detects | Levey-Jennings Chart Examples |
|------|---------|---------|-------------------------------|
| EWMA | EWMA for the current and previous results with newer results having more influence (weight). | Bias trend | 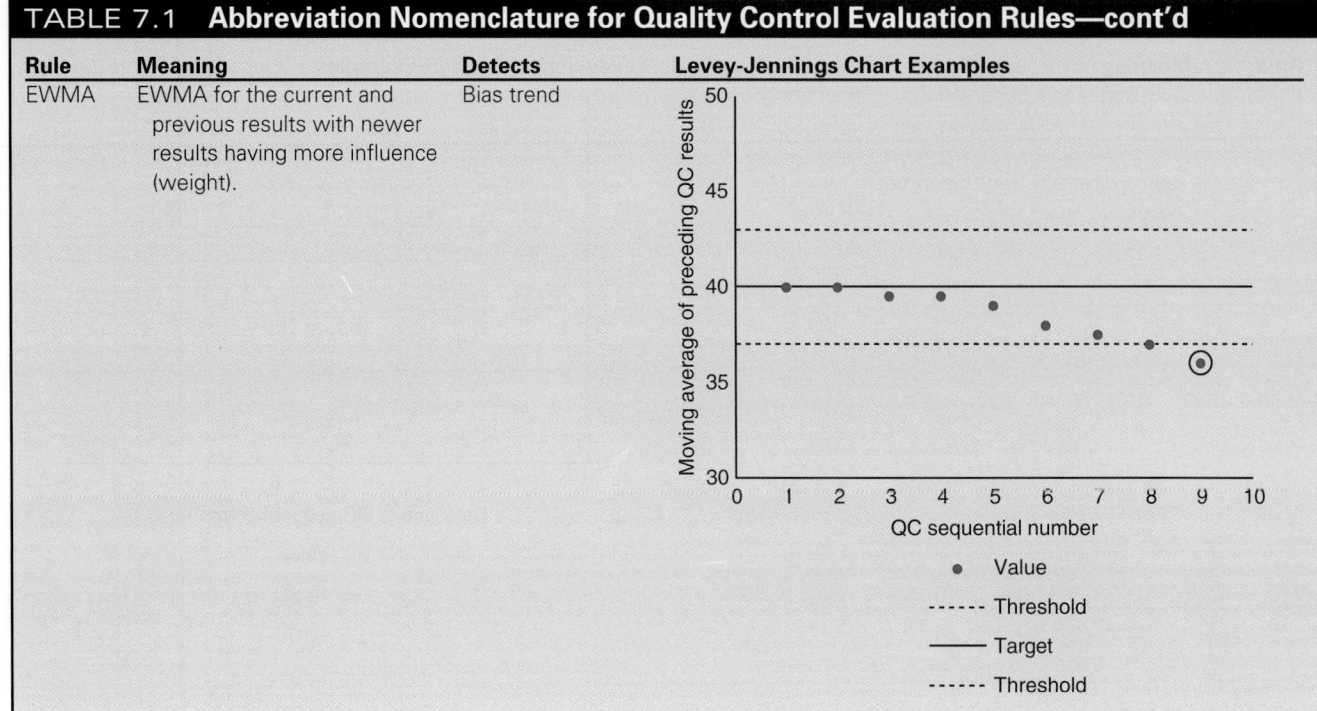 |

*CUSUM*, Cumulative sum; *EWMA*, exponentially weighted moving averages; *QC*, quality control; *SD*, standard deviation; *SDI*, standard deviation interval. Modified from Miller WG. Quality control. In: *Henry's Clinical Diagnosis and Management by Laboratory Methods*. 23rd ed. Philadelphia: Elsevier; 2016.

| Multirule Components | Type of Variability Detected |
|----------------------|------------------------------|
| $1_{3S}$ | Imprecision or bias |
| $2_{2.5S}$ | Bias |
| $R_{4S}$ | Imprecision |
| $8_{1.5S}$ | Bias trend |

**TABLE 7.2   Empirical Multirule for the Quality Control Data Presented in Fig. 7.2**

From Miller WG. Quality control. In: *Henry's Clinical Diagnosis and Management by Laboratory Methods*. 23rd ed. Philadelphia: Elsevier; 2016.

## Considerations for Point-of-Care Testing

Internal QC of POC instruments offers extra challenges compared with those addressed at the central laboratory. The main reasons are that POC instruments are often operated by persons without laboratory training; they often use methodologic principles that are different from those in the central laboratory; they often have "built-in" controls to reduce the risk of producing an erroneous result; and the number of measurements can be small, making the use of QC samples in the traditional way expensive. In cartridge-based and some strip-based instruments, the manufacturer often has placed the technology in the cartridge or strip together with QCs, and in some cases, QC rules are built in so that patient results cannot be reported unless the QC is "satisfactory." The instrument is then merely an electronic reader that often has incorporated an "electronic quality control" that verifies the electronics of the measurement procedure. The electronic instrument checks do not verify the reagents in the cartridges or strips, and unless each cartridge has internal QC materials, the

reagent cartridges or strips should be checked at delivery and then at intervals (e.g., with the arrival of a new shipment or lot or at a suitable interval such as weekly or monthly depending on the technology and stability of the cartridges/strips).

Not all POC instruments include enhanced QC features and in most of the POC instruments these features cannot replace conventional internal QC. In these cases, one must rely on liquid QC performed by the operator. The frequency must be determined based on the type of instrument, the risk of harm to a patient caused by an erroneous result, and the number of samples analyzed. The limitation of using the liquid QC sample in this situation is that it only checks if one disposable cartridge or strip meets the performance specifications. This limitation requires an assumption that all cartridges or strips in a lot were manufactured uniformly and will perform equivalently.

How internal QC should be performed and supervised also depends on the location of the POC instruments. In a hospital, it is now possible with real-time bidirectional connectivity

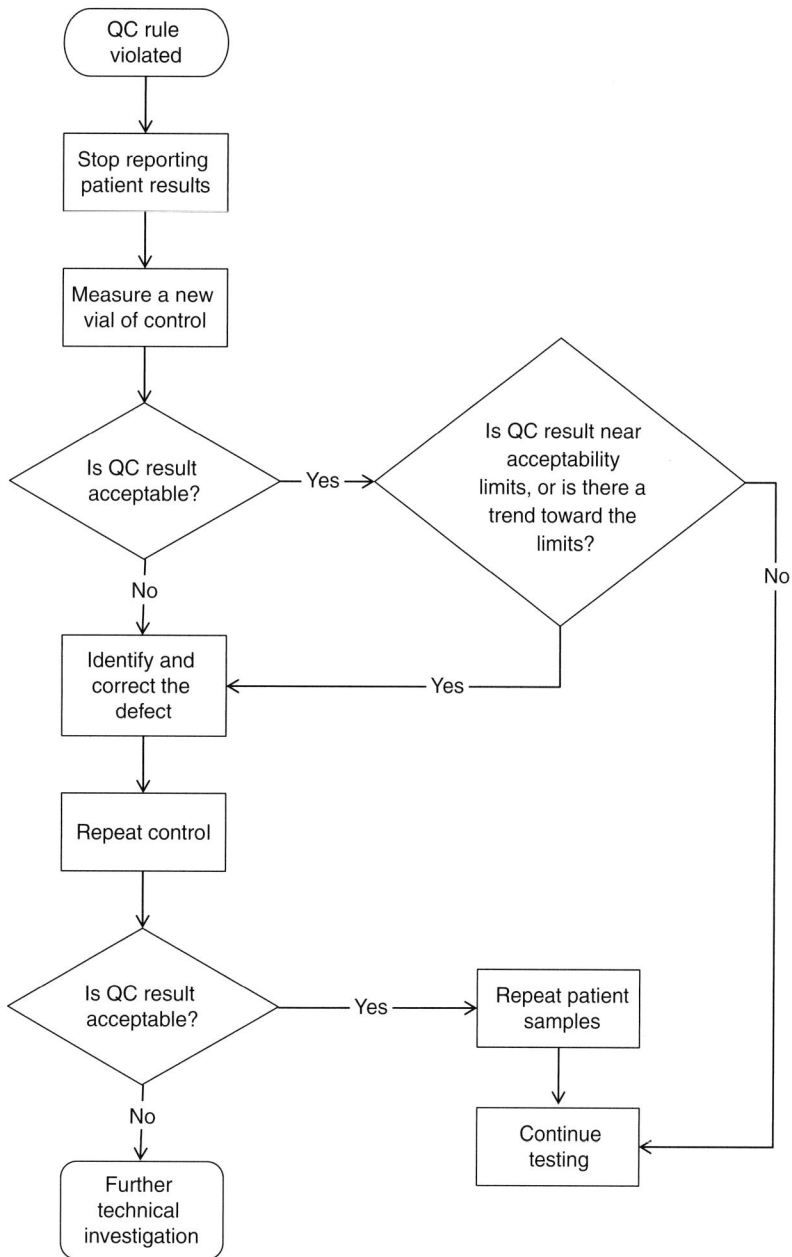

**Fig. 7.6** Generalized troubleshooting sequence showing the initial steps after an unacceptable quality control (QC) result. The details of troubleshooting the defect may be different for different rules violations or if more than one unacceptable QC result was obtained.

between the POC devices and the central laboratory to transfer both patient and QC results and to set lock-out parameters for conformance to a QC protocol. As technology advances, the general trend is for more sophisticated POC devices with built-in control systems to be incorporated to minimize or prevent the possibility for an incorrect result.

## Corrective Action When a Quality Control Result Indicates a Measurement Problem

A QC alert occurs when a QC result fails an evaluation rule, which indicates that an analytical problem may exist. A QC alert means there is a high probability that the measurement procedure is producing results that have the potential to be unreliable for patient care and testing must be stopped until the problem is resolved. Fig. 7.6 presents a generalized troubleshooting sequence. QC materials can deteriorate after opening because of improper handling and storage or because of unstable analytes. Thus, repeating the measurement on a new vial of the QC material is a useful step to determine if the alert was caused by deteriorated QC material rather than by a measurement procedure problem. In this situation, if the result for the new QC sample is acceptable, testing of patient samples can resume. One caution when the repeat QC result is near acceptability limits is to consider whether the repeat and original results are essentially the same. It is not acceptable to repeat the QC until a value happens to be just within the acceptable limit. In this situation the probability is high that a measurement problem exists, and this possibility should be investigated. In addition, current and preceding QC results should be examined for a trend in bias that indicates a measurement issue that needs to be corrected. These precautions in evaluating repeat results for a new QC sample can be challenging or impossible for automated evaluation by computer systems, thus requiring the laboratory technologist to be vigilant in reviewing results.

When repeat testing of a new QC sample does not resolve the alert situation, the instrument and reagents should be inspected for component deterioration, empty reagent containers, mechanical problems, and so on. In many cases, it will be necessary to recalibrate. When the problem is identified and corrected, QC samples should be measured to verify the correction, and all patient samples since the time of the last acceptable QC results, or the time when the error condition occurred, should be measured again. The laboratory director must establish acceptable criteria to determine if the repeat results agree adequately to permit reporting of original results without issuing a corrected report. Otherwise, corrected results must be reported. The criteria for acceptability of repeated tests are based mainly on the TE$_a$ described earlier with consideration of the measurement procedure performance characteristics.

It may be difficult to establish the time when an error condition occurred and repeating all samples since the last acceptable QC may be the simplest approach. One approach to establish the time when an error condition occurred is to repeat every few samples back to the time of the last acceptable QC results. The repeated results are then compared with acceptable criteria for repeated results agreement to identify a point in time when the error condition occurred. When selecting the samples to repeat, it is important to ensure that a substantial representation of the potentially erroneous samples is repeated and that samples at a concentration consistent with that of the unacceptable QC are represented. Alternatively, groups of 10 patient samples can be repeated, again ensuring that samples at a concentration consistent with that of the unacceptable QC are represented, until all repeat results in at least two sequential groups are within acceptable criteria for repeated results. When the point at which the error condition was likely to have occurred is identified, all patient samples must be repeated from that point until the unacceptable QC result was obtained. Any assessment of the point at which an error condition occurred by repeating selected patient samples has a risk to incorrectly identify that point, and laboratories are encouraged to repeat enough patient samples to have confidence in the assessment.

## Verifying Quality Control Evaluation Parameters After a Reagent Lot Change

Changing reagent lots can cause a shift in QC results when there is no change in results for patient samples. Because the matrix-related noncommutability between a QC material and a reagent can change with a different reagent lot, QC results are not a reliable indicator of a measurement

procedure's performance for patient samples after a reagent lot change. In the example in Fig. 7.7, QC values for the high-concentration control shifted after the change to a new lot of reagents, but there was no change in results for the low control. A comparison of results for a panel of patient samples measured using the new and old reagent lots showed equivalent results. Consequently, the change in QC values for the high-concentration material was due to a difference in matrix-related noncommutability bias between the QC material and each of the reagent lots.

It is necessary to use patient samples to verify the consistency of results between old and new lots of reagents because of the unpredictability of a matrix-related noncommutability bias being present for QC materials. Fig. 7.8 presents a protocol to verify or adjust QC material target values after a reagent lot change. A group of patient samples and the QC samples are measured using both the current (old) and new reagent lots. The first step is to verify that results for a group of patient samples measured with the new reagent lot are consistent with results from the current (old) lot. The patient sample results, not the QC results, provide the basis for verifying that the new reagent lot is acceptable for use. If a problem is identified, the calibration of the new reagent lot must be investigated and corrected, or the new reagent lot may be defective and should not be used. When evaluating the patient results, keep in mind that the calibration of the old reagent lot may have drifted and should be verified before concluding that the new reagent lot is not giving acceptable results for the patient samples.

The number of patient samples to use for verifying the performance of a new reagent lot will depend on the measuring interval, the imprecision of a measurement procedure, and the concentrations at which clinical decisions are made. CLSI document EP26 recommends a minimum of three patient samples and more patient samples depending on the number of important clinical decision concentrations and the imprecision of a measurement procedure. This CLSI guideline

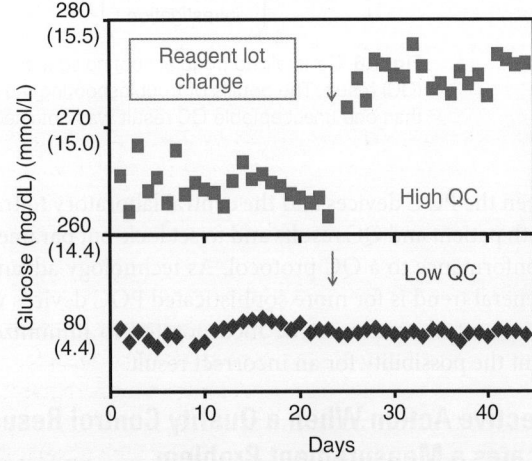

**Fig. 7.7** Levey-Jennings plot showing impact of a reagent lot change on matrix bias with quality control (QC) samples. (Modified with permission from Miller WG, Nichols JH. Quality control. In: Clarke WA, ed. *Contemporary Practice in Clinical Chemistry.* 2nd ed. Washington, DC: AACC Press; 2010.)

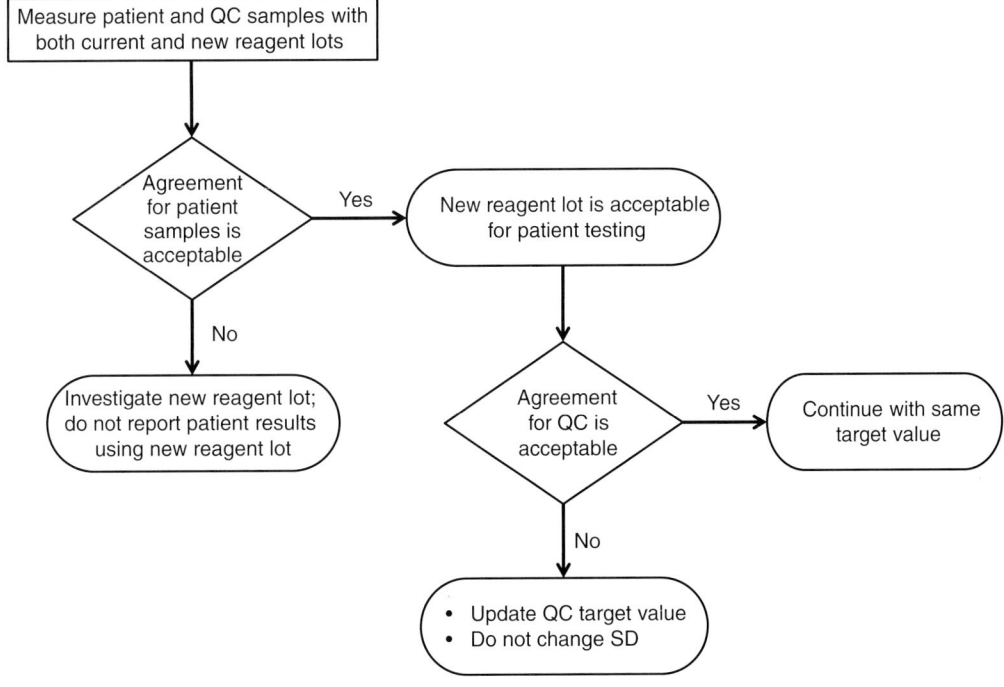

**Fig. 7.8** Process for assessment of potential matrix-related noncommutability bias on quality control (QC) samples after a reagent lot change. *SD*, Standard deviation. (From Miller WG. Quality control. In: *Henry's Clinical Diagnosis and Management by Laboratory Methods.* 23rd ed. Philadelphia: Elsevier; 2016.)

includes a statistical analysis to determine if a difference in patient results is less than a critical difference that would represent risk for an inappropriate patient care decision based on a particular laboratory test result. An alternate approach is to select 5 to 10 patient samples that span the measuring interval and use a difference plot to evaluate average performance over the interval of concentrations represented by the patient samples. The laboratory must establish acceptance criteria for the agreement of patient results for old and new lot measurements consistent with the relatively small number of samples used, the analytical performance characteristics of a measurement procedure, and the clinical requirements for interpreting results.

When the results for patients are acceptable, the second step in Fig. 7.8 evaluates results for each QC material to determine if its target value is correct for use with the new lot of reagent(s). If the target value has changed, it must be adjusted to correct for the change in matrix-related noncommutability bias between old and new lots of reagent(s). This adjustment keeps the expected variability centered around the QC target value so that QC interpretive rules will remain valid.

Failure to make a target value adjustment will cause subsequent QC results to be evaluated incorrectly, as illustrated in Fig. 7.9. The shift in target value would cause some of the results shown by *blue squares* to exceed the old upper QC rule limit, when in reality there is no defect in patient results because the increase in QC results is caused by the matrix-related noncommutability bias with the new reagent lot. Similarly, the increased magnitude of the gap to the old lower QC rule limit will permit a low bias condition, as shown by the *blue square* points at sequence number 29 and 30, to be

undetected. In most cases the SD for a QC material will be the same with any lot of reagent(s).

Note that a reagent lot induced matrix-related noncommutability bias change in the numeric values for the QC results will cause an incorrect increase in the cumulative SD if all results are used for the calculation. For this reason, it is recommended to use the cumulative SD from a single reagent lot or the pooled SD from more than one reagent lot when determining the SD to use for interpreting QC rules.

Experience in clinical laboratories has shown that there are changes, other than reagent lot changes, in measurement procedures that can also affect the QC values but not the results for patient samples. Such changes could be caused by instrument component replacement or other causes. In theory, there should be an assignable cause for such effects, but such a cause is not always identifiable. In practice, any condition that affects QC results but does not affect patient results is treated in the same manner as described for reagent lot changes. The important QC principle is that if the results for patient samples are consistent between the two conditions, then the target value for the QC sample should be adjusted, if necessary, to reflect its value under the new condition. Failure to adjust the QC target value will cause inappropriate acceptability criteria to be used for evaluating the QC results.

## Review of Quality Control Data and the Effectiveness of the Quality Control Plan

The immediate use of QC data is to determine if the results for patient samples can be reported for use in clinical care decisions, as described in the preceding sections. In addition, QC data must be reviewed by laboratory management

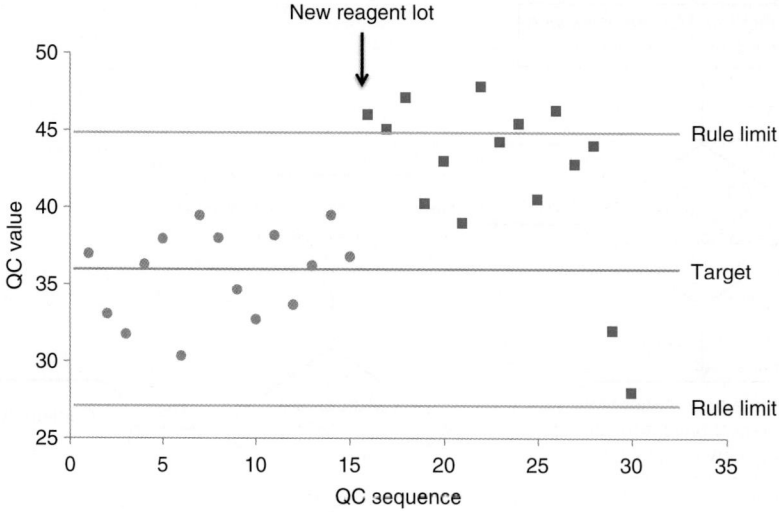

**Fig. 7.9** Illustration of the influence on the failure rate for a quality control (QC) rule when failing to adjust the target value for a matrix-related shift. QC results before a new reagent lot are shown as *gray circles* and after the new reagent lot as *blue squares*. (From Miller WG. Quality control. In: *Henry's Clinical Diagnosis and Management by Laboratory Methods*. 23rd ed. Philadelphia: Elsevier; 2016.)

on a regular schedule. Typical review schedules are weekly by senior technologists or supervisors and at least monthly by the laboratory director. However, the laboratory director or supervisor should promptly review items such as reagent or calibrator lot change validations, changes in QC target values associated with reagent lot or other changes, EQA/PT results review, and other occurrences that may affect quality of the laboratory results.

The weekly review process should determine that correct follow-up of any QC alerts was conducted, that all patient samples that may have had erroneous results were repeated, that any corrected reports were issued, and that the process was properly documented in QC records. The monthly review should include any issues identified by the weekly review process, as well as examination of the Levey-Jennings chart or a computer-based report, to identify trends or changes in assay performance that may need to be addressed before they have effects on clinical care decisions. Note that automated systems to assist in the review of QC data are acceptable, and individual Levey-Jennings charts do not need to be examined every month. The monthly review should also include any adjustments made to QC parameters or the QC plan for a measurement procedure during the month.

> **POINTS TO REMEMBER**
>
> - Internal QC samples are measured along with patient samples.
> - The target value and SD expected for a QC sample are established by the laboratory.
> - Results from QC samples are evaluated using interpretive rules that are established after considering the probability for false alerts and the probability for detecting errors that represent a risk of harm to a patient.

## EXTERNAL QUALITY ASSESSMENT OR PROFICIENCY TESTING

EQA/PT is used to evaluate measurement procedure performance by comparing a laboratory's results with those of other laboratories for the same set of samples. An EQA/PT provider circulates a set of samples among a group of laboratories that can be several thousand in larger programs. Each laboratory measures the EQA/PT samples as if they were patient samples and reports the results to the EQA/PT provider for evaluation. The EQA/PT provider establishes target values for the EQA/PT samples and determines if the results for an individual laboratory are in close enough agreement with the target value to be consistent with acceptable measurement procedure performance.

EQA/PT is not available for some analytes because a particular measurement procedure may be new to the clinical laboratory or is not commonly performed, or because analyte stability makes it difficult to include in an EQA/PT sample. In these situations, the laboratory should use an alternate approach to periodically verify acceptable performance of the measurement procedure. CLSI guideline GP27 provides approaches for verifying measurement procedure performance when formal EQA/PT is not available.

Internal QC material manufacturers may provide a data analysis service that compares results from different laboratories using the same QC material by calculating group statistics for performance evaluation. As with EQA/PT evaluation, this type of interlaboratory QC data analysis allows a laboratory to verify that it is producing QC results that are consistent with those of other laboratories using the same measurement procedure. This information can be helpful for troubleshooting measurement procedure issues and for assessing performance of a new measurement procedure being introduced to a laboratory.

## External Quality Assessment or Proficiency Testing Programs That Use Commutable Samples

EQA/PT programs that use commutable samples are preferred whenever available. Commutable samples are typically prepared by using an individual donor's specimen or by pooling clinical patient samples with minimal processing or additives to avoid alteration of the sample matrix. When commutable EQA/PT samples can be prepared, the results reflect what would be expected if individual patient samples were sent to each of the different laboratories. Thus, agreement among different laboratories and measurement procedures (harmonization) can be correctly evaluated. The agreement between an individual laboratory result and a reference measurement procedure result gives an assessment of correct calibration for the laboratory. The agreement between an individual laboratory result and an all-methods mean gives an assessment of harmonization of results with other measurement procedures. The agreement between a measurement procedure group mean value and the reference measurement procedure result gives an assessment of trueness and calibration traceability for the measurement procedure group. In addition, the agreement between a measurement procedure group mean value and an all results mean gives an assessment of harmonization of results. The information for measurement procedure groups is of particular interest to the producers of measurement procedures and can be used as part of a surveillance program for the calibration traceability scheme.

## External Quality Assessment or Proficiency Testing Programs That Use Noncommutable Samples

The materials commonly used for EQA/PT samples are derived from blood, urine, or other body fluids but are altered in the process to manufacture EQA/PT samples such that the matrix is modified, and the samples frequently do not have the same measurement characteristics as observed for unaltered clinical patient samples. In addition, some EQA/PT samples (e.g., urine, cerebrospinal fluid, or blood gas) are prepared as synthetic materials that are not derived from patient fluids. Consequently, many EQA/PT samples, as for QC samples, are noncommutable with authentic patient samples. The results for a noncommutable EQA/PT sample will have a different relationship in their numeric values between different measurement procedures and sometimes for different reagent lots within a measurement procedure than would be observed for patient samples.

It is a common practice for EQA/PT providers to organize results for noncommutable samples into "peer groups" of measurement procedures that represent similar technology expected to have the same result for a noncommutable EQA/PT sample. The mean or median value of the peer group results is the target value. Because the peer group mean value may be influenced by a matrix-related noncommutability bias, that mean value can be used only to evaluate laboratories using the same or very similar measurement procedures and cannot be used to evaluate laboratories using other measurement procedures or to evaluate if results from different measurement procedures agree with each other. If an individual laboratory's results agree with those of the peer group, the individual laboratory can conclude that the measurement procedure was performing similar to other measurement procedures in that group. An individual laboratory cannot use results for noncommutable EQA/PT samples to verify that a measurement procedure is calibrated correctly to be traceable to the reference system for an analyte.

However, even within a peer group using the same measurement procedure, differences can occur because of different reagent lots used by the measurement procedures in different laboratories, since the matrix of the EQA/PT material can influence the results from different reagent lots when the patient samples give similar results. Therefore, in some cases, reagent lots should be registered as part of the EQA/PT reporting, and even reagent lot–specific target values may need to be assigned.

## Reporting External Quality Assessment or Proficiency Testing Results When One Measurement Procedure Is Adjusted to Agree With Another Measurement Procedure

It is good laboratory practice to adjust the calibration of different measurement procedures for the same measurand used within a large hospital system that may have several satellite laboratories or within a collection of several hospitals with the same management structure, so that the results for patient samples are consistent, irrespective of which measurement procedure is used. Such harmonization of results is important for uniform use of reference intervals and decision thresholds within a hospital or clinic system. It is important to report EQA/PT results such that they can be properly evaluated against the peer group target value. The peer group target value will reflect the measurement procedure calibration established by the measurement procedure manufacturer. For an individual laboratory's EQA/PT result to be evaluated against the peer group mean, that individual result must be reported to the EQA/PT provider after removing any calibration adjustments so that the reported result is consistent with the manufacturer's nonadjusted calibration.

The most convenient way to remove a calibration adjustment is to first measure the EQA/PT samples with the calibration adjustment applied to the measurement procedure, as would be the usual measurement process for patient samples. After the measurement, the EQA/PT results should be adjusted "in reverse" by mathematically removing the calibration adjustment factors, and the results should be reported to the EQA/PT provider with any adjustment factors removed. One should not recalibrate the instrument with a new set of calibrators for the purpose of measuring the EQA/PT samples because this practice would violate regulations requiring the EQA/PT material to be measured in the same manner as patient samples. This process to remove adjustment factors permits the EQA/PT sample to be measured in the same manner as patient samples and the numeric result reported to the EQA/PT provider to reflect the measured result using the manufacturer's calibration settings.

## Interpretation of External Quality Assessment or Proficiency Testing Results

Many countries have regulations requiring EQA/PT and specifying the evaluation criteria for acceptable performance. When criteria are set by regulations, an EQA/PT provider is required to use them. When criteria are not set by regulations, the EQA/PT provider sets evaluation criteria on the basis of clinically acceptable performance, biological variation, or the analytical capability of the measurement procedures in use. EQA/PT evaluation criteria are usually designed to evaluate the total error of a single measurement. In some programs, measurements are made several times, and it is possible to separately assess the bias and the imprecision. The acceptability limits for EQA/PT include bias and imprecision components considered acceptable for clinical use of a result, plus other error components that are unique to EQA/PT samples such as between-laboratory variation in calibration; variable

matrix-related noncommutability bias with different lots of reagent within a peer group; uncertainty in the target value; stability variability in the EQA/PT material, both in storage and shipping, and after reconstitution or opening in the laboratory; and homogeneity of the EQA/PT material vials. Consequently, the acceptability limits for EQA/PT samples are frequently larger than what might be expected for clinically acceptable total error with patient samples.

Fig. 7.10 is an example of a typical evaluation report sent to a participating laboratory when noncommutable samples were used. Each reported result is compared with the mean result for the peer group using the same measurement procedure. The report also includes the SD for the distribution of results in the peer group, the number of laboratories in the peer group, and the SDI (also called a $z$-score), which expresses the reported result as the number of SDs it is from the mean value (SDI = [result − mean]/SD). The limits of

External Quality Assessment (Proficiency Testing) Participant Report
Shipment date: 1 May 2015
Evaluation date: 12 June 2015

| Analyte Units Method | Specimen | Reported Result | Mean | SD | Labs (n) | SDI | Limits of Acceptability Lower | Upper |
|---|---|---|---|---|---|---|---|---|
| Calcium | 1 | 9.6 | 9.92 | 0.23 | 587 | −1.4 | 8.9 | 11.0 |
| mg/dL | 2 | 8.8 | 8.86 | 0.26 | 592 | −0.2 | 7.8 | 9.9 |
| Arsenazo dye | 3 | 7.5 | 7.65 | 0.23 | 587 | −0.7 | 6.6 | 8.7 |
| Manufacturer A | 4 | 8.2 | 8.43 | 0.23 | 590 | −1.0 | 7.4 | 9.5 |
| | 5 | 10.8 | 10.87 | 0.25 | 589 | −0.3 | 9.8 | 11.9 |
| Iron | 1 | 190 | 192.5 | 7.0 | 397 | −0.4 | 154 | 232 |
| μg/dL | 2 | 65 | 65.0 | 3.4 | 394 | 0.0 | 51 | 78 |
| Pyridylazo dye | 3 | 74 | 69.2 | 3.2 | 395 | +1.5 | 55 | 83 |
| Manufacturer A | 4 | 124 | 107.9 | 4.6 | 395 | +3.5 | 86 | 130 |
| | 5 | 277 | 260.9 | 8.8 | 396 | +1.8 | 208 | 314 |

A

External Quality Assessment (Proficiency Testing) Participant Report
Shipment date: 1 May 2015
Evaluation date: 12 June 2015

| Analyte Units Method | Specimen | Reported Result | Mean | SD | Labs (n) | SDI | Limits of Acceptability Lower | Upper |
|---|---|---|---|---|---|---|---|---|
| Calcium | 1 | 2.40 | 2.48 | 0.06 | 587 | −1.4 | 2.22 | 2.74 |
| mmol/L | 2 | 2.20 | 2.21 | 0.06 | 592 | −0.2 | 1.95 | 2.47 |
| Arsenazo dye | 3 | 1.87 | 1.91 | 0.06 | 587 | −0.7 | 1.65 | 2.17 |
| Manufacturer A | 4 | 2.05 | 2.10 | 0.06 | 590 | −1.0 | 1.85 | 2.37 |
| | 5 | 2.69 | 2.71 | 0.06 | 589 | −0.3 | 2.45 | 2.97 |
| Iron | 1 | 34.0 | 34.5 | 1.3 | 397 | −0.4 | 27.6 | 41.5 |
| μmol/L | 2 | 11.6 | 11.6 | 0.6 | 394 | 0.0 | 9.1 | 14.0 |
| Pyridylazo dye | 3 | 13.3 | 12.4 | 0.6 | 395 | +1.5 | 9.8 | 14.9 |
| Manufacturer A | 4 | 22.2 | 19.3 | 0.8 | 395 | +3.5 | 15.4 | 23.3 |
| | 5 | 49.6 | 46.7 | 1.6 | 396 | +1.8 | 37.2 | 56.2 |

B

**Fig. 7.10** Example of an external proficiency testing evaluation report sent to a participating laboratory. Part (A) uses conventional units and (B) uses SI units. *SD,* Standard deviation; *SDI,* standard deviation interval. (From Miller WG. Quality control. In: *Henry's Clinical Diagnosis and Management by Laboratory Methods.* 23rd ed. Philadelphia: Elsevier; 2016.)

acceptability are shown. Acceptability criteria may be a number of SDs from the mean value, a fixed percent from the mean value, or a fixed concentration from the mean value. For example, in Fig. 7.10, calcium acceptability criteria are ±1 mg/dL (0.25 mmol/L) from the mean value, and iron criteria are ±20% from the mean value.

In Fig. 7.10 the calcium results are in close agreement with the peer group mean (SDI ranges from −0.2 to −1.4), and the laboratory can conclude that its results are consistent with those of others in the peer group using the same measurement procedure and that it is using the measurement procedure according to the manufacturer's specifications. However, the iron results show greater variability, with one result +3.5 SDI. Although all iron results are within the acceptability criteria, it is recommended to investigate the measurement procedure because a +3.5 SDI is more likely to be different from other participants in the peer group than to be in agreement with them.

Fig. 7.11 shows another type of evaluation report sent to a primary care office for hemoglobin $A_{1c}$ (HbA$_{1c}$) for one of two EQA/PT samples. In this situation the EQA/PT provider is communicating directly with the clinician or the coworker in the general practice office, and the feedback must be easy to understand for nonlaboratory professionals. The EQA/PT result is evaluated as "good," "acceptable," or "poor." The lot numbers of the reagent are registered so that the participant, in case of an aberrant result, can get information if the result was due to the measurement procedure used, the reagent lot used, or the performance of the user.

Fig. 7.12 shows a similar report from the same HbA$_{1c}$ survey provided to hospital laboratories. In addition to the figures about the distribution of results, information is provided on how different measurement procedures performed, as well as a historical overview of performance on consecutive EQA/PT samples and performance related to the concentration of the sample. The EQA/PT material used for the HbA$_{1c}$ is pooled fresh patient blood (commutable), and the target value is set by a reference measurement procedure and is therefore the same for all measurement procedures. Each sample was measured in duplicate (as requested by the EQA/PT provider), and the mean of the duplicate was used to estimate bias versus the reference measurement procedure. In the present example the performance was within the acceptability limits but with a generally high bias during the whole period. Because this observation was true for all the instruments using this measurement procedure, the EQA/PT organizer discussed the results with the manufacturer to solve the problem. Until the problem was solved (the manufacturer had to make a new calibrator), the participants were advised by the EQA/PT provider to use a correction factor when reporting their results for patient samples.

If an unacceptable EQA/PT result is identified, the measurement procedure must be investigated for possible causes and the necessary corrective and preventive action taken. Even when an EQA/PT result is within acceptability criteria, it is a good laboratory practice to investigate results that are more than approximately 2.5 SDI from the target value.

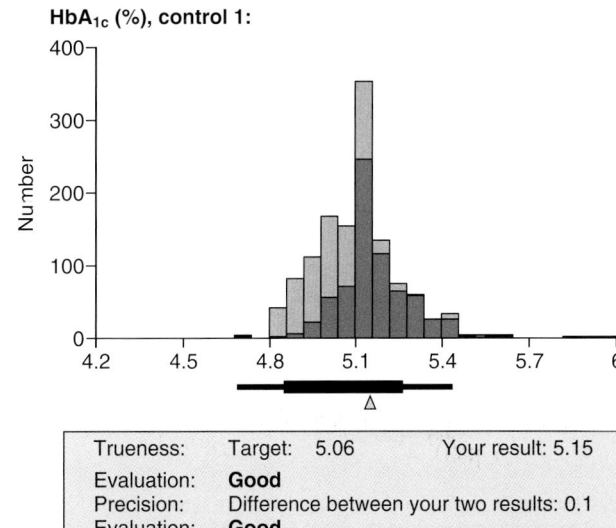

**HbA$_{1c}$ (%), control 1:**

| Trueness: | Target: | 5.06 | Your result: 5.15 |
|---|---|---|---|
| Evaluation: | **Good** | | |
| Precision: | Difference between your two results: 0.1 | | |
| Evaluation: | **Good** | | |

**Fig. 7.11** Example of part of a feedback report to hemoglobin A$_{1c}$ (HbA$_{1c}$) point-of-care (POC) users in a survey for general practitioners' offices and nursing homes. Commutable external quality assessment/proficiency testing material was circulated in two levels and measured in duplicate. The participant is informed about the bias (mean of the two results) compared with a reference measurement procedure target *(x-axis)* and "precision" as the difference between the two results. The histogram represents the distribution of results among all participants *(light blue)* and for the participant's method group *(dark blue)*. The thick black line represents the interval for "good" results, and the thin black line represents the interval for "acceptable" results. Results outside these limits are characterized as "poor." The triangle points to the result of the participant. (Modified with permission from the Norwegian Organization for Quality Improvement of Laboratory Exminations, the external quality assessment provider in Norway.)

When the SDI is 2.5, there is only a 0.6% probability that the result will be within the expected distribution of results; consequently, the probability is reasonable that a measurement procedure problem may need to be corrected.

Common causes for EQA/PT failure are listed in Box 7.1. Incorrect handling and reporting are unique to EQA/PT events and may not reflect the process used in the laboratory for patient samples. Because the influence of reagent lots on noncommutability related bias is well documented, a reagent lot-specific bias is a possible explanation when no other root cause can be identified.

---

## POINTS TO REMEMBER

- An independent external organization circulates EQA/PT samples with unknown target values.
- When commutable "patient-like" material is used, a laboratory can compare its results with results from all other measurement procedures and often with a true value from a reference measurement procedure.
- When noncommutable material is used, a laboratory can compare its results only with results from participants in a "peer group" using a similar measurement procedure.

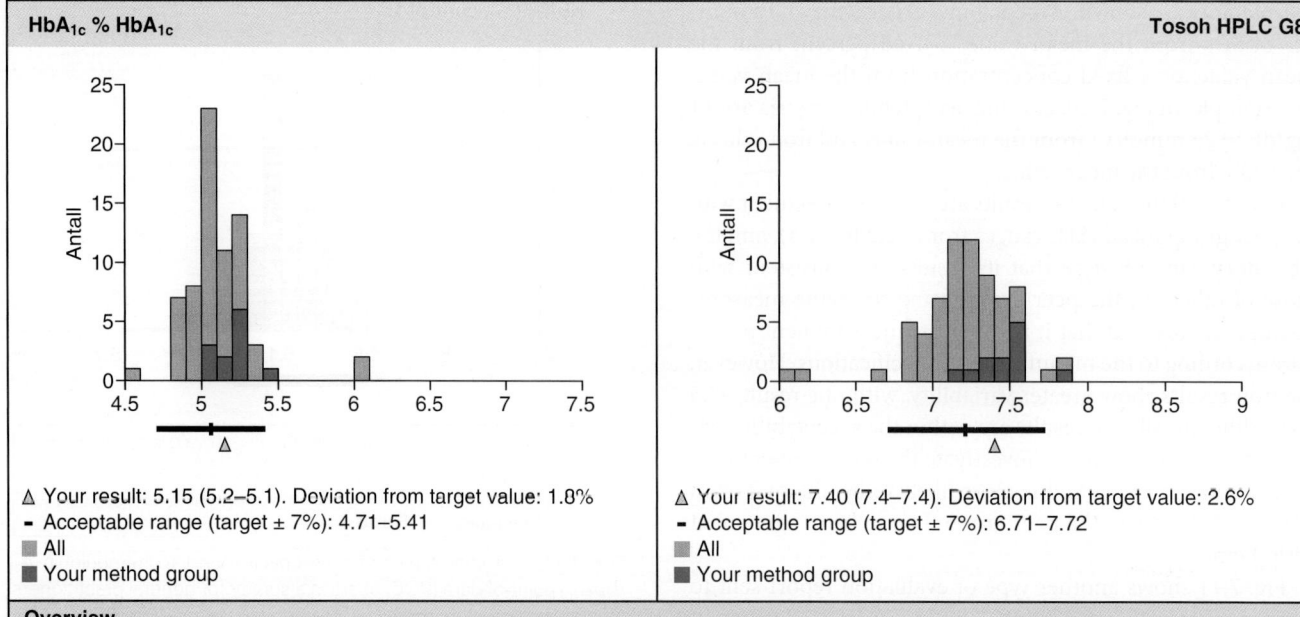

**HbA₁c % HbA₁c**                                                                 **Tosoh HPLC G8**

△ Your result: 5.15 (5.2–5.1). Deviation from target value: 1.8%
- Acceptable range (target ± 7%): 4.71–5.41
▪ All
▪ Your method group

△ Your result: 7.40 (7.4–7.4). Deviation from target value: 2.6%
- Acceptable range (target ± 7%): 6.71–7.72
▪ All
▪ Your method group

**Overview**

| Method group | 1-SHA115 | | | | | 2-SHA115 | | | | |
|---|---|---|---|---|---|---|---|---|---|---|
| | Median | SD | CV | n | nₓ | Median | SD | CV | n | nₓ |
| Afinion | 5.20 | | | 1 | 0 | 7.40 | | | 1 | 0 |
| Architect ci8200/c8000 | 5.00 | | | 4 | 1 | 7.18 | | | 4 | 1 |
| Biorad D10/Variant HPLC/Turbo | 5.00 | 0.107 | 2.1 | 8 | 0 | 7.23 | 0.113 | 1.6 | 8 | 0 |
| Cobas. Tina-quant | 5.00 | 0.200 | 4.0 | 21 | 2 | 7.20 | 0.268 | 3.7 | 21 | 2 |
| DCA 2000/2000+/Vantage | 5.00 | 0.130 | 2.6 | 20 | 0 | 7.08 | 0.216 | 3.1 | 20 | 0 |
| Dimension Vista 1500 | 5.25 | | | 1 | 0 | 7.70 | | | 1 | 0 |
| Tosoh HPLC G7/G8 | 5.20 | 0.108 | 2.1 | 12 | 0 | 7.45 | 0.186 | 2.5 | 12 | 0 |
| | | | | | | | | | | |
| | | | | | | | | | | |
| | | | | | | | | | | |
| | | | | | | | | | | |
| **Total** | **5.05** | **0.157** | **3.1** | **67** | **3** | **7.20** | **0.246** | **3.4** | **67** | **3** |

**History:  Deviation from target value (%)**                    **Deviation from target value (concentration)**

| Survey | Target | Result | Deviation | Instrument |
|---|---|---|---|---|
| 2015.1 | 5.06 | 5.15 | 1.8 | TOSG8 |
| 2015.1 | 7.21 | 7.40 | 2.6 | TOSG8 |
| 2014.4 | 5.71 | 5.85 | 2.5 | TOSG8 |
| 2014.4 | 7.46 | 7.80 | 4.6 | TOSG8 |
| 2014.3 | 5.04 | 5.20 | 3.2 | TOSG8 |
| 2014.3 | 7.46 | 7.80 | 4.6 | TOSG8 |
| 2014.2 | 5.57 | 5.65 | 1.4 | TOSG8 |
| 2014.2 | 7.13 | 7.30 | 2.4 | TOSG8 |
| 2014.1 | 6.34 | 6.35 | 0.2 | TOSG8 |
| 2014.1 | 6.78 | 7.00 | 3.2 | TOSG8 |
| 2013.4 | 5.08 | 5.10 | 0.4 | TOSG8 |
| 2013.4 | 6.84 | 7.10 | 3.8 | TOSG8 |
| 2013.3 | 5.76 | 6.00 | 4.2 | TOSG8 |
| 2013.3 | 6.83 | 7.15 | 4.7 | TOSG8 |
| 2013.2 | 5.06 | 5.20 | 2.8 | TOSG8 |
| 2013.2 | 7.14 | 7.50 | 5.0 | TOSG8 |

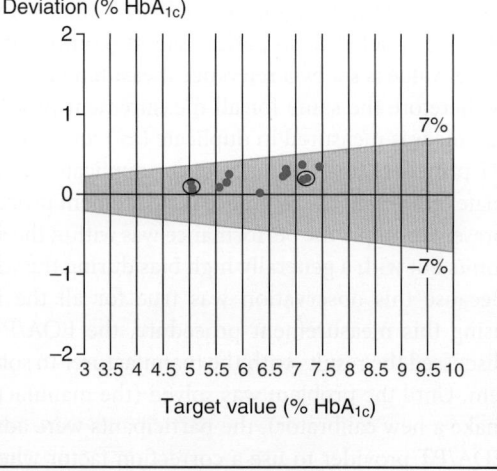

**Fig. 7.12** Example of a part of a feedback report to hemoglobin A₁c (*HbA₁c*) users in hospital laboratories. Same survey and same materials as presented in Fig. 7.11. The histogram represents the distribution of results among all participants *(light blue)* and for the participant's method group *(dark blue)*. Limits for "acceptable" results are given *(black lines in figures)*. Information about performance of measurement procedures is given in addition to a historical overview of percentage deviation from target values dependent on time and concentration of HbA₁c. *CV,* Coefficient of variation; *HPLC,* high-pressure liquid chromatography; *SD,* standard deviation. (Modified with permission from the Norwegian Organization for Quality Improvement of Primary Care Laboratory Examinations, the external quality assessment provider in Norway.)

## BOX 7.1 Classification of Potential Problems Identified When Investigating Unacceptable External Quality Assessment or Proficiency Testing Results[a]

1. Clerical errors
   Incorrectly transcribed EQA/PT result from the instrument read-out to the report form
   The EQA/PT sample was mislabeled in the laboratory
   Incorrect instrument or measurement procedure was reported on the results submission form
   Incorrect units were reported
   Decimal point was misplaced
2. Measurement procedure problems
   Inadequate SOP
   Problem with manufacture or preparation of reagents or calibrators (e.g., unstable)
   Lot-to-lot variation in reagents or calibrators
   Incorrect value assignment of calibrators
   Measurement procedure lacks adequate specificity for the measurand
   Measurement procedure lacks adequate sensitivity to measure the concentration
   Carry-over from a previous sample
   Inadequate QC procedures used
3. Equipment problems
   Obstruction of instrument tubing or orifice by clot
   Misalignment of instrument probes
   Incorrect instrument data processing functions
   Incorrect instrument setting
   Automatic pipetter not calibrated to acceptable precision and accuracy

   Equipment component malfunction (e.g., light source, membrane, fluidics, detector)
   Incorrect instrument conditions (e.g., water quality, surrounding temperature)
   Instrument maintenance not performed appropriately
4. Technical problems caused by personnel errors
   Did not operate equipment correctly or did not conform to measurement procedure SOP
   Incorrect storage, preparation, or handling of reagents or calibrators
   Delay causing evaporation or deterioration of the EQA/PT sample
   Failure to follow recommended instrument function checks or maintenance
   Pipetting or dilution error
   Calculation error
   Misinterpretation of test result
5. A problem with the EQA/PT material such as:
   Incorrect storage, preparation, or handling of EQA/PT materials
   Differences between EQA/PT samples and patient samples (e.g., matrix, additives, stabilizers)
   Sample deteriorated in transit or during laboratory storage
   Sample had weak or borderline reaction
   Sample contained interfering factors (which may be measurement procedure specific)
   Sample was not homogeneous among vials

[a]This classification scheme assists in developing an appropriate corrective action plan.
From Miller WG, Jones GR, Horowitz GL, et al. Proficiency testing/external quality assessment: current challenges and future directions. *Clin Chem.* 2011;57:1670–1680.
*EQA,* External quality assessment; *PT,* proficiency testing; *QC,* quality control; *SOP,* standard operating procedure.

## REVIEW QUESTIONS

1. Why should internal quality control be performed?
   a. To be sure that the quality control material is of good quality
   b. To examine if the control material is commutable—behaves like patient samples
   c. To have a high probability that correct patient results are released
   d. To be able to pass the accreditation inspection
   e. To examine if my measurement procedure gives results similar to other laboratories
2. How should I interpret results when an EQA/PT program uses noncommutable materials?
   a. When my result is within the performance specifications, I can be confident that I have no bias compared with a true value.
   b. When my result is outside the performance specifications, I have to recalibrate my measurement procedure.
   c. When my result is close to the target value for the peers in my measurement procedure group, I can be confident my laboratory is performing as well as my peers.

   d. I should compare my results with results from other measurement procedures to be confident my laboratory is not biased.
   e. I should compare my results with the average of all measurement procedure groups.
3. What is the advantage of using commutable EQA/PT materials? Select all that apply.
   a. They are similar to patient samples and should therefore not be used for QC.
   b. They are suitable for internal quality control but not for EQA/PT.
   c. They should be avoided since they are contagious.
   d. Their results provide information on the accuracy for patient samples if the target value is set by a reference measurement procedure.
   e. Their results can be compared among different measurement procedures to assess harmonization.
4. When should EQA/PT be used?
   a. To decide if patient results can be released
   b. Should be performed every second day

c. To assess the performance of your measurement procedure compared with other measurement procedures

d. Only when the provider uses commutable material

e. Is not necessary if you have documented traceability of your measurement procedure

5. How is the SD estimated for an internal QC material?

a. From measurements made during the target value assignment of a QC material

b. From the long-term SD that includes most types of variability expected to influence the measurement procedure

c. From the instructions for use provided by the measurement procedure manufacturer

d. From reports of interlaboratory summaries

e. From the range of acceptable results provided by the QC material manufacturer

## SUGGESTED READINGS

CLSI. *Laboratory Quality Control Based on Risk Management; Approved Guideline EP23-A*. Wayne, PA: Clinical and Laboratory Standards Institute; 2011.

CLSI. *Statistical Quality Control for Quantitative Measurement Procedures: Principles and Definitions; Approved Guideline C24-A4*. Wayne, PA: Clinical and Laboratory Standards Institute; 2016.

CLSI. *User Evaluation of Between-Reagent Lot Variation; Approved Guideline EP26-A*. Wayne, PA: Clinical and Laboratory Standards Institute; 2013.

CLSI. *Using Proficiency Testing to Improve the Clinical Laboratory; Approved Guideline GP27-A3*. Wayne, PA: Clinical and Laboratory Standards Institute; 2016.

Miller WG. Time to pay attention to reagent and calibrator lots for proficiency testing. *Clin Chem.* 2016;62:666–667.

Miller WG, Erek A, Cunningham TD, et al. Commutability limitations influence quality control results with different reagent lots. *Clin Chem.* 2011;57:76–83.

Miller WG, Jones GR, Horowitz GL, et al. Proficiency testing/external quality assessment: current challenges and future directions. *Clin Chem.* 2011;57:1670–1680.

Miller WG, Sandberg S. Quality control of the analytical examination process. In: Rifai N, Hovath AR, Wittwer CT, eds. *Tietz Textbook of Clinical Chemistry and Molecular Diagnostics*. Elsevier; 2017. chap 6.

Sandberg S, Fraser CG, Horvath AR, et al. Defining analytical performance specifications: Consensus Statement from the 1st Strategic Conference of the European Federation of Clinical Chemistry and Laboratory Medicine. *Clin Chem Lab Med.* 2015;53:833–835.

Stavelin A, Riksheim BO, Christensen NG, et al. The importance of reagent lot registration in external quality assurance/proficiency testing schemes. *Clin Chem.* 2016;62:708–715.

Vesper HW, Miller WG, Myers GL. Reference materials and commutability. *Clin Biochem Rev.* 2007;28:139–147.

# Principles of Basic Techniques and Laboratory Safety

*Stanley Lo and Tahir Pillay\**

## OBJECTIVES

1. Define the following:
   - Analyte
   - Centrifugation
   - Dilution
   - Evaporation
   - Filtration
   - Gravimetry
   - Lyophilization
   - Primary/secondary reference material
   - Relative centrifugal force/field (RCF)
   - Solution
   - Standard precautions
2. Describe three methods of preparing reagent-grade water; identify the criteria for determining when the purification process for Clinical Laboratory Reagent Grade Water is considered acceptable.
3. List and compare the different grades of reagents available, and state which are appropriate for use in a clinical laboratory.
4. Compare the two types of reference materials used in the clinical laboratory, and state the specific uses of each type.
5. List and describe three types of pipettes used in the clinical laboratory; state the proper use and the specific uses of each type.
6. For the process of centrifugation:

   - State the principle.
   - List six uses of centrifugation in the clinical laboratory.
   - Calculate RCF and revolutions per minute (rpm) when given the appropriate information.
   - Determine the time required for centrifugation using an alternate rotor.
   - Outline proper operation and operation practice of a centrifuge.
7. Compare serial dilutions with simple dilutions; state and calculate the formula used to prepare a solution of lesser concentration from one of greater concentration.
8. List and describe the elements of an Occupational Safety and Health Administration (OSHA)-approved chemical hygiene plan, a hazard exposure plan, and a tuberculosis control plan; describe the Standard Precautions document, including source and specific mandates; state the College of American Pathologists (CAP) requirements for a laboratory ergonomics program.
9. For the following hazard types, interpret laboratory hazard signage, and state the appropriate work practice used to control these hazards:
   - Biological
   - Chemical
   - Electrical
   - Fire

## KEY WORDS AND DEFINITIONS

**Analyte** A solute dispersed in a solution that is measured in laboratory practice; also referred to as a **measurand**.

**Buffer solution** A solution that contains either a weak acid and its salt or a weak base and its salt and is resistant to changes in pH.

**Centrifugation** The process of using centrifugal force to separate the lighter portions of a solution from the heavier portions; a centrifuge is a device by which centrifugation is affected.

**Chemical hygiene plan (CHP)** An Occupational Safety and Health Administration (OSHA)-required listing of responsibilities for laboratory employers, employees, and a chemical hygiene officer, and including a complete chemical inventory that is updated annually, along with a copy of the Safety Data Sheet (SDS) that defines each chemical as toxic, carcinogenic, or dangerous, and that must be on file and available to all employees 24 hours a day, 7 days a week.

**Clinical and Laboratory Standards Institute (CLSI)** The CLSI (formerly the National Committee for Clinical Laboratory Standards, or NCCLS) that guides the development and implementation of standards and guidelines that help all laboratories fulfill their goals.

*The authors gratefully acknowledge the original contributions of Drs. Edward W. Bermes, Stephen E. Kahn, Donald S. Young, Edward R. Powsner, and John C. Widman, on which portions of this chapter are based.

**Ergonomics**  The study of capabilities in relationship to work demands is completed by defining postures that minimize unnecessary static work and reduce the forces working on the body.

**Exposure control plan**  An OSHA-required plan that ensures the protection of laboratory workers against potential exposure to bloodborne pathogens, while ensuring that medical wastes produced by the clinical laboratory are managed and handled in a safe and effective manner.

**OSHA**  Occupational Safety and Health Administration, formed by the federal government of the United States to formally regulate the oversight of employee safety.

**Pipette**  Device used for the transfer of a volume of liquid from one container to another.

**Reagent**  Chemical used in many high-purity applications.

**Reference material**  A material or substance, one or more physical or chemical properties of which are sufficiently well established to be used for the calibration of an apparatus, the verification of a measurement method, or the assigning of values to materials. Certified, primary, and secondary are types of reference materials.

**Relative centrifugal force or field (RCF)**  Force required to separate two phases (liquid and solid) in a centrifuge.

**Safety Data Sheet (SDS)**  A technical bulletin that contains information about a hazardous chemical, such as chemical composition, chemical and physical hazard, and precautions for safe handling and use.

**Standard precautions**  Approach to infection control that treats all human blood and certain human body fluids as if they were known to be infectious for bloodborne pathogens.

---

An understanding of basic principles and techniques of analytical chemistry is necessary to appropriately interpret clinical laboratory tests and adequately validate assays. These are integral to understanding basic laboratory tasks such as making **buffer solutions,** performing dilutions, evaporation, and filtration. Safety is a constant concern for laboratory personnel. A comprehensive safety program consisting of a plan for the handling of chemicals, exposure to bloodborne pathogens, tuberculosis (TB), and other highly infectious agents, as well as training to handle various types of hazards is essential.

## CHEMICALS

The quality of the analytical results produced by the laboratory is directly affected by the purity of the chemicals used as analytical **reagents.** The availability and quality of the reference materials used to calibrate assays and to monitor their analytical performance are also important.

Laboratory chemicals are available in a variety of grades. The solutes and solvents used in analytical work are *reagent-grade chemicals,* among which water is a solvent of primary importance.

### Reagent-Grade Water

Preparation of many reagents and solutions used in the clinical laboratory requires "pure" water. Single-distilled water fails to meet the specifications for Clinical Laboratory Reagent Water (CLRW) established by the **Clinical and Laboratory Standards Institute (CLSI).** Because the terms *deionized water* and *distilled water* describe preparation techniques, they should be replaced by reagent-grade water, and, if appropriate, followed by the designation of CLRW, which better defines the specifications of the water and is independent of the method of preparation (Table 8.1).

### Preparation of Reagent-Grade Water

Distillation, ion exchange, reverse osmosis, and ultraviolet (UV) oxidation are processes used to prepare reagent-grade water. In practice, water is filtered before any of these processes are used.

*Distillation.* Distillation is the process of vaporizing and condensing a liquid to purify or concentrate a substance or to separate a volatile substance from less volatile substances. It is the oldest method of water purification. Problems with distillation for preparing reagent water include the carryover of volatile impurities and entrapped water droplets that may contain impurities in the purified water. This results in contamination of the distillate with volatiles, sodium, potassium, manganese, carbonates, and sulfates. As a result, water treated

**TABLE 8.1  Clinical and Laboratory Standards Institute Specifications for Clinical Laboratory Reagent Water**

|  | CLRW |
|---|---|
| Microbiological content[a] (cfu/mL) (maximum) | <10 |
| Resistivity[b] (MΩ/cm), 25°C | ≥10 |
| Particulate matter[c] | Water passed through 0.22-μm filter |
| Total organic content (ng/g) | <500 |

[a]Microbiological content. The microbiological content of viable organisms, as determined by total colony count after incubation at 36 ±1°C for 14 h, followed by 48 h at 25 ±1°C, and reported as colony-forming units per milliliters (cfu/mL).

[b]Specific resistance or resistivity. The electrical resistance in ohms measured between opposite faces of a 1-cm cube of an aqueous solution at a specified temperature. For these specifications, the resistivity will be corrected for 25°C and reported in megaohms per centimeters (MΩ/cm). The higher the quantity of ionizable materials, the lower will be the resistivity and the higher the conductivity.

[c]Particulate matter. When water is passed through a membrane filter with a mean pore size of 0.22 μm, nearly all microorganisms and particulates are removed.

*CLRW,* Clinical Laboratory Reagent Water.

From Clinical and Laboratory Standards Institute. *Preparation and Testing of Reagent Water in the Clinical Laboratory.* 4th ed. CLSI Document GP40-A4-AMD. Wayne, PA: CLSI; 2006.

by distillation alone does not meet the specific conductivity requirement of CLRW.

*Ion exchange.* Ion exchange is a process that removes ions to produce mineral-free deionized water. Such water is most conveniently prepared using commercial equipment, which ranges in size from small, disposable cartridges to large, resin-containing tanks. Deionization is accomplished by passing feed water through columns containing insoluble resin polymers that exchange hydrogen ($H^+$) and hydroxide ($OH-$) ions for the impurities present in the ionized form in the water. The columns may contain cation exchangers, anion exchangers, or a *mixed-bed resin exchanger*, which is a mixture of cation- and anion-exchange resins in the same container.

A single-bed deionizer generally is capable of producing water that has a specific resistance in excess of 1 M$\Omega$/cm. When connected in series, mixed-bed deionizers usually produce water with a specific resistance that exceeds 10 M$\Omega$/cm.

*Reverse osmosis.* Reverse osmosis is a process by which water is forced through a semipermeable membrane that acts as a molecular filter. The membrane removes 95% to 99% of organic compounds, bacteria, other particulate matter, and 90% to 97% of all ionized and dissolved minerals but has fewer of the gaseous impurities. Although this process is inadequate for producing reagent-grade water for the laboratory, it may be used as a preliminary purification method.

*Ultraviolet oxidation.* UV oxidation is another method that works well as part of a total system. The use of UV radiation at the biocidal wavelength of 254 nm eliminates many bacteria and cleaves many ionizing organics that are then removed by deionization.

## Quality, Use, and Storage of Purified Water

Autoclave or wash water (formerly type III water) may be used for glassware washing. However, final rinsing should be done with the water grade suitable for the intended glassware use. It may also be used for certain qualitative procedures, such as those used in general urinalysis. A variety of purification processes can be used to produce this type of water.

The CLRW, formerly described as type I or II water, is used for most routine clinical laboratory testing. Purification processes for CLRW must achieve specific targets for microbial content, resistivity, particulate matter, and total organic content (see Table 8.1). Storage and delivery systems should be constructed to ensure a minimum of chemical or bacterial contamination. The frequency of monitoring of water specifications and the purification system is to be determined by each laboratory.

Special reagent water is used for specific applications. At a minimum, the water should meet CLRW specifications; however, additional parameters may be needed for certain applications. For example, water used for DNA and RNA testing may have specifications for protease and nuclease activity. Water used in trace metal analysis should contain minimally detectable amounts of each metal being measured.

### Testing for Water Purity

At a minimum, water should be tested for microbiological content, particulates, resistivity, and total organic content. Protocols for testing the purity of water can be found in CLSI GP40-A4-AMD:2012. The frequency of monitoring water purity should be established by the laboratory, such that water purity is maintained for its intended purpose. It should be noted that measurements taken at the time of production may differ from those taken at the time and place of use. For example, if the water is piped a long distance, consideration must be given to deterioration en route to the site of use. To meet the specifications for high-performance liquid chromatography (HPLC), in some instances it may be necessary to add a final 0.1-$\mu$m membrane filter. The water can be tested by HPLC using a gradient program and monitored with a UV detector. No peaks exceeding the analytical noise of the system should be found.

### Reagent-Grade or Analytical Reagent-Grade Chemicals

Chemicals that meet specifications of the American Chemical Society are described as reagent or analytical reagent grade. These specifications have also become the de facto standards for chemicals used in many high-purity applications. These are available in two forms: (1) lot-analyzed reagents, in which each individual lot is analyzed and the actual amount of impurity reported, and (2) maximum impurities reagents, for which maximum impurities are listed. The Committee on Analytical Reagents of the American Chemical Society periodically publishes "Reagent Chemicals," which is a list of specifications (https://pubs.acs.org/isbn/9780841230460#). These reagent-grade chemicals are of very high purity and are recommended for quantitative or qualitative analyses.

### Ultrapure Reagents

Many analytical techniques require reagents whose purity exceeds the specifications of those described previously. Manufacturers offer selected chemicals that have been specially purified to meet specific requirements. There is no uniform designation for these chemicals and organic solvents. Terms such as *spectrograde*, *nanograde*, and *HPLC pure* have been used. Data of interest to the user (e.g., absorbance at a specific UV wavelength) are supplied with the reagent.

Other designations of chemical purity include chemically pure (CP), US Pharmacopeia (USP), and National Formulary (NF) grade (chemicals produced to meet specifications set down in the USP or the NF). Chemicals labeled purified, practical, technical, or commercial grade should not be used in clinical chemical analysis without previous purification.

## REFERENCE MATERIALS

A **reference material** is a material or substance with one or more physical or chemical properties that is sufficiently well established to be used for (1) calibrating instruments, (2) validating methods, (3) assigning values to materials, and (4) evaluating the comparability of results. Reference materials are of prime importance in establishing *metrologic transferability*, a term defined as "the property of a measurement result whereby the result can be related to a reference through a documented unbroken chain of calibrations, each contributing to the measurement uncertainty."

Primary, secondary, standard, and certified are types of reference materials.

### Primary Reference Materials

Primary reference materials are highly purified chemicals that are directly weighed or measured, and dissolved in a solvent with an exactly measured total volume after the chemical has gone completely into solution, to produce a solution whose concentration is exactly known. The International Union of Pure and Applied Chemistry (IUPAC) has proposed a degree of 99.98% purity for primary reference materials. These highly purified chemicals may be weighed out directly for the preparation of solutions of selected concentration or for the calibration of solutions of unknown strength. They are supplied with a certificate of analysis for each lot.

### Secondary Reference Materials

Secondary reference materials are solutions whose concentrations cannot be prepared by weighing the solute and dissolving a known amount into a volume of solution. The concentration of secondary reference materials is usually determined by analysis of an aliquot of the solution by an acceptable reference method, using a primary reference material to calibrate the method.

### Standard Reference Materials

Standard reference materials (SRMs) for clinical and molecular laboratories are available from the National Institute of Standards and Technology (NIST; http://www.nist.gov). Cholesterol, the first SRM developed by the NIST, was issued in 1967. It should be noted that not all SRMs have the properties and the degree of purity specified for a primary standard, but each has been well characterized for certain chemical or physical properties and is issued with a certificate that provides results of the characterization. These may then be used to characterize other materials.

### Certified Reference Materials

Certified reference materials (CRMs) are available for clinical and molecular laboratories from the Institute for Reference Materials and Measurents (IRMM) in Geel, Belgium (https://crm.jrc.ec.europa.eu/s/18/About-us). The IRMM

is one of the seven institutes of the Joint Research Centre (JRC), a Directorate-General of the European Commission (EC). Other acronyms used to label IRMM reference materials include European Reference Materials (ERM) and BCR (Community Bureau of Reference of the Commission of the European Communities). Reference materials are also available from the World Health Organization (WHO; http://www.who.int/biologicalshttps://www.who.int/teams/health-product-policy-and-standards/standards-and-specifications/catalogue).

---

**POINTS TO REMEMBER**

**Ultrapure Reagents**
There are several types of ultrapure reagents. For the clinical laboratory, they are referred to as reference materials. There are several different types of reference materials:
- Primary reference materials
- Secondary reference materials
- Standard reference materials
- Certified reference materials

---

## BASIC TECHNIQUES AND PROCEDURES

Basic practices used in clinical laboratories include (1) optical, (2) chromatographic, (3) electrochemical, (4) electrophoretic, (5) mass spectrometric, (6) enzymatic, and (7) immunoassay techniques. These techniques are discussed in detail in Chapters 9 through 15. This chapter discusses the basic techniques of volumetric sampling and dispensing, centrifugation, gravimetry, thermometry, and processing solutions.

### Volumetric Sampling and Dispensing

Clinical chemistry procedures require accurate volumetric measurements to ensure accurate results. For accurate work, only class-A glassware should be used. Class A glassware is certified to conform to the specifications outlined in NIST circular C-602.

#### Pipettes

**Pipettes** are used for the transfer of a volume of liquid from one container to another. They are designed either (1) to contain a specific volume of liquid or (2) to deliver a specified volume. Pipettes used in clinical laboratories include (1) manual transfer and measuring pipettes, (2) micropipettes, and (3) electronic and mechanical pipetting devices. Developments in improved design of pipetting systems include robotic automation, the capability to provide electronic and personal computer control of pipetting devices, and careful attention to advanced ergonomic design features. Automatic photometric pipette calibration systems are also available that reduce the time needed to periodically check pipettes and potentially allow more efficient use of personnel.

*Transfer and measuring pipettes.* A transfer pipette is designed to transfer a single known volume of liquid. Measuring and serologic pipettes are scored in units such that any volume up to a maximum capacity is delivered.

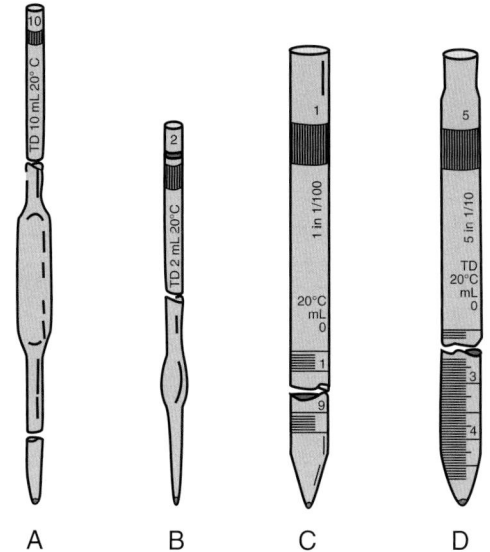

**Fig. 8.1** Pipettes. (A) Volumetric (transfer); (B) Ostwald-Folin (transfer); (C) Mohr (measuring); (D) serologic (graduated to the tip).

**Transfer pipettes.** Transfer pipettes include both volumetric and Ostwald-Folin pipettes (Fig. 8.1). They consist of a cylindrical bulb joined at both ends to narrower glass tubing. A calibration mark is etched around the upper suction tube, and the lower delivery tube is drawn out to a gradual taper. The bore of the delivery orifice should be sufficiently narrow to allow rapid outflow of liquid, without incomplete drainage causing measurement errors beyond the specified tolerances.

A volumetric transfer pipette (see Fig. 8.1A) is calibrated to accurately deliver a fixed volume of a dilute aqueous solution. The reliability of the calibration of the volumetric pipette decreases with decreased size, and therefore special micropipettes have been developed.

Ostwald-Folin pipettes (see Fig. 8.1B) are similar to volumetric pipettes, but they have the bulb closer to the delivery tip and are used for accurate measurement of viscous fluids, such as blood or serum. In contrast to a volumetric pipette, an Ostwald-Folin pipette has an etched ring near the mouthpiece, indicating that it is a blow-out pipette. Using a pipetting bulb, the liquid is blown out of the pipette only after the blood or serum has drained to the last drop in the delivery tip. When filled with opaque fluids, such as blood, the top of the meniscus must be read. Controlled slow drainage is required with all viscous solutions so that no residual film is left on the walls of the pipette.

**Measuring pipettes.** The second principal type of pipette is the graduated or measuring pipette (see Fig. 8.1C). This is a piece of glass tubing that is drawn out to a tip and graduated uniformly along its length. Two types are available. The Mohr pipette is calibrated between two marks on the stem, whereas the serologic pipette has graduated marks down to the tip. The serologic pipette (see Fig. 8.1D) must be blown out to deliver the entire volume of the pipette and has an etched ring (or pair of rings) near the bulb end of the pipette, signifying that it is a blow-out pipette. Mohr pipettes require controlled delivery of the solution between the calibration marks.

Serologic pipettes have a larger orifice than do Mohr pipettes and thus drain faster. In practice, measuring pipettes are used principally for measurement of reagents and generally are not considered sufficiently accurate for measuring samples and calibrators.

*Pipetting technique.* There are general pipetting techniques that apply to the pipettes described previously. For example, pipetting bulbs should always be used, and pipettes must be held in a vertical position when the liquid level is adjusted to the calibration line and during delivery. The lowest part of the meniscus, when it is sighted at eye level, should be level with the calibration line on the pipette. The flow of liquid should be unrestricted when volumetric pipettes are used, and the tips should be touched to the inclined surface of the receiving container for 2 seconds after the liquid has ceased to flow.

With graduated pipettes, the flow of liquid may have to be slowed during delivery. Serologic pipettes are calibrated to the tip, and the etched glass ring on top of the pipette signifies that it is to be blown out. First, the pipette is allowed to drain, and then the remaining liquid is blown out.

*Micropipettes.* Micropipettes are pipettes used for the measurement of microliter volumes. With such devices, the remaining volume that coats the inner wall of a pipette causes a notable error. For this reason, most micropipettes are calibrated to contain the stated volume rather than to deliver it. Proper use requires rinsing the pipette with the final solution after the contents are delivered into the diluent. Volumes are expressed in microliters (μL); the older term *lambda* is no longer recommended. Micropipettes generally are available in small sizes, ranging from 1 to 1000 μL; also, they are available for volumes as low as 0.2 μL.

**Semiautomatic and automatic pipettes and dispensers.** Fig. 8.2A and B illustrate two types of adjustable micropipetting devices that demonstrate unique ergonomic design features. These devices are programmable and are used with disposable plastic tips for simultaneously dispensing aliquots of liquid into multiple wells. Each channel is piston driven to allow the user to pipette with as few or as many tips as necessary. Aliquots of liquid as small as 0.2 μL are dispensed at three different aspiration or dispense rates.

Semiautomatic manual and electronic versions of pipettes and dispensers are available in sizes ranging from 0.5 μL to 10 mL or larger. Fig. 8.2C illustrates an electronically operated, positive-displacement multichannel pipettor. This device aspirates and dispenses its predefined volumes (from 0.5 to 200 μL) when its plunger is moved through a complete cycle. Its disposable, fluid containment tips are made of a plastic material that tends to retain less inner surface film than does glass. Such pipettes (1) avoid the risk of cross-contamination among samples, (2) eliminate the necessity for washing between samples, and (3) improve the precision of measurements. Models that allow for digital adjustment of the volume aspirated and dispensed are available.

Fig. 8.3A shows an automatic dispensing apparatus that aspirates and dispenses preset volumes of two different liquids by two motor-driven syringes, one for metering a volume

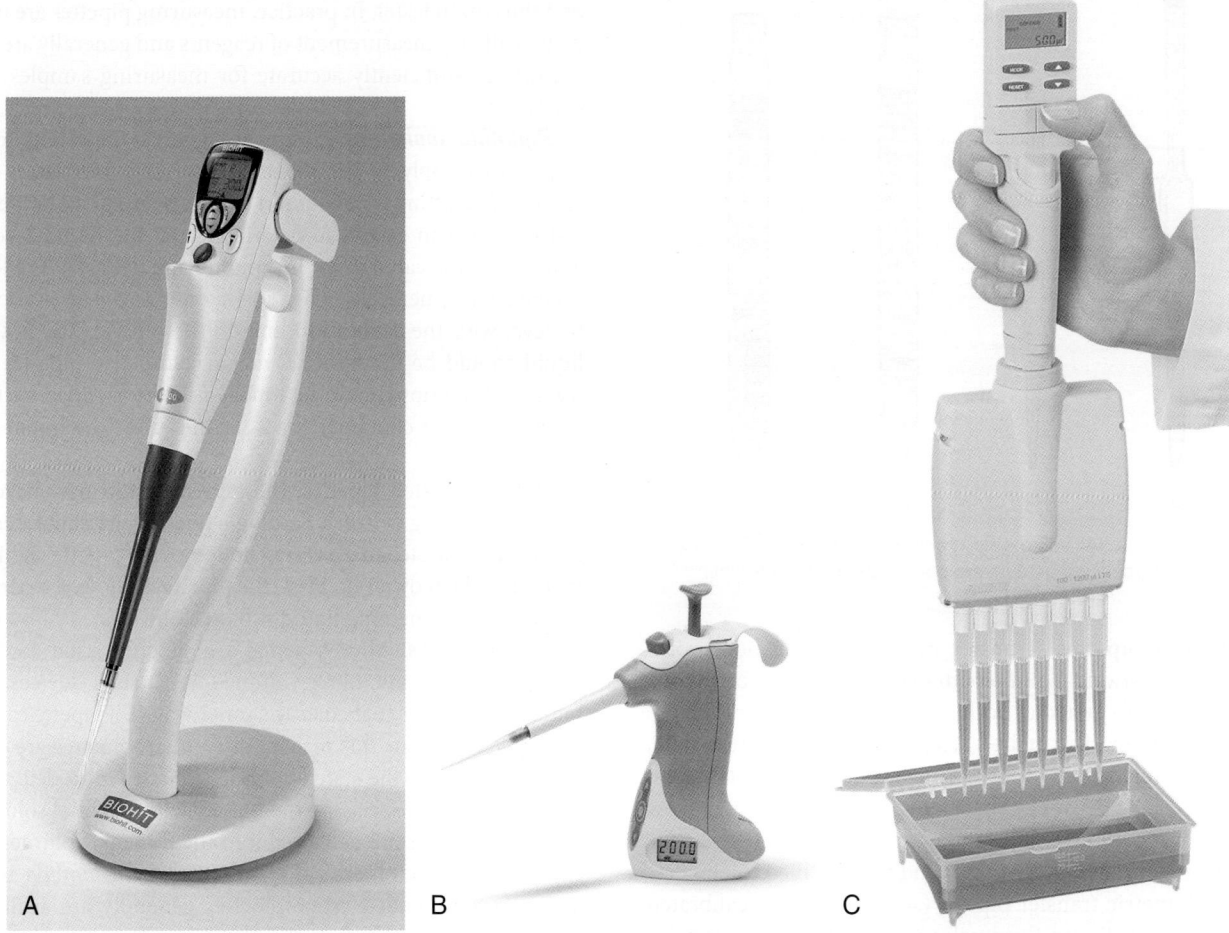

**Fig. 8.2** (A) Adjustable volume micropipetting device with ergonomic design. (B) Adjustable volume electronic micropipetting device with ergonomic design. (C) Electronic programmable multichannel pipette. (A, Courtesy Biohit Plc. B, Courtesy Vistalab Technologies, Inc. C, Courtesy Rainin Instrument LLC.)

of the sample and one for metering a volume of the diluent. It is possible to adjust this device to aspirate as little as 1 μL of one liquid and to deliver it with as much as 999 μL of the other. This type of device, available as a dilutor or dispenser, is obtainable as a manual, electronic, or computer-controlled device. The device is microprocessor-controlled and is easily programmed.

A more versatile piece of equipment is the robotic liquid handling workstation shown in Fig. 8.3B. This automated pipetting station is used with individual reaction tubes and also with 96- and 384-well microtiter plates. Depending on the design of the system, a single probe or multiple probes may be used to rapidly transfer programmed volumes of solution from one container to microtiter plates (e.g., so that the transfer to all 96 wells is complete in 1 minute). In some systems, liquid sensing is incorporated into the sample probes to minimize contact with samples and reagents, although automatic washing of the probes is performed between specimens. Two-dimensional (X-Y) movement of probes and tubes or microtiter plates is built into the pipetting stations to minimize the necessity for operator intervention. This device dispenses programmed volumes from 0.5 to 1000 μL in serial

dilutions from 4 to 16 channels using an autoloaded system with barcodes for positive identification.

## Volumetric Flasks

Volumetric flasks (Fig. 8.4) are used to measure exact volumes; they are commonly found in sizes varying from 1 to 4000 mL. In practice, they are used primarily to prepare solutions of known concentration, and they are available in various grades. The most accurate are certified as meeting standards set forth by the NIST.

An important factor in the use of a volumetric apparatus is the requirement for an accurate adjustment of the meniscus. A small piece of card that is half black and half white is most useful. The card is placed 1 cm behind the apparatus, with the white half uppermost and the top of the black area approximately 1 mm below the meniscus. The meniscus then appears as a clearly defined, thin black line. This device is also useful in reading the meniscus of a burette.

Volumetric equipment should be used with solutions equilibrated to room temperature. Solutions diluted in volumetric flasks should be repeatedly mixed during dilution so that the contents are homogeneous before the solution is

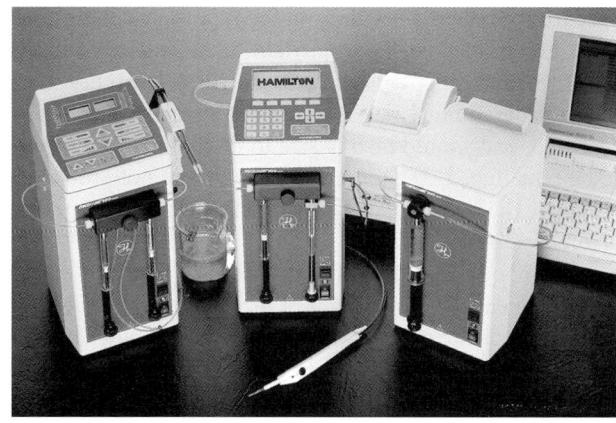

A

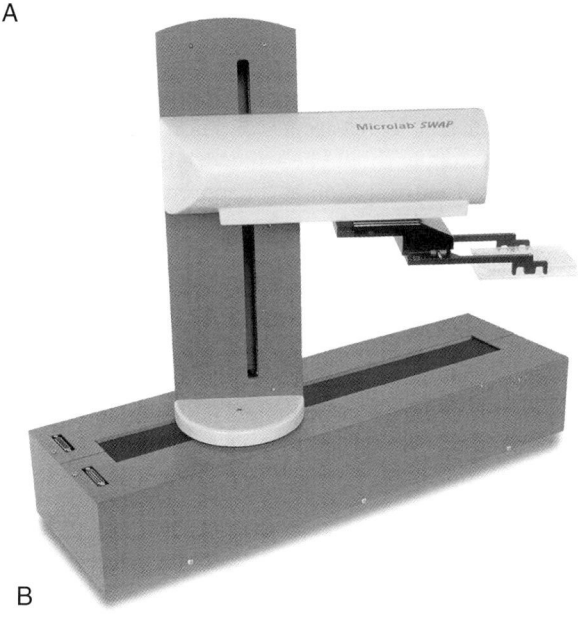

B

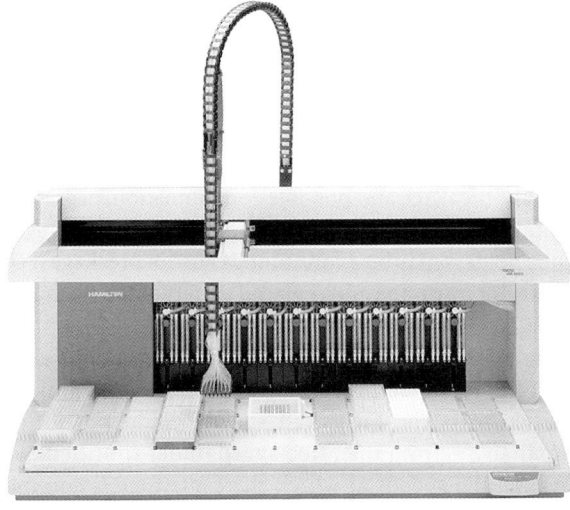

C

**Fig. 8.3** (A) Personal computer–controlled diluting and/or dispensing apparatus that aspirates and dispenses preset volumes of one or two different liquids, such as a diluent and sample, by motor-driven syringes. (B and C) Robotic liquid handling workstations. (A and B, Courtesy Hamilton Co.)

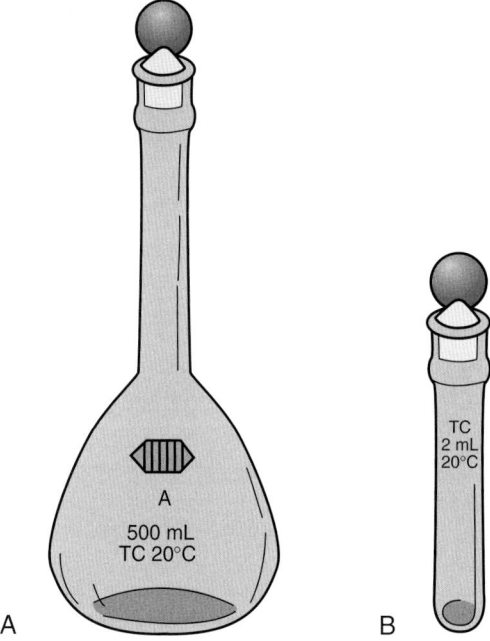

A                                                    B

**Fig. 8.4** Volumetric flasks. (A) Macro; (B) micro.

made up to final volume. Errors caused by expansion or contraction of liquids upon mixing are thereby minimized.

Volumetric flasks should be thoroughly cleaned and dried before calibration. The flask is then weighed and filled with carbon dioxide-free deionized water until just above the graduation mark. The neck of the flask just above the water level should be kept free of water. The meniscus mark is set at the graduation line by removing excess water, and the flask is reweighed. The final weight is corrected for the equilibrated water and air temperature to obtain the volume of the flask. Flasks also may be calibrated by the spectrophotometric technique described in the next section.

## Centrifugation

**Centrifugation** is the process of using centrifugal force to separate the lighter portions of a solution, mixture, or suspension from the heavier portions. A centrifuge is a device by which centrifugation is performed.

In the clinical laboratory, centrifugation is used to:
1. Remove cellular elements from blood to provide cell-free plasma or serum for analysis (see Chapter 6).
2. Concentrate cellular elements and other components of biological fluids for microscopic examination or chemical analysis.
3. Remove chemically precipitated protein from an analytical specimen.
4. Separate protein- or antibody-bound ligand from free ligand in immunochemical and other assays (see Chapter 15).
5. Extract solutes in biological fluids from aqueous to organic solvents.
6. Separate lipid components (e.g., chylomicrons) from other components of plasma or serum, and lipoproteins from one another (see Chapter 23).

## Types of Centrifuges

Several types of centrifuges are used in the clinical laboratory, including (1) horizontal head, (2) swinging bucket, (3) fixed-angle head, (4) angle head, (5) ultracentrifuge, and (6) axial units. In addition, the development of automatic balancing centrifuges has enabled centrifugation to be incorporated as an integral step in the total automation of laboratory testing (see Chapter 16).

## Principles of Centrifugation

The correct term to describe the force required to separate two phases in a centrifuge is **relative centrifugal force (RCF)**. Units are expressed as the number of times greater than gravity (e.g., $500 \times g$).

RCF is calculated as follows:

$$RCF = 1.118 \times 10^{-5} \times r \times rpm^2$$

where $1.118 \times 10^{-5}$ = empirical factor; $r$ = radius in centimeters from the center of rotation to the bottom of the tube in the rotor cavity or bucket during centrifugation; and rpm = the speed of rotation of the rotor in revolutions per minute.

The RCF of a centrifuge may also be determined from a nomogram distributed by manufacturers of centrifuges. RCF is derived from the distance from the rotor center to the bottom of the tube, whether the tube is horizontal to, or at an angle to, the rotor center.

The time required to sediment particles depends on the (1) rotor speed, (2) radius of the rotor, and (3) effective path length traveled by the sedimented particles (i.e., the depth of the liquid in the tube). Duplication of conditions of centrifugation is often desirable. The following is a useful formula for calculating the speed required of a rotor whose radius differs from the radius with which a prescribed RCF is originally defined:

$$rpm\ (alternate\ rotor) = 1000 \times \sqrt{\frac{RCF,\ original\ rotor}{11.18 \times [r\,(cm),\ alternate\ rotor]}}$$

The length of time for centrifugation is calculated so that running with an alternate rotor of a different size is equivalent to running with the original rotor:

$$Time\ (alternate\ rotor) = \frac{Time \times RCF\ (original\ rotor)}{RCF\ (alternate\ rotor)}$$

Note, however, that it may not be possible to reproduce conditions exactly when a different centrifuge is used. Descriptions of times of centrifugation include the time for the rotor to reach operating speed (which may vary from instrument to instrument) and do not include deceleration time, during which sedimentation is still occurring but is doing so less efficiently. Even with maximal braking, deceleration may take as long as 3 minutes in some centrifuges.

## Operation of the Centrifuge

For proper operation of a centrifuge, only those tubes recommended by their manufacturer should be used. The material used for the tube must withstand the RCF to which the tube is likely to be subjected. Polypropylene tubes generally are capable of withstanding RCFs of up to $5000 \times g$. The tubes should have a tapered bottom, particularly if a supernatant is to be removed, and should be of a size to fit securely into the rack to be centrifuged. The top of the tube should not protrude so far above the bucket that the swing into a horizontal position is impeded by the rotor.

For smooth operation of the centrifuge, the rotor must be properly balanced. The weight of racks, tubes, and their contents on opposite sides of a rotor should not differ by more than 1% or by an acceptable limit established by the manufacturer. Centrifuges that automatically balance their rotors are now available.

Tubes of collected blood should be centrifuged before they are unstoppered to reduce the probability of an aerosol being produced when the tube is opened. The practice of using a wooden applicator to release a clot stuck to the top of the tube or to its stopper should be avoided; it is a potential cause of hemolysis. Centrifugation at an appropriate RCF usually ensures that the clot is released from the tube wall and is drawn to the bottom of the tube.

Specific recommendations for each type of collection tube regarding RCF or times for centrifugation of blood specimens are usually provided by the manufacturer. Standards have not been established for centrifugation of other specimens, such as serum to which a protein precipitant has been added. Additional details pertaining to the handling and processing of blood specimens can be found in Chapter 6 and CLSI document GP44-A4.

## Operating Practice

Cleanliness of a centrifuge is important in minimizing the possible spread of infectious agents, such as hepatitis viruses. With proper operation of a centrifuge, fewer tubes will break. In case of breakage, the racks and chamber of the centrifuge must be carefully cleaned. Any spillage should be considered a possible bloodborne pathogen hazard. Gray dust arising from sandblasting of the chamber by fragments of glass indicates tube breakage and possible contamination, necessitating cleaning of the chamber. Broken glass embedded in cushions of tube holders may be a continuing cause of breakage if cushions are not inspected and replaced as part of the cleanup procedure.

The speed of a centrifuge should be checked according to the manufacturer's instructions or according to its intended use. The measured speed should not differ by more than 5% from the rated speed under specified conditions. All the speeds at which the centrifuge is commonly operated should be checked. The centrifuge timer should be checked weekly against a reference timer (such as a stopwatch), and the timer should not be more than 10% in error. Commutators and brushes should be checked depending on the frequency of use. Brushes (where used) should be replaced when they show considerable wear. However, in many modern induction-driven motors, brushes have been eliminated, thus removing a source of dust that causes motor failure.

Because centrifuges generate heat, the temperature in the chamber in many centrifuge models may increase by as much as 5°C after a single run. When the material to be centrifuged is thermolabile, a refrigerated centrifuge should be used. In the simplest form, a refrigerator unit is mounted beside the centrifuge, and cold air is blown into the rotor chamber. This approach is usually inadequate to stabilize the low temperature. In more sophisticated centrifuges, refrigeration coils around the chamber make it possible to maintain a preset temperature within ±1°C. The temperature of a refrigerated centrifuge should be measured monthly under reproducible conditions and should be within 2°C of the expected temperature.

## Gravimetry

Mass is an invariant property of matter. Gravimetry is the process used to measure the mass of a substance. Weight is a function of mass under the influence of gravity, a relationship expressed by the relationship

$$Weight = Mass \times Gravity$$

Two substances of equal weight and subject to the same gravitational force have equal mass. Mass is determined using a balance to compare the mass of an unknown with that of a known mass. This comparison is called weighing, and the absolute standards with which masses are compared are called weights. In practice, the terms mass and weight are used synonymously.

The classic form of a balance is a beam poised on an agate knife-edge fulcrum, with a pan hanging from each end of the beam and a rigid pointer hanging from the beam at the poised point. With the object to be weighed on one pan and weights of equal mass on the other pan, the pointer comes to rest at an equilibrium or balance point between the extremes of the path of excursion. The weight required to achieve the equilibrium is therefore equal to the weight of the substance being weighed.

### Principles of Weighing

Historically, one of two modes of weighing is used: (1) analytical weights are added to equal the weight of the object being weighed, or (2) the material to be weighed is added to a balance pan to achieve equilibrium with a preset weight. Currently, the electronic balance is most commonly used balance in the clinical laboratory. The electronic balance uses an electromagnetic force to return the balance beam to its null position. This force is proportional to the weight on the pan. Before a sample of the chemical is weighed, the weight of the container must be determined to subsequently allow for deducting the weight of the container from the gross weight of the container plus the sample to obtain the net weight of the sample. Most modern electronic balances allow for the readout to be set to "0" with an empty container on the pan. This is called *taring*. When taring is impractical, the weight of the empty container must be subtracted from the combined weight of the container and the material to obtain the weight of the material alone. In addition, in many modern balances,

a built-in computer compensates for changes in temperature and provides both automatic zero tracking and calibration.

### Analytical Weights

Analytical weights are used to verify the performance of balances. The NIST recognizes five classes of analytical weights. Class S weights are used for calibrating balances. In the clinical laboratory, balances should be calibrated based on frequency of use and before very accurate analytical work is conducted. These weights are typically made from brass or stainless steel and are lacquered or plated for protection. The fractional weights of a set of class S standards are usually made of platinum or aluminum. Tolerances of the different weights have been defined by the NIST. For class S weights from 1 to 5 g, the tolerance is ±0.054 mg; from 100 to 500 mg, it is ±0.025 mg; and from 1 to 50 mg, it is ±0.014 mg.

### Thermometry

In the clinical chemistry laboratory, measurements of temperature are made primarily to verify that devices measure within their prescribed temperature limits. Water baths and heated cells where reactions take place are examples of such devices, as are refrigerators, whose temperatures must be measured and recorded daily to meet laboratory regulatory requirements.

The two most popular types of thermometers in the chemistry laboratory are liquid-in-glass thermometers and thermistor probes.

All thermometers must be verified against a certified thermometer before they are placed into use. For example, the NIST SRM 934 is a mercury-in-glass thermometer with calibration points at 0°C, 25°C, 30°C, and 37°C. Some manufacturers supply liquid-in-glass thermometers that have ranges greater than the SRM thermometer and are verified to have been calibrated against the NIST thermometers. Details of verification of the calibration of a thermometer have been described. The NIST also supplies several materials that melt at a known temperature, including gallium (SRM 1968), which melts at 29.7723°C, and rubidium (SRM 1969), which melts at 39.3°C.

### Procedures for Processing Solutions

Several procedures are used routinely to process solutions in the clinical laboratory, including those used for diluting, concentrating, and filtering solutions.

### Dilution

Dilution is the process by which the concentration or activity of a given solution is decreased by the addition of a solvent. In laboratory practice, most dilutions are made by transferring an exact volume of a concentrated solution into an appropriate flask and then adding water or other diluent to the required volume, with appropriate mixing to ensure homogeneity. A serial dilution is a sequential set of dilutions in a mathematical sequence. A given dilution is expressed as the amount, either volume or weight, of a solute (**analyte**) in a specified volume. For example, a 1:5 volume-to-volume dilution contains one volume of an initial solution in a total of five volumes of the final solution (one volume plus four volumes). The dilution factor for a diluted solution is the reciprocal of the dilution of the initial solution. The dilution ratio is typically the ratio of the parts of volume ($V_1$) to the parts of another volume ($V_2$) or 1:4 in the previous example.

To prevent errors that arise when two liquids of different compositions are mixed, the technique of diluting to volume is used. Instead of adding 90 mL of water to 10 mL of concentrated solution, the 10 mL of concentrated solution should be pipetted into a 100-mL volumetric flask. Water is added to bring the volume to the 100-mL mark on the neck of the flask.

When a dilution is performed, the following equation is used to determine the final volume ($V_2$) necessary to dilute a given volume ($V_1$) of solution of a known concentration ($C_1$) to the desired lesser concentration ($C_2$):

$$C_1 \times V_1 = C_2 \times V_2 \qquad (8.1)$$

or

$$V_2 = \frac{C_1 \times V_1}{C_2} \qquad (8.2)$$

Likewise, Eq. 8.1 is also used to calculate the concentration of the diluted solution when a given volume is added to the starting solution.

### Evaporation

Evaporation is a process used to convert a liquid or a volatile solid into vapor. It is used in the clinical laboratory to remove liquid from a sample, thereby increasing the concentrations of analyte(s) left behind. A centrifugal evaporator is used to gently evaporate solvents from single or multiple samples. The components include a centrifuge, a vacuum pump, and a cold trap to collect evaporated solvent. A centrifugal force is applied to create a pressure gradient so samples boil from the top down to prevent "bumping." As the solvent is removed, the samples increase in concentration. The evaporation of solvent can also be accomplished by gently blowing a steady stream of gas, typically with its flow regulated through a needle, over the solution. Dry nitrogen gas is commonly used because it is relatively nonreactive.

### Lyophilization

Lyophilization (also known as *freeze drying*) is used in laboratory medicine for the preparation of (1) calibrators, (2) control materials, (3) reagents, and (4) individual specimens for analysis. Lyophilization entails first freezing a material at −40°C or less and then subjecting it to a high vacuum. Very low temperatures cause the ice to sublimate to a vapor state. The solid nonsublimable material remains behind in a dried state.

### Filtration

Filtration is defined as the passage of a liquid through a filter and is accomplished by gravity, pressure, or vacuum. Filtrate is the liquid that has passed through the filter, and the fraction that does not pass through the filter is the retentate. The purpose of filtration is to remove particulate matter from the liquid. Many filtrations in the clinical laboratory are carried out with filter paper and with plastic membranes of controlled pore size.

Membrane filters are used (1) under vacuum, (2) with positive pressure, or (3) with gravity. Filters have been incorporated into certain disposable tips for use with semiautomatic pipettes. These filters minimize the exchange of aerosol droplets between the tips and the pipette. This is of particular importance for DNA amplification and microbiological procedures. Other membrane filters are designed for ultrafiltration and are available with a variety of pore sizes for selective filtration. Ultrafiltration is a technique for removing dissolved particles using an extremely fine filter. It is used to concentrate macromolecules, such as proteins because smaller dissolved molecules pass through the filter.

## SAFETY

In the United States, the Federal Occupational Safety and Health Act of 1970 marked the beginning of formal regulatory oversight of employee safety. Since 1970, the **Occupational Safety and Health Administration (OSHA)** and the Centers for Disease Control and Prevention (CDC) have published numerous safety standards that apply to clinical laboratories. Each year, as The Joint Commission (JC) and CAP revise their guidelines, more attention is devoted to safety. Consideration for the health as well as responsibility for the safety of employees are now accepted as obligations of all employers and laboratory directors. In May 1988, OSHA expanded the Hazard Communication Standard to apply to hospital workers. Part of this standard is frequently referred to as the "Lab Right to Know Standard."

Outside of the United States, the regulations and practices regarding laboratory safety and quality are guided by ISO 15189:2012 Medical laboratories: Requirements for quality and competence. This comprehensive international standard provides guidance on management, staffing, customers, laboratory, quality control, and quality improvement.

There are many aspects to the safe operation of a clinical laboratory. Key elements for safety in the clinical laboratory include:

1. A formal safety program.
2. Documented policies and effective use of mandated plans and/or programs in the areas of chemical hygiene, control of exposure to bloodborne pathogens, TB control, and **ergonomics.**
3. Identification of significant occupational hazards, such as biological, chemical, fire, and electrical hazards, and clear identification and documentation of policies for employees to deal with each type of hazard (e.g., packaging and shipping of diagnostic specimens and infectious substances).
4. Recognition that there are additional important and relevant safety areas of concern. These areas include effective waste management and bioterrorism and chemical

terrorism response plans in the event of potential threats or casualties involving these types of agents.

## Safety Program

Every clinical laboratory must have and implement a comprehensive formal safety program. Regardless of the size of the clinical laboratory, a specific individual should be designated as the "Safety Officer" or "Chair of the Safety Committee" and given the responsibility to implement and maintain a safety program. Safety is each employee's responsibility, but responsibility for the entire program begins with the laboratory leadership (directors, administrative directors, supervisors, managers, and so on) and is delegated through the leadership to the safety officer or safety committee. This individual or committee then has the duties of providing guidance to laboratory leadership on matters related to the provision of a safe workplace for all employees. Although a small institution may have one individual who deals with all safety-related matters for all departments, including the laboratory, OSHA mandates that the laboratory specifically have a chemical hygiene officer, who is designated on the basis of training or experience to provide technical guidance in the development of the **chemical hygiene plan (CHP),** which is discussed later.

An integral part of the laboratory safety program is the education and motivation of all laboratory employees in all matters related to safety. All new employees should be given a copy of the general laboratory safety manual as part of their orientation. The continuing education program of the laboratory should include periodic talks on safety. Safety information is available from a variety of sources to support the continuing education element of the safety program.

Another important part of the laboratory safety program relates to ensuring that the laboratory environment meets accepted safety standards. This would include, but would not be limited to, attention to such items as (1) proper labeling of chemicals, (2) types and locations of fire extinguishers, (3) hoods that are in good working order, (4) proper grounding of electrical equipment, (5) ergonomic issues (which include equipment, such as pipetting devices, laboratory furniture, and prevention of musculoskeletal disorders), and (6) providing means for the proper handling and disposal of biohazardous materials, including all patient specimens.

## Safety Equipment

OSHA requires that institutions provide employees with all necessary personal protective equipment (PPE). Key important safety items are (1) clothing (such as laboratory coats, gowns, and/or scrubs), (2) gloves, and (3) eye protection. These safety items should be used in areas where they are appropriate. Eye washers or face washers should be available in every chemistry laboratory. Many types are available, and some simply connect to existing plumbing. A handheld eye and/or face safety spray is a requisite safety device and is typically placed in a position next to each sink using only a few inches of space. Safety showers, strategically located in the laboratory, must be available and should be tested on a regular schedule.

Heat-resistant (nonasbestos) gloves should be available for handling hot glassware and dry ice. Safety goggles, glasses, and visors, including some that fit conveniently over regular eyeglasses, are available in many sizes and shapes. Personnel wearing contact lenses should be aware of the danger of irritants getting under a lens, making it difficult to irrigate the eye properly. Shatterproof safety shields should be used in front of systems posing a potential danger because of implosion (vacuum collapse) or pressure explosions. Desiccator guards should be used with vacuum desiccators. Hot beakers should be handled with tongs. Inexpensive polyethylene pumps are available to pump acids from large bottles. Spill kits for acids, caustic materials, or flammable solvents come in various sizes. Such kits and the other appropriate safety materials should be located in convenient and appropriate sites in the laboratory.

A chemical fume hood is a necessity for every clinical chemistry laboratory. In practice, it is used for (1) opening any container of a material that gives off harmful vapors, (2) preparing reagents that produce fumes, and (3) heating flammable solvents. In the event of an explosion or a fire in the hood, closing its window contains the fire.

## Safety Inspections

It is good laboratory practice to organize a safety inspection team from the laboratory staff. This team is responsible for conducting periodic and scheduled safety inspections of the laboratory.

In the United States, several regulatory, private accreditation, state, and federal organizations may conduct a safety inspection of the laboratory. Some of these safety inspections may occur unannounced. From an external perspective, OSHA inspectors have the authority to enter a clinical laboratory unannounced, and on presentation of credentials, inspect it. The inspection may be regular or may occur as the result of a complaint or an accident in the lab. In addition, the Commission on Inspection and Accreditation of CAP inspects clinical laboratories and uses various safety checklists (available to the laboratory before inspection) when evaluating a laboratory for accreditation. Although the JC will accept CAP accreditation of a laboratory, it still may conduct a safety inspection of the laboratory when it inspects the hospital. The CAP and JC conduct their accreditation inspections, which may include a full laboratory or laboratory safety component, unannounced.

Depending on the group designated as responsible for accrediting a particular laboratory, selected laboratories may be subject to inspections for the purposes of accreditation and/or safety only by state agencies or local Centers for Medicare and Medicaid Services (CMS) groups. Inspections may be made on a regular basis by state or local health departments or by local fire departments to determine compliance with their particular safety requirements. Currently, a laboratory that meets federal or state OSHA requirements is likely to satisfy the standards of any other inspecting agency.

## Plans for the Clinical Laboratory

In 1991, OSHA mandated that all clinical laboratories in the United States must have a CHP and an **exposure control plan.**

OSHA has since updated their requirements for the exposure control plan to provide new examples of engineering controls and to place significantly greater responsibility on employers to minimize and manage employee occupational exposure to bloodborne pathogens. The CAP and other groups require that an accredited laboratory must have a documented TB exposure control plan that conforms to biosafety guidelines published by the CDC. Elements of the plan must include regularly defined intervals for employee exposure, as well as process controls, to minimize exposure to aerosolization of *Mycobacterium tuberculosis*.

In addition, it is now recognized that the workplace setting of a clinical laboratory exposes employees to the occupational risk of developing various musculoskeletal disorders. As a result, the focus of OSHA on laboratories that have an effective ergonomics program has led to federal, state, and private accreditation groups addressing this area of occupational safety. However, considerable controversy on this issue is ongoing, with a final ergonomics rule published and then withdrawn in 2001.

## Chemical Hygiene Plan

Major elements of a CHP include listing of responsibilities for employers, employees, and a chemical hygiene officer. Also, every laboratory must have a complete chemical inventory that is updated annually. A copy of the **Safety Data Sheet (SDS),** which defines each chemical as toxic, carcinogenic, or dangerous, must be on file, readily accessible, and available to all employees 24 hours a day, 7 days a week. The SDS contains important information for the benefit of laboratory employees. The chemical manufacturer's information, as supplied on the SDS, is used to ascertain whether a certain chemical is hazardous. Each SDS must give the product's identity as it appears on the container label and the chemical and common names of its hazardous components. The SDS also provides physical data on the product, such as boiling point, vapor pressure, and specific gravity. Easily recognized characteristics of the chemical are also listed on the line for "appearance and odor." Information about hazardous properties is given in detail on the SDS; this includes fire and explosion hazard data and health-related data such as the threshold limit value, exposure limits, and toxicity values. The threshold limit value is the exposure allowable for an employee during one 8-hour day. It also notes the effects of overexposure and details first-aid procedures. Each SDS also provides information on spill cleanup and disposal procedures, and protective personal gear and equipment requirements.

## Exposure Control Plan

OSHA regulations require that each laboratory develop, implement, adhere to, and maintain a plan that ensures the protection of laboratory workers against potential exposure to bloodborne pathogens and that medical wastes produced by the laboratory are managed and handled in a safe and effective manner. OSHA regulations also place responsibility on employers to implement new developments in exposure control technology, to solicit the input of employees directly involved in patient care in the identification, evaluation, and selection of these work practice controls, and in certain instances to maintain a log for employee percutaneous injuries from sharp devices such as syringe needles. Organizationally, the plan should include sections on (1) purpose, (2) scope, (3) applicable references, (4) applicable definitions, (5) definition of responsibilities, and (6) detailed procedural steps.

When implementing the plan, each laboratory employee must be placed into one of the following three groups:

Group I: a job classification in which all employees have occupational exposure to blood or other potentially infectious materials.

Group II: a job classification in which some employees have occupational exposure to blood or other potentially infectious materials.

Group III: a job classification in which employees do not have any occupational exposure to blood or other potentially infectious materials.

## Tuberculosis Control Plan

The purpose of the TB control plan is to prevent the transmission of TB, which occurs when an individual inhales a droplet that contains *M. tuberculosis*. *M. tuberculosis* is aerosolized when an infected individual sneezes, speaks or coughs, or when an infected sputum specimen is handled (http://www.cdc.gov/tb/publications/guidelines/control_elim.htm). Transmission of and exposure to TB are greatly diminished with (1) early identification and isolation of patients at risk, (2) environmental controls, (3) appropriate use of respiratory protection equipment, (4) education of laboratory employees, and (5) early initiation of therapy.

An effective TB control plan will include screening at the time of hire which includes a risk assessment, symptom evaluation, and a test. Annual testing is not recommended unless the risk for exposure is increased in the working environment. Engineering and work practice controls are particularly important in laboratory areas, such as surgical pathology and microbiology. However, there is a clear risk of exposure from specimens of patients with suspected or confirmed TB in every section of the laboratory, including chemistry.

## Pandemic Plan

A pandemic is an epidemic of infectious disease that spreads through populations across a large region or even worldwide. An influenza pandemic is a worldwide outbreak or epidemic caused by an influenza virus. For example, the influenza pandemic of 1918 to 1919 killed between 20 and 50 million people with more than 500,000 deaths reported in the United States alone (http://www.cdc.gov/flu/about/qa/1918flupandemic.htm). Other pandemic examples are the novel influenza A (H1N1) of swine origin detected in 2009 and SARS-CoV-2 identified in late 2019. Influenza and other viruses capable of causing a pandemic (1) must cause human disease, (2) have novel surface antigens, and (3) must be able to be spread effectively from person to person.

Because of the potential for exposure of individuals working in health care settings, the CDC has published recommendations for establishing infection control. These recommendations provide guidance for all individuals who may be processing or performing diagnostic testing on clinical specimens from patients with suspected pandemic-type viruses (i.e., influenza A [H1N1 or H5N1] virus, SARS-CoV-2, Ebola) or performing viral isolation. A highly contagious virus can easily become a pandemic situation if not controlled properly. Health care workers and laboratories need to be prepared for these types of infectious agents.

## Ergonomics Program

Several areas of occupational risk for development of musculoskeletal disorders have been identified in the clinical laboratory. These include (1) routine laboratory activity, (2) functionality of the workspace (including laboratory floor matting, bright lighting, and noise generation), and (3) equipment design (computer keyboards and displays, workstations, and chairs). One particular laboratory function, pipetting and related pipette design, has received considerable attention. As depicted in Fig. 8.2, pipettes are being designed with the goal of reducing an employee's risk of developing cumulative stress disorders caused by awkward posture, repetitive motion, and repeated use of force.

The CAP requires accredited laboratories to have a comprehensive and defined ergonomics program that is designed to prevent work-related musculoskeletal disorders through prevention and engineering controls. The documented ergonomics plan should include elements of employee training regarding the areas of risk, engineering controls to minimize or eliminate risks, and an assessment process to identify problematic issues for documentation and remediation.

## Hazards in the Laboratory

Various types of hazards are encountered in the operation of a clinical laboratory. These hazards must be identified and labeled, and work practices developed for dealing with them. The major categories of hazards encountered include (1) biological, (2) chemical, (3) electrical, and (4) fire hazards.

### Identification of Hazards

Clinical laboratories deal with each of the nine classes of hazardous materials. These are classified by the United Nations (UN) as (1) explosives, (2) compressed gases, (3) flammable liquids, (4) flammable solids, (5) oxidizer materials, (6) toxic materials, (7) radioactive materials, (8) corrosive materials, and (9) miscellaneous materials not classified elsewhere. Shipping and handling of class 6 toxic materials, specifically biological and potentially infectious materials, has received considerable attention. In 2002, the US Department of Transportation (DOT) released a revised rule with standards for infectious substance hazardous material handling. Warning labels aid in the identification of chemical hazards during shipment. Under the regulations of the DOT, chemicals that are transported in the United States must carry labels based on the UN classification. DOT placards or labels are diamond shaped with a digit imprinted on the bottom corner that identifies the UN hazard class (1 to 9). The hazard is

identified more specifically in printed words placed along the horizontal axis of the diamond. Color coding and a pictorial art description of the hazard supplement the identification of hazardous material on the label; the artwork appears in the top corner of the diamond (Fig. 8.5A).

The system is used by the DOT for shipping hazardous materials; however, when the hazardous material reaches its destination and is removed from the shipping container, this identification is lost. The laboratory must then label each individual container. Usually, the information necessary to classify the contents of the container appropriately is on the shipping label and should be noted. Important first aid information is usually provided on this label.

Although OSHA at present prescribes the use of labels or other appropriate warnings, no single uniform labeling system for hazardous chemicals exists for use by clinical laboratories. Appropriate hazard warnings include any words, pictures, symbols, or combinations that convey the health or physical hazards of the container's contents and must be specific as to the effect of the chemical and the specific target organs involved. The National Fire Protection Association

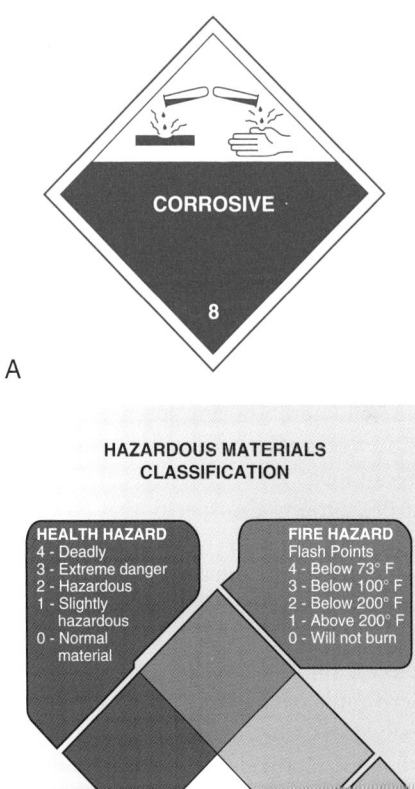

**Fig. 8.5** (A) US Department of Transportation label for corrosives. (B) Labeling identification system of the National Fire Protection Association. (Courtesy Lab Safety Supply Inc., Janesville, WI.)

(NFPA) has developed the 704-M Identification System, which classifies hazardous material from 0 to 4 (most hazardous) according to flammability and reactivity (instability). This system uses diamond-shaped labels (see Fig. 8.5B), which are available from most companies that sell laboratory safety equipment. The labels are color coded and are divided into quadrants. Three of the quadrants have a characteristic color and represent a type of hazard. A number in the quadrant indicates the degree of hazard. The fourth (lower) quadrant contains information of special interest to firefighters.

## Biological Hazards

It is essential to minimize the exposure of laboratory workers to infectious agents, such as the hepatitis viruses, HIV, and flu viruses. Exposure to infectious agents results from (1) accidental puncture with needles, (2) spraying of infectious materials by a syringe or spilling and splattering of these materials on bench tops or floors, (3) centrifuge accidents, and (4) cuts or scratches from contaminated vessels. Any unfixed tissue, including blood slides, must also be treated as potentially infectious material.

OSHA has mandated that all US laboratories have an exposure control plan. In addition, the National Institute for Occupational Safety and Health, a functional unit of the CDC, has prepared and widely distributed a document entitled **Standard Precautions** that specifies how US clinical laboratories should handle infectious agents. In general, it mandates that clinical laboratories treat all human blood and other potentially infectious materials as if they were known to contain infectious agents, such as hepatitis B virus (HBV), HIV, and other bloodborne pathogens. These requirements apply to all specimens of (1) blood, (2) serum, (3) plasma, (4) blood products, (5) vaginal secretions, (6) semen, (7) cerebrospinal fluid, (8) synovial fluid, and (9) concentrated HBV or HIV viruses. In addition, any specimen of any type that contains visible traces of blood should be handled using these Standard Precautions.

Standard Precautions also specify that barrier protection must be used by laboratory workers to prevent skin and mucous membrane contamination from specimens. These barriers, also known as PPE, include (1) gloves, (2) gowns, (3) laboratory coats, (4) face shields or mask and eye protection, (5) mouthpieces, (6) resuscitation bags, (7) pocket masks, and (8) other ventilator devices. A latex allergy is a problem for some individuals when latex gloves are used for barrier protection. For such individuals, medical-grade gloves made of materials such as vinyl, nitrile, neoprene, or thermoplastic elastomer are available. If latex gloves are to be used, they should be made of powder-free, low-allergen latex.

Products for increasing employee protection against needle sticks include an array of novel containers for sharps (e.g., needles, scalpels, glass) and biological safety disposal bags and needle sheaths that may be closed following venipuncture without physically touching the needle or the sheath. Although additional studies on their efficacy and effects on laboratory test results are required, microlaser devices are now available for piercing a patient's skin to collect a capillary blood specimen.

The CLSI has published a similar set of recommendations, several of which are specified as requirements in the OSHA exposure control plan. They include the following:

1. Never perform mouth pipetting and never blow out pipettes that contain potentially infectious material.
2. Do not mix potentially infectious material by bubbling air through the liquid.
3. Barrier protection, such as gloves, masks, and protective eyewear and gowns, must be available and used when drawing blood from a patient and when handling all patient specimens. This includes the removal of stoppers from tubes. Gloves must be disposable, nonsterile latex or of other material to provide adequate barrier protection. Phlebotomists must change gloves and adequately dispose of them between drawing blood from different patients.
4. Wash hands whenever gloves are changed.
5. Facial barrier protection should be used if there is a significant potential for the spattering of blood or body fluids.
6. Avoid using syringes whenever possible and dispose of needles in rigid containers (Fig. 8.6A) without handling them (see Fig. 8.6B).
7. Dispose of all sharps appropriately.
8. Wear protective clothing, which serves as an effective barrier against potentially infective materials. When leaving the laboratory, the protective clothing should be removed.
9. Strive to prevent accidental injuries.
10. Encourage frequent hand washing in the laboratory; employees must wash their hands whenever they leave the laboratory.
11. Make a habit of keeping your hands away from your mouth, nose, eyes, and any other mucous membranes. This reduces the possibility of self-inoculation.
12. Minimize spills and spatters.
13. Decontaminate all surfaces and reusable devices after use with appropriate US Environmental Protection Agency–registered hospital disinfectants. Sterilization, disinfection, and decontamination are discussed in detail in CLSI publication M29-A4.
14. No warning labels are to be used on patient specimens because all should be treated as potentially hazardous.
15. Biosafety level 2 procedures should be used whenever appropriate.
16. Before centrifuging tubes, inspect them for cracks. Inspect the inside of the trunnion cup for signs of erosion or adhering matter. Be sure that rubber cushions are free from all bits of glass.
17. Use biohazard disposal techniques (e.g., "Red Bag").
18. Never leave a discarded tube or infected material unattended or unlabeled.
19. Periodically, clean out freezer and dry-ice chests to remove broken ampoules and tubes of biological specimens. Use rubber gloves and respiratory protection during this cleaning.
20. OSHA requires that the hepatitis B vaccine be offered to all employees at risk of potential exposure as a regular or occasional part of their duties. The Advisory Committee

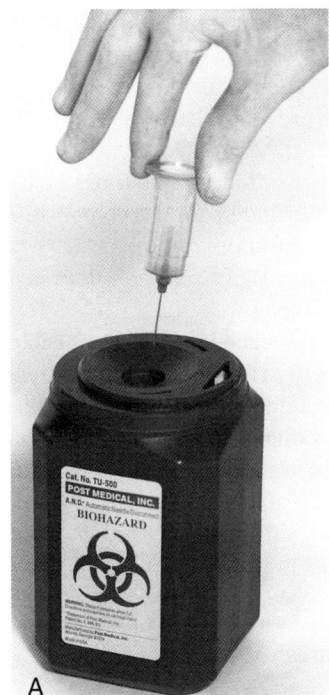

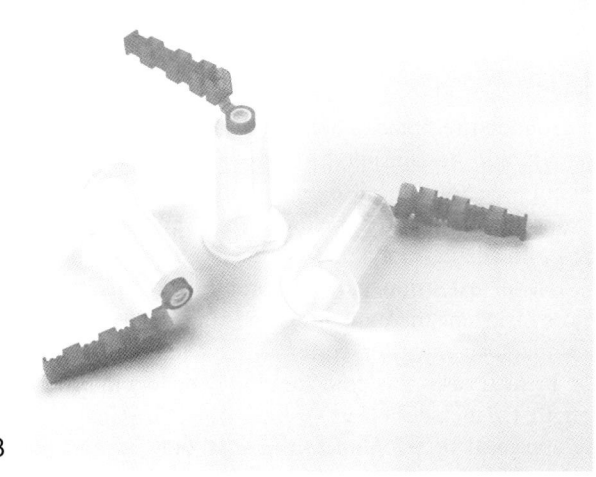

**Fig. 8.6** (A) Convenient needle disposal system for sharps. (B) Needle sheathing devices for prevention of body contact with needle. (B, Courtesy Marketlab Inc.)

on Immunization Practices of the CDC recommends that medical technologists, phlebotomists, and pathologists be vaccinated with the hepatitis B vaccine. It is a regulatory mandate that all of the previously mentioned laboratory employees at a minimum be given the option to receive a free hepatitis B vaccine.

Investigation of tragic air accidents in the late 1990s by the US National Transportation Safety Board led to the development of revised and strict requirements for the shipping and handling of hazardous materials by DOT, in cooperation with the International Air Transport Association and the International Civil Aviation Organization.

These regulations place particular emphasis on the hazardous material training that must be given to laboratory employees regarding the shipping and handling of infectious

substances. Elements include general awareness and familiarization, function-specific information, and safety training. Proper training, particularly in the areas of package labeling and documentation (including a shipper's declaration of contents for dangerous goods), is mandatory, and documented certification from employers that the relevant employees have had appropriate training programs is required. Although the adverse impact of improper training can be reflected most by potential human morbidity and mortality, identified violations of these regulations also carry large financial fines and penalties for both the infringing individual and the employer or institution.

## Chemical Hazards

Proper storage and use of chemicals is necessary to prevent dangers, such as burns, explosions, fires, and toxic fumes. Thus knowledge of the properties of the chemicals in use and of proper handling procedures greatly reduces dangerous situations. Bottles of chemicals and solutions should be handled carefully, and a cart should be used to transport heavy or multiple numbers of containers from one area to another. Glass containers with chemicals should be transported in rubber or plastic containers that protect them from breakage, and in the event of breakage, contain the spill. Appropriate spill kits should be available in strategic locations.

Spattering from acids, caustic materials, and strong oxidizing agents is a hazard to clothing and eyes and is a potential source of chemical burns. A bottle should never be held by its neck but instead firmly around its body with one or both hands, depending on the size of the bottle. Acids must be diluted by slowly adding them to water while mixing; water should never be added to concentrated acid. When working with acid or alkali solutions, safety glasses should be worn. Acids, caustic materials, and strong oxidizing agents should be mixed in the sink. This provides water for cooling and for confinement of the reagent in the event that the flask or bottle breaks.

All bottles containing reagents must be properly labeled. It is good practice to label the container before adding the reagent, thus preventing the possibility of having an unlabeled reagent. The label should bear the (1) name and concentration of the reagent, (2) initials of the person who made up the reagent, and (3) the date on which the reagent was prepared. When appropriate, the expiration date should also be included. The labels should be color-coded or an additional label added to designate specific storage instructions, such as the requirement for refrigeration or special storage related to a potential hazard. All reagents found in unlabeled bottles should be disposed of using appropriate procedures and precautions.

Strong acids, caustic materials, and strong oxidizing agents should be dispensed by a commercially available automatic dispensing device. Under no circumstances is mouth pipetting permitted.

In some instances, all waste materials are not collected in the same container. With certain pieces of equipment, strong acids or other hazardous materials are pumped directly into the drain. This should always be accompanied by a steady flow of water from the faucet. Safety glasses should be used by instrument operators when acids are pumped under pressure.

The Environmental Protection Agency controls the disposal of nonradioactive hazardous wastes. The Resource Conservation and Recovery Act of 1976 states that disposal of materials classifiable within any of the nine UN hazardous materials classes is enforced in such a way that health and safety professionals involved in the disposal of such materials are personally liable for each individual violation.

A CLSI publication (GP05-A3) covers hazardous waste disposal; however, many municipalities and states have their own regulations. These agencies should be contacted by the laboratory for specifics. Volatile chemicals and compressed gases pose specific hazards.

***Hazards from volatiles.*** The use of organic solvents in a clinical laboratory represents a potential fire hazard and hazards to health from inhalation of toxic vapors or skin contact. These solvents should be used in a fume hood. Storage of organic solvents is regulated by rules set down by OSHA. However, some local fire department rules are more stringent. Solvents should be stored in an OSHA-approved metal storage cabinet that is properly vented. The maximum working volume of flammable solvents allowed outside storage cabinets is 5 gallons per room. No more than 60 gallons of type I and II solvents may be stored in a single cabinet. No more than three cabinets may be located in each 5000 sq ft of laboratory space.

Vaporization is a major problem in the ignition and spread of fires. Vapors from flammable and combustible liquids and solids form a flammable mixture with air. They are characterized by their flash point, where the flash point is defined as the lowest temperature at which a solvent gives off flammable vapors in the close vicinity of its surface. The mixture at its flash point ignites when exposed to a source of ignition. At temperatures below the flash point, the vapor given off is considered too lean for ignition.

Disposal of flammable solvents in storm sewers or sanitary sewers generally is not allowed. Exceptions are small amounts of those materials that are miscible with water, but even disposal of these should be followed by large amounts of cold water. Other solvents should be collected in safety cans. Separate cans should be used for ether and for chlorinated solvents; all other solvents may be combined in a third can. The cans should be stored, in keeping with storage quantity rules, in a safety cabinet until pickup by a waste disposal firm. A more economical approach is to transfer the solvents to larger cans or drums in an outside storage facility so that pickup can be less frequent. Some large institutions have their own in-house disposal facilities.

***Hazards from compressed gases.*** DOT regulations cover the labeling of cylinders of compressed gases that are transported by interstate carriers. The diamond-shaped labels described previously are used on all large cylinders and on any boxes containing small cylinders. Some general rules for handling large cylinders of compressed gas are as follows:

1. Always transport cylinders using a hand truck to which the cylinder is secured.
2. Leave the valve cap on a cylinder until the cylinder is ready for use, at which time the cylinder should have been secured by a support around the upper one-third of its body. Disconnect the hose or regulator, shut off the valve, and replace the cap before the cylinder is completely empty to prevent the possibility of development of a negative pressure. Place an "empty" sign or label on the cylinder.
3. Chain or secure cylinders at all times even when empty.
4. Always check cylinders for the composition of their contents before connection.
5. Never force threads; if a regulator does not thread readily, something is wrong.

The precautions cited for large, refillable gas cylinders also apply to small cylinders that are not refillable. Propane cylinders and cylinders of calibrating gases for blood gas equipment are examples of disposable cylinders. Cylinders in floor-standing base supports require the additional security of a chain or strap attached to a wall or fixed piece of furniture. Local fire department regulations (which vary considerably from place to place) govern the disposal of exhausted cylinders.

## Electrical Hazards

Electrical wires or connections are potential shock or fire hazards. Worn wires on all electrical equipment should be replaced immediately, and all equipment should be grounded using three-prong plugs. OSHA regulations stipulate that the requirements for grounding of electrical equipment of the National Electrical Code (published by NFPA) be met. If grounded receptacles are not available, a licensed electrician should be consulted for proper alternative grounding techniques. Some local codes are more stringent than OSHA requirements and do not allow for two-pole mating receptacles with adapters for a three-pole plug.

Use of extension cords is prohibited. This standard is more stringent than any other existing regulation. In some instances, an extension cord may have to be used temporarily. In such cases, the cord should (1) be less than 12 feet in length, (2) include at least 16 American Wire Gauge wire, (3) be approved by the Underwriters Laboratory, and (4) have only one outlet at the end. If several outlets are necessary in a single area, a power strip with its own fuse or circuit breaker may be installed at least three in above the bench top level. Several manufacturers now sell devices to check for high resistance in neutral or ground wiring or excess voltage in neutral wiring.

Electrical equipment and connections should not be handled with wet hands, nor should electrical equipment be used after liquid has been spilled on it. The equipment must be turned off immediately and dried thoroughly. In case of a wet or malfunctioning electrical instrument that is used by several people, the plug should be pulled and a note cautioning coworkers against use should be left on the instrument.

## Fire Hazards

NFPA and OSHA publish standards covering subjects from emergency exits (including means of egress) to safety and firefighting equipment. NFPA also publishes the National

Fire Codes. Many state and local agencies have adopted these codes (some of which are more stringent than OSHA requirements), thus making them legally enforceable.

Every laboratory should have the necessary equipment to extinguish or confine a fire in the laboratory and to extinguish a fire on the clothing of an individual. Easy access to safety showers is essential. A safety shower should have a pull chain attached to the wall at a convenient height or hanging down from the shower head; the chain should have a large ring attached so that the shower may be easily activated, even with eyes closed. Fire blankets for smothering fire on clothing should be available in an easily accessible wall-mounted case. The blanket is unrolled from the case and is rolled around the body by taking hold of the rope that is attached to the blanket and turning the body around. The location of this equipment and the locations of fire alarms and maps of evacuation routes are dictated by the local fire marshal.

Various types of fire extinguishers are available. The type to use depends on the type of fire. Because it is impractical to have several types of fire extinguishers present in every area, dry chemical fire extinguishers are among the best all-purpose extinguishers for laboratory areas. An extinguisher should be provided near every laboratory door, and in a large laboratory, at the end of the room opposite the door. Everyone in the laboratory should be instructed in the use of these extinguishers and any other available firefighting equipment. All fire extinguishers should be tested by qualified personnel at intervals specified by the manufacturer. The three classes of fires and the type of fire extinguisher to be used for each are listed in Table 8.2. Every fire extinguisher is labeled as to the type of fire it should be used to extinguish.

Two additional types of fires, designated "D" and "E," should be handled only by trained personnel. Type D fires include those involving powdered metal materials (e.g., magnesium). A special powder is used to fight this hazard. A type E fire is one that cannot be put out or is liable to result in a detonation (such as an arsenal fire). A type E fire is usually allowed to burn out while nearby materials are appropriately protected.

Many clinical laboratories now have a computer that is housed in a temperature- and humidity-controlled room. The most popular automatic fire control system used for these rooms is Halon 1301 (bromotrifluoromethane). Although this is the least toxic of the halons, NFPA regulations require a warning sign at the entrance to the room and availability of self-contained breathing equipment.

Laboratory safety requirements defined by ISO 15190:2003 Medical laboratories-requirements for safety (Table 8.3).

ISO 15190: 2003 *Medical laboratories-requirements for safety* is a document from ISO that defines international standards and guidelines for enhancing safety in medical and clinical laboratories (summarized in Table 8.3). It should be used as a supplement to ISO 15189 Medical laboratories—Particular requirements for quality and competence. Adherence to the ISO 15190 standard will create a safe working environment and will enable laboratories to meet many of the OSHA standards.

---

**POINTS TO REMEMBER**

**Safety Elements**
Safety in the clinical laboratory contains many elements, including:
- A formal safety program
- A CHP
- A plan for exposure to bloodborne pathogens
- A plan for TB control
- An ergonomics plan
- Identification of significant occupational hazards
- A waste management plan
- A biochemical and chemical terrorism response plan

---

**TABLE 8.2   Classification of Fires and Fire Extinguisher Requirements**

| Type of Hazard | Class of Fire | Recommended Extinguisher Agents |
|---|---|---|
| Ordinary combustibles: wood, cloth, paper | A | Water, dry chemical foam, loaded steam |
| Flammable liquids and gases: solvents and greases, natural or manufactured gases | B | Dry chemical, carbon dioxide, loaded steam, Halon 1211 or 1301 foam |
| Electrical equipment: any energized electrical equipment; if electricity is turned off at source, this reverts to a class A or B | C | Dry chemical, carbon dioxide, Halon 1211 or 1301 foam |
| Combinations of ordinary combustibles and flammable liquids and gases | A and B | Dry chemical, loaded steam, foam |
| Combinations of ordinary combustibles and electrical equipment | A and C | Dry chemical |
| Combinations of flammable liquids and gases and electrical equipment | B and C | Dry chemical, carbon dioxide, Halon 1211 or 1301 foam |
| Combinations of ordinary combustibles, flammable liquids and gases, and electrical equipment | A, B, and C | Triplex dry chemical |

**TABLE 8.3    Summary of the Safety Standards of ISO 15190: 2003 Medical Laboratories-Requirements for Safety**

| | Item | Essential Elements | Additional Comments |
|---|---|---|---|
| 1 | Management requirements | Laboratory director is responsible for safety | Records of immunization kept according to ISO 15189[1a] |
| | | Document evidence of training related to potential work-related risks; records of immunization; hepatitis B vaccination should be offered | |
| 2 | Designing for safety | Adherence to building codes; general design requirements to cater for hazards and provide safe physical working environment (lighting, temperature, etc.), security | Designs of laboratories to ensure containment of microbiological, chemical, radiological and physical hazards |
| 3 | Staffing procedures and documentation | Designated safety officer and documented procedures for safety risk management, including safety audits, safety manuals, records; SOPs for dealing with risks | Records to be kept in accordance with ISO 15189 |
| 4 | Hazard identification | Systematic and clear physical identification of hazards | |
| 5 | Reporting of incidents and illnesses | Program for reporting incidents, injuries, illnesses | Regular review of reports |
| 6 | Training | As part of an established safety training program | |
| 7 | Personnel responsibilities | Adherence to rules pertaining to food, cosmetics, hair, jewelry, immunization status, personal property | |
| 8 | Clothing and personal protective equipment (PPE) | Protective clothing; face and body protection; first aid equipment and training | |
| 9 | Housekeeping practices | Cleaning, disinfecting, dealing with hazardous spills | Designated person to oversee this |
| 10 | Safe work practices | Safety with biological materials | |
| 11 | Aerosols | Reduce contact with aerosols | |
| 12 | Safety hoods and cabinets | For risk groups I and II[2b] | High-efficiency particulate air (HEPA) filtration and venting |
| 13 | Chemical safety | Avoiding chemical contamination; dealing with body contamination; disposal | |
| 14 | Radiation safety | Records of radionuclide acquisition, storage, use and disposal; regular monitoring of workplace | Radiation protection officer should be appointed |
| 15 | Fire precautions | Fire exits, alarm systems, fire risks, training program, emergency evacuation | |
| 16 | Emergency evacuation | Action plan for chemical, fire, microbiological emergencies; Annual fire drill | |
| 17 | Electrical equipment | Compliance with ISO/IEC 61010[3c] for electrical equipment | |
| 18 | Sample transport | Safe transport of samples from all sites | |
| 19 | Waste disposal | Comply with national, regional and local regulations; disposal of sharps and biological material | |

[a]ISO 15189: 2012 Medical laboratories—requirements for quality and competence.
[b]Risk group I (low risk)—microorganisms unlikely to cause disease; Risk group II (moderate risk) pathogens that can cause disease but not a serious hazard.
[c]IEC 61010-1:2010 specifies safety requirements for electrical equipment for measurement, control, and laboratory use.

## REVIEW QUESTIONS

1. One aspect of Standard Precautions, and an Occupational Safety and Health Administration (OSHA) requirement, involves the provision of personal protective equipment (PPE) to laboratory employees. PPE includes (but is not limited to) which of the following?
   a. Gloves only
   b. Gloves and a lab coat only
   c. Gloves, eye protection, and a lab coat
   d. Gloves, eye protection, a lab coat, and special footwear
2. Which of the following uses for analytical weights is false?
   a. Analytical weights are used for verifying performance of single pan balances.
   b. Class S weights are used for calibrating balances.

c. Balances must be calibrated each day of use for accurate analytical work.

d. Weights can be made of materials such as brass and platinum.

3. The organization that develops and implements standards and guidelines for laboratories in addition to setting certain safety guidelines is:
   a. CAP
   b. CLSI
   c. EPA
   d. DOT

4. The process by which the concentration or activity of a given solution is decreased by the addition of solvent is referred to as:
   a. solution.
   b. evaporation.
   c. lyophilization.
   d. dilution.

5. The formula used to determine the molarity of a solution is which of the following?
   a. $C_1V_1 = C_2V_2$
   b. number of moles of solute/number of liters of solution
   c. mg/L divided by mg molecular mass
   d. mass in grams/gram molecular weight in grams

6. Which type of highly purified material needs to minimally be 99.98% pure?
   a. Certified Reference Material
   b. Standard Reference Material
   c. Secondary Reference Material
   d. Primary Reference Material

7. Which of the following statements regarding water purification is *incorrect?*
   a. Water treated by distillation alone does not meet the specific conductivity requirement for Clinical Laboratory Reagent Water (CLRW).
   b. Reverse osmosis forces water through a semipermeable membrane.
   c. Only one purification process is necessary for obtaining CLRW.
   d. UV oxidation can eliminate many bacteria and cleave ionizing organics.

8. The two chemical grades that are suitable for use in a clinical chemistry laboratory are:
   a. technical and analytical reagent grades.
   b. ultrapure and technical grades.
   c. technical and National Formulary grades.
   d. ultrapure and analytical reagent grades.

9. Relative centrifugal force or field (RCF) is measured in which of the following units?
   a. Gravities (*g*)
   b. Centimeters (cm)
   c. rpm
   d. Forces (f)

10. Protection of laboratory workers against potential exposure to bloodborne pathogens and assurance that medical waste is handled safely are OSHA requirements that are part of which of the following plans?
    a. Chemical hygiene plan
    b. Exposure control plan
    c. Tuberculosis control plan
    d. Fire safety plan

## SUGGESTED READINGS

Armbruster D, Miller RR. The Joint Committee for Traceability in Laboratory Medicine (JCTLM): a global approach to promote the standardisation of clinical laboratory test results. *Clin Biochem Rev.* 2007;28:105–113.

Centers for Disease Control and Prevention. *Interim biosafety guidance for all individuals handling clinical specimens or isolates containing 2009-H1N1 influenza A virus (Novel H1N1), including vaccine strains.* http://www.cdc.gov/h1n1flu/guidelines_labworkers.htm. Accessed March 2022.

Clinical and Laboratory Standards Institute. *Clinical Laboratory Safety.* 3rd ed. CLSI Document GP17-A3. Wayne, PA: Clinical and Laboratory Standards Institute; 2012.

Clinical and Laboratory Standards Institute. *Clinical Laboratory Waste Management: Approved Guideline.* 3rd ed. CLSI Document GP5-A3. Wayne, PA: Clinical and Laboratory Standards Institute; 2011.

Clinical and Laboratory Standards Institute. *Laboratory Instrument Implementation, Verification, and Maintenance.* CLSI Document GP31-A. Wayne, PA: Clinical and Laboratory Standards Institute; 2009.

Clinical and Laboratory Standards Institute. *Preparation and Testing of Reagent Water in the Clinical Laboratory: Approved Guideline.* 4th ed. CLSI Document GP40-A4-AMD. Wayne, PA: Clinical and Laboratory Standards Institute; 2012.

Clinical and Laboratory Standards Institute. *Procedures for the Handling and Processing of Blood Specimens: Approved Guideline.* 4th ed. CLSI Document GP44-A4. Wayne, PA: Clinical and Laboratory Standards Institute; 2010.

Clinical and Laboratory Standards Institute. *Protection of Laboratory Workers From Occupationally Acquired Infections: Approved Guideline.* 4th ed. CLSI Document M29-A4. Wayne, PA: Clinical and Laboratory Standards Institute; 2014.

Davis DL. *Laboratory Safety.* Washington, DC: AACC Press; 2008.

De Bièvre P. The 2007 International Vocabulary of Metrology (VIM), JCGM 200:2008 (ISO/IEC Guide 99): meeting the need for intercontinentally understood concepts and their associated intercontinentally agreed terms. *Clin Biochem.* 2009;42:246–248.

Department of Health and Human Services, National Institutes of Health. *Centers for Disease Control and Prevention. Biosafety in Microbiological and Biomedical Laboratories.* 4th ed. Washington, DC: U.S. Government Printing Office; 1999.

Department of Transportation. 49 CFR, Part 171. Hazardous materials: revisions to standards for infectious substances. Final rule. *Fed Regist.* 2002;67(157).

International Standards Organization. *ISO 15189 Medical Laboratories—Particular Requirements for Quality and Competence*; 2003.

International Standards Organization. *ISO 15190 Medical Laboratories—Requirements for Safety*; 2003.

National Institute for Occupational Safety and Health (NIOSH). *Musculoskeletal Disorders and Workplace Factors: A Critical Review of Epidemiologic Evidence for Work-Related Musculoskeletal Disorders of the Neck, Upper Extremities, and Low Back.* Centers for Disease Control (NIOSH) Publication No. 97-141. Atlanta, GA: Centers for Disease Control; 1997.

National Institute for Occupational Safety and Health (NIOSH). Updated U.S. Public Health Service guidelines for the management of occupational exposures to HBV, HCV, and HIV and recommendations for postexposure prophylaxis. *MMWR Recommend Reports.* 2001;50:1–50.

Poon LLM, Chan KH, Smith GJ, et al. Molecular detection of a novel human influenza (H1N1) of pandemic potential by conventional and real-time quantitative RT-PCR assays. *Clin Chem.* 2009;55:1555–1558.

US Department of Labor. Occupational exposure to bloodborne pathogens: needlesticks and other sharps injuries. Final rule. Occupational Safety and Health Administration (OSHA). *Federal Register.* 2001;66:5318–5325.

US Department of Labor. Ergonomics program. Final rule: removal. Occupational Safety and Health Administration (OSHA). *Federal Register.* 2001;666:20403.

Vesper HW, Thienpont LM. Traceability in laboratory medicine. *Clin Chem.* 2009;55:1067–1075.

9

# Optical Techniques

*Khushbu Patel and Jason Y. Park\**

## OBJECTIVES

1. Define the following terms:
   Absorbance
   Atomic absorption
   Beer's law
   Electromagnetic radiation
   Flame emission spectrophotometry
   Fluorescence
   Fluorescence polarization
   Light
   Nephelometry
   Percent transmittance
   Photometry
   Spectral/natural bandwidth
   Spectrophotometry
   Stokes shift
   Transmittance
   Turbidimetry
   Visible/ultraviolet/infrared spectrum
   Wavelength
2. Describe the relationship between the light transmitted and the light absorbed by a solution of a compound; state this relationship as a mathematical formula.
3. Express Beer's law mathematically, and define each of the components of the formula; calculate the concentration of a substance in solution using Beer's law.
4. Explain how Beer's law is used to create a calibration curve, and list five conditions that must be met before Beer's law can be applied to a measurement.
5. State the principle of atomic absorption spectrophotometry; list the clinical laboratory applications of this technique.
6. List the components of an atomic absorption spectrophotometer and the role each component plays in measurement.
7. Describe and give examples of spectral and nonspectral interferences that might limit measurements made using atomic absorption.
8. Explain the basic concepts of chemiluminescence and electrochemiluminescence; list the clinical laboratory applications of these techniques.
9. Explain the basic concepts of light scattering, including six factors that affect light scattering.
10. Compare nephelometry and turbidimetry, and list the clinical laboratory applications of these techniques; describe a turbidimeter and a nephelometer.
11. List and describe two possible interferences that might limit light-scattering measurements.

## KEY WORDS AND DEFINITIONS

**Absorbance (A)** The amount of light absorbed as incident light passes through a sample, which is equivalent to $\log(1/T)$, where $T$ is transmittance. Absorbance and transmittance are inverse properties. For example, when absorbance is low (0.0), the transmittance is high (100%) ($A = \log(1/1.00)$). Conversely, when transmittance is low (10%), the absorbance is 1.0 ($A = 1.0 = \log(1/.10)$).

**Absorptivity (a)** A proportionality constant for a compound that is the measure of the absorption of radiant energy at a given wavelength as it passes through a solution of that compound at a concentration of 1 g/L; expressed mathematically as absorbance divided by the product of the concentration of a substance in g/L and the sample path length in centimeters ($a = A/bc$).

**Atomic absorption (AA) spectrophotometry** A technique in which an element in a sample is dissociated from its chemical bonds (atomized) and placed in an unexcited or ground state (neutral atom); the atom in the ground state is able to absorb radiation and the decrease in radiant energy from the light source transmitted through sample is measured.

*The authors gratefully acknowledge the original contributions by Drs. Larry J. Kricka, Merle A. Evenson, and Thomas O. Tiffany, upon which portions of this chapter are based.

**Bandpass** The range of wavelengths passed by a filter or a monochromator at one-half the peak transmittance of that filter.

**Beer's law** A mathematical equation stating that the concentration of a substance is directly proportional to the amount of light absorbed, mathematically expressed as $A = abc$ or $A = \varepsilon bc$.

**Blank** A solution used in photometry/spectrophotometry that is identical to the unknown solution except for the substance to be measured.

**Chemiluminescence** The emission of light when an electron returns from an excited or higher energy level to a lower energy level, in which the excitation event is caused by a chemical reaction and not by photo illumination, for example, by the oxidation of an organic compound.

**Electrochemiluminescence** The emission of light when an electron returns from an excited or higher energy level to a lower energy level, in which the excitation event is a reaction generated electrochemically on the surface of an electrode.

**Flow cytometry** The measurement of optical properties of cells or particles made while they pass singly through a measuring apparatus in a flowing fluid stream.

**Fluorescence** The emission of electromagnetic radiation that occurs when a molecule absorbs light at one wavelength and reemits light at a longer wavelength.

**Fluorometry** The measurement of emitted fluorescence light that occurs when a molecule absorbs light at one wavelength and reemits light at a longer wavelength.

**Light** Energy transmitted via electromagnetic waves that are characterized by frequency and wavelength; light is composed of photons whose energy is inversely proportional to the wavelength.

**Light scattering** Redirection of light that results from the interaction of light with molecules or particles in solution without absorption taking place.

**Molar absorptivity** ($\varepsilon$) A proportionality constant for a compound that is the measure of the absorption of radiant energy at a given wavelength as it passes through a solution of that compound at a concentration of 1 mol/L; expressed mathematically as absorbance divided by the product of the concentration of a substance in mol/L and the sample path length in centimeters ($\varepsilon = A/bc$).

**Nephelometry** The detection and measurement of light energy scattered or reflected toward a detector that is not in the direct path of the transmitted light; nephelometers may measure scattered light at right angles to the incident light, or at some angle other than 90 degrees.

**Photometry/spectrophotometry** The measurement of the luminous intensity of light or the amount of luminous light falling on a surface of a detector; spectrophotometry is the measurement of the intensity of light at varied wavelengths.

**Reflectance photometry** A spectrophotometric technique in which diffused light illuminates a reaction mixture in a carrier containing a substance of interest, and the intensity of the reflected light is measured and compared with a reference.

**Spectral bandwidth** The width in nanometers of the spectral transmittance curve at a point equal to one-half of the peak transmittance; used to describe the spectral purity of a filter or other monochromator.

**Transmittance** The intensity of a light beam that passes through a square cell containing a solution of a compound that absorbs light at a specific wavelength, divided by the intensity of an incident (incoming) light beam, stated as $T = I/I_0$.

**Turbidimetry** The detection and measurement of a decrease in intensity of an incident beam of light after it passes through a solution of molecules or particles.

**Wavelength** A characteristic of electromagnetic radiation; the distance between two adjacent maxima in a wave that is measured in nanometers.

---

Many determinations made in the clinical laboratory are based on measurements of radiant energy emitted, transmitted, absorbed, scattered, or reflected under controlled conditions. The principles involved in such measurements are considered in this chapter.

## NATURE OF LIGHT

Electromagnetic radiation includes radiant energy that extends from gamma rays with wavelengths less than 100 pm to long radio waves greater than 1000 km. However, in this chapter, the term **light** is used to describe radiant energy from the ultraviolet (UV; <380 nm) and visible portions of the spectrum (380 to 750 nm).

The **wavelength** of light is defined as the distance between two peaks as the light travels in a wavelike manner. This distance is expressed in nanometers (nm) for wavelengths commonly used in photometry. Other units include:

$$1\,nm = 1\,millimicron\,(m\mu) = 10\,Angstroms\,(\mathring{A}) = 10^{-9}\,m$$

In addition to possessing wavelength characteristics, light has properties of discrete energy packets called *photons*. The relationship between the energy of photons and their frequency is given by Planck's equation:

$$E = h\nu \tag{9.1}$$

where $E$ = energy in joules, $\nu$ = frequency of light in cycles per second, and $h$ = Planck's constant ($6.626 \times 10^{-34}$ joule seconds). The $\nu$ is related to the wavelength by an equation:

$$\nu = \frac{c}{\lambda} \tag{9.2}$$

where $c$ = speed of light in a vacuum ($3 \times 10^{10}$ cm/s), and $\lambda$ = wavelength in centimeters. Combining Eqs. (9.1) and (9.2) results in:

$$E = \frac{hc}{\lambda} \tag{9.3}$$

This equation shows that the energy of light is inversely proportional to the wavelength. For example, UV radiation at

200 nm possesses greater energy than infrared (IR) radiation at 750 nm.

The human eye detects radiant energy with wavelengths between approximately 380 and 750 nm, but modern instrumentation permits measurements at both shorter wavelength (UV) and longer wavelength (IR) portions of the spectrum. Sunlight, or light emitted from a tungsten filament, is a mixture of wavelengths or a spectrum of radiant energy of different wavelengths that the eye recognizes as "white." Table 9.1 shows approximate relationships between wavelengths and color characteristics for the UV, visible, and short IR portions of the spectrum.

### POINTS TO REMEMBER

**Radiant Energy**
- Wavelength size has a wide distribution, ranging from less than 10 pm to greater than 1000 km.
- The visible portion of the spectrum ranges from approximately 380 to 750 nm.
- The energy of light is inversely proportional to the wavelength; shorter wavelengths have greater energy.
- Light possesses both wavelength and energy packet characteristics; the packets are described as photons.

## SPECTROPHOTOMETRY

**Photometry** is defined as the measurement of light; **spectrophotometry** is defined as the measurement of the intensity of light at selected wavelengths. Spectrophotometric analysis is a widely used method of quantitative and qualitative analysis in the chemical and biological sciences. The method depends on the light-absorbing properties of the substance or a derivative of the substance being analyzed. The intensity of transmitted light passing through a solution containing an absorbing substance (chromogen) is decreased by the absorbed fraction. This fraction is detected, measured, and used to relate the light transmitted or absorbed to the concentration of the analyte in question.

### Basic Concepts

Consider an incident light beam with intensity $I_0$ passing through a square cell containing a solution of a compound that absorbs light of a certain wavelength, $\lambda$ (Fig. 9.1). Given the intensity of the transmitted light beam $I_S$, the **transmittance** $(T)$ of light is defined as:

$$T = \frac{I_S}{I_0} \qquad (9.4)$$

However, a portion of the incident light may be reflected by the surface of the cell or may be absorbed by the cell wall or solvent. To focus attention on the compound of interest, elimination of these factors is necessary. This is achieved using a reference cell identical to the sample cell, except that the compound of interest is omitted from the solvent in the reference cell (i.e., reference blank). The transmittance $(T)$ through this reference cell is $I_R$ divided by $I_0$; the transmittance for the compound in solution is then defined as $I_S$ divided by $I_R$. In practice, the light beam is blocked, the detector signal is set to zero transmittance, then a reference cell is inserted, and the detector signal is adjusted to an arbitrary scale reading of 100 (corresponding to 100% transmittance), followed by the cell containing the sample to be measured, and the percent transmittance reading is made on the sample. As the concentration of the compound in solution is increased, the transmittance varies inversely and logarithmically with the concentration. Consequently, it is more convenient to define a new term, **absorbance** *(A)*, which will be directly proportional to the concentration. Thus, the amount of light absorbed *(A)* as the incident light passes through the sample is equivalent to:

$$A = -\log\left(\frac{I_S}{I_R}\right) = -\log T \qquad (9.5)$$

| TABLE 9.1   Ultraviolet, Visible, and Short Infrared Spectrum Characteristics | | |
|---|---|---|
| **Wavelength (nm)** | **Region Name** | **Color Observed**[a] |
| <380 | Ultraviolet[b] | Invisible |
| 380–440 | Visible | Violet |
| 440–500 | Visible | Blue |
| 500–580 | Visible | Green |
| 580–600 | Visible | Yellow |
| 600–620 | Visible | Orange |
| 620–750 | Visible | Red |
| 800–2,500 | Near infrared | Not visible |
| 2,500–15,000 | Mid infrared | Not visible |
| 15,000–1,000,000 | Far infrared | Not visible |

[a]Because of the subjective nature of color, the wavelength intervals shown are only approximations.

[b]The ultraviolet (UV) portion of the spectrum is sometimes further divided into "near" UV (200 to 380 nm) and "far" UV (<220 nm). This arbitrary distinction has a practical basis because silica used to make cuvets transmits light effectively at wavelengths ≥220 nm.

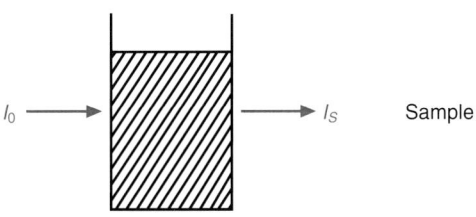
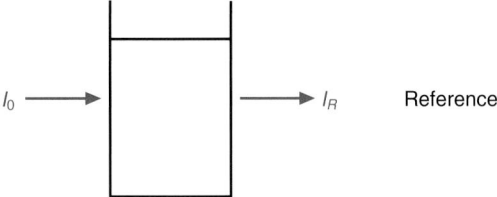

**Fig. 9.1** Transmittance of light through sample and reference cells. The transmittance of the sample versus the reference cell is then $I_S/I_R$. $I_0$, Intensity of incident light; $I_R$, intensity of transmitted light through a reagent blank in the reference cell; $I_S$, intensity of transmitted light for the compound in solution.

Analytically, the amount of light absorbed or transmitted is related mathematically to the concentration of the analyte in question by Beer's law.

## Beer's Law: Relationship Among Transmittance, Absorbance, and Concentration

**Beer's law** (also known as the Beer-Lambert law) states that the concentration of a substance is directly proportional to the amount of light absorbed or inversely proportional to the logarithm of the transmitted light (Fig. 9.2). Mathematically, Beer's law is expressed as:

$$A = abc \qquad (9.6)$$

where $A$ = absorbance; $a$ = proportionality constant defined as **absorptivity**; $b$ = light path (in centimeters); and $c$ = concentration of the absorbing compound (usually expressed in moles per liter).

This equation forms the basis of quantitative analysis by absorption photometry. When $b$ is 1 cm and $c$ is expressed in moles per liter, the constant $a$ is called the **molar absorptivity**. The value for $a$ is a constant for a given compound at a given wavelength under prescribed conditions of solvent, temperature, pH, and so forth. The nomenclature of spectrophotometry is summarized in Table 9.2. Values for $a$ are useful for characterizing compounds, establishing their purity, and comparing the sensitivity of measurements obtained on derivatives. For example, the molar absorptivity

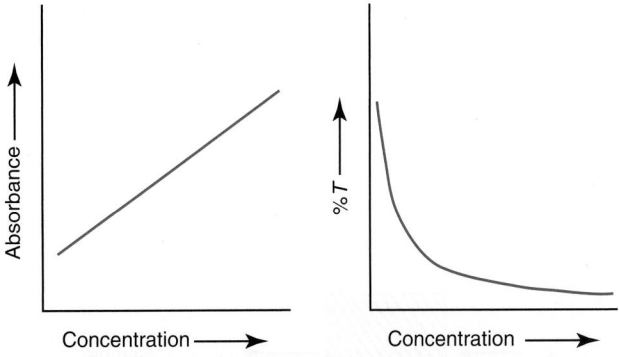

**Fig. 9.2** Absorbance and %*T* relationship.

## TABLE 9.2   Spectrophotometry Nomenclature

| Name | Symbol | Definition |
|---|---|---|
| Absorbance | $A$ | $-\log T$ or $\log I_0 / I$ |
| Absorptivity | $a$ | $A/bc$ ($c$ in g/L) |
| Molar absorptivity | $\varepsilon$ | $A/bc$ ($c$ in mol/L) |
| Path length | $b$ | Internal cell or sample length, in cm |
| Transmittance | $T$ | $I_s/I_0$[a] |
| Wavelength unit | nm | $10^{-9}$ m |
| Absorption maximum | λmax | Wavelength at which maximum absorption occurs |

[a]$I_s/I_0$ is the ratio of the intensity of transmitted light to incident light.

of the complex between ferrous iron and *s*-tripyridyltriazine is 22,600, whereas that with 1,10-phenanthroline is 11,000. Thus, for a given concentration of iron, *s*-tripyridyltriazine produces a complex with an absorbance approximately twice that of the complex with 1,10-phenanthroline. Consequently, *s*-tripyridyltriazine is a more sensitive reagent to use in the measurement of iron.

## Application of Beer's Law

In practice, a calibration relationship between absorbance and concentration is established experimentally for a given instrument under specified conditions using a series of reference solutions that contain increasing concentrations of analyte. Frequently, a linear relationship exists up to a certain concentration or absorbance. When this linear relationship exists, the solution is said to obey Beer's law up to this point. Within this limitation, a calibration constant may be derived and used to calculate the concentration of an unknown solution by comparison with a calibrating solution.

Certain precautions must be observed with the use of such calibration constants. For example, calibration constants cannot be used when the calibrator or unknown readings exceed the linear portion of the calibration relationship. In other words, calibration constants are used only when the curve obeys Beer's law. At least two and preferably more calibrators should be included in each series of determinations to permit direct comparison of unknown readings with calibrators or to calculate the calibration constant. Multiple calibrators are necessary because variations in reagents, working conditions, cell diameters, and deterioration or changes in instruments may result in day-to-day changes in the absorbance value for the calibrator. A nonlinear calibration curve may be used if enough calibrators of varying concentrations are included to cover the entire range encountered for readings of unknowns.

In some cases, a pure reference material may not be readily available, and constants may be provided that were obtained on pure materials and reported in the literature. In general, published constants should only be used if the method is followed in detail and readings are made on a spectrophotometer capable of providing light of high spectral purity at a verified wavelength. Use of broader band light sources usually leads to some decrease in absorbance. For example, the absorbance of nicotinamide adenine dinucleotide at 340 nm is frequently used as a reference for determination of enzyme activity, based on a molar absorptivity of 6220 cm$^{-1}$M$^{-1}$. This value is acceptable only under carefully controlled conditions and should not be used unless these conditions are met. Published values for molar absorptivities and absorption coefficients should be used only as guidelines until they are verified by readings on pure reference materials for a given instrument. In addition, Beer's law is followed only if the following conditions are met:

- Incident radiation on the substance of interest is monochromatic.
- The solvent absorption is insignificant compared with the solute absorbance.
- The solute concentration is within given limits.

- An optical interferent is not present.
- A chemical reaction does not occur between the molecule of interest and another solute or solvent molecule.

## INSTRUMENTATION

Modern instruments isolate a narrow wavelength range of the spectrum for measurements. Those that use filters for this purpose are referred to as *filter photometers;* those that use prisms or gratings are called *spectrophotometers.* Spectrophotometers are classified as single or double beam.

The major components of a single-beam spectrophotometer are shown in Fig. 9.3. In such an instrument, a beam of light is passed through a monochromator that isolates the desired region of the spectrum to be used for measurements. The light next passes through an absorption cell (cuvet), where a portion of the radiant energy is absorbed, depending on the nature and concentration of the substance in the solution. Light not absorbed can be transmitted to a detector, which converts light energy to electrical energy that is registered on a meter or recorder, or digitally displayed.

In operation, an opaque block is substituted for the cuvet, so that no light reaches the photocell, and the meter is adjusted to read 0% *T.* Next, a cuvet containing a reagent **blank** is inserted, and the meter is adjusted to read 100% *T* (zero absorbance). The composition of the reagent blank should be identical to that of the calibrating or unknown solutions except for the substance to be measured. Calibrating solutions containing various known concentrations of the substance are inserted, and readings are recorded. Finally, a reading is made of the unknown solution, and its concentration is determined by

comparison with readings obtained on the calibrators. In most spectrophotometers, digital hardware and software are integral components and perform these functions automatically.

Fig. 9.4 illustrates a typical double-beam instrument that uses a light-beam chopper (a rotating wheel with alternate silvered sections and cutout sections) inserted after the exit slit. A system of mirrors passes portions of the light reflected off the chopper alternately through the sample and a reference cuvet onto a common detector. The chopped-beam approach, using one detector, compensates for light source variation and for sensitivity changes in the detector.

### Components

The basic components of a spectrophotometer include (1) a light source, (2) a device to isolate light of a desired wavelength, (3) a cuvet, (4) a photodetector, (5) a readout device, and (6) a data system.

### Light Sources

Types of light sources used in spectrophotometers include incandescent lamps, xenon discharge lamps, lasers, and light-emitting diodes (LEDs).

***Incandescent, arc, and cathode lamps.*** The light source for measurements in the visible portion of the spectrum is usually a tungsten light bulb. The lifetime of a tungsten filament is greatly increased by the presence of a low pressure of iodine or bromine vapor within the lamp. An example is the quartz-halogen lamp, which has a fused-silica envelope and provides high-intensity light over a wide spectrum for extended operating periods (2000 to 5000 hours) before replacement is necessary.

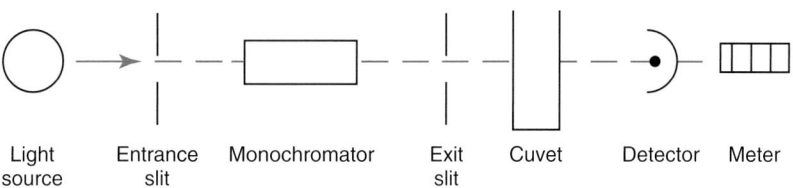

| Light source | Entrance slit | Monochromator | Exit slit | Cuvet | Detector | Meter |

**Fig. 9.3** Major components of a single-beam spectrophotometer.

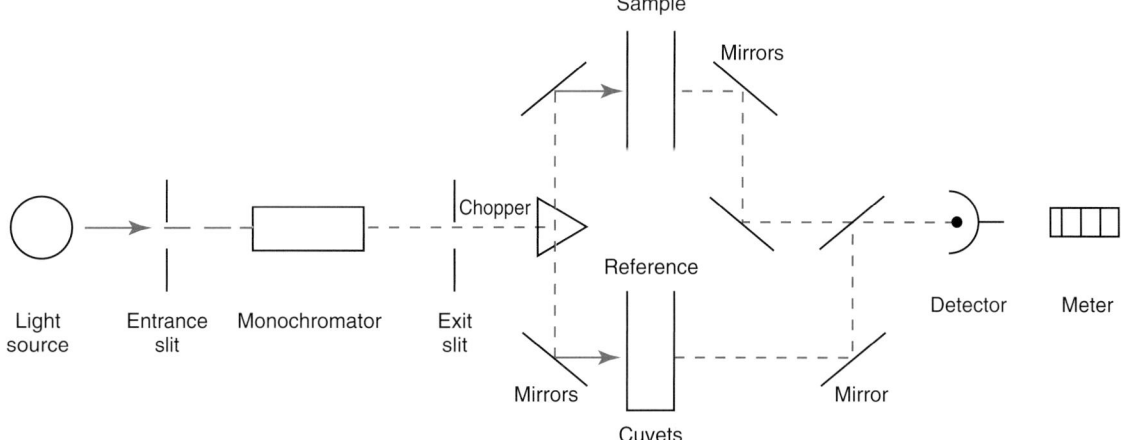

**Fig. 9.4** Major components of a double-beam spectrophotometer.

However, a tungsten light source does not supply sufficient radiant energy for measurements in the UV region (<320 nm). In the UV region of the spectrum, hydrogen and deuterium lamps, as well as high-pressure mercury and xenon arc lamps, are sources of continuous spectra with sharp emission lines. These sources are more commonly used in UV absorption measurements. Low-pressure mercury vapor lamps also provide spectra in the UV region and are useful for calibration purposes, but because of their limited wavelengths, they are not practical for absorbance measurements.

Mercury arc lamps emit an intense 254 nm resonance line and are widely used as detectors in high-pressure liquid chromatography (HPLC). Alternatively, some HPLCs use a miniature hollow cathode lamp as a very narrow wavelength intense source. For example, a zinc hollow cathode lamp emits a line at 214 nm that is close to the maximum wavelength of peptide bond absorption (206 nm); this emission property permits the usage of such lamps to measure peptides and proteins. Details on the hollow cathode lamp are found in the section on Atomic Absorption Spectrophotometry. The hollow cathode lamp also has a long, useful lifetime if a lower current, nonpulsed power supply is used.

*Laser sources.* A laser (light amplification by stimulated emission of radiation) is a device that controls the way that energized atoms release photons; lasers are used as light sources in spectrophotometers because they provide intense light of a narrow wavelength. Through selection of different materials, different wavelength(s) of light are emitted by different types of lasers.

Three properties of laser sources distinguish them from "conventional" sources: (1) spatial coherence is a property of lasers that allows beam diameters in the range of several micrometers; (2) lasers produce monochromatic light; and (3) lasers have pulse widths that vary from microseconds (flash lamp–pulsed lasers) to nanoseconds (nitrogen lasers) to picoseconds or less (mode-locked lasers) in duration. Air-cooled argon ion lasers produce approximately 25 mW of energy output at 488 nm and have plasma tube lifetimes of 6000 hours or longer. Continuous-wave dye lasers typically use an argon ion laser with an output of 1 W or less as an energy pump and use different fluorescent dyes to achieve excitation wavelength ranges of 400 to 800 nm. Helium-neon and helium-cadmium lasers are useful because of their low cost and ease of operation, and because they emit a number of excitation wavelengths; however, the power output of helium-neon lasers has been limited to approximately 2 mW at 594 nm.

Diode lasers are used in compact disc players and laser printers, and in bar code readers. They are solid-state devices, typically constructed of gallium arsenide, and energy is pumped into them at a low potential of −1.5 V. Depending on its construction, the wavelength output of the laser ranges from 350 to 29,000 nm. Development of inexpensive near-IR lasers has led to interest in using reflective techniques in the near-IR region of the spectrum (0.8- to 2.5-μm wavelength). Reflectance spectrophotometry is now used clinically for the transcutaneous measurement of bilirubin in neonates. Another application of reflectance spectrophotometry is measurement of blood oxygen saturation in near-IR and IR regions.

## Spectral Isolation

Radiant energy of a desired wavelength can be isolated and that of other wavelengths excluded in various ways, including the use of (1) filters (interference or dichroic filters), (2) prisms, and (3) diffraction gratings. Combinations of lenses and slits may be inserted before or after the monochromatic device to render light rays parallel or to isolate narrow portions of the light beam. Variable slits may be used to permit adjustments in total radiant energy to reach the photocell.

*Filters.* The simplest type of filter is colored glass. Certain metal complexes or salts, dissolved or suspended in glass, produce colors corresponding to the predominant wavelengths transmitted. The spectral purity of a filter or other monochromator is usually described in terms of its **spectral bandwidth**. This is defined as the width, in nanometers, of the spectral transmittance curve at a point equal to one half the peak transmittance. Glass filters have spectral bandwidths of approximately 50 nm, and are referred to as wide **bandpass** filters.

Other glass filters include narrow bandpass and sharp cutoff types. Operationally, a cutoff filter typically shows a sharp rise in transmittance over a narrow portion of the spectrum and is used to eliminate light below a given wavelength. Historically, narrow bandpass filters were constructed by combining two or more sharp cutoff filters or regular filters. Currently, however, the availability of high-intensity light sources now favors the use of narrow bandpass interference filters.

A narrow bandpass interference or dichroic filter uses a dielectric material of controlled thickness sandwiched between two thinly silvered pieces of glass. The thickness of the layer determines the wavelength of energy transmitted after constructive and destructive wavelength interference caused by reflections between the glass surfaces separated by the dielectric spacing. These filters have narrow spectral bandwidths, usually from 5 to 15 nm. Because they also transmit harmonics, or multiples, of the desired wavelength, accessory glass filters are required to eliminate undesired wavelengths. For example, an interference filter designed for 620 nm will also transmit some radiation at 310 and 1240 nm unless accessory cutoff filters are provided to absorb this undesired light.

*Prisms and gratings.* Prisms and diffraction gratings are widely used as monochromators. A prism separates white light into a continuous spectrum because shorter wavelengths are bent, or refracted, more than longer wavelengths as they pass through the prism. A diffraction grating is prepared by depositing a thin layer of aluminum-copper alloy on the surface of a flat glass plate, and then fabricating many small parallel grooves into the metal coating. Better gratings contain 1000 to 2000 lines/mm and must be made with great care. These are then used as molds to prepare less expensive replicas for general use in instruments.

Each line ruled on the grating, when illuminated, reflects light and gives rise to a tiny spectrum. An array of parallel wavefronts is formed that reinforce those wavelengths in phase and cancel those wavelengths not in phase. The net result is a uniform linear spectrum. Instruments contain diffraction gratings that produce spectral bandwidths in the range of 0.5 to 20 nm.

The flat surface grating discussed previously is called a plane transmission grating. Lines are engraved on the surface of a mirror, which may be a polished metal slab or a glass plate on which a thin, metallic film has been deposited. A grating may also be ruled at a specified angle, so that a maximum fraction of the radiant energy is directed into wavelengths diffracted at a selected angle.

*Selection of a wavelength isolation device.* The type of monochromator chosen depends on the analytical purpose for which it is to be used. For example, narrow spectral bandwidths are required in spectrophotometers for resolving and identifying sharp absorption peaks that are closely adjacent. Lack of agreement with Beer's law will occur when a part of the spectral energy transmitted by the monochromator is not absorbed by the substance being measured. This is more commonly observed with wide bandpass instruments. In practice, an increase in absorbance and improved linearity with concentration are usually observed with instruments that operate at narrower bandwidths of light. This is especially true for substances that exhibit a sharp peak of absorption.

The natural bandwidth of an absorbing substance is the bandwidth of the spectral absorbance at half the maximum absorbance. As a general rule, the spectral bandwidth should not exceed 10% of the natural bandwidth for peak absorbance readings to be within 99.5% of true values. For example, many chemistry procedures used in the clinical laboratory produce an absorbing species for which the natural bandwidth ranges from 40 to more than 200 nm. The natural bandwidth of nicotinamide adenine dinucleotide is 58 nm ($\lambda_{max}$ = 339 nm). Therefore, for accurate measurements of this compound, a spectral bandwidth of 6 nm or less should be used.

In practice, the wavelength selected is usually at the peak of maximum absorbance to attain the maximum measurement; however, it may be desirable to choose another wavelength to minimize interfering substances. For example, turbidity readings on a spectrophotometer are greater in the blue region than in the red region of the spectrum, but the latter region is chosen for turbidity measurements to avoid absorption of light by bilirubin (460 nm) or hemoglobin (417 and 575 nm). The absorbing species developed in the alkaline picrate procedure for creatinine produces a relatively flat peak in the visible region of the spectrum at approximately 480 nm, but the reagent blank itself absorbs light strongly at less than 500 nm. A compromise is made by selecting a wavelength at 520 nm to minimize the contribution of the blank. Blank readings should be kept to a minimum. A small difference between two large numbers is subject to greater uncertainty; hence, minimizing absorbance of the blank improves precision and accuracy. The linear working range of a method can be expanded by not measuring at the peak absorbance. However, measurements should not be taken on the steep slope of an absorption curve, because a slight error in wavelength adjustment will introduce a significant error in absorbance readings.

## Cuvets

A cuvet (also often termed a cuvette) is a small vessel used to hold a liquid sample to be analyzed in the light path of a spectrometer. Cuvets may be round, square, or rectangular, and are constructed from glass, silica (quartz), or plastic. Square or rectangular cuvets have plane-parallel optical surfaces and a constant light path. The most popular cuvets have a 1.0-cm light path, held to close tolerances. Ordinary borosilicate glass or plastic cuvets are suitable for measurements in the visible portion of the spectrum. However, quartz cells are usually required for readings at less than 340 nm. Some plastic cells have good clarity in both the visible and UV range, but they can present problems related to tolerances, cleaning, etching by solvents, and temperature deformations. Many plastic cuvets are designed for disposable, single-use applications. However, in many clinical analyzers, cuvets are cleaned and reused many times before optical degradation requires them to be replaced.

Cuvets must be clean and optically clear, because etching or deposits on the surface affect absorbance values. Cuvets used in the visible range are cleaned by copious rinsing with tap water and distilled water. Alkaline solutions should not be left standing in cuvets for prolonged periods, because alkali slowly dissolves glass and produces etching. Cuvets may be cleaned in mild detergent or soaked in a mixture of concentrated hydrogen chloride to water to ethanol (1:3:4). Cuvets should never be soaked in dichromate cleaning solution because the solution is hazardous and tends to adsorb onto and discolor the glass.

Cuvets used for measurements in the UV region should be handled with special care. Invisible scratches, fingerprints, or residual traces of previously measured substances may be present and may absorb significantly. A good practice is to fill cuvets with distilled water and confirm lack of absorbance against a reference blank over the wavelengths to be used.

## Photodetectors

A photodetector is a device that converts light into an electric signal that is proportional to the number of photons striking its photosensitive surface. The photomultiplier tube (PMT) is a commonly used photodetector for measuring light intensity in the UV and visible regions of the spectrum. Alternatively, photodiodes are solid-state devices that are also used in modern instruments. In older instruments, barrier layer cells (also known as photovoltaic cells) were used as photodetectors, because they were durable and inexpensive.

*Photomultiplier tubes.* A PMT contains a light-sensitive cathode, and a series of dynodes, all of which are enclosed in an evacuated glass enclosure. As many as 10 to 15 stages or dynodes are present in common photomultipliers. Photons that strike the photoemissive cathode emit electrons that are accelerated toward the dynodes. Additional electrons are generated at each dynode. Depending on the number of dynodes and the accelerating voltage, the cascading effect creates $10^5$ to $10^7$ electrons for each photon hitting the first cathode. This amplified signal is finally collected at the anode, where it can be measured.

PMTs (1) have extremely rapid response times, (2) are very sensitive, and (3) are slow to fatigue. Because these tubes are very sensitive and have a rapid response, they must be carefully shielded from all stray light. A PMT with the voltage applied should never be exposed to room light because it will burn out. Also, PMTs are sensitive over a wide range of wavelengths.

When voltage is applied to a PMT in the absence of any incident light, some current is usually produced. This current is called dark current. It is desirable to have the dark current of a PMT at its lowest level because this current appears as background noise.

*Photodiodes.* Photodiodes are solid-state photodetectors that are fabricated from photosensitive semiconductor materials such as silicon or gallium arsenide. These types of materials absorb light over a characteristic wavelength range (e.g., 250 to 1100 nm for silicon). Their development and use as detectors in spectrophotometers have resulted in instruments capable of measuring light at a multitude of wavelengths. When a photodetector consists of an array of diodes, it is known as a photodiode array. When light is spatially dispersed according to wavelength, each photodetector within the array responds to a specific wavelength. For example, spectrophotometers with photodiode arrays have been designed to have a 2-nm resolution per diode from 200 to 340 nm, and a 1-nm resolution per diode from 340 to 800 nm. The operation of photodiode arrays is complex but may include repeated scans of charging to a fixed voltage, followed by a discharge proportional to the quantity of incident light. Because scan time for diodes is in the millisecond range, many scans can be acquired. The resultant data are processed using a variety of algorithms, including signal averaging, background subtraction, and correction for scattered light. Consequently, an optical spectrum of an ongoing chemical reaction can be monitored as a function of time with a high degree of resolution and accuracy.

### Readout Devices

Electrical energy from a detector is displayed on a digital readout device that provides a visual or numerical display of absorbance or converted values of concentrations. Various types of software can be used in combination with computers to store data, perform calculations, and display data.

### Performance Parameters

In most spectrophotometric analytical procedures, the absorbance of an unknown is compared directly with that of a calibrator or a series of calibrators. Under these circumstances, minor errors in wavelength calibration, variation in spectral bandwidths, and the presence of stray light are compensated for and usually do not contribute serious errors. Using a series of calibrators covering a wide range of concentrations improves linearity (i.e., agreement with Beer's law for a given procedure and instrument). However, when calculations are based on published or previously determined values for molar absorptivities or absorption coefficients, the spectrophotometer should be checked more rigorously. Performance verification of spectrophotometers on a periodic basis also improves reliability of routine comparative analyses.

To verify that a spectrophotometer is performing satisfactorily, the following parameters should be tested: (1) wavelength accuracy, (2) spectral bandwidth, (3) stray light, (4) linearity, and (5) photometric accuracy.

The National Institute of Standards and Technology (NIST) provides several standard reference materials (SRMs) for spectrophotometry that are useful in the calibration or verification of the performance of photometers or spectrophotometers (e.g., SRM 930e is for the verification and calibration of the transmittance and absorbance scales of visible absorption spectrometers) (http://www.nist.gov/srm).

## REFLECTANCE PHOTOMETRY

In **reflectance photometry** reflected light is measured. The reaction mixture in a carrier is illuminated with diffused light, and the intensity of the reflected light from the chromogen is compared with the intensity of light reflected from a reference surface. The electro-optical components used in reflectance photometry are essentially the same as those required for absorbance photometry, except that the geometry of the system is modified so that the light source and the detector are located next to each other on one side of the sample, as opposed to on opposite sides of the sample cuvet, as in absorption photometry. Reflectance photometry is used as the measurement method with dry-film chemistry systems.

## FLAME EMISSION AND INDUCTIVELY COUPLED PLASMA SPECTROPHOTOMETRY

Flame emission spectrophotometry is based on the characteristic emission of light by atoms of many metallic elements when given sufficient energy, such as that supplied by a hot flame. The wavelength to be used for the measurement of an element depends on the selection of a line of sufficient intensity to provide adequate sensitivity and freedom from other interfering lines at or near the selected wavelength. For example, lithium produces a red, sodium a yellow, potassium a violet, rubidium a red, and magnesium a blue color in a flame. These colors are characteristic of the metal atoms that are present as cations in solution. Under constant and controlled conditions, the light intensity of the characteristic wavelength produced by each of the atoms is directly proportional to the number of atoms that are emitting energy, which in turn is directly proportional to the concentration of the substance of interest in the sample. Although this technique once was used widely for analysis of sodium, potassium, and lithium in body fluids, it now has been replaced largely by electrochemical techniques.

Inductively coupled plasma (ICP) atomic emission spectroscopy is a technique for elemental analysis (e.g., trace metals) that uses an ICP to produce excited species that emit light at wavelengths characteristic of a particular element present in the sample. An ICP spectrometer consists of an optical spectrometer and an ICP torch. The torch produces argon gas plasma (10,000°K) using a radiofrequency induction coil and an electric spark. A nebulized sample is injected into the argon gas plasma; elements in the sample become excited, and the electrons emit energy at a characteristic wavelength as they return to ground state. The emitted light is then measured by optical spectrometry.

## Atomic Absorption Spectroscopy

Atomic absorption (AA) spectroscopy is used in clinical laboratories to measure elements such as aluminum, calcium, copper, lead, lithium, magnesium, zinc, and other metals. AA is an absorption spectrophotometric technique in which a metallic atom in the sample absorbs light of a specific wavelength. However, the element is not appreciably excited in the flame, but is merely dissociated from its chemical bonds (atomized) and placed in an unexcited or ground state (neutral atom). Thus, the ground state atom absorbs radiation at a very narrow bandwidth corresponding to its own line spectrum. A hollow cathode lamp with the cathode made of the material to be analyzed is used to produce a wavelength of light specific for the atom. Thus, if the cathode were made of sodium, sodium light at predominantly 589 nm would be emitted by the lamp. When the light from the hollow cathode lamp enters the flame, some of it is absorbed by the ground-state atoms in the flame, resulting in a net decrease in the intensity of the beam from the lamp. This process is referred to as AA.

A specific hollow cathode lamp serves as the light source. The sample heated in the flame comprises the "cuvet" and its path length. Most of the atoms are in the ground state and are able to absorb light emitted by the cathode lamp. In general, AA methods are approximately 100 times more sensitive than flame emission methods. In addition, because of the unique specificity of the wavelength from the hollow cathode lamp, these methods are highly specific for the element being measured. A method for metal analysis that has begun to replace AA is inductively coupled plasma mass spectrometry (ICP-MS). AA retains advantages over ICP-MS in terms of overall cost and ease of use. However, a single ICP-MS instrument has greater flexibility in measuring multiple metals simultaneously and with greater sensitivity.

## Instrumentation

The components of an AA spectrophotometer are shown in Fig. 9.5. The hollow cathode lamp is made of the metal of the substance to be analyzed and is different for each metal analysis. In some cases, an alloy is used to make the cathode, resulting in a multielement lamp. The hollow cathode lamp usually contains argon or neon gas at a pressure of a few millimeters of mercury. An argon-filled lamp produces a blue-to-purple glow during operation, and the neon produces a reddish-orange glow inside the hollow cathode lamp. Quartz, or a special glass that allows transmission of the proper wavelength, is used as a window. A current is applied between the two electrodes inside the hollow cathode lamp, and metal is atomized from the cathode into the gases inside the glass envelope. When the metal atoms collide with the neon or argon gases, they lose energy and emit their characteristic radiation. Calcium has a sharp, intense, analytical emission line at 422.7 nm, which is used most frequently for calcium analysis. In an ideal interference-free system, only calcium atoms absorb the calcium light from the hollow cathode as it passes through the flame.

A pulsed hollow cathode lamp and a tuned amplifier are incorporated into most AA instruments. Operationally, the power to the hollow cathode lamp is pulsed, so that light is emitted by the lamp at a certain number of pulses per second. In contrast, all of the light originating from the flame is continuous. When light leaves the flame, it is composed of pulsed, unabsorbed light from the lamp and a small amount of nonpulsed flame spectrum and sample emission light. The detector senses all light, but the amplifier is electrically tuned to the pulsed signals and can subtract the background light measured when the lamp is off and the total light that includes both the lamp and flame background light. In this way, the electronics, in conjunction with the monochromator, discriminates between the flame background emission and the sample AA.

In flameless AA techniques (carbon rod or "graphite furnace"), the sample is placed in a depression on a carbon rod in an enclosed chamber. Strips of tantalum or platinum metal may also be used as sample cups. In successive steps, the temperature of the rod is raised to dry, char, and, finally, atomize the sample into the gas phase in the chamber. The atomized element then absorbs energy from the corresponding hollow cathode lamp. This approach is more sensitive than conventional flame methods and permits determination of trace metals in small samples of blood or tissue.

With flameless AA, a novel approach used to correct for background absorption is called the Zeeman correction. In Zeeman background correction, the atomizer and analyte are placed in a strong magnetic field. The intense magnetic field splits the atomic energy levels into two components that are

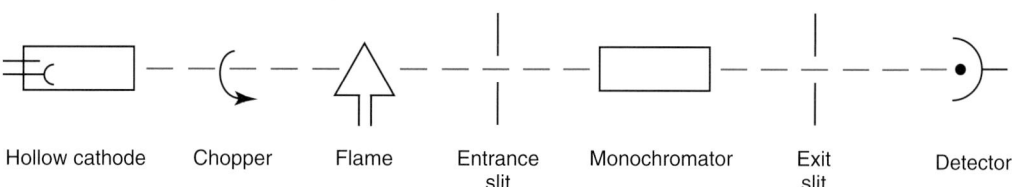

Hollow cathode    Chopper    Flame    Entrance
slit    Monochromator    Exit
slit    Detector

**Fig. 9.5** Basic components of an atomic absorption spectrophotometer.

polarized parallel and perpendicular to the magnetic field. The parallel component remains at the wavelength of the source, whereas the perpendicular components are shifted to different wavelengths. A polarizer is placed between the source and the atomizer, and two absorption measurements are taken at different polarizer settings. One measures both analyte and background absorptions, $A_t$, the other only the background absorption, $A_{bc}$. The difference between the two absorption readings is the corrected absorbance.

The major advantage of the Zeeman correction method is that the same light source at the same wavelength is used to measure the total and the background absorption. The implementation is complex and expensive, and the strength of the magnetic field needs to be optimized for every element, but the method gives more accurate results at higher background levels than those attained with the other correction techniques.

## Interferences in Atomic Absorption Spectrophotometry

Interferences in AA spectroscopy are divided into spectral and nonspectral interferences. Spectral interferences include absorption by other closely absorbing atomic species, absorption by molecular species, scattering by nonvolatile salt particles or oxides, and background emission (which can be electronically filtered). Absorption by other atomic species usually is not a problem because of the extremely narrow bandwidth (0.01 nm) used in the absorption measurements. Absorption and scattering by molecular species are particularly problematic with lower atomizing temperatures.

Nonspectral interferences may be nonspecific or specific. Nonspecific interference may arise from differences in sample viscosity, surface tension, or density that alter nebulization and the sample flow rate. Contaminants that decrease atomization efficiency can also interfere in a nonspecific manner. In contrast, specific interferences, also called chemical interferences, are analyte dependent. Specific interferences include solute volatilization, dissociation, ionization, and excitation interferences. Solute volatilization interference occurs when a contaminant alters the volatility of the analyte. For example, phosphate can interfere with calcium determinations because less volatile calcium–phosphate complexes are formed. The interference can be overcome by adding a cation, usually lanthanum or strontium that preferentially binds phosphate. In contrast, enhanced volatility is observed with aluminum in the presence of hydrofluoric acid that forms the more volatile aluminum fluoride. In dissociation interference, analyte dissociation is affected by, for example, the formation of oxides or hydroxides. In ionization interference, the presence of an easily ionized element, such as potassium, affects the degree of ionization of the analyte, which leads to changes in the analyte signal. Ionization interference is controlled by adding a relatively high concentration of an element that is easily ionized to suppress ionization of the analyte. In the case of excitation interference at higher temperatures, analyte atoms are excited in the atomizer with subsequent emission at the absorption wavelength.

## FLUOROMETRY

**Fluorescence** refers to the condition in which a molecule absorbs light at one wavelength and reemits light at a longer wavelength. An atom or molecule that fluoresces is termed a fluorophore. **Fluorometry** is defined as the measurement of emitted fluorescent light. Fluorometric analysis is widely used for quantitative measurement in the chemical and biological sciences due to its high accuracy and sensitivity.

### Basic Concepts

The relationship between absorption, fluorescence, and phosphorescence is shown in Fig. 9.6. As indicated, each molecule contains a series of closely spaced energy levels. Absorption of a quantum of light energy by a molecule causes the transition of an electron from the singlet ground state to one of a number of possible vibrational levels of its first excited singlet state. Once the molecule is in an excited state, it returns to its original energy state in several ways. These include (1) radiation-less vibrational equilibration, (2) the fluorescence process from the excited singlet state, (3) quenching of the excited singlet state, (4) radiation-less crossover to a triplet state, (5) quenching of the first triplet state, and (6) the phosphorescence process of light emission from the triplet state.

As shown in Fig. 9.6, vibrational equilibration before fluorescence results in some loss of the excitation energy. The emitted fluorescence is therefore of less energy or has a longer wavelength than the excitation light. The difference between the maximum wavelength of the excitation light and the maximum wavelength of the emitted fluorescence is a constant referred to as the Stokes shift. This constant is a measure of energy lost during the lifetime of the excited state (radiation-less vibrational deactivation) before returning to the ground singlet level (fluorescence emission).

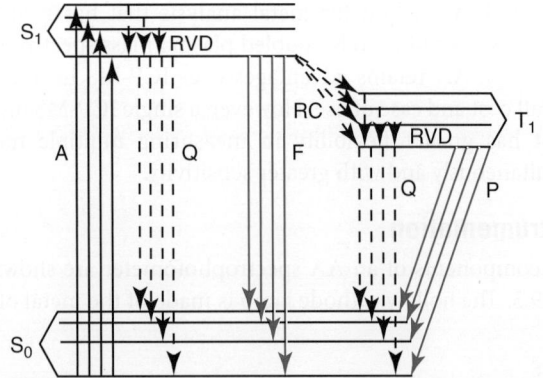

**Fig. 9.6** Luminescence energy-level diagram of a typical organic molecule. *A*, Absorption process; *F*, fluorescence process from the first excited singlet state; *P*, phosphorescence process from the first excited triplet state; *Q*, quenching of the excited singlet or triplet state; *RC*, radiation-less crossover from the first excited singlet state to the first excited triplet state; *RVD*, radiation-less vibrational deactivation; $S_0$, ground-level singlet state; $S_1$, first excited singlet state; $T_1$, first excited triplet state.

## Time Relationships of Fluorescence Emission

The time required for a molecule to absorb radiant energy and be raised to an excited state is approximately $10^{-15}$ s. The length of time for vibrational equilibration to occur to the lowest excited state is $10^{-14}$ to $10^{-12}$ s. The length of time required for fluorescence emission to occur is $10^{-8}$ to $10^{-7}$ s. Relatively speaking, there is a considerable time delay among the (1) absorption of light energy, (2) return to the lowest excited state, and (3) emission of light energy. This time relationship is shown in Fig. 9.7. In this figure, phase I represents the time period between the absorbance of light energy and the radiation-less loss of energy during vibrational rearrangement to the lowest excited energy state. This time period is represented by the up and down arrows in the diagram. Phase II shows the emission and decay of a *(b)* short- and *(a)* a long-lived fluorophore. If the fluorescence emission is measured over time following a pulse of light from an excitation source, such as a xenon lamp or laser, the intensity of the emitted light decays as a first-order process similar to radioactive decay (i.e., phase II of Fig. 9.7). The time required for the emitted light to reach $1/e$ of its initial intensity, where $e$ is the Naperian base 2.718, is called the average lifetime of the excited state of the molecule, or the fluorescence decay time.

The time delay between photon absorption and fluorescence emission is used in time-resolved fluorometers. Advantages of a time-resolved fluorometer include the elimination of background **light scattering** due to Rayleigh and Raman signals and a short-lived fluorescence background with a consequent dramatic increase in signal-to-noise and detection sensitivity.

Time-resolved fluorometry falls into one of two categories, depending on how the fluorescence emission response is measured: (1) pulse fluorometry, in which the sample is illuminated with an intense brief pulse of light and the intensity of the resulting fluorescence emission is measured as a function of time with a fast detector system; or (2) phase-resolved (frequency-domain) fluorometry, in which a sinusoidally modulated laser illuminates the sample, and the fluorescence emission response is monitored.

## Relationship of Concentration and Fluorescence Intensity

The relationship of concentration to the intensity of fluorescence emission is derived from the Beer-Lambert law. By expansion through a Taylor series, rearrangement, logarithm base conversion, and basic assumptions about dilute solutions, the following equation is obtained:

$$F = \varphi \; [I_o \, (2.3 - abc)] \qquad (9.7)$$

where $F$ = relative fluorescence intensity; $\varphi$ = fluorescence efficiency (i.e., the ratio between quanta of light emitted and quanta of light absorbed); $I_0$ = initial excitation intensity; $a$ = molar absorptivity; $b$ = volume element defined by geometry of the excitation and emission slits; and $c$ = the concentration in moles per liter.

Eq. (9.7) indicates that fluorescence intensity is directly proportional to the concentration of the fluorophore and the excitation intensity. This relationship holds only for dilute solutions, in which absorbance is less than 2% of the exciting radiation; the fluorescence intensity becomes nonlinear as the absorbance of the solution increases to greater than 2% of the exciting radiation. This phenomenon, called the inner filter effect, is discussed in more detail in a later section. Other factors influencing the measurement of fluorescence intensity include the sensitivity of the detector and the degree of background light scatter seen by the detector.

Fluorescence intensity measurements are more sensitive than absorbance measurements. The magnitude of absorbance of a chromophore in solution is determined by its concentration and the path length of the cuvet. The magnitude of fluorescence intensity of a fluorophore is determined by its concentration, the path length, and the intensity of the light source. The sensitivity of fluorescence measurements can be 100 to 1000 times greater than the sensitivity of absorbance measurements using more intense light sources, digital signal filtering techniques, and sensitive emission photometers. All of these are incorporated into conventional spectrofluorometric instrumentation, described later in this chapter.

Frequently, fluorescence measurements are expressed in units of relative intensity (relative fluorescence unit [RFU]). The word *relative* is used because the intensity measured is not an absolute quantity. It is a small part of the total fluorescence emission, and its magnitude is defined by the instrument slit width, detector sensitivity, monochromator efficiency, and excitation intensity. Because these are instrument-related variables, establishing an absolute intensity unit for a given concentration of a fluorophore that is valid from instrument to instrument is difficult, if not impossible.

## Fluorescence Polarization

Light is composed of electrical and magnetic waves at right angles to each other. Light waves produced by standard excitation sources have their electrical vectors oriented randomly. Light waves, passed through certain crystalline materials (polarizers), have their electrical vectors oriented in a single

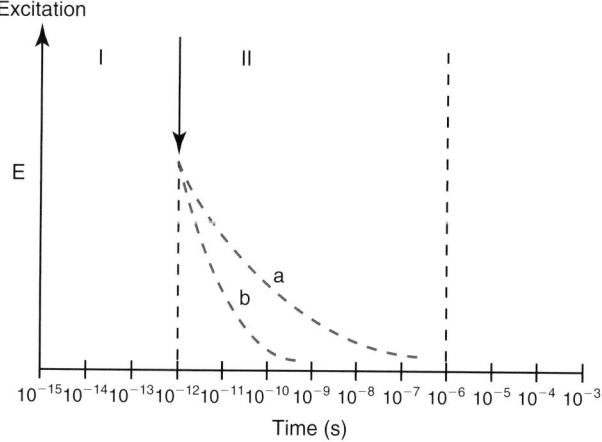

**Fig. 9.7** Fluorescence decay process. *a,* Long fluorescence decay time; *b,* short fluorescence decay time; *E,* absorption of energy; *I,* vibrational deactivation time phase; *II,* fluorescence emission time phase.

plane and are said to be plane-polarized. Fluorophores absorb light most efficiently in the plane of their electronic energy levels. If their rotational relaxation (brownian movement) is slower than their fluorescence decay time, as is the case for large fluorescent-labeled molecules, the emitted fluorescence light will remain polarized. Because small molecules have rotational relaxation times that are much shorter than their fluorescence decay time, their emitted fluorescence light is depolarized. However, if the small fluorescent molecule is attached to a macromolecule, or if it is placed in a viscous solution, the small molecule will emit polarized light. Fluorescence polarization, $P$, is defined by the following equation:

$$P = \frac{(I_v - I_h)}{(I_v + I_h)} \qquad \textbf{(9.8)}$$

where $I_v$ = intensity of the emitted fluorescence light in the vertical plane; and $I_h$ = intensity of the emitted fluorescence light in the horizontal plane.

As indicated, $P$ is the difference between the two observed intensities divided by their sum. Fluorescence polarization is measured by placing a mechanically or electrically driven polarizer between the sample cuvet and the detector. In the normal instrumentation mode, the sample is excited with polarized light to obtain maximum sensitivity. First, the polarization analyzer is positioned to measure the intensity of the emitted fluorescence light in the vertical plane ($I_v$); then the polarization analyzer is rotated 90 degrees to measure the emitted fluorescence light intensity in the horizontal plane ($I_h$). $P$ is then calculated manually or automatically by using Eq. (9.8).

Fluorescence polarization is used to quantitate analytes by using the change in fluorescence depolarization following immunologic reactions. Quantitation is accomplished by adding a known quantity of fluorescent-labeled analyte molecules to a reaction solution containing an antibody specific to the analyte. The labeled analyte binds to the antibody, and the slowed rotation and longer relaxation time results in an increased degree of fluorescence polarization. The addition of a nonlabeled analyte, such as an unknown quantity of a therapeutic drug in a serum specimen, will result in competition for binding to the antibody with the fluorescent-labeled analyte. This change in binding of the fluorophore-labeled analyte causes a change in fluorescence polarization that is inversely proportional to the amount of analyte contained in a given sample. Because the change in fluorescence polarization is a direct response to the reaction mixture, the bound fluorophore need not be separated from free fluorophore. Thus, fluorescence polarization is applicable to homogeneous assays of low-molecular-weight analytes, such as therapeutic drugs.

## Instrumentation

Fluorometers and spectrofluorometers are used to measure fluorescence and operationally have similar components with absorption spectrophotometers.

## Components

Basic components of fluorometers and spectrofluorometers include (1) an excitation source, (2) an excitation

monochromator, (3) a cuvet, (4) an emission monochromator (EmM), and (5) a detector. In Fig. 9.8, these components are shown as they would be configured in a 90-degree optical system.

With fluorometers and spectrofluorometers, placement of the cuvet and excitation beam relative to the photodetector is critical in establishing the optical geometry for fluorescence measurements. Because fluorescence is emitted in all directions from a molecule, several excitation and/or emission geometries are used to measure fluorescence (Fig. 9.9). Although the end-on approach allows the adaptation of a fluorescence detector to existing 180-degree absorption instruments, it is not widely used because its sensitivity is limited by the quality of the excitation and/or emission interference filter pair, the excitation and/or emission spectral band overlap, and the inner filter effect. In practice, most commercial spectrofluorometers and fluorometers use the right angle–detector approach because it minimizes the background signal that limits analytical sensitivity. The front surface approach provides the greatest linearity over a broad range of concentration because it minimizes the inner filter effect. The front surface approach shows similar sensitivity to the right-angle detectors but is more susceptible to background light scatter. Front surface fluorometry has been widely applied to heterogeneous solid-phase fluorescence immunoassay systems.

To accommodate these different geometries, the sample cell is oriented at different angles in relation to the excitation

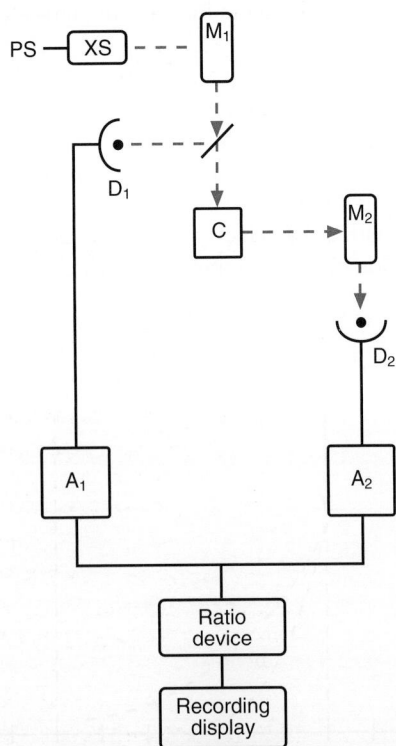

**Fig. 9.8** Block diagram of a typical spectrofluorometer. $A_1$ and $A_2$, Excitation signal and emission signal amplifiers, respectively; $C$, sample cell; $D_1$ and $D_2$, detectors ($D_1$ monitors the variation in excitation intensity and $D_2$ measures fluorescence emission intensity); $M_1$, excitation monochromator; $M_2$, emission monochromator; $PS$, power supply; $XS$, xenon source.

source and the detector. Major concerns related to the geometry of the sample cell include light scattering, the inner filter effect, and the sample volume element seen by the detector. Fig. 9.10A shows the sample cell and slit arrangement for a conventional fluorescence spectrophotometer, with the excitation and emission slits oriented at a right angle. Slit$_1$ and Slit$_2$ designate the excitation and emission slits, respectively. The position of the emission slit and the width of the slit are important. If the emission slit is located near the front edge of the sample cell, as shown in Fig. 9.10B, the inner filter effect is minimized. If the emission slit width is increased, sensitivity will increase, but specificity may decrease.

## Performance Verification

As with spectrophotometers, NIST provides a number of SRMs for use in calibration or verification of the performance of fluorometers or fluorospectrophotometers. These include SRM 936a (quinine sulfate dihydrate) for calibrating such instruments and SRM 1932 (fluorescein) for establishing a reference scale for fluorescence measurements (http://www.nist.gov/srm).

## Types of Fluorometers and Spectrofluorometers

Fluorometers and fluorescence spectrophotometers that offer a variety of features are available. These features include ratio

referencing, microprocessor-controlled excitation and EmMs, pulsed xenon light sources, photon counting, rhodamine cells for corrected spectra, polarizers, flow cells, front-surface viewing adapters, multiple cell holders, and microprocessor-based data reduction systems.

In addition to the basic spectrofluorometer discussed earlier, other types of fluorometric instruments include a ratio-referencing spectrofluorometer, a time-resolved fluorometer, and a flow cytometer.

***Ratio-referencing spectrofluorometer.*** The xenon lamp energy source in single-beam spectrofluorometers is unstable (i.e., arc flicker and lamp decay). This is a source of laboratory error and requires frequent calibration. The unstable energy source in single-beam spectrofluorometry can be addressed by ratio-referencing spectrofluorometry. The ratio-referencing spectrofluorometer splits the energy from the light source to energize both a sample PMT and a reference

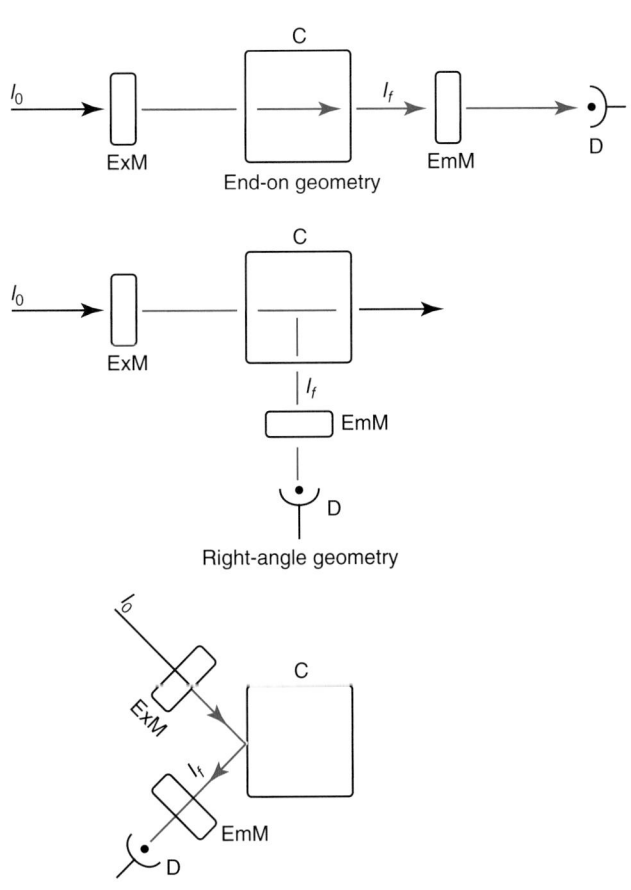

**Fig. 9.9** Fluorescence excitation/emission geometries. *C,* Sample cuvet; *D,* detector; *EmM,* emission monochromator; *ExM,* excitation monochromator; *I$_0$,* initial excitation energy; *I$_f$,* fluorescence intensity.

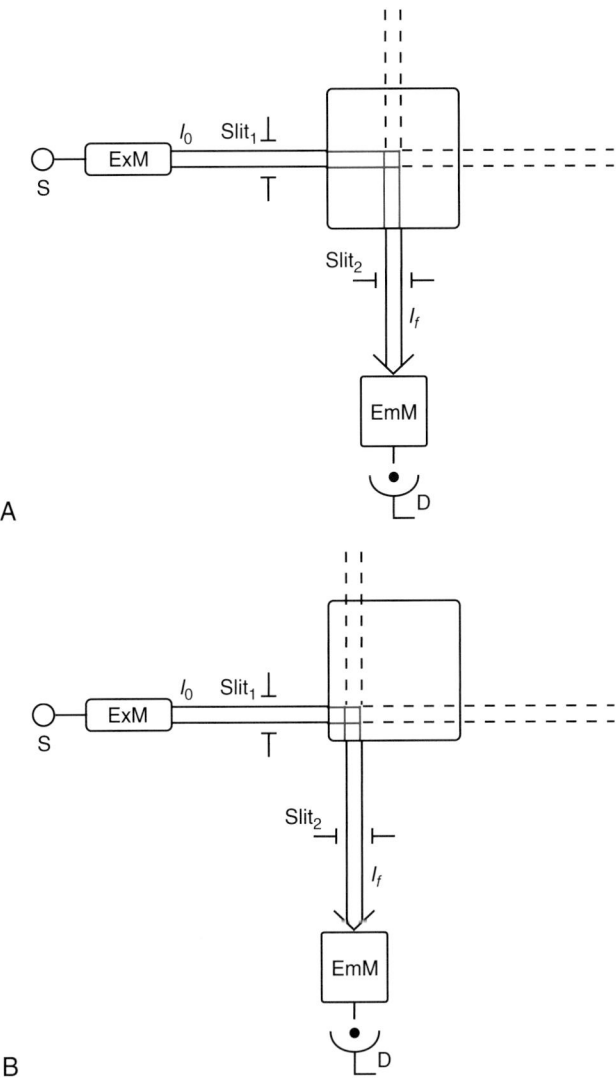

**Fig. 9.10** Two right-angle fluorescence sample cuvet positions. (A) The standard 90-degree configuration. (B) The offset positioning of the cuvet to minimize the inner filter effect. *D,* Detector; *ExM,* excitation monochromator; *EmM,* emission monochromator; *I$_0$,* initial excitation energy; *I$_f$,* fluorescence intensity; *S,* excitation source; *Slit$_1$,* excitation slit; *Slit$_2$,* emission slit.

PMT. Thus, any instability of the energy source will affect both the reference and sample PMT and reduce the possibility of measurement error.

A typical ratio-referencing spectrofluorometer is illustrated in Fig. 9.11. Basically, this is a right-angle instrument that uses two monochromators (ExM and EmM), two PMT detectors ($D_1$ and $D_2$, the reference, and sample PMTs), and a xenon lamp source. The light from the excitation monochromator (ExM) is split, and a small portion (10%) is directed to the reference PMT ($D_1$) for ratio-referencing purposes. The remaining excitation light is focused into the sample compartment. Emission optics are positioned at a right angle to the excitation optics. An EmM is used to select or scan the desired portion of the emission spectra, which is directed to the sample PMT ($D_2$) for measurement of emission intensity. Output signals from the reference and sample PMTs are amplified, and the ratio of the sample to the reference signal is provided by a digital display or a chart recorder. The operational mode of a ratio filter fluorometer is similar to that of a spectrofluorometer; however, only discrete excitation and emission wavelengths are available, and use of this type of instrument is precluded from scanning fluorophores to obtain emission and excitation spectra. The ratio filter fluorometer is most useful for obtaining concentration measurements at defined excitation and emission wavelengths.

The ratio-referencing spectrofluorometer is operated at fixed excitation and emission wavelength settings for concentration measurements; alternatively, it is used to measure the excitation or emission spectrum of a given compound. Measurement of the concentration of a specimen is accomplished in a similar manner as with a single-beam fluorometer. A blank and a calibrating solution are measured first; then the unknown specimens are measured. The ratio-referencing spectrofluorometer provides two advantages over single-beam spectrofluorometers. First, it eliminates short- and long-term xenon lamp energy fluctuations (i.e., arc flicker and lamp decay), thus minimizing the need for frequent calibration of the instrument during analysis. Second, it provides excitation spectra which are corrected for wavelength-dependent energy fluctuations.

***Time-resolved fluorometer.*** The time-resolved fluorometer is similar to the ratio-referencing fluorometer, with the exceptions that the light source is pulsed, and the detector monitors the exponential decay of the fluorescence signal after excitation in a fast photon-counting mode. Time-resolved fluorometry requires the use of long-lived fluorophores, such as the lanthanide (rare earth) metal ions europium ($Eu^{3+}$) and samarium ($Sm^{3+}$). Although most fluorescence compounds have decay times of 5 to 100 ns, $Eu^{3+}$ chelates decay in 0.6 to 100 seconds. Thus, time-resolved fluorescence assays take advantage of the difference in lifetimes of fluorophore and background fluorescence by measuring the decaying fluorescence signal. This eliminates background interferences and at the same time averages the signal to improve the precision of measurement. Detection limits of approximately $10^{-13}$ mol/L can be achieved with time-resolved fluorometry; this is an improvement of approximately four orders of magnitude compared with conventional fluorometric measurements.

***Flow cytometer.*** Cytometry is the measurement of physical and/or chemical characteristics of cells, or by extension,

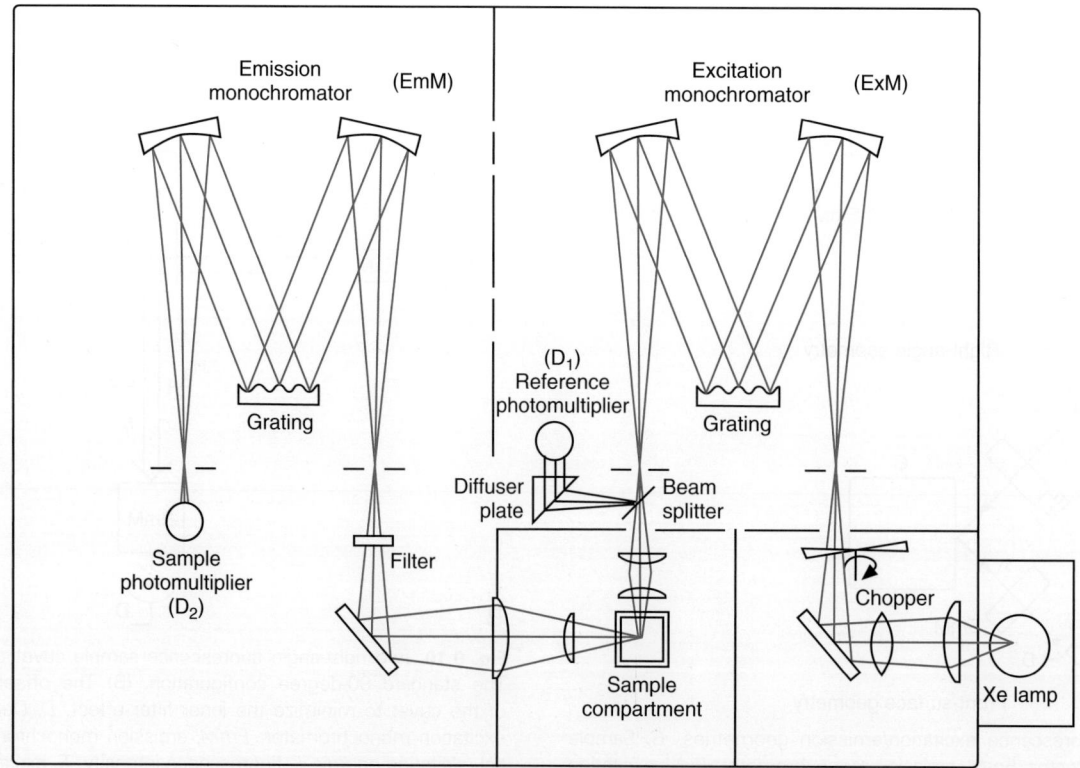

**Fig. 9.11** Diagram of a typical ratio-referencing spectrofluorometer. *Xe,* Xenon.

other biological particles. **Flow cytometry** is a process in which such measurements are made while cells or particles pass, preferably in single file, through the measuring apparatus in a fluid stream. Flow sorting extends flow cytometry by using electrical or mechanical means to divert and collect cells with one or more measured characteristics that fall within a range or ranges of values set by the user.

Operationally, flow cytometry combines laser-induced fluorometry with particle light scattering analysis that allows different populations of cells or particles to be differentiated by fluorescence, as well as size and shape using low-angle and right-angle light scattering. The use of a laser is ideally suited for low-angle light scattering. These cells or particles are typically labeled with specific antibodies that have attached fluorophores, such as β-phycoerythrin or fluorescein. As they move in a fluid stream through the flow cell, simultaneous fluorescence and light scattering measurements are automatically performed by the flow cytometer. Most flow cytometers incorporate two or more fluorescence channels, so that multiple fluorescent labels can be used. In this manner, cells or particles can be classified by size, shape, and type according to their light scattering and fluorescent properties. A schematic diagram of a flow cytometer is shown in Fig. 9.12. An optical stop is placed in the 180 degrees beam after the flow capillary to block the main laser beam and permit low-angle forward light scattering measurements. The 90 degrees emission signal is split and directed to multiple PMTs to determine right-angle light scattering and at least two separate fluorescence emission signals. Narrow bandpass interference filters are placed in front of the PMTs for fluorescence detection. A computer with substantial resident software is used to reduce the acquired data to appropriate histograms for final result reporting. Flow cytometers are able to measure multiple parameters, including cell size (forward scatter),

granularity (90 degrees; side scatter), DNA content, RNA content, antigens, and total protein content. Most commercial flow cytometers use one or more laser light sources. For example, the LSR II (BD Biosciences, Rockville, Maryland) can be equipped with seven lasers (355 nm [UV], 405 nm [violet], 488 nm [blue], 532 nm [green], 594 nm [yellow], 638 nm [red], and 785 nm [IR]), which are used to simultaneously measure 18 emission spectra. Cell-sorting electrodes are also shown in the schematic drawing, used for collecting cell populations within specific parameters.

Beyond cell-based measurements, particle-based flow cytometric assays use microspheres as the solid support for conventional immunoassays, affinity assays, or DNA hybridization assays. The plastic microspheres incorporate different proportions of two fluorescent dyes to generate 100 different signatures. Each of these signatures can be assigned to a specific analyte to multiplex 100 analytes in the same sample. The resultant system is flexible, and its use has led to the development of small volume assays that simultaneously assess a wide variety of analytes in the same sample.

## Limitations of Fluorescence Measurements

Factors that influence fluorescence measurements include concentration effects (e.g., inner filter effects, concentration quenching), background effects (due to Rayleigh and Raman scattering), solvent effects (e.g., interfering nonspecific fluorescence, quenching from the solvent), sample effects (e.g., light scattering, interfering fluorescence, sample adsorption), temperature effects, and photodecomposition (bleaching) of the sample.

### Inner Filter Effects

The linear relationship between concentration and fluorescence emission is valid when solutions absorb less than

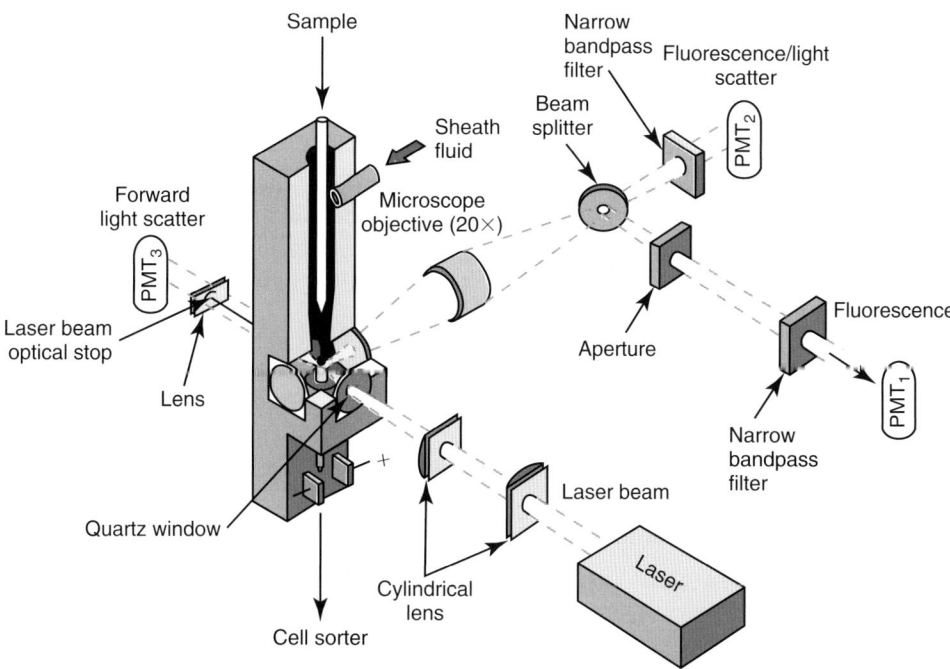

**Fig. 9.12** Schematic diagram of a flow cytometer. *PMT,* Photomultiplier tube.

2% of the exciting light. As the absorbance of the solution increases above this amount, the relationship becomes non-linear, a phenomenon known as the inner filter effect. It is primarily caused by loss of excitation intensity across the cuvet path length as excitation light is absorbed by the fluorophore. Thus, as the fluorophore becomes more concentrated, absorbance of the excitation intensity increases, and loss of the excitation light as it travels through the cuvet increases. This effect is most often encountered with a right-angle fluorescence instrument, in which the emission slits are set to monitor the center of the sample cell, where absorbance of excitation light is greater than that at the front surface of the cuvet. Therefore, it is less problematic if a front-surface fluorescence instrument is used. However, most fluorescence measurements are made on dilute solutions, and therefore, the inner filter effect is not a problem.

## Concentration Quenching

Another related phenomenon that results in a lower quantum yield than expected is called concentration quenching. This can occur when a macromolecule, such as an antibody, is heavily labeled with a fluorophore, such as fluorescein isothiocyanate. When this compound is excited, the fluorescence labels are in such close proximity that radiation-less energy transfer occurs. Thus, the resulting fluorescence is much lower than expected for the concentration of the label. This is a common problem in flow cytometry and laser-induced fluorescence when attempts are made to enhance detection sensitivity by increasing the density of the fluorescing label.

## Light Scattering

Light scattering—Rayleigh and Raman—limits the use of fluorescence measurements. Rayleigh scattering occurs with no change in wavelength. For fluorophores with small Stokes shifts, the excitation and emission spectra overlap and are particularly susceptible to loss of sensitivity because of background light scatter. Rayleigh-type light scatter is controlled by using well-defined emission and excitation interference filters or by appropriate monochromator settings and the use of polarizers.

Raman scattering occurs with lengthening of a wavelength. This type of light scattering is independent of excitation wavelength and is a property of the solvent. Because Raman light scattering appears at longer wavelengths than the exciting radiation, it is a difficult interference to eliminate when working at very low fluorophore concentrations.

## Cuvet Material and Solvent Effects

Certain quartz glass and plastic materials that contain UV absorbers will fluoresce. Some solvents, such as ethanol, are also known to cause appreciable fluorescence. It is therefore important when developing a fluorescence assay to assess the background fluorescence of all components of the reaction mixture.

## Sample Matrix Effects

A serum or urine sample contains many compounds that fluoresce. Thus, the sample matrix is a potential source of unwanted background fluorescence and must be examined when new methods are developed. The most serious contributors to unwanted fluorescence are proteins and bilirubin. However, because protein excitation maxima are in the spectral region of 260 to 290 nm, their contribution to overall background fluorescence is minor when excitation at more than 300 nm occurs.

Light scattering of proteins and other macromolecules in the sample matrix can cause unwanted background signal. For example, lipemic samples scatter light, and the relative contributions of lipids to the background signal of a fluorescence measurement should be investigated when setting up a new method.

In addition to background interferences, some fluorophores in the concentration range of $10^{-9}$ mol/L or less will adsorb to the walls of glass cuvets and other reaction vessels. Furthermore, dilute solutions of fluorophores are susceptible to photodecomposition by excitation light, proportional to its intensity and exposure time. Operationally, these problems are avoided by selecting proper reaction vessels, adding wetting agents, and minimizing the length of time a sample is exposed to the excitation light.

## Temperature Effects

The fluorescence quantum efficiency of many compounds is sensitive to temperature fluctuations. Therefore, the temperature of the reaction must be regulated to within ±0.1°C. In general, fluorescence intensity decreases with increasing temperature by approximately 1% to 5% per degree Celsius. Increased temperatures result in more frequent molecular collisions and quenching. Collisional quenching can be decreased by lowering the temperature or by increasing the viscosity.

## Photodecomposition

In conventional fluorometry, excitation of weakly fluorescing or dilute solutions with intense light sources will cause photochemical decomposition of the analyte (photobleaching).

The following steps help to minimize photodecomposition effects:

1. Always use the longest feasible wavelength for excitation that does not introduce light scattering effects.
2. Decrease the duration of excitation of the sample by measuring the fluorescence intensity immediately after excitation.
3. Protect unstable solutions from ambient light by storing them in dark bottles.
4. Remove dissolved oxygen from the solution.

In addition, fluorescence-based assays for analytes at ultralow concentrations require optimization of laser intensity and use of a sensitive detector. Highly intense laser light sources with an energy output greater than 5 to 10 mW have higher sensitivity and are used in applications that have low concentrations of analyte, such as flow cytometry, fluorescence microscopy, and laser-induced fluorescence measurements. However, these intense light sources rapidly photodecompose some fluorescence analytes. This decomposition introduces nonlinear response curves and loss of most of the sample fluorescence. Thus, optimization of laser intensity balances higher sensitivity with increased photodecomposition.

# CHEMILUMINESCENCE, BIOLUMINESCENCE, AND ELECTROCHEMILUMINESCENCE

Chemiluminescence, bioluminescence, and electrochemiluminescence are types of luminescence in which the excitation event is caused by a chemical, biochemical, or an electrochemical reaction, and not by photoillumination.

## Basic Concepts

The physical event of light emission in chemiluminescence, bioluminescence, and electrochemiluminescence is similar to fluorescence in that it occurs from an excited singlet state, and light is emitted when the electron returns to the ground state.

### Chemiluminescence and Bioluminescence

**Chemiluminescence** is the emission of light when an electron returns from an excited or higher energy level to a lower energy level. The excitation event is caused by a chemical reaction and involves the oxidation of an organic compound, such as luminol, isoluminol, acridinium esters, or luciferin, by an oxidant (e.g., hydrogen peroxide, hypochlorite, oxygen); light is emitted from the excited product formed in the oxidation reaction. These reactions occur in the presence of catalysts, such as enzymes (e.g., alkaline phosphatase, horseradish peroxidase), metal ions, or metal complexes (e.g., hemin).

Bioluminescence is a special form of chemiluminescence found in biological systems. In bioluminescence, an enzyme or a photoprotein increases the efficiency of the luminescence reaction. Luciferase and aequorin are two examples of these biological catalysts.

Chemiluminescence assays are ultrasensitive (attomole to zeptomole detection limits) and have wide dynamic ranges. They are now widely used in automated immunoassay and DNA probe assay systems.

### Electrochemiluminescence

**Electrochemiluminescence** differs from chemiluminescence in that the reactive species that produce the chemiluminescent reaction are electrochemically generated from stable precursors at the surface of an electrode. A ruthenium, tris(bipyridyl) chelate is the most commonly used electrochemiluminescent label, and electrochemiluminescence is generated at an electrode via an oxidation reduction–type reaction with tripropylamine. This chelate is stable and relatively small and has been used to label haptens or large molecules (e.g., proteins, oligonucleotides). The electrochemiluminescence process has been used in both immunoassays and nucleic acid assays. Advantages of this process include (1) improved reagent stability, (2) simple reagent preparation, and (3) enhanced sensitivity. With its use, detection limits of 200 fmol/L and a dynamic range extending over six orders of magnitude can be obtained.

## Instrumentation

Luminometers are instruments used to measure chemiluminescence and electrochemiluminescence. Basic components are (1) the sample cell housed in a light-tight chamber, (2) the injection system used to add reagents to the sample cell, and (3) the detector. The detector is usually a PMT. For electrochemiluminescence, the reaction vessel incorporates an electrode, at which electrochemiluminescence is generated.

## Limitations of Chemiluminescence and Electrochemiluminescence Measurements

Light leaks, light piping, and high background luminescence from assay reagents and reaction vessels (e.g., plastic tubes exposed to light) are common factors that degrade analytical performance. The extreme sensitivity of chemiluminescent assays requires stringent controls on the purity of reagents and the solvents (e.g., water) used to prepare reagent solutions. Efficient capture of light emission from reactions that produce a flash of light requires an efficient injector that provides adequate mixing when the triggering reagent is added to the reaction vessel. Chemiluminescent and electrochemiluminescent assays have a wide linear range that are usually several orders of magnitude, but high-intensity light emission can lead to pulse pile-up in PMTs, and this can lead to a serious underestimation of true light emission intensity.

**POINTS TO REMEMBER**

**Radiant Energy in Analytical Measurements**
- Fluorescence: light is absorbed by a molecule and subsequently emitted as light at a longer wavelength.
- Phosphorescence: light is absorbed by a molecule, but in contrast to fluorescence, the subsequently emitted light is from relaxation from an excited triplet state; compared with fluorescence, the emission time and wavelength of light are both much longer.
- Chemiluminescence: light is emitted as a result of chemical energy; no light is absorbed.
- Electrochemiluminescence: light is generated from precursor molecules at the surface of an electrode.

# NEPHELOMETRY AND TURBIDIMETRY

Light scattering is a physical phenomenon that results from the interaction of light with particles in solution. Nephelometry and turbidimetry are analytical techniques used to measure scattered light. Light scattering measurements have been applied to immunoassays of specific proteins and haptens.

## Basic Concepts

Light scattering occurs when radiant energy passing through a solution encounters a molecule in an elastic collision, which results in scattering of the light in all directions. Unlike fluorescence emission, the scattered light is of the same frequency as the incident light. Factors that influence light scattering include particle size, wavelength dependence, distance of observation, polarization of incident light, concentration of the particles, and molecular weight of the particles.

Light scattering from small particles is directly proportional to their concentration and molecular weight. Light scatter is inversely proportional to the fourth power of wavelength (blue light scatters more than red light) and inversely proportional to the square of the distance from the light scatter source to the detector. Thus, the detector should be located close to the analytical cell by combining the cell and the detector or by using good collection optics.

As the particles become larger than the incident light wave, the radiated light waves are no longer all in phase. Reinforcement of radiation occurs in some directions, and destructive interference occurs in others. The scattering patterns from these large particles are characteristic of the size and shape of the particle.

## Measurement of Scattered Light

Turbidimetry and nephelometry are methods used to measure scattered light. Such measurement has proven useful for the quantitation of serum proteins. The choice between turbidimetry and nephelometry depends on the application and the available instrumentation.

### Turbidimetry

Because of the light scattering that occurs with turbidity, the intensity of light reaching the detector at 180 degrees is reduced. Measurement of this decrease in intensity is called **turbidimetry**. Analogous to absorption spectroscopy, turbidity is defined as follows:

$$I = I_0 e^{-bt} \qquad \textbf{(9.9)}$$

where $t$ = turbidity; $b$ = path length of incident light through the solution of light scattering particles; $I$ = intensity of transmitted light; and $I_0$ = intensity of incident light.

Turbidity is measured at 180 degrees from the incident beam, or more simply, in the same manner as absorbance measurements are made in a spectrophotometer. Turbidity can be measured on most spectrophotometers and automated clinical chemistry analyzers. The stability and resolution of modern microprocessor-driven spectrophotometers and photometers have greatly improved their ability to measure turbidity with accuracy and precision.

Turbidimetric measurements are performed on photometers or spectrophotometers and require little optimization. The principal concern of turbidimetric measurements is signal-to-noise ratio. Photometric systems with electro-optical noise in the range of ±0.0002 absorbance unit or less are useful for turbidity measurements.

### Nephelometry

**Nephelometry** is defined as the detection of light energy scattered or reflected toward a detector that is not in the direct path of the transmitted light. Common nephelometers measure scattered light at right angles to the incident light. The ideal nephelometric instrument would be free of stray light, and neither light scatter nor any other signal would be seen by

the detector when the solution in front of the detector is free from particles. However, because of stray light-generating components in the optical system and in the sample cuvet or the sample itself, a truly dark field situation is difficult to obtain when making nephelometric measurements. Some nephelometers are designed to measure scattered light at an angle other than 90 degrees to take advantage of the increased forward scatter intensity caused by light scattering from larger particles (e.g., immune complexes).

Although light scattering can be measured with standard analytical fluorometers or photometers, the angular dependence of light scattering intensity has resulted in the design of special nephelometers. These devices place the PMT detector at appropriate angles to the excitation light beam. The design principle of a nephelometer is similar to the design principle applied in fluorescence measurement. The major operational difference between the fluorometer and the nephelometer is that the excitation and detection wavelengths will be set to the same value when operating a nephelometer. The principal concerns of light scatter instrumentation include excitation intensity, wavelength, distance of the detector from the sample cuvet, and minimization of external stray light. As shown in Fig. 9.13, the basic components of a nephelometer include (1) a light source, (2) collimating optics, (3) a sample cell, and (4) collection optics, which include light scattering optics, a detector optical filter, and a detector. The schematic diagram also shows the different angles from the incident light beam where the detector, filter, and optics are placed to measure light scattering. Fig. 9.13a shows the straight-through arrangement for turbidimetry, whereas Fig. 9.13b and c show arrangements frequently found in nephelometers. The detector arrangement shown in Fig. 9.13b is used for measurement

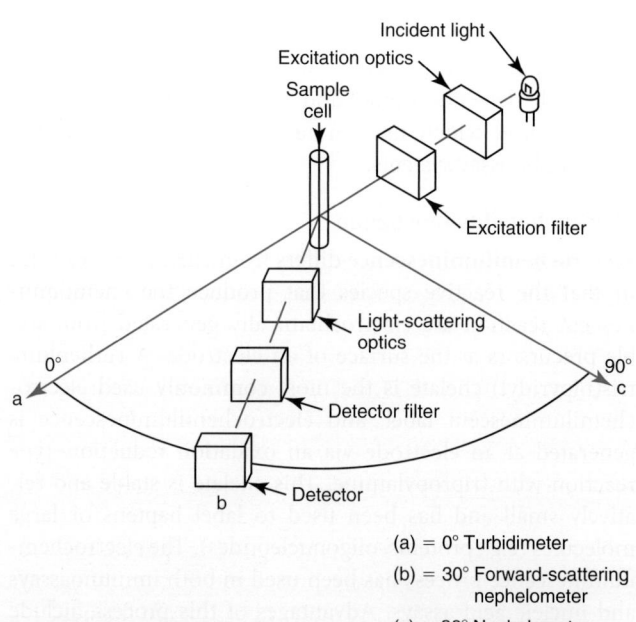

(a) = 0° Turbidimeter

(b) = 30° Forward-scattering nephelometer

(c) = 90° Nephelometer

**Fig. 9.13** Schematic diagram of light scattering instrumentation showing *(a)* the optics position for a turbidimeter, *(b)* the optics position for a forward scattering nephelometer, and *(c)* the optics position for a right-angle nephelometer.

of forward scatter at 30 degrees, which is the optical arrangement used with some commercial nephelometers.

Operationally, the optical components used in turbidimeters and nephelometers are similar to those used in fluorometers and photometers. For example, the light sources commonly used are quartz-halogen lamps, xenon lamps, and lasers. Helium-neon lasers, which operate at 633 nm, typically have been used for light scattering applications, such as nephelometric immunoassays, and particle size and shape determinations. The laser beam is used specifically in some nephelometers because of its high intensity; in addition, the coherent nature of laser light makes it ideally suited for nephelometric applications. In addition, ratio-referencing fluorometers are well suited for nephelometric measurements.

## Limitations of Light Scattering Measurements

Antigen excess and matrix effects are limitations encountered in the use of turbidimeters and nephelometers for measurement of analytes of clinical interest in some situations.

### Antigen Excess

Antigen–antibody reactions are complex and appear to result in a mixture of aggregate sizes. As turbidity increases during addition of antigen to antibodies, the signal increases to a maximum value and then decreases. The point at which the decrease begins marks the beginning of the phase of antigen excess. Consequently, light scattering methods for quantitation of antigen–antibody reactions must provide a method for detecting antigen excess. The kinetics of immune complex formation measured by nephelometry or turbidimetry is sufficiently different in each of the three phases—antibody excess, equivalence, and antigen excess—that computer

algorithms that detect antigen excess need to be included in a test system.

### Matrix Effects

Particles, solvent, and all serum macromolecules scatter light. Lipoproteins and chylomicrons in lipemic serum provide the highest background turbidity or nephelometric intensity. With appropriate dilutions, the relative intensity of light scattering from a lipemic sample is less than that of the antiserum blank. However, as the concentration of the antigen in serum decreases and correspondingly less dilute samples are used, background interference from lipemic samples becomes greater. An effective method for minimizing this background interference is the use of rate measurements, in which the initial sample blank is eliminated. Large particles, such as suspended dust, also cause significant background interference. This background interference is controlled by filtering all buffers and diluted antisera before analysis is attempted.

---

**POINTS TO REMEMBER**

**Light Scattering Assays**
- Turbidity assays measure light scattering to determine the formation of antigen–antibody complexes.
- Interferences in light scattering include:
  - an excess of antigen decreases the turbidity
  - macromolecules, such as lipoproteins, chylomicrons, and dust in the sample matrix, which will increase the background turbidity
- Macromolecule interference in light scattering can be decreased by using rate measurements rather than directly assessing light scattering.

---

## REVIEW QUESTIONS

1. Mathematically, Beer's law is expressed as $A = abc$. Which of the following statements is most correct?
   a. "$a$" is the absorptivity constant which is fixed for a given compound at a given wavelength under specific conditions.
   b. "$b$" is the light path measured in meters.
   c. The absorptivity constant is not affected by wavelength, solvent, temperature, and pH.
   d. If a compound formed with the substance of interest has a lower molar absorptivity, then it is more sensitively detected.
   e. Beer's law only applies when the radiant energy is white light.

2. Which of the following is true regarding light sources for laboratory instrumentation?
   a. Using ambient air to surround a tungsten filament will extend its operating life.
   b. Mercury arc lamps emit a resonance line at 750 nm and are used for wavelength calibration in spectrophotometers.

   c. Laser (light amplification by stimulated emission of radiation) is a device that provides coherent light of narrow wavelength.
   d. Light-emitting diode (LED) is a solid-state device that produces coherent and narrow wavelength of light.
   e. Ultraviolet light is in the visible spectrum from 800 to 900 nm.

3. Photodetectors convert light into electrical signals. Which of the following statements is most correct?
   a. Photomultiplier tubes are comprised of a photoemissive cathode enclosed in a glass chamber containing ambient air.
   b. Dark current is the current produced in a photomultiplier tube when there is incident light.
   c. Photodiodes are solid-state fabricated materials which can be assembled into an array with each photodiode designed to respond to multiple wavelengths.
   d. The human eye can be a sensitive photodetector from 900 to 1200 nm.

e. Charge-coupled detectors are solid-state devices with a superior high signal to noise ratio compared to photomultiplier tubes.

4. Which of the following statements best represents Rayleigh's description of the relationship between scattered and incident light?
   a. The intensity of light scattering is proportional to the wavelength of incident light.
   b. The intensity of light scattering is inversely proportional to the distance between the light scattering particles and the detector.
   c. Polarized light results in greater light scattering compared to nonpolarized light.
   d. When visible light is used at 600 nm, the upper limit on particle size that exhibit Rayleigh scattering is 30 nm.
   e. To minimize light scattering, the analytical detector should be as far a distance as possible from the cuvet.

5. What describes a major difference between laser diodes and LEDs?
   a. They are manufactured by different processes.
   b. Laser diodes provide coherent light, whereas LEDs provide incoherent light.
   c. Laser diodes emit in the infrared portion of the spectrum and LEDs emit in the ultraviolet portion of the spectrum.
   d. Laser diodes are used for applications requiring a wide range of wavelengths for excitation.
   e. LEDs are more useful for applications requiring narrow wavelengths of light.

6. What is the concentration of NADH in a solution if the absorbance at 340 nm in a 1 cm cuvette is 0.1? Use the NADH molar absorptivity 6220 L × mol$^{-1}$ × cm$^{-1}$.
   a. 1.6 μM
   b. 16 μM
   c. 6.2 μM
   d. 62 μM

7. Which of the following descriptions for an optical technique is correct?
   a. Chemiluminescence results from the excitation of a molecule at one wavelength resulting in the emission of light at a longer wavelength.
   b. Fluorescence results from the emission of light secondary to a chemical reaction.
   c. Electrochemiluminescence results from a chemical reaction generated at the surface of an electrode.
   d. Chemiluminescence results from excitation of molecules to form a chemical bond.
   e. Electrochemiluminescence results from excitation of molecules to form a chemical bond.

8. Which of the following characteristics of the light spectrum is true?
   a. The energy of light is proportional to the wavelength.
   b. Infrared wavelengths are higher in energy compared to ultraviolet wavelengths.
   c. The human eye is most sensitive in detecting changes in the ultraviolet range of the spectrum.
   d. A solution appears blue when it transmits light between 450 and 495 nm.
   e. A solid object appears blue when it absorbs light between 450 and 495 nm.

9. Which of the following statements are correct regarding analytical techniques for light scattering?
   a. Nephelometry is the measurement of light intensity at 180 degrees to the path of incident light.
   b. Turbidimetry is the measurement of light intensity at 180 degrees to the path of incident light.
   c. Nephelometry and turbidimetry have excellent performance in lipemic serum samples.
   d. Turbidimetry has increased light intensity at 180 degrees with increasing analyte concentration.
   e. Macromolecule interference of light scattering assays is worsened with the use of rate measurements.

10. Which of the following strategies are used to minimize photodecomposition (photobleaching) in fluorometry?
   a. Use the shortest excitation wavelength possible.
   b. Increase the time interval between excitation and measurement of fluorescence.
   c. Store fluorophores in protected (dark) containers to decrease exposure to ambient light.
   d. Increase the concentration of dissolved oxygen in the reaction.
   e. Use a higher energy laser for excitation.

## SUGGESTED READINGS

Cossarizza A, Chang HD, Radbruch A, et al. Guidelines for the use of flow cytometry and cell sorting in immunological studies. *Eur J Immunol.* 2017;47:1584–1797.

Gross EM, Maddipati SS, Snyder SM. A review of electrogenerated chemiluminescent biosensors for assays in biological matrices. *Bioanalysis.* 2016;8:2071–2089.

Lakowicz JR. *Principles of Fluorescence Spectroscopy.* 3rd ed. New York: Springer; 2017.

Nather RE, Mukadam AJ. A CCD time-series photometer. *Astrophys J.* 2004;605:846.

Rodríguez-Orozco AR, Ruiz-Reyes H, Medina-Serriteño N. Recent applications of chemiluminescence assays in clinical immunology. *Mini Rev Med Chem.* 2010;10:1393–1400.

Yamanishi CD, Chiu JH, Takayama S. Systems for multiplexing homogeneous immunoassays. *Bioanalysis.* 2015;7:1545–1556.

Zaydman MA, Brestoff JR, Logsdon N, et al. Kinetic approach extends the analytical measurement range and corrects antigen excess in homogeneous turbidimetric immunoassays. *J Appl Lab Med.* 2019;4:214–223.

# Electrochemistry and Chemical Sensors

*Prasad V.A. Pamidi\**

## OBJECTIVES

1. Define the following: (a) amperometry, (b) biosensor, (c) conductometry, (d) coulometry, (e) electromotive force, (f) indicator electrode, (g) ion activity, (h) molality, (i) potentiometry, (j) reference electrode, and (k) voltammetry.
2. State the major advantages of electrochemical sensors for whole blood measurements.
3. Describe the components of a basic potentiometric cell and their functions, including electrodes, filling solutions, and voltmeter.
4. State the principle, a clinical application, and a potential interfering substance for each of the following electrochemical measurement techniques: (a) potentiometry, (b) voltammetry/amperometry, (c) conductometry, and (d) coulometry.
5. Describe the fundamental differences between direct potentiometry for measurement of electrolytes in serum, plasma, and whole blood and analytical methods which measure ion concentration.
6. Describe a $PCO_2$ and $PO_2$ electrode, including components and internal reactions.
7. Define a biosensor; describe the two major categories of biosensors and a practical example of each type in the clinical laboratory.
8. Describe different transduction mechanisms used for enzyme-based biosensors and a practical example of each in the clinical laboratory.
9. Describe affinity biosensors and different bio-elements used in these sensors.
10. Introduce continuous glucose monitoring and different options for clinical use.

## KEY WORDS AND DEFINITIONS

**Amperometry** An electrolytic electrochemical process in which current is monitored at a fixed (controlled) voltage between working and reference electrodes in an electrochemical cell.

**Biosensor** A type of chemical sensor consisting of a biologic recognition element and a physicochemical transducer, often an electrochemical or an optical device.

**Conductometry** An electrochemical technique used to determine the quantity of an analyte present in a mixture by measuring its effect on the electrical conductivity of the mixture.

**Electrochemical cell** A device that consists of two electrodes (electron or metallic conductors) connected by an electrolyte solution that conducts ions (galvanic cell), or a device in which an external voltage is applied to a polarizable working electrode versus a reference electrode, with the resulting cathodic or anodic current of the cell being monitored (electrolytic cell).

**Electrode** A half-cell that consists of a single metallic conductor in contact with an electrolyte solution; the indicator (measuring) electrode is one half-cell and the reference electrode is the second half-cell.

**Electrode potential** The electromotive force (EMF) of a single half-cell measured with respect to the standard hydrogen electrode, set at zero by convention.

**Ion-selective electrode** An electrode that selectively interacts with a single ionic species; the potential produced at the membrane/sample solution interface is proportional to the logarithm of the ionic activity or the concentration of the ion in question.

**Nernst equation** The equation used to relate the potential of an electrochemical cell to the activity of a chemical species in solution.

**Potential difference** The work required to move an electrical charge that is measured in volts.

*The author gratefully acknowledges the contributions of Drs. Richard A. Durst, Ole Siggaard-Andersen, Mark E. Meyerhoff, and Paul D'Orazio to earlier versions of this chapter.

**Potentiometry** An electrochemical technique that measures an electrical potential difference between two electrodes (half-cells) in an electrochemical cell.

**Redox couple** A conjugate pair of substances that consists of any substance that accepts electrons (the oxidant) and any substance that donates electrons (the reductant); redox processes take place only between two redox couples, with electrons transferred from a reductant ($Red_1$) to an oxidant ($Ox_2$).

**Voltammetry** An electrolytic process in which a specific oxidation or reduction reaction occurs at the surface of the working electrode in response to an applied potential. The charge transfer at this interface (current flow) provides analytical information.

Recent advances in electro-mechanical, microfluidic, materials, and computer technologies have enabled the wider adoption of chemical sensors utilizing electrochemical methodologies in clinical analysis systems. Sensors for measurement of blood gases, electrolytes, metabolites, trace metals, and other important biomarkers are incorporated into automated, point-of-care and laboratory clinical analyzers. Miniaturization of sensors and the enabling technologies together with increasing demand for analyzers that are easy to use, portable, wireless capable, and offer low-skilled operation with minimal process steps are driving the growth of point-of-care testing. Biosensors that incorporate the same sensing principles together with biorecognition elements (such as enzymes, antibodies, aptamers, nucleic acids, etc.) have also been successfully applied for expanding the capabilities of these devices to measure or monitor different metabolites, coagulation reactions, biomarkers, detecting drugs, or toxic chemicals through ultrasensitive enzymatic or immunoassays, or genetic sequences in whole blood, plasma, serum, or urine samples.

In this chapter the fundamental electrochemical sensing principles of (1) potentiometry, (2) voltammetry/amperometry, (3) conductometry, and (4) coulometry will be summarized and clinical applications presented. Chemical sensors and biosensors, both biocatalytic and affinity based, will be introduced and practical examples including continuous glucose monitoring will be presented.

## POTENTIOMETRY

**Potentiometry** is used clinically for measurement of pH, $PCO_2$, and electrolytes ($Na^+$, $K^+$, $Cl^-$, $Ca^{2+}$, $Mg^{2+}$, $Li^+$) in whole blood, serum, plasma, and urine and as the basis for some biosensors for metabolites of clinical interest.

### Basic Concepts

**Potentiometry** is the measurement of an electrical potential difference between two electrodes (half-cells) in an **electrochemical cell** when the cell current is zero (Fig. 10.1). Such a cell consists of two electrodes, known as the indicator (measuring) and the reference electrodes, shown in Fig. 10.1 on the left and right, respectively. The two electrodes are connected by an electrolyte solution (sample). Each half-cell consists of an internal silver–silver chloride (Ag/AgCl) electrode, which is a specific type of potentiometric electrode known as a redox electrode. Each Ag/AgCl electrode is in contact with an internal electrolyte. The indicator electrode, also known as an **ion-selective electrode** (ISE), contains an inner electrolyte

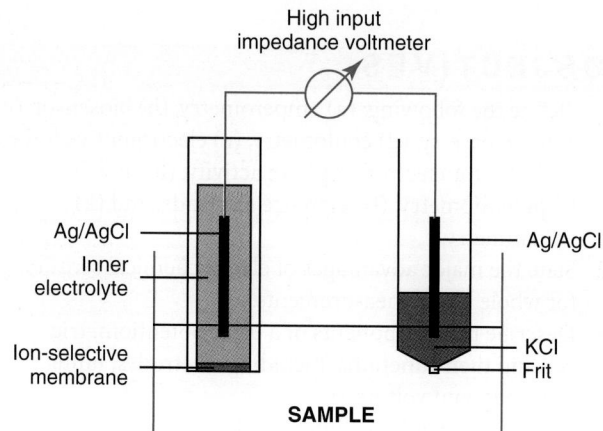

**Fig. 10.1** Schematic of an ion-selective membrane electrode–based potentiometric cell. *Ag/AgCl*, Silver–silver chloride; *KCl*, potassium chloride.

with a constant activity of the ion of interest in the form of a chloride salt. The reference electrode contains a high concentration of electrolyte, usually potassium chloride.

The electromotive force (E or EMF) is defined as the maximum difference in potential between the two electrodes when the cell current is zero. The cell potential is measured using a voltmeter, of which the common pH meter is a special type. To obtain an accurate potential measurement, it is necessary that no current flows through the cell. This is accomplished by incorporating a high input impedance of greater than $10^{12}$ Ω within the voltmeter.

The overall potential of a potentiometric cell is the sum of all potential gradients that exist between different phases of the cell. The potential of a single electrode with respect to the surrounding electrolyte and the absolute magnitude of the individual potential gradients between phases are unknown and cannot be measured. Only **potential differences** between two electrodes (half-cells) can be measured. Potential gradients can be classified as (1) redox potentials, (2) membrane potentials, or (3) diffusion potentials. In general, it is possible to devise a cell in such a manner that all potential gradients except one are constant. This potential then can be related to the activity of a specific ion of interest (e.g., hydrogen [$H^+$] or [$Na^+$]).

### Types of Electrodes

Different types of electrodes are used for potentiometric applications. They include (1) redox, (2) ion-selective membrane (glass and polymer), and (3) $PCO_2$ gas-sensing electrodes.

## Redox Electrodes

Redox potentials are the result of chemical equilibria involving electron transfer reactions:

$$\text{Oxidized form (Ox)} + ne^- \rightarrow \text{Reduced form (Red)} \quad (10.1)$$

where $n$ = the number of electrons involved in the reaction. Any substance that accepts electrons is an oxidant (Ox), and any substance that donates electrons is a reductant (Red). The two forms, Ox and Red, represent a **redox couple** (conjugate redox pair). Usually, homogeneous redox processes take place only between two redox couples. In such cases, electrons are transferred from $Red_1$ to an $Ox_2$. In this process, $Red_1$ is oxidized to its conjugate $Ox_1$, whereas $Ox_2$ is reduced to $Red_2$:

$$Red_1 + Ox_2 \leftrightarrow Ox_1 + Red_2 \quad (10.2)$$

The **electrode potential** for a redox couple is defined as the couple's potential measured with respect to the standard hydrogen ($H_2$) electrode, which by convention is set equal to zero. In such a cell, the standard $H_2$ electrode is the reference electrode and the given half-cell is the indicator electrode. The potential for the redox couple is shown by the Nernst equation:

$$E = E^0 - \frac{N}{n} \times \log\frac{a_{Red}}{a_{Ox}} = E^0 - \frac{0.0592 \text{ V}}{n} \times \log\frac{a_{Red}}{a_{Ox}} \quad (10.3)$$

where $E$ = electrode potential of the cell; $E^0$ = standard electrode potential when $\frac{a_{Red}}{a_{Ox}} = 1$; $n$ = number of electrons involved in the redox reaction; $N = (R \times T \times \ln 10)/F$ (the Nernst factor if $n = 1$); $N = 0.0592$ V if $T = 298.15$ K (25°C); $N = 0.0615$ V if $T = 310.15$ K (37°C); $R$ = gas constant (8.31431 joule $\times$ K$^{-1}$ $\times$ mol$^{-1}$); $T$ = absolute temperature (in kelvins); $F$ = faraday constant (96,487 coulombs $\times$ mol$^{-1}$); $\ln 10$ = natural logarithm of 10 = 2.303; $a$ = activity; and $\frac{a_{Red}}{a_{Ox}}$ = ratio between the chemical activities of the reduced and oxidized forms.

Redox electrodes currently in use include (1) inert metal electrodes immersed in solutions containing redox couples and (2) metal electrodes whose metal functions as a member of the redox couple.

### Inert Metal Electrodes

Platinum (Pt) and gold (Au) are examples of inert metals used to record the potential of a redox couple in a background electrolyte. The $H_2$ electrode is a special redox electrode for pH measurement. It consists of a Pt or Au electrode that is electrolytically coated (platinized) with highly porous Pt (Pt black) to catalyze the electrode reaction:

$$H^+ + e^- \leftrightarrow \frac{1}{2}H_2 \quad (10.4)$$

The electrode potential is given by:

$$E = E^0 - N \times \log\frac{(f_{H_2})^{1/2}}{a_{H^+}} \quad (10.5)$$

or

$$E = E^0 - N \times \left[\log (f_{H_2})^{1/2} - \log(a_{H^+})\right] \quad (10.6)$$

where $E^0$ = 0 at all temperatures (by convention); $f_{H_2}$ = fugacity of $H_2$ gas (the "effective" partial pressure of a gas under ideal conditions); $a_{H^+}$ = activity of $H^+$ ions; and $-\log a_{H^+}$ = negative log of $H^+$ activity ($pa_{H^+}$ or pH).

When fugacity $f_{H_2}$ in the solution is maintained constant by bubbling $H_2$, the potential is a linear function of $\log a_{H^+}$ ( $= -pH$). In the standard $H_2$ electrode, the electrolyte consists of an aqueous solution of HCl with activity of HCl equal to 1.000 (concentration of HCl = 1.2 mol/L) in equilibrium with a gas phase, and with $f_{H_2}$ equal to 1.000 ($PH_2 = 101.3$ kPa = 1 atm). The standard $H_2$ electrode is also used as a reference electrode.

### Metal Electrodes Participating in Redox Reactions

The Ag/AgCl electrode is an example of a metal electrode that participates as a member of a redox couple. The Ag/AgCl electrode consists of an Ag wire or rod coated with AgCl$_{(solid)}$ in contact with a Cl$^-$ solution of constant activity; this sets the half-cell potential. The Ag/AgCl electrode is itself considered a potentiometric electrode because its phase boundary potential is governed by an oxidation-reduction electron transfer equilibrium reaction that occurs at the surface of Ag:

$$AgCl_{(solid)} + e^- \leftrightarrow Ag^0_{(solid)} + Cl^- \quad (10.7)$$

The Nernst equation for the reference half-cell potential of an Ag/AgCl reference electrode is written as follows:

$$E_{Ag/AgCl} = E^0_{Ag/AgCl} + \frac{RT}{nF} \times \ln\frac{a_{AgCl}}{a_{Ag}a_{Cl^-}} \quad (10.8)$$

Because AgCl and Ag are both solids, their activities are equal to unity $\left(a_{AgCl} = a^0_{Ag} = 1\right)$. Therefore, from Eq. 10.8, the half-cell potential is controlled by the activity of the Cl$^-$ ion in solution $\left(a_{Cl^-}\right)$ contacting the electrode.

The Ag/AgCl electrode is used both as an internal reference element in potentiometric ISEs and as an external reference electrode half-cell of constant potential, which is required to complete a potentiometric cell (see Fig. 10.1). In both cases the Ag/AgCl electrode must be in equilibrium with a solution of constant Cl$^-$ ion activity.

The Ag/AgCl element of the reference electrode half-cell is in contact with a high-concentration solution of a soluble Cl$^-$ salt. Saturated KCl is commonly used. A porous membrane or frit is frequently used to separate the concentrated KCl from the sample solution. The frit serves both as a mechanical barrier to hold the concentrated electrolyte within the electrode and as a diffusional barrier to prevent proteins and other species in the sample from coming into contact with the internal Ag/AgCl element, which could poison and alter its potential. The interface between two dissimilar electrolytes (concentrated KCl/calibrator or sample) occurs within the frit and develops the liquid-liquid junction potential ($E_j$), a source of error in potentiometric measurements. The difference in $E_j$ between calibrator and sample (residual liquid junction potential) is responsible for this error and can be minimized and usually neglected in practice if the compositions of the calibrating solutions are matched as closely as possible to the sample with respect to ionic content and ionic strength. A reference electrolyte at high concentration, with equal cation and anion mobility, further helps to minimize the residual liquid junction potential. KCl at a concentration 2 mol/L or more is preferred.

## ION-SELECTIVE MEMBRANE ELECTRODES

Membrane potentials are produced by permeability of certain types of membranes to selected anions or cations. Such membranes are used to fabricate ISEs that selectively interact with a single ionic species. The potential produced at the membrane–sample solution interface is proportional to the logarithm of the ionic activity or concentration of the ion in question. Measurements with ISEs are simple, rapid, nondestructive, capable of being used directly in a turbid matrix such as whole blood and applicable to a wide range of concentrations.

The ion-selective membrane controls the selectivity of the electrode. Ion-selective membranes are typically composed of glass, crystalline, or polymeric materials. The chemical composition of the membrane is designed to achieve an optimal permselectivity (membrane or material's ability to selectively allow permeability to specific ions or analytes while blocking others) toward the ion of interest. In practice, other ions exhibit finite interaction with membrane sites and display some degree of interference for determination of an analyte ion. In clinical practice, if the interference exceeds an acceptable quantity, a correction is required.

The selectivity of an ISE for the ion of interest over interfering ions is:

$$E = E^0 + \left[ \frac{2.303RT}{z_i F} \right] \log \left( a_i + \sum_j K_{i/j} a_j^{z_i/z_j} \right) \quad \textbf{(10.9)}$$

where $a_i$ = activity of the ion of interest; $a_j$ = activity of the interfering ion; and $K_{i/j}$ = selectivity coefficient for the primary ion over the interfering ion. Low values indicate good selectivity for the analyte i over the interfering ion j; $z_i$ = charge of the primary ion; and $z_j$ = charge of the interfering ion. All other terms are identical to those in the Nernst equation (Eq. 10.3).

Glass membrane and polymer membrane electrodes are two types of ISEs that are commonly used in clinical chemistry.

### Glass Electrode

Glass membrane electrodes are used to measure pH and $Na^+$ and as an internal $H^+$ selective transducer for $PCO_2$ sensors. Glass electrode membranes are formulated from melts of

silicon and/or aluminum oxide ($Al_2O_3$) mixed with oxides of alkaline earth or alkali metal cations. By varying the glass composition, electrodes with selectivity for $H^+$, $Na^+$, $K^+$, $Li^+$, rubidium ($Rb^+$), cesium ($Cs^+$), $Ag^+$, thallium ($Tl^+$), and ammonium ($NH_4^+$) have been demonstrated. However, glass electrodes for $H^+$ and $Na^+$ are currently the only types with sufficient selectivity over interfering ions to allow practical application in clinical chemistry. A typical formulation for $H^+$ selective glass is 72% silicon dioxide ($SiO_2$), 22% $Na_2O$, and 6% calcium oxide ($CaO$), which has a selectivity order of $H^+$ $>>>$ $Na^+$ > $K^+$. This glass membrane has sufficient selectivity for $H^+$ over $Na^+$ to allow error-free measurements of pH in the range of 7.0 to 8.0 ($[H^+]$ = $10^{-7}$ to $10^{-8}$ mol/L) in the presence of greater than 0.1 mol/L $Na^+$. Glass pH electrodes with selectivity coefficients ($K_{H/Na}$) of $10^{-7}$ and better have been realized. By altering the formulation of the glass membrane slightly to 71% $SiO_2$, 11% $Na_2O$, and 18% $Al_2O_3$, its selectivity order becomes $H^+$ > $Na^+$ > $K^+$. Thus the preference of the glass membrane for $H^+$ over $Na^+$ is greatly reduced, resulting in a practical sensor for $Na^+$ at pH values typically found in blood.

### Polymer Membrane Electrodes

Polymer membrane ISEs are used for monitoring pH and for measuring electrolytes, including $K^+$, $Na^+$, $Cl^-$, $Ca^{2+}$, $Li^+$, $Mg^{2+}$, and carbonate ($CO_3^{2-}$) (for total $CO_2$ measurements). They are the predominant class of potentiometric electrodes used in clinical analysis instruments.

Response mechanisms of polymer membrane ISEs fall into three categories: (1) charged, dissociated ion exchanger; (2) charged associated carrier; and (3) neutral ion carrier (ionophore).

1. For charged, dissociated ion exchangers, selectivity is not controlled by any specific interaction between a ligand in the polymer membrane and an ion in solution but by extraction of ions into the membrane based on their lipophilic character. For example, dissociated anion exchanger–based electrodes using lipophilic quaternary ammonium salts as active membrane components are used commercially for the determination of $Cl^-$ in whole blood, serum, and plasma, despite some limitations. Selectivity for this type of ISE is controlled by extraction of the ion into the organic membrane phase and is a function of the lipophilic character of the ion because no direct binding interaction occurs between the exchanger site and the anion in the membrane phase. Thus, the selectivity order for a $Cl^-$ ISE based on an anion exchanger is fixed as lipophilic anion $R^-$ > perchlorate ($ClO_4^-$) > iodide ($I^-$) > nitrate ($NO_3^-$) > bromide ($Br^-$) > $Cl^-$ > fluoride ($F^-$), where $R^-$ represents anions with greater lipophilic character than $ClO_4^-$. Application of the $Cl^-$ ion-exchange electrode is therefore limited to samples without significant concentrations of anions more lipophilic than $Cl^-$. For example, blood samples containing salicylate or thiocyanate will produce positive interference for the measurement of $Cl^-$.

2. For charged, associated carriers, there is specific ion exchange or complexation between the carrier in the

polymer membrane and an ion in solution. An early charged-associated, ion-exchanger type ISE for $Ca^{2+}$ was developed and commercialized for clinical application in the 1960s based on the $Ca^{2+}$-selective, ion-exchange/complexation properties of 2-ethylhexyl phosphoric acid dissolved in dioctyl phenyl phosphonate. A porous membrane was impregnated with this cocktail and mounted at the end of an electrode body. This type of sensor was referred to as the "liquid membrane" ISE. Later, a method was devised in which these ingredients could be cast into a plasticized poly(vinyl chloride) (PVC) membrane that was more rugged and convenient to use.

3. For neutral ion carriers (ionophores), the ionophore molecule in the polymer membrane can reversibly and selectively complex an ion of interest in the sample. The interaction is not based on charge, but rather the ion is accommodated based primarily on size within a cavity in the structure of the molecule. A breakthrough in the development and routine application of PVC-type ISEs was the discovery that the neutral antibiotic valinomycin could be incorporated into organic liquid membranes (and later plasticized PVC membranes), resulting in a sensor with high selectivity for $K^+$ over $Na^+$ ($K_{K/Na}$ = $2.5 \times 10^{-4}$). The $K^+$ ISE based on valinomycin was the first example of a neutral carrier ISE and is now used extensively for the routine measurement of $K^+$ in blood. Fig. 10.2 shows the response of the valinomycin-based $K^+$ ISE in the presence of physiologic concentrations of $Na^+$, $Ca^{2+}$, and $Mg^{2+}$. The wide linear range and excellent selectivity of this ISE over three orders of magnitude makes it suitable for the measurement of $K^+$ in blood and urine. The $K^+$ range in blood is only a small portion of the electrode linear range and is spanned by a total $\Delta$EMF of approximately 9 mV. Interference from other cations, which is seen as deviation from linearity, is not

apparent at $K^+$ activities more than $10^{-4}$ mol/L. Other, less selective polymer-based ISEs based on neutral carriers (e.g., for the measurement of $Mg^{2+}$ and $Li^+$) are subject to interference from $Ca^{2+}/Na^+$ and $Na^+$, respectively, requiring simultaneous determination and correction for the presence of significant concentrations of these interfering ions. Studies regarding the relationship between molecular structure and ionic selectivity have resulted in the development of polymer-based ISEs using many naturally occurring and synthetic ionophores, with sufficient selectivity for application in clinical analysis. The chemical structures of several of these neutral ionophores are illustrated in Fig. 10.3.

High selectivity for the $CO_3^{2-}$ anion can be achieved using a neutral carrier ionophore that possesses trifluoroacetophenone groups doped within a polymeric membrane. Such ionophores form negatively charged adducts with $CO_3^{2-}$ anions, and the resulting electrodes have proven useful in commercial instruments for determination of total $CO_2$ in serum or plasma, after dilution of the sample to a pH value in the range of 8.5 to 9.0, where a significant fraction of total $CO_2$ exists as $CO_3^{2-}$.

## Electrodes for Partial Pressure of Carbon Dioxide

Electrodes have been developed to measure $PCO_2$ in body fluids. The first $PCO_2$ electrode, developed in the 1950s, used a glass pH electrode as the internal element in a potentiometric cell. This important development paved the way for commercial availability of the three-channel blood analyzer (pH, $PCO_2$, $PO_2$) providing a complete picture of oxygenation and acid-base status of blood.

Fig. 10.4 shows a diagram of a typical electrode for $PCO_2$. A thin membrane (approximately 20 µm), permeable only to gases and water vapor, is in contact with the sample. Membranes of silicone rubber, Teflon, and other polymeric materials are suitable for this purpose. On the opposite side of the membrane is a thin electrolyte layer consisting of a weak bicarbonate salt (approximately 5 mmol/L) and a $Cl^-$ salt. A pH electrode and an Ag/AgCl reference electrode are in contact with this solution. The $PCO_2$ electrode is a self-contained potentiometric cell. $CO_2$ gas from the sample or calibration matrix diffuses through the membrane and dissolves in the internal electrolyte layer. Carbonic acid is formed and dissociates, shifting the pH of the bicarbonate solution in the internal layer as follows:

$$CO_2 + H_2O \leftrightarrow H_2CO_3 \leftrightarrow H^+ + HCO_3^- \quad \textbf{(10.10)}$$

and

$$\Delta \log PCO_{2(sample)} \approx \Delta pH_{(internal\ layer)} \quad \textbf{(10.11)}$$

The relationship between the sample $PCO_2$ and the signal generated by the internal pH electrode is logarithmic and is governed by the Nernst equation. The electrode may be calibrated using precision gas mixtures or using solutions with stable $PCO_2$ concentrations. Although this style of electrode for $PCO_2$ has gained widespread use in modern blood gas analyzers, the format in which such sensors may be constructed

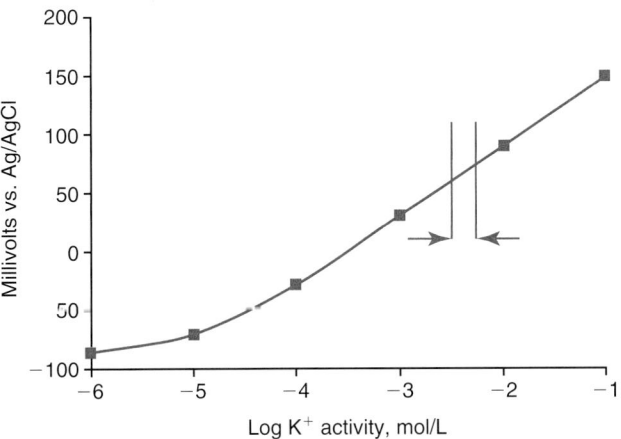

**Fig. 10.2** Typical electromotive force response of potassium ($K^+$) selective membrane electrode to changes in activity of $K^+$ in the sample solution. Bracketed interval represents the normal reference interval of $K^+$ concentration in blood. *Ag/AgCl*, Silver–silver chloride. (From D'Orazio P. In: Lewendrowski K, ed. *Clinical Chemistry: Laboratory Management and Clinical Correlations.* Philadelphia: Lippincott, Williams and Wilkins; 2002:455.)

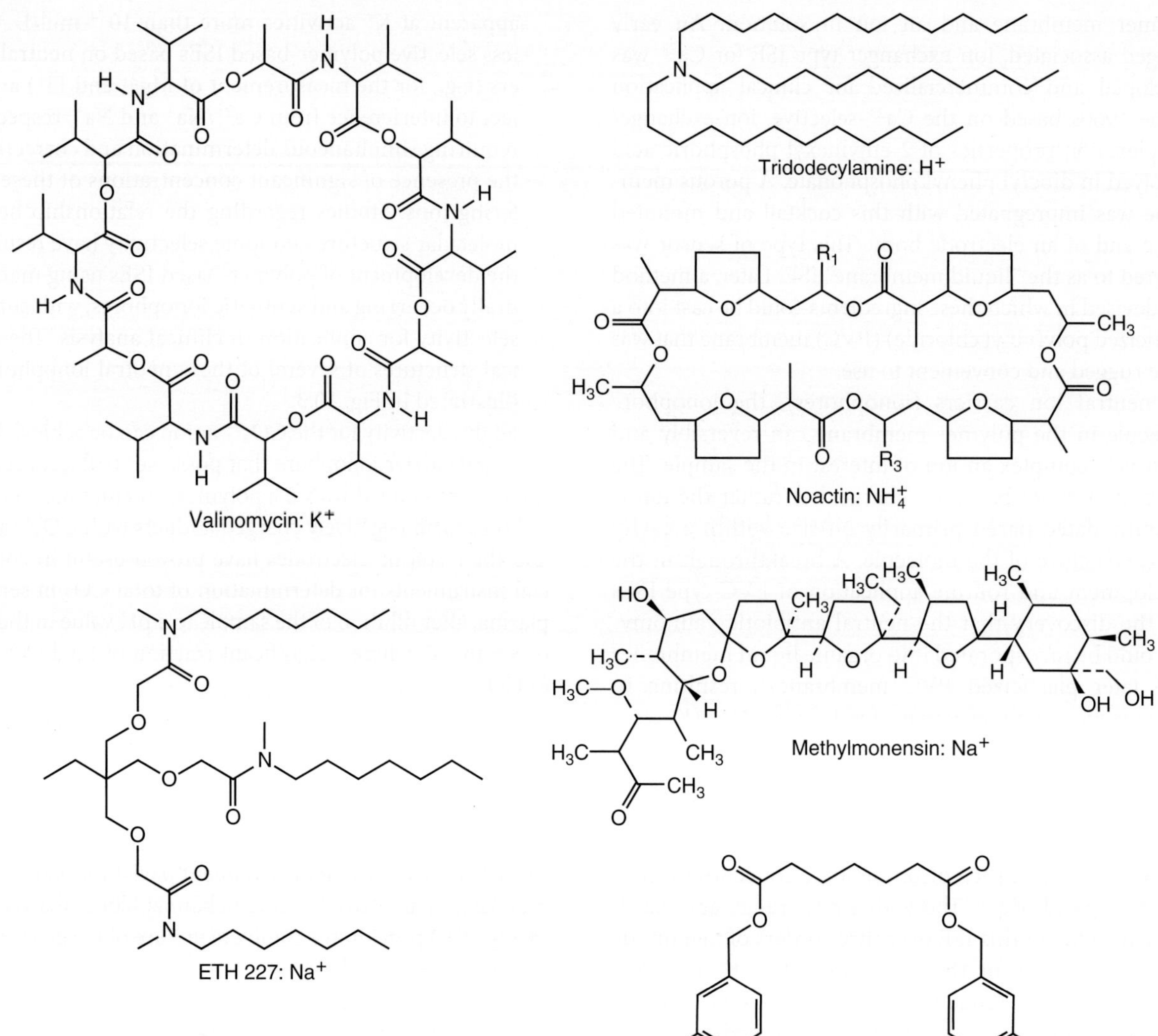

**Fig. 10.3** Structures of common ionophores used to fabricate polymer membrane–type ion-selective electrodes for clinical analysis.

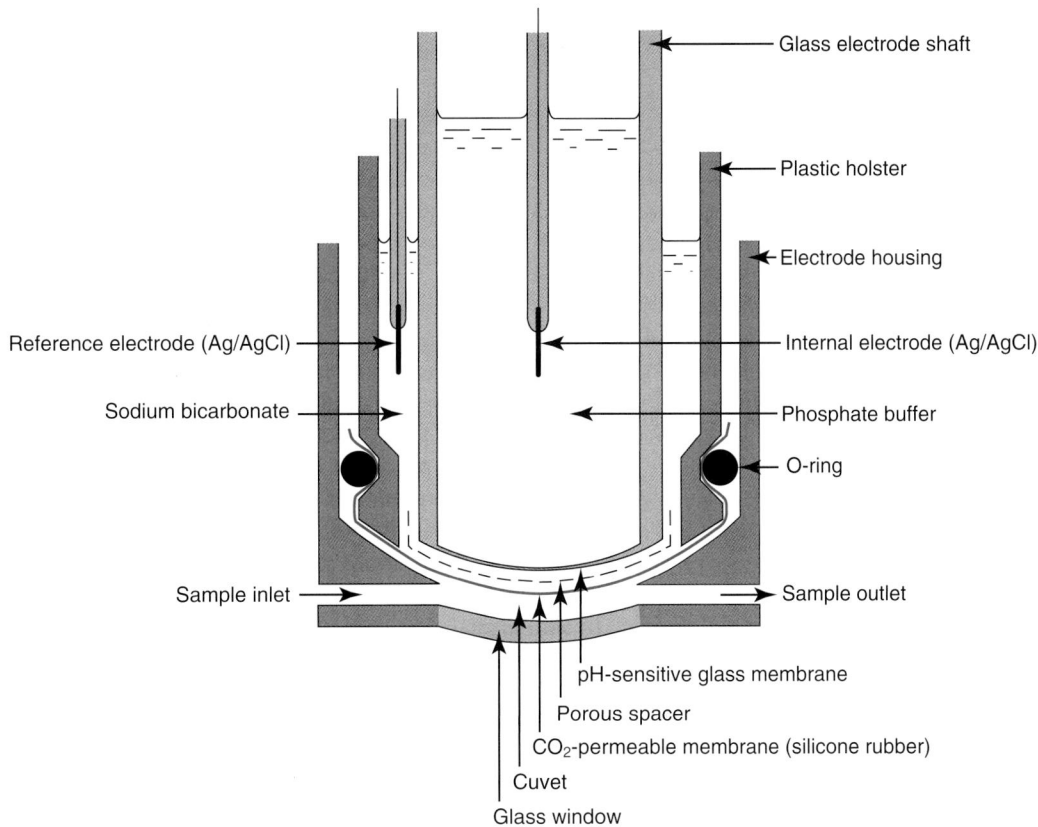

**Fig. 10.4** Partial pressure of carbon dioxide sensor used to monitor carbon dioxide *(CO₂)* concentrations in blood samples. *Ag/AgCl,* Silver–silver chloride. (From Siggard-Andersen O. *The Acid-Base Status of the Blood.* 4th ed. Baltimore, MD: Williams & Wilkins; 1974:172.)

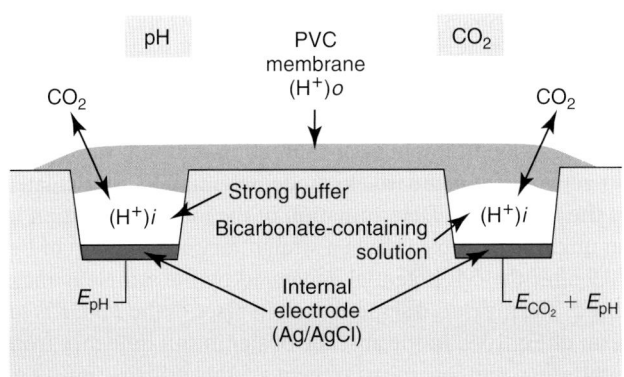

**Fig. 10.5** Differential planar partial pressure of carbon dioxide potentiometric sensor design, based on two identical polymeric membrane pH electrodes, but with different internal reference electrolyte solutions. Both pH sensing membranes are prepared with a hydrogen ($H^+$)-selective ionophore. *Ag/AgCl,* Silver–silver chloride; *PVC,* poly(vinyl chloride).

is limited by size, shape, and the ability to fabricate the internal pH sensitive element.

A slightly different potentiometric cell for $PCO_2$ is shown in Fig. 10.5. This cell arrangement uses two PVC-type, pH-selective electrodes in a differential mode. The electrode membranes contain tridodecylamine neutral ionophore exhibiting high selectivity for $H^+$ (see Fig. 10.3). One electrode has an internal layer that is buffered, and

the other is unbuffered, consisting of a low concentration of bicarbonate salt. $CO_2$ gas from the sample or calibration matrix diffuses across the outer $H^+$-selective PVC membranes of both sensors. On the unbuffered side, $CO_2$ diffusion produces a potential shift at the internal interface of the pH-responsive membrane proportional to the sample $PCO_2$ concentration. The signal at the electrode with the buffered internal layer is unaffected by the $CO_2$ that diffuses across the membrane. Consequently, one-half of the sensor responds to pH alone, and the other half responds to both pH and $PCO_2$. The signal difference between the two electrodes cancels any contribution of sample pH to the overall measured cell potential. The differential signal is proportional only to $PCO_2$. Unlike the prior electrode, this differential potentiometric cell $PCO_2$ sensor has been commercialized in a planar format and is more easily adaptable to mass production in sensor arrays.

### Direct Potentiometry by Ion-Selective Electrodes: Units of Measure and Reporting for Clinical Applications

Older analytical methods such as flame photometry for the measurement of electrolytes provide the total concentration *(c)* of a given ion in the sample, usually expressed in units of millimoles of ion per liter of sample. Molality *(m)* is a measure of the moles of ion per mass of water (millimoles per kilogram) in the sample. Using the $Na^+$ ion as an example, the relationship between concentration and molality is given by

$$c_{Na^+} = m_{Na^+} \times \rho H_2O \qquad (10.12)$$

where $\rho H_2O$ = mass concentration of water in kilograms per liter. For normal blood plasma, the mass concentration of water is approximately 0.93 kg/L, but in specimens with increased lipids or protein, the value may be as low as 0.8 kg/L. In these specimens the difference between concentration and molality may be as great as 20%. A significant advantage of direct potentiometry by ISE for the measurement of electrolytes is that the technique is sensitive to molality and therefore is not affected by variations in the concentration of protein or lipids in the sample. Techniques such as flame photometry, ISE methods that require sample dilution (indirect potentiometry), and other photometric methods requiring sample dilution are affected by the presence of protein and lipids. In these methods, only the water phase of the sample is diluted, which produces results lower than molality as a function of the concentration of protein and lipids in the sample. Thus there is a risk for error, such as a falsely low Na$^+$ concentration (pseudohyponatremia), in cases of extremely increased protein and lipid concentrations.

In addition to the difference between molality and concentration, measurement of ions by direct potentiometry provides yet another unit of measurement known as activity (a), the concentration of free, unbound ion in solution. Unlike methods sensitive to ion concentration, ISEs do not sense the presence of complexed or electrostatically "hindered" ions in the sample. The relationship between activity and concentration, using Na$^+$ ion as an example, is expressed as:

$$a_{Na^+} = \gamma_{Na^+} \times c_{Na^+} \qquad (10.13)$$

where $\gamma$ = dimensionless quantity known as the activity coefficient. The activity coefficient is primarily dependent on ionic strength of the sample as described by the Debye-Hückel equation:

$$\log \gamma = \frac{-Az^2 I^{0.5}}{1 + Ba I^{0.5}} \qquad (10.14)$$

where $A$ and $B$ = temperature-dependent constants ($A$ = 0.5213 and $B$ = 3.305 in water at 37°C); $a$ = ion size parameter for a specific ion; and $I$ = ionic strength ($I = 0.5\Sigma cz^2$, where $z$ is the charge number of the ions). Eq. 10.14 shows that a

decrease in the activity coefficient occurs with an increase in ionic strength. This effect is more pronounced when the charge ($z$) of the ion is higher. Activity coefficients for ions in biologic fluids, such as blood and serum, are difficult to calculate with accuracy because of the uncertain contribution of macromolecular ions, such as proteins, to the overall ionic strength. However, assuming that the normal ionic strength of blood plasma is 0.160 mol/kg, estimates of activity coefficients at 37°C are as follows: Na$^+$ = 0.75, K$^+$ = 0.74, and Ca$^{2+}$ = 0.31. Referring to Eq. 10.13, activity and concentration will differ greatly in samples of physiologic ionic strength, especially for divalent ions.

Physiologically, ionic activity is assumed to be more relevant than concentration when chemical equilibria or biologic processes are considered. Practically, however, ionic concentration is the more familiar term in clinical practice, forming the basis of reference intervals and medical decision concentrations for electrolytes. Early in the evolution of ISEs as practical tools in clinical chemistry, it was decided that changing clinical reference intervals to a system based on activity instead of concentration was impractical and carried risk for clinical misinterpretation. A pragmatic approach for using ISEs in modern analyzers without changing established concentration-based reference intervals is to formulate calibration solutions with ionic strengths and ionic compositions as close as possible to those of blood plasma. In this way, the activity coefficient of each ion in the calibrating solutions approximates that in the sample matrix, allowing calibration and measurement of electrolytes in units of concentration instead of activity.

A typical set of solutions for multi-ISE calibration in an analyzer is shown in Table 10.1. Two points may be used to calibrate each ISE. The difference in the cell potential generated by these two solutions ($\Delta E$) is used to calculate the response slope of the cell (slope = $\Delta E/\Delta \log c$), where $c$ is the concentration of ion in each calibrating solution, substituted for activity. The standard electrode potential, $E^0$, is calculated as the $y$-intercept. Determination of the ion concentration in an unknown sample is then a straightforward solution of Eq. 10.9 after the cell potential generated by the sample is measured. The measured slope is used in place of the $2.303RT/z_iF$ term of Eq. 10.9. In the absence of significant influence from interfering ions on measurement of the primary ion (e.g., ≤1% interference on the measured value), contributions from $a_j$ in Eq. 10.9 may be ignored.

## TABLE 10.1 Examples of Two-Value Calibrating Solutions for Measurement of pH and Electrolytes by Direct Potentiometry

| Analyte | Calibration Point (mmol/L) | Slope Point (mmol/L) | Expected Signal Δ (mV) |
|---|---|---|---|
| Na$^+$ | 140 | 110 | 6.6 |
| K$^+$ | 4.0 | 8.0 | 18 |
| Ca$^{2+}$ | 1.25 | 2.50 | 9 |
| Cl$^-$ | 100 | 80 | 6 |
| pH | 7.38 (pH units) | 6.84 (pH units) | 32.4 |

Ionic strength adjusted to 160 mmol/kg with buffer salts and inert electrolytes.
Ca$^{2+}$, Ionized calcium; Cl$^-$, chloride; K$^+$, potassium; Na$^+$, sodium.

Calibration of the cell is done in units of concentration; however, as mentioned earlier, direct potentiometry is sensitive to the molality of the ion, which is related to concentration by the water content of the sample (Eq. 10.12). The water content of the aqueous calibrating solutions shown in Table 10.1 is approximately 0.99 kg/L. The water content of normal blood plasma is approximately 0.93 kg/L. Molality is 7% greater than the concentration in this normal plasma specimen. The direct potentiometric cell will report results approximately 6% greater than the concentration in normal specimens because of this difference in water content between sample and the calibrator (0.99/0.93 = 1.06). Direct potentiometry presents an advantage in that the technique is not affected by the presence of protein and lipids in the sample; however, the application of clinical reference intervals based on concentration again poses a risk for confusion and clinical misinterpretation. Most manufacturers of electrolyte measurement systems have overcome this problem in a practical way by following Clinical and Laboratory Standards Institute (CLSI) guidelines that recommend the use of correlation factors to standardize ISE measurements to units of concentration. These factors may be obtained by standardizing the ISE measurement to certified reference materials based on human serum, with electrolyte values assigned in units of concentration. Appropriate correlation factors are then applied to sample calculations using algorithms resident in the instrument software.

---

### POINTS TO REMEMBER

**Advantages of Electrochemical Sensors for Whole Blood Measurements**
- Electrochemical sensors measure the most important critical care analytes (gases, electrolytes) directly in whole blood without need for sample pretreatment or dilution.
- Measurement is rapid and nondestructive.
- Measurement is not affected by sample turbidity (red cells, lipids); only the analyte present in the water phase of plasma is measured.
- Simultaneous measurement of multiple analytes in the same blood sample is possible.

---

## VOLTAMMETRY AND AMPEROMETRY

Voltammetric and amperometric techniques are among the most sensitive and widely applicable of all electroanalytical methods.

### Basic Concepts

In contrast to potentiometry, voltammetric and amperometric methods are based on electrolytic electrochemical cells in which an external voltage is applied to a polarizable working electrode versus a reference electrode and the resulting cathodic (for analytical reductions) or anodic (for analytical oxidations) measured current is proportional to the concentration of the analyte present in the sample. Current flows only if $E_{appl}$ is greater than a certain voltage (decomposition

voltage) determined by the thermodynamics for a given redox reaction of interest (Ox + $ne^-$ ↔ Red, which is defined by the $E^0$ value for that reaction [standard reduction potential]) and the kinetics for heterogeneous electron transfer at the interface of the working electrode. Often, slow kinetics of electron transfer for the redox reaction on a given inert working electrode (Pt, carbon, Au, etc.) mandates use of a much more negative (for reductions) or positive (for oxidations) $E_{appl}$ than predicted based on the $E^0$ for the redox reaction. This is called an overpotential ($\eta$). Regardless of whether an overpotential for electron transfer exists, a specific oxidation or reduction reaction occurs at the surface of the working electrode in **voltammetry** and/or **amperometry**, and it is the charge transfer at this interface (current flow) that provides the analytical information.

For electrolytic cells that form the basis of voltammetric and amperometric methods:

$$E_{appl} = E_{cell} + \eta - iR_{cell} \qquad (10.15)$$

where $E_{cell}$ = thermodynamic potential between the working and reference electrodes in the absence of an applied external voltage. When the external voltage is greater or less than this equilibrium potential, plus or minus any overpotential ($\eta$), current will flow because of an oxidation or reduction reaction at the working electrode. A voltammogram is simply the plot of observed current, $i$, versus $E_{appl}$ (Fig. 10.6). In **amperometry** (see later), a fixed voltage is applied, and the resulting current is monitored. The amount of current is inversely related to the resistance of the electrolyte solution and to any "apparent" resistance that develops because of mass transfer of the analyte species to the surface of the working electrode. Because electrochemical reactions are heterogeneous, occurring only at the surface of the working electrode, the amount of current observed is also dependent on the surface area ($A$) of the working electrode.

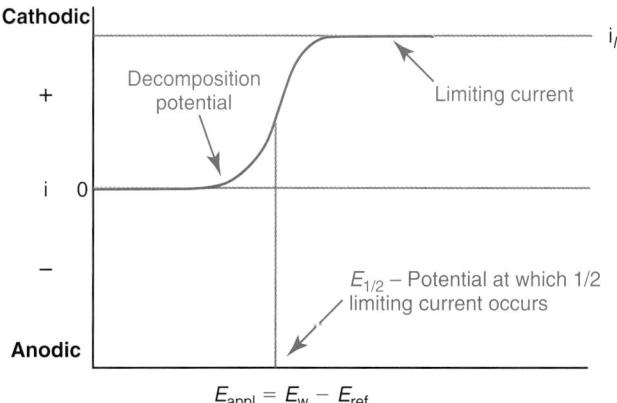

**Fig. 10.6** Current versus voltage curve (voltammogram) obtained for oxidized species that were reduced at the surface of the working electrode, as the $E_{appl}$ is scanned more negatively and the solution is stirred to yield a steady-state response. Decomposition potential is the applied potential where the oxidation or reduction reaction begins. Limiting current is the signal at steady state for the oxidation or reduction reaction and is proportional to the concentration of the analyte of interest. $E_{appl}$, Applied voltage; $E_{ref}$, potential at the reference electrode; $E_w$, potential at the working electrode.

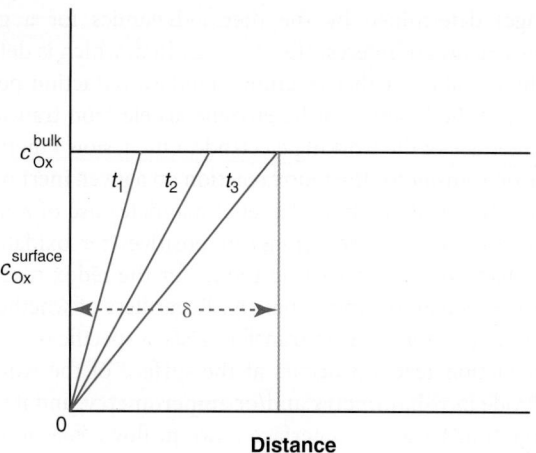

**Fig. 10.7** Diffusion layer thickness (concentration polarization) of analytes via reduction or oxidation *(Ox)* at the surface of the working electrode. As time increases ($t_1$, $t_2$, $t_3$, ...), the diffusion layer thickness at the surface of the working electrode *(δ)* grows quickly to a value determined by the degree of convection in the sample solution. $c_{Ox}^{bulk}$ and $c_{Ox}^{surface}$ are concentrations of oxidizable species in bulk solution and at the surface of the working electrode, respectively.

When a potential is applied to a working electrode that will oxidize or reduce a species in the solution phase contacting the electrode, the electrochemical reaction causes the concentration of electroactive species to decrease at the surface of the electrode (Fig. 10.7), a process termed concentration polarization. In turn, this causes a concentration gradient of analyte species between the bulk sample solution and the surface of the electrode. When the bulk solution is stirred, the diffusion layer of the analyte grows out from the surface of the electrode quickly to a fixed distance, which is controlled by how vigorously the solution is stirred. This diffusion layer is termed the Nernst layer and has a finite thickness *(δ)* after a relatively short time period when the solution is moving (convection). Voltammetry carried out in the presence of convection (by stirring the solution, rotating the electrode, flowing solution by the electrode, and so on) is called steady-state voltammetry. When the solution is not moving, the diffusion layer grows further and further with time (i.e., not constant), creating larger and larger δ values over time. This is termed non–steady state voltammetry and often results in peak currents in $i$ versus $E_{appl}$ plots for electrolytic cells.

In steady-state voltammetry, when the potential of the working electrode is scanned past a value that will cause an electrochemical reaction, the current will rise rapidly and then will plateau, even as $E_{appl}$ changes further. Fig. 10.6 illustrates such a wave for a hypothetical reduction of an oxidized species (Ox) via an $n$ electron reduction to a reduced species (Red). When the applied potential is much more negative than required, the current reaches a limiting value (termed the limiting current, $i_l$). This limiting current is proportional to the concentration of the electroactive species (Ox in this case) as expressed by the following equation:

$$i_l = nFA\left(\frac{D}{\delta}\right)c_{Ox} \qquad \text{(10.16)}$$

where $i$ = measured current in amperes; $n$ = the number of electrons in the electrochemical reaction (reduction in this case); $F$ = Faraday constant (96,487 coulombs/mol); $A$ = electrochemical surface area of the working electrode (in square centimeters, assuming a planar electrode geometry); $D$ = diffusion coefficient (in square centimeters per second) of the electroactive species (Ox in this case); $\delta$ = diffusion layer thickness (in centimeters); and $c$ = concentration of the analyte species (in moles per cubic centimeter). Note that Eq. 10.16 indicates a linear relationship for limiting current and concentration. The same equation applies for detecting reduced species by an oxidation reaction at the working electrode. In this case, by convention, the resulting anodic current is considered a negative current. As shown in Fig. 10.6, the potential of the working electrode that corresponds to a current that is exactly one-half the limiting current is termed $E_{\frac{1}{2}}$. This value is independent of analyte concentration. The $E_{\frac{1}{2}}$ is determined by the thermodynamics ($E^0$) of the given redox reaction, the solution conditions (e.g., if protons are involved in reaction, then pH will influence $E_{\frac{1}{2}}$), and any overpotential caused by slow electron transfer at a particular working electrode surface. The $E_{\frac{1}{2}}$ values are indicative of a given species undergoing an electrochemical reaction under specified conditions; hence the $E_{\frac{1}{2}}$ values enable distinguishing one electroactive species from another in the same sample. If the $E_{\frac{1}{2}}$ values for various species differ significantly (e.g., >120 mV), then measurements of several limiting currents in a given voltammogram yield quantitative results for several different species simultaneously.

Electrochemical cells used to carry out voltammetric or amperometric measurements can involve a two- or three-electrode configuration. In the two-electrode mode, external voltage is applied between the working electrode and a reference electrode, and the current is monitored. Because current passes through the reference electrode, such current can alter the surface concentration of electroactive species that poises the half-cell potential of the reference electrode, changing its value by a concentration polarization process. For example, if an Ag/AgCl reference electrode were used in a cell in which a reduction reaction for the analyte occurs at the working electrode, then an oxidation reaction would take place at the surface of the reference electrode:

$$Ag^0 + Cl^- \rightarrow AgCl_{(s)} + 1e^- \qquad \text{(10.17)}$$

Hence the activity and/or concentration of $Cl^-$ ions near the surface of the electrode would decrease, which would make the potential of the reference electrode more positive than its true equilibrium value based on the actual activity of the $Cl^-$ ion in the reference half-cell, because the Nernst equation for this half-cell is:

$$E_{Ag/AgCl} = E^0_{Ag/AgCl} - 0.059 \log\left(a_{Cl^-}^{surface}\right) \qquad \text{(10.18)}$$

Such concentration polarization of the reference electrode is prevented by keeping the current density (amperes per square centimeter) low at the reference electrode. This is achieved in practice by making sure that the area of the working electrode in the electrochemical cell is much smaller than the surface area of the reference electrode; hence the total current flow will be limited by this much smaller area, and current density values at the reference will be very small to prevent concentration polarization.

A three-electrode potentiostat is often used to completely eliminate changes in reference electrode half-cell potentials. In simple terms, the potentiostat applies a voltage to the working electrode, which is measured versus a reference electrode via a zero-current potentiometric-type measurement, but the current flow is between the working electrode and a third electrode, called the counter electrode. Thus, if reduction takes place at the working electrode, oxidation would occur at the counter electrode, but no net reaction would take place at the surface of the reference electrode because no current flows through this electrode. A potentiostat circuit is relatively simple to construct using modern operational amplifiers.

In voltammetric methods, $E_{appl}$ is varied via some waveform to alter the working electrode potential as a function of time and the resulting current measured. The current change occurs at the decomposition potential range, which is best when specific for a given analyte. However, the location of the current response as a function of $E_{appl}$ provides information on the nature of the species present (e.g., $E_{1/2}$), along with a concentration-dependent signal. This scan of $E_{appl}$ can be linear (linear sweep voltammetry), or it can have more complex shapes to enhance sensitivity for monitoring concentration of a given electroactive species (e.g., normal pulsed voltammetry, differential pulse voltammetry, square wave voltammetry).

Amperometric methods differ from voltammetry in that $E_{appl}$ is fixed, generally at a potential value in the limiting current plateau region of the voltammogram, and the resulting current is proportional to concentration. Amperometry can be more sensitive than common voltammetric methods because background charging currents, which arise from changing the $E_{appl}$ as a function of time in voltammetry, do not exist. Hence, when selectivity can be ensured at a given $E_{appl}$ value, amperometry may be preferred to voltammetric methods for more sensitive quantitative measurements.

## Applications

Molecular $O_2$ is capable of undergoing several reduction reactions, all with a significant overpotential at solid electrodes, such as Pt, Au, or Ag. For example, the following reaction

$$O_2 + 2H_2O + 4e^- \rightarrow 4OH^- \qquad \text{(10.19)}$$

$$\left(E^0 = +0.179\,vs.\,Ag/AgCl; 1\,mol/L\,Cl^-\right) \quad \text{(10.20)}$$

exhibits an $E_{1/2}$ at approximately $-0.500$ V on a Pt electrode (vs. a Ag/AgCl reference electrode), with a limiting current plateau beginning at approximately $-0.600$ V. This reaction is used to monitor the $PO_2$ in blood, which is the basis of the widely used amperometric $O_2$ sensor (Fig. 10.8). This device uses a small area planar Pt electrode as a working electrode (encased in insulating glass or other material) and an Ag/AgCl reference electrode, typically with a cylindrical design. This two-electrode electrolytic cell is placed within a sensor housing, on which a gas-permeable membrane (e.g., polypropylene, silicone rubber, Teflon) is held at the distal end.

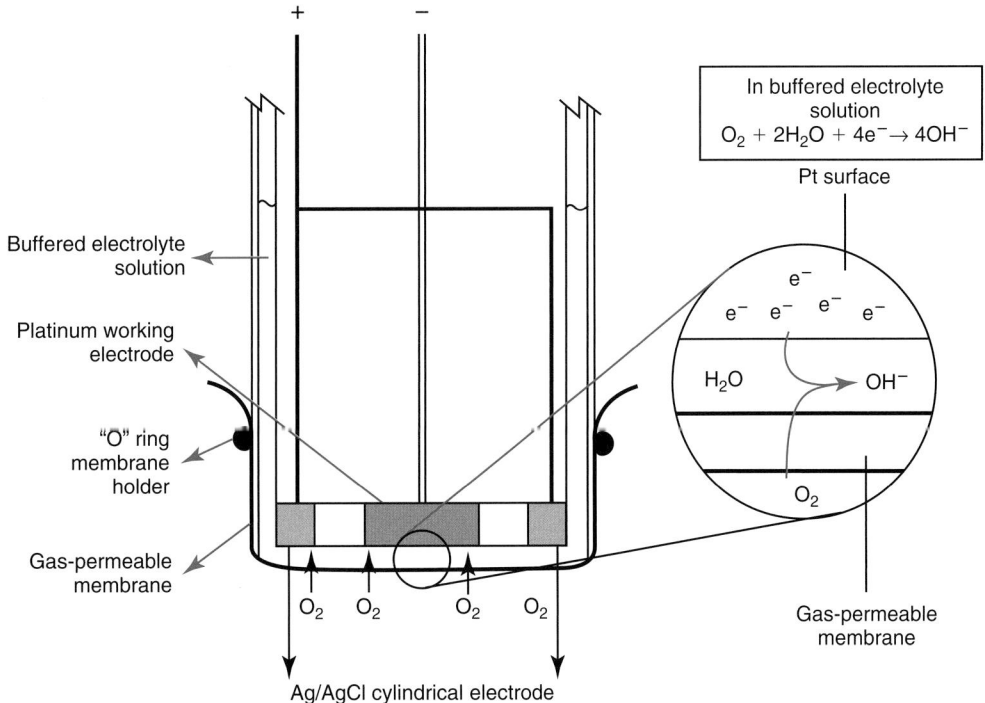

**Fig. 10.8** Design of an amperometric oxygen sensor used to monitor partial pressure of oxygen in blood. *Ag/AgCl*, Silver–silver chloride; *H2O*, water; *Pt*, platinum.

The inner working Pt electrode is pressed tightly against the gas-permeable membrane to create a thin film of internal electrolyte solution (usually buffer with KCl added). $O_2$ in the sample can permeate across the membrane and is reduced in accordance with the above electrochemical reaction. An $E_{appl}$ of −0.650 or −0.700 V versus Ag/AgCl (within the limiting current regime) to the Pt working electrode will result in an observed current that is proportional to $PO_2$ present in the sample (including whole blood). In the absence of any $O_2$, the current at this applied voltage under amperometric conditions will be near zero.

The outer gas-permeable membrane enables the electrode to detect $O_2$ with high selectivity over other easily reduced species that might be present in a given sample (e.g., metal ions, cystine). Only other gas species or highly lipophilic organic species can partition into and pass through such gas-permeable membranes. One type of interference in clinical samples can be caused by certain anesthesia gases, such as nitrous oxide, halothane, and isoflurane. These species can also diffuse through the outer membrane of the sensor, can be electrochemically reduced at the Pt electrode, and can yield a falsely high value for the measurement of $PO_2$. However, optimized gas-permeable membrane materials and appropriate control of the applied potential to the cathode of the sensor have greatly reduced this problem in modern instruments. The outer gas-permeable membrane also helps restrict diffusion of analyte to the inner working electrode; hence the membrane can control the mass transport of analyte ($D/\delta$ term in Eq. 10.16), such that in the presence or absence of sample convection, mass transport of $O_2$ to the surface of the Pt working electrode is essentially the same.

Amperometric $PO_2$ sensors can be used to detect other gas species by altering the applied voltage to the working electrode. For example, it is possible to detect nitric oxide (NO) with high selectivity using a similar gas electrode design in which the Pt is polarized at +0.900 versus Ag/AgCl to oxidize diffusing NO to nitrate at the Pt anode. Such NO sensors can be used for a variety of biomedically important studies to measure the amount of NO locally at or near the surface of various NO-producing cells.

Beyond amperometric devices, one specialized method of detecting trace concentrations of toxic metal ions in clinical samples is anodic or cathodic stripping voltammetry (ASV or CSV). In ASV a carbon working electrode is used (sometimes further coated with an Hg film), and the $E_{appl}$ is first fixed at a negative $E_{appl}$ voltage so that all metal ions in the solution will be reduced to elemental metals ($M^0$) within the Hg film and/or on the surface of the carbon. Then the $E_{appl}$ is scanned more positively, and reduced metals deposited in and/or on the surface of the working electrode are re-oxidized, giving a large anodic current peak proportional to the concentration of metal ions in the original sample. In CSV, the metal ions are held at an oxidizing potential and the oxidized ion are stripped from the electrode by sweeping potential negative. The potential at which these peaks are observed indicates which metal is present, and the height of the stripping peak current is directly proportional to the concentration of

the metal ion in the original sample. Such A/CSV techniques can be used to detect the total concentration of lead in whole blood samples, providing a rapid screening method for lead exposure and poisoning.

---

> **POINTS TO REMEMBER**
>
> **Predominant Types of Electrochemical Sensor Technologies Used in Whole Blood Analyzers**
> - Potentiometry: for measurement of pH, $PCO_2$, and electrolytes
> - Amperometry: for measurement of $PO_2$ and as the basis for whole blood glucose and lactate biosensors
> - Conductometry: for measurement of hematocrit

---

## CONDUCTOMETRY

**Conductometry** is an electrochemical technique used to determine the quantity of an analyte present in a mixture by measuring its effect on the electrical conductivity of the mixture. It is the measure of the ability of ions in solution to carry current under the influence of a potential difference. In a conductometric cell, potential is applied between two inert metal electrodes. An alternating potential with a frequency between 100 and 3000 Hz is used to prevent polarization of the electrodes. A decrease in solution resistance results in an increase in conductance, and more current is passed between the electrodes. The resulting current flow is also alternating. The current is directly proportional to solution conductance. Conductance is considered the inverse of resistance and may be expressed in units of $ohm^{-1}$ (siemens). In clinical analysis, conductometry is frequently used for measurement of the volume fraction of erythrocytes in whole blood (hematocrit) and as the transduction mechanism for some biosensors.

Erythrocytes act as electrical insulators because of their lipid-based membrane composition. This phenomenon was used first in the 1940s to measure the volume fraction of erythrocytes in whole blood (hematocrit) by conductivity and is used currently to measure hematocrit on multianalyte instruments for clinical analysis. The conductivity of whole blood depends not only on the volume fraction and shape of the erythrocytes but also on the conductivity of the surrounding plasma. An increase in the volume fraction of erythrocytes that are less conductive than the surrounding plasma leads to a decrease in conductivity shown by the following relationship:

$$G_b = \frac{a}{1 + \frac{H}{100 - H} \times c} \tag{10.21}$$

where $G_b$ = conductivity of whole blood; $a$ = plasma conductivity; $H$ = hematocrit in percent; and $c$ = factor for erythrocyte orientation. In practice, plasma conductivity also contains correction factors for $Na^+$ and $K^+$ concentrations. These cations are usually measured in conjunction with hematocrit on systems designed for clinical analysis.

Conductivity-based hematocrit measurements have limitations. Abnormal protein concentrations will change plasma conductivity and interfere with the measurement. Low protein concentrations resulting from dilution of blood with protein-free electrolyte solutions during cardiopulmonary bypass surgery will result in erroneously low hematocrit values by conductivity. Preanalytical variables, such as insufficient mixing of the sample, will also lead to errors. Hemoglobin is the preferred analyte to monitor blood loss and the need for transfusion during trauma and surgery. However, electrochemical measurement of hematocrit in conjunction with blood gases and electrolytes remains in use mainly because of its simplicity and convenience, despite some limitations.

Another clinical application of conductance is for electronic counting of blood cells in suspension. Termed the Coulter principle, it relies on the fact that the conductivity of blood cells is lower than that of a salt solution used as a suspension medium. The cell suspension is forced to flow through a tiny orifice. Two electrodes are placed on either side of the orifice, and a constant current is established between the electrodes. Each time a cell passes through the orifice, resistance increases; this causes a spike in the electrical potential difference between the electrodes. The pulses are then amplified and counted.

## COULOMETRY

Coulometry measures the electrical charge passing between two electrodes in an electrochemical cell. The amount of charge passing between the electrodes is directly proportional to oxidation or reduction of an electroactive substance at one of the electrodes. The number of coulombs transferred in this process is related to the absolute amount of electroactive substance by the Faraday law:

$$Q = nNF \qquad (10.22)$$

where $Q$ = amount of charge passing through the cell (unit: C = coulomb = ampere × second); $n$ = the number of electrons transferred in the oxidation or reduction reaction; $N$ = the amount of substance reduced or oxidized in moles; and $F$ = Faraday constant (96,487 coulombs/mol).

Current is the amount of charge passed per unit time (ampere = coulomb per second). Coulometry is used in clinical applications for the determination of $Cl^-$ in serum or plasma and as the mode of transduction in certain types of biosensors.

Coulometry is considered the "gold standard" for determination of $Cl^-$ in serum or plasma. However, the method is subject to interference from anions in the sample that have greater affinity for $Ag^+$ than $Cl^-$ (e.g., bromide) and is not commonly used currently in clinical laboratories.

## BIOSENSORS

A **biosensor** is a specific type of chemical sensor consisting of a biologic recognition element and a physicochemical transducer, often an electrochemical or an optical device. The biologic element is capable of recognizing the presence and activity and/or concentration of a specific analyte in solution. The recognition may be a *biocatalytic reaction (enzyme-based biosensor)* or a *binding process (affinity-based biosensor)* when the recognition element is, for example, an antibody, deoxyribonucleic acid (DNA) segment, or cell receptor. Interaction of the recognition element with a target analyte results in a measurable change in a solution property locally at the surface of the device, such as formation of a product or consumption of a reactant. The transducer converts the change in solution property into a quantifiable electrical signal. The mode of transduction may be one of several, including electrochemical or optical measurement and measurement of mass or heat. The present discussion is limited to biosensors based on electrochemical and optical modes of transduction because they constitute most biosensors used for clinical applications.

---

**POINTS TO REMEMBER**

**Biosensors**
- Biosensors measure substances lacking direct electroactive properties.
- Biosensors consist of a biologic recognition element and a physicochemical (e.g., electrochemical) transducer.
- Interaction of a biologic recognition element and an analyte results in either a biocatalytic reaction or a binding process, producing a measurable signal.
- Biosensors are used in most commercial blood glucose meters.
- Sensors for whole blood measurements without a biologic recognition element (e.g., ISEs) are not considered biosensors.

---

### Enzyme-Based Biosensors With Amperometric Detection

Enzyme-based biosensors based on electrochemical transducers, specifically amperometric electrodes, are most commonly used for clinical analyses and are frequently cited in the literature. Most of the current blood glucose meters are based on measurements using enzyme-based biosensors with amperometric detection, with glucose sensors produced in single-use formats. The first amperometric biosensor was used to measure glucose in blood and was based on immobilized glucose oxidase on the surface of an amperometric $PO_2$ sensor. A solution of glucose oxidase was physically entrapped between the gas-permeable membrane of the $PO_2$ electrode and an outer semipermeable membrane (Fig. 10.9). The outer membrane was of a low-molecular-weight cutoff to allow the substrate (glucose) and $O_2$ from the sample to pass, but not proteins and other macromolecules. In this way, enzymes could be concentrated at the sensor's surface. Oxidation of glucose, catalyzed by glucose oxidase as follows

$$Glucose + O_2 \xrightarrow{\text{Glucose oxidase}} Gluconic\ acid + H_2O_2 \quad \textbf{(10.23)}$$

consumes $O_2$ near the surface of the sensor. The rate of decrease in $PO_2$ is a function of the glucose concentration and is monitored by the $PO_2$ electrode. A steady-state $PO_2$ can be

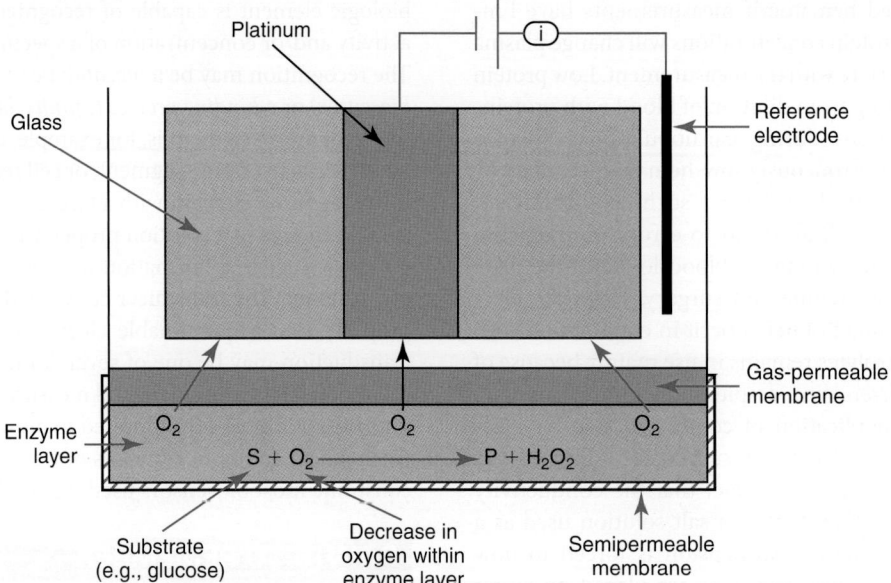

**Fig. 10.9** Illustration of an enzyme-based biosensor prepared using oxidase enzyme immobilized at the surface of an amperometric partial pressure of oxygen sensor. Increase in substrate concentration *(S)* reduces the amount of oxygen present at the surface of the sensor. $H_2O_2$, Hydrogen peroxide; *P*, product (e.g. gluconic acid).

achieved at the surface in a short period of time, yielding a steady-state current value that decreases as a function of glucose concentration in the sample.

If the polarizing voltage of the $PO_2$ electrode is reversed, making the Pt electrode positive (anode) relative to the Ag/AgCl reference electrode, and if the gas-permeable membrane is replaced with a hydrophilic outer membrane containing the immobilized enzyme, it is possible to oxidize the hydrogen peroxide ($H_2O_2$) produced by the glucose oxidase as follows:

$$H_2O_2 \rightarrow 2H^+ + O_2 + 2e^- \qquad (10.24)$$

The steady-state current produced is now directly proportional to the concentration of glucose in the sample.

In practice, a sufficiently high voltage (overpotential) must be applied to the Pt anode to drive the oxidation of the $H_2O_2$. An applied voltage of +0.7 V or greater (relative to Ag/AgCl) is typically used. Fig. 10.10A illustrates this basic $H_2O_2$ detection design, which is suitable for use in devising clinically useful sensors for glucose but also for a host of other substrates for which suitable oxidase enzymes generate $H_2O_2$.

Immobilization of enzymes in the early biosensors was a simple entrapment method behind a membrane of low-molecular-weight cutoff; this approach is still used in some commercial applications. Many other schemes for enzyme immobilization for biosensor development have been suggested. The most common are cross-linking of the enzyme with an inert protein (e.g., bovine serum albumin) using glutaraldehyde, simple adsorption of enzyme to electrode surfaces, and covalent binding of enzymes to insoluble carriers (e.g., nylon or glass). Another immobilization technique involves bulk modification of an electrode material, mixing enzymes with carbon paste, which serves as both

the enzyme immobilization matrix and the electroactive surface.

One of the first biosensor-based systems for the measurement of glucose in blood used amperometric detection of $H_2O_2$ as the measurement principle. Dependence of the measured glucose value on $O_2$ concentration in the sample was a problem because significantly less than the stoichiometric amount of dissolved $O_2$ is present in blood to support the glucose oxidase reaction and to produce a linear relationship of signal with glucose concentration. This is especially true at high concentrations of glucose found in samples from patients with diabetes (>500 mg/dL; 27.8 mmol/L). So, sample and calibration solutions were diluted at least 1:10 in buffer for equilibrium with atmospheric $PO_2$ to fix the $O_2$ concentration in the calibrator and sample to a constant value.

The problem of $O_2$ limitation for biosensors based on oxidase enzymes has been addressed by designing semipermeable membranes that restrict diffusion of the primary analyte (substrate) to the enzyme layer, which avoids saturation of the enzyme and keeps the ratio of $O_2$ to analyte always in excess of 1. This extends the linearity of response to analyte concentrations substantially higher than the $K_m$ of the enzyme and reduces the signal dependence on $O_2$. Outer track–etched polycarbonate membranes are commonly used, as are membranes of PVC, polyurethanes, and silicone emulsions. Another approach has been to use an $O_2$-rich electrode material as a reservoir of $O_2$ to support the bioreaction. A fluorocarbon (Kel-F Oil) has been used to formulate a carbon paste electrode to act as a source of $O_2$ and as the working electrode.

Electron acceptors other than $O_2$ can serve as mediators in the glucose oxidase reaction and completely eliminate

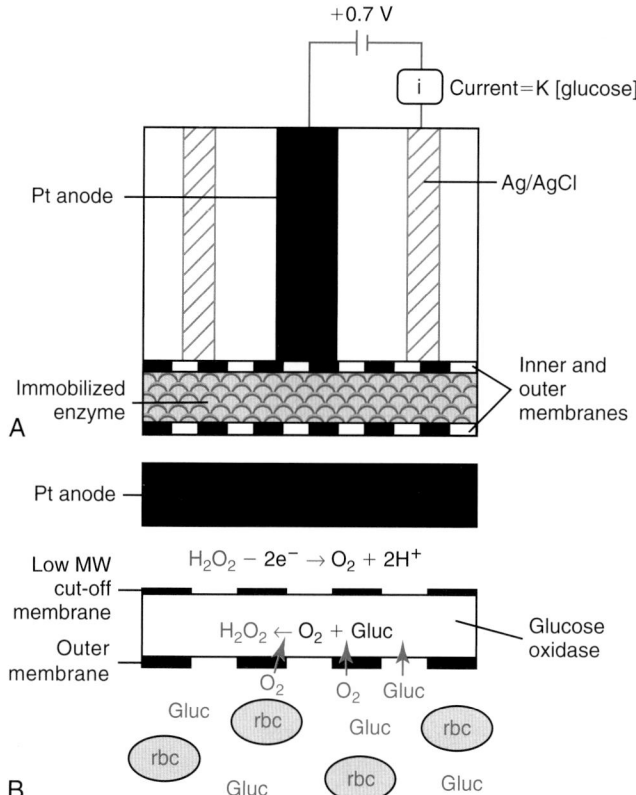

+0.7 V

i Current=K [glucose]

Pt anode

Ag/AgCl

Immobilized enzyme

Inner and outer membranes

A

Pt anode

Low MW cut-off membrane

$H_2O_2 - 2e^- \rightarrow O_2 + 2H^+$

Outer membrane

$H_2O_2 \leftarrow O_2 + Gluc$

Glucose oxidase

$O_2$  $O_2$  Gluc

Gluc  rbc  Gluc  rbc

rbc  rbc

Gluc  Gluc

B

Fig. 10.10 (A) Design of an amperometric enzyme-based biosensor based on anodic detection of hydrogen peroxide $(H_2O_2)$ generated from an oxidase enzymatic reaction (e.g., glucose oxidase). (B) Expanded view of the sensing surface shows the different membranes and electrochemical processes that yield the anodic current proportional to the substrate concentration in the sample. *Ag/AgCl,* Silver–silver chloride; *K,* proportionality constant; *MW,* molecular weight; *Pt,* platinum; *rbc,* red blood cells. (From Meyerhoff M. New in vitro analytical approaches for clinical chemistry measurements in critical care. *Clin Chem.* 1990;36:1570.)

any dependence of the amperometric response on the $O_2$ concentration of the sample. The mediator, which is usually coimmobilized with the enzyme, transports electrons to the anode surface, where it is reoxidized, resulting in a cyclic reaction mechanism (Fig. 10.11). Mediators with electron transfer kinetics (little or no overpotential) more favorable than that of $O_2$ allow operation of the sensor at lower applied potentials (+0.2 V vs. Ag/AgCl or lower) than those that are typically used for the oxidation of $H_2O_2$. This approach not only eliminates dependency of the reaction rate on $O_2$, the lower applied potential serves to reduce the contribution from oxidizable interfering substances (e.g., uric acid, ascorbic acid, acetaminophen) to the sensor response. Examples of mediators that have been used include quinones and conductive organic salts, such as tetrathiafulvalene-tetracyanoquinodimethane. Ferricyanide and ferrocene derivatives have also been used, including early commercial applications for home blood glucose monitoring. Dimethylferrocene is impregnated into a graphite electrode to which glucose oxidase has been immobilized. Reduced glucose oxidase from the enzymatic reaction is re-oxidized by the electrochemically generated ferricinium ion.

Electrode

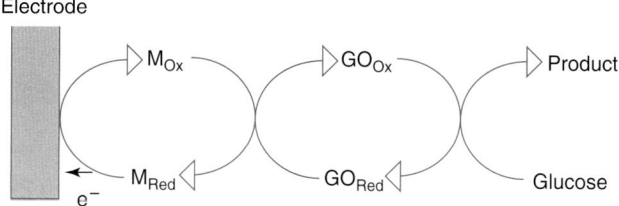

$M_{Ox}$  $GO_{Ox}$  Product

$M_{Red}$  $GO_{Red}$  Glucose

$e^-$

Fig. 10.11 The use of an electroactive mediator in the design of an amperometric enzyme-based biosensor. The mediator facilitates electron transfer between the enzyme and the electrode during the enzymatic conversion of glucose. The mediator $(M_{Ox})$ accepts electrons directly from the reduced enzyme $(GO_{Red})$ to form $M_{Red}$ and is oxidized at the surface of the working electrode to produce current proportional to glucose. In this process, reduced forms of enzyme and mediator are recycled back to their oxidized forms for continued reaction. Mediator and enzyme in oxidized form $M_{Ox}$ and $GO_{Ox}$, Mediator and enzyme in reduced form $M_{Red}$ and $GO_{Red}$. (From D'Orazio P. In: Lewendrowski K, ed. *Clinical Chemistry: Laboratory Management and Clinical Correlations.* Philadelphia: Lippincott, Williams & Wilkins; 2002:464.)

Current produced during this cycling mechanism is proportional to the concentration of glucose in the blood sample.

Another technique used to decrease interferences from easily oxidized species in a blood sample when traditional $H_2O_2$ electrochemical detection is used is to employ selectively permeable membranes in proximity to the electrode surface that allow transport of $H_2O_2$ to the electrode surface but reject the interfering substances based on size exclusion (see Fig. 10.10B). An example is as simple as a low-molecular-weight cutoff membrane, such as cellulose acetate, which is used in many commercial amperometric biosensors. Electropolymerized films, such as poly(phenylenediamine) formed in situ, are also used to reject interfering substances based on size. Another approach in a commercial application uses a second correcting electrode, identical to the working electrode but without enzyme that is sensitive only to the presence of oxidizable interfering substances. The resulting differential signal is proportional to the concentration of analyte.

A novel approach for elimination of electroactive interfering substances in a commercially available glucose sensor is to directly "wire" the redox center of the enzyme glucose oxidase to a metallic, amperometric electrode using an osmium (III/IV)-based redox hydrogel. Osmium sites effectively serve as mediators and can accept electrons directly from the entrapped enzyme, without need for $O_2$. This approach allows the operating potential of the electrode to be dramatically lowered to +0.2 V versus the saturated calomel reference electrode, where currents resulting from electrooxidation of ascorbate, urate, acetaminophen, and L-cysteine are negligible.

Substitution of other oxidoreductase enzymes for glucose oxidase allows amperometric biosensors for other substrates of clinical interest to be constructed. Practical sensors with commercial application in critical care analyzers for blood lactate have been realized. By using the multiple enzyme cascade shown in the reactions discussed here, amperometric biosensors for creatinine or lactate are also possible.

Electrochemical oxidation of $H_2O_2$ is the detection mechanism:

$$Lactate + O_2 \xrightarrow{\text{Lactate oxidase}} Pyruvate + H_2O_2 \quad (10.25)$$

$$Creatinine + H_2O \xrightarrow{\text{Creatine amidinohydrolase}} Creatine \quad (10.26)$$

$$Creatine + H_2O \xrightarrow{\text{Creatine amidinohydrolase}} Sarcosine + Urea \quad (10.27)$$

$$Sarcosine + O_2 \xrightarrow{\text{Sarcosine oxidase}} Glycine + Formaldehyde + H_2O_2 \quad (10.28)$$

The three-enzyme scheme for creatinine measurement suffers interference from endogenous creatine in the sample, requiring correction. Low concentrations of creatinine found in blood ($\leq 1.13$ mg/dL; $\leq 100$ µmol/L) must be measured in the presence of oxidizable interfering substances, which are sometimes present at higher concentrations than the analyte. Special electroactive layers within the biosensor have been proposed to remove redox-active interfering substances. Because the useful life of the creatinine or lactate biosensors requires enzyme(s) to retain activity, reusable commercial biosensors for creatinine or lactate typically have a short (few days) useful life, but improvements in enzyme immobilization methods and/or use of stabilizers and/or activators within calibrating reagents have yielded creatinine or lactate sensor devices with much longer lifetimes ($\geq 3$ weeks of continuous use after ambient storage for 6 months). Such improvements in stability and ability to measure directly in whole blood has resulted in commercial applications of these biosensors at the point of care.

## Enzyme-Based Biosensors With Potentiometric and Conductometric Detection

ISEs can be used as transducers in potentiometric biosensors. An example is a biosensor for urea (blood urea nitrogen [BUN]) based on a polymer membrane ISE for $NH_4^+$ ion (Fig. 10.12). The enzyme urease is immobilized at the surface of the $NH_4^+$-selective ISE based on the antibiotic nonactin (see structure of ionophore in Fig. 10.3) and catalyzes the hydrolysis of urea to $NH_3$ and $CO_2$:

$$Urea \xrightarrow{\text{Urease}} 2NH_3 + CO_2 \quad (10.29)$$

The ammonia ($NH_3$) produced forms $NH_4^+$, which is sensed by the ISE. The signal generated by the $NH_4^+$ produced is proportional to the logarithm of the concentration of urea in the sample. The response may be steady state or transient. Typically, correction for background $K^+$ is required because the nonactin ionophore has limited selectivity for $NH_4^+$ over $K^+$ ($K_{NH_4/K} = 0.1$). Potassium is measured simultaneously with urea and is used to correct the output of the urea sensor using Eq. 10.9.

The approach already described for measurement of urea using an enzyme-based potentiometric biosensor assumes

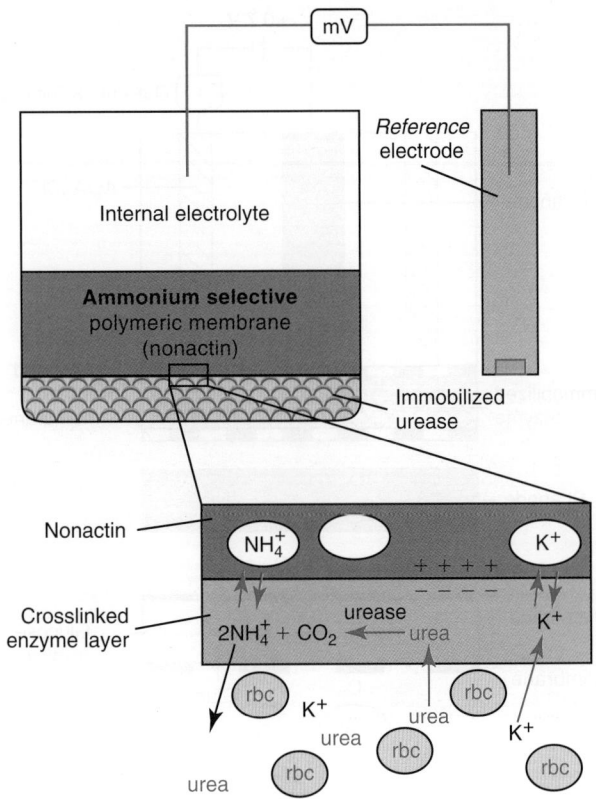

**Fig. 10.12** Potentiometric enzyme-based biosensor for determination of blood urea, based on urease immobilized on the surface of an ammonium ion–selective polymeric membrane electrode. An expanded view of the ammonium ion selective membrane and immobilized urease interface of the biosensor showing the enzymatic conversion of urea in blood to ammonium ion and its detection at a nonactin (ionophore for ammonium) based ion selective membrane. *CO₂*, Carbon dioxide; *K⁺*, potassium; *NH₄⁺*, ammonium; *rbc*, red blood cells.

that the turnover of urea to $NH_4^+$ at steady state provides a constant ratio of $NH_4^+$ to urea, independent of concentration. This is rarely the case, especially at higher substrate concentrations, which results in a nonlinear sensor response. The linearity of the sensor is also limited by the fact that hydrolysis of urea produces a local alkaline pH in the vicinity of the $NH_4^+$-sensing membrane, partially converting $NH_4^+$ to $NH_3$ ($pK_a = 9.3$). Ammonia is not sensed by the ISE. The degree of nonlinearity may be reduced by the placement of a semipermeable membrane between the enzyme and the sample to restrict diffusion of urea to the immobilized enzyme layer.

A change in solution conductivity has also been used as a transduction mechanism in enzyme-based biosensors. Examples include the measurement of glucose, creatinine, and acetaminophen using interdigitated electrodes. There are few practical applications of conductometric biosensors because of the variable ionic background of clinical samples and the requirement to measure small conductivity changes in media of high ionic strength. A commercial system for the measurement of urea in serum, plasma, and urine is based on the enzyme urease. Dissolution of products from Eq. 10.29 to $NH_4^+$ and $HCO_3^-$ produces a change in sample conductivity. The initial rate of change in conductivity is measured to compensate for the background conductivity of the sample. This approach is limited to the measurement of analytes at relatively high concentrations because of small changes in conductivity produced by low concentrations of analyte.

## Affinity Sensors

Affinity sensors are a special class of biosensors in which the immobilized biological recognition element is a binding protein, antibody (immunosensors), or oligonucleotide (e.g., DNA, aptamers) with high binding affinity and high specificity toward a clinically important analyte and/or partner. Such sensors are being developed as alternatives to conventional binding assays to enhance the speed and convenience of a wide range of assays that normally would be run on large, sophisticated instruments in a central laboratory. Affinity sensors may be more easily adaptable to systems developed for point-of-care testing for infectious disease, cardiac markers, or other applications where speed and ease of use are required. Ideally, direct binding of the immobilized species with its target in a clinical sample should yield a sensor signal proportional to the concentration of the analyte. However, direct sensing (without use of exogenous labels and/or tracers) of the binding events at analyte concentrations that would cover the full range for clinical applications is very difficult to achieve. Furthermore, high affinity of such binding reactions, which are required to achieve optimal sensitivity, also limits the reversibility of such devices (slow reverse rate constant). For repeated multiuse applications, some type of regeneration step (pH change, temperature change, and so on) to dissociate the tight binding between the biorecognition element and the target is generally required. Such regeneration steps can alter binding properties of bio-element and target and reduce sensor sensitivity or specificity. Unlike ISEs, $O_2$ sensors, and many of the enzyme-based biosensors described previously, affinity sensors based on electrochemical, optical, or other transduction modes are typically single-use devices.

Most affinity-type sensors appearing in the literature with a promise of clinical usefulness are based on labeled reagents, such as enzymes, fluorophores, and electrochemical tags, and hence, they function more like traditional binding and/or immunoassays, except that one recognition element is immobilized on the surface of a suitable electrode or another type of transducer. For example, electrochemical $O_2$ sensors have been used to carry out heterogeneous enzyme immunoassays (sandwich or competitive type), using catalase as a labeling enzyme (catalyzes $H_2O_2 \rightarrow 2H^+$ and $O_2$) and immobilizing capture antibodies on the outer surface of the gas-permeable membrane. After binding equilibration and washing steps, the amount of bound enzyme is detected by adding the substrate and following the increase in current generation caused by local production of $O_2$ near the surface of the sensor.

The number of research publications on affinity biosensors continues to increase, with potential application for detection of markers of cardiac disease, cancer, and autoimmune disease. Several commercial examples of immunosensors do exist, primarily in the unit-use, disposable format designed for point-of-care testing. One such example is a

cartridge-based device for cardiac troponin I, BNP, CK-MB, or β-hCG on the i-STAT handheld analyzer (Abbott Point of Care, Abbott Laboratories, Abbott Park, IL). This sensor uses a sandwich immunoassay format with electrochemical detection. A capture antibody is immobilized on an Au electrode for recognition and capture of specific analyte (antigen) in the blood sample. A second reporter antibody is labeled with alkaline phosphatase and binds with surface-captured antigen. Following incubation and washing steps, the substrate p-aminophenyl phosphate is introduced, and the product of the enzymatic reaction (p-aminophenol) is detected amperometrically by oxidation. The magnitude of the oxidative current is proportional to concentration of analyte in the sample.

The basic advantage of immobilizing affinity reagents on the surfaces of electrodes or sensing devices is somewhat diminished when separate washing steps are required to remove unbound label species. As discussed previously, true affinity biosensors should yield analytically useful responses in the presence of undiluted physiologic samples, without the need for discrete incubation and washing steps. One example of an electrochemical-based immunosensor method that partially achieves this goal is a technique termed nonseparation electrochemical enzyme immunoassay. The basic concept is illustrated in Fig. 10.13. As indicated, no separation or washing steps are required. This method was used to detect prostate-specific antigen (PSA) and human chorionic gonadotropin at nanogram per milliliter concentrations in undiluted plasma and whole blood. Direct affinity sensors eliminate the need for labeled reagents because the binding reaction results in a change in a property that may be monitored directly. Of these, few have adequate specificity to be used in complex clinical samples because of significant signals arising from nonspecific binding or electrochemical response. Direct immunosensors for sensitive assays of tumor markers have been reported. Examples include an electrochemical immunosensor for PSA with an enhanced lower limit of detection, based on an alternating current impedance measurement, and an assay for carcinoma antigen-125 using a quartz crystal microbalance. The former uses a control sensor with an immobilized immunoglobulin-G antibody instead of anti-PSA to subtract out effects from nonspecific binding to achieve a limit of detection of 1 pg/mL toward PSA.

## Affinity Sensors for Deoxyribonucleic Acid Analysis Using Electrochemical Labels

DNA sensors in which a segment of DNA complementary to a target strand is immobilized on a suitable electrochemical sensor have been demonstrated. These devices operate in direct (based on electrochemical oxidation of guanine in target DNA; Fig. 10.14A) or indirect (with exogenous electrochemical markers and/or labels, see later and Fig. 10.14B) transduction modes. Although most of the proposed electrochemical DNA biosensors require amplification methods, such as PCR, to multiply small amounts of DNA into measurable quantities, some are sensitive enough to eliminate the need for target amplification.

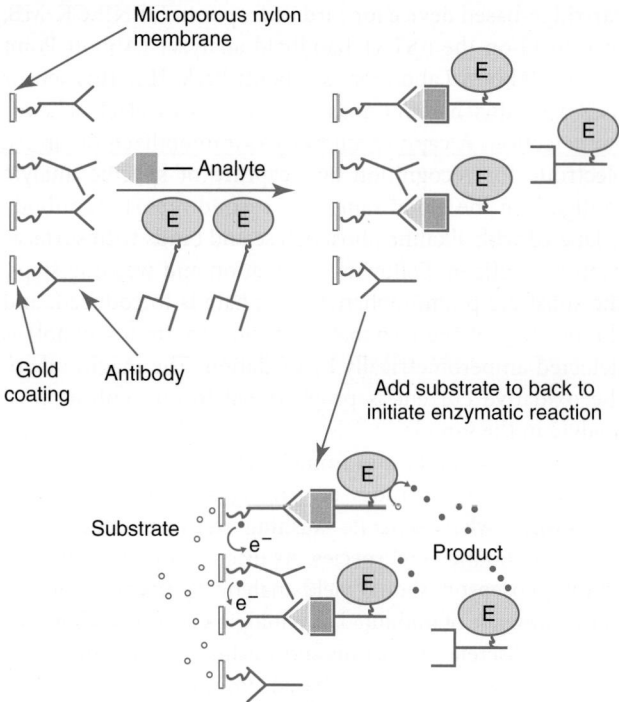

**Fig. 10.13** Homogeneous electrochemical enzyme immunoassay, shown as a sandwich immunoassay. A gold porous membrane electrode, installed as a separator in a diffusion cell in between two compartments, serves as a working electrode. Primary antibodies are immobilized on one surface of the electrode. Analyte and antibody labeled with an enzyme are then added to the same side of the porous gold electrode. The substrate for the enzyme is added to the other side of the porous gold electrode. During a short electrochemical measurement time (1 minute), substrate diffuses through the porous electrode and reacts only to surface-bound enzyme/antibody and not to the unbound complex in the bulk of the solution, producing an electroactive product.

Nanotechnology has been proposed, in the indirect format, for signal amplification. For example, a capture probe DNA is immobilized on an Au electrode. Reporter probes with electrostatically bound ruthenium complexes $(Ru[NH_3]_6)^{3+}$ are loaded onto Au nanoparticles (AuNP) and are capable of hybridizing with one of two sequences on target DNA. The other sequence on the target DNA is capable of hybridizing with the immobilized capture probe. Hybridization events on the electrode surface bring multiple reporter probes for each AuNP. Electroactive $(Ru[NH_3]_6)^{3+}$ is reduced at the electrode surface, and the coulometric signal is proportional to the concentration of target DNA. A commercial example of electrochemical DNA sensing, along with AuNP probes without need for PCR amplification, is the Verigene system (Nanosphere, Luminex), which is capable of detecting single-nucleotide polymorphisms related to common genetic disorders, such as (1) thrombophilia, (2) alterations of folate metabolism, (3) cystic fibrosis, and (4) hemochromatosis. Another commercially available, electrochemically based platform for nucleic acid detection without the need for sample purification or target amplification is from GeneFluidics (Irwindale, CA). The system uses a sensor array chip consisting of 16 nanoscale Au electrodes,

modified with thiol self-assembled monolayers, optimized for biomolecule immobilization. Horseradish peroxidase is the preferred target label because of its fast electron transfer kinetics, when used with amperometric detection.

Another example of an electrochemical "gene" sensor array uses electrochemical probes that are selectively inserted into hybridized DNA duplexes. In one approach, after the immobilized capture of oligo anchored to the electrode surface is allowed to bind the target sequence, hybridization is detected by exposing the surface of the electrode to an exogenous electroactive species (Co[III]tris-phenanthroline, ruthenium complexes, and so on) that intercalates within the duplex, but not to single-stranded DNA. After unbound electroactive species are removed by washing, the presence of hybridization is readily detected by voltammetry, scanning the potential of the underlying electrode to oxidize or reduce any intercalated electroactive species, with the current detected being proportional to the number of duplex DNA species on the surface of the electrode.

## Affinity Sensors Based on Aptamers (Aptasensors)

Aptamers have been explored as versatile recognition elements for a variety of biosensing applications, including small molecules, proteins, and cells. Aptamers are synthetic single-stranded nucleic acids capable of folding into three-dimensional structures to selectively bind target molecules. In practice, aptamers may be generated and selected in vitro to bind targets for which antibodies and other protein receptors are not easily obtained, using a process known as systematic evolution of ligands by exponential enrichment (SELEX). During the SELEX process, a large, random DNA or RNA library goes through an iterative process of selective binding toward a target analyte. After separation of bound and unbound DNA, the bound DNA is amplified using PCR for a subsequent round of selection and isolation of the optimum binding segment. The inherent advantage of aptamer-based affinity sensors is reduced nonspecific binding because of the conformational change of the aptamer during the binding event, making the aptamer less susceptible to recognition of many potential interfering substances in a complex sample matrix (e.g., blood serum). The same conformational change may optimize performance of a labeled target following a binding event; for example, by altering the local environment of a fluorescent label or changing the position of an electrochemical label with respect to a sensing electrode. Although few aptamer-based diagnostic products have been commercialized at present, reported practical applications for aptamer-based affinity sensors in clinical chemistry are increasing in the literature.

Aptamers have been demonstrated to function in biosensors using various transduction methods, including optical sensing (using fluorescently labeled aptamers), and acoustic, mass (cantilever-based), and electrochemical sensing, which use, for example, aptamer probes labeled with a redox species (e.g., ferrocene or methylene blue). As is the case with most affinity-based biosensors, electrochemical sensing for aptasensors may still be the preferred transduction mode because redox labels may be chosen to operate at an applied potential away from potentially interfering electroactive species in the

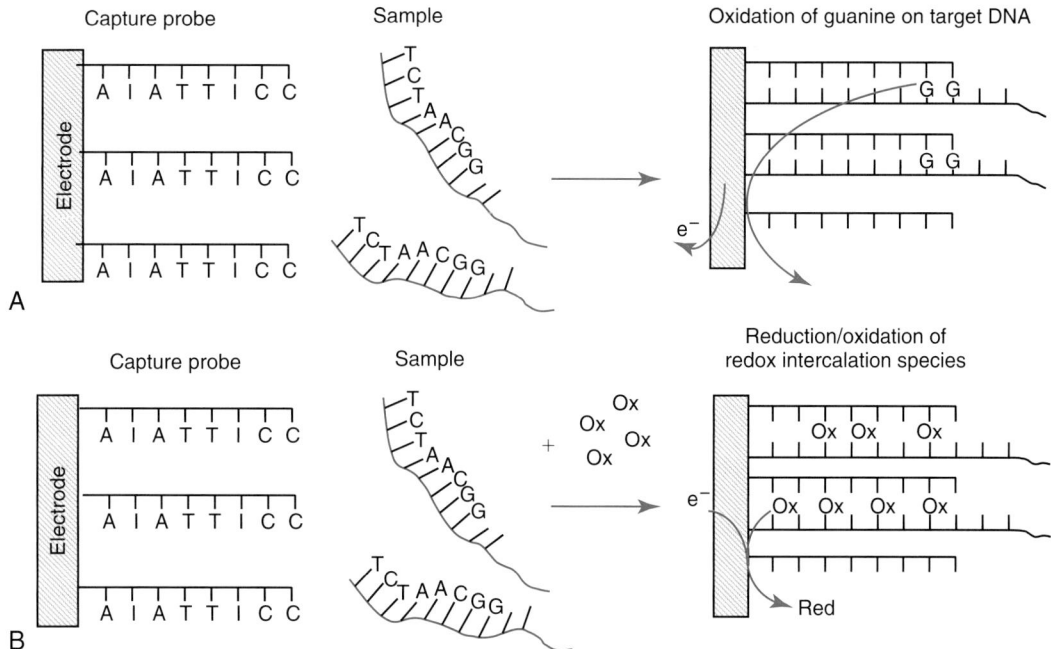

**Fig. 10.14** Examples of deoxyribonucleic acid (DNA) biosensor configurations. (A) Direct electrooxidation *(Ox)* detection of guanosine bases in target DNA after hybridization with immobilized capture probe on electrode surface. (B) Electrochemical detection of hybridization using exogenous redox *(Ox)* species that intercalate into hybridized complex between the immobilized capture DNA probe and target DNA.

sample matrix. By taking advantage of the conformational change of the aptamer during a binding event, it changes the relative proximity of an electrochemical label to an electrode surface. Using thrombin as a model analyte and methylene blue (MB) as an electroactive label, an aptasensor was constructed by immobilizing a MB-labeled, thrombin-binding aptamer to a thiol modified Au electrode. In the absence of thrombin, the aptamer chain is flexible, and the MB label is close to the electrode surface for high electron transfer efficiency. Upon binding to the thrombin target, the folding of the aptamer moves the label away from the electrode surface, inhibiting electron transfer. A sensitivity down to 6.4-nmol thrombin was demonstrated. The opposite transduction approach (in which target binding by the aptamer brings an electroactive label closer to an electrode surface) was demonstrated as a sensor for platelet-derived growth factor (PDGF) in blood serum. In this case, the MB label was attached at one end of the PDGF aptamer, and in the absence of a target, the label was relatively far from the electrode surface. Binding of the PDGF target brought the MB label close to the electrode surface in a stable configuration, enhancing an electron transfer. Detection of PDGF down to 50 pmol was shown.

Using a similar concept as the thrombin sensors described above, electrochemical aptamer-based sensors were developed for real-time, continuous, and multi-hour tracking of four drugs (doxorubicin, kanamycin, gentamicin, and tobramycin) in the bloodstream. These sensors were able to quickly respond (3 seconds) to different concentrations of these drugs following an injection into the bloodstream and recovered to baseline response after clearing of the drug from blood. Square wave voltammetry at high frequencies have been employed to achieve fast response. Such reusable fast-responding aptamer-based sensors can provide valuable insight to pharmacokinetic information including feedback-controlled drug delivery. Electrochemical aptamer sensors are growing rapidly in the scientific literature for different applications that are traditionally not feasible with ISE, enzyme, or antibody-based sensors. Examples include calibration-free sensors for phenylalanine concentrations, sensors for insulin monitoring, cocaine in undiluted blood, and sensors for toxins in food.

## Affinity Sensors for COVID

Different configurations of affinity-based electrochemical sensors discussed previously have been adapted in SARS-CoV-2 diagnostic assays. Three different testing strategies commonly are used for sensing SARS-CoV-2: (1) molecular tests based on viral DNA, (2) antigen tests based on viral proteins, and (3) antibody tests based on specific antibodies for viral proteins. Several electrochemical sensors have been reported on antigen or antibody tests for viral proteins. One example is an electrochemical sensor for SARS-CoV-2 N-protein antigen using nasopharyngeal samples and screen-printed carbon electrodes functionalized with immobilized capture antibodies. Following sample addition and horseradish peroxide conjugated detection antibodies, the concentration of virus in samples was assayed by chrono-amperometric detection in the presence of tetramethylbenzidine (TMB). Another example is an ultrasensitive detection of SARS-CoV-2 antibodies by a graphene field effect transistor (FET) with detection limit down to $10^{-18}$ M. The graphene modified FETs were immobilized with spike S1 protein and SARS-CoV-2 antibody binding with antigen generates conductance changes on graphene on the FET leading to ultrasensitive detection of the antibodies (150 antibodies in 100 μL serum). An aptamer-based electrochemical sensor was reported for rapid reagent-free and quantitative measurement was reported for SARS-CoV-2 spike protein. Similar to other electrochemical sensors described above, redox tag modified aptamers specific to SARS-CoV-2 spike protein change confirmation in the presence of spike protein causing the electrochemical tag to move further away from the electrode with a change in voltametric signal proportional to concentration in serum or saliva samples.

## Continuous Glucose Monitoring Sensors

Single-use electrochemical sensors test strips with capillary blood testing has been the routine methodology for frequent self-monitoring of blood glucose (SMBG) at home by diabetic patients. Recently, a new class of glucose sensors designed to help manage patients with diabetes by continuous monitoring of glucose in interstitial fluid (ISF) were introduced to the market. Although SMBG has been the standard of glucose testing at home, continuous glucose monitoring (CGM) is rapidly increasing in recent years due to the advances in wireless technologies, miniaturization, development of calibration-free sensing technologies, and a push for reducing finger pricks for self-monitoring.

Continuous monitoring of glucose in ISF first appeared commercially in the late 1990s. Currently, devices from multiple manufacturers are offered on the market. Subcutaneously implanted glucose sensors, in the earlier designs, required periodic calibration using results from fingerstick blood glucose and required replacement every 3 to 7 days. Despite limited commercial success in the early phase, continuous glucose monitors, based on subcutaneously implanted sensors, can detect and predict hypoglycemic events and reduce the time spent in the hypoglycemic range in patients with type 1 diabetes. Several clinical trials have shown significant reduction in glycosylated hemoglobin concentration among users of continuous glucose monitors.

Sensor technologies used in these ISF implanted devices are similar to glucose oxidase-based biosensors described in the biosensors section above with additional process steps to address biofouling during the use. To improve biocompatibility of these sensors when implanted in ISF, coatings were developed to minimize any biological response so that continuous analytical results closely matched those attained by conventional in vitro testing. Biocompatible polymeric and other coatings with anti-inflammatory drugs are often employed to address biofouling concerns.

In 2000, the Food and Drug Administration (FDA) approved the first CGM system from MiniMed (currently part of Medtronic, Northridge, CA) and had a mean absolute relative difference (MARD) of around 25% between glucose value measured by YSI (YSI, Inc, Yellow Springs, OH) glucose and the CGM sensor. Additionally, the MiniMed sensor required periodic calibration using an off-line fingerstick glucose from a single use blood glucose sensor to correlate the patient's glucose to the CGM signal. The FDA approved new devices from Abbott (Chicago, IL) in 2017 and from Dexcom (San Diego, CA) in 2018 that offer calibration-free or factory-calibrated sensors with MARD of 11.7% and 9.0%, respectively. The Abbott Freestyle CGM consists of a sensor patch that is worn on the upper arm and measures glucose in ISF every 15 minutes for up to 14 days. When users scan the monitor over the sensor patch, the current reading and an 8-hour glucose trend are reported. The Dexcom G6 CGM measures glucose every 5 minutes and the results are wirelessly communicated via Bluetooth technology to a monitor, cell phone, or an electronic watch for up to 10 days. A newer version of the Medtronic CGM, the Guardian Connect, has a 7-day useful life and requires calibration with finger-sticks every 12 hours. All three devices employ the same electrochemical glucose biosensor principles described in this chapter. One drawback of these ISF-based CGM sensors is that they are susceptible to erroneous glucose results from prolonged pressure on the sensor during sleep. Pressure on the sensor can induce changes in the interstitial space due to decreased tissue perfusion, oxygen tension, or change in temperature that alter the glucose response of the CGM sensor. Additionally, an adhesive patch is used for holding the sensor on the upper arm or on the abdomen and the adhesive patch can peel off from the skin. Another CGM with recent FDA approval is the Eversense (Senseonics, Germantown, MD) system. It has an optical sensor that requires surgical subcutaneous installation. This device measures glucose every 5 minutes and lasts 180 days. This new Eversense system provides the longest CGM with a MARD of less than 8.5% and eliminates the errors from localized pressures and patch adhesive issues. The Eversense CGM is based on fluorescence transduction and uses a non-enzymatic boronic acid–glucose binding polymer as the base principle for measuring glucose. Binding of glucose increases fluorescence proportionally to the concentration. However, the Eversense sensor assembly is bigger in size ($18.3 \times 3.5$ mm) than the typical electrochemical sensors that are micron-sized.

## Future Trends

Electrochemical sensor principles described in this chapter are increasingly finding applications in clinical diagnostics beyond ISEs and enzyme-based sensors in expanding the analyte menu in continuous monitoring, immunoassays, genetic testing, aptamers, and virus detection. Recent developments in CGM and the ability to continuously report results to external devices such as insulin pumps can lead to future devices that can provide automated insulin dosing using artificial intelligence and machine learning models to result in artificial pancreas systems. Development of enabling technologies for an artificial pancreas are underway at different CGM manufacturers and other medical devices companies.

Wearable devices (Apple Watch, Fitbit, Samsung Watch, etc.) for monitoring vital signs such as heart rate, steps, and mobility are gaining increased attention due to the emergence of mobile technology and digital medicine. The success of CGMs and wearable monitoring devices are driving innovations at academic and industry settings in developing sensors and other enabling technologies suitable as wearable devices to monitor non-invasively clinical parameters that are typically measured in body fluids (blood, plasma, urine) in clinical laboratories. Sensors for non-invasive measurements of electrolytes, metabolites, or other important analytes are being developed for use in saliva, sweat, tears, and ISF. Although these wearable sensing devices are at an early stage of development, progress is rapid and will enable the transition of clinical testing from central laboratories to the point of care. However, clinical and diagnostic correlations, such as normal and critical ranges in these body fluids (sweat, saliva, tears, etc.), are not currently available and are needed for the realization of these wearable devices for clinical and commercial applications.

> ## POINTS TO REMEMBER
>
> ### Affinity Biosensors
> - Affinity biosensors are a specific type of biosensor in which an immobilized recognition element exhibits a high binding constant for the analyte of interest.
> - Examples of recognition elements are antibodies and oligonucleotides (DNA segments).
> - Affinity biosensor binding reactions are typically irreversible and best suited to single-use sensors.
> - Most affinity biosensors for clinical application use indirect modes of transduction, including enzymatic, fluorescence, and electrochemical labels.

## REVIEW QUESTIONS

1. Ion-selective electrodes measure electrical potential difference across a membrane using the principles of:
   a. coulometry.
   b. potentiometry.
   c. amperometry.
   d. conductivity.
2. A basic component of an electrochemical cell is:
   a. enzyme
   b. whole blood
   c. antibody
   d. reference electrode
3. Voltammetry/amperometry measurements are based on which of the following electrochemical cell types?
   a. Ion-selective electrode cells
   b. Galvanic electrochemical cells
   c. Electromotive force cells
   d. Electrolytic electrochemical cells
4. A biosensor has the following biorecognition element:
   a. antibody
   b. ionophore
   c. whole blood
   d. plasma
5. A voltmeter that measures the potential across an electrochemical cell (between the two electrodes) is referred to as a:
   a. conductometer.
   b. amperometer.
   c. direct-reading potentiometer.
   d. redox meter.
6. Which of the following is an error source for blood hematocrit measurements based on conductivity-based methods?
   a. Glucose levels
   b. Abnormal protein levels
   c. Blood gases
   d. Hemoglobin
7. The maximum difference in potential between the two electrodes in an electrochemical cell obtained with the current at zero is the definition of:
   a. electrical potential.
   b. electromotive force.
   c. electrochemical gradient.
   d. Nernst equation.
8. What is the measurement principle used in glucose, lactate, and creatinine sensors?
   a. Amperometry.
   b. Voltammetry.
   c. Potentiometry.
   d. Conductometry.
9. The measurement of ions by direct potentiometry is based on the following equation:
   a. Nernst equation
   b. enzymatic reaction
   c. antigen and antibody binding
   d. oxygen reduction
10. Continuous glucose monitoring devices measure glucose in which of following fluids?
    a. Plasma
    b. Serum
    c. Interstitial fluid
    d. Arterial blood

## SUGGESTED READINGS

Apple FS, Koch DD, Graves S, et al. Relationship between direct-potentiometric and flame-photometric measurement of sodium in blood. *Clin Chem*. 1982;28:1931–1935.

Astrup P, Severinghaus JW. *The History of Blood Gases, Acids and Bases*. Copenhagen, Denmark: Munksgaard; 1986.

Bakker E, Bühlmann P, Pretsch E. Carrier-based ion-selective electrodes and bulk optodes. 1. General characteristics. *Chem Rev*. 1997;97:3083–3132.

Bates RG. *Determination of pH: Theory and Practice*. New York: John Wiley & Sons; 1973.

Buck RP, Lindner E. Recommendations for nomenclature of ion-selective electrodes. *Pure Appl Chem*. 1994;66:2527–2536.

Clark LC Jr, Lyons C. Electrode systems for continuous monitoring in cardiovascular surgery. *Ann N Y Acad Sci*. 1962;102:29–45.

D'Orazio P. Biosensors in clinical chemistry. *Clin Chim Acta*. 2003;334:41–69.

D'Orazio P. Biosensors in clinical chemistry—2011 update. *Clin Chim Acta*. 2011;412:1749–1761.

Faulkner LR. Understanding electrochemistry: some distinctive concepts. *J Chem Ed*. 1983;60:262–264.

Guilbault GG. *Handbook of Immobilized Enzymes*. New York: Marcel-Dekker; 1984.

Heller A. Amperometric biosensors. *Curr Opin Biotechnol*. 1996;7:50–54.

Lai RY, Plaxco KW, Heegar AJ. Aptamer-based electrochemical detection of picomolar platelet derived growth factor directly in blood serum. *Anal Chem*. 207;79:229–333.

Leiner MJP. Luminescence chemical sensors for biomedical applications: scope and limitations. *Anal Chim Acta*. 1991;255:209–222.

Luppa PB, Sokoll LJ, Chan DW. Immunosensors—principles and applications to clinical chemistry. *Clin Chim Acta*. 2001;314:1–26.

Mihai DA, Stefan DS, Stegaru D, et al. Continuous glucose monitoring devices: a brief presentation (review). *Exp Ther Med*. 2022;23:174.

Oesch U, Ammann D, Simon W. Ion-selective membrane electrodes for clinical use. *Clin Chem*. 1986;32:1448–1459.

Osswald HF, Wuhrmann HR. Calibration standards for multi ion analysis in whole blood samples. In: Lubbers DW, Acker H, Buck RP, et al., eds. *Progress in Enzyme and Ion-Selective Electrodes*. Berlin: Springer-Verlag; 1981:74–78.

Pioda LA, Simon W, Bosshard HR, et al. Determination of potassium ion concentration in serum using a highly selective liquid-membrane electrode. *Clin Chim Acta*. 1970;29:289–293.

Ronkainen NJ, Okon SL. Nanomaterial-based electrochemical immunosensors for clinically significant biomarkers. *Materials*. 2014;7:4669–4709.

Seitz WR. Chemical sensors based on fiber optics. *Anal Chem*. 1984;56:16A–34A.

Stott RAW, Hortin GL, Wilhite TR, et al. Analytical artifacts in hematocrit measurements by whole blood chemistry analyzers. *Clin Chem*. 1995;41:306–311.

Thevenot DR, Toth K, Durst RA, et al. Electrochemical biosensors: recommended definitions and classifications. *Biosens Bioelectron*. 2001;16:121–131.

# Electrophoresis

*Lindsay A.L. Bazydlo and James P. Landers*

## OBJECTIVES

1. Define the following:
   - Agarose
   - Ampholyte
   - Amphoteric
   - Blot/blotting
   - Densitometry
   - Electroendosmosis
   - Electrophoresis
   - Electrophoretic mobility
   - Polyacrylamide
   - Wick flow
2. State the theory of electrophoresis.
3. List and describe the components of an electrophoresis system, including buffers, support media, separation techniques, stains, and detection methods.
4. Identify the individual protein fractions of serum from an electropherogram.
5. Quantify the individual fractions of a scanned gel when given the total protein value.
6. Identify how each of the following affects electrophoresis: size and shape of molecule, heat and current produced by the power supply, buffer pH, and type of gel used.
7. Describe and compare the following types of electrophoretic techniques, including clinical utility, system components, and detection methods: (1) capillary, (2) isoelectric focusing, (3) microchip, (4) two-dimensional, and (5) zone.
8. Compare and contrast Southern, Northern, and Western blotting, including analyte, electrophoresis technique, and clinical utility.
9. State three advantages of capillary electrophoresis over conventional electrophoresis.
10. Explain how the following affect the performance of electrophoresis: endosmosis, buffer and stain integrity, sample type or appearance, and over-application or under-application of the sample.

## KEY WORDS AND DEFINITIONS

**Ampholyte**  A molecule that is positively or negatively charged on the basis of the pH of the solution in which it resides; proteins, because they contain many ionizable amino and carboxyl groups, behave as ampholytes in solution and are considered amphoteric.

**Capillary electrophoresis**  A method in which the classic techniques of electrophoresis are carried out in a small-bore, fused silica capillary tube coated with a polymeric covering.

**Densitometry**  A measuring technique that uses an optical system to scan and quantify electrophoretic fractions separated on a gel or other medium.

**Electropherogram**  A densitometric display of protein zones on a support material after separation and staining.

**Electrophoresis**  The migration of charged solutes or particles within a liquid medium under the influence of an electrical field.

**Electrophoretic mobility ($\mu$)**  The rate of migration (cm/s) of a charged solute in an electrical field, expressed per unit field strength (volts/cm).

**Endosmosis (electroendosmotic flow)**  Preferential movement of water in one direction through an electrophoresis medium due to selective binding of one type of charge on the surface of the medium.

**Isoelectric focusing**  An electrophoretic technique that separates amphoteric compounds within a medium that possesses a stable pH gradient.

**Isoelectric point (pI)**  The pH at which a molecule has no net charge and will not migrate during electrophoresis.

**Wick flow**  Movement of water from the buffer reservoirs toward the center of an electrophoresis gel or strip to replace water lost by evaporation.

**Zone electrophoresis**  Migration of charged molecules in an applied electric field.

## BASIC CONCEPTS

The first **electrophoresis** method used to study proteins was the free solution or moving boundary method devised by Tiseus in 1937. This technique was used in research to measure electrophoretic mobility and to study protein-protein interactions. It was able to resolve the serum proteins into only four component mixtures, with the $\alpha_1$ fraction incompletely separated from albumin.

Zone electrophoresis can be performed in a porous supporting medium, such as agarose gel film, such that each protein zone is sharply separated from neighboring zones by a protein-free area. Zones are visualized by staining with a protein-specific stain to produce an **electropherogram**, which is then scanned and quantified using a densitometer. The support medium can also be handled after drying and kept as a permanent record. This is the most commonly applied technique in clinical chemistry and is used to separate proteins in serum, urine, cerebrospinal fluid (CSF), and other physiologic fluids. Cellular proteins and nucleic acids can also be separated by electrophoresis after cell lysis.

Although electrophoretic separation of biologically relevant macromolecules in gels (or paper) has been the workhorse of modern biomedical research, the advent of **capillary electrophoresis** (CE) has revolutionized separations. Intense interest in carrying out electrophoretic separation in capillaries with inner diameters ranging from 20 to 75 μm has resulted from its unprecedented resolving power, separation speed, and small sample analysis capabilities. In addition to protein and polynucleic acid separations, CE can resolve a wide spectrum of analytes, including peptides, small drug-like molecules, and even ions.

---

**POINTS TO REMEMBER**

**Electrophoresis**
- Refers to the migration of ions in an electrical field
- Separation occurs based on the inherent electrophoretic mobility of an analyte
- Electrophoretic mobility is directly proportional to the net charge and inversely proportional to the size of the molecule and the viscosity of the electrophoresis medium

---

## THEORY OF ELECTROPHORESIS

Depending on the charge they carry, ionized solutes move toward either the cathode (negative electrode) or the anode (positive electrode) in an electrophoresis system. For example, positive ions (cations) migrate to the cathode, and negative ions (anions) to the anode. An **ampholyte** (a molecule that is either positively or negatively charged, formerly called a zwitterion) becomes positively charged in a solution that is more acidic than its **isoelectric point (pI)** and migrates toward the cathode. In a more alkaline solution, the ampholyte becomes negatively charged and migrates toward the anode. Because proteins contain many ionizable amino ($-NH_2$) and carboxyl ($-COOH$) groups, and because the bases in nucleic acids may also be positively or negatively charged, they both behave as ampholytes in solution.

The rate of migration of ions in an electrical field depends on the factors listed in Box 11.1. The equation expressing the driving force in such a system is given by:

$$F = (X)(Q) = \frac{(E)(Q)}{d} \qquad \textbf{(11.1)}$$

---

**BOX 11.1   Factors Affecting the Motility of Ions in an Electrophoretic System**

Net charge of the molecules
Size and shape of the molecules
Strength of the electrical field
Support medium properties
Ionic strength of the buffer
Temperature

---

where $F$ = the force exerted on an ion; $X$ = the current field strength (V/cm) (i.e., voltage drop per unit length of medium); $Q$ = the net charge on the ion; EMF = the electromotive force (voltage [V] applied); and $d$ = the length of the electrophoretic medium (cm).

Steady acceleration of the migrating ion is counteracted by a resisting force characteristic of the solution in which migration occurs. This force, expressed by Stokes' law, is:

$$F' = 6\pi r \eta v \qquad \textbf{(11.2)}$$

where $F'$ = the counter force; $\pi = 3.1416$; $r$ = the ionic radius of the solute; $\eta$ = the viscosity of the buffer solution in which migration is occurring; and $v$ = the rate of migration of the solute = velocity (length $[l]$ traveled per unit of time [cm/s]).

The force $F'$ counteracts the acceleration that would be produced by $F$ if no counter force were present, and the result of the two forces is a constant velocity. Therefore, when:

$$F = F' \qquad \textbf{(11.3)}$$

then:

$$6\pi r \eta v = (X)(Q) \qquad \textbf{(11.4)}$$

or:

$$v/X = l \times d/t \times E = Q/6\pi r \eta = \mu \qquad \textbf{(11.5)}$$

where $v/X$ is the rate of migration (cm/s) per unit field strength ($E$/cm), defined as the **electrophoretic mobility** and expressed by the symbol $\mu$.

Electrophoretic mobility is directly proportional to the net charge and is inversely proportional to the size of the molecule and the viscosity of the electrophoresis medium. Mobility may be positive or negative, depending on whether a protein migrates in the same or the opposite direction as the electrophoretic field (defined as extending from the anode to the cathode).

In addition to the factors listed in Box 11.1, other factors that affect electrophoretic mobility include electroendosmosis (endosmosis) and wick flow. Electroendosmosis affects mobility by causing uneven movement of water through the support medium. An electrophoretic support medium, such as a gel in contact with water, takes on a negative charge caused by the adsorption of hydroxyl ions. These ions are fixed to the surface and are immobile. Positive ions in solution cluster about the fixed negative charge sites, forming an ionic cloud of mostly positive ions. The number of negative ions in the solution increases with increasing distance from

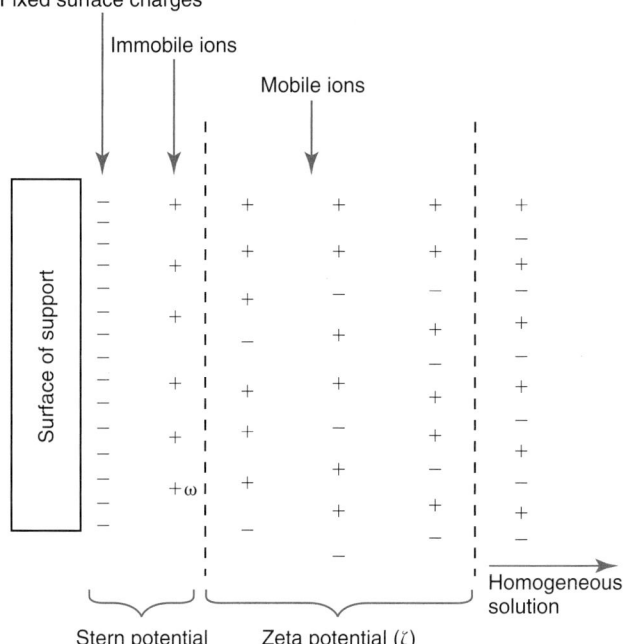

**Fig. 11.1** Distribution of + and − ions around the surface of an electrophoretic support. Fixed on the surface of the solid is a layer of − ions. A second layer of + ions is attracted to the surface. These two layers compose the Stern potential. The large, diffuse layer containing mostly + ions is the electrokinetic or zeta potential. Extending farther from the surface of the solid is homogeneous solution. The Stern potential plus the zeta potential equals the electrochemical potential, or epsilon potential.

the fixed negative charge sites until eventually positive and negative ions are present in equal concentrations (Fig. 11.1).

When current is applied to such a system, charges attached to the immobile support remain fixed, but the cloud of ions in solution moves to the electrode of opposite polarity. Because ions in solution are highly hydrated, this results in movement of the solvent as well. Movement of solvent and its solutes relative to the fixed support is referred to as **endosmosis** and causes preferential movement of water in one direction. Macromolecules in solution that move in the direction opposite to this flow may remain immobile or may even be swept back toward the opposite pole if they are insufficiently charged. In media in which endosmosis is strong, such as conventional cellulose acetate and unpurified agarose gel, γ-globulins are swept back from the application point. Because the inner surface of a glass capillary contains many such charged groups, endosmosis is very strong and is actually the primary driving force for migration in CE systems. However, the endosmosis in CE can be manipulated to modify the magnitude of the endosmotic effect. In electrophoretic media in which surface charges are minimal (starch gel, purified agarose gel, or polyacrylamide gel), endosmosis is minimal.

**Wick flow** results from the movement of buffer into the support medium. During electrophoresis, heat evolved because of the passage of current through a resistive medium can cause evaporation of solvent from the electrophoretic support. This drying effect draws buffer into the support, and, if significant, the flow of buffer can affect protein migration and hence the calculated mobility.

## CLINICAL ELECTROPHORESIS

In this section, focus will be on the electrophoresis methodology that is frequently used in the clinical laboratory. Refer to Chapter 18 for a thorough discussion on the various electrophoretic fractions present in clinical protein electrophoresis.

### Slab Gel Electrophoresis

Traditional methods, using a rectangular gel regardless of thickness, are referred to collectively by the term *slab gel electrophoresis*. Its main advantage is its ability to simultaneously separate several samples in one run. Starch, agarose, and polyacrylamide media have all been used in this format. It is the primary method used in clinical chemistry laboratories for the separation of various classes of serum or CSF proteins and deoxyribonucleic acid (DNA) and ribonucleic acid (RNA) fragments. Gels (usually agarose) may be cast on a sheet of plastic backing or completely encased within a plastic-walled cell, which allows horizontal or vertical electrophoresis and submersion for cooling, if necessary.

### General Operations

General operations performed in conventional electrophoresis include separation, detection, and quantification, as well as a number of "blotting" techniques.

#### Electrophoretic Separation

When electrophoresis is performed on precast microzone agarose gels, the following steps are typical: (1) excess buffer is removed from the support surface by blotting, taking care that bubbles are not present; (2) 5 to 7 μL of sample is applied using a comb or a plastic template and is allowed to diffuse into the gel; it is then blotted to remove the excess; (3) the gel is placed into the electrode chamber; (4) electrophoresis is performed at specified current, voltage, or power; (5) the gel is fixed, rinsed, and then dried; (6) the gel is stained and redried; and (7) the gel is scanned in a densitometer. If isoenzymes are to be determined, substrate dye solution is incubated on the gel to stain zones before fixing and drying. Alternative procedures can be used with the more sophisticated methods described later.

#### Detection

Once separated, proteins may be detected by staining followed by quantification using a densitometer, or by direct measurement using an optical detection system.

*Staining.* If staining is used to visualize separated proteins, the proteins usually are fixed first by precipitating them in the gel with a chemical agent such as acetic acid or methanol. This prevents diffusion of proteins out of the gel when submersed in the stain solution. The amount of dye taken up

**TABLE 11.1    Suggested Wavelengths for Quantitation of Protein Zones by Direct Densitometry**

| Separation Type | Stain | Nominal Wavelength (nm) |
|---|---|---|
| Serum proteins in general | Amido Black (Naphthol Blue Black) | 640 |
| | Coomassie Brilliant Blue G–250 (Brilliant Blue G) | 595 |
| | Coomassie Brilliant Blue R–250 (Brilliant Blue R) | 560 |
| | Ponceau S | 520 |
| Isoenzymes | Nitrotetrazolium Blue | 570 |
| Lipoprotein zones | Fat Red 7B (Sudan Red 7B) | 540 |
| | Oil Red O | 520 |
| | Sudan Black B | 600 |
| DNA fragments | Ethidium bromide (fluorescent) | 254 (Ex) |
| | | 590 (Em) |
| CSF proteins | Silver nitrate | — |

*CSF*, Cerebrospinal fluid; *DNA*, deoxyribonucleic acid; *Em*, emission; *Ex*, excitation.

by the sample is affected by many factors, such as the type of protein and the degree of denaturation of the proteins by fixing agents.

Table 11.1 lists dyes commonly used in electrophoresis, along with suggested wavelengths for quantification by **densitometry**. Most commercial methods for serum protein electrophoresis use Amido Black B or members of the Coomassie Brilliant Blue series of dyes for staining. Isoenzymes are typically visualized by incubating the gel in contact with a solution of substrate, which is linked structurally or chemically to a dye before fixing. Silver nitrate stains proteins and polypeptides with a sensitivity 10- to 100-fold greater than that of conventional dyes. Selective fixing and staining of protein subclasses can also be achieved by combining a stain molecule with an antiglobulin, as is done in immunofixation electrophoresis (IFE).

Sensitivity can be enhanced by linking an enzyme, such as alkaline phosphatase or peroxidase, to an antibody specific for particular proteins, such as oligoclonal immunoglobulin (Ig), or by spraying separated proteins with luminol and peroxide to develop chemiluminescence, which, in turn, exposes x-ray film to form a permanent image. Chemiluminescence has been used in this way to quantify IgE, and DNA fragments have been detected by linking with a fluorescent dye label.

In practice, a typical stain solution may be used several times before it is replaced. A good rule of thumb is that a stain solution of 100 mL may be used for a combined total of 387 cm² (60 in²) of agarose film. The stain solution may be considered faulty if leaching of stained protein zones occurs in the 5% acetic acid wash solution. Whenever protein zones appear too lightly stained, the stain or substrate reagent—in the case of isoenzymes—should always be suspected. Stain solution must be stored tightly covered to prevent evaporation.

*Quantification.* A densitometer is used to quantify stained zones. This instrument measures the absorbance of each fraction as the gel (or other medium) is moved past a photometric optical system and displays an electropherogram on a computer display. The software is able to automatically integrate the area under each peak and report each as a percent of total

or as absolute concentration or activity computed from the total protein or activity of enzyme in the sample.

Reliable densitometric quantification requires: (1) light of an appropriate wavelength; (2) linear response from the instrument; and (3) a transparent background in the medium being scanned. Linearity may be tested with a neutral density filter designed with separated or adjacent areas of linearly increasing density. The densities are permanent and have expected absorbance values. The very small sample sizes used and the transparency of agarose gels satisfy the requirement for a clear background. Nevertheless, problems can occur with densitometry because of differences in the quantity of stain taken up by individual proteins and differences in protein zone sizes.

Essential features of a densitometer include: (1) the ability to scan gels 25 to 100 mm in length; (2) electronic adjustment of the most intense peak to full scale; (3) automatic background zeroing (peaks are not lost or "cut off"); (4) variable wavelength control over the range of 400 to 700 nm; (5) variable slits to allow adjustment of the beam size; (6) an integrating device with both automatic and manual selection of cut points between peaks; and (7) automatic indexing, a feature that advances the electrophoresis strip from one sample channel to the next.

Desirable features of a densitometer include computerized integration and printout, built-in diagnostics for instrument troubleshooting, the choice of one of several scanning speeds, and the ability to measure in the reflectance mode. Models with a separate computer for data processing permit storage and reformatting of data, if desired, and reprinting or delayed transmission to a host computer.

DNA analysis requires the ability to scan larger gels, which may contain several dozen bands of DNA fragments of different length. Modern automated electrophoresis systems also use larger gels containing 30 or more samples, which are scanned on a new generation of densitometers referred to as *flatbed scanners* or *digital image analyzers*. These instruments are capable of scanning and storing digitized light intensity readings from large areas and use ultrasensitive charge-coupled device detectors having a resolution of up to 1200

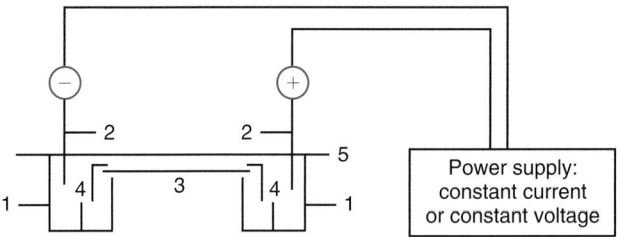

**Fig. 11.2** A schematic diagram of a typical electrophoresis apparatus showing two buffer boxes with: *(1)* baffle plates, *(2)* electrodes, *(3)* electrophoretic support, *(4)* wicks, *(5)* cover, and power supply.

dots per inch (21 μm). Sophisticated data processing software permits manipulation of stored image information to produce conventional scans and computations or more complex outputs, such as overlaying and subtraction of patterns from two different samples.

### Blotting Techniques

In 1975, Edward Southern developed a technique that is widely used to detect fragments of DNA. This technique, known as *Southern blotting*, first requires electrophoretic separation of DNA or DNA fragments by agarose gel electrophoresis (AGE). Next, a strip of nitrocellulose or a nylon membrane is laid over the agarose gel, and the DNA fragments are transferred or "blotted" onto it by capillary, electro, or vacuum blotting. They are then detected and identified by hybridization with a labeled, complementary nucleic acid probe. This technique is widely used in molecular biology for identifying a particular DNA sequence; determining the presence, position, and number of copies of a gene in a genome; and typing DNA.

*Northern* and *Western* blotting techniques, named by analogy to Southern blotting, were subsequently developed to separate and detect RNAs and proteins, respectively. Northern blotting is carried out identically to Southern blotting except that RNA species are separated by electrophoresis. Western blotting is used to separate, detect, and identify one or more proteins in a complex mixture. It involves first separating the individual proteins on a polyacrylamide gel and then transferring or "blotting" onto an overlying strip of nitrocellulose or a nylon membrane by electro-blotting. The strip or membrane is then reacted with a reagent that contains an antibody raised against the protein of interest.

### Instrumentation

Although modern electrophoresis equipment and systems vary considerably in form and degree of automation, the essential components common to all systems (Fig. 11.2) include: (1) two reservoirs that contain the buffer used in the process, (2) a means of delivering current from a power supply via platinum or carbon electrodes contacting the buffer, and (3) a support medium in which separation takes place connecting the two reservoirs. In some systems, wicks may connect the medium to the buffer solution or directly to the electrodes. The entire apparatus is enclosed to minimize evaporation and protect both the system and the operator.

The direct current power supply sets the polarity of the electrodes and delivers current to the medium.

### Power Supplies

The power supply drives the movement of ionic species in the medium and allows adjustment and control of the current or the voltage. With more sophisticated units, the power may be controlled as well, and conditions may be programmed to change during electrophoresis. Capillary systems use power supplies capable of providing voltages in the kilovolt range.

Current flowing through a medium that has resistance produces heat:

$$\text{Heat} = (E)(I)(t) \tag{11.6}$$

where $E$ = electromotive force (EMF) in volts (V); $I$ = current in amperes (A); and $t$ = time in seconds (s).

This heat is released into the medium and increases the thermal agitation of all dissolved ions, and therefore the conductance of the system (decreases resistance). With constant-voltage power supplies, the resultant rise in current increases both protein migration and evaporation of water from the medium. Any water loss increases the ion concentration and further decreases the resistance *(R)*. Under these circumstances, the current and therefore the migration rate will progressively increase. To minimize these effects, it is best to use a constant-current power supply. According to Ohm's law:

$$E = (I)(R) \tag{11.7}$$

Therefore, if $R$ decreases, the applied EMF also decreases, keeping the current constant. This in turn decreases the heat effect and stabilizes the migration rate.

### Buffers

Buffer ions have a twofold purpose in electrophoresis: they carry the applied current, and they fix the pH at which electrophoresis is carried out. Thus, they determine: (1) the type of electrical charge on the solute, (2) the extent of ionization of the solute, and therefore, (3) the electrode toward which the solute will migrate. The buffer's ionic strength determines the thickness of the ionic cloud (buffer and non-buffer ions) surrounding a charged molecule, the rate of its migration, and the sharpness of the electrophoretic zones. With increasing concentration of ions, the ionic cloud increases in size, and the molecule becomes more hindered in its movement.

According to Joule's law, power produced when current flows through a resistive medium is dissipated as heat. This heat increases in direct proportion to the resistance, but also in proportion to the square of the current. The reduction in resistance caused by a high ionic strength buffer therefore leads to increased current and excessive heat. These buffers yield sharper band separations, but the benefits of sharper resolution are diminished by the Joule (heat) effect that leads to denaturation of heat-labile proteins or the degradation of other components.

Ionic strength (also denoted by the symbol $\mu$) is computed according to the following:

$$\mu = 0.5 \sum c_i z_i^2 \qquad \text{(11.8)}$$

where $c_i$ = ion concentration in mol/L and $z_i$ = the charge on the ion.

The ionic strength $\mu$ of an electrolyte (buffer) composed of monovalent ions is equal to its molarity (mol/L). The ionic strength of a 1 mol/L electrolyte solution with one monovalent and one divalent ion is 3 mol/L, and for a doubly divalent electrolyte, it is 4 mol/L.

A relatively high ionic strength buffer used in *high-resolution electrophoresis* improves the separation of serum proteins into as many as 13 bands, with 2 or more bands in the $\alpha_1$, $\alpha_2$, and $\beta$-globulin regions and one or more additional bands seen in various pathologic conditions. Because of higher conductivity and the associated heat produced, it is necessary to reduce the temperature of the system to 10°C to 14°C. "Submarine" techniques, in which gels are submersed in circulating buffer cooled by an external cooling device, or are supported on an electrophoresis chamber cooled by circulating water or an integral Peltier plate, provide exact temperature control. Effective cooling with less precise temperature control may also be achieved using chambers designed with a sealed compartment of cooled ethylene glycol, which is in contact with the gel during running.

Because buffers used in electrophoresis are good culture media for the growth of microorganisms, they should be refrigerated when not in use. Moreover, a cold buffer is preferred in an electrophoretic run because it improves resolution and decreases evaporation from the electrophoretic support. Buffer used in a small-volume apparatus should be discarded after each run because of pH changes resulting from the electrolysis of water that accompany electrophoresis. If volumes used are larger than 100 mL, buffer from both reservoirs may be combined, mixed, and reused up to four times.

## Support Media

The support medium provides the matrix in which protein separation takes place. Various types of support media have been used in electrophoresis and range from pure buffer solutions in a capillary to insoluble gels (e.g., sheets, slabs, or columns of starch, agarose, or polyacrylamide) or membranes of cellulose acetate. Gels are cast in a solution of the same buffer to be used in the procedure and may electrophorese in a horizontal or vertical direction. In either case, maximum resolution is achieved if the sample is applied in a very fine starting zone. Separation is based on differences in charge-to-mass ratio of the proteins and, depending on the pore size of the medium, possibly molecular size.

***Cellulose acetate.*** Cellulose acetate, a thermoplastic resin made by treating cellulose with acetic anhydride to acetylate the hydroxyl groups, is primarily of historical interest. When dry, the membranes contain about 80% air space within the interlocking cellulose acetate fibers tend are opaque, brittle films. As the film is soaked in buffer, the air spaces fill with

liquid, and it becomes pliable. Samples are applied with a twin-wire applicator or the edge of a glass slide. Because of their opacity, stained membranes need to be made transparent (cleared) for densitometry by soaking in 95:5 methanol:glacial acetic acid. Cleared membranes are strong and could be stored as a permanent record, but because of the necessity for presoaking and clearing, cellulose acetate has largely been replaced by agarose in most clinical applications.

***Agarose.*** Agarose is a linear polymer containing alternating D-galactose and 3,6-anhydro-L-galactose monomers. It is the purified, essentially neutral fraction of agar obtained by separating agarose from agaropectin, a more highly charged fraction containing acidic sulfate and carboxylic side groups. Because the pore size in agarose gels is large enough for all proteins to pass through unimpeded, separation is based only on the charge-to-mass ratio of the protein. Advantages of agarose gel include its low affinity for proteins and its native clarity after drying, which permits excellent densitometry. It is essentially free of ionizable groups and so exhibits little endosmosis.

Most routine procedures for AGE are now performed using commercially produced, prepackaged microzone gels, and the sample is applied by means of a comb or a thin plastic template, with small slots corresponding to sample application points. The template is placed on the agarose surface, and 5 to 7 μL samples are placed on each slot. The serum sample is allowed to diffuse into the agarose for 5 minutes, the excess sample is removed by blotting, and the template is removed. AGE separation for most routine serum applications requires an electrophoresis time of 20 to 30 minutes.

***Polyacrylamide gel.*** Polyacrylamide is a polymeric matrix consisting of linear chains of acrylamide cross-linked with bis-acrylamide. It is thermostable, transparent, strong, and relatively chemically inert, and—depending on concentration—can be made in a wide range of pore sizes. Its average pore size in a typical 7.5% gel is about 5 nm (50 Å), which is large enough to allow most serum proteins to migrate unimpeded. However, proteins with a molecular radius and/or length that exceeds critical limits will be impeded in their migration. Some of these proteins are fibrinogen, $\beta$-lipoprotein, $\alpha_2$-macroglobulin, and $\gamma$-globulins; a schematic representation of serum protein electrophoresis by polyacrylamide gel electrophoresis (PAGE) is shown in Fig. 11.3. The separation is based on both charge-to-mass ratio

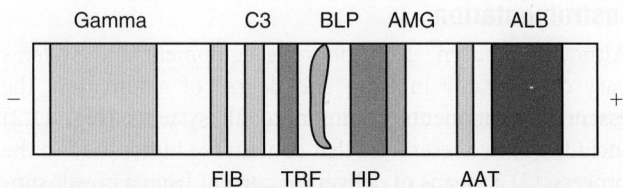

**Fig. 11.3** A simplified schematic drawing of a protein pattern from the serum of a subject with haptoglobin type 2-1 (separation by polyacrylamide gel electrophoresis). Some zones contain more than the one protein shown, as demonstrated by immunologic techniques. *AAT,* $\alpha_1$-Antitrypsin; *ALB,* albumin; *AMG,* $\alpha_2$-macroglobulin; *BLP,* $\beta$-lipoprotein; *C3,* complement 3; *FIB,* fibrinogen; *Gamma,* $\gamma$-globulin; *HP,* haptoglobin; *TRF,* transferrin.

and molecular size (a phenomenon referred to as *molecular sieving*), and serum proteins can be resolved into more individual fractions than with an agarose gel. Furthermore, these gels are uncharged, thus eliminating electroendosmosis. Precast minigels are available in a variety of concentrations and acrylamide-to-bis-acrylamide ratios suitable for most protein or nucleic acid separations. However, because of the known neurotoxicity of acrylamide, appropriate caution must be exercised when handling this material if the gels are prepared by hand.

Attempts to improve the hydrophilic nature of polyacrylamide have led to the development of mono- and di-substituted monomers, one of which is *N*-acryloyl-tris(hydroxymethyl) aminomethane, or Poly(NAT). This material is more hydrophilic than polyacrylamide, and its matrix has larger pores, thereby presenting less resistance to the passage of large molecules. It is ideally suited to the separation of DNA fragments up to 20 kilobases (kb) in size using a homogeneous (nonpulsed) electric field. Fragments that differ in size by as little as 2% can be resolved. Gels are submersed in buffer during use, allowing temperatures to be tightly controlled at values between 50°C and 60°C. Use of increased temperatures results in shorter run times and more reproducible band migration.

### Automated Systems

Because of increased volume of testing, primarily for serum proteins, many laboratories are converting to automated systems for electrophoresis. Such a system is the Helena SPIFE 4000 (Helena Laboratories, Beaumont, TX), an automated electrophoresis system providing automated reagent application and a variety of gel sizes that permit analysis of 10 to 100 samples simultaneously. It also features in-line sample application, automated electrophoretic separation and staining of analytes, multiple stain ports, and positive sample identification. The Interlab Microgel system (Interlab Srl, Rome, Italy) also fully automates the process and integrates sample application, temperature-controlled electrophoresis, staining, and densitometry into a single unit with the capability of managing four gels simultaneously. Other systems that have partially automated the procedure or incorporated the ability to process sequentially multiple gels of different compositions include the Phast System (Pharmacia LKB, Gaithersburg, MD), the HITE Fractoscan (Olympus, Invicon, München, Germany), the Hydragel-Hydrasys (Sebia Inc., Durham, NC), and the High-Performance Gel Electrophoresis (HPGE)-1000 system (LabIntelligence Inc., Belmont, CA). Most CE systems (see "Capillary Electrophoresis" section) have autosampling capability for sequentially processing specimens, but the Sebia CAPILLARYS permits simultaneous processing of seven samples by using multiple capillaries. Truly microfluidic-based analyzers, like the Agilent 2100 Bioanalyzer (Agilent Technologies Inc., Santa Clara, CA), significantly miniaturize the fluidics and increase the speed of the process for separating proteins, nucleic acids, or even entire cells. These advances substantially reduce the labor component associated with electrophoresis.

## CAPILLARY ELECTROPHORESIS

With CE, classic techniques are carried out in a small-bore (10- to 100-μm internal diameter) fused silica capillary tube, 20 to 200 cm in length.

Two distinct advantages of the capillary format include the ability to apply much higher voltages than in traditional electrophoresis and the ease of automation. Applications are also more extensive and include the separation of low molecular weight ions in addition to proteins and other macromolecules. Even uncharged molecules can be separated using CE in the micellar electrokinetic chromatography (MEKC) mode discussed later. CE has also proved useful for separation of inorganic ions, amino acids, organic acids, drugs, vitamins, porphyrins, carbohydrates, oligonucleotides, proteins, and DNA fragments.

### General Operations

A schematic diagram of a typical instrumental configuration for CE is shown in Fig. 11.4. As indicated, the capillary serves as an electrophoretic chamber, analogous to a lane on a gel, which is connected to buffer reservoirs at both ends, which, in turn, are connected to a high-voltage power supply. It is important to note that at some point along the length of the capillary (typically close to the end), a detector is interfaced for online detection. Improved heat dissipation from the capillary (as opposed to a slab gel) permits the application of voltages in the range of 10 to 30 kV, which enhances separation efficiency and reduces separation time—in some cases to less than 1 minute. Only a few microliters of the sample are required, with injected volumes in the nanoliter range. The small sample plug volume minimizes distortions in the applied field caused by the presence of analytes or other sample species.

In contrast to the cumbersome and time-consuming tasks of conventional electrophoresis, CE is easily automated. Analogous to high-performance liquid chromatography (HPLC) technology, samples typically are stored in a temperature-controlled environment and are automatically injected into the capillary, with a variety of detector types

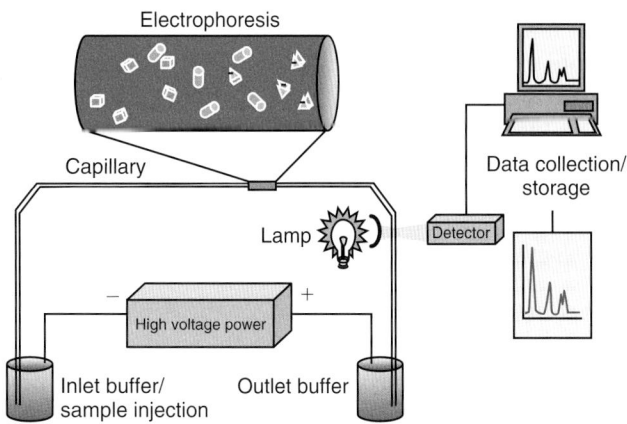

**Fig. 11.4** A schematic for capillary electrophoresis instrumentation.

available; the resulting electropherograms are analyzed and manipulated in much the same manner as chromatograms.

The capillaries used as separation columns in CE are most commonly made from fused silica (i.e., pure glass) coated with a thin exterior covering of polyimide to provide strength and flexibility. Although capillaries can be made from other materials, such as polyethylene or Teflon, such capillaries have seen limited use. The polyimide coating is usually removed from a small portion of the capillary close to the terminal end, creating a window for online optical detection. The outer diameter of the capillary tubing typically varies from 180 to 375 μm, the inner diameter from 20 to 180 μm, and the total length from 20 cm up to several meters. Noncylindrical capillary tubing suitable for CE is now available from some commercial providers. For example, rectangular capillaries (Polymicro Technologies, Phoenix, AZ) provide a flat surface that is more amenable to optical detection than that of their curved counterparts.

CE is distinguished from other forms of electrophoresis by the fact that extraordinarily high voltage (30,000 V) can be used to obtain rapid, high-efficiency separations. The problems encountered with noncapillary platforms (e.g., slab gels) are avoided because of the effective dissipation of Joule heat by forced air convection or liquid cooling of the narrow-bore capillary.

## Sample Injection

In CE, sample volumes of 1 to 50 nL are loaded into the capillary by hydrodynamic injection or electrokinetic (EK) injection. With hydrodynamic injection, an aliquot of a sample is introduced by applying positive pressure at the inlet vial or vacuum at the outlet vial. The volume of sample loaded is governed by a number of parameters, including (but not restricted to): (1) the inner diameter of the capillary; (2) buffer viscosity; (3) applied pressure; (4) temperature; and (5) time. With some earlier commercial or homemade systems, gravity was used as the source of pressure by raising the inlet vial (or lowering the outlet vial), thus allowing "siphoning" to occur for a timed interval. With EK injection, an aliquot of a sample is introduced by applying a voltage for a timed interval. The magnitude of the voltage is dependent on the analyte and buffer system used but typically involves field strengths three to five times lower than that used for separation. It is important to note that although hydrodynamic methods introduce a sample representative of the bulk specimen, EK injection favors the preferential movement of more electrokinetically mobile analytes into the capillary.

In practice, to maintain high separation efficiency, the sample plug length is usually less than 2% of the total capillary length.

## Direct Detection

With CE, separated analytes are detected and measured as they migrate past a point on the capillary that is optically interrogated. Optical detection is based on classical methods, such as photometric absorbance, refractive index, and fluorescence

(see Chapter 9). As with HPLC, ultraviolet-visible photometers are widely used as detectors to monitor CE separations. To interface such online detectors with the capillary, a detection window is created toward the outlet end of the capillary. This "window," which serves as an inline cuvette, typically is formed by burning off the polyimide with a small flame and cleaning the window with ethanol. Although this configuration allows high-efficiency separation, the inner diameter of the capillary tube defines the optical path length (OPL) of the inline cuvette. Because absorbance is directly proportional to the length of the cuvette used in an optical system, the 20 to 100 μm inner diameter of the capillary limits UV-visible absorbance detection limits to concentrations of $10^{-8}$ to $10^{-6}$ molar.

More sensitive optical techniques that have been used with CE include: (1) fluorescence, (2) refractive index, (3) chemiluminescence, (4) Raman spectrophotometry, and (5) circular dichroism. The most sensitive optical detection method used in CE is laser-induced fluorescence, which is capable of detection limits in the $10^{-9}$ to $10^{-12}$ molar (or better) range. This detection mode is easily accomplished with analytes that may be easily labeled with a fluorescent substrate (e.g., intercalators for double-stranded DNA) or may be naturally fluorescent (e.g., proteins or peptides containing tryptophan). CE systems have also been interfaced with mass spectrometers, and electrochemical detection methods have been developed, although such detectors must be isolated electrically from the electrophoretic voltages.

## Indirect Detection

When strong chromophores are lacking in the analyte of interest, absorbance and fluorescence detection have been used in an indirect mode. In this mode, a strongly absorbing ion is added to the running electrolyte and is monitored at a wavelength that gives a constant, high background absorbance. As solute ions move into their discrete zones during the electrophoretic process, they displace the indirect detection agent through mutual repulsion, and this produces a decrease in background absorbance as the zone passes through the detector. Reagents with appropriate fluorescence properties have been used in a similar manner. Indirect detection of amino acids by CE has been demonstrated, with the potential for use in the diagnosis of amino acidurias. Investigators have demonstrated the direct extrapolation of this technique to microchip detection when ultraviolet (UV) detection is difficult, if not impossible.

## Online Sample Concentration

Another technique used in CE systems to increase their limit of detection is preconcentration of the sample. One of the simplest methods for sample preconcentration is to induce a "stacking" effect with the sample components, which is easily accomplished by exploiting the ionic strength differences between the sample matrix and the separation buffer. This results from the fact that sample ions have decreased electrophoretic mobility in a higher conductivity environment. When voltage is applied to the system, sample ions in the sample plug instantaneously accelerate toward the adjacent separation buffer zone. Upon crossing the boundary, the higher conductivity environment induces a decrease in electrophoretic velocity and subsequent "stacking" of the sample components into a smaller buffer zone than the original sample plug. Within a short time, the ionic strength gradient dissipates and the charged analyte molecules begin to move from the "stacked" sample zone toward the cathode. Stacking has been used with hydrostatic or EK injection and typically yields a tenfold enhancement in sample concentration, resulting in a lower limit of detection.

An alternative approach to stacking is "focusing," which is based on pH differences between the sample plug and the separation buffer. This is very useful for the analysis of peptides, mainly because of their relative stability over a wide pH range. By increasing the pH of the sample to above that of the net pI of the analytes of interest and flanking the sample plug with low pH separation buffer zones (i.e., an equivalent volume of low pH separation buffer following introduction of the sample plug), negatively charged peptides are electrophoretically driven toward the anode. Upon entering the lower pH separation buffer, a pH-induced change in their charge state causes a reversal in their electrophoretic mobility, resulting in "focusing" of the peptides at the interface of the sample (high pH) and low pH buffer plugs (similar to those in isoelectric focusing). After the pH gradient dissipates, the peptides, again positively charged, migrate toward the cathode as a sharp zone. This approach has been applied to a variety of analytes, but it is limited to those that are able to withstand inherent changes in pH without substantial denaturation, and may yield as much as a fivefold enhancement of a system's limit of detection.

## TYPES OF ELECTROPHORESIS

### Capillary Zone Electrophoresis

CZE, also called *open-tube* or *free-solution* CE, is the simplest form of CE. It includes *capillary ion electrophoresis*, which refers to the analysis of inorganic ions by CZE, often using indirect detection. The power of the CZE mode is its ability to electrophoretically resolve charged species without a sieving matrix; this applies to a broad spectrum of analytes ranging from proteins, peptides, and amino acids to small molecules (e.g., drugs) and ions.

### Capillary Gel Electrophoresis

Capillary gel electrophoresis (CGE) is directly comparable with traditional slab or tube gel electrophoresis because the separation mechanisms are identical. Size separation is achieved with a suitable polymer, which acts as a molecular sieve or sizing mechanism. As charged analytes migrate through the polymer network, they become hindered to a degree that is governed by their size (larger molecules are hindered more than smaller ones). Macromolecules, such as DNA and sodium dodecyl sulfate (SDS)-saturated proteins,

cannot be separated without a gel or some other separation mechanism, because they have a mass-to-charge ratio that is size independent. The term *gel* in CGE is a misnomer, primarily because cross-linked "gels," as we know them in slab format, are not routinely used in CE. A more suitable term is a *sieving matrix* or *soluble polymer network*, a linear polymeric structure that is soluble, has reasonably low viscosity, and is capable of self-entangling in a manner that forms pores through which sieving can occur. A variety of polymeric matrices have been defined for DNA (e.g., polyacrylamide, cellulosic materials) and protein analysis (e.g., dextran-base matrices), provided that pores can be formed inherently that have diameters in the range of tens to hundreds of nanometers. One of the requirements that often accompany this type of analysis is reduction of electroosmotic flow. This is accomplished by covalently, adsorptively, or dynamically coating the surface. Cross-linked polyacrylamide was the main polymer of choice for this but recently has been supplanted by a host of polymeric matrices that not only provide effective molecular sieving but also adsorptively coat the capillary surface.

### Gel Technical Considerations

In performing electrophoretic separations, a number of technical and practical aspects need to be considered, as they affect the process.

### Sampling

To achieve a proper balance between sensitive measurements and resolution, the amount of serum protein applied to an electrophoretic support must be optimum. Albumin is about 10 times more concentrated in serum than the smallest fraction, the $\alpha_1$-globulins. Therefore, the amount of serum applied should prevent overloading with albumin but should still be adequate to quantify $\alpha_1$-globulin. For the separation of serum proteins using PAGE, 3 μL of serum containing approximately 210 μg of total protein is applied. For alkaline phosphatase isoenzymes, up to 25 μL of a normal serum may be applied (less may be used if activity is greatly increased). Urine specimens require 50- to 100-fold greater concentrations or extended application times for adequate sensitivity, and CSF may or may not require concentration, depending on the staining approach used.

### Unequal Migration Rates

Unequal migration of samples across the width of the gel may be caused by dirty electrodes, which may cause uneven application of the electric field, or by uneven wetting of the gel. If wicks are used to connect the gel to a power supply, uneven wetting of the wicks could cause unequal migration or bowing of sample lanes at the gel edges. Gels must be kept horizontal during storage to avoid sagging and uneven thickness. Finally, gels that may have been stored too close to heat sources (e.g., in a cabinet over a light fixture) could have partially and unevenly dried areas, contributing to similar problems.

## Capillary

Temperature and surface effects influence the separation capabilities of CE. Artifacts also have been known to arise with CE.

### Temperature Effects

In most slab or tube platforms for electrophoresis, moderate electric fields (up to 1000 V) are used, because the Joule heating that accompanies the use of higher field strengths causes nonuniform temperature gradients, local changes in viscosity, and subsequent zone broadening. CE is distinguished from other forms of electrophoresis by the fact that extraordinarily high fields (30,000 V) are used to obtain rapid, high-efficiency separations. The problems encountered with noncapillary platforms are prevented by effective dissipation of Joule heat by forced air convection or liquid cooling of the capillary, both of which are possible because of the narrow bore of the capillary. The Joule heat produced is a function of (1) buffer type, (2) concentration, (3) voltage applied, (4) capillary inner diameter, and (5) length, and can be determined for any given system by generating an *Ohm's law plot*, which allows easy determination of the maximum voltage that can be used effectively. Reducing the inner diameter of the capillary, the ionic strength of the running buffer, or the applied voltage will reduce the heat produced by the electrophoretic process. It should be noted that reducing the inner diameter will compromise the detection limit of UV measurements (smaller OPL); reducing the applied field is less desirable in that resolution is directly proportional to the applied field. Consequently, attempts should be made to alter other parameters before reducing inner diameter or the applied field.

### Surface Effects

As in electrophoresis in general, the flow of fluid (electroosmotic or electroendosmotic flow [EOF]) in CE is a consequence of surface charge on the solid support. In CE, EOF can play a significant role in the separation process. The charge on the inner surface of a fused silica capillary is determined by the ionization state of the silanol groups (SiOH) that populate it. Interaction of positively charged buffer species with bound surface anions generates a layer of mobile cations that move toward the cathode when voltage is applied. This induces a very strong EOF that mobilizes all analytes in the same direction, regardless of their charge. Separation is consequently achieved because of differences in the electrophoretic migration rates of analytes superimposed on this EOF.

Because the driving force of the flow is distributed along the wall of the capillary, the flow profile is nearly flat or plug-like, contrasting with the laminar or parabolic flow generated by a pressure-driven system caused by shear forces at the wall. A flat flow profile is beneficial because it does not contribute to the dispersion of solute zones. The magnitude and direction of the EOF are influenced by several parameters, including: (1) type of electrolyte used; (2) pH; (3) ionic strength; (4) use of additives (e.g., surfactants, organic solvents); and (5) polarity and magnitude of the applied electric field.

Although advantageous for the dissipation of Joule heat, the large surface area-to-volume ratio of the inner capillary space increases the likelihood of analyte adsorption onto the surface of its inner wall. This causes phenomena such as peak tailing and even total and irreversible adsorption of the analyte. Adsorption is typically noted between cationic solutes and the negatively charged inner wall of the capillary, primarily through ionic interactions (with deprotonated silanols), but also involves hydrophobic interactions (with siloxanes). Because of the numerous charges and hydrophobic regions, significant adsorptive effects have been noted, especially for highly cationic proteins. In practice, adsorption of substances, whether from the sample or from the buffer, to the inner surface of the capillary will alter migration times and other separation characteristics; unaddressed, the capillary eventually may become "fouled." Buffer components and/or additives, such as surfactants, can often render permanent changes to the inner surface of the capillary (through adsorption) and may warrant dedication of specific capillaries for use with particular surfactants.

To minimize these inner wall effects, capillaries are conditioned by chemical treatment, most commonly with base, to remove adsorbates and rejuvenate the surface. A typical wash method includes flushing the chamber with 10 to 20 capillary volumes of 0.1 to 1.0 mol/L NaOH, followed by flushing with "run" buffer. To prevent exposing the capillary surface to drastic fluctuations in pH, conditioning procedures for separations at low pH may be better served by using strong acids (e.g., $HNO_3$), surfactants (e.g., SDS), or organic solvents, such as acetonitrile or methanol.

***Serum protein analysis.*** Compared with AGE and cellulose acetate electrophoresis (CAE), capillary zone electrophoresis (CZE) is more advantageous for serum protein analysis. Fig. 11.5 shows a comparison of the separation of serum proteins by CAE, AGE, and CE. The presence of the classical zones with CE is apparent, albeit in reversed order, as is the identification of serum protein abnormalities in gamma regions. Retrospective studies have shown CE to be effective for detecting monoclonal proteins, which could then be immunotyped by conventional techniques (IFE and **isoelectric focusing** [IEF]). Moreover, CE can do both serum protein electrophoresis and immunotyping in hundreds of samples simultaneously. These and other studies put forth the same conclusion: that CE is more sensitive than AGE in identifying abnormalities. Furthermore, CZE can be used effectively in serum protein analysis.

With CE using online optical detection, artifacts can occur in the form of "system peaks." These often originate from the sample or from the interfaces between the sample and the separation buffer, because any species that absorbs at the detection wavelength will generate a response. This differs from protein slab gel electrophoresis, wherein detection specificity is governed by a protein-specific stain. It is not uncommon, for example, for buffer species present in the sample but not in the separation buffer to generate system peaks.

One problem associated with conventional electrophoresis of serum proteins is its proclivity for point-of-application artifacts. These are bands that result from the fact that

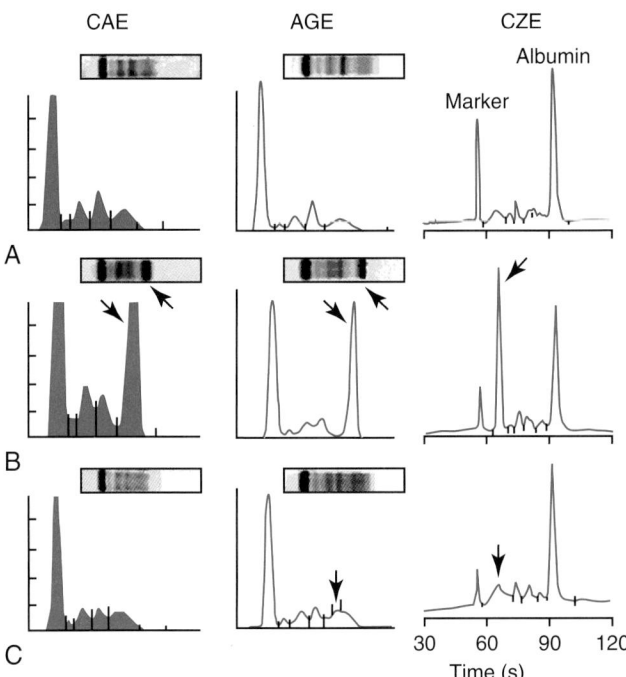

**Fig. 11.5** Rapid capillary zone electrophoresis of serum protein; comparison against scanning densitometry profiles obtained from cellulose acetate electrophoresis *(CAE)* and agarose gel electrophoresis *(AGE)*. (A) Normal serum. (B) Patient serum containing a large M-protein. (C) Patient serum containing a small monoclonal protein. Arrows indicate the position of the monoclonal proteins. *CZE*, Capillary zone electrophoresis.

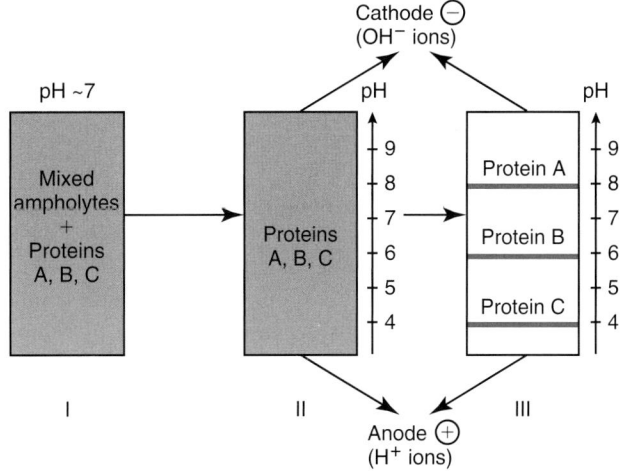

**Fig. 11.6** Schematic of an isoelectric focusing procedure. (I) A homogeneous mixture of carrier ampholytes, pH range 3 to 10, to which proteins A, B, and C, with isoelectric points (pI) of 8, 6, and 4, respectively, were added. (II) Current is applied and carrier ampholytes rapidly migrate to pH zones where the net charge is zero (the pI value). (III) Proteins A, B, and C migrate more slowly to their respective pI zones, where migration ceases. The high buffering capacity of the carrier ampholyte creates stable pH zones in which each protein may reach its pI.

electrophoretic mobility (e.g., with AGE) is bidirectional from the point of application. These precipitates may be euglobulin or cryoprecipitates and may or may not contain a monoclonal protein; only immunoelectrophoresis or IFE can identify the presence of monoclonal proteins. These bands must be immunotyped to distinguish real monoclonal proteins from artifacts—a process that is costly and time-consuming. CE prevents point-of-application artifacts in two ways. First, net mobility in CE results from the vectorial addition of both protein electrophoretic mobility and EOF. As a result of this unidirectional movement (toward the detector), the point of application remains removed from the detector. Second, unlike AGE, where precipitates cannot exit the loading well and enter the gel (thus appearing as a band in the scanned region of the gel), no gel matrix is present in CZE to impede electrophoretic migration because analysis occurs in free solution.

## SPECIALTY ELECTROPHORESIS TECHNIQUES

### Isoelectric Focusing Electrophoresis

IEF separates amphoteric compounds, such as proteins, with increased resolution in a medium possessing a stable pH gradient. The protein becomes "focused" at a point on the gel as it migrates to a zone where the pH of the gel matches the protein's pI. At this point, the charge of the protein becomes zero, and its migration ceases. Fig. 11.6 illustrates the procedure and shows the electrophoretic conditions before and

after current is applied. The protein zones are very sharp, because the region associated with a given pH is very narrow. Ordinary diffusion is also counteracted by the acquisition of a charge, as a protein varies from its pI position and subsequently migrates back because of electrophoretic forces. Proteins that differ in their pI values by only 0.02 pH unit have been separated by IEF.

The pH gradient is created with *carrier ampholytes*, a group of amphoteric polyaminocarboxylic acids that have slight differences in pKa value and molecular weights of 300 to 1000. Mixtures of 50 to 100 different compounds are added to the medium and create a "natural pH gradient" when individual ampholytes reach their pI values during electrophoresis. They establish narrow buffered zones, with stable but slightly different pHs, through which the slower-moving proteins migrate and stop at their individual pIs.

The anode is surrounded by a dilute acid solution and the cathode by a dilute alkaline solution. After focusing, the most negatively charged carrier ampholytes and proteins will be found at the anodal end, and the most positively charged near the cathodal end of the electrophoretic matrix. The other carrier ampholytes and proteins focus at intermediate points according to their pI values. Because carrier ampholytes are generally used in relatively high concentrations, a high-voltage power source (up to 2000 V) is necessary (power is in the vicinity of 2 to 50 W, depending on experimental conditions). As a result, the electrophoretic matrix must be cooled.

PAGE-IEF is widely used in analytical work, as it is essentially free of electroendosmosis. However, the polyacrylamide gel must have a large enough pore size so that protein migration will not be impeded by molecular sieving effects. In actual practice, impeded migration of some proteins, such as IgM, cannot be prevented. PAGE-IEF has the advantages that operating conditions are simple, and that large pore sizes make it unlikely that any proteins will be excluded on the basis of molecular size. IEF has been applied to the separation of alkaline phosphatase isoenzymes and is widely used in neonatal screening programs to test for variant hemoglobins. Off-gel techniques carry out the separation in free solution with sample containing ampholytes loaded into each of a linear series of wells separated by semipermeable membranes and in contact with a pH gradient strip. Electrophoresis separates sample proteins into different wells depending on their pI values. Separated fractions can be further resolved in a second similar focusing step or taken directly to further separation by two-dimensional electrophoresis or liquid chromatography-mass spectrometry. This technique has been useful in the study of the human proteome.

## Micellar Electrokinetic Chromatography

MEKC is a hybrid of electrophoresis and chromatography. MEKC, a mode that is separate and distinct from capillary electrokinetic chromatography, is an effective electrophoretic technique, because it can be used for the separation of neutral and charged solutes. The separation of neutral species is accomplished by exploiting micelles formed in the running buffer when the concentration of surfactant exceeds the critical micelle concentration (e.g., 8 to 9 mmol/L for SDS). During electrophoresis, neutral micelles can interact with analytes in a chromatographic manner through hydrophobic interactions in which analytes are micellized based on their degree of hydrophobicity. Under these conditions, partitioning into the micelle is the driving force for separation. With charged micelles (e.g., SDS), analytes can also interact through electrostatic interactions via the charge on the surface of the micelle.

### POINTS TO REMEMBER

**Capillary Zone Electrophoresis**
- Uses electroosmotic flow (EOF) to mobilize the sample plug pass the detector.
- The magnitude and direction of EOF can be manipulated through methodology.
- Higher voltages can be applied due to more efficient dissipation of heat; this can translate to faster separations.

## REVIEW QUESTIONS

1. For proteins to migrate on a gel during electrophoresis, the isoelectric point must be exceeded. The isoelectric point of an amino acid or protein is defined as the:
   a. ability of the amino acid or protein to carry both positive and negative charges.
   b. pH at which the amino acid or protein has a negative charge.
   c. pH at which a molecule has no net charge.
   d. point on an electrophoretic gel at which that specific protein migrates.

2. The term *amphoteric* means:
   a. the pH at which a protein has no net charge.
   b. that a protein will have a negative charge at a high pH.
   c. that a protein has both positive and negative charges because of its side chains.
   d. the positive electrode.

3. Unequal migration of samples down the gel in an electrophoresis assay is an interference usually caused by:
   a. dirty electrodes causing uneven application of the electrical field.
   b. dirty pipette tips or applicators.
   c. too much sample being applied.
   d. inappropriate binding of immunoglobulins to other proteins in a sample.

4. In serum protein electrophoresis, the greater the charge of a molecule:
   a. the slower it will migrate.
   b. the faster it will migrate.
   c. the less the migration rate will be affected.

5. Serum protein electrophoresis is what kind of basic technique?
   a. Immunoassay
   b. Standardization
   c. Qualitative technique
   d. Separation

6. Specimens with very low protein content sometimes require preconcentration before they are loaded onto an electrophoretic gel. An electrophoretic technique that *does not* require this concentration step is:
   a. disc electrophoresis.
   b. capillary electrophoresis.
   c. zone electrophoresis.
   d. two-dimensional gel electrophoresis.

7. What optical measuring technique allows for the scanning and quantification of electrophoretic fractions separated on a support medium?
   a. Spectrophotometry
   b. Chromatography
   c. Densitometry
   d. Nephelometry

8. A Southern blot is used to detect fragments of:
   a. RNA
   b. protein
   c. agarose
   d. DNA

9. A 1% agarose gel is best suited for separating DNA fragments in which one of the following size ranges:
   a. 500 bp (0.5 kbp) to 20 kbp
   b. 50 to 100 kbp
   c. 100 to 500 kbp
   d. larger than 500 kbp

10. The component of an electrophoresis system in which separation takes place is the:
   a. stain
   b. support medium
   c. densitometer
   d. zone

## SUGGESTED READINGS

Breadmore MC, Tubaon RM, Shallan AI, et al. Recent advances in enhancing the sensitivity of electrophoresis and electrochromatography in capillaries and microchips (2012-2014). *Electrophoresis*. 2015;36:36–61.

Dawod M, Arvin NE, Kennedy RT. Recent advances in protein analysis by capillary and microchip electrophoresis. *Analyst*. 2017;142:1847–1866.

Gassmann M, Grenacher B, Rohde B, et al. Quantifying Western blots: pitfalls of densitometry. *Electrophoresis*. 2009;30:1845–1855.

Gay-Bellile C, Bengoufa D, Houze P, et al. Automated multicapillary electrophoresis for analysis of human serum proteins. *Clin Chem*. 2003;49:1909–1915.

Herpol M, Lanckmans K, Van Neyghem S, et al. Evaluation of the Sebia Capillarys 3 Tera and the Bio-Rad D-100 systems for the measurement of hemoglobin A1c. *Am J of Clin Pathol*. 2016;146:67–77.

Kleparnik K. Recent advances in combination of capillary electrophoresis with mass spectrometry: methodology and theory. *Electrophoresis*. 2015;36:159–178.

Landers JP. Clinical capillary electrophoresis. *Clin Chem*. 1995;41:495–509.

Landers JP. Introduction to capillary electrophoresis. In: Landers JP, ed. *Handbook of Capillary and Microchip Electrophoresis and Associated Microtechniques*. 3rd ed. Boca Raton, FL: CRC Press; 2008:3–74.

Landers JP. Molecular diagnostics on electrophoretic microchips. *Anal Chem*. 2003;75:2919–2927.

Li SFY, Kricka LJ. Clinical analysis by microchip capillary electrophoresis. *Clin Chem*. 2005;52:37–45.

Ouimet CM, D'amico CI, Kennedy RT. Advances in capillary electrophoresis and the implications for drug discovery. *Expert Opin Drug Discov*. 2017;12:213–224.

Sharma K, Lee S, Han S, Lee S, et al. Two-dimensional fluorescence difference gel electrophoresis analysis of the urine proteome in human diabetic nephropathy. *Proteomics*. 2005;5:2648–2655.

Willrich MA, Ladwig PM, Andreguetto BD, et al. Monoclonal antibody therapeutics as potential interferences on protein electrophoresis and immunofixation. *Clin Chem Lab Med*. 2016;54:1085–1093.

Zhang W, Hankemeier T, Ramautar R. Next-generation capillary electrophoresis-mass spectrometry approaches in metabolomics. *Curr Opin Biotechnol*. 2017;43:1–7.

# 12

# Chromatography

*David S. Hage\**

## OBJECTIVES

1. Define the following terms:
   - Chromatogram
   - Chromatograph
   - Chromatography
   - Column chromatography
   - Mobile phase
   - Planar chromatography
   - Retention factor
   - Retention time and retention volume
   - Stationary phase
   - Void time and void volume
2. Evaluate a chromatogram and its peaks to determine their separation factor and resolution; list three ways to improve resolution.
3. Define and calculate the following terms for a chromatographic separation: number of theoretical plates and plate height. Explain how the plate height can vary with the linear velocity of the mobile phase.
4. Explain how external or internal calibration can be used for quantitative measurements in chromatography. Define *internal standard* and discuss how this can be used in quantitative measurements by chromatography.
5. Define gas chromatography (GC) and describe three types of GC based on the type of stationary phase that is present. List some stationary phases for each of these methods.
6. Summarize the components of a gas chromatograph and describe the function of each component.
7. Explain the differences between packed columns and capillary columns in GC.
8. Define the following terms and explain how they are used in GC: headspace analysis, isothermal elution, and temperature programming.
9. List and describe five types of detectors that are used in GC, including the advantages and disadvantages of each.
10. Define the terms *liquid chromatography* and *high-performance liquid chromatography*. List several ways in which liquid chromatography differs from GC.
11. Describe the following types of liquid chromatography, including the principles of separation, the types of stationary phases and mobile phases that are used, and some possible clinical applications of each.
    - Adsorption chromatography
    - Affinity chromatography
    - Hydrophilic interaction liquid chromatography
    - Ion-exchange chromatography
    - Ion-pair chromatography
    - Normal-phase chromatography
    - Reversed-phase chromatography
    - Size-exclusion chromatography
12. Summarize the components of a system that is used in high-performance liquid chromatography and describe the function of each component.
13. List and describe five types of detectors that are used in liquid chromatography, including the advantages and disadvantages of each.
14. Explain the principles of planar chromatography. Define the terms *paper chromatography* and *thin-layer chromatography*.
15. Know how to calculate and use the retardation factor to identify compounds in planar chromatography.

## KEY WORDS AND DEFINITIONS

**Adsorption chromatography** A type of liquid chromatography in which chemicals are retained based on their adsorption and desorption at the surface of an underivatized support.

**Affinity chromatography (AC)** A liquid chromatographic method that makes use of biologically related interactions for the retention and separation of chemicals.

*The author gratefully acknowledges the contributions of Drs. Glen L. Hortin, Bruce A. Goldberger, M. David Ullman, Carl A. Burtis, and Larry D. Bowers to this chapter in previous editions.

**Anion-exchange chromatography** A type of ion-exchange chromatography that uses positively charged groups as a stationary phase to bind and separate anions.

**Bonded phase gas chromatography** A type of gas chromatography in which the stationary phase is chemically linked or attached to the support.

**Carrier gas** A term often used to describe the mobile phase in gas chromatography.

**Cation-exchange chromatography** A type of ion-exchange chromatography that uses negatively charged groups as a stationary phase to bind and separate cations.

**Chiral stationary phase (CSP)** A stationary phase that is chiral and that can interact with compounds in a stereospecific manner.

**Chromatogram** A plot of detector response in chromatography as a function of the time or volume of the mobile phase that is needed to elute an analyte from a column.

**Chromatograph** The instrument that is used to perform a separation in chromatography.

**Chromatography** A method in which the components of a mixture are separated based on their differential interactions with two chemical or physical phases: a mobile phase and a stationary phase.

**Column chromatography** A type of chromatography that uses a column, or a tube, to contain the stationary phase and support.

**Gas chromatography (GC)** A type of chromatography that uses a gas as the mobile phase.

**Gas chromatography/mass spectrometry (GC/MS)** The use of a mass spectrometer as a detector for gas chromatography.

**Gas-liquid chromatography (GLC)** A type of gas chromatography in which the stationary phase is a liquid that is placed as a coating or layer on the support.

**Gas-solid chromatography (GSC)** A type of gas chromatography in which the same material acts as both the stationary phase and the support; chemicals are retained by their adsorption to the surface of the support.

**Headspace analysis** A sample introduction technique in which a portion of the vapor phase (or "headspace") that is above a liquid or solid sample is used in an analysis.

**Height equivalent of a theoretical plate (HETP or *H*)** A measure of efficiency in chromatography that is equal to length of a chromatographic system divided by the number of theoretical plates for the system, also known as the plate height.

**High-performance liquid chromatography (HPLC)** A type of liquid chromatography that uses small, efficient supports that produce narrow peaks.

**Hydrophilic interaction liquid chromatography (HILIC)** A type of partition chromatography that uses a polar stationary phase, and in which chemicals partition between an organic-rich region in the mobile phase and a more polar water-enriched layer that is at or near the surface of a polar support.

**Internal standard** A compound that is added in a constant amount to standard solutions and samples to help normalize the results for any variations that may occur during pretreatment steps or during injection into a chromatographic system.

**Ion-exchange chromatography (IEC)** A type of liquid chromatography in which ions are separated by their adsorption onto a support that contains fixed charges at its surface.

**Ion-pair chromatography (IPC)** A technique that combines columns that are used in reversed-phase chromatography with the ability to separate ionic compounds based on their charges, as achieved by adding an ion-pairing agent to the mobile phase.

**Isocratic elution** Use of a constant mobile phase composition throughout a separation.

**Isothermal elution** A chromatographic method that uses a constant temperature for elution.

**Liquid chromatography (LC)** A type of chromatography that uses a liquid as the mobile phase.

**Liquid chromatograph–electrochemical detection (LC-EC)** The combination of an electrochemical detector with liquid chromatography.

**Liquid chromatography–mass spectrometry (LC-MS)** A technique that combines liquid chromatography with mass spectrometry.

**Mobile phase** The phase that travels through a chromatographic system and carries sample components with it.

**Normal-phase chromatography** A type of partition chromatography that uses a polar stationary phase; also known as "normal-phase liquid chromatography," or NPLC.

**Number of theoretical plates *(N)*** A measure of efficiency and band-broadening that is given for a Gaussian-shaped peak by using either $N = 16 \, (t_R/W_b)^2$ or $N = 5.545 \, (t_R/W_h)^2$, where $t_R$ is the retention time for the peak, and $W_b$ or $W_h$ are baseline width or half-height width for the peak. The number of theoretical plates is also known as the plate number.

**Partition chromatography** A liquid chromatographic method in which solutes are separated based on their partitioning between the liquid mobile phase and a stationary phase that is coated or bonded onto a solid support.

**Planar chromatography** A type of chromatography in which the stationary phase is coated or placed onto a flat surface, or plane.

**Resolution ($R_s$)** A measure of the separation of two adjacent peaks in chromatography; the resolution equals the difference in retention time for the components in the two peaks divided by the average of the baseline widths for these peaks.

**Retardation factor ($R_f$)** In planar chromatography, the distance traveled by a chemical from its point of application divided by the distance traveled by the mobile phase in the same amount of time.

**Retention factor *(k)*** A measure of retention in chromatography, which is equal to the difference in the retention time and void time divided by the void time, or the difference in the retention volume and void volume divided by the void volume; also called the capacity factor.

**Retention time *($t_R$)*** The average time that is required for a particular chemical to pass through a chromatographic column.

**Retention volume *($V_R$)*** The average volume of mobile phase that is required for a particular chemical to pass through a chromatographic column.

**Reversed-phase chromatography** A type of partition chromatography that uses a nonpolar stationary phase; also known as reversed-phase liquid chromatography (RPLC).

**Separation factor *($\alpha$)*** A measure of the degree of separation in chromatography that is equal to the ratio of the retention factors for two neighboring peaks, where the larger retention factor appears in the numerator; also known as the selectivity factor.

**Size-exclusion chromatography (SEC)** A liquid chromatographic technique that separates analytes based on size through the use of a porous support that has an inert surface with little or no interactions with the sample components.

**Solvent programming** Use of a mobile phase composition that varies during a separation.

**Stationary phase** The phase in chromatography that is held within the system by a support and used to interact with and separate a sample's components as these components pass through the system.

**Temperature programming** A chromatographic method in which the temperature is changed over time.

**Ultra-high-performance liquid chromatography (UPLC or UHPLC)** A liquid chromatographic method that uses smaller diameter supports and pressures up to 15,000 psi.

**van Deemter equation** A relationship that shows how the overall value of plate height *(H)* for a chromatographic system is affected by the linear velocity of the mobile phase *(u)*, where $H = A + B/u + C\,u$ and the terms A, B, and C are constants that represent the contributions of several types of band-broadening processes.

**Void time *($t_M$)*** The elution time for a compound that is not retained in a chromatographic system.

**Void volume *($V_M$)*** The volume of mobile phase that is needed to elute a compound that is not retained in a chromatographic system.

# BASIC PRINCIPLES OF CHROMATOGRAPHY

## General Terms and Components of Chromatography

**Chromatography** is a method in which the components of a mixture are separated based on their differential interactions with two chemical or physical phases: a **mobile phase** and a **stationary phase** (Fig. 12.1). The mobile phase travels through the system and carries sample components with it once the sample has been applied or injected. The stationary phase is held within the system by a support. As a sample's components pass through this system, the components that have the strongest interactions with the stationary phase will be retained more and move through the system more slowly than components that have weaker interactions. This leads to a difference in the rate of travel for these components and their separation.

The type of chromatographic system that is shown in Fig. 12.1 is known as **column chromatography** because it uses a column (or a tube) to contain the stationary phase and support. The stationary phase may be the surface of the support, a coating on this support, or a chemical layer that is bonded to the support. In column chromatography, the support may be the interior wall of the column, or it may be a material that is placed or "packed" into the column. It is also possible to use a support and stationary phase that are present on a plane, or open surface. This second format is known as **planar chromatography**.

Besides being classified based on whether they use a column or plane, chromatographic methods can be classified based on the mobile phase. For instance, a chromatographic method that uses a mobile phase that is a gas is called **gas chromatography (GC)**, while a chromatographic method that uses a liquid mobile phase is known as liquid chromatography (LC). It is also possible to divide chromatographic methods according to the type of stationary phase that is present or the way in which this stationary phase is interacting with sample components. Examples include the GC methods of **gas-solid chromatography (GSC)** or **gas-liquid chromatography (GLC)**, and the LC methods of **adsorption chromatography** or **partition chromatography**.

The instrument that is used in chromatography is known as a **chromatograph**. This instrument can provide a response that is related to the amount of a compound that is exiting (or eluting) from a column as a function of the elution time or the volume of mobile phase that has passed through the system. The resulting plot of the response versus time or volume is known as a **chromatogram**, as illustrated in Figs. 12.1 and 12.2.

The average time or volume that is required for a chemical to pass through the column is known as that chemical's **retention time *($t_R$)*** or **retention volume *($V_R$)***. The elution time or volume for a compound that has no interaction with the stationary phase and is not retained is known as the **void time *($t_M$)*** or **void volume *($V_M$)***. In order for two chemicals to be separated by chromatography, it is necessary for these chemicals to have different values for $t_R$ and $V_R$. Retention times or retention volumes can be used to help identify the eluting compounds, while the area or height of the compound's peak can be used to measure the amount of the compound that is present.

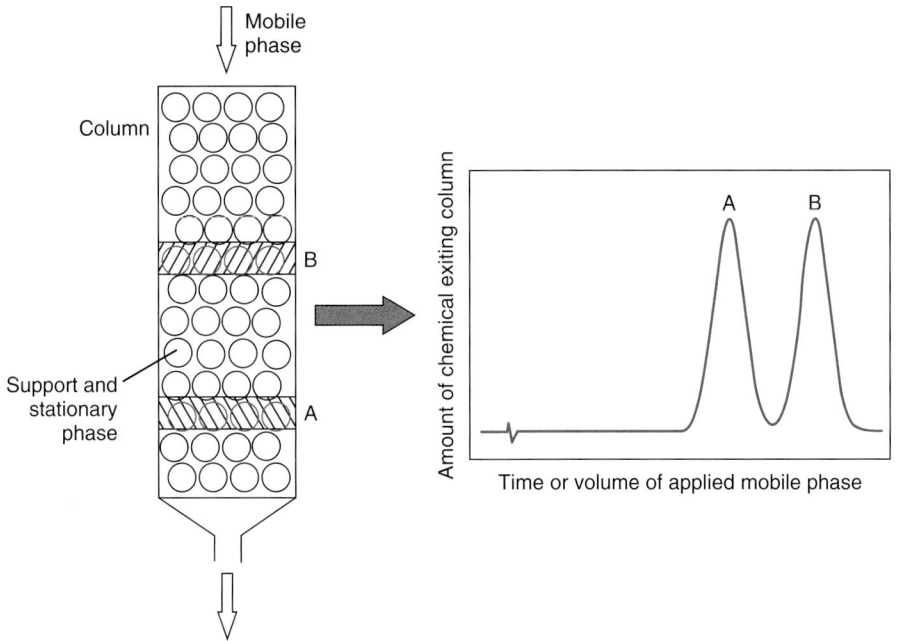

Fig. 12.1 The general components of a chromatographic system, as illustrated here by using a column to separate two chemicals, A and B.

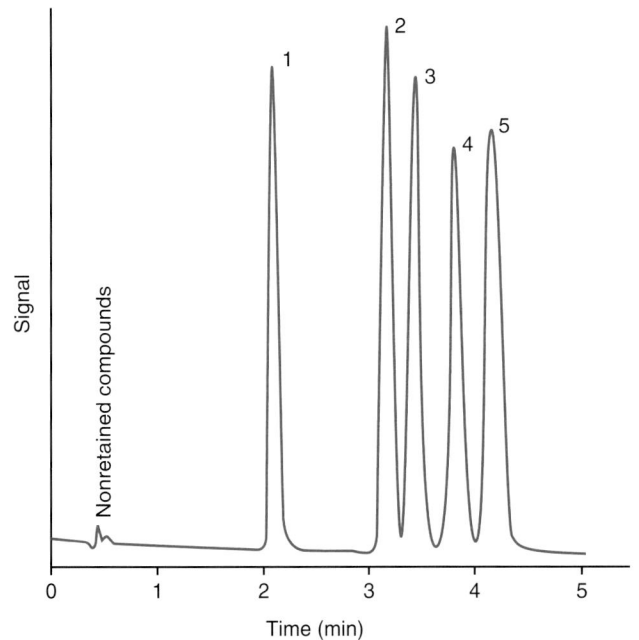

Column: C18, 3 μm, 0.46 ID × 10 cm
Eluent: Isocratic, 0.025 M phosphate
Buffer: pH 3.0 in 25% acetonitrile
Flow rate: 2 mL/min
Detection: 215 nm, 0.1 AUFS

Compounds:  1. Doxepin
            2. Desipramine
            3. Imipramine
            4. Nortriptyline
            5. Amitriptyline

Fig. 12.2 Chromatogram from a separation of tricyclic antidepressants based on reversed-phase chromatography and high-performance liquid chromatography. Detection was based on the use of an absorbance detector that monitored the column eluent at 215 nm. (Note: the signal is displayed at 0.1 AUFS [absorbance units-full scale].) (Courtesy Grace Vydac Separations Group Inc., Hesperia, CA.)

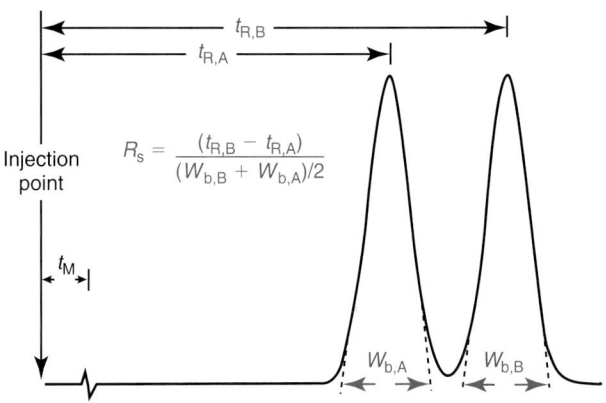

$$R_s = \frac{(t_{R,B} - t_{R,A})}{(W_{b,B} + W_{b,A})/2}$$

Fig. 12.3 An example of a general chromatogram that may be obtained when using a column. In this example, compound B is eluted later than compound A. $R_s$, Resolution; $t_M$, void time; $t_{R,A}$ and $t_{R,B}$, retention times for solutes A and B; $W_{b,A}$ and $W_{b,B}$, baseline peak widths for compounds A and B.

The width of each peak reflects the separating "performance" or "efficiency" of the chromatographic system. The width of a peak in a chromatogram is often represented by its baseline width ($W_b$) or its half-height width ($W_h$) (Fig. 12.3). As the widths of the peaks in a chromatogram decrease, and the peaks become sharper, it becomes easier for the chromatographic system to separate two neighboring peaks and to separate multiple peaks in a given amount of time. Sharper peaks are also easier to measure than broader peaks and tend to produce better limits of detection.

## Retention and Selectivity

For two chemicals to be separated by chromatography, these chemicals need to have some differences in how they are interacting with the stationary phase versus the mobile phase. These different interactions lead to differences in retention between the two chemicals. Besides using the retention time or retention volume, another way of representing retention in chromatography and identifying compounds is by using the **retention factor** ($k$), which is also sometimes called $k'$ or the "capacity factor." This value can be calculated from experimental data by using either of the following equivalent relationships:

$$k = (t_R - t_M) / t_M$$
$$\text{or } k = (V_R - V_M) / V_M$$

The retention factor is a unitless number, where a value of zero indicates that no interaction is occurring between a chemical and the stationary phase. As a chemical undergoes greater interactions with the stationary phase, this will result in longer retention times and an increased value of $k$. The value of $k$ is directly related to the strength of the interactions that are occurring between a chemical and the stationary phase or mobile phase, as well as the relative amount of stationary phase versus mobile phase that is present in the column.

Any separation in chromatography requires that there be some difference in retention for the chemicals of interest. One way of describing this difference is by using the **separation factor** or "selectivity factor" ($\alpha$). The separation factor for two compounds (A and B) is equal to the ratio of their retention factors ($k_A$ and $k_B$),

$$\alpha = k_B / k_A$$

where, the retention factor for the later eluting component ($k_B$) is given in the numerator. If two chemicals, A and B, have the same retention in a chromatographic system, the value of $\alpha$ will equal one. If A and B have different retention, the value of $\alpha$ will be greater than 1 and will increase as the degree of separation increases.

## Band-Broadening and Efficiency

The peaks for two sequentially eluting chemicals must also be sufficiently narrow to allow a difference in retention to be observed. The peaks observed from the injection of even a small sample will experience some increase in width, or band-broadening, as the chemical travels through a chromatographic system. This broadening is produced by various processes that are related to the rate of movement of the applied chemicals as they pass around or within the support and within or between the mobile phase and stationary phase.

The efficiency and degree of band-broadening in a chromatographic system are reflected by the width of a chemical's peak. This width can be described by using the $W_b$ or the $W_h$ of the peak. These values, in turn, can be used to find another measure of chromatographic efficiency that is known as the **number of theoretical plates** or *plate number* ($N$). The value of $N$ can be found for a Gaussian-shaped peak by using either of the following equivalent formulas:

$$N = 16(t_R / W_b)^2 \text{ or } N = 5.545(t_R / W_h)^2$$

where $t_R$ is the retention time for the peak, and the widths $W_b$ or $W_h$ are in the same units of time as $t_R$. The value of $N$ can

be thought of as representing the effective number of times that a chemical distributes between the mobile phase and stationary phase as the chemical passes through the chromatographic system. A larger value for $N$ represents many such steps, which makes it easier to separate two chemicals that have only small differences in their retention.

Another way to describe the efficiency of a chromatographic system is to use the **height equivalent of a theoretical plate** or "plate height" (HETP or $H$). The value of $H$ is found by dividing the length ($L$) of the chromatographic system by the number of theoretical plates for the system ($N$):

$$H = L / N$$

The value of $H$ represents the length of the column or chromatographic system that makes up one theoretical plate, or one distribution step, for a chemical between the mobile phase and stationary phase. A chromatographic system with high efficiency will have a small value for $H$.

A valuable feature of using $H$ to describe efficiency is that this term can be related directly to the parameters and processes that affect band-broadening. An example of this is the **van Deemter equation**, showing how $H$ is affected by the linear velocity of the mobile phase ($u$), which is directly related to the flow rate ($F$) through the relationship $u = (F \cdot L)/V_M$.

$$H = A + B / u + Cu$$

The terms A, B, and C in this equation are constants that represent the contributions of several types of band-broadening processes. The A term represents band-broadening processes that are independent of the linear velocity, the B term represents processes that produce more band-broadening at low linear velocities, and the C term represents processes that lead to an increase in $H$ as the linear velocity is increased. The van Deemter equation predicts that the combined effect of all these processes will be an optimum range of flow rates and linear velocities over which the lowest plate heights, and best efficiencies, will be obtained.

Several factors affect chromatographic efficiency. For instance, efficiency can be improved by using longer columns, which increases the value of $N$ but does not alter $H$. It is also possible to change the flow rate to its optimum value, use a smaller diameter or more efficient supports; or use a relatively narrow diameter capillary instead of a packed bed column. All of these latter factors help lower the value of $H$, which in turn increases the value of $N$ for a given length of column or chromatographic system.

## Resolution

The overall extent to which two peaks are separated in chromatography can be described by using the **resolution** ($R_s$), as illustrated in Fig. 12.3. The resolution between two neighboring peaks can be found by using the following formula:

$$R_s = \frac{(t_{R,B} - t_{R,A})}{(W_{b,B} + W_{b,A}) / 2}$$

In this equation, $t_{R,A}$ and $t_{R,B}$ are the average retention times for compounds A and B (where B elutes after A), while

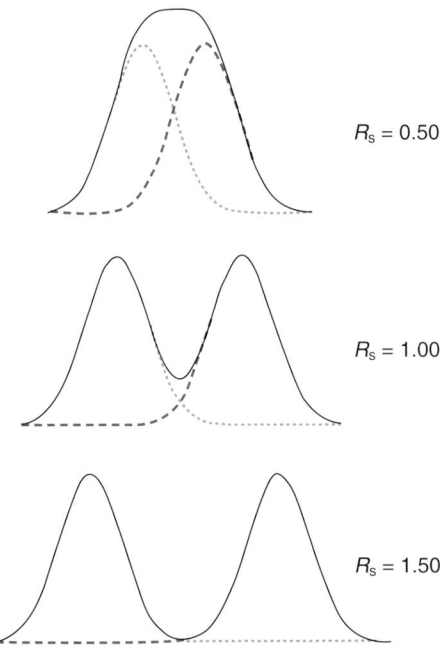

**Fig. 12.4** Degree of separation obtained for two chromatographic peaks that are present in a 1:1 area ratio as the resolution between these peaks ($R_s$) is varied.

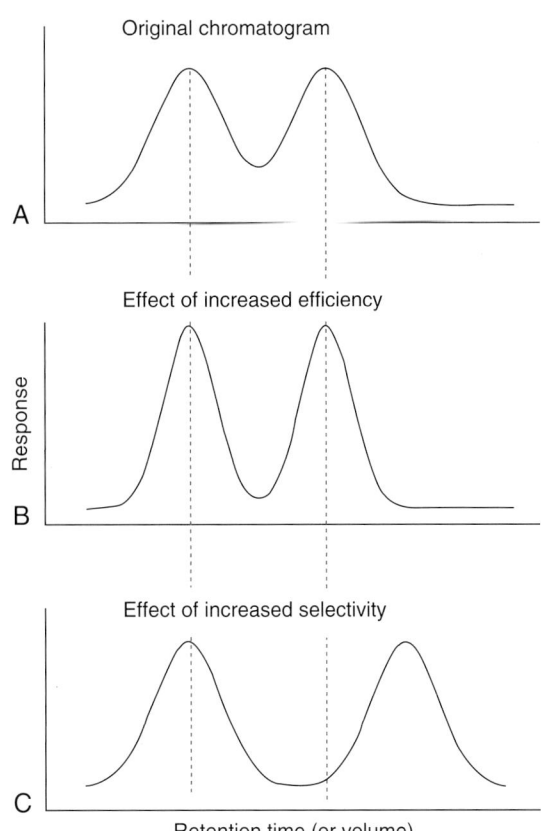

**Fig. 12.5** Effects of selectivity and efficiency on the resolution of peaks in chromatography. These three situations represent cases where there is poor or moderate resolution between two neighboring peaks (A), good resolution between the peaks as a result of high column efficiency (B), or good resolution between the peaks as a result of good column selectivity (C).

$W_{b,A}$ and $W_{b,B}$ are the baseline widths for the peaks of these compounds (in time units, in this case). An equivalent equation can be written in terms of retention volumes and baseline widths in volume units. Either approach will give a unitless value for $R_s$ that represents the average number of baseline widths that separate the centers of the two peaks.

Fig. 12.4 shows how the separation of two neighboring peaks increases as the value of $R_s$ increases for these peaks. An $R_s$ value of zero is obtained when there is no separation between the peaks and they have the exact same retention. An $R_s$ value of 1.5 or greater is often said to represent a complete separation between two equally sized peaks, or "baseline resolution." However, for many separations, resolution values between 1.0 or 1.25 and 1.5 may be adequate, especially if the peaks are about the same size and are to be measured by using their peak heights rather than their peak areas.

There are several approaches that can be used to improve the resolution between two peaks in chromatography (Fig. 12.5). These approaches are indicated by the following expression, which is sometimes known as the *resolution equation* of chromatography:

$$R_s = \left[ \left( N^{1/2} \right) / 4 \right] \cdot \left[ (\alpha - 1) / \alpha \right] \cdot \left[ k / (1 + k) \right]$$

In this equation, $k$ is the retention factor for the second of two neighboring peaks, $\alpha$ is the separation factor for the peaks, and $N$ is the number of theoretical plates for the chromatographic system. This relationship indicates that peak resolution can be increased in three ways: (1) by increasing the efficiency of the system, as represented by $N$; (2) by increasing the overall degree of retention, as represented by $k$; or (3) by increasing the selectivity of the column for one compound versus another, as represented by $\alpha$.

**POINTS TO REMEMBER**

**General Ways to Improve Peak Resolution in Chromatography**
- Increase the efficiency of the system.
- Increase the overall degree of peak retention.
- Increase the selectivity of the column for the peak of one compound versus another.

## Analyte Identification and Quantification

Chromatography is often used to identify analytes and/or to measure their concentrations. For example, the retention time, retention volume, and retention factor all reflect how an analyte is interacting within a particular chromatographic system. These retention values can be compared with those for a known sample of the same compound to confirm its identity. An alternative approach for identification is to use a detection method that provides structural information on the analyte, such as mass spectrometry (see Chapter 13).

The peak area or peak height can be used to produce quantitative information on an analyte. Peak areas tend to provide a more precise means for measuring an analyte, while peak heights are easier to use if there is not complete resolution between the analyte and its neighboring peaks. Both external

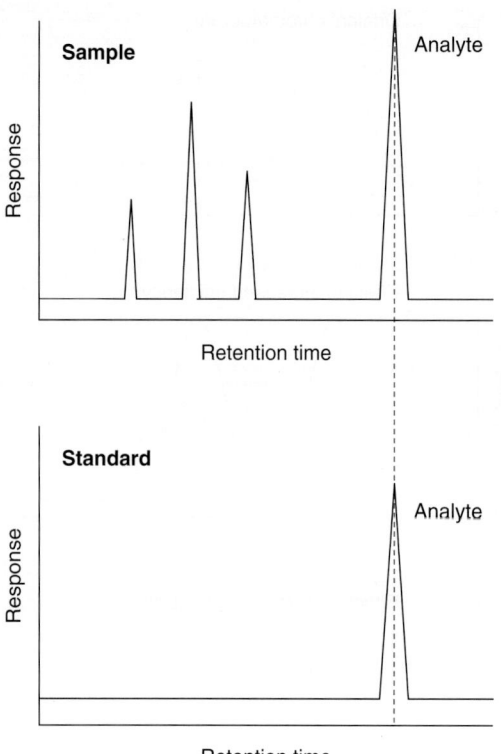

**Fig. 12.6** Use of external calibration and standards to quantify an analyte based on its peak height or area in a chromatogram for an injected sample.

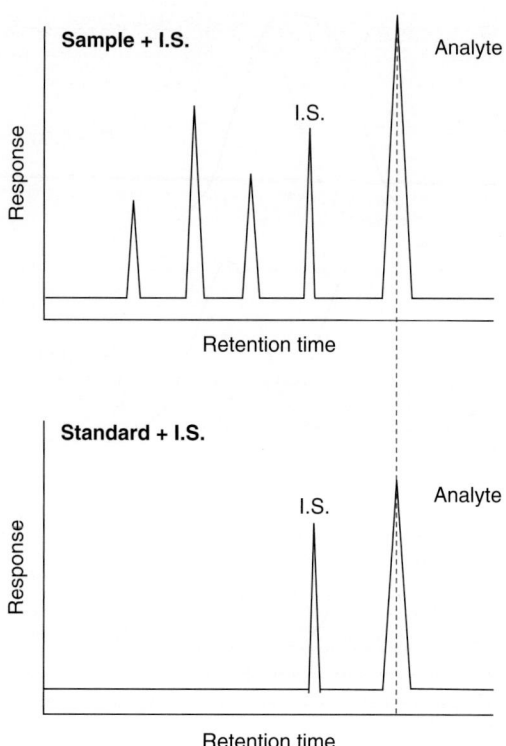

**Fig. 12.7** Use of internal calibration and samples or standards containing an internal standard (I.S.) to quantify an analyte based on its peak height or area in a chromatogram for an injected sample.

and internal calibration techniques can be used for such measurements. In external calibration, standard solutions containing known quantities of the analytes are processed and separated in the same manner as samples that contain one or more of these analytes (Fig. 12.6). A calibration curve is then constructed by plotting the peak height or peak area (or the spot density, in the case of planar methods) versus the concentration or mass of analyte that was applied in the standard solutions. This curve can then be used with the peak area or peak height that is determined for the same analyte in the samples to find the concentration or the amount of the analyte that was present.

In the method of internal calibration, standard solutions of the analyte are again prepared; however, a constant amount of a different compound known as the **internal standard** is also added to each standard solution and sample (Fig. 12.7). The internal standard should be a chemical that was not originally present in either the sample or the standard, that is similar in its chemical and physical properties to the analyte, and that can be measured independently from the analyte. This internal standard is typically added to the samples and standards before they are processed by any pretreatment steps. The addition of this agent can help normalize the results for any variations that may occur during the pretreatment steps or during injection onto the chromatographic system. This normalization is made by constructing a calibration curve in which the $y$-axis is based on the ratio of the peak height or peak area for the analyte in a given standard or sample divided by the peak height or peak area for the internal standard in the same

standard or sample. This ratio is plotted versus the concentration or amount of analyte that was in each standard. This calibration plot can then be used to find the concentration or the amount of the analyte in each sample.

# GAS CHROMATOGRAPHY

GC is a type of chromatography in which a gas is used as the mobile phase. This method can be used to separate and analyze compounds that either are naturally volatile or can be converted into a volatile form, such as through derivatization. The mobile phase is typically an inert gas such as nitrogen, helium, or argon, or a low mass gas such as hydrogen. Due to the low densities of gases, the compounds that are injected onto a GC column do not have any appreciable interactions with the mobile phase but are simply carried by this gas through the column. As a result, the term **carrier gas** is commonly used to refer to the mobile phase in GC. Separations in GC are instead based on differences in the vapor pressures of the injected compounds and in the interactions of these compounds with the stationary phase.

## Types of Gas Chromatography
### Gas-Solid Chromatography

There are several ways of classifying GC methods based on the type of stationary phase that is present. GSC is a type of GC in which the same material acts as both the stationary phase and the support. In this method, chemicals are retained by their adsorption to the surface of the support. This support is often an inorganic material like silica or alumina. Other supports that

**TABLE 12.1 Stationary Phases Commonly Used in Gas-Liquid Chromatography and as Bonded Phases in Gas Chromatography**

| Composition | Polarity | Commercial Examples | Typical Applications |
|---|---|---|---|
| 100% Methylpolysiloxane | Nonpolar | OV-1, SE-30 | Drugs, amino acid derivatives |
| 5% Phenyl–95% methylpolysiloxane | Nonpolar | OV-23, SE-54 | Drugs |
| 50% Phenyl–50% methylpolysiloxane | Intermediate polarity | OV-17 | Drugs, steroids, glycols |
| 50% Cyanopropylmethyl–50% phenylmethylpolysiloxane | Intermediate polarity | OV-225 | Fatty acid methyl esters, carbohydrate derivatives |
| Polyethylene glycol | Polar | Carbowax 20M | Acids, alcohols, glycols, ketones |

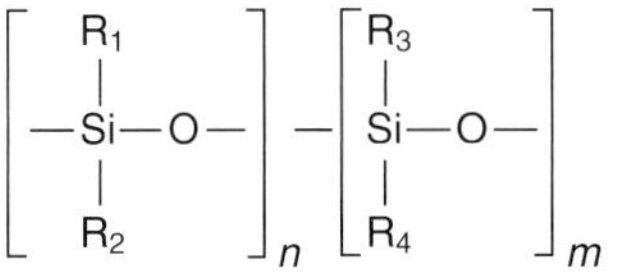

Fig. 12.8 General structure of a polysiloxane. The side groups are represented by $R_1$ through $R_4$, while $n$ and $m$ represent the relative lengths (or amounts) of each type of segment in the overall polymer.

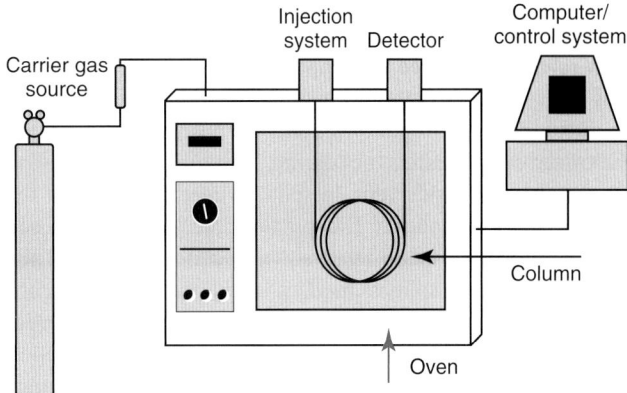

Fig. 12.9 General design of a gas chromatograph. (Modified from a figure courtesy Restek Corporation, Bellefonte, PA.)

can be used are molecular sieves, which are porous materials that are made from a mixture of silica and alumina, or organic polymers like porous polystyrene. The retention of an analyte on a GSC support will be affected by factors such as the surface area of the support, the size of the pores in this support, and the types of functional groups that are present on the support.

### Gas-Liquid Chromatography and Bonded Phases

In GLC the stationary phase is a liquid that is placed as a coating or layer on the support. This is the most common type of GC for chemical analysis. Various types of liquids can be used for this purpose (Table 12.1). Many GLC stationary phases are based on a polysiloxane (Fig. 12.8). The side chains in a polysiloxane can have structures that range from nonpolar methyl groups to polar cyanopropyl groups, and may be present in various ratios or as mixtures. The types of chemicals that will be retained by this type of stationary phase will be determined by the amounts and types of side chains that are present.

One issue in using a liquid as a stationary phase in GC is that some of this liquid will eventually leave the column over time in a process known as "column bleed." This process results in a change in the ability of the GC system to retain chemicals and may cause the signal of a detector to have a high background or to be noisy as the stationary phase leaves the column. Column bleed can be minimized by using a bonded phase (i.e., a stationary phase that is chemically linked or attached to the support) instead of a liquid as the stationary phase in the GC column. The resulting method is sometimes known as **bonded phase gas chromatography**.

### POINTS TO REMEMBER

**Types of Gas Chromatography Based on the Stationary Phase**
Gas-solid chromatography
Gas-liquid chromatography
Bonded phase gas chromatography

## Gas Chromatography Instrumentation
### Carrier Gas Sources and Flow Control

The typical components of a gas chromatograph are shown in Fig. 12.9. The carrier gas is usually supplied by a standard gas cylinder. However, a gas generator can also be connected to the GC system to isolate nitrogen from air or to produce hydrogen gas through the electrolysis of water. Good flow control is needed to maintain good column efficiency and provide reproducible retention times. The flow can be controlled by using a simple pressure regulator or a more sophisticated electronic device.

The choice of the carrier gas will depend on the expense, purity, and chemical or physical properties of the gas. Carrier gas impurities such as water, oxygen, and hydrocarbons can harm or alter the column and influence the performance of some detectors. Molecular sieves and traps are often used to remove water, hydrocarbons, oxygen, and particulate matter that may be present in the carrier gas.

Many GC detectors work best with certain types of carrier gases. For instance, nitrogen is often used as the carrier gas when working with a flame ionization detector (FID), electron capture detector (ECD), or thermal conductivity detector (TCD), as described in more detail later. Helium is often used with an FID or TCD, and nitrogen/argon-methane mixtures are used with an ECD.

### Injection Systems and Sample Derivatization

Most clinical GC methods make use of liquid-phase samples, from which the sample components are first extracted into a nonaqueous liquid or adsorbed onto a microextraction fiber. This liquid or microextraction fiber is then placed into the GC system by using a precise and rapid online injector (e.g., an autosampler or automated injection system). With packed columns, a glass microsyringe is used to inject a sample through a septum and into a heated injection port. *Volatile chemicals in the sample and the solvent are quickly vaporized in this heated port and swept into the column by the carrier gas.* Common problems during injection include septum leaks and the adsorption of sample components onto the septum. In addition, because the injection port is heated, thermal decomposition may occur and result in spurious peaks in the chromatogram for some compounds.

Because of the low sample capacities and slow carrier gas flow rates that are used with capillary columns, split and splitless injection techniques are used to introduce samples into such columns. For a split injection, only a small portion of the vaporized sample enters the column, with the remainder being passed through a side vent. In splitless injection, most of the sample enters the column. The split flow injection mode is used for samples that contain relatively high concentrations of the analytes, while the splitless mode is used for samples that contain lower concentrations. Temperature-programmable injection ports are also available and may be used in either injection mode to reduce the time that thermally unstable compounds are exposed to high temperatures in the port.

**Headspace analysis** is a sample introduction technique that can be used with aqueous solutions or samples that contain some nonvolatile components. In this method, a portion of the vapor phase (or "headspace") that is above a liquid or solid sample is used for the analysis. This vapor phase contains some of the more volatile sample components and can be directly injected onto a GC system. Headspace analysis can be carried out by using either a static method or a dynamic method. In the static method, the sample is placed in an enclosed container and allowed to reach equilibrium for the distribution of its components between the sample and the vapor phase above the sample. A portion of the vapor phase is then injected onto the GC system. In the dynamic method, an inert gas is passed through the sample and used to sweep away the volatile components. These components are then captured by a solid adsorbent or a cold trap and later injected onto the GC system.

Although a fairly large number of low-mass chemicals can be injected directly onto a GC system, many more are not sufficiently volatile or thermally stable for direct injection. A way to make a chemical more volatile and thermally stable is to alter its structure through derivatization. This usually involves replacing one or more polar groups on the analyte with less polar groups. A common example is the replacement of an active hydrogen on an alcohol, phenol, amine, or carboxylic acid group with a trimethylsilyl (TMS) group, producing a TMS derivative. Other examples include the use of alkylation (e.g., the formation of a methyl ester through the esterification of a carboxylic acid) or acylation (e.g., the production of an acetate derivative from an alcohol or amine). Some derivatization reactions can also be used to change the response of an analyte to certain detectors, such as an ECD through the addition of halogen atoms to a compound's structure.

## Columns and Supports

Both packed columns and capillary columns are used in GC. Packed GC columns are filled with support particles that contain the stationary phase and have typical inner diameters of 1 to 4 mm and lengths of 1 to 2 m. Packed GC columns are useful when it is necessary to apply a relatively large amount of a sample onto the GC system. However, packed columns also tend to have lower efficiencies than capillary columns, so they are mainly used in applications for which a relatively small number of compounds are to be separated.

Capillary columns, or open-tubular columns, consist of a column that has the stationary phase attached to or coated on its interior surface. Capillary columns have typical inner diameters of 0.1 to 0.75 mm and lengths that often range from 10 to 150 m. Capillary GC columns are usually made from fused silica capillaries that have a polyimide or aluminum coating on the outside to give the capillary sufficient strength and flexibility for use in a GC system. Although capillary columns have lower sample capacities than packed columns, they provide better peak resolution and higher efficiencies. These properties make capillary columns the most common type of support that is used in GC for analytical applications.

## Temperature Control

All GC systems require careful control of temperature with a column oven to obtain optimal performance and reliable results. The column may be maintained at a constant temperature (i.e., **isothermal elution**), or the temperature may be varied over time (i.e., **temperature programming**). Temperature programming is used for most clinical applications. In temperature programming, the sample components with the lowest boiling points and weakest interactions with the GC column will elute first, followed by chemicals that have higher boiling points and/or stronger interactions with the column. Temperature programming usually provides sharper and more distinct peaks in less time than can be obtained with isothermal elution. The main advantage of isothermal elution is that it can be faster for samples that do not contain a wide range of chemicals with different volatilities.

The thermal stabilities of the stationary phase and column are important to consider during the development of a GC method. Because each stationary phase has a specific temperature range over which it is stable, it is necessary to keep the column temperature within this usable range. Before any GC column is used for a routine analysis, it must be "thermally conditioned" by heating the column at various temperatures and for given lengths of time. This process helps remove volatile contaminants that may be initially present in the column or that have accumulated and can lead to unstable baselines. Preconditioned capillary columns are also available to minimize these problems.

## Gas Chromatography Detectors

*Flame ionization detector.* A variety of detectors can be used in GC systems (Table 12.2). An FID is commonly used with GC in clinical laboratories for the analysis of ethanol and other volatiles in blood or aqueous samples (Fig. 12.10). During the operation of an FID, the carrier gas that is leaving

## TABLE 12.2  Examples of Detectors Used in Gas Chromatography

| Type of Detector | Principle of Operation | Selectivity | Approximate Limit of Detection |
|---|---|---|---|
| Flame ionization detector (FID) | Production of gas phase ions from combustion of organic compounds | General—Organic compounds | $10^{-12}$ g carbon |
| Nitrogen-phosphorus detector (NPD) | Heated alkali bead selectively ionizes N- or P-containing compounds | Nitrogen- or phosphorus-containing compounds | $10^{-14}$ to $10^{-13}$ g nitrogen or phosphorus |
| Electron capture detector (ECD) | Capture of electrons by chemicals with electronegative groups | Chemicals with electronegative groups | $10^{-15}$ to $10^{-13}$ g |
| Mass spectrometry (MS) | Production of gas phase ions, followed by separation/analysis of these ions based on their mass-to-charge ratios | Universal—full-scan mode Selective—selected ion monitoring mode (SIM) | $10^{-10}$ to $10^{-9}$ g full-scan mode $10^{-12}$ to $10^{-11}$ g SIM mode |
| Thermal conductivity detector (TCD) | Measurement of change in thermal conductivity of carrier gas as compounds elute from the column | Universal | $10^{-9}$ g |
| Flame photometric detector (FPD) | P- and S-containing compounds emit light when burned in a flame; emitted light is detected | Phosphorus and sulfur-containing compounds | $10^{-12}$ g phosphorus $10^{-11}$ g sulfur |

Portions of this table are based on data from Hage DS, Carr JD. *Analytical Chemistry and Quantitative Analysis.* New York: Pearson; 2011, and references cited therein.

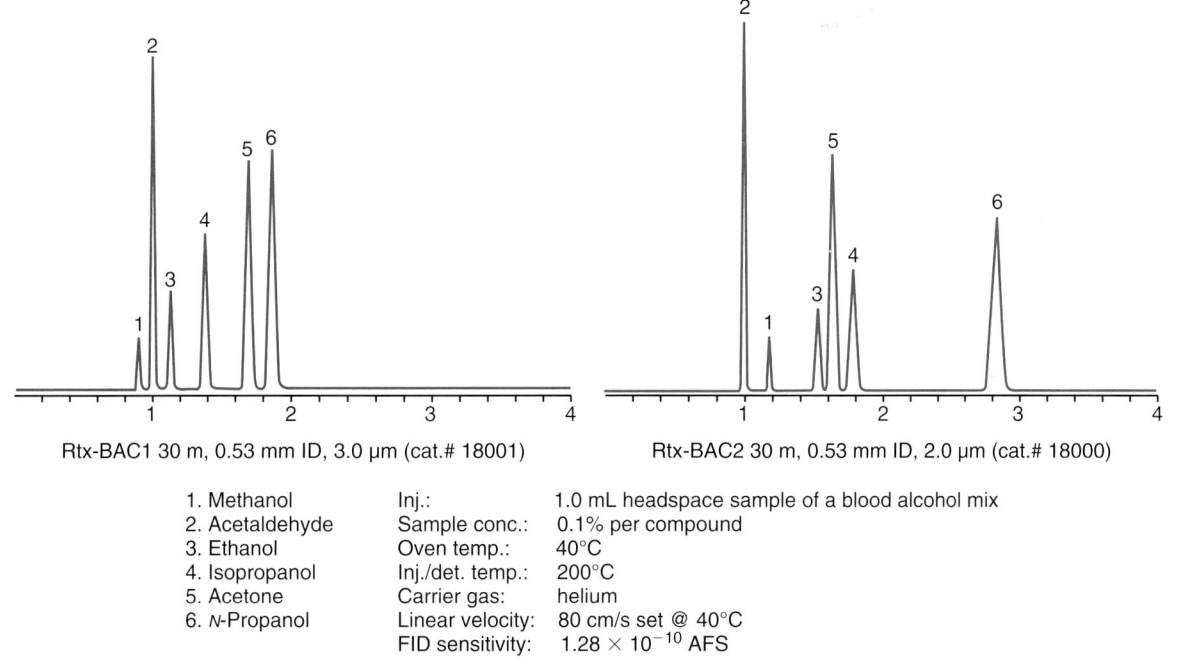

Rtx-BAC1 30 m, 0.53 mm ID, 3.0 μm (cat.# 18001)        Rtx-BAC2 30 m, 0.53 mm ID, 2.0 μm (cat.# 18000)

1. Methanol
2. Acetaldehyde
3. Ethanol
4. Isopropanol
5. Acetone
6. *N*-Propanol

Inj.: 1.0 mL headspace sample of a blood alcohol mix
Sample conc.: 0.1% per compound
Oven temp.: 40°C
Inj./det. temp.: 200°C
Carrier gas: helium
Linear velocity: 80 cm/s set @ 40°C
FID sensitivity: $1.28 \times 10^{-10}$ AFS

**Fig. 12.10** Chromatograms obtained during the analysis of volatile organic compounds when using headspace analysis and gas chromatography with a flame ionization detector *(FID)*. (Courtesy Restek Corporation, Bellefonte, PA.)

the column is mixed with hydrogen, and the eluting compounds are burned by a flame that is surrounded by air and an oxygen-rich environment. This process produces gas-phase ions from organic compounds, with these ions being detected and measured by an electrode that is positioned above the flame.

The advantages of an FID include its simplicity, reliability, and ease of operation. Another advantage of an FID is that this detector gives little or no signal for common carrier gases (e.g., He, Ar, or $N_2$) or typical contaminants in such gases (e.g., $O_2$ and $H_2O$). An FID is easy to use with temperature programming and is a good general detector for the routine

clinical analysis of organic compounds. One disadvantage of the FID is its destructive nature; additional downstream detectors cannot be used.

***Nitrogen-phosphorus detector.*** The nitrogen-phosphorus detector (NPD) is similar to an FID but instead creates gas-phase ions by using an electrically heated alkali bead that is generally made of rubidium. This heated bead is placed directly above the point where a mixture of the carrier gas and hydrogen enter the detector. Ions are generated at or above the surface of the heated alkali bead, which supplies electrons to electronegative compounds and leads to the formation of negatively charged ions, which are then measured at an electrode.

Nitrogen- or phosphorus-containing compounds are especially good at creating ions in an NPD. This feature makes the NPD useful for monitoring low concentrations of analytes that have nitrogen or phosphorus in their structures, such as many organic bases and acids. This type of detector does not respond to common GC carrier gases or their impurities. However, it is necessary to regularly change the alkali bead in this detector because this bead will degrade over time.

*Electron capture detector.* The ECD is a selective GC detector based on the capture of secondary electrons by electronegative compounds that are eluting from the column. High-energy electrons, or beta particles, are provided in an ECD by a radioactive source such as $^{63}$Ni or $^{3}$H. These beta particles collide with the carrier gas and lead to the release of a large number of secondary electrons. When only the carrier gas is passing through this detector, a consistent supply of the secondary electrons is created, which is collected at an electrode and measured. When a chemical with electronegative groups elutes from the column, some of these secondary electrons are captured and fewer reach the electrode, producing a change in the signal.

An ECD can provide both selective and sensitive detection for chemicals that contain electronegative groups. This includes chemicals that contain halogen atoms (I, Br, Cl, and F) or nitro groups ($-NO_2$). It also includes chemicals that are polycyclic aromatic hydrocarbons, anhydrides, or conjugated carbonyl compounds, among others. Derivatization with reagents containing chlorinated or fluorinated groups can be used with some chemicals to allow them to be monitored with an ECD. Large carrier gases such as argon and nitrogen are usually employed with an ECD because it is easy for them to collide with beta particles and to produce secondary electrons. Some methane is also usually combined with these carrier gases to produce a stable detector response. Because an ECD uses a radioactive source, this source needs to be replaced on a regular basis by a certified technician.

*Mass spectrometry.* Mass spectrometers are also used as detectors for GC. This combination is known as **gas chromatography/mass spectrometry (GC/MS)**. GC/MS is a powerful method for identifying and quantifying analytes. Ionization methods that are often used in GC/MS include electron impact ionization (EI) and chemical ionization (CI). Mass analyzers that are commonly used in GC/MS are quadrupole mass analyzers and ion traps (see Chapter 13).

In the "full-scan mode" of GC/MS, information is acquired on a wide range of ions. This mode is used when the goal is to detect many compounds in a single run or to provide data that can be used to identify an unknown compound from its mass spectrum. GC/MS can also examine specific analytes by using selected ion monitoring (SIM) to monitor only a few ions that are representative of the analytes of interest. SIM is used when selective detection and low detection limits are desired.

*Other gas chromatography detectors.* There are a variety of other detectors that can also be part of a GC system. A TCD is a general detector that can monitor both inorganic and organic compounds based on their ability to change how the carrier gas/analyte mixture will conduct heat away from a hot wire. The carrier gas used with a TCD is often helium or hydrogen, which have large differences in their ability to conduct heat when compared with most organic or inorganic compounds. The primary advantage of a TCD is its ability to detect many types of chemicals. This detector is nondestructive and can easily be combined with a second detector. However, a TCD can also respond to contaminants in the carrier gas and give a change in the background response during temperature programming. In addition, the TCD tends to have much higher detection limits than other common GC detectors.

Another group of GC detectors makes use of the interactions of chemicals with light. One example is a flame photometric detector (FPD). An FPD is a selective detector for phosphorus- or sulfur-containing compounds. Like an FID, an FPD passes the eluting chemicals into a flame, but the FPD then measures the release of light from excited-state phosphorus- or sulfur-containing species.

## Data Acquisition and System Control

Computers are used to control and automate GC systems, as well as to collect and process data. The computer can regulate parameters such as the (1) carrier gas composition and flow rate; (2) column back pressure; (3) temperature; (4) sample injection process; (5) detector selection and operation; and (6) timing steps during system operation. In terms of data acquisition, the computer can monitor and store the signals that are generated by the GC system's detectors. The computer system can also be used to search databases to aid in the identification of analytes based on their retention times or their response at the detector.

# LIQUID CHROMATOGRAPHY

**Liquid chromatography (LC)** is a type of chromatography in which the mobile phase is a liquid. Separations in LC are based on the distribution of chemicals between a liquid mobile phase and a stationary phase. LC is the dominant type of chromatography that is currently used for chemical analysis in clinical or biomedical laboratories. A key advantage of this method over GC is the ability of LC to work directly with liquid samples, as are often encountered with clinical or biological specimens.

The supports originally used in LC columns were based on large and irregularly shaped particulate supports like those used in packed columns for GC. These supports were useful in preparative work but were not suitable for many analytical applications because they tended to result in broad peaks and separations with low resolution. Work in the 1960s resulted in smaller, more mechanically stable and more efficient supports for LC, along with the instrumentation that could be used with such materials. This resulted in a method that is now known as **high-performance liquid chromatography (HPLC)**. The use of these more efficient supports made it possible to obtain narrower peaks, better separations, and lower limits of detection than traditional LC. These reasons, along with the ability of HPLC to be used as an automated method, have made this technique the method of choice for most routine chemical separations and analysis methods.

**Adsorption chromatography**
Separation based on adsorption of
chemicals to the surface of a support

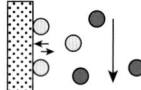

**Partition chromatography**
Separation based on partitioning of chemicals
into a layer of the stationary phase

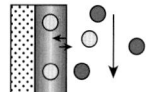

**Ion-exchange chromatography**
Separation of ions based on their binding to
fixed charges on a support

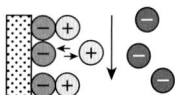

**Size-exclusion chromatography**
Separation of chemicals based on their size
and ability to enter a porous support

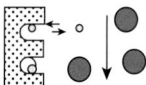

**Affinity chromatography**
Separation of chemicals based on their interactions
with a biologically related binding agent

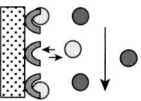

Fig. 12.11 Main types of liquid chromatography based on their separation mechanisms.

Because the pressure drop across a packed bed column increases with a decrease in the support particle's diameter, relatively high pressures can be required to pump liquids through HPLC columns. As a result, this technique has also been referred to as *high-pressure liquid chromatography*. Most modern HPLC systems can work at pressures up to 5000 to 6000 psi. Specialized systems that use even smaller diameter supports and that can operate at pressures up to 15,000 psi have recently been developed resulting in the technique called **ultra-high-performance liquid chromatography (UPLC or UHPLC)**.

One important difference between LC and GC is that the retention of chemicals in LC can depend on the interactions of these chemicals with both the mobile phase and stationary phase. This means the composition of the mobile phase is important to consider when adjusting the retention of a chemical in LC. The term *strong mobile phase* is used to describe a mobile phase that leads to weak retention for an analyte on a given type of stationary phase. The weakest retention for a chemical will occur when this substance favors staying in the mobile phase instead of the stationary phase. The term *weak mobile phase* refers to the opposite situation, in which a chemical favors the stationary phase versus the mobile phase and has its highest retention within a given column.

---

### POINTS TO REMEMBER

**Mobile Phase Strength in Liquid Chromatography**
- The mobile phase is important in liquid chromatography for determining chemical retention.
- A "strong mobile phase" is a mobile phase that leads to weak retention for an analyte on a given type of stationary phase and column.
- A "weak mobile phase" is a mobile phase in which a chemical favors the stationary phase and has a high retention on a given column.

## Types of Liquid Chromatography
### Adsorption Chromatography

Liquid chromatographic methods are classified according to the mechanisms by which they separate chemicals (Fig. 12.11). **Adsorption chromatography** is a type of LC in which chemicals are retained based on their adsorption and desorption at the surface of a support that is not derivatized (see Fig. 12.11). This method is sometimes referred to as *liquid-solid chromatography* (LSC). Retention in this method is based on the competition of the analyte with the mobile phase as both bind to the support. The degree of a chemical's retention in adsorption chromatography will depend on (1) the binding strength of this chemical to the support, (2) the surface area of the support, (3) the amount of mobile phase that is displaced from the support by the chemical, and (4) the binding strength of the mobile phase to the support.

Three types of adsorbents are generally used in adsorption chromatography: (1) polar acidic supports, (2) polar basic supports, and (3) nonpolar supports. The most common polar and acidic support is silica, which can adsorb polar compounds and works particularly well for basic substances. Alumina is a polar and basic adsorbent that also retains polar compounds, and especially polar acidic substances. Florisil is a polar and basic support that can be used in place of alumina. Nonpolar supports include charcoal and polystyrene.

### Partition Chromatography

**Partition chromatography** is an LC method in which solutes are separated based on their partitioning between the liquid mobile phase and a stationary phase that is coated or bonded onto a solid support (see Fig. 12.11). The support in most types of partition chromatography is silica. This method originally involved coating a liquid stationary phase onto such a support. However, most current columns in partition chromatography employ bonded stationary phases, which are more stable than coated stationary phases and provide better column efficiencies.

There are two main types of partition chromatography: normal-phase chromatography and reversed-phase chromatography. **Normal-phase chromatography** uses a polar stationary phase and is also known as *normal-phase liquid chromatography* (NPLC). The stationary phase in this method typically contains groups that can form hydrogen bonds or undergo dipole-related interactions. Examples of these bonded stationary phases are those that contain aminopropyl groups, cyano groups, and diol groups. Because this type of chromatography uses a polar stationary phase, it will have its highest retention for polar compounds. A weak mobile phase in this method will be a nonpolar liquid. A strong mobile phase is a more polar liquid, such as methanol or water.

Normal-phase chromatography can be used in many of the same applications as adsorption chromatography based on silica or alumina supports. These applications usually involve the separation or analysis of chemicals that are present in organic solvents and of substances that contain one or more polar functional groups. Examples of chemicals for which normal-phase chromatography has been used include steroids and sugars.

The second type of partition chromatography is **reversed-phase chromatography**, which is also known as *reversed-phase liquid chromatography* (RPLC). Reversed-phase chromatography uses a nonpolar stationary phase and is the most popular type of LC. One reason for this is that the weak mobile phase in reversed-phase chromatography is a polar solvent, such as water. This property makes this type of LC convenient for the analysis and separation of chemicals in aqueous-based systems, such as serum, urine, and blood. A strong mobile phase in this method is a liquid that is less polar than water, such as acetonitrile or methanol. Due to the presence of a nonpolar stationary phase, nonpolar compounds will have the highest retention in reversed-phase chromatography.

There are many applications for reversed-phase chromatography in clinical chemistry and biomedical research (see the example in Fig. 12.2). Examples of chemicals that can be separated or analyzed by this method include drugs, drug metabolites, amino acids, peptides, proteins, carbohydrates, lipids, and bile acids. It is important to consider both the type of analyte and support that are being used in these separations. For instance, large chemicals such as peptides or proteins will require reversed-phase supports with larger pore sizes than the supports that are used for separating small molecules.

The most common stationary phases used in reversed-phase chromatography are based on octadecyl ($C_{18}$), octyl ($C_8$), phenyl, or butyl ($C_4$) groups that are attached to a support such as silica. Alternative materials such as porous graphite, fluorinated hydrocarbons, and hydrophobic stationary phases with embedded polar groups can also be used. Silica tends to dissolve slowly at a pH greater than 8 or at a pH below 2, so separations that make use of silica supports are usually done in this pH range. Some of the other supports used in reversed-phase chromatography, such as polystyrene or porous graphite, are stable over a broader pH range (e.g., pH 2 to 13).

## Ion-Exchange Chromatography

**Ion-exchange chromatography** (IEC) is a type of LC in which ions are separated by their adsorption onto a support that contains fixed charges at its surface (see Fig. 12.11). Depending on the charge of the groups that make up the stationary phase, the types of ions that bind to the column may be either cations (i.e., positively charged ions) or anions (i.e., negatively charged ions). These two methods are referred to as **cation-exchange chromatography and anion-exchange chromatography**, respectively.

Supports for cation-exchange chromatography contain negatively charged groups. These groups may be the conjugate bases of strong acids, such as sulfonate ions that are formed by the deprotonation of sulfonic acid, or the conjugate bases of weak acids, such as those produced from carboxyl or carboxymethyl groups. The supports used in anion-exchange chromatography are usually the conjugate acids of strongly basic quaternary amines, such as triethylaminoethyl groups, or the conjugate acids of weak bases, such as aminoethyl (AE) or diethylaminoethyl (DEAE) groups. Supports that can be modified to contain these charged groups include silica, polystyrene, and carbohydrate-based materials such as agarose or cellulose.

A strong mobile phase in IEC is usually a mobile phase that contains a high concentration of competing ions. A weak mobile phase is one that contains few or no competing ions, or that otherwise promotes binding by charged analytes to the column. The retention of ions in this method may also be affected by (1) pH, (2) the type of competing ion that is used, (3) the type of fixed charges that are used as the stationary phase, and (4) the density of these fixed charges on the support.

IEC has a number of clinical applications. Examples are the separation and analysis of amino acids and hemoglobin variants. IEC is also frequently used as a preparative tool for purifying proteins, peptides, and nucleotides. A modified form of IEC known as *ion chromatography* can be used with a conductivity detector to analyze small inorganic and organic ions.

## Size-Exclusion Chromatography

**Size-exclusion chromatography** (SEC) is an LC technique that separates analytes based on size (see Figs. 12.11 and 12.12). In this method, a porous support is used that has an inert surface with little or no interactions with the sample components. This support should also have a range of pore sizes that are similar to the sizes of the compounds that are to be separated. As a sample travels through this type of column, small sample components can enter all or most of the pores while larger components may enter only a few or none of the pores. The result is a separation based on size or molar mass, in which the larger components elute first from the column.

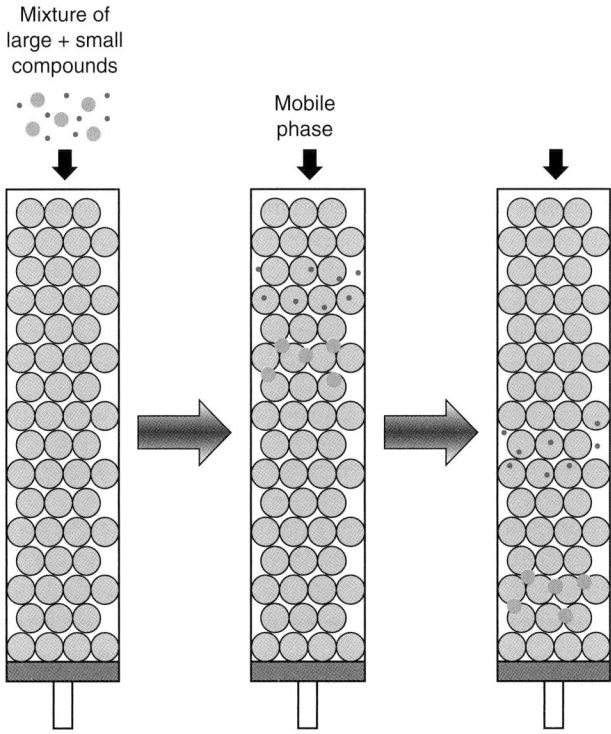

Fig. 12.12 General principle of size-exclusion chromatography. This method separates compounds based on their size by using a column that contains a porous support.

Many types of porous supports have been used in SEC. Cross-linked carbohydrate-based supports like dextran and agarose are often used for work with aqueous-based samples and biological compounds such as proteins or nucleic acids. Polyacrylamide gel and modified silica or glass beads can also be used for aqueous samples and biological compounds. Polystyrene is usually employed as the support when SEC is to be used with synthetic polymers and samples that are present in organic solvents. For each of these supports, the range of pore sizes that are present will determine the sizes of the injected compounds that can be separated.

The mobile phase in SEC can be a polar solvent, such as water, or a nonpolar solvent, which is usually tetrahydrofuran. Because the stationary phase is based on a physical difference in the accessible pore volume for the solutes, rather than being based on chemical interactions, there is no weak mobile phase or strong mobile phase in this method. The choice of the mobile phase is instead determined by the solubility and the stability of the analytes and of the support and the column. If water or an aqueous mobile phase is used in SEC, the resulting method is often called *gel filtration chromatography*. If an organic mobile phase is used, the size-exclusion method is referred to as *gel permeation chromatography*.

SEC in the form of gel filtration is useful for identifying intact complexes of agents such as lipoproteins, antibody-antigen complexes, and the binding of proteins with their target compounds. SEC is also often used to exchange buffers,

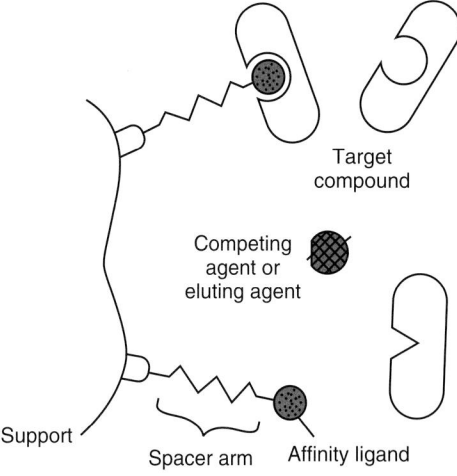

Fig. 12.13 General mechanism of separation in affinity chromatography. The target analyte is first allowed to bind to the immobilized affinity ligand in the column. After the non-retained sample components have been washed from the column, the retained analyte is later released by using an elution buffer. This elution may be based on a nonspecific method (e.g., the addition of a chaotropic agent or a change in pH), or it may be accomplished by adding a biospecific competing agent to the mobile phase to displace the analyte from the column.

to remove salts from large sample components, or to remove small molecules from large biomolecules (e.g., the isolation of drugs, fatty acids, and peptides from proteins). In addition, SEC can be used to estimate the molecular weight of a biomolecule, such as a protein or nucleic acid, or to characterize the distribution of molecular weights for a polymer.

## Affinity Chromatography and Chiral Separations

**Affinity chromatography (AC)** is an LC method that makes use of biologically related interactions for the retention and separation of chemicals (see Figs. 12.11 and 12.13). This method uses the selective, reversible interactions that are found in many biological systems, such as the binding of an antibody with an antigen or the interactions of an enzyme with a substrate or inhibitor. This type of binding is used in AC by immobilizing one of a pair of interacting compounds onto a support for use as the stationary phase. This immobilized agent is called the *affinity ligand* and creates a column that can bind and capture the complementary compound from samples.

AC is usually carried out by applying a sample to the column under conditions that allow strong and specific binding of the affinity ligand to its target compound. This is done in the presence of an application buffer, which mimics the pH and natural or preferred conditions for binding between the affinity ligand and the target. As the target binds to the column under these conditions, most other sample components are washed away. The retained target is then later released by using an elution buffer that either contains a competing agent that will displace the target from the affinity ligand or that uses a change in conditions such as pH, ionic strength, or polarity of the mobile phase to decrease the strength of binding between the target and affinity ligand. After the target has been eluted for detection or further use, the application buffer can be passed again through the column and the system is allowed to regenerate prior to the application of the next sample. For systems with weak-to-moderate binding strengths, it is also possible to use isocratic elution for both sample application and target elution. This second type of elution is usually employed in chiral separations.

There are various types of AC. Bioaffinity chromatography is the most common type of AC and involves the use of a biological binding agent as the affinity ligand. Examples of bioaffinity chromatography are the purification of an enzyme by using an immobilized inhibitor, and the use of lectins (i.e., nonimmune system proteins that can bind carbohydrate residues) such as concanavalin A for the isolation of glycopeptides, glycoproteins, and glycolipids. Immunoaffinity chromatography (IAC) is a type of bioaffinity chromatography that uses an antibody or antibody-related agent as the affinity ligand. The selectivity of this method has made it popular for the isolation and analysis of many targets, as well as a tool for sample pretreatment prior to analysis by other methods.

Another group of methods in AC are those that use nonbiological binding agents. Immobilized metal-ion affinity chromatography (IMAC) is a method in which the affinity ligand is a metal ion, such as $Ni^{2+}$, that is complexed with an immobilized chelating agent. This technique is frequently used to isolate recombinant histidine-tagged proteins and has been used for the isolation or analysis of phosphorylated proteins in proteomics. Boronate affinity chromatography uses an affinity ligand that is boronic acid or a related derivative, which is useful in binding to compounds that contain *cis*-diol groups, such as polysaccharides, glycoproteins, and catecholamines. An important clinical application of boronate AC is its use in the analysis and isolation of glycosylated hemoglobin in blood from diabetic patients.

Many biological molecules (including amino acids, peptides, and proteins) occur as stereoisomers, or in specific chiral forms. As a result, it is not unusual for the different chiral forms of a drug to have some variations in their interactions with these biological agents. The two mirror-image chiral forms of a drug (or enantiomers) generally have identical physical and chemical properties and cannot be separated by most types of chromatography, which tend to use nonstereoselective (or achiral) stationary phases. However, it may be possible to separate the enantiomers and stereoisomers of a drug or target compound if the stationary phase is also chiral and can interact with these compounds in a stereospecific manner. This type of medium is known as a **chiral stationary phase (CSP)**. Carbohydrates, peptides, enzymes, and other proteins have all been used as CSPs. Cyclodextrins, which are cyclic polymers of glucose, are an important set of carbohydrates that have been used for separating many types of chiral compounds in both LC and GC.

### Hydrophilic Interaction Liquid Chromatography and Mixed-Mode Methods

There are a number of LC methods that combine several separation modes. One example is **hydrophilic interaction liquid chromatography (HILIC)**. HILIC is a type of partition chromatography that uses a polar stationary phase, and in which

chemicals partition between an organic-rich region in the mobile phase and a more polar water-enriched layer that is at or near the surface of a polar support. The surface of the support, which can often undergo hydrogen bonding or dipole-related interactions with the applied solutes, may also have charged groups that can interact with these compounds. These features make HILIC a variation of normal-phase chromatography that is combined with some of the characteristics of reversed-phase chromatography and IEC. HILIC and related methods have become popular in areas such as proteomics and glycomics. Advantages of these methods include (1) their ability to give better separations for polar compounds than can be obtained by reversed-phase chromatography, (2) the greater ease with which they can be used with aqueous samples and in solubilizing polar compounds compared with normal-phase chromatography, and (3) the ability to couple these methods with mass spectrometry.

**Ion-pair chromatography (IPC)** is a technique that combines columns that are used in reversed-phase chromatography with the ability to separate ionic compounds based on their charges, as is done in IEC. This method is carried out by adding an ion-pairing agent to the mobile phase for a reversed-phase column. The ion-pairing agent is usually a surfactant that has a charged group at one end and a nonpolar tail or group at the other end. The purpose of the ion-pairing agent is to combine with ions of the opposite charge in the sample, thus also allowing their retention on the reversed-phase column through the ion-pairing agent's nonpolar tail or through the formation of a neutral complex. IPC is useful in separating charged compounds that are poorly resolved by IEC. Applications of IPC include the separation and analysis of catecholamines, drugs, and nucleic acids.

## Liquid Chromatography Instrumentation
### Mobile Phase Reservoirs and Delivery Systems

The major components of a system used in HPLC are shown in Fig. 12.14. The mobile phases in LC are contained in solvent reservoirs, which are often glass bottles or flasks into which "feed lines" to the pump are inserted. Filters are often placed at the inlets of these feed lines to prevent any particles in the mobile phase from moving on to the rest of the system. Most mobile phase reservoirs also have a means of "sparging" the mobile phase by bubbling through a gas such as helium or nitrogen to remove dissolved air or oxygen that may interfere with the response of some detectors. The removal of air and oxygen, or "degassing," can also be achieved by applying a vacuum to the reservoir by placing gas exchange devices or gas filters in the flow path leading from the reservoir. Degassing the mobile phase is important to avoid dissolved gases coming out of solution and forming bubbles as the pressure drops from the column to the detector.

The composition and "strength" of the mobile phase are factors that can be used to adjust and control a separation in LC. If the same mobile phase is used throughout the separation, this approach is known as **isocratic elution**. If the composition of the mobile phase is varied over time, the method is called **solvent programming** or gradient elution (Fig. 12.15). Solvent programming begins with a weak mobile

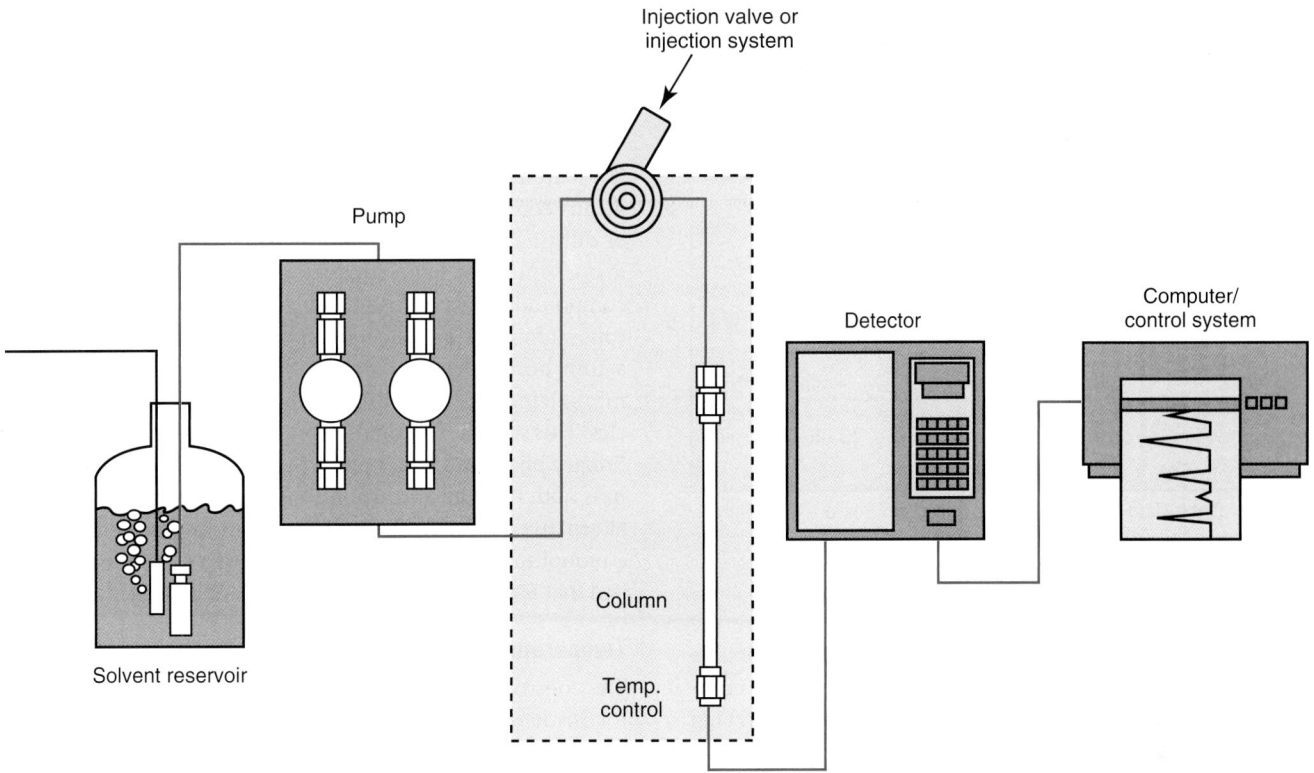

**Fig. 12.14** General design of a liquid chromatograph, as used in high-performance liquid chromatography. (Modified from a figure courtesy Restek Corporation, Bellefonte, PA.)

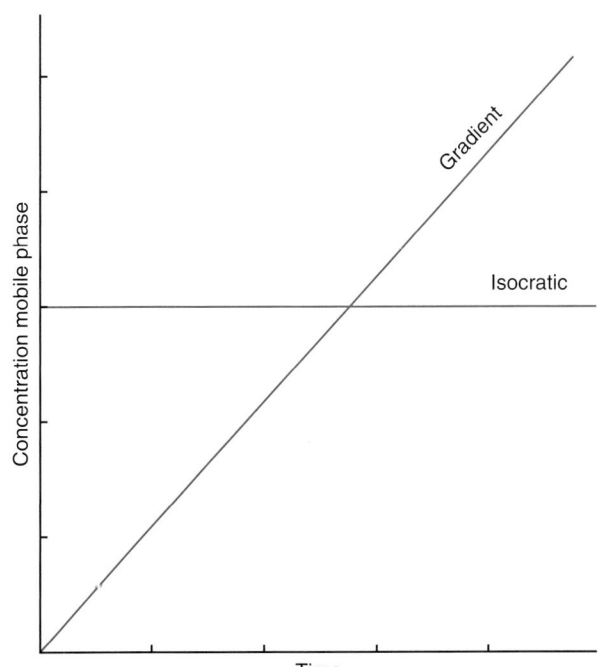

**Fig. 12.15** Examples of isocratic elution (i.e., constant mobile phase composition) or linear gradient elution based on solvent programming (i.e., varying mobile phase composition).

phase, to allow chemicals with weak retention to interact with the column, and then goes to a stronger mobile phase to elute chemicals with moderate or high retention. This change in the mobile phase can be made in one or more steps and may involve a linear or nonlinear change over time.

Several types of pumps have been used in LC. Peristaltic and diaphragm-type pumps can be used with columns that are operated at low pressures, as are encountered in classic and low-to-medium performance LC. Reciprocating pumps and syringe pumps are used to achieve the higher pressures that are needed to deliver the mobile phase in HPLC. Reciprocating pumps are used at flow rates in the mL/min range and have a piston that moves in and out of the solvent chamber, with check valves being used to keep the flow of the mobile phase moving from the pump inlet to the outlet. The reciprocating action of the piston does generate some pulsation in the pressure and mobile phase flow, which can increase the baseline noise at the detector but can be minimized by electronic control of the pump and by placing pulse dampers in the flow path. Syringe pumps use a solvent chamber in a syringe to continuously deliver the mobile phase to the rest of the system. These pumps can deliver essentially pulse-free flow and can be used at much lower flow rates than reciprocal pumps (e.g., flow rates in the μL/min range).

## Injection Systems and Sample Derivatization

Various approaches can be used to introduce a sample into an LC system. Important characteristics to consider when selecting an injection system are its (1) reproducibility, (2) the amount of sample carryover from one injection to the next, and (3) the range of volumes that can be injected. The most widely used approach in HPLC is a fixed-loop injector that is switched into or out of the flow path by manual control or through the use of an autoinjector.

**TABLE 12.3  Typical Column Sizes Used in Analytical High-Performance Liquid Chromatography**

| Type of Column | Typical Inner Diameter (I.D.) and Lengths | Typical Flow Rate Range |
| --- | --- | --- |
| Conventional packed column | 4–5 mm I.D. × 5–30 cm | 1–3 mL/min |
| Narrow bore column | 2–3 mm I.D. × 5–15 cm | 0.2–0.6 mL/min |
| Microbore column | 1–2 mm I.D. × 10–100 cm | 0.05–0.2 mL/min |
| Packed capillary | 0.1–0.5 mm I.D. × 20–200 cm | 0.1–20 µL/min |
| Open tubular column | 0.01–0.075 mm I.D. × 1–100 cm | 0.05–2 µL/min |

Portions of the data in this table are based on Poole CF, Poole SK. *Chromatography Today.* New York: Elsevier; 1991.

Derivatization is sometimes used in LC to improve the response of compounds to the detector. It is also possible to use derivatization in LC to alter the retention of a compound on the column. There are two main ways of carrying out derivatization in LC: (1) precolumn derivatization and (2) postcolumn derivatization. Precolumn derivatization is done before the sample is injected and can be used to alter a compound's retention or to increase the signal it generates at the detector. Postcolumn derivatization is carried out online as compounds elute from a column and is used only to improve the response of the detector to those compounds.

### Columns and Supports

The columns in LC can have various combinations of packing materials and diameters or lengths. In the clinical laboratory, most packed HPLC columns are made of tubes based on stainless steel or pressure-resistant polymers with internal diameters that range from 4 to 5 mm and lengths that range from 5 to 30 cm (Table 12.3). An inlet filter may be present to remove particulate matter, and a short guard column that contains the same packing material may be placed before the longer analytical HPLC column to protect and extend the usable life of the HPLC column.

Better efficiencies and lower detection limits are achieved with HPLC columns that have longer lengths and smaller inner diameters, including narrow bore columns (with approximate inner diameters of 2 to 3 mm) and microbore columns (with approximate inner diameters of 1 to 2 mm). These small-diameter columns may also require lower flow rates and smaller volumes of the mobile phase for their operation than the longer conventional packed columns. Capillary columns may also sometimes be used in LC for work with flow rates in the mid-to-low µL/min range.

The most common type of support in LC is a packed bed of small particles, which are usually porous supports with diameters in the range of 1.8 to 10 µm. A smaller diameter for these supports, as is used in UPLC, provides better efficiency but also leads to an increase in back pressure across the column.

Low to medium performance separations, which have much lower operating pressures than HPLC, typically use packing materials such as cross-linked dextran or agarose, which consist of particles with diameters of 50 to 200 µm.

When using porous support particles, the mobile phase flows around the support but not through the particle. This means compounds must travel within the particle by means of diffusion, which is a relatively slow process that can be a major source of band-broadening. The distance that these compounds must diffuse can be reduced by using a nonporous support or a pellicular support, in which the latter has a thin porous layer or porous shell. Another approach for minimizing this band-broadening is to use perfusion particles. This support has small pores that contain most of the stationary phase and larger pores that allow the mobile phase to pass both through and around the support particles. Another alternative support that can be used to improve efficiency is a monolithic support, which consists of a continuous porous bed that is usually prepared from silica or an organic polymer.

### Temperature Control

The control of column temperature can be an important factor in determining the reproducibility and efficiency of an LC separation. Temperature control of an LC column can be achieved by using temperature-controlled column chambers, water jackets, blankets, and heating/cooling blocks.

### Liquid Chromatography Detectors

There are many types of detectors that can be used in LC (Table 12.4). A key component for most of these detectors is the flow cell through which the mobile phase and eluting compounds from the column must pass to provide a response. A postcolumn reactor may also be present between the column and detector to derivatize some of the eluting compounds and to generate products that give a stronger and more specific signal at the detector.

*Absorbance detectors.* The absorption of ultraviolet (UV) or visible (vis) light is often used to detect compounds as they elute from an LC column. Many of the absorbance detectors that are used in LC can measure the absorption of UV light at wavelengths in the range of 190 to 400 nm or of visible light in the range of 400 to 700 nm. Many organic compounds with aromatic groups or double or triple bonds absorb light between 250 and 300 nm. Other organic compounds, such as those containing amide bonds or carboxylic acids, can absorb in the range of 190 to 220 nm. In addition, some ions, inorganic compounds, and metal complexes can be detected by their absorption of light in the UV or visible range.

There are several types of absorbance detectors that can be used in LC. Fixed-wavelength absorbance detectors have the simplest design and are used to monitor absorbance at a particular wavelength or wavelength band. A variable-wavelength absorbance detector has a more flexible design that can operate at a wavelength that is selected from a broad wavelength range. A photodiode array detector (PDA) is an absorbance detector that uses an array of small detector cells

## TABLE 12.4  Examples of Detectors Used in Liquid Chromatography

| Type of Detector | Principle of Operation | Range of Application | Detection Limit |
|---|---|---|---|
| Absorbance detector | Measures absorbance of light at a given wavelength or set of wavelengths | Compounds with chromophores that can absorb ultraviolet or visible light | $10^{-10}$ to $10^{-9}$ g |
| Fluorescence detector | Measures ability of chemicals to absorb and reemit light through fluorescence | Compounds with fluorophores | $10^{-12}$ to $10^{-9}$ g |
| Electrochemical detector | Measures current or charge as a result of chemical oxidation or reduction | Electrochemically active compounds | $10^{-11}$ to $10^{-9}$ g |
| Conductivity detector | Measures change in conductivity of the mobile phase as ions elute from the column | General for ionic solutes | $10^{-9}$ g |
| Refractive index detector | Measures change in refractive index of the mobile phase as compounds elute the column | Universal | $10^{-7}$ to $10^{-6}$ g |
| Mass spectrometry | Production of gas phase ions, followed by separation/analysis of these ions based on their mass-to-charge ratios | Universal—full-scan mode Selective—selected ion monitoring (SIM) mode | $10^{-10}$ to $10^{-9}$ g (full-scan mode) $10^{-12}$ g or lower (SIM mode) |

Portions of the data in this table are based on Poole CF, Poole SK. *Chromatography Today.* New York: Elsevier; 1991.

to measure the change in absorbance at many wavelengths simultaneously, which can be valuable in identifying overlapping peaks or in identifying analytes in complex samples such as urine and serum.

The use of an absorbance detector requires solvents and mobile phase components that have little or no absorption of light at the wavelengths of interest. Effective degassing of the mobile phase is important to minimize bubble formation, which can interfere with absorbance measurements. The use of some back pressure across the detector can further reduce bubble formation. However, care must be taken with this approach to avoid exceeding the usable pressure range of the detector.

***Fluorescence detectors.*** Fluorescence detectors measure the ability of a chemical to absorb light at one wavelength and reemit the light at a different, longer wavelength. Fluorescence detectors in LC are generally much more selective and have better limits of detection than absorbance detectors for chemicals that are naturally fluorescent or that can be converted into a fluorescent derivative. Both precolumn and postcolumn derivatization have been used to modify chemicals (e.g., amino acids, peptides, and proteins) for this type of detector.

***Electrochemical and conductivity detectors.*** The combination of an electrochemical detector with LC is often known as **liquid chromatography–electrochemical detection (LC-EC)**. In an amperometric electrochemical detector (see Chapter 10), an electroactive chemical that enters the flow cell may be oxidized or reduced at an electrode that is held at a constant potential. The current needed for or generated by this process is then measured, with the magnitude of the current being proportional to the concentration of the analyte. Electroactive compounds of clinical interest and that can be examined by this process include catecholamines, ascorbic acid, and thiol-containing compounds such as homocysteine. In addition, electrochemically active tags (e.g., bromine) can be added to compounds such as

unsaturated fatty acids or prostaglandins for use with this type of detector.

Coulometric detectors measure the amount of charge that is required for a given electrochemical reaction. These detectors are selective, sensitive, and have reasonably wide linear ranges. Coulometric detectors are used in clinical laboratories for the analysis of metanephrines, vanillylmandelic acid, homovanillic acid, and 5-hydroxyindole acetic acid in human urine.

A conductivity detector measures the ability of the mobile phase and its contents to conduct a current when they are placed in an electrical field. This type of detector is often used in combination with IEC to monitor salt gradients, or in ion chromatography to monitor the elution of charged analytes. Conductivity detectors have been used to measure compounds such as sulfate in biological fluids.

***Refractive index detectors.*** A refractive index (RI) detector in LC measures the change in the refraction of light as chemicals pass within the mobile phase through a flow cell. An important advantage for this type of detector is that it can monitor substances such as alcohols, salts, and sugars that do not absorb light at usable wavelengths or fluoresce. One disadvantage of this type of detector is it does not have limits of detection as low as absorbance or fluorescence detectors, and it has a response that can be sensitive to changes in the mobile phase composition and temperature.

***Mass spectrometry.*** LC can be combined with mass spectrometry, giving a combined technique known as **liquid chromatography–mass spectrometry (LC-MS)**. This combination makes it possible to both measure chemicals and to identify them based on the masses of their molecular ions or fragment ions. When used in the full-scan mode, the mass spectrometer in LC-MS acts as a general detector. If the mass spectrometer is instead used for looking at particular ions, this device then acts as a selective detector. It is also possible to add another dimension based on mass spectrometry, as occurs in LC-MS/MS, to look at fragment ions that are

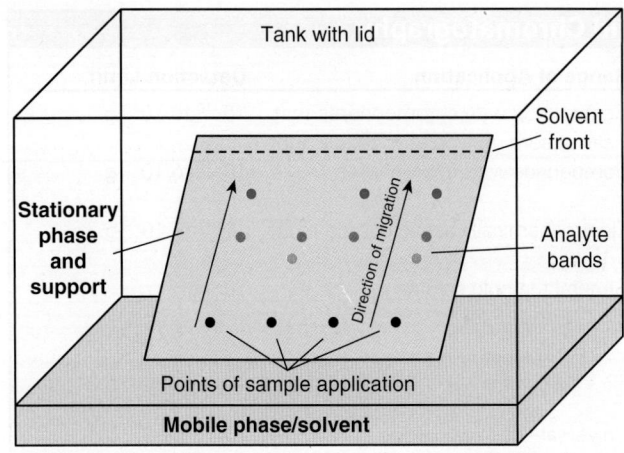

**Fig. 12.16** General operation and system components of thin-layer chromatography. In this particular example, the mobile phase moves up the glass plate and a thin layer of adsorbent by means of capillary action.

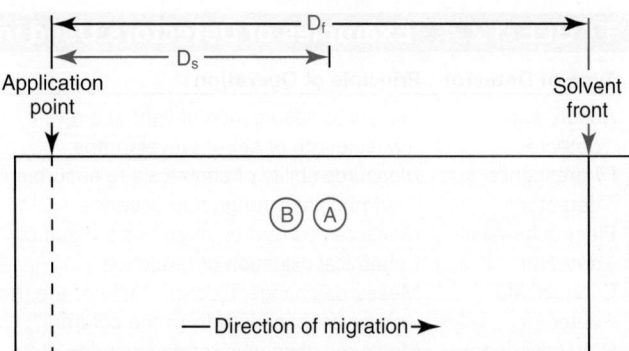

**Fig. 12.17** General example of a separation obtained by planar chromatography. In this example, compound *B* is more strongly retained and migrates a shorter distance than compound *A*. $D_s$, Distance travelled by an analyte (*A*, in this example) from the point of sample application; $D_f$, distance travelled by the mobile phase, or solvent front, from the point of sample application in the same amount of time as allowed for sample migration.

produced from a given precursor ion. This addition can further increase the ability of the method to resolve or detect multiple components and can enable the analysis of hundreds or thousands of components in a sample.

Several types of ionization methods and mass analyzers can be employed in LC-MS (see Chapter 13). A common combination is the use of electrospray ionization with a quadrupole mass analyzer. Other possible ionization methods that can be used are CI or photoionization. The interface in LC-MS has to remove solvent from the mobile phase and place the sample components in a charged form in the gas phase that can be analyzed by the mass spectrometer. This process requires that the buffers used in LC-MS be sufficiently volatile to avoid overloading and contaminating the interface.

### Data Acquisition and System Control

The system controller for an HPLC will often manage (1) sample injections, (2) solvent delivery, (3) the system flow rate and temperature, as well as (4) control the detectors, and (5) acquire data from these detectors. Data acquisition systems can collect thousands of data points from an individual run. These data can then be used to identify and measure the eluting compounds based on the retention times and areas or heights of their peaks. The hardware and software that are used for data analysis can become particularly important as the amount of collected data becomes large, as can often occur with the use of a PDA or LC-MS. Libraries of spectra or other databases can be searched to aid in the identification of chemicals based on the chromatograms and signals that are generated during the separation.

## PLANAR CHROMATOGRAPHY

In planar chromatography, the stationary phase is coated or placed onto a flat surface, or plane. The sample is added as a small spot or band on this surface. This support is then placed into an enclosed container with one edge in contact with

the mobile phase and the sample band located just beyond this point of contact (Fig. 12.16). The mobile phase is usually allowed to travel across the plane by means of capillary action. After this movement has occurred for a given period of time, the support is removed from the mobile phase and dried prior to the analysis or measurement of the separated sample components.

The planar surface that is used in this method may be a sheet of paper, known as *paper chromatography*, or some other type of surface, resulting in a method known as *thin-layer chromatography* (TLC). In paper chromatography, the stationary phase is the surface of the paper or a layer of a solvent or chemical that is coated or placed onto the paper. In TLC, a thin layer of particles (such as silica or alumina) is spread on a glass plate, plastic sheet, or aluminum sheet.

In planar chromatography, retention is described by the distance that compounds have traveled in a given amount of time (Fig. 12.17), rather than the time or volume of mobile phase required for elution, as is used in column chromatography. The distance traveled by a chemical from its point of application ($D_s$) in paper chromatography and TLC is often compared with the distance that has been traveled by the mobile phase in the same amount of time ($D_f$). This information can be used to calculate a measure of retention that is known as the **retardation factor** ($R_f$).

$$R_f = D_s / D_f$$

The value for $R_f$ will always be between zero and one. Chemicals that have high retention with the stationary phase will have low values $R_f$, and chemicals that have low retention will have $R_f$ values that approach one. Chemicals can be identified in planar chromatography by comparing their retention and $R_f$ values with those for reference compounds that have been examined on the same stationary phase and support and mobile phase. The detection characteristics of the reference compounds can also be compared with the chemicals in the unknown sample (e.g., the color of their bands or their response to a color-forming reagent). Additional confirmation can be obtained by comparing the unknown compound and the reference compound under a different set of separation conditions.

The separated components in planar chromatography can often be detected by their natural color, by their response to UV light or through their fluorescence, or by their visualization with reagents that form colored products. In some cases, these chemicals may be allowed to react with labeled antibodies for their detection, or they may be detected by using radiolabels and autoradiography. Their bands may also be removed from the planar surface for analysis by a method such as mass spectrometry or nuclear magnetic resonance spectroscopy.

Paper chromatography and TLC tend to be used primarily for qualitative analysis. One application of these techniques is their use in the analysis of amniotic fluid to determine lecithin-to-sphingomyelin ratios. Another application is in the screening of urine for drugs or metabolites such as amino acids that accumulate during hereditary disorders.

## REVIEW QUESTIONS

1. Which component in a chromatographic system carries the sample?
   a. Stationary phase
   b. Mobile phase
   c. Support
   d. Column

2. Which of the following is *not* an approach that can be used to improve the separation of two compounds by a chromatographic system?
   a. Increase the degree of peak retention
   b. Increase the selectivity of the system for one compound versus another
   c. Increase the amount of sample that is applied
   d. Increase the efficiency of the system

3. In column chromatography, unknown analytes are identified as they pass through the detector. Comparison of the _____ of unknown analytes with that of standard compounds can be used for identification of the analytes.
   a. separation factor
   b. retention factor
   c. resolution
   d. plate height

4. Before it can be used in a separation by GC, a compound must:
   a. be volatile or be converted into a volatile form.
   b. not be volatile.
   c. be water soluble.
   d. be present in a large quantity in a sample.

5. Which type of GC might use alumina particles as the stationary phase?
   a. Gas-liquid chromatography
   b. Gas-solid chromatography
   c. Bonded phase gas chromatography
   d. Capillary gas chromatography

6. Which of the following common detectors for GC can be used in more than one mode to either detect many compounds or examine specific analytes?
   a. Nitrogen-phosphorus detector
   b. Electron capture detector
   c. Mass spectrometer
   d. Flame ionization detector

7. Which of the following statements concerning LC is *not* correct?
   a. HPLC is the form of LC used in most routine chemical separation or analysis methods.
   b. Normal-phase chromatography uses a nonpolar stationary phase and is one of the most popular types of LC.
   c. Cation-exchange chromatography uses negatively charged groups as the stationary phase.
   d. A porous support is used in size-exclusion chromatography.

8. Some point-of-care tests use chromatography as a processing step in the assay. In point-of-care pregnancy testing, for example, the stationary phase is nitrocellulose paper and the hCG antigen is present in a urine sample, which is considered the mobile phase. The antigen in the mobile phase binds with an antibody in the stationary phase. This is an example of planar chromatography using which of the following as the separation mechanism?
   a. Partition chromatography
   b. Ion-exchange chromatography
   c. Size-exclusion chromatography
   d. Affinity chromatography

9. Which statement is true about the mobile phase in LC?
   a. The strength of the mobile phase is varied during solvent programming.
   b. A strong mobile phase gives strong retention for compounds on an LC column.
   c. An organic solvent is a weak mobile phase in reversed-phase chromatography.
   d. The mobile phase has few interactions with the injected compounds in LC.

10. Which of the following statements is *not* true about planar chromatography?
   a. Compounds may be identified by using their retardation factors.
   b. Paper may be used as a support in this method.
   c. This method is mainly used for quantitative analysis.
   d. Thin-layer chromatography is one form of this method.

## SUGGESTED READINGS

Allenmark S. *Chromatographic Enantioseparations: Methods and Applications*. 2nd ed. New York: Ellis Horwood; 1991.

Drozd J. *Chemical Derivatization in Gas Chromatography*. Amsterdam: Elsevier; 1981.

Ewing GW, ed. *Analytical Instrumentation Handbook*. 2nd ed. New York: Marcel Dekker; 1997.

Gross ML, Capriol RM, Niessen W. *Hyphenated Methods. The Encyclopedia of Mass Spectrometry*. Vol. 8. Amsterdam: Elsevier; 2006:1–1068.

Hage DS, ed. *Handbook of Affinity Chromatography*. 2nd ed. Boca Raton: CRC Press; 2006.

Hage DS, Carr JD. *Analytical Chemistry and Quantitative Analysis*. New York: Pearson; 2011.

Janson JC, ed. *Protein Purification: Principles, High Resolution Methods and Applications*. 3rd ed. Hoboken: Wiley; 2011.

Jorgenson JW. Capillary liquid chromatography at ultrahigh pressures. *Ann Rev Anal Chem*. 2010;3:129–150.

Karger BL, Snyder LR, Horvath C. *An Introduction to Separation Science*. New York: Wiley; 1973.

Lough WJ, Wainer IW. *High Performance Liquid Chromatography: Fundamentals Principles and Practice*. New York: Blackie Academic; 1995.

Lunn G, Hellwig GC. *Handbook of Derivatization Reactions for HPLC*. New York: Wiley-Interscience; 1998.

Majors RE. A review of HPLC column packing technology. *Am Lab*. 2003;3:46–54.

McNair HM, Miller JM. *Basic Gas Chromatography*. 2nd ed. Malden: Wiley Interscience; 2009.

Miller JM. *Chromatography: Concepts and Contrasts*. 2nd ed. Malden: Wiley Interscience; 2009.

Ravindranath B. *Principles and Practice of Chromatography*. New York: Wiley; 1989.

Sherma J, Fried B, eds. *Planar Chromatography*. New York: Taylor & Francis; 2003.

Shushan B. A review of clinical diagnostic applications of liquid chromatography-tandem mass spectrometry. *Mass Spectrom Rev*. 2010;29:930–944.

Snyder LR, Kirkland JJ, Dolan JW. *Introduction to Modern Liquid Chromatography*. 3rd ed. New York: Wiley; 2009.

Svec F, Huber CG. Monolithic materials: promises, challenges, achievements. *Anal Chem*. 2006;78:2100–2108.

# Mass Spectrometry

*Mark M. Kushnir, Nigel J. Clarke, and Alan L. Rockwood\**

## OBJECTIVES

1. Define the following terms:
   - Base peak
   - Ion trap
   - Mass analysis
   - Mass spectrometry (MS)
   - Mass-to-charge ratio *(m/z)*
   - Molecular ion
   - Product ion
   - Fragment ion
   - Quadrupole
   - Triple quadrupole
   - Tandem mass spectrometry
   - Time-of-flight (TOF)
   - Matrix-assisted laser desorption/ionization (MALDI)-TOF

2. Describe the main components of a mass spectrometer, their functions, and principles of operation.
3. For the following ionization methods, state the principle and specific uses of each type:
   - Electron
   - Chemical
   - Electrospray
   - Atmospheric pressure chemical
   - Inductively coupled plasma (ICP)
   - MALDI
4. State the principles of operation of quadrupole, triple quadrupole, ion trap, and TOF mass analyzers and describe the principle of operation of electron multiplier detectors.
5. Explain the role of mass spectrometry in clinical laboratories.

## KEY WORDS AND DEFINITIONS

**Base peak** The most abundant peak in the mass spectrum; it is assigned a relative abundance of 100%.

**Electrospray ionization** Using this ionization technique, a sample is passed through a capillary to which a high voltage is applied, resulting in expulsion of ions from a spray of fine droplets.

**Extracted ion chromatogram** A plot consisting of a sum of abundances of ions of selected mass-to-charge ratios displayed as a function of chromatographic elution time.

**Fragment ion** An ion formed by fragmentation of a molecular ion.

**Gas chromatography–mass spectrometry (GC-MS)** A technique that uses a gas chromatograph coupled to a mass spectrometer.

**Internal standard** A structural analog of a substance that is added to calibrators, controls, and unknown samples at a constant amount. An internal standard corrects for variable recovery among samples during the sample preparation and instrumental analysis. The internal standard should have similar physical and chemical properties to the targeted molecule, with a distinct mass spectrometry (MS) signal. Internal standards used in MS-based methods typically have the same molecular structure as the compound of interest but contain stable isotopes of atoms (e.g., $^{13}C$ or $^{2}H$ [deuterium]) to distinguish the internal standard from the compound of interest by a mass difference.

**Ion** An atom or a molecule that has acquired an electrical charge by losing or gaining one or more electrons or other charged species (e.g., protons).

**Ionization** Required for all MS techniques; "ionization" describes the production of ions from neutral atoms or molecules using various techniques, including but not limited to electron ionization, chemical ionization, or electrospray ionization.

**Ion trap** Type of mass analyzer in which ions are held in a spatially confined region using a radiofrequency electric field or a combination of magnetic and electrostatic fields.

**Isotope** A variant of a chemical element; each variant differs in the number of neutrons in the nucleus, and therefore differs in atomic weight.

**Isotope dilution mass spectrometry (IDMS)** An analytical technique that is used to quantify a compound relative to its isotopic analog (internal standard).

*The authors gratefully acknowledge the original contributions by Thomas M. Annesley and Nicholas E. Sherman on which portions of this chapter are based.

**Liquid chromatography–mass spectrometry (LC-MS)** A technique that uses a liquid chromatograph coupled to a mass spectrometer.

**Mass analysis** The process of resolving ionic species based on their mass-to-charge ratios.

**Mass spectrometer** An analytical instrument that ionizes atoms or molecules, separates the ions, and detects the $m/z$ of these ionized atoms or molecules or their ion fragments. Mass spectrometers are often interfaced with other instruments, including, but not limited to, a second mass spectrometer, a liquid chromatograph, or a gas chromatograph.

**Mass spectrometry** An analytical technique that is used to measure $m/z$ of ions and their abundances. Other physiochemical properties may sometimes also be inferred through interpretation of the mass spectrum and/or combining MS with other techniques.

**Mass spectrum** A plot of the relative abundance of ions as a function of their mass-to-charge ratio.

**Mass-to-charge ratio** *(m/z)* The ratio formed by dividing the molecular mass of an ion by its charge.

**Matrix-assisted laser desorption/ionization (MALDI)** A soft ionization technique allowing analysis of organic molecules, biomolecules (proteins, peptides, DNA, polysaccharides), and microorganisms. MALDI ionization is performed by irradiation of samples mixed with a matrix, using a pulsed laser.

**Product ion** A fragment ion formed when a molecular ion breaks into smaller pieces. In a tandem mass spectrometer, the fragmentation process takes place after molecular ions have been separated in the first stage MS.

**Selected ion monitoring (SIM)** A MS technique where signal is acquired only from ions of a specified $m/z$.

**Tandem mass spectrometer** A mass spectrometer capable of separating ions according to $m/z$ values in two (or more) stages. The stages can be separated by geometry (tandem in space) or by time (tandem in time.)

**Torr** A non-SI unit of pressure with 760 torr equal to 101.3 kPa. One torr is equal to the pressure exerted by a one-millimeter-high column of mercury.

**Total ion chromatogram (TIC)** A chromatogram created by summing up intensities of all $m/z$ responses acquired by a mass analyzer during chromatographic separation, displayed as a function of time.

## BASIC CONCEPTS

A **mass spectrometer** is an analytical instrument that ionizes atoms or molecules and then separates and measures the **mass-to-charge ratio** *(m/z)* of the ionized atoms or molecules, and in the case of molecules, also their fragments. **Mass analysis** is the process of identification of the $m/z$ of the ions. **Mass spectrometry** (MS) can be used for qualitative analysis (identifying and determining elemental composition and structure of compounds), as well as for performing quantitative analysis of components of samples.

A **mass spectrum** plots the relative abundance of **ions** as a function of their $m/z$ (Fig. 13.1). The unfragmented ion of a molecule is called the *molecular ion*. **Fragment ions** are formed when a molecular ion breaks into smaller pieces. The ion with the highest abundance in the mass spectrum is assigned a relative value of 100% and is called the **base peak**. The base peak may be the molecular ion or a fragment ion. Fragmentation of ions at specific bonds depends on their chemical nature; in some cases, it is possible to determine the structure of a molecule from the fragment ions observed in the mass spectrum. Because patterns of relative abundance among the fragment ions of a given compound are often unique to that compound, computer-based mass spectral libraries can be used to identify analytes from their mass spectra. This is often used in screening methods in toxicology, environmental and agricultural analyses.

In **tandem mass spectrometry** fragmentation takes place after ions have been separated by their $m/z$ values in a first stage of MS; these fragment ions are named **product ions** (the term "daughter ion" was often used in the older literature).

Mass spectrometers are often informally called "universal detectors" because most molecules can be ionized and can therefore be detected. When interfaced with a liquid or a gas chromatograph, the MS can provide highly specific detection, as well as structural information. In such instruments, multiple mass spectra are acquired across the chromatographic peaks, and the sum of the signal from all the ions detected across the acquisition time can be displayed as a function of time. Such plots represent a **total ion chromatogram (TIC)**. It is possible to program the data analysis system to display the sum of ions over a narrow mass range, rather than the full acquired mass range, or to display the selected $m/z$ values. The resultant chromatogram is called an **extracted ion chromatogram (EIC**; Fig. 13.2). Both TICs and EIC are displayed as signal intensity plotted as a function of time.

In targeted quantitative analysis, when only a few analytes are of interest, and their mass spectra are known, the MS is typically set up to monitor only the ions of interest; this mode of MS operation is known as **selected ion monitoring (SIM)**. In the SIM mode, the mass spectrometer cycles repeatedly and rapidly through a list of the specified $m/z$ values, monitoring the abundance of each $m/z$ for a specified time. Because SIM focuses only on specified ions, the signal-to-noise ratios for the targeted analytes increases, resulting in the lower limits of detection.

Mass spectra of most molecules contain a series of peaks; in the case of singly charged molecules, they differ by approximately one $m/z$ unit. These peaks are attributed to

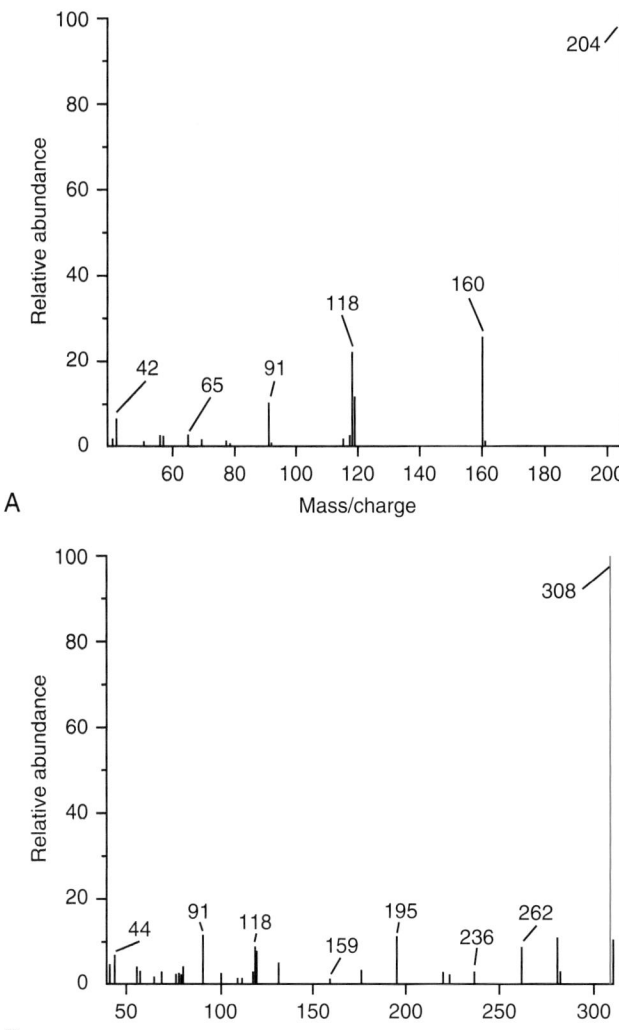

A

B

**Fig. 13.1** Mass spectrum of (A) pentafluoropropionyl, and (B) carbethoxyhexafluorobutyryl derivatives of D-methamphetamine.

the presence of atoms of different elemental isotopes within the molecule; they are referred to as isotope peaks or isotopic peaks. For example, the mass spectrum of $C_2H_7O^+$ consists primarily of three isotopic peaks at nominal $m/z$ values of 47, 48, and 49, with relative abundances of 100%, 2.4%, and 0.2%, respectively. The isotopic peaks of $C_2H_7O^+$ contain contributions from $^{12}C$, $^{13}C$, $^1H$, $^2H$, $^{16}O$, $^{17}O$, and $^{18}O$ in various combinations. For example, the $m/z$ 48 peak of $C_2H_7O^+$ is composed of $^{12}C^{13}C^1H_7^{16}O^+$, $^{12}C_2^1H_6^2H^{16}O^+$, and $^{12}C_2^1H_7^{17}O^+$ (Fig. 13.3). Calculation of isotopic patterns can be challenging, particularly for high-molecular-weight compounds. Methods for calculation of isotopic distributions corresponding to a molecular formula have been developed and discussed in the literature.

Molecules can be isotopically labeled by substituting atoms with stable isotope atoms (typically $^2H$, $^{13}C$, $^{15}N$) at selected positions within a molecule. During the MS analysis a labeled molecule is observed at a different $m/z$ than the unlabeled molecule, and relative abundances of labeled vs. unlabeled molecules can be measured. Relative abundance of the peaks

of unlabeled vs. labeled molecules is used in isotope dilution mass spectrometry (IDMS), which serves as basis for quantitative analysis using MS detection. With IDMS, a known amount of stable isotope-labeled analog (internal standard) of the targeted analyte is added to calibrators, controls, and unknown samples and quantitation is performed using the ratio of abundances of the signal from the targeted analyte and the internal standard. This technique compensates for variable analyte recovery during sample preparation and instrumental analysis (e.g., incomplete recovery of the target analyte during sample preparation, sample-to-sample, or day-to-day variations in instrument response).

## INSTRUMENTATION

All mass spectrometers include the following components: (1) ion source, (2) vacuum system, (3) mass analyzer, (4) detector, and (5) computer (Fig. 13.4). Usually a chromatograph is used as a sample introduction device.

### Ion Source

All MS techniques require an ionization step, in which an ion is produced from a neutral atom or molecule, or ions present in solution get transferred into the gas phase. The most frequently utilized ionization methods include (1) electron ionization (EI), (2) electrospray ionization (ESI), and (3) atmospheric pressure chemical ionization (APCI). Less frequently used ionization techniques are (1) inductively coupled plasma (ICP), (2) matrix-assisted laser desorption/ionization (MALDI), (3) chemical ionization (CI), and (4) atmospheric pressure photoionization (APPI).

### Electron Ionization

EI and CI are techniques used when gas phase molecules are introduced directly into the mass analyzer, usually from a gas chromatograph. In EI, gas phase molecules are bombarded by electrons emitted from a heated filament (Fig. 13.5). This process must occur in a vacuum to prevent filament oxidation and attenuation of the electron beam. Electrons emitted from a hot filament by thermionic emission are accelerated through a potential difference of ~70 V and directed to a vaporized sample. The kinetic energy of the electrons is sufficient to eject an electron from the analyte molecule, producing radicals (denoted here with asterisks) and cations. In most cases, these radical ions then undergo unimolecular rearrangements and fragmentation to produce other cations and radicals, for example:

$$AB^{+*} \rightarrow A^+ + B^*$$

In this process, positive ions (cations) are drawn out of the ionization chamber by an electrical field and introduced into the mass analyzer. The fragmentation pattern, relative intensity of the molecular ion, and the fragment ions are reasonably reproducible within and among the instruments. In EI, the mass spectral pattern in most cases is dominated by fragment ions and can be matched to the entries in a mass spectral library. EI ionization is most commonly used in gas

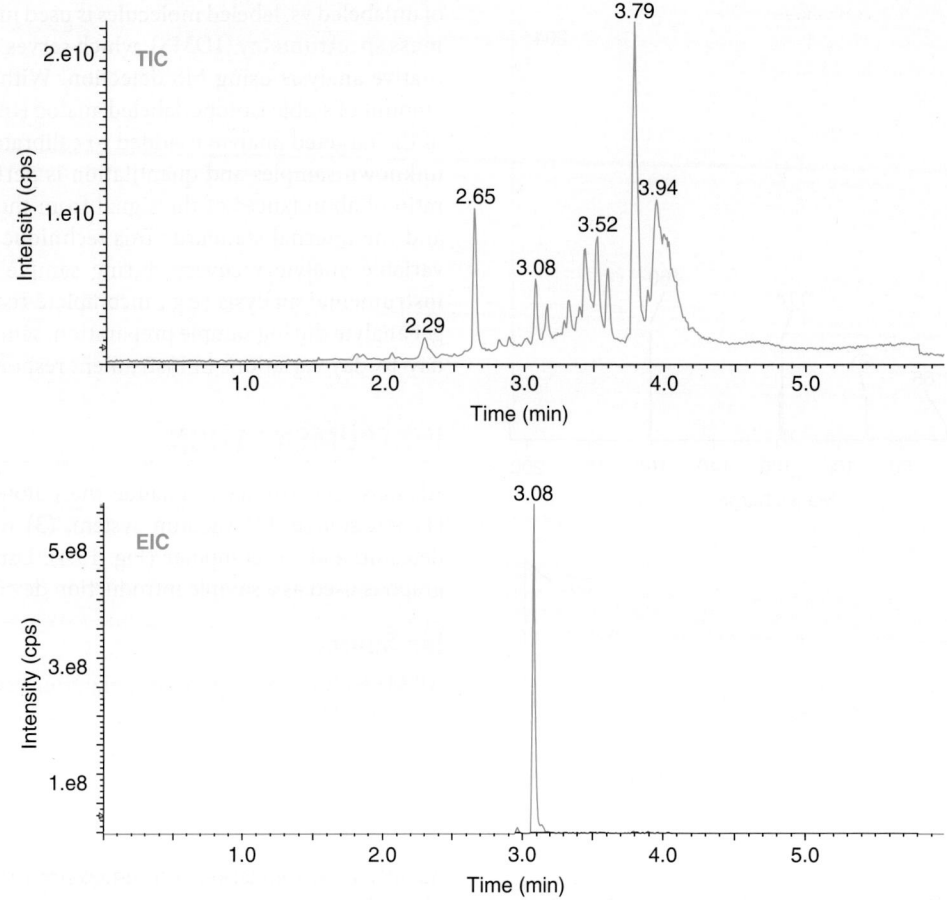

Fig. 13.2 An example of total ion chromatogram *(TIC)*, scanning *m/z* between 100 and 500) is shown in the top panel, and an extracted ion chromatogram *(EIC)*, *(m/z* range 415.0 and 416.0) is shown in the bottom panel. *cps*, Counts per second.

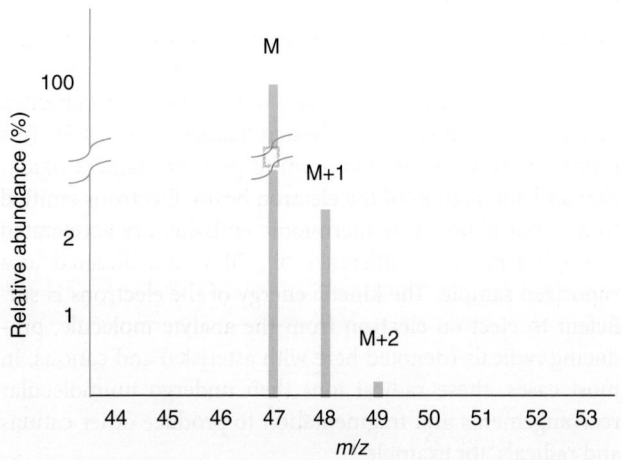

Fig. 13.3 Monoisotopic and isotopic peaks of the ion $C_2H_7O^+$ and their composition. *M* is the monoisotopic ion $C_2H_7O^+$ composed of $^{12}C_2{}^1H_7{}^{16}O^+$. *M+1* is the first isotopic ion of $C_2H_7O^+$ that could be composed of $^{13}C^{12}C^1H_7{}^{16}O^+$, $^{12}C_2{}^1H_6{}^2H^{16}O^+$, or $^{12}C_2{}^1H_7{}^{17}O^+$. *M+2* is the second isotopic ion of $C_2H_7O^+$ that could be composed of $^{13}C_2{}^1H_7{}^{16}O^+$, $^{12}C^{13}CH_7{}^{17}O^+$, $^{12}C_2{}^1H_6{}^2H_1{}^{17}O^+$, $^{12}C_2{}^1H_5{}^2H_2{}^{16}O^+$, or $^{13}C^{12}C^1H_7{}^{17}O^+$.

chromatography–mass spectrometry (GC-MS) instruments, and the reproducibility and uniqueness of the mass spectral patterns serves as the basis for identification of constituents of samples, provided that mass spectra of the constituents exist in the utilized mass spectral library.

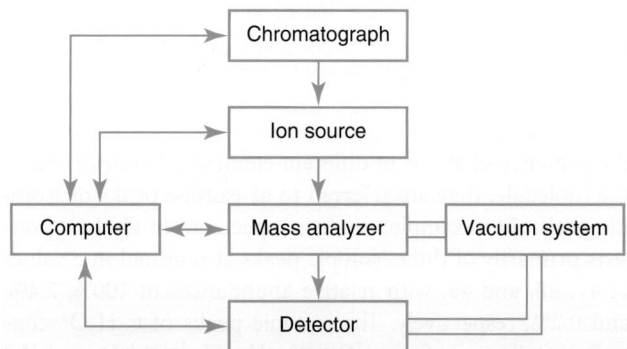

Fig. 13.4 Block diagram of the components of a chromatograph-mass spectrometer system.

An important limitation of GC-MS is the requirement that compounds be sufficiently volatile to allow transfer from the liquid phase to the gas phase, and transfer from the chromatographic column to mass spectrometer. Since volatility is required for GC analysis, many biological compounds need to be derivatized before they can be analyzed using GC-MS.

Derivatization is a technique that transforms a chemical compound into a different compound of related, though not identical chemical structure. In GC-MS methods, derivatization involves the reaction of chemically active functional

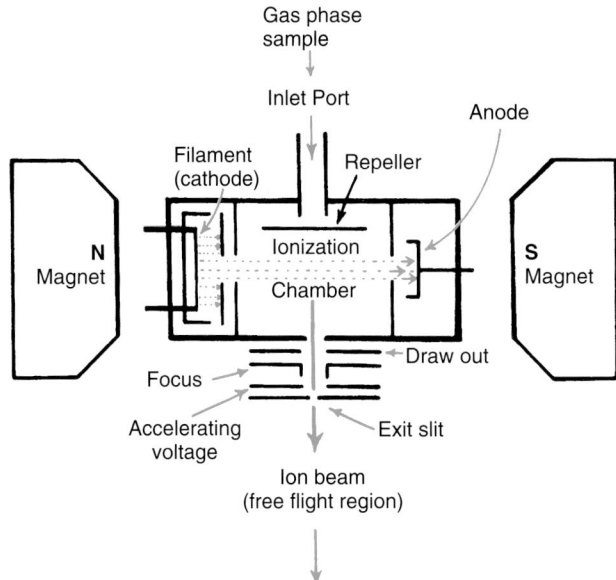

Fig. 13.5 Electron impact ion source. The magnets are used to collimate a dense electron beam which is drawn from a heated filament placed at a negative potential. The electron beam is positioned in front of a repeller, which is at a slight positive potential compared with the ion source. The repeller sends any positively charged fragment ions toward the opening at the front of the ion source. The accelerating plates strongly attract the positively charged fragment ions.

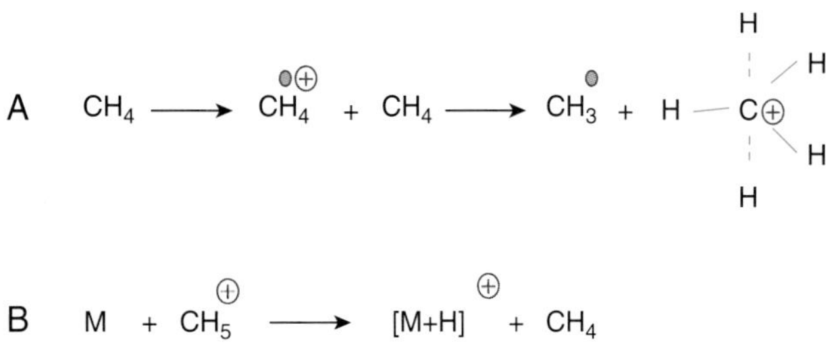

Fig. 13.6 Proposed mechanism of a chemical ionization process. In (A), an electron beam ionizes a reagent gas ($CH_4$) and produces reactive species ($CH_5^+$). In (B), positive ions are produced by proton transfer to an analyte molecule.

takes place through generation of ions from reagent gas, through bombardment of the reagent gas with a beam of electrons, which result in production (sometimes indirectly via ion-molecule reactions) of reactive species, followed by proton transfer from or to the analyte molecule. CI is a low-energy process that typically results in a mass spectrum dominated by the (unfragmented) molecular ion (Fig. 13.6). Ions produced by accepting a proton are typically closed-shell ions (i.e., not radical ions). Because of the lack of fragmentation, CI is advantageous for the determination of molecular mass of the constituents of samples, and in quantitative analysis. Because CI does not produce fragment ions, this type of ionization does not allow confirmation of the identity of the molecules based on compound-specific mass spectral patterns.

A variation of CI is negative ion electron capture CI; this type of ionization is used in analysis of molecules containing electronegative functional groups (e.g., chlorine, fluorine, nitro). Since the number of compounds capable of negative ionization is relatively small, the background noise signal in the mass spectra is typically low, and because the entire signal corresponds to a molecular ion, negative ion CI could provide lower limits of detection than EI and positive ion CI.

## Electrospray Ionization

ESI is a technique in which a molecule of interest is ionized at atmospheric pressure before it is introduced into the mass analyzer. In ESI, effluent from a chromatographic column is passed through a capillary to which 1.5 to 5 kV is applied (Fig. 13.7A). In the process, electrostatic forces applied to the effluent result in formation of charged droplets. A coaxially applied nebulizing gas helps to nebulize the liquid and direct the charged droplets toward a counter-electrode. As droplets evaporate and shrink, the field strength on the surface increases and solvated ions are expelled from the droplets. In positive ion mode, the proton adducts of the molecule (typically clustered with solvent molecules) are "desolvated" to form "bare" ions, which then pass through an aperture inside the vacuum region of the mass analyzer.

ESI depends mainly on solution phase chemistry. Basic compounds tend to be efficiently detected in positive ion mode because they are easily protonated. Less commonly, positive ions are formed by adduction with positively charged ions, such as an ammonium ion or an alkali metal ion (e.g., $K^+$, $Na^+$). In some cases, the ion may arise from a permanently

groups within the targeted molecule, with formation of a product, which has improved volatility and stability at elevated temperatures, different boiling temperatures, and/or more favorable fragmentation patterns during mass analysis. The resulting new chemical and its physical properties (e.g., improved volatility, stability at elevated temperatures, more favorable fragmentation patterns than the parent molecule) enable GC-MS analysis, and often enhance sensitivity and specificity of analysis.

Liquid chromatography separations are useful for compounds that are not suited to gas chromatography-based separation, and methods where a simpler sample preparation and higher throughput of the testing could be beneficial. It is more difficult to interface liquid chromatographs with mass spectrometers, as compared to gas chromatographs, because the mobile phase is a liquid rather than a gas. Several interface techniques for coupling liquid chromatographs to mass spectrometers have been developed (ESI, APCI, APPI), which led to liquid chromatography–mass spectrometry (LC-MS) and liquid chromatography–tandem mass spectrometry (LC-MS/MS) instruments becoming routine methodologies in analytical laboratories.

## Chemical Ionization

CI is a "soft" ionization technique, meaning that relatively little fragmentation occurs during the ionization process. In the ionization process, taking place in a gas phase, a proton is transferred to (or abstracted from) analyte by a reagent gas molecule. Commonly used reagent gases are (1) methane, (2) ammonia, (3) isobutane, and (4) water vapor. The ionization

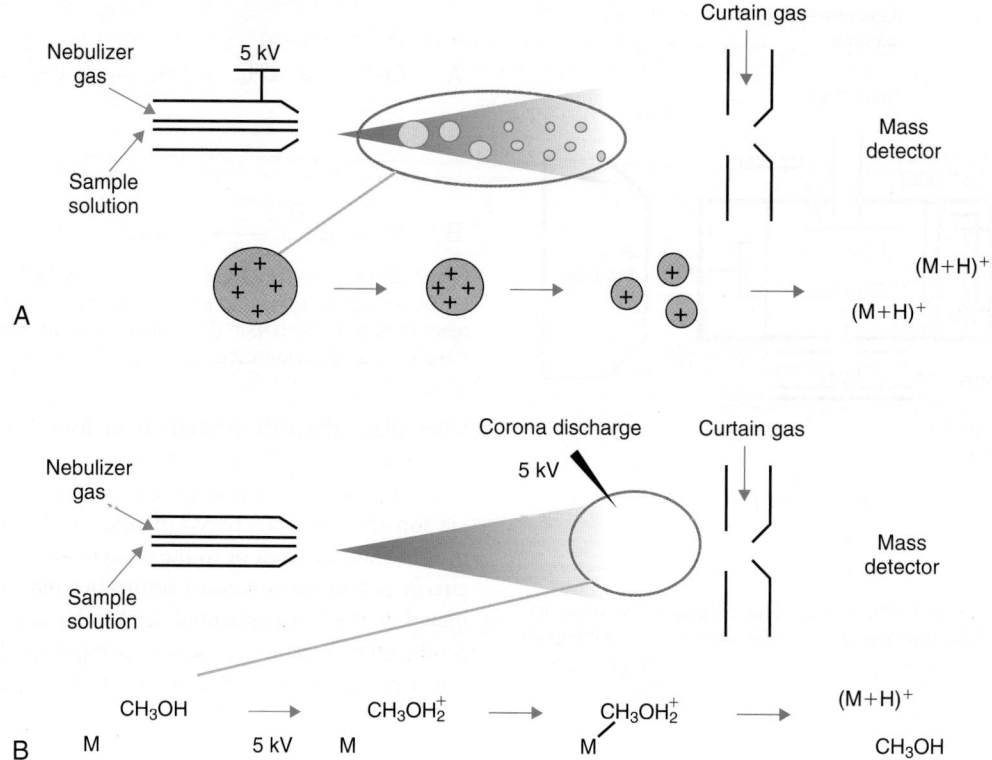

**Fig. 13.7** Schematics of (A) electrospray, and (B) atmospheric pressure chemical ionization ion sources. Note the different points where ionization occurs.

charged functional group within the targeted molecule, such as a quaternary ammonium group (e.g., acylcarnitines, choline). Acidic compounds (e.g., carboxylic acids) may lose a proton to form negatively charged ions, which can be detected in negative ion mode of instrument operation.

ESI is different from other ionization techniques in its ability to produce multiply charged ions. This effectively extends the instrument's mass range by a few orders of magnitude, allowing detection of proteins and peptides. It is common to observe approximately one charge for every ~10 amino acid residues in a protein. For example, a protein molecule of mass 20,000 could have 20 charges and could be detected at $m/z$ 1,001.0 ([20,000+20]/20). In most cases where multiple charging occurs, a series of charge states are observed appearing at a series of $m/z$ values (e.g., for a molecule with mass 20,000, $m/z$ 1121.1, 1053.6, 1001.0 will be observed, which correspond to ions of charges +18, +19, +20, respectively). In most cases, ions are produced by proton adduction, and peaks are observed at $m/z = (M + n)/n$, where $M$ is the molecular weight and $n$ is the charge (equal to the number of attracted protons).

Although Fig. 13.7A shows the sample introduction probe directed toward the sampling orifice of the MS, in some designs the ESI probe is offset (or orthogonal) relative to the sampling cone to enhance the performance and to minimize contamination of the mass analyzer.

### Atmospheric Pressure Chemical Ionization

APCI (see Fig. 13.7B), similarly to ESI, takes place at atmospheric pressure, involves nebulization, de-solvation of ions,

and uses the same sampling and extraction cones as ESI. However, with APCI, voltage is not applied to the inlet capillary; instead, a corona discharge needle is positioned on the path of the evaporated stream of the effluent from a chromatographic column. The corona discharge initiates a cascade of gas phase reactions that ionize compounds through a series of ion-molecule reactions, similar to the reactions occurring in CI (see Fig. 13.6), with evaporated constituents of the mobile phase (e.g., water, methanol) serving as reagent gas molecules. Products of these secondary reactions typically contain clusters of solvent and analyte molecules, so a heated transfer tube or a countercurrent flow of an inert gas (e.g., nitrogen) and an electric potential are used to de-cluster the ions. APCI is the second most commonly used ion source in **liquid chromatography–mass spectrometry (LC-MS)** and liquid chromatography–tandem mass spectrometry (LC-MS/MS).

### Inductively Coupled Plasma

Similar to ESI and APCI, ICP is an atmospheric pressure ionization method. However, unlike most atmospheric pressure ionization methods, which are "soft" and produce little fragmentation, ICP is the ultimate in "hard" ionization, typically used to completely atomize the introduced molecules in a plasma of ionized gas generated by a radio frequency (RF) field. Consequently, its primary use is for elemental analysis. In clinical laboratories ICP-MS is used for trace metal and heavy metal analysis in tissues or body fluids. ICP-based instruments are extremely sensitive (e.g., parts per trillion) and are capable of a wide dynamic range. The sample is typically prepared by acid digestion and is introduced into the ion source via a nebulizer fed by a peristaltic pump. The nebulized sample is transmitted into hot plasma, maintained at atmospheric pressure by inductively coupling power using a high-power RF generator. A fraction of the generated ions are transmitted through an orifice into the vacuum region of a mass analyzer through a series of differential pumping stages.

Because with ICP ionization the molecules fragment to atoms, ICP-MS is typically free from interferences. The most common types of interferences in ICP-MS are polyatomic species, produced in the plasma via ion-molecule reactions when isobaric molecules (of the same molecular mass) with the elements of interest are present. For example, $^{40}Ar^{35}Cl^+$, $^{59}Co^{16}O^+$, $^{36}Ar^{38}Ar^1H^+$, $^{38}Ar^{37}Cl^+$, and $^{36}Ar^{39}K$ are all isobaric to $^{75}As$. One approach to overcome interference from the polyatomic species is to position a dynamic reaction cell between the ion source and mass analyzer where a reactant gas (e.g., ammonia) is introduced, which fragments the polyatomic species.

### Matrix-Assisted Laser Desorption/Ionization

MALDI is a soft ionization technique using a laser energy absorbing matrix to create ions. Sample is mixed with a solution of matrix (typically a low-molecular-weight UV-absorbing compound), placed on a target, and allowed to dry under controlled conditions. As the liquid evaporates, the matrix crystallizes and incorporates analyte molecules in the crystals. A pulsed laser irradiates the sample, triggering rapid vaporization and desorption of the sample and matrix material; the analyte molecules are ionized in the plume of ablated gases and ions enter the mass analyzer (Fig. 13.8). Because MALDI produces discrete, pulsed ion packets, it is often coupled with a time-of-flight (TOF) mass analyzer. During the last 10 years, MALDI–TOF instruments have become widely adopted in clinical laboratories for bacterial identification.

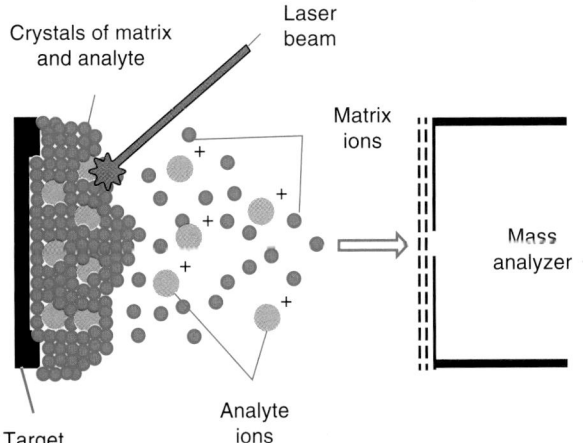

**Fig. 13.8** Matrix-assisted laser desorption ionization. Co-crystallized matrix and analyte are irradiated with an ultraviolet laser, resulting in formation of a plume of matrix ions and analyte ions. Gas phase ions are directed into a mass analyzer.

### Vacuum System

With the exception of certain ion trap mass spectrometers, ion separation in a mass analyzer requires that the ions do not collide with other ions and molecules during $m/z$ analysis. This requires the use of a vacuum ranging from $10^{-3}$ to $10^{-9}$ torr, depending on the mass analyzer type. To reach this level of vacuum, mass spectrometers use a combination of low-vacuum and high-vacuum pumps. The mechanical pump allows to achieve vacuum, at which the high-vacuum pump is effective. The low-vacuum pumps in addition act as a backing pump to the high-vacuum pump. Turbomolecular pumps are the most commonly used type of high-vacuum pumps.

## MASS ANALYZERS, ION DETECTORS, AND TANDEM MASS SPECTROMETERS

### Types of Mass Spectrometers

Mass spectrometers are broadly classified as (1) beam and (2) trapping type instruments. In beam-type instruments, ions make one trip through the instrument and are destructively detected when striking a detector. The entire process, from the time an ion enters the analyzer, until the time it is detected, generally takes microseconds to milliseconds.

In a trapping-type analyzer, ions are held in a spatially confined region by RF or magnetic plus electrostatic fields. The trapping fields are manipulated to allow $m/z$ measurements to be performed. Trapping times vary from a fraction of a second to minutes; most applications use trapping time at the low end of this range.

*Beam-type designs.* Beam-type mass spectrometers include (1) quadrupole, (2) magnetic sector, and (3) TOF instruments. It is convenient to categorize beam-type instruments into two broad categories: those that produce a mass spectrum by scanning the $m/z$ range over a period of time (quadrupole and magnetic sector) and those that acquire successive instantaneous snapshots of the mass spectra (TOF).

**Quadrupole.** Quadrupole mass spectrometers (QMSs) are the most widely used type of mass analyzers. They offer a number of attractive and practical features, including (1) ease of use, (2) flexibility, (3) adequate performance for most practical applications, (4) relatively low cost, (5) relatively small size, and (6) non-critical site requirements (as compared to some other types of mass analyzers).

A QMS consists of four parallel, electrically conductive rods, arranged in a square array (Fig. 13.9). The ion beam is introduced near the axis at one end of the array, passes through the array in a direction parallel to the axis, and exits at the far end of the array. The ion beam entering the

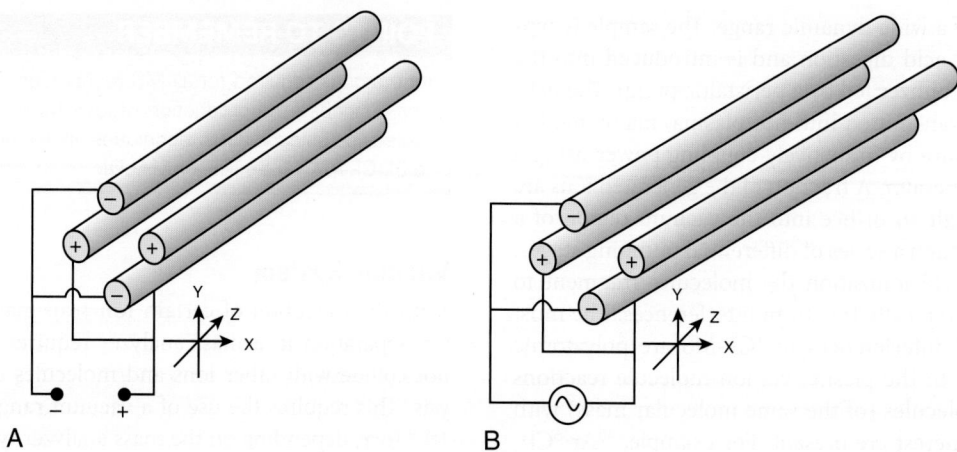

**Fig. 13.9** Diagram of a quadrupole mass analyzer, showing (A) direct current and (B) radio frequency voltages applied to a quadrupole rod assembly.

quadrupole array may contain a mixture of ions of various $m/z$ values; by adjusting voltages applied to the quadrupoles and the lenses, it is possible to allow ions of a narrow $m/z$ range (typically $\Delta m/z \leq 1$) to be transported through the device to reach the detector. Ions with $m/z$ outside of this narrow range are ejected radially.

The principle of operation of QMS is based on a superposition of RF and direct current (DC) potentials applied to the rods. DC voltages are applied to the electrodes in a quadrupolar pattern. For example, a positive DC potential is applied to electrodes 1 and 3, as indicated in Fig. 13.9, and an equivalent negative DC potential is applied to electrodes 2 and 4. The DC potentials are relatively small, on the order of a few volts. Superimposed on the DC potentials are the RF potentials, also applied in a quadrupolar fashion. The RF potentials are of a few kilovolts in magnitude with a fixed frequency of ~1 MHz.

The device may be operated in a SIM mode or in a scanning mode. For example, the mass spectrometer may be set to pass ions of $m/z$ 363.2 ± 0.5; both the center $m/z$ (363.2) and the $\Delta m/z$ (0.5) are adjusted by the appropriate choice of DC and RF, which establish the passband ($\Delta m/z$) and the resolution [$(m/z)/(\Delta m/z)$]. Typical mass resolution of quadrupole instruments is up to several thousand. Because of the relatively small size and simplicity of operation, QMS are commonly interfaced with gas and liquid chromatographs.

**Time-of-flight.** TOF mass spectrometers (TOF-MS) are widely used and offer a number of advantages, as compared to the other types of mass analyzers, including (1) nearly unlimited $m/z$ range, (2) high acquisition speed, (3) high mass accuracy, (4) moderately high resolution, (5) high sensitivity, (6) absence of peak skew in the mass spectrum, and (7) reasonable cost. They are often used with ESI ion sources, while also well adapted to pulsed ionization sources, which is an advantage in some applications, particularly with MALDI and related techniques.

Modern TOF-MSs are capable of single-digit parts per million (ppm) mass accuracy, which in some cases may

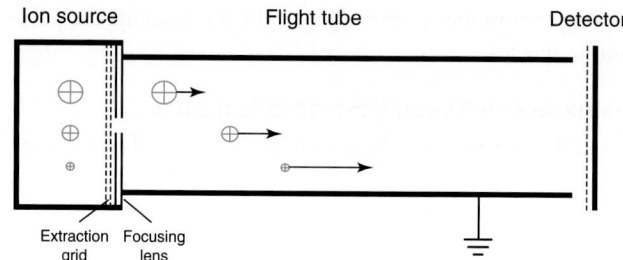

**Fig. 13.10** Diagram of a time-of-flight mass analyzer.

allow to confirm the compound's molecular formula. TOF-MSs are conceptually simple to understand, as they are based on the principle that lighter ions travel faster in vacuum than heavier ions, provided that both have the same kinetic energy. A TOF-MS resembles a long pipe (Fig. 13.10); ions are created or injected at the ion source end of the pipe and accelerated by a potential of several kilovolts. The ions travel through the flight tube and strike the detector at the far end of the tube. The time it takes for an ion to traverse the tube is proportional to the square root of the $m/z$, is known as the *flight time*, and serves as the basis for determining the $m/z$ of the ion. Because of the short flight time the data recording system must operate on a nanosecond time scale. Advances in signal processing electronics have made TOF-MS practical and relatively modest cost mass analyzers, and this has been a major factor in the rise in popularity of TOF-MS.

TOF-MS is often used with continuous flow ion sources (ESI, EI), but because it is inherently a pulsed technique, it couples more easily to pulsed ionization sources, with MALDI being the most common type. MALDI-TOF makes its biggest impact in protein, peptide, and microbiology related applications.

Another area where TOF-MS excels is in analyses of macromolecules (e.g., intact proteins) because its mass range is potentially unlimited. In MALDI-TOF, for example, proteins with molecular weights exceeding 100,000 Da can be detected.

Absence of peak skew is another advantage of TOF-MS, when it is used as a chromatographic detector. Peak skew is a distortion of the relative abundances of peaks in different parts of a mass spectrum, and this in turn distorts the shape of chromatographic peaks derived from the mass spectral data. Peak skew is related to interaction between the scanning function of the instrument and the changing concentrations of analytes over the elution profile of a chromatographic peak. TOF-MS instruments are essentially free of this artifact.

*Trapping mass spectrometers.* These mass spectrometers are based on trapping and holding ions for an extended time in a confined space, with the trapping times varying from a fraction of a second to minutes. The division between scanning and non-scanning instruments has less meaning for ion-trapping instruments than for beam-type instruments. The main practical difference between scanning and non-scanning instruments is related to the peak skew, as discussed in the above section on TOF mass analyzers. In terms of producing skewed mass spectra, trapping devices are more like non-scanning instruments, such as TOF. This is related to the fact that capture of the ions takes place in an instant, and the mass analysis performed at leisure. Because the sample is captured in an instant, no skewing of the spectra occurs, regardless of whether the $m/z$ analysis is performed by a scanning or by a non-scanning procedure.

Classes of ion traps include (1) quadrupole ion traps (QITs); (2) linear ion traps; (3) ion cyclotron resonance (ICR) mass spectrometers (not discussed in this chapter); and (4) Orbitrap mass spectrometers.

**Quadrupole ion trap.** QITs are (1) relatively compact, (2) relatively inexpensive, and (3) versatile. QITs are useful for exploratory studies, structural characterization, and identification of unknown components present in samples.

Operation of the QIT is based on the same physical principle as the QMS because both types of the devices use RF fields to confine ions. However, the RF field of an ion trap is designed to trap ions in three dimensions rather than to allow the ions to pass through as in a QMS, which confines ions in two dimensions. A diagram of an ion trap mass spectrometer is shown in Fig. 13.11. In QIT, ions are trapped and selectively ejected to generate a mass spectrum.

Although QITs and QMS were first described around the same time, the QMS achieved greater popularity as an analytical device, especially for quantitative analysis. Later, two discoveries allowed wider implementation of QIT. First, addition into the trap of low-molecular-weight gas (e.g., helium at ~$10^{-3}$ torr) which improved mass resolution and detection limits; second, the development of mass-selective ejection, which improved QIT scanning performance. When no DC voltage is applied and low RF voltage is used, ions of all $m/z$ are stored in the QIT field. When the RF voltage is increased, ions of increasing $m/z$ become axially unstable and leave the QIT sequentially according to their $m/z$. Ions leaving the QIT through the end cap are detected by an electron multiplier.

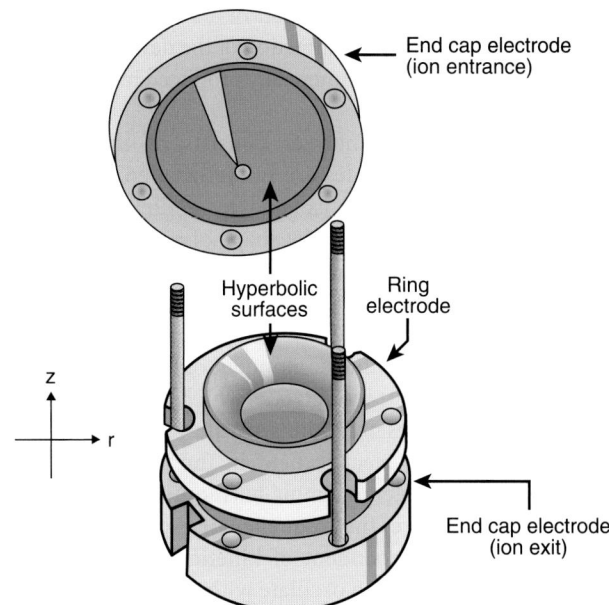

**Fig. 13.11** Diagram of a quadrupole ion trap (QIT) mass analyzer. The QIT consists of a ring electrode and two hyperbolic end-electrodes. Ions enter the QIT through the entrance endcap electrode and are trapped in the space between the electrodes by AC (oscillating) and DC (non-oscillating) electric fields. Voltages are applied to the electrodes to trap and eject ions according to their $m/z$. The ring electrode RF potential produces a quadrupolar potential field within the trapping space, which traps ions in a stable oscillating trajectory. The electrode system potentials are altered to produce instability in the ion trajectories, causing the ions to be axially ejected in order of increasing $m/z$ values.

In addition to the oscillating voltage mode of operation, the QIT can be operated in other modes. For example, a mass-selective storage mode involves selecting a combination of RF and DC that only allows ions of a specified $m/z$ to be stored in the QIT.

One unique capability of QIT, not available in most other types of mass analyzers, is that multiple stage tandem MS experiments (MS/MS/MS, or MS$^n$) can be performed with these instruments.

**Linear ion trap.** The linear ion trap is based on a modified linear QMS. Rather than serving as a pass-through device, in a linear ion trap electrostatic fields are applied to the ends of the quadrupoles to prevent ions from exiting the device. While trapped, ions are manipulated in the same ways as in a QIT. An advantage of the linear quadrupole trap is that it allows more ions to be stored and consequently has a higher dynamic range than a QIT. Commercial triple QMS are available, in which the third quadrupole is modified so it can function either as a QMS or as a linear trap.

**Orbitrap.** The physical principles of orbital ion trapping were described by Kingdon in his seminal work published in 1923. However, during the next 80 years no practically useful mass spectrometers based on this principle were developed. The orbital trapping technology was further developed by Alexander Makarov, who made several significant technological advances, notably the superposition of a static quadrupolar electrostatic field in the axial direction of the device, enabling development of a line of commercially produced instruments, Orbitrap.

The Orbitrap mass analyzer consists of three electrodes. Two outer electrodes are funnel-shaped, face each other, and are electrically isolated by a dielectric ring. A third central electrode has the shape of a spindle. When voltages are applied to the outer and the central electrodes, the resulting electric field enables harmonic oscillations of ions in a direction roughly parallel to the axis of the spindle-shaped electrode. The radial component of the electric field attracts ions to the central electrode, which in combination with centrifugal forces traps ions in the radial direction. A static quadrupolar electric field in the axial direction causes the ions to undergo simple harmonic motion along that axis. Furthermore, the frequency of oscillation in the axial direction is independent of kinetic energy, causing the ions of different $m/z$ to oscillate with different frequencies. This results in ions of different $m/z$ values to oscillate at different frequencies. The outer electrodes of the Orbitrap mass analyzer serve as receiver plates for image current detection (measuring charge, induced on a nearby electrode) of the axial oscillations of the ions. The detected image currents are Fourier-transformed into a frequency domain and then mathematically transformed into a mass spectrum.

Compared to other commonly used mass analyzers, Orbitrap MS have greater mass accuracy and mass resolution, and are more-and-more commonly used in research applications and clinical laboratories.

## Tandem Mass Spectrometers

Tandem mass spectrometry (MS/MS) has become an important technique in clinical and analytical laboratories. In addition to quantitative analysis, MS/MS instruments are useful for compound identification and structural characterization. When coupled with chromatographic techniques, well-designed MS/MS assays are typically characterized by high specificity, low consumable costs, and high sample throughput.

The physical principle of tandem mass spectrometers is best understood for beam-type instruments. In these instruments, two mass spectrometers are arranged sequentially, with a "collision cell" placed between the two mass analyzers. The first analyzer is used to select ions of a particular $m/z$, called *precursor ions*. The precursor ion is directed into the collision cell, where ions collide with background gas molecules and are fragmented into smaller ions, called product ions. The second analyzer acquires the mass spectrum of the product ions.

The key to the high selectivity of MS/MS is that it characterizes compounds by two properties: precursor ion mass and product ion mass. Chromatographic separation adds a third dimension of selectivity. Use of these three compound-specific properties allows highly specific analysis and eliminates most interferences that are often encountered using less selective detection techniques.

As illustrated in Fig. 13.12, a variety of scan functions are possible with tandem mass spectrometers. A product ion scan involves setting the first mass spectrometer, MS1, to select a given $m/z$ and scanning through the full mass spectrum of product ions using the second mass spectrometer (MS2). This mode of instrument operation is often used for structural characterization of unknown compounds. In precursor ion scan mode, the MS2 is set to select $m/z$ of a specific product ion, and MS1 is working in a scanned mode. Peaks in the precursor ion scan are indicative of parent ions producing a specific product ion, a capability that is often used to analyze for specific classes of compounds, such as acylcarnitines.

A constant neutral loss scan consists of scanning both mass spectrometers synchronously, with a constant mass offset between the two mass analyzers. This scan function is selective for ions that lose a neutral fragment of a specific mass, corresponding to the value of the offset between the two mass spectrometers. This mode of operation is useful for analyses of certain classes of compounds, such as amino acids.

In multiple reaction monitoring (MRM) acquisition, the instrument cycles through a list of precursor/product ion pairs. Both mass analyzers, MS1 and MS2, are set in a static mode, whereby only selected precursor ions of the targeted compounds (and their internal standards) are passed through MS1. These preselected precursor ions are then fragmented in the collision cell, and the fragment ions derived from the compounds of interest are passed by MS2 to the detector. In methods for quantitative analysis utilizing MRM data acquisition, the precursor ion is typically the molecular ion of the targeted analyte, and product ions are unique fragments of the analyte generated in the collision cell.

As with single-stage mass spectrometers, tandem mass spectrometers are categorized as beam-type and trapping instruments. The most popular beam-type instrument is the triple quadrupole. In this instrument, the first quadrupole (Q1) functions as MS1, and the third quadrupole (Q3) functions as MS2. Between these two quadrupoles is another quadrupole, Q2, which functions as the collision cell rather than as a QMS.

So-called hybrid mass spectrometers include a combination of two different types of mass spectrometers in a tandem arrangement. Popular types of such instruments are a combination of a quadrupole for MS1 and an Orbitrap, TOF, or ion trap for MS2. These instruments are widely used in proteomics and metabolomics research where high specificity detection could be provided through use of high mass accuracy,

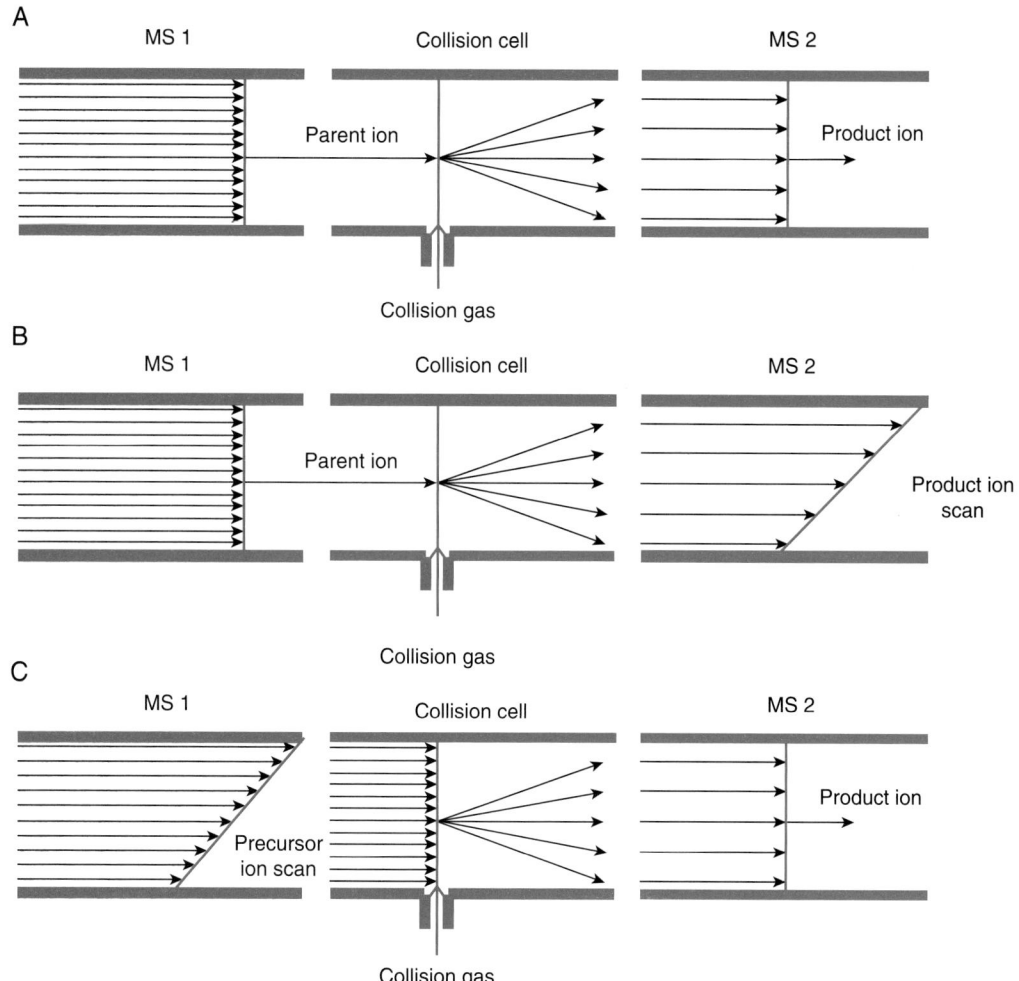

**Fig. 13.12** Scan modes in triple quadrupole mass spectrometry (MS/MS). (A) Single reaction monitoring (SRM) mode. The first mass analyzer (MS1) is fixed to monitor a single *m/z*, and the second mass analyzer (MS2) is fixed to monitor a single *m/z*. In cases when multiple mass transitions are monitored, this scan type is named "multiple reaction monitoring." (B) Product ion scan mode. MS1 is fixed to monitor a single *m/z*, and MS2 scans through a range of *m/z*. (C) Precursor ion scan mode. MS2 is fixed to monitor a single *m/z*, and MS1 is scanned through a range of *m/z* values.

high mass resolution, or incorporation of additional stages of fragmentation.

## Detectors

With the exception of Orbitrap type instruments, nearly all mass spectrometers use electron multipliers for ion detection. Three main types of electron multipliers are (1) discrete dynode multipliers; (2) continuous dynode electron multipliers (also known as *channel electron multipliers)*; and (3) microchannel plate electron multipliers. Although they are different in design, the principle of operation of all three is based on a multiplication process that is repeated through a chain of dynodes. Most designs of electron multipliers have 12 to 24 discrete dynodes. Both channel electron multipliers and continuous dynode electron multipliers use a continuous semiconducting layer rather than discrete dynodes.

The multiplication process typically produces a gain of $10^4$ to $10^8$, where the generation of one electron at the first dynode produces a pulse of $10^4$ to $10^8$ electrons at the end of the cascade. This first electron is generated by collision of an ion with the surface of the first dynode, causing ejection of an electron from the surface, with the duration of the pulse (after multiplication) of typically less than 10 nanoseconds. The combination of the number of electrons in a pulse and duration of a pulse is sufficient to allow single ion detection events.

Another type of detector used in mass spectrometers is the Faraday cup. This detector collects the ion current directly without going through a multiplication step. The Faraday cup is most commonly used in ICP-MS instruments, when the ion abundance is so high that it would saturate the output of an electron multiplier.

## Data Acquisition and Data Analysis Software

The signal produced by an instrument is digitized, and the digital signal is recorded and processed by computers. Modern MS instruments generate immense quantities of raw data, requiring high computing power. For example, in toxicology and biochemical genetics laboratories, one important function of the data analysis is library searching, which assists in compound identification. Several commercial libraries are available, including (1) Wiley Registry of Mass Spectral Data (https://sciencesolutions.wiley.com/solutions/technique/gc-ms/wiley-registry-12th-edition-nist-2020/; accessed on September 12, 2022); (2) the US National Institute of Standards and Technology (NIST) Mass Spectral Database, and the (3) Mass Spectral Library of Drugs, Poisons, Pesticides, Pollutants and Their Metabolites. In addition, many laboratories generate custom libraries. Important factors in the utility of such libraries include (1) the quality of cataloged mass spectra, (2) the search algorithm, and (3) the number of entries in the library. Several library search algorithms are available; the most popular are probability-based matching and the dot product matching approaches. All approaches allow assessment of match quality between the observed spectra and the library spectra.

The computer and software are used for (1) controlling the instrument and data acquisition, (2) signal processing, (3) quantitative calibration, (4) calculation of concentrations in quantitative analysis, (5) database searches, and (6) generating reports.

## CLINICAL APPLICATIONS

Mass spectrometers coupled with gas and liquid chromatographs (GC-MS and LC-MS) are versatile analytical instruments that allow development of high specificity, high sensitivity, and high throughput methods for the analysis of complex samples. In addition, many MS-based methods do not require specialized and/or expensive reagents, other than small quantities of isotopically labeled analogs of the analytes targeted in the methods (internal standards).

## Gas Chromatography-Mass Spectrometry

Gas chromatography–mass spectrometry (GC-MS) has been used for decades in the analysis of biological samples. One of the most common applications of GC-MS is in drug testing for clinical or forensic purposes. Because many drugs have low molecular weights and are sufficiently volatile, they are suitable for analysis by GC. EI with full-scan mass acquisition is a widely used approach for comprehensive drug screening and organic acid profiling in screening newborns for inborn errors of metabolism. Identification of unknown compounds is achieved by comparison of the acquired mass spectra with entries in a mass spectral library. "Unknown" in this sense means a compound that is not specifically targeted by the analysis, although its mass spectrum exists in a mass spectral library. In addition to identifying unknown constituents, MS-based techniques are the gold standard methodology for confirming drugs found by immunochemical analyses and as a reference methodology for many diagnostically important biomarkers. Additional clinical uses for GC-MS include analysis of xenobiotic compounds, fatty acids, steroids, pesticides, and pollutants.

## Liquid Chromatography-Mass Spectrometry

LC-MS/MS methods are widely used in clinical laboratories in the areas of newborn screening for metabolic disorders, toxicological drug screening and confirmation, endocrinology and metabolism, therapeutic drug monitoring, analysis of biogenic amines and vitamins, cancer biomarkers, protein and peptide biomarkers, and other applications. The majority of methods for targeted analysis in clinical laboratories use MRM data acquisition (see Fig. 13.12A).

An important area in which tandem MS is used clinically is newborn screening and confirmation of genetic and metabolic disorders. The ability to analyze multiple compounds in a single analysis makes this technique a highly efficient tool for screening purposes. For example, electrospray tandem MS is the most commonly used methodology for analysis of acylcarnitines and amino acids to screen for disorders of fatty acid oxidation, organic acid metabolism, amino acid, and the urea cycle defects.

One difficulty in measuring diagnostically important acylcarnitines and amino acids relates to the different instrument sensitivities required among the analytes included in the panels. To address this issue, a butyl ester derivatization of carboxyl groups can be used to make the molecules more ionizable, thus yielding more uniform ionization efficiency and sensitivity. Methods for amino acid analysis by MS/MS have been developed that utilize esterification to form butyl esters of amino acids. Collision-induced dissociation of the butyl ester derivatives result in the loss of a neutral fragment, butyl formate ($m/z$ 102 Da), enabling sensitive detection with uniform sensitivity among the diagnostically important amino acids (using constant neutral loss scanning.) The same derivatization strategy based on formation of butyl derivatives can be used for analysis of acylcarnitines, with detection (using precursor ion scan mode) of the molecules, which have a common characteristic fragment ion of *m/z* 85 Da. In many cases an analysis is performed on extracts from dried blood spots (collected on filter paper cards), without performing chromatography, particularly in the case of screening for hereditary metabolic defects.

Quantification of targeted compounds using LC-MS/MS is most commonly performed using MRM data acquisition (see Fig. 13.12). Because only molecule-specific ions are transmitted through MS1 and typically two molecule specific fragment ions (per analyte) are transmitted through MS2, the MRM data acquisition provides very high specificity and a greater sensitivity than could be achieved using other acquisition modes of triple quadrupole MS, as well as any other type of mass analyzers.

## Matrix-Assisted Laser Desorption/Ionization–Time-of-Flight Mass Spectrometry

MALDI is typically coupled with TOF mass analyzers (Fig. 13.13). During the last 10 years, identification of microorganisms using MALDI-TOF has become widely accepted for routine use in clinical laboratories. The fact that different bacteria express unique mixtures of proteins and peptides serves as the basis of bacteria identification. When culture samples are analyzed using MALDI-TOF, the bacteria-specific mass spectra are observed in the mass range of *m/z* 2000 to 20,000 Da, allowing the use of mass spectral libraries for matching mass spectra of unknown samples to the entries in the mass spectral library (fingerprints of the peaks in the mass spectra correspond to the bacteria-specific proteins and peptides).

Advantages of MALDI-TOF for microorganism identification include: (1) accuracy of identification at the species level that is comparable to traditional microbiology methods; (2) fast turnaround time; (3) ease and speed of sample preparation; (4) high-throughput data acquisition and data analysis;

and (5) relatively low cost per sample. Some of the disadvantages of the technique are related to the lack of information on the identity of most of the observed mass spectral peaks, inability to distinguish some strains of the bacteria, and that the mass spectral libraries are typically specific to the sample preparation method used.

Some limitations of MALDI as a technique are (1) MALDI cannot be directly interfaced with online separations (e.g., HPLC, capillary electrophoresis), (2) there is a high background noise in MALDI mass spectra, and (3) poor reproducibility among individual scans. Because of the above, MALDI-TOF MS is predominantly a qualitative technique. Progress has been made toward MALDI-TOF use for quantitative analysis; however, such applications often require off-line sample preparation and fractionation prior to instrumental analysis.

## Inductively Coupled Plasma Mass Spectrometry

In clinical laboratories, ICP-MS is used for quantification of trace elements in whole blood, urine, plasma, serum, and tissue biopsy samples. Clinical reasons for analyzing biological samples for trace elements include screening and confirmation of suspected heavy metal poisoning and diagnosing/monitoring patients with metabolic disorders (e.g., Wilson disease). In some cases, toxicity depends on the presence of the metal within specific molecules. This requires elemental speciation that is performed to separate and quantify an element incorporated in various organic or inorganic molecules (e.g., arsenic speciation), rather than determining the total element concentration. These applications use sample fractionation with HPLC, or capillary electrophoreses to separate various metal-containing molecules before sample introduction in an ICP-MS instrument.

## Proteomics and Metabolomics

In the mid-1990s MS came to the forefront of analytical techniques used to study proteins, and the term *proteomics* was coined. Currently MS is routinely used to accomplish many tasks in proteomics. Traditionally proteomics referred to the identification and quantification of proteins and their posttranslational modifications. A common approach to identify proteins is known as bottom-up analysis, wherein proteins are enriched and then enzymatically digested, usually with trypsin. The resulting digests are then analyzed, and the detected peptides are matched to the theoretical digests using mass spectral databases.

Partial sequencing and therefore potential identification of intact proteins may be achieved without prior digestion, using top-down techniques or using partially digested proteins (a middle-down approach). Approaches used for protein top-down characterization include extraction of the proteins from samples followed by fractionation and analysis of the samples using high resolution MS/MS with collision induced dissociation, higher energy collision dissociation (HCD), electron capture dissociation (ECD), or electron transfer dissociation (ETD) fragmentation. The main benefits of the top-down and middle-down analyses are the ability to

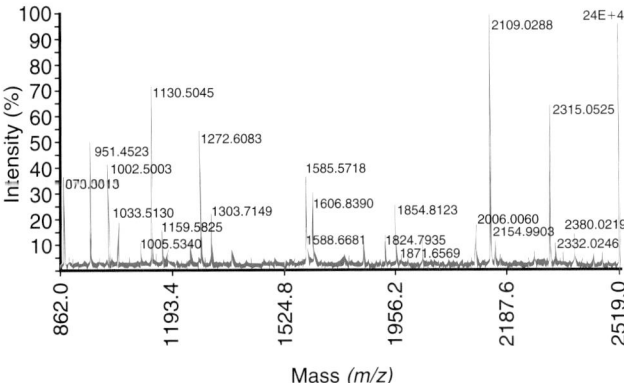

**Fig. 13.13** An example of a matrix-assisted laser desorption/ionization–time-of-flight spectrum showing peptides generated in a tryptic digest of a spot from a two-dimensional sodium dodecyl sulfate-polyacrylamide gel.

detect proteins containing posttranslational modifications and sequence variants.

Most often the term *proteomics* is used in the context of biomarker discovery. In clinical diagnostic testing, it also includes qualitative and quantitative analysis of known protein and peptide biomarkers. One of methods recently introduced in routine testing is quantitative analysis of thyroglobulin, a marker of the recurrence of thyroid cancer. Measurement of thyroglobulin is commonly used for the follow-up of patients treated for differentiated thyroid carcinoma. Because thyroid tissue is the only source of thyroglobulin, after total thyroidectomy serum concentrations of thyroglobulin should decrease to very low or undetectable concentrations; a rise in the serum concentration of thyroglobulin is indicative of cancer recurrence. The presence of endogenous anti-thyroglobulin autoantibodies (Tg-AAb) can mask the epitopes used by reagent antibodies in immunoassays, and this may lead to false negative results. The LC-MS/MS based methods for measurement of thyroglobulin overcome interference of Tg-AAb. The published methods use enzymatic digestion of proteins present in samples; during the digestion, thyroglobulin and Tg-AAb get digested to peptides, thus removing the interference and allowing accurate, quantitative measurement of thyroglobulin based on the concentration of thyroglobulin-specific peptides present in the digested samples. Currently, LC-MS/MS methods

for thyroglobulin are offered in several commercial laboratories; these methods provide an important tool for physicians monitoring patients for the recurrence of thyroid cancer. Introduction of these methods for measurement of thyroglobulin in clinical practice is one example of the application of MS for routine quantitative measurement of proteins. LC-MS/MS methods have also been used for identification of hemoglobin variants, insulin analogs, and for quantification of insulin-like growth factor, parathyroid hormone (PTH), parathyroid hormone-related protein (PTHrP), and a number of other clinically relevant protein biomarkers.

Another area where MS plays an important role is in the field of *metabolomics*. This scientific area investigates and characterizes intermediates and products of metabolism that are present in biological fluids under various conditions. Some areas of interest in metabolomics include (1) normal homeostasis, (2) disease states, (3) metabolic diseases, (4) stress, (5) dietary modification, (6) treatment protocols, and (7) aging. In a similar fashion to a mass spectrum, a fingerprint signature for specific molecules and patterns of compounds can be identified for different metabolomic and physiologic states.

MS provides great potential for highly specific measurements, but in order to realize this potential, all MS-based methods should be extensively validated and standardized.

## REVIEW QUESTIONS

1. Which of the following types of mass spectrometers involve a single path for ions through the instrument, followed by the ions striking a detector where they are destructively detected?
   a. Trapping type
   b. Beam type
   c. Mass-selective ejection type
   d. Ion-cyclotron resonance type
2. In mass spectrometry, the sum of abundances of all ions produced, displayed as a function of time, represents:
   a. product ion.
   b. extracted ion profile.
   c. mass spectrum.
   d. total ion chromatogram.
3. Which type of ionization technique uses an electron beam to ionize the reagent gas and produce a reactive species as a result of gas-phase ion-molecule reactions?
   a. Electron ionization
   b. Chemical ionization
   c. Electrospray ionization

   d. Inductively coupled plasma ionization
4. Inductively coupled plasma mass spectrometry is typically used for:
   a. determination of trace elements.
   b. identification of a protein.
   c. drug identification.
   d. isotopic labeling of molecules.
5. The ionization technique most commonly used in mass analyzers coupled with gas chromatography is:
   a. electrospray ionization.
   b. chemical ionization.
   c. matrix-assisted laser desorption/ionization.
   d. electron ionization.
6. The type of mass spectrometer most commonly used for quantitative analysis is the:
   a. quadrupole mass spectrometer.
   b. time-of-flight instrument.
   c. Orbitrap.
   d. linear ion trap mass spectrometer.

## SUGGESTED READINGS

Anderson NL, Anderson NG, Pearson TW, et al. A human proteome detection and quantitation project. *Mol Cellular Proteom.* 2009;8:883–886.

Bystrom CE, Sheng S, Clarke NJ. Narrow mass extraction of time-of-flight data for quantitative analysis of proteins: determination of insulin-like growth factor-1. *Anal Chem.* 2011;83(23):9005–9010.

Ceglarek U, Lembcke J, Fiedler GM, et al. Rapid simultaneous quantification of immunosuppressants in transplant patients by turbulent flow chromatography combined with tandem mass spectrometry. *Clin Chim Acta.* 2004;346:181–190.

Cherkaoui A, Hibbs J, Emonet S, et al. Comparison of two matrix-assisted laser desorption ionization-time of flight mass spectrometry methods with conventional phenotypic identification for routine identification of bacteria to the species level. *J Clin Microbiol.* 2010;48:1169–1175.

Clarke NJ, Hoofnagle AN. Mass spectrometry continues its march into the clinical laboratory. *Clin Lab Med.* 2011;31, ix–xi.

Clarke NJ, Zhang Y, Reitz RE. A novel mass spectrometry-based assay for the accurate measurement of thyroglobulin from patient samples containing antithyroglobulin autoantibodies. *J Invest Med.* 2012l;60:1157–1163.

Covey TR, Thomson BA, Schneider BB. Atmospheric pressure ion sources. *Mass Spectrom Rev.* 2009;28:870–897.

Dilillo M, Heijs B, McDonnell LA. Mass spectrometry imaging: how will it affect clinical research in the future? *Expert Rev Proteomics.* 2018;15:709–716.

Feider CL, Krieger A, DeHoog RJ, Eberlin LS. Ambient ionization mass spectrometry: recent developments and applications. *Anal Chem.* 2019;91:4266–4290.

Fenn JB. Electrospray wings for molecular elephants (Nobel lecture). *Angewandte Chem Intl Ed Engl.* 2003;42:3871–3894.

Hoofnagle AN, Roth MY. Clinical review: improving the measurement of serum thyroglobulin with mass spectrometry. *J Clin Endocrinol Metab.* 2013;98:1343–1352.

Kuhara T. Gas chromatographic-mass spectrometric urinary metabolome analysis to study mutations of inborn errors of metabolism. *Mass Spectromet Rev.* 2005;24:814–827.

Kushnir MM, Rockwood AL, Bergquist J. Liquid chromatography-tandem mass spectrometry applications in endocrinology. *Mass Spectromet Rev.* 2010;29:480–502.

Kushnir MM, Rockwood AL, Nelson GJ, et al. Assessing analytical specificity in quantitative analysis using tandem mass spectrometry. *Clin Biochem.* 2005;38:319–327.

Mbughuni MM, Jannetto PJ, Langman LJ. Mass spectrometry applications for toxicology. *EJIFCC.* 2016;27:272–287.

Rockwood A, Palmblad M. Isotopic distributions. *Methods Mol Biol.* 2013;1007:65–99.

Sandalakis V, Goniotakis I, Vranakis I, et al. Use of MALDI-TOF mass spectrometry in the battle against bacterial infectious diseases: recent achievements and future perspectives. *Expert Rev Proteomics.* 2017;14:253–267.

Villoria JG, Pajares S, López RM, et al. Neonatal screening for inherited metabolic diseases in 2016. *Sem Pediatr Neurol.* 2016;23:257–272.

Whitehouse CM, Dreyer RN, Yamashita M, et al. Electrospray interface for liquid chromatographs and mass spectrometers. *Analyt Chem.* 1985;57:675–679.

Zubarev RA, Makarov A. Orbitrap mass spectrometry. *Analyt Chem.* 2013;85:5288–5296.

# Enzyme and Rate Analyses

*Ilenia Infusino and Mauro Panteghini\**

## OBJECTIVES

1. Explain how enzyme measurements are used in laboratory medicine.
2. Delineate how enzymes are classified in the Enzyme Commission (EC) system and give an example.
3. Give examples of primary, secondary, tertiary, and quaternary structures of enzymes.
4. Describe the importance of the relationship of structure to enzyme function.
5. Give an example of how enzymes carry out their reactions at the active site.
6. Write an equation for the formation of an enzyme-substrate complex.
7. Describe how enzymatic reactions are influenced by changes in:

   a. Enzyme concentration
   b. Substrate concentration
   c. Ionic concentration
   d. Temperature
   e. Inhibitors and activators
8. Give an example of an enzyme assay and describe how it works.
9. Write an equation that delineates how the velocity of an enzyme reaction depends on substrate concentration.
10. Describe three different kinds of enzyme inhibition.
11. Explain how enzyme measurements can be standardized by using metrological traceability concepts.
12. Describe the use of enzymes as analytical reagents.

## KEY WORDS AND DEFINITIONS

**Activator** Small molecule or ion that increases the rate of an enzyme-catalyzed reaction by promoting formation of the most active state of the enzyme, substrate, or other reactant.

**Active center/active site** That part of an enzyme formed by the tertiary structure at which the noncovalent binding of substrate occurs to form the intermediate enzyme-substrate complex.

**Analytical selectivity** Property of a measurement procedure, whereby it provides measured quantity values for one or more measurands such that the values of each measurand are independent of other measurands or other quantities in the sample being investigated.

**Catalyst** A substance that modifies and increases the rate of a chemical reaction without being permanently changed or consumed; an enzyme is a protein catalyst of biological origin.

**Clinical enzymology** The branch of medical science that deals with the biochemical nature and activity of enzymes of clinical relevance.

**Coenzyme** A small molecule (some contain structures derived from vitamins) that is required for some enzyme-catalyzed reactions to occur. Coenzymes are temporarily or permanently bound to the enzyme.

**Commutability** The ability of an enzyme (reference or control) material to show inter-assay catalytic activity changes comparable to those of the same enzyme in human serum.

**Enzyme** A protein with catalytic properties.

**First-order kinetics** A phase in an enzymatic reaction where substrate concentration is limiting and the reaction rate is proportional to the concentration of substrate.

**Inhibitor** A substance that reduces the rate of an enzymatic reaction.

**International unit** The quantity of enzyme that catalyzes the conversion of one micromole of substrate to product per minute.

**Isoenzyme** A form of an enzyme that originates at the level of the gene that encodes the structure of the enzyme protein and is distinguished by certain physical properties.

**Isoform** A form of an enzyme that is modified by posttranslational processing.

**Katal** The quantity of an enzyme that catalyzes the conversion of one mole of substrate to product per second.

**Lineweaver-Burk plot** A plot of the reciprocal of the velocity of an enzyme-catalyzed reaction (ordinate; y-axis) against the reciprocal of the substrate concentration (abscissa; x-axis).

**Michaelis-Menten constant ($K_m$)** A constant for a given enzyme acting under given conditions; the experimentally determined substrate concentration at

*The authors gratefully acknowledge the original contributions of R. Bais on which portions of this chapter are based.

which the enzymatic reaction velocity equals one-half of the maximum velocity of the enzymatic reaction.

**Product** The substance produced by an enzyme-catalyzed conversion of a substrate.

**Substrate** A reactant in an enzyme-catalyzed reaction that binds to the active center of an enzyme.

**Zero-order kinetics** A phase in an enzymatic reaction when the substrate concentration is saturating and the reaction rate is maximal; the reaction rate depends only on the enzyme concentration and is independent of substrate concentration.

---

Enzymes are biological catalysts that can be used in the diagnosis and monitoring of disease. Some enzymes have remarkable properties that make them sensitive indicators of pathologic change. Metabolism can be regarded as an integrated series of enzymatic reactions, and some diseases as a derangement of the physiologic pattern of metabolism. Many enzymes exist in multiple forms and differences in their properties help in differentiating them and understanding organ-specific pathophysiology. Genetically determined variations in enzyme structure between individuals are used to account for such characteristics as differences in sensitivity to drugs and differences in metabolism, which manifest themselves as hereditary metabolic diseases.

## ENZYME NOMENCLATURE

Historically, individual enzymes were identified using the name of the **substrate** or group on which they act and then adding the suffix *-ase*. For example, the enzyme hydrolyzing urea was ur*ease*. Later, the type of reaction involved was identified, as in carbonic anhydrase, D-amino acid oxidase, and succinate dehydrogenase. In addition, some enzymes were given empirical names such as trypsin, diastase, ptyalin, pepsin, and emulsin.

Because this combination of trivial common names and semisystematic names was found to be inadequate, in 1955 the International Union of Biochemistry (IUB) appointed an Enzyme Commission (EC) to study the problem of enzyme nomenclature. Its subsequent recommendations, with periodic updating, provide a rational and practical basis for identifying all enzymes now known and enzymes that will be discovered in the future.

With the IUB system, a systematic and trivial name is provided for each enzyme. The systematic name describes the nature of the reaction catalyzed and is associated with a unique numeric code. The trivial or practical name, which may be identical to the systematic name but is often a simplification of it, is suitable for everyday use. The unique numeric designation for each enzyme consists of four numbers, separated by periods (e.g., 2.2.8.11), and is prefixed by the letters *EC*, denoting *Enzyme Commission*. The first number defines the class to which the enzyme belongs. All enzymes are assigned to one of six classes, characterized by the type of reaction they catalyze: (1) oxidoreductases, (2) transferases, (3) hydrolases, (4) lyases, (5) isomerases, and (6) ligases. The next two numbers indicate the subclass and the sub-subclass to which the enzyme is assigned. For example, these may differentiate the amino-transferring subclass from the phosphate-transferring subclass, or the sub-subclass accepting ethanol from those accepting acyl groups. The last number is the specific serial number given to each enzyme within its sub-subclass.

Table 14.1 lists selected enzymes of clinical interest, identified by trivial, abbreviated, and systematic names and by their code numbers.

Although not recommended by the EC, it is a common and convenient practice to use capital letter abbreviations for the names of certain enzymes, such as ALT for alanine aminotransferase, AST for aspartate aminotransferase, LDH for lactate dehydrogenase, and CK for creatine kinase (see Table 14.1).

## ENZYMES AS PROTEINS

Enzymes are proteins and thus possess the primary, secondary, and tertiary structural characteristics of proteins (see Chapter 18). Many enzymes also exhibit quaternary structure. The *primary* structure, the linear sequence of amino acids linked through their α-carboxyl and α-amino groups by peptide bonds, is specific for each type of enzyme molecule. Each polypeptide chain is coiled into three-dimensional (3D) secondary and tertiary structures. Secondary structure refers to the conformation of limited segments of the polypeptide chain, namely α-helices, β-pleated sheets, random coils, and β-turns. The combination of secondary structural elements and amino acid side chain interactions that define the 3D structure of the folded protein is referred to as its tertiary structure. In many cases, biological activity, such as the catalytic activity of enzymes, requires two or more folded polypeptide chains (subunits) to associate to form a functional molecule. The specific combination of these subunits defines the quaternary structure. The subunits may be multiples of the same polypeptide chain (e.g., the MM isoenzyme of CK, the $H_4$ isoenzyme of LDH), or they may be combinations of distinct polypeptides (e.g., the MB isoenzyme of CK).

No feature of primary structure is common to all enzyme molecules. However, considerable homologies of amino acid sequences are found between enzymes that appear to share a common evolutionary origin, such as the proteases trypsin and chymotrypsin. Similarities of sequence are even more marked among the members of a family of isoenzymes. The amino acid sequence in the immediate neighborhood of the **active center** of the enzyme (discussed later) is often similar in enzymes with related function (e.g., the *serine proteases* are so called because they all have this amino acid in the active center).

**TABLE 14.1   Enzyme Commission Numbers, Systematic and Trivial Names, and Frequently Adopted Abbreviations of Enzymes of Major Clinical Importance**

| EC Number | Systematic Name | Trivial Name | Abbreviation |
|---|---|---|---|
| 1.1.1.27 | L-Lactate: NAD$^+$ oxidoreductase | Lactate dehydrogenase | LDH |
| 1.4.1.3 | L-Glutamate: NAD(P)$^+$ oxidoreductase (deaminating) | Glutamate dehydrogenase | GLD |
| 2.3.2.2 | ($\gamma$-Glutamyl)-peptide: amino acid $\gamma$-glutamyltransferase | $\gamma$-Glutamyltransferase | GGT |
| 2.6.1.1 | L-Aspartate: 2-oxoglutarate aminotransferase | Aspartate aminotransferase (transaminase) | AST |
| 2.6.1.2 | L-Alanine: 2-oxoglutarate aminotransferase | Alanine aminotransferase (transaminase) | ALT |
| 2.7.3.2 | ATP: creatine N-phosphotransferase | Creatine kinase | CK |
| 3.1.1.3 | Triacylglycerol acylhydrolase | Lipase | LIP |
| 3.1.1.7 | Acetylcholine acetylhydrolase | Acetylcholinesterase, true cholinesterase, choline esterase I | — |
| 3.1.1.8 | Acetylcholine acylhydrolase | Pseudocholinesterase, butyryl cholinesterase, choline esterase II (serum cholinesterase) | CHE |
| 3.1.3.1 | Orthophosphoric-monoester phosphohydrolase (alkaline optimum) | Alkaline phosphatase | ALP |
| 3.1.3.2 | Orthophosphoric-monoester phosphohydrolase (acid optimum) | Acid phosphatase | ACP |
| 3.1.3.5 | 5'-Ribonucleotide phosphohydrolase | 5'-Nucleotidase | NTP |
| 3.2.1.1 | 1,4-$\alpha$-D-Glucan glucanohydrolase | Amylase | AMY |
| 3.4.21.4 | No systematic name | Trypsin | TRY |

*EC,* Enzyme Commission; *NAD,* nicotinamide adenine dinucleotide; *NAD(P),* NAD phosphate.

Enzyme molecules differ in the proportion of secondary structures—such as α-helices—that they contain, although no enzyme molecule studied thus far approaches the large proportion of α-helices found in myoglobin and hemoglobin. The tertiary structures of different types of enzyme molecules are as individually characteristic as their primary structures; nevertheless, some common features exist. Enzyme molecules are roughly globular in overall shape, with a preponderance of polar amino acid side chains on the outside of the molecule and nonpolar side chains in the interior. The ionizable residues in contact with the surrounding medium are responsible for many of the properties of the enzyme molecules in solution, such as their migration in an electric field and their solubility. Covalent disulfide bridges may link different parts of the polypeptide chains in some enzyme molecules, but the 3D structure is mainly stabilized by the large number of hydrophobic interactions formed between the nonpolar side chains in the interior of the molecule.

The application of physical methods, such as x-ray crystallography and multidimensional nuclear magnetic resonance, has provided structural insights from which enzyme mechanisms have been proposed. Furthermore, the tools of molecular biology, such as molecular cloning, have enabled the

purification and characterization of enzymes that previously were available only in minute amounts. Molecular biology also enables the manipulation of the amino acid sequence of enzymes. Site-directed mutagenesis (substituting one amino acid residue for another) and deletion mutagenesis (eliminating sections of the primary structure) have enabled the identification of chemical groups that participate in ligand binding and specific chemical steps during catalysis. The biological activity of a protein molecule depends generally on the integrity of its structure, and any disruption of its secondary, tertiary, or quaternary structure will likely be accompanied by a loss of activity, a process known as *denaturation.* If the process of denaturation is minimal, it may be reversed with the recovery of enzyme activity on removal of the denaturing agent. However, prolonged or severe denaturing conditions result in an irreversible loss of activity. Denaturing conditions include increased temperatures, extremes of pH, and exposure to certain chemicals. Heat inactivation of most enzymes takes place at an appreciable rate at room temperature, and in most cases becomes very fast above 60°C. However, certain enzymes, most notably some polymerases, can retain activity at temperatures as high as 95°C. This property has been exploited in the polymerase chain reaction (see Chapter 48).

Extremes of pH also cause the unfolding of enzymes and, with few exceptions, should be avoided when enzyme samples are preserved. Addition of chemicals, such as urea and detergents, disrupts hydrogen bonding and hydrophobic interactions, also resulting in enzyme inactivation.

## SPECIFICITY AND THE ACTIVE CENTER

With the exception of enzymes such as proteases, nucleases, and amylases, which act on macromolecular substrates, enzyme molecules are considerably larger than their substrate molecules. Consideration of the structure of an enzyme's active site and its substrate(s) in their ground and transition states is necessary to understand the rate enhancement and specificity of chemical reactions catalyzed by an enzyme. The active site of an enzyme will vary among enzymes, but in general, the following statements hold:

1. The active site of an enzyme is relatively small compared with the total size of the enzyme molecule and may involve less than 5% of its amino acids.
2. The active sites of enzymes are 3D structures that are formed as a result of the overall tertiary structure of the protein. This results in the amino acids and cofactors in the active site of an enzyme being spatially structured in an exact, 3D relationship with respect to one another and to the structure of the substrate molecule.
3. Typically, the binding of substrate molecules to the active site of an enzyme is noncovalent, and is stabilized by hydrogen bonding, electrostatic, hydrophobic, and van der Waals interactions.
4. Active sites of enzymes typically occur in clefts and crevices in the protein's tertiary structure.

The specificity of substrate binding is a function of the exact spatial arrangement of atoms in the enzyme active site that complements the structure of the substrate molecule.

## ISOENZYMES AND OTHER MULTIPLE FORMS OF ENZYMES

Isoenzymes are enzymes that can catalyze the same reaction, but that differ in some aspect of their structure. They may occur within a single organ or even within a single type of cell. The forms can be distinguished on the basis of differences in various properties, such as electrophoretic mobility, immunological reactivity, and resistance to chemical or thermal inactivation. They often have significant quantifiable differences in catalytic properties, but all forms of a particular enzyme retain the ability to catalyze its characteristic reaction.

The existence of multiple forms of enzymes in human tissue has important implications in the study of human disease. The presence in different organs of isoenzymes with distinctive properties helps in understanding organ-specific patterns of metabolism. Genetically determined variations in enzyme structure among individuals account for such characteristics as differences in sensitivity to drugs and differences in metabolism, which manifest themselves as hereditary metabolic diseases. For diagnostic enzymology, the existence of multiple forms of enzymes, whether the result of genetic or nongenetic causes, provides opportunities to increase the diagnostic specificity and sensitivity of enzyme assays in body fluid samples.

Similar to other proteins, enzymes usually elicit the production of antibodies when they are injected into animals of a species other than those in which they originate. Even small structural differences among closely similar molecules, such as the members of a family of isoenzymes, are often sufficient to render them antigenically distinct, allowing antibodies to be produced specific to a single isoenzyme. The availability of immunochemical methods has been particularly important in the analysis of isoenzyme mixtures with many commercial immunoassays using monoclonal antibodies to increase specificity.

### Genetic Origins of Enzyme Variants

True isoenzymes result from the existence of more than one gene coding for the structure of the enzyme protein. Many human enzymes (more than one-third) are known to be determined by more than one structural gene. Similar but distinct genes have undergone differential modifications during the course of evolution so that the enzyme proteins coded by them no longer have identical structures, although they can catalyze the same reaction; in other words, they are isoenzymes.

The multiple genes that determine a particular group of isoenzymes are not necessarily closely linked on one chromosome. For example, the structural genes that code for human salivary and pancreatic amylases both are located on chromosome 1, whereas the genes that code for cytoplasmic and mitochondrial malate dehydrogenase are on chromosomes 2 and 7, respectively. Among the enzymes of clinical importance that exist as isoenzymes because of the presence of multiple-gene loci are LDH, CK, α-amylase, and some forms of alkaline phosphatase (ALP).

An enzyme can exist in molecular forms that differ from one individual to another because of the existence of alternative alleles that are inherited according to Mendelian laws. These alleles give rise to gene products, enzymes, with the same function. Isoenzymes that result from the existence of different alleles are termed *allozymes*. Many human genes have allelic variation and the probability that individuals will differ in their isoenzyme patterns is high.

The number of allelic variants and the frequency with which variants occur within the population vary considerably across enzymes. For example, mutations at either of the two principal loci that determine human LDH are extremely rare, but a high incidence of mutant alleles occurs at the single locus that determines the structure of placental ALP. More than 400 mutations in the glucose-6-phosphate dehydrogenase gene have now been identified on the X chromosome. When isoenzymes, because of variation at a single locus, occur with appreciable frequency in a human population, the population is said to be *polymorphic* with respect to the isoenzymes in question.

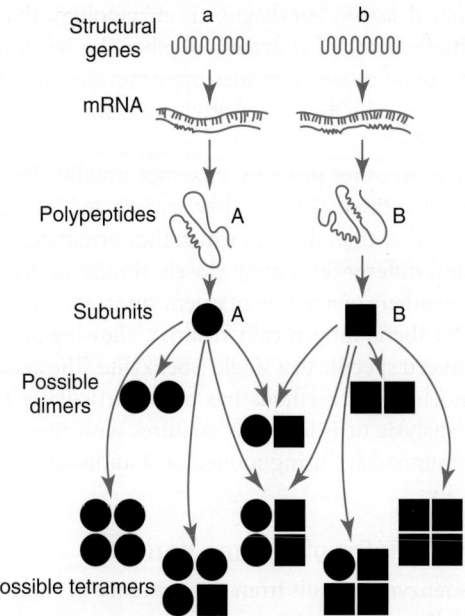

**Fig. 14.1** Diagram showing the origin of isoenzymes, assuming the existence of two distinct genes. When the active enzymes are polymers containing more than one subunit, hybrid isoenzymes consisting of mixtures of different subunits may be formed. One such isoenzyme can be formed in the case of a dimeric enzyme, such as creatine kinase, and three if the enzyme is a tetramer (e.g., lactate dehydrogenase). In both cases, two homopolymeric isoenzymes can also exist. (From Moss DW. *Isoenzyme Analysis.* London: The Chemical Society. Reproduced by permission of The Royal Society of Chemistry; 1979.)

Another category of multiple molecular forms can arise when enzymes are oligomeric and possess quaternary structure. The association of different subunits in various combinations gives rise to a range of active enzyme molecules. When the subunits are derived from different structural genes—multiple genes or multiple alleles—the hybrid molecules so formed are called *hybrid isoenzymes*. The ability to form hybrid isoenzymes is evidence of considerable structural similarities among the different subunits. Hybrid isoenzymes can be formed in vitro, but they are also formed in vivo when different types of constituent subunits are present in the same subcellular compartment.

The number of different hybrid isoenzymes that can form from two nonidentical protomers depends on the number of subunits in the complete enzyme molecule. For a dimeric enzyme, one mixed dimer (hybrid isoenzyme) can be formed. If the enzyme is a tetramer, three heteropolymeric isoenzymes may be formed (Fig. 14.1). Examples of hybrid isoenzymes include the mixed MB (muscle-brain) dimer of CK and the three hybrid isoenzymes, LDH-2, LDH-3, and LDH-4 of LDH.

## Nongenetic Causes of Multiple Forms of Enzymes

Posttranslational modifications of enzyme molecules give rise to multiple forms known as **isoforms** (Fig. 14.2). For example, removal of amide groups accounts for some of the heterogeneity of amylase and carbonic anhydrase (each of these enzymes also exists as a true isoenzyme). Modification also can take place as a result of extraction procedures. Many erythrocyte enzymes, including adenosine deaminase, acid

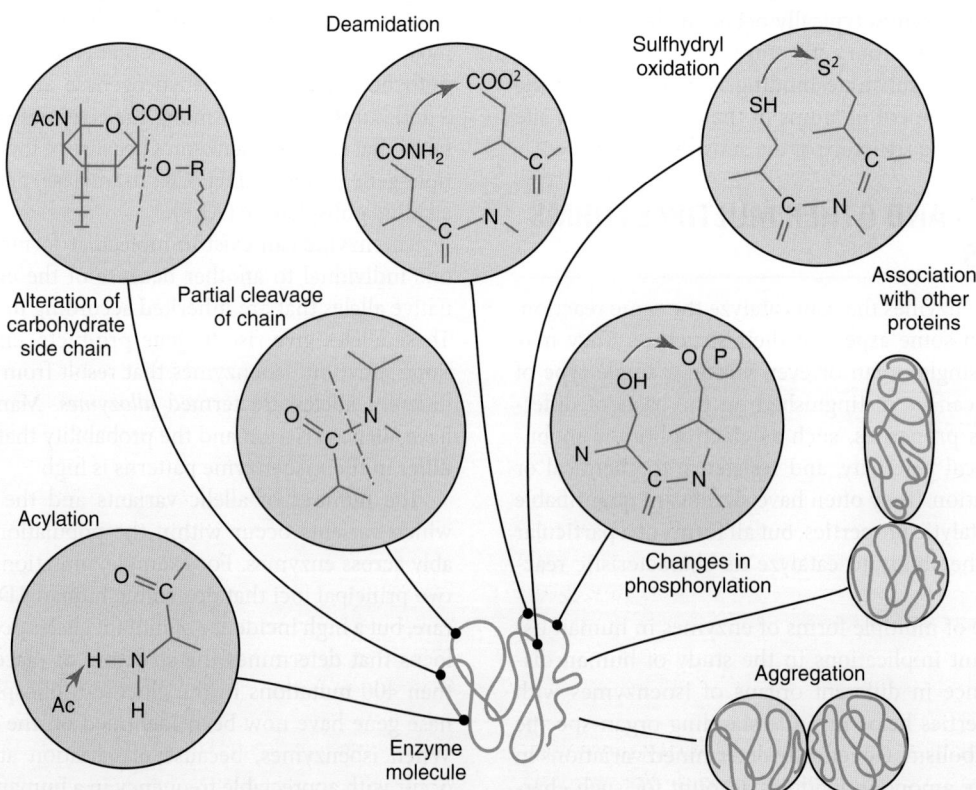

**Fig. 14.2** Nongenetic modifications that may give rise to multiple forms of enzymes. (From Moss DW. *Isoenzymes.* London: Chapman & Hall; 1982.)

phosphatase, and some forms of phosphoglucomutase, contain sulfhydryl groups that are susceptible to oxidation. In hemolysates, oxidation may be brought about by the action of oxidized glutathione, although in intact cells, this compound is present in its reduced form.

Serum isoforms of CK are formed as part of the normal clearance process of the cell. Human myocardial and skeletal muscle tissues have the CK-MM and CK-MB isoenzymes, which are modified on release into the circulation by removal of the C-terminal amino acid lysine from the M subunits by the action of carboxypeptidase.

Modifications of enzyme molecules also may include nonprotein components that lead to molecular heterogeneity. Many enzymes are glycoproteins, and variations in carbohydrate side chains are a common cause of nonhomogeneity. Some carbohydrate moieties, notably N-acetylneuraminic acid (sialic acid), are strongly ionized and consequently have a profound effect on some enzyme molecules. For example, removal of terminal sialic acid groups from the human liver and/or bone ALP with neuraminidase greatly reduces the electrophoretic heterogeneity of the enzyme.

Aggregation of enzyme molecules with each other or with nonenzymatic proteins may give rise to multiple forms that can be separated by techniques that depend on differences in molecular size. For example, four catalytically active cholinesterase components with molecular weights ranging from approximately 80,000 to 340,000 are found in most sera, with the heaviest component, $C_4$, contributing most of the enzyme activity. Other enzyme forms are also occasionally present, but it appears that the principal serum cholinesterase fractions can be attributed to different states of aggregation of a single monomer.

A specific form of interaction between enzymatic and nonenzymatic proteins, such as immunoglobulins, results in the formation of an enzyme-protein complex (macrocomplex). Enzyme–immunoglobulin complexes have been observed involving amylase, LDH, CK, ALP, and other enzymes.

A single polypeptide chain, in theory, exists in an infinite number of different conformations. However, one specific conformation generally appears to be the most stable for any given sequence of amino acids, and this conformation is assumed by the chain as it is synthesized within the cell. Thus the primary structure of the polypeptide chain also determines its 3D secondary and tertiary structures. It is conceivable that, in some cases, several alternative conformations (conformers) of a single chain that are almost equally stable may be present, and therefore these alternative forms may coexist. However, multiple-enzyme forms that demonstrate conformational isomerism have not been shown unequivocally.

## Changes in Isoenzyme Distribution During Development and Disease

The patterns of many isoenzymes change during physiologic development in tissues from many species. For example, during the embryonic development of skeletal muscle, the proportions of more cationic isoenzymes—both LDH and CK—progressively increase until approximately the sixth month of intrauterine life when the pattern resembles that of differentiated muscle.

The liver also shows characteristic changes in the patterns of several isoenzymes during embryogenesis. In early fetal development, three aldolase isoenzymes—A, B, and C—together with various hybrid tetramers, can be detected in extracts of liver. However, at birth, as in the adult liver, aldolase B is the predominant isoenzyme. Striking changes in the distribution of isoenzymes of alcohol dehydrogenase also occur in the human liver during prenatal development.

Changes in isoenzyme patterns during development result from changes in the relative activities of different genes within developing cells of a particular type (e.g., muscle cells). Other alterations in the balance of isoenzymes within the whole organism may derive from changes in the number or activity of cells that contain large amounts of a characteristic isoenzyme. An example of this is the increased number and activity of the osteoblasts, which are responsible for mineralization of the skeleton between the early postnatal period and the beginning of the third decade of life. An excess of ALP from active osteoblasts enters the circulation, where its presence can be recognized by its characteristic properties and where it increases the total serum ALP activity of young individuals to values higher than in skeletally mature adults. An ALP from the liver also contributes to the total activity of this enzyme in the plasma of healthy individuals, and the amount of this form in plasma shows a small, progressive increase with age. The reason for the latter age-dependent change is not known, but it may result from increased synthesis of the enzyme by hepatocytes in response to continuing exposure to inducing factors.

The distributions of isoenzymes of aldolase, LDH, and CK in the muscles of patients with progressive muscular dystrophy are similar to those in the early development of fetal muscle. Isoenzyme abnormalities in dystrophic muscle have been interpreted as failure to reach or maintain a normal degree of differentiation. Isoenzyme patterns seen in regenerating tissues also may show some tendency to approach fetal distributions. This tendency may result from relaxation or modification of control systems in rapidly dividing cells and may account for some of the isoenzyme changes noted (e.g., in muscle in acute polymyositis).

Cancer cells show progressive loss of the structure and metabolism of the healthy cells from which they arise. Therefore, the pattern of isoenzymes of mature, differentiated tissue may be lost or modified if normal differentiation is arrested or reversed; and many examples of isoenzyme changes accompanying cancer have been reported. Reemergence of fetal patterns of isoenzyme distribution is a feature of malignant transformation in many tissues. This phenomenon was first studied extensively in the case of LDH isoenzymes. Malignant tumors in general show a significant shift in the balance of isoenzymes toward LDH-4 and LDH-5. The decline in activity of the LDH-1 and LDH-2 isoenzymes results in patterns that are reminiscent of those occurring in embryonic tissues. Tumors of prostate, cervix, breast, brain, stomach, colon, rectum, bronchus, and lymph nodes are among those that show this transformation. In contrast, comparatively benign gliomas show a relative increase in LDH-1 and LDH-2. A relative increase in the proportion of LDH-4 and LDH-5 has been observed in tissue adjacent to malignant tumors (e.g., the colon), although the cells in these regions are morphologically normal.

## Differences in Properties Among Multiple Forms of Enzymes

Structural differences among the multiple forms of an enzyme give rise to differences in physicochemical properties, such as electrophoretic mobility, resistance to inactivation, and solubility, or in catalytic characteristics, such as preferential reactions with substrate analogs or natural substrates, or relative susceptibility to inhibitors. Methods of isoenzyme analysis have therefore been designed to investigate a wide range of catalytic and structural properties of enzyme molecules. However, it is usually possible to make only limited deductions about the nature of the underlying structural differences between isoenzymes that are responsible for the dissimilar properties. Equally, the changes in properties that may result from specific structural alterations in enzyme molecules are difficult to predict.

Techniques of molecular biology, such as gene cloning and sequencing, have revolutionized the investigation of the primary structures of isoenzymes. Differences in primary structures among isoenzymes, whether derived from multiple genes or from different alleles, are now known to exist in a growing number of cases. Furthermore, many questions have been answered about whether multiple-enzyme forms represent true (genetically determined) isoenzymes or result from posttranslational modification.

Isoenzymes caused by the existence of multiple genes usually differ quantitatively in catalytic properties. These differences may be manifested in such characteristics as molecular activity, $K_m$ values for substrate(s), sensitivity to various inhibitors, and relative rates of activity with substrate analogs (when the specificity of the isoenzymes allows the substrate to be varied), underscoring the biological importance of isoenzymatic variation. In contrast, multiple-enzyme forms that arise by posttranslational modifications such as aggregation usually have similar catalytic properties.

Multigene isoenzymes also usually differ in terms of antigenic specificity, although these differences may be less pronounced among isoenzymes that have emerged relatively recently in evolutionary history and are closely related in structure. Immunologic cross-reaction is not uncommon among multigene isoenzymes. Multiple-enzyme forms caused by posttranslational modification frequently have common antigenic determinants. Isoenzymes derived from different alleles of the same gene (allozymes) are also often antigenically similar, even to the extent that they may cross-react with antisera to the common isoenzyme, despite a mutation having abolished enzyme activity altogether. The capacity for detecting differences among antigenically similar isoenzyme molecules depends on the extent of monoclonal antibody specificity.

Differences in resistance to denaturation (e.g., by heat, concentrated urea solutions, detergents) are commonly found among true isoenzymes, whether these are the products of multiple genes or multiple alleles. Other multiple forms of enzymes often do not differ or differ only slightly in this respect. The most commonly exploited difference among isoenzymes is the difference in net molecular charge that results from the altered amino acid compositions of the molecules; this forms the basis of separation by zone electrophoresis, ion-exchange chromatography, or isoelectric focusing. Separation methods that depend on differences in molecular size, such as gel filtration, do not distinguish among the small size differences that often exist among true isoenzyme molecules but are important in the detection of multiple forms that involve aggregation or association of enzyme molecules with other proteins, such as immunoglobulins.

## ENZYMES AS CATALYSTS

A catalyst is a substance that modifies and increases the rate of a particular chemical reaction without being consumed or permanently altered. Enzymes are protein catalysts of biological origin. Metabolism is a coordinated series of chemical reactions that occur within a living cell to provide energy and accomplish biosynthesis. The process can be regarded as an integrated series of enzymatic reactions, whereas some diseases can be viewed as a derangement of the normal pattern of metabolism. The remarkable properties of enzymes make them sensitive indicators of pathologic change.

Because of their catalytic activity, enzymes convert an enormous number of substrate molecules into products within a short time. This property is used to measure increased amounts of enzymes in the bloodstream, although the amount of enzyme protein released from damaged cells is small compared with the total quantity of nonenzymatic proteins in blood.

## UNITS FOR EXPRESSING ENZYME ACTIVITY

When enzymes are measured by their catalytic activities, the results are expressed as *units of activity*. The unit of activity is defined by the rate at which the reaction proceeds (e.g., the quantity of substrate consumed or product formed in a chosen unit of time). In clinical enzymology, enzyme activity is generally reported as units of activity per unit of volume, such as units per liter of serum or per 1.0 mL of packed erythrocytes. Because the rate of the reaction depends on experimental parameters, such as pH, type of buffer, temperature, nature of substrate, ionic strength, concentration of activators, and other variables, these parameters must be specified in the definition of the unit.

To standardize how enzyme activities are expressed, the EC proposed that the unit of enzyme activity should be defined as the quantity of enzyme that catalyzes the conversion of 1 µmol of substrate to product per minute and that this unit should be termed the international unit (U). Catalytic concentration is expressed in terms of units per liter (U/L) or kilounits (kU/L), whichever gives the more convenient numeric value. In this chapter, the symbol U is used to denote the international unit. In those instances in which there is some uncertainty about the exact nature of the substrate, or when difficulty is encountered in calculating the number of micromoles reacting (as with macromolecules such as starch, protein, and complex lipids), the unit is expressed in terms of the chemical group or residue produced in the reaction (e.g., μmol/min glucose or amino acid formed).

Contrary to the previously noted EC recommendation, the International System of Units (SI) recommends that enzyme activity be expressed in moles per second or katals. Enzyme concentration can then be expressed in terms of katals per liter (kat/L). The relationship between the EC and SI measures of enzymatic activity is:

$$1 \text{ SI unit (katal)} = 1 \text{ mol/s} = 10^6 \, \mu\text{mol/s}$$
$$= 6 \times 10^7 \, \mu\text{mol/min} = 6 \times 10^7 \text{ EC units}$$

The katal is so large that it is difficult to use and, therefore, the EC units of enzyme activity (μmol/min) are commonly employed.

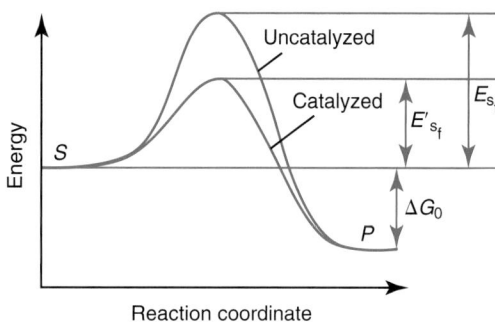

Fig. 14.3 Activation energy barrier and reaction course, with and without enzyme catalysis. $E_{S_f}$ is the activation energy for the forward reaction ($S \to P$) in the absence of a catalyst, and $E'_{S_f}$ is the activation energy in the presence of a catalyst. $\Delta G_0$ is the change in free energy for the reaction.

---

### POINTS TO REMEMBER

- Enzymes are biological catalysts that can be used in the monitoring and diagnosis of disease.
- Enzymes are proteins with the ability to accelerate or catalyze chemical reactions.
- The characteristics of the reactions catalyzed by an enzyme depend on the structure of its active site and its relationship to substrates.
- Enzymes exist in multiple forms, isoenzymes and isoforms, the properties and distribution of which are often important in diagnosis.

---

## ENZYME KINETICS

### Enzyme-Substrate Complex

Enzymes act through the formation of an enzyme–substrate (ES) complex, in which a molecule of substrate is bound to the active center of the enzyme molecule. The binding process transforms the substrate molecule to its activated state. The energy required for this transformation is provided by the free energy of binding of S to E. Therefore, activation takes place without the addition of external energy, so that the energy barrier to the reaction is lowered and the conversion to products is accelerated (Fig. 14.3). The ES complex dissociates to give the reaction products (P) and free enzyme (E):

$$E + S \leftrightarrow ES \to P + E \qquad (14.1)$$

All reactions catalyzed by enzymes are in theory reversible. However, under the conditions found in the human body in vivo, or in the clinical lab in vitro, the reaction is usually more rapid in one direction than in the other, so that an equilibrium is reached in which the product of the forward or the backward reaction predominates, sometimes so markedly that the reaction is virtually irreversible.

If the product of the reaction in one direction is removed as it is formed (e.g., because it is the substrate of a second enzyme present in the reaction mixture), the equilibrium of the first enzymatic process will be displaced so that the reaction will proceed to completion in that direction. Reaction sequences in which the product of one enzyme-catalyzed reaction becomes the substrate of the next enzyme and so on, often through many stages, are characteristic of biological processes. In the laboratory also, several enzymatic reactions may be linked together to provide a means of measuring the activity of the first enzyme or the concentration of the initial substrate in the chain. For example, the activity of CK is usually measured by coupling the adenosine triphosphate (ATP) formed in the CK-catalyzed reaction to the phosphorylation of glucose catalyzed by hexokinase, and then coupling the glucose-6-phosphate product to oxidation by glucose-6-phosphate dehydrogenase, with the formation of a photometrically measurable product, nicotinamide adenine dinucleotide phosphate (NADPH).

When a secondary enzyme-catalyzed reaction, known as an indicator reaction, is used to determine the activity of a different enzyme, the primary reaction must be the rate-limiting step. Reaction conditions must ensure that the rate of reaction catalyzed by the indicator enzyme is directly proportional to the rate of product formation in the first reaction.

## FACTORS GOVERNING THE RATE OF ENZYME-CATALYZED REACTIONS

Factors that affect the rate of enzyme-catalyzed reactions include enzyme and substrate concentration, pH, temperature, and the presence of inhibitors, activators, coenzymes, and prosthetic groups.

### Enzyme Concentration

The simplest enzymatically catalyzed reaction for converting substrate S into product P with the intermediate formation of an ES complex is as follows:

$$E_f + S \underset{k_1}{\overset{k_1}{\rightleftharpoons}} ES \xrightarrow{k_2} E_f + P \qquad (14.2)$$

where $E_f$ = free enzyme; $k_1$ = rate constant for the association of the complex; $k_{-1}$ = rate constant for the dissociation of the complex; ES = enzyme–substrate complex; $k_2$ = rate constant for breakdown of ES to $E_f$ and $P$; and $P$ = product.

Michaelis and Menten assumed that equilibrium is attained rapidly among $E$, $S$, and ES, with the effect of product formation (ES → $P$) on the concentration of ES being negligible. In addition, the formation of product is written as an irreversible process because there is no product in the solution under initial conditions. Therefore, the overall rate of the reaction under otherwise constant conditions is proportional to the concentration of the ES complex.

Provided that an excess of free substrate molecules is present, addition of more enzyme molecules to the reaction system increases the concentration of the ES complex and thus the overall rate of reaction. This accounts for the observation that the rate of reaction is generally proportional to the concentration of enzyme present in the system and is the basis for the quantitative determination of enzymes by measurement of reaction rates. Reaction conditions are selected to ensure that the observed reaction rate is proportional to enzyme concentration over as wide a range as possible.

## Substrate Concentration

In addition to explaining the dependence of reaction rate on enzyme concentration under conditions in which excess substrate is present, the formation of an ES complex accounts for the hyperbolic relationship between reaction velocity and substrate concentration (Fig. 14.4A).

## Single-Substrate Reactions

If the enzyme concentration is fixed and the substrate concentration is varied, the rate of reaction is first order and proportional to substrate concentration when the substrate concentration is low. Under these conditions, only a fraction of the enzyme is associated with substrate, and the rate observed reflects the low concentration of the ES complex. At high substrate concentrations, variation in substrate concentration has no effect on rate, and the reaction is in zero order with respect to substrate concentration. Under these conditions, all the enzyme is bound to the substrate and a much higher rate of reaction is obtained. Moreover, because all the enzyme is now present in the form of the complex, no further increase in complex concentration and no further increment in reaction rate are possible. The maximum possible velocity for the reaction has been reached. The significance of substrate-rate curves was first emphasized by Michaelis and Menten, and such curves are referred to as Michaelis-Menten plots.

Referring again to Eq. 14.2, the overall rate of the reaction ($v$) is determined by the rate at which product is formed:

$$v = \frac{d[P]}{dt} = K_2 [ES] \quad \textbf{(14.3)}$$

The formation of ES will depend on the rate constant $k_1$ and the availability of enzyme and substrate. If it is assumed that the system is in a steady state with the ES complex being

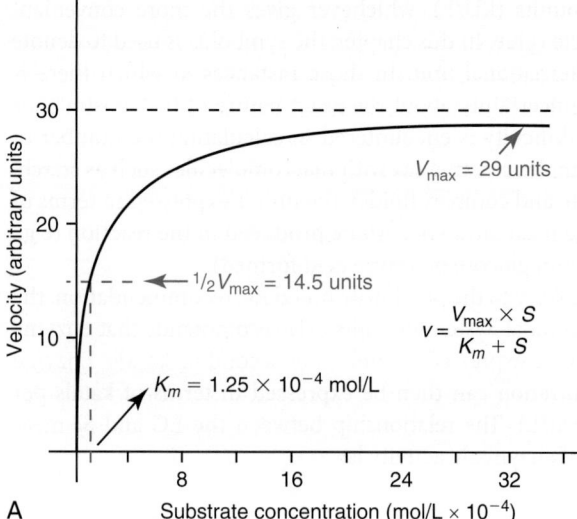

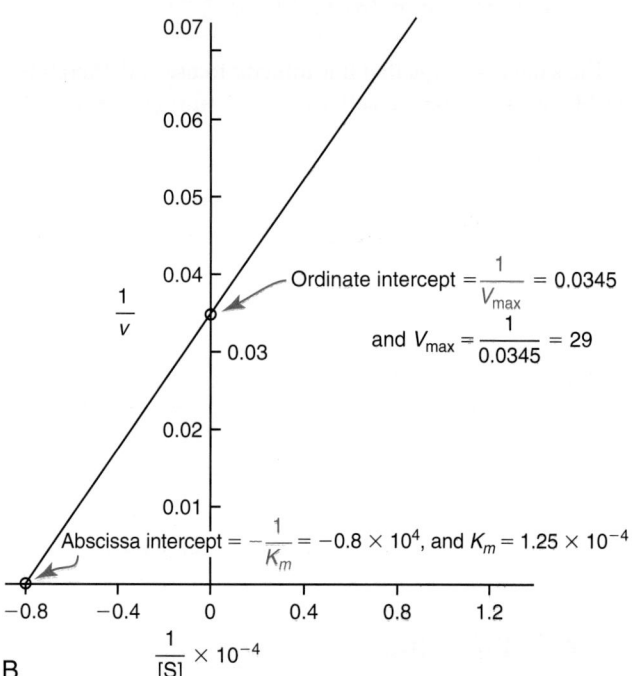

**Fig. 14.4** (A) Michaelis-Menten curve relating the velocity (rate) of an enzyme-catalyzed reaction to substrate concentration. The value of $K_m$ is given by the substrate concentration at which one-half of the maximum velocity is obtained. (B) Lineweaver-Burk transformation of the curve in (A), with $1/v$ plotted on the ordinate ($y$-axis), and $1/[S]$ on the abscissa ($x$-axis). The indicated intercepts permit calculation of $V_{max}$ and $K_m$.

formed and broken down at the same rate so that overall (ES) is constant, then the steady-state equation is:

$$k_1 [E] [S] = k_{-1} [ES] + k_2 [ES] \quad \textbf{(14.4)}$$

This equation can be rearranged to:

$$[ES] = \frac{k_1 [E] [S]}{k_{-1} + k_2} \quad \textbf{(14.5)}$$

when these rate constants are combined into a single term; writing the **Michaelis-Menten constant (Km)** as:

$$K_m = \frac{k_{-1} + k_2}{k_1} \qquad (14.6)$$

and then substituting this into Eq. 14.5 gives:

$$[ES] = \frac{[E][S]}{K_m} \qquad (14.7)$$

Because the total amount of enzyme in the system does not change:

$$[E_t] = [ES] + [E] \qquad (14.8)$$

and on substituting Eq. 14.3 into Eq. 14.7 and solving for [ES] using Eq. 14.8 gives:

$$v = \frac{k_2 \times [E_t] \times [S]}{K_m + [S]} \qquad (14.9)$$

For a given amount of enzyme, the maximum reaction velocity ($V_{max}$) is reached when all of the enzyme is saturated with substrate (i.e., $[ES] = [E_t]$), and therefore $V_{max} = k_2 \times [E_t]$. Substituting this in Eq. 14.9 gives:

$$v = \frac{V_{max}[S]}{K_m + [S]} \qquad (14.10)$$

A plot of $v$ against [S] gives a section of a rectangular hyperbola (see Fig. 14.4A), and this is the shape of the curve that is found experimentally for most enzyme reactions. When $[S] = K_m$, $K_m$ is the substrate concentration at which the reaction proceeds at half of its maximum velocity. In practice, it is now customary to restrict $K_m$ to the experimentally determined substrate concentration at which $v = 0.5 V_{max}$ and to use the symbol $K_s$ to represent the true ES association constant, where this is known.

Although it is simple to set up an experiment to determine the variation of $v$ with [S], the exact value of $V_{max}$ is not easily determined from hyperbolic curves. Furthermore, many enzymes deviate from ideal behavior at high substrate concentrations and may even be inhibited by the excess of substrate, so the calculated value of $V_{max}$ cannot be achieved in practice. In the past, it was common practice to transform the Michaelis-Menten equation (Eq. 14.10) into one of several reciprocal forms (Eqs. 14.11 and 14.12), and either $1/v$ was plotted against $1/[S]$, or $[S]/v$ was plotted against [S]:

$$\frac{1}{v} = \left( \frac{K_m}{V_{max}} \times \frac{1}{[S]} \right) + \frac{1}{V_{max}} \qquad (14.11)$$

$$\frac{[S]}{v} = \left( \frac{1}{V_{max}} \times [S] \right) + \frac{K_m}{V_{max}} \qquad (14.12)$$

Eq. 14.11, for example, when plotted, results in a Lineweaver-Burk plot that gives a straight line with intercepts at $1/V_{max}$ on the ordinate and $-1/K_m$ on the abscissa. The data for Fig. 14.4A are replotted in Lineweaver-Burk form in Fig. 14.4B.

It is now routine practice to determine kinetic constants such as $K_m$ and $V_{max}$ using software packages. Free and commercial packages are available; these vary from specialized routines for kinetic simulations or for data fitting, to general mathematical, statistical, or graphical packages.

The value of $K_m$ is to compare the binding of homologous or related substrates to the same enzyme. Also, if measured against the same substrate under defined conditions, the $K_m$ value can be used to compare the properties of similar enzymes from different sources. Isoenzymes determined by distinct genes typically differ in their $K_m$ (e.g., the isoenzymes of LD).

When setting up methods of enzyme assay, it is necessary to (1) explore the relationship between reaction velocity and substrate concentration over a wide range, (2) determine $K_m$, and (3) detect any inhibition at high substrate concentrations. Zero-order kinetics is maintained if the substrate is present in large excess (i.e., concentrations at least 10 and preferably 100 times that of the value of $K_m$). When $[S] = 10 \times K_m$, $v$ is approximately 91% of the theoretical $V_{max}$. The $K_m$ values for the majority of enzymes are on the order of $10^{-5}$ to $10^{-3}$ mol/L; therefore, substrate concentrations are usually chosen to be in the range of 0.001 to 0.10 mol/L. On occasion, the optimal concentrations of substrate cannot be used, for example, when the substrate has limited solubility or when the concentration of a given substrate inhibits the activity of another enzyme needed in a coupled reaction system.

## Two-Substrate Reactions

Most enzymes catalyze reactions with two or more interacting substrates symbolized by the following equation:

$$\text{Substrate 1} + \text{Substrate 2} \overset{E}{\longleftrightarrow} \text{Product 1} + \text{Product 2}$$
$$\text{S1} \qquad\qquad \text{S2} \qquad\qquad \text{P1} \qquad\qquad \text{P2}$$
$$(14.13)$$

The concentrations of both substrates may be variable and both may affect the rate of reaction. Among the bisubstrate reactions important in clinical enzymology are the reactions catalyzed by dehydrogenases, in which the second substrate is a specific coenzyme, such as the oxidized or reduced forms of nicotinamide adenine dinucleotide (NADH), or NADPH, and the amino-group transfers catalyzed by the aminotransferases.

If a bisubstrate reaction proceeds by way of intermediate ES complexes, then:

$$E + S_1 \leftrightarrow ES_1 \qquad (14.14)$$

followed by:

$$ES_1 + S_2 \leftrightarrow ES_1S_2 \rightarrow P_1 + P_2 + E \qquad (14.15)$$

and if $S_1$ and $S_2$ bind to separate sites on the enzyme molecule, the rate of reaction is given by:

$$v = \frac{V_{max} \times [S_1][S_2]}{[S_1][S_2] + [S_2]K_m^1 + [S_1]K_m^2 + K_S^1 K_m^2} \qquad (14.16)$$

$K_m^1$ and $K_m^2$ are the $K_m$ values for the two substrates, and $[S_1]$ and $[S_2]$ are their concentrations. $K_s^1$ is the equilibrium constant for the reversible reaction between the enzyme and $S_1$. If the equation is rearranged into the double reciprocal form:

$$\frac{1}{v} = \frac{1}{[S_1]} \left( \frac{K_m^1}{V_{max}} + \frac{K_m^2 K_S^1}{[S_2] V_{max}} \right) + \frac{1}{V_{max}} \left( 1 + \frac{K_m^2}{[S_2]} \right)$$

(14.17)

a plot of $1/v$ against $1/[S_1]$ gives a straight line, but both the slope of the line and its intercept on the ordinate are dependent on $[S_2]$, the concentration of the second substrate. A plot of $1/v$ against $1/[S_2]$ is rectilinear but with the slope and intercept dependent on $[S_1]$.

In some bisubstrate reactions, no ternary complex $ES_1S_2$ is formed, because the binding of the first substrate is followed by release of the first product before the second substrate is bound and the second product is released. This sequence is described as a *ping-pong bi-bi* type of reaction. This occurs in reactions catalyzed by aminotransferases.

Values of $K_m$ and $V_{max}$ for each substrate are derived from experiments in which the concentration of the first substrate is held constant at saturating quantities while the concentration of the second substrate is varied, and vice versa. The selection of reaction conditions for the measurement of enzymatic activity involving two substrates is approached similarly by varying the concentration of the first substrate and keeping the concentration of the second substrate constant until maximum activity is reached. The process is then repeated with the concentration of the first substrate held at the value thus determined, whereas the concentration of the second substrate is varied.

## Consecutive Enzymatic Reactions

As discussed previously, an enzymatic reaction is usually found to be more rapid in one direction than the other, so that the reaction is essentially irreversible. If the product of the reaction in one direction is removed as it is formed (i.e., because it is the substrate of a second enzyme present in the reaction mixture), the equilibrium of the first enzymatic process is displaced so that the reaction may continue to completion in that direction. Analytically, several enzymatic reactions may be linked together to provide a means of measuring the activity of the first enzyme or the concentration of the initial substrate in the chain.

When a linked enzyme assay, known as an *indicator reaction*, is used to determine the activity of a different enzyme, it is essential that the primary reaction be the rate-limiting step. For example, in the determination of AST activity, the indicator reaction is the reduction of the 2-oxoglutarate formed in the aminotransferase reaction to malate by malate dehydrogenase and NADH. The activity of the indicator enzyme must be sufficient to ensure the immediate removal of the product of the first reaction so as to prevent significant reversal of the first reaction. The measured enzyme typically acts

under conditions of saturation with respect to its substrate; however, the concentration of the substrate of the indicator enzyme (i.e., the product of the first reaction) remains in the region of the Michaelis-Menten curve, in which $v$ is directly proportional to $[S]$. Therefore the rate of reaction catalyzed by the indicator enzyme is directly proportional to the rate of product formation in the first reaction.

During a lag period that occurs after the start of the first reaction, the concentration of its product reaches a steady state. Because the rate of the second reaction depends on the activity of the indicator enzyme and on the concentration of its substrate (the product of the primary reaction), the duration of the lag period is reduced by increasing the concentration of the indicator enzyme, thus lowering the steady-state concentration of the product of the primary reaction.

The rate of the indicator reaction, $v_i$, is related to substrate concentration and therefore to the product concentration $[P]$ by the Michaelis-Menten equation:

$$v_i = \frac{V_{max}^i \times [P]}{[P] + K_m^i}$$

(14.18)

in which $V_{max}^i$ and $K_m^i$ are the maximum velocity and $K_m$ of the indicator enzyme, respectively. For the rate of the indicator reaction not to be the rate-limiting factor, $v_i$ must at least equal the limiting velocity of the primary reaction, $v_t$, which the assay system is expected to measure. Therefore, the minimum activity of the indicator enzyme needed is given by:

$$v_t = \frac{V_{max}^i \times [P]}{[P] + K_m^i}$$

(14.19)

which can be rearranged to:

$$V_{max}^i = v_t \left( 1 + \frac{K_m^i}{[P]} \right)$$

(14.20)

The ratio of activities of the indicator and primary enzymes varies from one assay method to another, depending on (1) the range of activity measured, (2) the $K_m$ of the indicator enzyme, and (3) the lag period that is considered acceptable. Nevertheless, the catalytic concentration of the indicator enzyme in the reaction mixture must always be much greater than that of the enzyme being determined.

## Effect of pH

The rate of an enzyme-catalyzed reaction typically shows a marked dependence on pH (Fig. 14.5). Many of the enzymes in blood plasma show maximum activity in vitro in the pH range from 7 to 8. However, activity has been observed at pH values as low as 1.5 (pepsin) and as high as 10.5 (ALP). The optimal pH for a given forward reaction may be different from the optimal pH found for the corresponding reverse reaction. The form of the pH-dependence curve is the result of a number of separate effects, including ionization of the substrate and the extent of dissociation of certain key amino acid side chains in the protein molecule, both at the active

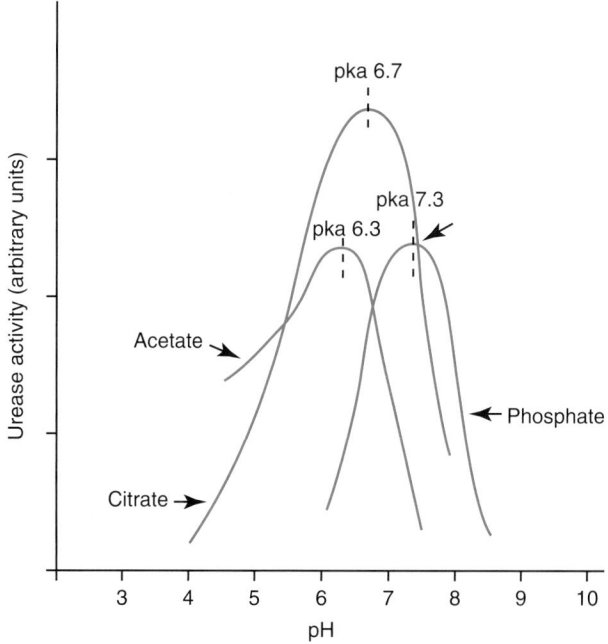

Fig. 14.5 The pH activity curves for urease show the effects of buffer species on pH optimum. (Modified from Howell SF, Sumner JB. The specific effects of buffers upon urease activity. *J Biol Chem*. 1934:104;619.)

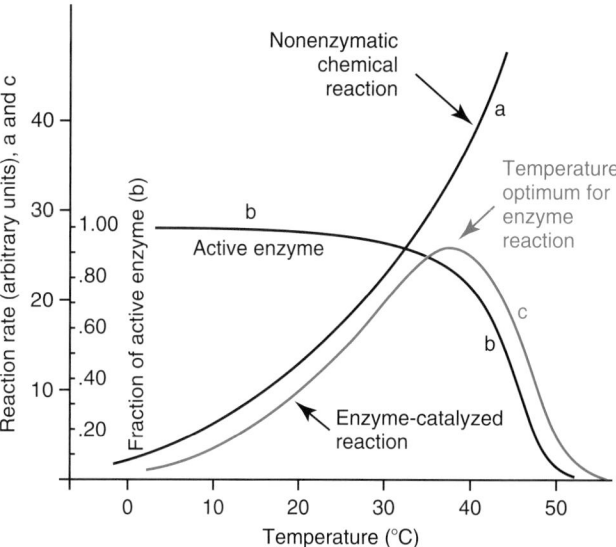

Fig. 14.6 Schematic diagram showing the effects of temperature on the rate of non-enzyme-catalyzed and enzyme-catalyzed reactions.

center and elsewhere in the molecule. The pH and ionic environment will also have an effect on the 3D conformation of the protein and therefore on enzyme activity to such an extent that enzymes may be irreversibly denatured at extreme pH values.

The pronounced effects of pH on enzyme reactions emphasize the need to control this variable by means of adequate buffer solutions. Enzyme assays should be carried out at the pH of optimal activity because the pH-activity curve has its minimum slope near this pH, and a small variation in pH will cause a minimal change in enzyme activity. The buffer system must be capable of counteracting the effect of adding the specimen (e.g., serum itself is a powerful buffer) to the assay system, as well as the effects of acids or bases formed during the reaction (e.g., formation of fatty acids by the action of lipase). Because buffers have their maximum buffering capacity close to their $pK_a$ values, whenever possible a buffer system should be chosen with a $pK_a$ value within 1 pH unit of the desired pH of the assay. Interaction between buffer ions and other components of the assay system (e.g., the chelation of activating metal ions) may eliminate certain buffers from consideration.

## Temperature

The rate of an enzymatic reaction is proportional to its reaction temperature, but only up to a certain point. For most enzymatic reactions, values of $Q_{10}$ (the relative reaction rates at two temperatures differing by 10°C) vary from 1.7 to 2.5. However, an increase in the rate of the catalyzed reaction is not the only effect of increasing temperature on an enzymatic reaction. Enzyme inactivation, due to protein denaturation as the temperature increases, accounts for the existence

of an apparent optimal temperature for enzyme activity (Fig. 14.6).

At some critical temperature, an enzyme will undergo thermal inactivation influenced by the presence of substrate and its concentration, the pH, and the nature and ionic strength of the buffer. The presence of other proteins, as in serum samples, may help to stabilize enzymes. Storage of serum samples at low temperatures is usually necessary to minimize loss of enzyme activity while awaiting analysis, although repeated freezing and thawing should be avoided. However, individual enzymes vary in their stability characteristics, and appropriate storage conditions vary correspondingly. Serum amylase, for example, is stable at room temperature (22°C to 25°C) for 24 hours, whereas acid phosphatase is exceedingly unstable, even when refrigerated, unless kept at a pH below 6.0. ALP exhibits an unusual property; in sera stored at refrigerated temperatures, ALP increases slowly (2% per day), which is thought to be due to the reincorporation of cations required for full activity. Frozen specimens should be thawed and kept at room temperature for 18 to 24 hours before measurement to achieve full enzyme reactivation. This effect is shared by reconstituted, lyophilized preparations of the enzyme and affects their use for quality control purposes. A few enzymes are inactivated at refrigerator temperatures; a clinically important example is the liver isoenzyme of LDH, LDH-5, which appears to be less stable at lower temperatures. As a result, sera for LDH determinations should be kept at room temperature and not refrigerated.

Most analytical systems operate at 37°C, and reference methods for several clinically relevant enzymes have now been developed at this temperature. Accurate temperature control to within ±0.1°C during the enzymatic reaction is essential, and it is achievable by modern instruments.

## Inhibitors and Activators

The rates of enzymatic reactions are often affected by substances other than the enzyme or substrate. These modifiers may be **inhibitors** that reduce the reaction rate, or **activators** that increase the rate of reaction. Activators and inhibitors are usually small molecules (compared with the enzyme itself) or even ions. They vary in specificity from modifiers that exert similar effects on a wide range of different enzymatic reactions, to substances that affect only a single reaction. The activity of some enzymes depends on the presence of particular chemical groups, such as reduced sulfhydryl (–SH) groups, in the active center. Reagents that alter these groups (e.g., oxidizing agents) therefore act as general inhibitors of such enzymes.

Some phenomena of enzyme activation or inhibition are caused by interactions between the modifier and a non-enzymatic component of the reaction system, such as the substrate (e.g., magnesium [$Mg^{2+}$] combining with ATP to form MgATP, a required substrate for the CK reaction). In most cases, however, the modifier binds to the enzyme itself, either to the active site or to some other part of the enzyme's structure.

## Inhibition of Enzyme Activity

Inhibitors are classified as reversible or irreversible. *Reversible inhibition* implies that the activity of the enzyme is fully restored when the inhibitor is removed from the system by some physical separative process, such as dialysis, gel filtration, or chromatography. An *irreversible inhibitor* combines covalently with the enzyme so that physical methods are ineffective in separating the two. For example, organophosphorus compounds are extremely potent irreversible inhibitors of esterases, including acetylcholinesterase, which is the mechanism for organophosphate poisoning. The enzyme breaks one of the bonds in the inhibitor, but part of the molecule is left bound to the active center of the enzyme, preventing further activity. In some cases, enzymes that have combined with irreversible inhibitors can be reactivated by a chemical reaction that removes the blocking group (e.g., the phosphoryl enzymes formed with organophosphorus compounds can sometimes be reactivated by treatment with oximes or hydroxamic acids).

*Reversible inhibition.* Reversible inhibition is characterized by the existence of equilibrium between enzyme, E, and inhibitor, I:

$$E + I \leftrightarrow EI \qquad (14.21)$$

The equilibrium constant of the reaction, $K_i$ (the *inhibitor constant*), is a measure of the affinity of the inhibitor for the enzyme, just as $K_m$ generally reflects the affinity of the enzyme for its substrate.

A *competitive* inhibitor is usually a structural analog of the substrate that can combine with the free enzyme in such a way that it competes with the normal substrate for binding at the active site. The rate of the reaction in the presence of a reversible inhibitor is strictly dependent on the relative concentrations of substrate and inhibitor. Two equilibriums are therefore possible:

$$E + S \leftrightarrow ES \rightarrow E + Products \qquad (14.22)$$

and:

$$E + I \leftrightarrow EI \qquad (14.23)$$

The equation that relates the observed reaction velocity to the concentrations of substrate, [S], and inhibitor, [I], is as follows:

$$v = \frac{V_{max}[S]}{[S] + K_m \left(1 + \frac{[I]}{K_i}\right)} \qquad (14.24)$$

This is the Michaelis-Menten equation, but with $K_m$ modified by a term including the inhibitor concentration and the inhibitor constant, while $V_{max}$ remains unaltered. Therefore, curves of $v$ against [S] in the presence and absence of the inhibitor reach the same limiting value at high substrate concentrations, but when the inhibitor is present, $K_m$ is accordingly greater. Plots of $1/v$ against $1/[S]$ with and without inhibitor intersect the ordinate at the same point but have different slopes and intercepts on the abscissa (Fig. 14.7).

Competitive inhibition is responsible for the inhibition of some enzymes by excess substrate because of competition between substrate molecules for a single binding site. In two-substrate reactions, high concentrations of the second substrate may compete with binding of the first substrate. For example, AST is inhibited by excess concentrations of the substrate 2-oxoglutarate, and this inhibition is competitive with respect to L-aspartate. Therefore, to maintain a given velocity at high 2-oxoglutarate concentrations, the concentration

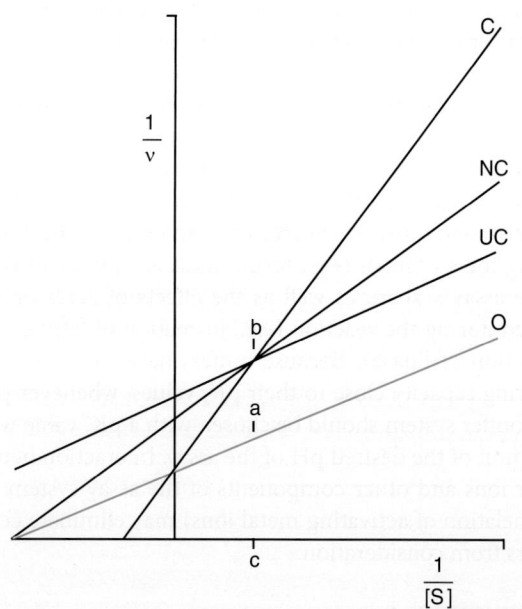

**Fig. 14.7** Effects of different types of inhibitors on the double-reciprocal plot of $1/v$ against $1/[S]$. Each of the inhibitors has been assumed to reduce the activity of the enzyme by the same amount, represented by the change in $1/v$ from *a* to *b* at a substrate concentration of *c*. Line *O* is the plot for enzyme without inhibitor, *C* with a competitive inhibitor, *NC* with a noncompetitive inhibitor, and *UC* with an uncompetitive inhibitor. (From Moss DW. Measurement of enzymes. In: Hearse DJ, de Leiris J, eds. *Enzymes in Cardiology: Diagnosis and Research.* New York: John Wiley & Sons; 1979. Reprinted by permission of John Wiley & Sons.)

of L-aspartate has to be increased above the value needed at lower concentrations of 2-oxoglutarate.

Competitive inhibition also contributes to the reduction in the rate of an enzymatic reaction over time. For example, rate reduction can occur because increasing concentrations of reaction products tend to drive the reaction backward if it is freely reversible. A product may be an inhibitor of the forward reaction, so even if the reaction is not readily reversible, it slows down in the presence of a rising concentration of the inhibitor. A familiar example of product inhibition is the release of the competitive inhibitor inorganic phosphate by the action of ALP on its substrates. In this case, both organic phosphates and inorganic phosphates bind to the active center of the enzyme with similar affinities (i.e., $K_m$ and $K_i$ are of the same order of magnitude).

Product inhibition is a cause of nonlinearity of reaction progress curves during fixed-time methods of enzyme assay. For example, oxaloacetate produced by the action of AST inhibits the enzyme, particularly the mitochondrial isoenzyme. The inhibitory product may be removed as it is formed by a coupled enzymatic reaction; malate dehydrogenase converts the oxaloacetate to malate and at the same time oxidizes NADH to NAD$^+$.

Competitive inhibition by metal ions occurs when two metal ions compete for the same binding site on the enzyme. Sodium and lithium are potent inhibitors of pyruvate kinase, for which potassium is an obligatory activator.

A noncompetitive inhibitor is usually structurally different from the substrate. It is assumed to bind at a site on the enzyme molecule that is different from the substrate-binding site; thus, there is no competition between inhibitor and substrate, and a ternary enzyme substrate–inhibitor (ESI) complex is formed. Attachment of the inhibitor to the enzyme does not alter the affinity of the enzyme for its substrate (i.e., $K_m$ is unaltered), but the ESI complex does not break down to give products. Because the substrate does not compete with the inhibitor for binding sites on the enzyme molecule, increasing the substrate concentration does not overcome the effect of a noncompetitive inhibitor. Thus $V_{max}$ is reduced in the presence of such an inhibitor, whereas $K_m$ is not altered, as the Lineweaver-Burk plot shows (see Fig. 14.7).

Uncompetitive inhibition is produced by a combination of the inhibitor with the ES complex. It is more common in two-substrate reactions, in which a ternary ESI complex forms after the first substrate combines with the enzyme. In uncompetitive inhibition, parallel lines are obtained when plots of $1/v$ against $1/[S]$ with and without the inhibitor are compared (see Fig. 14.7); that is, both $K_m$ and $V_{max}$ are decreased.

*Irreversible inhibition.* Irreversible inhibitors render the enzyme molecule inactive by covalently and permanently modifying a functional group required for catalysis. An irreversible inhibitor is not in equilibrium with the enzyme. Its effect is progressive with time, becoming complete if the amount of inhibitor present exceeds the total amount of enzyme. The rate of the reaction between the enzyme and the inhibitor is expressed as the fraction of the enzyme activity

that is inhibited in a fixed time by a given concentration of inhibitor. The velocity constant of the reaction of the inhibitor with the enzyme is a measure of the effectiveness of the inhibitor.

When the inhibitor is added to the enzyme in the presence of its substrate, the reaction between the enzyme and the inhibitor may be delayed because some of the enzyme molecules are combined with the substrate and are therefore protected from reacting with the inhibitor. However, when the substrate molecules react chemically, the active centers become available, and inhibition will eventually become complete, even though an excess of substrate may have been present initially. Furthermore, the addition of more substrate is ineffective in reversing the inhibition in contrast to its effect on reversible competitive inhibition.

Irreversible inhibitors have been useful in mapping active sites by covalently modifying different types of functional groups in the enzyme molecule to establish whether such groups are necessary for catalytic activity.

A physiologically important category of irreversible enzyme inhibition is exemplified by various trypsin inhibitors. These are proteins that bind to trypsin irreversibly, nullifying its proteolytic activity. One such inhibitor is present in the $\alpha_1$-globulin fraction of serum proteins; others are found in soybeans and lima beans. Similar proteolysis inhibitors present in plasma prevent the accumulation of excess thrombin and other coagulation enzymes, thus keeping the coagulation process under control.

*Inhibition by antibodies.* The combination of enzyme molecules with specific antibodies often has no effect on catalytic activity, which is retained by the enzyme-antibody complex. However, in some cases, the reaction of the enzyme and antibody reduces or even abolishes enzymatic activity. The most probable explanation for this type of inhibition is that the antibody molecule restricts access of the substrate molecules to the active center by steric hindrance or, in extreme cases, completely masks the substrate-binding site. However, it appears that some examples of enzyme inhibition by combination with antibodies are caused by a conformational change induced in the enzyme molecule.

Inhibition of the activity of an enzyme molecule labeled with a hapten (e.g., morphine) as a result of combination with a specific antibody forms the basis for a homogeneous enzyme immunoassay (see Chapter 15).

## Enzyme Activation

Activators increase the rates of enzyme-catalyzed reactions by promoting formation of the most active state of the enzyme or of other reactants, such as the substrate. This generalization covers a wide variety of mechanisms of activation.

Many enzymes contain metal ions as an integral part of their structures (e.g., zinc in ALP and carboxypeptidase A). The function of the metal may be to stabilize tertiary and quaternary protein structures. Removal of divalent metal ions by treatment with an appropriate quantity of ethylenediaminetetraacetic acid (EDTA) solution is accompanied by conformational changes and inactivation of the enzyme. The enzyme can often be reactivated by dialysis against a solution of the appropriate metal ion or simply by addition of the ion to the reaction mixture. Reactivation may take some time because rearrangement of polypeptide chains into the active conformation is not instantaneous.

When the activator ion is an essential part of the functional enzyme molecule, whether as a purely structural element or with an additional catalytic role, it is usually incorporated quite firmly into the enzyme molecule. Therefore, it is not usually necessary to add the activator to reaction mixtures and an excess of the ion may even have an inhibitory effect. However, in some cases, the activating ion is attached only weakly or transiently to the enzyme (or its substrate) during catalysis. Enzyme samples may therefore be deficient in the ion so that addition of the ion increases the reaction rate or indeed may be essential for the reaction to take place. For example, all phosphate transfer enzymes (kinases), such as CK, require the presence of $Mg^{2+}$ ions. Other common activating cations are manganese ($Mn^{2+}$), iron ($Fe^{2+}$), calcium ($Ca^{2+}$), zinc ($Zn^{2+}$), and potassium ($K^+$). More rarely, anions may act as activators. Amylase functions at its maximal rate only if chloride ($Cl^-$) or other monovalent anions, such as bromide ($Br^-$) or nitrate ($NO_3^-$), are present. Addition of 5 mmol/L of chloride increases amylase activity almost threefold, at the same time shifting the pH optimum from 6.5 to 7.0. The $Cl^-$ ion may combine with a positively charged group in the enzyme, changing the ionization constant of a group important in catalysis. Some enzymes require the presence of two activating ions. $K^+$ and $Mg^{2+}$ are essential for the activity of pyruvate kinase, and both $Mg^{2+}$ and $Zn^{2+}$ are required for ALP activity.

The velocity of the reaction depends on the concentration of a reversible activator in a fashion similar to its dependence on substrate concentration. An activator constant, $K_a$, analogous to $K_m$, can be determined from data relating enzyme activity to increasing activator concentration in the presence of excess substrate. The simplest interpretation of $K_a$ is that it is the dissociation constant of the equilibrium between E and the activator, A. However, this is true only when the combination of enzyme and activator is independent of the reaction between E and S, and the same value for $K_a$ is obtained at all concentrations of the substrate. If the free enzyme and the ES complex have different affinities for the activator, the value for $K_a$ varies with [S].

Apparent activation of an enzyme may be observed whenever a substance that can counteract the presence of some inhibiting agent is added.

## Coenzymes and Prosthetic Groups

Coenzymes are usually more complex molecules than activators, although they are smaller molecules than the enzyme proteins. Some compounds, such as the dinucleotides NAD and NADP, are classified as coenzymes and are specific substrates in two-substrate reactions. Their effects on the rate of reaction follow the Michaelis-Menten pattern of dependence on substrate concentration. The structures of these two coenzymes are identical except for the presence of an additional phosphate group in NADP; nevertheless, individual dehydrogenases, for which these coenzymes are substrates, are predominantly or even absolutely specific for one or the other form.

Coenzymes such as NAD and NADP are bound only momentarily to the enzyme during the course of the reaction, as is the case for substrates in general. Therefore, no reaction takes place unless the appropriate coenzyme is present in solution (e.g., by adding it to the reaction mixture in the assay of dehydrogenase activity). In contrast to these entirely soluble coenzymes, some coenzymes are more or less permanently bound to the enzyme molecules, where they form part of the active center and undergo cycles of chemical change during the reaction. In this case, the coenzyme is known as a prosthetic group. Prosthetic groups, such as activators with a structural role, do not usually have to be added to elicit full catalytic activity of the enzyme unless previous treatment has caused the prosthetic group to be lost from some enzyme molecules.

The active *holoenzyme* results from the combination of the inactive *apoenzyme* with the prosthetic group. An example of a prosthetic group is pyridoxal-5′-phosphate (P-5′-P), a component of AST and ALT. The P-5′-P prosthetic group undergoes a cycle of conversion of the pyridoxal moiety to pyridoxamine and back again during the transfer of an amino group from an amino acid to an oxoacid. However, both normal and pathologic serum samples contain appreciable quantities of apoaminotransferases, which are converted to active holoenzymes through a suitable period of incubation with P-5′-P.

A study of the formulas of coenzyme and prosthetic groups shows that many contain structures derived from vitamins (see Chapter 27). Thus, the nicotinamide portion of NAD and NADP derives from the vitamin niacin, whereas the P-5′-P prosthetic group of the aminotransferases is a derivative of pyridoxine, vitamin $B_6$.

---

### POINTS TO REMEMBER

- The catalytic properties of enzymes can be described by equations based on the formation of an ES complex.
- Enzyme reactions are affected by temperature, pH, enzyme concentration, substrate concentration, and the presence of any inhibitors or activators.

---

## ANALYTICAL ENZYMOLOGY

Analytically, the clinical laboratorian is concerned with measuring the activity or mass of enzymes in serum or plasma that are predominantly intracellular, and that are physiologically present in the serum in low concentrations only. By measuring changes in the concentrations of these enzymes in disease, it is possible to infer the location and nature of pathologic changes in body tissues.

## Measurement of Reaction Rates

Both *fixed-time* and *continuous-monitoring* methods are used to measure reaction rates. In the fixed-time method, the amount of product produced from substrate by the enzyme is measured after the reaction is stopped at the end of a fixed-time interval. In the continuous-monitoring method, the rate of product formation is monitored as the reaction is proceeding. These two methods have different advantages and limitations. To appreciate them, it is necessary to consider the way in which the rate of an enzymatic reaction varies with time.

The progress of conversion of the substrate into products in the presence of an enzyme is monitored by measuring the decreasing concentration of the substrate or the increasing concentration of the products. Measurement of product formation is preferable because determination of the increase in concentration of a substance above an initially zero or low concentration is analytically more reliable than measurement of a decline from an initially high concentration.

At the moment when the enzyme and the substrate are mixed, the rate of the reaction is zero. The rate then typically rises rapidly to a maximum value, which remains constant for a period of time (Fig. 14.8). During the period of constant reaction rate, the rate depends only on enzyme concentration and is completely

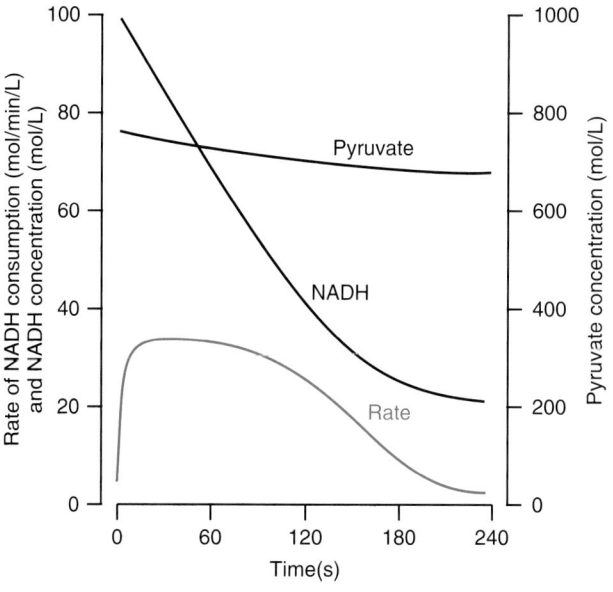

**Fig. 14.8** Changes in substrate concentrations and rates of reaction during an assay of lactate dehydrogenase activity at 37°C in phosphate buffer, with pyruvate and nicotinamide adenine dinucleotide (NADH) as substrates. The reaction is followed by observing the fall in absorbance at 340 nm as NADH is oxidized to $NAD^+$. The rate of reaction rises rapidly to a maximum value, from which it declines only slightly until about half the NADH has been used up. During this phase of the reaction, the rate is essentially zero order with respect to substrate concentration. At the point at which the rate falls below about 90% of its maximum value, NADH concentration is approximately $10 \times K_m$. The $K_m$ for NADH is on the order of $5 \times 10^{-6}$ mol/L, whereas for pyruvate it is $9 \times 10^{-5}$ mol/L. Thus an initial pyruvate concentration of approximately 10 times that of NADH is used. (Concentrations are per liter of reaction mixture.) (From Moss DW. Measurement of enzymes. In: Hearse DJ, de Leiris J, eds. *Enzymes in Cardiology: Diagnosis and Research*. New York: John Wiley & Sons; 1979. Reprinted by permission of John Wiley & Sons.)

independent of substrate concentration. The reaction is said to follow zero-order kinetics because its rate is proportional to the zero power of the substrate concentration. Ultimately, however, as more substrate is consumed, the reaction rate declines and enters a phase of first-order dependence on substrate concentration. Other factors that contribute to the decline in reaction rate include accumulation of products that may be inhibitory, the growing importance of the reverse reaction, and even enzyme denaturation. Enzyme assays are usually made under conditions that are initially saturating with respect to substrate concentration. The rate of reaction during the zero-order phase is determined by measuring the product formed during a fixed period of incubation in which the rate remains constant. This is illustrated in Fig. 14.9. Measurement of reaction rates at any portion of *curve A* gives results that are identical to the true *initial rate*. However, *curve B* deviates from linearity over its entire course, and rates fall off with time. From *curve C*, correct results are obtained only if the rate is measured along segment II. Incorrect results are obtained if the rate is measured during the lag phase (I) or during the phase of substrate depletion (III).

Careful selection of reaction conditions, such as the concentrations of substrates and cofactors, improves the reaction progress curves, eliminates lag phases, and prolongs the period of zero-order kinetics so that fixed-time methods of analysis become feasible. Improvements in optical techniques, leading to more reliable and sensitive measurement of product formation, also have allowed the duration of incubation to be shortened compared with that of older assays. Nevertheless, an upper limit of activity exists in all fixed-time methods, above which progress curves will no longer be linear. In this case, the amount of change measured over the fixed-time interval no longer represents true zero-order rate conditions.

The upper limit of activity must be chosen so samples with activities below it give linear progress curves; alternatively, if the limit is set too low, many samples will have to be diluted and reanalyzed unnecessarily. Samples that are above the limit should ideally be assayed again after shortening the incubation period until a constant reaction rate is obtained. However, this is difficult or impossible in some automated methods, in which the duration of incubation is fixed by the configuration of the apparatus. It then becomes necessary to dilute the specimen to obtain valid results. However, some diluents can cause matrix-related alterations to the reaction kinetics and may not always result in a proportional change in activity.

The initial rate of reaction theoretically increases without limit as enzyme concentration increases, as long as no other factor, such as substrate concentration, becomes limiting. In practice, the reaction rate becomes so rapid at high enzyme activities that it is impossible to measure the initial rate of reaction, even with continuous monitoring methods. Therefore, an upper limit of activity that is measurable without modification of the assay procedure exists even in continuous monitoring methods; but this limit is usually much higher than those observed in fixed-time methods. Therefore, fewer samples require special treatment when using continuous monitoring methods. Furthermore, continuous monitoring allows identification of the appropriate zero-order portion of the progress curve for each sample and identification of samples

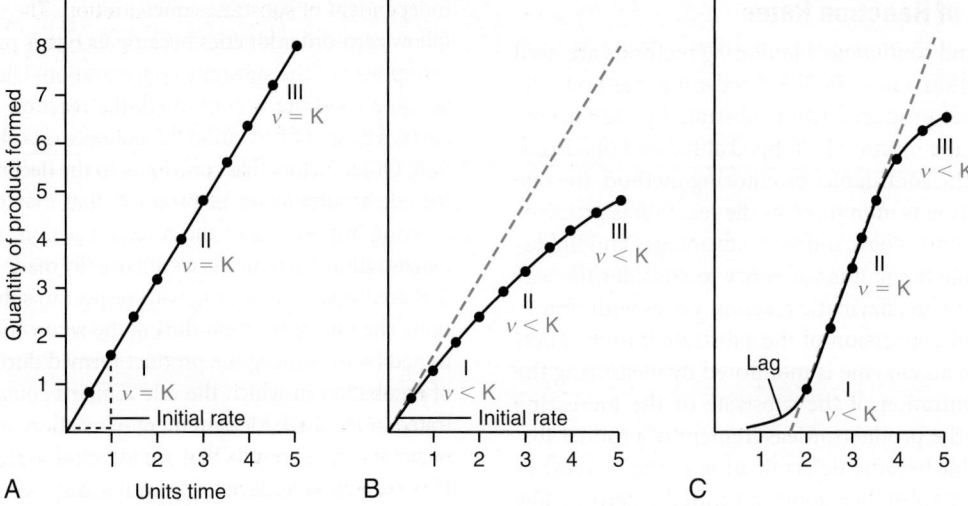

**Fig. 14.9** Graphs showing change in enzyme reaction rate as a function of time. (A) The rate is constant during the entire run, and rates calculated as I, II, and III will be identical to the initial rate. (B) The rate falls off continuously; rates calculated at I, II, and III will be different and less than the true initial rate. (C) A measurement at II will be representative of the maximum rate, but at I (lag period) and III (substrate depletion), it will be less than at II.

that require special treatment. Continuous-monitoring methods, therefore, provide a decisive advantage in enzyme assay and should be used whenever possible.

## Measurement of Substrates

The amount of substrate transformed into products during an enzyme-catalyzed reaction can be measured with any appropriate analytical method, such as spectrophotometry, fluorometry, or chemiluminescence (see Chapter 9). *Self-indicating* reactions of this type are particularly valuable because they allow continuous monitoring. Important examples of self-indicating reactions are determination of dehydrogenase activity by monitoring the change in absorbance at 339 (340) nm of the coenzyme NADH or NADPH during oxidation or reduction, and measurement of ALP activity by the generation of the yellow *p*-nitrophenolate ion from the substrate *p*-nitrophenyl phosphate in alkaline solution. These indicator reactions are so versatile that dehydrogenase reactions are frequently coupled to the product of a primary reaction, to provide a measurable absorbance change when the primary product does not possess a strong specific absorptivity.

The introduction of prism or diffraction-grating spectrophotometers capable of isolating a narrow beam of monochromatic light in the ultraviolet or visible spectrum, and stable and sensitive photomultipliers as detectors, greatly improved the reproducibility of photometric measurements (see Chapter 9). Consequently, it is customary to make use of the known molar absorptivity of well-defined reaction products (such as NADH) when calculating changes in their concentrations based on measurements made with spectrophotometers.

## Optimization and Standardization

To measure enzyme activity reliably, all factors that affect the reaction rate—other than the concentration of active enzyme—need to be optimized and rigidly controlled. When the reaction velocity is at or near its maximum under optimal conditions, a larger analytical signal is obtained, making more accurate results possible than with the smaller signal obtained under suboptimal conditions. Much effort, therefore, has been devoted to determining optimal conditions for measuring the activities of enzymes of clinical importance.

### Optimization

Optimization of reaction conditions for enzyme assays traditionally has been carried out by varying a single factor and studying its effect on the reaction rate, then repeating the experiment with a second factor and so on, until the effects of all the variables have been tested. An optimal combination of variables is selected on the basis of these experiments, and the validity of the chosen conditions is verified. Not only is this approach labor intensive, it is also difficult to adapt in situations in which the effects of different variables are interdependent, as is frequently the case in enzyme analysis. This traditional empirical approach to optimization has been replaced by techniques of simplex co-optimization and response surface methodology.

### Standardization

Despite considerable effort, the goal of a single universally used procedure to measure the catalytic activity of a given enzyme has not been achieved. As a practical alternative, enzyme standardization efforts have been focused on the development of a system that allows comparability of results for human serum samples, independent of the test kits and instruments used. To achieve this, the *reference measurement system* approach, based on the concepts of metrological traceability and on a hierarchy of measurement procedures and calibrator materials, has been proposed. In applying the reference system theory, enzymes represent a special class of analytes, because the numerical results of catalytic concentration measurements depend entirely on the experimental conditions under which measurements are made. Thus, the reference measurement procedure, which defines the conditions under which a given enzyme activity is measured, occupies the highest level of the traceability chain (Fig. 14.10). The International Federation of Clinical Chemistry and Laboratory Medicine (IFCC) established and validated reference procedures at 37°C for the measurement of the majority of clinically important enzymes, that is, AST, ALT, γ-glutamyltransferase, LDH, CK, ALP, and α-amylase. In addition to the development of primary reference measurement procedures, the system also requires materials acting as calibrators for the intermediate transfer of trueness from the reference procedure to the field assays. The reference procedure is used to assign a certified value to a reference material, and this certified material should then be used by the manufacturer to assign values to commercial calibrators. Medical laboratories that use commercial measuring systems with validated calibrators to measure clinical samples may obtain values that are traceable to the reference procedure, independently of the method or instrument employed, finally permitting comparability of enzyme results.

For a reference measurement system to be capable of standardizing the results of different assays of a given enzyme catalytic concentration, some conditions must be satisfied. First, the reference procedure used to assign the value of the reference (calibrator) material and the field assay(s) to be calibrated should have similar, if not identical, selectivity for the measurand (enzyme or isoenzyme) under study. Second, the properties of the reference (calibrator) material must be the same as or closely similar to those of the analyte enzyme in its natural matrix, that is, must be commutable. If commutable reference materials suitable for direct calibration of field methods are lacking, manufacturers may approach standardization by splitting a panel of native clinical samples with a laboratory performing the reference measurement procedure and then calibrate their commercial measuring systems in accordance with correlation results obtained using the reference measurement procedure-assigned values of clinical samples.

An aspect associated with standardization efforts is the possibility to define globally useful reference intervals for serum enzyme catalytic concentrations once standardized. Reference intervals obtained with analytical procedures that produce results traceable to the corresponding reference measurement system can be transferred between laboratories (becoming "common"), providing that served populations have the same biological characteristics, and the specific enzyme is not influenced by ethnicity or environmental factors. The definition of traceable reference intervals should lead to the disappearance of different intervals employed for the same enzyme, providing more effective and less confusing information to clinicians.

In addition to the definition of reference measurement systems, the analytical performance specifications (APS) for enzyme measurements should be established to make their determination clinically suitable and to ensure that the measurement error does not prevail on the result. Among proposed models, the one based on the biological variability has been used to derive APS for enzymes. Table 14.2 reports the APS for bias and measurement uncertainty at desirable and optimal quality levels derived from the biological variability data of standardized enzymes (European Federation of Clinical Chemistry and Laboratory Medicine [EFLM ] Database. http://biologicalvariation.eu; accessed January, 2022).

## Measurement of Enzyme Mass Concentration

Immunoassays for human enzymes and isoenzymes that measure protein mass instead of catalytic concentration have been described. To develop such assays, purified enzyme protein has to be prepared to (1) act as a calibrator, (2) be labeled, and (3) be used to raise the enzyme-specific antibody. These methods identify all molecules with the antigenic determinants necessary for recognition by the antibody so that inactive enzyme molecules that are immunologically unaltered are measured along with active molecules. In the majority of cases, however, no degradation or changes in the active enzyme occur in blood so that the clinical equivalence of the different measurement approaches (i.e., estimation of catalytic and mass concentration) is obtained.

Immunoassays typically are not used for determination of total activities for the more important diagnostic enzymes because these assays generally cannot compete in terms of full automation and cost with measurements of catalytic activity concentration. Furthermore, several enzyme activities in serum are due to mixtures of immunologically distinct forms, so an assay using a single type of antibody usually determines only one of the enzyme forms. However, this disadvantage in the determination of total enzyme activity becomes a marked advantage in the measurement of specific isoenzymes and isoforms, and immunologic methods have been used routinely in the isoenzyme analysis of CK, amylase, and ALP.

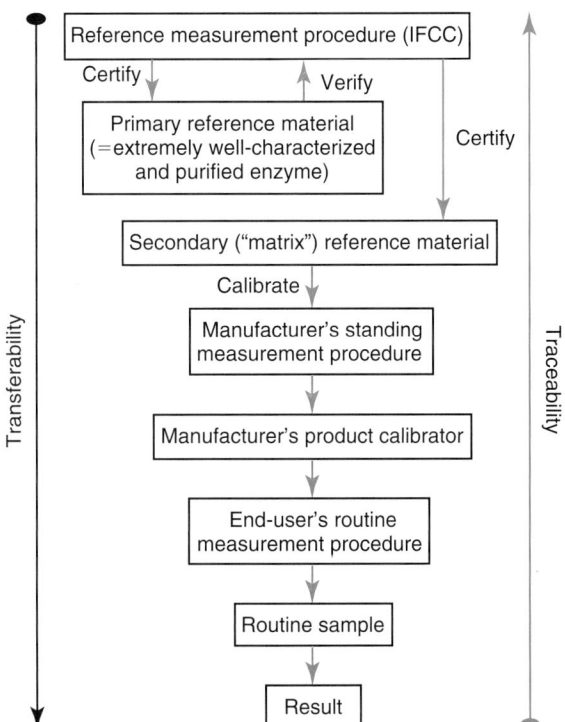

Fig. 14.10 The reference system for enzyme measurement showing the traceability of the laboratory result to the reference measurement procedure. (From Panteghini M, Ceriotti F, Schumann G, et al. Establishing a reference system in clinical enzymology. *Clin Chem Lab Med.* 2001;39:795–800. Reprinted with permission of Walter de Gruyter.)

**TABLE 14.2 Analytical Performance Specifications at Desirable and Optimal Quality Levels for Bias and Uncertainty of Enzyme Measurements, Derived From Biological Variation Data**

| Enzyme | ALLOWABLE BIAS[a] | | ALLOWABLE MEASUREMENT UNCERTAINTY[b] | |
|---|---|---|---|---|
| | Desirable (%) | Optimum (%) | Desirable (%) | Optimum (%) |
| ALT | ±7.7 | ±3.9 | ±10.1 | ±5.1 |
| ALP | ±5.5 | ±2.8 | ±6.0 | ±3.0 |
| AST | ±5.7 | ±2.9 | ±9.6 | ±4.8 |
| CK | ±10.2 | ±5.1 | ±15.0 | ±7.5 |
| γGT | ±11.4 | ±5.7 | ±9.1 | ±4.6 |
| LDH | ±3.4 | ±1.7 | ±5.2 | ±2.6 |
| AMY | ±7.7 | ±3.9 | ±6.6 | ±3.3 |

[a]Calculated as $0.250\ (CV_I^2 + CV_G^2)^{0.5}$ (desirable) and $0.125\ (CV_I^2 + CV_G^2)^{0.5}$ (optimum).
[b]Calculated as standard uncertainty as $0.50\ CV_I$ (desirable) and $0.25\ CV_I$ (optimum), and expanded by multiplying by a coverage factor of 2 (95.45% level of confidence).
All biological variation information (i.e., within-subject CV [$CV_I$] and between-subject CV [$CV_G$]) is derived from the EFLM database (https://biologicalvariation.eu), except for ALP derived from Infusino I, Frusciante E, Braga F and Panteghini M. Progress and impact of enzyme measurement standardization. *Clin Chem Lab Med.* 2017;55:334–340.

## Enzymes as Analytical Reagents

Enzymes are used as analytical reagents for measurement of several metabolites and substrates and in immunoassays to detect and quantify immunologic reactions.

### Measurement of Metabolites

The use of enzymes as analytical reagents to measure metabolites frequently offers the advantage of great specificity for the substance being determined. This high specificity typically removes the need for preliminary separation or purification steps, so the analysis can be carried out directly on complex mixtures such as serum. Uricase (urate oxidase), urease, and glucose oxidase are examples of highly specific enzymes used in clinically important assays, such as the measurement of uric acid, urea, and glucose in biological fluids. However, high specificity cannot always be achieved in practice, and knowledge of the substrate specificities of reagent enzymes is essential to identify possible interferences with the assay, and to correct for them if possible. Coupled reactions are often necessary to construct an enzymatic assay for a specific compound. For example, in the enzymatic determination of glucose, hexokinase converts a number of sugars to their 6-phosphate esters. However, the indicator reaction used to monitor this change uses glucose-6-phosphate dehydrogenase, which is highly specific for glucose-6-phosphate, rendering the assay highly specific for glucose.

*Equilibrium methods.* Most assays used to determine the amount of a substance enzymatically are allowed to continue to completion so that all substrate has been converted into a measurable product. These methods are called *end point* or, more correctly, *equilibrium* methods because the product concentration no longer increases when equilibrium is reached. Reactions in which the equilibrium point corresponds virtually to complete conversion of the substrate to product are obviously preferable for this type of analysis. However, an unfavorable equilibrium often can be overcome by additional enzymatic or nonenzymatic reactions that convert or trap a product of the first reaction. Removing one of the products of the reaction keeps the system in disequilibrium, allowing for nearly total conversion of substrate into product. For example, when measuring lactate with LD, the pyruvate formed can be trapped by the addition of hydrazine, with which it forms an irreversible hydrazone, preventing the pyruvate from causing product inhibition of the LD reaction.

Theoretically, the time required to transform a fixed quantity, $Q$, of substrate into products is inversely proportional to the amount of enzyme, [E], present:

$$Q = k_1 \times [E] \times t \qquad (14.25)$$

and:

$$[E] = \frac{Q}{K_1} \times \frac{1}{t} \qquad (14.26)$$

where $k_1$ is the rate constant and $t$ is the elapsed time. Equilibrium methods may therefore require the use of appreciable amounts of enzyme for each sample, to avoid inconveniently long incubation periods. As the substrate concentration falls to low quantities toward the end of the reaction, the $K_m$ of the enzyme becomes important in determining the reaction rate. Enzymes with high affinities for their substrates (low $K_m$ values) are most suitable for equilibrium analysis. Equilibrium methods are largely insensitive to minor changes in reaction conditions, so it is not necessary to have exactly the same amount of enzyme in each reaction mixture or to maintain the pH or temperature absolutely constant, provided that the variations are not so great that the reaction is not completed within the fixed time allowed.

*Kinetic methods.* First-order or pseudo–first–order reactions are the most important reactions for the kinetic determination of substrate concentration. For any first-order reaction, the substrate concentration [S] at a given time $t$ after the start of the reaction is given by:

$$[S] = [S_0] \times e^{-kt} \qquad (14.27)$$

where [$S_0$] is the initial substrate concentration, e is the base of the natural log, and $k$ is the rate constant.

The change in substrate concentration $\Delta[S]$ over a fixed time interval, $t_1$ to $t_2$, is related to $[S_0]$ by the equation:

$$[S_0] = \frac{-\Delta[S]}{e^{-kt_1} - e^{kt_2}} \qquad (14.28)$$

As this equation indicates, the change in substrate concentration over a fixed time interval is directly proportional to its initial concentration. This is a general property of first-order reactions.

For an enzymatic reaction, first-order kinetics is followed when [S] is small compared with $K_m$. Thus:

$$v = \frac{V_{max}}{K_m} \times [S] \qquad (14.29)$$

or:

$$v = k[S] \qquad (14.30)$$

Therefore, the first-order rate constant, $k$, is equal to $\frac{V_{max}}{K_m}$.

Methods in which some property related to substrate concentration (e.g., absorbance, fluorescence, chemiluminescence) is measured at two fixed times during the course of the reaction are known as *two-point* kinetic methods. Theoretically, they are most accurate for the enzymatic determination of substrates. However, these methods are technically more demanding than equilibrium methods and all factors that affect reaction rate, such as pH, temperature, and amount of enzyme, must be kept constant from one assay to the next, as must the timing of the two measurements. These conditions can be readily achieved in automated analyzers. A reference solution of the analyte (substrate) is used for calibration. To ensure first-order reaction conditions, the substrate concentration must be low compared with the $K_m$ (i.e., in the order of less than $0.2 \times K_m$). Enzymes with high $K_m$ values are therefore preferred for kinetic analysis to obtain a wider usable range of substrate concentrations.

## Immunoassay

In enzyme immunoassay, enzyme-labeled antibodies or antigens are first allowed to react with a ligand; then an enzyme substrate is added. Enzymes such as ALP have been used as enzyme labels. A modification of this methodology is the enzyme-linked immunosorbent assay (ELISA), in which one of the reaction components is bound to a solid-phase surface. In this technique, an aliquot of sample is allowed to interact with the solid-phase antibody. After washing, a second antibody labeled with enzyme is added to form an Ab–Ag–Ab–enzyme complex. Excess free enzyme-labeled antibody is then washed away, and the substrate is added; the conversion of substrate is proportional to the quantity of antigen. In immunoassays, it is not the specificity of labeled enzymes that is important, but rather their sensitivity.

## Measurement of Isoenzymes and Isoforms

A number of analytical techniques have been used to measure specific isoenzymes or isoforms including (1) electrophoresis (see Chapter 11), (2) chromatography (see Chapter 12), (3) chemical inactivation, and (4) differences in catalytic properties, but the most widely used methods are now based on immunochemical principles (see Chapter 15).

### Electrophoresis

Various forms of electrophoresis have been used to separate isoenzymes. The methods are time-consuming, difficult to quantify, relatively expensive, and currently only available from a few laboratories.

### Chromatography

Ion-exchange chromatography makes use of differences in net molecular charge at a given pH to separate isoenzymes. A typical ion-exchange material is diethylaminoethyl (DEAE) cellulose, in which ionizable DEAE groups are attached to an inert cellulose matrix. Ion-exchange chromatography, in general, lacks the resolving power of electrophoresis, but relatively large quantities of proteins can be separated with good recovery of enzymatic activity; the method is of great value in enzyme purification.

Other forms of chromatography that have been applied to fractionation of isoenzyme mixtures include high-performance liquid chromatography and affinity chromatography. The latter makes use of differences between isoenzymes in their affinities for a specific ligand that is attached to an inert insoluble support used as the stationary phase in a chromatography column or in a batch technique.

### Immunochemical Assays

Immunochemical methods of isoenzyme analysis are particularly applicable to isoenzymes derived from multiple genes because these are usually most clearly antigenically distinct. However, the greater discriminating power of monoclonal antibodies has potentially brought all multiple forms of an enzyme within the scope of immunochemical analysis. Some of these methods detect catalytic activity of the isoenzymes. For example, residual activity may be measured after reaction with antiserum. The preferred method for measuring isoenzymes in the medical laboratory is based on a solid-phase sandwich ELISA assay, which is today fully automatable. These methods do not depend on the catalytic concentration of the isoenzyme being determined.

The choice and application of various methods of isoenzyme analysis in clinical enzymology in relation to specific isoenzyme systems are discussed in Chapter 19.

---

### POINTS TO REMEMBER

- Because of their specificity, enzymes can be used as analytical reagents to measure compounds such as metabolites in complex mediums.
- The measurement of isoenzymes may increase the diagnostic specificity and sensitivity of enzyme assays in body fluid samples.

## REVIEW QUESTIONS

1. The enzyme 2.2.8.11 is a(n):
   a. oxidoreductase.
   b. transferase.
   c. hydrolase.
   d. lyase.
   e. isomerase.
   f. ligase.

2. A disulfide bond in a protein is an example of:
   a. primary structure.
   b. secondary structure.
   c. tertiary structure.
   d. quaternary structure.

3. The active site of an enzyme is:
   a. small compared to the entire enzyme.
   b. usually in the center of the enzyme.
   c. not specific for inhibitors.
   d. typically only involves a few continuous bases along the primary structure.

4. Which of the following can affect the rate of an enzyme-catalyzed reaction?
   a. Enzyme concentration
   b. Substrate concentration
   c. pH
   d. Reaction temperature
   e. All of the above

5. $K_m$ is:
   a. the enzyme concentration that results in 50% of the maximal reaction rate.
   b. a property of an enzyme and substrate under certain conditions.
   c. a property of an enzyme irrespective of the substrate.
   d. a property of a substrate irrespective of the enzyme.

6. Which statement is correct?
   a. Either the enzyme or the coenzyme, but not both, are consumed during an enzymatic reaction.
   b. An enzyme without a prosthetic group attached is referred to as a coenzyme.
   c. Coenzymes may be derivatives of vitamins.
   d. All of the above statements are correct.

7. An enzyme assay determined by a single measurement taken at the termination of the enzymatic reaction is referred to as a:
   a. fixed-time assay.
   b. terminator assay.
   c. kinetic assay.
   d. continuous-monitoring assay.

8. A reactant in a catalysis reaction that binds to the enzyme's active site is the:
   a. enzyme.
   b. product.
   c. substrate.
   d. coenzyme.

9. An international unit (U) of enzyme activity is the amount of enzyme that will catalyze the reaction of:
   a. one micromole of substrate per minute.
   b. one mole of substrate per second.
   c. one micromole of enzyme per hour.
   d. one millimole of substrate per minute.

10. In what kind of inhibition is the inhibitor usually a structural analog of the substrate?
    a. Competitive
    b. Noncompetitive
    c. Uncompetitive
    d. Racemic mirroring

11. In an analytical enzymatic measurement of substrate, an enzyme reaction is accompanied by a change in absorbance of one component of the assay system. If this change is continuously monitored while it is occurring, the reaction is referred to as a(n):
    a. fixed-time reaction.
    b. end point assay.
    c. rate-limiting reaction.
    d. self-indicating reaction.

## SUGGESTED READINGS

Aloisio E, Frusciante E, Pasqualetti S, et al. Traceability validation of six enzyme measurements on the Abbott Alinity c analytical system. *Clin Chem Lab Med.* 2020;58:1250–1256.

Braga F, Panteghini M. Commutability of reference and control materials: an essential factor for assuring the quality of measurements in Laboratory Medicine. *Clin Chem Lab Med.* 2019;57:967–973.

Canalias F, Camprubí S, Sánchez M, et al. Metrological traceability of values for catalytic concentration of enzymes assigned to a calibration material. *Clin Chem Lab Med.* 2006;44:333–339.

Copeland RA. *Enzymes: A Practical Introduction to Structure, Mechanism, and Data Analysis.* 2nd ed. New York: Wiley-VCH; 2000.

Cook PF, Cleland WW. *Enzyme Kinetics and Mechanism.* 1st ed. New York: Garland Science; 2007.

Harris TK, Keshwani MM. Measurement of enzyme activity. *Methods Enzymol.* 2009;463:57–71.

Infusino I, Bonora R, Panteghini M. Traceability in clinical enzymology. *Clin Biochem Rev.* 2007;28:155–161.

Infusino I, Frusciante E, Braga F, et al. Progress and impact of enzyme measurement standardization. *Clin Chem Lab Med.* 2017;55:334–340.

Infusino I, Schumann G, Ceriotti F, et al. Standardization in clinical enzymology: a challenge for the theory of metrological traceability. *Clin Chem Lab Med.* 2010;48:301–307.

Moss DW. *Isoenzyme Analysis.* London: The Chemical Society; 1979.

Nomenclature Committee of the International Union of Biochemistry and Molecular Biology (NC-IUBMB). *Enzyme Nomenclature: Recommendations.* San Diego: Academic Press; 1992:862. with Supplement 1 (1993), Supplement 2 (1994), Supplement 3 (1995), Supplement 4 (1997), Supplement 5 (1999) (in *Eur J Biochem*. 1994;223:1–5; *Eur J Biochem* 1995;232:1–6; *Eur J Biochem*. 1996;237:1–5; *Eur J Biochem*. 1997;250;1–6, and *Eur J Biochem*. 1999;264;610–650; respectively, and subsequent Supplements 6–19 at http://www.chem.qmul.ac.uk/iupac/bibliog/jcbn.html.

Okotore RO. *Essentials of Enzymology*. Bloomington, IN: Xlibris Corporation; 2015.

Panteghini M, Ceriotti F, Schumann G, et al. Establishing a reference system in clinical enzymology. *Clin Chem Lab Med*. 2001;39:795–800.

Price NC, Stevens L. *Fundamentals of Enzymology: The Cell and Molecular Biology of Catalytic Proteins*. 3rd ed. Oxford: Oxford University Press; 2000.

Rautela GS, Snee RD, Miller WK. Response-surface co-optimization of reaction conditions in clinical chemical methods. *Clin Chem*. 1979;25:1954–1964.

Siekmann L, Bonora R, Burtis CA, et al. IFCC primary reference procedures for the measurement of catalytic activity concentrations of enzymes at 37 degrees C. Part 1. The concept of reference procedures for the measurement of catalytic activity concentrations of enzymes. *Clin Chem Lab Med*. 2002;40:631–634.

# 15

# Immunochemical Techniques

*Jason Y. Park and Khushbu Patel**

## OBJECTIVES

1. Define the following:
   - Affinity
   - Antibody
   - Antigen
   - Avidity
   - Hapten
   - Immunoassay
   - Immunogen
   - Monoclonal antibody
   - Polyclonal antiserum
   - Sandwich immunoassay
2. Diagram, label, and state the function of the components of an immunoglobulin G (IgG) antibody molecule.
3. List three binding forces that act to produce antigen/antibody binding.
4. Explain how the following factors affect antigen/antibody binding:
   - Addition of a linear polymer
   - Ion species
   - Precipitin reaction
5. For each of the following qualitative immunochemical techniques, state the principle and clinical use:
   - Immunofixation
   - Western blotting

6. For each of the following quantitative immunochemical techniques, state the principle and clinical use:
   - Nephelometry
   - Turbidimetry
7. List five types of nonisotopic labels used in a labeled immunochemical assay, and provide one example of each type of label.
8. Compare competitive with noncompetitive immunoassays, including procedure, assay components, and uses in the clinical laboratory. Do the same for heterogeneous and homogeneous immunoassays.
9. For each of the following immunochemical techniques, state the principle, the components of each assay, the type of assay, and the clinical uses:
   - Cloned enzyme donor immunoassay
   - Enzyme-linked immunosorbent assay
   - Enzyme-multiplied immunoassay
   - Fluoroimmunoassay
   - Immunocytochemistry
10. Describe three factors that can adversely affect immunoassay results.

## KEY WORDS AND DEFINITIONS

**Affinity** Energy of interaction of a single antibody-combining site and its corresponding epitope on the antigen.

**Antibody** Immunoglobulin (Ig) class of molecule (e.g., IgA, IgG, IgM) that binds specifically to an antigen or hapten.

**Antigen** Any material capable of reacting with an antibody without necessarily being capable of inducing antibody formation.

**Avidity** Overall strength of binding of antibody and antigen; includes the sum of the binding affinities of all individual combining sites on the antibody.

**Competitive immunoassay** An immunoassay in which all reactants are simultaneously or sequentially mixed

together and unlabeled antigen competes with labeled antigen for binding sites on the antibody.

**Hapten** A chemically defined determinant that, when conjugated to an immunogenic carrier, stimulates the synthesis of antibody specific for the hapten.

**Heterogeneous immunoassay** An immunochemical reaction in which it is assumed that the formation of the antigen/antibody complex occurs more quickly than the breakdown of the complex into antigen and antibody; in this assay, the antigen is labeled and separation of the free from the bound-labeled antigen is required.

**Homogeneous immunoassay** An immunochemical reaction in which the activity of the label attached to the

*The authors gratefully acknowledge the original contributions by Dr. Larry J. Kricka, upon which portions of this chapter are based.

antigen is modulated directly by antibody binding; this assay does not require a separation.

**Hook effect**   A phenomenon occurring with certain immunoassays due to very high concentrations of a particular analyte; it results in a false-negative result. The hook effect mostly affects one-step immunometric assays.

**Immunoassay**   An assay based on the reaction of an antigen with an antibody specific for the antigen.

**Immunogen**   A substance capable of inducing an immune response.

**Label**   Any substance with a measurable property attached to an antigen, antibody, or binding substance.

**Noncompetitive immunoassay**   An immunoassay in which a capture antibody is bound to a surface with subsequent antigen binding, followed by the addition of a second labeled antibody that reacts with the initial antigen/antibody complex.

**Western blotting**   Membrane-based assay in which proteins are separated by electrophoresis, which is followed by transfer to a membrane and probing with a labeled antibody.

## BASIC CONCEPTS AND DEFINITIONS

An **antigen** is any material capable of reacting with an antibody. With **immunoassays**, the antigen is the analyte of clinical interest that is being measured. **Antibodies** are immunoglobulins that bind specifically to a wide array of natural and synthetic antigens, such as (1) proteins, (2) carbohydrates, (3) nucleic acids, (4) lipids, and (5) other molecules. Analytically, immunoglobulin (Ig)G is the most prevalent immunochemical reagent in use. It is a glycoprotein that has a molecular weight (MW) of 158,000 Da and is composed of two duplex chains, with each set composed of a heavy ($\gamma$) and a light ($\lambda$ or $\kappa$) chain joined by disulfide bonds (Fig. 15.1). Interchain disulfide bonds hold the duplex chains together and create a symmetrical molecule. The variable amino acid sequence at the amino terminal end of each chain determines the antigenic specificity of the particular antibody. Each unique amino acid sequence is a product of a single plasma cell line or clone, and each plasma cell line produces antibodies with single specificities. A complex antigen elicits a multiplicity of antibodies with different specificities derived from different cell lines. An antibody developed in this manner is termed *polyclonal* and exhibits diverse specificities in its reactivity with the immunogen. Each unique region of the molecular antigen that binds a complementary antibody is termed an *epitope* (antigenic determinant).

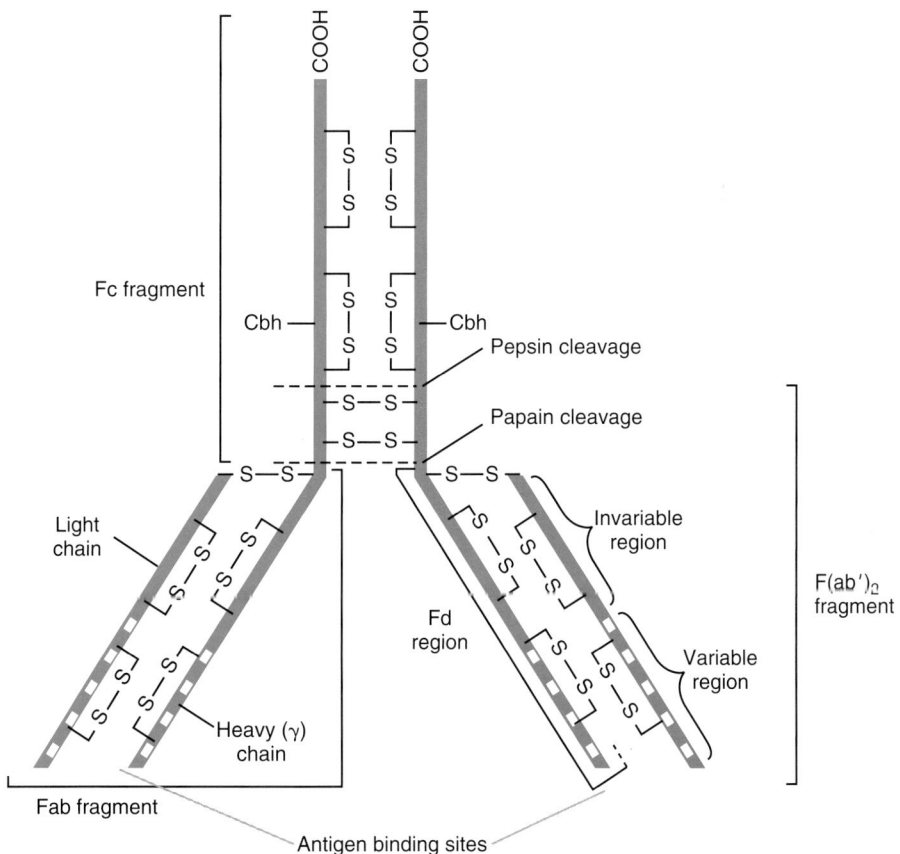

**Fig. 15.1** Schematic diagram of immunoglobulin G (IgG) antibody molecule showing carbohydrate *(Cbh)*, disulfide bonds *(SS)*, and major fragments produced by proteolytic enzyme treatment (F[ab']₂, Fc, Fab, Fd).

An **immunogen** is a protein or a substance coupled to a carrier, usually a protein. Introduction of an immunogen into a foreign host induces the formation of an antibody. A **hapten** is a chemically defined determinant that, by itself, will not stimulate an immune response. However, when conjugated to an immunogenic carrier, the conjugated molecule stimulates the synthesis of antibody specific for the hapten. Some general properties required for immunogenicity include the following:

1. Areas of structural stability within the molecule
2. Randomness of structure
3. Minimum MW of 4000 to 5000 Da
4. Ability to be metabolized (a necessary but insufficient criterion for some classes of antigens)
5. Accessibility of a particular immunogenic configuration to the antibody-forming mechanism
6. Structurally foreign quality

The strength or energy of interaction between the antibody and the antigen is described in two terms. **Affinity** refers to the thermodynamic quantity defining the energy of interaction of a single antibody-combining site and its corresponding epitope on the antigen. The affinity can be influenced by thermodynamic factors such as pH and temperature. **Avidity** refers to the overall strength of the binding of antibody and antigen and includes the sum of the binding affinities of all individual combining sites on the antibody. The avidity is also dependent on the valency and structural arrangements of the antibody and antigen. For example, IgG has two antigen binding sites, whereas IgM has 10 antigen binding sites per antibody molecule.

*Polyclonal antiserum* is produced in a normal animal host in response to immunogen administration. In contrast, a *monoclonal antibody* is the product of a single clone or plasma cell line rather than a heterogeneous mixture of antibodies produced by many cell clones in response to immunization. Monoclonal antibodies now are used widely as reagents in immunoassay techniques.

Monoclonal antibodies provide an analytical advantage in that two different antibody specificities can be used in a single assay. For example, a solid-phase antibody specific for a unique epitope and another labeled antibody specific for a different epitope are reacted with antigen in a single incubation step. This combination eliminates (1) the two-step sequential addition of antigen and labeled antibody to the solid phase, (2) one incubation step, and (3) one washing step, which would be necessary when polyclonal antibodies binding to both sites are used.

## ANTIGEN-ANTIBODY BINDING

In this section, several of the factors that affect the binding of antigens and antibodies are discussed.

### Binding Forces

Several forces act cooperatively to produce antigen-antibody binding. The three major contributing forces are (1) electrostatic van der Waals–London dipole-dipole interactions, (2)

hydrophobic interactions, and (3) ionic coulombic bonding (primarily between carboxylate and protonated amino groups on the antigen and the antibody).

### Reaction Mechanism

The binding of antigen to an antibody is not static but is an equilibrium reaction that proceeds in three phases. The initial reaction (phase 1) of a multivalent antigen ($Ag_n$) and a bivalent antibody (Ab) occurs very rapidly in comparison with subsequent growth of the complexes (phase 2) and is depicted by the following equation:

$$Ag_n + Ab \underset{k_{-1}}{\overset{k_1}{\rightleftharpoons}} Ag_n \ Ab \underset{k_{-2}}{\overset{k_2}{\rightleftharpoons}} Ag_a Ab_b \quad (15.1)$$

where $k_1 \ggg k_2$, $n$ is the number of epitopes per molecule, and $a$ and $b$ are the numbers of antigen and antibody molecules per complex, respectively. Phase 3 of the reaction involves the precipitation of the complex after a critical size is reached. The speed of these reactions depends on electrolyte concentration, pH, and temperature, as well as on antigen and antibody types and the binding affinity of the antibody.

### Precipitin Reaction

The curve shown in Fig. 15.2 is a schematic diagram of the classic precipitin curve. Although the concentration of total antibody is constant, the concentration of free antibody, $[Ab]_f$, and of free antigen, $[Ag]_f$, varies for any given Ag/Ab ratio. A low Ag/Ab ratio exists in Fig. 15.2A (zone of antibody excess). Under these conditions, excess Ab is free

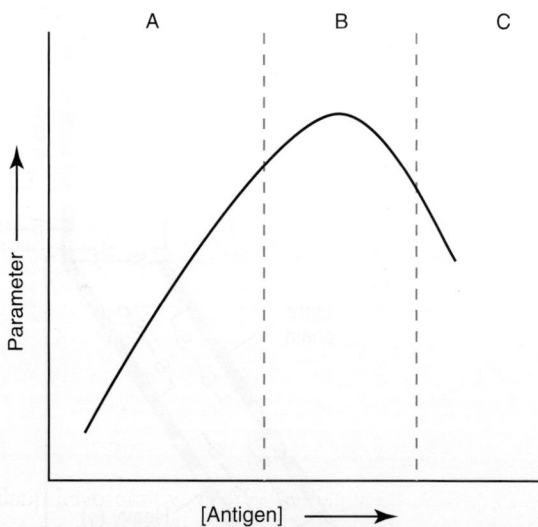

**Fig. 15.2** Schematic diagram of precipitin curve illustrating different antigen concentration zones. *A,* Antibody excess. *B,* Equivalence. *C,* Antigen excess. The parameter measured may be the quantity of protein precipitated, light scattering, or another measurable parameter. Antibody concentration is held constant in this example.

in solution, but all Ag is bound and immune complexes are small. As total antigen increases, the size of the immune complexes increases up to equivalence (see Fig. 15.2B), and little or no $[Ab]_f$ or $[Ag]_f$ exists. This is the zone of equivalence, and it is the optimal combining ratio for cross-linking. As Ag/Ab further increases (see Fig. 15.2C), the immune complex size decreases and $[Ag]_f$ increases (zone of antigen excess).

## Chemical Factors

Chemical factors that influence antibody-antigen binding include ionic species, ionic strength, and polymeric molecules.

### Ion Species and Ionic Strength Effects

Cationic salts inhibit antibody binding to a cationic hapten. The order of inhibition by various cations corresponds to their decreasing ionic radius and the increasing radius of hydration (e.g., $Cs^+ > K^+ > Li^+$). For anionic haptens and anionic salts, the order of inhibition of binding again follows the order of decreasing ionic radius and increasing radius of hydration (e.g., $SCN^-$ [thiocyanate] $> I^- > F^-$).

### Polymer Effect

The addition of a linear polymer to a mixture of antigen and antibody causes a significant increase in the rate of immune complex growth and enhances the precipitation of immune complex, especially with low-avidity antibody. This is due to the increased probability of contact between the antigen and antibody caused by the presence of large polymer molecules in solution (steric exclusion). The most desirable characteristics of the polymer are high (1) MW, (2) degree of linearity (minimum branching), and (3) aqueous solubility. Polyethylene glycol 6000 has these characteristics and is particularly useful in immunochemical methods at concentrations of 3 to 5 g/dL.

## QUALITATIVE METHODS

Immunochemical techniques used for qualitative purposes include (1) immunofixation (IF) and (2) Western blotting.

IF has gained widespread acceptance as an immunochemical method used to identify proteins. With this technique, electrophoresis is first performed in an agarose gel to separate the proteins in the mixture. Subsequently, antiserum spread directly on the gel causes the protein(s) of interest to precipitate. The immune precipitate is trapped within the gel matrix, and all other nonprecipitated proteins are then removed by washing of the gel. The gel then is stained for identification of the proteins. The utility of IF, which now is used widely for the evaluation of myeloma proteins, is illustrated in Fig. 15.3.

## Blotting

The previously discussed technique uses direct examination of immunoprecipitation of the protein(s) in the gel. However, certain media, such as polyacrylamide, do not lend themselves to direct immunoprecipitation, nor does sufficient antigen concentration always exist to produce an immunoprecipitate that is

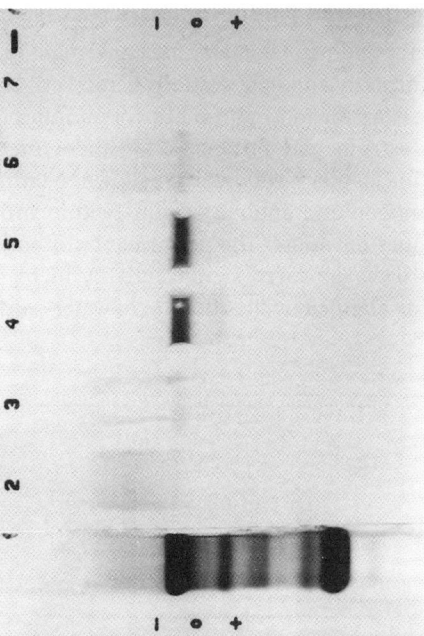

Fig. 15.3 Immunofixation of a serum containing an immunoglobulin (Ig)M kappa paraprotein. *Lane 1*, Serum electrophoresis stained for protein; *lane 2*, anti-IgG, Fc piece specific; *lane 3*, anti-IgA, α-chain specific; *lane 4*, anti-IgM, α-chain specific; *lane 5*, anti-κ light chain; *lane 6*, anti-λ light chain. (Courtesy Katherine Bayer, Philadelphia, PA.)

retained in the gel during subsequent processing. Under these circumstances, the technique of **Western blotting** is used. This technique involves an electrophoresis step, followed by transfer of the separated proteins onto an overlying strip of nitrocellulose or nylon membrane by a process called *electroblotting*. Once the proteins are fixed to the membrane, they are detected with antibody probes labeled with molecules such as enzymes. With the use of such probes, the limits of detection are 10 to 100 times lower than the values obtained through direct immunoprecipitation and staining of proteins.

An example of blotting analysis for human immunodeficiency virus type 1 (HIV-1) antibodies is shown in Fig. 15.4. When applied to antigen assays, concentrations of antigen as low as 500 ng/mL or 2.5 ng per band in the gel have been detected. The detection limit of the technique is lowered even farther to approximately 100 pg by chemiluminescent detection of the enzyme-labeled antibody.

A simpler technique that bypasses the electrophoretic separation step is known as *dot blotting*. A protein sample to be analyzed is applied to a membrane surface as a small "dot" and is dried. The membrane then is exposed to a labeled antibody specific for the test antigen contained in the dotted mixture. After the membrane is washed, bound-labeled antibody is detected with a photometric or chemiluminescent detection system.

## QUANTITATIVE METHODS

Immunochemical techniques have been used to develop quantitative methods and include turbidimetric and nephelometric assays and labeled immunochemical assays.

## Turbidimetric and Nephelometric Assays

Turbidimetry and nephelometry are convenient techniques, based on turbidity and light scattering, respectively, that are used to measure the rate of formation of immune complexes in vitro. Instrumental principles for these methods are described in Chapter 9. Studies have shown that the reaction between antigen and antibody begins within milliseconds and continues for hours. The performance of both types of assays has been improved significantly by increases in the reaction rate attained by the addition of water-soluble linear polymers.

Both turbidimetric and nephelometric immunochemical methods using rate and pseudoequilibrium protocols have been described for (1) proteins, (2) antigens, and (3) haptens. In rate assays, measurements are made early in the reaction because the largest change ($dI_s/dt$) in intensity of scattered light ($I_s$) with respect to time is attained during this time interval. For pseudoequilibrium assays, waiting 30 to 60 minutes is necessary so that the $dI_s/dt$ is small relative to the time required to make the necessary measurements. Such assays are termed *pseudoequilibrium* rather than *equilibrium* because true equilibrium is not reached within the time allowed for these assays.

Nephelometric methods are generally more sensitive than turbidimetric assays and have a lower limit of detection of approximately 1 to 10 mg/L for a serum protein. Lower limits of detection are attained in fluids such as cerebrospinal fluid and urine because of their lower lipid and protein concentrations, which result in a higher signal-to-noise ratio. In addition, for low-molecular-weight proteins such as myoglobin (MW 17,800 Da), limits of detection have been lowered through a latex-enhanced procedure based on antibody-coated latex beads.

Nephelometric and turbidimetric assays have also been applied to the measurement of drugs (haptens). An example of this type of assay is the particle-enhanced turbidimetric inhibition immunoassay (PETINIA see Fig. 15.5) that measures decreasing agglutination in the presence of increasing concentrations of analyte (e.g., digoxin). The reagents comprise an antibody to the analyte of interest and a reagent containing the analyte of interest linked to a latex bead. In the absence of analyte in a specimen, reagent antibody binds to the reagent containing the analyte linked to the latex bead, resulting in increased turbidity. When a specimen with high analyte concentrations is added to the reagent mixture, the reagent antibody is bound by the analyte in the specimen and not to the reagent containing the analyte linked to the latex bead. Thus, the presence of specimen analyte results in less turbidity.

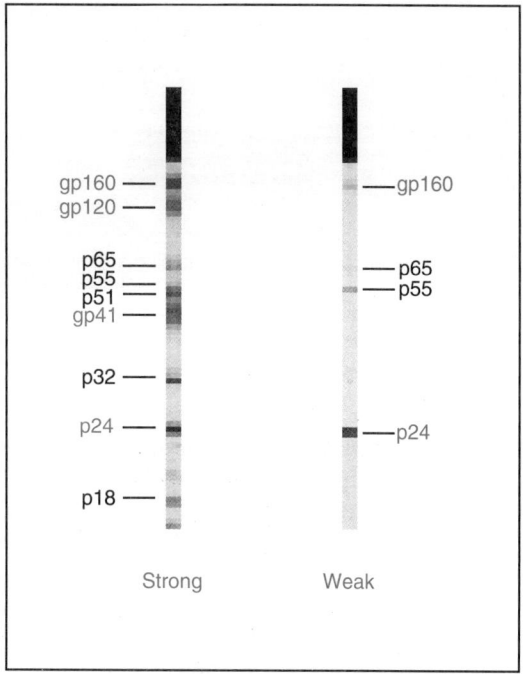

**Fig. 15.4** Blot analysis of serum samples strongly positive and weakly positive for human immunodeficiency virus-1 antibody. Core proteins (GAGs, group-specific antigens) p18, p24, and p55; polymerase p32, p51, and p65; and envelope proteins gp41, gp120, and gp160. (Courtesy Bio-Rad Laboratories Diagnostics Group, Hercules, CA.)

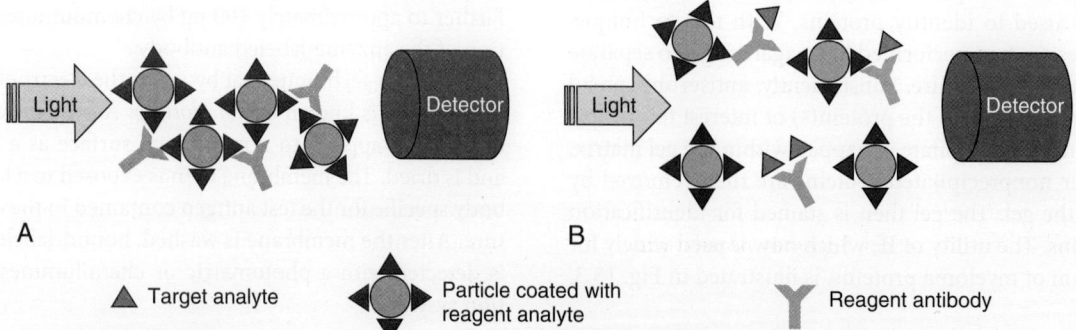

**Fig. 15.5** PETINIA (particle-enhanced turbidimetric inhibition immunoassay). PETINIA measures decreased agglutination in the presence of increasing analyte. The absence of analyte results in agglutination of the reagent particles and antibodies and decreased light transmission to the detector (A). When the target analyte is introduced, it binds the reagent antibody, resulting in less agglutination of the reagent particles and, therefore, decreased turbidity with increased light transmission (B). (From Park JY, Patel K. Immunochemical techniques. In: Rifai N, ed. *Tietz Textbook of Laboratory Medicine.* 7th ed. St. Louis: Elsevier; 2022.)

## Surface Plasmon Resonance–Based Immunoassay

Surface plasmon resonance (SPR) is a label-free immuno-assay based on an optical phenomenon that enables detection of unlabeled reactants in real time based on changes in the index of refraction at the surface where the binding interaction occurs. The assay is conducted on an electrically conducting gold-coated glass slide mounted on a prism. The binding agent is immobilized on the gold surface over which reactant is flowed. Polarized light is directed underneath the glass slide and interacts with the gold surface to produce electron charge density waves called plasmons at the sample and gold surface interface. This results in a reduction in the intensity of the reflected light. Slight changes in the refractive index at the interface lead to a change in the signal, thus facilitating real-time detection of surface molecular interactions (e.g., association and dissociation of biomolecules with the binder immobilized on the gold surface). SPR assays are used to characterize binding reactions (e.g., antibody affinity, kinetics, cross-reactivity).

## Labeled Immunochemical Assays

The previously discussed methods rely on examination of immune complex formation as an index of antigen-antibody reaction. As demonstrated in Eq. 15.1, the overall reaction occurs in sequential phases, and only the final phase consists of formation of the immune complex. However, initial binding of antibody and antigen has been used with antigens and antibodies that have labels to develop many sensitive and specific immunochemical assays. The reaction describing this initial binding and the kinetic constant for the overall reaction are shown in Eqs. 15.2a and 15.2b, respectively.

$$Ab + Ab \underset{k_{-1}}{\overset{k_1}{\rightleftharpoons}} AbAg \qquad (15.2a)$$

$$K = \frac{[AbAg]}{[Ab][Ag]} \qquad (15.2b)$$

where $k_1$ = rate constant for the forward reaction; $k_{-1}$ = rate constant for the reverse reaction; and $K$ = equilibrium constant for the overall reaction.

As predicted from the law of mass action, the concentrations of Ab, Ag, and Ab:Ag are dependent on the magnitude of $k_1$ and $k_{-1}$. For polyclonal antiserum, the average avidity of the antibody populations determines $K$, and the magnitude of $k_1$ in comparison with $k_{-1}$ determines the ultimate limit of detection attainable with a given antibody population.

### Types of Labels

In the decade following the pioneering developments of Yalow and Berson in 1960, all immunoassays used radioactive labels in competitive assays. Since the introduction of enzyme immunoassays (EIAs) in the 1970s, sophisticated assays with various nonisotopic labels (Table 15.1) have been developed.

### TABLE 15.1 Labels Used for Nonisotopic Immunoassay

| | |
|---|---|
| Chemiluminescent | Acridinium ester, sulfonyl acridinium ester, isoluminol |
| Enzyme | Alkaline phosphatase, marine bacterial luciferase, β-galactosidase, firefly luciferase, glucose oxidase, glucose-6-phosphate dehydrogenase, horseradish peroxidase, lysozyme, malate dehydrogenase, microperoxidase, urease, xanthine oxidase |
| Fluorophore | Europium chelate, fluorescein, phycoerythrin, terbium chelate |
| Metal | Gold sol, selenium sol, silver sol |
| Particle | Bacteriophage, erythrocyte, latex bead, dyed latex bead, liposome, quantum dot, magnetic particle |
| Phosphor | Upconverting lanthanide-containing nanoparticle |
| Polynucleotide | DNA |

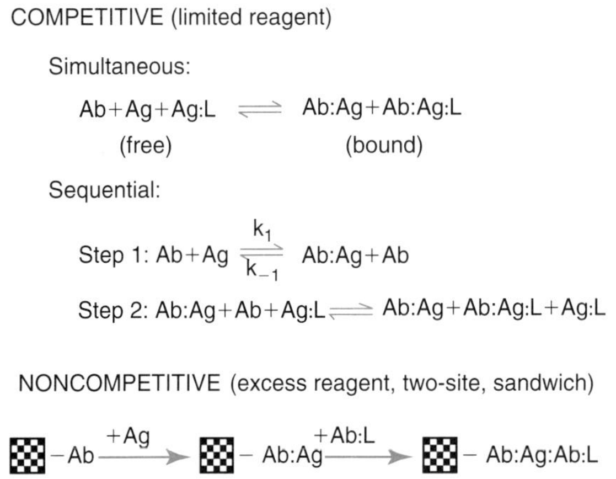

Fig. 15.6 Immunoassay designs. *Ab*, Antibody; *Ag*, antigen; $k_1$, forward rate constant; $k_{-1}$, reverse rate constant; *L*, label.

## Methodologic Principles

As shown in Fig. 15.6, the two major types of reaction formats used in immunochemical assays are termed *competitive* (limited reagent assays) and *noncompetitive* (excess reagent, two-site, or sandwich assays).

## Competitive Immunoassays

In a competitive immunochemical assay, all reactants are simultaneously or sequentially mixed together. In the simultaneous approach, labeled antigen (Ag:L) and unlabeled antigen (Ag) compete to bind with the antibody. In such a system, the avidity of the antibody for labeled and unlabeled antigens must be the same. Under these conditions, the probability of the antibody binding the labeled antigen is inversely proportional to the concentration of unlabeled antigen; hence, bound label is inversely proportional to the concentration of unlabeled antigen.

In a sequential competitive assay, unlabeled antigen is mixed with excess antibody and binding is allowed to reach equilibrium (see Fig. 15.6, Step 1). Labeled antigen is then added sequentially (see Fig. 15.6, Step 2) and allowed to equilibrate. After separation, the bound label is measured and is used to calculate the unlabeled antigen concentration. With this two-step method, a larger fraction of unlabeled antigen is bound by the antibody than in the simultaneous assay, especially at low antigen concentrations. Consequently, a twofold to fourfold lower detection limit is seen in a sequential immunoassay, compared with that in a simultaneous assay, provided $k_1 \gg k_{-1}$. This improvement in detection limit results from an increase in AgAb binding (and thus a decrease in Ag:L binding), which is favored by the sequential addition of Ag and Ag:L. If $k_1 \geq k_{-1}$, dissociation of AgAb becomes more probable, resulting in increased competition between Ag:L and Ag. A typical immunochemical binding curve is shown in Fig. 15.7.

## Noncompetitive Immunoassays

In a typical noncompetitive assay, the "capture" antibody is first passively adsorbed or covalently bound to the surface of a solid phase. Next, the antigen from the sample is allowed to react and is captured by the solid phase antibody. Other proteins are then washed away, and a labeled antibody (conjugate) is added that reacts with the bound antigen through a second and distinct epitope. After additional washing to remove the excess unbound labeled antibody, the bound label is measured, and its concentration or activity is directly proportional to the concentration of antigen.

In noncompetitive assays, either polyclonal or monoclonal antibodies are used as capture and labeled antibodies. If monoclonal antibodies with specificity for distinct epitopes are used, simultaneous incubation of the sample and the conjugate with the capture antibody is possible, thus simplifying the assay protocol.

Noncompetitive immunoassays are performed in simultaneous or sequential mode. The sequential mode is described above. In the simultaneous mode, a high concentration of analyte saturates both capture and labeled antibodies. Under these conditions, the analyte is present in such high concentrations that it reacts simultaneously with the capture and labeled antibodies, reducing the number of complexes formed and producing a falsely low result. Thus, the calibration curve of the assay exhibits a **hook effect**, in which the assay response drops off at high analyte concentrations in assays for analytes for which the normal pathologic concentration range is very wide. For example, assays for chorionic gonadotropin (CG) and alpha fetoprotein (AFP) are particularly prone to this problem. Dilutions of a sample usually are reanalyzed to check for this type of analytical interference. In practice, the hook effect is eliminated if a sequential assay format is adopted and the concentrations of capture and labeled antibodies are sufficiently high to cover analyte concentrations over the entire analytical range of the assay.

Noncompetitive immunoassays rely on different epitopes on a large analyte molecule so as to provide a binding site for both the capture antibody and the labeled antibody. In the past, a small molecule could not be measured using the conventional sandwich format because it had too few epitopes. One strategy developed to expand the scope of the sandwich assay to small molecules is exemplified by a 25-hydroxy vitamin D (25OH-D) assay. In this assay format, 25OH-D binds to an immobilized capture antibody and a second antibody (an antimetatype antibody) specifically recognizes the immunocomplex formed between the 25OH-D molecule and the capture antibody, hence facilitating a sandwich assay design.

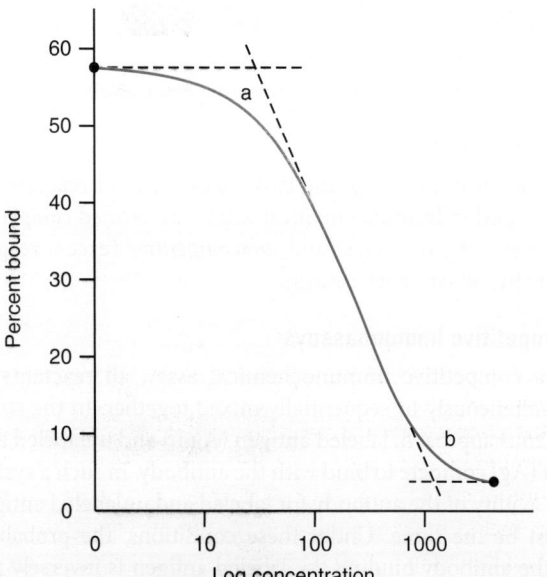

Fig. 15.7 Schematic diagram of the dose-response curve for a typical immunoassay. The analytically useful portion of the curve is bracketed by points *a* and *b*.

## POINTS TO REMEMBER

- Competitive immunoassays are primarily for small molecules.
- Sandwich immunoassays can be designed for both small and large molecules.
- The sandwich type of immunoassay is more sensitive than the competitive immunoassay.
- Noncompetitive immunoassays performed in simultaneous mode are prone to a hook effect.

## Heterogeneous Versus Homogeneous Immunochemical Assays

Immunochemical assays that require separation of the free label from the bound label are termed **heterogeneous immunoassays**. These assays use labeled antigen where the measurable property of the label is the same, whether it is bound to an antibody or not; thus, bound and free label must be physically separated to measure how much is bound to an antibody. **Homogeneous immunoassays** do not require separation because the measurable property of the label depends on whether it is bound to an antibody or not.

***Heterogeneous immunoassays.*** Heterogeneous immunoassays implicitly assume that $k_1 \gg k_{-1}$, and solid phase adsorption is widely used to separate the free, labeled (Ag:L) from the bound, labeled antigen (Ag:L:Ab).

Solid phase adsorption is the separation technique that currently is the most popular and widely used in both manual and automated heterogeneous immunoassays. In this technique, the binding and competition of labeled and unlabeled antigens for the binding sites of the antibody occur on the surface of a solid support onto which the capture antibody has been attached by physical adsorption or covalent bonding. Several different types of solid supports have been used, including the inner surface of plastic tubes or wells of microtiter plates, and the outer surface of insoluble materials such as cellulose or magnetic latex beads or particles. With tubes and microtiter plates, the solid surface containing the attached antibody and the bound antigen is washed "in place," and indicator reagents are subsequently added to complete the assay. When beads or particles are used, they are added directly to the reaction mixture and, after incubation, are removed by centrifugation or magnetic separation. After the supernatant has been removed by siphoning or decanting, the beads or particles are washed, and indicator reagents are subsequently added to complete the assay.

***Homogeneous immunoassays.*** Homogeneous immunoassays do not require separation of bound and free labeled antibody or antigen. In this type of assay, the activity of the label attached to the antigen is modulated directly by antibody binding. The magnitude of the modulation is proportional to the concentration of the antigen or antibody being measured. Consequently, it is necessary only to incubate the sample containing the analyte antigen with the labeled antigen and antibody and then directly measure the activity of the label "in place," making these assays technically easier and faster.

### POINTS TO REMEMBER

Important nonseparation (homogeneous) immunoassays include:
- Enzyme-multiplied immunoassay technique (EMIT)
- Cloned enzyme donor immunoassay (CEDIA)
- Luminescent oxygen channeling immunoassay (LOCI)
- Fluorescence resonance energy transfer (FRET)

Homogeneous immunoassays that use enzyme labels that are performed on spectrophotometric analyzers (see subsequent descriptions of the enzyme-multiplied immunoassay technique [EMIT] and the cloned enzyme donor immunoassay [CEDIA]) are in routine use for a range of small molecules. A homogeneous sandwich format chemiluminescent immunoassay has also been developed that expands the scope of homogeneous assays to large molecules (see subsequent description of the luminescent oxygen channeling immunoassay [LOCI]). In addition, a diverse range of homogeneous fluoroimmunoassays (FIAs) based on fluorescence resonance energy transfer (FRET) between fluorescent donor dye– and

fluorescent acceptor dye–labeled assay components represent a further expansion of the scope of homogeneous immunoassays (see subsequent descriptions of FRET).

### Immunoassay Calibration

Calibration of an immunoassay involves assaying a series of calibrators with known values and fitting a straight line or curve to the resulting data to determine the relationship between the measurable signal and the analyte concentration. This dose-response curve is then used to determine the concentration of analyte in the patients' samples. Joining successive points in a calibration curve is usually achieved by means of an appropriate mathematical equation. Several curve-fitting methods are in use. Interpolation methods join successive points by straight lines (linear interpolation) or curved lines (curvilinear interpolation). When the latter approach is used, a cubic polynomial ($y = a + bx + cx^2 + dx^3$) links the response ($y$) to the calibrator concentration ($x$), and the best fit is attained through a series of recalculations (iterations) that smooth the joints between the curves linking successive points on the curve. The resulting equation is called a *spline function*. Empirical curve-fitting methods use different mathematical models, including (1) hyperbolic, (2) polynomial, and (3) log-logit and its variants (e.g., four-parameter log-logistic), to calculate a curve to fit the calibration data.

It should be appreciated that a source of error with all curve-fitting methods is the uncertainty of the shape of the curve between successive calibrators and the imprecision in the measurement of each calibrator. Imprecision may not be constant over the concentration range represented by the calibrators, and in this case the response variable is termed *heteroscedastic*.

### Analytical and Functional Sensitivity

The analytical limits of detection of **competitive immunoassays** are determined principally by the affinity of the antibody. A lower limit of detection of 10 fmol/L (i.e., 600,000 molecules of analyte in a typical sample volume of 100 μL) is possible in a competitive assay when an antibody with an affinity of $10^{12}$ mol/L is used.

For noncompetitive immunoassays, the ability of the detector to measure the label determines the detection limit of an assay. A radioactive label, such as $^{125}$I, has low specific activity (7.5 million labels are necessary for detection of 1 disintegration/s) compared with enzyme labels and chemiluminescent and fluorescent labels. Enzyme labels provide an amplification (each enzyme label producing many detectable product molecules), and the detection limit for an enzyme is lowered if the conventional photometric detection is replaced with chemiluminescent or bioluminescent detection. The combination of amplification and an ultrasensitive detection reaction makes noncompetitive chemiluminescent EIAs among the most sensitive types of immunoassays. Fluorescent labels also have high specific activity; a single high–quantum-yield fluorophore is capable of producing 100 million photons/s. In practice, several factors degrade the detection limit of an immunoassay. These include (1) background signal from the detector, (2) assay reagents, and (3) nonspecific binding of the labeled reagent.

Secondary labels, such as biotin, are used to introduce amplification into an immunoassay. The binding constant of the biotin/avidin complex is extremely high ($10^{15}$ mol/L). This high binding allows for the design of immunoassay systems that are even more sensitive than simple antibody systems. Such a biotin/avidin system uses a biotin-labeled first antibody. Biotin is attached to the antibody in a relatively high proportion without loss of immunoreactivity of the antibody. When an avidin-conjugated label is added, a complex of Ag:Ab-biotin:avidin label is formed. Further amplification is achieved by a biotin:avidin:biotin linkage because the binding ratio of biotin:avidin is 4:1 (e.g., Ag:Ab-biotin:avidin:[3 biotin labels]). If the label is an enzyme, large numbers of enzyme molecules in the complete complex provide a large increase in enzymatic activity, coupled with the small amount of antigen being determined, and the antigen assay is correspondingly more sensitive.

Another type of sensitivity is termed "functional sensitivity." This is defined as the lowest concentration that can be measured in an assay with an interassay coefficient of variation of 20% (see also Chapter 2). This is used to establish a more realistic and robust detection limit for an assay used in patient care. Functional sensitivity is associated with the concept of assay generations, with each successive generation representing a one-log concentration improvement in sensitivity (e.g., for a thyroid-stimulating hormone [TSH] immunoassay, first generation 1 mIU/L, second generation 0.1 mIU/L, etc.).

## Examples of Labeled Immunoassays

Specific examples of different types of labeled immunoassays are discussed in the following section.

*Radioimmunoassay.* Radioimmunoassays (RIAs) use radioactive isotopes of iodine, $^{125}I$ and $^{131}I$, and tritium ($^3H$) as labels. In practice, competition between radiolabeled and unlabeled antigen or antibody in an antigen-antibody reaction is used to analytically determine the concentration of the unlabeled antigen or antibody. It takes advantage of the specificity of the antigen-antibody interaction and the ability to measure very low quantities of radioactive elements. RIAs have been used to determine the concentration of antibodies or any antigen against which a specific antibody is produced. When used to measure the concentration of an antigen, RIA requires that the antigen be available in a pure form and be labeled with a radioactive isotope. An alternative assay design uses labeled antibody (e.g., immunoradiometric assay [IRMA]) and does not require purified antigen because the antigen need not be labeled. This obviates potential problems that may be caused by iodination of labile antigens. Antibodies are more stable proteins and are easier to label without damage to the function of the protein.

Nonseparation RIAs have also been developed that are based on the modulation of a tritium or $^{125}I$ label by microparticles loaded with a scintillant. These scintillation proximity assays (SPAs) have found routine application in high-throughput screening assays for drug discovery.

Although they were once popular, the use of RIAs in clinical laboratories has declined primarily because of concerns over safe handling and disposal of radioactive reagents and waste.

*Enzyme immunoassay.* EIAs use the catalytic properties of enzymes to detect labeled antigens or antibodies, discriminate between bound and free label, and quantify immunological reactions. Alkaline phosphatase (ALP), horseradish peroxidase (HRP), glucose-6-phosphate dehydrogenase (G6PDH), and β-galactosidase labels predominate in EIA.

Various detection systems have been used to monitor and quantify EIAs. Assays that produce compounds that can be monitored photometrically are very popular because compact, high-performance photometers are available. However, EIAs that use fluorescent- or chemiluminescent-labeled substrates or products are often preferred to photometry-based assays, owing to the inherent sensitivity of fluorescent and chemiluminescent measurements. Immunoassays that incorporate HRP as a label can be assayed by chemiluminescence using a mixture of luminol, peroxide, and an enhancer such as *p*-iodophenol (Fig. 15.8A), or by using an acridan derivative. A very sensitive assay for ALP labels uses a chemiluminescent adamantyl 1,2-dioxetane aryl phosphate substrate (see Fig. 15.8B). The enzyme dephosphorylates the substrate, which decomposes with a concomitant long-lived glow of light (detection limit for ALP using this assay is 10 zeptomoles [$10^{-20}$ moles]).

Types of EIA include (1) enzyme-linked immunosorbent assay (ELISA), (2) EMIT, and (3) CEDIA.

**Enzyme-linked immunosorbent assay.** ELISA is a heterogeneous EIA technique. With this type of assay, one of the reaction components is attached to the surface of a solid phase, such as that of a microtiter well. This attachment

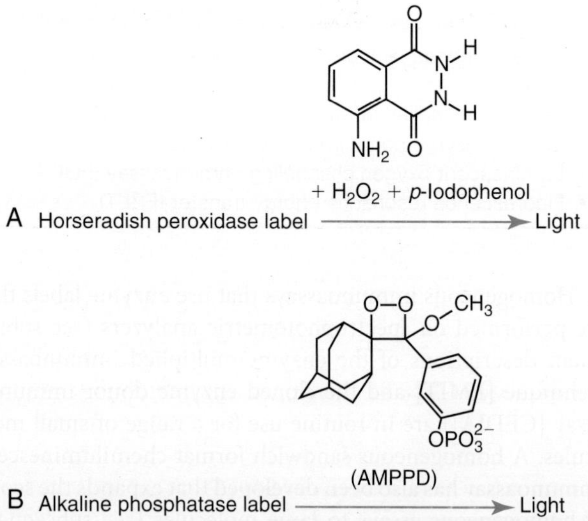

A  Horseradish peroxidase label  ⟶  Light

B  Alkaline phosphatase label  ⟶  Light

**Fig. 15.8** Ultrasensitive assays using horseradish peroxidase and alkaline phosphatase labels. (A) Chemiluminescent assay for horseradish peroxidase label using luminol. (B) Chemiluminescent assay for an alkaline phosphatase label using AMPPD (disodium 3-(4-methoxyspiro[1,2-dioxetane-3,2′-tricyclo[3.3.1.1]-decan]4-yl)phenyl phosphate).

may consist of nonspecific adsorption or chemical or immunochemical bonding and facilitates separation of bound and free labeled reactants. Typically with ELISA, an aliquot of sample or calibrator containing the antigen to be measured is added to and allowed to bind with a solid-phase antibody. After the solid phase has been washed, an enzyme-labeled antibody different from the bound antibody is added and forms a "sandwich complex" of solid phase–Ab:Ag:Ab enzyme. Excess (unbound) antibody then is washed away, and enzyme substrate is added. The enzyme label then catalyzes the conversion of substrate to product(s), the amount of which is proportional to the quantity of antigen in the sample. Antibodies in a sample also are quantified through the use of an ELISA procedure in which antigen instead of antibody is bound to a solid phase, and the second reagent is an enzyme-labeled antibody specific for the analyte antibody. For example, in a microtiter plate format, ELISA assays have been used extensively for detection of antibodies to viruses and parasites in serum or whole blood. In addition, enzyme conjugates coupled with substrates that produce visible products have been used to develop ELISA-type assays with results that are interpreted visually.

**Enzyme-multiplied immunoassay technique.** EMIT is a homogeneous EIA that is very widely used in clinical analyses, an illustration of this is shown in Fig. 15.9. Because EMIT does not require a separation step, it is simple to perform and has been used to develop a wide variety of small molecule (drug, hormone, or metabolite) assays. Because of their operational simplicity, EMIT-type assays are easily automated and are included in the repertoire of many automated clinical and immunoassay analyzers. In this technique, the patient's sample is incubated with (1) an enzyme conjugated to the antigen (drug, hormone, or metabolite), (2) antibody against the antigen, and (3) the enzyme substrate. Antigen in the patient's sample competes with the enzyme-conjugated antigen for the antibody. Binding of the antibody to the enzyme-antigen conjugate affects enzyme activity by physically blocking access of the substrate to the active site of the enzyme or by changing the conformation of the enzyme molecule and thus altering its activity. The relative change in enzyme activity resulting from the formation of the antigen-antibody complex is proportional to the antigen concentration in the patient's sample. The concentration of the antigen is calculated from a calibration curve prepared by analyzing calibrators that contain known quantities of the antigen in question.

**Cloned enzyme donor immunoassay.** As shown in Fig. 15.9, CEDIA is a homogeneous EIA; it was the first EIA designed and developed through the use of genetic engineering techniques. Two inactive fragments (the enzyme "donor" and "acceptor") of β-galactosidase are prepared by manipulation of the Z gene of the *lac* operon of *Escherichia coli*. These two fragments spontaneously reassemble to form active enzyme even if the enzyme donor is attached to an antigen. However, binding of antibody to the enzyme donor–antigen conjugate inhibits reassembly, and no active enzyme is formed. Thus, competition between the antigen and the enzyme donor–antigen conjugate for a fixed amount of antibody in the presence of the enzyme acceptor modulates the measured enzyme activity. High concentrations of the antigen result in the greatest enzyme activity; low concentrations result in the least enzyme activity.

*Fluoroimmunoassay.* Fluoroimmunoassay (FIA) uses a fluorescent molecule as an indicator label to detect and quantify immunologic reactions. Examples of fluorophores used as labels in FIA and their properties are listed in Table 15.2. An early problem with FIA was that background fluorescence from within the sample limited its utility. This problem has been overcome by the use of time-resolved immunoassay techniques that use chelates of rare earth (lanthanide) elements as labels (see Chapter 9). These techniques are based on the fact that fluorescent emissions from lanthanide chelates such as (1) europium, (2) terbium, and (3) samarium have long lives (>1 μs) compared with the typical background fluorescence encountered in biologic specimens. In a time-resolved FIA, a europium chelate label is excited by a pulse of excitation light (0.5 μs), and the long-lived fluorescence emission from the label is measured after a delay (400 to 800 μs). The measurement after the delay ensures that any short-lived background signal has decayed.

Fluorescence polarization immunoassay (FPIA) is a type of homogeneous FIA that is widely used to measure drugs and other small molecules (Fig. 15.10). The polarization of the fluorescence from a fluorescein-antigen conjugate is determined by its rate of rotation during the lifetime of the excited state in solution. When the fluorescein-antigen conjugate is bound to the large antibody molecule, the fluorophore is constrained from rotating in the time between absorption of the incident radiation and emission of fluorescence; hence, the fluorescence emission is still highly polarized. In contrast, when the fluorescein-antigen conjugate is free in solution, it can rotate more rapidly and the emitted light is depolarized.

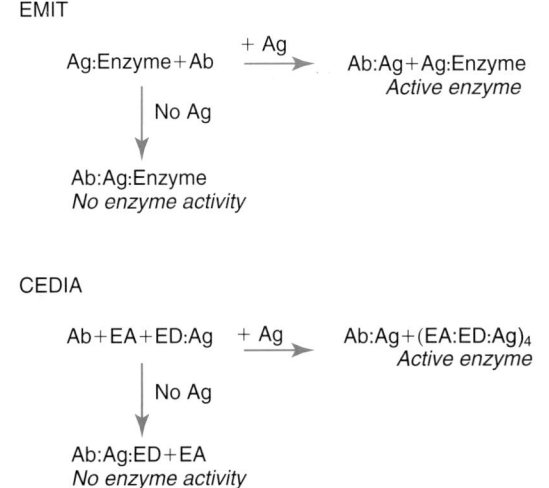

Fig. 15.9 Enzyme-multiplied immunoassay technique *(EMIT)* and cloned enzyme donor homogeneous immunoassay *(CEDIA)*. *Ab,* Antibody; *Ag,* antigen; *EA,* enzyme acceptor; *EA:Ag,* antigen labeled enzyme acceptor; *(EA:ED:Ag)₄,* enzymatically active tetrameric β-galactosidase; *ED,* enzyme donor.

## TABLE 15.2   Properties of Fluorescent Labels

| Fluorophore | Excitation (nm) | Emission (nm) | Fluorescence Quantum Yield[a] | Lifetime (ns) |
|---|---|---|---|---|
| Cy3 (cyanine dye) | 550 | 570 | 0.15 | — |
| Cy5 (cyanine dye) | 650 | 670 | 0.28 | — |
| Europium (β-naphthoyl trifluoroacetone) | 340 | 590,613 | — | 500,000 |
| Fluorescein isothiocyanate | 492 | 520 | 0.0–0.85 | 4.5 |
| NN382 | 778 | 806 | 0.59 | — |
| Phycobiliprotein | 550–620 | 580–660 | 0.5–0.98 | — |
| Rhodamine B isothiocyanate | 550 | 585 | 0.0–0.7 | 3.0 |
| Umbelliferone | 380 | 450 | — | — |

[a]Fluorescence quantum yield: fraction of molecules that emit a photon.

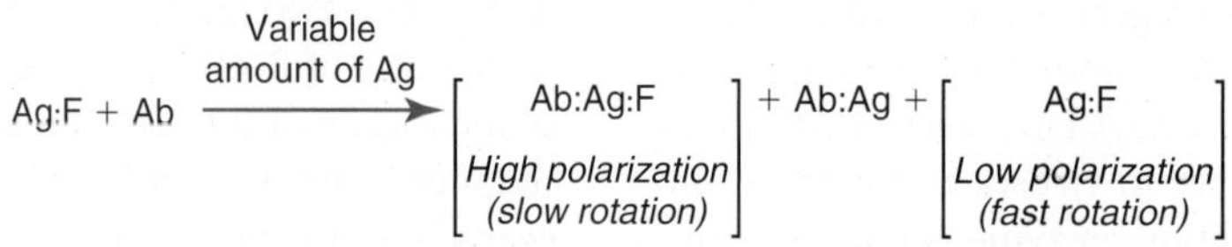

Fig. 15.10 Homogeneous polarization fluoroimmunoassay. *Ab,* Antibody; *Ag,* antigen; *F,* fluorescein.

Thus, binding to antibody modulates polarization, and a homogeneous assay is possible.

Förster or FRET is the distance-dependent transfer of energy from a fluorescent donor dye to a fluorescent acceptor dye. Distances at which there is 50% transfer efficiency are typically 1 to 20 nm, and up to approximately 20 nm is possible for some donor-acceptor pairs (e.g., lanthanide chelates and quantum dots). In, for example, a sandwich FRET immunoassay format used in the time-resolved amplified cryptate emission (TRACE) assay, an antibody labeled with a europium chelate (donor) is matched with an antibody labeled with an allophycocyanin dye (XL665; acceptor). The two antibodies form a sandwich immunocomplex with the antigen, and following irradiation with a pulsed excitation light (337 nm), energy transfer occurs from the donor europium chelate to the XL665 acceptor. In the absence of immunocomplex formation, the XL665 fluorescence is short-lived (nanoseconds). However, with immunocomplex formation, the europium chelate on the first antibody provides sustained energy to excite and prolong the normally short-lived fluorescence of the XL665 dye on the second antibody (microseconds). Intensity of the 665-nm emission is proportional to antigen concentration. Another strategy used in a system for cardiac markers uses an antibody-coated latex particle containing a donor dye (a silicon phthalocyanine derivative) and a second antibody–coated latex particle containing an acceptor dye (a different silicon phthalocyanine dye). Analyte in the sample binds to create donor particle:analyte:acceptor particle complexes. Excitation at 670 nm excites the donor dye, and energy transfer to the acceptor dye occurs due to the proximity of the two differently dyed particles. The acceptor particle then emits light at 760 nm (long wavelength in the red portion of the spectrum). An advantage of this red emission is that scattering and fluorescence from blood plasma are minimized.

***Phosphor immunoassay.*** Phosphor is a material that emits light (phosphorescence) over a relatively long time scale following exposure to excitation energy. A particular type of phosphor, an upconverting phosphor nanoparticle, can be used as a label in immunoassays (e.g., to label an antibody in a sandwich immunoassay). In one application, the upconverting phosphor nanoparticle (200- to 400-nm diameter) can be a crystalline lanthanide oxysulfide. This nanoparticle absorbs two or more photons of infrared light (980 nm) and produces light emission at a shorter wavelength (anti-Stokes shift). The phosphorescence is not influenced by reaction conditions (e.g., temperature, buffer), and no upconverted signal is obtained from biologic components in the sample (low background). Multiplexing is possible because different types of particles produce different wavelengths of phosphorescence (e.g., yttrium/erbium oxysulfide particles are green [550 nm], yttrium/thulium oxysulfide particles are blue [475 nm]).

***Chemiluminescent immunoassay.*** Chemiluminescence is the name given to light emission produced during a chemical reaction. Isoluminol and acridinium esters are important examples of chemiluminescent labels used in chemiluminescent immunoassays. Oxidation of isoluminol by hydrogen peroxide in the presence of a catalyst, such as microperoxidase, produces a relatively long-lived light emission at 425 nm, and oxidation of an acridinium ester by alkaline hydrogen peroxide in the presence of a detergent (e.g., Triton X-100) produces a rapid flash of light at 429 nm. Acridinium and sulfonyl acridinium esters are high specific activity labels (detection limit for the label is 800 zeptomoles) that can be used to label both antibodies and haptens (Fig. 15.11A).

LOCI is a particularly important type of chemiluminescent immunoassay. It is one of the few homogeneous immunoassays that operate in a noncompetitive ("sandwich") format and can be used to assay large molecules. LOCI uses two reagent particles (sensitizer and chemiluminescent

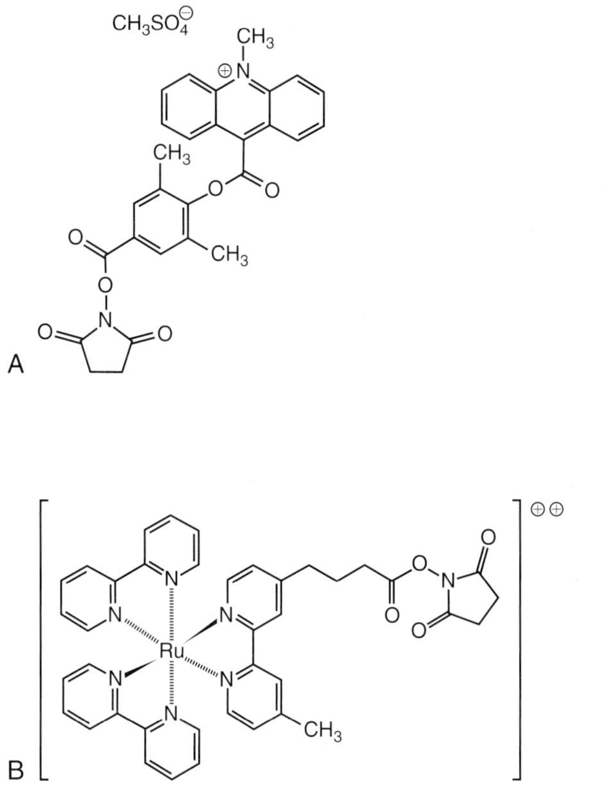

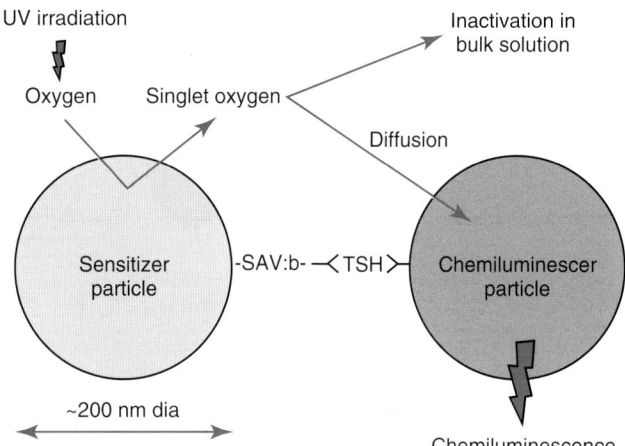

Fig. 15.12 Example of luminescent oxygen channeling immunoassay for thyroid-stimulating hormone *(TSH)*. In this assay, TSH links two latex microbeads—one containing a photosensitive reagent and the other, a precursor of a chemiluminescent reagent. *b*, Biotin; *SAV*, streptavidin; *UV*, ultraviolet.

**Fig. 15.11** Luminescent labels. (A) Chemiluminescent acridinium ester label. (B) Electrochemiluminescent ruthenium (II) tris(bipyridyl) NHS (*N*-hydroxysuccinimide) ester label. (A, From Law S-J, Miller T, Piran U, et al. Novel poly-substituted aryl acridinium esters and their use in immunoassay. *J Biolumin Chemilumin*. 1989;4:88–98.)

particles) that form a complex with the analyte of interest. The presence of analyte links the two reagent latex particles in close proximity. The first particle contains a photosensitizer (e.g., phthalocyanine) and, in the presence of light, converts oxygen to singlet oxygen. The second chemiluminescent particle contains a chemiluminescent agent (e.g., olefin) that reacts with singlet oxygen to form a dioxetane that decomposes and emits light. This reaction occurs only if the two particles are in close proximity and the singlet oxygen can diffuse efficiently from the sensitizer particle to the chemiluminescent particle. Singlet oxygen does not react with unbound chemiluminescent particles because of the short lifetime of this transient species in an aqueous environment. An example of a LOCI assay for TSH is illustrated in Fig. 15.12. TSH binds to a biotinylated anti-TSH antibody, and this complex links the streptavidin-coated sensitizer particle to the anti-TSH antibody–coated chemiluminescer particle. Exposure to light results in emission of singlet oxygen from the photosensitive particle. The singlet oxygen activates the chemiluminescent particle to emit light that is then measured.

*Electrochemiluminescence immunoassay.* Ruthenium (II) tris(bipyridyl) (see Fig. 15.11B) undergoes an electrochemiluminescent reaction (620 nm) with tripropylamine at an electrode surface, and this chelate is now used as a label in competitive and sandwich electrochemiluminescence

immunoassays. Using this label, various assays have been developed with magnetic beads as the solid phase. Beads are captured by a magnet at an electrode surface in a flow cell, and unbound label is washed out of the cell by a wash buffer. Label bound to the bead undergoes an electrochemiluminescent reaction, and the light emission is measured by an adjacent photomultiplier tube.

**Particle immunoassay.** Various micro- and nano-sized particles can be used as labels. For example, dyed-latex particles and gold sols are visible to the naked eye and have found wide application in simplified immunoassays based on the lateral flow principle (see Chapter 17). A magnetic particle, detected via its reflective and light scattering properties, is used in an optogenetic sandwich immunoassay. Magnetic nanoparticles coated with detection antibody bind to captured antigens and are detected using frustrated total internal reflection. An advantage of this assay format is speed (external fields are used to manipulate the magnetic particles), and it has been applied to a fast turnaround intraoperative parathyroid hormone assay.

Nuclear magnetic resonance detection of magnetic particle labels facilitates a homogeneous immunoassay design. The assay uses magnetic nanoparticles (~20-nm diameter) coated with antibody that binds to and clusters around analyte in solution. A consequence of the binding and clustering is that the microscopic environment of water in the reaction mixture is altered, and this can be detected by nuclear magnetic resonance as a change in the T2 relaxation signal (Fig. 15.13). An advantage of this type of immunoassay is that the signal is unaffected by the sample matrix (e.g., opacity), and this allows direct detection in various types of specimens (e.g., whole blood and sputum).

**Immuno-polymerase chain reaction and bio-barcode immunoassay.** DNA has been used in a number of different immunoassay designs. Immuno-PCR is a heterogeneous immunoassay in which a piece of single- or double-stranded DNA is used as a label for an antibody in a sandwich assay. Bound DNA label is amplified using the polymerase chain

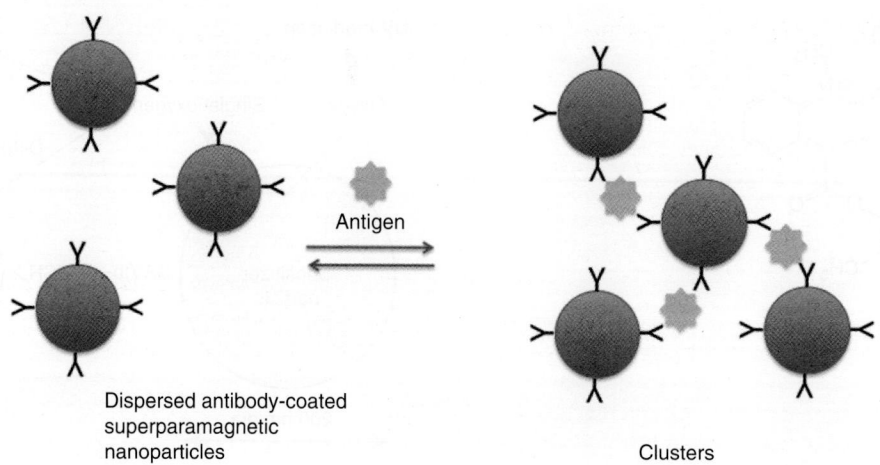

**Fig. 15.13** Magnetic particle immunoassay. Antigen binds to magnetic nanoparticles (~20-nm diameter) coated with antibody. The binding and resulting clustering of the particles alters the microscopic environment of water in the reaction mixture, and this can be detected by nuclear magnetic resonance (change in the T2 relaxation signal).

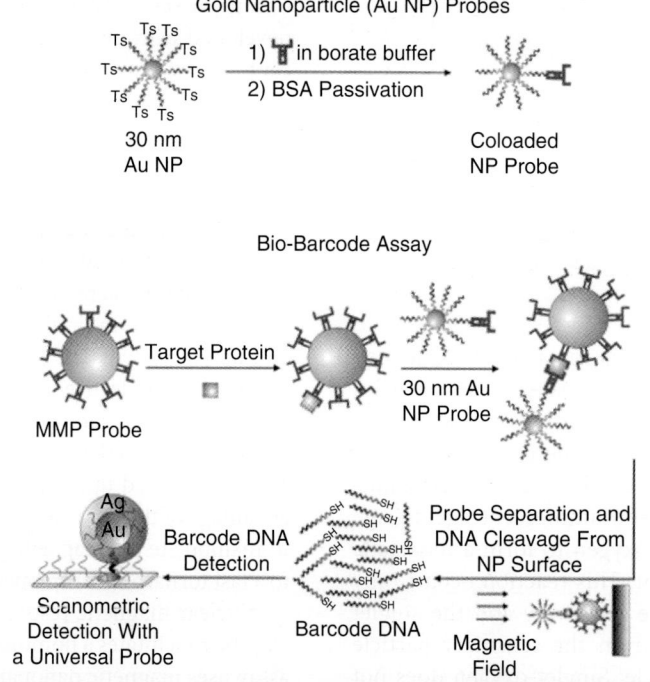

**Fig. 15.14** Bio-barcode assay for a protein target. Barcode DNA–functionalized gold nanoparticles *(Au NP)* (30-nm diameter) are conjugated to target protein–specific antibodies (via tosyl *[Ts]* groups) to generate the coloaded target protein Au NP probes that are then passivated with bovine serum albumin *(BSA)*. The next steps in the sandwich immunoassay are reaction of the target protein with 1-μm magnetic microparticle probes *(MMPs)* coated with monoclonal antibodies to target protein, washing to remove excess serum components, and then reaction with the Au-NP. After magnetic separation and wash steps, the target protein–specific DNA barcodes are released into solution (thiolated *[SH]* barcode DNA) and detected using the scanometric assay (includes an Au-NP–catalyzed silver enhancement step). Approximately one-half of the barcode DNA sequence is complementary to the "universal" scanometric Au NP probe DNA, and the other half is complementary to a surface immobilized DNA sequence that is responsible for sorting and binding barcodes complementary to the target protein barcode sequence. (From Thaxton CS, Elghanian R, Thomas AD, et al. Nanoparticle-based bio-barcode assay redefines "undetectable" PSA and biochemical recurrence after radical prostatectomy. *Proc Natl Acad Sci U S A.* 2009;106:18437–18442, with permission.)

reaction (PCR). The amplified DNA product is separated by gel electrophoresis and quantitated by densitometric scanning of an ethidium-stained gel.

In a bio-barcode assay, capture antibody immobilized on a magnetic particle binds to the analyte (e.g., a protein) and the bound analyte is reacted with a gold particle (30-nm diameter) decorated with detection antibody and barcode dsDNA (Fig. 15.14; refer to the figure legend for details). Following complex formation and washing, one strand of the barcode dsDNA is released from the gold particle. Next, the released barcode dsDNA is hybridized to an immobilized capture DNA probe and to a gold particle-labeled detection probe. The bound gold particle–labeled detection probe is first decorated with silver and then detected scanometrically. This type of assay has achieved very low detection limits (e.g., pg/mL range for serum prostate-specific antigen).

**Multiplexed immunoassays and protein microarrays.** Multiplexed immunoassays, in which two or more analytes are detected/measured in a single assay, improve the efficiency of detecting/measuring multiple analytes. Two important strategies are based on discrete reaction zones on a planar surface (microarray) and on optically coded microspheres ("liquid array").

Arrays of hundreds or thousands of micrometer-sized dots of antigens or antibodies immobilized on the surface of a glass or plastic chip are emerging as an important tool in proteomic studies and in assessing protein-protein interactions. This format facilitates simultaneous multianalyte immunoassays using (e.g., fluorophore-labeled conjugates). The arrays are made by printing or spotting 1-nL drops of protein solutions onto a flat surface, such as a glass microscope slide. In a typical sandwich assay, the array on the surface of the slide is incubated first with sample and then with conjugate. The fluorescence of the bound conjugate is detected using a scanning device. The pattern of the signal provides information on the presence and amount of individual analytes in the sample or the reactivity of a single analyte with the range of proteins arrayed on the surface of the slide.

Another type of microarray, the so-called liquid array, is based on collections of microbeads optically coded with fluorescent dyes. Each type of fluorescent bead is coated with a different antibody, and following the immunologic reaction with sample and labeled antibody, the formation of an immunocomplex on each bead is assessed using flow cytometric or fluorescence imaging principles. Up to 500 different signatures can be created, allowing multiplexing of up to 500 different assays in a single assay vessel.

**Digital immunoassay.** A long-cherished goal in immunoassay has been single-molecule sensitivity. A new digital immunoassay design has led to dramatic improvements in sensitivity (Fig. 15.15). This ELISA type of assay is performed on small antibody-coated paramagnetic microbeads. At the end of the incubation of the capture antibody–coated beads with sample and β-galactosidase labeled antibody, the beads, in the presence of a fluorogenic substrate, are distributed into an array of 216,000 wells (one bead per well), each with a volume of 40 fL. A single target molecule captured onto the bead in an fL-sized well generates sufficient fluorescence signal for detection. The signal from the array of wells is imaged using a charge-coupled device (CCD) camera, and the number of fluorescent wells is counted (a digital read-out), thus counting the number of molecules in the sample. At the 10:1 bead-to-molecule ratio used in the assay, the number of beads that carry a labeled immunocomplex follows a Poisson distribution, such that at low protein concentrations each bead will capture one labeled immunocomplex or none. The combination of the sensitive label detection method and the low background achieved by the signal counting leads to protein assays with fg/mL sensitivity.

FIA can also be operated in a digital mode by combining a magnetic microparticle-based sandwich FIA and single-molecule counting technology. It integrates capillary flow, laser-induced fluorescence, and a highly sensitive detection optics module for sample analysis. Upon completion of sandwich formation, the fluorescent dye–labeled detection antibody is released from the captured antigen and is eluted into a very small volume (20 μL) for counting. Fluorescence

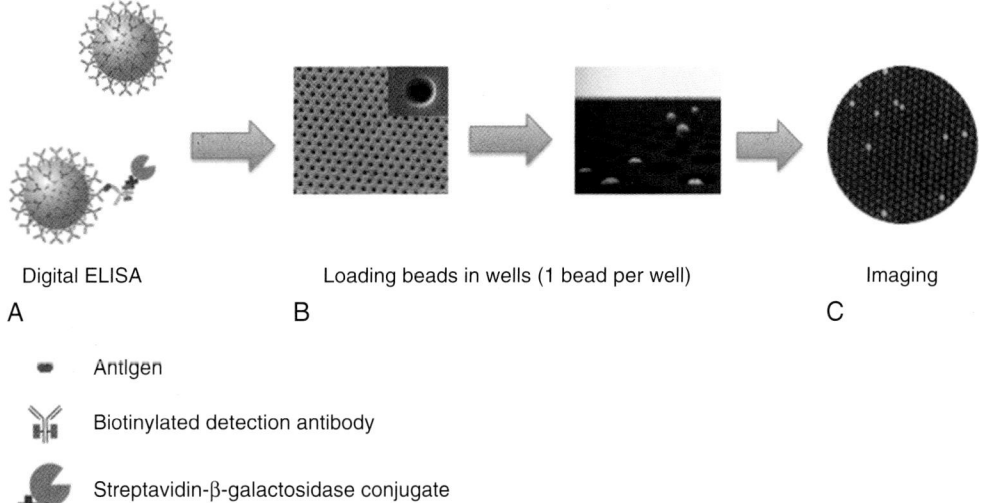

Digital ELISA          Loading beads in wells (1 bead per well)          Imaging

A                      B                                                 C

⬤ Antigen

Ⲩ Biotinylated detection antibody

⬤ Streptavidin-β-galactosidase conjugate

**Fig. 15.15** Design of a digital immunoassay (Simoa). (A) Reaction of the antigen with capture antibody–coated magnetic beads and biotinylated detection antibody. This is then followed by reaction of the bound complex with streptavidin–β-galactosidase conjugate to form single immunocomplexes of the magnetic beads. (B) The beads are loaded into wells, one bead per well, and then treated with a fluorometric substrate for β-galactosidase. (C) Fluorescence from the beads in the array detected by imaging. *ELISA*, Enzyme-linked immunosorbent assay. (Images used with permission of Quanterix Corporation.)

detection occurs in a flow system in a very small interrogation space (5 μm) that is illuminated by a laser. Signals above the background are counted as digital events, and the sum of the digital events is related to the original concentration of the analyte in the sample.

*Interferences.* Immunologic assays are prone to interferences, in spite of the use of highly specific antibodies for molecular recognition of the analyte. Falsely low results can occur because of the hook effect at high antigen concentrations (see earlier discussion). False-negative or false-positive results are encountered if the sample contains anti–animal Ig antibodies. For example, in a two-site sandwich assay for human chorionic gonadotropin (hCG) based on mouse antibodies, any human anti-mouse antibodies (HAMAs) present in the specimen will recognize the immobilized mouse capture and mouse conjugate antibodies and will form a complex that is indistinguishable from an immobilized capture antibody:hCG:conjugate complex. This leads to a false-positive result. A false-negative result will be obtained if the HAMAs react with the capture antibody or the conjugate to such an extent that specific antibody binding to hCG is prevented. Many different types of circulating anti–animal Ig antibodies have been detected (e.g., human anti-goat, human anti-bovine antibodies) and shown to interfere in immunoassays. In practice, this

type of interference is minimized by including additives in the immunoassay reagents such as nonimmune serum or IgG from the species used to raise the antibodies used in the assay. In practice, this type of interference can sometimes be uncovered by performing dilution studies (nonlinear response) or from changes in values following incubation of the sample in a heterophile blocking tube.

## CELL-BASED AND TISSUE-BASED IMMUNOCHEMICAL TECHNIQUES

Other analytical methods of clinical interest that use antibodies include immunocytochemistry and agglutination assays. In immunocytochemical assays, labeled (e.g., HRP) antibody reagents are used as specific probes for protein and peptide antigens to evaluate single cells or pieces of tissue for their synthetic capability and/or phenotypic identity. In an agglutination method, the visible clumping of particulates, such as cells and latex particles, is used as an indicator of the primary reaction of antigen and antibody.

Hemagglutination, agglutination reactions in which the antigen is located on an erythrocyte, is used in the direct testing of erythrocytes for blood group, Rh, and other antigenic types.

## REVIEW QUESTIONS

1. What does a strong signal in a microtiter well–based competitive enzyme immunoassay (EIA) for thyroxine signify?
   a. A low concentration of thyroxine in the sample
   b. A high concentration of thyroxine in the sample
   c. Enzyme substrate not added to the well
   d. Enzyme inhibitor present in the sample
   e. Bound antibody has detached from the surface of the well

2. What does a very weak signal in a microtiter well–based sandwich EIA for thyroid-stimulating hormone (TSH) signify?
   a. A low concentration of TSH in the sample
   b. A high concentration of TSH in the sample
   c. A hook effect
   d. Effective competition between the conjugate and the TSH for capture antibody
   e. Capture antibody saturated with TSH:conjugate complexes

3. The energy of interaction of a single antibody-combining site and its corresponding epitope on the antigen is referred to as:
   a. sensitivity.
   b. specificity.
   c. immunogenicity.
   d. affinity.

4. Which one of the following immunochemical assays requires separation of the free label from the bound labeled substance?
   a. Enzyme-multiplied immunoassay technique (EMIT)
   b. Enzyme-linked immunosorbent assay (ELISA)

   c. Cloned enzyme donor immunoassay (CEDIA)
   d. Luminescent oxygen channeling immunoassay (LOCI)
   e. Fluorescence polarization immunoassay (FPIA)

5. The addition of a linear polymer such as polyethylene glycol to a mixture of antigen and antibody causes_____ in the rate of immune complex formation and precipitation.
   a. a decrease
   b. an increase
   c. no change

6. Transferring electrophoretically separated proteins into a strip of nylon membrane by electroblotting is the second step in:
   a. radial immunodiffusion.
   b. enzyme-linked immunosorbent assay.
   c. Western blotting.
   d. immunofixation.
   e. crossed immunoelectrophoresis.

7. In a two-site antibody-based sandwich immunoassay, the presence of human anti-mouse antibodies produces a false-negative result by:
   a. binding a mouse immunoglobulin capture antibody and the mouse immunoglobulin conjugate to form a bridge.
   b. mimicking the specific analyte being assessed.
   c. binding to the mouse monoclonal capture antibody reagents.
   d. reacting with one of the assay reagents to prevent formation of the sandwich.

8. Which one of the following immunoassay procedures does not involve the coating of a solid phase with antibody or antigen?
   a. Enzyme-multiplied immunoassay technique (EMIT)
   b. Luminescent oxygen channeling immunoassay (LOCI)
   c. Enzyme-linked immunosorbent assay (ELISA)
   d. Particle-enhanced turbidimetric inhibition immunoassay (PETINIA)
   e. Bio-barcode immunoassay

9. The immunoglobulin most often used in immunochemical assays is:
   a. IgG.
   b. IgA.
   c. IgM.
   d. IgE.

10. Which one of the following statements is false?
    a. Dyed-latex microparticles are effective labels in simplified immunoassays because they are visible to the naked eye.
    b. Binding of an antigen to an antibody involves van der Waals–London dipole-dipole interaction.
    c. Addition of polymers to an antigen-antibody reaction increases the rate of immune complex growth.
    d. The functional sensitivity of an immunoassay is the lowest concentration that can be measured with a within-assay coefficient of variation of 20%.
    e. Fluorescence resonance energy transfer from donor to acceptor dye is distance dependent.

## SUGGESTED READINGS

Blackburn GF, Shah HP, Kenten JH, et al. Electrochemiluminescence detection for development of immunoassays and DNA probe assays for clinical diagnostics. *Clin Chem*. 1991;37:1534–1539.

Kricka LJ. Chemiluminescent and bioluminescent techniques. *Clin Chem*. 1991;37:1472–1481.

Luo ZX, Fox L, Cummings M, et al. New frontiers in in vitro medical diagnostics by low field T2 magnetic resonance relaxometry. *TrAC Trends Anal Chem*. 2016;83:94–102.

Omi K, Ando T, Sakyu T, et al. Noncompetitive immunoassay detection system for haptens on the basis of antimetatype antibodies. *Clin Chem*. 2015;61:627–635.

Rissin DM, Fournier DR, Piech T, et al. Simultaneous detection of single molecules and singulated ensembles of molecules enables immunoassays with broad dynamic range. *Anal Chem*. 2011;83:2279–2285.

Templin MF, Stoll D, Schrenk M, et al. Protein microarray technology. *Trends Biotechnol*. 2002;20:160–166.

Todd J, Freese B, Lu A, et al. Ultrasensitive flow-based immunoassays using single-molecule counting. *Clin Chem*. 2007;53:1990–1995.

Turgeon ML. *Immunology and Serology in Laboratory Medicine*. 5th ed. St Louis: Elsevier; 2014.

Wild D, ed. *The Immunoassay Handbook*. 4th ed. Amsterdam: Elsevier; 2013.

# Automation in the Clinical Laboratory

*Jonathan R. Genzen and Carl T. Wittwer\**

## OBJECTIVES

1. List four benefits of using automation in the clinical laboratory.
2. State four advantages of using barcoded labels to identify specimens.
3. List and describe the considerations that must be evaluated when an automated laboratory system is selected.
4. List the advantages and potential problems encountered when automated laboratory processes are used and integrated for:
   - Specimen identification
   - Specimen delivery
   - Reagent identification
   - Chemical reaction phases
5. Compare the following analyzer configurations with regard to specimen and reagent handling and processing:
   - Random-access
   - Continuous flow
   - Sequential
   - Multiple-channel
   - Discrete
   - Single-channel
6. Compare an "open" versus a "closed" automated analyzer with regard to reagent usage.
7. Describe how automation has been applied to the polymerase chain reaction (PCR) and deoxyribonucleic acid (DNA) sequencing.
8. Describe the trade-offs between automating complex processes and developing simpler processes that do not require automation.

## KEY WORDS AND DEFINITIONS

**Automation** The process whereby an analytical instrument performs many tests with only minimal involvement of an analyst; also defined as the controlled operation of an apparatus, process, or system by mechanical or electronic devices without human intervention.

**Batch analysis** Type of analysis in which multiple specimens are grouped in the same analytical session.

**Carryover** The transport of a quantity of analyte or reagent from one specimen reaction into and contaminating a subsequent one.

**Continuous-flow analysis** Type of analysis in which each specimen in a batch passes through the same continuous stream at the same rate and is subjected to the same analytical reactions.

**Molecular diagnostics** Using the presence, quantity, or sequence of DNA or RNA to identify the nature of an illness.

**Multiple-channel analysis** Type of analysis in which each specimen is subjected to multiple analytical processes so that a set of test results is obtained on a single specimen; similar to random-access analysis.

**Polymerase chain reaction (PCR)** A molecular biology method to amplify a segment of DNA by repeated temperature cycles for primer annealing, polymerase extension, and product denaturation.

**Random-access analysis** The most common configuration of an automated analyzer, in which analyses are performed on a collection of specimens sequentially and each specimen is analyzed for a different selection of tests.

**Real-time PCR** A variant of PCR where fluorescence is measured during amplification, allowing quantification of the initial template.

**Sequential analysis** Type of analysis in which each specimen in a batch enters the analytical process one after another, and each result or set of results emerges in the same order as the specimens are entered.

**Single-channel analysis** Type of analysis in which each specimen is subjected to a single process so that only results for a single analyte are produced; similar to batch analysis.

**Throughput** The number of specimens processed by an analyzer during a given period of time, or the rate at which an analytical system processes specimens.

**Workstation** An area in the clinical laboratory dedicated to a defined task and containing appropriate laboratory instrumentation to carry out that task.

\*The authors would like to acknowledge the original contributions of Ernest Maclin, PE; Donald S. Young, MB, PhD; James C. Boyd, MD; and Charles D. Hawker, PhD, upon which portions of this chapter are based.

The term automation in clinical chemistry describes the process whereby an analytical instrument performs many tests with only minimal involvement of an analyst. However, the term also applies to the automation of nonanalytical processes (preanalytical and postanalytical) that have become very important to the performance of laboratories over the past two decades. This chapter covers both nonanalytical and analytical automation in clinical laboratories.

The availability of automation systems and automated instruments enables laboratories to process larger workloads without comparable increases in staff. The evolution of automation in clinical laboratories has paralleled that in the manufacturing industry, progressing from fixed automation, whereby an instrument performs a single repetitive task by itself, to programmable automation, which allows one instrument to perform a variety of different tasks. Intelligent automation further allows individual instruments or systems to self-monitor and respond appropriately to changing conditions.

One benefit of automation is a reduction in the variability of results and errors of analysis through the elimination of tasks that are repetitive and monotonous for most individuals. Better reproducibility gained by automation, in turn, improves the quality of laboratory tests.

Small laboratories may consolidate into larger, more efficient entities in response to market trends involving cost reduction. The drive to automate these mega-laboratories has led to new avenues in laboratory automation. No longer is automation simply used to assist the medical laboratory scientist in test performance; it now includes (1) processing and transport of specimens, (2) loading of specimens into automated analyzers, (3) assessment of the results of the tests performed, and (4) storage of specimens. Automation is crucial to the future prosperity of clinical laboratories of all sizes.

# NONANALYTICAL AUTOMATION FOR THE CLINICAL LABORATORY

Integrating and automating pre- and post-analytical activities has rapidly progressed in the clinical laboratory. Preanalytical automated systems range from robotics that perform a single function such as aliquoting or sorting (also called *task-targeted automation systems*) to more complex workstations that perform several preanalytical functions. Several options are also available as modules in total laboratory automation (TLA) systems, which are discussed later in this section.

Preanalytical automation begins with automation of operations in the specimen processing area where specimens are (1) identified, (2) labeled, (3) scheduled for analysis, (4) centrifuged, and (5) sorted. After this initial processing, specimens are transported to appropriate workstations in the laboratory, either manually or using conveyors, where they can then be analyzed with minimal or no human intervention. Rules-based expert system software (1) assists with the review of laboratory results by automatically releasing results that have no associated problems and (2) identifies any problematic results to bring to the attention of trained medical laboratory scientists. All specimens are catalogued after analysis and stored in a central storage facility, which may include automated storage and retrieval functions. The following sections describe various aspects of nonanalytical process automation.

## Specimen Identification

Typically, the identifying link (identifier) between the patient and specimen is created at the patient's bedside. Maintenance of this connection throughout (1) transport of the specimen to the laboratory, (2) subsequent specimen analysis, and (3) preparation of a report, is essential. Several technologies are available for automatic identification and data collection (Box 16.1). Automatic identification typically detects a unique characteristic or unique data string associated with a physical object. For example, identifiers such as (1) serial number, (2) part number, (3) color, (4) manufacturer, (5) patient name, (6) medical record number, and (7) accession number have been used to identify an object or patient through the use of electronic data processing. In the clinical laboratory, labeling with a barcode has become the technology of choice for automatic identification.

### Labeling

In many laboratory information systems (LIS), electronic entry of a test order in the laboratory or at a nursing station for a uniquely identified patient generates a specimen label bearing a unique laboratory accession number. A record is established that remains incomplete until a result (or a set of results) is entered into the computer against the accession number. The unique label is affixed to the specimen collection container when the specimen is obtained and the patient is properly identified. This may be at the bedside using preprinted labels carried from the laboratory or using a portable label printer connected wirelessly through the network to the laboratory computer. Many companies now provide these portable barcode labeling systems, and many hospitals are now using them. Proper alignment of the label on a specimen tube can be critical for correct processing of barcoded labels, although newer imaging systems can be more tolerant. The Clinical and Laboratory Standards Institute (CLSI) published a standard in 2011 (*Specimen Labels: Content and Location,*

---

**BOX 16.1 Technologies Used for Automatic Identification and Data Collection**

Barcoding
Optical character recognition
Magnetic stripe and magnetic ink character recognition
Voice identification
Radiofrequency identification
Touch screens
Light pens
Hand print tablets
Optical mark readers
Smart cards

*Fonts, and Label Orientation*) that was intended to standardize specimen labels in clinical laboratories to reduce errors such as patient misidentification. The focus of this standard was not the barcode itself, but rather the human-readable content of the label, particularly the location and appearance of the patient name.

An electronic or paper requisition form typically initiates specimen acquisition. Labels to identify the patient and the date and time of collection are typically applied to specimen containers and tubes at the time of collection. Many systems also assign a laboratory accession number at this time. Alternatively, accession numbers may be assigned upon arrival of the sample in the laboratory during a log-in procedure that includes date, time, and condition of the specimen.

After receipt by the laboratory, specimens undergo various technical handling processes. Some automated analyzers sample directly from the original collection tube, simultaneously reading the accession number from the barcode label on the tube; other analyzers require an aliquot of the serum or plasma from the original tube. When physical removal of serum or plasma from the original tube is required, secondary labels bearing essential information from the original label must be affixed to any secondary tubes. Secondary barcode labels, if necessary, may be generated at the time of accessioning or at the time the aliquots are prepared. This aliquoting step may be automated.

## Barcoding

A major advance in the automation of specimen identification in clinical laboratories is the incorporation of barcoding technology into analytical systems. A barcoding system consists of a barcode printer and a barcode reader, or scanner. In clinical laboratories, one-dimensional or linear barcode systems have historically been used. CLSI published a standard (AUTO02-A) in 2000 and updated it (AUTO02-A2) in 2003, specifying that clinical laboratories should only use the Code 128B symbology on specimen labels. CLSI has been working to develop a new standard (AUTO14) for the use of two-dimensional barcodes in clinical and anatomic pathology laboratories. Two-dimensional barcodes offer the prospect of encoding more data in smaller formats and having greater reliability than one-dimensional barcodes.

In practice, a barcode label (often generated by the LIS and bearing the sample accession number) is placed onto the specimen container and is subsequently "read" by one or more barcode readers placed at key positions in the analytical sequence. Examples of these key positions are a handheld barcode reader in a laboratory section, a task-targeted automation system, the loading unit for a TLA system, and an automated analyzer. The resultant identifying and ancillary information is then transferred to and processed by the system software. Generating barcodes prior to specimen acquisition with identification at a patient's bedside ensures greater integrity of the specimen's identity throughout these processes.

Unequivocal positive identification of each specimen is achieved in analyzers with barcode readers. Advantages of the use of barcode labels include the following:
1. Elimination of work lists for the system
2. Avoidance of mistakes made in the placement of tubes in the analyzer or during sampling
3. Avoidance of the need for analysis of specimens in a defined sequence
4. Decrease in identification errors

A best practice to reduce errors caused by barcode misreads is to set the barcode readers on analyzers and automation systems to only read the symbology expected on the specimen labels (e.g., Code 128B). This prevents reading errors in the event that a second barcode of a different symbology might be visible on an underlying label (e.g., a tube vendor's barcode that indicates the tube type and its additive).

### Identification Errors

Many opportunities arise for the mismatch of specimens and results. These risks begin at the bedside and are compounded with each processing step a specimen undergoes between collection from the patient and analysis by the instrument. The risks are particularly great when hand transcription is invoked for accessioning, labeling and relabeling, and creation of lists of samples for analysis in one **batch analysis**, also referred to as a "load list." An incorrect accession number, one in which the digits are transposed, or a load list with transposed accession numbers, may cause test results to be attributed to the wrong patient. An additional hazard exists when specimens must be inserted into certain positions in the loading zone defined by a load list. Human misreading of the specimen label or the loading list may cause misplacement of specimens, calibrators, or controls. Automatic reading of barcode labels reduces the error rate from 1 in 300 characters (for human entry) to about 1 in 1 million characters barring (1) imperfections in printed bar codes, (2) improper barcode scanner resolution, or (3) skewed orientation of barcode labels on containers, all of which can result in read errors.

### Specimen Preparation

Some tests may be performed on whole blood, although, more commonly, serum is required. The clotting of blood in specimen collection tubes, subsequent centrifugation, and the transfer of serum to secondary tubes all require time. To eliminate the delays associated with specimen preparation, systems are being developed to automate this process. Alternatively, whole blood can be used for some analysis.

#### Use of Whole Blood for Analysis

When whole blood is used in an assay system, specimen preparation time is essentially eliminated. Automated or semiautomated ion-selective electrodes, which measure ion activity in whole blood rather than ion concentration, have been incorporated into automated systems to provide test results within minutes of collecting a specimen. Comparable electrode-based methods can be used for glucose, creatinine, and lactate. Another simple approach involves manual or automated application of whole blood to dry reagent films, and visual or instrumental observation of a quantitative change.

## Specimen Delivery

Automated methods are often used to deliver specimens to the laboratory instead of more manual methods (e.g., phlebotomist transport, courier service, nurse delivery). Pneumatic tube systems have been used in many hospitals, but mobile robots can also transport specimens and other laboratory supplies within a laboratory or to the laboratory from other locations in the facility. Some hospitals are now incorporating radiofrequency identification (RFID) tags to track preanalytic transport of specimens. Additional, RFID-based systems are increasingly being used by vendors to assist with reagent management and inventory monitoring.

### Pneumatic Tube Systems

Pneumatic tube systems provide rapid specimen transport and are reliable when installed as point-to-point services. However, when switching mechanisms are introduced to allow carriers (the bullet-shaped containers used to hold specimens) to be sent to various locations, mechanical problems may occur and may cause misrouting. In addition, close attention to the design of the pneumatic tube system is necessary to prevent hemolysis of the specimen. Avoidance of sudden accelerations and decelerations and the use of proper packing material inside the carriers can help to minimize hemolysis. Pneumatic tube systems should be validated prior to use in order to ensure that analytical results are not impacted by hemolysis.

### Mobile Robots

Automated guided vehicles, also called mobile robots, have been used successfully to transport laboratory specimens both within a laboratory and outside a central laboratory. They are easily adapted to carry various sizes and shapes of specimen containers and are reprogrammable with changes in laboratory geometry. In addition, in a busy laboratory setting, delivery of specimens to laboratory benches by a mobile robot can be more frequent than human pickup and is cost-effective. Inexpensive models follow a line on the floor, but others have more sophisticated guidance systems. Some mobile robots have been integrated with robotic systems that automate loading and unloading of specimens; others initiate an audible or visual signal of their arrival at a specified station so that employees are able to load or unload the specimens being transported.

### Single-Function Workstations

Some laboratories have gained efficiency, improved quality, and lowered turnaround time by implementing an automated system that performs a single task. This automation is also referred to as *task-targeted automation*. Examples of such automation include automated centrifuges, decappers, recappers, aliquoters, and sorters. Box 16.2 lists a number of vendors offering one or more single-function workstations.

Fig. 16.1 is an example of a sorter, one of the different types of single-function workstations that are available. A laboratory could use a sorter for both preanalytical sorting for different testing areas and postanalytical sorting for archival storage.

## Multifunction Workstations (Automated Specimen Processing)

Although the manual operations carried out in a specimen processing area may look simple, considerable complexity underlies them. Consequently, specimen processing has been one of the most difficult areas of the clinical laboratory to automate. Each specimen passing through a specimen processing area has to undergo a series of operations, including (1) receiving the specimen; (2) inspecting it for appropriateness (labeling, container type, temperature, and quantity of specimen); (3) logging the specimens into the LIS; (4) recording the date and time of collection and phlebotomist ID, if not already entered; (5) labeling the specimen with an accession number if not already there; and (6) separating urgent and stat specimens from routine specimens. Also, specimens may have to be sorted for centrifugation and aliquoting.

An example of a stand-alone specimen processing system is shown in Fig. 16.2. Such systems place processed specimens into racks that must be transported manually to the testing areas, with some exceptions. They may be a good choice for laboratories (1) with daily workloads of 500 to 1500 specimens, (2) with space limitations, or (3) that desire ease of use with different analyzers from different vendors. Some laboratories may choose to use multiples of a stand-alone specimen processing system based on higher daily volumes or to automate postanalytical archiving in addition to preanalytical specimen processing.

Box 16.3 lists vendors offering multifunction or specimen processing workstations. Although there may be some variation in the functions that are included, these systems will typically (1) receive incoming specimens, (2) sort, (3) decap, (4) aliquot, and (5) label aliquoted specimen containers with barcodes. All may be interfaced to the laboratory's LIS. Some systems may also include automated centrifugation. Some of the systems sort into instrument-specific racks for analyzers from a number of different vendors. In addition, some users apply these systems to aliquot and sort reference or "send-out" testing.

## Total Laboratory Automation Systems

Several manufacturers offer integrated or modular automation systems that use conveyor belts to connect preanalytical

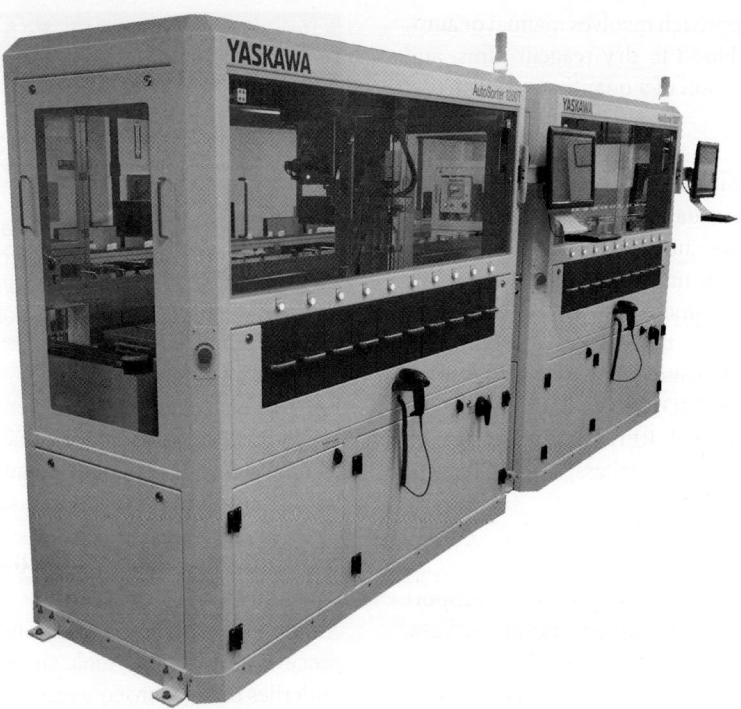

**Fig. 16.1** Example of a single-function nonanalytical automated workstation. Pictured is a Motoman Auto-Sorter 1200, which has sorting speeds of up to 2000 specimens per hour, several different options for deck configurations, and the possibility of different analyzer-specific output racks. Photo shows two units side by side. (Courtesy Yaskawa America, Motoman Robotics Division, Waukegan, IL.)

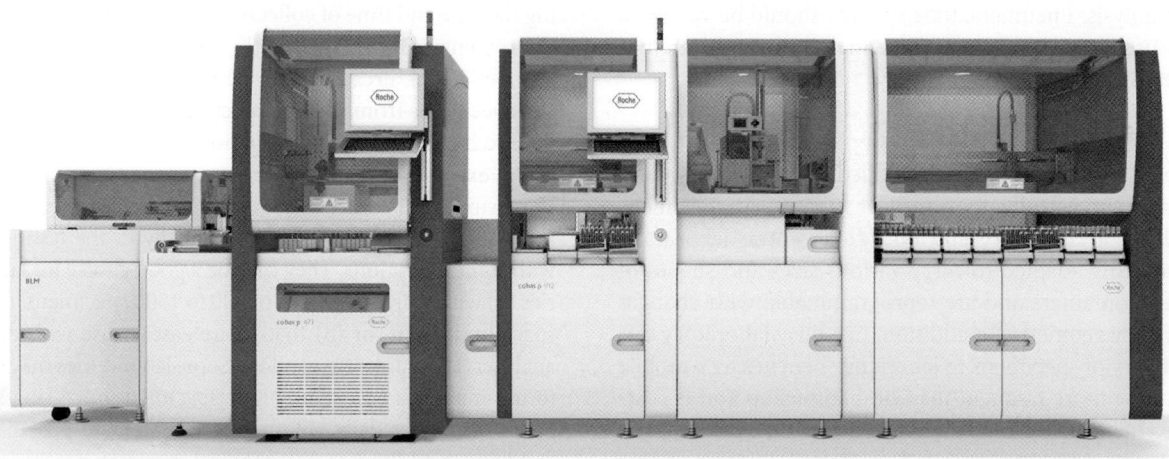

**Fig. 16.2** Example of a multifunction nonanalytical automated workstation. Pictured is a Roche Cobas p 612 system with automated centrifugation, decapping and recapping, aliquoting, and barcode labeling of secondary tubes, including sample quality inspection. (Courtesy Roche Diagnostics, Indianapolis, IN.)

specimen processing and other functions directly to analyzers. A list of automation vendors offering TLA systems can be found in Box 16.4; Fig. 16.3 illustrates a large TLA system with a variety of connected nonanalytical and analytical modules.

In addition to the nonanalytical functions listed in the preceding section, TLA systems typically add (1) conveyor transport; (2) interfacing to automated analyzers; (3) more sophisticated process control; and, in some cases, (4) a specimen storage and retrieval system. Some systems use an open design, which permits interfaces to analyzers from a variety of vendors, but other systems are of a closed design and are interfaced only to the vendor's own (or a limited number of other) analyzers. Closed systems typically do not have process control software that is independent of the instruments or system; rather, the automation process control is integrated to work with the vendor's analyzers.

To achieve maximum effectiveness of an automation system, process control software should be able to read the specimen's ID barcode and obtain information from the LIS about specimen type and ordered tests. This process control software is usually referred to as the Laboratory Automation System (LAS), not to be confused with the actual hardware of the laboratory automation. The software determines the processes required and the exact route or course of action for each specimen. It should be able to (1) calculate the number of aliquots and the proper volume for each specimen depending on the tests requested, (2) route the specimens to preanalytical processing equipment and then to analyzers, (3) command the recapping of specimens after testing, and (4) retain the specimens for automatic recall. The software monitors analyzers for in-control production status and automatically make decisions if a test is not available. Specimen integrity for hemolysis, icterus, and lipemia can be performed by automatic spectrophotometric methods. Rules-based decisions from analysis at multiple wavelengths may correct the effects of interferents for some assays and alert the laboratory on others. Finally, most process control software should include (1) "autoverification," which is validation of analyzer results by making rules-based decisions that flag exceptions for medical laboratory scientist review and (2) automated retrieval of specimens for repeat, reflex, and dilution testing.

Although most of these systems are restricted to handling specific types of specimen containers, they are capable of processing much of the daily workload of a large clinical laboratory. In addition to process control software and an LIS interface, each of these systems incorporates some or all of the following components:

1. *Specimen input area:* This is a holding area where barcode-labeled specimens are introduced into the system.
2. *Barcode reading stations:* Multiple barcode readers are placed at critical locations in the processing system to track specimens and provide information for their proper routing to various stations. Alternately, barcode readers may only be required at limited locations in the system if each transport carrier (puck) has a unique ID such as an RFID chip, and the specimen's barcode ID is "married" to the puck's ID when first placed in the puck.
3. *Transport system:* Segments of a conveyor belt line that move specimens to the appropriate location.
4. *A high-level device to sort or route specimens:* A device that separates specimens based on processing requirements or order code and passes them to the transport system or to a system using racks. A high-level sorter is often used to separate specimens that require centrifugation or other processing steps.
5. *Automated centrifuge:* An area of the specimen processor in which specimens requiring centrifugation are removed from the conveyor belt, introduced into a centrifuge that is automatically balanced, centrifuged (refrigerated or at room temperature), removed from the centrifuge, and placed back on the transport system.
6. *Liquid level detection and evaluation of specimen adequacy (specimen integrity):* An area where sensors are used to evaluate the volume of specimen in each specimen container and to look for the presence of hemolysis, lipemia, or icterus (HIL indices). Spectrophotometric methods to assess HIL indices are commonly included as functionality within automated chemistry analyzers. Liquid level detection sensors are commonly incorporated into most chemistry analyzers and immunoanalyzers.
7. *Decapper station:* An area or device in the automated system where specimen caps or stoppers are automatically removed and discarded into a waste container.
8. *Recapper station:* An area or device in the automated system where specimen tubes are automatically recapped with new screw caps, stoppers, or an alternate air-tight closure (such as a foil seal).
9. *Aliquoter:* A machine that aspirates appropriately sized aliquots from each original specimen container and places them into barcoded secondary specimen containers for sorting and transport to multiple analytical workstations.
10. *Physical interfaces to automated analyzers:* A direct physical connection to an automated analyzer that permits the analyzer's sampling probe to aspirate directly from an open specimen container while the container is still on the conveyor, or which may robotically lift the container from the conveyor and place it onto the analyzer.

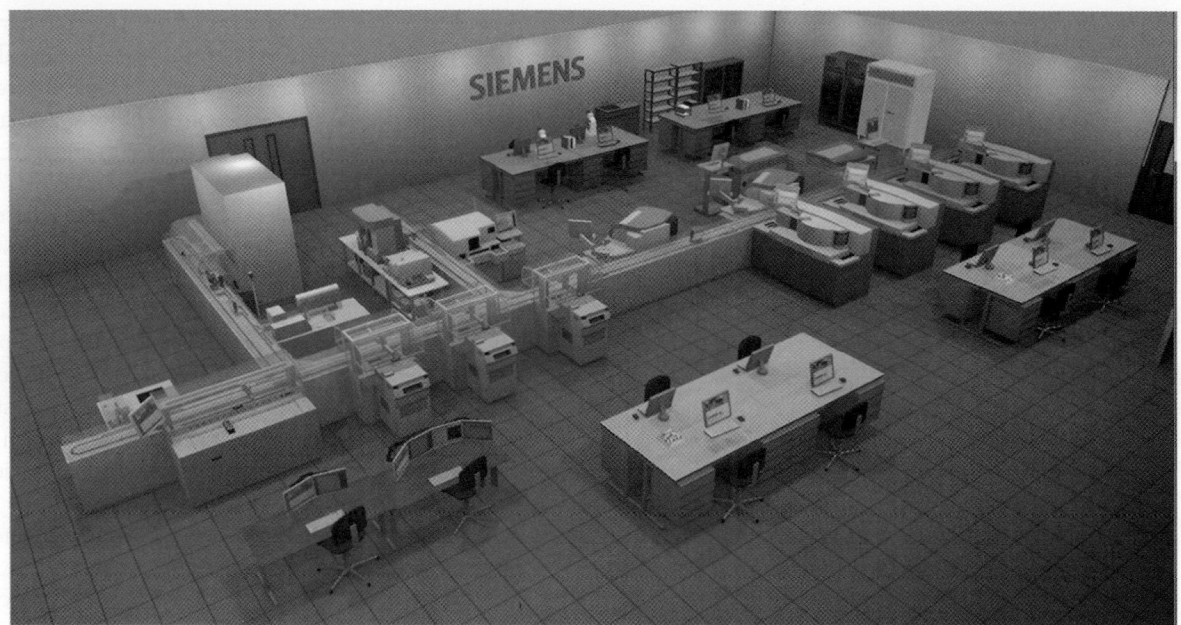

**Fig. 16.3** Example of a total laboratory automation system. Pictured is a Siemens Aptio Automation System, which can include options such as a hematology analyzer with autoslide maker or stainer, hemostasis analyzer, clinical chemistry and immunoassay systems, integrated chemistry systems, and data management system laboratory information systems (workstation and the following pre- and postanalytical modules: tube inspection, centrifuge, refrigerated storage, aliquoter, bulk input, rack input, input and output, sealer, desealer, decapper, and aliquoter recapper). (Courtesy Siemens Healthineers. Copyright Siemens Healthcare Diagnostics, Inc., 2016.)

11. *Sorter:* An automated output, used to sort specimens to a rack or tray for delivery to an analyzer or workstation not physically attached to the automation, or for a specific workflow. Such a sorter typically sorts into 30 to 100 different sort groups in racks or carriers. In some systems, the racks may be specific to certain analyzers for convenience. Some automation systems may use a sorter as a temporary holding area for specimens that may require a repeat test.

12. *Take-out stations:* Temporary storage areas for specimens before or after analysis. The take-out station may be the same as the sorter described earlier, where specimens are sorted for manual delivery. However, it may also serve as a holding area (stockyard) for specimens awaiting autoverification of results.

13. *Storage and retrieval system:* This unit may serve the same function as the take-out station or stockyard—that of holding specimens after analysis in case a specimen is necessary for a repeat test—but it has one major difference. These units are typically refrigerated and hold many more specimens (3000–30,000) than the typical take-out station or stockyard. Specimen containers are loaded and retrieved with a robot. Some storage systems include automated specimen discard directly into biohazard waste bins after a predetermined storage duration has been reached.

## Conveyor Belts

One main feature of integrated TLA systems is the use of conveyor belts. Ordinary industrial conveyor belts have been used successfully when only transportation is required. To increase the variety of types of specimen containers that are carried on a conveyor belt system, specimens are placed into specially designed carriers that fit on a conveyor belt line. Sometimes known as "pucks" or "racks" (depending on whether they carry individual specimens or groups of specimens), the carriers have receptacles for variously sized tubes, generally ranging from 13 × 75 mm to 16 × 100 mm—sizes that are consistent with the CLSI Standard AUTO01-A. The industrial, motor-driven conveyor belts used in typical LASs have transport rates ranging from a few hundred pucks per hour up to 2000 per hour. In addition, linear synchronous motors and magnetic pucks are now being used in some automation systems.

Two types of conveyor belt systems are typically used as illustrated in Fig. 16.4. Fig. 16.4A depicts a loop conveyor that has a single module for both input of new specimens and removal of completed specimens. The flow around the loop takes specimens to the processing and analytical modules. Specimens may be sampled directly by the analytical instrument while on the conveyor, or a robot attached to the workstation may remove selected specimens from the conveyor for analysis. Fig. 16.4B depicts a unidirectional conveyor in which specimens are inputted at one end of the belt, flow past various processing and analytical modules, and arrive at the opposite end where they are removed. Analyzers access specimens in the same way as the loop conveyor. Depending on the vendor, both of these conveyor types can have bypass lanes that enable specimens not designated to stop at certain modules to bypass them entirely and proceed to other modules.

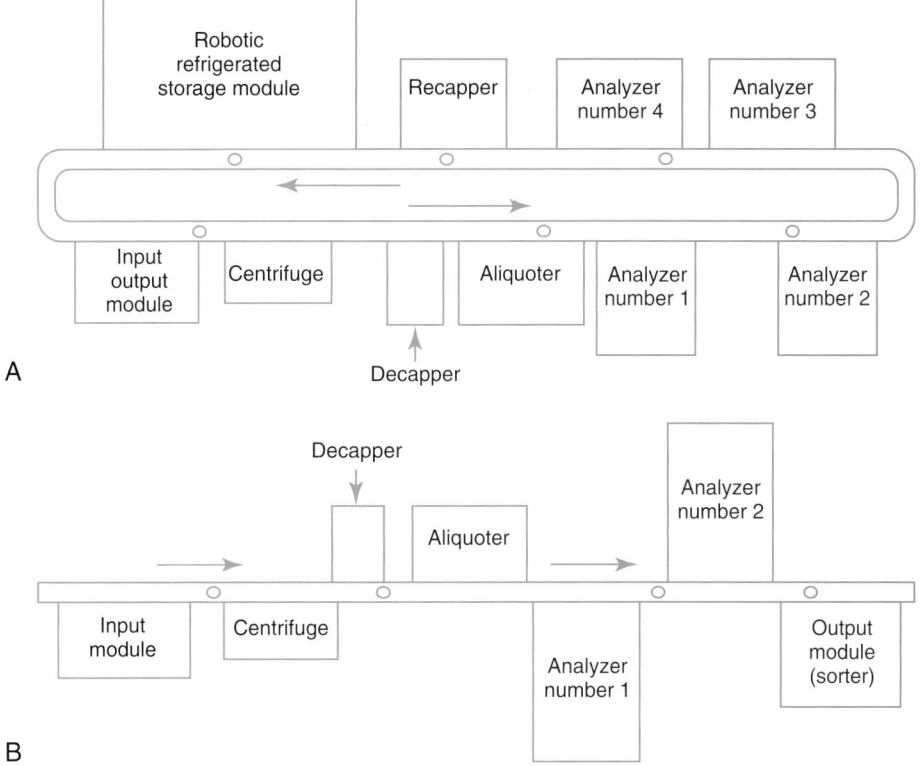

Fig. 16.4 (A) A depiction of a laboratory automation system using a continuous loop–type conveyor. In this concept, a single module is used for loading of new specimens and unloading of completed specimens. Depending on the needs of the laboratory, all other modules illustrated are options that can be included or not. (B) A depiction of a laboratory automation system using a unidirectional conveyor. In this concept, separate modules are required for loading of new specimens and unloading of completed specimens. The output module may also perform sorting of specimens for other testing. Other modules can be included, depending on the laboratory's needs.

This approach has the advantage that it does not require that specimens be aliquoted because specimens pass by workstations where tests are not performed. If specimens are robotically removed from their carriers on the line for testing, systems for queuing empty carriers to return the tubes back to the conveyor and to identify which specimen is in each carrier are required.

Transfer of specimens from the conveyor belt to the laboratory workstation has been implemented in various ways. For example, specimen containers may be moved from the conveyor belt onto the analyzers, or the analyzer may sample directly from specimen containers remaining on the conveyor. In practice, the automation system must stop the tube in the exact location required by the analyzer for sample transfer and barcode identification. Depending on the automation system, specimens for immediate short turnaround testing (STAT) (specimen with a high medical priority i.e., stat specimen) may or may not be processed and analyzed at speeds that are faster than if manually handled. Laboratories that are purchasing LASs are advised to learn how each system being considered handles stat specimens.

## Automated Specimen Storage and Retrieval

The automated capability to store and retrieve specimens on demand and with readily known exact storage locations is an important aspect of automated specimen delivery systems. In addition to automated storage and retrieval options in some of the integrated systems described earlier, several automated or semiautomated options for storage and retrieval, as well as LIS modules and PC-based software systems, permit laboratories to track trays or racks of specimens in their own freezers or refrigerators.

## PRACTICAL CONSIDERATIONS

In this section, the practical considerations that influence a laboratory's decision to automate part or all of its operations are discussed. Some of the suggested readings provide more insights and details about these practical considerations, including workflow mapping.

### Evaluation of Requirements

Any consideration of total or modular laboratory automation should start with an evaluation of requirements. Such an evaluation begins with mapping of the current laboratory workflow from the arrival of patient specimens through completion of testing and reporting of results. Box 16.5 lists potential workflow steps that should be mapped. Workflow mapping of material (specimen) flows and data flows is directly related to process flow and assists the laboratory in

## BOX 16.5  Clinical Laboratory Steps for Workflow Mapping

Unpacking from transport containers
Presorting
Temperature preservation
Order entry
Document management (e.g., requisitions)
Labeling
Sorting
Centrifugation
Labeling of aliquot tubes
Decapping
Pouring of aliquots
More sorting
Delivery to laboratory sections
More sorting
Preparing work lists
Labeling analyzer-specific tubes for specimens
Pouring or pipetting analyzer-specific specimens
Loading tubes on analyzers
Performing tests (steps such as extraction, centrifugation, precipitation, and dilution are not specifically listed)
Unloading analyzers
Recapping
Data manipulations (calculations)
Results review and verification
Reporting of results
Delivery of specimens to archival storage system
Archival storage of specimens
Reflexive testing
Repeat testing, diluting, if necessary
Additional physician-ordered testing
Specimen retrieval for additional or repeat testing
Disposal of expired specimens

## POINTS TO REMEMBER

When considering new automation or expansion of existing automation:
- Understand the laboratory's needs (moving from the current state to the desired state).
- Review the laboratory's specimen volumes by hour and by day (determine peaks and troughs).
- Review the percentages that are centrifuged, aliquoted, refrigerated or frozen, and shared among lab sections.
- Consider logistics, handling, facilities, and space issues.
- Map the laboratory's workflow. (What are the paths for all specimens?)
- Time the workflow to find bottlenecks.
- Rank the laboratory's needs in order of importance and differentiate needs that are "must haves" from needs that are "desired."
- Identify possible solutions that will meet the identified needs.
- Evaluate alternatives that will meet those needs.
- Use performance measures for productivity, turnaround time, and quality to establish baselines against which post-automation performance can be measured.
- Cost justification will likely be required by management, but the performance measures, if credibly predicted, will likely provide the basis for justification.

determining process steps that (1) are bottlenecks, (2) waste labor, and (3) are prone to error.

Some laboratorians use an "80% rule" in guiding decisions about automation. Clinical laboratories have many exceptional tests, specimen containers, and handling situations. Nevertheless, if 80% of the daily workload of specimen containers, covering most routine handling situations, can be standardized and automated, the laboratory will achieve a dramatic reduction in its labor usage and costs, which should be sufficient to justify the investment in automation and the planning and evaluation time involved.

After the laboratory's existing workflow has been mapped and its requirements have been identified, alternative solutions are considered. Consideration of lean processing and efficiency can help to ensure that automated solutions ultimately improve operations. Vendors are invited to make presentations and to host visits of the laboratory management team to other laboratories where vendors have successful installations. Key points to remember when a laboratory is considering either new automation or an addition to existing automation are listed in the following Points to Remember box.

## Problems of Integration

Building a highly integrated laboratory generates many potential problems. Most vendors of clinical LASs prefer customer settings in which the integrated analyzers are their own brand. However, many laboratories may prefer to use analyzers from multiple vendors, including the automation system vendor, making integration of instruments and robotic devices from different manufacturers necessary. Decisions must be made concerning which device will be the master controller and which vendor will develop the software that provides overall control of the automation scheme. In the past two decades, automation vendors have gained considerable experience implementing integrated systems.

### Device Integration

One objective in developing an integrated laboratory is to link laboratory instruments and devices into an automated system to maximize the number of functions automated. Automatic specimen introduction requires the development of mechanical interfaces between each laboratory analyzer and devices such as conveyor belts, mobile robots, or robot arms. Some systems have added enhancements such as electronic interfaces for laboratory instruments to allow remote computer control of front-panel functions, notification of instrument status information, and coordination of the distribution of specimens between instruments. In the ideal integrated clinical LAS, the LAS is a process controller that would integrate, automate, and monitor many of the decision-making tasks that occur in the daily activity of a laboratory. The LAS would also control and schedule nonanalytical modules such as automated centrifuges, aliquoters, decappers, and so forth. Most existing LISs have no process control capability, and their interfaces with laboratory analyzers provide only the ability to download accession numbers and the tests requested on each specimen and to upload results generated by the analyzer. The distribution of tasks must be carefully specified in developing such a communications network.

## AUTOMATION OF THE ANALYTICAL PROCESSES

The following sections describe basic concepts inherent to automating the analytical process, with a focus on how these concepts have been integrated into clinical chemistry and immunochemistry instrumentation. Advances in analytical automation in clinical chemistry, immunochemistry and immunology, urinalysis, hematology, coagulation, transfusion medicine, microbiology, mass spectrometry (MS), and molecular diagnostics are then discussed separately.

### Basic Concepts

The individual steps required to complete all phases of laboratory analysis are referred to as *unit operations* (Box 16.6). Automated analyzers are generally designed to perform mechanized versions of previous manual laboratory techniques and procedures. Analytical automation provides opportunities for efficiency, reproducibility, and throughput that may not be possible with manual processes. As such, modern instrumentation is engineered in a wide variety of configurations that are influenced by the manufacturer's hardware design, the testing to be performed, the testing environment, and the instrument and LIS connectivity that are ultimately required.

The most common automated instrument configuration is the random-access analyzer. In random-access analysis, testing is performed sequentially (or prioritized, i.e., STAT) on a set of specimens, with each specimen analyzed for a different selection of tests based on its respective clinical orders. Tests in random-access analysis are performed through the use of different vials, packs, or kits of reagents stored onboard the analyzer. This approach permits measurement of both a variable number and variety of analytes in each specimen loaded onto the instrument.

---

### BOX 16.6   Unit Operations in an Analytical Process

Specimen identification
Specimen delivery
Specimen processing
Sample introduction and internal transport
Sample loading and aspiration
Reagent handling and storage
Reagent delivery
Chemical reaction phase
Measurement phase
Signal processing, data handling, and process control
Result delivery to the laboratory information system

---

Other analyzer configurations include continuous-flow analysis and centrifugal analyzers. *Continuous-flow analyzers* (e.g., the Technicon AutoAnalyzer) were the first automated analyzers used in clinical laboratories. Initially, these analyzers were used in a single-channel analysis configuration and carried out a sequential analysis of a set number of tests (e.g., a basic metabolic panel) on each specimen. Subsequently, multiple-channel analysis versions were developed in which analysis of each specimen was performed on every channel in parallel. Results from nonrequested tests in the test profile were discarded as unnecessary after the analysis was complete. Inflexibility of the test menu and specimen-to-specimen carryover on these analyzers eventually led to their replacement in the marketplace by more versatile, discrete processing configurations.

*Centrifugal analyzers* used discrete pipetting to load aliquots of specimens and reagents sequentially into discrete chambers in a rotor. The specimens subsequently were analyzed in parallel *(parallel analysis)* by spinning the rotor to exert centrifugal force to mix the specimens and reagents and to drive the mixtures into cuvettes located on the periphery of the rotor. Such analyzers could be operated in a multiple-specimen/single-chemistry or a single-specimen/multiple-chemistry mode. Although such technology was developed as part of the space program and is suitable for application in a zero-gravity environment, it was not sufficiently versatile to compete with other random-access analyzers and has largely been abandoned for use in high-volume routine laboratory testing. Centrifugal microfluidics, however, is an important component in near-patient testing in which whole-blood specimen processing on small instrumentation enables plasma separation and multiple analyses into separate micro wells.

### Specimen Loading

The loading zone of an analyzer is the area where specimens are held in the instrument before they are analyzed. This holding area is often a circular tray, a rack, a series of racks built into a cassette, or an array of individual containers ("pucks") into which tubes are inserted. Although most automated instrumentation is now able to identify tubes through techniques such as barcode scanning, some instruments may still require loading of specimens in a defined sequence as specified by a load list. For some analyzers, specimens designated for a subsequent run may be placed on a separate tray while an existing run is already in progress. In most large-scale automated analyzers, specimens may be added continuously by the operator as they become available. This configuration is also most compatible with modular automation and TLA solutions in which specimens are automatically distributed to component instruments.

A desirable feature of any automated analyzer is the ability to insert new specimens ahead of specimens already in place in the loading zone. This feature allows the timely analysis of a specimen with a high medical priority (i.e., STAT specimens). When specimen identification is machine read, it is usually possible for the operator to reposition specimens in the loading zone. When specimen identification is tied to a loading list, however, insertion or repositioning of specimens must be accompanied by revision of the loading list. The ability to perform add-on testing when a specimen is present on the instrument is another characteristic that can improve efficiency and decrease manual interventions.

In clinical chemistry testing, the specimen for automatic analysis is often serum or plasma. Most automated chemistry analyzers are able to directly aspirate specimens from primary collection tubes of common container sizes. Instrument manufacturers typically specify acceptable specimen container types to ensure physical compatibility of the tube and to prevent inadvertent damage to the instrument. Although the outer tube diameter is most frequently evaluated for instrument compatibility, the inner tube diameter (e.g., double-walled collection tubes) may also impact compatibility with instrument probes or pipettes. The inner tube diameter may also impact accurate estimations of sample volume in systems with automated volume detection. Many primary collection tubes contain gel separator materials (i.e., separator tubes) that form a barrier after centrifugation between serum or plasma and the cellular elements underneath. Sample aspiration in automated analytical systems must be designed to prevent or withstand probe crashes with the bottom of the tube, as well as crashes or plugging due to gel separators in the specimen container.

Many analyzers also sample from secondary containers (cups or aliquot tubes) filled with sample transferred from an original specimen tube. Often the design of the sampling cup is unique for a particular analyzer. Each cup should be designed to minimize *dead volume*, that is, the excess specimen that must be present in a cup to permit aspiration of the full volume required for testing. Many instruments use *short-sample cups* or *false-bottom tubes* to help facilitate testing by automated analyzers with minimal dead volume. When the creation and placement of aliquots or pour-offs into secondary containers is not automated, careful attention is required to prevent specimen mix-ups, particularly when the secondary container is too small to be directly labeled with appropriate patient identifiers. Secondary containers must be made of inert material so they do not interact with the analytes being measured. They should be disposable to minimize cost and the potential for cross-contamination, and their shape should, even without a cap, limit evaporation by minimizing the surface area of sample exposed to air.

Specimens may undergo other forms of degradation in addition to evaporation. For example, specimens that contain thermolabile constituents may undergo degradation if held at ambient temperatures. Thermolability is minimized when both specimens and calibrators are held in a refrigerated loading zone. Other constituents such as bilirubin are photolabile. Photodegradation is reduced by the use of semi-opaque cups and placement of smoke- or orange-colored plastic covers over the specimen cups. The potential effects of both thermolability and photolability, however, can be minimized by automated instrumentation that tests specimens promptly and efficiently.

## Specimen Sampling

The instrument sampling mechanism aspirates specimen from a loaded container for subsequent testing. Automated analyzers may sample fixed or variable volumes depending on the instrument and assay configuration. Sampling takes place using either fixed reusable probes or disposable pipettes. Fixed probes limit disposable costs, reduce the need for supply management, and eliminate ongoing operator loading of disposable pipettes. Onboard wash stations for fixed probes are required, however, to reduce the risk of sample or reagent carryover.

Many automated analyzers incorporate *liquid-level sensing* to detect potential short samples, ensure appropriate specimen aspiration, and minimize the risk of probe crashes. Liquid-level sensing is typically conducted using either pressure or capacitive (radiofrequency) methods. Disposable capacitive pipette tips are available for processes that are vulnerable to carryover. Automated analyzers may also integrate methods for *clot detection* because clots may result in inadequate specimen volumes being aspirated, as well as plugging of the probe, tubing, or fluidic channels. Instrument "clot errors" that occur in specimens without evidence of detectable clots should raise the suspicion for potential specimen hyperviscosity, which is a clinically urgent finding.

*Closed-container sampling* systems have also been developed for use in automated chemistry and hematology analyzers. In these systems, the specimen probe passes through a hollow needle that initially penetrates the primary container's rubber stopper. This configuration prevents damage or plugging of the specimen probe while allowing the level sensor to remain active. After the specimen probe is withdrawn, the outer hollow needle also is withdrawn, so the stopper reseals, and no specimen escapes. Closed-container sampling is used widely in hematology analyzers because specimen mixing through gentle tube inversion is commonly required before analysis. Such mixing may even be incorporated into instrument functionality. Closed-container sampling also reduces the risk of contamination or splatter associated with removing the specimen container stopper.

Transmission of infectious diseases by automated equipment is a concern in clinical laboratories. The potential method of transmission by automated equipment is primarily through splatter of specimens during the acquisition of samples from rapidly moving specimen probes. The use of level sensors, which restrict the penetration of sample probes into specimens, and provision of software for smoother motion control, greatly reduce the possibility of splatter. Additional engineering controls include closed-tube sampling, covers over the specimen probe sampling areas, automated discard to waste bins for disposable sample probes, specimen cups, reaction cuvettes, direct-line plumbing of instrument liquid waste, and appropriate decontamination protocols before routine maintenance or service.

## Specimen Introduction and Internal Transport

The method used to introduce sample into the analyzer and its subsequent transport within the analyzer is the major difference between *continuous-flow* and *discrete processing* systems. In continuous-flow systems, the sample is aspirated through the sample probe into a stream of flowing liquid, whereby it is transported to analytical stations in the instrument. In discrete systems, the sample is aspirated into the sample probe and is then delivered, often with reagent, through the same orifice into reaction cups or other containers where the chemical reaction and analysis takes place. Carryover is a potential problem with both types of systems.

## Continuous-Flow Systems

Peristaltic pumps and plastic tubing are used to advance the sample and reagents in continuous-flow analysis. Peristaltic pumps trap a "slug" of fluid between two rollers that occlude the tubing. As the rollers travel over the tubing, the trapped fluid is pushed forward and, as the leading roller lifts from the tubing, is added to the fluid beyond it. Peristaltic pumps are seldom used today because of their inherent risk of specimen hemolysis and cross-contamination (i.e., carryover of specimen or reagent, as described in a following section).

## Discrete Processing Systems

Air- or positive-liquid displacement pipettes are used for sampling in most discrete automated systems in which specimens, calibrators, and controls are delivered by a single pipette. A pipette may be designed for one of two operational modes: (1) to dispense only aspirated sample into the reaction receptacle or (2) to flush out sample together with diluent. Both systems use a plastic or glass syringe with a plunger, the tip of which usually is made of Teflon. Instrument pipettes may be designed as (1) fixed, (2) variable, or (3) selectable volume. Selectable-volume pipettes allow the selection of a limited number of predetermined volumes. Whereas pipettes with unlimited or selectable volumes are typically used in systems that allow many different applications, fixed-volume pipettes are used for samples and reagents in instruments dedicated to the performance of only a small variety of tests.

## Carryover

Carryover is defined as the transfer of a quantity of analyte or reagent from one specimen or reaction into a subsequent one. Because it interferes with analytical results from subsequent reactions, carryover should be minimized or eliminated. In discrete systems with disposable reaction vessels and measuring cuvettes, carryover is generally caused by the pipetting system. In instruments with reusable cuvettes or flow cells, carryover may also arise from incomplete cleaning of the cuvettes or flow cells between assays.

Most manufacturers of discrete systems reduce sample-to-sample carryover by using disposable pipette tips or by incorporating wash stations for the sample probe that flush the internal and external surfaces of the probe with copious amounts of wash solution. An adequate ratio of flush and rinse to specimen volume controls carry over in many cases to acceptable limits. Many instruments separate the pipetting steps for specimens from pipetting steps used for reagents to further minimize risk of carryover. Appropriate choice of

sample probe material, geometry, and surface conditions also influences carryover. Some systems clean the outside of the sample probe to prevent transfer of a portion of the previous specimen into the next specimen cup. Use of disposable sample probe tips eliminates the risk of contamination of one sample by another inside the probe, as well as the risk of carryover of one specimen into a specimen in the next cup, because a new pipette tip is used for each pipetting.

Although many high-volume automated chemistry analyzers have fixed reusable probes, instrumentation associated with processes that are more vulnerable to carryover and contamination (e.g., serology and molecular diagnostics) generally incorporate disposable pipettes for sample aspiration. For example, the reduction of sample-to-sample carryover is a more stringent requirement for automated analyzers that perform immunoassays in which some analytes (e.g., human chorionic gonadotropin) have a wide range of concentrations. Some systems use extra steps, such as additional washes, or an additional washing device to reduce carryover for selected tests to acceptable limits. Because extra steps reduce overall throughput, additional rinsing functions may be included for assays with large analytical measurement ranges (AMRs).

Sample-to-sample carryover can be detected by the preparation of two sample pools—one having a very high analyte concentration (H), the other having a low concentration (L). By running sequences of tests (e.g., HHHLLLHHLLHHLL) if sample-to-sample carryover is present, higher results will be noted in the low-concentration sample analyses that immediately follow a high-concentration sample.

Reagent-to-reagent carryover can also occur on discrete systems that use a common probe for pipetting reagents. Its minimization or elimination requires use of the same approaches described for sample-to-sample carryover. Detection of reagent-to-reagent carryover can be difficult for end users and usually requires involvement of the instrument vendor.

## Sample Pretreatment

Analytical procedures sometimes require the capability to remove proteins or other interferents from specimens to ensure the specificity of an analytical method. Dialysis, column chromatography, extraction, filtration, and solid-phase nucleic acid binding have been used for this purpose. Additional pretreatment processes include specimen concentration and/or dilution to bring an analyte of interest into an assay's AMR. Automation of pretreatment processes through offline or integrated specimen processing systems can improve the efficiency of these procedures. Sample pretreatment steps may also be integrated into assays designed for automated platforms. Examples include the addition of reagents that displace analytes from their endogenous binding proteins and instrument addition of red blood cell (RBC) lysing reagents in automated glycated hemoglobin (e.g., HbA1c) measurements.

## Reagents
### Reagent Management and Configuration

Reagent management is an important consideration in choosing automated instrumentation. Analytical systems may require that different reagents be stored at ambient, refrigerated (4°C), or frozen (−20°C or −80°C) temperatures. Availability of adequate reagent storage close to instrumentation is an important consideration in implementing efficient analytical systems. Reagents, calibrators, and quality control (QC) material that are supplied as lyophilized (dry) powder requiring reconstitution can require significant ongoing manual processing on the part of instrument operators. Some analytical systems have the capacity for onboard reconstitution of certain reagents, QC, or calibrators.

Many automated systems use liquid reagents stored in plastic or glass containers. For analyzers with a working inventory maintained in the system, the volumes of reagents stored onboard are often optimized based on the desired number of tests to be performed without operator intervention. Such analyzers often track the amount of reagent that is currently onboard and notify the operators when a replacement is required. In larger systems, reagent storage compartments may be maintained at refrigerated temperatures to increase onboard stability. Some analyzers have the ability to cap reagents while not in use to decrease evaporation and reagent degradation. Larger automated analyzers may have the ability to load new reagent packs (and discard empty packs) without interrupting the testing process or placing the instrument in a "standby" mode. Additionally, many automated instruments allow the loading of more than one similar type of reagent pack so that testing is not delayed when the first pack runs empty. Having an excess number of available reagent positions on automated instrumentation allows for optimization of reagent management to match the laboratory's daily workflow with minimal operator involvement. For analyzers in which specimens are not processed continuously, in-use reagents are often stored in laboratory refrigerators and are only introduced onto instruments when required for testing. Some automated analyzers (particularly point-of-care [POC] and near-patient devices) may use dry reagents that are built into disposable single-use cartridges.

## Reagent Identification

Labels on reagent containers include information such as (1) reagent identification, (2) volume of the contents or the number of tests in each container, (3) expiration date, and (4) lot number. Many reagent containers carry barcodes or RFID tags that contain some or all of this information. Advantages of using reagent barcodes include (1) facilitation of inventory management, (2) the ability to insert reagent containers in random sequence, and (3) the ability of the system to track in-use reagent lot numbers and document that appropriate calibration and QC was performed on a specific lot or pack before testing. Furthermore, when a barcode reader is coupled with a level-sensing system on the reagent probe, it alerts the operator as to whether a sufficient quantity of reagent exists to complete a workload. Barcodes on reagent containers may also contain information about calibrators, such as the definition of a calibration curve algorithm and values of curve constants defined at the time of reagent manufacture. Accompanying calibrator materials provided in their own

barcoded tubes at the time of manufacture ensure that calibration functions are integrated properly into the analysis. Inventory management systems (tied to barcodes or RFID tags) can be used to track reagent usage and reorder reagent to prevent depletion of inventory and corresponding test delays. Such systems (combined with vendor reagent lot sequestering programs) can decrease the need for new-lot workups and therefore maximize instrument and operator productivity.

## Vendor-Supplied Versus User-Defined Reagents

Automated analyzers can be classified as "open" or "closed" with respect to reagent compatibility. A "closed" system analyzer is one in which reagents or calibrators (or both) are provided only by the instrument manufacturer and other reagents or methods cannot be used. Closed systems can be restricted based on proprietary licensing or technical restrictions of reagent components, reagent pack size and shape, or software restrictions associated with compatibility of vendor barcodes or the ability to configure custom test parameters. In an "open" analyzer, the operator is able to change the parameters related to an analysis and to load user-defined reagents (UDRs), either by preparing "in-house" reagents or using reagents from alternative suppliers. Open systems usually have considerable flexibility and adapt readily to new methods and analytes. Many vendors of automated analyzers allow a limited number of UDRs on an otherwise closed system, with restrictions based on technical (instrument-related) or contractual limitations. Some types of assays (e.g., general chemistry) are far more amenable to UDRs than others (e.g., antibody-based chemiluminescence). Advantages of UDRs include decreased cost, increased flexibility, and the ability to optimize assay performance. Disadvantages of UDRs may include additional regulatory requirements for laboratory-developed tests, manual processes associated with reagent preparation, lack of manufacturer-associated barcode information on reagent packs, and smaller peer group sizes in proficiency testing challenges.

## Reagent Delivery and Mixing

Liquid reagents are often acquired and delivered to mixing and reaction chambers by pumps (through tubes) or by positive-displacement syringe devices. In analyzers in which more than one reagent is acquired and dispensed by the same syringe, washing or flushing of the probe is essential to prevent reagent carryover. Reagent carryover may interfere with subsequent reactions depending on which combinations of tests were sequentially performed on the instrument. Reagent carryover experiments are particularly important when considering UDR kits because UDRs would not have been evaluated by the instrument vendor for potential interference because of reagent carryover.

## Chemical Reaction Phase

Sample and reagents react in the chemical reaction phase. Factors that are important in this phase include (1) the vessel where the reaction occurs; (2) the cuvette where the reaction is monitored; (3) the timing of the reaction(s); (4) the mixing and transport of reactants; (5) the thermal conditioning of fluids; and (6) for some immunoassay systems, the separation of bound and unbound fractions.

## Type of Reaction Vessels and Cuvettes

In continuous-flow systems, each specimen passes through the same continuous stream and is subjected to the same analytical reactions as every other specimen and at the same rate. In such systems, the reaction occurs in the flow-through component. In discrete systems, each specimen has its own physical and chemical reaction space, separate from every other specimen. Discrete analyzers use either individual (disposable or reusable) reaction vessels transported through the system after sample and reagent have been dispensed, or they use stationary reaction chambers.

Reaction vessels (typically cuvettes) are reused in many instruments. The replacement interval for reusable reaction vessels depends on their composition and the washing mechanisms used. Some manufacturers have computer algorithms that automatically control when individual reaction vessels should be replaced, depending on how many assays and what types of assays have been performed in a given cuvette.

## Mixing of Reactants

Various techniques are used to mix reactants. In discrete systems, these include (1) forceful dispensing, (2) magnetic stirring, (3) vigorous lateral displacement, and (4) physical stirring. Dry reagent systems obviate the need for mixing because the specimen completely interacts with the dry chemicals as it flows through the matrix of the reaction unit. However, regardless of the technique used, mixing can be a difficult process to automate and one that may contribute to reaction-to-reaction carryover among reused components. Inadequate mixing can lead to erroneous test results that may be detectable by QC failures, error flags, or unusual specimen results.

## Thermal Regulation

Thermal regulation requires the establishment of a controlled-temperature environment in close contact with the reaction container and efficient heat transfer from the environment to the reaction mixture. Various technologies have been used for temperature regulation, including air baths, water baths, and Peltier devices. Onboard water baths often require specific maintenance and cleaning, particularly if the reaction monitoring system involves passage of light through the water bath to a reaction cuvette. Automated analyzers may also be influenced by external operating temperatures in the laboratory. Most vendors define acceptable temperature (and humidity) limits for their instruments.

## Separation in Immunoassay Systems

Automation of heterogeneous immunoassays requires wash steps to separate free and bound fractions, whereas homogeneous immunoassays do not. Several approaches can accomplish this separation. For example, these automated heterogeneous assays may use bound antibodies or proteins in a solid-phase format. With this approach, the binding of antigens and antibodies occurs on a solid surface to which the antibodies or other reactive proteins have been adsorbed or chemically bonded. Different types of solid phases are used, including (1) beads, (2) coated tubes, (3) microtiter plates, (4) magnetic and nonmagnetic microparticles, and (5) fiber matrices.

## Measurement Approaches

Automated chemistry analyzers traditionally have relied on photometers and spectrophotometers to measure the absorbance of the reaction produced in the chemical reaction phase. Alternative approaches now incorporated into analyzers include reflectance photometers, fluorometers, and luminometers. Immunoassay reactions that produce fluorescence, chemiluminescence, and electrochemiluminescence may enhance sensitivity. Ion-selective electrodes and other electrochemical techniques also are quite common. Many of these methods are discussed in detail elsewhere in this textbook (see Chapters 9, 10, 14, and 15).

## Postanalytic Processing

After a test is performed on a specimen, additional automated or manual specimen processing may still be required to obtain a final, clinically reportable result. Two such processes that are commonly performed are dilutions and repeat testing before reporting.

## Dilutions

If initial results are above the assay's AMR, dilutions may be required to bring the analyte concentration into the linear range. Dilutions may also be used to exclude the possibility of antigen excess ("hook effect"; see Chapter 15). Some instruments have the capability to perform automated dilutions by (1) pipetting less specimen volume into the reaction mixture, (2) pipetting more reagent into the reaction mixture, or (3) using onboard dilution vessels. Dilution functionality may be limited to certain assays on the instrument based on results of validation studies by the vendor. Instrument dilutions may be performed automatically (based on analyzer settings) or triggered by operator request. Some instruments also allow the operation to input a dilution manually. Analyzers that are unable to perform dilutions may still notify operators when an offline dilution is required. Many analyzers will then allow the operator to input the dilution factors so that final results are calculated automatically to limit the chance of error.

## Repeat Testing

Many laboratories have protocols such that certain assays are automatically repeated before reporting. Some examples include critical results, medically improbable results, or tests for life-altering diagnoses. Improved analytical methods and instrumentation have challenged the need for routine repeat testing. Regardless, many automated analyzers allow configurations for repeat testing without operator intervention, thus decreasing the time for result availability and communication to the ordering provider.

## Instrument Clusters (Workcells)

To reduce labor costs, instrument manufacturers have developed approaches that allow a single medical laboratory scientist to simultaneously control and monitor the functions of several instruments or modules. Initially, such workstations were configured with clusters of identical instruments from the same manufacturer. Advanced instrument clusters may incorporate different chemistry, immunochemistry, or hematology analyzers into the same cluster or combine different types of detection systems into a platform (see Figs. 16.3, 16.5, and 16.6). These instrument clusters are also commonly known as workcells.

A cluster of analyzers has its own central computer control module with software designed to assist the operator in monitoring the functions of each analyzer and to aid in the review of laboratory results generated by the cluster. Access to the many front-panel functions of each analyzer is provided by the interface between the analyzer and the central control module. Thus, the operator loads specimens onto each instrument (or a shared input module) and then monitors subsequent operation of, and reviews results from, all the instruments in the cluster. By incorporating the activities of multiple instruments into a single integrated workstation, this approach can improve overall efficiency.

## Microtiter Plate Systems

Microtiter plate systems are commonly used in immunoassays and nucleic acid analyses. Microtiter plates (as used for enzyme-linked immunosorbent assays [ELISAs]) are usually made of polystyrene and have 48 or 96 wells coated with antibody specific for an antigen of interest. After incubation of specimen in the microtiter plate well, the well is washed to remove unbound antigen, and a second antibody with conjugated indicator enzyme is added. After a second incubation period, the well is washed to remove the unbound conjugate. A color-producing product is developed by the addition of enzyme substrate, and the reaction is terminated at a specific time. With the development of automated pipetting stations (see next section), the liquid handling steps have been fully automated to make microtiter plate assays a viable technology for carrying out large numbers of immunoassays. Measurement of absorbance and data processing are also automated in many instruments.

## Automated Pipetting Stations

Automated pipetting stations have a Cartesian robot with a pipette fixed to the end of a probe that moves in three-dimensional space. The probe is capable of moving in the $x$-, $y$-, and $z$-axes. Liquids may be aspirated and dispensed in any location within the space. Pipetting stations may be used to automate custom analytical procedures for which an automated analyzer does not exist or cannot be cost justified, such as mixing and distributing reagents including multiple primer pairs for multiplex PCR or sequencing. Pipetting robots should (1) be relatively easy to program, (2) rarely malfunction, and (3) be capable of delivering aliquots of liquids with high precision and accuracy. Multiple-channel pipetting robots allow parallel processing of specimens with 8- or 12-channel probes to handle microtiter plates.

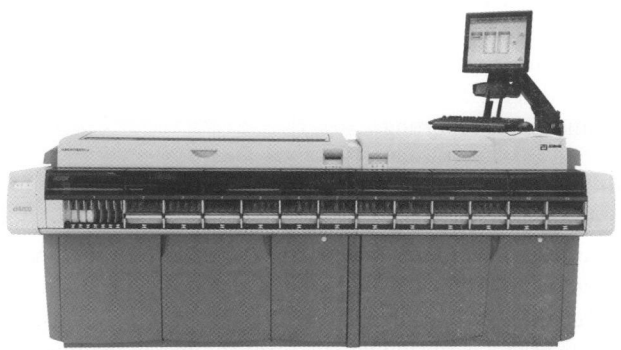

**Fig. 16.5** Example of an integrated chemistry and immunoassay system. The ARCHITECT *ci*8200 (Abbott Diagnostics) combines a c8000 clinical chemistry module *(left)* with an *i*2000SR immunoassay module *(right)* in one connected platform. (Courtesy Abbott Diagnostics, Lake Forest, IL.)

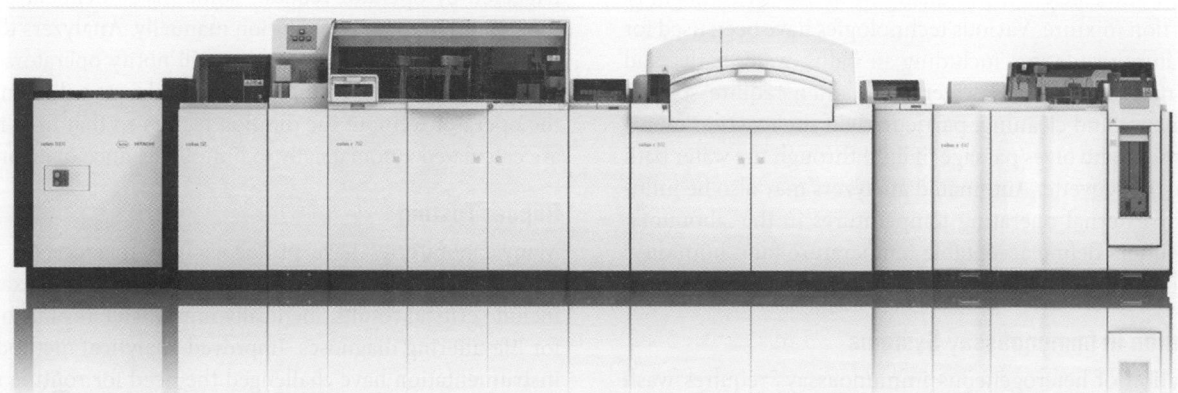

**Fig. 16.6** Example of an integrated chemistry and immunoassay system. The Cobas 8000 (Roche Diagnostics) modular analyzer series configuration shows (from *left* to *right*) a core unit, an ion-selective electrode module, as well as c702 and c502 chemistry and e602 immunoassay instruments. Module sample buffers allow additional capacity and random-access distribution of racks. (Courtesy Roche Diagnostics, Switzerland.)

## Signal Processing, Data Management, and Laboratory Information

The interfacing and integration of computers into automated analyzers and analytical systems has had a major impact on the acquisition and processing of analytical data. Analog signals from detectors are converted to digital signals. Computer software then processes the digital data into useful and meaningful output. Data processing has allowed automation of complex calibration relationships. Computer workstations provide a central point of communication with the user regarding (1) instrument status, (2) sample queues, (3) display of preliminary results, (4) QC tracking, (5) troubleshooting and maintenance records, and (6) result release to the LIS.

### Laboratory Information System

Traditional LISs were designed to track patient orders, manage result reporting, and facilitate billing. The LIS can be a standalone program or a module integrated into a broader health information system. A modern LIS provides the infrastructure required to manage all information directly related to specimen testing in the clinical laboratory, and includes order and result tracking, data storage, operational data for billing, and transmission of information to and from the electronic health record (EHR). Discipline-specific information systems are often necessary to address unique workflows and data requirements in areas such as anatomic pathology, digital pathology, molecular pathology, and transfusion medicine. For small laboratories with only a few instruments, direct connection of instruments to the LIS may be feasible. For laboratories with multiple analyzers (often from different vendors), the process becomes more complicated. Middleware can be used to address functionality and connectivity needs that are not included within the LIS. Laboratory information management systems (LIMS) are also increasingly being used to track overall activities, operations, and specimen processes that cannot otherwise be managed by the LIS. The LIMS is a distinct system not to be confused with the LAS software described previously.

### Test Autoverification

Autoverification is the process whereby patient results generated from interfaced instruments are compared by computer software against laboratory-defined acceptance parameters. If results fall within these defined parameters, the results are automatically released for reporting with no additional laboratory staff intervention. Any data that fall outside the defined parameters are reviewed by laboratory staff before reporting. Autoverification has been implemented in a variety of ways, such as by using the LIS to compare results against acceptance parameters. Alternatively, autoverification can be performed by an additional computer system or software between the analyzer and LIS (termed "middleware"). Most autoverification systems use rule-based decision logic. For example, if the QC for a test is outside allowable limits, do not report test results and alert the operator. More complex rules may incorporate critical values or other metrics. The rules applied require careful development and validation by laboratories before and after they are implemented. Regulations regarding autoverification are incorporated into most laboratory accreditation programs.

## AREAS OF ANALYTICAL AUTOMATION

Although the automation principles discussed earlier focus primarily on clinical chemistry applications, the following sections describe aspects of analytical automation that are unique to individual disciplines, including (1) clinical chemistry, (2) immunology and immunochemistry, (3) urinalysis, (4) hematology, (5) coagulation, (6) transfusion, (7) microbiology, (8) MS, and (9) molecular diagnostics.

### Clinical Chemistry

Automated systems in clinical chemistry can be differentiated based on (1) the volume of testing that is performed on the instrument(s) and (2) the capability for connectivity into instrument clusters or a larger LAS, such as TLA.

Laboratories that perform a lower volume of testing or have limited available floor space may choose smaller analyzers to minimize cost, complexity of maintenance, and instrument footprint. Many low-volume laboratory automated chemistry instruments include similar functionalities to those seen on high-volume instruments, including a diverse assay menu, multiple methods of analytical detection, compatibility with UDRs, onboard QC management, and LIS connectivity. Smaller instruments may also be used in large-volume laboratories for specialized methods, where test order volume or assay compatibility is either not supported or cost-effective on higher volume instruments (Fig. 16.7). For example, use of smaller instruments for esoteric testing may be amenable to batch processing with less reagent wastage.

Automated instruments for large-volume laboratories typically improve efficiency by handling more tests per hour with a larger capacity for both specimens and reagents (Fig. 16.8).

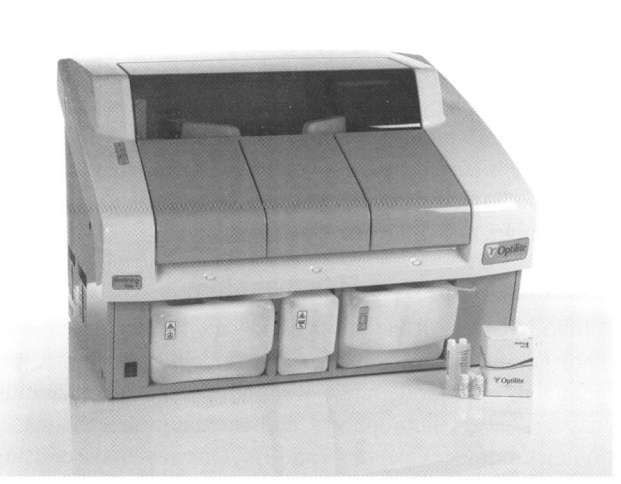

Fig. 16.7 Example of an automated bench-top special protein analyzer (Optilite, The Binding Site Group). (Courtesy The Binding Site Group Ltd., Birmingham, United Kingdom.)

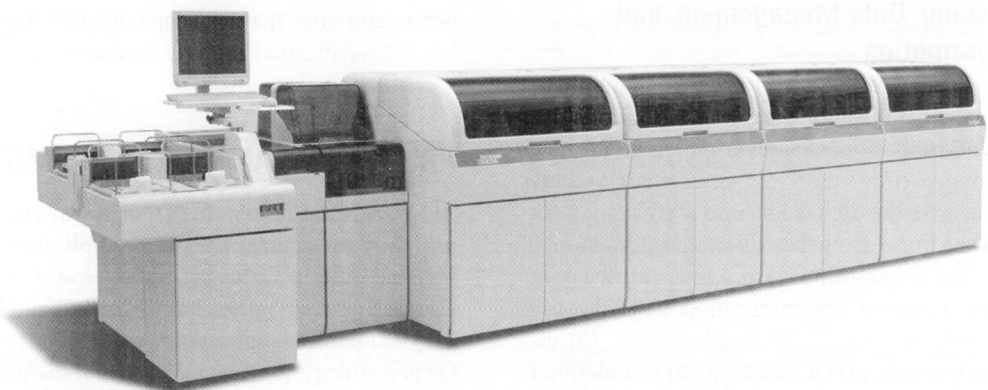

**Fig. 16.8** Example of a high-throughput automated clinical chemistry system. Shown is a Beckman Coulter AU5840 Clinical Chemistry System, which includes loading and rack buffer units, dual ion-selective electrodes, and four analytical modules. (AU 5800 Copyright 2016 Beckman Coulter, Inc. All rights reserved. Used with permission.)

Larger instruments may have more physical plant (infrastructure) requirements than their smaller counterparts, including floor space, ventilation, water supply, electrical, and drainage. Although these requirements may place greater initial costs on a larger automated system, when they are in place, they support greater efficiency of instrument operation. Larger automated instruments also typically offer greater options for connectivity in both instrument clusters and TLA solutions.

Larger systems may also have more complex maintenance procedures. Furthermore, instrument downtime for service may have a significant impact on clinical operations with high-volume consolidated platforms. For this reason, many high-volume laboratories are designed to incorporate instrument and assay redundancy so that if one analyzer is down for service, clinical testing can still be conducted on separate instruments. This is particularly important for laboratories that support acute-care, inpatient, and emergency department operations.

Along with routine chemistry analyzers that perform traditional photometric and ion specific measurements, automation in clinical chemistry also includes specialized instrumentation for specific clinical needs. Blood gas analysis (including instrumentation in clinical laboratories, STAT laboratories, and POC) is conducted on automated instrumentation. These platforms may include built-in QC assessment; single- or multiple-use reagent systems; and quantification of additional analytes that may be useful to near-patient testing, including electrolytes, glucose, ionized calcium, lactate, hemoglobin, or hematocrit.

## Immunochemistry and Immunology

Antibody-based detection methods are incorporated into many automated instruments and include nephelometry, turbidimetry, and a wide range of immunoassays incorporating enzymes, labels, fluorophores, and chemiluminescent detection methods (see Chapters 9 and 15). One advantage of using antibodies in automated instrumentation is that by varying reagents (antibodies), the same instrumentation may be used for the detection and quantification of many different analytes.

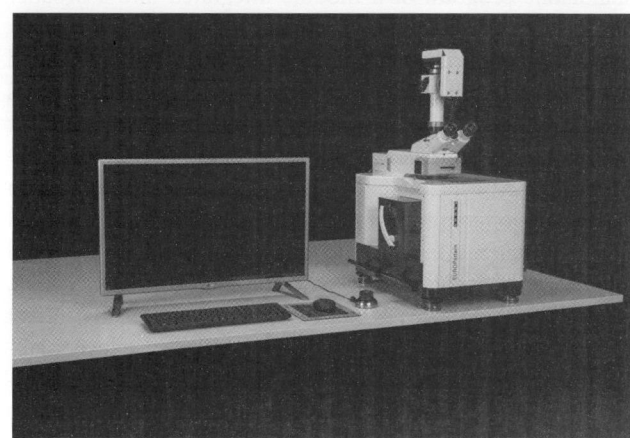

**Fig. 16.9** Example of an automated immunofluorescence microscopy system (EUROPattern, EUROIMMUN). (Courtesy EUROIMMUN US, Mountain Lakes, NJ.)

Along with discrete processing systems, automated immunoassay platforms may also be designed for microplates and microwells, including ELISAs and cell-based immunofluorescence assays. Automated indirect immunofluorescence microscopy systems are also available (Fig. 16.9). Automated systems are offered for processing of Western blots and immunoblots, techniques that have otherwise been very manually intensive. Finally, bead-based multiplex systems allow for the detection of multiple analytes in the same reaction mixture. The beads are typically analyzed by flow cytometry, and multiple antigens, antibodies, or nucleic acids can be measured. For example, HLA genotyping and specific human leukocyte antigen (HLA) antibodies are often performed on beads by flow cytometry. Such systems can decrease the specimen volume and analytic time otherwise required for parallel analyses.

## Urinalysis

Although many of the same analytical principles are used for the quantification of serum and urine chemical constituents, traditionally it has been more challenging to fully automate urinalysis. Nevertheless, several automated urinalysis

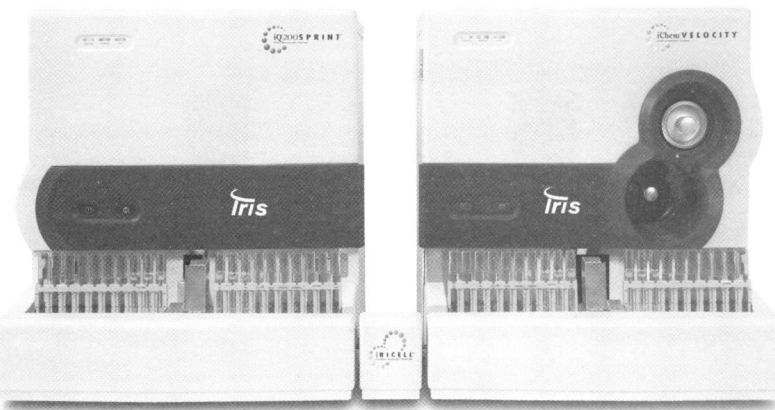

**Fig. 16.10** Example of an automated urinalysis system. The Iris iRICELL3000 (Beckman Coulter) combines urine chemistry analysis (iChemVELOCITY, *right*) with a digital flow morphology module (iQ200SPRINT, *left*). (iRICELL Copyright 2016 Beckman Coulter, Inc. All rights reserved. Used with permission.)

instruments are now commercially available for chemical analyses (automated and semiautomated test strip reading by reflectometry) as well as analysis of sediment, particles, or cellular elements using flow cytometric and microscopic analysis. Many systems combine both chemical and particle analysis modules into a workcell (Fig. 16.10) such that particle analysis may be conducted automatically on specimens with abnormal test strip results. Instruments for microscopic urine analysis have also been applied to automating the process of body fluid cell counting. Finally, although manual reading of urine test strips is still commonly performed as a POC test, small semiautomated instruments are available for Clinical Laboratory Improvement Amendments (CLIA)-waived automated reagent strip interpretation. Furthermore, interfacing such instruments to the LIS mitigates the risk of transcription errors versus manual entry of results.

## Hematology

Analyzers that perform a complete blood count have been automated through the use of (1) the "Coulter principle," which is based on cell conductivity, (2) light scatter, (3) flow cytometry, and, more recently, and (4) digital microscopic analysis. Individual blood cells are analyzed by application of one or more of these techniques. The Coulter principle is based on changes in electrical impedance produced by nonconductive particles suspended in an electrolyte as they pass through a small aperture between electrodes. RBCs, white blood cells (WBCs), and platelets are identified by their sizes.

When abnormal cells or cell counts that are outside of predetermined limits are observed in automated counting methods, it may be necessary to generate a blood smear for additional microscopic review or generation of a manual differential. Integrated hematology systems may include automated slide makers and slide stainers to limit the manual intervention involved in creating and labeling slides (Fig. 16.11). Additionally, advances in slide imaging have enabled the development of automated systems to classify and count cell types based on a digital scan of the slide or regions of interest. Automated digital imaging systems may also offer electronic review of categorizations by an operator, as well as electronic storage and sharing of images with clinicians outside the laboratory (i.e., digital pathology).

Flow cytometry analyzes individual cells as they travel in suspension one by one past a laser light source at a rate of about 1000 cells/s. The cells are typically stained with multiple fluorescently labeled antibodies of different colors that identify different cellular antigens. Each cell also scatters light in all directions. Light scattered in the forward direction is correlated to cell size, while light scattered at right angles correlates with internal granularity. Using a combination of light scatter and fluorescence, different cell populations can be identified and selected or "gated on" to accurately quantify subpopulations of clinical interest. Modern flow cytometry is a fine example of the power of both serial (cell by cell) and parallel (multiple markers on many cells) automation that is applied clinically in the classification of leukemias.

## Coagulation

Most coagulation testing is now performed on automated analyzers. A variety of methodologies are used, including optical and mechanical clot detection, as well as turbidimetric, chromogenic, and antibody-based analyses. Many instruments permit use of UDRs for more specialized coagulation testing. Connectivity to TLA systems is an option with some instrumentation, and this allows for automated specimen handling and centrifugation before coagulation testing. Cap piercing technology is also available with some analyzers. Additional instrumentation and methods used in coagulation testing include aggregometers, platelet function analyzers, and thromboelastography. Automated POC and near-patient devices are also available for many coagulation tests including prothrombin time, activated partial thromboplastin time, and activated clotting time.

## Transfusion Medicine

Advances in laboratory automation have also impacted most areas of blood banking and transfusion medicine. Robust

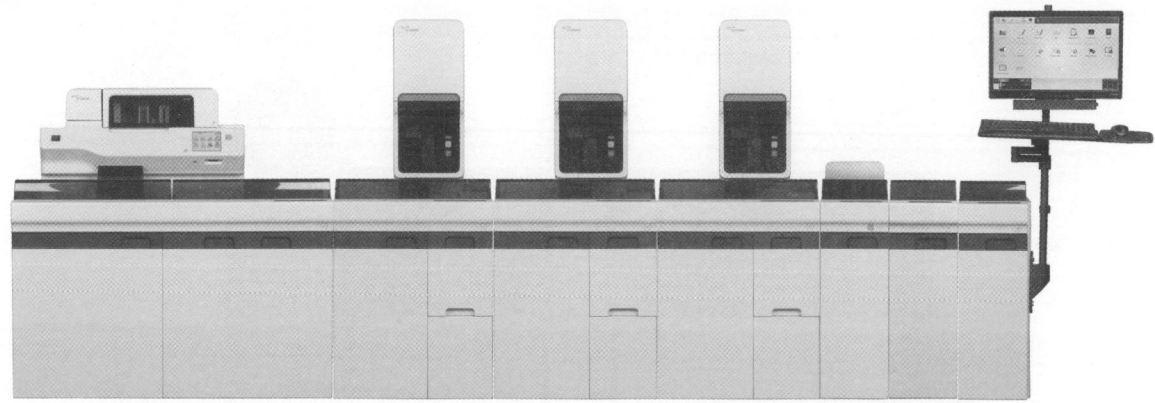

**Fig. 16.11** Example of an automated hematology system. A scalable Sysmex XN-9000 Automated Hematology System, including three XN-10 hematology test modules and one SP-10 module for slide making and staining *(left)*. (Courtesy Sysmex America, Inc., Lincolnshire, IL.)

information technology systems to track donor history, blood component traceability, barcoding, transfusion-transmissible diseases, immunohematological testing, inventory management, and component administration all work to improve the safety and traceability of transfused blood products. Automation at blood collection sites through apheresis donations helps to maximize the yield of specific blood component donations. Automated component processing systems at blood centers improve the efficiency of post-donation handling of blood products, thus enabling fresh components of blood products (with less chance of processing errors) to ultimately be distributed for transfusion.

Traditionally, immunohematological testing in the blood bank was conducted manually by RBC agglutination techniques in individual test tubes. Both small- and large-scale systems are now available to automate many of these techniques, including RBC typing (ABO, Rh), antigen typing, screening and identification of alloantibodies, direct antiglobulin testing (DAT), dilutions, titrations, reflex testing, and crossmatching of potential products for transfusion (Fig. 16.12). In general, automated blood bank systems are as reliable and sensitive as routine manual testing. Advantages include less opportunity for processing and transcription errors. The decision to automate immunohematology testing includes the same factors discussed previously in connection with adopting TLA, such as staffing and expertise, test volumes, variation in orders between day and night shifts, workflow considerations, and overall expense. Finally, RBC molecular typing (genotyping) may further refine how donor and recipient screening is automated within the blood bank.

## Microbiology

Clinical microbiology has recently undergone a transition toward far greater automation. Although standalone instrumentation for aseptic plate preparation, blood culture incubation and microbial detection, biochemical identification, and antimicrobial susceptibility have all been commercially available for years, much of the processing and interpretation steps within the microbiology workflow remained largely

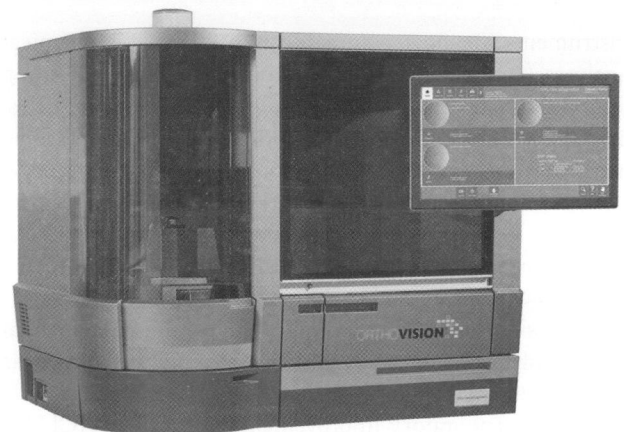

**Fig. 16.12** Example of an automated transfusion medicine analyzer. The ORTHO VISION Analyzer (Ortho Clinical Diagnostics) offers automated immunohematology testing. (Courtesy Ortho Clinical Diagnostics, Raritan, NJ.)

manual. Both standalone and TLA solutions are now available to automate many of these processes.

TLA microbiology solutions with tracking systems have been designed to handle preanalytical, analytical, and postanalytical steps (Fig. 16.13), and may include specimen decapping and recapping; Petri dish barcode labeling; plate inoculation and streaking; Gram stain preparation; automated incubation ($O_2$ and $CO_2$); high-resolution digital imaging of plates; and colony sampling for biochemical identification, antibiotic susceptibility testing, and seeding of plates for subsequent matrix-assisted laser desorption ionization time-of-flight (MALDI-TOF) mass spectrometric analysis. Organism identification by MALDI-TOF is a rapidly growing area of microbiology.

## Mass Spectrometry

Advances in MS are impacting all areas of laboratory diagnostics. These applications are therefore discussed in greater detail in Chapter 13. Although both the instrumentation and preanalytical processes have benefitted tremendously by automation, easy-to-operate MS modules that are more amenable

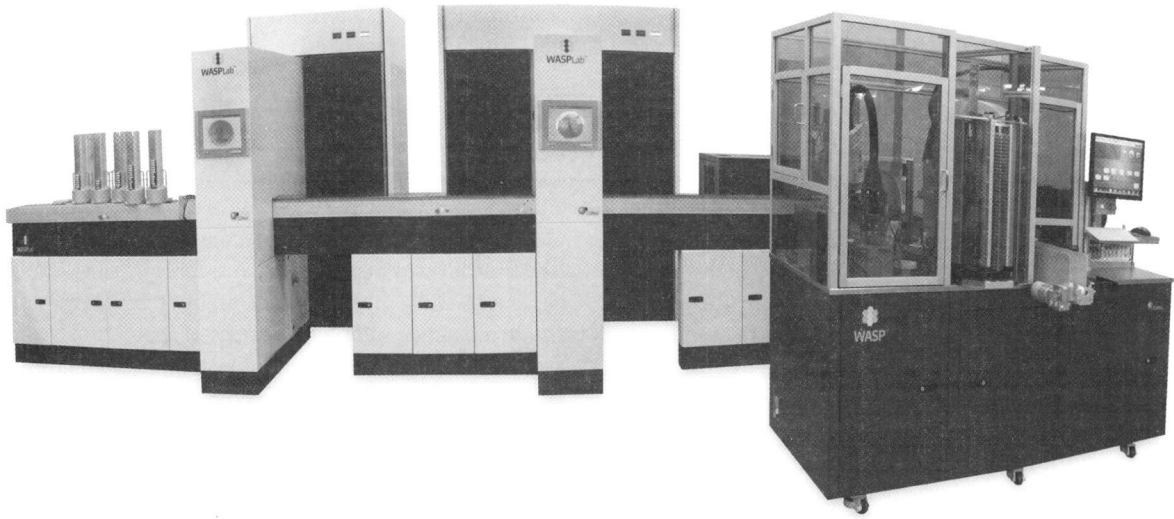

**Fig. 16.13** Example of an automated microbiology system. The WASPLab system (Copan) includes automated specimen processing, management, incubation, and digital imaging. (Courtesy Copan Diagnostics, Murrieta, CA.)

to TLA integration or moderate-complexity settings remain a challenge. Differences in preanalytical processes (e.g., extraction) may vary based on the analyte of interest and are one important barrier toward achieving TLA with MS systems.

## Molecular Diagnostics

Automation has been crucial for the expansion of molecular diagnostics into the clinical laboratory. Once a guaranteed money sink that only academic laboratories could afford, the realm of DNA and RNA analysis is now a cherished part of most laboratories, large or small. "Molecular diagnostics" has come to mean analysis of DNA or RNA, unfairly excluding proteins, electrolytes, small molecules, and other polymers.

Molecular diagnostics is a relatively new field, with the structure of DNA only described in 1953. Automation has had major impacts in (1) nucleic acid preparation, (2) liquid handling, (3) amplification, and (4) analysis of molecular diagnostic assays. Nucleic acid preparation typically involves (1) cell lysis, (2) separation from proteins, and (3) purification from interfering substances. Sample preparation instruments today often rely on reversible binding to silica-coated paramagnetic beads that can easily be washed to remove impurities. Most molecular methods require several mixing or transfer steps that can be automated by liquid handling. For example, PCR requires mixing reaction components together before thermal cycling. Although many components are common to all reactions and can be combined as a "master mix," template DNA and primers are unique and must be pipetted individually for each reaction. One common use for the Cartesian pipetting stations mentioned previously is to automate the setup of such reactions when large numbers of samples or assays need to be processed. Instead of onsite automation just before the assay, another alternative is to perform the automation well before the assay is performed. For example, primer plates can

be made, dried, and stored by a Cartesian automation station that patterns different primer pairs on a 96-well plate when multiple assays are performed together, greatly reducing the complexity for the medical laboratory scientist. Commercial vendors can provide one- or two-dimensional arrays of targets, including millions of hybridization targets on a chip for expression profiling, genotyping, or copy number assessment. The commercial use of automation can provide products to the laboratory that greatly reduce the complexity at the site where the assay is performed, albeit often with a loss in flexibility.

Although single-molecule techniques are now available, most molecular methods require target or signal amplification for visualization. For example, PCR requires repetitive temperature cycling of multiple reactions between two or three temperatures, a task begging for automation that has resulted in many different instruments. Isothermal methods of amplification were developed many years later and nicely match rapid, near-patient testing. Automated analysis of molecular assays can be as simple as viral or bacterial detection with self-contained rapid diagnostic kits, or as complicated as whole genome sequencing. Whole genome analysis is only possible because of the computer storage and computational speed enabled by modern computers.

### Sequencing Automation

Nucleic acid sequencing is a complicated multistep process, whether performed by conventional capillary electrophoresis or on modern massively parallel sequencers. Although some steps can be automated, sample preparation, data analysis, and clinical interpretation are manual in most clinical laboratories. Future progress toward automated integration of sample preparation and analysis into massively parallel sequencing is sure to come because of the promise and power of the technology.

## Polymerase Chain Reaction Automation

Polymerase chain reaction (PCR) was first automated before thermostable polymerases were available. Because the enzyme was inactivated in each cycle at the high temperatures needed for DNA denaturation, enzyme needed to be replenished in each cycle. Automation required not only temperature cycling but also the addition of reagents in each cycle. The combination of thermal control and repetitive reagent addition was complex and expensive. Although the liquid handling could be automated, it was made obsolete by the use of thermostable polymerases that could withstand the required DNA denaturation temperatures. A simple change in the process greatly simplified the automation requirements.

The thermal cycling provided by PCR instruments was at first slow, requiring 4 hours for amplification. Most common platforms used metal blocks that hold samples in tubes or plates that are convenient to handle, although circulating air or water systems allow better thermal control and faster cycling. Rapid-cycle PCR was developed in the early 1990s and reduced PCR amplification times down to 10 to 15 minutes. More recently, extreme PCR amplifies small products in as little as 15 seconds, indicating that the speed of PCR is limited by the instrumentation, not the biochemistry. Often, physical automation cannot keep up with the speed of molecular reactions.

## Real-Time PCR, Melting Analysis, and Digital PCR

Real-time PCR combines fluorimetry with thermal cycling, allowing fluorescence monitoring of double-stranded DNA production during PCR. Nucleic acid quantification, previously very difficult to obtain by PCR, is greatly simplified and used extensively for messenger RNA quantification and viral load assessment. Automated melting analysis and its more precise sibling, high-resolution DNA melting, have replaced manual gels in many applications and provide closed-tube genotyping, scanning, and relative quantification without probes. Digital PCR uses many small partitions that become either positive or negative, converting the analog signal of real-time PCR into a multitude of cells that are either "on" or "off." The partitioning and readout are automated.

## Throughput and Molecular Applications

*Throughput* is defined as the number of samples processed in a given period of time. Automation can improve throughput either by increasing the batch size of a run (the number of samples analyzed at once) or by decreasing the turnaround time (the time it takes to process each sample or run). Automation has successfully improved throughput by increasing batch size, from single samples, to strips of 8 or 12, to 96 and 384-well plates. Large automated molecular microbiology systems are used for infectious disease testing for HIV, hepatitis C virus, and several other major infections. Less emphasis has focused on decreasing turnaround time, although rapid (15–60 minutes) sample-to-answer systems for molecular targets are now approved by the Food and Drug Administration and some are CLIA waived. COVID-19 has emphasized the importance of rapid SARS-CoV-2 testing by both antigen and molecular means. Future developments in POC and at-home testing requiring simplicity and automation are sure to follow.

---

### POINTS TO REMEMBER

**Analytical Automation**
- Analytical automation has impacted all areas of laboratory medicine.
- Along with automating the testing phase, analyzers may incorporate specimen handling, reagent management, QC, and result review.
- Automated processes, including liquid-level sensing, clot detection, closed-container sampling, and instrument auto-dilution, help to improve the efficiency of laboratory testing.
- Analytical systems can be organized into clusters or TLA solutions, allowing operators to control multiple instruments.
- Analytical automation is increasing testing options and decreasing TAT in POC settings

---

## REVIEW QUESTIONS

1. Which type of specimen label has resulted in a reduction in preanalytical specimen identification errors and is used extensively in automated specimen identification?
   a. Social Security numbers stamped on all individual specimen containers
   b. Hospital identification numbers written on tubes of blood
   c. Labels containing barcodes that are unique identifiers
   d. Medical accounting numbers written on the lids of all containers
2. One serious issue with the use of accelerating/decelerating pneumatic tube systems to deliver specimens to the laboratory is the occurrence of:
   a. Clot formation
   b. Hemolysis
   c. Specimen breakage
   d. Specimen volume loss
3. Which of the following activities are important in the evaluation of the need for automation and in identifying the solution?
   a. Workflow mapping
   b. Plotting the volumes of arriving specimen by the hour of the day
   c. Vendor analyses and presentations of findings
   d. Visiting laboratories with installed systems and asking frank questions
   e. All of the above
4. The transport of a quantity of analyte or reagent from one specimen reaction into a subsequent one is referred to as:
   a. Batching
   b. Carryover

c. Misdelivery

d. Indiscrete handling

5. Which type of software would likely apply to the control of specimen routing/motion on a total laboratory automation (TLA) system?

 a. Laboratory automation system (LAS)

 b. Laboratory information system (LIS)

 c. Electronic health record (EHR)

d. Middleware

6. The greatest benefit of automation in terms of method performance relates to:

 a. Speed of throughput

 b. Reproducibility of process

 c. Detection of problematic specimens

 d. Reduction of cost

## SUGGESTED READINGS

Armbruster DA, Overcash DR, Reyes J. Clinical chemistry laboratory automation in the 21st century—amat victoria curam (victory loves careful preparation). *Clin Biochem Rev*. 2014;35(3):143–153.

Bailey AL, Ledeboer N, Burnham CD. Clinical microbiology is growing up: the total laboratory automation revolution. *Clin Chem*. 2019;65(5):634–643.

Boyd JC, Felder RA. Preanalytical automation in the clinical laboratory. In: Ward-Cook KM, Lehmann CA, Schoeff LE, et al., eds. *Clinical Diagnostic Technology: The Total Testing Process*. The Preanalytical Phase; Vol. 1. Washington, DC: AACC Press; 2002:107–129.

Dorak MT, ed. *Real-Time PCR*. New York: Taylor and Francis; 2006.

Farnsworth CW, Webber DM, Krekeler JA, et al. Parameters for validating a hospital pneumatic tube system. *Clin Chem*. 2019;65(5):694–702.

Genzen JR, Burnham CD, Felder RA, et al. Challenges and opportunities in implementing total laboratory automation. *Clin Chem*. 2018;64(2):259–264.

Hawker CD. Laboratory automation: total and subtotal. In: Friedberg RC, Weiss RL, eds. *Clinics in Laboratory Medicine*. Philadelphia, PA: Elsevier; 2007:749–770.

Hawker CD. Nonanalytic laboratory automation: a quarter century of progress. *Clin Chem*. 2017;63(6):1074–1082.

Hawker CD, Garr SB, Hamilton LT, et al. Automated transport and sorting system in a large reference laboratory. Part 1: evaluation of needs and alternatives and development of a plan. *Clin Chem*. 2002;48(10):1751–1760.

Hawker CD, Genzen JR, Wittwer CT. Automation in the clinical laboratory. In: Rifai N, Horvath AR, Wittwer CT, eds. *Tietz Textbook of Clinical Chemistry and Molecular Diagnostics*. Philadelphia, PA: Elsevier; 2018:370.e1–370.e24.

Landegren U, Kaiser R, Caskey T, et al. DNA Diagnostics—molecular techniques and automation. *Science*. 1988;242(4876):229–237.

Lyon E, Wittwer CT. LightCycler technology in molecular diagnostics. *J Mol Diagn*. 2009;11(2):93–101.

Melanson SEF, Lindeman NI, Jarolim P. Selecting automation for the clinical chemistry laboratory. *Arch Pathol Lab Med*. 2007;131(7):1063–1069.

Mullins GR, Harrison JH, Bruns DE. Smartphone monitoring of pneumatic tube system-induced sample hemolysis. *Clin Chim Acta*. 2016;462:1–5.

Smith LM, Sanders JZ, Kaiser RJ, et al. Fluorescence detection in automated DNA sequence analysis. *Nature*. 1986;321(6071):674–679.

Yu HE, Lanzoni H, Steffen T, et al. Improving laboratory processes with total laboratory automation. *Lab Med*. 2019;50(1):96–102.

# 17

# Point-of-Care Testing

*Ping Wang*

## OBJECTIVES

1. Define point-of-care testing (POCT) and other terms (e.g., near-patient testing, bedside testing) used to describe this process.
2. Describe the analytical requirements and technological considerations for POCT.
3. Describe examples of POCT devices.
4. Describe the relationship between informatics and POCT.
5. Describe key factors in the implementation and management of POCT programs.
6. Discuss types of evidence that can be used to demonstrate the effectiveness of POCT.

## KEY WORDS AND DEFINITIONS

**Accreditation** The formal recognition by an independent body that the process or service operates according to defined standards.

**Analyte** The substance that is to be measured (also known as a measurand).

**Aptamer** Short, single-stranded DNA or RNA molecules that can selectively bind to a target, such as proteins, peptides, carbohydrates, and small molecules.

**Audit** The examination of the quality of performance of a process measured against a predetermined standard.

**Connectivity** The property of a device that enables it to communicate with an information system (e.g., a laboratory information system) for the primary purposes of transmitting patient data and order information, and for monitoring the performance of the device.

**Effectiveness** Demonstrating through evidence that POCT brings benefits to patients and the overall clinical care process.

**Fluidics** Process by which liquid moves within a confined space, as in the case of a narrow channel or a porous matrix. Such processes include surface tension, diffusion, and the use of pumps.

**Informatics** The structure, creation, management, storage, retrieval, dissemination, transfer, and analysis of information.

**Operator interface** The part of a device that the operator is required to use in order for the device to work (e.g., a reader switch, a keypad for patient or sample identification, or calibration mechanism).

**Point-of-care testing (POCT)** A mode of testing in which the analysis is performed close to the patient rather than in a laboratory.

**Quality management** The act of overseeing all activities and tasks needed to maintain a desired level of excellence.

**Recognition element** A molecule that is used for the recognition (and sometimes capture) of the analyte of interest (e.g., enzyme, antibody, aptamer, nucleic acid, affinity ligand).

**Sensor** A device that receives and responds to a signal or stimulus. There are many examples in life, including the receptors of the tongue, the ear, and so on.

**Transducer** A substance or device that converts input energy in one form into output energy of another form.

**Point-of-care testing (POCT)** can be simply defined as "medical testing at the site of patient care" that therefore allows more rapid clinical decision-making with the possibility of improved health outcomes. Many other terms have been used to describe POCT, including "bedside," "near patient," "physician's office," "extra-laboratory," "decentralized," "off-site," "satellite," "kiosk," "ancillary," and "alternative site" testing. POCT also includes "self-testing," where the patients perform the tests themselves. Self-monitoring for blood glucose and prothrombin time or international normalized ratio (INR) together form the largest segment of the POCT market.

Advances in a range of technologies and manufacturing processes such as thin film sensors, semiconductor engineering, plastic molding, microfluidics, nanotechnology, and consumer electronics, make it possible to adapt many methods used in the laboratory to the point-of-care setting. In turn, these advances have now enabled healthcare providers and patients to make a choice about where testing is conducted (Box 17.1).

Clinical needs met by POCT can include more rapid clinical decision-making (especially in situations of clinical urgency), with the possibility of improved clinical outcomes. POCT can also reduce the complexity of the testing process—so-called process needs—which include improving the immediate patient/clinician/caregiver interaction, as well as expediting the patient journey, improving the patient's experience and patient empowerment, and decreasing healthcare resource utilization. The patient testing process is shown in

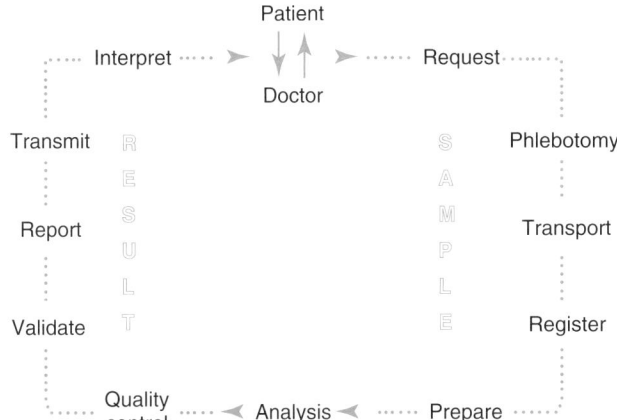

**Fig. 17.1** Schematic representation of the key steps in requesting, delivering, and using a diagnostic test result.

Fig. 17.1, while the advantages and disadvantages of POCT are summarized in Box 17.2.

## TECHNOLOGY

The technology used to measure analytes outside of the conventional laboratory setting has come about partly through the long-term trend of miniaturization—that is, reducing the size of electronic devices, as in the case of mobile phones. Advances in information and communication technologies have also played an important role. Starting with instruments to measure electrolytes, blood gases, and glucose, it is now possible to measure many other analytes using increasingly smaller devices. Accompanying the process of miniaturization has been the development of dry, stable reagents that can be incorporated in disposable unit-dose devices. While the throughput of tests for these devices is low (e.g., typically <10 samples per hour depending on test type), the time required to produce the results is usually short (e.g., may vary from

seconds for capillary blood glucose testing to minutes for immunoassay-based tests).

## Required Features of Point-of-Care Testing Devices

As with any device, it is important that designers first consider the needs of users, and these depend to some extent on the clinical setting or application. Some simply stated but critical requirements are as follows:

1. Devices should be simple to use.
2. Reagents and consumables must be robust over extended periods of time.
3. Results from POCT devices should be concordant with established laboratory methods, and the analytical quality of results should be appropriate to the intended clinical purpose.
4. The device together with its associated reagents and consumables must be safe to use.

Design criteria become more specific for particular clinical settings. For example, criteria exist for devices designed for use in the developing world for sexually transmitted infections (STIs), a major unmet medical need that is just beginning to be addressed effectively. Provided by the World Health Organization (WHO), the so-called ASSURED criteria are as follows:

- Affordable—for those at risk of infection
- Sensitive—minimal false negatives
- Specific—minimal false positives
- User-friendly—minimal steps to carry out test
- Rapid and robust—short turnaround time (TAT) and no need for refrigerated storage
- Equipment-free—no complex equipment
- Delivered—to end users

In addition, target product profile (TPP) (scope, performance, operational characteristics, and price) has been developed to guide and support the development of POCT

## TABLE 17.1   Classification of Types of Point-of-Care Testing Instruments

| POCT Class | Analytical Principles | Example Analytes |
|---|---|---|
| Small handheld, single use | Reflectance | Urine and blood chemistry |
| | Lateral-flow or flow-through immunoassays | Infectious disease agents, cardiac markers, human chorionic gonadotropin (hCG) |
| Small handheld, single use, with a monitoring device | Reflectance | Glucose |
| | Electrochemistry | Glucose |
| | Reflectance | Blood chemistry |
| | Light scattering, optical motion | Coagulation |
| | Lateral-flow, flow-through, or solid phase immunoassays | Cardiac markers, drugs, C-reactive protein (CRP), allergy, and fertility tests |
| | Immunoturbidimetry | HbA1C, urine albumin |
| | Spectrophotometry | Blood chemistry |
| | Electrochemistry | pH, blood gases, electrolytes, metabolites |
| | Fluorescence, electrochemistry with polymerase chain reaction (PCR) | Infectious agents |
| Larger cartridge-type and bench-top | Electrochemistry | pH, blood gases, electrolytes, metabolites |
| | Fluorescence | pH, blood gases, electrolytes, metabolites |
| | Multiwavelength spectrophotometry | Hemoglobin species, bilirubin |
| | Time-resolved fluorescence | Cardiac markers, drugs, CRP |
| | Electrical impedance | Complete blood count |
| | Polymerase chain reaction | Bacteria and viruses |

diagnostic tools of several infectious diseases such as tuberculosis and hepatitis C.

**Connectivity** to information systems, including the patient health record, is a growing requirement in modern healthcare systems.

A more recent design challenge is the need to simultaneously measure multiple analytes in the same cartridge—so-called multiplexing. The Piccolo chemistry analyzer (Abaxis, Union City, CA) and blood gas or critical care analyzers are examples of such technologies. The main benefit is the reduced overall time to result.

## Design

There is a great diversity of devices being used for POCT (Table 17.1), the majority relying on technologies devised more than two decades ago. Many of the devices use the same analytical principles as those found in conventional laboratory analyzers, but newer technologies are starting to appear, some of which will be described.

Irrespective of the type of technology, all POCT devices should have several key components, which include (1) the operator interface, (2) barcode identification systems, (3) sample and reagent delivery mechanisms, (4) reaction cell, (5) sensors, (6) control and communications systems, and (7) data management and storage. The main objectives of the design are to (1) enable the required reaction to take place that allows measurement of the analyte of interest, (2) ensure reliable and stable performance of the device over a period of time, and (3) minimize the risk of operator error.

### Operator Interface

The **operator interface** for a POCT device should (1) require minimal operator interaction; (2) guide the user through the operation; (3) indicate whether any key steps have failed; and (4) allow identification of the (A) operator, (B) patient, and (C) test to be measured.

Advances in information technology (IT) and electronics have had a major impact on this area. Types of user interfaces include (1) keypads, (2) barcode readers, (3) printers, and (4) touch screens.

### Barcode Identification Systems

Many POCT devices incorporate barcode reading systems for a number of purposes. These include (1) identifying the reagent package to the system—whether it be a single-use disposable or a multiuse reagent pack, (2) incorporating factory calibration data, and in some cases, (3) programming the instrument to process a particular test or group of tests. Some POCT devices use magnetic strips as a way of storing similar information, such as lot-specific calibration data. Other functions of the barcode reader include the capability to identify both the operator and the patient sample to the system.

### Sample Types and Sample Delivery

The vast majority of POCT devices use whole blood or urine specimens; in the case of blood, this commonly involves a capillary or finger-stick sample. In this way the sample can be introduced to the POCT device directly. Alternatively, a venous or arterial blood specimen can be collected and a small sample removed for POCT; in some cases the blood collection container can be inserted directly into the POCT instrument.

Sample access and delivery to the actual sensing component of the strip, cassette, cartridge, or fluidic cell are also key processes that are prone to error. Ideally, following the addition of the sample, there should be no further need for operator intervention. Devices are now available that minimize the degree of interaction to the point where a closed tube simply has to be placed in a holder and the instrument automatically performs all other functions.

## Reaction Cell

Where the analytical reaction takes place varies from a simple porous pad to a microfluidic cartridge, or surface within a cartridge. Advances in **fluidics** and fabricating techniques have been critical to the development of POCT devices. As analytical reactions have increased in complexity, more reaction cells/zones have been added. Thus, in the case of molecular tests, different reaction zones may be required for deoxyribonucleic acid (DNA) extraction, amplification, and probe detection. Another consideration in the design of reaction cells is to ensure that the requisite mixing of sample and reagents occur, which is critical when using very small volumes.

## Sensors

Much of the development focus in POCT devices is in **sensor** design of which there are various types. A chemosensor is one where the analyte has an intrinsic property, such as electrochemical, that enables it to be detected without a specific **recognition element**. More commonly, chemosensors used in many POCT devices have a transducing element such as a chemical indicator or binding molecule that recognizes the analyte to be measured and produces a signal, usually electrical or optical. A biosensor is distinguished from a chemosensor by having a biological or biochemical component as the recognition element. Enzymes are the most common biological elements used as recognition elements, followed by antibodies; transduction typically is via an optical or electrical signal, although there is now an increasing use of **aptamer** and nucleic acid recognition elements.

## Control and Communications Systems

In even the smallest device, there is a control subsystem that coordinates all the other systems and ensures that the required processes for an analysis take place in the correct order. Operations that require control include (1) insertion or removal of the strip, cartridge, cassette, or reagent; (2) temperature control; (3) sample injection or aspiration; (4) sample detection; (5) reagent addition—especially in a fluidic-based system; (6) mixing; (7) timing of the detection process; (8) detection of measurement signal; and (9) waste removal. Fluid movement is often accomplished by mechanical means through pumps or centrifugation, and by fluidic properties, such as surface tension; the latter is often a critical element in the design of simple strip tests and in microfabricated systems.

## Data Management and Storage

Information technology is crucial to POCT devices and may include rules-based assessment of internal quality control results, computing, and reporting of patient results. Increasingly devices use wireless technology for communication. These and other devices include communication protocols that allow data to be transferred to other data management systems, electronic medical records, and mobile computing devices.

## Types of Existing Point-of-Care Testing Technology

POCT devices can be classified into small, handheld devices that often use qualitative or quantitative reagent strips (or similar technology with a reading device), and larger, benchtop devices that are often variants of ones used in conventional laboratories. This classification is somewhat arbitrary since there is no sharp demarcation. There are gradations in both size and internal complexity of devices, although differentiation can sometimes be made on the need for external power. The clear trend is toward devices becoming smaller and with greater functionality.

### Small Handheld, Single Use Point-of-Care Testing Devices

Many POCT devices fall into this category, including (1) single- or multi-pad tests that are read visually, by reflectance photometry or electrochemically; (2) more complex pads that use light reflectance for measurement; and (3) fabricated cassettes or cartridges that incorporate methodologies such as immunochromatography and are used as immunosensors. All these devices are truly portable and for that reason their operational mode (i.e., proximity to the patient) differs from larger bench-top devices. For example, devices that require application of a whole blood sample such as glucose strips obviate the need for sample containers, labeling or transport, as compared with larger POCT instruments that may be some distance from the patient.

*Single- and multi-pad strip tests.* These are relatively simple in construction and are composed of a pad of porous material, such as cellulose, that is impregnated with reagent and then dried. Samples are added to the device either by dipping (e.g., in urine analysis) or by spotting (e.g., in blood glucose analysis). In the latter case, there has been a gradual transition from optical to electrochemical detection, avoiding the need to wipe the strip to remove surplus specimen prior to measurement. A critical operator factor when spotting the sample onto the pad is the need to cover the whole pad with the sample. In addition, because the reactions often do not proceed to completion, it is necessary for visually-read tests to be timed between placing the sample on the pad and comparing the resulting color to a color chart. More complex pads are composed of several layers, the uppermost of which is a semipermeable membrane that prevents cells from entering the matrix.

*ImmunoStrips.* These are biological sensors in which the recognition agent is an antibody that binds to the analyte. Detection of the binding event or signal **transducer** is usually via an optical mechanism, either reflectance or fluorescence spectrophotometry, although visual inspection has also been used. Immunosensors typically use solid phase technologies in conjunction with (1) flow-through, (2) lateral-flow, or (3) immunochromatography processes. In the flow-through format, a heterogeneous immunoassay takes place in a porous matrix that acts as the solid phase and requires an additional reagent to wash and separate bound and unbound label. In lateral flow, the separation stage takes place as the sample passes along the porous matrix, and no additional wash solution is required. In all these different formats, uniform and predictable flow of the sample through or along the solid phase matrix is a major determinant of the reproducibility of the technique.

In a typical example of an ImmunoStrip for cardiac troponin T (cTnT), the blood sample is added and first flows through a glass fiber fleece, which separates the plasma from whole blood. Simultaneously, two monoclonal antihuman cTnT antibodies, one conjugated to biotin and one labeled with gold particles as the signal antibody, bind to troponin T in the sample to form a sandwich complex. The antibody-troponin sandwich complex then flows in a lateral direction along the cellulose nitrate test strip until it reaches the capture zone, which contains streptavidin bound to a solid phase. The biotin in the antibody troponin complex binds to the streptavidin and immobilizes the complex. The complex is then visualized as a purple band by the gold particles attached to the signal antibody. The unreacted gold-labeled antibody moves farther down the strip, where it is captured by a zone containing a synthetic peptide consisting of the epitope of human cTnT and is visualized as a separate but similar colored band. The presence of this second band serves as an internal quality indicator because it shows that the sample has flowed along the test strip and the device has performed correctly.

While the majority of quantitative lateral flow immunoassay devices only measure a single analyte at a time, some can measure a panel of analytes, such as cardiac markers, fertility tests, and drugs of abuse.

### Small Handheld, Single Use Point-of-Care Testing Devices With a Monitoring Device

*Glucose Measurement.* In clinical practice, capillary glucose measurement is the most common POCT application. These devices are biosensors because they all use an enzyme as the recognition agent—glucose oxidase (GO), hexokinase (HK), or glucose dehydrogenase (GDH)—with photometric (reflectance) or, now increasingly, electrochemical detection.

Modern glucose strips use *thick-film* technology with several layers, each having a specific function. These are shown diagrammatically for a reflectance-based strip in Fig. 17.2. When blood is added to a strip, both water and glucose pass into the analytical layer. For some photometric systems, erythrocytes are excluded by a spreading or separating layer that contains various components, including glass fibers, fleeces, membranes, and special latex formulations. In photometric systems, a spreading layer is also important for the fast, homogeneous distribution of the sample. In contrast, electrochemical strips use systems that rely on capillary action to move the blood sample over the electrodes. The support layer is usually a thin plastic material that in the case of reflectance-based strips may also have reflective properties. Additional reflectance properties have been achieved through the inclusion of substances such as titanium oxide, barium sulphate, and zinc oxide.

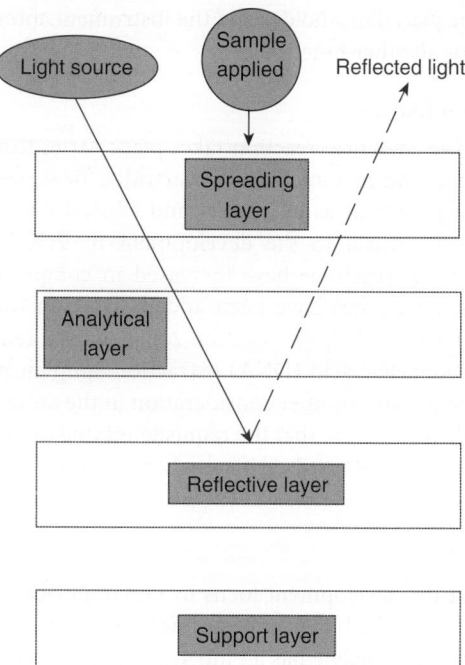

**Fig. 17.2** Schematic diagram of the components that make up a typical reflectance-based glucose strip.

Glucose strips are produced in large batches, and after extensive quality assurance procedures by the manufacturer, each batch is given a code that is stored in a magnetic strip on the underside of each test strip. This code describes the performance of the batch, including the calibrating relationship between the photometric or electrochemical signal and the concentration of glucose. More recently, electrochemical glucose strips that do not require coding have become more commonplace. These are composed of a silver-silver chloride (Ag-AgCl) reference electrode and a carbon-based active electrode, both manufactured using screen-printing technology with ferrocene or its derivatives contained in the printing ink. The conversion of glucose is accompanied by the reduction of ferrocene and the release of electrons. Continuing innovations have also facilitated the production of smaller meters, nonwipe strips, less need to clean instrument optics, more rapid results, and smaller sample volume requirements.

Although electrochemical systems have enabled the design of strips that are less subject to interferences, problems still persist. Strips that use GO are more substrate specific but are affected by oxygen tension, with high $PO_2$ values leading to falsely low results. Blood oxygen tension does not affect GDH based strips, and genetically engineered GDH are free from interference by maltose. Hematocrit is another important interference, the effects of which have been reduced in newer strip designs.

*INR Measurement.* Another common meter-type device used by patients at home and by healthcare professionals in clinics are those employed to monitor warfarin (Coumadin) therapy and measure prothrombin time (reported as INR levels). First devised some two decades ago, a number of different technologies have been developed to measure INR at

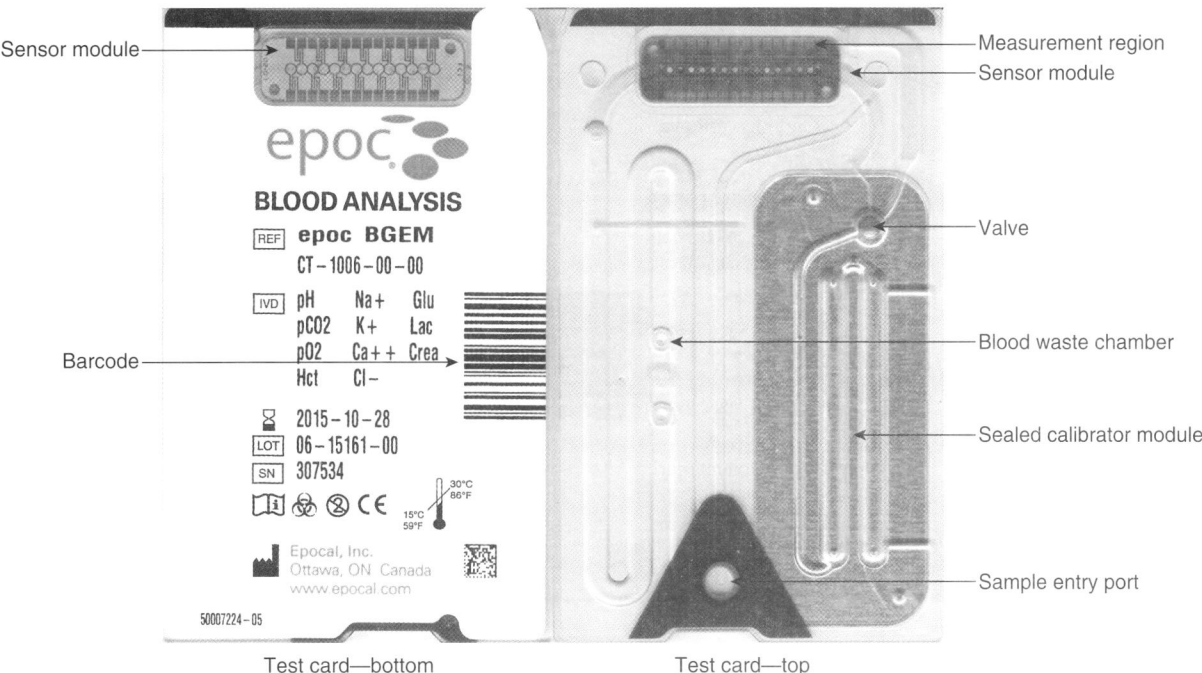

**Fig. 17.3** Epoc test card for blood gas analysis. (Courtesy Alere.)

the point of care, including optical and electrochemical detection. Innovation has been applied both to the strip, where a drop of blood is placed, and to the meter into which the strip is placed. In the HemoSense device (Alere, Waltham, MA), clotting is detected by change in impedance, while in a Roche device (Roche Diagnostics, Basel, Switzerland), a change in current is detected. Both devices incorporate quality control (QC) systems that are activated when a patient sample is placed on the strip. In the case of HemoSense, the strip has three channels: one for the patient test and the other two for different concentrations of internal QC material.

*Handheld integrated cartridge technology.* The prime example of this type of technology is the i-STAT analyzer (Abbott Point of Care, Princeton, NJ), a handheld device originally designed to measure blood gases but now with a considerably extended menu that includes electrolytes, glucose, creatinine, coagulation parameters, and cardiac markers. In contrast to the thick-film technology described above, the single-use sensors are constructed using *thin-film* technology. The latter involves microlithographic processes to deposit thin layers of 1 to 10 μm (as opposed to 10 to 50 μm layers in thick-film technology), similar to the construction of computer chips and other silicon-based devices. Each single use i-STAT cartridge contains an array of electrochemical sensors for a set of particular analytes, and it is operated in conjunction with a handheld reading device. Because the sensor layer is very thin, analytes permeate to this layer quickly, and the sensor cartridge, once it reaches room temperature (if it has been refrigerated), can be used immediately. This is an advantage over some thick-film sensors that require an equilibration or "wet-up" time before they are used.

A disadvantage of thin-film technology is that manufacturing costs are high due to the need for special clean air facilities. Thus, more recent technology to measure blood gases and related parameters utilizes less costly, so-called smart card technology. An example is the Epoc system (Siemens Healthineers, Ottawa, Canada), which is used in conjunction with a handheld analyzer to provide a range of critical care tests, including immunoassay measurement. Fig. 17.3 shows two views of the Epoc test card, which is manufactured on a 35 mm tape on reel format; on the right is the top view of the test card showing the sample entry port, the sealed calibrator reservoir, and the sensor module at the top; on the left is the bottom view of the card with the sensor module, where measurements take place, and below this are details of the test panel.

## Larger Cartridge Type and Bench-Top Point-of-Care Testing Devices

This section includes a wide range of devices that are all quantitative, not handheld but varying considerably in size. The smaller ones typically incorporate small, compact detectors, such as a charge-coupled device (CCD) camera that is a multichannel light detector, similar to a photomultiplier tube in a spectrophotometer. This type of technology enables quantitative measurements of lateral-flow immunoassay strips and is incorporated in the many different POCT devices available on the market.

*Cartridge-type devices.* A number of single-use, quantitative POCT devices are available that employ a cassette or cartridge rather than lateral-flow strips. Several cassette-based systems have been developed for the measurement of hemoglobin. In one such system, red cells are lysed in a mini-cuvette, hemoglobin is converted to methemoglobin, and the methemoglobin is measured at 570 nm; an additional measurement at 880 nm corrects for turbidity.

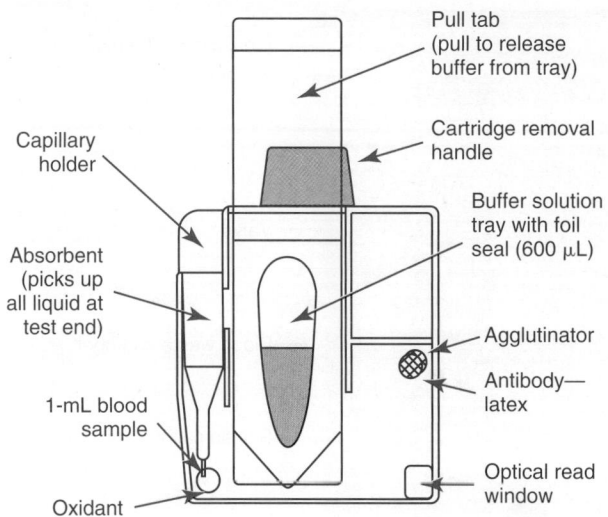

**Fig. 17.4** Schematic diagram of the Bayer DCA 2000 HbA1C immunoassay cartridge. (Courtesy Siemens Medical Diagnostics.)

Another type of cartridge design uses a light-scattering immunoassay to measure glycated hemoglobin, together with a photometric assay for total hemoglobin. The cartridge is a relatively complex structure that contains all the reagents required for the immunoassay, as well as lysing reagents and potassium ferricyanide reagent for measurement of total hemoglobin (Fig. 17.4). Agglutination takes place between the latex bound antibody and a synthetic polymer that contains the immunoreactive portion of HbA1C that leads to increased scattering of light. Addition of HbA1C in the patient sample reduces the agglutination by competing for the latex bound antibody, and the reduction in light scattering is proportional to the concentration of HbA1C. Measurement takes place when the cartridge is placed into a temperature-controlled reader, and the analytical performance of the Siemens DCA device (Siemens Healthineers, Munich, Germany) is sufficient for quantitative monitoring of glycemic control, and can also be used for measurement of urinary albumin and creatinine. Following placement into the instrument, the analysis proceeds without further involvement of the operator. The most recent of these types of instruments is also considerably smaller, and that trend is likely to continue.

*Multianalyte desktop analyzers.* A typical example of these is the Piccolo (Abaxis), which can measure a wider range of general chemistry analytes on a very small sample volume. Piccolo uses a small disposable rotor that contains all the required reagents and diluents to perform a battery of related tests such as liver function tests.

The Radiometer AQT90 (Radiometer Medical, DK-2700, Bronshoj, Denmark) bench-top, random access immunoassay analyzer utilizes a proprietary dry-chemistry concept and a detection method based on europium nonenhanced time-resolved fluorescence (TRF) technology. The europium-based chelates have certain natural advantages that allow sensitive and rapid detection methods. Analysis takes place in a small reagent cup on which are immobilized biotinylated capture antibodies, as well as streptavidin and europium-labeled tracer antibodies. Following addition of the patient sample and incubation, an antibody-antigen-antibody "sandwich" complex is formed, and after washing and drying, the europium response to excitation light is measured, the amount of which is directly proportional to the antigen present. The AQT90 also has a unique, walk-away, closed-tube sampling device from which the instrument dispenses a sample into a cup containing dried reagents including antibodies to the analytes of interest and europium lanthanide chelate as the signal reagent. The menu includes troponin, brain natriuretic peptide (BNP), D-dimer, beta human chorionic gonadotropin (hCG), and C-reactive protein (CRP).

*Critical care testing analyzers.* These remain the most commonly used type of POCT bench-top analyzers; the expanded menu of analytes allows use in many clinical areas. These devices use the same type of thick-film sensors or electrodes in strips, as described above, but in this case the sensors are reusable. They are manufactured from thick films of paste and inks using screen-printing techniques to produce individual or multiple sensors for metabolites, blood gases, and electrolytes. Further details of the analytical principles behind these sensor technologies can be found in Chapter 10 of this textbook. The sensors have been incorporated with reagents and calibrators into a single cartridge or pack, which is placed in the body of a small- to medium-sized, portable critical care analyzer. Each pack contains reagents sufficient to test a certain number of samples during a specific time period, after which it is relatively simple to replace. An example of such a device is the GEM Premier 5000 (Werfen—IL/Instrumentation Laboratory, Bedford, MA; Fig. 17.5).

Other key developments in critical care instruments include liquid calibration systems that use a combination of aqueous base solutions and conductance measurements to calibrate the pH and $PCO_2$ electrodes, with oxygen being calibrated with an oxygen-free solution and room air. In addition, automated QC packages are integrated into these instruments to ensure that QC samples are analyzed at regular intervals. These comprise packs or bottles of QC material that are contained within the instrument and sampled at predetermined intervals with on-board software, interpreting the results and generating alerts, if necessary. Box 17.3 shows the various features that are incorporated into a critical care analyzer that contribute to its ease of use and reduce the potential for errors.

*Hematologic and immunologic analyzers.* Small bench-top devices are now available to perform hematologic and immunologic analysis at point of care. Again, they are often scaled-down versions of laboratory instruments but have been reduced in complexity, thus reducing the risk of operator error by nontechnically trained staff. The range of hematology instruments includes those that measure just hemoglobin and white cell counts to the Sysmex pocH-100i (Sysmex, Lincolnshire, IL), which can measure up to 17 parameters.

Another relatively new product is the PIMA flow cytometer device (Abbott Point of Care) that can be used for measurement of T-helper cells, or CD4 counts. The PIMA uses the same imaging and cell counting technology

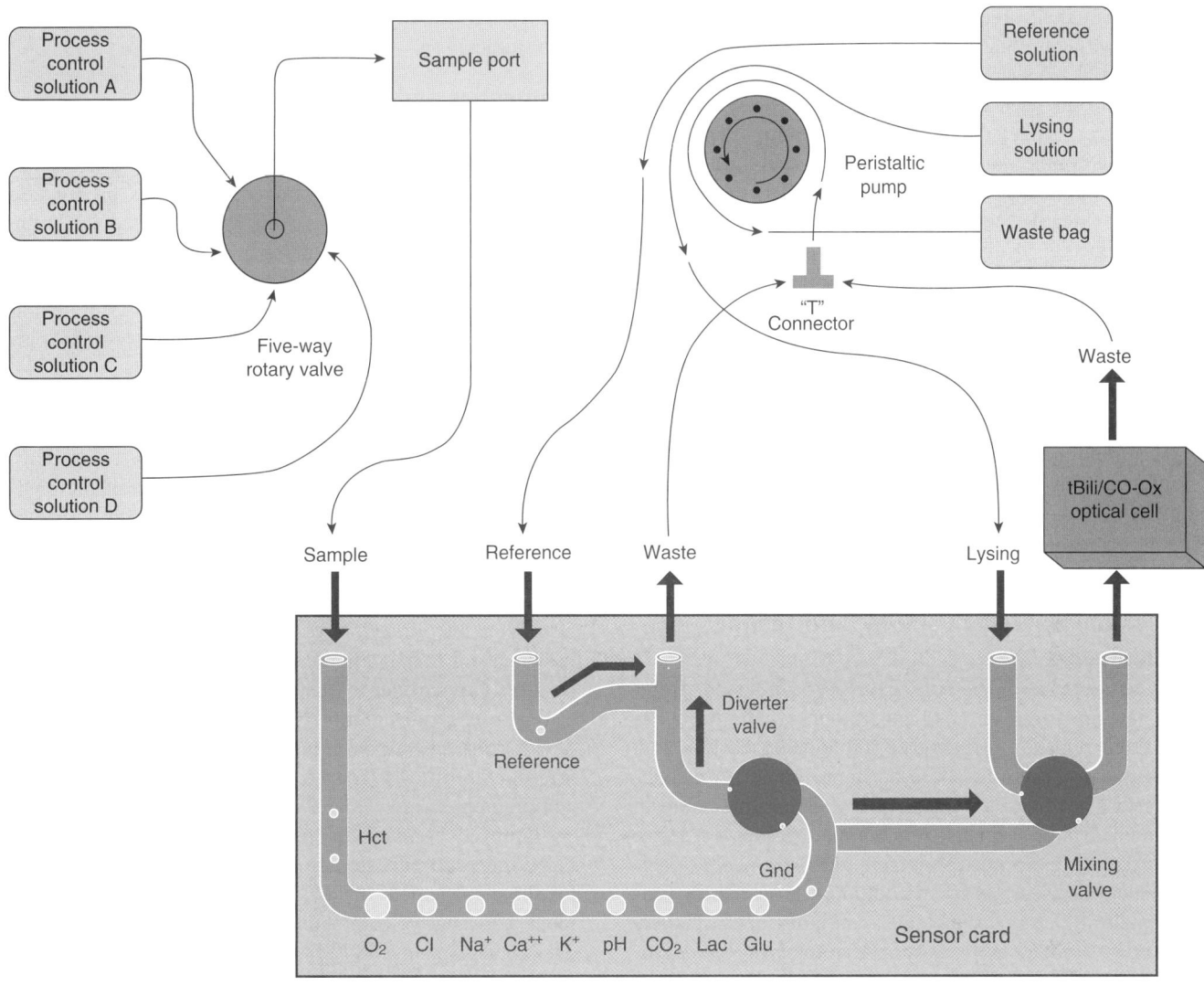

**Fig. 17.5** Schematic diagram of the components and patient sample fluidic pathways of the GEM Premier 3000 critical care analyzer. (Courtesy Instrumentation Laboratory.)

---

### BOX 17.3 Features of Critical Care Analyzers That Contribute to Ease-of-Use and Reduce the Risk of Errors

Long-life, maintenance-free electrodes or disposable sensor packs
Touch screens as the user interface
Software that can demand user and patient identification
Built-in barcode scanners
Sample aspiration instead of injection
Reduced sample sizes
Clot detection within analysis chamber
Sample detection to prevent short samples
Liquid calibration systems instead of gas bottles
Automated calibrations
Automated quality control sampling
Sophisticated QC programs including interpretation of data
Connectivity to information systems allowing remote monitoring and control
Built-in videos for training purposes

---

employed in laboratory instruments but redesigned into a smaller, more compact instrument, which is simple to operate. Following mixing of the sample with the reagents and incubation, fluorescence is measured in the stained sample by a CCD camera and the results are displayed on the screen.

## Molecular Diagnostic Analyzers

The so-called Lab on a Chip (LOC) concept has been translated into devices for targeted measurement of nucleic acids at the point-of-care, particularly for detection of infectious agents. LOC devices have grown from the microelectronics industry through techniques of miniaturization and microfabrication, incorporate features such as microfilters, microchannels, microarrays, micropumps, microvalves, and bioelectronic chips, and perform analysis at microscopic scales (i.e., 1 to 500 μm). One such LOC device is the Cepheid GeneXpert system (Cepheid, Sunnyvale, CA). This bench-top device can perform real-time quantitative polymerase chain reaction (PCR) in approximately 90 minutes with minimal operator interaction, thus enabling the potential to perform rapid molecular testing in situations where the need for results is urgent. The system uses single-use cartridges that each contain multiple chambers to hold the sample, various purification and elution buffers, and all the PCR reagents, including enzymes; in addition, all waste is retained within the cartridge. Through a series of valves in the syringe, the sample is moved through the various stages of the PCR process using the reagents stored in the cartridge, and culminating in real-time detection of the amplified products. Due to the sensitivity conferred by nucleic acid amplification, molecular diagnostic analyzers are able to overcome the limited sensitivity of traditional lateral flow assays, which is an advantage for some clinical applications, including infectious disease detection. As an example, such molecular diagnostic devices with relatively short turn-around-times have been used extensively in the testing of respiratory pathogens such as SARS-CoV-2 and influenza.

## Newer and Emerging Point-of-Care Testing Technologies

Many of the technologies that have been discussed earlier were devised several decades ago. The intervening time has seen them refined and packaged into smaller devices and, in many cases, there has been an improvement in analytical performance and a reduced risk of error. That trend in incremental improvements will continue because no device is risk free, and, in some cases, there remains a need for better analytical performance. In addition, the search for fundamentally different technologies continues because there are known limitations to existing technologies. For example, lateral flow strip technology continues to dominate the POCT market, but lateral flow strips have a number of limitations, including inadequate sensitivity and difficulty with multiplexing (measurement of more than two or three analytes on the same strip). Some emerging and growing POCT technologies encompass innovations across multiple aspects, including specimen types and acquisition methods, testing methods, fabrication, detection technologies, connectivity and integration of analyzers, choice of materials, data processing methods, and testing menu. The overall trend of the innovations in the POCT field is to facilitate more convenient, accurate, and cost-efficient measurement of a broader range of analytes near the patient. Another notable trend is to transition from in vitro and snapshot-based analysis to more continuous and real-time monitoring. Continuous glucose monitoring systems are already available, in which glucose measurements performed on interstitial fluid are fed back to a monitor linked to an insulin pump. Contact lens sensors that detect glucose in tears have also been described, and other promising technologies include tattoo-based sensors and smart holograms. Clearly, changes in analyte concentrations may vary in different body fluid compartments, so this will have to be taken into account when designing and developing

analytical technologies, as well as performing clinical validation studies.

## Informatics and Point-of-Care Testing

Most analytical devices used in clinical laboratories are directly linked or connected via an electronic interface to a laboratory information system (LIS). In this progression, many different informatics functions are used, including the electronic transfer of data from the analyzers to the LIS and ultimately into a patient's electronic medical record. This provides healthcare professionals with quick, accurate, and appropriate access to the patient's medical history and clinical information.

Considerable effort has been expended to incorporate these same processes into POCT devices because of the vital importance of capturing analytical data in a patient's medical record in order to avoid the errors associated with manual transcription of data. Thus, newer POCT devices have addressed this problem by incorporating the prerequisite hardware and software into their design, and in the last decade so-called connectivity standards have also been introduced, which facilitate linking devices to information management systems. Adherence to these connectivity standards ensures that POCT devices meet critical user requirements, such as (1) bi-directionality, (2) device connection commonality, (3) commercial software interoperability, (4) security, and (5) QC and/or regulatory compliance.

Improved connectivity has enabled two major trends. First, and primarily due to demand from those responsible for the management of POCT, there has been the development of a range of commercial and specialized products for data management of POCT results with software devoted to ensuring compliance with procedures and managing data. These systems offer a range of features and benefits that include the ability of central laboratories to both monitor and remotely control their instruments in locations outside of the main laboratory.

The second trend is that connectivity standards, together with less expensive network technology and widespread access to the internet and smart mobile phones, have provided the capability to establish POCT networks across major secondary and tertiary care institutions and, perhaps more importantly, in the community or primary care where POCT has the potential to make a much bigger impact than in the hospital setting. The structure of such a typical community POCT network is shown in Fig. 17.6.

The most important benefit of connectivity remains that of facilitating the transfer and capture of patient POCT and quality-related data into permanent medical records. Additional benefits include that of providing alerts of abnormal results, particularly those that may be critical. However, the increasing ability to interface devices more easily to other information systems should also enable the development of applications, which add value to patient data such as the use of decision support software to assist with interpretation and

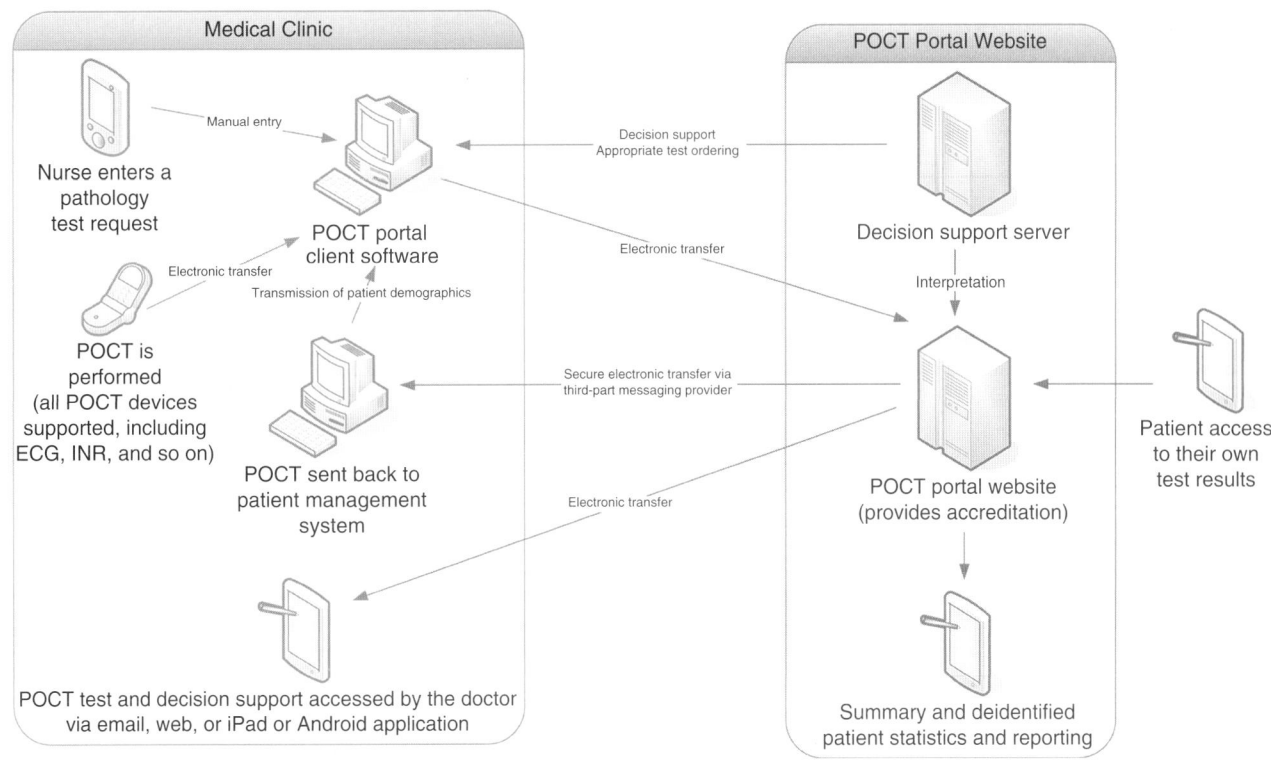

**Fig. 17.6** Schematic diagram of a point-of-care testing (POCT) network showing the relationships between the user, POCT device, other health information systems, and the patient's caregiver. *INR*, International normalized ratio. (Courtesy R. Tirimacco, ICCNET.)

clinical decision-making. One such example is the use of dosing software in combination with POCT INR measurements to manage warfarin treatment.

---

**POINTS TO REMEMBER**

**Point-of-Care Testing Technology**
- POCT devices need to be simple to use, and the reagents and consumables need to be robust over extended periods of time.
- Analytical results need to have an analytical quality appropriate for the clinical requirement.
- Glucose strips and lateral flow immunosensors remain the most common type of POCT technology.
- Newer technologies and POCT molecular techniques are now emerging.
- All devices should either have a means of data storage or be interfaced to an information system so that data can be stored, transmitted, and recalled.

---

## QUALITY MANAGEMENT

Management and maintenance of a POCT service requires planning, oversight, inventory control, and assurance of the reliability of test results through adequate training and QC. Several guidelines document these requirements, based on the ISO standard 22870 ("Point-of-Care Testing [POCT]—Requirements for Quality and Competence"), and are available from various professional laboratory organizations.

### Establishment of Need

The decision to implement a POCT service requires (1) establishment of the unmet need, (clinical, operational, or economic); (2) critical appraisal of the evidence supporting the claimed clinical, operational, and economic benefits; and (3) examination of the costs and changes in the clinical process involved. Addressing the questions listed in Box 17.4 is useful for establishing the requirement for a POCT service.

When organizing and implementing a POCT service, it is important to consult with all the stakeholders, by establishing a POCT coordinating committee. Membership should include representatives of those who use the service and those who deliver the service, together with a representative of the organization's management team. The users may include (1) physicians, (2) physician assistants, (3) family nurse practitioners, (4) nurses, (5) other health care providers, and (6) patients. Typically, a laboratory professional will chair such a committee, and it is also recommended that the committee report to the medical director of the hospital or other care provider organization. The work of the committee should be governed by the organization's policy on POCT.

### Point-of-Care Testing Policy and Accountability

Implementation of a POCT service requires a POCT policy that establishes all of the procedures required to ensure the

### BOX 17.4    Assessing the Need for a Point-of-Care Testing Service

Which tests are required?
What is the desired turnaround time?
What clinical question is being asked when requesting this test?
What clinical decision is likely to be made upon receipt of the result?
What action is likely to be taken upon receipt of the result?
What outcome should be expected from the action taken?
Why isn't the laboratory able to deliver the required service?
Will point-of-care testing (POCT) provide the required accuracy and precision of result?
Are there staff available to perform the test?
Are there adequate facilities to perform the test and store the equipment and reagents?
Will you abide by the organization's POCT policy?
Are there operational benefits to this POCT strategy?
Are there economic benefits to this POCT strategy?
Will a change in practice be required to deliver these benefits?
Is it feasible to deliver the change in practices that might be required?

### BOX 17.5    Elements of a Point-of-Care Testing Policy

**General Information**
- Approved by
- Original distribution
- Related policies
- Further information
- Replacement of previous policies

**Introduction**
- Background
- Definitions
- Accreditation of services
- Audit of services

**Laboratory Services in the Organization**
- Locations
- Logistics
- Policy on diagnostic testing

**POCT Committee and Accountability**
- Officers
- Committee members
- Terms of reference
- Responsibilities
- Meetings

**Equipment and Consumable Procurement**
- Criteria for procurement
- Process of procurement

**Standard Operating Procedures**
- Training
- Certification
- Recertification

**Quality Control and Quality Assurance**
- Procedures
- Documentation and review

**Health and Safety Procedures**
**Bibliography**

*POCT,* Point-of-care testing.

delivery of a high-quality service, together with the responsibility and accountability of all staff associated with the POCT. This may be (1) part of the organization's total **quality management** system, or (2) part of its clinical governance policy, and will be required for **accreditation** purposes. The elements of a POCT policy are listed in Box 17.5.

## Equipment Procurement and Evaluation

After identifying a requirement for POCT, developing a POCT policy, and establishing a coordinating committee, the next stage in the process is equipment procurement. This involves identifying candidate POCT equipment having the prerequisite analytical and operational capabilities to meet the clinical requirements of the POCT service. A CLSI protocol (Clinical Laboratory Standards Institute, Document POCT09-P. Selection Criteria for Point of Care Testing Devices) describes the features of the evaluation process, and further guidance can be sought from other evaluations described in the literature. In addition, the educational and certification requirements of the device operator also have to be identified, and the potential for operator error determined. Independent validation of these analytical and operational characteristics is obtained from (1) the manufacturer, (2) published evaluations performed by government agencies, (3) reports in the peer-reviewed literature, and (4) discussions with colleagues.

## Training, Competency, and Certification

Many of the agencies involved in the regulation of healthcare delivery now require that all personnel associated with the delivery of diagnostic test results demonstrate their competence, and this applies equally to operators of POCT equipment. The elements of a training program are listed in Box 17.6. Clearly the extent of this program will, to a certain extent, depend on how well the complexity of the analytical

method has been engineered to minimize operator requirements. In practice, such a program is tailored to meet the needs of the individual and the organization.

Training may include formal presentations, self-directed learning, or computer-aided learning. It is important to document the satisfactory completion of training, and that the individual has been tested and found competent, with a combination of questions probing the understanding and practical demonstration of the skills gained. The latter is achieved by performing tests on a series of QC materials and repeat testing of patient samples that have recently been analyzed in the laboratory or on another device—so-called parallel testing.

Competence on a long-term basis is maintained through regular practice of skills and continuing education, and it is important to build these features into any POCT program.

Regular review of performance in QC and quality assurance programs will provide a means of overseeing the competence of operators. The error log may also highlight when problems are arising. However, it is important to encourage an open approach to the assessment of competence so that operators themselves seek help if they believe that problems are occurring.

## Quality Control, Quality Assurance, and Audit

Quality control, external quality assurance (EQA), or proficiency programs and **audits** provide a formal means of monitoring the quality of a service. The QC program gives a relatively short-term view and typically compares the current performance of a device with prior analyses. EQA is a more comprehensive process that includes comparing testing performance of different sites and/or different pieces of equipment or methods. Audit measures the performance of all aspects of the testing process against predetermined standards. However, the foundation to ensuring good quality remains a successful training and competency scheme.

Classically, quantitative QC involves the analysis of a sample for which the analyte concentration is known, and the mean and range of acceptable results is quoted for the method used. There are several challenges to the classical approach with POCT. The first concern is the frequency of testing—should a QC sample be analyzed every time that (1) a sample is analyzed, (2) a new operator uses the system, (3) a new lot number of reagents is used, or (4) the system is recalibrated? There is no consistent agreement on the correct approach, and one probably has to be guided by the reproducibility and overall analytical performance of the system, but it should never be less than what is recommended by

the manufacturer or what is necessary to meet regulatory requirements.

For single-use POCT disposable devices, the above strategy does not completely monitor the quality of the test system. For example, when conventional QC material is analyzed on a unit-use or single-test POCT system, only that testing unit is monitored. Under these circumstances, there is greater dependence placed on the manufacturing reproducibility of the devices to ensure a good quality service.

There are also other QC approaches, but many do not test the whole process. For example, the use of a plastic surrogate reflectance pad as a QC sample will only test the performance of the reflectance meter and so on. Similarly, some forms of electronic internal QC also do not test the sampling technique, but simply the functionality of the cassette and the associated reader. As with conventional QC, any electronic process checks should not be less than those recommended by the manufacturer.

EQA, or proficiency testing, is a systematic approach to QC monitoring in which samples are analyzed by one or more laboratories to determine the capability of each participant. In this approach, the operator has no knowledge of the analyte concentration, and therefore it is considered closer to a "real testing situation." The results are transmitted to a central authority, which then prepares a report and returns a copy to each participating laboratory. More details of quality management as applied to POCT can be found in Chapter 7 of this textbook.

## Maintenance and Inventory Control

The implementation and maintenance of a POCT service require that a supply of devices and associated consumables be maintained at all times and that a formal program for doing so is employed. The key points in this process are to (1) adhere to the recommended storage conditions, (2) be aware of the stated shelf life of the consumables, and (3) ensure that stocks are released in time for any preanalytical preparation to be accommodated (e.g., thawing).

Clear guidelines should be available from the manufacturer and should be adhered to rigorously. Issues that usually require particular vigilance include expiration dates, biocontamination, electrical safety, maintenance of optics, and inadvertent use of inappropriate consumables.

## Documentation

It is critically important to keep an accurate record of the (1) test request, (2) result, and (3) action taken, in the medical record. Some of the issues concerning documentation are now being resolved with the advent of the patient electronic record, electronic requesting, and better connectivity of POCT instrumentation to information systems and the patient record.

## Accreditation and Regulation of Point-of-Care Testing

Regulatory and/or accrediting bodies of medical laboratories generally require compliance to minimum standards,

**TABLE 17.2  Outcome Measures That Can Be Used to Assess Point-of-Care Testing Technologies**

| OUTCOME MEASURE | | | |
| Clinical | Process | Application | Test |
| --- | --- | --- | --- |
| Reduce antibiotic use | Reduce the need for laboratory tests | Rule out UTI | Urinalysis |
| Early detection of renal disease | Advise the patient at the clinic visit | Rule out albuminuria | Urine albumin: creatinine ratio |
| Faster and earlier diagnosis | Reduced clinic visits Use of echocardiography | Rule out heart failure | Natriuretic peptide |
| Reduced complication rate | Reduced nonattendance at the clinic Reduced clinic visits | Screening for infection | *Chlamydia* |
| Increased period within the therapeutic window Reduced complication rate | Reduced clinic visits Reduced hospitalization | Self-monitoring Self-dose adjustment | INR |
| Improved glycemic control indicated by HbA1C | Reduced clinic visits | Primary care management of diabetes | HbA1C in primary care |
| Faster triage to therapeutic intervention | Reduced length of stay in ED | Rule out acute coronary syndrome | Troponin I or T in ED |
| Faster diagnosis and treatment | Reduced clinic visits | Rule out DVT | D-dimer in primary care |

*DVT*, Deep venous thrombosis; *ED*, emergency department; *INR*, international normalized ratio; *UTI*, urinary tract infection.

and this applies equally to POCT services. Thus, the Clinical Laboratory Improvement Amendments of 1988 (CLIA) legislation in the United States stipulates that all POCT must meet certain minimum standards. In the United States, the Centers for Medicare and Medicaid Services, the Joint Commission on Accreditation of Healthcare Organizations, and the College of American Pathologists are among those responsible for inspecting sites, and each is committed to ensuring compliance with testing regulations for POCT.

---

**POINTS TO REMEMBER**

**Quality Management**
- Any point-of-care testing (POCT) service should be based on satisfying a documented clinical or operational need.
- A POCT policy agreed by all stakeholders should determine how the service is run within an institution.
- All POCT equipment should be evaluated by those responsible for the service.
- Training and assessment of competency of POCT users is essential since many will not be trained in laboratory science.
- POCT needs to be accredited to the same levels as the laboratory.

---

# EVIDENCE OF EFFECTIVENESS

The objective of employing POCT is to enable clinical decisions to be made at the time of the consultation with the patient, where the decisions may relate to screening, diagnosis, treatment, or monitoring. The outcomes of these decisions should lead to clinical, operational, and/

or economic benefits if implementation is to be considered. Typically, those involved in the management decisions to implement POCT will look for evidence of clinical and cost **effectiveness**; those involved in implementation will, in addition, look for evidence of operational effectiveness, as that evidence will inform the implementation plan. It follows therefore that the evidence of effectiveness is employed in business cases proposing the adoption of POCT, and that it informs the implementation plan. The needs of all stakeholders involved in delivering the care package must be addressed. This can be challenging, as stakeholder perspectives may differ across a care pathway, for example, the current desire to shift care closer to home may have an adverse impact on the revenue received by the hospital.

## Clinical Effectiveness

The core outcome measures of clinical effectiveness are mortality and morbidity. Surrogate or intermediate outcome measures are generally used for evidence of effectiveness in both the generation of evidence, as well as in performance management and audit. Some examples of outcome measures are given in Table 17.2. The generation of evidence of clinical effectiveness in the field of diagnostics including POCT is challenging, primarily because (1) the timely delivery of a result in itself does not lead to improved outcomes (i.e., outcomes are dependent on the clinical management decision based on the test result), (2) variability can occur with both the decisions made and the action taken on receipt of the result, and (3) it is difficult to design studies that minimize the generally accepted risks of introducing bias (e.g., operator bias; see Chapter 2).

Examples of tests where there is good evidence for the clinical effectiveness of POCT include (1) rapid diagnosis of *Chlamydia* infection, (2) managing warfarin treatment with INR self-monitoring, (3) ruling out a diagnosis of deep vein thrombosis, and (4) managing patients with diabetes using HbA1C.

## Cost-Effectiveness

Economic assessment is becoming more important because of the growing debate around "value-for-money" in health care, and consequently healthcare economics is seen as an integral part of evidence-based practice. An economic assessment of POCT should ask the question: What are the complete consequences and costs of using POCT compared with testing done in the laboratory? The consequences would include any operational changes involved with introducing POCT—particularly in the clinical setting, in addition to the impact on clinical outcomes. The reality is that relatively few economic assessments have been conducted in this way for laboratory tests and even fewer for POCT.

Instead of robust economic studies, there has been a focus in the past on simplistic comparisons of the cost of POCT technology to that used in the central laboratory without any consideration of the patient outcomes from using the tests. Thus, many studies in the literature are of the cost minimization type and not surprisingly have shown that POCT is more expensive than the central laboratory, where economies of scale can deliver obvious efficiencies. However, this situation is changing to one that moves beyond a comparison of testing costs to one that includes assessment of the complete process of patient care and identification of the economic outcomes that can be achieved with POCT. Some of the economic benefits may result from a clinical impact upon the patient, but others may be operational benefits such as more rapid treatment, or reduction in length of stay.

> ## POINTS TO REMEMBER
>
> ### Effectiveness of Point-of-Care Testing
> - Point-of-care testing (POCT) may offer increased operational efficiency, for example, more rapid patient triage in an emergency department.
> - POCT may be associated with improved clinical outcomes, for example, reduced morbidity and mortality for home INR monitoring of Coumadin treatment.
> - POCT may offer increased patient accessibility and convenience, for example, testing and treatment in one visit for sexually transmitted infections.

Consideration of cost-effectiveness must examine the impact of POCT on the entire care pathway, including patient outcomes.

## REVIEW QUESTIONS

1. Which of the following statements best describes the value of point-of-care testing (POCT) compared to standard laboratory testing?
   a. More accurate results
   b. Lower reagent costs per test
   c. Testing that enables the clinician or caregiver to make a decision at the point-of-care
   d. Better quality control

2. The benefits of using POCT are best assessed by:
   a. comparing the analytical results of the device with those obtained by the central laboratory.
   b. performing a study of clinical and cost effectiveness.
   c. assessing the performance of the device in an external quality assurance program.
   d. asking the patients what they think.

3. The technical performance of a POCT device is best assessed by:
   a. comparing the results obtained by the person(s) who will be operating the device in the intended setting.
   b. reviewing the manufacturer's literature.
   c. testing the device in the laboratory.
   d. looking for information on the Internet.

4. Quality control of POCT for lateral flow strips read with a reflectance meter is best achieved by:
   a. analysis of a designated QC specimen on at least one occasion in each shift.
   b. use of the reflectance control strip supplied by the manufacturer.
   c. comparison of analysis of a specimen using the POCT with the results from sending the same specimen to the laboratory.
   d. analysis of an aqueous solution prepared for the purpose.
   e. reliance on the manufacturer to provide a quality control product.

5. The first step to be considered in the implementation of a POCT solution is:
   a. the analytical imprecision of the POCT device.
   b. the analytical bias of the POCT device.
   c. the unmet clinical need.
   d. the cost of each test.

## SUGGESTED READINGS

Adams EJ, Ehrlich A, Turner KM, et al. Mapping patient pathways and estimating resource use for point of care versus standard testing and treatment of Chlamydia and gonorrhoea in genitourinary medicine clinics in the UK. *BMJ Open*. 2014;4:e005322.

Attia UM, Marson S, Alcock JR. Micro-injection molding of polymer microfluid devices. *Microfluid Nanofluid*. 2009;7:1–29.

Clinical Laboratory Standards Institute. *Clinical Laboratory Standards Institute. Point-of-Care Connectivity: Approved Standard—Second Edition. CLSI Document POCT01–A2*. Wayne, PA: CLSI; 2006.

International Organization for Standardization. ISO 22870:2006. *Point-of-Care Testing (POCT) Requirements for Quality and Competence. Clinical Laboratory Standards Institute. Selection Criteria for Point of Care Testing Devices, CLSI Document POCT09-P.* Wayne, PA: CLSI; 2009.

International Organization for Standardization. ISO 22870:2016. Point-of-care testing (POCT)—Requirements for quality and competence; 2016. https://www.iso.org/standard/71119.html. Accessed June 2022.

Kost GJ, ed. *Principles and Practice of Point-of-Care Testing.* Philadelphia, PA: Lippincott Williams & Wilkins; 2002.

Oliver NS, Toumazou C, Cass AE, et al. Glucose sensors: a review of current and emerging technology. *Diabet Med.* 2009;26:197–210.

Peeling RW, Holmes KK, Mabey D, et al. Rapid tests for sexually transmitted infections (STIs): the way forward. *Sex Transm Infect.* 2006;82(suppl 5):v1–v6.

Posthuma-Trumpie GA, Korf J, van Amerongen A. Lateral flow (immuno)assay: its strengths, weaknesses, opportunities and threats. A literature survey. *Analyt Bioanalyt Chem.* 2009;393:569–582.

Price CP, St John A. *Point-of-Care Testing. Making Innovation Work for Patient-Centred Care.* Washington, DC: AACC Press; 2012.

Price CP, St John A, Kricka LJ, eds. *Point-of-Care Testing Needs, Opportunities and Innovation.* 3rd ed. Washington, DC: AACC Press; 2010.

Raja S, Ching J, Xi L, et al. Technology for automated, rapid, and quantitative PCR or reverse transcription-PCR clinical testing. *Clin Chem.* 2005;51:882–890.

St John A, Price CP. Economic evidence and point-of-care testing. *Clin Biochem Rev.* 2013;34:61–74.

Tonyushkina K, Nichols JH. Glucose meters: a review of technical challenges to obtaining accurate results. *J Diabetes Sci Technol.* 2009;3:971–980.

Turner APF. In: Karube I, Wilson GS, eds. *Biosensors: Fundamentals and Applications.* Oxford: Oxford University Press; 1987:1–770.

US Department of Health and Human Services. Medicare, Medicaid and CLIA programs: regulations implementing the clinical laboratory improvement amendments of 1988 (CLIA). *Fed Regist.* 1992;57:7002–7018.

US Department of Health and Human Services. Medicare, Medicaid and CLIA programs: regulations implementing the clinical laboratory improvement amendments of 1988 (CLIA) and clinical laboratory act program fee collection. *Fed Regist.* 1993;58:5215–5237.

Walter B. Dry reagent chemistries. *Anal Chem.* 1983;55:498A–514A.

Wang P, Kricka L. Current and emerging trends in point-of-care technology and strategies for clinical validation and implementation. *Clin Chem.* 2018;64(10):1439–1452.

Wong R, Tse H. *Lateral Flow Immunoassay.* New York: Humana Press; 2009:223.

# Amino Acids, Peptides, and Proteins

*Dennis J. Dietzen and Maria Alice V. Willrich*

## OBJECTIVES

1. Define the following:
   - Acute-phase response
   - Bence Jones proteins
   - The complement system
   - Essential amino acid
   - Immunoglobulin
   - Isoelectric point
   - Paraprotein
   - Peptide bond
2. Diagram and describe the basic chemical structure of an amino acid.
3. Diagram the formation of a peptide bond from two adjacent amino acids.
4. Describe amino acid and protein analyses, including specimen requirements and quantitative analytical techniques.
5. Describe how amino acid carbon contributes to energy production.
6. Match the peptide(s) to the physiologic function:
   Peptide:
   Hepcidin
   Natriuretic peptides
   Angiotensins
   Vasopressin

Function:
   Promote Na retention and increased blood pressure
   Inhibit iron mobilization
   Promote water retention in collecting duct
   Promote Na and water excretion
7. Discuss primary, secondary, tertiary, and quaternary protein structure.
8. Compare plasma and serum with regard to protein concentration.
9. List the acute-phase response proteins and the negative acute-phase response proteins.
10. List the various classes of protease molecules and representative members of each class.
11. List the various protein posttranslational modifications and cite specific examples of proteins modified by each of the modifications.
12. Discuss the complement pathways triggers, and describe the proteins involved in each of the three cascades.
13. List the immunoglobulin classes. Describe their biochemistry, function, and clinical significance, and explain how they are affected by disease.
14. Explain the presence of protein in cerebral spinal fluid (CSF) and the significance of increased CSF protein.

## KEY WORDS AND DEFINITIONS

**Acute-phase response** Body's response to injury or inflammation.

**Amino acid** An organic compound containing both amino (−NH2) and carboxyl (−COOH) functional groups.

**Complement system** Complex system of proteins found in blood that combines with antibodies to destroy pathogenic bacteria and other foreign cells.

**Immunoglobulins** A family of proteins also known as antibodies that contain highly specific antigen-binding sites consisting of two identical heavy (H) chains and two identical light (L) chains.

**Monoclonal gammopathy of undetermined significance (MGUS)** A pre-malignant condition in which a paraprotein is found in an individual's blood with undetermined significance.

**Multiple myeloma** A cancer in which a single clone of an antibody-producing plasma cell grows in an uncontrolled and malignant manner.

**Paraprotein** A monoclonal immunoglobulin produced in excessive amounts in disorders such as multiple myeloma or MGUS.

**Peptide** A compound consisting of two or more amino acids linked in a chain via peptide bonds.

**Protein** A polymer of amino acids linked by peptide bonds with a specific sequence that folds into a defined structure; any of a group of complex organic compounds that contain carbon, hydrogen, oxygen, nitrogen, and usually sulfur (the characteristic element being nitrogen).

**Proteome** The total complement of proteins expressed by the genetic material of an organism under a given set of environmental conditions.

Amino acids, peptides, and proteins are crucial for virtually all biologic processes. **Amino acids** serve as structural subunits of peptides and proteins but also play diverse roles in metabolism, neurotransmission, and intercellular signaling. **Peptides** serve as autocrine and endocrine signaling molecules that control appetite, vascular tone, and electrolyte homeostasis, as well as carbohydrate and mineral metabolism. **Proteins**, longer peptide chains with molecular mass typically greater than approximately 6000 daltons (Da), serve as (1) intracellular and extracellular structural components, (2) biologic catalysts, (3) mediators of contractility and motility, (4) agents of molecular assembly, (5) ion channels and pumps, (6) molecular transporters, (7) mediators of immunity, and (8) components of intracellular and intercellular signaling networks.

The human genome contains more than 20,000 open-reading frames that encode proteins. The actual number of proteins is far greater, however, because of alternative splicing of messenger RNA (mRNA), somatic recombination, mutation, proteolytic processing, and posttranslational modification. The **proteome** represents the complete set of proteins in an organism or compartment of an organism such as the plasma space. Efforts to catalog the proteome include those by the Human Proteome Organization (hupo.org), the National Center for Biotechnology Information (ncbi.nlm.nih.gov), the Swiss Institute of Bioinformatics (expasy.org), and the Healthy Human Individual's Integrated Plasma Proteome Database (bio.informatics.iupui.edu/HIP2). Most databases were designed mainly to assist with peptide and protein identification, but efforts have shifted to characterizing the abundance of specific protein components in healthy and diseased populations, the usual basis for diagnostic applications.

This chapter begins with a discussion of the chemistry, metabolism, and analysis of amino acids. Inherited disorders of amino acid metabolism are discussed in Chapter 45. A description of the chemistry and biochemistry of the peptide bond is then followed by a description of several clinically relevant peptide systems and methods for in vitro assessment. The protein narrative begins with an account of protein structure and cellular compartmentalization followed by discussion of co- and post-translational modifications. Constituents of the proteome in body fluids are also addressed, followed lastly by a description of methods for specific and global assessment of the proteome for clinical purposes. More in-depth treatment of other specific proteins and protein networks may be found in Chapters 19 (serum enzymes), 20 (tumor markers), 23 (lipoproteins), and 28 (hemoglobin), as well as other chapters dedicated to the specific pathophysiology of cardiac, liver, renal, bone, pituitary, thyroid, and adrenal disease. In-depth treatment of measurement modalities for amino acids, peptides, and proteins such as electrophoresis, chromatography, mass spectrometry (MS), and immunoassay may be found in Chapters 11–13 and 15, respectively.

## AMINO ACIDS

Amino acids were likely among the first organic molecules to emerge from the mix of methane, hydrogen, ammonia, and water in earth's primordial atmosphere. Only 20 of the hundreds of known amino acids account for the vast majority of residues in human polypeptide chains. Their structure and molecular properties are summarized in Table 18.1. These 20 along with dozens of non–protein-forming amino acids are critical to the form and function of the human body. Disrupted amino acid metabolism is not surprisingly associated with a multitude of pathologic processes.

### Basic Biochemistry

Amino acids are organic compounds containing both an amino group ($-NH_2$) and a carboxyl group ($-COOH$) or another acidic group such as a sulfonate group ($-SO_3$). In a majority of biologically relevant amino acids, the amine moiety is primary ($-NH_2$), but some (e.g., sarcosine) are secondary ($-NH-$) amines, and others containing tertiary amines (e.g., proline) are referred to as imino ($=N-$) acids. With the exception of proline, the amino acids that occur in protein are $\alpha$-amino acids (Fig. 18.1).

The R group represents the unique side chains responsible for the chemical properties of individual amino acids. Not all biologic amino acids are $\alpha$ amino acids. $\beta$ amino acids such as $\beta$-alanine and taurine as well as $\gamma$-amino acids such as $\gamma$-aminobutyric acid (GABA) also play key biochemical roles.

With the exception of glycine, all $\alpha$ amino acids contain four distinct moieties asymmetrically arranged around the $\alpha$ carbon. As a consequence, amino acids may exist as mirror images (enantiomers) referred to as the *D* or *L* configuration. With few exceptions, the biologically relevant amino acids exist in the *L* configuration. Small quantities of *D*

## TABLE 18.1 Structure and Chemical Properties of the 20 Proteogenic Amino Acids

| Amino Acid | MW (Da) | Structure (pH 7.0) | pK₁ | pK₂ | pK₃ | pI | HI |
|---|---|---|---|---|---|---|---|
| Alanine (ALA, A) | 89.09 | | 2.4 | 9.7 | | 6.0 | 1.8 |
| Arginine (ARG, R) | 174.20 | | 2.2 | 9.0 | 12.5 | 10.8 | −4.5 |
| Asparagine (ASN, N) | 132.12 | | 2.0 | 8.8 | | 5.4 | −3.5 |
| Aspartate (ASP, D) | 133.10 | | 2.1 | 9.8 | 3.9 | 2.9 | −3.5 |
| Cysteine (CYS, C) | 121.16 | | 1.7 | 10.8 | 8.3 | 5.1 | 2.5 |
| Glycine (GLY, G) | 75.07 | | 2.3 | 9.6 | | 6.0 | −0.4 |
| Glutamate (GLU, E) | 147.13 | | 2.2 | 9.7 | 4.3 | 3.2 | −3.5 |
| Glutamine (GLN, Q) | 146.15 | | 2.2 | 9.1 | | 5.7 | −3.5 |
| Histidine (I IIS, H) | 155.16 | | 1.8 | 9.2 | 6.0 | 7.6 | −3.2 |
| Isoleucine (ILE, I) | 131.17 | | 2.4 | 9.7 | | 6.0 | 4.5 |
| Leucine(LEU, L) | 131.17 | | 2.4 | 9.6 | | 6.0 | 3.8 |
| Lysine (LYS, K) | 146.19 | | 2.2 | 9.0 | 10.5 | 9.7 | −3.9 |
| Methionine (MET, M) | 149.21 | | 2.3 | 9.2 | | 5.8 | 1.9 |

*Continued*

## TABLE 18.1    Structure and Chemical Properties of the 20 Proteogenic Amino Acids—cont'd

| Amino Acid | MW (Da) | Structure (pH 7.0) | pK₁ | pK₂ | pK₃ | pI | HI |
|---|---|---|---|---|---|---|---|
| Phenylalanine (PHE, F) | 165.19 | 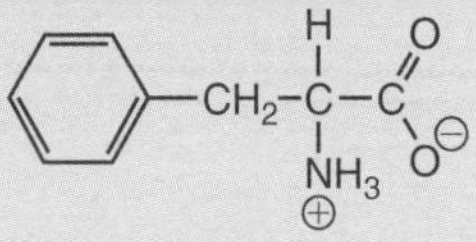 | 1.8 | 9.1 | | 5.5 | 2.8 |
| Proline (PRO, P) | 115.13 | 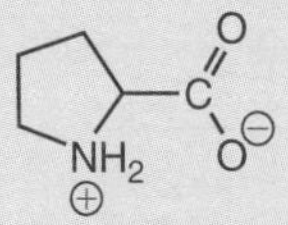 | 2.1 | 10.6 | | 6.1 | 1.6 |
| Serine (SER, S) | 105.09 | 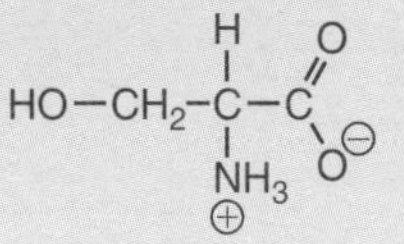 | 2.2 | 9.2 | | 5.7 | −0.8 |
| Threonine (THR, T) | 119.12 | 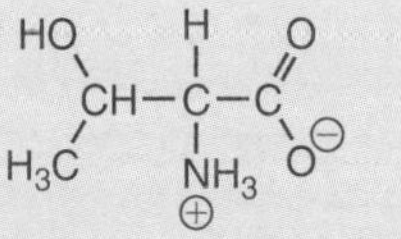 | 2.6 | 10.4 | | 6.5 | −0.7 |
| Tryptophan (TRP, W) | 201.22 | 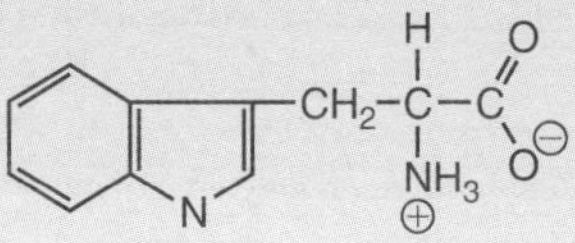 | 2.5 | 9.4 | | 5.9 | −0.9 |
| Tyrosine (TYR, Y) | 181.19 | 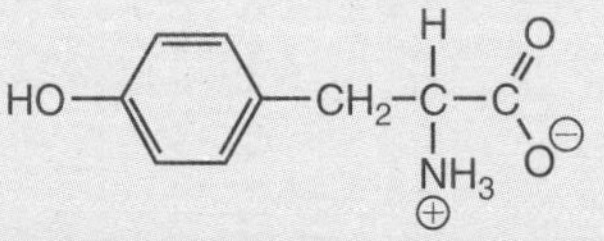 | 2.2 | 9.2 | 10.5 | 5.7 | −1.3 |
| Valine (VAL, V) | 117.17 | 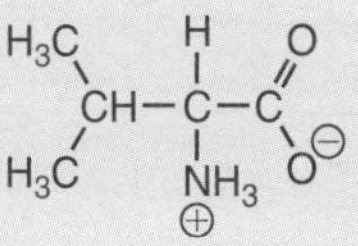 | 2.3 | 9.6 | | 6.0 | 4.2 |

*HI*, Hydropathy index; *MW*, molecular weight; *pk*, acid ionization constant; *pl*, isoelectric p.

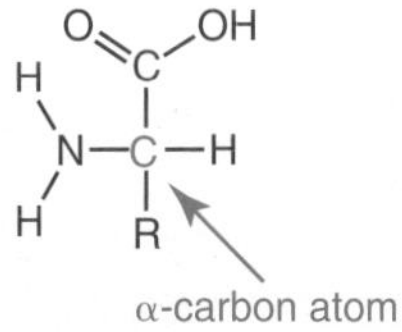

Fig. 18.1 Planar representation of an α-amino acid.

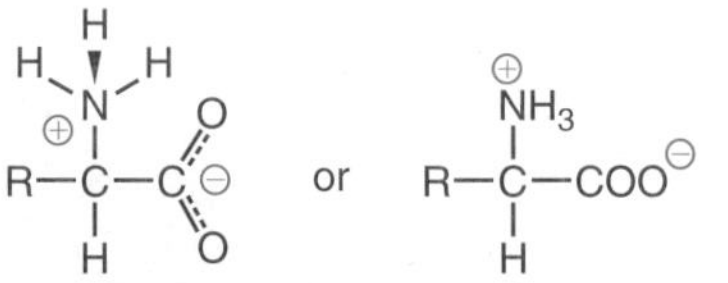

Fig. 18.2 Planar structure of an α-amino acid as a zwitterion.

amino acids occur in physiological fluids but typically do not have specific functions. An exception is *D* serine, which represents 5% to 20% of total serine in cerebrospinal fluid (CSF) and may serve as a neurotransmitter. Two amino acids, threonine and isoleucine, have a second asymmetric carbon, and their stereoisomers are referred to as *allothreonine* and *alloisoleucine*. The latter compound has utility in the diagnosis of maple syrup urine disease (see Chapter 45 and Online Mendelian Inheritance in Man; https://www.omim.org/entry/248600).

Acid–base properties of amino acids depend on the amino– and carboxyl groups attached to the α carbon and on the basic or acidic groups occurring on some side chains. At physiologic pH near 7.4, the α-carboxyl group is ionized and carries a negative charge, and the α amino group is protonated and carries a positive charge. Molecules existing simultaneously as cations and anions

are referred to as zwitterions or ampholytes (diagrammed in Fig. 18.2).

The pH at which ionizable groups exist equally as charged and uncharged forms is referred to as the pK. Amino acids thus have two or more pKs—one for the carboxyl, one for the amino group, and an additional one in the presence of an ionizable side chain. The isoelectric point (pI) is the pH at which an amino acid or other molecule has a net charge of 0. For a typical neutral amino acid such as glycine, the pI of 5.97 is midway between the pK of 2.34 for the carboxylic acid and the pK of 9.60 for the amino group. The pKs of amino acid side chains in proteins vary somewhat from those in free amino acids because of the influence of neighboring amino acids.

The structural diversity of side chains permits formation of proteins with a variety of structure and function. Side chain diversity is dictated not only by pK but by size and hydrophobicity. Amino acids with longer aliphatic or aromatic side chains such as isoleucine, leucine, and phenylalanine have greater hydrophobicity than shorter side chains such as the methyl group found in alanine. Neutral amino acids with polar groups such as hydroxyl or amide groups in their side chains are more hydrophilic. Acidic amino acids have side chains with carboxylic acids, and basic amino acids have side chains with amino, guanidino, or imidazole groups. The thiol side chain (–SH) of cysteine oxidizes easily and may become linked to other molecules via disulfide bonds. In plasma, cysteine occurs as cystine (cysteine homodimer linked via a disulfide) or as a mixed disulfide with heterogeneous thiol compounds, albumin, or other proteins.

With some exceptions, amino acids are water soluble and stable in plasma. Amino acid solubility is rarely limiting in vivo except in some metabolic disorders. Deposition of tyrosine crystals in the eye and skin is common in tyrosinemia, particularly type II (https://www.omim.org/entry/276600). Likewise, cystine may crystallize in the renal parenchyma in patients with cystinuria (https://omim.org/entry/220100). Structural and chemical details for the 20 protein-forming amino acids are displayed in Table 18.1.

## Amino Acid Supply and Transport

Amino acids participate in many metabolic pathways in addition to serving as substrates for protein synthesis. In the healthy state, women require approximately 46 g/day and men approximately 56 g/day of dietary protein (0.8 g/kg body weight), and substantial increases in demand occur during growth and in many disease states. Dietary protein is digested by proteases in the stomach (e.g., pepsin) and small intestine (e.g., trypsin, chymotrypsin) to yield amino acids. Endogenous protein turnover serves as another source of free amino acids. Eight amino acids used for protein synthesis (isoleucine, leucine, lysine, methionine, phenylalanine, threonine, tryptophan, and valine) are not synthesized by humans and therefore are considered "essential" constituents of the diet. Meat, milk, eggs, and fish contain a full range of essential amino acids. Gelatin is deficient in tryptophan, and some plant sources of protein may be additionally deficient in lysine or methionine. Therefore, diets based on a single source of plant protein may be nutritionally inadequate. When liver function is compromised, cysteine and tyrosine become essential because they are not produced from their usual precursors, methionine and phenylalanine. Arginine may be conditionally essential as well because endogenous rates of synthesis may be insufficient to meet requirements in adults under metabolic stress or in growing children.

Requirements for dietary protein to maintain nitrogen balance increase in infancy and childhood when there are increased demands for growth. Daily requirements increase by up to 3.5 to 4 g protein/kg body weight for premature infants, for example. Protein demand is also increased in pregnancy, lactation, and states of protein loss or catabolic states (e.g., burn patients). Persistent negative nitrogen balance results in a number of undesirable phenotypic features. A diet severely deficient in protein and consisting primarily of high-starch foods can lead to kwashiorkor, a disorder characterized by decreased serum albumin, immune deficiency, edema, ascites, growth failure, apathy, and many other symptoms. Marasmus results when protein and energy sources such as carbohydrates are deficient, causing wasting of muscles and subcutaneous tissues. Albumin or prealbumin concentrations are sometimes used to assess the adequacy of the amino acid supply. The shorter biologic half-life of prealbumin compared with albumin (2 vs. 20 days) makes it a valuable marker for acute dietary assessment.

Homeostasis of cellular amino acid concentrations is dependent on supply, catabolism, and excretion. Supply and excretion are regulated by a series of transport systems with overlapping substrate specificity, strategic tissue expression, and polarized cellular distribution. Amino acids are derived from dietary protein precursors through the action of proteolytic enzymes in the stomach and small intestine that produce shorter oligopeptides and individual amino acids. Enteral absorption of di- and tripeptides is mediated by a single proton-coupled transport system termed peptide transporter 1 or PEPT1 (encoded by *SLC15A1*). Transport of individual amino acids across the intestinal and renal epithelium as well as the blood-brain barrier is far more specialized.

A diverse array of transport systems consisting of multiple polypeptide subunits has evolved for both inter- and intracellular amino acid transport. At least 400 genes belonging to 65 *SLC* (solute carrier) gene families are required for comprehensive, functional transporter function. Some transporters require energy (often in the form of a Na gradient), while others rely on established amino acid concentration gradients. The substrate specificity of these systems is often broad. For example, distinct systems are responsible for transporting branched-chain, cationic, anionic, or hydrophobic amino acids. Multiple systems cooperate to achieve amino acid absorption across the gut or renal epithelia. Molecular defects in these systems are responsible for a number of disease states such as cystinuria (https://omim.org/entry/220100), cystinosis (https://omim.org/entry/219800), lysinuric protein intolerance (https://omim.org/entry/227100), or HHH (**H**yperornithinemia, **H**yperammonemia, **H**omocitrullinuria) syndrome (https://omim.org/entry/238970).

## Amino Acid Metabolism

Amino acids serve as scaffolds for the synthesis of many hormones, nucleotides, lipids, signaling molecules, and metabolic intermediates that play a role in energy production. The transformation of amino acid carbon to energetic intermediate typically begins with transamination. Excess nitrogen is excreted as urea. Resulting α-ketoacids may enter the Krebs cycle, undergo conversion to ketone bodies, fatty acids, or glucose, or be completely oxidized to $CO_2$ depending on cellular energy demands.

## Amino Acid Concentrations

Plasma amino acid concentrations collectively span 4 orders of magnitude from very low micromolar quantities (e.g., β-alanine, cystathionine) to near 1 mmol/L (e.g., glutamine, glycine). With protein intake of 1 to 2 g/kg, daily concentrations vary by approximately 30% in healthy adults. Amino acid concentrations tend to peak between 12 and 8 p.m. with a nadir between midnight and 4 a.m. After an ingested protein bolus, dietary amino acids rise and tend to return to preprandial levels in 3 to 6 hours. Determination of "fasting" amino acid concentrations, therefore, requires extended periods of dietary abstinence.

Most amino acids in blood undergo glomerular filtration but are efficiently reabsorbed in proximal renal tubules by saturable transport systems. Increased renal excretion of amino acids (aminoaciduria) results from filtration of excessive plasma concentrations, generalized tubular impairment, or heritable defects in amino acid transport systems. Glycine tends to be most abundant in normal urine followed by histidine, glutamine, and serine. Increased concentrations of proteogenic amino acids in plasma tend to precipitate only mildly elevated excretion because of efficient reabsorption. Other amino acids that accumulate in plasma secondary to metabolic errors (e.g., argininosuccinate, homocitrulline) demonstrate pronounced excretion because of the absence of specific tubular mechanisms enabling reclamation from the filtrate.

With the exception of glutamine, CSF amino acid concentrations are typically less than 10% of those found in plasma. This high plasma-to-CSF gradient suggests active net brain-to-blood transport across the blood-brain barrier. Glutamine concentrations in CSF are generally equal to those in plasma, suggesting a bidirectional facilitative transport process. Insofar as CSF concentrations reflect synaptic concentrations, regulation of neurotransmitter amino acid concentrations is critical for normal neural action potential propagation. Glutamate is the most abundant amino acid in the brain and is the primary excitatory transmitter. Glycine and GABA are the predominant inhibitory transmitters. Lumbar puncture to access the CSF amino acid pool must be done with great care to avoid overestimation of central amino acid concentrations secondary to contamination with peripheral blood.

Assessment of amino acid concentrations in blood, urine, and spinal fluid has been historically applied to the detection of inborn errors of metabolism. These are comprehensively covered in Chapter 45. Aside from the measurement of homocysteine as a marker of vitamin $B_{12}$ and folate status, clinical applications of amino acid measurement beyond metabolic diseases are limited.

## Analysis of Amino Acids

For decades, the standard method of amino acid analysis was cation-exchange chromatography with postcolumn spectrophotometric or fluorescent detection of various primary amine derivatives. The earliest commercial systems required as long as 2 to 3 hours to quantitate 30 to 50 physiologic amino acids in a single patient specimen. These systems have given way to smaller bench-top systems that still require 90 to 120 minutes for full sample analysis.

MS is increasingly being adopted for amino acid profiling. Newborn screening programs quantitate amino acid butyl esters derived from dried blood spots using flow-injection MS protocols. These methods do not use chromatographic separation and so cannot distinguish between isomeric or isobaric amino acids such as leucine, isoleucine, alloisoleucine, and hydroxyproline. Liquid chromatography-tandem mass spectrometry (LC-MS/MS) methods for detection of amino acids in plasma and other body fluids have also been developed. Advantages of MS-based techniques include improved analytic specificity, a 3- to 4-order-of-magnitude dynamic range, and rapid (20-minute) throughput. MS methods may also be optimized for profiling multiple molecular species in addition to amino acids. Such approaches promise to improve the scope of metabolic disorders detectable with a single patient specimen in a single analytic run.

# PEPTIDES

This section describes the basic biochemistry of peptides. In general, the term *peptide* applies to relatively short polymers of amino acids with molecular weights less than 6000 Da (<~50 amino acid residues). The chemistry of the peptide bond and the physical characteristics of the peptide backbone are discussed in this section along with a number of clinically relevant peptide systems.

## Peptide Bond

A peptide bond, also referred to as an amide bond, is formed between the α-nitrogen atom of one amino acid and the carbonyl carbon of a second (Fig.18.3). So-called isopeptide bonds refer to amide bonds between sidechain amines or carbonyl carbons rather than α-amine or α-carbonyl. In glutathione, for example, the γ-carboxyl group of glutamic acid is linked to the α-amino group of cysteine. During translation, peptide bonds are formed from the amino (N) to the carboxyl (C) terminus by removal of water (also referred to as dehydration or condensation) and catalyzed by RNA (referred to as a ribozyme) that forms part of the ribosome. Cleavage of peptide bonds may be achieved nonspecifically via acid hydrolysis or specifically by a host of proteolytic enzymes with affinity for bonds between specific amino acid residues. These protease systems are described later in this chapter.

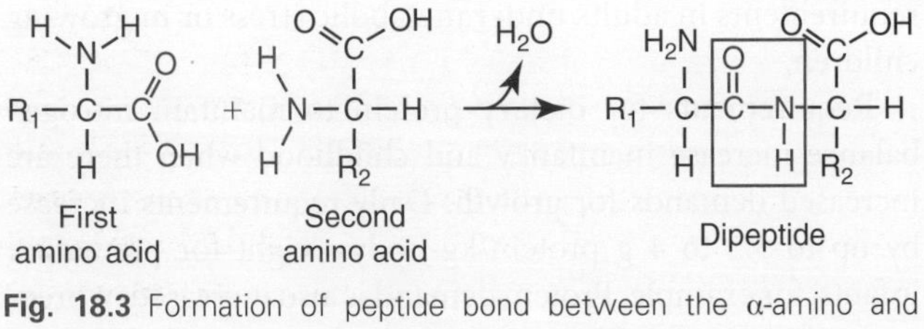

**Fig. 18.3** Formation of peptide bond between the α-amino and α-carbonyl of adjacent amino acids.

## Peptide Heterogeneity and Analysis

Assessment of circulating peptide concentrations has a number of limitations. In the absence of enzymatic activity, peptide measurements have been historically limited to immunologic techniques (discussed in more detail in Chapter 15). Antibodies may recognize linear sequence epitopes or discontinuous, conformational epitopes. These epitopes typically involve 10 to 20 amino acids binding exposed areas of 600 to 1000 $\text{Å}^2$. Measurement of short peptides (<20 to 30 amino acids) are therefore limited to single-site, competitive assays that lack the analytic specificity of two-site (sandwich) immunoassays. The molecular specificity issues may be addressed using MS as an alternative. Small peptides may be ionized via electrospray (ESI) or matrix-assisted laser desorption (MALDI) and interfaced to tandem quadrupole mass analyzers (see Chapter 13).

Absolute analytic specificity is not always ideal when applied to biologic peptide systems. Peptide populations may consist of species with a variable number of amino acid residues possessing sometimes unknown biologic potency. Hepcidin, for example, is an iron transport regulatory peptide that circulates principally as a 25–amino acid peptide but also as shorter peptides of 22 and 20 amino acids with diminished biologic activity. Likewise, dozens of truncated forms of the mature 32–amino acid B-type natriuretic peptide ranging from 24 to 31 amino acids are detectable in heart failure patients. Some of these truncated forms are present in vivo, and others likely develop in vitro. Thus, narrowly targeted MS assays may exclude active peptide species and run the risk of underestimating bioactive peptide. Cross-reactive immunoassays, on the other hand, may stoichiometrically detect both active and inactive peptide, thus running the risk of overestimating bioactive peptide concentrations. Examples of several important biologic peptide systems and their analytic considerations follow.

## Selected Clinically Relevant Peptide Systems

### Pro-Opiomelanocortin System

The pro-opiomelanocortin (POMC) gene on chromosome 2 is expressed primarily in the pituitary gland, the hypothalamus, and melanocytes. The gene produces a 241–amino acid prohormone that can yield as many as 10 distinct biologically active peptides depending on patterns of cleavage in specific tissue types. The POMC peptides have diverse effects on glucose and electrolyte homeostasis, body mass and appetite, pigmentation, and pain.

### Natriuretic Peptides

This peptide family consists of atrial natriuretic peptide (ANP), B-type natriuretic peptide (BNP, formerly brain natriuretic peptide), and C-type natriuretic peptide (CNP). ANP and BNP are highly expressed in cardiac tissue. The mature forms of these peptides contain a 17–amino acid loop stabilized by an intramolecular disulfide bond. Each peptide acts via a specific guanylate cyclase-coupled receptor to promote sodium and water excretion, blunt activation of the renin-angiotensin system, and decrease vascular resistance. Circulating concentrations of ANP and BNP (but not CNP) increase rapidly in response to increased cardiac filling pressures that are characteristic of heart failure.

### Hepcidin

Hepcidin is a 25 amino acid peptide derived from the *HAMP* gene on chromosome 19 and was initially described as an antimicrobial peptide. The role of hepcidin in iron metabolism was noted by Nicolas et al in 2001. Hepcidin binding promotes the internalization and degradation of ferroportin, thus inhibiting mobilization of iron stores. Physiologic states such as chronic inflammation are characterized by microcytic anemia with paradoxically adequate iron stores known as anemia of chronic disease. Increased hepcidin expression is at the pathologic root of this condition.

### Angiotensins

Renin is secreted by the afferent arterioles of the kidney in response to decreased blood flow and sodium delivery. Renin catalyzes the conversion of angiotensinogen to vasoactive peptides that act to reestablish glomerular flow. The N-terminal decapeptide cleaved from angiotensinogen is referred to as angiotensin I. Angiotensin-converting enzyme (ACE) cleaves 2 C-terminal residues from angiotensin I to form the octapeptide, angiotensin II, which promotes contraction of vascular smooth muscle and stimulates proximal tubular sodium reabsorption to increase blood pressure. ACE inhibitors (e.g., captopril, enalapril, quinapril) are important pharmacologic tools used to treat hypertension.

### Vasopressin

Vasopressin (arginine vasopressin [AVP]), also known as antidiuretic hormone (ADH), is a nonapeptide stored in and secreted from the posterior pituitary gland. Its primary target organ is the distal convoluted tubule and collecting duct, where it acts to promote water reabsorption. ADH circulates at very low concentrations (<40 pmol/L) and has a very short half-life (15 to 20 minutes), making routine diagnostic measurement impractical. Copeptin, a prohormone form of ADH, exhibits a longer half-life and is an attractive alternative target for measurement. Diabetes insipidus (DI) may result from faulty secretion (central DI) or from end-organ resistance (nephrogenic DI). Head injury, tumors, and some medications may also induce pathologic secretion of ADH, resulting in fluid overload referred to as the syndrome of inappropriate antidiuretic hormone secretion (SIADH). A synthetic analog referred to as DDAVP (1-desamino, 8-D-arginine vasopressin) is used therapeutically to treat DI and some forms of coagulopathy. In patients with some forms of von Willebrand disease and hemophilia, DDAVP stimulates the release of von Willebrand factor from endothelial cells and extends the half-life of circulating factor VIII, thereby mediating improved hemostasis.

### Glutathione

Glutathione consists of a glutamate residue linked to cysteine via its γ-carboxyl rather than the α-carboxyl group and followed by a conventional peptide bond between cysteine and glycine. This ubiquitous tripeptide is the most abundant intracellular thiol (1 to 10 mmol/L) and circulates in the blood at micromolar concentrations. The cellular ratio of reduced glutathione (GSH) to oxidized glutathione (GSSG) ranges from 10 to 100. Intracellular glutathione performs a variety of important functions. It plays an important role in maintaining the proper ratio of oxidized to reduced forms of metabolically important thiols such as coenzyme A. It also provides reducing equivalents that detoxify reactive oxygen species such as peroxides (catalyzed by glutathione peroxidase). Through the activity of glutathione-S-transferase, glutathione also serves to detoxify other xenobiotic compounds via formation of a thioether derivative, which can then be excreted. Amino acids are sometimes transported across the plasma membrane via the γ-glutamyl moiety of glutathione, a reaction catalyzed by γ-glutamyl-transpeptidase.

# PROTEINS

The structural diversity of proteins may be described using the following features:

1. Primary structure is the linear sequence of amino acids in a peptide or protein. Posttranslational modifications of amino acids contribute to increased diversity.
2. Secondary structure describes the nature of the peptide backbone. Examples of secondary structure include α-helix, β-sheet, and β-turn. An α-helix has about 3.6 residues per turn and is stabilized by hydrogen bonds between the N–H and C=O group of the fourth following amino acid. A β-sheet involves hydrogen bonds between the peptide bonds of adjacent peptide chains arranged in parallel or antiparallel configurations. Random coils refer to segments of peptide that lack a defined secondary structure.
3. Tertiary structure refers to the folding of the polypeptide chain and elements of secondary structure into a compact three-dimensional (3D) shape. Folding is a complex process driven by energy minimization of intramolecular and solvent interactions. Hydrophobic groups tend to fold into the interior with less exposure to solvent, while charged and polar sidechains tend to be located on the surface. The 3D structure is stabilized by intramolecular hydrogen bonds, van der Waals forces, and hydrophobic interactions. Disulfide bonds between cysteine residues also stabilize 3D structure. Denaturation of protein refers to unfolding that occurs with temperature change or in the presence of organic solvents, detergents, or reagents that disrupt hydrogen bonds. Limited denaturation can be reversible, but extensive unfolding and denaturation of proteins often lead to irreversible aggregation and precipitation.
4. Quaternary structure refers to the incorporation of two or more polypeptide chains or subunits into a larger multimeric unit. Examples range from the relatively simple creatine kinase, a heterodimer of M and B subunits, to branched chain α-ketoacid dehydrogenase, which is a heteromeric complex of 12 E1, 24 E2, and 6 E3 subunits.
5. Ligands and prosthetic groups provide additional functional and structural elements, such as metals in metalloenzymes, heme in hemoglobin and cytochromes, and lipids in lipoproteins. Proteins without their associated ligands are often referred to as apoproteins. For example, apotransferrin lacks bound iron and apolipoproteins lack a full complement of lipid.

## Physical Properties of Proteins

The diverse structural features of proteins result in unique physical properties that can be exploited for analysis. For example, tyrosine and tryptophan residues absorb light at 280 nm, and the abundance of these amino acids determines the extinction coefficient of a peptide or protein. A pure protein, therefore, may be quantitated using $A_{280}$. Some prosthetic groups such as heme also possess intrinsic absorbance that may be monitored to assess the presence of specific proteins. Automated clinical analyzers assess the presence of hemoglobin at 540 to 570 nm, for example, to detect hemolyzed plasma or serum specimens. Ionizable groups exert a strong effect on physical properties depending on the pH of the surrounding solution. Differing physical properties serve as the basis of methods to separate proteins. Some important characteristics include the following:

1. *Differential solubility.* The solubility of proteins is affected by pH, ionic strength, temperature, and the characteristics of the solvent. Changing solvent pH affects the net charge of a protein. Changing ionic strength affects the hydration and solubility of proteins.
2. *Molecular size.* Separation of small and large molecules is commonly achieved by differential migration through molecular filters. Examples are size exclusion chromatography (also known as gel filtration), ultracentrifugation, and electrophoresis. These techniques may be used under conditions when proteins and peptides are in native globular states or under denaturing conditions. Addition of reducing agents allows separation of disulfide-linked components.
3. *Molecular mass.* Advances in MS allow the determination of masses of peptides and proteins with increasing accuracy. Peptides and proteins can be ionized by laser desorption (MALDI) or electrospray (ESI) ionization.
4. *Electrical charge.* Ion-exchange chromatography, isoelectric focusing, and electrophoresis separate peptides and proteins based on charge.
5. *Surface adsorption.* The affinity of peptides and proteins for a variety of physical surfaces may also be used as the basis for separation. Reverse-phase chromatography, for example, exploits the interaction of hydrophobic molecular moieties with hydrophobic surfaces (C8 or C18 alkyl chains) when the ratio of water to organic solvent is high but not when organic content is increased.
6. *Affinity chromatography.* Specific ligands, antibodies, and other recognition molecules have been used to separate peptides or proteins selectively.

## Protein Formation

### Folding

Proteins are synthesized by ribosomes reading from the 5′-end of mRNA. Triplet codons in mRNA are matched with a complementary sequence in transfer RNA carrying specific amino acids. Protein synthesis begins with an AUG codon encoding methionine, and the polypeptide chain is synthesized from the N-terminus.

Instructions for folding are largely contained in the primary amino acid sequence of the growing polypeptide chain. The rate of elongation (typically 5 to 10 amino acids per second in eukaryotes) may have a significant impact on folding. Pauses in translation may enhance formation of secondary structural elements. Protein folding is an error-prone process, and many molecular chaperones work to refold, prevent aggregation, or degrade misfolded proteins.

Despite these protective mechanisms, many age-related, genetic, and infectious diseases appear connected to faulty protein folding or protein aggregation. Prion diseases are infectious diseases in which the transmissible protein agent may catalyze misfolding of endogenous proteins. In Alzheimer disease, deposits of insoluble amyloid may contribute to pathogenesis. Polyglutamine expansion in the huntingtin protein leads to protein aggregation and the clinical sequelae of Huntington disease. In $\alpha_1$-antitrypsin deficiency, liver injury results from aggregation and accumulation of misfolded protein. The most common cause of cystic fibrosis results from a single amino acid deletion ($\Delta$F508), which results in rapid degradation of the cystic fibrosis transmembrane conductance regulator (CFTR). Small molecule therapeutics capable of modulating protein folding have shown some promise in mitigating disease caused by abnormal protein aggregation.

### Targeting

Proteins that are secreted, located in vesicular compartments, or oriented on the external surface of cell membranes usually contain a hydrophobic N-terminal signal peptide about 15 to 30 amino acids in length. Signal peptides interact with signal recognition particles (SRPs) and mediate interaction with the endoplasmic reticulum (ER). Nascent peptide chains are inserted through the membrane of the ER as the protein is synthesized. Signal peptides of most secretory proteins are removed even before synthesis of the entire protein chain is completed. Co-translational membrane retention may be achieved via an uncleaved signal sequence, by one or more hydrophobic transmembrane domains, or by lipid modifications such as N-myristoylation.

Newly synthesized proteins ultimately reside in a number of membranous or soluble compartments, including the nucleus, lysosome, peroxisome, mitochondrion, or plasma membrane. Plasma membrane sorting is further complicated in polarized epithelial cells where proteins may be targeted to basolateral or apical environments.

### Posttranslational Modifications

After translation, proteins may be subject to a number of further covalent modifications. Some of these modifications are reversible and mediate location, activity, or half-life of the modified protein. A list of the more common modifications follows below.

### Acetylation

Eighty to 90% of eukaryotic cellular proteins are acetylated. Acetyl-CoA is the typical substrate for a variety of acetyl transferase enzymes localized to the nucleus, cytoplasm, and mitochondria. Most acetylation occurs on the N-terminal $\alpha$-amino group of methionine or another exposed N-terminal residue after excision of the initiator methionine. Acetylation targeting the $\varepsilon$-amino group of lysine is reversible. Acetylation contributes to control of gene expression, cell motility and division, metabolism, and oncogenesis.

### Fatty Acylation

The activity and localization of a variety of proteins are modulated by covalent attachment of fatty acyl chains. Attachment of myristate via a glycine residue provides a mechanism for membrane association. Thioester linkage of palmitate to membrane proximal cysteine residue controls subcellular membrane localization.

### Phosphorylation

Reversible phosphorylation may impact as many as one-third of all human cellular proteins. O-phosphorylation occurs at serine, threonine, and tyrosine residues. The human genome encodes approximately 1000 kinases, enzymes responsible for phosphorylation, and about 500 phosphatases responsible for removal of covalent phosphate groups. Serine and threonine phosphorylation acutely modifies enzyme activity (e.g., glycogen phosphorylase) and subcellular localization (e.g., cAMP (cyclic adenosine monophosphate)-dependent protein kinase). Tyrosine phosphorylation regulates a plethora of signaling pathways (e.g., mitogen-activated protein kinase, Janus kinase pathways) in part by providing docking site proteins that propagate a transmembrane signal.

### Prenylation

Isoprenoid compounds such as farnesyl pyrophosphate (15 carbons) and geranylgeranyl pyrophosphate (20 carbons) are hydrophobic moieties formed from 3-hydroxy-3-methylglutaryl CoA (HMGCoA). These groups modify more than 300 members of the human proteome. Isoprenylation regulates membrane and molecular association of a number of proteins important for signal transduction, vesicular trafficking, cytoskeletal function, and the integrity of the nuclear membrane.

### Glycosylphosphatidylinositol Anchor

The GPI anchor is a glycoglycero-phospholipid construct that mediates membrane attachment for a variety of proteins. GPI-anchored proteins associate with the lipid bilayer via interdigitation of two fatty acyl chains with a single membrane leaflet. Notable examples of GPI-anchored proteins include decay accelerating factor (DAF, CD55), membrane inhibitor of reactive lysis (MIRL, CD59), and alkaline phosphatase. Defects in the *PIGA* gene product that mediates GPI synthesis are responsible for paroxysmal nocturnal hemoglobinuria (PNH), a disorder characterized by abnormal complement-mediated lysis of erythrocytes deficient in CD55 and CD59.

## γ-Carboxylation

Glutamic acid is a five-carbon α-amino dicarboxylic acid. Vitamin K acts as a cofactor facilitating enzymatic addition of a second carboxyl group to the γ-carbon. A cluster of γ-carboxylated glutamyl residues is referred to as a "gla" domain. This modification mediates calcium-dependent membrane association and is required for full functional activity. Many proteins of the coagulation cascade contain the gla domain, including thrombin, factors VII, IX, and X, and protein C, S, and Z. Warfarin exerts its anticoagulant effect by abrogating the activities of the vitamin K–dependent factors.

## Glycosylation

Secreted proteins and the extracellular domains of transmembrane proteins are commonly modified with carbohydrate. Carbohydrate plays an important role in folding, secretion, and stability of the modified polypeptide. Sugar chains are added in the ER and Golgi apparatus via O-linkage to serine and threonine residues or N-linkage to the amide nitrogen of asparagine residues. O-linked sugar modifications are typically simple and consist of one to four residues. N-linked sugars are far more complex. More than 200 human gene products are involved in editing the core glycan structure and more than 100 genetic defects in this process, collectively known as congenital disorders of glycosylation (CDG), have been documented.

## Sulfation

Sulfation of proteins on tyrosine residues was described in 1954. Nearly 50 secreted and transmembrane proteins carry this irreversible modification. Examples of sulfated proteins include coagulation factors V, VIII, and IX, fibrinogen, thyroglobulin, and α-fetoprotein. The function of sulfation is likewise not well understood beyond its capacity to enhance the affinity of molecular recognition events. A naturally occurring Tyr → Phe at position 1680 of factor VIII, for example, prevents sulfation and weakens its interaction with von Willebrand factor, causing a mild form of hemophilia.

## Hydroxylation

Hydroxylation is the most prevalent posttranslational modification of human proteins. Hydroxylation most commonly occurs at the 4-position of the proline ring. Approximately 30% of proline residues in collagen are modified in this way. Hydroxyproline residues are, therefore, more common in proteins than many other common amino acid residues, including cysteine, histidine, methionine, phenylalanine, tryptophan, and tyrosine. Hydroxylation is thought to alter the flexibility of proline, thereby stabilizing the triple helical structure of collagen and other connective tissue proteins (e.g., elastin).

## Nitrosylation

Nitric oxide is a volatile free radical produced from arginine via three human NOS enzyme systems: neuronal (nNOS), endothelial (eNOS), and an inducible form (iNOS). NO forms covalent nitrosothiol (S–N=O) derivatives with free cysteine thiol groups. Thousands of proteins are reversibly modified in this way. The role of protein nitrosylation in health and disease remains to be fully clarified.

## Ubiquitination

Ubiquitin is a highly conserved 76–amino acid polypeptide containing seven lysine residues. Intracellular polypeptide chains may be modified with ubiquitin through the concerted action of three ubiquitin ligase enzymes (E1 to E3). Target proteins may be modified by a single ubiquitin moiety, or multiple molecules may be added to the original ubiquitin at one or more of the seven ubiquitin lysine residues. Limited ubiquitination of target proteins generally modifies their subcellular location or intermolecular interactions, and poly-ubiquitination targets the protein for destruction.

## Sumoylation

Small Ubiquitin-like MOdifier (SUMO) proteins consist of approximately 100 amino acids (~12 kDa) and exhibit 15% to 20% homology with ubiquitin. At least 2500 sumoylated proteins have been identified. SUMO is attached via C-terminal glycine and forms an isopeptide bond with lysine in the target protein. Sumoylation has a significant impact on protein survival as it antagonizes protein modification by ubiquitin. Altered sumoylation has been implicated in numerous pathologic states including cancer as well as Parkinson, Alzheimer, and Huntington disease.

# PROTEIN CATABOLISM

The steady-state concentration of any specific intra- or extracellular protein reflects its rate of synthesis relative to its rate of degradation. The degradative process is much more than a passive, nonspecific mechanism for disposing of unwanted cellular material. It is highly specific and tightly controlled. As supporting evidence, consider that the human genome encodes more than 500 proteases. These proteases belong to one of four families based on the catalytic mechanism for hydrolyzing peptide bonds. Representative members of the four protease families are detailed in Table 18.2.

## Protease Families

### Serine Proteases

The serine proteases are the most abundant family in humans and are so named because serine serves as the nucleophilic residue at the active site of the enzyme. Serine protease inhibitors (serpins) include α₁-antitrypsin, antithrombin, plasminogen activator inhibitor-1, and protein C. Some members of the serpin family, including angiotensinogen and thyroxine-binding globulin, do not possess known protease activity.

### Cysteinyl Proteases

This group of proteases uses a cysteine thiol in nucleophilic attack on the peptide bond. In humans, cysteine proteases mediate apoptosis via a series of enzymes referred to as caspases. Other notable cysteine proteases include some in the cathepsin

## TABLE 18.2   Selected Members of the Four Protease Families

| Protease/Family | Gene Loci | Tissue Expression | Subcellular Localization | Substrate, Function, Pathology |
|---|---|---|---|---|
| **Serine** | | | | |
| Corin | 4p13 | Broad | Plasma membrane | Natriuretic peptides (heart failure) |
| Trypsin | 7q34 | Pancreas | Secreted | Promiscuous (cleavage of LYS-X, ARG-X) |
| Chymotrypsin | 16q23 | Pancreas | Secreted | Promiscuous (cleavage of TRP-X, PHE-X, TYR-X) |
| Neutrophil elastase | 19p13 | Myeloid cells | Cytoplasm, secreted | Promiscuous (cleavage of VAL-X, ALA-X) |
| Factor IX | Xq27 | Liver | Secreted, plasma membrane | Conversion of factor X to Xa (hemophilia B) |
| Activated protein C | 2q14 | Liver | | Factor $V_a$, factor $VIII_a$ (coagulopathy) |
| PSA (prostate-specific antigen) (kallikrein) | 19q13 | Prostate | Secreted | Semen liquefaction; marker of prostate mass and cancer |
| **Cysteinyl** | | | | |
| Caspase-3 | 4q34 | Broad | Cytosol, nucleus, mitochondria | ASP-X-X-ASP (apoptosis) |
| Cathepsin C | 8p23 | Broad | Lysosome | Amyloid precursor (Alzheimer disease) |
| **Aspartyl** | | | | |
| Renin | 1q32 | Ovary, broad | Secreted | Angiotensinogen (hypertension) |
| Pepsin | 6p21 | GI tract, lung | Secreted | Cleavage at adjacent hydrophobic residues (PHE-VAL, ALA-LEU, LEU-TYR) |
| Presenilin | 14q24 | Broad | Endoplasmic reticulum/Golgi | Amyloid precursor (Alzheimer disease) |
| **Metallo** | | | | |
| ADAMTS13 | 9q34 | Liver, erythroid precursors, broad | Secreted | von Willebrand factor (thrombotic thrombocytopenic purpura) |
| MMP-1 | 11q22 | Muscle | Secreted | Collagen (tissue remodeling, embryogenesis, metastasis) |
| Angiotensin I converting enzyme | 17q23 | Testes, broad | Secreted | Angiotensin I (hypertension) |

family and interleukin 1β converting enzyme (ICE). Cystatins are endogenous inhibitors of cysteine protease activities.

## Aspartyl Proteases

Peptide bond lysis by aspartyl proteases is achieved in a single step through the coordination of a water molecule between two highly conserved aspartate residues. Human aspartyl protease enzymes include members of the pepsin, cathepsin, and renin families. The target for HIV protease inhibitors (e.g., indinavir, ritonavir) is also an aspartyl protease.

## Metalloproteases

Members of this protease family, commonly referred to as MMPs (matrix metalloproteases), include approximately 25 $Zn^{2+}$-dependent enzymes sub-classified by their reactivity to collagen, gelatin, and other extracellular matrix proteins. MMPs play an important role in wound healing and repair, pathogen defense, cancer metastasis, and rheumatoid arthritis. MMP activity is controlled by an endogenous group of

four proteins referred to as tissue inhibitors of matrix metalloproteases (TIMPs).

## Proteins in Human Serum and Plasma

The circulating proteome is a complex mixture of thousands of gene products. The 12 most abundant proteins represent more than 95% of total protein mass. Albumin alone represents more than 50% of the total mass of protein and an even higher proportion of the number of **molecules**, making it the main contributor to colloid osmotic pressure (oncotic pressure). The distinction between mass and molar concentrations of circulating proteins may be significant in considering oncotic pressure, protease inhibition, and the binding capacity for ions, drugs, or small molecules. Table 18.3 lists the 30 most abundant proteins by mass and molecular abundance. An exhaustive list of the contents of the circulating proteome would exceed 12,000 entries.

The range of protein concentrations measured in clinical assays spans more than 10 orders of magnitude and thus poses

## TABLE 18.3   Abundant Plasma Proteins

| | RANKED BY MASS ABUNDANCE (mg/L) | | RANKED BY MOLECULAR ABUNDANCE (µmol/L) | |
|---|---|---|---|---|
| Rank | Protein | Concentration | Protein | Concentration |
| 1 | Albumin | 35,000–52,000 | Albumin | 500–800 |
| 2 | Immunoglobulin G | 7000–16,000 | Immunoglobulin G | 40–120 |
| 3 | Transferrin | 2000–3600 | Apolipoprotein A-I | 30–70 |
| 4 | Immunoglobulin A | 700–4000 | Apolipoprotein A-II | 30–60 |
| 5 | $\alpha_2$-Macroglobulin | 1300–3000 | Transferrin | 25–45 |
| 6 | Fibrinogen | 2000–4000 | $\alpha_1$-Antitrypsin | 18–40 |
| 7 | $\alpha_1$-Antitrypsin | 900–2000 | Haptoglobin | 6–40 |
| 8 | Apolipoprotein A-I | 910–1940 | $\alpha_1$-Acid glycoprotein | 15–30 |
| 9 | C3 | 900–1800 | $\alpha_2$HS-glycoprotein | 9–30 |
| 10 | IgM | 400–2300 | Immunoglobulin A | 5–30 |
| 11 | Haptoglobin | 300–2000 | Hemopexin | 9–20 |
| 12 | Apolipoprotein B | 600–1550 | Apolipoprotein C III | 6–20 |
| 13 | $\alpha_1$-Acid glycoprotein | 500–1200 | Fibrinogen | 5–18 |
| 14 | $\alpha_2$HS-glycoprotein | 400–1300 | Gc-globulin | 8–14 |
| 15 | Hemopexin | 500–1150 | Apolipoprotein C-I | 6–12 |
| 16 | Gc-globulin (vitamin D–BP) | 400–700 | C3 | 5–10 |
| 17 | Factor H | 240–740 | $\alpha_1$-Antichymotrypsin | 4–9 |
| 18 | $\alpha_1$-Antichymotrypsin | 300–600 | Apolipoprotein D | 2–10 |
| 19 | Inter-$\alpha$-trypsin inhibitor | 200–700 | Prealbumin | 4–8 |
| 20 | Apolipoprotein A-II | 260–510 | $\beta_2$-Glycoprotein I | 3–6 |
| 21 | C4b-binding protein | 200–530 | Apolipoprotein A-IV | 3–6 |
| 22 | Ceruloplasmin | 200–500 | Apolipoprotein C-II | 2–7 |
| 23 | Factor B | 180–460 | Serum amyloid A4 | 3–6 |
| 24 | Prealbumin | 200–400 | Inter-$\alpha$-trypsin inhibitor | 3–5 |
| 25 | Gelsolin | 200–400 | Antithrombin III | 3–5 |
| 26 | Fibronectin | 300 | $\alpha_1$B-glycoprotein | 3–5 |
| 27 | C1 inhibitor | 190–370 | Gelsolin | 3–5 |
| 28 | C4 | 100–400 | Ceruloplasmin | 2–5 |
| 29 | Plasminogen | 150–350 | Factor H | 2–5 |
| 30 | Antithrombin III | 170–300 | Factor B | 2–5 |

*IgM*, Immunoglobulin M.
Data from Hortin GL, Sviridov D, Anderson L. High-abundance polypeptides of the human plasma proteome comprising the top 4 logs of polypeptide abundance. *Clin Chem*. 2008;54:1608–1616.

a significant analytic challenge. In decreasing order of abundance, the source of circulating proteins include (1) proteins secreted directly into plasma, (2) proteins associated with the cell membrane and shed into the circulation, (3) secretory proteins in exocrine secretions, (4) high-abundance cytoplasmic proteins, (5) low-abundance cytoplasmic proteins, (6) transmembrane proteins, and (7) organellar proteins that must traverse more than one membrane to exit cells. Many of these serve as useful markers of physiology and disease.

Circulating concentrations of proteins depend not only on rates of production and efficiency of entry to the circulation but also on rates of clearance. Proteins and peptides substantially smaller than albumin are cleared from the circulation by glomerular filtration unless they are bound to larger carrier molecules. Peptides and small proteins not bound to carriers are cleared with half-lives of about 2 hours under conditions of normal kidney function and accumulate in kidney failure. Other proteins and peptides are cleared by receptor-mediated uptake or by peptidases.

For all circulating proteins, the choice of measurement using plasma or serum is not without consequence. Plasma refers to the fluid portion of blood in the presence of an anticoagulant **after** the cells are removed by centrifugation. Common anticoagulants include dry heparin or ethylenediaminetetraacetic acid (EDTA) or solutions containing citrate. Small molecular weight additives such as EDTA may introduce osmotic effects on plasma volume, and citrate solutions introduce some specimen dilution. Serum is the fluid component of blood after blood is allowed to clot. It differs from plasma in several respects. An approximate 4% decrease in total protein content caused by conversion of fibrinogen to insoluble thrombin during coagulation. Serum has a lower viscosity than plasma because fibrinogen is absent. Intact clotting factors are consumed during the clotting process and in their place, proteolytic fragments and the contents of platelet granules produced by the clotting process may be recovered in serum.

## Abundant Components of the Circulating Proteome
### Prealbumin (Transthyretin)

Prealbumin (molecular weight, 35 kDa) transports 10% of circulating triiodothyronine ($T_3$) and thyroxine ($T_4$).

Prealbumin concentrations are often used as an indicator of adequacy of **protein** nutrition because of its relatively short half-life (~2 days) and high proportion of essential amino acids. When compared with albumin, prealbumin is a minor component of plasma but is a proportionately greater component of CSF. Prealbumin is most commonly measured using immunonephelometric or immunoturbidimetric methods, and in protein electrophoresis migrates anodally to albumin.

## Albumin

The name *albumin* (*L. albus,* meaning white) originated from the white precipitate formed during the boiling of acidic urine from patients with proteinuria. Albumin has an approximate molecular weight of 66 kDa and circulates with a half-life of 15 to 19 days. It is the most abundant plasma protein from the fetal period onward, accounting for about half of the plasma protein mass and is a major component of most body fluids, including interstitial fluid, CSF, urine, and amniotic fluid. Albumin serves as the major component of colloid osmotic pressure. and as a transporter for a diverse range of substances, including fatty acids and other lipids, bilirubin, foreign substances such as drugs, thiol-containing amino acids, tryptophan, calcium, and metals. Most clinical laboratories assay albumin in plasma or serum samples by dye-binding methods, which rely on a shift in the absorption spectrum of dyes such as bromocresol green (BCG) or purple (BCP) upon albumin binding. BCP is slightly more specific for albumin and yields lower values than BCG, particularly for patients with kidney failure.

## $\alpha_1$-Antitrypsin

$\alpha_1$-antitrypsin (AAT) is a serpin and also known as $\alpha_1$-proteinase inhibitor (or Pi). AAT is synthesized by hepatocytes and contains 394 amino acid residues and 3 *N*-linked oligosaccharides, yielding a total molecular weight of approximately 51 kDa. AAT deficiency is inherited in an autosomal codominant fashion with a prevalence of 1 in 3000 to 5000 in the United States resulting in liver and pulmonary disease. Assessment of circulating AAT concentrations is usually performed by immunoturbidimetry or immunonephelometry. Concentrations typically range from 70 to 200 mg/dL (14 to 50 µmol/L) in healthy adults but are higher in patients with inflammatory disorders, malignancy, or trauma and in women who are pregnant, on estrogen therapy, or taking oral contraceptives.

## Ceruloplasmin

Ceruloplasmin (Cp) is an $\alpha_2$-globulin that contains 95% of circulating copper. Failure to incorporate copper into Cp results in an unstable protein and is the cause of Wilson disease.

## Haptoglobin

Haptoglobin (Hp) scavenges hemoglobin in the vascular space. The normal plasma half-life of Hp is about 5.5 days. Hp depletion is usually a sensitive biochemical indicator of intravascular hemolysis. Measurement of Hp is performed typically by immunoturbidimetry or immunonephelometry and is a part of the assessment of possible transfusion reactions or other causes of hemolysis.

## Transferrin

Transferrin (originally named *siderophilin*) is the principal plasma transport protein for iron ($Fe^{3+}$). Transferrin has a molecular weight of 79.6 kDa, including 5.5% carbohydrate and circulates with a half-life of 8 to 10 days. Clinical indications for direct measurement of transferrin are few. Indirect assessment of transferrin concentration may be inferred by total iron-binding capacity (TIBC). Transferrin glycan structure is widely used to detect congenital disorders of glycosylation. Transferrin with altered glycans is generically referred to as carbohydrate-deficient transferrin (CDT). A desialylated version of transferrin, termed tau-transferrin or $\beta_2$-transferrin, is a substantial component of CSF but not serum or plasma and may be used as a CSF leakage marker.

## $\beta_2$-Microglobulin

$\beta_2$-microglobulin (BMG) is a small, nonglycosylated 99 residue protein with a molecular weight of 11.8 kDa. It is the noncovalently bound light chain subunit of class I major histocompatibility complex molecules present on the surface of all nucleated cells. Its small size allows efficient glomerular filtration, resulting in a plasma half-life of approximately 100 minutes. In addition to renal failure, therefore, high plasma concentrations occur in inflammation and neoplasms, especially those associated with B lymphocytes.

## C-Reactive Protein

C-reactive protein (CRP) consists of five identical, nonglycosylated 23 kDa subunits and aids in nonspecific host defense against infectious organisms by activating the classical complement pathway. CRP is one of the strongest acute-phase reactants with plasma concentrations rising up to 1000-fold after myocardial infarction, stress, trauma, infection, inflammation, surgery, or neoplastic proliferation. Concentrations are generally higher in bacterial than viral infection. Mildly increased CRP concentrations are associated with an elevated risk of cardiovascular disease. The use of CRP for these purposes requires assays with detection limits below 0.3 mg/L that generally are referred to as high-sensitivity CRP assays.

## Complement

The complement system consists of more than 50 soluble proteins synthesized primarily by the liver, as well as cell-bound receptors and control proteins. A basic schematic of the complement cascade is presented in Fig. 18.4. The basic functions of the complement cascade are to recruit effector phagocytes for opsonization and clearance of foreign pathogens as well as trigger direct destruction of foreign organisms. Activation of the cascade proceeds by three different molecular recognition systems responsive to different threats:

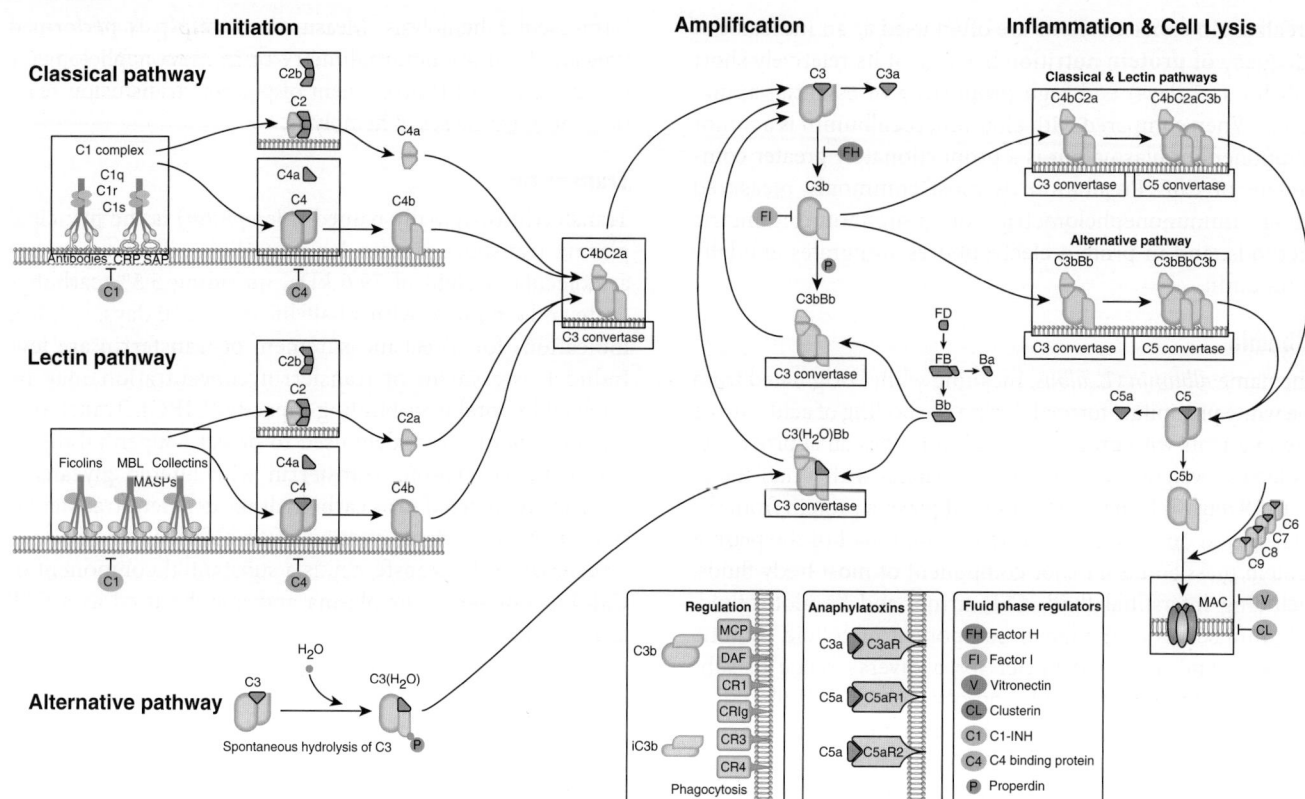

**Fig. 18.4** Complement initiation, amplification, regulation, and formation of the terminal complement complex (TCC). *Initiation, top*: Classical pathway (CP) initiation via C1q and the C1 complex to form the C3 convertase (C4bC2a). *Initiation, middle*: Lectin pathway (LP) initiation via ficolins, MBL and collectins to form the C3 convertase (C4bC2a). The roles of C1-INH, C4BP, and FI in regulating CP and LP initiation are shown. *Initiation, bottom*: Alternative pathway (AP) initiation via the "tick-over" mechanism (spontaneous hydrolysis of C3) to form the AP C3 convertase C3$_{H2O}$Bb. *Amplification*: The amplification loop shows the role of properdin in complement initiation and amplification. The roles if FI, FH, CFHR1 (HR-1) in regulation of complement amplification are highlighted along with the role of FD and FB in complement cascade amplification. *Inflammation and cell lysis:* The role of the amplification loop in generating the C5 convertases is shown along with the C5 convertase formation of the TCC. (Used with permission of the Mayo Foundation for Medical Education and Research, all rights reserved.)

1. The classical pathway (CP) is activated primarily by immune-complex formation. A single immunoglobulin M (IgM) or two immunoglobulin G (IgG) molecules binding to antigens are sufficient to activate a complex consisting of C1q, C1r, and C1s. CP components are numbered consecutively from C1 to C9.
2. The alternative pathway (AP) is not triggered by antibodies but rather, by foreign pathogenic surfaces such as lipopolysaccharides from microbes or it can be spontaneously activated in a surveillance role. AP components are commonly identified with letters and include Factors B, D, H, I, and P.
3. The lectin pathway (LP) is activated after recognition of danger-associated molecular patterns (DAMPs) and pathogen-associated molecular patterns (PAMPs), by binding of mannan-binding lectin (MBL), ficolins or collectins to mannose-rich oligosaccharides that are present in the cell walls of many microorganisms. This event triggers activation of MBL-associated serine proteases termed MASP-1 and MASP-2, which are homologous to C1r and C1s in the CP.

During activation of the cascades, many complement components are enzymatically cleaved into two or more fragments. The cascades converge at C3, and the terminal complement cascade has three main effects:

1. cell lysis via generation of the C5b-9 or membrane attack complex,
2. inflammation via generation of anaphylatoxins such as C3a and C5a fragments, and
3. opsonization, the process of tagging molecules with C3b fragments to facilitate phagocytosis.

The constant slow, chronic activation of complement components would have devastating consequences were it not for a host of regulatory proteins designed to limit complement activity. Deficiency of DAF and CD59 can lead to abnormal lysis of RBCs, such as observed in paroxysmal nocturnal hemoglobinuria. Defects in C1 inhibitors are linked to hereditary angioedema. Factor H plays a role in age-related macular degeneration, atypical hemolytic uremic syndrome and C3 glomerulopathies. Proper function of complement regulatory proteins prevents the destruction of endogenous cells at the same time that foreign cells are destroyed by complement.

Laboratory analyses of the complement system can be divided into five different types of testing. The oldest and most widely available type of testing is the assessment of **(1) complement function or activity**. Measurement of complement activity is a screening test that demonstrates an intact pathway from activation to formation of the MAC for the study of complement deficiencies or over-activation. The classic version of this assay is a hemolytic assay, which tests the capacity of patient sera to lyse sheep RBCs coated with rabbit anti-sheep antibodies. CH50 refers to the amount of serum required to lyse 50% of the added erythrocytes. Many new versions of the test have become available in the past decades, including ones amenable to automation, which utilize liposomes coated with immune-complexes instead of RBCs. ELISA versions of the test, which can assess CP, AP, or LP function, depending on the type of trigger coated on the ELISA plate (Fig. 18.5), made the functional tests relatively simple to adopt. An abnormal result will be low, suggesting poor complement proteins synthesis or increased consumption.

The second most common type of complement test is **(2) measurement of individual component concentrations**, such as the assessment of circulating C3 and C4. C3 and C4 are typically determined with immunoturbidimetry or immunonephelometry. Measurement of C3 and C4 are used to assess activation of the AP and CP, respectively. Low concentrations are observed in complement deficiency, glomerulonephritis, systemic lupus erythematosus, and sepsis.

More recently, the availability of assays to measure **(3) activation fragments of complement components** has helped to differentiate complement deficiencies from complement consumption in which the parent molecules are being cleaved constantly due to an auto-immune or infectious process. Measurement of the more stable activation fragments such as C4d, Bb, sC5b-9 (the soluble MAC) using ELISA are part of complex evaluations performed for a full picture of the complement cascade.

The detection of **(4) autoantibodies against complement components** may help elucidate if complement dysregulation has a genetic or acquired cause. Acquired causes of complement dysregulation may be treated with immunosuppressants and plasma exchange. Autoantibodies against the complement convertases, called C3, C4, and C5 nephritic factors (for the AP and CP C3 convertases, respectively, and the C5 convertases) are present in kidney diseases such as the

## ELISA–Based Complement Functional Assays

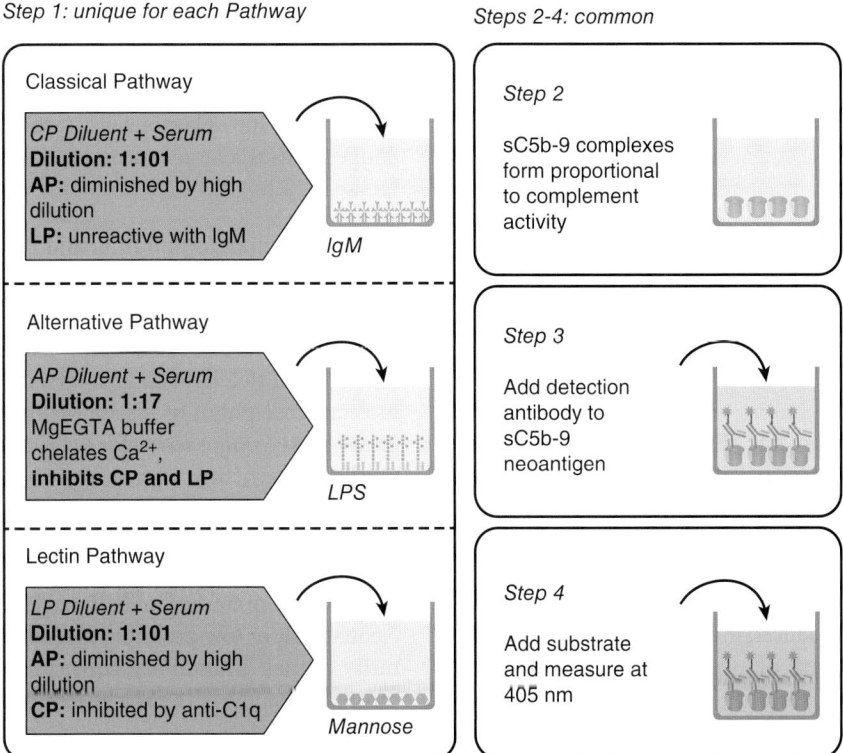

**Fig. 18.5** ELISA (enzyme-linked immunosorbent assay) assays are available to measure function of Classical, Lectin and Alternative pathways of complement. For the classical pathway (CP) function assessment, the plate is coated with immunoglobulin M *(IgM)*. For the lectin pathway (LP) function the plate has mannose, and for the alternative pathway (AP) function there are lipopolysaccharides from Gram negative bacteria coated on a solid-phase support ELISA plate. The CP and LP assays are run with diluted serum at 1:101, and the AP assay uses 1:18 dilution. In addition, the buffer used for the LP uses antibodies to C1q to block initiation of CP. The high dilution makes it difficult to trigger the AP. The buffer used in the AP assay uses magnesium EGTA to chelate calcium, necessary for the activity of CP and LP but not the AP. Function is tested when the complement system in patient's serum is activated by the plate triggers, and its cascades amplified to create C3 and C5 convertases, and ultimately the membrane attack complex (MAC). The conjugate antibody for all assays targets neoepitopes generated after the formation of the MAC. (Created with biorender.com.)

C3 glomerulopathies, a rare type of membranoproliferative glomerulonephritis where the AP damages kidney structures. Antibodies to Factor H have also been described as an acquired cause of atypical hemolytic uremic syndrome and C3 glomerulopathies.

**Genetic studies of complement genes (5)** support differentiation between hereditary or acquired causes of deficiency or disease, and testing frequently helps clinicians in determining prognosis, course of therapy and potential risk of relapses. Known pathogenic genetic variants may require specific treatment with complement inhibitors such as eculizumab or ravulizumab, monoclonal antibody therapies that block the terminal pathway component C5 and the subsequent lytic effects of complement.

## Immunoglobulins

**Immunoglobulins** (antibodies) are generated against foreign immunogens and initiate clearance of the foreign molecule or organism. Human immunoglobulin molecules (commonly depicted in the shape of a Y, Fig. 18.6) consist of one or more basic units built of two identical heavy (H) chains and two identical light (L) chains. L chains have one variable and one constant domain while H chains have one variable and three to four constant domains, with the variable region involved in antigen recognition and binding (see Chapter 15). Extensive diversity in the variable domains is generated by somatic recombination and mutation of the immunoglobulin genes. Individual plasma cells or clonally expanded cells are committed to synthesis of a single variable domain sequence for heavy and light chains. The amino acid sequences of the variable domains at the N-terminal ends of the four chains form two antigen-binding sites with a high degree of variation in binding specificity. The constant domains are the same for every immunoglobulin molecule of a given subclass and carry sites for binding to complement receptors and activation of complement.

Cleavage of immunoglobulins with pepsin or papain can yield antigen-binding fragments (Fab) and constant region fragments (Fc). Variations in the constant domains of heavy chains (Fc region) result in the classes and subclasses into which immunoglobulins are grouped: IgM, IgG (four subclasses), immunoglobulin A (IgA) (two subclasses), immunoglobulin D (IgD), and immunoglobulin E (IgE), respectively. Light chains, which are produced independently and in slight excess of heavy chains, are of two types—kappa (κ) and lambda (λ).

Immunoglobulins are synthesized by plasma cells, the progeny of B-lymphocyte stem cells in bone marrow. More mature B lymphocytes, found mainly in lymph nodes and in blood, develop receptor immunoglobulins on their surface membranes. Upon binding a target antigen, these B lymphocytes proliferate and develop into a clone of plasma cells, producing antibodies to the target antigen. Somatic mutation of immunoglobulins leads to further diversity of immunoglobulin variable region and antibody maturation, generally leading to antibodies with higher affinity. B lymphocytes at first have IgM surface receptors and secrete IgM as the first

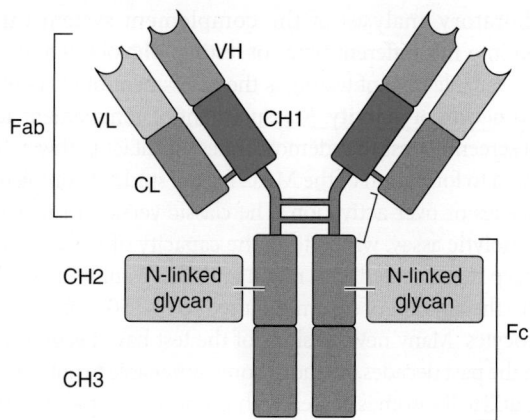

**Fig. 18.6** Human immunoglobulin's basic structure composed of two identical heavy chains and two light chains. *CH*, Constant region of heavy chain; *CL*, constant region of light chains; *Fab*, antigenic binding fragment; *Fc*, crystallizable region fragment; *VH*, variable region of heavy chain; *VL*, variable region of light chain. The hinge region is located in between Fab and Fc. (Created with biorender.com.)

or "primary" response to an antigen. Membrane and secreted forms of the antibody arise from differential splicing of the messenger RNA for heavy chains, which adds a transmembrane segment to the membrane-bound form. Heavy chains of the IgM surface receptor molecules undergo class switching to produce immunoglobulins with γ- or α-heavy chains (IgG or IgA), but the variable regions remain unchanged; as the cells change into plasma cells, second exposure to the same antigen causes a larger secondary or anamnestic response of IgG secretion.

### Individual Immunoglobulins and Light Chains

*Immunoglobulin G.* IgG accounts for 70% to 75% of the total immunoglobulins in plasma. Only 35% is found in the plasma space, and 65% is extravascular. IgG consists of two γ-heavy and two light chains, linked by disulfide bonds. The molecular weight of IgG is approximately 150 kDa, including one N-linked oligosaccharide on each heavy chain. The oligosaccharide structure may change in inflammatory states and affect interactions with receptors.

IgG has four subclasses: $IgG_1$, $IgG_2$, $IgG_3$, and $IgG_4$. $IgG_1$ is the principal IgG to cross the placenta, and neonatal concentrations are similar to maternal concentrations (Fig. 18.7). Neonates have low production of IgG as the result of immaturity of their immune systems, and IgG concentrations fall through infancy as the maternally acquired antibody repertoire is cleared.

*Immunoglobulin M.* IgM is produced at earlier stages of B-cell development. In the immature immune systems of neonates, IgM is the major immunoglobulin synthesized. In adult serum, it is the third most abundant immunoglobulin, usually accounting for 5% to 10% of total circulating immunoglobulins. IgM as a membrane receptor molecule is monomeric, but most of the serum IgM is a pentamer containing five monomers linked via disulfide bonds to the small J (joining) chain. Plasma cell malignancies may secrete monomeric IgM in addition to, or instead of, pentamers.

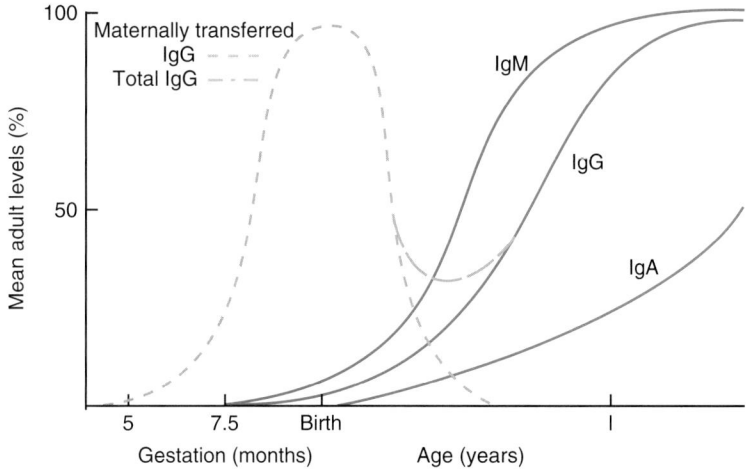

**Fig. 18.7** Serum immunoglobulin concentrations as percent of mean adult concentrations before birth and for the first year of life. *IgA,* Immunoglobulin A; *IgG,* immunoglobulin G; *IgM,* immunoglobulin M.

The high molecular weight of IgM (970 kDa; approximately 10% carbohydrate) prevents its ready passage into extravascular spaces. IgM is not transported across the placenta and therefore is not involved in hemolytic disease of neonates. It activates complement even more efficiently than IgG. Binding of one IgM molecule may be adequate to activate the complement classical pathway. In rare hyper-IgM syndromes, class switching to IgG and IgA is deficient. Affected patients have deficiency of IgG and IgA and increased susceptibility to infection.

*Immunoglobulin A.* IgA has a molecular weight of 160 kDa, including about 10% carbohydrate derived from both N- and O-linked oligosaccharide chains. IgA accounts for about 10% to 15% of serum immunoglobulin and has a half-life of 6 days. In its monomeric form, its structure is similar to that of IgG, but 10% to 15% of IgA in serum is dimeric, particularly IgA$_2$, which is more resistant to destruction by pathogenic bacteria than IgA$_1$. On electrophoresis, IgA migrates in the β-γ region, anodal to most IgG. IgA is an important component of mucosal immunity. Secretory IgA is found in tears, sweat, saliva, milk, colostrum, and gastrointestinal (GI) and bronchial secretions. Secretory IgA has a molecular weight of 380 kDa and consists of two molecules of IgA: a secretory component (70 kDa) and a J chain (15.6 kDa). It is synthesized mainly by plasma cells in the mucous membranes of the gut and bronchi and in the ductules of the lactating breast. The secretory component assists with transport of secretory IgA across mucosal epithelium and into secretions. Secretory IgA in colostrum and milk is more abundant than IgG and may aid in protection of neonates from intestinal infection. IgA can activate complement by the AP, but the exact role of IgA in serum is not clear.

*Immunoglobulin D.* IgD accounts for less than 1% of serum immunoglobulin. It is monomeric, contains about 12% carbohydrate, and has a molecular weight of 184 kDa. Its structure is similar to that of IgG. Similar to IgM, IgD is a surface receptor for antigens on B lymphocytes, but its primary function is unknown. A condition named hyperimmunoglobulin D syndrome is a rare, autosomal recessive genetic disorder characterized by recurrent episodes of fever with lymphadenopathy, abdominal pain, and increased serum IgD concentration above 14 mg/dL or 100 IU/mL. The IgD increase in hyper IgD syndrome is polyclonal. IgD monoclonal gammopathies can occur and have a worse prognosis than other monoclonal gammopathies.

*Immunoglobulin E.* IgE contains 15% carbohydrate and has a molecular weight of 188 kDa. IgE is so rapidly and firmly bound to specific IgE receptors on mast cells that only trace amounts are normally present in serum. IgE binds to mast cells via sites on its Fc region. When the antigen (allergen) cross-links two of the attached IgE molecules, the mast cell is stimulated to release histamine and other vasoactive amines that increase vascular permeability and smooth muscle contraction, mediating type 1 hypersensitivity reactions such as hay fever, asthma, urticaria, and eczema. Rare regulatory disorders with hyperproduction of IgE lead to a primary immunodeficiency disorder referred to as Job syndrome, characterized by eczema, recurrent infection, and markedly increased IgE. IgE molecules specific for particular allergens are commonly assessed to identify the specificity of allergies. The total serum concentration of IgE may be increased in individuals with allergic disorders.

*Free immunoglobulin light chains.* Light chains are usually synthesized in excess of heavy chains beyond quantities required for intact immunoglobulins. Consequently, small amounts of free light chains (FLCs), representing only about 0.1% of total immunoglobulin, are present in serum or plasma. Amounts in plasma are kept low by renal clearance and FLCs have a half-life of 2 to 6 hours. Free κ-light chains (23 kDa) are cleared about two to three times faster than free λ-light chains (frequently a disulfide-linked dimer of 46 kDa). Consequently, even though production of κ-light chains is about twice as great as that of λ-light chains, the plasma concentration of free λ-light chains is usually higher, except in renal failure. Immunoassays specific for FLCs are employed to study plasma cell disorders.

Quantitative FLC assays use antisera directed against epitopes that are exposed only when the light chains are free (unbound to heavy chain) in solution. These cryptic sites are involved in the very tight, non-covalent binding of light chains to heavy chains. FLC immunoassays can be used to specifically quantitate FLCs even in the presence of large concentrations of polyclonal serum immunoglobulins. The approach is to quantitate the κ FLC and the λ FLC and use the ratio of κ/λ FLC to detect unbalanced light chain synthesis, for an estimation of monoclonality, which has proven surprisingly sensitive for detecting clonal-free light chain diseases.

## Clinical Utility of Immunoglobulin Measurement

Serum normally contains a diverse, polyclonal mixture of antibodies with varying amino acid sequences, which represent multiple "idiotypes" (i.e., the products of many different clones of plasma cells, each producing a specific immunoglobulin molecule). Disease states may be associated with a decrease or an increase in normal polyclonal immunoglobulins or an increase in one or more monoclonal immunoglobulins. These disease states are detailed below.

*Immunoglobulin deficiency.* Immunodeficiency states may be due to a single factor or combinations affecting multiple systems of immune defense. Severe combined immune deficiency (SCID) is a disorder of B-cell development or activation affecting 1 in 100,000 newborns and resulting in broad-spectrum immunoglobulin deficiency. The more common primary deficiencies involve only one or two immunoglobulin classes (IgA) or subclasses (IgA or IgG subclasses) or ability to generate antibodies against polysaccharide antigens. IgA deficiency may lead to false-negative assays for celiac disease detection, and some affected individuals are at risk for anaphylaxis if they receive blood products containing IgA. Selective deficiency of IgG subclasses is not rare, but it is unclear whether it is an important risk for infection. Deficiency of IgG2 may be related to poorer responses to polysaccharide antigens and increased risk of infection with encapsulated organisms.

The diagnosis of major deficiencies in immunoglobulin production is clinically important to avoid infection, particularly in neonates, as their maternally acquired antibodies decline. Infants have transient physiologic deficiency of IgG, with a nadir at about 3 months of age (Fig. 18.8). Prolonged or severe physiologic deficiency may be associated with increased infection rates, especially with encapsulated bacteria. Concentrations of maternal IgG, transferred across the placenta, rise rapidly in the fetus during the last half of pregnancy but then drop over a few months after birth. Two groups of neonates are at risk for clinically significant IgG deficiency: premature infants who begin life with less maternal IgG and

infants with delayed initiation of IgG synthesis. Monitoring of IgG concentrations can identify this problem. Rising IgM and normal salivary IgA concentrations at 6 weeks of age suggest a favorable prognosis. Contact of the neonate with environmental antigens normally causes B lymphocytes to begin to multiply and IgM concentrations to start to rise, followed weeks to months later by IgA and IgG.

*Polyclonal hyperimmunoglobulinemia.* Polyclonal increases in plasma immunoglobulins are the normal response to infection. IgG predominates in autoimmune responses. IgA is increased in skin, gut, respiratory, and renal infections, and IgM is increased in primary viral infections and bloodstream infection with parasites such as malaria. Chronic bacterial infection may cause increased concentrations of all immunoglobulins. Measurements of total IgE are used in the management of asthma and other allergic conditions, especially in children. Measurements of allergen-specific IgE assist in identifying the stimulus for hypersensitivity responses.

*Monoclonal immunoglobulins (paraproteins).* A single clone of plasma cells produces immunoglobulin molecules with a single defined amino acid sequence. If the clone expands greatly, it may produce a discrete band on electrophoresis, often referred to as an M-spike or M-protein. These monoclonal immunoglobulins, termed **paraproteins**, may be polymers, monomers, individual immunoglobulin chains such as FLC or heavy chains, or fragments of immunoglobulins. Clinical, epidemiologic, and biochemical characteristics of monoclonal paraprotein isotypes found in **multiple myeloma** are summarized in Table 18.4. About 60% of paraproteins are associated with plasma cell malignancies (light chain amyloidosis, multiple myeloma, or solitary plasmacytoma), and approximately 15% are caused by overproduction by B lymphocytes, mainly in lymph nodes (lymphomas, chronic lymphocytic leukemia, Waldenström macroglobulinemia, or heavy-chain disease). Virtually every multiple myeloma is preceded by the premalignant condition **monoclonal gammopathy of undetermined significance (MGUS)**. The incidence of MGUS increases with age, with a 1% incidence for people 50 to 70 years of age and a 3% incidence for people older than 70. The occurrence of MGUS is associated with increased risk of progression to multiple myeloma that should be monitored after the initial diagnosis is made. MGUS is the most commonly diagnosed monoclonal gammopathy, followed by multiple myeloma and primary light-chain amyloidosis, also known as AL amyloidosis.

The primary clinical interest in identifying paraproteins is to detect or monitor proliferative disorders of B cells. However, from the laboratory standpoint, paraproteins are

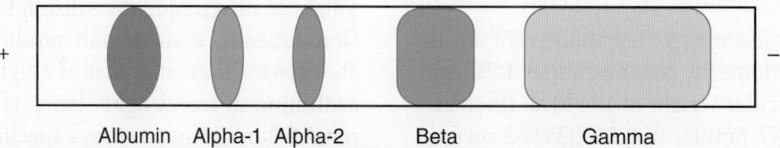

Fig. 18.8 Schematic of protein migration and regional annotation in serum protein electrophoresis. The anode is depicted on the left and cathode on the right. Blue shading represents the relative protein concentration (darker is higher) in each region of a normal individual.

## TABLE 18.4   Monoclonal Immunoglobulins (Paraproteins) in Multiple Myeloma

| Plasma Paraprotein | Incidence[a] (%) | Mean Age of Occurrence[a] (Years) | Incidence of Free Light Chain in Urine (%) | Comments |
|---|---|---|---|---|
| IgG | 50 | 65 | 60 | Patients more susceptible to infection; paraproteins reach highest concentrations |
| IgA | 25 | 65 | 70 | Tend to have hypercalcemia and amyloidosis |
| Free light chain only | 20 | 56 | 100 | Often renal failure; bone lesions; amyloidosis; poor prognosis |
| IgD | 2 | 57 | 100 | 90% λ type; often have extraosseous lesion, amyloidosis, renal failure; poor prognosis |
| IgM | 1 | — | 100 | May or may not have hyperviscosity syndrome |
| IgE | 0.1 | — | Most | Rare, less than 50 cases described |
| Biclonal | 1 | — | — | Prognosis not more serious due to biclonality |
| None detected | <1 | — | 0 | Usually found with reduction of normal immunoglobulins (hypogammaglobulinemia on PEP); increased plasma cells in bone marrow biopsy or plasmacytomas |

[a]Approximate.

*Ig*, Immunoglobulin; *PEP*, protein electrophoresis.

also significant as a potentially unpredictable source of interference with many assays. Paraproteins may aggregate or precipitate, causing interference in a variety of photometric reactions and in light-scattering hematology analyzers.

Many patients with paraproteins have nonspecific presentations such as anemia or infection. Identification of paraproteins in serum usually is based on serum protein electrophoresis and immunofixation electrophoresis (IFE) (described in a later section), along with measurement of FLCs. Urine protein electrophoresis and urine IFE are helpful mainly in identifying patients with free immunoglobulin light chains and amyloidosis. Urinary FLCs, as described by Bence Jones in the 1850s, were the first tumor marker. FLC are often referred to as *Bence Jones proteins.*

## Acute Phase Response

Systemic inflammation in response to infection, tissue injury, or inflammatory disease triggers changes in hepatic production of multiple plasma proteins. This process, mediated by the action of interleukin-6 (IL-6) and other cytokines has been termed the acute-phase response (APR). It is a nonspecific reaction to inflammation, analogous to the increase in temperature or leukocyte count. In the APR, synthesis of a few proteins, including albumin, transferrin, and prealbumin, is downregulated. These proteins are termed *negative acute-phase reactants*. Production of a number of proteins, including AAT, $\alpha_1$-acid glycoprotein (AAG), Hp, Cp, C4, C3, fibrinogen, and CRP, increases severalfold. Plasma concentrations of these individual *positive acute-phase reactants* rise at different rates, and all reach maxima within 2 to 5 days after an acute insult (Box 18.1).

## Methods for Analyzing Proteins
### Determination of Total Protein

Plasma normally contains about 6.5 to 8.5 g/dL protein and serum about 4% less. Determination of total protein in biologic fluids in some respects represents a greater challenge than analysis of a specific protein because variable protein composition of biologic fluids leads to variable carbohydrate composition, charge, and physical characteristics of proteins in the mixture. Many methods of protein analysis respond differentially to different proteins and present problems when applied to specimens of varying protein composition. The Biuret method is the most commonly employed technique for clinical assessment of total protein. Under strongly alkaline conditions, $Cu^{2+}$ ions form multivalent complexes with peptide bonds in proteins. Binding shifts the absorption spectrum of $Cu^{2+}$ ions to shorter wavelengths, leading to a color change from blue to violet that has been termed the *biuret reaction.* Absorbance attributable to protein is measured at 540 nm. Biuret reagent is commonly thought to react equally with all proteins and peptides longer than two amino acids. Protein concentration in more dilute fluid compartments like CSF and urine is typically determined with dye-binding methods (e.g., pyrogallol red) or light-scattering (e.g., benzethonium chloride, precipitation).

*Variables affecting measured protein concentrations.* Calibration of biuret methods commonly uses bovine or human albumin. Protein mixtures with specific albumin-to-globulin ratios have been recommended for calibration of other methods. Hemodilution and dehydration along with a change in position (standing vs. recumbent) also alters plasma protein

## BOX 18.1 The Acute Phase Response

**Changes in Plasma Protein Concentrations**

*Positive Acute Phase Response*

C-reactive protein (extreme)
Serum amyloid A (extreme)
$\alpha_1$-Acid glycoprotein
$\alpha_1$-Antitrypsin
$\alpha_1$-Antichymotrypsin
Antithrombin III
C3, C4, and C9
C1 inhibitor
C4b-binding protein
Ceruloplasmin
Factor B
Ferritin
Fibrinogen
Haptoglobin
Hemopexin
Lipopolysaccharide-binding protein
Mannan-binding protein (lectin)
Plasminogen
Procalcitonin

*Negative Acute Phase Response*

Albumin
Apolipoprotein A-I
Apolipoprotein B
Insulin-like growth factor I
Prealbumin
Retinol-binding protein
Thyroxine-binding globulin
Transferrin

Data from Craig WY, Ledue TB, Ritchie RF. *Plasma Proteins: Clinical Utility and Interpretation.* Scarborough, ME: Foundation for Blood Research, 2001; Gabay C, Kushner I. Acute-phase proteins and other systemic responses to inflammation. *N Engl J Med.* 1999;340:448–454; and Vollmer T, Piper C, Kleesiek K, Dreier J. Lipopolysaccharide-binding protein: a new biomarker for infectious endocarditis? *Clin Chem.* 2009;55:295–302.

concentration. A recumbent position decreases total protein concentration by 0.3 to 0.5 g/dL. This reflects the redistribution of extracellular fluid from the extravascular space to the intravascular space and therefore dilution of a constant amount of plasma protein in a larger volume.

## Immunochemical Techniques for Specific Proteins

Nephelometric and turbidimetric methods are performed as equilibrium or rate methods for measuring the amount of light scattering by antigen–antibody complexes. Limits of detection of approximately 10 mg/L can be achieved with routine nephelometric and turbidimetric methods using antibodies in solution. Binding antibodies to particles of latex or other materials enhances light scattering and can lower limits of detection by 10- to 100-fold. Such assays may be described as latex-enhanced or as particle-enhanced assays. Turbidimetric methods can be applied on most automated chemistry analyzers capable of performing photometric methods. Nephelometry requires instrumentation capable of measuring light scattering at an angle to the incident light.

## Electrophoresis

Electrophoresis is used to separate proteins by charge. Electrophoretic techniques commonly performed in clinical laboratories include non-denaturing electrophoresis on cellulose acetate strips or agarose gels, capillary electrophoresis (CE). Subsequent detection of separated protein is achieved using dyes, antibodies, or increasingly, MS.

*Serum protein electrophoresis.* An idealized representation of serum protein electrophoresis is shown in Fig 18.8. Generally, serum rather than plasma is used for electrophoresis of proteins on agarose gels to avoid the fibrinogen band at the $\beta$-$\gamma$ interface. Abundant proteins within gels are visualized with a variety of dyes including amido black, Ponceau S, acid violet, and Coomassie blue. Intensity of staining and linearity of protein detection vary. Only a few of the most abundant proteins are visualized, and intensities of bands with protein stains usually relate to the mass of peptide. Quantitation of individual components is typically achieved using densitometry.

The major clinical application of serum protein electrophoresis is the detection of monoclonal immunoglobulins (paraproteins) to assist in the diagnosis and monitoring of multiple myeloma and related disorders. Most monoclonal immunoglobulins are observed in the $\beta$-region or $\gamma$-region. Quantitation of monoclonal components serves as a means of monitoring disease progression and response to therapy. Protein electrophoresis may also aid in the diagnosis of other conditions unrelated to monoclonal gammopathies, however, for these uses, specific tests are available. Changes in the $\alpha_1$-region are typically related to AAT. Decreases are associated with AAT deficiency or protein-losing disorders. Increases are related to inflammation. Changes in the $\alpha_2$-region usually relate to changes in Hp and $\alpha_2$ macroglobulin (AMG). Bands in the $\beta$-region are related to transferrin, C3, and LDL. An increase between $\beta$- and $\gamma$-bands, so-called bridging of $\beta$- and $\gamma$-bands, suggests an increase in IgA as seen with cirrhosis, respiratory tract or skin infection, and rheumatoid arthritis. Finally, increases or decreases in the $\gamma$-region suggest changes in immunoglobulin concentrations. Fig. 18.9 provides multiple examples of serum electrophoretic patterns in normal and pathologic specimens.

*Immunofixation electrophoresis.* IFE employs antisera targeted to specific proteins rather than nonspecific dyes. Examples of IFE from two patients with monoclonal gammopathies are shown in Fig. 18.10. Specific lanes of the gel are overlaid with antisera against $\kappa$ and $\lambda$ light chains or $\gamma$, $\mu$, and $\alpha$-immunoglobulin heavy chains. Paraproteins characteristically yield sharper precipitin bands than the heterogeneous polyclonal immunoglobulins. IFE helps identify the immunoglobulin type of the paraprotein. Sometimes more than one clone may be expanded, or a monoclonal free light chain may occur concurrently with a monoclonal intact immunoglobulin. Uncommonly, paraproteins may be of the IgD or IgE class. These paraproteins should be detected by standard

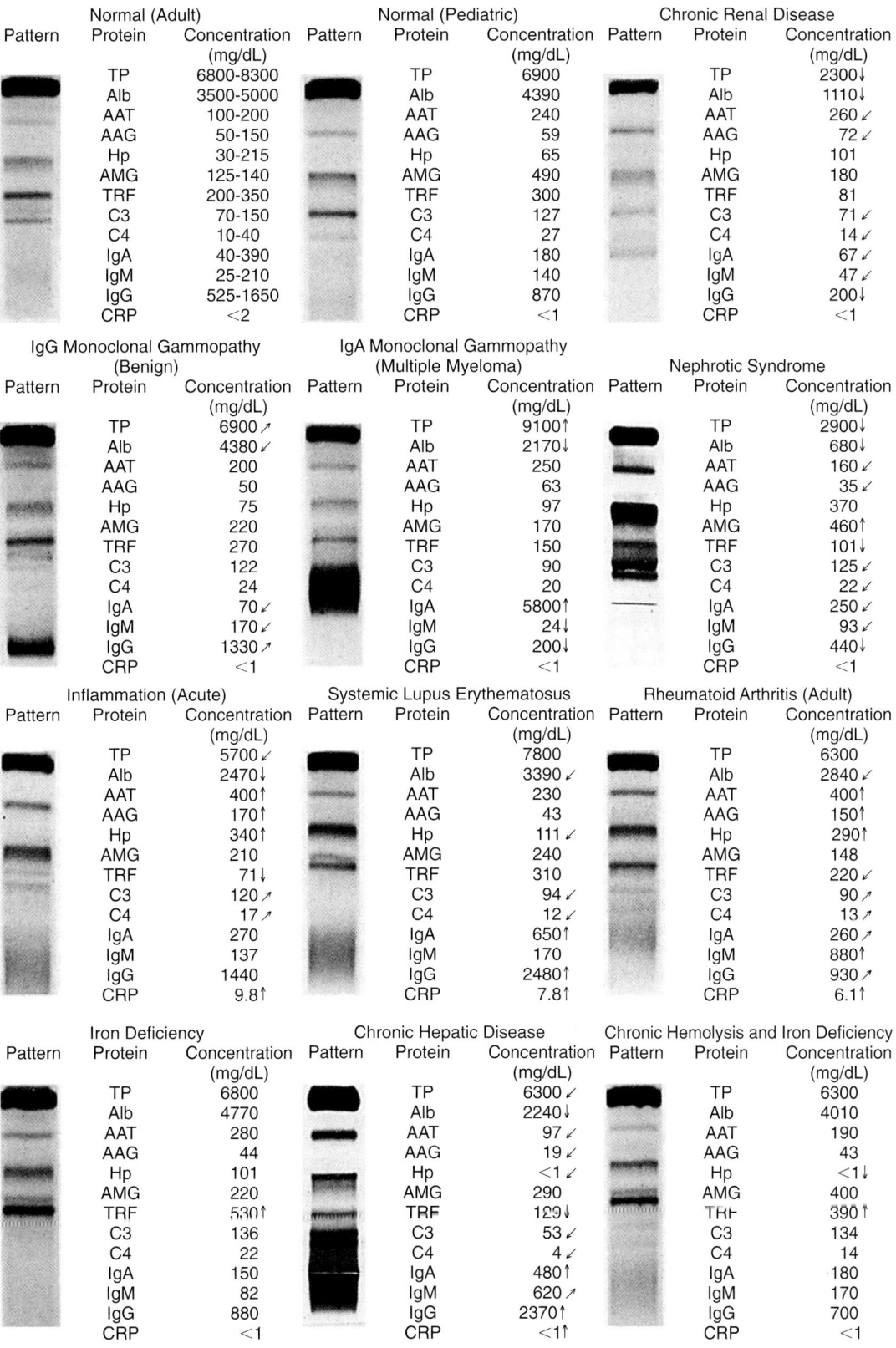

| Normal (Adult) | | |
|---|---|---|
| Pattern | Protein | Concentration (mg/dL) |
| | TP | 6800-8300 |
| | Alb | 3500-5000 |
| | AAT | 100-200 |
| | AAG | 50-150 |
| | Hp | 30-215 |
| | AMG | 125-140 |
| | TRF | 200-350 |
| | C3 | 70-150 |
| | C4 | 10-40 |
| | IgA | 40-390 |
| | IgM | 25-210 |
| | IgG | 525-1650 |
| | CRP | <2 |

| Normal (Pediatric) | | |
|---|---|---|
| Pattern | Protein | Concentration (mg/dL) |
| | TP | 6900 |
| | Alb | 4390 |
| | AAT | 240 |
| | AAG | 59 |
| | Hp | 65 |
| | AMG | 490 |
| | TRF | 300 |
| | C3 | 127 |
| | C4 | 27 |
| | IgA | 180 |
| | IgM | 140 |
| | IgG | 870 |
| | CRP | <1 |

| Chronic Renal Disease | | |
|---|---|---|
| Pattern | Protein | Concentration (mg/dL) |
| | TP | 2300↓ |
| | Alb | 1110↓ |
| | AAT | 260↙ |
| | AAG | 72↙ |
| | Hp | 101 |
| | AMG | 180 |
| | TRF | 81 |
| | C3 | 71↙ |
| | C4 | 14↙ |
| | IgA | 67↙ |
| | IgM | 47↙ |
| | IgG | 200↓ |
| | CRP | <1 |

| IgG Monoclonal Gammopathy (Benign) | | |
|---|---|---|
| Pattern | Protein | Concentration (mg/dL) |
| | TP | 6900↗ |
| | Alb | 4380↙ |
| | AAT | 200 |
| | AAG | 50 |
| | Hp | 75 |
| | AMG | 220 |
| | TRF | 270 |
| | C3 | 122 |
| | C4 | 24 |
| | IgA | 70↙ |
| | IgM | 170↙ |
| | IgG | 1330↗ |
| | CRP | <1 |

| IgA Monoclonal Gammopathy (Multiple Myeloma) | | |
|---|---|---|
| Pattern | Protein | Concentration (mg/dL) |
| | TP | 9100↑ |
| | Alb | 2170↓ |
| | AAT | 250 |
| | AAG | 63 |
| | Hp | 97 |
| | AMG | 170 |
| | TRF | 150 |
| | C3 | 90 |
| | C4 | 20 |
| | IgA | 5800↑ |
| | IgM | 24↓ |
| | IgG | 200↓ |
| | CRP | <1 |

| Nephrotic Syndrome | | |
|---|---|---|
| Pattern | Protein | Concentration (mg/dL) |
| | TP | 2900↓ |
| | Alb | 680↓ |
| | AAT | 160↙ |
| | AAG | 35↙ |
| | Hp | 370 |
| | AMG | 460↑ |
| | TRF | 101↓ |
| | C3 | 125↙ |
| | C4 | 22↙ |
| | IgA | 250↙ |
| | IgM | 93↙ |
| | IgG | 440↓ |
| | CRP | <1 |

| Inflammation (Acute) | | |
|---|---|---|
| Pattern | Protein | Concentration (mg/dL) |
| | TP | 5700↙ |
| | Alb | 2470↓ |
| | AAT | 400↑ |
| | AAG | 170↑ |
| | Hp | 340↑ |
| | AMG | 210 |
| | TRF | 71↓ |
| | C3 | 120↗ |
| | C4 | 17↗ |
| | IgA | 270 |
| | IgM | 137 |
| | IgG | 1440 |
| | CRP | 9.8↑ |

| Systemic Lupus Erythematosus | | |
|---|---|---|
| Pattern | Protein | Concentration (mg/dL) |
| | TP | 7800 |
| | Alb | 3390↙ |
| | AAT | 230 |
| | AAG | 43 |
| | Hp | 111↙ |
| | AMG | 240 |
| | TRF | 310 |
| | C3 | 94↙ |
| | C4 | 12↙ |
| | IgA | 650↑ |
| | IgM | 170 |
| | IgG | 2480↑ |
| | CRP | 7.8↑ |

| Rheumatoid Arthritis (Adult) | | |
|---|---|---|
| Pattern | Protein | Concentration (mg/dL) |
| | TP | 6300 |
| | Alb | 2840↙ |
| | AAT | 400↑ |
| | AAG | 150↑ |
| | Hp | 290↑ |
| | AMG | 148 |
| | TRF | 220↙ |
| | C3 | 90↙ |
| | C4 | 13↗ |
| | IgA | 260↗ |
| | IgM | 880↑ |
| | IgG | 930↗ |
| | CRP | 6.1↑ |

| Iron Deficiency | | |
|---|---|---|
| Pattern | Protein | Concentration (mg/dL) |
| | TP | 6800 |
| | Alb | 4770 |
| | AAT | 280 |
| | AAG | 44 |
| | Hp | 101 |
| | AMG | 220 |
| | TRF | 530↑ |
| | C3 | 136 |
| | C4 | 22 |
| | IgA | 150 |
| | IgM | 82 |
| | IgG | 880 |
| | CRP | <1 |

| Chronic Hepatic Disease | | |
|---|---|---|
| Pattern | Protein | Concentration (mg/dL) |
| | TP | 6300↙ |
| | Alb | 2240↓ |
| | AAT | 97↙ |
| | AAG | 19↙ |
| | Hp | <1↙ |
| | AMG | 290 |
| | TRF | 129↓ |
| | C3 | 53↙ |
| | C4 | 4↙ |
| | IgA | 480↑ |
| | IgM | 620↗ |
| | IgG | 2370↑ |
| | CRP | <1↑ |

| Chronic Hemolysis and Iron Deficiency | | |
|---|---|---|
| Pattern | Protein | Concentration (mg/dL) |
| | TP | 6300 |
| | Alb | 4010 |
| | AAT | 190 |
| | AAG | 43 |
| | Hp | <1↓ |
| | AMG | 400 |
| | TRF | 390↑ |
| | C3 | 134 |
| | C4 | 14 |
| | IgA | 180 |
| | IgM | 170 |
| | IgG | 700 |
| | CRP | <1 |

Fig. 18.9 Electrophoretic patterns typical of normal conditions and of some pathologic conditions (agarose gel). The *upward-* and *downward-pointing arrows* indicate increase and decrease from the reference interval, respectively. *Right-* and *left-slanting arrows* indicate variation from normal to an increase or from normal to a decrease from the reference interval, respectively. *AAG,* Alpha-1 acid glycoprotein; *AAT,* alpha-1 antitrypsin; *Alb,* albumin; *AMG,* alpha-2 macroglobulin; *C3,* complement component 3; *C4,* complement component 4; *CRP,* C-reactive protein; *Hp,* haptoglobin; *Ig,* immunoglobulin; *TP,* total protein concentration; *TRF,* transferrin.

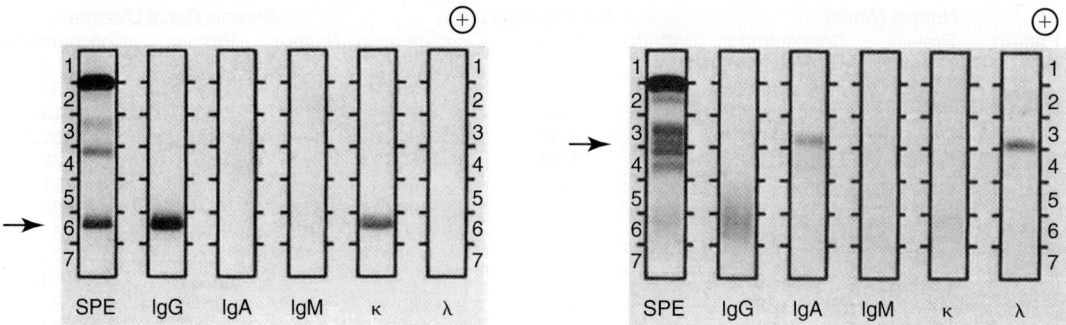

Fig. 18.10 Immunofixation electrophoresis (IFE). *Left,* Patient specimen with an immunoglobulin G (IgG; κ) monoclonal protein. *Right,* Patient specimen with an immunoglobulin A (IgA; λ) monoclonal protein. The *arrow* indicates the position of monoclonal protein. *IgA,* Immunoglobulin A; *IgG,* immunoglobulin G; *IgM,* immunoglobulin M.

antisera directed against κ and λ light chains but require δ or ε heavy chain–specific antisera to distinguish them from FLC.

***Capillary electrophoresis.*** CE of proteins relies on zone electrophoresis in small-bore (10 to 100 μm), fused silica capillary tubes 20 to 200 cm in length (see Chapter 11). Electrokinetic or hydrostatic injection introduces a small amount of protein that is resolved rapidly under high voltage. One of the challenges is to avoid the adsorption of proteins to the surface of the capillary. CE is suitable for automation and offers rapid analysis with no need for gel handling or staining. Direct UV detection offers slightly different specificity than protein staining and offers better reproducibility of quantitation than densitometry. Immunofixation cannot be performed with CE. Immunosubtraction with specific antisera is used as an alternative procedure to identify paraproteins, with similar sensitivity.

***Mass spectrometry.*** Multiple types of MS instrumentation provide qualitative or quantitative information about proteins (see Chapter 13). An advantage of MS is the ability to analyze a large number of components in a single analysis, including rapid-sequence analysis of peptides. MS, therefore, has been an enabling technology in *proteomics,* defined as the effort to study the complete set of proteins in an organism or in subcompartments of an organism such as plasma. Ionization of peptides and proteins is accomplished by electrospray or MALDI sources. Electrospray is better suited to analyzing small peptides rather than larger intact proteins. After ionization, proteins can be separated by quadrupoles, ion traps, time-of-flight, and other types of mass analyzers. Use of tandem MS with an intermediate fragmentation step between two stages of MS separation offers high sensitivity and specificity for the quantitative analysis of peptides, as it does for most small molecules.

Advantages of using MS for quantitative analysis include the ability to analyze components without developing specific antibodies and the ability to multiplex a large number of measurements. MS can provide information about posttranslational modifications that is difficult to assess by immunoassays and chromatographic or electrophoretic techniques. Examples of clinical applications include identification of genetic variants of prealbumin and CDT. The use of MS is likely to increase for accurate determination of protein

concentrations as recently applied for standardization of hemoglobin $A_{1c}$, insulin, and C-peptide. Likewise, MS is also able to distinguish peptides differing in length by one or two amino acids or by a posttranslational modification. For these reasons, MS is likely to find increased use for clinical laboratory analysis of bioactive peptides and other components of the peptidome.

In the setting of proteomics, several MS assays have been implemented in the past decade for large proteins. For immunoglobulins, MALDI-TOF has been applied to the detection and characterization of monoclonal proteins. The methods combine immunoenrichment coupled to MALDI-TOF MS to identify and isotype paraproteins. This method has equal or improved limits of detection in comparison to immunofixation. It is capable of quantitating paraproteins when coupled to nephelometry or turbidimetry. Given the automation potential, rapid analysis time and improved lower limit of quantitation, this method could be a cost-competitive replacement for electrophoresis and immunofixation in the near future.

## Proteins in Other Body Fluids

Complex mixtures of proteins are present in all biologic fluids; analysis of a variety of other specimens is diagnostically useful, including analyses of urine, CSF, pleural and peritoneal fluids, amniotic fluid, saliva, and feces.

### Saliva

Saliva has a very different protein composition than plasma. Protein composition varies with the site and method of sampling. In addition to the well-known presence of amylase, proteomic approaches have detected sequences from hundreds of different proteins in saliva. Proteins involved in host defense against pathogens such as immunoglobulins, lysozyme, and lactoferrin are particularly abundant. Efforts are underway to exploit the salivary proteome to detect and characterize susceptibility to dental caries, periodontal disease, head and neck cancers, diabetes, and cystic fibrosis. Patients with Sjögren syndrome exhibit increased concentrations of BMG and other inflammatory proteins compared with unaffected patients. Interrogation of saliva for the presence of secretory IgA is common in the diagnostic workup of hypogammaglobulinemia.

## Cerebrospinal Fluid

CSF is the extracellular fluid around the brain and spinal column. CSF usually has total protein concentrations about 100-fold lower than plasma and a different protein composition because most proteins have limited passage across the blood-brain barrier. CSF for testing is most frequently obtained by lumbar puncture. The blood-brain or blood-CSF barrier limits exchange of large compounds, so low to intermediate molecular weight plasma proteins such as prealbumin, albumin, and transferrin normally predominate in CSF. Analyses of total protein and specific proteins in CSF are used primarily to detect increased permeability of the blood-CSF barrier, increased intrathecal protein synthesis, or increased release of proteins from neural and glial tissue. Conditions such as viral meningitis, encephalitis, increased intracranial pressure, trauma, and hemorrhage may all compromise the blood-brain barrier, resulting in increased CSF protein. Protein concentrations associated with these conditions are displayed in Table 18.5. Increased intrathecal synthesis of immunoglobulins, particularly IgG, occurs in demyelinating diseases of the central nervous system (CNS), especially multiple sclerosis.

*Total protein in cerebrospinal fluid.* The protein concentration of CSF usually is more than 100-fold lower than plasma, so methods with greater sensitivity or increased specimen volume are required for CSF applications. The usual reference interval for CSF total protein in adults is 15 to 45 mg/dL. Total CSF protein concentrations are considerably higher in neonates and in healthy elderly adults. In CSF from premature and full-term neonates, concentrations up to 400 mg/dL are observed. In term newborns, a progressive decline in CSF protein is seen over the first few weeks of life, with values approaching adult concentrations by 4 months of age.

*Assessment of specific cerebrospinal fluid proteins.* The electrophoretic pattern of normal CSF has two striking features—a prealbumin band and two transferrin bands—one at $\beta_2$ in addition to the usual $\beta_1$ position. $\beta_2$-transferrin has decreased charge because its glycosyl chains lack terminal sialic

## TABLE 18.5  Cerebrospinal Fluid Total Protein in Various Diseases

| Clinical Condition | Appearance and Cells × $10^6$/L | Total Protein, mg/dL |
|---|---|---|
| Normal | Clear, colorless; 0–5 lymphocytes | 15–45[a] |
| **Increased Admixture of Proteins From Blood** | | |
| *Increased Capillary Permeability* | | |
| • Bacterial meningitis | Turbid, opalescent, purulent, usually >500 polymorphs | 80–500 |
| • Cryptococcal meningitis | Clear or turbid; 50–150 polymorphs or lymphocytes | 25–200 |
| • Leptospiral meningitis | Clear to slight haze; polymorphs early, then 5–100 lymphocytes | 50–100 |
| • Viral meningitis | Clear or slight haze, colorless; usually ≤500 lymphocytes | 30–100 |
| • Encephalitis | Clear or slight haze, colorless; usually ≤500 lymphocytes | 15–100 |
| • Poliomyelitis | Clear, colorless; ≤500 lymphocytes | 10–300 |
| • Brain tumor | Usually clear; 0–80 lymphocytes | 15–200 (usually normal) |
| *Mechanical Obstruction* | | |
| • Spinal cord tumor[b] | Clear, colorless, or yellow | 100–2000 |
| *Hemorrhage* | | |
| Cerebral hemorrhage | Colorless, yellow, or bloody; blood cells | 30–150 |
| *Local Immunoglobulin Production* | | |
| • Neurosyphilis | Clear, colorless; 10–100 lymphocytes | 50–150 |
| • Multiple sclerosis[c] | Clear, colorless; 0–10 lymphocytes | 25–50 |
| *Both Increased Capillary Permeability and Local Immunoglobulin Production* | | |
| • Tuberculous meningitis | Colorless, fibrin clot, or slightly turbid; 50–500 lymphocytes | 50–300 (occasionally ≤1000) |
| • Brain abscess | Clear or slightly turbid | 20–120 |
| After myelography (inflammatory reaction) | | Slight increase |

[a]Premature infants: ≤400 mg/dL; children: 30–100 mg/dL; older adults: ≤60 mg/dL.
[b]Froin syndrome: Lumbar fluid values are much higher than cisternal fluid values.
[c]Similar values may occur in certain other chronic inflammatory conditions of the nervous system.

acid residues. Both $\beta_2$-transferrin and another relatively abundant CSF protein, prostaglandin D synthase or $\beta$-trace, have been used to determine whether clear fluids from nasal or ear passages represent leakage of CSF, so-called CSF rhinorrhea and otorrhea. CSF immunoglobulin concentrations and oligoclonal immunoglobulin bands on electrophoretic separations of CSF are helpful in the diagnosis of multiple sclerosis and other inflammatory diseases of the CNS. A number of other proteins such as S100B and neuron-specific enolase are potential markers of traumatic or ischemic brain injury. Concentrations of tau, phospho-tau, and $\beta$-amyloid isoforms have proven useful in the diagnosis and prognosis of Alzheimer disease.

### Peritoneal and Pleural Fluids

Pathologic accumulations of fluid in the peritoneal and pleural cavities or elsewhere vary greatly in protein content. These fluids may be ultrafiltrates with low-protein concentrations relative to plasma and scant amounts of large proteins (transudates). Alternatively, fluids may have protein concentrations approaching those of plasma and significant amounts of large proteins such as immunoglobulins and AMG (exudates) in response to local inflammation and increased vascular permeability. Distinction between transudates and exudates assists in diagnosing the cause of fluid accumulation. The major cause of pleural transudates is congestive heart failure. Exudates occur with infection, pleuritis, pulmonary embolism, and cancer.

### Fecal Material

The use of fecal material for protein analysis is indicated in some specific clinical circumstances. Assessment of protein content in feces is fraught with a number of limitations. Results of fecal protein content are often normalized to fecal weight. Thus, watery stool specimens generally provide decreased estimates of protein concentration. Extraction is likewise dependent on stool consistency and homogeneity, leading to considerable within- and between-subject variability.

Protein loss in the gastrointestinal tract may be assessed using an assay of fecal AAT. The amount of fecal AAT excreted over time is determined as a function of the serum AAT concentration. Correction for serum AAT concentration is necessary because of variation in serum AAT from severe enteric losses or from acute-phase responses. Inflammatory bowel disease (IBD) includes Crohn disease and ulcerative colitis. Although gastrointestinal histology remains the gold standard for diagnosis, fecal protein markers have been employed as tools for screening and response to therapy. These are indicators of inflammation rather than leakage of plasma proteins. Fecal products secreted by white blood cells (WBCs), such as lactoferrin and calprotectin, have been used as a measure of disease activity in IBD. Exocrine pancreatic disease occurs in the setting of multiple pathologic states, including chronic alcoholism, diabetes, HIV, celiac disease, and cystic fibrosis. Determination of fecal elastase derived from pancreatic secretions provides an alternative for the diagnosis of pancreatic insufficiency compared with gold standard duodenal sampling after secretin administration.

## POINTS TO REMEMBER

### Amino Acids

Amino acid homeostasis depends on enteral extraction, broad-specificity transport systems, and catabolism.

Amino acids are the building blocks of protein but also serve as substrates for energy generation and other important biomolecules.

Amino acids such as glycine, glutamate, and $\gamma$-aminobutyric acid are important neurotransmitters.

### Peptides

An array of small peptide systems derived from larger protein precursors dictate control of numerous physiologic processes, including glucose and electrolyte homeostasis (ACTH), fluid retention (natriuretic peptides, vasopressin), iron metabolism (hepcidin), and vascular tone (angiotensins, endothelins)

Broad specificity immunoassays may detect both active and inactive peptides, overestimating active peptide concentrations.

Narrowly targeted mass spectrometry assays may underestimate the concentration of active peptides by excluding detection of some molecules with substantial biologic potency

### Proteins

Current catalogs of the circulating human proteome contain more than 12,000 components.

The human proteome includes more than 500 different proteases, classified into four families according to the catalytic mechanism employed to cleave peptide bonds.

Complement activation is triggered by direct detection of lipopolysaccharide or oligosaccharide components of foreign organisms (alternative and lectin pathways) or via antibody recognition of microbes (classical pathway).

Pathologic conditions such as cystic fibrosis, sickle cell disease, Alzheimer disease, and amyloidosis result largely from protein folding defects.

Protein diversity is derived from linear amino acid sequence and an array of cotranslational and posttranslational modifications, including acylation, prenylation, phosphorylation, and glycosylation.

More than 100 congenital disorders of glycosylation have been documented among the nearly 200 human gene products involved in protein glycosylation.

Immunoglobulin abundance is ranked as IgG, IgA, IgM, IgD, and IgE. Immunoglobulin deficiencies, polyclonal increases associated with infectious or autoimmune processes, and

## POINTS TO REMEMBER—cont'd

Monoclonal proteins which are characteristic of pre-malignant or malignant plasma cell disorders such as multiple myeloma are indications for measurement of immunoglobulins in the clinical laboratory.

Infants typically manifest a transient IgG deficiency with a nadir at about 3 months of age coinciding with the decline of maternally-acquired antibodies.

Proteins in CSF are available in concentrations approximately 100-fold lower than plasma. CSF protein testing is performed primarily to evaluate the integrity of the blood-brain barrier and the intrathecal synthesis of proteins.

## REVIEW QUESTIONS

1. Which of the following amino acids participates in formation of new polypeptide chains?
   a. Desmosine
   b. Ornithine
   c. Histidine
   d. Taurine
2. Which of the following amino acids is the most hydrophobic at physiologic pH?
   a. Glutamate
   b. Lysine
   c. Isoleucine
   d. Threonine
3. The pH at which a molecule such as a protein has a net charge of zero is referred to as the:
   a. isoelectric point.
   b. dissociation constant.
   c. isosbestic point.
   d. solubility point.
4. A paraprotein is a:
   a. membrane-bound protein.
   b. denatured/unfolded protein.
   c. protein-prosthetic group.
   d. monoclonal immunoglobulin.
5. Which of the following is a ketogenic amino acid?
   a. Glycine
   b. Leucine
   c. Glutamate
   d. Proline
6. Which of the following is a positive acute-phase reactant?
   a. Transferrin
   b. Albumin
   c. Ferritin
   d. Prealbumin
7. Covalent modification of proteins with ubiquitin leads to:
   a. altered folding.
   b. catabolism/destruction.
   c. enhanced activity.
   d. increased calcium binding.
8. The plasma protein that serves to transport a large number of compounds including bilirubin, calcium, drugs, and free fatty acids is:
   a. prealbumin.
   b. ceruloplasmin.
   c. haptoglobin.
   d. albumin.
9. $\alpha_1$ Antitrypsin inhibits which class of protease?
   a. Metalloproteases
   b. Aspartyl proteases
   c. Cysteinyl proteases
   d. Serine proteases
10. The most abundant circulating immunoglobulin in adult serum is:
    a. IgA.
    b. IgD.
    c. IgG.
    d. IgM.

## SUGGESTED READINGS

Brown DA, Rose JK. Sorting of GPI-anchored proteins to glycolipid-enriched membrane subdomains during transport to the apical cell surface. *Cell.* 1992;68(3):533–544.

Cohen P. The regulation of protein function by multisite phosphorylation—a 25 year update. *Trends Biochem Sci.* 200025(12):596–601.

Dietzen DJ, Weindel AL, Carayannopoulos MO, et al. Rapid comprehensive amino acid analysis by liquid chromatography/ tandem mass spectrometry: comparison to cation exchange with post-column ninhydrin detection. *Rapid Commun Mass Spectrom.* 2008;22(22):3481–3488.

Dobson CM. Protein folding and misfolding. *Nature.* 2003;426(6968):884–890.

Ganz T, Nemeth E. Hepcidin and iron homeostasis. *Biochim Biophys Acta.* 2012;1823(9):1434–1443.

Hall C. Essential biochemistry and physiology of (NT-pro)BNP. *Eur J Heart Fail.* 2004;6(3):257–260.

Hoofnagle AN. Peptide lost and found: internal standards and the mass spectrometric quantification of peptides. *Clin Chem.* 2010;56(10):1515–1517.

Kandasamy P, Gyimesi G, Kanai Y, et al. Amino acid transporters revisited: new views in health and disease. *Trends Biochem Sci.* 2018;43(10):752–789.

Keren DF, Bocsi G, Billman BL, et al. Laboratory detection and initial diagnosis of monoclonal gammopathies: guideline from the College of American Pathologists in Collaboration with the American Association for Clinical Chemistry and the American Society for Clinical Pathology. *Arch Pathol Lab Med.* 2022;146(5):575–590. https://doi.org/10.5858/arpa. 2020-0794-cp.

Knight V, Heimall JR, Chong H, et al. A toolkit and framework for optimal laboratory evaluation of individuals with suspected primary immunodeficiency. *J Allergy Clin Immunol Pract.* 2021;9(9):3293–3307.

Laterza OF, Modur VR, Ladenson JH. Biomarkers of tissue injury. *Biomark Med.* 2008;2(1):81–92.

Law RH, Zhang Q, McGowan S, et al. An overview of the serpin superfamily. *Genome Biol.* 2006;7(5):216.

Lingappa VR, Blobel G. Early events in the biosynthesis of secretory and membrane proteins: the signal hypothesis. *Recent Prog Horm Res.* 1980;36:451–475.

McGinley MP, Goldschmidt CH, Rae-Grant AD. Diagnosis and treatment of multiple sclerosis: a review. *JAMA.* 2021;325(8):765–779.

Mills JR, Kohlhagen MC, Dasari S, et al. Comprehensive assessment of M-proteins using nanobody enrichment coupled to MALDI-TOF mass spectrometry. *Clin Chem.* 2016;62(10):1334–1344.

Miller SL. A production of amino acids under possible primitive earth conditions. *Science.* 1953;117(3046):528–529.

Murray JD, Willrich MA, Krowka MJ, et al. Liquid chromatography-tandem mass spectrometry-based alpha1-antitrypsin (AAT) testing. *Am J Clin Pathol.* 2021;155(4):547–552.

Rodnina MV, Beringer M, Bieling P. Ten remarks on peptide bond formation on the ribosome. *Biochem Soc Trans.* 2005;33(Pt 3):493–498.

Williams AJ, Paulson HL. Polyglutamine neurodegeneration: protein misfolding revisited. *Trends Neurosci.* 2008;31(10):521–528.

Willrich MAV, Braun KMP, Moyer AM, et al. Complement testing in the clinical laboratory. *Crit Rev Clin Lab Sci.* 2021;58(7):1–51.

# Serum Enzymes

*Mauro Panteghini*

## OBJECTIVES

1. Define the following and give an example of each type:
   - Hydrolase
   - Phosphotransferase
   - Lyase
   - Transferase
   - Oxidoreductase
2. List the factors that affect enzyme activity and appearance in blood.
3. For each of the following enzymes, state and describe the biochemistry, physiological actions (if known), tissue distribution, clinical significance, method of laboratory analysis, and possible analytical interferences:
   - 5′-Nucleotidase
   - Aspartate aminotransferase (AST)
   - Alanine aminotransferase (ALT)
   - Creatine kinase (CK)
   - Alkaline phosphatase (ALP)
   - γ-Glutamyltransferase (GGT)
   - Amylase (AMY)
   - Lactate dehydrogenase (LDH)
   - Lipase (LIP)
   - Tartrate-resistant acid phosphatase
   - Serum cholinesterase
4. List the isoenzymes, the clinical significance of the isoenzymes (if any), and methods of laboratory analysis used to assess the isoenzymes of each of the following:
   - ALP
   - Amylase
   - Tartrate-resistant acid phosphatase
   - CK
5. Assess and solve case studies involving serum enzymes and isoenzymes and describe the laboratory methods for their analysis.

## KEY WORDS AND DEFINITIONS

α-Amylase  An enzyme that catalyzes the hydrolysis of 1,4-alpha-glycosidic linkages in starch, glycogen, and related polysaccharides and oligosaccharides.

Alkaline phosphatase  A hydrolase that catalyzes the alkaline hydrolysis of a large variety of naturally occurring and synthetic substrates.

Cholinesterase  An enzyme of the hydrolase class that catalyzes the cleavage of the acyl group from various esters of choline, including acetylcholine, and some related compounds.

Coenzyme  An organic nonprotein molecule that binds with the protein molecule (apoenzyme) to form the active enzyme (holoenzyme).

Creatine kinase  A dimeric transferase enzyme that catalyzes the reversible phosphorylation of creatine by adenosine triphosphate (ATP). Creatine kinase (CK) has four isoenzymes CK-MM, CK-MB, CK-BB, and mitochondrial CK.

γ-Glutamyltransferase  A transferase enzyme that reversibly catalyzes the transfer of a glutamyl group from a glutamyl-peptide and an amino acid to a peptide and a glutamyl-amino acid.

Holoenzyme  Active enzyme formed by combination of a coenzyme and an apoenzyme.

Isoenzyme  A molecular form that originates at the level of the genes that encode the structures of the enzyme proteins in question.

Isoform  An enzyme molecular form that has been posttranslationally modified.

Lactate dehydrogenase  An oxidoreductase enzyme that reversibly catalyzes the reduction of pyruvate to (L)-lactate, using NADH (reduced form of nicotinamide adenine dinucleotide) as an electron donor.

Lipase  A hydrolase that hydrolyzes glycerol esters of long-chain fatty acids.

The basic principles of enzyme and rate analyses are discussed in Chapter 14. Enzymes of clinical utility are discussed in this chapter. To better clarify their clinical use, the individual enzymes are discussed relative to the organs or tissues in which their measurements are clinically most important. However, overlap may occur for this classification because the same enzyme may be used for investigating disease in different organs.

## BASIC CONCEPTS

For a substance to serve as a biochemical marker of damage to a specific organ or tissue, it must arise predominantly from the organ or tissue of interest. Injury to tissue releases cellular substances such as enzymes, which can be used as plasma markers of tissue damage. Some enzymes are found predominantly in specialized tissues (e.g., lipase [LIP] in the pancreas); others, more widely distributed, have tissue-specific isoenzymes or isoforms (e.g., the pancreatic isoenzyme of α-amylase) that can be evaluated to enhance tissue and organ specificity.

In general, laboratory medicine uses changes in activity of the serum enzymes that are predominantly intracellular and physiologically present in the blood at relatively low concentrations. Increases in the serum activities of these enzymes are used to infer the location and nature of pathological changes in tissues of the body. Therefore, an understanding of the factors that affect the rate of release of enzymes from their cells of origin and the rate at which they are cleared from the circulation is necessary to correctly interpret changes in activity that occur with disease.

Knowledge of the intracellular location of enzymes can assist in determining the nature and severity of a pathological process if suitable enzymes are assayed in the blood. For instance, a mild inflammation of the liver, such as a mild attack of viral hepatitis, is likely to increase only the permeability of the liver cell membrane, allowing cytoplasmic enzymes to leak out into the blood. In contrast, a severe attack causing cell necrosis also disrupts the mitochondrial membrane, and both cytoplasmic and mitochondrial enzymes are detected in the blood.

The timing of the enzyme's diagnostic window is another important aspect to be considered when these markers are used to evaluate acute injury. The diagnostic window for an injury marker is the interval of time after an episode of injury during which blood concentrations of the marker are increased, thereby demonstrating the occurrence of injury.

### POINTS TO REMEMBER

The pattern of appearance of an enzyme in blood after an acute injury depends on:
- The intracellular location
- Molecular weight (because larger molecules enter the circulation at a slower rate)
- Local blood and lymphatic flow
- The rate and the route of elimination from blood

The main enzymes of established clinical value, together with their tissues of origin and their major clinical applications, are listed in Table 19.1.

## MUSCLE ENZYMES

Enzymes in this category include **creatine kinase** and aldolase.

### Creatine Kinase

**Creatine kinase** (CK) (EC 2.7.3.2; adenosine triphosphate [ATP]: creatine $N$-phosphotransferase) is a dimeric enzyme (82 kDa) that catalyzes the reversible phosphorylation of creatine (Cr) by ATP.

Physiologically, when muscle contracts, ATP is converted to adenosine diphosphate (ADP), and CK catalyzes the rephosphorylation of ADP to ATP using creatine phosphate (CrP) as the phosphorylation reservoir.

Optimal pH for the forward (Cr + ATP → ADP + CrP) and reverse (CrP + ADP → ATP + Cr) reactions is 9.0 and 6.7, respectively. $Mg^{2+}$ is an obligate activating ion that forms complexes with ATP and ADP. The optimal concentration range for $Mg^{2+}$ is narrow, and excess $Mg^{2+}$ is inhibitory. Many metal ions, such as $Mn^{2+}$, $Ca^{2+}$, $Zn^{2+}$, and $Cu^{2+}$, inhibit enzyme activity, as do iodoacetate and other sulfhydryl-binding reagents.

The enzyme in serum is relatively unstable, with activity being lost because of sulfhydryl group oxidation at the active site of the enzyme. Activity can be partially restored by incubating the enzyme preparation with sulfhydryl compounds, such as $N$-acetylcysteine, dithiothreitol (Cleland reagent), or glutathione.

### Biochemistry

CK activity is highest in striated muscle and heart tissue, which contain approximately 2500 and 550 U/g of protein, respectively. Other tissues, such as (1) brain, (2) gastrointestinal tract, and (3) urinary bladder, contain significantly less activity (Table 19.2).

CK is a dimer composed of two subunits (B and M), each with a molecular weight of about 40 kDa. These subunits are the products of loci on chromosomes 14 and 19, respectively.

## TABLE 19.1  Distribution of Clinically Important Enzymes

| Enzyme | Principal Sources of Enzyme in Blood | Principal Clinical Applications |
|---|---|---|
| Alanine aminotransferase | Liver | Hepatic parenchymal disease |
| Alkaline phosphatase | Liver, bone, intestinal mucosa, placenta | Hepatobiliary disease, bone disease |
| Amylase (pancreatic isoenzyme) | Pancreas | Pancreatic disease |
| Aspartate aminotransferase | Heart, liver, skeletal muscle, erythrocytes | Hepatic parenchymal disease |
| Creatine kinase | Skeletal muscle, heart | Muscle disease |
| γ-Glutamyltransferase | Liver, pancreas | Hepatobiliary disease |
| Lactate dehydrogenase | Heart, erythrocytes, lymph nodes, skeletal muscle, liver | Hemolytic and megaloblastic anemias, leukemia and lymphoma, oncology |
| Lipase | Pancreas | Pancreatic disease |

## TABLE 19.2  Approximate Concentrations of Tissue Creatine Kinase Activity (Expressed as Multiples of Creatine Kinase Activity Concentrations in Serum) and Cytoplasmic Isoenzyme Composition

| Tissue | Relative CK Activity | ISOENZYMES (%) | | |
|---|---|---|---|---|
| | | CK-BB | CK-MB | CK-MM |
| Skeletal muscle (type I, slow twitch, or red fibers) | 50,000 | <1 | 3 | 97 |
| Skeletal muscle (type II, fast twitch, or white fibers) | 50,000 | <1 | 1 | 99 |
| Heart | 10,000 | <1 | 22 | 78 |
| Brain | 5,000 | 100 | 0 | 0 |
| Gastrointestinal tract smooth muscle | 5,000 | 96 | 1 | 3 |
| Urinary bladder smooth muscle | 4,000 | 92 | 6 | 2 |

CK, Creatine kinase.

Because the active form of the enzyme is a dimer, three different pairs of subunits can exist: BB (or CK-1), MB (or CK-2), and MM (or CK-3). The distribution of these isoenzymes in the various tissues of humans is shown in Table 19.2. All three of these isoenzyme species are found in the cytosol of the cell or are associated with myofibrillar structures. However, a fourth isoenzyme exists that differs from the others both immunologically and by electrophoretic mobility. This isoenzyme (CK-Mt) is located between the inner and outer membranes of mitochondria, and it can constitute (e.g., in the heart) up to 15% of total CK activity. The gene for CK-Mt is located on chromosome 15.

CK in serum may also be found in macromolecular forms—the so-called macro-CK. Two types of macro-CK exist. Type 1 is a complex of CK, typically CK-BB, and an immunoglobulin, often IgG. Type 1 macro-CK is not pathologically significant, but it can be the cause of increased measured CK results, leading to diagnostic confusion and unnecessary further investigation. Prevalence of macro-CK type 1 in the general population has been estimated between 0.8% and 2.3%, and more than 80% of positive individuals are female. Macro-CK type 2 is oligomeric CK-Mt, with a reported prevalence of between 0.5% and 2.6% in hospitalized patients. It is found predominantly in adults who are severely ill with malignancy or liver disease, and in children who have notable tissue distress. The appearance of macro-CK type 2 in serum is usually associated with a poor prognosis. Macro-CKs can interfere with the assay of CK-MB by some immune-inhibition methods and should be

considered when measured CK results are not consistent with clinical presentation.

## Clinical Significance

Measurement of CK enzyme activity is the preferred laboratory test in cases of suspected muscle damage. Serum CK activity is increased in nearly all patients when (1) injury, (2) inflammation, or (3) necrosis of skeletal (or heart) muscle occurs.

Increased serum CK activity may be the only sign of subclinical neuromuscular disorders. About 30% to 44% of asymptomatic subjects with persistently elevated CK activity have myopathy. Serum CK activity is greatly elevated in all types of muscular dystrophy. In progressive muscular dystrophy (particularly Duchenne sex-linked muscular dystrophy), enzyme activity in the serum is highest in infancy and childhood and may be increased long before the disease is clinically apparent. Serum CK activity characteristically falls as patients get older and as the mass of functioning muscle diminishes with progression of the disease. About 50% to 80% of asymptomatic female carriers of Duchenne dystrophy show three- to sixfold increases in CK activity. High values of CK (up to 50-fold the upper reference limit [URL] in active disease) are noted in viral myositis, polymyositis, immune-mediated myopathy, and other inflammatory myopathies. However, in neurogenic muscle diseases, such as (1) myasthenia gravis, (2) multiple sclerosis, (3) poliomyelitis, and (4) Parkinsonism, serum CK enzyme activity is not increased.

In acute rhabdomyolysis caused by crush injury, there is severe muscle destruction, which causes serum CK release, and serum CK enzyme activity results exceeding 200 times the URL may be found. In this condition, a very high serum CK, mirroring myoglobinuria and its heme-induced mechanism of renal injury, has been associated with the risk of development of acute kidney injury (AKI). If the CK activity remains below 5000 U/L during the first 3 days after the insult, the probability of developing AKI appears to be low. Milder increases in serum CK activity can be observed after other direct trauma to muscle, including intramuscular injection and surgical intervention. Finally, a number of drugs can increase serum CK activities. The drugs principally responsible are (1) statins, (2) fibrates, (3) antiretrovirals, and (4) angiotensin II receptor antagonists. Up to 5% of statin users develop CK elevation. The clinical spectrum of statin-induced myotoxicity includes (1) asymptomatic rise in serum CK activity, (2) myalgia, (3) myopathy/myositis, and rarely (0.02%) (4) rhabdomyolysis. Routine monitoring of CK in asymptomatic subjects taking statins is not recommended; however, CK must be assessed in patients presenting with muscle pain and weakness, and statin treatment stopped if values increase above a threshold defined in local guidelines.

Hypothyroidism is a common cause of endocrine myopathy. Because up to 60% of hypothyroid subjects show an increase of CK activity in serum, subjects with unexplained persistent CK elevation should also obtain a thyroid function assessment.

Changes in serum CK and its MB isoenzyme after acute myocardial infarction were used for diagnosis for many years. However, because the MB isoenzyme of CK is also found in skeletal muscle, it is now more clinically appropriate to use more cardiac-specific troponin I or T for this application (see Chapter 34).

During physiologic childbirth, a sixfold increase in maternal serum CK activity occurs. Surgical intervention during labor further increases the activity of CK in the serum.

### Determination of Creatine Kinase Activity

Currently, all commercial assays for total CK are based on the reverse reaction (Cr ← CrP), which proceeds about six times faster than the forward reaction. CK catalyzes the conversion of CrP to Cr with concomitant phosphorylation of ADP to ATP. The ATP produced is measured by hexokinase (HK)/glucose-6-phosphate dehydrogenase (G6PD)—coupled reactions that ultimately convert $NADP^+$ to NADPH, which is monitored spectrophotometrically at 340 nm. The assay is optimized by adding (1) N-acetylcysteine to activate CK, (2) ethylenediaminetetraacetic acid (EDTA) to bind $Ca^{2+}$ and increase the stability of the reaction mixture, and (3) adenosine pentaphosphate ($Ap_5A$) in addition to AMP to inhibit adenylate kinase (AK), which may otherwise interfere in the CK activity measurement. The International Federation of Clinical Chemistry and Laboratory Medicine (IFCC) developed a reference measurement procedure based on this reaction principle for the measurement of CK at 37°C.

Specimens for CK analysis include serum and heparinized plasma. Anticoagulants other than heparin should not be used in collection tubes because they inhibit CK activity. CK activity in aliquoted serum is relatively unstable and is rapidly lost during storage. Average CK stabilities are less than 8 hours at room temperature, 48 hours at 4°C, and 1 month at −20°C. Therefore, the serum specimen should be chilled to 4°C if the sample is not analyzed immediately and stored at −80°C if analysis is delayed for longer than 30 days. A moderate degree of hemolysis is tolerated because erythrocytes contain no CK activity. However, severely hemolyzed specimens are unsatisfactory because enzymes and intermediates (AK, ATP, and glucose-6-phosphate) liberated from the erythrocytes may affect the lag phase and side reactions occurring in the assay system.

Serum CK activity is influenced by a number of physiological factors, such as (1) sex, (2) age, (3) ethnicity, (4) muscle mass, and (5) physical activity. Men have higher CK activity values than women, and Black subjects have higher values than non-Black subjects. One set of proposed reference intervals, based on European residents from different backgrounds, was: 47 to 322 and 29 to 201 U/L for White men and women, 47 to 641 and 37 to 313 U/L for Asian men and women, and 71 to 801 and 48 to 414 U/L for Black men and women, respectively. Newborns generally have higher CK activity than older infants, resulting from skeletal muscle trauma during birth. Physical exercise, particularly if unaccustomed, can increase serum CK activity, which may ascend as high as 10 times the URL within 24 hours of activity. Accordingly, in assessing asymptomatic CK elevations, the test should be repeated after a week of rest.

### Separation and Quantification of Creatine Kinase Isoenzymes

Electrophoretic methods are useful for the separation of all CK isoenzymes, but they are no longer routinely used. The isoenzyme bands are visualized by incubating the support (e.g., agarose or cellulose acetate) with a concentrated CK assay mixture using the reverse reaction. NADPH formed in this reaction is then detected by observing the bluish-white fluorescence after excitation by long-wave (360 nm) ultraviolet light.

Though currently considered clinically outmoded, "sandwich" immunoassays are available for the direct (i.e., mass) measurement of CK-MB.

### Aldolase

Aldolase (ALD) (EC 4.1.2.13; D-fructose-1,6-diphosphate D-glyceraldehyde-3-phosphate-lyase) catalyzes the splitting of D-fructose-1,6-diphosphate to D-glyceraldehyde-3-phosphate and dihydroxyacetone-phosphate, an important reaction in the glycolytic breakdown of glucose to pyruvate. ALD is probably present in all cells, but it is found in large quantities in muscles, liver, and brain.

Serum ALD determinations have been proposed for diagnosing diseases of skeletal muscle. In general, however, measurement of ALD activity in the serum of subjects with suspected muscle disease does not add information to that available more readily from measurement of CK. Accordingly,

ALD measurement is now considered redundant and obsolete and should be discouraged.

## LIVER ENZYMES

Enzymes in this category include (1) alanine aminotransferase (ALT), (2) aspartate aminotransferase (AST), (3) alkaline phosphatase (ALP), (4) γ-glutamyltransferase (GGT), and (5) 5′-nucleotidase (NTP). The aminotransferases, ALP and GGT, are widely used and available on automated analyzers. They have often been mistakenly considered as a part of liver "function" tests. They are not, of course, tests of liver function, but the habit sometimes persists.

The most common alterations in liver enzyme activities encountered in clinical practice are divided into two major pathophysiology subgroups: (1) hepatocellular damage (increased aminotransferase activities) and (2) cholestasis (increased ALP and GGT activities), although certain liver diseases may display a mixed biochemical picture (Fig. 19.1).

### Aminotransferases

The aminotransferases constitute a group of enzymes that catalyze the interconversion of amino acids to 2-oxo-acids by transfer of amino groups. ALT (EC 2.6.1.2; L-alanine: 2-oxoglutarate aminotransferase) and AST (EC 2.6.1.1; L-aspartate: 2-oxoglutarate aminotransferase) are the aminotransferases of clinical interest.

The 2-oxoglutarate/L-glutamate couple serves as one amino group acceptor and donor pair in all amino-transfer reactions; the specificity of the individual enzymes derives from the particular amino acid that serves as the other donor of an amino group. Thus, AST catalyzes the following reaction:

L-Aspartate   2-Oxoglutarate   Oxaloacetate   L-Glutamate

ALT catalyzes the analogous reaction as follows:

L-Alanine   2-Oxoglutarate   Pyruvate   L-Glutamate

The reactions are reversible, but the equilibria of the AST and ALT reactions favor formation of aspartate and alanine, respectively.

Pyridoxal-5′-phosphate (P-5′-P) and its amino analogue, pyridoxamine-5′-phosphate, function as **coenzymes** in in vivo amino-transfer reactions. The P-5′-P is bound to the inactive apoenzyme and serves as a true prosthetic group. P-5′-P bound to the apoenzyme accepts the amino group from the first substrate, aspartate or alanine, to form enzyme-bound pyridoxamine-5′-phosphate and the first reaction product, oxaloacetate or pyruvate, respectively. The coenzyme in amino form then transfers its amino group to the second substrate, 2-oxoglutarate, to form the second product, glutamate. P-5′-P is thus regenerated.

Both coenzyme-deficient apoenzymes and **holoenzymes** may be present in the serum. Therefore, addition of P-5′-P under measurement conditions that allow recombination with the enzymes usually produces an increase in aminotransferase activity. For clinical assays, in accordance with the principle that all factors affecting the rate of reaction must be optimized and controlled, the addition of P-5′-P in aminotransferase assays is mandatory to ensure that all enzymatic activity is measured.

### Biochemistry

Whereas AST is found primarily in the (1) heart, (2) liver, (3) skeletal muscle, and (4) kidney, ALT is found primarily in the liver and kidney (Table 19.3). ALT is exclusively cytoplasmic, but both mitochondrial and cytoplasmic forms of AST are found in cells. These are genetically distinct AST isoenzymes. About 5% to 10% of the activity of total AST in serum from healthy individuals is of mitochondrial origin.

### Clinical Significance

Liver disease is the most important cause of increased aminotransferase activity in the serum and represents the indication for serum ALT and AST activity measurements. Although serum activities of both ALT and AST increase whenever disease processes affect liver cell integrity, ALT is the more liver-specific enzyme. Serum increases of ALT activity are rarely observed in conditions other than parenchymal liver disease. Moreover, increases of ALT activity persist longer than those of AST activity. Thus, the incremental benefit of routine determination of AST, in addition to ALT, is limited, making the routine requesting of both enzymes of little value. Laboratories reporting abnormal ALT results (e.g., >URL) may choose to offer AST as an automatic reflex test and calculate the AST-to-ALT ratio (AAR) because it provides useful diagnostic and prognostic information in clinical hepatology.

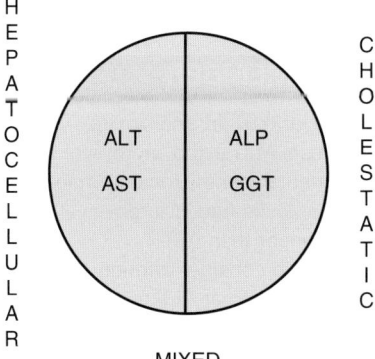

Fig. 19.1 Liver enzymology patterns. *ALP*, Alkaline phosphatase; *ALT*, alanine aminotransferase; *AST*, aspartate aminotransferase; *GGT*, γ-glutamyltransferase.

### TABLE 19.3  Aminotransferase Activities in Human Tissues, Relative to Serum as Unity

|  | Aspartate Aminotransferase | Alanine Aminotransferase |
| --- | --- | --- |
| Heart | 7,800 | 450 |
| Liver | 7,100 | 2,850 |
| Skeletal muscle | 5,000 | 300 |
| Kidneys | 4,500 | 1,200 |
| Pancreas | 1,400 | 130 |
| Spleen | 700 | 80 |
| Lungs | 500 | 45 |
| Erythrocytes | 15 | 7 |
| Serum | 1 | 1 |

In most types of liver disease, ALT activity is higher than that of AST; exceptions may be seen in (1) alcoholic hepatitis, (2) advanced liver fibrosis, and (3) liver neoplasia. An AAR of ≥2 is suggestive and an AAR of ≥3 is highly suggestive of alcoholic liver disease, as mitochondrial injury caused by alcohol results in more AST leakage. An AAR of 1 or greater has a high positive predictive value for diagnosing the presence of advanced fibrosis in patients with chronic liver disease. Furthermore, the amount of increase in the AAR can reflect the grade of fibrosis in these patients. It is worth mentioning that before interpreting the AAR, contributions to AST from other nonhepatic tissues should be excluded.

In viral hepatitis and other forms of liver disease associated with acute hepatic necrosis, serum AST and ALT activities are increased even before the clinical signs and symptoms of disease (e.g., jaundice) appear. Activities for both enzymes may reach values as high as 100 times the URL, although 10-fold to 40-fold increases are most frequently encountered. The most efficient ALT threshold for diagnosing acute liver injury lies at seven times the URL (sensitivity and specificity >95%). Peak values of aminotransferase activity occur between the 7th and 12th days; activities then gradually decrease, reaching physiological concentrations by the 3rd to 5th week if recovery is uneventful. Peak enzyme activities bear no relationship to prognosis and may fall with worsening of the patient's condition due to cumulative losses of functional hepatocytes to continue enzyme release.

Persistence of increased ALT for longer than 6 months after an episode of acute hepatitis is used to diagnose chronic hepatitis. Therefore, in patients with acute hepatitis, ALT should be measured periodically over the next 1 to 2 years to determine if it becomes and stays normal.

Nonalcoholic fatty liver disease (NAFLD) is the most common cause of aminotransferase increases other than viral and alcoholic hepatitis. NAFLD includes a spectrum of liver pathology, from simple steatosis to nonalcoholic steatohepatitis (NASH), in which inflammatory changes and focal necrosis may progress to (1) liver fibrosis, (2) cirrhosis, and (3) hepatic failure. NAFLD is now considered to be an additional feature of metabolic syndrome (aka, syndrome X) with serum aminotransferase elevation associated with (1) higher body mass index (BMI), (2) increased waist circumference, (3) elevated serum triglycerides, (4) elevated fasting insulin, and (5) lower HDL cholesterol—all features characteristic of this syndrome.

Slight or moderate elevations of aminotransferase activities have been observed after administration of various medications, such as (1) nonsteroidal antiinflammatory drugs, (2) antibiotics, (3) antiepileptic drugs, (4) statins, or (5) opiates. Over-the-counter medications and herbal preparations are also implicated. A helpful resource that is available to ascertain whether a drug or supplement may be hepatotoxic is the website livertox.nih.gov. In patients with increased aminotransferase activities, negative viral markers and a negative history for drugs or alcohol ingestion, the diagnostic workup should include less common causes of chronic hepatic injury, such as (1) autoimmune hepatitis, (2) primary biliary cholangitis (cirrhosis), (3) primary sclerosing cholangitis, (4) celiac disease, (5) hemochromatosis, (6) Wilson disease, and (7) $\alpha_1$-antitrypsin deficiency.

As might be expected from the high AST concentration in muscles, AST activity also is increased in patients with primary muscular diseases such as muscular dystrophy and myositis, but normal in muscular diseases of neurogenic origin such as amyotrophic lateral sclerosis and neurogenic atrophy. Finally, significant AST activity increases are noted in hemolytic disease because erythrocytes contain abundant AST and cell lysis releases the AST to the serum/plasma compartment.

Several studies have described AST-bound immunoglobulins, which are commonly called macro-AST. Typical findings include a persistent increase in serum AST activity with normal ALT concentrations in an asymptomatic subject, and the absence of any demonstrable pathology in organs rich in AST. In such cases, the increased AST activity likely reflects decreased clearance of AST-antibody complexes from circulation. Macro-AST has no known clinical relevance. However, identification is important to avoid unnecessary diagnostic procedures in these subjects. The presence of macro-AST in serum is confirmed with differential precipitation using polyethylene glycol (PEG) 6000 (see the Amylase section later in this chapter).

### POINTS TO REMEMBER

- Routine testing of AST in addition to ALT is not recommended, because ALT is the more liver-specific enzyme and the incremental benefit of determination of AST, in addition to ALT, is limited. Moreover, increases of ALT activity persist longer than AST.
- Laboratories should consider offering AST as a reflex test in samples with abnormal ALT results (e.g., greater than the URL), and report the AST-to-ALT ratio when enzyme activities are abnormal because this ratio provides useful diagnostic and prognostic information.

## Methods of Analysis

Continuous-monitoring methods are used to measure aminotransferase activity by coupling aminotransferase reactions to specific dehydrogenase reactions. The oxo-acids formed in the aminotransferase reaction are measured indirectly by enzymatic reduction to corresponding hydroxy acids, and the accompanying change in NADH concentration is monitored spectrophotometrically. Thus oxaloacetate, formed in the AST reaction, is reduced to malate in the presence of malate dehydrogenase (MD).

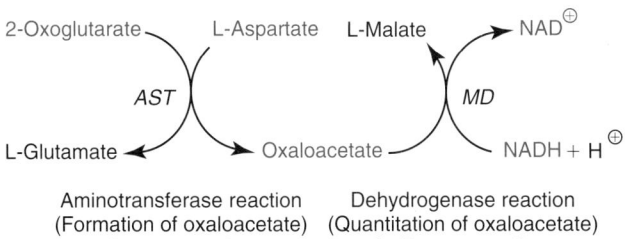

Aminotransferase reaction
(Formation of oxaloacetate)
**Assay reaction**

Dehydrogenase reaction
(Quantitation of oxaloacetate)
**Indicator reaction**

Pyruvate formed in the ALT reaction is reduced to lactate by **lactate dehydrogenase (LDH)**. The substrate, NADH, and an auxiliary enzyme, MD or LDH, are present in sufficient quantities, so that the reaction rate is limited only by the amounts of AST and ALT, respectively. As the reactions proceed, NADH is oxidized to NAD+. The conversion of NADH to NAD+ is followed by measuring the decrease in absorbance at 340 nm. The change in absorbance per minute ($\Delta A$/min) is proportional to the micromoles of NADH oxidized and in turn to micromoles of substrate transformed per minute. A preliminary incubation period is necessary to ensure that NADH-dependent reduction of endogenous oxo-acids in the sample is completed before 2-oxoglutarate is added to start the aminotransferase reaction. As already mentioned, supplementation with P-5'-P ensures that all aminotransferase activity of the sample is measured.

Primary IFCC reference measurement procedures are available for the measurement of catalytic activity concentrations of AST and ALT. Values assigned to the manufacturers' product calibrators and measurement results obtained with commercial measuring systems in daily practice should be traceable to these top-level reference measurement procedures, thus assuring the inter-assay comparability of patient results (see Chapter 14). It should be remembered that this may be obtained only if the reference procedure and corresponding commercial procedures have identical, or at least very similar, selectivity for the measured enzyme. Thus, it will not be possible to calibrate procedures for aminotransferases that do not incorporate P-5'-P using a procedure that does, such as the IFCC reference procedure, because the ratio of preformed holoenzyme to apoenzyme differs among specimens. Consequently, the lack of P-5'-P addition in commercial reagents is the most frequent cause of unacceptably biased results of aminotransferase activity.

AST activity in serum is stable for up to 48 hours at 4°C. Conversely, ALT activity should be assayed on the day of sample collection because activity is lost at room temperature, at 4°C, and at −25°C. ALT stability is better maintained at −70°C. Hemolyzed specimens should not be used, especially when AST is measured, because of the large amount of this enzyme present in erythrocytes.

Using assays traceable to the IFCC reference procedures, the AST URL for adults, calculated as the 97.5th percentile of the reference distribution, is 34 U/L, with no significant sex-related differences. Conversely, a clear difference in ALT activities has been noted between men and women. Corresponding ALT URLs are 49 U/L and 33 U/L, respectively. ALT does not reveal a distinct age dependency during childhood, but serum AST activity in neonates and in children younger than 3 years old is twice that expected in adults.

## Alkaline Phosphatase

**Alkaline phosphatase (ALP)** (EC 3.1.3.1; orthophosphoric-monoester phosphohydrolase [alkaline optimum]) catalyzes the alkaline hydrolysis of a large variety of naturally occurring and synthetic substrates. Some divalent ions, such as $Mg^{2+}$, $Co^{2+}$, and $Mn^{2+}$, are activators of the enzyme, and $Zn^{2+}$ is a constituent metal ion. Inhibitors of ALP activity include (1) phosphate, (2) borate, (3) oxalate, and (4) cyanide ions. The type of buffer present affects the rate of enzyme activity. Accordingly, buffers can be classified as (1) inert (carbonate and barbital), (2) inhibiting (glycine and propylamine), or (3) activating (2-amino-2-methyl-1-propanol [AMP], tris [hydroxymethyl] aminomethane [TRIS], and diethanolamine [DEA]).

### Biochemistry

ALP activity is present in most organs of the body; it is located on cell surfaces, anchored on the cell membrane by glycosylphosphatidylinositol ("ectoenzyme"). ALP is most commonly associated with the mucosa of the small intestine and the lining of the proximal convoluted tubules of the kidney, bone (osteoblasts), liver, and placenta. Although the exact metabolic function of the enzyme is not yet understood, it appears that ALP is associated with lipid transport in the intestine, the calcification process in bone, and host defense through endotoxin dephosphorylation.

ALP exists in multiple homodimeric forms, some of which are true isoenzymes, encoded at separate genetic loci. Bone, liver, and kidney ALP forms share a common primary structure encoded by the same genetic locus (as tissue-nonspecific ALP), but they differ in their unique carbohydrate content via posttranslational modifications.

The ALP activity present in the sera of healthy adults originates mainly from the liver and bone, with a ratio of approximately 1:1. Minimal amounts of intestinal ALP may also be present, particularly in the sera of individuals of blood group B or O (i.e., those who are secretors of blood group substances). Because intestinal ALP activity in the serum may increase after a meal, fasting specimens should be collected for ALP measurement.

### Clinical Significance

Increases in serum ALP activity commonly originate from one or both of two sources: liver and bone. Consequently, serum ALP measurements are of interest in the investigation of hepatobiliary disease and bone disease associated with increased osteoblastic activity.

*Hepatobiliary disease.* Any form of biliary tree obstruction induces the hepatocellular synthesis of ALP. The newly formed ectoenzyme is released from the cell membrane by the detergent action of bile salts and enters the circulation to increase the enzyme activity in the serum. The increase tends to be more notable in extrahepatic obstruction (e.g., by stones or cancer of the head of the pancreas) than in intrahepatic obstruction, and the degree of ALP activity abnormality is proportional to the amount of obstruction. Serum enzyme activities return to baseline after 1 week of surgical removal of the obstruction. A similar increase is seen in patients with advanced primary liver cancer or widespread secondary hepatic metastases. GGT activity is co-elevated with ALP in cases of obstructive intrahepatic or posthepatic biliary disease and can help differentiate the source of an ALP elevation.

Liver diseases that principally affect parenchymal cells, such as infectious hepatitis, typically show only moderately (less than threefold) increased or normal serum ALP activities. Increases in ALP activity may also be a consequence of a reaction to drug therapy, and ALT/ALP-based criteria help detect and qualify the type of liver injury in drug-induced liver injury (DILI) (Table 19.4). Intestinal ALP isoenzyme, an asialoglycoprotein normally cleared by the hepatic asialoglycoprotein receptors, is often elevated in patients with liver cirrhosis.

*Bone disease.* Bone ALP (BAP) is produced by the osteoblast and has been demonstrated in matrix vesicles deposited as "buds" derived from the cell's membrane. The enzyme

therefore is an excellent indicator of global bone formation activity. A genetic inability to produce tissue-nonspecific ALP (including bone isoform) results in a rare inherited disorder known as hypophosphatasia, which results in severe bone disease and impaired bone growth.

Among the bone diseases, the highest BAP activities are encountered in **Paget disease** (osteitis deformans) as a result of the action of osteoblastic cells as they try to rebuild bone that is being resorbed by uncontrolled activity of osteoclasts. Values from 10 to 25 times the URL are not unusual, and in broad terms, the increase reflects the extent of disease. In vitamin D deficiency (osteomalacia and rickets), enzyme concentrations two to four times the URL may be observed, and these return to baseline with treatment. Hyperparathyroidism (primary and secondary) is associated with slight to moderate increases of BAP in serum, with the existence and degree of increase reflecting the presence and extent of skeletal involvement. Very high enzyme concentrations are present in patients with osteogenic bone cancer. Increased ALP indicates bone metastasis in 70% of prostate cancers, and its measurement is included in the European Association of Urology guidelines for the diagnostic work-up of this neoplasia. The 2017 Kidney Disease: Improving Global Outcomes (KDIGO) clinical practice guideline for the diagnosis, evaluation, prevention, and treatment of chronic kidney disease-mineral and bone disorder (CKD-MBD) recommends monitoring ALP activity (together with serum calcium, phosphate, and parathyroid hormone concentrations) in adults with glomerular filtration rate (GFR) less than 60 mL/min/1.73 m$^2$. In dialysis patients, BAP measurement can be used to evaluate bone disease because markedly high or low values may predict underlying bone turnover. BAP can be slightly increased in osteoporosis, but individuals with osteoporosis are not clearly distinguished from age-matched controls. Transient increases of ALP may be found during the healing of bone fractures. Physiological bone growth increases BAP in serum, and this accounts for the fact that in the sera of growing children, the enzyme concentration is 1.5 to 7 times that in healthy adult serum, the maximum being reached earlier in girls than in boys.

*Other conditions that increase alkaline phosphatase.* An increase in ALP activity of up to two to three times URL is observed in women in the third trimester of pregnancy, with the additional enzyme activity contributed by placental ALP. This makes ALP an unreliable marker of hepatobiliary disease in pregnancy. Additionally, reports have described a benign familial increase in serum ALP activity caused by increased concentrations of intestinal ALP. Transient, benign increases in serum ALP may also be observed in infants and children, with changes often more than 10 times the URL. These changes seem to reflect a reduction in the removal of ALP from blood caused by transient modifications of enzyme glycosylation. Complexes between ALP and immunoglobulins (macro-ALP) occur occasionally in serum, giving abnormal ALP values,

### TABLE 19.4 Enzyme-Based Criteria for Drug-Induced Liver Injury (Enzyme Values Expressed as Multiples of the Upper Reference Limit in Serum)

| Injury Type | ALT | ALP | R Value[a] |
|---|---|---|---|
| Hepatocellular | >2 × URL | <URL | ≥5 |
| Cholestatic | <URL | >2 × URL | ≤2 |
| Mixed | >2 × URL | >2 × URL | 2–5 |

[a]Ratio of ALT to ALP relative to their URLs [R = (ALT/URL)/(ALP/URL)]. Note: In 2011, the International DILI Expert Working Group recommended to raise the cutoff level of ALT elevation to 5 URL to exclude clinically unimportant and self-limited drug-related hepatocellular events.

*ALT,* Alanine aminotransferase; *ALP,* alkaline phosphatase; *DILI,* drug-induced liver injury; *URL,* upper reference limit.

Data from the Council of International Organizations of Medical Sciences, 1990.

but they do not provide specific diagnostic information in the present state of knowledge.

ALP forms essentially identical to the normal placental or germ cell isoenzymes appear in the sera of some patients with malignant disease. This appears to result from de-repression of the corresponding genes in tumors. The presence of these isoenzymes can be readily detected in the serum by their typical stability at 65°C.

## Methods of Analysis for Total Alkaline Phosphatase Activity and Isoenzyme Content

The most popular of the chromogenic substrates for ALP is 4-nitrophenyl phosphate (usually abbreviated 4-NPP, or PNPP from the older name, *p*-nitrophenyl phosphate). This ester is colorless, but the final product is yellow at the pH of the reaction:

4-Nitrophenyl phosphate (colorless)

4-Nitrophenoxide (colorless, benzenoid form)

4-Nitrophenoxide (yellow, quinonoid form)

ALP, $Mg^{2+}$
pH 10.3

Rearranges at alkaline pH

The enzyme reaction is continuously monitored by observing the rate of formation of the 4-nitrophenoxide ions at 405 nm. The liberated phosphate group is transferred to water, and the rate of phosphatase action is enhanced if certain amino alcohols are used as phosphate-accepting buffers. Among these activators are compounds such as (1) AMP, (2) DEA, and (3) TRIS. The IFCC-recommended reference procedure uses 4-NPP as the substrate and AMP as the phosphate-acceptor buffer.

Serum or heparinized plasma, free of hemolysis, should be used. Complexing anticoagulants—such as citrate and EDTA—must be avoided because they bind cations, such as $Mg^{2+}$ and $Zn^{2+}$, which are necessary cofactors for ALP activity. Freshly collected serum samples should be kept at room temperature and assayed as soon as possible, but preferably within 4 hours after collection. In sera stored at a refrigerated temperature, ALP activity increases slowly (2% per day). Frozen specimens should be thawed and kept at room temperature for 18 to 24 hours before measurement to achieve full enzyme reactivation.

ALP activities in the serum vary with age and, to a minor extent, with sex. Using assays traceable to the IFCC reference procedure, the following reference intervals (central 95th percentiles) can be employed: 33 to 98 U/L for premenopausal women and 43 to 115 U/L for adult men. For women, a progressive increase in ALP activity after menopause is described, with a reference interval between 53 and 141 U/L. Infants and peripubertal children show higher ALP activity (up to fivefold) than healthy adults as a result of the leakage of BAP from osteoblasts during bone growth. The decrease in ALP activity to typical adult ranges occurs on average 2 years earlier in females than in males.

Criteria that have been used to differentiate the isoenzymes and other multiple forms of ALP in serum include (1) electrophoretic mobility, (2) stability to denaturation by heat or chemicals, (3) response to specific pretreatments, and (4) immunochemical characteristics.

After electrophoresis, ALP zones are made visible by incubating the gel in a solution of buffered substrate. The liver ALP typically moves most rapidly toward the anode. BAP, which typically gives a more diffuse zone than the liver form, has slightly reduced anodal mobility, although the two zones usually overlap to some extent. A short (15 minutes at 37°C) sample pretreatment with neuraminidase to remove a portion of the terminal sialic acid residues can be used to improve the electrophoretic separation between bone and liver ALPs, exploiting differences in the carbohydrate portions of the two forms of ALP. Whereas intestinal ALP migrates more slowly than the bone enzyme, the placental isoenzyme commonly appears as a discrete band overlying the diffuse bone fraction. An additional band, which is frequently present in the serum of patients with various hepatic diseases, contains a high-molecular-weight form of ALP that is strongly negatively charged. This form corresponds to the main liver form attached to the cell membrane moiety. Macro-ALP can be identified as abnormally migrating bands in the γ-globulin zone. PEG precipitation (see the Amylase section later in this chapter) may represent a suitable alternative for macro-ALP detection.

As an alternative to electrophoretic fractionation of ALP, measurement of GGT, which is increased in liver disease but not in bone disease, may be a useful rapid tool to distinguish between the two diseases as the explanation for increased serum ALP.

Immunoassays for direct determination of BAP, which measure enzyme activity or mass concentration, are commercially available; cross-reactivity with the liver form by 6% to 20%, however, has been established.

## γ-Glutamyltransferase

Peptidases are enzymes that catalyze the hydrolytic cleavage of peptides to form amino acids or smaller peptides. They constitute a broad group of enzymes of varied specificity. The constituents of one group of peptidases act as amino acid transferases and catalyze the transfer of amino acids from one peptide to another amino acid or peptide. For example, γ-Glutamyltransferase (GGT) (EC 2.3.2.2; γ-glutamyl-peptide:

amino acid γ-glutamyltransferase) catalyzes the transfer of the γ-glutamyl group from peptides and compounds to an acceptor. The γ-glutamyl acceptor is (1) the substrate itself, (2) an amino acid or peptide, or (3) water, in which case simple hydrolysis takes place. The enzyme acts only on peptides or peptide-like compounds containing a terminal glutamate residue joined to the remainder of the compound through the terminal (-γ-) carboxyl group. Glycylglycine is five times more effective as an acceptor than glycine or the tripeptide (gly-gly-gly). An example of a reaction catalyzed by the GGT is shown here:

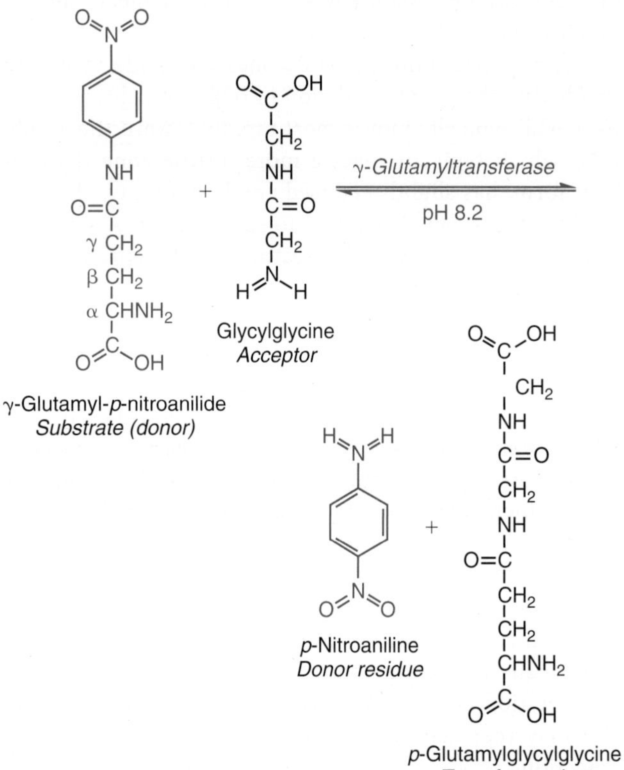

## Biochemistry

Mature GGT has a molecular weight of 68 kDa and consists of two subunits: a 46-kDa subunit responsible for enzyme anchorage on cellular membranes through a hydrophobic transmembrane domain and a 22-kDa subunit that carries the catalytic center. GGT is present (in decreasing order of abundance) in (1) proximal renal tubule, (2) liver, (3) pancreas, and (4) intestine. While cellular GGT is present in cytoplasmic microsomes, the larger fraction is anchored to the outer surface of the plasma membranes and may transport amino acids and peptides into the cell across the cell membrane in the form of γ-glutamyl peptides. GGT is critical for the maintenance of adequate intracellular concentrations of reduced glutathione, a major antioxidant agent.

## Clinical Significance

Even though renal tissue has the highest concentration of GGT, the enzyme present in serum originates primarily from the hepatobiliary system. GGT is a sensitive indicator of the presence of hepatobiliary disease, but its usefulness is limited by lack of specificity. Like ALP, GGT activity is highest in cases of posthepatic biliary obstruction, reaching activities 10 to 30 times the URL. High increases of GGT (>5 URL) are also noted in patients with a primary or metastatic liver neoplasm, presumably caused by intrahepatic obstruction. Moderate increases (<3 URL) occur in infectious hepatitis. In pancreatitis and in some pancreatic malignancies (especially if associated with hepatobiliary obstruction), enzyme activity may be 5 to 15 times the URL.

Increased activities of GGT are found in the sera of patients with alcoholic-related liver disease and in sera from people who are heavy drinkers in which this increase can be used as a marker of occult alcohol abuse. Even occasional drinking is associated with higher GGT activity than is observed in alcohol abstainers. GGT activity is also increased with increased body weight and obesity. Increased concentrations of the enzyme are also found in the serum of subjects receiving anticonvulsant drugs such as phenytoin and phenobarbital. Such an increase in GGT activity in serum may reflect induction of new enzyme activity by the action of the alcohol and drugs or their toxic effects on microsomal structures in liver cells.

Epidemiologic evidence has shown that serum GGT activity possesses an independent prognostic value for cardiovascular morbidity and mortality. However, the addition of GGT to conventional risk factors is unlikely to substantially improve prediction of cardiovascular events.

## Methods of Analysis

Early GGT assays used L-γ-glutamyl-p-nitroanilide (GGPNA) as the substrate, with glycylglycine serving as the γ-glutamyl residue acceptor. The p-nitroaniline produced in the reaction is determined by its yellow color, which is monitored at 405 nm. However, GGPNA has limited solubility in the reaction mixture, and it is therefore difficult to obtain saturating substrate concentrations. To obviate this problem, derivatives of GGPNA, in which various groups have been introduced into the benzene ring to increase solubility in water, have been used. The most useful of these substrates is L-γ-glutamyl-3-carboxy-4-nitroanilide, which is readily soluble in water and is split by GGT at a rate comparable with that observed with GGPNA. In the IFCC reference measurement procedure for GGT, L-γ-glutamyl-3-carboxy-4-nitroanilide serves as the substrate, with glycylglycine serving as an acceptor. Buffering is provided by glycylglycine itself.

GGT activity is stable for at least 1 month at 4°C and for 1 year at −20°C. Nonhemolyzed serum is the preferred specimen, but EDTA plasma has also been used. Heparin may produce turbidity in the reaction mixture; citrate, oxalate, and fluoride depress GGT activity by 10% to 15%.

In adults, the URL for GGT activity in serum is 40 U/L for females and 68 U/L for males, when measured with an assay traceable to the IFCC reference procedure. Reference limits are approximately twofold higher in people of African ancestry. In normal full-term neonates, GGT activity at birth is approximately six to seven times the adult reference interval; the activity then declines, reaching stable values by the age of 6 months.

## 5′-Nucleotidase

5′-Nucleotidase (NTP) (EC 3.1.3.5; 5′-ribonucleotide phosphohydrolase) is a phosphatase that acts only on nucleoside-5′-phosphates, such as adenosine-5′-phosphate (AMP) and adenylic acid, releasing inorganic phosphate.

NTP is a glycoprotein that is widely distributed throughout the tissues of the body and is principally localized in the cytoplasmic membrane of the cells in which it occurs. Despite its ubiquitous distribution, serum NTP activities appear to reflect hepatobiliary disease with considerable specificity. Particularly, NTP is increased in hepatobiliary diseases with associated impairment of bile secretion. This may be due to extrahepatic causes (a stone or tumor occluding the bile duct), or it may arise from intrahepatic conditions, such as cholestasis caused by malignant infiltration of the liver or biliary cholangitis. When parenchymal cell damage is predominant, as in infectious hepatitis, serum NTP activity is only moderately increased.

The assay of NTP activity has been considered of value as an addition to the measurement of total ALP in patients with suspected hepatobiliary disease, and increased NTP activity is interpreted as evidence of a hepatic origin of increased ALP activity in serum. However, approximately half of individuals in whom liver ALP activity is increased in serum may simultaneously show a normal NTP. On the other hand, increased NTP in the serum of patients with normal liver ALP is very often associated with the presence of liver disease. Thus, the frequent dissociation of the two enzyme activities supports the usefulness of determining both ALP and NTP to enhance diagnostic efficiency in patients with suspected liver disease.

In a commercially available assay, serum NTP catalyzes the hydrolysis of inosine-5′-phosphate (IMP) to yield inosine, which is then converted to hypoxanthine by purine-nucleoside phosphorylase. Hypoxanthine is oxidized to urate with xanthine oxidase. Two moles of hydrogen peroxide are produced for each mole of hypoxanthine liberated and converted to uric acid. The formation rate of hydrogen peroxide is monitored at 510 nm by the oxidation of a chromogenic system. The effect of ALP on IMP is inhibited by β-glycerophosphate. Using this method, the reference interval for NTP activity at 37°C is from 3 to 9 U/L, with no sex-related differences.

NTP activity in serum or plasma heparin is stable for at least 4 days at 4°C and 4 months at −20°C.

# PANCREATIC ENZYMES

The most used serum biomarkers for investigation of pancreatic disease, and more specifically acute pancreatitis, are LIP and P-type amylase (see Chapter 38).

## Lipase

Human pancreatic **lipase** (LIP) (EC 3.1.1.3; triacylglycerol acylhydrolase) is a single-chain glycoprotein with a molecular weight of 48 kDa. For full catalytic activity and greatest specificity, the presence of bile salts and a cofactor called *colipase*, which is a small protein secreted by the pancreatic acinar cells, are required.

### Biochemistry

LIPs are defined as enzymes that hydrolyze glycerol esters of long-chain fatty acids.

Only ester bonds at carbons 1 and 3 (α-positions) are cleaved, and products of the reaction include 2 moles of fatty acids and 1 mole of 2-acylglycerol (β-monoglyceride) per mole of substrate. The latter is resistant to hydrolysis, but it can spontaneously isomerize to the α-form (3-acylglycerol). The isomerization permits the third fatty acid to be split off, but at a much slower rate.

LIP acts only when the substrate is present in an emulsified form at the interface between water and the substrate. Thus, the rate of LIP action depends on the surface area of the dispersed substrate. Bile acids ensure that the surface of the dispersed substrate remains free of other proteins, by lining the surface of the insoluble substrate and the aqueous medium.

Most LIP activity found in serum derives from pancreatic acinar cells, but some is secreted by gastric and intestinal mucosa. LIP concentration in the pancreas is approximately 5000-fold greater than in other tissues, and the concentration gradient between the pancreas and serum is approximately 20,000-fold. LIP is a small enough molecule to be filtered through the glomerulus, but it is totally reabsorbed by the renal tubules, and it is not detectable in urine.

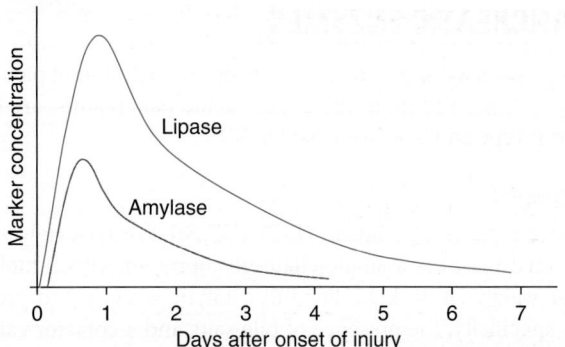

**Fig. 19.2** Time-dependent changes in serum amylase and lipase after uncomplicated acute pancreatitis.

## Clinical Significance

LIP measurement in serum is the recommended laboratory test to diagnose acute pancreatitis. The clinical sensitivity is 80% to 100%, depending on the selected diagnostic cutoff, and the clinical specificity is 85% to 100%, depending on the mix of the patient population studied. After an attack of acute pancreatitis, serum LIP activity increases within 4 to 8 hours, peaks at about 24 hours, and returns to baseline within 7 to 14 days (Fig. 19.2). The increase in serum LIP activity observed in acute pancreatitis is not necessarily proportional to the severity of the attack.

Acute pancreatitis is sometimes difficult to diagnose because it must be differentiated from other acute intra-abdominal disorders with similar clinical findings, such as (1) acute cholecystitis, (2) perforated gastric or duodenal ulcer, (3) intestinal obstruction, or (4) ruptured abdominal aortic aneurysm. A correct diagnosis of pancreatitis is vitally important, as the treatment for the other conditions mimicking pancreatitis typically involves surgery, while surgery is generally contraindicated in pancreatitis. In differential diagnosis, increase of serum LIP activity to greater than three times the URL, in the absence of severe renal failure, is a more specific diagnostic finding than increases in serum α-amylase activity. Furthermore, LIP concentrations remain increased longer than those of α-amylase do, which is another advantage over α-amylase measurement in patients with delayed presentation (see Fig. 19.2). Therefore, it is recommended that LIP should definitively replace α-amylase as the initial diagnostic test for acute pancreatitis in the emergency department; routine measurement of both serum α-amylase and LIP is not warranted and represents a source of redundant test duplication.

In patients with a marked reduction of GFR, serum LIP activity may be increased; this is likely because the LIP filtration by glomeruli is decreased. Thus, care should be exercised when interpreting increased serum LIP values in patients with CKD.

## Methods of Analysis

Many LIP methods have been described; they have used both triglyceride and nontriglyceride substrates. In general, long-chain triglyceride (and some diglyceride) substrates have demonstrated better correlation of results with the clinical state. Spectrophotometric methods have the advantage of ease of automation.

In the enzymatic reaction rate diglyceride assay for LIP, the following sequence of indicator and auxiliary enzymes is used:

$$\text{1,2-Diacylglycerol} + H_2O \xrightarrow[\text{pH 8.7}]{\substack{\text{Pancreatic lipase} \\ \text{Colipase}}} \text{2-Monoacylglycerol} + \text{Fatty acid}$$

$$\text{2-Monoacylglycerol} + H_2O \xrightarrow{\text{Monoglyceride lipase}} \text{Glycerol} + \text{Fatty acid}$$

$$\text{Glycerol} + \text{ATP} \xrightarrow{\text{Glycerol kinase}} \text{L-}\alpha\text{-glycerophospate} + \text{ADP}$$

$$\text{L-}\alpha\text{-glycerophospate} + O_2 \xrightarrow{\text{L-}\alpha\text{-glycerophospate kinase}} \text{Dihydroxyacetone phosphate} + H_2O_2$$

$$2\,H_2O_2 + \text{4-Aminoantipyrine} + \text{TOOS} \xrightarrow{\text{Peroxidase}} \text{Quinonediimine dye (colored)} + 2\,H_2O$$

TOOS is sodium *N*-ethyl-*N*-(2-hydroxyl-3-sulfopropyl)-m-toluidine, and its oxidation produces an intensely colored dye detectable at 550 nm.

In another method, a synthetic substrate (1,2-*O*-dilauryl-rac-glycero-3-glutaric acid-[4-methyl-resorufin]-ester) consisting of two glycerol ether bonds and one ester bond is used. LIP hydrolyzes the ester bond in an alkaline medium to an unstable dicarbonic acid ester that spontaneously hydrolyzes to yield glutaric acid and methylresorufin; this is a bluish-purple chromophore with peak absorption at 580 nm. The rate of methylresorufin formation is directly proportional to the LIP activity of the sample.

1,2-O-Dilauryl-rac-glycero-3-glutaric acid-
(4 methyl-resorufin)-ester

*Lipase*
+ OH $\ominus$

*Spontaneous*      OH $\ominus$

Glutarate

Red, $\lambda$ = 580 nm

LIP activity in serum is stable at room temperature for 1 week; sera may be stored for 3 weeks at 4°C and for several years at −25°C.

LIP is among the more poorly standardized laboratory tests, so reference intervals for LIP activity are largely method dependent. For the enzymatic reaction rate diglyceride assay, the suggested URL is 45 U/L. The URL is 64 U/L for methylresorufin assay. There are no sex- or age-related URLs.

## Amylase

α-Amylases (AMYs) (EC 3.2.1.1; 1,4-α-D glucan glucanohydrolase) are enzymes that catalyze the hydrolysis of 1,4-α-glucosidic linkages in polysaccharides. Both straight-chain (linear) polyglucans (amylose) and branched polyglucans (amylopectin and glycogen) are hydrolyzed, but at different rates. AMYs do not attack the α-1,6-linkages at the branch points. AMYs are calcium metalloenzymes, with the calcium essential for functional integrity. However, full AMY activity is displayed only in the presence of various anions, with chloride and bromide being the most effective activators.

### Biochemistry

AMYs have molecular weights varying from 54 to 62 kDa. These enzymes are thus small enough to pass through the glomeruli of the kidneys, and AMY is the only plasma enzyme normally found in urine. AMYs are present in many organs and tissues. The greatest concentration is noted in the salivary glands, which secrete a potent AMY

(S-type) to initiate hydrolysis of starches while the food is still in the mouth and esophagus. In the pancreas, the enzyme (P-type) is synthesized by acinar cells and then secreted into the intestinal tract by way of the pancreatic duct system. AMY activity is also found in extracts from (in decreasing amounts) the (1) ileum, (2) jejunum, (3) duodenum, (4) colon, (5) lungs, and (6) fallopian tubes. Epithelial tumors of the lung and ovary may contain considerable AMY activity (usually S-type) and produce hypcramylasemia. Cases of AMY-producing multiple myeloma have also been described.

The enzyme present in serum and urine is predominantly of pancreatic (P-AMY) and salivary gland (S-AMY) origin. In healthy adults, P-AMY represents approximately 40% to 50% of total AMY activity in serum. AMY isoenzymes also undergo posttranslational modification of (1) deamidation, (2) glycosylation, and (3) deglycosylation to form a number of isoforms.

### Clinical Significance

Blood AMY activity is physiologically low and greatly increases in acute pancreatitis and salivary gland inflammation. In acute pancreatitis, a rise in serum AMY activity occurs within 5 to 8 hours of symptom onset; activities typically return to baseline by the third or fourth day (see Fig. 19.2). The specificity of AMY for the diagnosis of acute pancreatitis is, however, low because increased values are also found in a number of acute intra-abdominal disorders and in several nonpancreatic conditions (Table 19.5).

## TABLE 19.5    Causes of Hyperamylasemia

| | |
|---|---|
| Pancreatic disease | Pancreatitis, any cause (P-AMY↑)[a] |
| | Pancreatic trauma (P-AMY↑) |
| Intra-abdominal diseases other than pancreatitis | Biliary tract disease (P-AMY↑) |
| | Intestinal obstruction (P-AMY↑) |
| | Mesenteric infarction (P-AMY↑) |
| | Perforated peptic ulcer (P-AMY↑) |
| | Gastritis, duodenitis (P-AMY↑) |
| | Ruptured aortic aneurysm |
| | Acute appendicitis (perforated) |
| | Peritonitis |
| | Trauma |
| Genitourinary disease | Ectopic, ruptured tubal pregnancy |
| | Salpingitis (S-AMY↑) |
| | Ovarian malignancy (S-AMY↑) |
| | Renal insufficiency (Mixed) |
| Miscellaneous | Salivary gland lesions (S-AMY↑) |
| | Acute alcoholic abuse (S-AMY↑) |
| | Diabetic ketoacidosis (S-AMY↑) |
| | Macroamylasemia (S-AMY↑ or P-AMY↑) |
| | Septic shock (S-AMY↑) |
| | Cardiac surgery (S-AMY↑) |
| | Tumor (usually S-AMY↑) |
| | Drugs (usually S-AMY↑) |

[a]Predominant isoenzyme type is shown in parentheses.
*Mixed,* Either or both isoenzymes may be present; *P-AMY,* pancreatic; *S-AMY,* salivary.

Lack of specificity of total AMY measurement has resulted in the promotion of the direct measurement of P-AMY instead of total enzyme activity for the differential diagnosis of patients with acute abdominal pain, making the measurement of total AMY a less preferred option. By applying the best decision limit (an activity equal to three-fold the URL), the specificity of P-AMY for the diagnosis of acute pancreatitis is close to 90%. Sensitivity in late detection of this condition is also notably improved with P-AMY. This long-standing increase in P-AMY activity in serum also makes redundant the traditional measurement of total AMY in urine—a test traditionally performed to achieve better diagnostic sensitivity in the late phase of pancreatitis.

Various intra-abdominal nonpancreatic events, such as biliary tract disease, can lead to a significant increase in serum P-AMY activities. In renal insufficiency, serum P-AMY activity is increased in proportion to the extent of renal impairment.

In 1% of the population, macroamylases are present in sera and may cause hyperamylasemia; these are complexes of ordinary AMY (usually S-type) and IgG or IgA. These macroamylases cannot be filtered through the glomeruli of the kidneys because of their large size (>200 kDa molecular weight) and are thus retained in the plasma, where their presence may increase AMY activity some two- to eightfold above the URL, typically stable over time. No clinical symptoms are associated with this condition.

### POINTS TO REMEMBER

Pancreatic enzymes in acute pancreatitis:
- The diagnostic performance of pancreatic enzymes is greatly improved by restricting their use to a population with suspected disease.
- LIP measurement is superior to P-AMY in terms of diagnostic performance. Therefore, it is recommended that LIP replaces P-AMY as initial test for acute pancreatitis in emergency departments.
- Measuring both serum LIP and P-AMY routinely is not warranted.
- The measurement of total AMY should be discouraged.

## Methods of Analysis

The use of defined substrates in the AMY assay has improved the reaction stoichiometry and led to more controlled and consistent hydrolysis conditions. Substrates used include (1) small oligosaccharides and (2) 4-nitrophenyl (4-NP)-glycoside substrates prepared by bonding 4-NP to the reducing end of a defined oligosaccharide. If the oligosaccharide is maltoheptaose (G7), the substrate is then 4-NP-G7. AMY splits this substrate to produce free oligosaccharides (G5, G4, and G3) and 4-NP-G2, 4-NP-G3, and 4-NP-G4. Combined hydrolysis by AMY in the specimen and by the reagent α-glucosidase results in free NP production, which is detected by its absorbance at 405 nm. Problems arose with the use of the 4-NP-glycoside assay with regard to the poor stability of the reconstituted assay mixture because of slow hydrolysis of the 4-NP-glycoside by α-glucosidase. This effect has been reduced by covalently linking a "blocking" group (i.e., a 4,6-ethylidene group; ethylidene-protected substrate [EPS]) to the nonreducing end of the molecule. The blocked substrate also shows a more advantageous hydrolysis pattern, thus increasing the liberation of 4-NP. The IFCC has recommended this method as reference measurement procedure for AMY.

$$5 \text{ Ethylidene-4-NP-G}_7 + 5 \text{ H}_2\text{O} \xrightarrow{\alpha\text{-Amylase}}$$
$$2 \text{ Ethylidene-G}_5 + 2 \text{ 4-NP-G}_2 +$$
$$2 \text{ Ethylidene-G}_4 + 2 \text{ 4-NP-G}_3 +$$
$$\text{Ethylidene-G}_3 + \text{ 4-NP-G}_4$$

$$2 \text{ 4-NP-G}_2 + 2 \text{ 4-NP-G}_3 + 10 \text{ H}_2\text{O} \xrightarrow{\alpha\text{-Glucosidase}} 4 \text{ 4-NP} + 10 \text{ G}$$

Only methods based on selective S-AMY inhibition by monoclonal antibodies have shown sufficient (1) precision, (2) reliability, (3) practicability, and (4) analytical speed to allow the introduction of P-AMY determination into clinical practice. After the S-AMY activity is inhibited by the addition of antibodies, uninhibited P-AMY activity is measured using EPS-4-NP-G7 as a substrate. This assay is available in full automation today on clinical chemistry platforms with reagent costs similar to total AMY, which permits laboratories

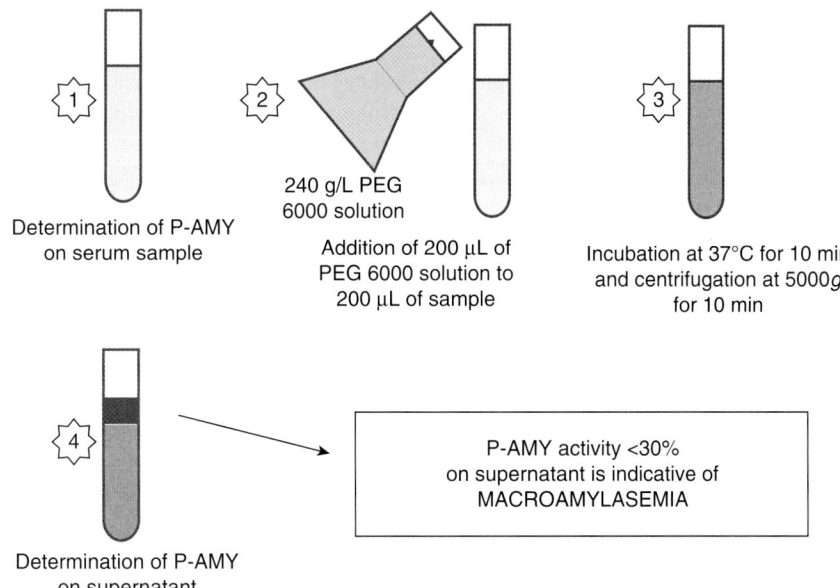

Fig. 19.3 Demonstration of macroamylasemia by polyethylene glycol (PEG) 6000 solution. *P-AMY*, Pancreatic amylase.

to abandon the latter. Using this method, falsely increased P-AMY results have been reported in subjects with macroamylasemia, in whom immunoglobulin complexed to AMY forms diminishes or voids the ability of monoclonal antibodies included in the test to efficiently inhibit S-AMY. In this condition, precipitation of the macrocomplex by a PEG 6000 solution (240 g/L) presents an easy and effective approach to confirm the suspicion of macroamylasemia. Residual P-AMY activity of less than 30% in the supernatant is indicative of macroamylasemia (Fig. 19.3).

Except for heparin, all common anticoagulants inhibit AMY activity because they chelate calcium. Therefore, P-AMY assay should be performed only on serum or heparinized plasma. AMY is quite stable; activity is fully retained during storage for 4 days at room temperature, for 2 weeks at 4°C, and for 1 year at −25°C.

Using the immunoinhibition method, the reference interval for P-AMY activity in sera from adults is 13 to 53 U/L. Serum P-AMY activity is not demonstrable in most children younger than 6 months, but activity rises slowly thereafter to reach adult concentrations by 5 years of age, reflecting the postnatal development of exocrine pancreatic function.

## OTHER CLINICALLY IMPORTANT ENZYMES

### Lactate Dehydrogenase

LDH (EC 1.1.1.27; l-lactate: NAD+ oxidoreductase) catalyzes the oxidation of l-lactate to pyruvate with the mediation of NAD+ as a hydrogen acceptor.

As indicated, the reaction is reversible, and the reaction equilibrium strongly favors the reduction of pyruvate to lactate (P → L)—the "reverse reaction." Both pyruvate and lactate in excess inhibit enzyme activity, although the effect of pyruvate is greater. EDTA inhibits the enzyme—perhaps by binding zinc ions, which are postulated as LDH activator.

### Biochemistry

LDH has a molecular weight of 134 kDa and is composed of four peptide chains of two types, M and H, each under separate genetic control. The subunit compositions of the five isoenzymes are LDH-1 (HHHH; $H_4$), LDH-2 (HHHM; $H_3M$), LDH-3 (HHMM; $H_2M_2$), LDH-4 (HMMM; $HM_3$), and LDH-5 (MMMM; $M_4$).

LD activity is present in many cells of the body and is invariably found in the cytoplasm. Different tissues show different isoenzyme composition. In the heart, kidneys, and erythrocytes, isoenzymes LDH-1 and LDH-2 predominate, while LDH-4 and LDH-5 isoenzymes account for the enzyme activity in the liver and skeletal muscle.

### Clinical Significance

Because of its wide tissue distribution, serum LDH increases occur in a variety of diseases, but its clinical utility is now relegated to hematology and oncology. Hemolytic anemias significantly increase LDH concentrations in the serum. Marked increases of LDH activity—up to 50 times the URL—have been observed in the megaloblastic anemias, usually resulting from the deficiency of folate or vitamin $B_{12}$. These increases rapidly return to normal after appropriate treatment. For monitoring purposes, LDH is relevant in predicting disease activity in leukemia, and the probability of survival and duration in Hodgkin disease and non-Hodgkin lymphoma. In multiple myeloma, a Revised International Staging System

(RISS) has been developed, which combines markers of tumor burden (albumin, beta-2 microglobulin) with markers of aggressive disease biology (high-risk cytogenetics and elevated serum LDH).

Patients with solid tumors often show increased LDH activity in their serum; up to 60% to 70% of patients with liver or lymph node metastases have increased LDH activity. Therefore, LDH elevation is harbinger of poor outcome in patients with several types of solid tumors. Elevated LDH (LDH-1) is observed in germ cell tumors (≈60% of cases) such as seminoma of the testis and dysgerminoma of the ovary.

LDH measured in pleural fluid (in combination with serum LDH) is part of the Light's criteria for distinguishing exudative from transudative effusions. Macro-LDH, which occurs as a result of the formation of an autoantibody-enzyme complex leading to a persistent increase in the amount of circulating enzyme, is present in fewer than 1 in 10,000 people without any pathologic significance.

## Methods of Analysis

Methods for quantitation of LDH activity use kinetic spectrophotometry to measure the interconversion of the coenzymes $NAD^+$ and NADH at 340 nm. Procedures employing the L → P reaction are recommended because there is less dependence on the $NAD^+$ and lactate concentrations and less contamination of $NAD^+$ with inhibiting products. A reference measurement procedure based on this reaction has been recommended by the IFCC.

Serum is the preferred specimen for measuring LDH activity. Plasma samples may be contaminated with platelets, which contain high concentrations of LDH. Hemolyzed serum must not be used because erythrocytes contain 4000 times more LDH activity than does serum. LDH-4 and LDH-5 isoenzymes are very sensitive to cold. Thus, serum specimens should be stored at room temperature, at which no loss of activity occurs for at least 3 days.

The reference interval for LDH activity in adults, applicable for assays traceable to the IFCC reference procedure, is 125 to 220 U/L. LDH reference intervals are higher in children, with a gradual decrease noted throughout childhood and adolescence.

Electrophoretic separation is the only procedure commercially available to demonstrate LDH isoenzymes. However, considering the limited clinical use of the enzyme in hematology and oncology, LDH isoenzyme measurement is not routine.

## Cholinesterase

Two related enzymes can hydrolyze acetylcholine. One is acetylcholinesterase (EC 3.1.1.7; acetylcholine acetylhydrolase), which is called *true cholinesterase* or *choline esterase I*. True **cholinesterase** is found in (1) erythrocytes, (2) the lungs and spleen, (3) nerve endings, and (4) the gray matter of the brain. It is responsible for the prompt hydrolysis of acetylcholine

released at the nerve endings to mediate transmission of the neural impulse across the synapse. The other cholinesterase is acylcholine acylhydrolase (EC 3.1.1.8; acylcholine acylhydrolase), also called *pseudocholinesterase*, *serum cholinesterase* (CHE), *butyrylcholinesterase*, or *choline esterase II*. CHE is found in the (1) liver, (2) pancreas, (3) heart, (4) white matter of the brain, and (5) serum. Its exact biological role is unknown.

The type of reaction catalyzed by both cholinesterases is shown:

## Biochemistry

The atypical (genetic) variants of CHE, characterized by diminished activity against acetylcholine and other substrates, are of clinical interest and are found in the sera of a small fraction of apparently healthy people. The gene controlling the synthesis of CHE can exist in many allelic forms. Four of the most common forms are designated as $E^u$, $E^a$, $E^f$, and $E^s$. These four allelic genes can be combined to form one normal and nine abnormal genotypes. The normal, most common genotype is designated as $E^u E^u$, or $UU$ (u for usual). The gene $E^a$ is referred to as the *atypical* gene; the sera of people homozygous for this gene ($E^a E^a = AA$) are only weakly active toward most substrates for CHE and demonstrate increased resistance to inhibition of enzyme activity by dibucaine. The $E^f$ gene (f for *fluoride resistant*) gives rise to a weakly active enzyme but with increased resistance to fluoride inhibition. The $E^s$ gene (s for *silent*) is associated with the absence of enzyme or the presence of a protein with minimal or no catalytic activity. Homozygous forms, *AA* and *FF*, are found in 0.3% to 0.5% of the White population; their incidence among Black populations is even lower.

## Clinical Significance

Measurements of CHE activity in the serum are used (1) as a test of liver function, (2) as an indicator of possible insecticide poisoning, and (3) for the detection of patients with atypical forms of the enzyme who are at risk for prolonged responses to certain muscle relaxants [succinylcholine (suxamethonium) and mivacurium] used in surgical procedures to aid in endotracheal intubation.

In the absence of genetic causes or known inhibitors, any decrease in CHE activity reflects impaired synthesis of the enzyme by the liver. Among the organic phosphorous compounds that inhibit CHE activity are many insecticides, such as (1) parathion, (2) sarin, and (3) tetraethyl pyrophosphate. Workers in agriculture and organic chemical industries may be subject to poisoning by inhalation of these materials or by direct cutaneous contact with them. Muscle-relaxant drugs used in surgical procedures are hydrolyzed by CHE, and in individuals with low enzyme activities or in those with a weakly active variant, destruction of the drug will not occur rapidly enough, and the subject may enter a period of prolonged paralysis of the respiratory muscles (apnea) requiring mechanical ventilation until the drug effects gradually wear off. Preoperative screening of CHE activity has been advocated in the past to identify these individuals; however, this is not currently recommended because every individual undergoing succinylcholine treatment should be managed as potentially at-risk. Measurements of total CHE activity and determination of "dibucaine number" and "fluoride number" are needed to characterize CHE variants. The latter values indicate the percentage inhibition of enzyme activity in the presence of standard concentrations of dibucaine or fluoride. Mutation genotyping may confirm CHE gene abnormalities.

## Methods of Analysis

Historically, many methods were proposed to measure CHE, using different acyl(thio)choline esters as substrates. At present, however, most automated measuring systems use butyrylthiocholine for determining the CHE activity as this substrate provides the best reproducibility. After the substrate hydrolysis, the thiocholine formed can be measured by reaction with chromogenic disulfide agents, such as 5,5′-dithio-bis(2-nitrobenzoate) (DTNB). The reaction of the thiocholine product with colorless DTNB forms colored 5-mercapto-2-nitro-benzoic acid, which is measured spectrophotometrically at 410 nm. Another colorimetric principle, in which the thiocholine formed reduces yellow hexacyanoferrate(III) to colorless hexacyanoferrate(II) and the decrease of absorbance at 405 nm is directly proportional to the CHE activity in the sample, is also used.

Based on differences in sensitivity to inhibition by the local anesthetic dibucaine, a simple test ("dibucaine number") was developed to classify the type of CHE as (1) usual, (2) intermediate, or (3) atypical. Characteristically, the usual CHE is inhibited by 80%, but the atypical CHE is inhibited by only 20%. Subjects heterozygous for the normal and the atypical gene show about 60% inhibition of CHE. Molecular methods that can be used to identify various CHE genetic defects have been developed and are being used increasingly in clinical laboratories.

Serum is the sample of choice. Enzyme activity in serum is stable for several weeks if the specimen is stored under refrigeration and for several years if stored at −20°C.

Using butyrylthiocholine as substrate at 37°C, a value of 6.6 kU/L was calculated as the threshold with 100% sensitivity in detecting succinylcholine-sensitive individuals. The significant CHE decrease (≈30%) during pregnancy and early puerperium is explained by hemodilution.

## Bone Acid Phosphatase (Tartrate-Resistant 5b Isoform)

Under the name of acid phosphatase (ACP; EC 3.1.3.2; orthophosphoric-monoester phosphohydrolase [acid optimum]) are included all phosphatases with optimal activity below a pH of 7.0. ACP is present in lysosomes, which are organelles present in all cells except erythrocytes. Extralysosomal ACPs are also present in many cells. The greatest concentrations of ACP activity occur in (1) prostate, (2) bone (osteoclasts), (3) spleen, (4) platelets, and (5) erythrocytes. At least four ACP-determining genes have been identified and mapped; the lysosomal and prostatic isoenzymes are strongly inhibited by dextrorotatory tartrate ions, but the erythrocyte and bone isoenzymes are not. The tartrate-resistant type (TR-ACP) expressed in osteoclasts and other tissue macrophages, such as alveolar macrophages and Kupffer cells (type 5 ACP), consists of two structurally related isoforms that differ by their carbohydrate content: TR-ACP 5a, which derives mainly from macrophages and dendritic cells, and type 5b, a more specific marker of osteoclastic activity. Most of the physiologically low ACP activity of (unhemolyzed) serum is a TR-ACP and probably originates mainly in osteoclasts. Activities of this fraction are increased physiologically in growing children and pathologically in conditions of increased osteolysis and bone remodeling.

Serum TR-ACP 5b is a potentially useful marker of conditions with a marked osteolytic component. Unlike blood concentrations of other markers of bone resorption (e.g., C-telopeptide of type I collagen), TR-ACP 5b is not affected by renal dysfunction. This makes TR-ACP 5b the only useful resorption marker for CKD-MBD. However, TR-ACP 5b appears to show relatively small dynamic changes in comparison with markers of bone resorption related to type I collagen metabolism. This may be attributable to the fact that the enzyme is released into the sealed osteoclast microenvironment, rather than directly into the circulation.

Immunoassays for serum TR-ACP have been developed that preferentially detect isoform 5b and are now commercially available. However, they are not entirely bone-specific.

Serum should be immediately separated from erythrocytes and stabilized by the addition of 50 μL of acetic acid (5 mol/L) per milliliter of serum to lower the pH to 5.4, at which the enzyme is stable. Under these conditions, TR-ACP activity is maintained at room temperature for several hours, for up to 1 week if the serum is refrigerated, and for 4 months if stored at −20°C. Hemolyzed serum specimens are contaminated with the erythrocyte isoenzyme and should be rejected.

In the sera of healthy adults, the reference intervals for TR-ACP 5b activity are 2.7 to 5.1 U/L for men, 2.3 to 5.7 U/L for premenopausal women, and 2.6 to 6.8 U/L for postmenopausal women, respectively.

## REVIEW QUESTIONS

1. The enzyme that demonstrates highest serum activity in Paget disease (osteitis deformans) and is also elevated in hepatobiliary disease is:
   a. alkaline phosphatase (ALP).
   b. creatine kinase (CK).
   c. amylase (AMY).
   d. γ-glutamyltransferase (GGT).

2. Activity of which of the following isoenzymes of lactate dehydrogenase (LDH) is highest in the serum of individuals with seminoma of the testis?
   a. LDH-1
   b. LDH-2
   c. LDH-4
   d. LDH-5

3. The serum enzyme that demonstrates an increase in activity 4 to 8 hours after an attack of acute pancreatitis, peaks at 24 hours, and then returns to baseline within a week is:
   a. AMY.
   b. lipase (LIP).
   c. ALP.
   d. serum cholinesterase (CHE).

4. Which of the following enzymes catalyzes the reaction of glutamate and pyruvate to form 2-oxoglutarate and an amino acid?
   a. ALP
   b. Aspartate aminotransferase (AST)
   c. Alanine aminotransferase (ALT)
   d. CK

5. In the laboratory measurement of ALP, a chromogenic assay forms the basis of almost all current methods used for ALP analysis. The substrate in this assay is:
   a. acid phosphatase.
   b. 4-nitrophenyl phosphate.
   c. *p*-nitroaniline.
   d. butyrylthiocholine.

6. Measurement of decreased activity of which of the following enzymes is used to determine possible insecticide poisoning?
   a. CK
   b. ALP
   c. ALT
   d. CHE

7. Children have higher ALP activity than healthy adults because:
   a. ALP leaks from osteoblasts during physiological bone growth.
   b. developing hepatocytes produce excess ALP during physiologic growth.
   c. striated muscle contains the greatest activity of ALP, and children are more energetic than adults with concomitant release of excess ALP from muscle.
   d. the presence of ALP in the pancreas is elevated during childhood.

8. The isoenzyme of AMY that is synthesized by acinar cells of the pancreas and that remains elevated in most individuals for at least 1 week after the onset of pancreatitis is:
   a. S-AMY.
   b. macro-AMY.
   c. P-AMY.
   d. S-AMY + P-AMY.

9. Which of the following enzymes demonstrates an increase in activity with progressive Duchenne muscular dystrophy, followed by a decrease as muscle mass decreases?
   a. ALP
   b. ALT
   c. CHE
   d. CK

10. The oxidoreductase that is increased significantly during megaloblastic anemia is:
    a. LDH.
    b. CK.
    c. ALP.
    d. Tartrate-resistant acid phosphatase.

## SUGGESTED READINGS

Dufour DR, Lott JA, Nolte FS, et al. Diagnosis and monitoring of hepatic injury. II. Recommendations for use of laboratory tests in screening, diagnosis, and monitoring. *Clin Chem.* 2000;46:2050–2068.

Gomez D, Addison A, De Rosa A, et al. Retrospective study of patients with acute pancreatitis: is serum amylase still required? *BMJ Open.* 2012;2:e001471.

Kim WR, Flamm SL, Di Bisceglie AM, et al. Serum activity of alanine aminotransferase (ALT) as an indicator of health and disease. *Hepatology.* 2008;47:1363–1370.

Kristensen SR. Mechanisms of cell damage and enzyme release. *Dan Med Bull.* 1994;41:423–433.

Lilford RJ, Bentham LM, Armstrong MJ, et al. What is the best strategy for investigating abnormal liver function tests in primary care? Implications from a prospective study. *BMJ Open.* 2013;3:e003099.

Lippi G, Panteghini M, Bernardini S, et al. Laboratory testing in the emergency department: an Italian Society of Clinical Biochemistry and Clinical Molecular Biology (SIBioC) and Academy of Emergency Medicine and Care (AcEMC) consensus report. *Clin Chem Lab Med.* 2018;56:1655–1659.

McQueen MJ. Clinical and analytical considerations in the utilization of cholinesterase measurements. *Clin Chim Acta.* 1995;237:91–105.

Mohammed-Ali Z, Brinc D, Kusalingam V, et al. Defining appropriate utilization of AST testing. *Clin Biochem.* 2020;79:75–77.

Morandi L, Angelini C, Prelle A, et al. High plasma creatine kinase: review of the literature and proposal for a diagnostic algorithm. *Neurol Sci.* 2006;27:303–311.

Moss DW. Perspectives in alkaline phosphatase research. *Clin Chem.* 1992;38:2486–2492.

Moss DW, Raymond FD, Wile DB. Clinical and biological aspects of acid phosphatase. *CRC Crit Rev Clin Lab Sci.* 1995;32:431–467.

Pagani F, Panteghini M. 5'-Nucleotidase in the detection of increased activity of the liver form of alkaline phosphatase in serum. *Clin Chem.* 2001;47:2046–2048.

Panteghini M. Lactate dehydrogenase: an old enzyme reborn as a COVID-19 marker (and not only). *Clin Chem Lab Med.* 2020;58:1979–1981.

Panteghini M, Ceriotti F, Pagani F, et al. Recommendations for the routine use of pancreatic amylase measurement instead of total amylase for the diagnosis and monitoring of pancreatic pathology. *Clin Chem Lab Med.* 2002;40:97–100.

Phillip V, Steiner JM, Algül H. Early phase of acute pancreatitis: assessment and management. *World J Gastrointest Pathophysiol.* 2014;5:158–168.

Pimentel A, Ureña-Torres P, Zillikens MC, et al. Fractures in patients with CKD—-diagnosis, treatment, and prevention: a review by members of the European Calcified Tissue Society and the European Renal Association of Nephrology Dialysis and Transplantation. *Kidney Int.* 2017;92:1343–1355.

Pratt DS, Kaplan MM. Evaluation of abnormal liver-enzyme results in asymptomatic patients. *N Engl J Med.* 2000;342:1266–1271.

Sprague SM, Bellorin-Font E, Jorgetti V, et al. Diagnostic accuracy of bone turnover markers and bone histology in patients with CKD treated by dialysis. *Am J Kidney Dis.* 2016;67:559–566.

Tenner S, Baillie J, DeWitt J, et al. American College of Gastroenterology guideline: management of acute pancreatitis. *Am J Gastroenterol.* 2013;108:1400–1415.

Whitfield JB. Gamma glutamyl transferase. *CRC Crit Rev Clin Lab Sci.* 2001;38:263–355.

# Tumor Markers

*Catharine Sturgeon*

## OBJECTIVES

1. List the requirements of the "ideal" tumor marker.
2. Describe how to validate a "new" tumor marker.
3. Describe the major applications of tumor markers, providing specific examples as recommended in clinical guidelines.
4. Outline requirements of an optimal tumor marker service from test request to laboratory report.
5. Describe pitfalls and caveats in the use and interpretation of tumor markers.

## KEY WORDS AND DEFINITIONS

**Cancer** Heterogeneous but related diseases characterized by uncontrolled division of cells.

**Diagnostic accuracy** The ability of a test to correctly identify patients who have malignancy.

**Heterophilic antibodies** Antibodies that may react with immunoassay reagents, yielding inappropriately high or low results.

**High-dose "hooking"** Interference leading to inappropriately low results for specimens of high analyte concentrations.

**Serial monitoring** Post-treatment tumor marker measurement enabling early detection of disease progression.

**Therapy prediction** Identification of patients likely to benefit from a particular treatment.

**Prognosis** Prediction of the likely outcome of disease with respect to risk of relapse or progression.

**Screening** Detection of unsuspected disease in asymptomatic subjects.

**Tumor marker** Substances found in cells or body fluids that may be a sign of cancer. Tumor markers include proteins that are usually present in abnormally high concentrations in body fluids or tissue from cancer patients and genetic changes in tumor DNA and RNA.

---

Tumor markers are substances that may be present in abnormally high concentrations or in altered forms in body fluids, tissue, or cells from patients with cancer. They can be measured either qualitatively or quantitatively using chemical, immunologic, or molecular biological methods. They range from simple molecules (e.g., catecholamines) through relatively well-characterized proteins (e.g., hormones) to much more heterogeneous glycoproteins and mucins (e.g., CA125), which may be defined by the antibodies used to measure them. Tumor markers also include DNA mutations and altered forms or levels of RNA expression.

Several important tumor markers (e.g., α-fetoprotein [AFP], carcinoembryonic antigen [CEA], and human chorionic gonadotropin [hCG]) are oncofetal antigens, which are present in the fetus in a normal pregnancy but may be expressed at high concentrations in tissue or body fluids of adults with some cancers. Reflecting the heterogeneous nature of cancer, tumor markers encompass a variety of molecular species. Many tumor markers are produced by a variety of different tumors and few tumor markers are organ- or cancer-specific.

Although their structures and properties vary widely, the broad principles underpinning their evidence-based clinical use are common to all tumor markers. They can contribute to cancer management in a number of ways, including in screening, diagnosis, assessment of prognosis, therapy prediction, and/or post-treatment monitoring (Table 20.1).

This chapter provides a brief overview of cancer and tumor marker development followed by a review of these principles. Clinically relevant tumor markers for a number of malignancies are then discussed.

## CANCER—AN OVERVIEW

Cancer is the name given to a collection of heterogeneous but related diseases which can start in most parts of the body and are characterized by uncontrolled division of cells that ultimately may spread into surrounding tissues. Causative factors include exposure to carcinogens, which may be physical (e.g., radiation), chemical (e.g., polycyclic hydrocarbons), or biological (e.g., viral). Excess weight, physical inactivity, and poor nutrition may also contribute.

| TABLE 20.1 **Current Clinical Applications of Tumor Markers** | | |
| --- | --- | --- |
| **Clinical Application** | **Requirements** | **Examples** |
| Screening for cancer | An acceptable test in asymptomatic patients for a disease that poses an important health problem for which the natural history is well-understood, and the test identifies treatable early-stage cancers for which early intervention with effective treatment improves outcome. High clinical sensitivity (few false negatives) and specificity (few false positives) are essential prerequisites as the population screened is asymptomatic. | *Population screening:* Fecal occult blood testing for colorectal cancer. *Screening of high-risk groups:* Serum hCG testing for choriocarcinoma in women who have had a molar pregnancy. |
| Diagnosing cancer | High clinical sensitivity and specificity as for screening. Most serum tumor markers are not cancer-specific and/or organ-specific and are raised in different cancers and/or in nonmalignant disease, severely limiting their use in diagnosis. | *As a diagnostic aid in high-risk groups:* Serum AFP testing as an adjunct to ultrasound for hepatocellular carcinoma (HCC) in patients with cirrhosis who are at high risk of developing HCC. *Differential diagnosis:* CA125 contributes (with menopausal status and ultrasound findings) to calculation of the Risk of Malignancy index which is used to differentiate patients with benign and malignant pelvic masses. |
| Assessing prognosis | A test that can provide a probability estimate of outcome (risk of relapse or disease progression) and/or differentiate indolent from aggressive disease for a heterogeneous population of patients, thereby influencing treatment decisions. | Serum AFP, hCG and lactate dehydrogenase (LDH) measurements are mandatory for determining prognosis and selection of chemotherapy in patients with metastatic non-seminomatous germ cell tumors. Gene expression profiles such as the Oncotype Dx test which measures expression of 21 genes in breast tumor tissue enable calculation of a recurrence score that predicts the risk of distant disease at 10 years in a specific sub-set of breast cancer patients. |
| Prediction of treatment response | A test that can identify whether or not a potential treatment is likely to be effective and of benefit to the patient. | Measurement of estrogen receptors (ER) is mandatory for all newly diagnosed invasive breast cancer to predict response to treatment with anti-estrogen therapy (i.e., aromatase inhibitors and tamoxifen). Measurement of human epidermal growth factor receptor 2 (HER2) is essential to identify patients with HER2-positive breast cancer who are likely to benefit from treatment with anti-HER2 monoclonal antibody therapy. |
| Monitoring response during and/or shortly after treatment | A test that assesses whether the tumor is responding to treatment, enabling withdrawal and/or change of ineffective treatment. | In patients receiving for ovarian cancer a reduction of at least 50% in CA125 concentrations from a pre-treatment sample has been defined as a response provided it is confirmed and maintained for at least 28 days and if a pre-treatment CA125 concentration was greater than twice the upper limit of the reference interval and measured within 2 weeks of the start of chemotherapy. |
| Monitoring disease post-treatment to detect progression | A test that reliably indicates earlier than clinical symptoms whether disease is progressing in patients with no evidence of disease post-therapy and/or in patients with detectable disease. Whether this information is helpful crucially depends on whether alternative therapies are available. | Inclusion of CEA measurements in intensive follow-up strategies for patients with nonmetastatic colorectal cancer patients following curative surgery has been shown to improve overall survival and increase the detection of asymptomatic recurrences and curative surgery attempted at recurrence. Such follow-up is also associated with earlier detection of recurrence. |

Genetic predisposition to some cancers is increasingly identifiable due to advances in molecular techniques. Simple genetic analysis of mutations within cancerous cells may be too simplistic to explain a complex process but increased understanding of such interactions is already leading to more finely targeted therapies.

Cancer remains a leading cause of death in the United States, second only to heart disease, although death rates have decreased significantly over the last three decades. Early detection and more effective treatment combined with prevention (e.g., decreased smoking, improved diet) may further reduce the cancer mortality rate. However, identification of smaller more indolent cancers with newer techniques and screening programs may also contribute to the perceived increase in survival.

Reflecting advances in treatment over recent decades, many patients survive for much longer than previously. While surgical removal of a primary tumor is the only curative therapy for almost all cancers, new chemotherapeutic and biological therapies that prevent progression are increasingly available. Some relatively indolent cancers are now almost regarded as chronic diseases like diabetes, to be controlled rather than cured. Breast and prostate cancers are among the best examples. However, for these and other cancers, distinguishing cancers that are likely to progress rapidly from those that are slow-growing or indolent is critical and remains a challenge.

Early detection of malignancy optimizes any opportunities for curative surgery for some in situ cancers. Unfortunately, most cancers do not produce symptoms until tumors are too large to be removed surgically or until cancerous cells have spread to other tissue either by invading local lymph nodes or by distant spread (metastasis) to other organs. Systemic treatments (chemotherapy, endocrine therapy, or immunotherapy) are then usually the only options but are not curative. Any residual viable cancerous cells remaining after treatment may proliferate, develop resistance to further therapy, and ultimately cause the death of the patient.

## HISTORICAL BACKGROUND

The introduction of new tumor markers has mirrored developments in analytical techniques and, more recently, the availability of new therapies, many of which are effective only in subsets of cancer patients.

The first tumor marker to be used clinically was Bence Jones protein, identified in 1847 and still the basis of many diagnoses of multiple myeloma. In the first half of the 20th century, the presence or absence of other hormones, enzymes and isoenzymes, and blood group antigens were recognized to be associated with malignancy, but it was not until development of the technique of radioimmunoassay (RIA) in the 1960s that these observations could be translated into routine clinical practice. Monoclonal antibody technology subsequently enabled the development of two-site immunometric assays of complex cancer-associated mucins identified primarily by their reactivity with given monoclonal antibody pairs (e.g., the cancer-associated antigens CA125 and CA15-3). As automated methods became available, many more laboratories added tumor markers to their test repertoires.

Advances in molecular genetics, including the study of oncogenes, suppressor genes, and genes involved in DNA repair, have led to improved understanding and use of tumor markers at both the molecular and cellular levels, particularly in high-risk individuals. Genetic predisposition to some cancers, including some familial cancers (e.g., MEN2, BRCA1), is facilitated by these developments and is already leading to more finely targeted therapies. As the choice of therapy may be influenced by molecular results, it is essential that mutation analysis is always carried out in accredited laboratories that have robust quality assurance practices in place.

Mass spectrometry is also increasingly used both as a discovery and a diagnostic tool, albeit with limited success thus far in translating new tumor marker tests into clinical practice. These developments require sophisticated bioinformatics support, which encourage multiparametric analysis for cancer diagnosis, prognosis, and therapy prediction.

## GENERAL PRINCIPLES GUIDING THE USE OF ALL TUMOR MARKERS

Tumor markers can help make or confirm a cancer diagnosis, monitor treatment effectiveness and the course of disease, estimate prognosis, and/or predict whether a specific therapy is likely to be successful (see Table 20.1). Their measurement should permit more efficient application of therapies, by ensuring that these are applied only to those patients most likely to benefit and reducing exposure to unnecessary toxicity for those patients unlikely to benefit. Tumor markers should be measured only after considering whether the result is likely to provide information that may improve outcome for the individual patient or as part of a clinical trial.

An evidence-based approach to clinical decision-making is therefore essential and careful consideration must be given to whether an individual tumor marker can fulfill requirements in selected clinical circumstances. Guidelines published by the National Comprehensive Cancer Network (NCCN) in the United States include patient pathways that clearly indicate which tumor markers should be measured and when. Complementing these clinically oriented guidelines, those published by the National Academy of Clinical Biochemistry (NACB) focus on the use of tumor markers, considering in detail requirements for their appropriate use in all phases of both the patient pathway and laboratory provision, helpfully comparing recommendations made with those of other groups. These are summarized later in this chapter.

More commonly requested serum tumor markers are shown in Table 20.2. Some less commonly requested serum tumor markers with an established clinical role are shown in

## TABLE 20.2    Properties and Applications of More Commonly Requested Serum Tumor Markers

| Tumor Marker | Biochemical Properties | Molecular Weight | Main Clinical Applications |
|---|---|---|---|
| Alpha-fetoprotein (AFP) | Glycoprotein, 4% carbohydrate; considerable homology with albumin | ~70 kDa | Diagnosis and monitoring of primary hepatocellular carcinoma, hepatoblastoma, and germ cell tumors. Prognosis of germ cell tumors |
| Calcitonin | 32 amino acid peptide | ~3.5 kD | Monitoring medullary carcinoma of the thyroid |
| Cancer antigen 125 (CA125) | Mucin identified by monoclonal antibodies OC125 and M11. Developed from serous cystadenocarcinoma cell line | ~200 kD | Monitoring ovarian carcinoma. Measurement required for determination of the Risk of Malignancy Index (RMI) for ovarian carcinoma |
| Cancer antigen 15.3 (CA15.3), BR 27.29 | Mucin (MUC-1 glycoprotein peptide) identified by monoclonal antibodies | >250 kD | Monitoring breast cancer |
| Cancer antigen 19.9 (CA19.9) | Glycolipid carrying the Lewis$^a$ blood group determinant | ~1000 kD | Monitoring pancreatic carcinoma following curative resection |
| Carcinoembryonic antigen (CEA) | Family of glycoproteins, 45%–60% carbohydrate | ~180 kD | Monitoring colorectal cancers |
| Paraproteins | Monoclonal immunoglobulins | Variable | See Chapter 18 |
| Prolactin | Pituitary hormone | ~22 kD but high molecular forms also exist | See Chapter 40 |
| Prostate-specific antigen (PSA) | Glycoprotein; member of the kallikrein family with serine protease activity. Circulates as free enzyme or complexed to $\alpha_1$-antichymotrypsin (measurable) or $\alpha_2$-macroglobulin (not detected by most immunoassays) | ~30 kD (free enzyme) | Diagnosis, risk assessment and monitoring of prostate carcinoma. Lower concentrations of free PSA relative to complexed PSA (i.e., free: total ratio) found in prostatic cancer as compared with benign prostatic hypertrophy |

Table 20.3. Table 20.4 lists some tissue markers essential to inform selection of endocrine and immunotherapy in individual patients.

The broad principles guiding the validation of any new tumor marker and its subsequent introduction into routine clinical practice are similar and are considered in detail in the following sections. Rigorous validation of analytical performance is essential. Objective assessment of the potential clinical value of a proposed new tumor marker together with an estimate of the magnitude of its benefit and effect on outcome in the patient populations in whom the test will be used is a pre-requisite for introducing any new test into routine practice. Establishing how its measurement will fit into the patient pathway should be carefully considered, as is ensuring that the new test will provide information that adds to that already available from existing tests. Three key issues requiring evaluation are clinical utility, magnitude of effect and reliability. Only when these have been established and regulatory requirements fulfilled should a tumor marker be adopted in clinical practice. It is then essential to ensure that the new test is requested appropriately, that those requesting the test are aware of any pre-analytical requirements, that these are met in routine practice, that analytical performance is reliable as confirmed by rigorous internal quality control and proficiency testing, and that

post-analytical reporting of results to clinical users is both informed and informative.

## Tumor Marker Validation

Assuming there is preliminary evidence that the marker has clinical potential, requirements for validation prior to introduction into routine use include:

1. *Protocols for sample collection and processing.* Availability of clinical specimens (e.g., serum, plasma, tissue) that have been collected, processed and stored following validated standard operating procedures (SOP). The panel should include samples from patients with a variety of malignant and nonmalignant conditions. Specimens from biobanks may be appropriate provided their provenance is well-documented.

2. *Analytical/technical validation and verification.* Development and validation of each specific assay to be used in the clinic, having regard to the requirements described below including biological variation of the marker where feasible, followed by its verification (acceptance testing) prior to introduction into routine use. Validation is primarily the responsibility of the diagnostic company manufacturing the test and verification the responsibility of the laboratory undertaking its routine measurement.

**TABLE 20.3   Properties and Applications of Less Commonly Requested Serum Tumor Markers**

| Tumor Marker | Biochemical Properties | Molecular Weight | Main Clinical Applications |
|---|---|---|---|
| Catecholamines | Biogenic amines | ~0.2 kD | *See Chapter 26* |
| Chromogranin A | Member of the granin family of acid secretory glycoproteins | ~49 kD | Monitoring neuroendocrine tumors. *See Chapter 26* |
| CYFRA 21-1 | Fragments of cytokeratin 19 | ~30 kD | Monitoring lung carcinoma. |
| Gut hormones | Small peptide hormones including vasoactive intestinal peptide (VIP), pancreatic polypeptide (PP), somatostatin, gastrin | - | *See Chapter 26* |
| Human epididymis protein 4 (HE4) | Product of the WFDC2 (HE4) gene that is overexpressed in patients with ovarian carcinoma | ~25 kD | Monitoring ovarian cancer. Potentially an aid in diagnosis as part of the risk of malignancy algorithm (ROMA). Under evaluation |
| Inhibin A ($\alpha$-$\beta_A$) Inhibin B ($\alpha$-$\beta_B$) | Heterodimeric glycoproteins composed of an $\alpha$- and a $\beta$-subunit. There are several forms of the $\beta$-subunit, as indicated | 32 kDa | Monitoring of ovarian granulosa cell tumors and testicular Sertoli and Leydig tumors |
| Neuron specific enolase (NSE) | Dimer of the enzyme enolase | ~87 kD | Monitoring small cell lung carcinoma, neuroblastoma, and neuroendocrine tumors |
| Pro-gastrin releasing peptide (proGRP) | More stable precursor of gastrin releasing peptide | ~16 kD | Monitoring small cell lung carcinoma |
| Prostate cancer gene 3 protein (PCA3) | Protein product of PCA3 gene in urine or prostate cancer patients | ~86 kD | Potentially an aid to diagnosis of prostate cancer particularly in biopsy-negative men. Under evaluation |
| Prostate marker algorithm | PHI | Not applicable | An algorithm combining serum measurements of total PSA, free PSA and proPSA in serum |
| Squamous cell carcinoma antigen (SCCA) | Serine protease inhibitor isolated from glycoprotein sub-fraction of tumor antigen TA-4 | 48 kD | Monitoring squamous cell carcinomas (e.g., cervix) |
| S100 proteins | Family of proteins characterized by two calcium-binding sites that have helix-loop-helix confirmations | ~20 kD | Monitoring advanced melanoma |
| Thyroglobulin (Tg) | Glycoprotein dimer of two identical subunits | 670 kDa | Monitoring differentiated thyroid cancer |

**TABLE 20.4   Tissue Markers Whose Measurement Informs Selection of Endocrine and Immunotherapy in Individual Patients**

| Tumor Marker | Biochemical Properties | Molecular Weight | Main Clinical Applications |
|---|---|---|---|
| Anaplastic lymphoma receptor tyrosine kinase *(ALK)* | Enzyme encoded by the *ALK* gene | ~176 kD | Predicting response to the thymidine inhibitor (TKI) crizotinib in non–small cell lung cancer |
| *BRA* mutation | Proto-oncogene that encodes the serine/threonine protein kinase B-Raf | ~87 kD | Predicting response to inhibitors of BRAF-mutated protein including vemurafenib and dabrafenib in melanoma |
| Estrogen receptor (ER) | Nuclear transcription factor | ~5 kD | Predicting response to endocrine therapy in breast cancer |
| Human epidermal growth factor receptor-2 (HER-2 or c-erb2) | Transmembrane glycoprotein encoded from HER-2/neu oncogene | ~185kDa | Predicting response to trastuzumab (Herceptin) in breast cancer. Predicting response to TKIs in non–small cell lung cancer |
| *KRAS* mutation | Guanosine-nucleotide-(GTP)-binding protein | ~23 kD | Predicting response to TKIs in non–small cell lung cancer and reducing need for testing for *HER2* and *ALK* alterations |
| Progesterone receptor | Nuclear transcription factor | A form ~4 kD B form: ~120 kD | Predicting response to endocrine therapy in breast cancer |

3. *Clinical validation.* Definition of the specific context in which the tumor marker is to be used so as to identify the type of specimens to be used in the clinical validation step, the informative statistics and the acceptability criteria. Clinical validation should be reported in terms of **diagnostic accuracy** for tests intended for use in diagnosis. The risk of pitfalls including study bias, over-fitting of data and other statistical problems can be reduced by strict adherence to a written protocol and rigorous reporting of all work.

4. *Demonstration of clinical value.* Strong evidence that the test will benefit the patient, e.g., by increasing overall survival or leading to fewer invasive procedures or hospital visits. Ideally, this should include high level evidence from a prospective or retrospective randomized clinical trial or systematic review of the literature.

5. *Achieving regulatory approval.* Requirements vary but, in the US, involve either clearance approval by the Food and Drug Administration (FDA) and/or evaluation in a CLIA-certified laboratory or by a laboratory-developed test pathway.

6. *Post-market evaluation.* Analytical performance of the test in the routine clinical setting should be subject to continued evaluation, through rigorous implementation of internal quality control and proficiency testing procedures. On-going clinical audit to ensure that the marker retains its value in the clinical setting is also essential. When a newly introduced tumor marker replaces an earlier one, it is important to ensure that the first test is discontinued.

## The "Ideal" Tumor Marker

An "ideal" tumor marker should be:
1. Detectable only in a given malignancy and absent in the healthy population or in nonmalignant conditions, i.e., have clinical specificity and clinical sensitivity approaching 100%.
2. Present in a convenient biological matrix (e.g., serum, urine, tumor tissue).
3. Present at concentrations proportional to tumor burden.
4. Conveniently measured by a readily available, simple, reproducible, and inexpensive procedure.
5. Beneficial to clinical care with a measurable effect on patient outcome.

No such tumor marker has yet been identified. However, measurement of hCG approaches ideal in the screening and monitoring of women who have had a molar pregnancy and are at risk of developing gestational trophoblastic neoplasia (GTN) (choriocarcinoma). Other tumor markers can also contribute usefully to patient management provided they are used intelligently and with regard to requirements of the clinical application (see Tables 20.2–20.4) as outlined below.

## Clinical Applications of Tumor Markers
### Screening for Cancer

Screening for disease differs fundamentally from diagnosis or "case finding" because the aim of screening is to detect unsuspected disease in asymptomatic subjects (see Table 20.1). The World Health Organization (WHO) criteria for screening programs originally proposed by Wilson and Jungner in 1968 remain valid. High clinical sensitivity and specificity of the test for the target disease are both essential, with the success of a screening program dependent on the prevalence of the condition in the population being screened.

Diagnostic accuracy is established by studying test performance at different decision (cut-off) concentrations in appropriately selected diseased and disease-free populations. The relationship between these parameters is most conveniently depicted graphically as a receiver operating characteristic (ROC) plot. Changing the decision concentration selected alters both sensitivity and specificity but cannot improve both concurrently. These parameters define the characteristics of the test and, together with the prevalence of the disease in the population studies, yield its positive predictive value. The low prevalence of the majority of cancers, even in age groups most at risk, together with the low sensitivity and specificity of most tumor markers, generally precludes their use in screening.

### Diagnosis of Cancer

The lack of sensitivity and specificity that limit the application of tumor markers in screening also apply to diagnosis and case finding (see Table 20.1). Tumor markers are not helpful for diagnosis in patients with nonspecific symptoms and cannot replace biopsy for establishing a cancer diagnosis. However, in carefully selected undiagnosed patients at high risk of malignancy, raised concentrations of tumor markers may contribute to diagnosis, e.g., when the patient is unable or unwilling to undergo more invasive testing such as colonoscopy. In general, the higher the serum tumor marker value the greater the likelihood of malignancy, but results within the reference interval never necessarily exclude malignancy. Requests for panels of tumor marker measurements should be actively discouraged.

### Assessing Prognosis

Prognostic markers predict the likely outcome of disease with respect to risk of relapse or disease progression (see Table 20.1). They are generally most useful at the time of initial diagnosis, when a marker of good prognosis is suggestive of prolonged survival and/or the possibility of cure. A marker of poor prognosis indicates an increased probability of early recurrence. Prognostic markers can help identify patients with aggressive tumors that require further treatment (e.g., with systemic adjuvant chemotherapy following surgery) while minimizing the risk of over-treatment of patients with indolent disease that is unlikely to progress. Few prognostic markers are used in routine clinical practice as they provide a probability estimate of outcome for a heterogeneous population rather than for an individual patient. Most of those used are measured in tissue. Exceptionally, measurement of AFP, hCG, and LDH in serum or plasma following primary surgery in patients with non-seminomatous germ cell tumors (GCTs) is mandatory. These well-validated markers provide strong independent prognostic information complementing that of conventional prognostic factors.

### Prediction of Treatment Response

Even cancers of the same histological type may vary widely in response to a particular treatment and for most cancers, only a subset of patients will respond (see Table 20.1). Predictive markers that can identify such patients are therefore critical in treatment planning so that treatment can be offered to patients who will benefit, and alternative treatment can be offered to those who will not, sparing them unnecessary side-effects. Both clinically and economically, predictive markers, most of which are measured in tissue rather than serum, are increasingly essential to identify patients likely to benefit from new and costly molecularly targeted treatments. Several important predictive markers are already well established in clinical use.

### Monitoring Response During and/or Shortly After Treatment

The main application of most serum tumor markers is in monitoring the course of disease. Generally, it is helpful to measure the relevant tumor marker pre-treatment to provide a baseline for subsequent interpretation and for some cancers measurements made during and immediately after treatment are also desirable. In general, a decrease in marker concentrations to within expected population ("normal") limits following treatment is a favorable sign. In some cases, subnormal or absent post-treatment values should be achieved.

### Monitoring Disease Post-treatment to Detect Progression or Recurrence

Serial monitoring of tumor marker concentrations post-treatment provides early indication of disease progression or recurrence, often months before there are clinical signs and symptoms. Whether this information is of benefit depends crucially on whether the increase will prompt clinical action (e.g., early ultrasound, CT, or MRI scanning), whether alternative treatment is available and/or whether that treatment can be implemented without confirmatory scan evidence. If not, and if the patient is not enrolled in a clinical trial, whether tumor marker monitoring is likely to be of benefit should be discussed with the patient before the test is requested.

## QUALITY REQUIREMENTS FOR TUMOR MARKER USE IN THE CLINIC

The clinical laboratory should provide readily available information to those requesting tumor markers to encourage selection of the correct test or tests (and, importantly, to discourage inappropriate requesting) and to ensure that specimen timing is appropriate and other pre-analytical requirements met. Ensuring that results are analytically correct and that accurate and informative reports are returned to the requesting clinician are also laboratory responsibilities. Laboratory-oriented guidelines for tumor markers that outline quality requirements for provision of a high-quality tumor marker service have been developed by the NACB and form the basis of the following discussion.

### Pre-analytical Requirements
#### Test Ordering

Although numerous serum tumor markers can be measured (see Tables 20.2–20.4), those in Table 20.2 are most commonly requested. Table 20.5 summarizes current NACB recommendations for their appropriate clinical use while typical clinical presentations that might prompt such requests are described in Table 20.6.

Requests for tumor markers may be for diagnosed cancer patients who have already been referred to specialist centers and are being or have been treated, for patients who have been referred to hospital for investigation of suspected malignancy, and for patients who have presented to their family doctor with symptoms suspicious for malignancy. Requests in the first category (with a baseline measurement prior to therapy always desirable) are most likely to be appropriate.

Nonspecialist users should always consider carefully whether a tumor marker result is likely to be of benefit to the patient before making a request. Requestors should be aware of the lack of sensitivity of most tumor markers, particularly for early-stage disease, their lack of specificity, and the numerous nonmalignant conditions in which they may be increased (Table 20.7). Nonspecialist users should also be aware that increased tumor marker concentrations do not necessarily indicate malignancy. Attempting to identify the reason for an increased tumor marker that should never have been requested and may not be associated with malignancy can be expensive and time-consuming, and psychologically stressful for the patient. Conversely, requestors should be reminded that a result within the reference interval never necessarily excludes malignancy or progressive disease. Clinical biochemists should also think carefully before requesting additional tests that might lead to a diagnosis of malignancy and should seek the agreement of the clinician caring for the patient before doing so.

Unfocused requests such as "tumor marker screen" or "malignancy?" should be actively discouraged and met with offers for educational support. Advice about appropriate test selection should be made readily available at the time of requesting, ideally electronically.

### Specimen Timing

Timing of specimens within the day for tumor marker measurement is not usually critical, as there is little evidence of diurnal variation for most markers. A pre-treatment specimen is always helpful when interpreting subsequent results. Specimens should be taken before some procedures that may transiently release tumor markers into the circulation (e.g., CA125 following abdominal surgery, CEA following colonoscopy and PSA after prostatic biopsy or digital rectal examination [DRE]). Awareness of benign conditions that may cause transient increases in tumor marker

## TABLE 20.5  National Academy of Clinical Biochemistry (NACB) Recommendations for Appropriate Clinical Use of Commonly Requested Serum Tumor Markers

| | Relevant Cancer | CURRENTLY RECOMMENDED CLINICAL APPLICATIONS | | | | |
|---|---|---|---|---|---|---|
| | | Screening or Early Detection | Diagnosis or Case Finding | Prognosis (With Other Factors) | Detecting Recurrence | Monitoring Therapy |
| Alpha fetoprotein (AFP) | Germ cell/testicular tumor | ✓a | ✓ | ✓ | ✓ | ✓ |
| | Hepatocellular carcinoma | | ✓b | ✓ | ✓ | ✓c |
| Calcitonin | Medullary thyroid carcinoma | | ✓ | | ✓ | ✓ |
| Cancer antigen 125 (CA125) | Ovarian cancer | ✓d | ✓e | ✓ | ✓ | ✓f |
| Cancer antigen 15-3 (CA15-3) | Breast cancer | | | | ✓g | ✓h |
| Cancer antigen 19-9 (CA 19-9) | Pancreatic cancer | | ✓i | ✓ | ✓ | ✓j |
| Carcinoembryonic antigen (CEA) | Colorectal cancer | | | ✓ | ✓c | ✓c |
| Human chorionic gonadotrophin (hCG) | Germ cell and testicular cancers; gestational trophoblastic neoplasiak | | ✓ | ✓ | ✓ | ✓ |
| Paraproteins (Bence Jones protein) [In urine also] | Multiple myeloma | | ✓ | | ✓ | ✓ |
| Prostate specific antigen (PSA) | Prostate cancer | | ✓ | ✓ | ✓ | ✓ |
| Thyroglobulin | Thyroid cancer (follicular or papillary) | | | | ✓ | ✓ |

aOnly for subjects in high-risk groups (e.g., with chronic HBV, HCV or cirrhosis) and only in conjunction with ultrasound (impact on mortality unclear).

bIn conjunction with liver imaging, AFP levels greater than 200 μg/L are regarded as virtually diagnostic of HCC in patients with hypervascular lesions.

cEspecially for disease that cannot be evaluated by other modalities.

dOnly for women at high risk of ovarian cancer and only in conjunction with transvaginal ultrasound.

eOnly for differential diagnosis of pelvic masses, especially in post-menopausal women.

fPreliminary results of a randomized trial show no survival benefit from early treatment based on a raised serum CA125 level alone so this recommendation may be modified to exclude asymptomatic patients.

gPost-surgery when may provide lead-time for early detection of metastasis but clinical value unclear.

hEspecially in patients with nonevaluable disease (for which CEA is also recommended in carefully selected patients).

iIn patients in whom pancreatic disease is strongly suspected, CA19-9 may complement other diagnostic procedures.

jEspecially after chemotherapy and in combination with imaging.

kUse of hCG in screening for gestational trophoblastic neoplasia, a rare malignancy that may develop following a molar pregnancy provides an excellent example of "best practice" in screening. Further information is available from the Trophoblastic Tumour Screening and Treatment Centre (http://www.hmole-chorio.org.uk/).

concentrations (see Table 20.7) and avoiding inappropriate timing reduces the risk of misinterpreting spuriously raised results that may cause undue distress to the patient and also decrease confidence in laboratory testing.

### Specimen Handling

Serum and/or plasma specimens are appropriate for most tumor marker measurements. Gel tubes may not be suitable for some assays and requirements should be checked in the product information supplied. Tumor markers are generally stable (refer to Chapter 47 for information regarding the processing of samples for DNA and/or RNA analysis), but serum or plasma should be separated from the clot as soon as possible and then stored at 4°C (short-term) or −30°C or below. For longer-term storage, specimens should be stored at −70°C or below. Standardized conditions of specimen collection and fixation are crucial for immunohistochemical analyses.

### Analytical Requirements
### Assay Validation

Prior to introduction into routine clinical practice, both immunoassays and immunohistochemical methods must be validated as described above using defined and well-characterized protocols that meet regulatory guidelines (e.g., FDA approval in the United States and CE marking in Europe). Individual laboratories should verify analytical performance prior to introduction into routine use. Internationally recognized guidelines for the performance

## TABLE 20.6   Typical Clinical Presentations Which Might Prompt a Request for the Most Frequently Used Tumor Markers[a]

| Tumor Marker | Relevant Cancer | Typical Clinical Presentation | Other Cancers in Which Marker May Be Raised[b] |
|---|---|---|---|
| Alpha fetoprotein (AFP) | Germ cell/testicular tumor | Diffuse testicular swelling; hardness | Gastric; colorectal; biliary; pancreatic; lung |
| | Hepatocellular carcinoma | Ascites, encephalopathy, jaundice; upper abdominal pain; weight loss; early satiety in high-risk subjects (i.e., hepatitis B or C related cirrhosis) | |
| Cancer antigen 125 (CA125) | Ovarian cancer | Pelvic mass; persistent, continuous or worsening unexplained abdominal or urinary symptoms; bloating; early satiety[c] | Breast; endometrial; cervix; peritoneal; uterus; lung; pancreas; hepatocellular; non-Hodgkin lymphoma |
| Cancer antigen 19-9 (CA 19 9) | Pancreatic cancer | Progressive obstructive jaundice with profound weight loss and/or pain in the abdomen or mid-back; anemia; nausea; vomiting; pruritis | Colorectal; gastric; hepatocellular; esophageal; ovary |
| Carcinoembryonic antigen (CEA) | Colorectal cancer | Altered bowel habit; intermittent abdominal pain, nausea, vomiting or bleeding; palpable abdominal mass; passing blood or mucus | Breast; gastric; lung; mesothelioma; esophageal; pancreas |
| Human chorionic gonadotrophin (hCG) | Germ cell/testicular tumor | Diffuse testicular swelling, hardness and pain | Lung cancer |
| | Gestational trophoblastic neoplasia | Hyperemesis; persistent irregular vaginal bleeding; previous history of hydatidiform mole | |
| Paraproteins (M protein/Bence Jones protein) (Also measured in urine) | Multiple myeloma | Combination of symptoms including some/all of the following: anemia; back pain; weakness or fatigue; osteopenia; osteolytic lesions; raised ESR or globulins; spontaneous fractures; recurrent infections | |
| Prostate specific antigen (PSA) | Prostate cancer | Frequency, urgency, nocturia, dysuria; acute retention; back pain, weight loss, anemia; enlarged prostate | None |

[a]Tumor markers are often not helpful in diagnosis (see text).
[b]This list is not comprehensive. The marker may be raised in other cancers.
[c]Women may develop some of these nonspecific symptoms several months before diagnosis.

of immunohistochemical tests should be adopted if available and methods described in detail if appropriate high quality reference materials are not available.

### Internal Quality Control

Robust procedures for internal quality control should be established. Within-run variability less than 5% and between-run variability less than 10% should be readily achievable for automated tumor marker methods. Some newer techniques may perform significantly better than this, although manual and/or research assays may be less precise. Appropriate action should be taken immediately if an assay run fails to meet objective criteria for assay acceptance so that no potentially erroneous results are reported. Criteria for acceptance should be pre-defined and preferably based on logical criteria such as those of Westgard (Chapter 7). Given the long-term monitoring involved in cancer care, assay stability should be assured over prolonged periods.

Quality control material not provided by the method manufacturer is preferable as kit controls may provide an overly optimistic impression of performance. At least one authentic serum matrix control from an independent source should be included in addition to quality control materials provided by the manufacturer. Negative and low positive controls should be included for all tumor markers and should include concentrations close to important decision points (e.g., 0.1 and 3 or 4 µg/L for PSA; 4 to 7 µg/L for AFP; 5 U/L for hCG). The broad concentration range should be covered and ideally a high concentration control should occasionally be included to check the accuracy of dilution, whether manual or on-board.

### Proficiency Testing/External Quality Assessment

Proficiency testing specimens should ideally be prepared from authentic patient sera, which for tumor markers may require dilution of high concentration patient sera into a normal serum base pool. Proficiency testing specimens should be commutable with patient specimens to ensure valid between-method comparisons. Specimens prepared by spiking purified analyte into serum base pools are likely to provide an overly optimistic impression of between-method performance. Specimens should assess performance over the working range and include assessment of linearity on dilution, baseline security and stability of results over time.

## TABLE 20.7 Nonmalignant Conditions That May Cause Increases (Some Transient) in Serum Tumor Marker Concentrations That May Lead to Incorrect Interpretation[a]

| | |
|---|---|
| Acute cholangitis | CA19-9 |
| Acute hepatitis | CA125, CA15-3 |
| Acute and/or chronic pancreatitis | CA125, CA19-9 |
| Acute urinary retention | CA125, PSA |
| Arthritis/osteoarthritis/rheumatoid arthritis | CA125 |
| Benign prostatic hyperplasia (BPH) | PSA |
| Biliary obstruction | CA19-9 |
| Catheterization | PSA |
| Cholangitis | CA19-9 |
| Cholestasis | CA19-9 |
| Chronic liver diseases (e.g., cirrhosis, chronic active hepatitis) | CEA, CA125, CA15-3, CA19-9 |
| Chronic renal failure | CA125, CA15-3, CEA, hCG |
| Colitis | CA125, CA15-3, CEA |
| Congestive heart failure | CA125 |
| Cystic fibrosis | CA125 |
| Dermatological conditions | CA15-3 |
| Diabetes | CA125, CA19-9 |
| Diverticulitis | CA125, CEA |
| Endometriosis | CA125 |
| Heart failure | CA125 |
| Hypogonadism | hCG |
| Irritable bowel syndrome | CA125, CA19-9, CEA |
| Jaundice | CEA, CA19-9 |
| Leiomyoma | CA125 |
| Liver regeneration | AFP |
| Marijuana use | hCG |
| Menopause | hCG |
| Menstruation | CA125 |
| Mesothelioma | CEA |
| Nonmalignant ascites | CA125 |
| Ovarian hyperstimulation | CA125 |
| Pancreatitis | CA125, CA19-9 |
| Pericarditis | CA125 |
| Peritoneal inflammation | CA125 |
| Pregnancy | AFP, CA125, hCG |
| Prostatitis | PSA |
| Recurrent ischemic strokes in patients with metastatic cancer | CA125 |
| Respiratory diseases (e.g., pleural inflammation, pneumonia) | CA125, CEA |
| Sarcoidosis | CA125 |
| Systemic lupus erythematosus | CA125 |
| Urinary tract infection | PSA |
| Viral hepatitis | AFP |

[a]This list is not comprehensive; these markers may be raised in other nonmalignant conditions.

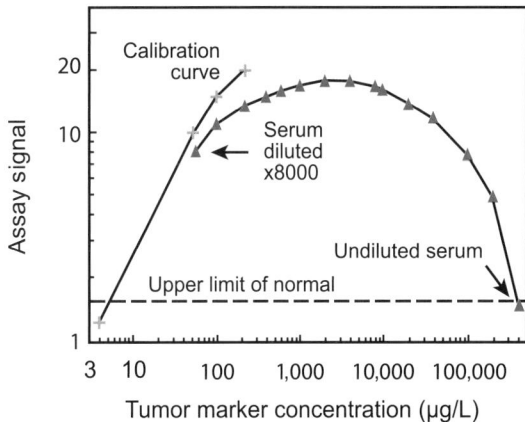

Fig. 20.1 Schematic illustration of high-dose hooking in tumor marker immunoassays. The extremely high tumor marker concentration blocks antibody-binding sites in the immunoassay such that the apparent result "hooks" back onto the calibration curve and an erroneously low result may be reported. (See text and Chapter 15 for further details.)

## Standardization

Major international initiatives continue to be directed towards encouraging manufacturers to calibrate their methods accurately in terms of commutable International Standards (IS) or Reference Reagents where available. Improved understanding of what is being measured is also critical if improved comparability is to be achieved. Manufacturers should provide clear information about the specificity of the antibodies used in their methods and data on cross-reactivity that is readily comparable with that of other methods so that users are aware of the differences.

Despite these efforts to improve comparability, the molecular heterogeneity of most tumor markers means that results obtained using different methods are not interchangeable and considerable care is required in the interpretation of serial results obtained using more than one method.

### Clinically Relevant Interferences

Tumor marker measurements are subject to the same interferences as all immunoassays (see Chapter 15), but the following are particularly relevant:

*High-dose "hooking."* As tumor marker concentrations can range over several orders of magnitude, protocols enabling identification of **high-dose "hooking"** are essential to minimize the risk of reporting erroneously low results, particularly in patients for whom markers are being measured for the first time, especially babies and children. An example is shown in Fig. 20.1. The risk of "hooking" is reduced by using solid-phase antibodies of higher binding capacity, by using sequential assays that include a wash step, and by assaying specimens at two dilutions. Methods vary in their vulnerability to this interference (see Chapter 15).

*Specimen carry-over.* Specimen carry-over is possible whenever high concentration specimens are assayed so it is desirable to check periodically for this possibility. Serum concentrations of hCG can be greater than 1,000,000 U/L so carry-over as low as 1/10,000 can still lead to a falsely positive result in the following sample.

*Interference from heterophilic or human anti-mouse antibodies.* Some patient sera contain anti-immunoglobulin antibodies (most often IgG) that may react with immunoassay reagent antibodies (see Chapter 15). High concentrations of human anti-mouse antibodies (HAMA) may also be present in serum from cancer patients who have received treatment with mouse monoclonal antibodies for imaging or therapeutic purposes. For either interference, results may be falsely high or low. Identifying such interference requires a high degree of clinical suspicion, which is facilitated by availability of relevant clinical details. Possible interference can be investigated by assaying the specimen at several dilutions, by re-assaying after treatment with a commercially available blocking agent, by adding further non-immune mouse serum to the reaction mixture and re-assaying, and/or by re-assaying the specimen using a different method and preferably a different methodology. Caution should be applied in interpretation. For example, linearity on dilution does not always exclude the presence of HAMA.

## Post-analytical Requirements

Brief information on the request form about the source of the suspected or diagnosed malignancy and the treatment stage (e.g., preoperative, postoperative, pre-chemotherapy) is highly desirable. This information should be recorded both in the laboratory computer and on the laboratory report. Trends in tumor marker results are generally most informative, so reports should include cumulative and, if possible, graphical presentation of results. Such reporting facilitates interpretation and also helps to identify occasional errors in requesting or in the laboratory (e.g., incorrect sample identification or mis-sampling on an analyzer) as well as highlighting unexpected results (e.g., sudden changes that are out-of-accord with the clinical picture) that require confirmation and further investigation. Brief comments relating to interpretation of the analytical results (e.g., whether an increase is likely to be clinically significant or not) and advice about the frequency of monitoring and the need for confirmatory specimens are also desirable.

Urgent results that may be required for immediate patient management should be identified by the reporting biochemist so as to ensure that these reach the relevant clinician promptly, e.g., by telephone. These include tumor marker results that can be used to diagnose advanced disease in critically ill but treatable patients (e.g., AFP in hepatoblastoma, hCG in choriocarcinoma, AFP and hCG in non-seminomatous GCTs and PSA in men with advanced prostate cancer). The consequences of failure to telephone such results can be severe.

In view of the method-related differences discussed above, and as recommended by the NACB, the method used should be stated on the clinical report so that changes in method are readily identifiable. If there has been a method change, it is highly desirable that the laboratory indicates whether this is likely to influence interpretation of the trend in results. There should be a defined protocol for method changes, and the likely effect clearly communicated to clinical users. Managing method changes may necessitate analyzing the previous specimen by the new method or requesting a further specimen to re-establish the baseline and/or confirm the trend in marker concentrations.

Reference intervals should be derived using an appropriate healthy population and should ideally be specific to the method used. They are usually most relevant for cancer

patients pre-treatment as subsequently, the patient's individual "baseline" results provide the most important reference point for most marker results. Provided "baseline" marker concentrations are well-established in diagnosed patients post-treatment, sustained increases even within the reference interval may be significant and the patient investigated for possible relapse.

The percentage increase or decrease that constitutes a significant change should be defined and should take account of analytical and biological variation, as well as the time between samples. For tumor markers a confirmed increase or decrease of ±25% is frequently considered to be clinically significant.

Laboratories should be able to provide calculated tumor marker half-lives or doubling-times for markers for which these are relevant (e.g., AFP and hCG). Half-lives are defined as the time to 50% reduction of circulating tumor marker concentration following complete removal of tumor tissue. Their calculation may be irrelevant if a 50% reduction does not represent a significant change. (See Germ Cell Tumor section for calculation details.)

Proactive provision of a high-quality tumor marker service helps to encourage good communication between laboratory and clinical staff and is likely to encourage appropriate use of tumor marker tests as well as early identification of any results that are not in accord with the clinical picture and require investigation. An example of a laboratory report that fulfills many of these requirements is shown in Fig. 20.2.

### POINTS TO REMEMBER

- Cancer is a heterogeneous disease that is a leading cause of death, although death rates for individual cancers vary markedly and there have been considerable advances in treatment over recent decades.
- Tumor markers are surrogate indicators that can help make or confirm a cancer diagnosis, monitor treatment effectiveness and the course of disease, estimate prognosis and/or predict whether a specific therapy is likely to be effective.
- Optimal use of tumor markers requires an evidence-based approach to clinical decision-making and knowledge of the limitations of these tests particularly in relation to clinical sensitivity and specificity.
- Tumor marker results are rarely diagnostic and cannot replace biopsy for the primary diagnosis of cancer.
- Tumor marker measurements are not recommended for patients with vague symptoms when the population likelihood of cancer is low.
- A raised tumor marker result never necessarily indicates malignancy and a result within the reference interval never necessarily excludes malignancy.
- In diagnosed patients, a pre-treatment result is essential and provides the baseline against which subsequent results can be assessed.
- Tumor marker results should be confirmed on a repeat specimen if decisions about therapy depend on the result.
- Tumor marker results should be interpreted in the context of all available information and the possible influence of other factors (e.g., medication, analytical effects) considered.

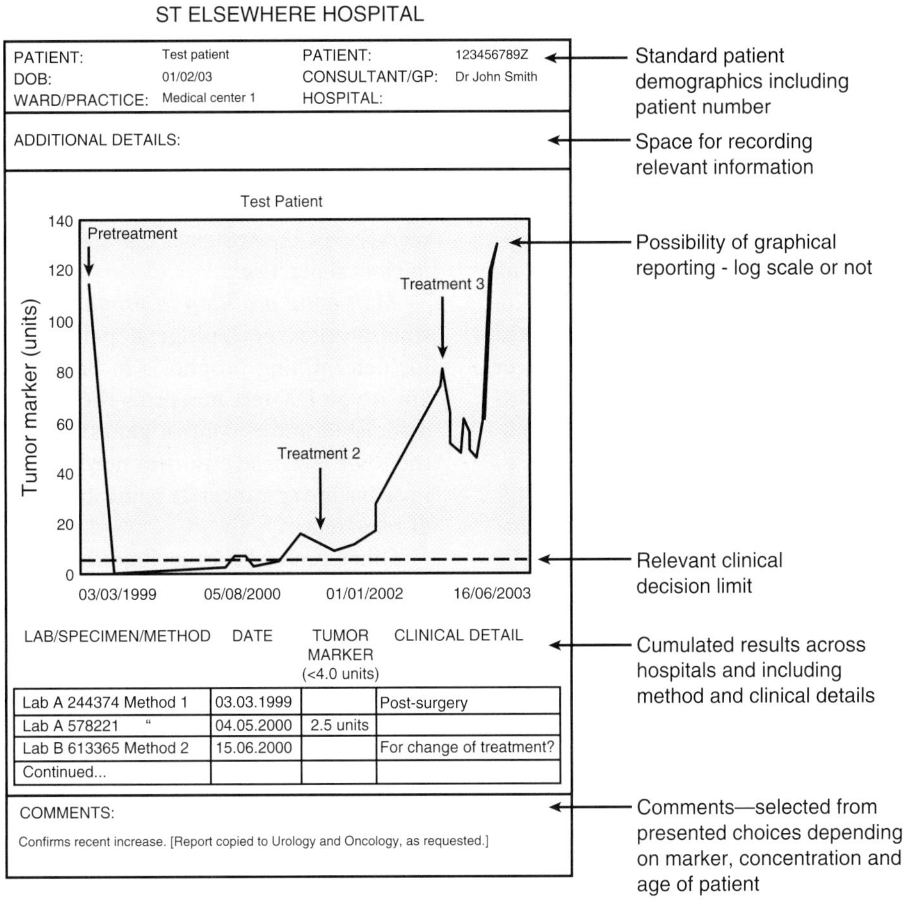

ST ELSEWHERE HOSPITAL

| PATIENT: | Test patient | PATIENT: | 123456789Z |
| DOB: | 01/02/03 | CONSULTANT/GP: | Dr John Smith |
| WARD/PRACTICE: | Medical center 1 | HOSPITAL: | |

ADDITIONAL DETAILS:  ← Space for recording relevant information

← Standard patient demographics including patient number

Test Patient

← Possibility of graphical reporting - log scale or not

*(graph: Tumor marker (units) vs dates, markers Pretreatment, Treatment 2, Treatment 3)*

← Relevant clinical decision limit

| LAB/SPECIMEN/METHOD | DATE | TUMOR MARKER (<4.0 units) | CLINICAL DETAIL |
|---|---|---|---|
| Lab A 244374 Method 1 | 03.03.1999 | | Post-surgery |
| Lab A 578221 " | 04.05.2000 | 2.5 units | |
| Lab B 613365 Method 2 | 15.06.2000 | | For change of treatment? |
| Continued... | | | |

← Cumulated results across hospitals and including method and clinical details

COMMENTS:
Confirms recent increase. [Report copied to Urology and Oncology, as requested.]

← Comments—selected from presented choices depending on marker, concentration and age of patient

**Fig. 20.2** Schematic diagram of a desirable clinical laboratory report for tumor markers that fulfills current reporting recommendations.

# USE OF TUMOR MARKERS IN SPECIFIC MALIGNANCIES

The extent to which tumor markers currently contribute to the management of a number of important malignancies is briefly reviewed in the following sections.

## Bladder Cancer

More than 700,000 Americans are currently affected by bladder cancer, with 81,000 new cases diagnosed each year. The most common symptom is intermittent hematuria, which is present in 80% to 85% of patients, with voiding problems or dysuria also common. Transitional cell carcinomas (TCC) account for the majority of bladder cancers, but adenocarcinomas, squamous cell carcinomas, and sarcomas occur. Diagnosis is usually established by cystoscopic evaluation. Primary treatment is complete surgical resection, usually by transurethral resection with or without additional immunotherapy, chemotherapy, or radiotherapy. There is a high risk of recurrence and 50% to 70% of patients will develop tumor recurrence within 5 years, depending on the stage of disease. Lifelong surveillance with cystoscopy and urine cytology is therefore required.

## Tumor Markers Relevant to Bladder Cancer

Markers evaluated for bladder cancer include nuclear matrix proteins (NMPs), human complement factor H-related protein, fibronectin, telomerase, cytokeratins, and survivin. NMPs make up the internal structure of the nucleus and contribute to the regulation of some of the key functions that occur in the nucleus.

The FDA has approved an enzyme-linked immunosorbent assay (ELISA) for the measurement of nuclear mitotic apparatus protein, a component of the nuclear matrix which is over-expressed in bladder cancer. Approved uses of the NMP-22 test are as an aid in the diagnosis of symptomatic patients or those with risk factors suggesting TCC and in the management and monitoring of patients with TCC. A qualitative point-of-care version of the test is available as an aid in monitoring patients with a history of bladder cancer.

The bladder tumor associated antigens (BTA), human complement factor H-related protein and related proteins are involved in the regulation of the alternative pathway of complement activation that prevents complement-mediated damage to healthy cells. The BTA-Trak and BTA–Stat tests have been approved by the FDA for use in conjunction with cystoscopy in the management of bladder cancer patients.

# Breast Cancer

Breast cancer is the most common cancer in women worldwide, affecting 10% to 12% of women. In symptomatic women, the main presenting features include a lump in the breast, nipple change or discharge and skin contour changes. Worldwide the incidence appears to be increasing, but in some Western countries mortality rates are declining. This decrease has been attributed to earlier detection by systematic screening with mammography, greater awareness among women of early signs of breast cancer and availability of adjuvant treatment for newly diagnosed cases. In the United States, breast cancer represents about 15% of all new cancer cases and nearly four million women are living with the disease. For the approximately 60% of breast cancer patients in the United States who have localized disease at diagnosis (i.e., confined to the primary site), the 5-year survival rate is 99.1% as compared with 30.0% for the 6% of patients who have distant metastases at diagnosis.

Primary treatment for localized breast cancer is either breast-conserving surgery and radiation or mastectomy. Following primary treatment, most women with invasive breast cancer receive systemic adjuvant such as chemotherapy, hormone therapy or immunotherapy or a combination of these. Depending on estrogen receptor status and other factors, not all patients with breast cancer require adjuvant treatment.

## Tumor Markers Used in the Management of Breast Cancer

Tissue tumor marker measurements essential for the management of breast cancer include those for receptors for estrogen, progesterone, and HER-2, while CA15-3 and the closely related BR27.29 are the serum markers of choice. Measurement of CEA may also be helpful in patients with metastatic breast cancer. In early-stage disease, concentrations of CA15-3 may be similar to those found in healthy women or women with benign breast disease.

*Screening and diagnosis.* Early detection undoubtedly improves 5-year survival but the low specificity and sensitivity of currently available serum tumor markers, especially in early-stage disease, precludes their use in screening for breast cancer and x-ray imaging with mammography remains the only screening modality.

Women at increased risk of breast cancer because of a strong family history of breast cancer (e.g., relatives diagnosed at a young age) or because they are carriers of the *BRCA1, BRCA2,* or *TP53* genetic mutations are likely to benefit from additional screening with magnetic resonance imaging (MRI), which is current policy in the United Kingdom.

Definitive diagnosis of breast cancer requires biopsy and histology. Serum tumor markers do not contribute to this but preoperative measurements of CA15-3 and/or CEA are desirable if either marker is going to be used for post-treatment monitoring. A high CA15-3 concentration (e.g., >40 to 50 kU/L) in a patient with apparently localized breast cancer should prompt further investigation to exclude the possibility of metastatic disease.

*Prognosis.* Accurate assessment of prognosis is essential for optimal management of breast cancer patients so as to avoid under-treatment of patients with advanced disease and over-treatment of patients with indolent disease. The extracellular serine protease urokinase plasminogen activator (uPA) and its endogenous inhibitor plasminogen activator inhibitor 1 (PAI-1) are the best validated tissue prognostic markers for breast cancer but are not currently widely used in clinical practice.

*Multigene profiling in prognosis.* Several gene expression profiles or multigene panels have been proposed for determining prognosis in breast cancer patients. The Oncotype DX test measures the expression of 16 cancer-associated and 5 control genes in breast tumor tissue at the RNA level and stratifies newly diagnosed patients with invasive breast cancer as being at low, medium or high risk of recurrence.

Other gene profiles include the MammaPrint test which measures the expression of 70 genes involved in signal transduction pathways responsible for breast cancer metastasis. MammaPrint is approved by the FDA to assist in assignment of women with ER-positive or ER-negative breast cancer into high or low risk groups for recurrence.

Preoperative serum concentrations of CA15-3 predict shortened disease-free or overall survival in breast cancer patients and can provide additional prognostic information, perhaps because the marker is detecting micrometastases or occult disease that is not clinically evident. As CA15-3 measurement is relatively convenient and inexpensive, it may be appropriate to use it when planning optimal treatment of newly diagnosed patients with breast cancer but further evaluation is required.

*Therapy prediction.* Measurement of ER, the longest-established molecular marker for breast cancer, is mandatory in all newly diagnosed invasive breast cancer patients to determine whether anti-estrogen endocrine therapy is likely to be effective. Patients with ER-positive tumors tend to respond to hormonal therapy while those with ER-negative tumors will be treated using chemotherapy or other therapies. The negative predictive value of ER is high, i.e., patients who are ER-negative are very unlikely to benefit from endocrine therapy. However, in both early and advanced breast cancer its positive predictive value is less accurate.

Patients with breast cancers that over-express the *HER2* gene are candidates for treatment with anti-HER2 immunotherapies, which have been cleared by the US FDA. As amplification of the *HER2* gene occurs in only 20% of patients with invasive breast cancers, it is important to identify these patients so as to avoid treating patients unlikely to respond.

Detailed recommendations and good practice guidelines for measurement of ER and progesterone receptors (PR) have been published by the American Society for Clinical Oncology (ASCO) and the College of American Pathologists (CAP) and endorsed by the NCCN.

*Monitoring.* Most women who have been treated for breast cancer, with or without adjuvant therapy and/or curative surgery, are subsequently evaluated at regular intervals with history, physical examination, and annual mammography. The aim of follow-up is to identify early recurrence or metastatic disease on the assumption that early intervention will improve survival. If serum tumor markers are measured, CA15-3, CEA, and/or BR27.29 are the markers of choice.

The clinical value of serial measurements of CA15-3 and other tumor markers is however unclear. Their regular measurement can provide a lead time of 5 to 6 months, but whether early intervention based solely on tumor marker increase alone improves outcome is still not known and guideline recommendations vary. The NACB states that tumor markers can be measured where other methods of evaluation are not possible. The NCCN includes rising CA15-3, CEA, and/or BR27.29 in its definition of disease progression and states that marker increases raise the suspicion of tumor progression, while cautioning that such increases may be seen in responding disease, while ASCO states that these markers may be used as adjunctive assessments, but not alone, to contribute to decisions regarding therapy in women with metastatic breast cancer. The Southwest Oncology Group is undertaking a prospective clinical trial to evaluate the impact of serial testing.

## Cervical Cancer

Cervical cancer is the fourth most common cancer in women worldwide and a leading cause of cancer death in women in the developing world, where 85% of cases occur. In the United States, an estimated 14,000 new cases will be diagnosed in 2022 and nearly 4300 patients will die of the disease. The most important factor in the development of cervical cancer is persistent infection with human papilloma viruses (HPV). Primary prevention is therefore feasible with prophylactic vaccination.

Most women are asymptomatic and are frequently diagnosed only after abnormal cervical cytology is identified in a screening program. Introduction of widespread cytology screening in the United States decreased the incidence of cervical cancer from 14.8 per 100,000 women in 1975 to 6.6 per 100,000 in 2008, with a similar reduction in mortality. HPV testing is gradually being added to screening programs in a number of countries. Women with higher grade abnormalities identified by cytology are referred immediately for colposcopy while for low-grade or borderline cell abnormalities, the sample is automatically tested for HPV.

Treatment planning of patients with cervical cancer is primarily determined by the clinical stage of the disease and histological type. Early-stage disease can be treated by radical hysterectomy and pelvic lymphadenectomy or radiotherapy. For more advanced disease, chemoradiation or neoadjuvant chemotherapy may also be required.

## Tumor Markers Used in the Management of Cervical Cancer

Squamous cell carcinoma antigen (SCCA) is the serum tumor marker of choice for squamous cell cervical carcinoma, while CEA and CA125 may have possible utility in patients with cervical adenocarcinoma. Serum SCCA concentrations correlate with tumor stage, tumor size, residual tumor post-treatment, recurrent or progressive disease, and survival in patients with squamous cell cervical carcinoma. However, whether serum SCCA measurements are useful in clinical practice remains uncertain. There is no evidence that earlier detection of recurrent disease through tumor marker monitoring influences outcome or prognosis. Consequently, no currently available serum tumor markers are recommended for routine clinical use in patients with cervical cancer.

## Colorectal Cancer

Colorectal cancer is the second leading cause of cancer-related death both worldwide and in the United States, where it is also the fourth most frequently diagnosed cancer. Some typical presenting symptoms are listed in Table 20.6. The natural history of the disease involves slow multi-stage progression from mucosal cell hyperplasia through adenoma formation, growth and dysplasia followed by malignant transformation and invasive cancer. In the United States, 5-year survival is ~91% for locally confined tumors, ~73% for those that have spread regionally, but only ~15% if distant metastases are present, highlighting the importance of detecting early-stage disease.

## Tumor Markers Used in the Management of Colorectal Cancer

CEA, an oncofetal antigen first identified as being associated with colorectal cancer in the 1960s, remains the most relevant serum tumor marker for colorectal cancer.

*Screening for colorectal cancer using tumor markers.* Several randomized controlled trials have shown that population-based screening using fecal occult blood tests can reduce mortality from colorectal neoplasia, with an average reduction in mortality of at least 16%. Follow-up colonoscopy is required for positive tests.

Based on this evidence, a number of countries have introduced screening for colorectal cancer, replacing the early guaiac-based tests with newer fecal immunochemical tests (FIT) which detect the globin component of hemoglobin.

Typically patients collect fecal samples at home on a card which is mailed to a central testing laboratory for either test. FITs are easier to use than guaiac-based tests and provide quantitative rather than qualitative results with adjustable cut-off points, are less vulnerable to interference (e.g., due to diet or drugs), have greater analytical specificity and better clinical sensitivity for cancers and advanced adenomas, are cost-effective and can be automated. Ease of use is particularly important as the uptake of any screening program depends on its acceptability to the population being screened.

Individuals with a strong family history of colorectal cancer, hereditary non-polyposis colon cancer (Lynch syndrome), or familial adenomatous polyposis (FAP) are at high risk of developing colorectal cancer and should be referred for risk assessment and endoscopic screening according to agreed protocols. Genetic counseling and germline gene testing for Lynch syndrome should be offered to patients for microsatellite instability (MSI) or mismatch repair (MMR) gene mutations.

*Diagnosis.* The low clinical sensitivity of CEA, particularly for early-stage disease, precludes its use in diagnosis. It is increased in only 30% to 50% of patients at the time of diagnosis and cannot be used in isolation to diagnose even advanced disease. Its specificity is also low as it can be increased in nonmalignant liver and renal disease as well as in other malignancies. However, clearly increased concentrations can assist in diagnosis in certain clinical circumstances and are suggestive of metastatic disease, although they do not necessarily indicate a colorectal primary.

*Prognosis, staging, and therapy prediction.* Increased preoperative CEA concentrations at the time of initial presentation of patients with colorectal cancer are associated with adverse outcome and can provide both prognostic information and a baseline value for interpreting subsequent results.

Patients with advanced colorectal cancer may be treated with anti-epidermal growth factor (EGFR) monoclonal antibodies which bind to the extracellular domain of EGFR. Patients with a specific mutation of the *K-RAS* gene appear to benefit most from such treatment and modeling studies suggest that administering anti-EGFR antibody treatment only to patients with wild-type *K-RAS* would result in significant net cost savings.

*Monitoring.* Meta-analyses of a number of randomized controlled trials designed to compare intensive follow-up with either control or minimal follow-up colorectal cancer patients following curative resection have demonstrated that intensive follow-up which includes CEA improves overall survival. It is now recommended that CEA testing should be performed every 3 to 6 months for 5 years following curative surgery for colorectal cancer. CEA results within the reference interval do not exclude recurrence.

An increase in CEA should prompt referral for early investigation of possible recurrence, but any increase should be confirmed by a second sample taken within approximately 1 month. What constitutes a significant increase in CEA is not yet well-established. An elevation at least 30% over that of the previous concentration is regarded by some groups as significant while smaller consecutive increases (e.g., 15% to 20%) observed on at least three successive occasions with intervals of at least 2 weeks between them may also prompt intervention.

Resection of metastatic deposits in the liver can prolong survival for a small but increasing number of patients with Dukes' stage B or C disease, provided deposits are detected before symptoms develop. It is therefore recommended that CEA is measured every 3 months for at least 3 years following surgery in patients with Dukes' stage B or C disease who would be candidates for liver resection. Measurement of CEA following liver resection provides a helpful indication of its success.

Its measurement is also recommended during chemotherapy for metastatic disease, although care in interpretation is required as CEA concentrations may be affected by factors other than tumor progression (e.g., liver damage). CEA-defined responses agree well with radiologic responses (the "gold standard") in greater than 90% of cases, suggesting that use of CEA is as accurate as CT imaging for assessing the response of colorectal cancer liver metastases to chemotherapy.

Monitoring of colorectal cancer outside a clinical trial should only be undertaken if it is likely to benefit the patient. CEA concentrations in individual patients should be monitored using the same methods because results obtained in two methods may not be the same. If a change of method is unavoidable, re-baselining may be necessary as described above. Coordination of follow-up monitoring should ideally be supported by an automatic computer system.

## Gastric Cancer

Gastric cancer is relatively rare, although it is the second most common gastrointestinal cancer worldwide. Approximately 26,000 new cases are diagnosed in the United States each year, about 80% of which will have already spread to regional lymph nodes or metastasized. Survival is closely related to stage at diagnosis, with 5-year survival approximately 70% for localized disease and ≤6% for patients with distant metastases.

### Tumor Markers Used in the Management of Gastric Cancer

Although CEA and CA19-9 are increased in 20% to 50% of patients with advanced disease and AFP in 20% to 25%, these markers are raised in less than 20% of patients with early-stage disease and consequently cannot be used for screening or diagnosis of gastric cancer. Measurement of serum CEA or CA19-9 may provide early indication of recurrence in a proportion of patients, but their use is not recommended as there is currently no evidence that this improves clinical outcome.

This may change with availability of more effective systemic treatment as 10% to 25% of patients overexpress HER2. As patients with advanced HER2-positive gastric tumors benefit from treatment with the anti-HER2 antibody, if such patients are being considered for systemic therapy, HER2 should be measured.

## Germ Cell Tumors

Representing only 1% of all male tumors, GCTs are the solid tumor most frequently diagnosed in men between the age of 20 and 34 years and account for about 95% of malignant tumors arising in the testes. They also occur elsewhere, particularly along the "midline," i.e., the mediastinum, retroperitoneum, or perineal gland. The incidence of GCTs has increased over the last few decades with 9.910 new cases predicted in the United States in 2022. Risk factors include positive family history, cryptorchidism, testicular dysgenesis, Klinefelter's syndrome and a prior history of GCT. Some typical presenting symptoms are listed in Table 20.6.

GCTs are usually aggressive but respond well to treatment with surgery and, where appropriate, adjuvant chemotherapy and/or radiotherapy. The anticipated 5-year survival rate for localized disease is 99% in the United States although only 73% for patients presenting with advanced disease. There are well-established national and international guidelines relating to the management of patients with GCTs. Treatment in specialist centers is advantageous and all patients should be discussed at multidisciplinary team meetings at which a clinical biochemist is present.

### Tumor Markers Used in the Management of Germ Cell Tumors

Measurements of hCG, AFP, and LDH are integral to the management of patients with GCTs. Tumor marker results should be reviewed together with histological immunostaining and radiological results and any inconsistencies noted when treatment decisions are considered.

*Screening.* The low prevalence of GCTs in the general population, together with the relatively low sensitivity and specificity of AFP, hCG, and LDH, preclude the use of tumor markers in screening.

*Diagnosis.* Although rare, the possibility of a GCT should be considered in any patient with a poorly defined epithelial malignancy, especially young individuals with mid-line masses. Plasma or serum AFP and hCG should be measured in any male with a suspicious lump in the testes and in any patient with malignancy of unknown origin. Hyperthyroidism may be a presenting feature if the hCG concentration is very high as hCG shares structural similarities with TSH. Patients with clinical findings consistent with GCTs (e.g., testicular lump, lung metastases, and/or abdominal mass) and markedly increased serum concentrations of AFP and/or hCG should be urgently discussed with physicians at the regional cancer center. Referral for immediate chemotherapy may be appropriate before later surgery to remove residual tumor.

Measurement of serum tumor markers is essential for the differential diagnosis of GCTs as treatment differs according to whether the GCT is seminomatous, non-seminomatous (NSGCT) (with yolk sac elements) or a combined tumor with both seminomatous and non-seminomatous elements. Serum or plasma concentrations of AFP and/or hCG are increased in 80% to 85% of men with NSGCT, while less than 25% of those with seminomas have raised hCG and none have raised AFP. Non-seminomas are more clinically aggressive so tumors with both elements are managed as for non-seminomas. Marker measurements can sometimes modify histopathological diagnoses. Increased AFP in a patient diagnosed with seminoma suggests that the AFP may not be related to the tumor (e.g., may be of liver origin) or that yolk sac elements were overlooked.

hCG and AFP should be measured before surgery for a suspected GCT in order to allow the rate of fall of the markers to be monitored post-treatment.

As for all tumor markers, it is important to remember that concentrations within the reference interval do not necessarily exclude malignancy. Only a small proportion of seminomas or dysgerminomas (the female equivalent of seminomas) produce hCG and up to 25% of NSGCT do not produce AFP or hCG.

As for other oncology applications the hCG method used should recognize both intact hCG and its free beta-subunit (hCGβ). Some immunoassay methods for hCG may be vulnerable to interference from heterophilic antibodies and high dose "hooking" is always a possibility (see Interferences discussion above). AFP and/or hCG can be increased in nonmalignant diseases and other malignancies and both are increased in normal pregnancy.

*Prognosis.* The lowest tumor marker concentration reached post-surgery, the primary tumor site and the sites of metastatic disease all contribute to the prognostic classification of GCTs using criteria established by the International Germ Cell Cancer Collaborative Group. Treatment depends on whether the tumor is classified as having good, intermediate, or poor prognosis.

*Monitoring.* Provided disease is confined to the testis or ovary, serum AFP and/or hCG should decline to normal with respective apparent half-lives of 5 to 6 days for AFP and 1 to 2 days for hCG. Fig. 20.3 shows the decrease in AFP observed in a patient with widespread metastatic disease who had a

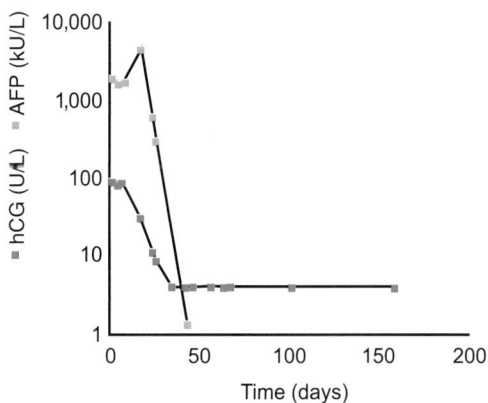

Fig. 20.3 Tumor marker responses in a patient with widespread metastatic disease who had a complete radiologic and marker response to chemotherapy. *AFP,* α-Fetoprotein; *hCG,* human chorionic gonadotropin.

complete radiological and marker response to chemotherapy. The equation used to calculate the apparent half-life ($t_{1/2}$) of the tumor marker is

$$t_{1/2} = \frac{-0.3t}{\log_{10}\dfrac{[M]_T}{[M]_{T_0}}}$$

where $[M]_T$ and $[M]_{T_0}$ are tumor marker concentrations at time $T$ and $T_0$, respectively, and $t$ is the difference in days between $T$ and $T_0$.

Further treatment with chemotherapy of radiation is required if AFP and/or hCG remain increased following surgery or if imaging identifies residual or metastatic disease.

*Long-term surveillance.* Following treatment, tumor markers should be measured regularly following defined clinical protocols which depend on prognostic category and treatment and any significant increases reported immediately to the relevant clinical team. The importance of careful monitoring of tumor markers is illustrated in Fig. 20.4. After an initially very good response to a number of different chemotherapy agents, the patient required surgery, further chemotherapy and ultimately a successful bone marrow transplant.

## Gestational Trophoblastic Disease

Gestational trophoblastic disease (GTD) are rare and previously fatal diseases of pregnancy that develop in the trophoblast cells that surround the embryo immediately after conception. They may occur following a molar pregnancy, a nonmolar pregnancy or a live birth. Some typical presenting symptoms are listed in Table 20.6. A urine hCG pregnancy test should be performed in any woman presenting with such symptoms. Diagnosis requires histological examination of the products of conception following surgical evacuation. If there is any evidence of persistence of GTD, which is most commonly defined as a persistent increase of serum hCG, the condition is referred to as GTN.

Characteristics of the main forms of GTD are briefly described below.

### Hydatidiform Moles

Hydatidiform moles ("molar pregnancies") are the most common form of GTD and are nonmalignant. They may develop when a sperm fertilizes an "empty" egg containing no nucleus (a "complete" mole) or when two sperm fertilize a normal egg ("partial" mole). Fetal tissue is not present in complete moles. Following surgical removal, few patients with a partial mole require further treatment and these moles rarely become malignant.

### Invasive Moles

Following surgical removal of a complete mole, about 20% of women develop invasive moles. The tumor metastasizes to other sites (most often lung) in about 15% of patients. The risk of metastasis is increased if more than 4 months elapse between cessation of periods and treatment, if the uterus has

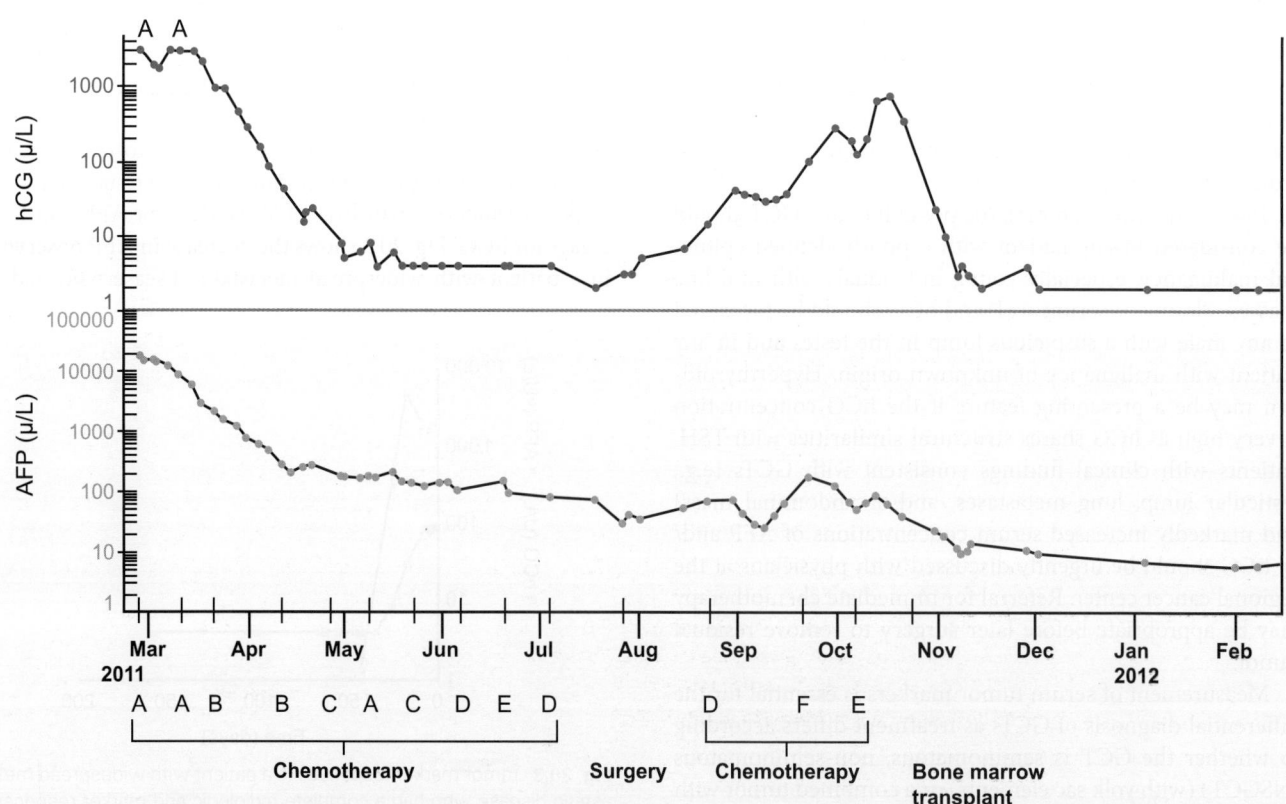

Fig. 20.4 Tumor marker monitoring of a patient who required a number of chemotherapy treatments prior to surgery, further chemotherapy and a bone marrow transplant. *AFP*, α-Fetoprotein; *hCG*, human chorionic gonadotropin.

### Choriocarcinoma

Choriocarcinoma most frequently develops from a complete hydatidiform mole but can occur after normal pregnancy or after early fetal loss in pregnancy. Metastasis to distant organs is more likely than for invasive moles but can be treated highly effectively with chemotherapy.

### Tumor Markers in Gestational Trophoblastic Disease

Successful clinical management of GTD depends on accurate measurement of hCG, which has ~99% specificity and sensitivity for this disease in the clinical setting described above, achieving almost ideal tumor marker performance in this application. Measurement of hCG using a method that recognizes both hCG and hCGβ is essential.

### Human Chorionic Gonadotropin in Screening for Gestational Trophoblastic Disease

Screening of women at high risk of developing GTD, i.e., women who have had a partial or complete hydatidiform mole in a previous pregnancy, is conveniently performed by measuring hCG in urine collected by the patient in her own home and sent by mail to a central screening center. In the United Kingdom, there is a well-established registration system that enables life-time follow-up, which is recommended as the disease can occur years after the affected pregnancy. Three specialist centers provide hCG testing in urine, with all patients with increasing hCG referred for treatment to a specialist unit in London. Costs of the program are relatively low compared with the social cost avoided per life saved.

*Human chorionic gonadotropin as an aid to diagnosis of gestational trophoblastic disease.* Definitive diagnosis requires histological examination of the products of conception but hCG serum measurements may be helpful in diagnosing molar pregnancies as values greater than two multiples of the median for the gestational date are suggestive of GTD.

*Human chorionic gonadotropin in prognosis.* Prognosis is assessed according to the International Federation of Gynaecology and Oncology staging system for GTN, which includes pre-treatment hCG concentration as one of eight prognostic factors used for scoring. Women at high risk of recurrence are treated with multi-agent chemotherapy until the hCG concentration returns to normal and then for a further 6 weeks.

*Monitoring.* Post-treatment monitoring is essential in the follow-up of molar pregnancy and involves serial measurements of hCG in either blood or urine. A urinary hCG pregnancy test should be performed 3 weeks after medical management of failed pregnancy if products of conception are not sent for histological examination. Following a diagnosis of GTD and surgical evacuation, if hCG has reverted to normal within 56 days then follow-up will be for 6 months from the date of uterine evacuation. If hCG has not reverted to normal within 56 days, then follow-up will be for 6 months from normalization of the hCG concentration. In the United Kingdom, women who had GTD in a previous pregnancy are requested to notify the screening center following any future pregnancies, whatever the outcome of the new pregnancy. hCG concentrations are then checked 6 to 8 weeks after the end of that pregnancy to exclude disease recurrence.

### Hepatocellular Carcinoma (Primary Liver Cancer)

Hepatocellular carcinoma (HCC), the 13th most commonly diagnosed cancer in the United States, is the 5th most common cause of cancer death. Worldwide, however, HCC is the second leading cause of cancer death with an incidence that has increased exponentially in recent decades. Asia and sub-Saharan Africa account for almost 85% of more than 800,000 new cases of HCC reported annually worldwide. The single largest risk factor for development of HCC is cirrhosis of any etiology. Major causative factors in these countries are chronic infection with hepatitis B virus (HBV) and ingestion of food contaminated with aflatoxin B, a fungal toxin that is genotoxic and carcinogenic. Nonviral causes associated with increased risk for HCC in Western countries and include alcoholic cirrhosis, Wilson disease and stage IV primary biliary cirrhosis. Primary prevention by eliminating risk factors clearly represents the most realistic approach to decreasing the incidence of HCC (see Chapter 37).

Typical symptoms suggestive of HCC are shown in Table 20.6. CT, MRI and/or biopsy are required for diagnosis. Depending on imaging results, biopsy confirmation of a diagnosis may not be required for liver nodules greater than 1 cm in size.

Potentially curative treatment options include liver transplantation (for which only about 5% of patients are suitable), surgical resection (which requires very good liver function and has a recurrence rate of 50% to 60% after 5 years), ablative therapy (with alcohol, radiofrequency and/or microwaves), chemoembolization and chemotherapy. Eligibility for these treatments depends on diagnosing early-stage disease, which is often asymptomatic. In developed countries, only 30% to 40% of HCC patients are diagnosed early enough for curative treatment.

### Tumor Markers for Hepatocellular Carcinoma

AFP is the most clinically useful tumor marker for HCC. AFP concentrations may range from within the reference interval to as high as $10 \times 10^6$ μg/L ($8.3 \times 10^6$ kU/L) but may not be increased in up to 20% of untreated patients with HCC, especially in early-stage disease. AFP concentrations may be transiently raised during recovery from viral hepatitis and in some benign conditions (see Table 20.7).

### Screening for Hepatocellular Carcinoma in High-Risk Groups Using α-Fetoprotein

Clinical outcome can be improved by early detection of HCC through well-organized screening of high-risk populations with abdominal ultrasound and 3- or 6-monthly AFP measurement. Studies suggest that serial AFP testing more accurately identifies those patients with HCV and/or advanced fibrosis or cirrhosis who are most likely to develop HCC. If serum AFP is rising or if a liver mass nodule is identified on ultrasound, the NCCN recommends additional CT or MRI imaging. According to the NACB, AFP concentrations ≥20 µg/L (i.e., ≥17 kU/L) and rising should prompt further investigation even if ultrasound is negative.

*α-Fetoprotein as an aid to diagnosis.* The same caveats that apply to use of AFP for screening apply to its use as an aid to diagnosis. Generally, nodules of less than 1 cm detected by ultrasound scanning should be monitored at 3-monthly intervals but those of 1 to 2 cm in cirrhotic livers should be investigated by two imaging modalities (e.g., CT and MRI) and treated as HCC if imaging results are consistent with this. For liver lesions greater than 2 cm in size where ultrasound scanning is typical of HCC and AFP is greater than 200 µg/L (i.e., ~170 kU/L), a diagnosis of HCC can be made without biopsy. If no mass is detected, AFP testing and liver imaging should be continued every 3 months.

*α-Fetoprotein in prognosis.* AFP concentrations may provide prognostic information in untreated HCC patients and in those being considered for liver resection or transplantation, with high concentrations generally associated with poor prognosis. Preoperative AFP decision limits ranging from 200 to 1000 µg/L (i.e., ~170 to 830 kU/L)[a] have been suggested to predict outcome after liver transplantation but there is no international agreement about the decision concentration. In the UK, current National Health Service (NHS) Blood and Transplant guidelines state that patients with serum AFP greater than 1200 µg/L (i.e., >1000 kU/L) should be de-selected from eligibility for transplant.

*α-Fetoprotein in post-treatment monitoring.* Measurement of AFP for detection of recurrence is recommended to monitor disease status after liver resection or liver transplantation, after ablative therapies and/or during palliative treatment. This reflects the general consensus that earlier identification of disease may enable alternative treatments to be instituted or patients entered into a clinical trial. Current practice suggests monitoring patients with AFP every 3 months for 2 years and then every 6 to 12 months. Rising AFP concentrations should be confirmed with a repeat specimen within 3 months. Re-evaluation, including AFP measurement, should be instituted earlier if there is clinical suspicion of disease recurrence.

## Lung Cancer

Lung cancer has been the most common cancer and cause of cancer death worldwide for several decades, accounting for nearly 20% of all cancer deaths. Survival rates depend strongly on tumor stage at diagnosis. Trends in incidence

and mortality generally reflect smoking habits and/or exposure to other environmental or occupational carcinogens. Public health campaigns to discourage smoking and to minimize other risk factors should ultimately reduce incidence.

Early symptoms are nonspecific and include dyspnea, cough, and thoracic pain, with hemoptysis often indicating advanced disease. Investigations for suspected lung cancer include CT and/or MRI, bronchoscopy, and biopsy. Histological differentiation and staging of lung cancer is essential as the two major histological types have different clinical behaviors and sensitivity to chemo- and radiotherapy.

About 75% to 85% of lung cancers are non–small cell lung cancers (NSCLCs) and require surgery as first-line treatment, with subsequent adjuvant radio- and/or chemotherapy if appropriate. Several molecularly targeted therapies are available, targeting EGFR, VEGF and other mutations. Small cell lung cancers (SCLCs) account for the other 15% to 25% of lung cancers and often have neuroendocrine components (see Chapter 26). They are aggressive tumors that double rapidly and metastasize early but respond initially to chemotherapy and/or radiotherapy.

### Tumor Markers in the Management of Lung Cancer

The serum tumor markers most frequently associated with SCLC are neuron specific enolase (NSE) and progastrin-releasing peptide (ProGRP), while Cyfra 21-1 and CEA are primarily associated with NSCLC. SCCA may be raised in the subset of NSCLC patients with squamous cell carcinoma.

*Screening and diagnosis.* No serum tumor markers are sufficiently sensitive or specific, singly or in combination, for use in screening for lung cancer, even in high-risk groups such as smokers.

In patients in whom inoperable lung cancer is suspected but for whom histology is not available, clearly increased serum NSE and/or ProGRP support a diagnosis of SCLC, while clearly raised serum SCC concentrations are consistent with squamous cell cancer.

*Prognosis.* Measurements of Cyfra 21-1, CEA and/or LDH may provide prognostic information for NSCLC while NSE and LDH can be used similarly in SCLC.

*Therapy prediction.* Serum tumor markers cannot be used to predict therapy response in lung cancer patients. However, with the increasing availability of molecularly targeted therapies, measurement of molecular biomarkers to identify the most appropriate treatment of lung cancer patients eligible for these treatments is now essential to ensure that these treatments are given to those most likely to benefit. Recommended molecular biomarkers include EGFR and BRF V600E mutations and ALK or ROS1 translocations.

*Monitoring.* Monitoring of lung cancer patients with serum tumor markers is controversial in view of the often aggressive nature of the disease. Serial determinations following surgery may provide an indication of the completeness of tumor removal and an early indication of subsequent recurrence. The latter is only likely to benefit the patient if

---

[a]1 µg/L of AFP is equivalent to 0.83 kU/L. This factor applies to most current immunoassays but Instructions for Use provided by the manufacturer should always be consulted to confirm this.

alternative treatment is available and there is as yet no evidence to suggest that monitoring improves outcome.

## Melanoma

Melanoma is a skin cancer that can occur anywhere on the body but is most common in skin that is frequently exposed to sunlight. The incidence of melanoma has steadily increased over the last 30 years. Signs of melanoma include changes in the appearance of moles or pigmented areas of the skin. Surgery is curative in early-stage disease, but the prognosis is poor in metastatic disease. However, increasing availability of systemic targeted therapies and immunotherapies has revolutionized therapy for melanoma, markedly improving survival as compared with chemotherapy regimens.

### Tumor Markers Used in the Management of Melanoma

Diagnosing malignant melanoma in pathological specimens involves staining with antibodies to S100, a family of multifunctional proteins with regulatory roles in a number of cellular processes. S100 is increased in serum in patients with malignant melanoma but its clinical utility has yet to be established and it lacks sensitivity in early disease. Rising concentrations are specific and sensitive for progression in patients with advanced disease but its measurement is only appropriate if further treatment options are available. Although very nonspecific, LDH is sometimes used to monitor patients with melanoma and may have prognostic value in advanced disease.

*Therapy prediction.* Biomarker measurements for mutations of the *BRAF, NRAS,* and *cKit* genes are now mandatory for effective management of advanced melanoma and other molecular predictive markers are likely to be identified. However, their clinical use is currently limited, other than in selecting patients for clinical trials.

## Neonatal and Pediatric Tumors

In children under 19 years old, cancer is the leading cause of death in the United States, but advances in treatment mean that greater than 80% of children diagnosed with cancer are now cured. Tumor markers can contribute significantly to the management of childhood neuroblastomas, malignant hepatic tumors and GCTs. The general principles are the same as for adults with some additional caveats.

### Tumor Markers Used in the Management of Childhood Malignancies

AFP and hCG are the tumor markers most frequently used in childhood malignancies. Plasma AFP is markedly increased at birth and then declines steadily to adult concentrations by 6 to 12 months. Age-related reference intervals are therefore essential. AFP is higher in pre-term infants and may remain increased for longer in children with delayed development. Serial measurements are more useful than isolated results, particularly in neonates in whom acute hepatocellular damage may result in marked increases in AFP concentrations.

Additional care must be taken to avoid reporting results that are inappropriately low due to high dose "hooking" as tumor marker concentrations may be very high in some childhood cancers. Considerable care is also required to ensure that dilutions of serum are made and recorded correctly. As AFP and hCG requests for young children are relatively infrequent, it is highly desirable that all such samples are routinely assayed at more than one dilution.

### Childhood Germ Cell Tumors

Measurement of AFP and hCG is mandatory as either or both are frequently increased at the time of diagnosis. Yolk sac tumors are the most common pure malignant GCTs in childhood. Dysgerminomas are the most common pure malignant GCT occurring in the ovary and central nervous system in girls, who may present with precocious puberty.

### Hepatoblastoma

Hepatoblastoma and HCC are the most frequent malignant hepatic tumors in childhood and differential diagnosis is essential. More than 80% of children with hepatoblastoma and about 50% of those with HCC have tumors that produce AFP, often at extremely high concentrations [e.g., $1.2 \times 10^6$ µg/L ($1.0 \times 10^6$ kU/L)]. Children with hepatoblastomas that secrete hCG may develop precocious puberty. Complete surgical resection is the treatment of choice for hepatoblastomas and HCC with adjuvant chemotherapy is also important for hepatoblastomas.

### Neuroblastoma

Neuroblastomas are malignant embryonal tumors that may exhibit extremely malignant behavior or may regress spontaneously. They account for 8% to 10% of childhood cancers, with about 80% of cases occurring in children less than 4 years old. Treatment includes surgery, chemotherapy, and radiotherapy. The diagnosis can be confirmed and the success of treatment monitored by measuring urinary catecholamines which are increased in greater than 90% of cases (see Chapter 26).

## Ovarian Cancer

Ovarian cancer is relatively rare (approximately 1.0% of all new cancer cases per year in the United States). Five-year survival rates are greater than 90% for women diagnosed with disease confined to the ovary but approximately 28% for women with advanced disease at diagnosis. Early detection is difficult due in part to the relative rarity and heterogeneity of the disease and as many as 30% of women with ovarian cancer may present for the first time at the Emergency Department.

Most malignant ovarian tumors (80% to 85%) are surface epithelial carcinomas that occur in five distinct histological sub-types, predominantly serous. When evaluating the clinical utility of tumor markers in ovarian cancer, the different clinical behavior of the different sub-types must be considered.

GCTs account for about 15% of malignant ovarian tumors (see above) or sex cord stromal tumors, two-thirds of which are granulosa cell tumors.

### Tumor Markers Used in the Management of Ovarian Cancer

CA125 is the most widely used serum tumor marker for all epithelial ovarian cancers but is most sensitive for serous adenocarcinomas. CA125 is raised in many nonmalignant conditions (see Table 20.7), so careful interpretation of results in the clinical context is essential. Occasional and sometimes transiently raised concentrations of CA125 greater than 5000 kU/L may be seen in patients with nonmalignant ascites and CA125 is increased in other malignancies, particularly adenocarcinomas. Some methods are vulnerable to interference, particularly from heterophilic antibodies (see Chapter 15).

Human epididymal protein 4 (HE4) has recently emerged as a promising serum tumor marker that could potentially complement measurement of CA125 in ovarian cancer patients. Serum HE4 is less sensitive than CA125 for detecting early-stage ovarian cancers among asymptomatic women but has better sensitivity and specificity for differentiating malignant from nonmalignant pelvic masses, especially in pre-menopausal patients.

The serum markers of choice for ovarian GCTs are AFP, hCG and LDH, while for granulosa cell tumors inhibin is the appropriate tumor marker. An inhibin method that detects all forms of inhibin, including inhibin A, B, and pro-αC, is required.

*Screening for ovarian cancer.* A reliable screening test for early ovarian cancer could make a major difference to outcome since most patients with advanced disease die of it. Assuming a disease prevalence of 40 per 100,000 in women over 50 years old, very high specificity (99.7%) is required to achieve an acceptable positive predictive value of 10% for ovarian cancer. The feasibility of screening women over 50 years of age using CA125 and ultrasound has been investigated extensively in several large major randomized controlled trials, two of which demonstrated no significant difference in deaths due to ovarian cancer between the screen and no screen arms. Routine screening is not recommended by any professional society.

The situation is different for women with a strong family history of ovarian, breast, or colon cancer, who should be referred for formal genetic counseling to assess their cancer risk, as recommended by the American College of Obstetricians and Gynecologists and the NCCN.

*Diagnosis.* CA125 measurement in isolation is not recommended for diagnosis due to its low sensitivity and specificity for ovarian cancer. A level within the reference interval does not necessarily exclude ovarian cancer and an increased concentration does not necessarily indicate it, particularly in premenopausal women. Nevertheless, extremely high CA125 values may be helpful in evaluating pre-menopausal women provided other potential causes are excluded.

In post-menopausal women, CA125 measurement can help in differentiating malignant from nonmalignant pelvic masses using well-established "Risk of Malignancy" (RMI) algorithms that incorporate ultrasound, menopausal status and CA125. At an RMI cut-off value of 200, the positive predictive value for malignancy is about 80%.

Women with ovarian cancer may develop nonspecific symptoms several months before diagnosis of early-stage disease (see Table 20.6). Reflecting this, UK National Institute for Health and Clinical Excellence (NICE) guidelines recommend that serum CA125 be measured in women presenting with persistent, frequent (>12 times a month) and continuous symptoms including abdominal bloating or distension, early satiety and/or loss of appetite, pelvic or abdominal pain and/or increased urinary urgency and/or frequency. If CA125 is ≥35 kU/L, an ultrasound scan of the abdomen is arranged and the RMI calculated. Women with RMI greater than 250 are referred urgently to a specialist team. An audit will be required to assess the cost-effectiveness of this approach.

*Prognosis.* Higher preoperative CA125 concentrations are generally associated with a worse prognosis. Five-year survival rates in patients with a preoperative CA125 concentration greater than 65 kU/L have been found to be significantly lower than those for patients with CA125 less than 65 kU/L. CA125 values greater than 500 kU/L may predict the occurrence of difficult or complex surgery, potentially aiding treatment planning.

Following primary treatment with surgery and/or chemotherapy, the rate and extent of fall of CA125 during the initial two cycles of platinum-based chemotherapy generally reflect prognosis. Factors influencing CA125 concentrations postsurgery must be taken into account to minimize the risk of misinterpreting results.

*Monitoring.* Criteria used to evaluate changes in CA125 during treatment and follow-up in the "Response Evaluation Criteria in Solid Tumors" (RECIST). A CA125 response is defined as a 50% decrease from the pre-treatment concentration provided the decrease is maintained for at least 28 days. The RECIST criteria enable objective assessment of response which can influence decisions to continue effective treatment or change ineffective treatment.

Results of a European randomized trial to evaluate posttreatment monitoring with CA125 indicated that early intervention based on CA125 conferred no survival advantage but resulted in earlier deterioration in quality of life. It was concluded that the value of routine measurement of CA125 in the follow-up of patients with ovarian cancer who attain a complete response after first-line treatment is not proven and that these patients should be told that routine CA125 monitoring is not necessary until or unless they are worried or develop any signs suspicious of tumor relapse. The NCCN considers the European trial to have limitations and recommends that patients should discuss with their clinician the pros and cons of having CA125 measurements made

## Pancreatic Cancer

Pancreatic cancer is the 10th most common cancer in the United States, representing 3.2% of all new cancer cases but is the third leading cause of cancer death. Most patients with pancreatic cancer present with symptoms that may include jaundice, weight loss, abdominal pain, nausea or vomiting, and/or pruritus (see Table 20.6). Only 12% are diagnosed when the tumor is confined to the primary site and may be resectable.

### Tumor Markers Used in the Management of Pancreatic Cancer

The most clinically useful serum tumor marker for pancreatic cancer is CA19-9, a sialylated Lewis a antigen (Le[a])

commonly produced in pancreatic and hepatobiliary disease but also increased in many other conditions (see Table 20.7). CA19-9 is undetectable and therefore uninformative in the 5% to 10% of the general population who are Le$^a$-negative.

## Clinical Applications of CA19-9 in Pancreatic Cancer

*Screening and diagnosis.* The low positive predictive value of CA19-9 means it cannot be used in screening, but in symptomatic patients it can contribute to diagnosis. It should only be measured in patients in whom pancreatic cancer is suspected and with the usual caveats that a result within the reference interval does not exclude pancreatic malignancy and vice versa. CA19-9 is frequently increased in patients with biliary obstruction due to benign pancreatobiliary and other conditions and is best measured after complete biliary decompression (if necessary) and when bilirubin is normal.

*Prognosis and therapy prediction.* Preoperative CA19-9 concentrations correlate with staging and disease burden so can complement information from imaging, laparoscopy and biopsy when assessing whether a pancreatic tumor is resectable. In patients without biliary obstruction, a high CA19-9 concentration can be used as an indication for staging laparoscopy, with concentrations greater than 130 kU/L strongly associated with sub-radiographic unresectable disease. Low postoperative CA19-9 concentrations at 3 months and before adjuvant chemotherapy are independently prognostic, with normalization of CA19-9 following neoadjuvant therapy associated with longer median survival. Postoperative CA19-9 concentrations may also help to predict the benefit of adjuvant therapy.

*Monitoring.* Rising CA19-9 concentrations suggest progression and can be used, together with radiographic and clinical data, to influence decisions to initiate palliative treatment in a patient whose disease progresses after surgery or to change (or discontinue) chemotherapy in patients progressing during treatment. Obtaining a CA19-9 measurement immediately before each therapeutic intervention is essential in order to have a baseline with which to compare subsequent results. ASCO does not recommend the routine use of serum CA19-9 alone to monitor response to treatment but states that in advanced disease CA19-9 can be measured at the start of treatment for locally advanced metastatic disease and every 1 to 3 months during active treatment. An increase may indicate progression and should prompt confirmation with other modalities.

It is particularly important that the same CA19-9 method be used for serial monitoring since results are not interchangeable between methods.

## Prostate Cancer

Prostate cancer is most frequently diagnosed in men aged 65 to 74 years old. It is predicted to account for approximately 14% of all new cancer cases in the United States in 2022, but for only 5.7% of all cancer deaths. While many more men with prostate cancer die with, rather than of their cancer (autopsy studies show that approximately 80% of men have some cancer cells in their prostate by the age of 80 years), some prostate cancers are lethal. Developing a reliable and noninvasive means of differentiating aggressive cancers from indolent cancers remains a major challenge.

Common symptoms at presentation include frequency, urgency, nocturia, dysuria, acute retention, prostatic enlargement, back pain, weight loss and anemia (see Table 20.6). The first six of these are also associated with benign prostatic hyperplasia (BPH), a nonmalignant condition reflecting increased prostate size with advancing age. The last three symptoms tend to be symptomatic of more advanced prostate cancer.

Treatment options for early-stage disease include curative surgery (prostatectomy), brachytherapy, and radiotherapy, while "active surveillance" without intervention is also a realistic option. In advanced metastatic disease endocrine (anti-androgen) therapy is effective as prostate cancers are dependent on testosterone. Eventually, however many advanced cancers no longer respond to traditional androgen-reducing treatments and other treatment options including chemotherapy are required.

Widespread measurement of serum prostate-specific antigen (PSA), which can identify potential prostatic disease in both asymptomatic and symptomatic patients, informs decisions to proceed to prostatic biopsy, and probably accounts for an apparent increased incidence of prostate cancer. However, many of the cancers identified are indolent and such over-diagnosis is a major issue for health systems.

## Tumor Markers Used in the Management of Prostate Cancer

*Prostate specific antigen.* Optimal treatment of patients with prostate cancer relies on PSA measurements. Unlike many other tumor markers, PSA is essentially organ-specific. However, PSA is not cancer-specific as increased serum concentrations occur in men with benign prostatic disease and/or urinary tract infections and following intervention involving the prostate. Prostatic biopsy is therefore required for a definitive diagnosis.

A member of the kallikrein serine protease family, 70% to 90% of immunoreactive PSA protein in blood is bound to protease inhibitors, primarily alpha-1-antichymotrypsin (ACT). The remaining 10% to 30% of the immunoreactive protein circulates in a free or unbound form, thought to be biologically inactive and known as "free PSA." Multiple forms of free PSA and its precursor forms exist in serum and have been proposed as new markers for prostate cancer. In clinical practice, methods measuring total PSA (i.e., free PSA and the PSA-ACT complex) are most often used.

Several strategies to improve the diagnostic accuracy of PSA with the primary aim of decreasing the number of unnecessary biopsies have been proposed. These include use of age- and/or race-related reference intervals (PSA may be higher in older men and in African Americans), measurement of the ratio of free to total PSA when total PSA is ≤10 µg/L (the ratio is lower in men with prostatic cancer compared with men with BPH), PSA density (calculated as total PSA divided by prostate volume can differentiate men with high PSA from a large prostate from those with prostate cancer), PSA velocity when total PSA is ≤10 μg/L (the rate of change over time may reflect aggressiveness of prostate cancer). These approaches all have some important caveats.

## Other Tumor Markers for Prostate Cancer

Tests that are not at present widely used in clinical practice include PCA3 (a noncoding, prostate tissue-specific RNA measured in urine), PHI (an algorithmic combination of total PSA, free PSA and proPSA measured in serum) and the 4K score (a combination of free and total PSA, human kallikrein 2 and intact PSA measured in serum).

*Prostate-specific antigen in screening for prostate cancer.* Screening asymptomatic men for prostate cancer with PSA remains controversial, primarily because its inability to differentiate aggressive and indolent prostate cancers can inevitably lead to over-diagnosis and over-treatment of some men. In two of these, outcomes were similar in the screened and unscreened groups while the third concluded that PSA-based screening reduced mortality by 21%.

Most published guidelines do not recommend population screening but are in accord with the ACS view that asymptomatic men who have at least a 10-year life expectancy should have an opportunity to make an informed decision with their health care provider about whether to have PSA measured after receiving information about the associated potential benefits, risks, and uncertainties before undergoing the test.

*Prostate-specific antigen as an aid to diagnosis of prostate cancer.* Men with symptoms suggestive of prostate cancer should be offered a PSA test and a DRE before referral for specialist care. A PSA result within the reference interval does not necessarily exclude prostatic disease and an increased PSA does not necessarily indicate malignancy. In general, however, the higher the PSA result the greater the likelihood of prostate cancer, providing prostatitis, urinary tract infection, catheterization and other possible confounding factors that may increase PSA have been excluded (see Table 20.7). Results above the upper limit of the reference interval but less than 10 μg/L are considered to be within a "gray zone" where additional testing (e.g., percent free PSA) may be undertaken in some centers before proceeding to biopsy. A second specimen to confirm a raised PSA result is always desirable.

Generally, diagnosis of prostate cancer requires biopsy and pathological confirmation unless clinical suspicion of malignancy is high, there is evidence of bone metastases and the PSA concentration is clearly increased (e.g., >100 μg/L). Prior to prostatic biopsy, the benefits and potential side-effects should be discussed with the patient, and individual risk factors (e.g., age and ethnicity) and comorbidities carefully considered.

*Prostate-specific antigen in prognosis and therapy prediction of prostate cancer.* In patients with immunohistochemically confirmed prostate cancer, treatment depends on whether the disease is confined to the prostate or has spread to other organs, so accurate pre-treatment staging is crucial. The higher the PSA value the greater the risk of extra-prostatic extension and lymph node involvement but PSA should not be used in isolation to assess prognosis. Predictive tables or method-specific nomograms are available that combine pre-treatment PSA concentrations with information on clinical stage and the immunohistochemical Gleason score which assesses the degree of cellular differentiation in the prostate tissue examined and ranges from 2 in well-differentiated tumors to 10 in completely anaplastic tumors. Such nomograms can provide a reasonable indication of whether disease is localized to the prostate and aid in predicting treatment outcome.

Pre-treatment PSA can contribute to assessment of the need for bone, CT, and/or MRI scans for staging asymptomatic men with localized prostate cancer. Bone scans are generally not necessary in patients with newly diagnosed prostate cancer who have a PSA less than 20.0 μg/L unless history or clinical examination suggests bony involvement and/or if the patient has a Gleason score greater than 8. Similarly, CT is rarely positive when pre-treatment PSA less than 20.0 μg/L unless disease is locally advanced or the Gleason score is ≥8.

Following radical prostatectomy, PSA should decrease to and remain at undetectable concentrations, with measurable concentrations indicative of residual disease or possibly the presence of benign glands. A confirmed post-prostatectomy PSA value of ≥0.2 μg/L is likely to indicate residual disease or recurrence and should be actively investigated.

PSA decreases more slowly after radiotherapy, rarely falling to less than 0.2 μg/L. However, the level should remain stable. Any rise in PSA value ≥2.0 μg/L predicts treatment failure with great sensitivity and specificity after radiotherapy with or without androgen deprivation.

Following hormonal therapy, a low PSA nadir can be linked to survival. Failure to achieve a PSA nadir of less than 4.0 μg/L 7 months after initiation of therapy is associated with very poor prognosis (median survival approximately 1 year) while patients achieving a nadir of <0.2 μg/L have relatively good prognosis (median survival >6 years).

*Prostate-specific antigen in monitoring of prostate cancer.* Sustained increases in PSA after treatment provide objective evidence of disease progression, often months before other diagnostic procedures. Consistently rising PSA usually, although not always, indicates recurrence. Conversely, a stable PSA does not necessarily exclude progression if clinically suspected. An increase in PSA should always be confirmed, taking into account intra-individual biological variation in PSA of up to 20% to 30% before concluding an increase is clinically significant. For patients in whom it can be calculated PSA doubling time can provide valuable information about the likely time to progression. Patients with a PSA doubling time greater than 15 months have a low likelihood of prostate cancer-specific mortality over a 10-year period. In some patients, knowledge of increasing PSA concentrations may have adverse psychological consequences, and monitoring with PSA may be undesirable, particularly if effective alternative treatments are not available.

## Testicular Cancer

GCTs account for more than 90% of testicular tumors in adults (see Germ Cell section). Leydig and Sertoli cell tumors develop in the stroma, the hormone-producing tissue of the testicles, and represent 4% of adult testicular tumors and 20% of childhood tumors. Leydig cell tumors normally produce androgens. They usually do not spread and can be cured by surgical removal. Those that do spread are usually resistant to both chemotherapy and radiation. Sertoli cell tumors are very similar and are also difficult to treat if they spread beyond the testes.

As for granulosa cell tumors of the ovary, the marker of choice for both Sertoli and Leydig cell tumors is inhibin and the same analytical requirements apply.

## Thyroid Cancer

Thyroid cancers represent approximately 2% to 4% of cancers in all age groups, with women more than three times likely to be affected. There are four histological types: papillary, follicular, and anaplastic thyroid cancer and medullary thyroid carcinoma (MTC). The diagnosis is often made when a patient presents to the thyroid clinic with a painless neck lump. As the major differential diagnosis required is between benign and malignant thyroid nodules the reader is referred to Chapter 42 but use of the relevant tumor markers is described briefly here.

### Tumor Markers Used in the Management of Thyroid Cancers

Papillary and follicular thyroid cancers are differentiated thyroid cancers and can be monitored post-treatment by measuring serum thyroglobulin. A large complex glycoprotein synthesized by the follicular cells of the thyroid and stored in the colloid space, thyroglobulin is present in benign and malignant thyroid tissue. Its production is stimulated by thyroid-stimulating hormone (TSH). In patients with an intact thyroid, thyroglobulin reflects thyroid volume and injury and also TSH receptor stimulation. It should be undetectable in serum in the absence of thyroid cells.

MTC is a rare and challenging malignancy that often presents as a lump in the neck, with dysphagia or systemic effects such as diarrhea or flushing. The 10-year survival is approximately 75% but patients may survive for many more years even with a significant tumor burden. Most appropriately managed in specialist centers, MTC has a hereditary component in about 25% of cases and can be associated with multiple endocrine neoplasia (MEN 2b) (see Chapter 26). Germline testing for the RET proto-oncogene distinguishes hereditary from sporadic MTC and should be offered to all patients with a family history consistent with MEN2 or familial MTC. Prophylactic thyroidectomy may be indicated in children and screening for other endocrine tumors (e.g., pheochromocytoma, pituitary, parathyroid) is essential. Calcitonin is an excellent tumor marker for MTC. CEA is also a very good marker of tumor burden in MTC.

*Screening, diagnosis and prognosis.* Serum thyroglobulin measurement is not helpful in screening for or diagnosis of thyroid cancer and has no value as a prognostic marker. Basal calcitonin measurements can contribute to the diagnosis of C-cell hyperplasia and MTC and CEA should be measured preoperatively.

*Monitoring.* Thyroglobulin has an important role in monitoring patients with papillary or follicular thyroid cancer after treatment with surgery and/or radioiodine. Following either of these treatments, TSH is usually kept suppressed by adjusting the replacement dose of thyroxine in order to minimize the risk of stimulating the growth of any remaining thyroid cancer cells. If TSH is suppressed, serum thyroglobulin should be undetectable following complete ablation. A confirmed rise in thyroglobulin is consistent with recurrence.

Calcitonin and CEA should be measured before surgery and 6 weeks post-surgery. Any increase should be confirmed with an early repeat determination using the same analytical method. Provided the concentrations fall to within reference limits following treatment, annual monitoring may be adequate after the first year (see Chapter 26).

*Analytical and reporting requirements for thyroglobulin.* There are several potential pitfalls in thyroglobulin measurement. Analytically, RIA and immunometric methods for thyroglobulin are vulnerable to interference from anti-thyroglobulin autoantibodies which may be present in some patient sera. Results obtained may be falsely low or falsely high, with immunometric methods being particularly prone to giving falsely low results. Appropriate cautions should be added to reports.

## Cancers of Unknown Primary

When cancer is found in one or more metastatic sites, but the primary site of origin cannot be determined, the diagnosis made is of cancer of unknown primary or occult primary cancer. Such cancers account for 2% of all new cancer diagnoses, with approximately 31,000 cases diagnosed per year in the United States. Symptoms vary according to the sites of metastases and may include swollen lymph nodes, abdominal mass, shortness of breath, pain in the chest or abdomen, bone pain, skin tumors, anemia, weakness, fatigue, poor appetite, and/or weight loss. The average survival time is about 9 to 12 months after diagnosis.

Routine clinical investigations to demonstrate the organ of origin are generally unproductive, with an approximate 30% rate of identification which has not been associated with significant improvement in survival. However, for a small subset of patients with cancer of unknown primary (possibly <1%) tumor marker measurements can contribute to diagnosis of an unsuspected but potentially treatable malignancy that has presented in an atypical manner. These include gestational choriocarcinoma, GCTs of the testis or ovary, prostate cancer, ovarian cancer, and breast cancer.

### Tumor Markers Used in the Management of Cancers of Unknown Primary

Measurement of AFP and hCG is recommended in patients with midline metastatic disease (mediastinal nodes or presence of a retroperitoneal mass) to assess the possibility of a GCT. CA125 measurement is recommended in women with symptoms that could be consistent with an occult non-germ cell ovarian malignancy, together with a gynecologic-oncologic consultation if indicated. Men presenting with

bone metastases or multiple sites of involvement should have PSA levels assessed. Chromogranin A measurement is recommended in patients with features of neuroendocrine tumors. Measurement of estrogen and PRs may identify hormone-sensitive tumors amenable to specific therapy. In patients in whom a pancreatic tissue origin is suspected, measurement of CA19-9 is recommended by the NCCN. The usual caveats apply to the use of these tumor markers in diagnosis. If their measurement identifies a likely primary source of malignancy (e.g., a GCT) then monitoring protocols, if required, should be according to established protocols for these cancers and tumor markers.

## CONCLUSION

Tumor marker measurements contribute significantly to the management of cancer patients, but considerable care is required to ensure that their use is appropriate. The clinical laboratory should proactively encourage correct test selection, sample handling, analysis, reporting and interpretation of tumor marker results, taking particular care to remind users of the caveats associated with these tests. This is essential not only for the well-established tumor markers but also for the new generation of molecular and genetic tumor markers on which clinicians increasingly will rely in order to provide optimal care. Involvement of laboratorians in developing clinical pathways that will enable optimal use of tumor markers—both the well-established and the newly developing—in routine practice provides new and exciting challenges which clinical laboratories are well positioned to meet.

## REVIEW QUESTIONS

1. Which of the following best describes appropriate use for most serum tumor marker measurements?
   a. Diagnosing or excluding a diagnosis of malignancy.
   b. Providing definitive information about likely prognosis in individual patients.
   c. Monitoring treatment effectiveness and the course of disease.
   d. Identifying the primary cancer by testing panels of serum tumor markers.
   e. Testing that is essential in the follow-up of all cancer patients.
2. For which of the following has measurement of a serum tumor marker been unequivocally demonstrated to be essential for early detection of disease in the appropriate screening population?
   a. Breast cancer
   b. Prostate cancer
   c. Ovarian cancer
   d. Malignant melanoma
   e. Choriocarcinoma
3. Which of the following is mandatory for the clinical management of the majority of breast cancer patients?
   a. Estrogen receptors

b. CA15-3
c. CEA
d. uPA
e. Gene profiling
4. Age-related reference intervals for most tumor markers are either not relevant and/or are not universally applied for most clinical applications, but are mandatory for which of the following age groups?
   a. AFP in men >30 years old
   b. AFP in neonates and infants under 12 months old
   c. hCG in men >30 years old
   d. hCG in neonates and infants under 12 months old
   e. CEA in men >30 years old
5. In women with suspected ovarian cancer the risk of malignancy index (RMI) is used primarily for which of the following?
   a. To exclude the need for pelvic ultrasound
   b. To identify whether a colorectal surgeon should be present at the time of operation
   c. To identify women with stage I disease where clear cell and endometrioid histologies predominate
   d. To assist in triaging women with pelvic masses
   e. To determine menopausal status

6. Which of the following statements best describes the contribution of International Standards and Reference Reagents to tumor marker measurements?
   a. They ensure that results are reported worldwide in the same units of measurement
   b. They can be used as kit standards by manufacturers
   c. Their introduction guarantees improved between-method agreement
   d. They enable accurate calibration of all the most widely used serum tumor markers
   e. They provide a benchmark against which the accuracy of calibration can be assessed

## SUGGESTED READINGS

American Cancer Society. *Cancer Facts and Figures 2022.* https://www.cancer.org/content/dam/cancer-org/research/cancer-facts-and-statistics/annual-cancer-facts-and-figures/2022/2022-cancer-facts-and-figures.pdf. Accessed September 2022.

Dalton-Fitzgerald E, Tiro J, Kandunoori P, et al. Practice patterns and attitudes of primary care providers and barriers to surveillance of hepatocellular carcinoma in patients with cirrhosis. *Clin Gastroenterol Hepatol.* 2015;13:791–798.e1.

Duffy MJ. PSA in screening for prostate cancer: more good than harm or more harm than good? *Adv Clin Chem.* 2014;66:1–23.

Duffy MJ, Crown J. Precision treatment for cancer: role of prognostic and predictive markers. *Crit Rev Clin Lab Sci.* 2014;51:30–45.

Duffy MJ, Sturgeon CM, Sölétormos G, et al. Validation of new cancer biomarkers: a position statement from the European Group on tumor markers. *Clin Chem.* 2015;61:809–820.

International Germ Cell Consensus Classification: a prognostic factor-based staging system for metastatic germ cell cancers. International Germ Cell Cancer Collaborative Group. *J Clin Oncol.* 1997;15:594–603.

Jassam N, Jones CM, Briscoe T, et al. The hook effect: a need for constant vigilance. *Ann Clin Biochem.* 2006;43:314–317.

NACB. National Academy of Clinical Biochemistry Laboratory Medicine Practice Guidelines for use of tumor markers. *Clin Chem.* 2008;54:e1–e10; *Clin Chem.* 2008;54:e11–e79; *Clin Chem.* 2010;56:e1–48.

NCCN. *National Comprehensive Cancer Network Clinical Practice Guidelines in Oncology.* https://www.nccn.org/professionals/physician_gls/f_guidelines.asp. Accessed September 2022.

Sturgeon CM, Lai LC, Duffy MJ. Serum tumour markers: how to order and interpret them. *BMJ.* 2009;339:b3527.

Sturgeon CM, Viljoen A. Analytical error and interference in immunoassay: minimizing risk. *Ann Clin Biochem.* 2011;48:418–432.

# Kidney Function Tests

*Edmund J. Lamb and Graham R.D. Jones\**

## OBJECTIVES

1. Define the following:
   - Creatinine
   - Urea
   - Uric acid
   - Gout
2. Diagram the pathway that results in the formation of creatinine.
3. State the clinical usefulness of measuring serum and urine creatinine.
4. State the principle of the Jaffe reaction and list five interferences that affect this method.
5. List and describe three enzymatic assays used to measure creatinine in serum.
6. Describe "compensated assays" in relation to the measurement of creatinine.
7. Diagram the catabolic pathway that results in the formation of urea.
8. State the clinical usefulness of measuring serum urea; list the causes of increased and decreased serum urea.
9. Describe the urease approach for measuring urea in serum; list one interference that affects this method.
10. Convert serum urea nitrogen given in milligrams per deciliter to urea nitrogen in millimoles per liter.
11. Diagram the pathway that results in the formation of uric acid.
12. State the clinical usefulness of measuring serum uric acid.
13. List the causes of hyperuricemia; explain the pathogenesis of gout and urinary tract uric acid stones.
14. Compare and contrast primary and secondary gout.
15. List the causes of hypouricemia.
16. Describe the uricase method of measuring uric acid in serum; list two interferences that affect this method.
17. List and describe the proteins found in urine, including their characteristics, how they are affected in disease, and the laboratory methods of protein measurement.

## KEY WORDS AND DEFINITIONS

**BUN (blood urea nitrogen)** Obsolete term used to report results of a urea assay, but still used in some countries, including the United States.

**Creatinine** A nonprotein nitrogen compound derived from the spontaneous hydrolysis of creatine or the cyclization of phosphocreatine; creatinine production is relatively constant, is related to muscle mass, and is used as a marker of the glomerular filtration rate of the kidneys.

**Gout** A condition caused by precipitation of uric acid in joints causing arthritis.

**Hyperuricemia** An excess of uric acid or urates in the blood with many causes; it is the major risk factor for the development of gout and may lead to kidney disease.

**Hypouricemia** Decreased uric acid concentration in the blood, secondary to a number of underlying conditions such as severe hepatocellular disease and defective renal tubular reabsorption.

**Jaffe reaction** The reaction of creatinine with alkaline picrate to form a colored compound; this type of creatinine assay is subject to numerous interferences.

**Urea** The major nitrogen-containing metabolic product of protein catabolism in humans.

**Urease methods** Enzymatic assays that measure urea concentration by hydrolysis of urea by urease to generate ammonia, which is quantified by a variety of methods.

**Uric acid** A nitrogenous compound derived from the catabolism of purine nucleosides.

**Uricase methods** A group of enzymatic assays for uric acid that initially involve oxidation of uric acid by uricase to eventually produce a chromogen that is spectrophotometrically measured to determine uric acid concentration.

\*Data on current creatinine method usage in the United Kingdom were provided by Finlay Mackenzie from the United Kingdom National External Quality Assessment Scheme (UKNEQAS), Birmingham, United Kingdom. Further information about the UKNEQAS estimated glomerular filtration rate (GFR) scheme may be found at https://birminghamquality.org.uk. We are grateful to the College of American Pathologists and the Royal College of Pathologists of Australasia Quality Assurance Program for data on current creatinine method usage and performance in the United States and Australasia, respectively. We also acknowledge the input of Professor Christopher Price to previous editions of this chapter.

Creatinine, urea, and uric acid are nonprotein nitrogen-containing metabolites that are cleared from the body by the kidney following glomerular filtration. Measurements of plasma or serum concentrations of these metabolites are commonly used as indicators of kidney function and other conditions. In particular, creatinine is most commonly measured to assess kidney function, and it is now widely used in equations to estimate the glomerular filtration rate (GFR). Cystatin C, a low-molecular-weight protein, is also increasingly being used to estimate the GFR. The measurement of total protein and/or albumin in urine can give useful information regarding the integrity of the glomerular filter and tubular function.

## PROTEINURIA: TOTAL PROTEIN AND ALBUMIN

Higher molecular weight proteins are retained within the circulation by the glomerular filter, and lower molecular weight proteins are freely filtered and reabsorbed and catabolized within the tubular cells. Consequently, the appearance of notable amounts of protein in the urine suggests kidney disease of either the glomerulus, the tubules, or both. The association between kidney disease and proteinuria dates as far back to at least the early 19th century, when Bright first described albuminous nephritis. Proteinuria can be classified as either tubular or glomerular, depending on the pattern of proteinuria observed. A third category, overflow proteinuria, is also recognized in which filtration of excessive amounts of low-molecular-weight protein exceeds the tubular capacity for reabsorption. Examples of the latter include Bence Jones proteinuria and myoglobinuria. Proteinuria is a potent risk marker for progressive kidney disease, and reduction of protein excretion is a therapeutic target. Proteinuria may be detected and measured using reagent strip devices or laboratory measurements of either total protein or albumin.

### Sample Collection for Urinary Total Protein and Albumin Measurement

It is generally recognized that a 24-hour sample is the definitive means of demonstrating and quantifying the presence of proteinuria, but this is a difficult procedure to control effectively, and inaccuracies in urinary collection may contribute to errors in estimation of protein losses. Overnight, first void in the morning (early morning urine [EMU]), second void in the morning, or random sample collections have also been used. Because creatinine excretion in the urine is fairly constant throughout the 24-hour period, measurement of the albumin-to-creatinine ratio (ACR) or protein-to-creatinine ratio (PCR) allows the use of a spot sample, providing correction for variations in urinary concentration in an individual. Spot samples for ACR or PCR measurement generally have good diagnostic performance and correlation with the 24-hour collection and are widely recommended for routine clinical use. An EMU sample is often preferred because it is unaffected by orthostatic (postural) proteinuria.

The diagnosis of albuminuria requires the demonstration of increased albumin loss (either increased ACR or increased albumin in a timed collection) in at least two out of three urine samples collected in the absence of infection or an acute medical illness (Fig. 21.1). Establishing the diagnosis of albuminuria or proteinuria has both prognostic and management implications. In the setting of diabetes, the best possible metabolic control should be achieved before patients are examined for albuminuria, and patients should not be screened during other transitory illnesses. Screening should commence 5 years after diagnosis in patients with type 1 diabetes mellitus and at diagnosis in patients with type 2 diabetes, and should continue on an annual basis up to the age of 75 years. Patients demonstrating an ACR of 3.0 mg/mmol or greater should have EMU samples sent to the laboratory on two other occasions (ideally within 2 months) for ACR measurement. Patients demonstrating increased ACRs in one or both of these additional samples are said to have persistent albuminuria. Diabetic nephropathy is uncommon in patients who have had type 1 diabetes for less than 5 years, and other causes of kidney disease should be considered.

Samples for urinary albumin (or total protein) measurement may be analyzed fresh, stored at 4°C for up to 1 week, or stored at −70°C for longer periods. Freezing at −20°C appears to result in loss of measurable albumin and is not recommended. For analysis, stored samples should be allowed to reach room temperature and be thoroughly mixed prior to testing.

### Analytical Methods and Traceability: Urinary Total Protein

Numerous methods can be used for the measurement of protein in urine, including the original Lowry method, turbidimetry after mixing with trichloroacetic or sulfosalicylic acid, turbidimetry with benzethonium chloride (benzyl dimethyl {2-[2-(p-1,1,3,3-tetramethyl butylphenoxy)ethoxy]ethyl} ammonium chloride), and dye binding with Coomassie Brilliant Blue, pyrogallol red molybdate, and pyrocatechol violet-molybdate, which is used in dry-slide applications.

Total protein measurement is more difficult in urine than in serum. The concentration of urinary protein is normally low (100 to 200 mg/L) and large sample-to-sample variation in the amount and composition of proteins is common. The concentration of nonprotein potentially interfering substances is high relative to the protein concentration and is highly variable, and the inorganic ion content is high. All these factors affect the precision, accuracy, and comparability of the various methods.

Because of the need for automation, the benzethonium chloride and dye-binding methods have become the most popular in current clinical use but they do not provide equal analytical specificity and sensitivity for all proteins. Concerns about different responses to different proteins have led to many variants of the published methods. Most methods tend to react more strongly with albumin than with globulin and other nonalbumin proteins. As different methods are responding to different properties of proteins and the abundance of these properties varies between the proteins found in urine, the measurand ("the quantity intended to be measured") is not the same for different assays. For those reasons, there is no reference measurement procedure

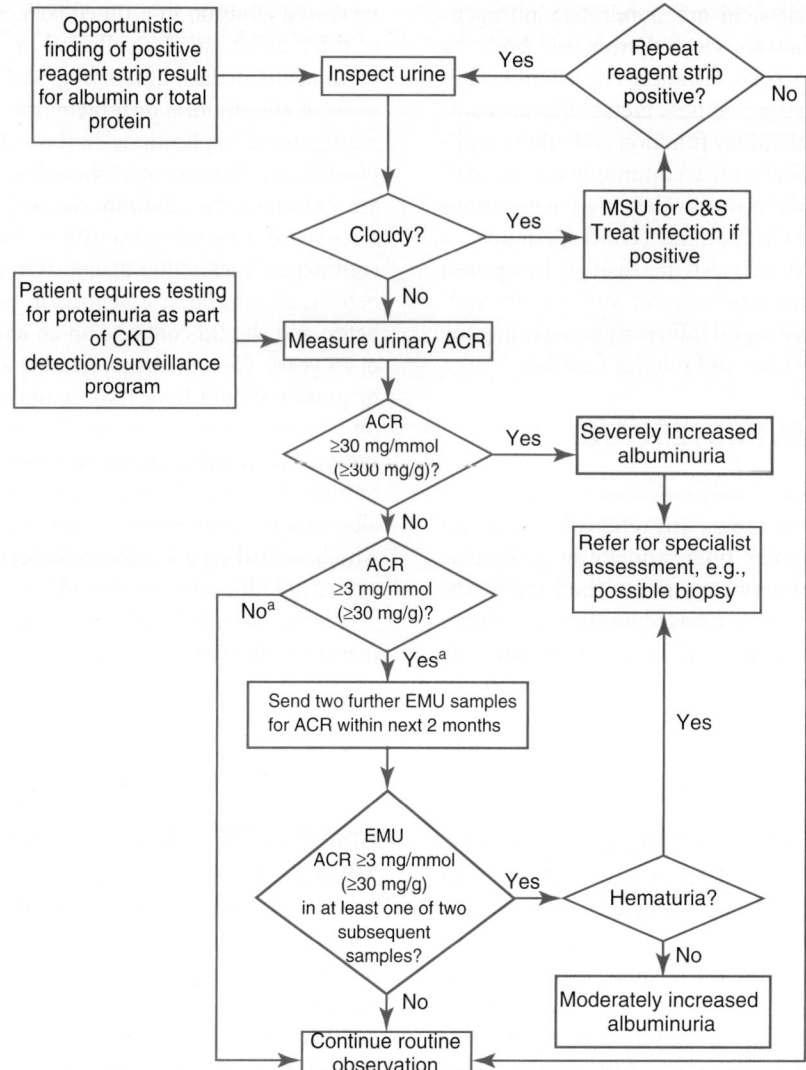

**Fig. 21.1** Suggested protocol for the further investigation of an individual demonstrating a positive reagent strip test for albuminuria/proteinuria or quantitative albuminuria/proteinuria test. Reagent strip device results should be confirmed using laboratory testing of the albumin-to-creatinine ratio (ACR) on at least two further occasions. Patients with two or more positive (≥3 mg albumin/mmol creatinine) tests on early morning samples 1 to 2 weeks apart should be diagnosed as having persistent albuminuria. (The possibility of postural proteinuria should be excluded by the examination of an early morning urine.) Protein-to-creatinine ratio (PCR) measurement can be substituted for the ACR but is insensitive in the detection of mild to moderately increased albuminuria/proteinuria: Approximate PCR equivalent to an ACR of 30 mg/mmol is 50 mg/mmol. *Note:* US guidelines express albuminuria or proteinuria as mg/g creatinine, whereas other guidelines use mg/mmol creatinine. An approximate conversion factor of 0.1136 can be used to convert results in mg/g to mg/mmol. However, for clarity and pragmatism, recent guidelines have accepted decision points that are approximately equivalent: hence, when using this protocol in the United States, 300 mg/g should be substituted for 30 mg/mmol and 30 mg/g for 3 mg/mmol.
[a]Consider other causes of increased ACR (e.g., menstrual contamination, uncontrolled hypertension, symptomatic urinary tract infection, heart failure, other transitory illnesses, and strenuous exercise), especially in the case of type 1 diabetes present for less than 5 years. The presence of hematuria may indicate nondiabetic renal disease. *C&S,* Culture and sensitivity; *CKD,* chronic kidney disease; *EMU,* early morning urine; *MSU,* midstream urine.

or standardized reference material for urinary total protein. The variety of methods in use means that significant between-laboratory variation is inevitable. This variation tends to diminish at higher concentrations of urinary total protein, presumably in part as albumin becomes the predominant protein and thus reduces a component of the between-sample variation. These methodological problems

are a major reason why urine albumin is a preferred analyte for the assessment of proteinuria.

## Analytical Methods and Traceability: Urinary Albumin

Urinary albumin has been measured using immunoassay since the 1960s when the first such assays became available. Urinary

## TABLE 21.1    Characteristics of Some Clinically Important Urinary Proteins

| Protein | Mr (kDa) | Free Plasma Concentration (g/L) | Diameter (nm) | pI | Glomerular Sieving Coefficient | Filtered Load >(mg/L)[a] | Urinary Concentration (mg/L)[b] | % Reabsorbed |
|---|---|---|---|---|---|---|---|---|
| IgG | 150 | 10 | 5.5 | 7.3 | 0.0001 | 1 | 0.1 | 99 |
| Albumin | 66 | 40 | 3.5 | 4.7 | 0.0002 | 8 | 5 | 99 |
| α₁-Microglobulin | 31 | 0.025 | 2.9 | 4.5 | ~0.3 | 7.5 | 5 | 99 |
| Retinol-binding protein | 22 | 0.025 | 2.1 | 4.5 | ~0.7 | 17.5 | 0.1 | 99 |
| Cystatin C | 12.8 | 0.001 | 3.0 | 9.2 | ~0.7 | 0.7 | 0.1 | 99 |
| β₂-Microglobulin | 11.8 | 0.002 | 1.6 | 5.6 | 0.7 | 1.1 | 0.1 | 99 |

[a]Concentration in the glomerular filtrate.
[b]Typical concentrations observed in health.
*IgG*, Immunoglobulin G; *pI*, isoelectric point.

albumin is predominantly measured using quantitative immunoturbidimetric or immunonephelometric approaches capable of detecting albumin at low concentrations. No Joint Committee for Traceability in Laboratory Medicine (JCTLM) listed reference measurement procedure or higher order reference material is currently available for urinary albumin. To date, most urinary albumin assays have been standardized against a serum-based calibrant (ERM-DA-470k/IFCC) distributed by the Institute for Reference Materials and Measurements of the European Commission.

### Reference Intervals, Definitions of Proteinuria and Albuminuria

There is no consistent definition of *proteinuria*. The upper limit of the reference interval for urinary total protein loss varies between 150 and 300 mg/day, depending on the source.[†] Given average daily creatinine excretion of about 10 mmol (0.11 g), an upper limit of normal protein loss of 150 mg/day is equivalent to a urinary PCR of approximately 15 mg/mmol (130 mg/g). The protein in the urine of healthy individuals is made up of albumin (<30 mg/day) and some smaller proteins, together with proteins secreted by the tubules, of which Tamm-Horsfall glycoprotein (THG) predominates. Typical concentrations of proteins found in urine are listed in Table 21.1. Readers should note that the units of expression used for ACR and PCR differ depending on geographical location, typically whether it is inside or outside the United States.[‡]

Proteinuria is often detected at the point of care (POC) using urine reagent strip devices, and clinical proteinuria has sometimes been defined as equivalent to a color change of "+" or greater on the relevant pad on the strip. This equates to approximately 300 mg/L of total protein or a PCR of 50 mg/mmol, or protein loss of approximately 500 mg/day (assuming an average urine volume of 1.5 L/day). Indeed, the limits for proteinuria and albuminuria are best described as clinical decision points because they are generally described or defined by expert groups rather than as the product of formal reference interval studies.

In health, relatively small amounts of albumin (<30 mg/day) are lost in the urine. In the international classification of kidney disease (see Chapter 35), proteinuria is categorized based on levels of albumin loss: A1 normal to mildly increased, less than 3.0 mg/mmol (approximately equivalent to <30 mg/g); A2 moderately increased, 3 to 30 mg/mmol (approximately equivalent to 30 to 300 mg/g); and A3 severely increased, greater than 30 mg/mmol (approximately equivalent to ≥300 mg/g). These categories are approximately equivalent to what would have formerly been considered normoalbuminuria, microalbuminuria, and macroalbuminuria (sometimes referred to as "clinical" or "significant" proteinuria), respectively. *Microalbuminuria* is a term that has been widely used to describe an increase in urinary albumin loss above the reference interval for healthy nondiabetic subjects, but at a level that is not generally detectable by less sensitive clinical tests such as reagent strips designed to measure total protein. The term *microalbuminuria* is somewhat misleading in that the albumin being measured is identical in form to that circulating in plasma, and the so-called microalbuminuric range refers to increased, not "micro-," albumin losses. Current guidelines do not support the continuing use of this term, and the term *albuminuria* is used in this chapter.

### Clinical Significance

The physiology and pathophysiology of renal protein handling and the clinical significance of proteinuria in specific clinical situations are discussed in more detail in Chapter 35; more general considerations follow. While reagent strip tests are commonly used in clinical practice, false negative and positive results are common. Most authors agree that positive tests require confirmation by laboratory measurement of the PCR or ACR on an early morning or random urine sample (see Fig. 21.1).

---

[†]Laboratories should select and verify appropriate ranges for use in their own settings.

[‡]USA guidelines express albuminuria or proteinuria as mg/g creatinine, whereas other guidelines generally use mg/mmol creatinine. A conversion factor of 0.1136 can be used to convert ACR or PCR results in mg/g to mg/mmol (e.g., 200 mg/g = 23 mg/mmol, 30 mg/g = 3.4 mg/mmol). Results in mg/mmol are multiplied by 8.80 to give mg/g.

Most commonly, proteinuria reflects albuminuria, and it is suggested that urinary total protein measurement can be replaced by urine albumin measurement. Strong evidence has linked increased urinary albumin loss to mortality and morbidity, including kidney disease progression, in people both with and without diabetes: albuminuria is generally held to be a more sensitive indicator of kidney disease than increased total protein loss. However, increases in albumin loss may also reflect overall changes in vascular permeability, and therefore may not indicate explicit deterioration in renal function. Increased urinary albumin loss is a common indicator of renal damage in the general population and is not only due to the presence of diabetes.

---

### POINTS TO REMEMBER

**Urinary Albumin**

- Albumin (Mr 66 kDa) is predominantly retained in the circulation by the glomerular basement membrane due to its size and negative charge.
- In health, only small amounts of albumin are filtered. This is largely reabsorbed in the proximal tubule.
- Albuminuria may arise due to both glomerular (increased filtration) and tubular (decreased reabsorption) disease.
- Albumin is the predominant urinary protein in the setting of proteinuria.
- Due to high biological variability and nonrenal influences, albuminuria should be confirmed on at least two occasions, preferably with first morning samples.
- Measurement of the ACR allows the use of a spot sample with correction for variations in urinary concentration in an individual.

---

## CREATININE

### Biochemistry and Physiology

Creatine, the immediate precursor of creatinine, is synthesized in the kidneys, liver, and pancreas and is then transported in blood to other organs, such as muscle and brain, where it is phosphorylated to phosphocreatine, a high-energy compound.

Interconversion of phosphocreatine and creatine is a particular feature of the energy supply for the processes of muscle contraction. A proportion of free creatine in muscle (thought to be between 1% and 2%/day) spontaneously and irreversibly converts to its anhydride waste product, creatinine. Thus, the amount of creatinine produced each day in an individual is fairly constant and is related to the muscle mass. In health, the serum concentration of creatinine is also fairly constant over time although it may be influenced by diet (see later). Creatinine (Mr approximately 113 Da) is present in all body fluids and secretions and is freely filtered by the glomerulus. Although it is not reabsorbed to any great extent by the renal tubules, a small but notable tubular secretion is present, as well as concentration-related losses in the gut.

### Sample Collection

Creatinine in serum, heparin plasma, or urine is stable for at least 7 days at 4°C, and is stable during long-term frozen storage (at −20°C and below) and after repeated thawing and refreezing. However, it should be noted that delayed separation (beyond 14 hours) of serum from erythrocytes leads to a significant increase in apparent serum creatinine concentration using some kinetic Jaffe (but not enzymatic) assays, possibly as the result of release of noncreatinine chromogens from the red cells (see later). Creatinine concentration increases in blood after meals containing cooked meat or fish, due to the conversion of creatine in the meat to creatinine, and ideally blood for serum creatinine measurement should be obtained in the fasting state.

### Analytical Methods

Serum creatinine is measured in virtually all clinical laboratories as a test of kidney function. Most laboratories use adaptations of the same assay for measurements in both serum and urine. Both chemical and enzymatic methods are used to measure creatinine in body fluids.

Most chemical methods for measuring creatinine are based on its reaction with alkaline picrate. As first described by Jaffe in 1886, creatinine reacts with picrate ion in an alkaline medium to yield an orange-red complex which is measured spectrophotometrically.

A serious analytical problem with the **Jaffe reaction** is its lack of specificity for creatinine. For example, many compounds have been reported to produce a Jaffe-like chromogen (also known as noncreatinine chromogens), including (1) ascorbic acid, (2) blood-substitute products, (3) cephalosporins, (4) glucose, (5) guanidine, (6) ketone bodies, (7) protein, and (8) pyruvate. The degree of interference from these compounds is dependent on the specific reaction conditions chosen. The effect of glucose, ketones, and ketoacids is probably of the greatest significance clinically, although the effect is very method dependent. Thus, reports on acetoacetate interference vary from a negligible increase to an increase of 3.5 mg/dL (310 μmol/L) in the apparent creatinine concentration at an acetoacetate concentration of 8 mmol/L. Bilirubin is a negative interferant with the Jaffe reaction. Of note these factors are generally not relevant to measurement of urine creatinine as they are often not present in the urine, or their concentrations relative to the amount of creatinine in urine makes the effects negligible.

There are many variations in the format of Jaffe creatinine assays which have been developed to minimize the effect of interferences. These variations include the following: the use of kinetic assays measuring the rate of color change rather than endpoint assays; the selection of the time period of measuring the reaction to minimize the effect of so-called fast and slow acting chromogens; the concentrations of picrate and hydroxide to provide a wide linear range; the choice of buffering ions; the use of surfactants; the selection of measurement wavelengths; the reaction temperature; the use of rate-blanking to minimize bilirubin interference and calibration compensation. The important message behind these factors is that Jaffe creatinine assays from different manufacturers often have different assay formats and so will react differently to various interferences. Also, laboratorians should not adjust the assay formats as there may be unexpected consequences for the assay performance. In summary, there is not a single Jaffe creatinine assay, there are many different Jaffe creatinine assays.

The issue of assay compensation requires special attention because of its relevance to assay traceability. As a result of reaction with noncreatinine chromogens, Jaffe methods often have historically overestimated true serum creatinine concentrations by up to 20% compared with high-performance liquid chromatography (HPLC) or isotope dilution mass spectrometry (IDMS) methods, at physiologic concentrations. In an attempt to adjust for this, some manufacturers have introduced so-called "compensated" Jaffe assays, in which a fixed concentration is automatically subtracted from each result. For example, Roche Diagnostics Ltd. (Lewes, Sussex, United Kingdom) has realigned its assays on the Cobas systems by −0.30 mg/dL (−26 µmol/L). Such assays produce lower results more closely aligned with IDMS reference measurement procedures at concentrations within the reference interval. However, they make an assumption that the noncreatinine chromogen interference is a constant between samples; this is clearly an oversimplification, especially when adult and pediatric samples are compared.

## Enzymatic Methods

Enzymes from a number of metabolic pathways have been investigated for the measurement of creatinine with the aim of increased analytical specificity. The methods involve a multistep approach leading to a photometric equilibrium with the two main approaches, described below.

### Creatininase and Creatinase

The most commonly used methods involve the use of creatininase (EC 3.5.2.10; creatinine amidohydrolase) to catalyze the conversion of creatinine to creatine, and creatinase (EC 3.5.3.3; creatine amidinohydrolase) to convert creatine to sarcosine and urea. Sarcosine is then measured with further enzyme-mediated steps using sarcosine oxidase (EC 1.5.3.1)

to produce glycine, formaldehyde, and hydrogen peroxide with the latter being detected and measured with a variety of methods. This final step may be subject to interference from a number of endogenous (e.g., bilirubin) and exogenous (e.g., medications), and manufacturers have taken a range of measures to reduce these interferences.

### Creatinine Deaminase

Creatinine deaminase (EC 3.5.4.21; creatinine iminohydrolase) catalyzes the conversion of creatinine to N-methylhydantoin and ammonia. One of these products is then determined by an additional reaction, e.g., the use of the enzyme N-methylhydantoin amidohydrolase.

### Dry Chemistry Systems

A number of multilayer dry reagent methods have been described for the measurement of creatinine using variations of the enzyme-mediated reactions listed above. In these methods, the color produced in the film is quantified by reflectance spectrophotometry.

### Other Methods

Gas or liquid chromatography-IDMS (GC-IDMS, LC-IDMS) are now accepted as the methods of choice for establishing the true concentration of creatinine in serum because of its excellent specificity and low imprecision. GC- and LC-IDMS methods have been approved by the JCTLM as reference measurement procedures for serum creatinine.

## Creatinine Methods: General Quality Issues and Preanalytical Considerations

Assessment of the methods used for the measurement of creatinine is complex by virtue of the number of variants of the Jaffe reaction and the innovations attempted using enzymatic procedures to overcome the limitations of the former. Although enzymatic methods are more expensive, they are used in dry chemistry systems, including some POC testing devices. Any laboratorian assessing a new creatinine method (e.g., as part of an analyzer purchase) should review the data for that method on common interferences recognizing that no method, Jaffe or enzymatic, is completely free from interferences and that each individual method may be affected in different ways. Where possible, it is recommended that enzymatic assays are implemented as they generally have fewer common interferences and also achieve better assay standardization due to more robust assay calibration.

Different methods for assaying serum creatinine have varying degrees of accuracy and imprecision. Mean within-individual biological variation for serum creatinine has been reported as approximately 4.5%, indicating a desirable analytical performance goal of less than 2.3%. External Quality Assurance (EQA) data using commutable samples and current methods from major manufacturers has delivered a total CV (including within and between method variation) of less than 5% for over 200 laboratories for values within the reference interval and average within-laboratory

CVs of 2.7%. This data indicates that acceptable analytical performance is possible; however, other EQA data indicates that there is room for improvement in many laboratories. However within- and between-laboratory agreement deteriorates as serum creatinine concentration falls within and to below the reference interval; the exponential relationship between serum creatinine and GFR means that imprecision at lower creatinine concentrations contributes to greater error in GFR estimation than at higher creatinine concentrations, a matter of particular concern with pediatric creatinine testing.

Over the past 20 years, appreciation of chronic kidney disease (CKD) as a major public health issue and of its identification, staging and monitoring using GFR-estimating equations has led to increased focus on the measurement of creatinine. Creatinine-based estimates of GFR (see later) will clearly vary, depending on how accurate the creatinine measurement used in the calculation is. The more a method overestimates "true" creatinine, the greater will be the underestimation of GFR, and vice versa (see later).

## Traceability of Serum Creatinine Measurement

In response to the known positive bias of historical creatinine assays there has been active work to improve the metrological traceability of these measurements. Standardized serum matrix reference materials (SRM 967) with known creatinine concentrations (0.80 mg/dL [71 µmol/L] and 4.00 mg/dL [354 µmol/L]) were prepared by the National Institute of Standards of Technology (NIST). The material was value-assigned using mass spectrometry and issued in 2007, and included in a list of higher order reference materials by the JCTLM. This material, in combination with GC-IDMS reference methodology, was used by most major reagent manufacturers to restandardize their methods and since 2009 most clinical laboratory methods have had calibration traceable to the reference measurement procedure and standard. As a shorthand this is often referred to as producing results which are "traceable to IDMS," however reference materials are the true top of the traceability chain. The original SRM 967 is no longer available. However, since that time other pure and matrix matched materials as well as reference laboratories are listed on the JCTLM database.

Although undoubtedly desirable, it must be recognized that standardization is only one arm of the problem. Standardization will not solve the problems of noncommutable calibrator materials and differential reactivity with noncreatinine chromogens across different patient samples, which can be resolved only by the use of highly specific creatinine methods. Wider adoption of enzymatic methods should further improve between-laboratory agreement in creatinine measurement.

## Reference Intervals

Data for establishing reference intervals for serum creatinine should be limited to that produced using IDMS traceable methods. A systematic review of creatinine reference intervals in which studies were included only if their calibration was traceable to the reference IDMS procedure proposed adult reference intervals of 0.72 to 1.18 mg/dL (64 to 104 µmol/L) in men and 0.55 to 1.02 mg/dL (49 to 90 µmol/L) in women. These data were derived using an enzymatic (Roche Diagnostics Ltd) assay. Serum creatinine concentration in patients with untreated kidney failure may exceed 11 mg/dL (1000 µmol/L). In addition to reference intervals, clinical decision points based on estimated GFR (eGFR) values derived from serum creatinine measurements play a major role in the clinical utility of these measurements (see below).

Urinary creatinine excretion is higher in men (14 to 26 mg/kg/day, 124 to 230 µmol/kg/day) than in women (11 to 20 mg/kg/day, 97 to 177 µmol/kg/day). Creatinine excretion decreases with age. Typically, for a 70 kg man, creatinine excretion will decline from approximately 1640 to 1030 mg/day (14.5 to 9.1 mmol/day) with advancing age from 30 to 80 years. These sex differences and changes with age are related to variations in average muscle mass. The measurement of urinary creatinine excretion is a useful indication of the completeness of a timed urine collection. Creatinine excretion is often used as a method of normalizing the urinary excretion of analytes, that is, the excretion of the test analyte (in millimoles or grams) is divided by the total amount of creatinine (in millimoles or grams) excreted in the same urine specimen. This is most commonly used as a method of adjusting for urinary concentration differences in random ("spot") urine samples.

## Clinical Significance

Serum creatinine concentration in health is maintained within narrow limits by the balance between production and removal, largely by glomerular filtration. As production in an individual is constant over time, both serum creatinine concentration and its renal clearance ("creatinine clearance") have been used as markers of the GFR. The application and limitations of these tests are discussed later in this chapter.

### POINTS TO REMEMBER

**Creatinine**
- Creatinine is produced at a fairly constant rate within an individual as a result of a breakdown of creatine within muscle tissue.
- Creatinine is freely filtered at the glomerulus and also secreted in the tubules to a lesser extent.
- Because it is predominantly excreted by the kidneys, plasma creatinine concentration is approximately inversely proportional to GFR (halving the GFR approximately doubles the serum creatinine).
- In addition to GFR, other factors related to creatinine production affect plasma creatinine concentration, including age, gender, race, muscularity, certain drugs, diet, and nutritional status.
- Estimated GFR (eGFR) based on plasma creatinine is a major use for these measurements (see Table 21.2).

# CYSTATIN C

## Biochemistry and Physiology

Cystatin C is a low-molecular-weight (12.8 kDa) protein synthesized by all nucleated cells whose physiologic role is that of a cysteine protease inhibitor. The gene has been sequenced, and the promoter region has been identified as that of the housekeeping type, with no known regulatory elements. Consequently, the rate of cystatin C release into the circulation was initially considered to be constant. Over time a number of factors have been identified that can affect cystatin C production and thus the circulating concentration (e.g., thyroid hormone concentration, obesity, inflammation). Unlike creatinine, muscle mass does not have a major effect on cystatin C concentration.

Cystatin C is removed from the circulation by the kidneys with no known extrarenal routes of elimination. Due to its small size and high isoelectric point (pI 9.2), it is more freely filtered than some other putative protein markers of GFR (see Table 21.1). Following filtration, cystatin C is essentially fully resorbed and broken down in the tubules usually leading to very low concentrations in the urine.

In addition to renal function and pathophysiological factors, serum cystatin C concentrations are also affected by age and sex, and these factors are taken into account with some cystatin C-based GFR estimating equations (see later).

## Analytical Methods

Cystatin C is measured by immunoassay, the most practical approaches being particle-enhanced turbidimetric or nephelometric immunoassay, which can run on automated chemistry analyzers or specific nephelometers. Using these assays, a between-day imprecision of CV 3% to 6% can be expected at the upper limit of the reference interval ($\cong 1.00$ mg/L) and less than 3% at higher values. The use of immunoassays makes cystatin C relatively free of the interferences that affect Jaffe creatinine assays although the reagents are markedly more expensive than those used for creatinine measurement.

## Traceability of Cystatin C Measurement

An international standard, ERM-DA471/IFCC Cystatin C in human serum, has been developed by an International Federation of Clinical Chemistry and Laboratory Medicine (IFCC) working party. The material has verified commutability and is listed on the JCTLM database. Most manufacturers have restandardized their assays against this material, and the use of these traceable assays in research and in the routine laboratory is recommended to improve comparability of results.

## Reference Intervals

While single reference intervals for adult males and females of all ages are commonly used, typically of the order 0.6 to 1.1 mg/L, it is known that cystatin C concentrations are higher in males than females and climb throughout adult life, reflecting the fall in GFR with advancing age seen in most populations. In a similar manner to serum creatinine, clinical decisions based on cystatin C are more likely to be made using GFR values estimated from cystatin C than on the serum cystatin C concentration itself, making the reference interval less relevant as a decision support tool.

## Clinical Significance

Because cystatin C is produced at a relatively constant rate, freely filtered at the glomerulus and neither secreted nor reabsorbed intact in the proximal tubule, its concentration in serum can serve as a marker of GFR, with GFR being approximately related to the reciprocal of serum cystatin C. In a similar manner to serum creatinine, equations have been developed to estimate GFR based on serum cystatin C with or without added demographic variables and with or without serum creatinine; some of these equations are given in Table 21.2. The Chronic Kidney Disease-Epidemiology Collaboration (CKD-EPI) cystatin C equations are well validated in adults.

Generally, the use of cystatin C equations provides some, albeit modest, improvement over equations based on serum creatinine alone. Some evidence suggests that the use of cystatin C GFR-estimating equations gives improved risk prediction of death and kidney failure unrelated to the accuracy of the GFR estimation; this improved predictive ability may relate to non-GFR determinants of serum cystatin C concentration. A specific recommendation from the international guideline group, Kidney Disease Improving Global Outcomes (KDIGO), suggests that, if confirmation of CKD is required, a cystatin C eGFR should be determined in adults who have creatinine-eGFR between 45 and 59 mL/min/1.73 m² and who do not have other markers of kidney damage.

---

**POINTS TO REMEMBER**

**Cystatin C**
- Cystatin C is a low-molecular-weight protein (12.8 kDa) produced at a fairly constant rate from most body cells.
- A modest increase in production is seen in obesity, hyperthyroidism, and inflammation.
- Cystatin C is removed from the circulation by the kidneys. It is freely filtered at the glomerulus and largely destroyed in the tubules.

---

# UREA

## Biochemistry and Physiology

Urea ($CO[NH_2]_2$, Mr 60 Da) is the major nitrogen-containing metabolic product of protein catabolism in humans. During the process of protein catabolism, nitrogen derived from amino acids enters the urea cycle via intermediates, which include aspartate and ammonia. Urea is synthesized exclusively in the liver by the enzymes of the urea cycle (Fig. 21.2). The rate of urea production is dependent on the rate of protein catabolism from both dietary and endogenous sources, the latter being largely from muscle. Urea is distributed evenly throughout the total body water due to its ability to diffuse through most cell membranes facilitated by urea transporter

TABLE 21.2  **Representative Glomerular Filtration Rate Estimating Equations for Use in Adults**

| Abbreviation | Glomerular Filtration Rate Equation |
|---|---|
| Cockcroft and Gault | $([(140 - \text{age}) \times \text{weight})] \times 1.23)/(\text{Scr}) \times 0.85$ (if female) |
| MDRD (ID-MS traceable) | GFR (mL/min/1.73 m$^2$) = $175 \times (\text{Scr} \times 0.01131)^{-1.154} \times (\text{age})^{-0.203} \times (1.210$ if patient is Black$) \times (0.742$ if patient is female$)$ |
| CKD-EPI$_{creat}$ (2009) | $141 \times \min(\text{Scr} \times 0.01131/\kappa, 1)^{\alpha} \times \max(\text{Scr} \times 0.01131/\kappa, 1)^{-1.209} \times 0.993^{age} \times 1.018$ (if female) $\times 1.159$ (if Black), where Scr is serum creatinine, $\kappa$ is 0.7 for females and 0.9 for males, $\alpha$ is $-0.329$ for females and $-0.411$ for males, min indicates the minimum of Scr/$\kappa$ or 1, and max indicates the maximum of Scr/$\kappa$ or 1. |
| CKD-EPI$_{cys}$ | $133 \times \min(\text{Scys}/0.8, 1)^{-0.499} \times \max(\text{Scys}/0.8, 1)^{-1.328} \times 0.996^{age} \times 0.932$ (if female), where min indicates the minimum of Scys/$\kappa$ or 1, and max indicates the maximum of Scys/$\kappa$ or 1. |
| CKD-EPI$_{creat-cys}$ (2009) | $135 \times \min(\text{Scr} \times 0.01131/\kappa, 1)^{\alpha} \times \max(\text{Scr} \times 0.01131/\kappa, 1)^{-0.601} \times \min(\text{Scys}/0.8, 1)^{-0.375} \times \max(\text{Scys}/0.8, 1)^{-0.711} \times 0.995^{age} \times 0.969$ (if female) $\times 1.08$ (if Black), where Scr is serum creatinine, Scys is serum cystatin C, $\kappa$ is 0.7 for females and 0.9 for males, $\alpha$ is $-0.248$ for females and $-0.207$ for males, min indicates the minimum of Scr/$\kappa$ or 1, and max indicates the maximum of Scr/$\kappa$ or 1. |
| CKD-EPI$_{creat}$ (2021) | $142 \times \min(\text{Scr} \times 0.01131/\kappa, 1)^{\alpha} \times \max(\text{Scr} \times 0.01131/\kappa, 1)^{-1.200} \times 0.9938^{age} \times 1.012$ (if female), where Scr is serum creatinine, $\kappa$ is 0.7 for females and 0.9 for males, $\alpha$ is $-0.241$ for females and $-0.302$ for males, min indicates the minimum of Scr/$\kappa$ or 1, and max indicates the maximum of Scr/$\kappa$ or 1. |
| BIS1 | $3736 \times (\text{Scr} \times 88.4)^{-0.87} \times \text{age}^{-0.95} \times 0.82$ (if female) |
| BIS2 | $767 \times \text{Scys}^{-0.61} \times \text{Scr}^{-0.40} \times \text{age}^{-0.57} \times 0.87$ (if female) |
| CAPA cystatin C equation | $130 \times \text{cystatin C}^{-1.069} \times \text{age}^{-0.117} - 7$ |

Age is given in years, serum creatinine in micromoles per liter, serum cystatin C (Scys) in milligram per liter, and weight in kilograms.
*BIS,* Berlin Initiative Study; *CAPA,* Caucasian, Asian, pediatric, and adult; *CKD-EPI,* Chronic Kidney Disease–Epidemiology Consortium; *GFR,* glomerular filtration rate; *ID-MS,* isotope dilution-mass spectrometry; *MDRD,* modification of diet in renal disease; *Scr,* serum creatinine; *Scys,* serum cystatin C.

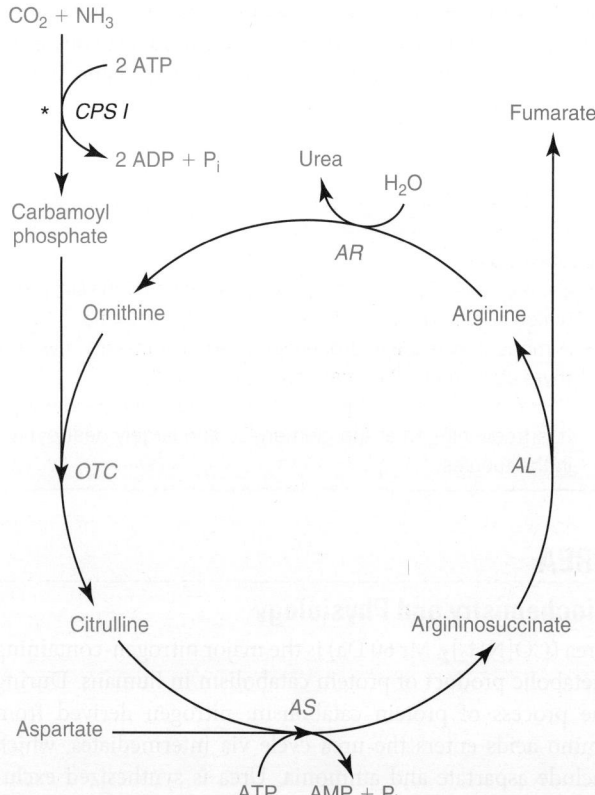

Fig. 21.2 The urea cycle pathway. *ADP,* Adenosine diphosphate; *AL,* argininosuccinate lyase; *AMP,* adenosine monophosphate; *AR,* arginase; *AS,* argininosuccinate synthetase; *ATP,* adenosine triphosphate; *CPS I,* carbamoyl phosphate synthetase I (*N-acetylglutamate as positive allosteric effector); *OTC,* ornithine transcarbamylase; *P$_i$,* inorganic phosphate.

proteins, and is therefore described as having a volume of distribution equal to the total body water.

Renal excretion accounts for more than 90% of urea removal from the body, with some losses through the gastrointestinal tract and skin. Urea is freely filtered at the glomerulus and, while it is neither actively reabsorbed nor secreted by the tubules, over 50% of urea moves passively out of the renal tubule, into the renal interstitium and back into the plasma. The back-diffusion of urea is dependent on urine flow rate, with less entering the interstitium in high-flow states (e.g., pregnancy) and more with low-flow situations (e.g., prerenal reduction in GFR due to fluid losses). Because water is resorbed to a far greater extent than the urea back-diffusion, urea is markedly concentrated during the process of urine formation, being present in urine at about 20 to 100 times the plasma concentration and is therefore the major contributor to urine osmolality. The role of urea in the functioning of the kidney is complex, involving specific urea transporters under the action of vasopressin.

## Analytical Methods

The vast majority of urea measurements in clinical laboratories are undertaken using enzymatic methods based on preliminary hydrolysis of urea with urease to generate ammonium ion, which then is quantitated. This approach has been used in end-point, kinetic, conductimetric, and dry chemistry systems and are collectively described as **urease methods**.

The analytical specificity of all routine methods is good and typical assay precision is usually small compared with the biological variation of serum urea indicating good analytical performance. Pure reference materials, as well as reference methods and laboratories using IDMS are available for urea and are listed on the JCTLM database, and assays from different providers generally provide acceptably consistent results.

## Reference Intervals

Serum urea concentrations are higher in men than in women, and there is an increase in the upper reference limit throughout adult life by a factor of about 50% from the 20s to the 70s. Pregnancy is associated with lower urea concentrations compared with age-matched nonpregnant women due to the associated glomerular hyperfiltration. In the pediatric age range, from after the first 2 weeks, the first year of life is associated with low serum urea, followed by a rise to slightly above adult concentrations to the age of about 10 years, then falling to young adult values by the late teens.

A reference interval for serum urea in healthy adults is 2.1 to 7.1 mmol/L (6 to 20 mg/dL expressed as urea nitrogen). Specific reference intervals will depend on the age, diet, and gender balance of the reference population. For example, in adults older than 60 years of age, a higher reference interval (e.g., 2.9 to 8.2 mmol/L [8 to 23 mg/dL]) may be used. On an average protein diet, urinary urea excretion expressed as urea nitrogen is 12 to 20 g/day (430 to 710 mmol/day).

The term **blood urea nitrogen (BUN)** is used in some countries to refer to serum urea tests, with results reported as mg/dL of BUN. The SI system recommends the use of the term urea, expressed in mmol/L. To convert mg/dL BUN to mmol/L urea multiply the value by 2.8 (or by 0.357 for the reverse).

## Clinical Significance

Measurement of blood and serum urea has been used for many years as an indicator of kidney function. However, it is generally accepted that creatinine measurement provides better information in this respect. Serum and urinary urea measurement may still provide useful clinical information in particular circumstances, for example, in patients with muscle wasting disorders where the serum creatinine concentration may be extremely low. The measurement of urea in dialysis fluids is widely used in assessing the adequacy of dialysis (see Chapter 35).

Urea concentration in serum is significantly affected by the rate of production as well as the rate of removal, which not only limits its value as a test of kidney function, but also allows its use for a range of other factors. For example, urea production, and therefore high plasma concentration, is increased by a high-protein diet, increased endogenous protein catabolism, such as occurs in many hospitalized patients, reabsorption of blood proteins after gastrointestinal hemorrhage, and treatment with cortisol or its synthetic analogues.

Urea removal from the circulation can be reduced due to any cause of reduced glomerular filtration, including prerenal, renal, or postrenal factors. The differential response of urea relative to creatinine can be useful diagnostically. In obstructive postrenal conditions (e.g., malignancy, nephrolithiasis, and prostatism), both serum creatinine and urea

concentrations will be increased, although in these situations the increase in serum urea is greater than that of creatinine because of increased back-diffusion. These considerations give rise to the main proposed clinical use of serum urea—namely, its measurement in conjunction with that of serum creatinine and subsequent calculation of the urea to creatinine ratio. This can be used as a crude discriminator between prerenal and intrinsic causes of reduced GFR. For a normal individual on a normal diet, the reference interval for the ratio is between about 0.049 and 0.081 mmol urea/μmol creatinine (12 and 20 mg urea/mg creatinine). In the setting of known acute kidney injury (AKI), a raised urea to creatinine ratio (>0.081 mmol/μmol, which can be rounded up to >0.1 for convenience) is thought to be more indicative of a prerenal cause than an intrinsic renal cause, such as acute tubular necrosis. This test is far from an absolute diagnostic test and must be placed with the clinical findings and consideration to other factors which may influence the urea and creatinine concentrations.

A low serum urea concentration occurs in the setting of low protein intake—for example, starvation or anorexia nervosa. This is less commonly seen among hospital inpatients who, although often do not consume adequate nutrients, do not exhibit a low serum urea due to the presence of significant catabolism of endogenous protein. Low serum urea concentration can also be seen with end-stage liver disease due to decreased urea synthesis and in pregnancy.

Measurement of urinary urea output provides a crude index of overall nitrogen balance and may be used as a guide to replacement in patients receiving parenteral nutrition.

# URIC ACID (URATE)

## Biochemistry and Physiology

Uric acid ($C_5H_4N_4O_3$, Mr 168) is the major product of catabolism of the purine nucleosides, adenosine, and guanosine in humans (Fig. 21.3). These precursors are metabolized into uric acid in a series of metabolic steps finishing with the conversion of xanthine to uric acid by the action of xanthine oxidase. The bulk of excreted uric acid arises from the degradation of endogenous nucleic acids (approximately 400 mg/day) with a lesser contribution from dietary sources (300 mg/day). Overproduction of uric acid may result from increased synthesis of purine precursors. In humans, approximately 75% of uric acid excreted is lost in the urine; most of the remainder is secreted into the gastrointestinal tract, where it is degraded to allantoin and other compounds by bacterial enzymes.

Renal handling of uric acid is complex and involves four sequential steps: (1) glomerular filtration of virtually all the uric acid in capillary plasma entering the glomerulus; (2) near complete reabsorption in the proximal convoluted tubule; (3) secretion into the distal portion of the proximal tubule; and (4) further reabsorption in the distal tubule. The net urinary excretion of uric acid is 6% to 12% of the amount filtered.

The physicochemical properties of uric acid are important in considering uric acid concentrations in the circulation, in

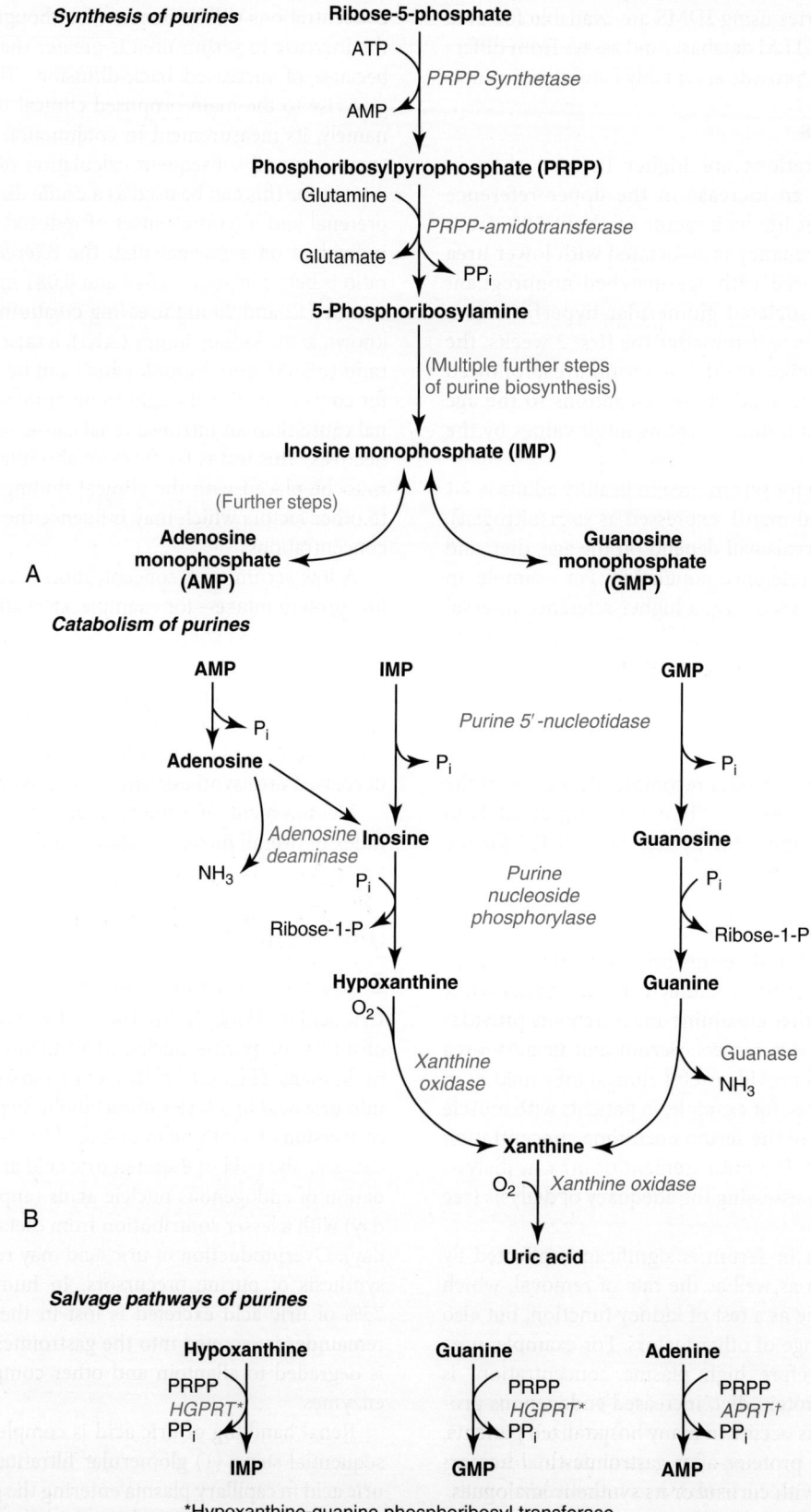

**Fig. 21.3** Metabolism of purines: (A) Synthesis. (B) Catabolism. (C) Salvage pathways. *ATP*, Adenosine triphosphate; $P_i$, inorganic phosphate; $PP_i$, inorganic pyrophosphate.

tissue, and in the kidneys. The first pKa of uric acid is 5.75; above this pH, uric acid exists chiefly as urate ion, which is more soluble than uric acid. At a urine pH below 5.75, uric acid is the preponderant form. On the basis of the ionization form in the circulation, it has been proposed that urate should be the preferred term rather than uric acid when describing serum measurements.

## Sample Collection

Most blood collection tubes are suitable for sample collection, and urate is sufficiently stable that no special collection or sample handling conditions are required. Traditionally, urinary uric acid excretion is determined in a 24-hour urine sample. If analysis is not undertaken promptly, alkalinization of the sample is recommended to maintain uric acid in solution.

## Analytical Methods

Methods based on the enzyme uricase (urate:oxygen oxidoreductase; EC 1.7.3.3) are the most commonly used routine methods for measuring uric acid and are collectively known as **uricase methods**. Uricase acts on uric acid to produce allantoin, hydrogen peroxide, and carbon dioxide. The reaction can be observed in either the kinetic or the equilibrium mode. Most current enzymatic assays for serum urate involve a peroxidase system coupled with one of a number of oxygen acceptors to produce a chromogen. The step for quantitation of the hydrogen peroxide produced is sometimes referred to as a Trinder reaction. One common method measures hydrogen peroxide with the aid of horseradish peroxidase and an oxygen acceptor to yield a chromogen in the visible spectrum. The most common oxygen acceptor used is 4-aminophenazone, together with phenol or a substituted phenol. The JCTLM lists pure substance and matrix matched certified reference materials for uric acid as well as IDMS reference methods and reference measurement services for analysis in serum and urine. Evidence suggests that most routine methods are meeting clinical needs. Interference in Trinder assays can be caused by antioxidants such as ascorbate (e.g., intravenous vitamin C), bilirubin, and unspecified interferants in serum from patients with kidney failure. Rasburicase is a urate-consuming enzyme (urate oxidase) used to treat patients with tumor lysis syndrome. Rasburicase can lower serum urate concentrations in blood collection tubes ex vivo unless both whole blood and serum are cooled before and after separation or treated by acidification.

## Reference Intervals

The serum urate concentration increases gradually with age, rising about 10% between the ages of 20 and 60 years. A significant rise is seen in women after menopause, reaching concentrations similar to those found in men. Additionally, higher concentrations of serum urate are found with increases in waist circumference, body mass index, and other components of the metabolic syndrome. A population reference interval may require partitioning on the basis of gender and age, and will be affected by the metabolic status of the population. It can be argued that a clinical decision

point for the relevant clinical question may be more useful than a population reference interval given the interaction with common comorbidities. A reference interval for serum urate has been reported to be 3.5 to 7.2 mg/dL (0.21 to 0.43 mmol/L) for males and 2.6 to 6.0 mg/dL (0.16 to 0.36 mmol/L) for females.

During pregnancy, serum urate concentrations fall during the first trimester and until about 24 weeks' gestation, when values begin to rise and eventually exceed nonpregnant concentrations. Urinary uric acid excretion in individuals on a diet containing purines is 250 to 750 mg/day (1.5 to 4.5 mmol/day). Excretion may decrease by 20% to 25% on a purine-free diet to less than 400 mg/day (2.4 mmol/day).

## Clinical Significance

The most common clinical use for urate assessment is risk assessment for gout and determination of therapy adequacy. Other clinical conditions where serum urate measurements have potential utility include cardiovascular risk assessment and a diagnosis of preeclampsia. Urine uric acid measurements may play a role in assessing the cause of hyperuricemia and in assessing the risk of renal stone formation.

### Hyperuricemia

The major causes of hyperuricemia are summarized in Box 21.1. Asymptomatic hyperuricemia is frequently

---

**BOX 21.1 Causes of Hyperuricemia**

**Increased Formation**
*Primary*
Idiopathic
Inherited metabolic disorders

*Secondary*
Excess dietary purine intake
Increased nucleic acid turnover (e.g., leukemia, myeloma, radiotherapy, chemotherapy, trauma)
Psoriasis
Altered ATP metabolism
Tissue hypoxia
Preeclampsia
Alcohol

**Decreased Excretion**
*Primary*
Idiopathic

*Secondary*
Acute or chronic kidney disease
Increased renal reabsorption
Reduced secretion
Lead poisoning
Preeclampsia
Organic acids (e.g., lactate and acetoacetate)
Salicylate (low doses)
Thiazide diuretics
Trisomy 21 (Down syndrome)

*ATP, Adenosine triphosphate.*

detected through biochemical screening, although there is no evidence for clinical benefit resulting from this practice.

## Gout

**Gout** occurs when monosodium urate precipitates in joints and tissues from supersaturated body fluids. These deposits of urate are responsible for the clinical signs and symptoms. Gouty arthritis is caused by urate crystal formation in joint fluid and may be associated with deposits of crystals (tophi) in tissues surrounding the joint. The deposits may occur in other soft tissues as well, and wherever they occur they elicit an intense inflammatory response. The first metatarsophalangeal joint (big toe) is the classic site for gout. Gout is a condition characterized by occasional attacks and long periods of remission. It is important to appreciate that the serum uric acid concentration is often normal during an acute attack and is not a component of the diagnostic criteria. The demonstration of uric acid crystals in joint aspirate fluid is the pathognomonic sign for gout. For details on the diagnostic criteria and associated evidence base, readers are referred to the European League Against Rheumatism (EULAR) guidelines. This report also provides information on the risk factors for the development of gout, which represent those for increasing concentrations of serum uric acid; of these, the major ones are male gender, CKD, hypertension, and obesity.

Gout may be classified as primary or secondary. Primary gout is associated with essential hyperuricemia, which has a polygenic basis. In more than 99% of cases, the cause is uncertain, but the condition is probably due to a combination of metabolic overproduction of purines, decreased renal excretion, and increased dietary intake. Very rarely, primary gout is attributable to inherited defects of enzymes in the pathways of purine metabolism.

Secondary gout is a result of hyperuricemia attributable to several identifiable causes such as CKD; as a consequence of administration of drugs (in particular diuretics); and ketoacidosis or to lactic acidosis (by reducing tubular secretion of urate). Increased nucleic acid turnover and a consequent increase in catabolism of purines may be encountered in rapid proliferation of tumor cells and in massive destruction of tumor cells on therapy with certain chemotherapeutic agents.

Management of an acute attack of gout can be divided into broad strategies: management of the attack and the prevention of subsequent attacks. The main focus for acute management is pain relief. Avoidance of subsequent attacks is based on lifestyle and pharmacotherapy with the aim of reducing plasma urate, which is monitored to assess therapeutic success. An evidence-based treatment target for prevention of gout recurrence is a serum urate concentration less than 0.36 mmol/L (6.0 mg/dL).

## Kidney Disease

Kidney disease associated with hyperuricemia may take one or more of several forms: (1) gouty nephropathy with urate deposition in renal parenchyma, (2) acute intratubular deposition of urate crystals, and (3) urate nephrolithiasis.

## Kidney Stones

Uric acid kidney stones occur in approximately one in five patients with clinical gout. Although serum and urinary uric acid should be measured in stone formers, many uric acid stone formers do not demonstrate hyperuricosuria or hyperuricemia. Uric acid stone formation is promoted by the passage of a persistently acid urine with undissociated uric acid (pKa 5.57) being relatively insoluble, whereas urate at pH 7.0 is greater than 10 times more soluble. Pure uric acid stones account for approximately 8% of all urinary tract stones and, unlike many of the calcium-containing stones, are radiolucent. Allopurinol is the mainstay of treatment of uric acid stones.

## Preeclampsia

Preeclampsia is pregnancy-induced hypertension associated with proteinuria (>0.3 g/day) and often edema and may become life threatening for the mother or the fetus (see Chapter 44). The role of uric acid measurement in the management of preeclampsia is uncertain: measurement recommendations appear in some guidelines but not others. If assessing urate concentrations in this setting, it is important to use pregnancy-specific reference intervals.

## Inherited Diseases

Hyperuricemia can be a feature of several inherited disorders of purine metabolism, most of which are rare, and the diagnosis requires support from a specialist purine laboratory. Readers are referred to specialist textbooks for further information.

## Hypouricemia

**Hypouricemia,** often defined as serum urate concentrations less than 2.0 mg/dL (0.12 mmol/L), is much less common than hyperuricemia. It may be secondary to severe hepatocellular disease with reduced purine synthesis or xanthine oxidase activity, or defective renal tubular reabsorption of uric acid. Defective reabsorption may be congenital, as in generalized Fanconi syndrome, or acquired. Overtreatment of hyperuricemia with allopurinol or uricosuric drugs and cancer chemotherapy with 6-mercaptopurine or azathioprine (inhibitors of de novo purine synthesis) may also cause hypouricemia.

## Cardiometabolic Outcomes and Urate

Recent publications have highlighted positive associations between serum urate concentrations and a range of important cardiovascular and health outcomes that are generally associated with the metabolic syndrome (e.g., obesity and insulin resistance, hypertension and renal disease, cardiovascular disease, type 2 diabetes, and all-cause and cardiovascular mortality). More important, as well as indicating risk for patients with hyperuricemia, these relationships occur within the usually described "normal range" with the higher urate values associated with increasing risk. While these associations appear to be robust, it is less clear whether or not there is a causal association or whether urate-lowering therapy may be beneficial. Of note, recent work has demonstrated that reducing plasma urate does not slow the progression of CKD. The role of measurement of urate in the routine laboratory, validated clinical decision points, and appropriate management of patients based on the results remains to be determined; however, it is likely that there will be more roles for this analyte in the future.

---

**POINTS TO REMEMBER**

**Urate**
- Urate (uric acid) is the major end product of catabolism of the purine nucleosides.
- Excretion of urate is predominantly renal.
- Expected values for urate are influenced by many factors, including age, gender, menopausal status, diet, and waist circumference.
- Gout occurs when monosodium urate precipitates in joints and tissues from supersaturated body fluids, eliciting an intense inflammatory response.
- When treating gout, a target urate concentration of less than 6.0 mg/dL (<0.36 mmol/L) is used.

---

# ASSESSMENT OF KIDNEY FUNCTION: GLOMERULAR FILTRATION RATE

GFR is the amount of fluid filtered by the glomerulus in a fixed period of time and is widely accepted as the best overall measure of kidney function. Progressive decrease in GFR is associated with the clinical signs and laboratory changes of kidney damage in all forms of kidney disease. Measuring GFR in established disease is useful in targeting treatment, monitoring progression, and predicting the point at which renal replacement therapy (dialysis or transplantation) will be required. It is also used as a dosage guide to prevent toxicity by drugs excreted by the kidneys. There are a range of methods available to measure and estimate the GFR.

## The Concept of Clearance

All tests for GFR are based on the clearance of a substance from the circulation by the kidneys. Renal clearance of a substance is defined as the volume of plasma from which the substance is completely cleared (removed) by the kidneys per unit of time. Provided a substance S is freely filtered in the glomerulus and not secreted, resorbed, nor metabolized in the tubules, the renal clearance of S is equal to the GFR, and carries the same unit dimension (volume/time). Under these conditions the following equations apply.

$$GFR \times PS = US \times V \qquad (21.1)$$

$$GFR = (US \times V) / PS \qquad (21.2)$$

where GFR = the flow rate in mL per minute of plasma through the glomerular membranes, equivalent to a clearance in units of mL of plasma cleared of a substance per minute; US = urinary concentration of the substance; V = volumetric flow rate of urine in milliliter per minute; and PS = plasma (or serum) concentration of the substance (in the same units as the urinary concentration of the substance).

The units of milliliter per minute is the most commonly used unit for GFR and is recommended for universal adoption to avoid confusion from the use of different units.

Kidney size and GFR are roughly proportional to body size, with larger people having a higher GFR and vice versa; to remove this effect it is conventional to adjust GFR to a standard body surface area (BSA) of 1.73 m². There are a number of formulae available to estimate BSA (e.g., Du Bois and Du Bois, Haycock). A variety of markers, both exogenous (radioisotopic and nonradioisotopic) and endogenous, have been used to measure or estimate GFR with the choice of marker and procedure based on cost and availability as well as accuracy.

## Exogenous Markers of Glomerular Filtration Rate

Protocols for direct measurement of GFR are based on exogenous markers, with urinary clearance of inulin considered to be the "gold standard." There are many other exogenous markers and also different protocols for GFR determination. Markers may be given intravenously either by continuous infusion or single bolus and measured in serial urine or blood collections. The nonradioisotopic markers include inulin and iohexol, and the radiolabeled markers include labeled EDTA, DTPA, and iothalamate. Determination of GFR with exogenous markers is available in many hospitals and should be considered for clinical use when accurate GFR determination is required (e.g., prior to kidney donation, when dosing particularly toxic medications). There are guidelines recommending protocols for this type of testing; however, there are no EQA programs to assess overall performance. In general, a service needs to perform a significant number of these tests to gain proficiency.

## Endogenous Markers of Glomerular Filtration Rate

The most widely used endogenous marker of GFR is creatinine, expressed as its serum concentration, as renal clearance or included in eGFR equations. Although a range of other low-molecular-weight compounds have been investigated for clinical use, only creatinine and cystatin C are recommended for routine use.

## Creatinine

Serum creatinine concentration is by far the most commonly measured analyte for the purpose of assessing renal function and testing is widely available, cheap, and convenient. While there are methods to estimate GFR from serum creatinine (see below), creatinine alone plays an important role, especially with assessing changes in GFR. For example, a rise in serum creatinine of greater than 50% is one of the diagnostic criteria for AKI.

When interpreting creatinine concentrations, or the results of calculations based on serum creatinine, consideration needs to be given to factors that may affect the rate of release into the circulation as well as the rate of removal. As stated above, creatinine is produced in muscle from creatine at a fairly constant rate proportional to the amount of muscle present. Because muscle mass is affected by age, gender, race, nutrition, exercise, and other factors, the rate of production is variable between different people. The major route of creatinine removal from the circulation is by free filtration at the renal glomerulus although there is some additional loss into the urine by tubular secretion and by loss through the bowel. Due to the key role of glomerular filtration in creatinine removal, the concentration of creatinine in the circulation is approximately inversely related to GFR—that is, for the same creatinine production, a halving of the GFR will lead to an approximate doubling of the serum creatinine concentration.

A range of other factors affect creatinine metabolism and measurement, which are important when they are used to assess renal function. Drug effects can be due to blockage of tubular secretion (e.g., cimetidine, trimethoprim) or interference in creatinine assays. In patients with CKD, extrarenal clearance of creatinine becomes important when caused by degradation as a result of bacterial overgrowth in the small intestine, further blunting the anticipated increase in plasma creatinine in response to falling GFR. An important factor for any creatinine-based interpretation is that serum creatinine can remain within the reference interval until considerable kidney function has been lost. Additionally, serum creatinine measurement will not detect people with mildly reduced GFR (60 to 89 mL/min/1.73 m$^2$) and will fail to identify many patients with CKD and category 3A GFR (45 to 59 mL/min/1.73 m$^2$) (Fig. 21.4). Thus, although an increased serum creatinine concentration generally equates with impaired kidney function, a normal serum creatinine does not necessarily equate with normal kidney function. However, while the interpretation of creatinine concentration against population-based decision points is insensitive for the detection of CKD, changes in serum creatinine within an individual may be used as a sensitive tool for detecting changes in kidney function, whether the results are within or outside population reference intervals. In this setting, changes greater than expected by chance (i.e., that due to biological and analytical variation) are likely to indicate a significant change in GFR in a patient. Recent guidance from the American Association for Clinical Chemistry (AACC) recommends further assessment if the serum creatinine rises by the greater of 20%, or 20 µmol/L (rounded to 0.2 mg/dL). This has been referred to as the 20/20 rule and applies to all starting creatinine concentrations, even within or below the population reference interval.

## Creatinine Clearance

A measured creatinine clearance, performed using a 24-hour urine collection and serum collection during this period, has been used for many years as a marker of GFR. However, the difficulty in obtaining a complete, timed 24-hour urine collection, together with a high within-subject biological

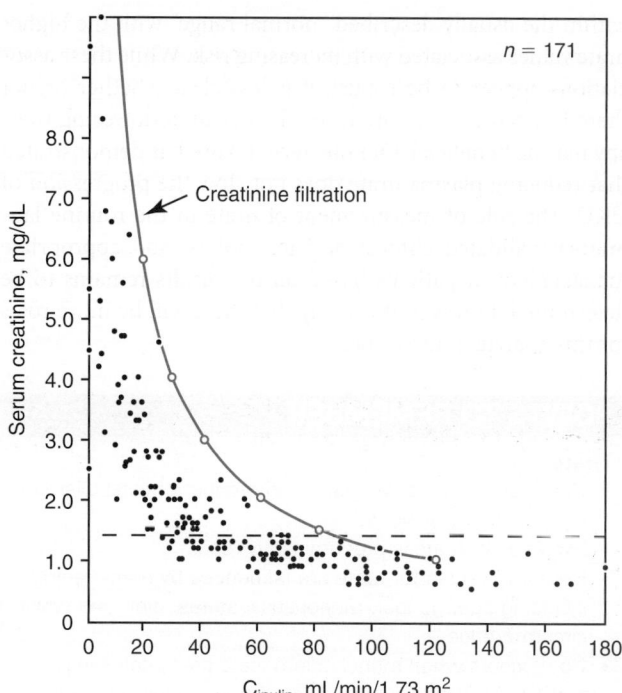

**Fig. 21.4** The relationship between serum creatinine concentration and glomerular filtration rate (GFR), measured as the clearance of inulin, in 171 patients with glomerular disease. The hypothetical relationship between GFR and serum creatinine is shown as a *continuous line*, assuming that only filtration of creatinine takes place. The *dashed horizontal line* represents an upper limit of normal for serum creatinine (1.4 mg/dL, 124 µmol/L) widely used at the time of publication. Because of creatinine secretion and/or a creatinine deficit through gut excretion, the serum creatinine consistently overestimates the GFR. (From Shemesh O, Golbetz H, Kriss JP, et al. Limitations of creatinine as a filtration marker in glomerulopathic patients. *Kidney Int.* 1985;28:830–838.)

variation in creatinine excretion and the known overestimation of GFR due to creatinine tubular secretion make this test both inaccurate and imprecise as a measure of GFR. In spite of these limitations, creatinine clearance remains in common use in recommendations for drug dosing decisions (see later).

## Estimating Glomerular Filtration Rate

The approximate mathematical relationship between serum creatinine and GFR (GFR $\alpha_1$/serum creatinine) can be improved by correcting for some of the variables that influence this relationship. Many different equations have been derived that estimate GFR using serum creatinine and inputs of some or all of gender, body size, race, and age. These generally produce a better estimate of GFR than serum creatinine alone or measured creatinine clearance, and professional societies throughout the world have recommended that such estimates should be used in association with serum creatinine. In adults, several such equations have been widely used, including the Cockcroft and Gault equation, the Modification of Diet in Renal Disease (MDRD) Study equations, and the CKD-EPI equations.

The Cockcroft and Gault equation is one of the earliest of these equations (see Table 21.2). It remains widely used in the context of assessing drug dosages for patients with kidney impairment (see later). However, the requirement for the measurement of body weight, the lack of a version validated for standardized creatinine assays, and the availability of demonstrably better equations have limited its ongoing use.

The era of GFR estimation as a widely used simple clinical tool began with publication of the four variable (creatinine, age, gender, race [African American/non-African American]) MDRD Study equation in 2000. The MDRD equation was updated in 2006 to a version suitable for IDMS traceable creatinine assays and this was widely endorsed by national organizations. Generally, the MDRD equation was found to provide a more accurate assessment of GFR than the Cockcroft and Gault equation, with the important advantage of not requiring knowledge of weight, allowing automatic reporting of eGFR with the results for serum creatinine.

In 2009, the CKD-EPI described a further equation (CKD-EPI$_{creat}$), again based on serum creatinine, gender, race (African American/non-African American), and age (see Table 21.2). This equation showed some improvement over MDRD, especially at higher levels of GFR (>60 mL/min/1.73 m$^2$).

Because the relationship between creatinine and kidney function varies among individuals, disease conditions, and populations, no GFR equation to date has found universal applicability. This remains an intense area of ongoing research. Other equations that have been developed are the CKD-EPI equations based on cystatin C, either alone or in combination with creatinine, and the Berlin Initiative Study (BIS) Group equations with claimed superior performance in older people (see Table 21.2).

There is a clear benefit to the use of the same equation by all laboratories in a country or region so that individual patients will get similar results if attending different laboratories, and so that CKD guidelines can be uniformly applied. This also affects research into treatments and prevalence of CKD. However, the relationship between creatinine and GFR has been shown to vary between some ethnicities, possibly due to differences in body habitus and dietary pattern. For example, the MDRD and CKD-EPI$_{creat}$ equation publications showed a clear distinction between subjects identifying as African American and non-African American. The requirement to adjust GFR estimating equations for race is a potential limitation to their global application and local implementation. In 2012, KDIGO recommended that the CKD-EPI$_{creat}$ equation from 2009 should be used to estimate GFR. However in 2021, following concern over race-based health inequalities, the 2009 CKD-EPI equation was revised to produce a "race neutral" version. This is now recommended for use in the United States and is being considered for use in other countries.

Limitations to creatinine-based GFR estimating equations include interferences in creatinine measurement and patient-specific factors. Any factor affecting creatinine measurement, such as bias, imprecision, drug effects, hemolysis, icterus, or lipemia, will directly affect the eGFR. Any relevant way in which a patient is different from those included in the trials to establish the equations will also affect the accuracy of the equation at an individual level. These include patients with AKI, in whom serum creatinine concentrations may change rapidly and with extremes of muscularity (e.g., bodybuilders, amputees, and people with muscle wasting disorders). The equations are also not suitable for patients on dialysis and for use during pregnancy; adult equations should not be used with patients under 18 years of age. Notwithstanding this, in general, equations improve the estimation of GFR compared with serum creatinine alone.

## Glomerular Filtration Rate and Drug Dosing Decisions

One key use for estimates of renal function is adjustment of renally excreted medication doses. Historically much of the data for drug dosing has been based on creatinine clearance or its estimate based on the Cockcroft and Gault formula (sometimes referred to as "eCrCl"). It is now known that these measurements are less accurate estimates of GFR than newer calculations, with the additional benefit that eGFR can be reported with all serum creatinine results making the result immediately available to clinicians. There are moves to update drug information to use eGFR results, but these changes need to be considered with attention to the risks and benefits to patient care. One aspect that is important in this area is the process of normalization of GFR for BSA. Creatinine clearance and Cockcroft and Gault results are in mL/min, that is, not corrected for BSA. This is thought to be appropriate for drug dosing decisions as the amount of drug lost in the urine is related to this raw value. With this in mind, for patients with large or small body size, it can be appropriate to remove the BSA normalization of eGFR calculations reported in mL/min/1.73 m$^2$, irrespective of the eGFR formula used. To remove the in-built BSA normalization of eGFR result multiply the result by the patient's BSA/1.73.

## Reference Intervals

An average GFR in young healthy individuals is 110 mL/min/1.73 m$^2$ (5th to 95th percentiles approximately 90 to 140 mL/min/1.73 m$^2$) with a gradual fall with increasing age. The age-related changes are also seen in outputs of eGFR equations. Age-related reference intervals are not widely used in clinical medicine with decision points based on CKD staging or advice for drug dosing providing the usual clinical support.

## Glomerular Filtration Rate Measurement and Estimation: Future Considerations

Evaluation of kidney function remains an essential component of medical practice, and much has been achieved in recent years to improve and standardize estimates of GFR. However, there remains room for improvement, and research into new and better markers, equations, and procedures for the measurement of kidney function will continue. The challenge to the clinical laboratory is to use the best available tools in a coordinated manner so that evidence-based clinical decisions can be made. One particular focus should be collaboration between laboratories so that patients and doctors obtain the same clinical information irrespective the laboratory selected.

## REVIEW QUESTIONS

1. The plasma concentration of creatinine is maintained within narrow limits predominantly by what process or factor?
   a. The constant catabolism of purines
   b. The constant rate of protein metabolism
   c. The glomerular filtration rate
   d. An individual's diet

2. What causes the symptoms of gout?
   a. Decreased renal perfusion as in heart failure
   b. Precipitation of excessive uric acid in joints and the urinary tract
   c. A low-protein diet
   d. Liver dysfunction as in hepatitis

3. What is the main nitrogen-containing compound that accounts for more than 75% of urinary nonprotein nitrogen?
   a. Uric acid
   b. Creatinine
   c. Creatine
   d. Urea

4. What is the effect of a deficiency of the enzyme xanthine oxidase due to severe hepatocellular disease?
   a. Increased urea concentration
   b. Decreased creatinine concentration
   c. Hypouricemia
   d. Hyperuricemia

5. During protein breakdown, the amino acid nitrogen groups are converted to urea through the urea cycle in which of the following organs?
   a. Liver
   b. Kidneys
   c. Heart
   d. GI tract

6. What is the process involved in compensated Jaffe assays for creatinine assessment?
   a. Add a fixed value to the assay result to compensate for interferants
   b. Subtract a fixed value from each result to compensate for noncreatinine interference
   c. Use a special formula that involves body mass and urine production to "normalize" creatinine results
   d. Involve averaging of values to remove possible discrepancies between two samples obtained at different times of the day

7. A value of 8.4 mg/dL of urea converts to what in mmol/L?
   a. 2.99
   b. 29.9
   c. 3.92
   d. 39.2

8. Ascorbic acid and bilirubin are interferants in which of the following assays?
   a. Jaffe reaction and uricase methods
   b. Jaffe reaction only
   c. Jaffe reaction, urease methods, and uricase methods
   d. Urease methods only

9. What are the main interferants in the uricase method of uric acid measurement that must be minimized?
   a. Phenol and bilirubin
   b. Ascorbic acid and bilirubin
   c. Endogenous ammonia and oxidizing agents
   d. Ketone bodies and protein

10. What is uric acid?
    a. The major product of protein catabolism
    b. A derivative of muscle creatine
    c. A metabolite of urinary nitrogen
    d. The major product of purine catabolism

## SUGGESTED READINGS

Atkins RC, Briganti EM, Zimmet PZ, et al. Association between albuminuria and proteinuria in the general population: the AusDiab study. *Nephrol Dial Transplant*. 2003;18:2170–2174.

Bachmann LM, Nilsson G, Bruns DE, et al. State of the art for measurement of urine albumin: comparison of routine measurement procedures to isotope dilution tandem mass spectrometry. *Clin Chem*. 2014;60:471–480.

Ceriotti F, Boyd JC, Klein G, et al. Reference intervals for serum creatinine concentrations: assessment of available data for global application. *Clin Chem*. 2008;54:559–566.

Chronic Kidney Disease Prognosis Consortium, Matsushita K, van der Velde M, et al. Association of estimated glomerular filtration rate and albuminuria with all-cause and cardiovascular mortality in general population cohorts: a collaborative meta-analysis. *Lancet*. 2010;375:2073–2081.

Earley A, Miskulin D, Lamb EJ, et al. Estimating equations for glomerular filtration rate in the era of creatinine standardization: a systematic review. *Ann Intern Med*. 2012;156:785–795.

El-Khoury JM, Hoenig MP, Jones GRD, et al. AACC guidance document on laboratory investigation of acute kidney injury. *JALM*. 2021;6:1316–1337.

Greenberg N, Roberts WL, Bachmann LM, et al. Specificity characteristics of 7 commercial creatinine measurement procedures by enzymatic and Jaffe method principles. *Clin Chem*. 2012;58:391–401.

Grubb A, Blirup-Jensen S, Lindström V, et al. First certified reference material for cystatin C in human serum ERM-DA471/IFCC. *Clin Chem Lab Med*. 2010;48:1619–1621.

Inker LA, Schmid CH, Tighiouart H, et al. Estimating glomerular filtration rate from serum creatinine and cystatin C. *N Engl J Med*. 2012;367:20–29.

KDIGO 2012 clinical practice guideline for the evaluation and management of chronic kidney disease. *Kidney Int*. 2013;3:1–150.

Lamb EJ, Mackenzie F, Stevens PE. How should proteinuria be detected and measured? *Ann Clin Biochem*. 2009;46:205–217.

Levey AS, Stevens LA, Schmid CH, et al. A new equation to estimate glomerular filtration rate. *Ann Intern Med*. 2009;150:604–612.

McTaggart MP, Newall RG, Hirst JA, et al. Diagnostic accuracy of point-of-care tests for detecting albuminuria: a systematic review and meta-analysis. *Ann Intern Med.* 2014;160:550–557.

Miller WG, Bruns DE, Hortin GL, et al. Current issues in measurement and reporting of urinary albumin excretion. *Clin Chem.* 2009;55:24–38.

Miller WG, Kaufman HW, Levey AS, et al. National Kidney Foundation Laboratory Engagement Working Group recommendations for implementing the CKD-EPI 2021 race-free equations for estimated glomerular filtration rate: practical guidance for clinical laboratories. *Clin Chem.* 2022;68:511–520.

Myers GL, Miller WG, Coresh J, et al. Recommendations for improving serum creatinine measurement: a report from the Laboratory Working Group of the National Kidney Disease Education Program. *Clin Chem.* 2006;52:5–18.

National Institute for Health and Care Excellence. Chronic kidney disease: assessment and management; 2021. https://www.nice.org.uk/guidance/ng203.

Peralta CA, Shlipak MG, Judd S, et al. Detection of chronic kidney disease with creatinine, cystatin C, and urine albumin-to-creatinine ratio and association with progression to end-stage renal disease and mortality. *JAMA.* 2011;305:1545–1552.

Price CP, Newall RG, Boyd JC. Use of protein:creatinine ratio measurements on random urine samples for prediction of significant proteinuria: a systematic review. *Clin Chem.* 2005;51:1577–1586.

Soveri I, Berg UB, Björk J, et al. Measuring GFR: a systematic review. *Am J Kidney Dis.* 2014;64:411–424.

# 22

# Carbohydrates

*David B. Sacks*

## OBJECTIVES

1. Define the following:
   Carbohydrate
   Gluconeogenesis
   Glycogen
   Glycogen storage disease
   Glycogenesis
   Glycogenolysis
   Glycolysis
   Glycoprotein
   Hypoglycemia
   Monosaccharide, disaccharide, and polysaccharide
2. Provide two examples each of a monosaccharide, a disaccharide, and a polysaccharide; describe the chemical structure of each.
3. Summarize the regulation of glucose concentration in the blood, including two hormones involved in this process.
4. Explain the relationship between glucose, lactate, and pyruvate.
5. Discuss the brain's dependence on glucose, including how the brain is affected in a hypoglycemic state and the alternative energy source used.
6. State the blood glucose concentration at which hypoglycemia is typically diagnosed.
7. List three causes of fasting hypoglycemia and three causes of postprandial (nonfasting) hypoglycemia;

describe the 72-hour fast test for diagnosing hypoglycemia.
8. List two causes of hypoglycemia in persons with type 1 diabetes.
9. Compare glucose values in fasting whole-blood, capillary, and venous blood specimens; state the reasons for the discrepant values.
10. State the effects of glycolysis on glucose in whole blood; list two ways in which glycolysis can be inhibited.
11. Describe the hexokinase method for measurement of glucose in blood; state the specimen requirements and the principle of the reaction; and list the known interferences.
12. Describe the glucose oxidase method for measurement of glucose in blood, state the specimen requirements and the principle of the reaction, and list the known interferences.
13. Describe the chemical reaction used to assess lactate concentrations in blood; describe the chemical reaction used to assess pyruvate concentrations in blood.
14. State the specimen collection and storage requirements for blood lactate and pyruvate analyses.
15. Analyze and resolve case studies regarding carbohydrate disorders; correlate the results of carbohydrate analysis with carbohydrate disorders.

## KEY WORDS AND DEFINITIONS

**Aldehyde** An organic compound with a carbonyl group (a carbon atom double-bonded to an oxygen) at the end of the carbon chain bonded to hydrogen and an R group (usually an alkyl group).

**Carbohydrate** Aldehyde or ketone derivatives of polyhydroxy alcohols are composed of carbon, hydrogen, and oxygen in a ratio of 12:1.

**Diabetes mellitus** A group of metabolic disorders of carbohydrate metabolism in which glucose is underutilized, producing hyperglycemia.

**Glucose** A six-carbon monosaccharide derived from the breakdown of carbohydrates in the diet or in body stores;

can also be endogenously synthesized from protein or the glycerol moiety of triglycerides.

**Glycogen** An extensively branched polysaccharide containing many glucose residues and found particularly in muscle and liver cells for glucose storage.

**Hypoglycemia** Blood glucose concentration in the blood decreased below a healthy reference interval.

**Insulin** A protein hormone that maintains blood glucose concentration by decreasing blood glucose through cellular uptake.

**Ketone**  An aldehyde that has a carbonyl group (a carbon atom double-bonded to an oxygen atom) at any position other than at the end of the carbon chain.

**Lactate**  An intermediary product in glucose metabolism that accumulates in the blood predominantly when tissue

oxygenation is decreased, as during strenuous exercise; an increased blood lactate concentration is called lactic acidosis.

**Pyruvate**  An organic acid formed from glucose through glycolysis.

---

Carbohydrates, including sugar and starch, are widely distributed in plants and animals. They perform multiple functions, such as serving as structural components in RNA and DNA (ribose and deoxyribose sugars) and providing a source of energy (glucose). Glucose is derived from (1) the breakdown of carbohydrates in the diet (grains, starchy vegetables, and legumes) or in body stores (glycogen), and (2) endogenous synthesis from protein or from the glycerol moiety of triglycerides. When energy intake exceeds expenditure, the excess is converted to fat and glycogen for storage in adipose tissue, and liver or muscle, respectively. When energy expenditure exceeds caloric intake, endogenous glucose formation occurs from the breakdown of carbohydrate stores and from noncarbohydrate sources (e.g., amino acids, lactate, glycerol).

The glucose concentration in the blood is maintained within a fairly narrow interval under diverse conditions (feeding, fasting, or severe exercise) by hormones such as insulin, glucagon, and epinephrine (see details in Chapter 33). Measurement of glucose is one of the most commonly performed procedures in hospitals and other health care chemistry laboratories, and glucose measurement by point-of-care and home-use meters is a multi-billion-dollar industry. The most frequently encountered disorder of carbohydrate metabolism is high blood glucose concentration due to diabetes mellitus, which affects approximately 11% of the US adult population. The incidence of hypoglycemia (low blood glucose) is unknown but is low (excluding patients who use exogenous insulin to control blood glucose).

## CHEMISTRY OF CARBOHYDRATES

Carbohydrates are aldehyde or ketone derivatives of polyhydroxy (more than one –OH group) alcohols or compounds that yield these derivatives on hydrolysis.

### Monosaccharides

A monosaccharide is a simple sugar that consists of a single polyhydroxy aldehyde or ketone unit and is unable to be hydrolyzed to a simpler form. The backbone is made up of several carbon atoms. Sugars containing three, four, five, six, and seven carbon atoms are known as *trioses, tetroses, pentoses, hexoses,* and *heptoses,* respectively. One of the carbon atoms is double-bonded to an oxygen atom to form a carbonyl group. An aldehyde has the carbonyl group at the end of the carbon chain, whereas if the carbonyl group is at

any other position, a ketone is formed (Fig. 22.1). The simplest carbohydrate is glycol aldehyde, the aldehyde derivative of ethylene glycol. The aldehyde and ketone derivatives of glycerol are, respectively, glyceraldehyde and dihydroxyacetone (see Fig. 22.1). Monosaccharides are termed *aldoses* or *ketoses* according to the position of the carbonyl group (Fig. 22.2).

Compounds that are identical in composition but differ only in spatial configuration are called *stereoisomers.* The carbon atoms in the unbranched chain are numbered 1 to 6, as shown by the numbers at the left of the formula for D-glucose in Fig. 22.2. The designation D- or L- refers to the position of the hydroxyl group on the carbon atom adjacent to the last (bottom) $CH_2OH$ group. In general, designations of D- and L- for a sugar molecule refer to the stereoisomeric forms of the highest-numbered asymmetrical carbon atom.[a] By convention, the D-sugars are written with the hydroxyl group on the right, and the L-sugars are written with the hydroxyl group on the left (see Fig. 22.2). Most sugars in the human body are of the D-configuration. Several different structures exist, depending on the relative positions of the hydroxyl groups on the carbon atoms.

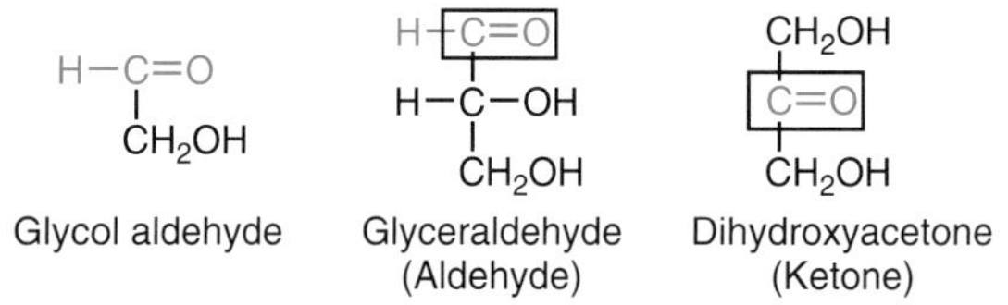

Fig. 22.1 Two- and three-carbon carbohydrates.

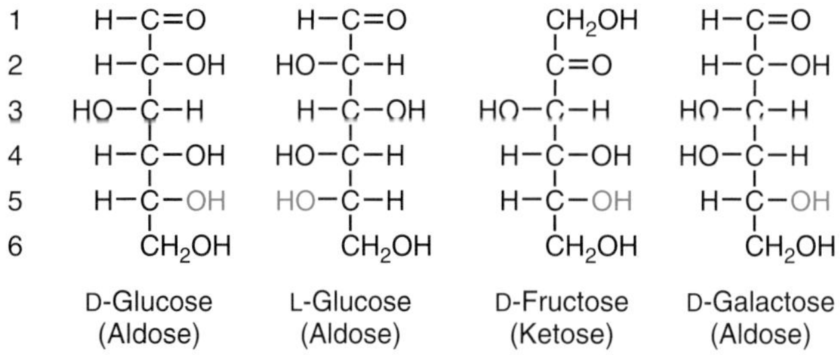

Fig. 22.2 Typical six-carbon sugars.

---

[a]Although the D and L designations are used in this chapter, readers should be aware that in the Cahn-Ingold-Prelog system, a series of rules determine configurations. In this new system, the symbols R and S are used to designate configurations.

The formula for glucose can be written in the form of aldehyde or enol, a short-lived reactive species. A shift to the enol anion is favored in alkaline solution, as follows:

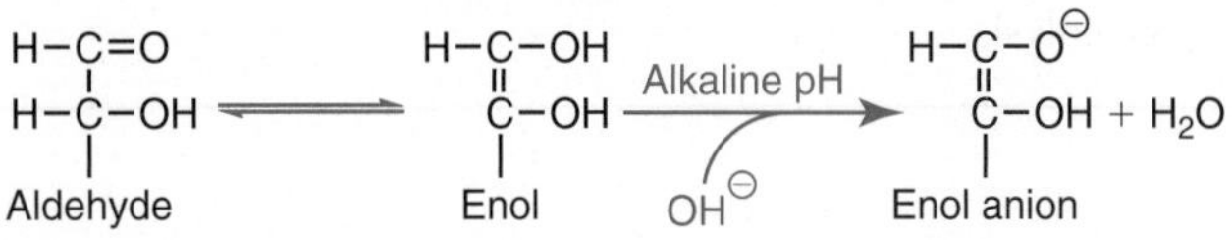

H–C=O          H–C–OH                    H–C–O⁻
H–C–OH   ⇌    C–OH    —Alkaline pH→     C–OH + H₂O
|              ||                         |
Aldehyde       Enol      OH⁻            Enol anion

The presence of a double bond and a negative charge in the enol anion makes glucose an active reducing substance that is oxidized by relatively mild oxidizing agents, such as cupric and ferric ions. Glucose in hot alkaline solution readily reduces cupric ions to cuprous ions. The color change has been used as a presumptive indication for the presence of glucose; for many years, blood and urine glucose concentrations were measured this way. Some other sugars also reduce cupric ions in alkaline solution; these are collectively referred to as *reducing sugars.*

The aldehyde group reacts with the hydroxyl group on carbon 5, represented by a symmetrical ring structure and depicted by the Haworth formula, in which glucose is considered as having the same basic structure as pyran (Fig. 22.3). In this formula, the plane of the ring is considered to be perpendicular to the plane of the paper, with the heavy lines pointing toward the reader. Hydroxyl groups in position 1 are then below the plane (α-configuration) or above the plane (β-configuration). A six-member ring sugar containing five carbons and one oxygen is a derivative of pyran and is called a *pyranose.* When linkage occurs with the formation of a five-member ring containing four carbons and one oxygen, the sugar has the same basic structure

as furan and is called a *furanose.* Fructose is shown in two cyclical forms. Fructopyranose is the configuration of the free sugar, and fructofuranose occurs whenever fructose exists in combination with disaccharides and polysaccharides, as in sucrose and inulin.

## Disaccharides

Two monosaccharides join covalently by an *O*-glycosidic bond, with loss of a molecule of water, to form a disaccharide. The chemical bond between the sugars always involves the aldehyde or ketone group of one monosaccharide joined to an alcohol group (e.g., maltose) or an aldehyde or ketone group (e.g., sucrose) of the other monosaccharide (Fig. 22.4). The most common disaccharides are as follows:

  Maltose = glucose + glucose
  Lactose = glucose + galactose
  Sucrose = glucose + fructose

If the linkage between two monosaccharides is between the aldehyde or ketone group of one molecule and a hydroxyl group of another molecule (as in maltose and lactose), one potentially free ketone or aldehyde group remains on the second monosaccharide. Consequently, the second glucose residue can be oxidized and is capable of existing in α- or β-pyranose form. Thus, the disaccharide is a reducing sugar, but its reducing power is only approximately 40% of the reducing power of the two single monosaccharides added together.

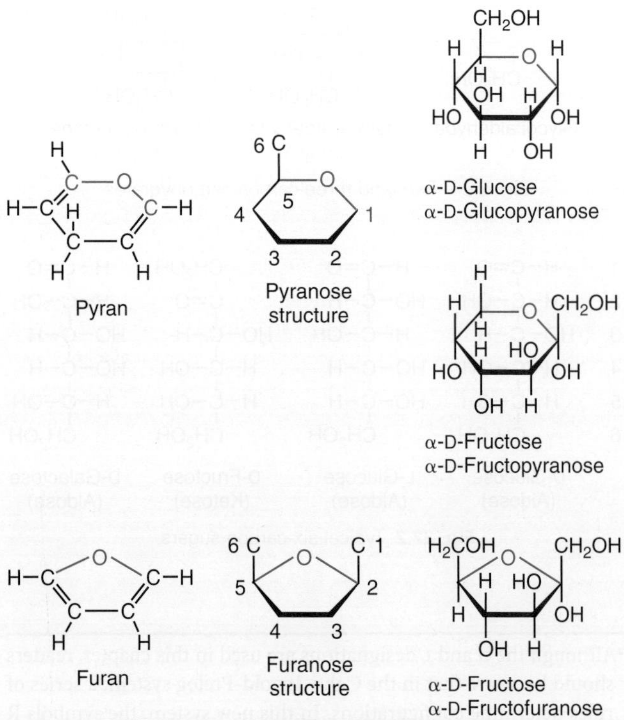

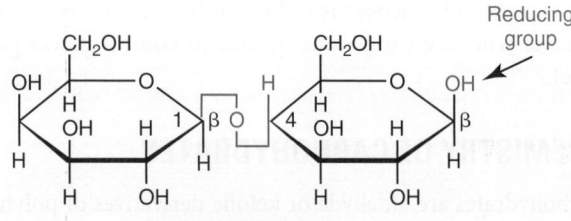

**Fig. 22.3** The Haworth formula for sugars.

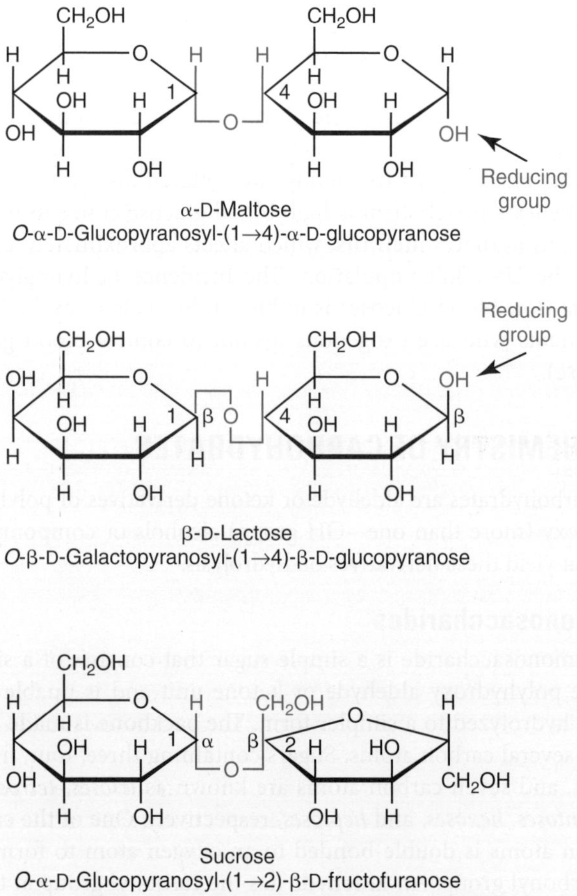

**Fig. 22.4** Structural formulas of disaccharides.

Alternatively, if the linkage between two monosaccharides involves the aldehyde or ketone groups of both molecules (as in sucrose), a nonreducing sugar is formed because no free aldehyde or ketone group remains.

## Polysaccharides

The linkage of multiple monosaccharide units results in the formation of polysaccharides. The major storage carbohydrates are starch in plants and glycogen in animals, both of which form granules inside cells. Polysaccharides can provide structural support. Cellulose is used by plants, whereas chitin is the principal component of the exoskeleton of arthropods (insects and crustacea).

### Starch and Glycogen

Most starches are composed of a mixture of amyloses and amylopectins. Amylose consists of one long, unbranched chain of glucose units linked together by α-1,4-linkages, with only the terminal aldehyde group free. In amylopectin, most of the units are joined by α-1,4-links, but α-1,6-glycosidic bonds also exist every 24 to 30 residues, producing sidechains. Amylopectin contains up to 1 million glucose residues. The structure of **glycogen** is similar to that of amylopectin, but branching is more extensive and is evident every 8 to 12 glucose residues. These branches enhance the solubility of glycogen and allow the glucose residues to be more readily mobilized. Glycogen is most abundant in the liver and is also found in skeletal muscle. The difference in structure between amylose and amylopectin is important in the selection of the appropriate starch substrate for amylase determinations (see Chapter 19). The rate of hydrolysis is affected by structural differences in the starch.

### Cellulose

Cellulose is an important structural polysaccharide in plants. It is an unbranched polymer of glucose residues joined by β-1,4-linkages. The β-configuration facilitates the formation of long, straight chains, producing fibers of high tensile strength. The β-1,4-linkages are not hydrolyzed by α-amylases. Because humans do not have cellulases, they are unable to digest vegetable fiber.

### Glycoproteins

Many integral membrane proteins have oligosaccharides covalently attached to the extracellular region, forming glycoproteins. In addition, most proteins that are secreted, such as antibodies, hormones, and coagulation factors, are glycoproteins. The number of attached carbohydrate residues varies among proteins and constitutes 1% to 70% of the weight of the glycoprotein. The oligosaccharides are attached by *O*-glycosidic linkages to the sidechain oxygen of serine or threonine residues or by *N*-glycosidic linkages to the sidechain nitrogen of asparagine residues.

One of the biological functions of the carbohydrate chains is to regulate the life span of proteins. Loss of sialic acid residues from the ends of oligosaccharide chains on erythrocytes results in the removal of red blood cells from the circulation. Carbohydrates have also been implicated in cell-cell recognition, in secretion, and in targeting of proteins to specific subcellular domains.

## BIOCHEMISTRY AND PHYSIOLOGY

Glucose is the primary energy source for the human body. After absorption (see Chapter 38), the metabolism of all hexoses proceeds according to the body's requirements. This metabolism results in (1) energy production by conversion to carbon dioxide and water, (2) storage as glycogen in the liver or as triglyceride in adipose tissue, or (3) conversion to keto acids, amino acids, or protein.

The complete picture of intermediary metabolism of carbohydrates is complex and interwoven with the metabolism of lipids and amino acids. For details, readers should consult a biochemistry textbook.

### Regulation of Blood Glucose Concentration

The concentration of glucose in the blood is regulated by a complex interplay of multiple pathways, modulated by several hormones. *Glycogenesis* is the name for the conversion of glucose to glycogen, the most important storage polysaccharide in liver and muscle. The reverse process, namely, the breakdown of glycogen to glucose and other intermediate products, is termed *glycogenolysis*. The formation of glucose from noncarbohydrate sources, such as amino acids, glycerol, or lactate, is termed *gluconeogenesis*. The conversion of glucose or other hexoses into lactate or pyruvate is called *glycolysis*. Further oxidation to carbon dioxide and water occurs through the Krebs (citric acid) cycle and the mitochondrial electron transport chain coupled to oxidative phosphorylation, which generates the adenosine triphosphate (ATP) that provides chemical energy for many bodily processes. Oxidation of glucose to carbon dioxide and water also occurs through the hexose monophosphate shunt pathway, which produces the reduced form of nicotinamide-adenine dinucleotide phosphate (NADPH).

### Hypoglycemia

**Hypoglycemia** is a blood glucose concentration below the fasting value, but the definition of a specific limit is difficult. The most widely used cutoff is 50 mg/dL (2.8 mmol/L), but some authors suggest 60 mg/dL (3.3 mmol/L). A glucose concentration of 70 mg/dL (3.9 mmol/L) or below should be an alert for hypoglycemia in an individual with diabetes mellitus. A transient decline may occur 1.5 to 2 hours after a meal, and it is not uncommon for plasma glucose concentrations as low as 50 mg/dL (2.8 mmol/L) to be observed 2 hours after ingestion of an oral glucose load. Similarly, extremely low fasting blood glucose values may be occasionally noted without symptoms or evidence of underlying disease. Hypoglycemia is rare in persons who do not have drug-treated diabetes mellitus.

Symptoms of hypoglycemia vary among individuals, and none is specific. Epinephrine produces the classic signs and symptoms of hypoglycemia, namely, trembling, sweating, nausea, rapid pulse, light-headedness, hunger, and epigastric discomfort. These autonomic symptoms are nonspecific and may be noted in other conditions, such as hyperthyroidism, pheochromocytoma, or even anxiety. Although controversial, some investigators have proposed that a rapid decrease in blood glucose concentrations may trigger the symptoms even though the blood glucose itself may not reach hypoglycemic values, whereas gradual onset to a similar glucose concentration may not produce symptoms.

The brain is completely dependent on blood glucose for energy production under physiological conditions, and approximately half of the glucose used in resting adults is in the central nervous system (CNS). Very low concentrations of blood glucose (<20 or 30 mg/dL; 1.1 or 1.7 mmol/L) cause severe CNS dysfunction. During prolonged fasting or hypoglycemia, ketones may be used as an energy source. The broad spectrum of symptoms and signs of CNS dysfunction range from headache, confusion, blurred vision, and dizziness to seizures, loss of consciousness, and even death; these symptoms are known as *neuroglycopenia*. Restoration of blood glucose usually produces prompt recovery, but irreversible damage may occur.

The age of onset of hypoglycemia is a convenient way to classify the disorder, but some overlap occurs among the various groups. For example, some glycogen storage disorders may arise in the third decade of life, and hormone deficiencies may occur in childhood.

## Hypoglycemia in Neonates and Infants

Neonatal blood glucose concentrations are much lower than those of adults (mean, ~35 mg/dL; 2.0 mmol/L) and decline shortly after birth when liver glycogen stores are depleted. Glucose concentrations as low as 30 mg/dL (1.7 mmol/L) in a term infant and 20 mg/dL (1.1 mmol/L) in a premature infant may occur without clinical evidence of hypoglycemia. The more common causes of hypoglycemia in the neonatal period include prematurity, maternal diabetes, gestational diabetes mellitus (GDM), and maternal toxemia/preeclampsia. These are usually transient. Hypoglycemia with onset in early infancy is usually less transitory and may be due to inborn errors of metabolism or ketotic hypoglycemia; this type of hypoglycemia usually develops after fasting or a febrile illness.

## Fasting Hypoglycemia in Adults

Hypoglycemia results from a decreased rate of hepatic glucose production or an increased rate of glucose use. Symptoms suggestive of hypoglycemia are fairly common, but hypoglycemic disorders are rare. However, true hypoglycemia usually indicates a serious underlying disease and may be life-threatening. An exact threshold for the establishment of hypoglycemia is not always possible, and values as low as 30 mg/dL (1.7 mmol/L) may be encountered in healthy, premenopausal women during the classic test—a 72-hour fast. Symptoms usually begin at plasma glucose concentrations below 55 mg/dL (3 mmol/L), and impairment of cerebral function begins when glucose is less than 50 mg/dL (2.8 mmol/L).

The 72-hour fast should be conducted in a hospital. During the fast, the patient should be allowed a liberal intake of calorie-free and caffeine-free fluids. Samples are typically drawn every 6 hours for analysis of plasma glucose, insulin, C-peptide, and proinsulin. When the plasma glucose concentration is 60 mg/dL (3.3 mmol/L) or less, analyses are performed every 1 to 2 hours. The fast should be concluded when the plasma glucose concentration falls to a predetermined concentration (such as 45 mg/dL [2.5 mmol/L] or less) or the patient exhibits signs or symptoms of hypoglycemia, or after 72 hours. Most patients with true hypoglycemia show an abnormally low value within 12 hours of beginning a fast. Women exhibit significantly lower glucose concentrations than men. Low plasma glucose alone is not sufficient to establish the diagnosis, and the absence of signs or symptoms of hypoglycemia during the fast excludes the diagnosis of a hypoglycemic disorder as the cause of such symptoms.

## Causes of Hypoglycemia

More than 100 causes of hypoglycemia have been reported. Drugs are the most prevalent cause, and many widely used drugs, including propranolol, salicylates, and disopyramide, produce hypoglycemia. Oral hypoglycemic agents, which have long half-lives (35 hours for chlorpropamide), are the most frequent cause of drug-induced hypoglycemia and may be directly measured in blood or urine. Surreptitious administration of insulin is detected by the discovery of low C-peptide concentrations with increased insulin concentrations.

Ethanol produces hypoglycemia by inhibiting gluconeogenesis, and this inhibition is aggravated by malnutrition (low glycogen stores) in individuals with chronic alcoholism. Individuals with hepatic failure (e.g., viral hepatitis, ingestions of toxins) have impaired gluconeogenesis or glycogen storage, which may result in hypoglycemia. Decreased hepatic glucose production requires dysfunction of more than 80% of the liver. Deficiencies of growth hormone (especially with coexistent adrenocorticotropic hormone [ACTH] deficiency), glucocorticoids, thyroid hormone, or glucagon may also produce hypoglycemia. Although a deficiency of glucocorticoids (e.g., Addison disease) is most consistently associated with hypoglycemia, most glucocorticoid-deficient adults are not hypoglycemic. Hormonal deficiency causes hypoglycemia in children more frequently than in adults.

Demonstration of a low plasma glucose concentration in the presence of a high plasma insulin value is highly suggestive of an insulin-producing pancreatic islet cell tumor. Because healthy people exhibit a wide range of insulin concentrations, absolute hyperinsulinemia occurs in less than 50% of individuals with insulinomas. Serum insulin concentrations inappropriately high for concurrent plasma glucose values denote autonomous insulin secretion. Provocative tests (glucagon, tolbutamide, or calcium) or suppression tests (infusion of insulin and measurement of C-peptide), although strongly recommended in the past, generally are not necessary.

Nonpancreatic neoplasms that cause hypoglycemia are rare, but when present, they are often extremely large mesenchymal neoplasms. No single mechanism explains the hypoglycemia in all cases, but secretion of a precursor of insulin-like growth factor 2 is the most commonly encountered finding. Glucose utilization is increased, especially in muscle, presumably reflecting activity of the hormone.

Hypoglycemia caused by septicemia should be relatively easy to diagnose. The mechanism is not well defined, but depleted glycogen stores, impaired gluconeogenesis, and increased peripheral use of glucose may all be contributing factors. Glucose tolerance is commonly depressed in individuals with renal disease, and hypoglycemia may occur in those with end-stage renal failure.

Some of the conditions that produce fasting hypoglycemia are readily apparent, but others require a lengthy diagnostic workup. Once fasting hypoglycemia is demonstrated, specific tests should be performed to establish the underlying cause. The oral glucose tolerance test (OGTT) is not an appropriate study for evaluation of a patient suspected of having hypoglycemia.

## Postprandial Hypoglycemia

Drugs, antibodies to insulin or the insulin receptor, inborn errors (e.g., fructose-1,6-diphosphatase deficiency), and *reactive hypoglycemia* (also referred to as *functional hypoglycemia*) produce hypoglycemia in the postprandial (fed) state. It has been proposed that for individuals with vague symptoms after food ingestion, the preferred terminology should be *idiopathic reactive hypoglycemia* or *idiopathic postprandial syndrome*.

At the Third International Symposium on Hypoglycemia, reactive hypoglycemia was defined as a "clinical disorder in which the patient has postprandial symptoms suggesting hypoglycemia that occur in everyday life and are accompanied by a blood glucose concentration less than 45 to 50 mg/dL (2.5 to 2.8 mmol/L) as determined by a specific glucose measurement on arterialized venous or capillary blood, respectively." Patients complain of autonomic symptoms that occur approximately 1 to 3 hours after eating and seem to obtain relief, lasting 30 to 45 minutes, by food intake. These symptoms are rarely due to low blood glucose concentrations. A 5- or 6-hour glucose tolerance test had been the standard procedure to establish the presence of postprandial hypoglycemia, but that has been discredited. Consequently, an *OGTT should not be used in the diagnosis of reactive hypoglycemia.*

Postprandial hypoglycemia is infrequent, and demonstration of hypoglycemia during spontaneously occurring symptomatic episodes is necessary to establish the diagnosis. If this is not possible, a 5-hour meal tolerance test (which simulates the composition of a normal diet) or a "hyperglucidic" (high-glucose) breakfast test has been proposed.

The diagnosis of hypoglycemia has also been used to explain a wide variety of disorders that appear unrelated to blood glucose abnormalities. These nonspecific symptoms include fatigue, muscle spasms, palpitations, numbness, tingling, pain, sweating, mental dullness, sleepiness, weakness, and fainting. Behavioral abnormalities, poor school performance, and delinquency have been incorrectly attributed to low blood glucose concentrations. A diagnosis of hypoglycemia should not be made unless a patient meets the criteria of *Whipple's triad of low blood glucose concentration:* (1) symptoms known or likely to be caused by hypoglycemia, (2) low glucose measured when symptoms occur, and (3) relief of symptoms when glucose is increased to normal. Demonstration of normal plasma glucose concentration

when the patient exhibits symptoms excludes the possibility of a hypoglycemic disorder.

## Hypoglycemia in Diabetes Mellitus

Hypoglycemia occurs frequently in individuals with type 1 or type 2 diabetes. The American Diabetes Association (ADA) classifies hypoglycemia in diabetes into three levels: level 1, glucose less than 70 mg/dL (3.9 mmol/L) and ≥54 mg/dL (3.0 mmol/L); level 2, glucose less than 54 mg/dL (3.0 mmol/L); and level 3, a severe event with altered mental/physical status that requires assistance for treatment of hypoglycemia. Patients using insulin experience approximately one to two episodes of symptomatic hypoglycemia per week, and severe hypoglycemia that requires assistance from others or is associated with loss of consciousness (level 3) affects about 10% of this population per year. In patients practicing intensive insulin therapy (e.g., multiple injections, continuous subcutaneous insulin infusion), these figures are increased twofold to sixfold. The chief adverse event associated with intensive therapy in the Diabetes Control and Complications Trial (DCCT) was a threefold increase in the incidence of severe hypoglycemia. Similarly, hypoglycemia occurs in patients with type 2 diabetes (caused by oral hypoglycemic agents or insulin) but is less frequent than in type 1 diabetes. Defective glucose counterregulation (ability to increase glucose counter to the effect of insulin) and hypoglycemia unawareness are two pathophysiological mechanisms that contribute to hypoglycemia in patients with diabetes.

*Defective glucose counterregulation.* Counterregulatory responses become impaired in patients with type 1 diabetes, increasing the risk of hypoglycemia. The secretion of glucagon in response to hypoglycemia is impaired by an unknown mechanism early in the course of type 1 diabetes. The secretory response of epinephrine to hypoglycemia becomes deficient later in the course of the disease. These defects are selective because other stimuli continue to elicit glucagon and epinephrine secretion. Glucose counterregulation does not appear to be notably defective in patients with type 2 diabetes.

*Hypoglycemia unawareness.* Up to 50% of patients with long-standing (longer than 30 years) type 1 diabetes do not experience neurogenic warning symptoms and are prone to more severe hypoglycemia. The mechanism is thought to be associated with a decreased epinephrine response to hypoglycemia. Intensively treated patients with type 1 diabetes require lower plasma glucose concentrations to elicit symptoms of hypoglycemia. Some authors have claimed that therapeutic use of human insulin rather than other insulins results in an increased incidence of ignorance of hypoglycemia, but analysis of 45 studies revealed no significant differences in hypoglycemic episodes among insulin species.

## Lactate and Pyruvate

Lactic acid, an intermediary in carbohydrate metabolism, is predominantly derived from white skeletal muscle, brain, skin, renal medulla, and erythrocytes. The blood lactate concentration depends on the rate of production in these tissues and the rate of metabolism in the liver and kidneys. The liver uses approximately 65% (75 g/day) of the total basal lactate produced, predominantly in gluconeogenesis. The Cori cycle is the conversion of glucose to lactate in the periphery and reconversion of lactate to glucose in the liver. Extrahepatic removal of lactate occurs by oxidation in red skeletal muscle and the renal cortex. A moderate increase in lactate production results in increased hepatic lactate clearance, but uptake by the liver is saturable when concentrations exceed 18 mg/dL (2 mmol/L). During strenuous exercise, for example, lactate concentrations may increase significantly, from an average concentration of about 8 mg/dL (0.9 mmol/L) to more than 180 mg/dL (20 mmol/L) within 10 seconds. No concentration of lactate is uniformly accepted for the diagnosis of lactic acidosis, but lactate concentrations exceeding 45 mg/dL (5 mmol/L) with a pH less than 7.25 indicate significant lactic acidosis.

Pyruvate is one of the critical metabolites in cells, most of which originates from anaerobic glycolysis. It is further metabolized by four enzyme systems, namely (1) alanine aminotransferase (alanine production), (2) pyruvate carboxylase (the major regulatory enzyme in gluconeogenesis), (3) lactate dehydrogenase (lactate formation), and (4) pyruvate dehydrogenase. The last is a complex of enzymes that decarboxylate pyruvate in the presence of oxygen to acetyl coenzyme A (CoA), allowing entry into the citric acid cycle.

Measurement of pyruvate is useful in the evaluation of patients with inborn errors of metabolism who have increased serum lactate concentrations. A lactate-to-pyruvate ratio of less than 25 suggests a defect in gluconeogenesis, whereas an increased ratio (≥35) indicates reduced intracellular conditions found in hypoxia. Inborn errors associated with an increased lactate-to-pyruvate ratio include pyruvate carboxylase deficiency and defects in oxidative phosphorylation. Pyruvate is also measured in clinical studies evaluating reperfusion after myocardial ischemia and increased cerebrospinal fluid (CSF) pyruvate was reported in patients with Alzheimer disease.

## Lactic Acidosis

Lactic acidosis occurs in two clinical settings: (1) type A (hypoxic), associated with decreased tissue oxygenation, such as shock, hypovolemia, and left ventricular failure; and (2) type B (metabolic), associated with disease (e.g., diabetes mellitus, neoplasia, liver disease), drugs/toxins (e.g., ethanol, methanol, salicylates), or inborn errors of metabolism. Lactic acidosis is not uncommon and occurs in approximately 1% of those admitted to the hospital. It has a mortality rate greater than 60%, which approaches 100% if hypotension is also present. Type A is much more common.

The mechanism of type B lactic acidosis is not known but is speculated to be a primary defect in mitochondrial function with impaired oxygen use. This leads to reduced stores of ATP and nicotinamide adenine dinucleotide ($NAD^+$), with accumulations of NADH and $H^+$. In the presence of decreased liver perfusion or liver disease, lactate removal from the blood is reduced, thereby aggravating the lactic acidosis.

An uncommon but often undiagnosed cause of lactic acidosis is D-lactic acidosis. Humans were initially thought to be unable to produce D-lactate, but normal individuals have a large capacity to metabolize D-lactate. Absorption and accumulation of D-lactate from abnormal intestinal bacteria may cause systemic acidosis. This condition occurs after jejunoileal bypass surgery and manifests as altered mental status (from mild drowsiness to coma) with increased blood concentrations of D-lactate. With the acceptance of gastric bypass surgery for the treatment of type 2 diabetes and obesity, D-lactic acidosis is likely to become more common. Virtually all the commonly used laboratory assays for lactate use L-lactate dehydrogenase, which does not detect D-lactate. D-Lactate can be measured by gas-liquid chromatography or enzymatically with a specific D-lactate dehydrogenase.

Lactate in CSF normally parallels blood concentrations. With biochemical alterations in the CNS, however, CSF lactate values change independently of blood values. Increased CSF concentrations are noted in individuals with cerebrovascular accidents, intracranial hemorrhage, bacterial meningitis, epilepsy, and other CNS disorders. In aseptic (viral) meningitis, lactate concentrations in CSF are not usually increased; hence, CSF lactate has been used to help discriminate between viral and bacterial meningitis, but the clinical utility has been questioned. In a few children with inherited metabolic diseases, CSF lactate concentrations may be increased despite plasma lactate in the reference interval.

## Inborn Errors of Carbohydrate Metabolism

Deficiency or absence of an enzyme that participates in carbohydrate metabolism may result in accumulation of monosaccharides, which can be measured in the urine. Most of these conditions are inherited as autosomal recessive traits. Sugars frequently appear in the urine as a result of excessive consumption, without the presence of underlying disease.

Techniques used to separate and identify sugars have included fermentation, optical rotation, osazone formation with phenylhydrazine, specific chemical tests, and paper or thin-layer chromatography. The availability of glucose oxidase test strips, specific for glucose, has greatly simplified the differentiation of glucose from other reducing substances. For practical purposes, the urinary sugars of clinical interest are glucose and galactose. Urine from infants and children should be tested by both the glucose oxidase and copper reduction tests to identify individuals with inborn errors of metabolism. Reducing substances other than glucose should be further identified by chromatographic procedures.

## Glycogen Storage Disease

Glycogen, although present in most tissues, is stored predominantly in the liver and skeletal muscle. During fasting, liver glycogen is converted to glucose to provide energy for the whole body. In contrast, skeletal muscle lacks glucose-6-phosphatase, and muscle glycogen can be used only locally for energy. Glycogen storage disease is a generic name encompassing at least 12 rare inherited disorders of glycogen storage in tissues. The different forms of glycogen storage disease are categorized by numerical type in the chronological sequence in which these defects were identified. Each form is due to a deficiency of a specific enzyme in glycogen metabolism, producing a quantitative or qualitative defect in glycogen storage. Numerous mutations have been identified in patients with these conditions.

Because liver and skeletal muscle have the highest rates of glycogen metabolism, these tissues are most affected. The liver forms (types I, III, IV, VI, and IX), which comprise approximately 80% of the total, are marked by hepatomegaly (due to increased liver glycogen stores) and hypoglycemia (caused by inability to convert glycogen to glucose). Hypoglycemia manifests with autonomic clinical symptoms (sweating, shakiness, and a light-headed feeling), growth retardation, and laboratory findings of decreased insulin and increased glucagon concentrations in the blood. By contrast, the muscle forms (types II, V, and VII) have mild symptoms that usually appear in young adulthood during strenuous exercise as a result of the inability to provide energy for muscle contraction. Other muscle disorders may exhibit similar symptoms, but are readily differentiated through evaluation of glycogen stores. The specific diagnosis of each type is made directly by demonstrating the enzyme defect in tissue.

## ANALYTICAL METHODOLOGY

Analytical methods for measuring glucose, lactate, and pyruvate are discussed in this section. Methods for measuring insulin, proinsulin, and glucagon are discussed in Chapter 33.

### Measurement of Glucose in Body Fluids

Several methods are used to measure glucose in blood, serum, plasma, and urine. The College of American Pathologists (CAP) surveys demonstrate that all methods exhibit a coefficient of variation (CV) among laboratories that is less than 3.0% for glucose values on lyophilized serum.

### Specimen Collection and Storage

In individuals with a normal hematocrit, the fasting whole-blood glucose concentration is approximately 10% to 12% lower than plasma glucose. Although the glucose concentrations in the water phases of red blood cells and plasma are similar (the erythrocyte plasma membrane is freely permeable to glucose), the water content of plasma (93%) is approximately 11% greater than that of whole blood at a normal hematocrit. In most clinical laboratories, plasma or serum is used for most glucose determinations; methods for self-monitoring of glucose use whole-blood samples but may measure the glucose concentration in the plasma phase. During fasting, the capillary blood glucose concentration is only 2 to 5 mg/dL (0.1 to 0.3 mmol/L) higher than that of the venous blood. After a glucose load, however, capillary blood glucose concentrations are 20 to 70 mg/dL (1.0 to 3.9 mmol/L; mean, ≈30 mg/dL [1.7 mmol/L]; equivalent to 20% to 25%) higher than the concentrations in concurrently drawn venous blood samples, probably due to glucose consumption in the tissues.

Glycolysis decreases serum glucose by approximately 5% to 7% in 1 hour (5 to 10 mg/dL; 0.3 to 0.6 mmol/L) in normal uncentrifuged coagulated blood at room temperature. The rate of in vitro glycolysis is higher in the presence of leukocytosis or bacterial contamination. In separated, nonhemolyzed sterile serum, the glucose concentration is generally stable for as long as 8 hours at 25°C and up to 72 hours at 4°C; variable stability is observed with longer storage periods. Plasma, removed from the cells after moderate centrifugation, contains leukocytes that also metabolize glucose, although cell-free sterile plasma has no glycolytic activity.

Sodium fluoride or, less commonly, sodium iodoacetate is used to inhibit glycolysis. Fluoride ions prevent glycolysis by inhibiting enolase, an enzyme that requires $Mg^{2+}$. Inhibition is due to the formation of an ionic complex consisting of $Mg^{2+}$, inorganic phosphate, and fluoride ions; this complex interferes with the interaction of enzyme and substrate. Fluoride is also a weak anticoagulant because it binds calcium; however, clotting may occur after several hours, and it is therefore advisable to use a *combined fluoride-oxalate mixture,* such as 2 mg of potassium oxalate ($K_2C_2O_4$) and 2 mg of NaF/mL of blood, to prevent late clotting. Other anticoagulants (e.g., ethylenediaminetetraacetic acid or EDTA, citrate, heparin) can also be used. Fluoride ions in high concentration inhibit the activity of urease and certain other enzymes; consequently, the specimens may be unsuitable for determination of urea in procedures that require urease and for direct assay of some serum enzymes. $K_2C_2O_4$ causes a loss of cell water, thereby diluting the plasma. Samples collected in these tubes should therefore not be used for measurement of other analytes.

Although fluoride has been widely used to inhibit glycolysis, the rate of decline in the first 1 to 2 hours after sample collection is not altered, and glycolysis continues for up to 4 hours. Tubes with only fluoride-oxalate are not adequate to inhibit glycolysis. Moreover, inhibitors of glycolysis are necessary in patients with greatly increased leukocyte counts because differences of up to 65 mg/dL (3.6 mmol/L) have been observed between glucose values with and without glycolytic inhibitors after 1 to 2 hours of contact with the blood cells.

Acidification of blood with a sodium citrate buffer inhibits in vitro glycolysis more effectively than fluoride. Therefore, a tube containing a rapidly effective inhibitor, such as granulated citrate buffer (pH 5.3 to 5.9) with sodium fluoride and EDTA, should be used. While these are commercially available in several countries, especially in Europe, they are not available in the United States at the time of writing. When citrate tubes are not available, the sample tube should immediately be placed in an ice-water slurry and subjected to centrifugation to remove the cells within 15 to 30 minutes. Tubes with only fluoride do not adequately impair glycolysis.

CSF may be contaminated with bacteria or other cells and should be analyzed immediately for glucose. If a delay in measurement is unavoidable, the sample should be centrifuged and stored at 4°C or at −20°C.

In 24-hour collections of urine, glucose may be preserved by adding 5 mL of glacial acetic acid to the container before starting the collection. The final pH of the urine is usually between 4 and 5, which inhibits bacterial activity. Other preservatives that have been proposed include 5 g of sodium benzoate per 24-hour specimen, or chlorhexidine and 0.1% sodium nitrate with 0.01% benzethonium chloride. These may be inadequate, and urine should be stored at 4°C during collection. Urine samples may lose as much as 40% of their glucose after 24 hours at room temperature.

## Measurement of Glucose in Blood

Hexokinase (HK), or glucose oxidase, is widely used in assays to measure the concentration of glucose in body fluids.

*Hexokinase methods.* HK methods are based on a coupled enzyme assay that uses HK and glucose-6-phosphate dehydrogenase.

$$\text{Glucose} + \text{ATP} \xrightleftharpoons{\text{Hexokinase}} \text{Glucose-6-phosphate} + \text{ADP}$$

$$\text{Glucose-6-phosphate} \xrightleftharpoons[\phantom{xx}]{\text{G-6-PD}} \text{6-Phosphogluconate}$$

$$\text{NADP}^{\oplus} \quad\quad \text{NADPH} + \text{H}^{\oplus}$$
$$(\text{or NAD}^{\oplus}) \quad\quad (\text{or NADH})$$

As indicated, glucose is first phosphorylated by ATP in the presence of HK and $Mg^{2+}$. The glucose-6-phosphate formed is oxidized by G6PD to 6-phosphogluconate in the presence of $NADP^+$ or $NAD^+$. The amount of reduced NADP (NADPH) or NADH produced is directly proportional to the amount of glucose in the sample and is measured by the increase in absorbance at 340 nm. $NADP^+$ is the cofactor when G6PD derived from yeast is used in the assay; $NAD^+$ is the cofactor when bacterial *(Leuconostoc mesenteroides)* G6PD is used. A reference method based on this principle has been developed and validated. In the reference method, serum or plasma is deproteinated by the addition of solutions of barium hydroxide and zinc sulfate. The clear supernatant is mixed with a reagent containing ATP, $NAD^+$, HK, and G6PD, incubated at 25°C until the reaction is complete, and NADH is measured. Calibrators and blanks are carried through the entire procedure, including the deproteination step.

Although highly accurate and precise, the reference method is too exacting and time-consuming for routine use in a clinical laboratory. An alternative approach is to apply the reaction directly to serum or plasma and use a specimen blank to correct for interfering substances that absorb at 340 nm.

Serum or plasma may be used. Sodium fluoride (NaF), with an anticoagulant such as EDTA, heparin, oxalate, or citrate, may be used. Hemolyzed specimens containing more than 0.5 g of hemoglobin/dL are unsatisfactory because phosphate esters and enzymes released from red blood cells interfere with the assay. Other sources of interference include drugs, bilirubin, and lipemia (triglycerides of 500 mg/dL [~5.7 mmol/L] or greater causing a positive interference).

Absorbances of sample or calibrator reaction mixtures are measured after the reactions have continued to completion (steady-state reaction, "end-point" method) or at a fixed time after initiation of the reaction (fixed-time kinetics). In the steady state, end-point methods for glucose concentrations may be calculated directly, based on the molar absorptivity of NADPH or NADH, but inclusion of a set of calibrators is recommended to detect possible deterioration of enzymes, ATP, $NADP^+$, or $NAD^+$—all of which are unstable. Reagents may also contain substances that react with the coenzymes. The presence of these substances is evaluated by measurement of the increase in absorbance observed in a reagent blank. The highest calibrator provides a check on the linearity of the response and the adequacy of the enzyme reagent. The procedures typically show a linear relation between absorbance and glucose concentrations of 0 to 500 mg/dL (0 to 28 mmol/L). Serum or plasma samples with glucose concentrations that exceed 500 mg/dL (28 mmol/L) should be diluted (usually with isotonic saline) and reassayed.

Also available are HK procedures in which indicator reactions produce colored products, enabling absorbance measurements in the visible range. An oxidation-reduction system containing phenazine methosulfate and a substituted tetrazolium compound, 2-(*p*-iodophenyl)-3-*p*-nitrophenyl-5-phenyltetrazolium chloride (INT), is reacted with NADPH formed in the reaction. The reduced INT is colored, with maximal absorbance at 520 nm.

*Glucose oxidase methods.* Glucose oxidase catalyzes the oxidation of glucose to gluconic acid and hydrogen peroxide:

$$\text{Glucose} + \text{H}_2\text{O} + \text{O}_2 \xrightarrow{\text{Glucose Oxidase}} \text{Gluconic acid} + 2\text{H}_2\text{O}_2$$

Addition of the enzyme peroxidase and a chromogenic oxygen acceptor, such as *o*-dianisidine, results in the formation of a colored compound that is measured:

$$o-\text{Dianisidine} + \text{H}_2\text{O}_2 \xrightarrow{\text{Peroxidase}} \text{Oxidized } o-\text{Dianisidine} + \text{H}_2\text{O} \text{ (Colored)}$$

Glucose oxidase is highly specific for β-D-glucose. Because 36% and 64% of glucose in solution are in the α- and β-forms, respectively, complete reaction requires mutarotation of the α-form to the β-form. Some commercial preparations of glucose oxidase contain an enzyme, mutarotase, which accelerates this reaction. Otherwise, extended incubation time allows spontaneous conversion.

The second step, involving peroxidase, is much less specific than the glucose oxidase reaction. Various substances, such as uric acid, ascorbic acid, bilirubin, hemoglobin, tetracycline, and glutathione, inhibit the reaction (presumably by competing with the chromogen for $H_2O_2$), producing lower values. Some glucose oxidase preparations contain catalase as a contaminant; catalase activity decomposes peroxide and decreases the intensity of the final color obtained. Calibrators and unknowns should be simultaneously analyzed under conditions in which the rate of oxidation is proportional to the glucose concentration.

Glucose oxidase methods are suitable for measurement of glucose in CSF. Urine, however, contains high concentrations of substances (such as uric acid) that interfere with the peroxidase reaction, producing falsely low results. Therefore, the glucose oxidase method should not be used for urine. A method in which the urine is first pretreated with an ion exchange resin to remove interfering substances has been described.

Some instruments use a polarographic oxygen electrode that measures the rate of oxygen consumption after the sample is added to a solution containing glucose oxidase. Because this measurement involves only the glucose oxidase reaction, interferences encountered in the peroxidase step are eliminated. To prevent formation of oxygen from $H_2O_2$ by catalase present in some preparations of glucose oxidase, $H_2O_2$ is removed by two additional reactions:

$$H_2O_2 + C_2H_5OH \xrightarrow{\text{Catalase}} CH_3CHO + 2H_2O$$

$$H_2O_2 + 2H^+ + 2I^- \xrightarrow{\text{Molybdate}} I_2 + 2H_2O$$

The latter reaction is effective even when catalase activity has diminished on storage of reagents. The procedure has been applied directly to urine, serum, plasma, or CSF. However, this approach should not be used for determination of glucose in whole blood because blood cells consume oxygen.

In dry, multilayer, slide-automated systems, glucose is measured by a glucose oxidase procedure. A 10-µL sample of serum, plasma, urine, or CSF is placed on a porous film on top of the layer containing the reagents. Glucose diffuses through the film and reacts with the reagents to produce a colored end product or dye. The intensity of this dye is measured through a lower transparent film by reflectance spectrophotometry. Advantages include small sample sizes, no liquid reagents, and improved stability on storage.

*Glucose dehydrogenase method.* The enzyme glucose dehydrogenase (β-D-glucose: NAD oxidoreductase, EC 1.1.1.47) catalyzes the oxidation of glucose to gluconolactone with concomitant reduction of $NAD^+$ to NADH. Mutarotase is added to shorten the time necessary to reach equilibrium. The amount of NADH generated is proportional to the glucose concentration. The reaction appears to be highly specific for glucose, shows no interference from common anticoagulants and substances normally found in serum, and provides results in close agreement with HK procedures. The glucose dehydrogenase procedure is not widely used in the United States, except in a glucose meter.

## Measurement of Glucose in Urine

Examination of urine for glucose is rapid, inexpensive, and noninvasive and has been used to screen large numbers of samples. Monitoring of urine glucose lacks sensitivity and specificity and provides no information about blood glucose concentrations below the renal threshold (usually 180 mg/dL; 10 mmol/L). Older screening tests detect all sugars that reduce copper. Unfortunately, these tests also react with reducing substances other than glucose. Qualitative, quantitative, and semiquantitative methods are widely available for

measuring glucose in urine and have essentially replaced the nonspecific tests in adults. Note that a reducing sugar method other than an enzymatic method for glucose must be used when neonates or infants are screened for inborn errors of metabolism that result in the appearance of reducing sugars other than glucose (e.g., galactose, fructose) in the urine.

*Qualitative method for measurement of total reducing substances.* Benedict qualitative reagent contains cupric ion complexed to citrate in alkaline solution. Reducing substances convert cupric to cuprous ions, forming yellow cuprous hydroxide or red cuprous oxide. A convenient adaptation of the procedure marketed in tablet form (Clinitest) has been discontinued.

*Semiquantitative measurement of glucose in urine.* Convenient paper test strips are commercially available from several manufacturers. Examples are Clinistix, Diastix, and Chemstrip. All use the glucose-specific enzyme glucose oxidase in a chromogenic assay. For example, Clinistix has filter paper impregnated with glucose oxidase, peroxidase, and the dye o-toluidine. Other dyes, such as tetramethylbenzidine, can be used. The test end of the strip is moistened with freshly voided urine and is examined after 10 seconds. A blue color develops if glucose is present at a concentration of 100 mg/dL or greater. Results are read by comparing the test color with a standard color chart. Automated urinalysis systems capable of analyzing 300 strips per hour are commercially available. The test is more sensitive for glucose than is the copper reduction test (Clinitest), which has a detection limit of 250 mg/dL (~14 mmol/L).

False-positive results may be produced by contamination of urine with $H_2O_2$ or a strong oxidizing agent, such as hypochlorite (bleach). False-negative results may occur with large quantities of reducing substances, such as ketones, ascorbic acid, and salicylates. For routine examinations, a negative result by the strip test is usually interpreted to mean that the urine specimen is negative for glucose.

Other strip tests (such as Multistix 10 SG) are designed for the semiquantitative estimation of 10 analytes, including glucose and ketone bodies. The glucose portion of the strip uses the glucose oxidase–peroxidase method. The hydrogen peroxide produced oxidizes iodide to iodine, yielding various intensities of brown that correspond to increasing concentrations of glucose in the urine. The detection limit is 100 mg/dL (5.5 mmol/L).

*Quantitative methods for determination of glucose in urine.* Applications of various procedures for quantitative determination of glucose in urine were previously discussed in the section on the determination of glucose in body fluids. HK or glucose dehydrogenase procedures are recommended for greatest accuracy and specificity. Glucose oxidase procedures that depend only on the consumption of oxygen or the production of $H_2O_2$ are also reliable. Glucose oxidase procedures that include the $H_2O_2$-peroxidase reaction are not used for urine.

## Reference Intervals

Although glucose is assayed by several different analytical procedures, reference intervals do not vary significantly among methods. The following values are representative of glucose assays:

## Sample Reference Intervals for Fasting Glucose

Plasma/Serum
| | |
|---|---|
| Adults | 74–99 mg/dL (4.1–5.5 mmol/L) |
| Children | 60–100 mg/dL (3.5–5.5 mmol/L) |
| Premature neonates | 20–60 mg/dL (1.1–3.3 mmol/L) |
| Term neonates | 30–60 mg/dL (1.7–3.3 mmol/L) |
| Whole blood | 65–95 mg/dL (3.6–5.3 mmol/L) |
| Cerebrospinal fluid | 40–70 mg/dL (60% of plasma value) (2.2–3.9 mmol/L) |

Urine
| | |
|---|---|
| 24 h | 1–15 mg/dL (0.1–0.8 mmol/L) |

Note that the ADA and World Health Organization (WHO) criteria of fasting glucose of 126 mg/dL (7.0 mmol/L) or greater—not the reference interval—are used for the diagnosis of diabetes. Moreover, the threshold for diagnosis of hypoglycemia is variable and is considerably less than the lower limit of the reference interval. No sex difference exists. Plasma glucose concentrations increase with age from the third to sixth decade—fasting approximately 2 mg/dL (0.1 mmol/L) per decade; postprandial 4 mg/dL (0.2 mmol/L) per decade; and after a glucose challenge, 8 to 13 mg/dL (0.4 to 0.7 mmol/L) per decade.

CSF glucose concentrations should be approximately 60% of plasma concentrations and must always be compared with concurrently measured plasma glucose for adequate clinical interpretation.

## Measurement of Lactate and Pyruvate in Body Fluids

### Determination of Lactate in Whole Blood

Lactate is oxidized to pyruvate by lactate dehydrogenase in the presence of $NAD^+$. The NADH formed in this reaction is measured spectrophotometrically at 340 nm and serves as a measure of the lactate concentration:

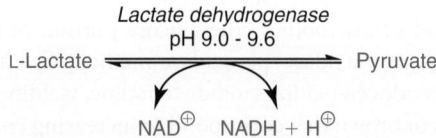

The equilibrium of the reaction normally lies far to the left. However, by buffering the pH between 9.0 and 9.6, adding an excess of $NAD^+$, and trapping the reaction product pyruvate with hydrazine, the equilibrium can be shifted to the right. Pyruvate can also be removed through a reaction with L-glutamate in the presence of alanine aminotransferase.

Because of its high specificity and simplicity, the enzymatic method is the method of choice for the measurement of lactate, although other methods may also be used (e.g., gas chromatography).

The Vitros analyzer, formerly the Ektachem, uses an assay in which lactic acid is oxidized to pyruvate by lactate oxidase. The $H_2O_2$ generated oxidizes a chromogen system, and the absorbance of the resulting dye complex, measured

spectrophotometrically at 540 nm, is directly proportional to the lactate concentration in the specimen. Each mole of lactate that is oxidized produces 0.5 mol of dye complex.

***Specimen collection and storage.*** Careful techniques are necessary to prevent changes in lactate concentration while blood is drawn and afterward. Patients should be fasting and at complete rest for at least 2 hours to allow lactate concentrations to reach a steady state.

Venous specimens should be obtained without the use of a tourniquet or immediately after the tourniquet has been applied. Alternatively, the tourniquet should be removed after the puncture has been performed, and the blood should be allowed to flow for several minutes before the sample is withdrawn. Arterial blood sampling, which prevents these potential pitfalls, may also be used. Patients should avoid exercise of the hand or arm immediately before and during the procedure.

Both venous and arterial blood may be collected in heparinized syringes and immediately delivered into a premeasured amount of chilled protein precipitant, such as trichloroacetic acid, metaphosphoric acid, or perchloric acid. The clear supernatant, after centrifugation, is stable at 4°C for as long as 8 days. Meticulous attention to sample preparation is required. If blood is not preserved as directed, lactate rapidly increases in the blood as a result of glycolysis. Increases may be as great as 20% within 3 minutes and 70% within 30 minutes at 25°C. Specimens collected as described in this section are also suitable for the determination of pyruvate.

If a plasma specimen is required, blood should be collected in a tube containing 10 mg of NaF and 2 mg of $K_2C_2O_4$ per milliliter of blood. Ideally, the specimen should be immediately cooled and the cells separated within 15 minutes, but reasonable stability of volunteers' lactate is seen at room temperature for 30 minutes in whole blood with NaF. Once the plasma is separated from the cells, lactate is stable.

***Reference intervals.*** The reference intervals for lactate in adults are as follows:

| | **LACTATE** | |
|---|---|---|
| **Specimen** | **mmol/L** | **mg/dL** |
| Venous Blood | | |
| At rest | 0.3–2.0 | 2.7–18 |
| Arterial Blood | | |
| At rest | 0.3–1.5 | 2.7–13.5 |

Laboratories should verify that these ranges are appropriate for use in their own settings.

Individuals in the hospital exhibit a wider range of values. Lactic acidosis occurs with blood lactate concentrations exceeding 5 mmol/L (45 mg/dL). Severe exercise dramatically increases lactate concentrations, and even movement of leg muscles by individuals at bed rest may result in significant increases. Plasma values are about 7% higher than those in whole blood, although differences depend on the procedure used. CSF values are usually similar to blood concentrations but may change independently in CNS disorders. Age-related reference intervals for CSF lactate (and lactate-to-pyruvate ratios) have been established in children. The upper limit of the reference interval (90th percentile) for CSF lactate in children in hospitals from birth to 15.5 years varies continuously from 16 to 17 mg/dL (1.78 to 1.88 mmol/L). Normal 24-hour urine output of lactate is 5.5 to 22 mmol/dL.

### Determination of Pyruvate in Whole Blood

The reaction involved in the determination of pyruvate is essentially the reverse of the reaction used in the lactate procedure:

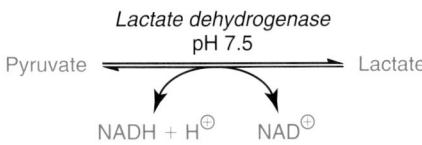

At about pH 7.5, the equilibrium constant strongly favors the reaction to the right. The method is very specific, and 2-oxoglutarate, oxaloacetate, acetoacetate, and β-hydroxybutyrate do not interfere as with colorimetric methods. Pyruvate is extremely unstable in blood, more so than lactate; immediate use of a chilled protein precipitant is recommended.

Fasting venous blood, drawn when the individual is at rest, has a pyruvate concentration of 0.3 to 0.9 mg/dL (0.03 to 0.10 mmol/L). Arterial blood contains 0.2 to 0.7 mg/dL (0.02 to 0.08 mmol/L). Values for CSF are 0.5 to 1.7 mg/dL (0.06 to 0.19 mmol/L). Urine output of pyruvate is normally 1 mmol/dL or less. Few clinical indications warrant the measurement of blood or urine pyruvate concentrations.

## REVIEW QUESTIONS

1. What is the formation of glucose from noncarbohydrate sources termed?
   a. Gluconeogenesis
   b. Glycogenesis
   c. Glycolysis
   d. Glycogenolysis
2. Which of the following hormones decreases blood glucose?
   a. Epinephrine
   b. Glucagon
   c. Cortisol
   d. Insulin
3. Which additive to blood collection tubes is considered the best for serum glucose analysis because it most effectively inhibits glycolysis?
   a. Sodium iodoacetate
   b. Combined fluoride-oxalate
   c. Combined citrate-fluoride-EDTA
   d. Heparin
4. Which is an example of a disaccharide?
   a. Glucose
   b. Starch
   c. Lactose
   d. Fructose
5. What is the conversion of glucose into its storage form termed?
   a. Glycogenesis
   b. Glycolysis
   c. Glycogenolysis
   d. Gluconeogenesis
6. Which of the following statements concerning carbohydrates is *incorrect*?
   a. Individuals diagnosed with type 1 diabetes mellitus can display hypoglycemic symptoms because of the impairment of glucagon secretion.
   b. Ethanol produces hypoglycemia by inhibiting gluconeogenesis.
   c. Monosaccharides are formed from the breakdown of starches and disaccharides within the small intestine.
   d. The brain functions normally with a low concentration of plasma glucose (<20 to 30 mg/dL).
7. The formation of 6-phosphogluconate with concomitant production of NADH is the final step in which of the following coupled-enzyme assays for glucose?
   a. Hexokinase method
   b. Glucose oxidase method
   c. Glucose dehydrogenase method
   d. Polarographic method

8. What is the typical cause of an inborn error of carbohydrate metabolism?
   a. Lack of insulin production
   b. Glucagonoma
   c. Absence of an enzyme involved in carbohydrate metabolism
   d. Chronic alcoholism with hepatic failure
9. What is the most widely used cutoff blood glucose concentration that indicates hypoglycemia in an individual with diabetes?
   a. 100 mg/dL
   b. 80 mg/dL
   c. 70 mg/dL
   d. 25 mg/dL
10. What condition will result from the deficiency of a specific enzyme involved in glycogen metabolism?
    a. Glycogen storage disease
    b. Lactic acidosis
    c. Insulin deficiency
    d. Glycolysis

## SUGGESTED READINGS

Adeva-Andany M, López-Ojén M, Funcasta-Calderón R, et al. Comprehensive review on lactate metabolism in human health. *Mitochondrion.* 2014;17:76–100.

American Diabetes Association. Classification and diagnosis of diabetes. *Diabetes Care.* 2022;45(suppl 1):S17–S38.

Chan AY, Swaminathan R, Cockram CS. Effectiveness of sodium fluoride as a preservative of glucose in blood. *Clin Chem.* 1989;35:15–317.

Chen YT. Glycogen storage diseases. In: Scriver CR, Beaudet AL, Sly WS, et al., eds. *The Metabolic and Molecular Bases of Inherited Disease.* Vol 8. New York: McGraw-Hill; 2001:1521–1551.

Cryer PE, Axelrod L, Grossman AB, et al. Evaluation and management of adult hypoglycemic disorders: an endocrine society clinical practice guideline. *J Clin Endocrinol Metab.* 2009;94:709–728.

Diabetes Control and Complications Trial Research Group, Nathan DM, Genuth S, et al. The effect of intensive treatment of diabetes on the development and progression of long-term complications in insulin-dependent diabetes mellitus. *N Engl J Med.* 1993;329:977–986.

Gambino R, Piscitelli J, Ackattupathil TA, et al. Acidification of blood is superior to sodium fluoride alone as an inhibitor of glycolysis. *Clin Chem.* 2009;55:1019–1021.

Gerich JE. Physiology of glucose homeostasis. *Diabetes Obes Metab.* 2000;2:345–350.

Koeberl DD, Kishnani PS, Bali D, et al. Emerging therapies for glycogen storage disease type I. *Trends Endocrinol Metab.* 2009;20:252–258.

Kraut JA, Madias NE. Lactic acidosis. *N Engl J Med.* 2014;371:2309–2319.

Martin-Rendon E, Blake DJ. Protein glycosylation in disease: new insights into the congenital muscular dystrophies. *Trends Pharmacol Sci.* 2003;24:178–183.

Pithukpakorn M. Disorders of pyruvate metabolism and the tricarboxylic acid cycle. *Mol Genet Metab.* 2005;85:243–246.

Robinson BH. Lactic acidemia (disorders of pyruvate carboxylase, pyruvate dehydrogenase). In: Scriver CR, Beaudet AL, Sly WS, et al., eds. *The Metabolic and Molecular Bases of Inherited Disease.* 7th ed. New York: McGraw-Hill; 1995:1479–1499.

Sacks DB. Carbohydrates. In: Rifai N, Chiu RW, Young IS, et al., eds. *Tietz Textbook of Laboratory Medicine.* 7th ed. St Louis: Elsevier Saunders; 2022:353.e1–e23.

Sacks DB, Arnold M, Bakris GL, et al. Guidelines and recommendations for laboratory analysis in the diagnosis and management of diabetes mellitus. *Clin Chem.* 2011;57:e1–e47.

Seaquist ER, Anderson J, Childs B, et al. Hypoglycemia and diabetes: a report of a workgroup of the American Diabetes Association and the Endocrine Society. *Diabetes Care.* 2013;36:1384–1395.

Shapiro ET, Bell GI, Polonsky KS, et al. Tumor hypoglycemia: relationship to high molecular weight insulin-like growth factor-II. *J Clin Invest.* 1990;85:1672–1679.

UK Prospective Diabetes Study (UKPDS) Group. Intensive blood-glucose control with sulphonylureas or insulin compared with conventional treatment and risk of complications in patients with type 2 diabetes (UKPDS 33). *Lancet.* 1998;352:837–853.

# Lipids and Lipoproteins

*Jeffery W. Meeusen, Jing Cao, Leslie Donato, and Alan T. Remaley*

## OBJECTIVES

1. Define the following terms:
   a. Apolipoprotein
   b. Basic lipid panel
   c. Cholesterol
   d. Cholesteryl ester
   e. Fatty acid
   f. Glycerol
   g. Ketone bodies
   h. Lipid
   i. Lipoprotein
   j. Lipoprotein lipase
   k. Phospholipid
   l. Prostaglandin
   m. Sphingolipid
   n. Triglyceride
2. Describe the six major classes of lipids based on chemical structure and function.
3. Discuss the metabolism of cholesterol, fatty acids, and triglycerides, including synthesis, esterification, absorption, and catabolism.
4. Compare and contrast the major lipoprotein classes on the basis of their physical characteristics, functions, and clinical significance.
5. Describe the following processes of lipid metabolism:
   a. Exogenous pathway
   b. Endogenous pathway
   c. Reverse cholesterol transport
   d. Intracellular cholesterol transport
6. State the clinical features of the following disorders and any association with cardiovascular disease:
   a. Hyperchylomicronemia
   b. Familial hypercholesterolemia
   c. Familial combined hyperlipidemia
   d. Dysbetalipoproteinemia
   e. Familial hypertriglyceridemia
   f. Type V hyperlipoproteinemia
   g. Hypoalphalipoproteinemia
7. Describe how lipid testing is used to manage cardiovascular disease risk in adults and children.
8. Draw a diagram showing the typical enzymatic reactions used in the laboratory to measure cholesterol and triglycerides.

## KEY WORDS AND DEFINITIONS

**Acylglycerol (glycerol ester)** A three-carbon alcohol that contains a hydroxyl group on each of its carbons and is classified by the number of fatty acyl groups present; triglycerides are the predominant form of glycerol ester in plasma.

**Amphipathic** A molecule (e.g., lipid, protein) with both hydrophilic and hydrophobic parts.

**Apolipoproteins** The major protein components of lipoproteins.

**Atherosclerosis** A pathogenic build-up of plaque containing lipids and inflammatory mediators on and within artery walls.

**Atherosclerotic cardiovascular disease** Deformation of blood vessels caused by atherosclerotic plaque that impairs the supply of blood to tissues.

**Cholesterol** A 27 carbon alcohol arranged in a tetracyclical sterane ring system, synthesized by all cells and tissues.

**Fatty acid** A carboxylic acid containing an alkyl-chain with variable length of 2–26 carbons that may contain none, one, or many unsaturated carbon–carbon bonds.

**Lipids** A class of compounds that are nearly insoluble in water and contain nonpolar carbon-hydrogen bonds.

**Lipoprotein(a)** An atherogenic lipoprotein structurally similar to low-density lipoprotein (LDL) but containing a plasminogen-like protein called *apo(a)*.

**Lipoproteins** Spherical micelle-like particles involved in the transport of lipids.

**Phospholipid** A polar amphipathic lipid located on the surface of a lipoprotein and at the aqueous interface of biologic membranes.

**Triglyceride** A glycerol ester consisting of three fatty acids esterified to glycerol and constituting 95% of tissue storage fat.

# INTRODUCTION

**Lipids** have important roles in virtually all aspects of life, including hormonal signaling, energy storage, and structural components in cell membranes. In addition, lipids and **lipoproteins**, the particles that transport lipids in the blood, are directly involved in the development of **atherosclerosis**—a common disorder that occurs when fat, cholesterol, and other substances build up in the walls of arteries and form atherosclerotic plaques in the vessel wall. Atherosclerosis is the underlying cause of coronary heart disease, cerebrovascular disease, and peripheral vascular disease. In this chapter, the basic biochemistry, clinical significance, and laboratory analysis of major lipids and lipoproteins are discussed.

# LIPID BIOCHEMISTRY

The term *lipid* applies to a class of compounds that are soluble in organic solvents but nearly insoluble in water. Lipids primarily contain nonpolar carbon–carbon (C–C) and carbon–hydrogen (C–H) bonds. Some lipids also contain charged or polar groups, which makes these lipids **amphipathic** with affinity for both water and organic solvents. Amphipathic lipids, such as **phospholipids**, are found at the aqueous interface of biologic membranes and lipoproteins. Most phospholipids contain a diglyceride, a phosphate group, and a simple organic molecule, such as choline, as the head group. One exception to this rule is sphingomyelin, which is derived from sphingosine instead of glycerol. Overall, lipids are broadly subdivided into six groups on the basis of their chemical structure: (1) cholesterol, (2) fatty acids, (3) acylglycerols, (4) sphingolipids, (5) prostaglandins, and (6) terpenes.

## Cholesterol

**Cholesterol** is found almost exclusively in animals and is a key membrane component of all cells. It is a steroid alcohol with 27 carbon atoms arranged in a tetracyclic ring system, with an aliphatic side chain (Fig. 23.1). Although it is relatively hydrophobic, cholesterol does contain a polar hydroxyl (OH) group, making it amphipathic and accounting for surface orientation in cell membranes.

## Cholesterol Absorption

The average Western diet contains approximately 300–450 mg of cholesterol per day, which is derived mostly from meat and dairy products, but only 30%–60% of it is absorbed. Cholesterol esters are formed by combination of fatty acid attached to the hydroxyl group (see Fig. 23.1). Dietary esterified cholesterol is rapidly hydrolyzed in the intestine to release free cholesterol and fatty acids by cholesterol esterases secreted from the pancreas and small intestine.

Before it is absorbed, cholesterol is first solubilized through a process called *emulsification*, which involves the formation of micelles that contain: (1) unesterified cholesterol, (2) fatty acids, (3) monoglycerides, (4) phospholipids, and (5) conjugated bile acids. Bile acids, by acting as detergents, are the most critical factor in micelle formation.

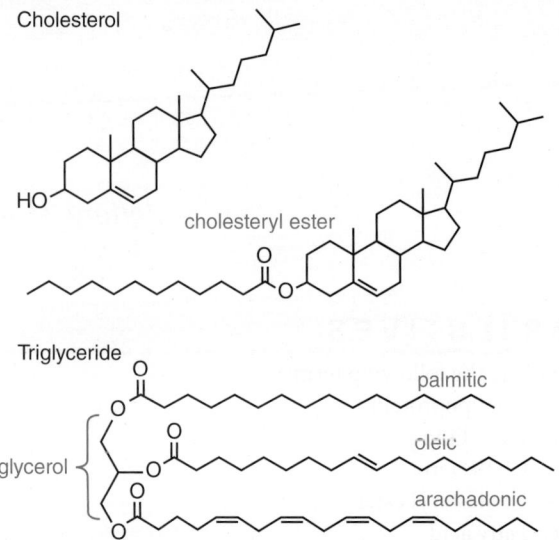

**Fig. 23.1** Cholesterol, cholesteryl esters, and triglycerides are the primary lipids in lipoproteins.

Increased amounts of fat favor the absorption of cholesterol by the formation of more micelles. Most cholesterol absorption occurs in the middle jejunum and the terminal ileum of the small intestine and is mediated by the enterocyte protein NPC1L1 (Niemann-Pick C1-like 1). The cholesterol lowering drug, ezetimibe blocks cholesterol absorption by targeting NPC1L1. Once cholesterol enters the intestinal mucosal cell, it is packaged with **triglycerides**, phospholipids, and a large protein called **apolipoprotein** (apo) B-48 into large lipoprotein particles called *chylomicrons*. Chylomicrons are secreted directly into the lymph and eventually enter the circulation, where they deliver the absorbed dietary lipid to the liver and peripheral tissues.

## Cholesterol Synthesis

Cholesterol is synthesized by all cells in the body, but particularly by the liver and the intestine. The biosynthesis of cholesterol involves multiple enzymes and occurs in three stages redundant to all tissues (Fig. 23.2). In the first stage, three molecules of acetyl coenzyme A (CoA) are combined to form the six-carbon thioester 3-hydroxy-3-methyl-glutaryl (HMG)-CoA. In the second stage, HMG-CoA is reduced to mevalonate and decarboxylated to form a series of five-carbon isoprene molecules. Three of these isoprenes are combined to form a 15-carbon intermediate (farnesyl pyrophosphate). Two of these 15-carbon molecules then combine to produce squalene, the final product of the second stage. The second stage is important because it contains the microsomal enzyme HMG-CoA reductase, the rate-limiting enzyme in cholesterol biosynthesis. HMG-CoA reductase is inhibited by statins, the most effective class of cholesterol-lowering drugs. The third stage occurs in the endoplasmic reticulum, with many of the intermediate products bound to a specific carrier protein. In a series of oxidation–decarboxylation reactions, side chains are removed from the tetracyclic sterane ring structure to form the 27-carbon molecule of cholesterol.

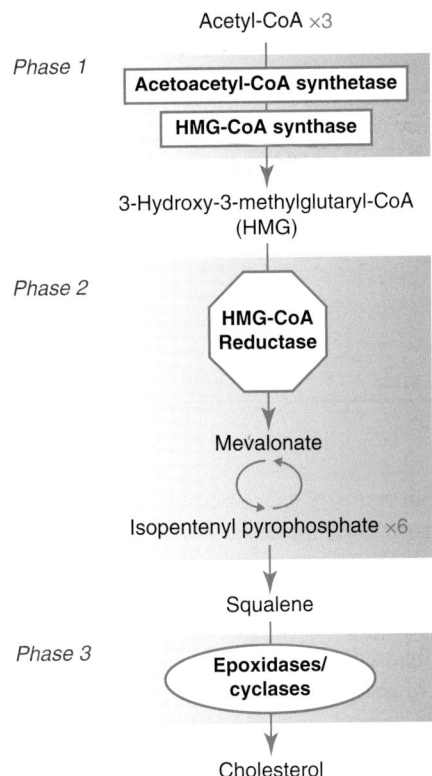

*Phase 1*

Acetyl-CoA ×3

Acetoacetyl-CoA synthetase

HMG-CoA synthase

3-Hydroxy-3-methylglutaryl-CoA (HMG)

*Phase 2*

HMG-CoA Reductase

Mevalonate

Isopentenyl pyrophosphate ×6

Squalene

*Phase 3*

Epoxidases/ cyclases

Cholesterol

**Fig. 23.2** Cholesterol biosynthesis occurs in three phases. *Phase 1* combines three acetyl-CoA molecules to form 3-Hydroxy-3methylglutaryl-CoA (HMG-CoA). *Phase 2* begins with a rate-limiting enzyme HMG-CoA reductase and combines six HMG-CoA to form squalene. *Phase 3* rearranges squalene to form cholesterol.

## Cholesterol Esterification

Cholesterol is esterified with a fatty acid to form a cholesteryl ester by two different enzymes. In cells, excess cholesterol is esterified by acylcholesterol acyltransferase (ACAT), which helps reduce the cytotoxicity of excess free cholesterol. Once esterified, cholesteryl esters are stored in intracellular lipid drops. Cholesteryl esters also are formed in the circulation by the action of a plasma enzyme called *lecithin cholesterol acyltransferase* (LCAT), which is bound to lipoproteins, particularly high-density lipoproteins (HDLs). The reaction involves the transfer of a fatty acid from the second carbon position of phosphatidylcholine (lecithin) to cholesterol. Cholesteryl esters account for approximately 70% of the total cholesterol in plasma. Once cholesterol is esterified, it loses its free hydroxyl group and becomes much more hydrophobic, moving from the surface of lipoprotein particles to its hydrophobic core.

## Cholesterol Catabolism

Except for specialized endocrine cells that use cholesterol as a precursor for steroid hormones, most peripheral cells have limited ability to further metabolize cholesterol. Cholesteryl esters are hydrolyzed to free cholesterol by various lipases in all cells, but thereafter most cholesterol must be returned to the liver to undergo any further catabolism. About one-third of the daily production of cholesterol, or ~400 mg/day, is converted in the liver into bile acids. Nearly 90% of bile acids are reabsorbed in the ileum and returned to the liver by the enterohepatic circulation. Bile acids that enter the large intestine can be further altered by bacterial enzymes into secondary bile acids.

Most cholesterol delivered to the liver is not converted to bile salts but is re-packaged into lipoproteins and secreted into the circulation. A small portion is directly excreted into the bile unchanged, where it is solubilized into micelles by bile acids and phospholipids. When the amount of cholesterol in bile exceeds the capacity of the solubilizing agents, cholesterol can precipitate, forming gallstones.

## Fatty Acids

RCOOH is the general chemical formula for a *fatty acid*, where "R" stands for an alkyl chain. Fatty acid chain lengths vary and are commonly classified as short-chain (2–4 carbon atoms), medium-chain (6–10 carbon atoms), or long-chain (12–22 carbon atoms) fatty acids. Some fatty acids in the retina and the brain can have chain lengths of up to 40 carbons and are called *very long chain fatty acids*. Those of most importance in human nutrition and metabolism are included in the long-chain class and typically contain an even number of carbon atoms.

Fatty acids are further classified according to their degree of saturation. Saturated fatty acids have no double bonds (C=C) between their carbon atoms; monounsaturated fatty acids contain one double bond; and polyunsaturated fatty acids contain multiple double bonds (see Fig. 23.1). The double bonds in polyunsaturated fatty acids are usually three carbon atoms apart, and therefore fatty acids do not have a color, unlike Vitamin A, which contains a conjugated electron system. Fatty acids from fish, such as salmon, possess up to six unsaturated double bonds and can be more than 22 carbon atoms long. Unsaturated fatty acids are prone to oxidation by the nonenzymatic reaction of oxygen with their double bonds.

Numbering of the carbon atoms in fatty acids can be done from the carboxyl terminal end (Δ-numbering system) or from the methyl terminal end (ω-numbering system; Table 23.1). In addition, carbon atoms may be labeled with Greek symbols, with α being adjacent to the carboxyl group and ω being farthest away. In the Δ-system, fatty acids are abbreviated according to the: (1) number of carbon atoms, (2) number of double bonds, and (3) position(s) of double bond(s). For example, linoleic acid would be written as C18:2⁹,¹² and contains 18 carbons and two unsaturated bonds between carbons 9 and 10 and carbons 12 and 13. When the ω-system is used, linoleic acid would be abbreviated as C18:2(n-6), where only the first carbon from the methyl terminal end forming the unsaturated pair is written. The *Geneva* or *systematic* classification, which is based on their chemical names, is a third common nomenclature system for fatty acids (see Table 23.1).

In saturated fatty acids, the chain is extended and flexible; the carbon atoms rotate freely around their longitudinal axis. However, unsaturated fatty acids have a fixed 30° bend in their chains at each double bond. Depending on the plane in which this bend occurs, the *cis* or the *trans* isomer is produced. In

## TABLE 23.1   Fatty Acids Commonly Found in Human Tissue

| Common Name | Systematic Name | Δ-Numbering | (ω)-Numbering |
|---|---|---|---|
| Lauric | Dodecanoic | 12:0 | 12:0 |
| Myristic | Tetradecanoic | 14:0 | 14:0 |
| Palmitic | Hexadecanoic | 16:0 | 16:0 |
| Palmitoleic | 9-Hexadecanoic | 16:19 | 16:1n-7 |
| Stearic | Octadecanoic | 18:0 | 18:0 |
| Oleic | 9-Octadecanoic | 18:19 | 18:1n-9 |
| Linoleic[a] | 9,12-Octadecadienoic | 18:29,12 | 18:2n-6 |
| Linolenic[a] | 9,12,15-Octadecatrienoic | 18:39,12,15 | 18:3n-3 |
| Arachidic | Eicosanoic | 20:0 | 20:0 |
| Arachidonic | 5,8,11,14-Eicosatetraenoic | 20:45,8,11,14 | 20:4n-6 |

[a]Essential fatty acids.

mammals, all naturally occurring unsaturated fatty acids are of the *cis* variety. *Trans* fatty acids in our diet primarily come from catalytic hydrogenation, which reduces the unsaturated double bonds to raise their melting point. This process is used to "harden" or solidify fats in the manufacture of certain foods, such as margarine.

Most fatty acids are also synthesized by the body except for essential fatty acids, such as linoleic acid (C18:29,12), which is made only by plants. Linoleic acid is also converted to arachidonic acid (C20:45,8,11,14), which is a precursor for prostaglandin synthesis.

Unesterified of "free" fatty acids in blood plasma are primarily bound to albumin. Esterified fatty acids exist as triglycerides, phospholipids, or cholesteryl esters. The free fatty acid carboxyl group has a pKa of approximately 4.8; thus, free fatty acid molecules exist primarily in their ionized forms. The normal concentration of free fatty acids in human plasma is 0.3–1.1 mmol/L (8–31 mg/dL) and is very sensitive to physiological energy demands and the availability of alternative forms of metabolic fuel, such as glucose. Most of the free fatty acids in the circulation are derived from intracellular lipolysis of triglycerides by adipose tissue but some are produced by lipolysis of triglycerides in lipoproteins by lipoprotein lipase.

### Fatty Acid Catabolism

Fatty acids are catabolized in the mitochondria and produce energy by a series of reactions known as β-oxidation (Fig. 23.3). This process is repeated to shorten the fatty acid chain by two carbon atoms at a time from the carboxy terminal end of the molecule. For example, one mole of palmitic acid (C16) is eventually converted to eight moles of acetyl CoA. Acetyl CoA does not normally accumulate in the cell but is condensed enzymatically with oxaloacetate, derived largely from carbohydrate metabolism, to yield citrate, an intermediate of the tricarboxylic acid cycle (Krebs cycle). The Krebs cycle is a common pathway for the oxidation of nearly all metabolic fuels, whether derived from carbohydrate, fat, or protein. It ultimately results in the production of adenosine triphosphate (ATP), the main energy storage molecule in the body. Triglycerides contain three fatty acid molecules and are therefore a relatively efficient storage form of metabolic energy. Furthermore, energy storage by triglycerides

is efficient in terms of space because it does not require any water for hydration, unlike carbohydrates.

### Ketone Formation

During prolonged starvation, or when carbohydrate metabolism is impaired, as in uncontrolled diabetes mellitus, the formation of acetyl-CoA exceeds the supply of oxaloacetate. The resulting acetyl-CoA excess is diverted to an alternative pathway in the mitochondria for the formation of: (1) acetoacetate, (2) β-hydroxybutyrate, and (3) acetone—the three compounds known collectively as *ketone bodies* (see Fig. 23.3). Ketosis develops from excessive production of acetyl-CoA, as the body attempts to obtain necessary energy from stored fat in the absence of an adequate supply of carbohydrate metabolites (see Chapter 22).

### Acylglycerols (Glycerol Esters)

Glycerol is a three-carbon alcohol that contains a hydroxyl group on each of its carbon atoms.

The class of acylglycerol is determined by the number of fatty acyl groups present: (1) one fatty acid—monoacylglycerols (monoglycerides); (2) two fatty acids—diacylglycerols (diglycerides); and (3) three fatty acids—triacylglycerols (triglycerides).

Triglycerides constitute 95% of tissue storage fat and are the predominant form of glyceryl esters found in plasma. The fatty acid residues found in triglycerides vary considerably and usually include different combinations of long-chain fatty acids (see Table 23.1). In general, triglycerides from plant sources, such as corn, sunflower, and safflower, tend to be enriched in unsaturated fatty acids, particularly in the C-2 position, and are liquid oils at room temperature. Triglycerides from animals, especially ruminants, tend to have saturated acids and are solids at room temperature.

Dietary triglycerides are digested in the duodenum and are efficiently absorbed in the proximal ileum. Through the action of pancreatic and intestinal lipases and in the presence of bile acids, they are first hydrolyzed to glycerol, monoglycerides, and fatty acids. After absorption, these components of triglycerides are reassembled into triglycerides in the intestinal epithelial cells and then are packaged with cholesterol into chylomicrons.

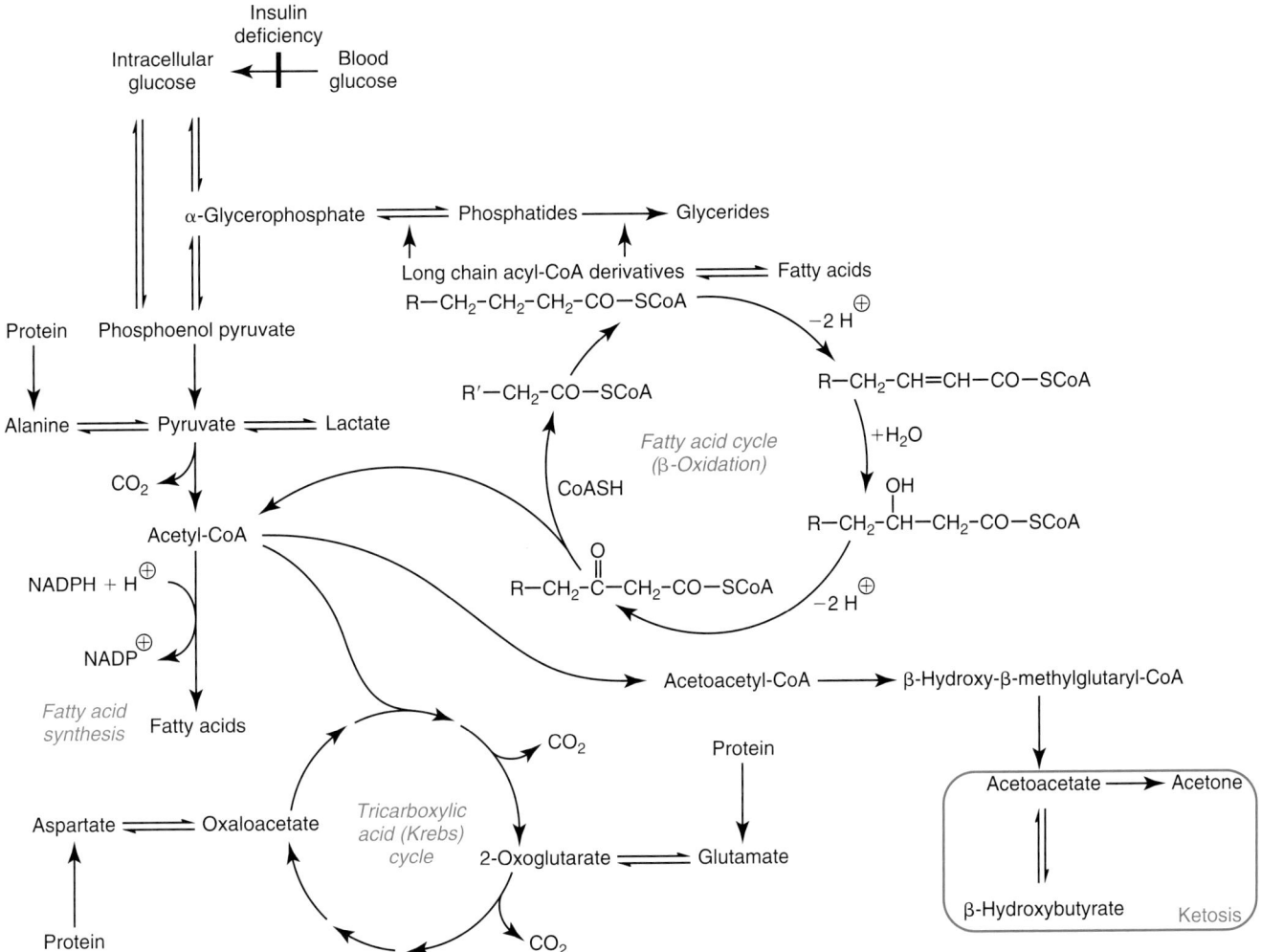

**Fig. 23.3** Metabolic pathway interactions among intermediates of carbohydrate, fat, and protein metabolism. Note that acetyl-coenzyme A (*CoA*) is produced from both carbohydrate and fat. The glucogenic amino acids, derived from protein metabolism, enter glycolytic paths as α-keto acids. Ketogenic amino acids enter as acetyl-CoA.

Another major class of acylglycerols includes those containing a phosphate, which are referred to as phosphoglycerides (Fig. 23.4).

## Sphingolipids

Sphingolipids make up a fourth class of lipids derived from the amino alcohol sphingosine (see Fig. 23.4). A fatty acid containing 18 or more carbon atoms is attached to the amino group through an amide linkage to form *ceramide*. Ceramides can be further modified by the addition of phosphate or carbohydrate groups (see Fig. 23.4). Carbohydrate-containing ceramides can have additional moieties leading to sulfatides and gangliosides. Gangliosides are especially abundant in the membranes of the gray matter of the brain, whereas glycosphingolipids have a more general role in cell membranes and can also be a source of blood group and tumor antigens.

## Prostaglandins

Prostaglandins and related compounds, such as thromboxanes and leukotrienes, are derivatives of fatty acids, primarily from arachidonate. These potent bioactive lipids exert diverse physiological actions at concentrations as low as 1 μg/L. The prostaglandins are a series of C20 unsaturated fatty acids that contain a cyclopentane ring; the parent fatty acid has been given the trivial name prostanoic acid. By convention, prostaglandins are abbreviated PG, with the class designated by a capital letter (A, B, E, F, G, H, and I), followed by a number and in some cases a Greek letter (see Fig. 23.4). The number after the capital letter is usually written as a subscript and is used to designate the number of unsaturated bonds in the PG side chains and not within the ring structure itself. Sixteen naturally occurring prostaglandins have been described, but only seven, along with two thromboxanes, are commonly found in the body. These are termed *primary prostaglandins*.

Although prostaglandins have hormone-like action, they are different from conventional hormones in that they are synthesized at their site of action and are made in almost all tissues. Linoleic acid (C18:2(n-6)) and linolenic acid (C18:3(n-3)) are essential fatty acids and precursors to form prostaglandins. Prostaglandins are not stored; once formed they have short-lived effects and are catabolized within

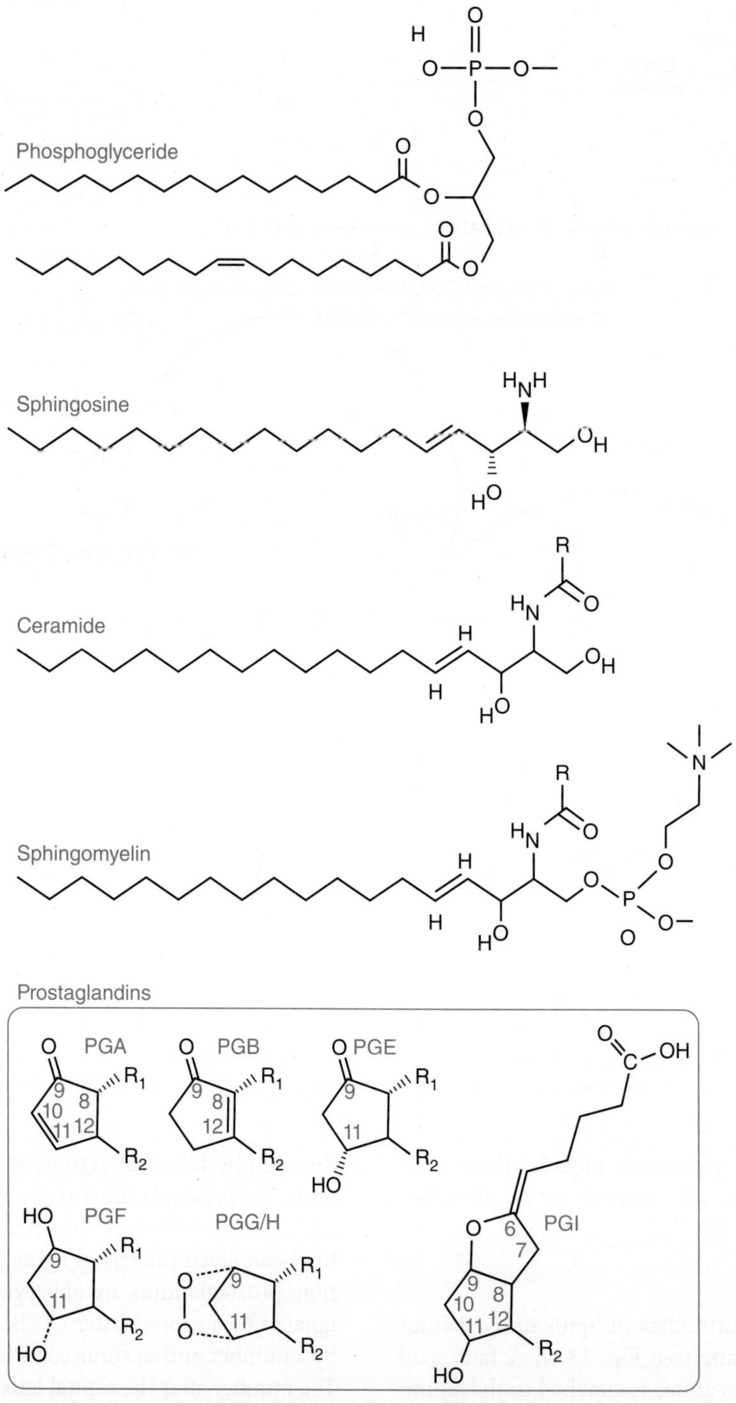

**Fig. 23.4** Structure of phosphoglycerides, sphingolipids, and prostaglandins. "R" stands for various carbon chains.

seconds. Inactivation of prostaglandin appears to be mediated by two enzymes: 15α-hydroxy-prostaglandin dehydrogenase and Δ13-prostaglandin reductase. When prostaglandin synthesis is stimulated, the C20 precursor is hydrolyzed from phospholipids by phospholipase A2. Release of the C20 fatty acid appears to be the rate-limiting step in prostaglandin synthesis and is stimulated by various mediators, such as bradykinin, thrombin, or angiotensin II.

Once released, arachidonic acid follows one of two pathways. The lipoxygenase route leads to leukotriene production, while cyclooxygenase (COX) generates prostaglandins. Nonsteroidal antiinflammatory drugs (NSAIDs; such as aspirin, ibuprofen, naproxen, and indomethacin) inhibit the COX enzymes, thereby decreasing prostaglandin synthesis.

## Terpenes

Terpenes are polymers of the five-carbon isoprene unit and include vitamins A, E, and K, and the dolichols, which play important roles in protein glycosylation (see Chapter 27).

# LIPOPROTEINS

Lipids synthesized in the liver and in the intestine are transported in the plasma in macromolecular complexes known as *lipoproteins*. Lipoproteins are typically spherical micelle-like particles with nonpolar neutral lipids (triglycerides and cholesterol esters) in their core and more polar amphipathic lipids (phospholipids and free cholesterol) at their surface (Fig. 23.5). They also contain one or more specific proteins, called apolipoproteins, on their surface.

## Classification

Lipoproteins have different physical and chemical properties derived from their differing size and composition (Table 23.2). Traditionally, lipoproteins have been categorized according to density as determined by ultracentrifugation. The density categories include: (1) chylomicrons, (2) very-low-density lipoprotein (VLDL), (3) intermediate-density lipoprotein (IDL), (4) low-density lipoprotein (LDL), and (5) HDL. In general, the larger lipoproteins contain more core lipids, such as triglycerides and cholesteryl esters and hence are lighter in density. Larger lipoproteins also contain a smaller relative percentage of protein. In the fasting state, most plasma triglycerides are present in VLDL, but 2–6 hours after a meal,

most triglycerides are transported on chylomicrons. LDL carries approximately 70% of total plasma cholesterol but very little triglyceride (see Table 23.2). HDL typically contains approximately 20%–30% of plasma cholesterol.

**Lipoprotein(a) [Lp(a)]** is biochemically unique with density that overlaps both LDL and HDL. Lp(a) is a distinct class of lipoprotein that is structurally related to LDL because both lipoproteins possess one molecule of apo B-100 per particle, with similar lipid compositions. Unlike LDL, Lp(a) also contains a carbohydrate-rich protein called *apo(a)*, which is covalently bound to the apo B-100 through a disulfide linkage. Apo(a) exhibits a significant sequence homology with plasminogen and a high degree of variation in polypeptide chain length (Fig. 23.6). Apo(a) contains a tandem array of a protein motif called a *kringle domain* with different-sized apo(a) molecules (polymorphisms) reflecting the inclusion of variable numbers of kringle 4 type 2 domains. The plasma level of Lp(a) is mostly genetically determined and is relatively invariant and thus does not need to be repeatedly measured. The mechanism is unclear, but Lp(a) is particularly proatherogenic, based on recent genetic studies, and has also been associated with aortic stenosis. There is currently no adequate drug or dietary therapy for lowering Lp(a), but a promising new therapy based on antisense oligonucleotides is being developed.

Lipoproteins can be electrophoretically separated, and this forms the basis for one system of nomenclature. For example, at pH 8.6, HDL migrates with the α-globulins, LDL with the β-globulins, and VLDL and Lp(a) between the α- and β-globulins, in the pre-β-globulin region. IDL forms a broad band between β- and pre-β-globulins. Chylomicrons remain at the application point. Traditionally, lipoprotein classes were referred to by their electrophoretic locations as pre-β-lipoprotein, VLDL; β-lipoprotein, LDL; and α-lipoprotein, HDL. Electrophoresis provided the foundation for an early original phenotypical classification system (types 1–5) for familial dyslipidemias (for further discussion on electrophoresis, refer to Chapter 11).

## Apolipoproteins

Apolipoproteins are the major protein components of lipoproteins (Table 23.3). Each class of lipoprotein carries several apolipoproteins in differing proportions. Apo A-I is the major

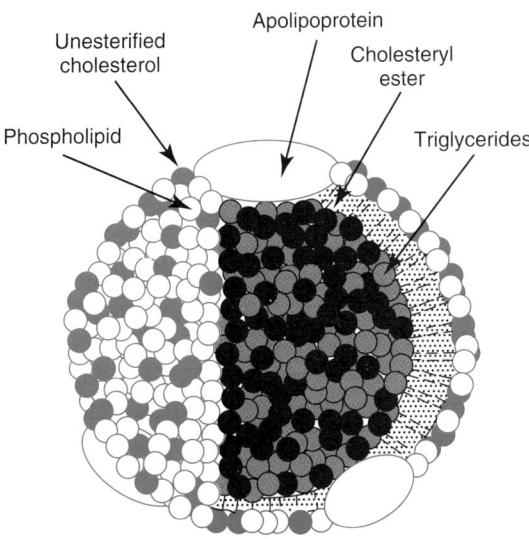

**Fig. 23.5** Structure of a typical lipoprotein particle.

| TABLE 23.2 | **Characteristics of Human Plasma Lipoproteins** | | | | | |
|---|---|---|---|---|---|---|
| **Characteristic** | **Chylomicron** | **VLDL** | **IDL** | **LDL** | **HDL** | **Lp(a)** |
| Density (g/mL) | <0.95 | 0.95–1.006 | 1.006–1.019 | 1.019–1.063 | 1.063–1.210 | 1.040–1.130 |
| Diameter (nm) | >70 | 26–70 | 22–24 | 19–23 | 4–10 | 26–30 |
| Composition (%) | | | | | | |
| Triglyceride | 86 | 55 | 23 | 6 | 5 | <10 |
| Cholesterol | 5 | 19 | 38 | 50 | 22 | 50 |
| Phospholipid | 7 | 18 | 19 | 22 | 33 | 20 |
| Protein | 2 | 8 | 19 | 22 | 40 | 10–20 |

*HDL*, High-density lipoprotein; *IDL*, intermediate-density lipoprotein; *LDL*, low-density lipoprotein; *Lp(a)*, lipoprotein(a); *VLDL*, very-low-density lipoprotein.

protein in HDL. Apo B-100 is the main protein on LDL and Lp(a), and apo B-48, which is produced from apo B-100 messenger RNA (mRNA) by an RNA editing process, is found on chylomicrons. Both apo B-100 and apo B-48 are found at one molecule per particle, are firmly bound, and do not exchange between particles, as the other apolipoproteins do. Apolipoproteins perform the following major functions: (1) modulate the activity of enzymes that act on lipoproteins; (2) maintain the structural integrity of the lipoprotein complex; and (3) facilitate the uptake of lipoprotein by acting as ligands for specific cell-surface receptors. Most apolipoproteins contain amphipathic helices, which are α-helices with one face containing hydrophobic amino acids and the other face containing polar or charged amino acids. This feature enables apolipoproteins to bind to lipids and still interact with the surrounding aqueous environment.

## LIPOPROTEIN METABOLISM

Lipoprotein metabolism is commonly divided into: (1) exogenous, (2) endogenous, (3) reverse cholesterol transport pathways, and (4) intracellular cholesterol transport.

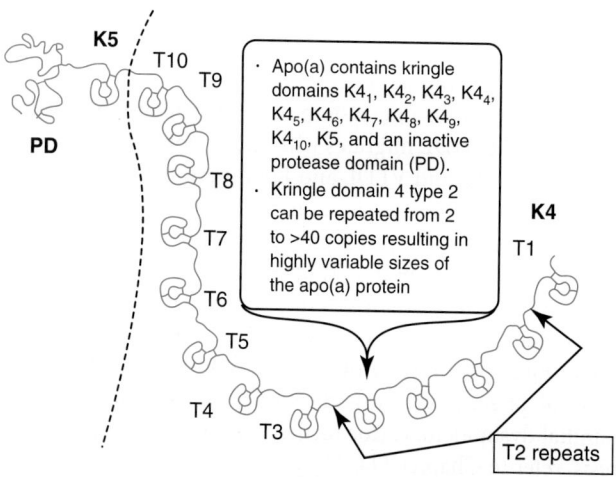

· Apo(a) contains kringle domains K4$_1$, K4$_2$, K4$_3$, K4$_4$, K4$_5$, K4$_6$, K4$_7$, K4$_8$, K4$_9$, K4$_{10}$, K5, and an inactive protease domain (PD).
· Kringle domain 4 type 2 can be repeated from 2 to >40 copies resulting in highly variable sizes of the apo(a) protein

Fig. 23.6 Structure of apolipoprotein(a).

### Exogenous Pathway

The exogenous pathway of lipoprotein metabolism transports dietary lipids from the intestine to the liver and peripheral tissues (Fig. 23.7). After cholesterol and fatty acids are absorbed in the intestine, cholesterol and fatty acids are esterified to form cholesteryl esters and triglycerides in enterocytes. Esterified cholesterol, triglycerides, fat soluble vitamins, and other lipids such as phospholipids are packaged with apo B-48 to form nascent chylomicrons. The triglyceride-rich (>90% in mass) chylomicrons are then secreted into the lymphatic channels and enter the circulation. They further acquire other apolipoproteins including apo E, apo C-III, and apo C-II from interaction with HDL.

Lipoprotein lipase (LPL) attached to the luminal surface of capillary endothelial cells hydrolyzes the triglycerides on chylomicrons to free fatty acids. Liberated fatty acids are taken up by muscle cells and other peripheral tissues as an energy source, with any excess being stored as triglycerides predominantly in the adipocytes, and also in the liver. Apo C-II is a potent activator of LPL whereas apo C-III inhibits LPL and hepatic clearance of lipoproteins. Due to lipolysis and triglyceride loss, chylomicron particles become smaller and denser. These chylomicron remnant particles are rapidly taken up by the liver delivering cholesterol and fat soluble vitamins.

### Endogenous Pathway

The endogenous pathway of lipoprotein metabolism transfers lipids derived from liver to peripheral cells for energy metabolism. Lipids synthesized by the liver and dietary lipids transferred to the liver via the exogenous pathway are combined with apo B-100 to form very low-density lipoproteins (VLDL) (see Fig. 23.7). Once in the plasma, VLDL acquires apoE, apoC-II, and apoC-III from HDL. Triglycerides account for approximately 55% of the VLDL mass, and VLDL and chylomicrons are often referred to as triglyceride-rich lipoproteins. VLDL interaction with LPL leads to release of free fatty acids and transforms VLDL into smaller particles with higher density. VLDL remnants are cleared rapidly, however, continued

| TABLE 23.3 | Classification and Properties of Major Human Plasma Apolipoproteins | | | |
|---|---|---|---|---|
| **Apolipoprotein** | **Molecular Weight (kDa)** | **Exchangeable** | **Function** | **Lipoprotein Carrier(s)** |
| apoAl | 29 | No | Cofactor LCAT | Chylomicron, HDL |
| apo B-100 | 513 | No | Secretion of triglycerides from liver, binding LDL receptor | VLDL, IDL, LDL |
| apo B-48 | 241 | No | Secretion of triglycerides from intestine | Chylomicron |
| apoC-II | 8.9 | Yes | Cofactor LPL | Chylomicron, VLDL, HDL |
| apoC-III | 8.8 | Yes | Inhibition of apoC-II activation of LPL | Chylomicron, VLDL, HDL |
| apoE | 34 | Yes | Binding to LDL receptor and LRP | Chylomicron, VLDL, IDL, HDL |
| apo(a) | 187–662 | No | Unknown | Lp(a) |

*HDL,* High-density lipoprotein; *IDL,* intermediate-density lipoprotein; *LCAT,* lecithin cholesterol acyltransferase; *LDL,* low-density lipoprotein; *Lp(a),* lipoprotein(a); *LPL,* lipoprotein lipase; *LRP,* LDLR-related protein; *VLDL,* very-low-density lipoprotein.

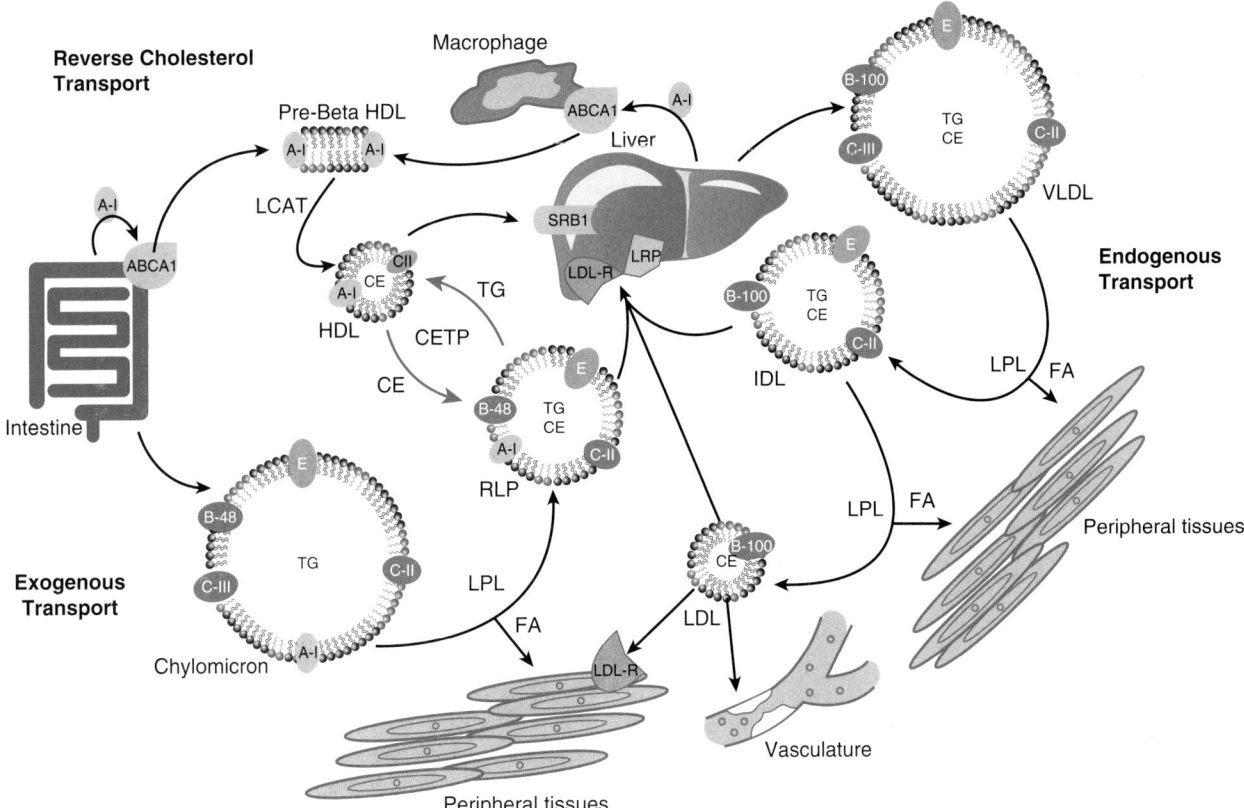

**Fig. 23.7** Lipoprotein metabolism. The *Exogenous Pathway* transports dietary lipids to the liver. The *Endogenous Pathway* redistributes lipids from the liver to other tissues. *Reverse Cholesterol Transport* facilitates transport of cholesterol from peripheral tissues to the liver. A-1, Apolipoprotein A-I; *ABCA1*, ATP-binding cassette transporter A1; *B-48*, apolipoprotein B-48; *B/E*, ApoB- and ApoE-dependent receptors; *C-II*, apolipoprotein C-II; *CE*, cholesterol ester; *CETP*, cholesterol ester transfer protein; *E*, apolipoprotein E; *FA*, fatty acid; *FC*, free cholesterol; *HDL*, high-density lipoprotein; *LCAT*, lecithin cholesterol acyltransferase; *LDLR*, low-density lipoprotein receptor; *LPL*, lipoprotein lipase; *LRP*, LDLR-related protein; *TG*, triglyceride.

LPL activity leads to intermediate density lipoproteins (IDL) and ultimately low-density lipoproteins (LDL). Triglycerides within LDL are further depleted by the cholesterol ester transfer protein (CETP), which exchanges HDL cholesteryl esters for LDL triglycerides, further reducing LDL size and increasing density.

Plasma clearance of VLDL, IDL, and LDL is dependent on apoE and its strong affinity toward the LDL receptor (LDLR). VLDL remnants and IDL retain sufficient apoE for rapid clearance. However, smaller particles contain fewer apoE and LDL is too small to contain any apoE. Thus, plasma clearance of LDL relies on the single apo B-100 ligand and its relatively weak affinity interaction with LDLR. Unsurprisingly, the circulation half-life of LDL is 3–5 days; considerably longer than the 1–12 hours for VLDL, IDL, or chylomicrons. Most cholesterol secreted via VLDL is eventually returned to the liver to be: (1) reused for lipoprotein secretion, (2) converted to bile salts, or (3) direct excretion into the bile.

## Reverse Cholesterol Transport Pathway

The reverse cholesterol transport pathway removes excess cholesterol from peripheral tissues and returns it to the liver for reuse or excretion (see Fig. 23.7). The main lipoprotein involved in this process is high-density lipoprotein (HDL).

Unique among lipoproteins, the structure of HDL is maintained around apoA-I. apoA-I is synthesized by the liver and intestine where it is secreted as a lipid-poor "pre-beta HDL". Cholesterol is actively pumped by ABCA1 transporter outside of the cell where it is incorporated into pre-beta HDL, forming disc-shaped nascent HDL. HDL acquires and exchanges various lipids and serves as a dynamic reservoir for exchangeable apolipoproteins in the plasma and interstitial space. CETP and lecithin:cholesterol acyltransferase (LCAT) play a key role in the remodeling of nascent discoidal HDL into mature particles. LCAT esterifies cholesterol on HDL into cholesterol esters, which form a hydrophobic core for mature HDL. CETP transfers cholesteryl esters from HDL onto LDL to be cleared from the circulation by hepatic LDLR. Triglyceride-poor and cholesterol-rich HDL particles are recycled in the liver through binding with the scavenger receptor class B type I (SR-BI) receptor. Cholesterol and cholesterol esters are removed, then the lipid-depleted HDL returns to the circulation for additional rounds of cholesterol removal from peripheral cells.

## Intracellular Cholesterol Transport Pathway

The intracellular cholesterol transport pathway utilizes, stores, and clears cholesterol in the cell. LDLR on the cell

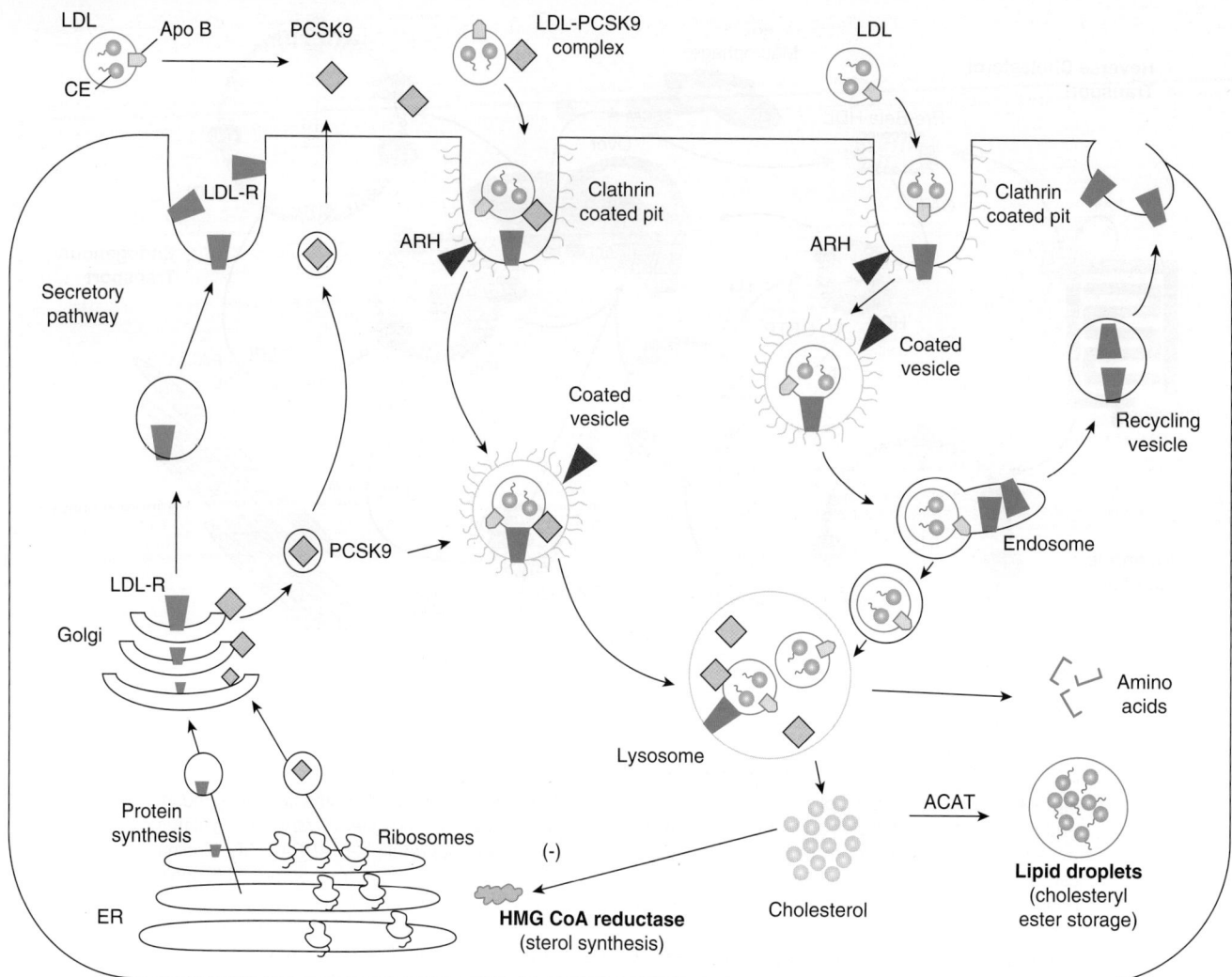

**Fig. 23.8** Intracellular cholesterol transport pathway. *ACAT*, Acyl-CoA cholesterol acyltransferase; *Apo B*, apolipoprotein B-100; *ARH*, autosomal recessive hypercholesterolemia adaptor protein; *HMG-CoA reductase*, 3-hydroxy-3-methylglutaryl coenzyme A reductase; *LDL*, low-density lipoprotein; *LDL-R*, low-density lipoprotein receptor; *PCSK9*, proprotein convertase subtilisin/kexin type 9.

surface inter-reacts with lipoproteins to internalize cholesterol and deliver intact lipoprotein particles to lysosomes for degradation. Lysosomal acid lipase de-esterifies cholesteryl esters to free cholesterol to go through one of these routes, membrane biogenesis, storage in intracellular lipid drops after re-esterification by acyl-CoA:cholesterol acyltransferase (ACAT) or removal by the reverse cholesterol transport pathway. Enterocytes also secrete cholesterol directly into intestinal lumen. Excessive intracellular cholesterol is toxic. Accumulation of intracellular cholesterol inhibits cellular cholesterol biosynthesis and downregulates expression of LDLR (Fig. 23.8).

## INHERITED DISORDERS OF LIPOPROTEIN METABOLISM

Nutritional, lifestyle, and genetic factors all influence the concentration and composition of plasma lipids and lipoproteins. Genetic causes of dyslipidemias include both inherited monogenic or polygenic mutations and common polygenic

variants with individually small contributions to the phenotype.

Inherited genetic disorders of lipoprotein metabolism rise from defects in pathways in the production of lipoproteins, intravascular processing and cellular uptake of lipoproteins, and removal of lipoproteins, that result in either hyper- or hypolipoproteinemia.

### Hyperlipoproteinemia

Based on the lipoprotein electrophoretic separation patterns, the Fredrickson nomenclature of hyperlipoproteinemias (HLP) classifies major groups of HLP according to elevations of one or more different lipoprotein subclasses (Table 23.4). Type I, Chylomicrons; IIa, LDL; IIb, LDL and VLDL; III, remnants of VLDL and chylomicrons; IV, VLDL; V, chylomicrons and VLDL.

### Chylomicronemia: Type I

In type I HLP chylomicrons and correspondingly triglyceride levels are elevated. The major causes of type I HLP include

## TABLE 23.4 Classical Fredrickson Phenotypes for Hyperlipoproteinemias

| Phenotype | Elevated Lipoprotein(s) | Triglycerides | Cholesterol | Electrophoresis Pattern | Clinical Significance |
|---|---|---|---|---|---|
| I | Chylomicrons | Very high | Normal | Staining at application point | High pancreatitis risk; monogenic hereditary |
| IIA | LDL | Low | High | Increased β band | High ASCVD risk |
| IIB | LDL and VLDL | High | High | Increased β and pre-β band | High ASCVD risk |
| III | IDL/RLP | High | High | Broad β/pre-β band | High ASCVD risk |
| IV | VLDL | Very high | Low | Increased pre-β band | Moderate ASCVD risk |
| V | Chylomicrons, VLDL | Very high | Normal | Application point and pre-β bands | Pancreatitis risk; low ASCVD risk; acquired |

*ASCVD*, Atherosclerotic cardiovascular disease; *HDL*, high-density lipoprotein; *IDL*, intermediate-density lipoprotein; *LDL*, low-density lipoprotein; *RLP*, remnant lipoprotein; *VLDL*, very-low-density lipoprotein.

deficiency in lipoprotein lipase (LPL) and deficiency in apolipoprotein C-II (apo C-II) that activates LPL.

***Deficiency in lipoprotein lipase activity.*** LPL hydrolyzes triglyceride and converts chylomicrons to chylomicron remnants. Deficiency in LPL activity prolongs the lifetime of chylomicrons and leads to hyperchylomicronemia. Insertions or deletions in the LPL gene (*LPL*) lead to reduced LPL protein quantity or defective LPL catalytic activity. This deficiency is inherited in an autosomal-recessive pattern affecting about 1 per 1 million individuals. Patients with this disorder are unable to catabolize fat from dietary sources and may present with eruptive xanthomas and lipemia retinalis with extremely high triglyceride levels >23 mmol/L (2000 mg/dL). The concentration of triglycerides often shows great fluctuation in response to diet. Individuals with this disorder are not predisposed to atherosclerotic disease, most likely because the chylomicron particles are too large to enter the vessel wall. Episodes of abdominal pain from acute pancreatitis is the most common symptom that leads to the detection of this disorder. The diagnosis is made by determination of *LPL* activity in plasma collected after heparin is injected into patients to release the LPL that is bound to heparin sulfate and other glycosaminoglycans on the surface of endothelial cells.

***Defects in apolipoprotein C-II.*** Mutations in the apolipoprotein C-II gene (*APOC2*) also result in impairment of chylomicron catabolism associated with less severe conditions than with LPL mutations. Apo C-II is the apolipoprotein cofactor that activates LPL activity. Structural defects in the apo C-II gene result in the absence of apo C-II or a defective apo C-II. Reduced activity of apo C-II impairs the clearance of chylomicrons and raises plasma chylomicrons as well as triglycerides. This disorder is inherited in an autosomal-recessive mode, at a frequency lower than 1 in 1 million. Heterozygotes of the apo C-II genetic defect do not exhibit abnormality in lipid levels because 10% of normal concentration of apo C-II is sufficient to activate LPL activity. Triglyceride levels in patients with apo C-II deficiency vary from 5.65 to 113 mmol/L (500–10,000 mg/L). Abdominal

pain from pancreatitis is the predominant symptom. These patients often are not predisposed to high risk of atherosclerotic diseases. Immunoassays for apo C-II detect lower than normal concentrations of apo C-II but do not recognize nonfunctional apo C-II. Therefore, measurement of LPL activity after heparin infusion is the preferred diagnostic method for apo C-II deficiency. The definitive diagnosis of this rare autosomal recessive condition is made by demonstrating low LPL activity in post-heparin plasma that is restored after the addition of apo C-II to the LPL assay mixture.

### Familial Hypercholesterolemia: Type IIa

Familial hypercholesterolemia (FH) is a genetically inherited disorder of cholesterol metabolism with a prevalence between 1:500 to 1:200 in its heterozygous form. FH is caused by defects in the LDLR pathway, which binds and removes LDL from the circulation. In cases of reduced or absent LDLR function, LDL accumulates at high levels in the plasma. The severe excess LDL leads to increased deposition in the skin, tendons, and arteries, where it causes atherosclerosis (see Chapter 34) and premature atherosclerotic cardiovascular disease (ASCVD) if untreated. Both LDL and its precursor, VLDL, show a rise in concentration as the result of impaired LDL clearance, and to a lesser extent, decreased IDL clearance. LDL particles tend to be larger and carry increased amounts of cholesterol. Triglyceride concentration may be normal or only slightly increased, and HDL-C concentration is slightly decreased.

The majority of these patients have gene defects in the LDLR gene (*LDLR*). Less commonly, defects in two other genes, *RHOA* (formerly called *ARH1*) and *PCSK9*, which code for proteins involved in internalization or processing of the LDLR, may cause FH.

LDLR is present on most tissues and is responsible for cellular uptake of apoB and apoE-containing lipoproteins. LDLRs on the liver account for clearing the vast majority of LDL particles from the plasma. The recycling and degradation of LDLRs is regulated by the peptide PCSK9. Several hundred mutations in the LDLR gene have been described. Mutations of *LDLR* found in FH patients include defects that result in the absence of LDLR, reduced LDL binding, or inefficient LDL internalization.

There is geographical variation of the mutations, except in populations that have been genetically isolated. Mutations in *LDLR* and in *PCSK9* are inherited in an autosomal codominant pattern. Homozygous FH patients are severely affected, whereas heterozygotes usually have a milder phenotype but are still clinically affected usually at a later age. Defects in *RHOA* are inherited in an autosomal recessive pattern.

Patients that are heterozygous for FH usually have total cholesterol >10 mmol/L (400 mg/dL). Cutaneous xanthomas result from cholesterol deposition and start to develop in the late 20s and clinical symptoms of atherosclerotic cardiovascular diseases can occur in the fourth decade of life in male patients. Homozygotes of FH show total cholesterol >20 mmol/L (800 mg/dL) with cutaneous xanthomas developed at birth or in the first few years of life. Tendon xanthomas and atherosclerotic complications, such as myocardial infarction, also begin in early childhood. If aggressive lipid-lowering therapies are not made available to the patient, death from cardiovascular events typically occurs in the second or third decade of life. Increased plasma concentration of LDL-C is suggestive but not diagnostic for FH. A definitive diagnostic method that commonly is accepted is the sequencing of the LDLR gene to identify one or more of the more than 150 different mutations.

*Familial defective apolipoprotein B-100.* Familial defective apo B-100 is an autosomal dominant disorder, the result of mutations in the gene *APOB*, which reduce its affinity for the LDL receptor. LDL-C is increased, but triglycerides and HDL-C are usually within reference intervals. Like those with FH, these individuals have an increased incidence of CHD, but overall, the dyslipidemia in this disorder is less aggressive than in FH. Clinical differentiation between this disorder and heterozygous FH is sometimes difficult, but management of the two disorders is similar. The frequency of this mutation is 1:500 to 1:600 in hypercholesterolemic individuals from populations of European descent, but it is very rare in non-Europeans.

## Familial Combined Hyperlipidemia: Type IIb

Familial combined hyperlipidemia (FCHL) is an autosomal dominant disorder that accounts for as many as 10%–15% of individuals with premature CHD. Families with FCHL often have increased plasma concentrations of total and LDL-C (type IIa) or triglyceride/VLDL (type IV), or both (type IIb). Lipoprotein patterns also vary within an individual over time. In all cases, apo B-100 concentrations are increased because of overproduction. LDL particles in these patients tend to be small and dense because of a decreased lipid-to-protein ratio. LDL-C is usually only modestly increased to approximately 4.9 mmol/L (190 mg/dL), which is less than LDL-C typically observed in heterozygous FH of 9 mmol/L (350 mg/dL). The concentration of triglycerides usually is between 2.3 and 4.5 mmol/L (200 and 400 mg/dL) but may be significantly higher. The underlying genetic basis of FCHL is not known; it is mostly likely a polygenetic disorder.

## Familial Dysbetalipoproteinemia: Type III

Type III HLP is also called "familial dysbetalipoproteinemia," which is an autosomal-recessive disorder that affects the clearance of IDL and other remnant lipoproteins, such as intestinal chylomicrons and hepatic VLDL. It is therefore also called *remnant removal disorder*. The remnant clearance process is mediated through apo E on the surface of lipoprotein remnant particles and its interaction with hepatic receptors. ApoE exists in three common polymorphisms or variants, named E2, E3, and E4.

Patients with dysbetalipoproteinemia either have a rare mutation in apo E that results in apo E deficiency, or a combination of homozygous apoE2 superimposed with metabolic syndrome, insulin resistance or obesity. The inefficient binding of apo E to hepatic receptors leads to accumulation of cholesterol-rich lipoprotein remnants. The remnant particles that accumulate are enriched in cholesterol, have a density less than 1.006 g/mL, and are commonly referred to as β-VLDL or "floating β"-lipoproteins. This condition is shown as a broad beta band on lipoprotein electrophoresis and usually presents with simultaneous and equal elevations of cholesterol and triglycerides. Patients have a ratio of VLDL cholesterol/ triglyceride generally ≥0.3.

The incidence of dysbetalipoproteinemia is approximately 0.1% in the general population. It has a late onset and may manifest in patients with a secondary cause of dyslipidemia or obesity. Premature atherosclerosis commonly develops, particularly in the lower extremities.

## Familial Hypertriglyceridemia: Type IV

Familial hypertriglyceridemia (FHTG) is an autosomal dominant disease characterized by a moderate increase in serum triglycerides. The cause is thought to be overproduction of large VLDL particles with abnormally high triglyceride content, but decreased lipolysis is possibly another contributory factor. Together with hypertriglyceridemia, plasma HDL-C is often notably decreased. This disorder is a polygenic disorder, with an estimated population frequency of approximately 1 in 500. It is inherited in an autosomal dominant pattern with delayed clinical onset. FHTG is often associated with insulin resistance, metabolic syndrome, hypertension, and obesity, as well as increased risk for acute pancreatitis.

## Mixed Hyperlipidemia: Type V

Type V hyperlipoproteinemia is characterized by an increase in both chylomicrons and VLDL triglycerides typically in the range of 11.3–22.6 mmol/L (1000–2000 mg/dL). Acute pancreatitis commonly develops due to hypertriglyceridemia. The inherited Type V HLP has an incidence of approximately 1 in 500, which is an autosomal dominant disorder with increased production and/or decreased removal of VLDL. The activity of LPL in these individuals may be normal or low, and the plasma concentration of apo C-II is normal. Clinical presentations include eruptive xanthomas, lipemia retinalis, pancreatitis, and abnormal glucose tolerance. Most of these patients have a modestly increased risk of cardiovascular disease.

## Lipoprotein(a)

Lipoprotein(a), abbreviated to "Lp(a)," is an HLP not covered by the Fredrickson classification. The size variation in Lp(a) and consequently the plasma concentration of Lp(a) is largely determined genetically. A large variation in "kringle" motif repeats in the APOA gene that encodes apo(a) leads to very heterogenous intra-individual variation in size of Lp(a). However, the density of Lp(a) is similar to that of LDL and most clinical methods will include Lp(a) with LDL quantification.

Elevated Lp(a) concentrations impose increased risk of ASCVD and calcific aortic valve diseases. Markedly elevated Lp(a) also tends to run in certain families, but the inheritance pattern is not clearly defined.

## Lipoprotein X

Lipoprotein X (LpX) is not a directly hereditary disorder. LpX is an abnormal mis-formed lipoprotein produced in severe obstructive biliary tract diseases. The density of LpX is similar to LDL and consequently most methods quantify it as LDL cholesterol. LpX can be distinguished from LDL clinically due to its sudden onset of elevated cholesterol and elevated bilirubin.

A likely mechanism for LpX formation is that when the neutral cholesteryl esters are insufficient to form a lipid core in lipoproteins, LpX is generated. It has a phospholipid bilayer instead of the single phospholipid layer in normal lipoproteins, and it lacks apo B-100 that is present on other lipoproteins in the endogenous pathway, which may confound the measurement or calculation of cholesterol fractions. LpX is characterized by sudden onset of extreme elevation in measured total cholesterol and LDL cholesterol.

## Sitosterolemia

Sitosterolemia is another HLP not covered by Fredrickson classification. It is a rare inherited disease characterized by overabsorption of dietary plant sterols. As a result, cholesterol synthesis and elimination are altered, and cholesterol levels are increased. Homozygotes for this defect have increased plasma sitosterol concentrations (requiring highly specialized laboratory measurement), xanthomas, and very early onset of atherosclerotic cardiovascular disease.

## Hypolipoproteinemia

Causes of hypolipidemia include malnutrition, malabsorption, chronic liver diseases, or genetic defects that manifest with decreased concentrations of triglycerides and cholesterol.

## Hypoalphalipoproteinemia

Several rare genetic defects lead to hypoalphalipoproteinemia. Mutations or deletions of *APOA1* that translate to apo

A-I deficiency or inactivity result in a profoundly low level of HDL. LCAT deficiency is also associated with low HDL. These patients often have cloudy corneas as a consequence of infiltration of lipid, as well as renal disease due to lipids trapped in the glomerulus.

*Tangier disease.* Tangier disease is a rare disorder associated with a notable reduction in HDL, which is inherited in an autosomal co-dominant pattern. Tangier disease is caused by mutations in the ATP-binding cassette A1 gene (*ABCA1*). ABCA1 transporter mediates the first step of the reverse cholesterol transport pathway, efflux of cholesterol from cells and is present in macrophages, liver, and intestine. Homozygous patients with Tangier disease have total cholesterol levels <1.8 mmol/L (70 mg/dL) and undetectable HDL-C and apo A-I. The major clinical signs of Tangier disease are hyperplastic orange tonsils, splenomegaly, and peripheral neuropathy. Deposition of cholesteryl esters is increased in various tissues of the body, particularly macrophages, which form foam cells.

*Lecithin-cholesterol acyltransferase deficiency.* Another cause of hypoalphalipoproteinemia is mutations in the gene encoding lecithin-cholesterol acyltransferase (*LCAT*), which are inherited as an autosomal-recessive disorder. LCAT esterifies cholesterol and is essential for the maturation of HDL (see Fig. 23.7). Absence of LCAT leads to the predominant presence of a nascent discoidal form of HDL, which is rich in phospholipid but poor in cholesterol. This form of HDL has a small size and is rapidly catabolized, resulting in the low HDL concentration found in patients.

## Hypobetalipoproteinemia

Hypobetalipoproteinemia is caused by mutations in *APOB*, and abetalipoproteinemia is caused by mutations in the microsomal triglyceride transfer protein gene (*MTTP*). Hypobetalipoproteinemia is an autosomal-co-dominant disorder, and heterozygotes for a single mutation are asymptomatic. In contrast, heterozygotes for the abetalipoproteinemia mutation have decreased lipid concentrations. In both diseases, homozygosity of the mutated allele leads to the absence of apo B.

# CLINICAL MANAGEMENT OF LIPOPROTEIN DISORDERS

Diagnosis and management of dyslipoproteinemia are based largely on total cholesterol, triglycerides, HDL-C, LDL-C, and non-HDL-C. These five values are reported in the *basic lipid panel* (Box 23.1). Medical history and other laboratory test results are important for determining whether a dyslipoproteinemia is the result of a hereditary lipoprotein disorder (see above) or is a consequence of one or more secondary causes of hyperlipidemia. In most cases, the primary indication for lipid assessment is ASCVD risk management.

In contrast to most other laboratory tests, elevations of lipids are defined based on epidemiologic studies of ASCVD risk. Consequently, while reference intervals for most lab tests are based on the central 95th percentile of normal individuals, lipid values are interpreted in a context of "desirable" versus "increased risk" values, which are typically between the 50th and 75th percentiles of otherwise healthy populations (Table 23.5 and Table 23.6).

---

### BOX 23.1 The Basic Lipid Panel

**Reported Components**
- Measured Parameters:
  - Total cholesterol
  - Triglycerides
  - High-Density Lipoprotein Cholesterol (HDL-C)
- Calculated Parameters:
  - Non-HDL cholesterol = [Total cholesterol – HDL-C]
  - Low-Density Lipoprotein cholesterol (LDL-C)
- [Multiple equations available]

**Pre-analytical Considerations**
- Non-fasting is acceptable for screening and establishing baseline values
- Fasting is preferred when triglycerides are elevated

**Indications for Testing**
- Management of atherosclerotic cardiovascular disease (ASCVD) risk
- Diagnosis and management of lipid-related hereditary disorders

**Frequency of Assessment**
- At least once for children aged 2–19 years
- Screening every 5 years for adults ≥20 years
- Follow-up assessment every 3–12 months for patients on lipid-lowering therapy

---

## Lipids and Atherosclerotic Cardiovascular Disease Risk in Adults

Elevated serum cholesterol is recognized as the primary causal risk factor for ASCVD. The casual association between serum cholesterol and ASCVD is based on overwhelming evidence from randomized controlled trials, longitudinal observation cohorts, and Mendelian randomization studies. Major recommendations for cholesterol and dyslipidemia management have been cooperatively published by multiple medical societies and summarized as follows:

1. All patients are advised to adopt a healthy lifestyle, which includes appropriate nutrition and adequate exercise.
2. Pharmacological LDL-C lowering therapy is advised to patients with:
   a. History of ASCVD
   b. LDL-C >4.9 mmol/L (190 mg/dL)
   c. Diabetes mellitus (type I or II)
   d. ASCVD 10-year predicted risk of ≥7.5%.

Lipid screening is recommended every 4–6 years for all adults >20 years and without any history of ASCVD. International guidelines state that *non-fasting specimens* are reasonable for lipid panels. In the absence of any severe lipid abnormalities suggestive of hereditary dyslipoproteinemia (as mentioned above), lipid screening should be accompanied by risk assessment for ASCVD. The US multi-society guidelines recommend the pooled cohort equation (PCE) for ASCVD risk assessment, which combines a patient's age, sex, race, smoking status, systolic blood pressure, diabetes history, and serum total cholesterol and HDL-cholesterol. The PCE output is a 10-year risk for ASCVD displayed as a percentage.

---

### TABLE 23.5 Guideline Recommended Clinical Decision Thresholds for Basic Lipids in Adults

| Lipid | Threshold (mg/dL) | Description |
|---|---|---|
| **Total cholesterol** | <200 | Desirable |
| | 200–239 | Borderline high |
| | ≥240 | High |
| **LDL cholesterol** | <100 | Desirable |
| | 100–129 | Above desirable |
| | 130–159 | Borderline high |
| | 160–189 | High |
| | ≥190 | Very high |
| **Non-HDL cholesterol** | <130 | Desirable |
| | 130–159 | Above desirable |
| | 160–189 | Borderline high |
| | 190–219 | High |
| | ≥220 | Very high |
| **HDL cholesterol** | <50 Female | Low |
| | <40 Male | Low |
| **Triglycerides** | <150 | Normal |
| | 150–199 | Borderline high |
| | 200–499 | High |
| | ≥500 | Very high |

*HDL*, High-density lipoprotein; *LDL*, low-density lipoprotein.
For conversion to SI units multiply cholesterol by 0.02586 and triglycerides by 0.0113.

**TABLE 23.6 Guideline Recommended Clinical Decision Thresholds for Basic Lipids in Pediatric Patients**

| Lipid | THRESHOLD (PEDIATRIC) (mg/dL) | | Description |
|---|---|---|---|
| Total cholesterol | <170 | | Acceptable |
| | 170–199 | | Borderline high |
| | ≥200 | | High |
| LDL cholesterol | <110 | | Acceptable |
| | 110–129 | | Borderline high |
| | ≥130 | | High |
| Non-HDL cholesterol | <120 | | Acceptable |
| | 120–144 | | Borderline high |
| | ≥145 | | High |
| HDL cholesterol | <40 | | Low |
| | 40–45 | | Borderline low |
| | >45 | | Acceptable |
| Triglycerides | *0–9 YEARS* | *10–17 YEARS* | |
| | <75 | <90 | Normal |
| | 75–99 | 90–129 | Borderline high |
| | ≥100 | ≥130 | High |

For conversion to SI units multiply cholesterol by 0.02586 and triglycerides by 0.0113.

## Lipids and ASCVD Risk in Children and Adolescents

In 2019, the American Heart Association (AHA) issued a scientific statement on cardiovascular risk reduction in high-risk pediatric patients. Childhood conditions that have lifelong impact on an individual's risk of developing ASCVD include both familial inherited conditions (e.g., homozygous or heterozygous FH, hypertension, or severe obesity), and acquired medical conditions (e.g., chronic kidney disease, chronic inflammatory conditions). These conditions confer varying degrees of increased future ASCVD risk and the statement categorizes patients into three tiers of risk for development of cardiovascular disease—tier 1: high risk, tier 2: moderate risk, and tier 3: at risk. Annual non-fasting lipid assessment is recommended for all categories to be followed-up with a fasting lipid panel if triglycerides are elevated. Maintaining blood pressure ≤90th percentile for age and sex (or <120/70 mm Hg), fasting glucose <5.6 mmol/L (100 mg/dL), hemoglobin $A_{1c}$ <5.7%, triglycerides <1.7 mmol/L (150 mg/dL) and non-HDL cholesterol <3.8 mmol/L (145 mg/dL) is recommended for all risk categories. Risk-dependent BMI and LDL-C targets are further recommended.

Children with a family history of premature cardiovascular disease or significant hypercholesterolemia should be screened for FH using a fasting lipid profile beginning at 2 years of age and then every 3–5 years through adulthood, even if previous profiles are within normal ranges. The diagnosis of FH can be considered confirmed if there is a positive genetic testing for an LDL-C-raising gene defect in a first-degree relative. As with all cases of hypercholesterolemia, secondary causes of hypercholesterolemia should be excluded, including hypothyroidism, nephrotic syndrome, or liver diseases. Treatment for heterozygous FH should include statins, low saturated fat diet high in fiber, adequate physical activity, and a smoke-free environment. Bariatric surgery likely has a role in the management of children with severe obesity and serious comorbidities. Children with chronic inflammatory diseases including, but not limited to, rheumatoid arthritis, psoriasis, inflammatory bowel disease, and systemic lupus erythematosus, should be screened on a periodic basis for cardiovascular risk factors. Childhood cancer survivors are at increased risk of death from cardiovascular disease as compared with age-matched controls. The increased risk likely originates from multiple factors, such as radiation exposure, hematopoietic stem cell transplantation, and increased risk of traditional cardiovascular disease risk factors. All childhood cancer survivors should have a lipid profile and fasting glucose or hemoglobin $A_{1c}$ performed every 2 years.

## ANALYSIS OF LIPIDS, LIPOPROTEINS, AND APOLIPOPROTEINS

As risk-related cutoff points (see Tables 23.5, 23.6) were developed, much effort has gone into improvement and standardization of lipid and lipoprotein assays to ensure their proper performance and to ensure comparability of test results between different methods and different clinical laboratories, thus reducing misclassification of patients' ASCVD risk.

Historically, worldwide, the policy that most laboratories follow is an overnight fast of a minimum of 8 hours prior to obtaining samples for testing the lipid profile to decrease the variability in TG concentration that occurs post-prandially. However, the need for patient fasting prior to lipid panel testing has been questioned. This is particularly true when the primary clinical indication for testing is ASCVD risk assessment. In fact, most clinical practice guidelines and expert consensus statements agree that routine measurement of lipids can be performed using blood samples obtained from non-fasting individuals. The European Atherosclerosis Society/European Federation of Clinical Chemistry and Laboratory Medicine

(EAS/EFLM) recently published a consensus statement promoting the use of non-fasting lipid profiles for the assessment of cardiovascular disease risk. There are several reasons for this change in recommendations. First is the observation that the differences in basic lipid panels measures are considered clinically negligible in the post-prandial state compared with the fasting state. Moreover, there is no change in HDL-C, apoB, or Lp(a) concentrations. The minimal changes in lipid concentrations translate into essentially no change in ASCVD risk assessment using results obtained from fasting versus non-fasting samples. Not requiring fasting eases the burden on clinical, laboratory, and phlebotomy workflows by allowing for more varied collection and testing times. In addition to convenience and comfort, direct patient benefit of non-fasting lipid assessment is observed in decreased risk of hypoglycemia induced by fasting.

## Cholesterol Assays

Enzymatic methods are the assay of choice for the routine measurement of cholesterol. Enzyme reagents are mixed with serum or plasma and are incubated under controlled conditions to generate molar equivalents of hydrogen peroxide and ultimately a chromophore (4-aminoantipyrineperoxidase) for color development (Fig. 23.9).

Enzymatic methods are subject to interference from other colored compounds or from those that compete with the oxidation reaction, such as: (1) bilirubin, (2) ascorbic acid, and (3) hemoglobin. Assays are usually linear, up to approximately 20 mmol/L (800 mg/dL).

## Triglyceride Assays

Triglycerides are also routinely measured with enzyme reagents. The first step is the lipase-catalyzed hydrolysis of triglycerides to glycerol and fatty acids, followed by a series of enzymatic conversions to generate an equimolar amount of hydrogen peroxide for each glycerol (see Fig. 23.9).

Enzymatic triglyceride methods are specific in that they do not detect glucose or phospholipids. They are linear in

the concentration range up to approximately 10 mmol/L (900 mg/dL) and have analytical coefficients of variation (CVs) in the range of approximately 2%–3%. Because glycerol is a product of normal metabolic processes, it is present in serum. Thus, the measured quantity of triglycerides in serum is overestimated slightly, if not corrected for endogenous glycerol. In healthy individuals, endogenous glycerol represents the equivalent of less than 0.1 mmol/L (10 mg/dL) of triglyceride; therefore, the error due to glycerol is not usually clinically significant. Some laboratories use an alternative triglyceride assay, in which the endogenous glycerol is first "blanked out" by adjustment of the calibrators to compensate for an average bias or by enzymatic consumption of glycerol in a pre-reaction step before triglycerides are measured. However, many of these glycerol blanked triglyceride assays have recently been discontinued making the identification of *pseudohypertriglyceridemia* from elevated glycerol more challenging.

## High-Density Lipoprotein Cholesterol Assays

HDL methods utilize the same enzymatic cholesterol measurement described above, however, prior to analysis the non-HDL lipoproteins are physically removed or effectively masked. Historically, non-HDL lipoproteins—VLDL, IDL, Lp(a), LDL, and chylomicrons—were precipitated with polyanions. Polyanions react with positively charged groups on lipoproteins, and this interaction is further facilitated in the presence of divalent cations, such as magnesium, to create a precipitate. The precipitate is removed by centrifuging for at least 45,000 $g$-min, and cholesterol is measured enzymatically in the supernatant. Several polyanion-divalent cation combinations have been used, including: (1) heparin sulfate-MnCl$_2$, (2) dextran sulfate-MgCl$_2$, and (3) phosphotungstate-MgCl$_2$. HDL-C measurements using the precipitation method are considered inaccurate in samples containing triglyceride concentrations >4.5 mmol/L (400 mg/dL). Despite this limitation, the precipitation method is considered the gold-standard.

1. CE + H$_2$O $\xrightarrow{\text{Cholesteryl ester hydrolase}}$ Cholesterol + Fatty acid
2. Cholesterol + O$_2$ $\xrightarrow{\text{Cholesterol oxidase}}$ Cholest–4–en–3–one + H$_2$O$_2$
3. H$_2$O$_2$ + Phenol + 4–aminoantipyrine $\xrightarrow{\text{Peroxidase}}$ Quinoneimine dye + 2H$_2$O

A

1. Triglyceride + 3 H$_2$O $\xrightarrow{\text{Lipase}}$ Glycerol + 3 fatty acids
2. Glycerol + ATP $\xrightarrow{\text{Glycerokinase}}$ Glycerophosphate + ADP
3. Glycerophosphate + O$_2$ $\xrightarrow{\text{Glycerophosphate oxidase}}$ Dihydroxyacetone + H$_2$O$_2$
4. H$_2$O$_2$ + Phenol + 4–aminoantipyrine $\xrightarrow{\text{Peroxidase}}$ Quinoneimine + 2H$_2$O

B

Fig. 23.9 Enzymatic methods used in routine clinical chemistry analysis for (A) cholesterol and (B) triglycerides.

Direct HDL-C assays, also known as *homogeneous assays*, are most commonly used in clinical laboratories. In contrast to precipitation-based assays, no physical separation of HDL from non-HDL fractions occurs. Instead, HDL-C is selectively measured by effective masking or promoting the consumption of cholesterol from non-HDL fractions so that it does not react with the enzymes used to measure cholesterol on HDL. This is achieved by a variety of methods, depending on the type of assay. For example, some assays involve the use of antibodies or various polymers or complexing agents, such as cyclodextrin, that shield the cholesterol in the non-HDL fractions from reacting with cholesterol-measuring enzymes. Some assays depend on modifications of cholesteryl esterase and cholesterol oxidase that make them more selective for HDL-C. Finally, some assays use a blanking step that enzymatically consumes cholesterol from non-HDL fractions. Unlike the precipitation HDL-C assays, no sample pretreatment step is performed with direct assays and thus they can be fully automated. However, these assays sometimes show relatively poor performance compared with reference methods on dyslipidemic samples, particularly those with high triglycerides.

## Low-Density Lipoprotein Cholesterol

The gold-standard method for LDL cholesterol measurement is referred to as "beta-quantification" and relies on separating lipoproteins with density <1.006 g/mL (VLDL and chylomicrons) followed by precipitation of HDL and enzymatic cholesterol measure (Box 23.2). This process requires extensive time and labor. Most clinical laboratories report estimated LDL-C concentrations obtained from a calculation using more easily measured total cholesterol, triglycerides, and HDL-C.

Until recently, the most widely used calculation was the Friedewald equation (see Box 23.2). The VLDL cholesterol concentration is estimated as total triglycerides divided by 5 (in mg/dL) and is based on the average ratio of triglycerides to cholesterol in VLDL. The ratio of triglycerides to VLDL cholesterol can be altered in several commonly encountered situations including: (1) presence of chylomicrons (nonfasting specimens); (2) triglycerides 4.5 mmol/L (>400 mg/dL); (3) presence of IDL and remnant lipoproteins (dysbetalipoproteinemia); and (4) in patients with low LDL cholesterol <1.8 mmol/L (70 mg/dL). The Friedewald equation was established based on measured values from about 500 patients. Alternative calculations have been established using data from hundreds of thousands of measurements to account for the variation in triglyceride to VLDL cholesterol (see Box 23.2).

Several direct methods for measurement of LDL-C are also used in clinical practice. In general, these assays yield results similar to those obtained by calculating LDL-C and performing the β-quantification reference method. However, evidence suggests that different direct assays may not be specific and quantify cholesterol from other lipoproteins or miss some LDL subfractions. Despite these limitations, direct LDL-C methods are widely routinely used.

---

## BOX 23.2  Clinical Methods for Low-Density Lipoprotein Cholesterol

**Estimated Methods**
*Friedewald*

$$TC - HDL - C - \frac{TG}{5}$$

*Martin/Hopkins*

$$TC - HDL - C - \frac{TG}{X}$$

*Sampson/NIH*

$$\frac{TC}{0.948} - \frac{HDL-C}{0.971} - \left(\frac{TG}{8.56} + \frac{TG \times NonHDL-C}{2140} - \frac{TG^2}{16100}\right) - 9.44$$

where *TC* = total cholesterol; *HDL-C* = high-density lipoprotein cholesterol; *TG* = triglycerides; *X* = an empirically determined variable factor (see *JAMA*. 2013;310:2061–2068).

**Direct Homogeneous Methods**
- Multiple methodological approaches with varying specificity for LDL are available:
  - LDL solubilization (Kyowa Medex)
  - LDL protected/deprotected by surfactants (Daiichi, Wako)
  - Non-HDL catalase/LDL azide (Denka Seiken)

**Beta-Quantification Method**
- Not commonly performed
- Restricted to work-up of hereditary dyslipidemias or clinical trials

  Method:
  1. Separate serum lipoproteins at density (d) 1.006 g/mL
  2. Remove d <1.006 g/mL fraction (VLDL and chylomicrons)
  3. Measure cholesterol in d >1.006 g/mL fraction (LDL-C + HDL-C)
  4. Precipitate apoB-lipoproteins with heparin/$Mn^{2+}$ or $Mg^{2+}$/dextran
  5. Measure cholesterol in supernatant (this equals HDL-C)
  6. Subtract HDL-C from d >1.006 g/mL cholesterol

---

## Measurement of Apolipoproteins

Immunoturbidimetric and immunonephelometric assays are typically used in measuring apo A-I and apo B-100 (see Chapter 15). Considerable effort has been expended to standardize apo A-I and B-100 measurements, leading to significant improvement in the overall performance of these assays, but they are still not widely used for ASCVD risk assessment. Immunoassays for total apo E are not commonly performed for clinical evaluation, but genotyping of apo E is used to identify the apo E4 isoform, which is associated with increased cholesterol and risk for Alzheimer disease.

### Lipoprotein(a)

Although Lp(a) particles typically carry only a relatively small fraction of total cholesterol, these lipoprotein particles are particularly proatherogenic and are an independent and causal risk factor for ASCVD and aortic stenosis. Additionally, in randomized cholesterol lowering treatment trials, ASCVD events are higher when Lp(a) is elevated independent of any achieved LDL-C concentration. Therefore Lp(a) is often measured in individuals with a normal lipid panel but with a history of premature ASCVD and/or a strong family history of ASCVD. Turbidimetric, nephelometric, RIA, and ELISA methods are all currently used for Lp(a) measurement. Most of these assays, except for ELISA, are based on the use of polyclonal antibodies. Sandwich-type ELISAs are usually based on the use of a combination of monoclonal and polyclonal antibodies to apo B and apo(a). Lp(a) is both unique and a challenge to measure accurately in all patients because the size of the lipoprotein particle varies due to allelic heterogeneity of isoform lengths for the apo(a) protein. The immunoreactivity of antibodies directed to the repeat kringle 4 type 2 domain in apo(a) makes the results obtained from Lp(a) assays vary as a function of apo(a) size. All currently available immunoassays suffer from some degree of inaccuracies when measuring Lp(a) of different sizes, but some assays are more susceptible than others. These assays tend to underestimate apo(a) concentration in samples with apo(a) of smaller size than the apo(a) present in the assay calibrator and to overestimate the apo(a) concentration in samples with larger apo(a). Traditionally, Lp(a) concentrations have been reported in terms of total Lp(a) particle mass (mg/dL) or, alternatively, in terms of Lp(a) protein. Most population analyses and clinical cut-points for increased ASCVD risk have been performed using assays that report in mg/dL. However, to provide Lp(a) values that are less biased by apo(a) size, it is recommended that the Lp(a) assay use antibodies directed to an apo(a) domain other than kringle 4 type 2, or to the apo B-100 component of Lp(a). This would allow the values to be expressed in nanomoles per liter. At present, Lp(a) measurements are not well standardized, but a value of approximately 30 mg/dL of total Lp(a) particle mass has traditionally been used as a cutoff, above which increased concentrations of Lp(a) are associated with increased risk of ASCVD. Higher clinical cut-points for patient care decisions have been proposed in various professional society guidelines. When using an assay that reports in molar units, increased risk starts at 75 nmol/L with specific higher clinical cut-points suggested in the various guidelines.

While the standard method to measure Lp(a) is the immunoassays described above, it should be noted that the cholesterol within Lp(a) is reported as LDL-C in nearly all methods for measuring LDL-C including calculations and even beta quantification. The Lp(a) particle is the same size and density and contains apoB just like LDL, therefore most methods that measure LDL-C will include Lp(a)-cholesterol. While both are proatherogenic, distinguishing LDL-C from Lp(a)-C

may be clinically important when physicians are considering a diagnosis for an observed hypercholesterolemia that may lead to genetic testing or family cascade testing. Additionally, patients with high Lp(a)-C may not respond to standard lipid lowering treatments to the same extent as those with high LDL-C. Some have advocated for an estimate of Lp(a)-C using the Lp(a) concentration measured by the immunoassay using a conversion factor. However, given the heterogeneity of Lp(a) size, these estimates can be quite inaccurate. Methods to measure cholesterol within Lp(a) specifically often require the separation of Lp(a) from LDL and subsequent cholesterol measurements. Those assays are typically only offered at referral laboratories.

## Sources of Variation and Bias in Test Measurement

Concentrations of various lipoproteins and their constituent parts—lipids and apolipoproteins—vary within individuals (see Chapter 4). Analytical variations for such measurements are relatively small—generally approximately 2%–3% CVs for cholesterol—but some direct measurements of LDL-C and HDL-C do not meet National Cholesterol Education Program (NCEP) guidelines for analytical performance on dyslipidemic samples. In contrast, physiological variations are much larger and contribute to most of the overall variation in lipid and lipoprotein concentrations.

## ADVANCED LIPID AND LIPOPROTEIN TESTING FOR ASCVD RISK ASSESSMENT

Despite the strong association of plasma lipid concentrations with ASCVD risk, it has been long recognized that half of all myocardial infarctions occur among individuals with a normal lipid panel. Consequently, there is a constant search for enhanced biomarkers of altered lipid metabolism and ASCVD risk. Measurement of lipoprotein particle number, and size by advanced methods such as nuclear magnetic resonance (NMR) spectroscopy or by mass spectrometry are commonly ordered by clinicians. Other tests are based on oxidized lipids, sphingolipids, or inflammatory proteins. While these measures can be predictive of disease, the association is largely diminished after accounting for basic lipid panel results. No advanced lipoprotein particle number, size or oxidation methods have been endorsed or recommended by any medical society. High-sensitivity C-reactive protein (hsCRP), which measures within the normal range of the acute phase reaction protein CRP, is considered a risk-enhancing factor for ASCVD. Several large clinical trials have supported this use for CRP and it is the one enhanced biomarker with multisociety guideline approval.

## REVIEW QUESTIONS

1. The Friedewald formula for estimating LDL-C is not accurate in which of the following conditions?
   a. Elevated triglycerides
   b. The presence of chylomicrons
   c. Dysbetalipoproteinemias
   d. Very low LDL-C
   e. All the above

2. The protein component of a lipoprotein is referred to as:
   a. terpene
   b. apolipoprotein
   c. prostaglandin
   d. phospholipid
3. The lipoprotein that contains a carbohydrate-rich protein covalently bound to apo B-100 and a special protein motif called the "kringle" domain is:
   a. LDL
   b. HDL
   c. chylomicron
   d. lipoprotein(a)
4. Which lipoprotein transports mostly cholesteryl esters through the blood?
   a. LDL
   b. VLDL
   c. Chylomicrons
   d. IDL
5. The enzyme that is critical for hydrolysis of triglycerides on chylomicrons for their conversion to chylomicron remnants is:
   a. cholesterol oxidase
   b. glycerol kinase
   c. lipoprotein lipase
   d. HMG-CoA reductase
6. The rate-limiting enzyme in cholesterol biosynthesis that is inhibited by statin drugs is:
   a. cholesterol oxidase
   b. glycerol kinase
   c. lipoprotein lipase
   d. HMG-CoA reductase
7. Which of the following lipid metabolic pathways has a role in transferring excess cholesterol from peripheral tissues to the liver?
   a. Exogenous pathway
   b. Endogenous pathway
   c. Intracellular cholesterol transport pathway
   d. Reverse cholesterol transport pathway
8. The basic lipid panel includes which of the following parameters?
   a. Total cholesterol, VLDL-C, HDL-C, Lp(a), and LDL-C
   b. Total cholesterol, triglycerides, HDL-C, non-HDL-C, and LDL-C
   c. HDL-C and LDL-C
   d. Total cholesterol, HDL-C and hsCRP
9. Regarding lipids, a carboxyl (–COOH) with a long side chain (R) containing an even number of carbon atoms that is important in human nutrition and metabolism is referred to as a(n):
   a. acylglycerol
   b. ester
   c. fatty acid
   d. terpene
10. In the laboratory analysis of triglycerides, the initial step in all methods is:
    a. phosphorylation of glycerol catalyzed by glycerokinase
    b. oxidation of cholesterol by cholesterol oxidase
    c. hydrolysis of triglyceride to form free glycerol
    d. reduction of phenol and $H_2O_2$ by peroxidase

## SUGGESTED READINGS

Davidson MH, Ballantyne CM, Jacobson TA, et al. Clinical utility of inflammatory markers and advanced lipoprotein testing: advice from an expert panel of lipid specialists. *J Clin Lipidol.* 2011;5:338–367.

Expert panel on integrated guidelines for cardiovascular health and risk reduction in children and adolescents: summary report. *Pediatrics.* 2011;128:S1–S44.

Grundy SM, Stone NJ, Bailey AL, et al. 2018 AHA/ACC/AACVPR/AAPA/ABC/ACPM/ADA/AGS/APhA/ASPC/NLA/PCNA Guideline on the Management of Blood Cholesterol: A Report of the American College of Cardiology/American Heart Association Task Force on Clinical Practice Guidelines. *Circulation.* 2019;139:e1082–e1143.

Havel RJ, Kane JP. Introduction: structure and metabolism of plasma lipoproteins. In: Scriver CR, Beaudet AL, Sly WS, Valle D, eds. *The Metabolic and Molecular Basis of Inherited Diseases.* 8th ed. New York: McGraw-Hill; 2001:2705–2716.

Mahley RW, Innerarity TL, Rall Jr SC, et al. Plasma lipoproteins: apolipoprotein structure and function. *J Lipid Res.* 1984;25:1277–1294.

Nordestgaard BG, Langsted A, Mora S, et al. Fasting is not routinely required for determination of a lipid profile: clinical and laboratory implications including flagging at desirable concentration cutpoints—A Joint Consensus Statement from the European Atherosclerosis Society and European Federation of Clinical Chemistry and Laboratory Medicine. *Clin Chem.* 2016;62:930.

Vesper HW, Wilson PW, Rifai N. A message from the laboratory community to the National Cholesterol Education Program Adult Treatment Panel IV. *Clin Chem.* 2012;58:523–527.

Wilson DP, Jacobson TA, Jones PH, et al. Use of lipoprotein(a) in clinical practice: A biomarker whose time has come. A scientific statement from the National Lipid Association. *J Clin Lipidol.* 2019;13:374.

Wilson PWF, Jacobson TA, Martin SS, et al. Lipid measurements in the management of cardiovascular diseases: Practical recommendations a scientific statement from the national lipid association writing group. *J Clin Lipidol.* 2021;15:629–648.

# Electrolytes and Blood Gases

*Mark D. Kellogg and Mark A. Cervinski*

## OBJECTIVES

1. Define the following terms:
   - Anion
   - Blood gas
   - Cation
   - Colligative properties
   - Electrolyte
   - Electrolyte exclusion effect
   - Osmolality
   - Oxygen dissociation curve
   - Oxygen saturation
   - pH
   - Partial pressure
   - Co-oximetry
   - Sweat chloride test
2. For each of the following electrolytes, state and describe the biochemistry, physiological functions, localization, clinical significance, method of analysis, and potential analytical interferences:
   a. Bicarbonate
   b. Chloride
   c. Potassium
   d. Sodium
3. Compare direct and indirect ion-selective electrode testing, including uses of and interferences in each method.
4. Discuss the measurement of sweat chloride, including reasons for performing, details of the phases of testing, and specimen requirements.
5. Describe the following methods of electrolyte/blood gas measurement, including which analytes are measured with each technique, the principle of the method, specimen requirements, and possible interferences:
   a. Coulometry-amperometry
   b. Osmometry
   c. Potentiometry
   d. Sweat testing
6. List and describe the four colligative properties of a solution.
7. State the formula that demonstrates the relationship between total concentration of $CO_2$, bicarbonate, and hydrogen ion concentration.
8. State the Henderson-Hasselbalch equation and explain each of its components.
9. List the three essential properties of arterial blood required for adequate oxygen delivery to tissues.
10. For blood gas determinations, describe each of the following:
    a. Specimen requirements
    b. Preferred anticoagulant
    c. Collection technique
    d. Specimen transport conditions
11. List the analytical problems that arise in the analysis of pH, $pO_2$, and $pCO_2$ with inappropriate specimen collection or transport.
12. Diagram a generic blood gas analyzer; state and describe the methods or calculations used to measure pH, $pO_2$, and $pCO_2$, including noninvasive and continuous monitoring methods.

## KEY WORDS AND DEFINITIONS

**Anemic hypoxia** Hypoxia (a reduced supply of oxygen to the tissues) resulting from a decrease in the amount of hemoglobin or number of erythrocytes in the blood.

**Blood gases** $pCO_2$ and $pO_2$ (partial pressures of carbon dioxide and oxygen), usually in whole blood.

**Colligative properties** Properties of solutions that depend on the number of particles in the solution; examples include (1) osmotic pressure, (2) boiling point elevation, (3) freezing point depression, and (4) vapor pressure lowering.

**Cystic fibrosis (CF)** Inherited disorder of a transmembrane conductance regulator protein (CFTR) that leads to chronic pancreatic and obstructive pulmonary disease.

**Cystic fibrosis transmembrane conductance regulator (CFTR)** A transmembrane protein produced by the *CFTR* gene.

**Electrolytes** Charged low-molecular-mass molecules or elemental ions are present in plasma and in cells, usually ions of (1) sodium, (2) potassium, (3) calcium, (4) magnesium, (5) chloride, (6) bicarbonate, (7) phosphate, (8) sulfate, and (9) lactate.

**Electrolyte exclusion effect** Electrolytes are excluded from the fraction of total plasma volume that is occupied by solids, which leads to an underestimation of electrolyte concentration by some methods.

**Extracellular fluid compartment (ECF)** Compartment comprised of the intravascular and interstitial spaces. The fluids in these compartments comprise about 1/3rd of the total body water.

**Hemoglobin (Hb)** An oxygen-carrying, heme-containing protein abundant in red blood cells.

**Henderson-Hasselbalch equation** Equation that defines the relationship between pH, bicarbonate, and the partial pressure of dissolved carbon dioxide gas

$$pH = pK + \log\left(\frac{cHCO_3^-}{\alpha \times pCO_2}\right)$$

**Ion-selective electrode (ISE)** A type of special-purpose, potentiometric electrode consisting of a membrane selectively permeable to a single ionic species. The potential produced at the membrane–sample solution interface is proportional to the logarithm of the ionic activity or concentration.

**Intracellular fluid** Fluid found inside cells, accounting for approximately 2/3rds of total body water.

**Osmolal gap** A difference between the observed and calculated osmolalities in serum analysis. The formula for calculated osmolality is $2 \times Na$ (mmol/L) + glucose (mmol/L) + blood urea nitrogen (mmol/L); or $2 \times Na$ (mmol/L) + glucose (mg/dL)/18 + urea (mg/dL)/2.8.

**Osmometry** Technique for measuring the concentration of dissolved solute particles in a solution.

**Osmotic pressure** The pressure required to stop osmosis through a semipermeable membrane between a solution and a pure solvent.

**Oximetry** A technique used to determine the oxygen saturation of arterial blood.

**Oxygen dissociation curve** The sigmoidal curve obtained when $SO_2$ of blood is plotted against $pO_2$.

**Oxygen saturation ($SO_2$)** The fraction (percentage) of functional hemoglobin that is saturated with oxygen.

**Oxyhemoglobin** Hemoglobin that contains bound $O_2$.

**$P_{50}$** $pO_2$ for a given blood sample, at which the hemoglobin of the blood is half saturated with $O_2$; $P_{50}$ reflects the affinity of hemoglobin for $O_2$.

**Partial pressure** The substance (mole) fraction of gas times the total pressure, for example, the partial pressure of oxygen, $pO_2$, is the fraction of oxygen gas times the barometric pressure.

**pH** The negative logarithm of hydrogen ion activity.

**Pilocarpine iontophoresis** Noninvasive method that uses electricity to force the drug pilocarpine into the skin for the purpose of inducing localized sweating at the site of iontophoresis.

**Sweat chloride** The concentration of chloride in sweat; increased sweat chloride is characteristic of cystic fibrosis.

**Water homeostasis** The body process that maintains a balance of water intake and output.

Maintenance of water homeostasis is paramount to life for all organisms. In humans, the maintenance of water homeostasis in various body fluid compartments is primarily a function of the four major electrolytes: $Na^+$, $K^+$, $Cl^-$, and $HCO_3^-$. These electrolytes also have a role in acid-base balance and heart and muscle function and serve as cofactors for enzymes. Abnormal electrolyte concentrations may be the cause or the consequence of a variety of medical disorders. Because of their physiologic and clinical interrelationships, this chapter discusses determination of (1) electrolytes, (2) osmolality, (3) sweat testing, (4) blood gases and pH, and (5) oxygen hemodynamics.

## ELECTROLYTES

Electrolytes may be classified as *anions*, negatively charged ions that move toward an anode, or *cations*, positively charged ions that move toward a cathode. Important physiologic electrolytes include $Na^+$, $K^+$, $Ca^{2+}$, $Mg^{2+}$, $Cl^-$, $HCO_3^-$, $H_2PO_4^-$, $HPO_4^{2-}$, $SO_4^{2-}$, and some organic anions, such as lactate. At physiologic pH, proteins in serum are usually anions, and albumin accounts for most of the difference between the commonly measured cations ($Na^+$, $K^+$) and anions ($Cl^-$, $HCO_3^-$), also known as the anion gap. Hydrogen ion ($H^+$) concentration is routinely measured as pH, but its concentration is so low relative to other ions ($10^{-9}$ vs. $10^{-3}$ mol/L) that

its role as an electrolyte is negligible for clinical purposes. The major electrolytes ($Na^+$, $K^+$, $Cl^-$, $HCO_3^-$) occur primarily as free ions, whereas significant amounts (>40%) of $Ca^{2+}$, $Mg^{2+}$, and trace elements are bound by proteins, mainly albumin. Determination of body fluid concentrations of the four major electrolytes ($Na^+$, $K^+$, $Cl^-$, and $HCO_3^-$) is commonly referred to as an *electrolyte profile*.

## SODIUM

Sodium is the major cation of extracellular fluid. Because it represents approximately 90% of the ≈154 mmol of inorganic cations per liter of plasma, $Na^+$ is responsible for almost one-half the osmotic strength of plasma. It therefore plays a central role in maintaining the normal distribution of water and osmotic pressure in the extracellular fluid compartment (ECF).

Sodium is freely filtered by renal glomeruli. Seventy to 80% of the filtered $Na^+$ load is actively reabsorbed in the proximal tubules, with $Cl^-$ and water passively following in an iso-osmotic and electrically neutral manner. Another 20% to 25% is reabsorbed in the loop of Henle, along with $Cl^-$ and more water. In the distal tubules, interaction of the adrenal hormone aldosterone with the coupled $Na^+$-$K^+$ and $Na^+$-$H^+$ exchange systems results directly in the reabsorption of $Na^+$, and indirectly of $Cl^-$, from the remaining 5% to 10%

of the filtered load. It is the regulation of this latter fraction of filtered Na+ that primarily determines the amount of Na+ excreted in the urine. These processes are discussed in detail in Chapter 35.

## Specimens

Serum, plasma, and urine may be stored at 4°C or frozen. Erythrocytes contain only 1/10th of the Na+ present in plasma, so hemolysis does not cause significant errors in serum or plasma Na+ values. Lipemic samples should be ultracentrifuged, and the infranatant analyzed unless a direct ISE is used (see the section "Electrolyte Exclusion Effect").

Fecal and GI fluid specimens require preparation before assay. Because significant electrolyte loss in feces only occurs in diarrhea, only liquid stool samples may be justified for analysis. Immediately after collection, liquid stool specimens should be clarified of particulate matter by filtration through gauze or filter paper and by centrifugation. If not analyzed immediately, fecal and GI fluids should be stored frozen to prevent microbial growth.

## Reference Intervals

A typical reference interval for *serum* or plasma Na+ is 135 to 145 mmol/L. The interval for premature newborns at 48 hours is 128 to 148 mmol/L, and the value for umbilical cord blood from full-term newborns is ≈127 mmol/L.

*Urinary sodium* excretion varies with diet, but for an adult male consuming 7 to 14 g of NaCl per day, an interval of 120 to 240 mmol/L is typical. A large diurnal variation in Na+ excretion has been noted, with the rate of Na+ excretion during the night being only 20% of the peak rate during the day. The Na+ concentration of cerebrospinal fluid is 136 to 150 mmol/L. Mean fecal Na+ excretion is less than 10 mmol/L.

# POTASSIUM

Potassium is the major intracellular cation, with an average concentration in tissue cells of ~150 mmol/L, and in erythrocytes, the concentration is ~105 mmol/L. High intracellular concentrations are maintained by the Na+, K+ adenosine triphosphate (ATP)ase pump, which continually transports K+ into the cell against a concentration gradient. Diffusion of K+ out of the cell into the ECF and plasma occurs whenever pump activity is decreased because of (1) depletion of metabolic substrates such as glucose; (2) competition for ATP between the pump and other energy-consuming activities of the cell; or (3) slowing of cellular metabolism (as occurs with refrigeration). The importance of these considerations on sample integrity for analysis of K+ is discussed later.

Potassium absorbed from the GI tract is rapidly distributed, with a small amount taken up by cells and most excreted by the kidneys. Potassium filtered through the glomeruli is almost completely reabsorbed in the proximal tubules and is then secreted in the distal tubules in exchange for Na+ under the influence of aldosterone. Aldosterone enhances K+ secretion and Na+ reabsorption in the distal tubules by a Na+-K+ exchange mechanism. The kidneys respond to K+ loading with an increase in K+ output, so that urine collected during or after a period of high K+ intake may have K+ concentrations as high as 100 mmol/L. In contrast, the tubular response to conserve K+ is very slow in the initial stages of depletion. Unlike the prompt response to conserve Na+ in deficit states, it can take up to 1 week for the tubules to reduce K+ excretion to 5 to 10 mmol/day from the typical 50 to 100 mmol/day.

Factors that regulate distal tubular secretion of K+ include intake of Na+ and K+, mineralocorticoid concentration, and acid-base balance. Because renal conservation mechanisms are slow to respond, K+ depletion can be an early consequence of restricted K+ intake or loss of K+ by extrarenal routes such as diarrhea. A diminished glomerular filtration rate is typical of renal failure, and the consequent decrease in distal tubular flow rate is an important factor in the hyperkalemia associated with renal failure.

## Specimens

Comments made earlier on specimens for Na+ analysis are generally applicable to those for K+ analysis, with some caveats. Potassium concentrations in plasma and whole blood are 0.1 to 0.7 mmol/L lower than those in serum. The extent of this difference depends on the platelet count because additional K+ in serum is primarily a result of platelet rupture during clotting. This variability in the amount of additional K+ in serum makes plasma the specimen of choice.

Specimens for determining K+ concentrations in whole blood, serum, or plasma must be collected by methods that minimize hemolysis because the release of K+ from as few as 0.5% of erythrocytes can increase K+ values by 0.5 mmol/L. An increase in K+ of 0.6% has been estimated for every 10 mg/dL of plasma **hemoglobin** caused by hemolysis. Thus slight hemolysis (Hb ≈ 50 mg/dL) can be expected to raise K+ values by ≈3%, marked hemolysis (Hb ≈ 200 mg/dL) by 12%, and gross hemolysis (Hb > 500 mg/dL) by as much as 30%. The use of correction factors based on a hemolysis index has been suggested for estimating K+ in hemolyzed samples, but their use has been questioned. Regardless, it is imperative that if the laboratory chooses to report K+ concentrations on hemolyzed samples that the presence of hemolysis is noted with a comment that results are falsely elevated, whether an estimate of the extent of elevation is provided or not. It is important to remember that if K+ concentrations are determined by ISE on whole blood specimens, hemolysis is not readily visible. When hemolysis is suspected, as in the case of an unexpected increase in K+, a portion of the specimen should be centrifuged, and the plasma visually inspected.

Clinically significant preanalytical errors can occur for K+ determinations if blood samples are not processed quickly. Maintenance of the intracellular-extracellular K+ gradient depends on the activity of the energy-dependent Na+-K+-ATPase. If a whole blood specimen is maintained at 4°C versus 25°C before separation, glycolysis is inhibited, and the energy-dependent Na+-K+-ATPase cannot maintain the Na+/K+ gradient. An increase in plasma K+ will occur as a result of K+ leakage from erythrocytes and other cells. The increase of K⁺ in serum is on the order of 0.2 mmol/L by 1.5 hours at 25°C, and is as high as 2 mmol/L after 4 hours at 4°C.

A falsely decreased K⁺ value can be observed if an unseparated sample is stored at 37°C, because glycolysis occurs and K⁺ shifts intracellularly. Even at room temperature, extreme leukocytosis can initially cause falsely decreased K⁺ concentrations. The extent of this decrease depends on leukocyte count, temperature, and glucose concentrations, but has been reported to be as much as 0.7 mmol/L at 37°C. In addition to causing pseudohypokalemia, samples from leukemic patients with very high white blood cell (WBC) counts ($>300 \times 10^9$ cells/L) can result in pseudohyperkalemia due to WBC rupture. Taken together, the recommendation for reliable K⁺ determinations is to collect blood with heparin and to maintain it near 25°C, and then separate the plasma within minutes by high-speed centrifugation. In practical terms, separation within 1 hour when samples are maintained at room temperature is unlikely to introduce great error.

Finally, skeletal muscle activity causes K⁺ efflux from muscle cells into plasma and can cause a marked elevation in plasma K⁺ values. A common example occurs when an upper arm tourniquet is not released before beginning to draw blood after a patient has repeatedly clenched their fist. This combination of tourniquet-induced venostasis and muscular activity can artificially raise plasma K⁺ values as much as 2 mmol/L.

## Reference Intervals

Reported reference intervals for the serum of adults vary from 3.5 to 5.1 mmol/L and from 3.7 to 5.9 for newborns. For plasma, a frequently cited adult interval is 3.3 to 4.9 mmol/L. Urinary excretion of K⁺ varies with dietary intake, but a typical range observed is 42 to 86 mmol/L for males and 33 to 70 mmol/L for females. In severe diarrhea, GI loss may be as much as 60 mmol/L.

## METHODS FOR THE DETERMINATION OF SODIUM AND POTASSIUM

Sodium and potassium are most commonly determined in the clinical laboratory by potentiometric ion-selective electrodes (ISE). Historically, sodium and potassium were also determined via atomic absorption spectrophotometry, flame ionization spectrophotometry, or spectrophotometrically via enzymatic methods. See Chapter 10 for detailed explanations of the methodologies utilized in electrolyte analysis.

Two types of ISE methods, indirect ISE and direct ISE, are in use and must be distinguished. With *indirect ISE methods,* the sample is first mixed with a large volume of diluent of low ionic strength prior to introduction into the measurement chamber. Indirect ISE is most commonly used on automated, high-throughput clinical chemistry systems. Indirect methods were developed early in the history of ISE technology, when dilution was necessary to present a small sample in a volume large enough to adequately cover a large electrode and to minimize the concentration of protein at the electrode surface. With *direct ISE methods,* the sample is presented to the electrodes without dilution. Direct ISE methods became possible with electrode miniaturization and are available on a few automated laboratory instruments. Direct ISE electrodes are primarily used in blood gas analyzers and point-of-care devices where whole blood is directly presented to the electrodes.

Errors observed in the use of ISEs fall into three categories. First are errors caused by a lack of selectivity. For instance, many Cl⁻ electrodes lack selectivity against other halide anions such as I⁻ or SCN⁻ from the metabolism of sodium nitroprusside. Second are errors introduced by repeated protein coating of the ISE membranes, or by contamination of the membrane or salt bridge by ions that compete or react with the selected ion and thus alter the electrode response. Such errors in ISE measurements necessitate periodic changes of the membrane as part of routine maintenance. Finally, the **electrolyte exclusion effect**, which applies only to indirect methods and is caused by the solvent-displacing effect of lipids and proteins in the sample, results in falsely decreased values.

## Spectrophotometric Methods

Spectrophotometric methods are based on Na⁺ or K⁺-specific enzyme activation. However, the higher cost of these methods and the fact that few problems exist with ISE methods have resulted in "niche" uses of spectrophotometric analysis, primarily with smaller instruments used in physicians' offices and more recently in "isolation" laboratories for patients with emerging infectious diseases.

Kinetic spectrophotometric assays for Na⁺ are based on the activation of the enzyme β-galactosidase by Na⁺ to hydrolyze *o*-nitrophenyl-β-D-galactopyranoside. The rate of production of *o*-nitrophenol (the chromophore) is measured at 420 nm.

*o*-Nitrophenyl-β-D-galactopyranoside    Galactose + *o*-Nitrophenol ($\lambda_{max}$ = 420 nm)

Spectrophotometric K⁺ assays rely upon the K⁺ activation of pyruvate kinase for the conversion of phosphoenolpyruvate to pyruvate, which is then reduced to lactate by lactate dehydrogenase, in the process of oxidizing NADH to NAD⁺.

## ELECTROLYTE EXCLUSION EFFECT

The major plasma electrolytes, Na⁺, K⁺, Cl⁻, and $HCO_3^-$, have minimal protein binding and are carried in the water phase of plasma. The composition of plasma is approximately 93% water and 7% solids such as proteins and lipids. When the fixed volume of plasma (e.g., 10 μL) is pipetted for dilution into a buffer of low ionic strength before indirect ISE analysis, only 9.3 μL of *plasma water* that contains the electrolytes is added to the diluent. However, when we report plasma electrolyte concentrations, we report the values in mmol/L of total plasma volume, not plasma water volume. Thus in the absence of increased plasma protein or lipid concentrations, a reported $Na^+$ concentration of 140 mmol/L of plasma volume would equal a $Na^+$ concentration in plasma water of 150 mmol/L (140 × [100/93]). This negative "error" or bias in plasma electrolyte analysis has been recognized for many years.

All electrolyte reference intervals are based on the assumption that plasma is reliably ~93% water and reflect concentrations in total plasma volume and not in water volume. Even though it is the electrolyte concentration in plasma water that is physiologically relevant (the $Na^+$ concentration of normal saline is 150 mmol/L), it was assumed that the volume fraction of water in plasma is sufficiently constant that this difference could be ignored. This electrolyte exclusion effect, however, becomes problematic when pathophysiologic conditions are present that alter the plasma water volume, such as hyperlipidemia or hyperproteinemia. In these settings, falsely low electrolyte values are obtained whenever samples are diluted before analysis.

In certain settings, such as ketoacidosis with severe hyperlipidemia or multiple myeloma with severe hyperproteinemia, the negative exclusion effect may be so large that laboratory results lead clinicians to believe that electrolyte concentrations are normal or low, when in fact the concentration in the water phase may be high or normal, respectively, leading to pseudohyponatremia (Fig. 24.1).

In severe hypoproteinemia, the effect works in reverse, resulting in falsely high (2% to 4%) $Na^+$ or $K^+$ values. As with the indirect ISE, the original method for measuring plasma electrolytes, flame photometry, also required dilution of the sample prior to analysis and, as such, is also subject to pseudohypo- and hypernatremia.

Direct ISE methods do not require sample dilution, and as there is no dilution, ion activity is directly proportional to the concentration in the water phase, not the concentration in the total plasma volume. Therefore, direct ISE methods are free of electrolyte exclusion effects. To make results from direct ISEs equivalent to those from indirect ISEs (and flame photometry), direct ISE methods operate in what is commonly referred to as the "flame mode." In this mode, the directly measured concentration in plasma water is multiplied by the average water volume fraction of plasma (0.93). Although the actual water volume fraction of plasma may vary widely, as long as the activity of the specific ion is constant, the concentration of the ion in the water phase becomes *independent* of the relative proportions of water and total solids if the ion is not bound by proteins. Most clinical chemists and physicians have reached the conclusion that direct ISE methods for electrolyte analysis are the methods of choice. However, results from direct ISE methods will continue to be converted to total plasma volume concentrations by use of the "flame mode," as greater than 80% of laboratories continue to use indirect ISE methods.

## CHLORIDE

Chloride is the major extracellular anion and, similar to $Na^+$, is significantly involved in the maintenance of water distribution, osmotic pressure, and anion-cation balance in the ECF. In contrast to its high ECF concentrations (≈103 mmol/L), the concentration of $Cl^-$ in the **intracellular fluid** of erythrocytes is 45 to 54 mmol/L, and in the intracellular fluid of most other tissue cells it is only ≈1 mmol/L. In gastric and intestinal secretions, $Cl^-$ is the most abundant anion.

Chloride ions are almost completely absorbed from the intestinal tract. In the kidneys, they are filtered from plasma at the glomeruli and are passively reabsorbed, along with $Na^+$, in the proximal tubules. In the thick ascending limb of the loop of Henle, $Cl^-$ is actively reabsorbed by the chloride pump, which promotes passive reabsorption of $Na^+$. Loop diuretics such as furosemide inhibit the chloride pump. Chloride concentrations are not homeostatically controlled and passively reflect the concentration of the major ions sodium and bicarbonate. In addition, chloride concentrations will decrease to maintain the electroneutrality of body fluids when pathological levels of other anions (e.g., ketoacids and lactate) are present.

### Specimens

Chloride can be measured in whole blood, serum, plasma, urine, and sweat. Fecal determination of $Cl^-$ may also be useful for the diagnosis of congenital hypochloremic alkalosis with hyperchloridorrhea (increased $Cl^-$ in stool). Chloride is stable in serum and plasma, and hemolysis does not significantly alter whole blood, serum, or plasma $Cl^-$ concentrations because the erythrocyte concentration of $Cl^-$ is approximately half of that in plasma.

### Reference Intervals

Reported reference intervals for serum or plasma $Cl^-$ vary from 98 to 107 mmol/L to 100 to 108 mmol/L. Urinary excretion of $Cl^-$ varies with dietary intake, but an interval of 110 to 250 mmol/24 h is typical.

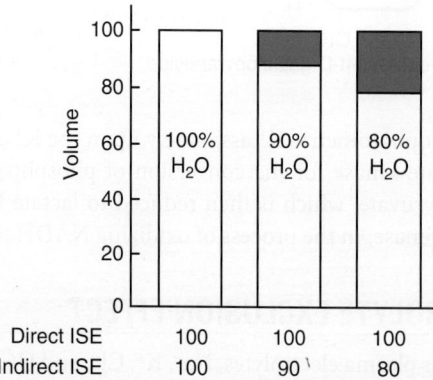

**Fig. 24.1** Predicted influence of water content on sodium measurements for a 100 mmol/L NaCl solution by direct ion-selective electrode (*ISE*) versus indirect ISE. *Blue areas* represent the volumes of nonaqueous components that are suspended in the solution. In plasma, these consist of lipids or proteins. (Modified from Apple FS, Koch DD, Graves S, et al. Relationship between direct-potentiometric and flame-photometric measurement of sodium in blood. *Clin Chem.* 1982;28:1931–1935.)

# METHODS FOR DETERMINATION OF CHLORIDE IN BODY FLUIDS

Chloride is determined largely using ISE methods, with some laboratories performing coulometric-amperometric titration for sweat chloride testing.

## Ion-Selective Electrode Methods

Chloride ISEs are composed of solvent polymeric membranes incorporating quaternary ammonium salt anion exchangers. Although they are by far the most common methods for measuring $Cl^-$ in clinical laboratories, these electrodes may suffer from membrane instability and lot-to-lot inconsistency in terms of selectivity to other anions. Anions that tend to be problematic include other halides and organic anions (e.g., $SCN^-$), which can be particularly problematic because of their ability to solubilize in the polymeric organic membrane of these electrodes.

# SWEAT CHLORIDE

## Sweat Collection

Sweat chloride ion concentration is used to confirm the diagnosis of cystic fibrosis (CF). CF is caused by dysfunction of the cystic fibrosis transmembrane conductance regulator (CFTR). Sweat collection is a two-step procedure involving (1) localized sweating stimulated by iontophoresis of the cholinergic drug pilocarpine nitrate into an area of skin (pilocarpine iontophoresis), and (2) collection of sweat from the stimulated area into plastic microbore tubing or gauze.

The macroduct (microbore tubing) iontophoresis system uses a small electric current to deliver pilocarpine from a pilocarpine-impregnated agar disk at the positive electrode (anode) and an electrolyte-containing agar disk at the negative electrode (cathode) to complete the circuit. Both electrodes are ideally placed on the inner flexor surface of the same forearm; however, the inner thigh may also be used but frequently yields lower sweat volume.

Following stimulation of sweat production, a plastic disk containing a coil of small plastic tubing is tightly placed on the spot where the positive electrode was previously, and sweat is collected via capillary action.

The filter paper/gauze method, sometimes referred to as the Gibson-Cooke method, is carried out in the same manner, except reagent-soaked filter paper or gauze is used for sweat stimulation. Following stimulation, a new pre-weighed piece of filter paper or gauze is applied to the spot where the positive electrode was placed, in order to absorb sweat.

Of the two methods, the technique utilizing plastic microbore tubing has become the dominant method (~90% of laboratories), with the remainder using pre-weighed filter paper or gauze.

## Sufficient Sample Collection

The Cystic Fibrosis Foundation (CFF) requires 15 μL or 75 mg of sweat, if collected by Macroduct or filter paper/gauze methods, respectively. CFF-accredited centers are required to monitor the rate of their "quantity not sufficient" (QNS) specimens and must review sample collection steps should the QNS rate exceed acceptable limits. Collecting an adequate amount of sweat can be more challenging in patients younger than 1 month of age. For this reason, it is recommended that sweat testing in asymptomatic individuals be performed when the infant is at least 2 weeks of age, is more than 36 weeks' gestation at birth, and weighs more than 2 kg. To increase the chances of an adequate collection, two sites can be stimulated at one patient encounter. If the laboratory collects sweat from two sites (bilateral testing), the collection is considered QNS only when both sites are inadequate.

### Storage and Handling of Sweat Chloride Samples

The most common cause of falsely elevated sweat chloride is evaporation. Sweat samples should be analyzed soon after collection on the same day but may be stored up to 72 hours at 4°C if necessary. For samples collected in microbore tubing, the sweat sample should be transferred to a 0.2 mL microcentrifuge tube with a tight-fitting cap for transportation and storage. If sweat is collected into gauze, the weight of the gauze should be determined promptly and then stored in a small container with a tightly fitting lid.

### Quantitative Analysis of Sweat Chloride
#### Coulometric-Amperometric Titration

Sweat chloride concentration is determined by coulometric titration using a device referred to as a chloridometer, as this method can precisely measure chloride concentrations as low as 10 mmol/L. ISEs cannot be used to measure sweat chloride, as they lack precision at the chloride concentrations found in normal subjects.

Coulometric-amperometric determinations of $Cl^-$ depend on generation of $Ag^+$ from a silver electrode at a constant rate, and on the reaction of $Ag^+$ with $Cl^-$ in the sample to form insoluble silver chloride (AgCl):

$$Ag^+ + Cl^- \rightarrow AgCl$$

After the stoichiometric point is reached, excess $Ag^+$ in the mixture triggers shutdown of the $Ag^+$ generation system. A timing device records elapsed time between the start and stop of $Ag^+$ generation. Because the time interval is proportional to the amount of $Cl^-$ in the sample, the concentration of $Cl^-$ can be determined by comparing the time elapsed against a calibration curve.

This method is subject to interferences by other halide ions, by $CN^-$ and $SCN^-$ ions, by sulfhydryl groups, and by heavy metal contamination. Maintenance of the systems is crucial for proper operation.

### Reference Intervals for Sweat Chloride

For all individuals, including newborns with a positive newborn screen for CF, a sweat chloride concentration of less than 30 mmol/L indicates that CF is unlikely. The following reference intervals are recommended for all patients, regardless of age:

≤29 mmol/L: CF unlikely
30 to 59 mmol/L: intermediate
≥60 mmol/L: indicative of CF

The functional upper limit for sweat chloride is 160 mmol/L. A sweat chloride concentration greater than 160 mmol/L represents specimen contamination or analytical error. A sweat chloride concentration less than 30 mmol/L alone is insufficient to rule out the diagnosis; the value should be interpreted in regard to the clinical presentation and with the knowledge that "normal" concentrations have been associated with CF. Some mutations of the *CF* gene are associated with intermediate or normal sweat chloride concentrations. For example, according to the CFF registry, 3.5% of CF patients had sweat chloride concentrations less than 60 mmol/L, and 1.2% had concentrations less than 40 mmol/L.

## BICARBONATE (TOTAL CARBON DIOXIDE)

Total carbon dioxide is used here to describe the quantity that is measured most often in automated clinical chemistry analyzers by acidification of a serum or plasma sample and measurement of carbon dioxide released by the process, or by alkalization and measurement of total bicarbonate. Under certain conditions of collection and specimen handling, total carbon dioxide values determined in this manner will be almost identical to values for the calculated concentration of total carbon dioxide obtained in blood gas analysis (see the later section in this chapter on blood gas methods).

### Specimens

The same sample types used for $Na^+$ or $K^+$ may be assayed. Given a specimen collected in an evacuated tube, the concentration of total $CO_2$ is most accurately determined when the test is done as soon as possible after collection and centrifugation of the blood in a fully filled, unopened tube. Ambient air contains far less $CO_2$ than plasma, and gaseous dissolved $CO_2$ will escape from the specimen into the air, with a consequent decrease in the $CO_2$ value of up to 2 to 3 mmol/L in the course of 1 hour. In practical terms, the logistics of high-volume processing and automated analysis of specimens almost ensure that most $CO_2$ measurements are done on specimens that have lost some dissolved gaseous $CO_2$, simply because preservation of anaerobic conditions is not practical between the time plasma is placed on an instrument and the time it is sampled. Thus the term *bicarbonate* may be preferable to *total CO_2*.

### Methods for Determination of Serum or Plasma Total Carbon Dioxide

Methods for total $CO_2$ measurement with modern automated instruments may be electrode based or enzymatic. In indirect electrode-based methods, the plasma sample is acidified to convert the various forms of $CO_2$ present in the sample to gaseous $CO_2$. The amount of gaseous $CO_2$ released after acidification is determined by a $pCO_2$ electrode in the reaction chamber of the $CO_2$ module. *Direct ISE methods* for total $CO_2$

are no longer common on automated analyzers due to problems with specificity.

In *enzymatic methods* for $CO_2$, the specimen is first alkalinized to convert all $CO_2$ and carbonic acid to $HCO_3^-$. The enzymatic reactions are as follows:

The decrease in absorbance at 340 nm, as NADH is oxidized to $NAD^+$, is proportional to the total $CO_2$ content. The enzymatic method is more common than the electrode-based method, with approximately 80% of laboratories utilizing an enzymatic method.

### Reference Intervals

The reference interval for total carbon dioxide in adults is 22 to 28 mmol/L but can be method and instrument dependent. The reference interval for $CO_2$ also varies with age, with pediatric patients exhibiting lower values due to a higher respiratory rate.

### POINTS TO REMEMBER

- Sodium, potassium, and chloride concentrations in biological fluids are predominantly quantified using ion-selective electrodes.
- Sweat chloride concentrations are quantified utilizing coulometric-amperometric titration, and elevated concentrations are used to diagnose cystic fibrosis.
- Indirect ion-selective electrodes used for measuring serum/plasma sodium concentrations are prone to the electrolyte exclusion effect in samples containing high concentrations of lipids and/or proteins.
- Total serum/plasma $CO_2$ concentrations will decrease when samples are uncapped and exposed to room air.

## PRINCIPLES OF OSMOTIC PRESSURE AND OSMOSIS

**Osmometry** is a technique for measuring the concentration of solutes that contribute to the osmotic pressure of a solution. Osmotic pressure governs the movement of solvent (water in biological systems) across semipermeable membranes that separate two solutions. Examples of biologically important selective membranes are those enclosing the glomeruli and capillary vessels that are permeable to water and to essentially all *small* molecules and ions, but not to large protein molecules. Differences in the concentrations of osmotically active molecules that cannot cross a membrane cause those molecules that can cross the membrane (such as water in the descending loop of Henle) to move to equalize the concentrations on both sides of the membrane. The force driving this movement of solute and permeable ions is known as **osmotic pressure**. As a simple example, consider an aqueous solution of sucrose placed within a sac made up of a membrane permeable only to water, with an open vertical glass tube attached to the sac. If the sac is placed in a beaker of distilled water, water will move from the beaker across the membrane into the sucrose solution. The pressure of this solvent movement will cause the sucrose solution to rise up the tube. At equilibrium, the gravitational pressure of the column of solution in the tube equals the osmotic pressure and prevents further net movement of water from the beaker. The height of the rise of the sucrose solution in the glass tube is a measure of the *osmotic pressure* of the sucrose solution. This is the pressure that would have to be exerted on the sucrose side of the membrane to prevent the flow of water across the membrane.

If the sucrose solution in the above example was replaced with a solution of NaCl at the same molarity, the solution in the glass tube would reach equilibrium at a point almost twice as high as that observed with sucrose. This is because NaCl dissociates into two ions per molecule and would thus have twice as many osmotically active solutes (osmoles) for the same molar concentration as the sucrose solution. In reality, the number of active particles in a solution of NaCl is less than this (~0.93 for NaCl), as explained later in this chapter. The total number of individual solutes present in a solution per given mass of solvent, regardless of their chemical nature (i.e., nonelectrolyte, ion, or colloid), determines the total osmotic pressure of the solution. In blood plasma, for example, nonelectrolytes such as glucose and urea and, to a much lesser extent, proteins contribute to the osmotic pressure.

## Colligative Properties

In addition to the osmotic pressure being raised when a solute is dissolved in a solvent, the *vapor pressure* of the solution is *lowered* below that of the pure solvent. As a result of the change in vapor pressure, the *boiling point* of the solution is *raised* above, and the *freezing point* of the solution is *lowered* below that of the pure solvent.

These four properties of solutions—(1) increased osmotic pressure, (2) lowered vapor pressure, (3) increased boiling point, and (4) decreased freezing point—are called **colligative properties**. All are directly related to the total number of dissolved solutes per mass of solvent. For example, a 1-molal (mol/kg) aqueous solution boils at a temperature 0.52°C higher than and freezes at a temperature 1.858°C lower than pure water. The vapor pressure of this solution is 0.3 mm Hg lower than the vapor pressure of pure water, which is 23.8 mm Hg at 25°C. The term *osmolality* expresses concentrations relative to *mass* of the solvent (1 osmolal solution is defined to contain 1 Osmol/kg $H_2O$), whereas the term *osmolarity* expresses concentrations per volume of solution (1 osmolar solution is defined to contain 1 Osmol/L). Osmolality (Osmol/kg $H_2O$) is a thermodynamically more exact expression because solution concentrations expressed on a weight basis are temperature independent, whereas those based on volume vary with temperature. Although the term *osmolarity* is often used in the medical literature, *osmolality* is what the clinical laboratory measures.

An electrolyte in solution dissociates into two (in the case of NaCl) or three (in the case of $CaCl_2$) dissolved ions; therefore the colligative effects of such solutions are multiplied by the number of dissociated ions formed per molecule. However, because of incomplete electrolyte dissociation and associations between solute and solvent molecules, many solutions do not behave as the ideal case, and a 1-molal solution may give an osmotic pressure lower than theoretically expected. The osmotic activity coefficient is a factor used to correct for deviation from the "ideal" behavior of the system:

$$osmolality = \frac{osmol}{kgH_2O} = \Phi nC$$

where $\Phi$ = osmotic coefficient, $n$ = number of solutes into which each molecule in the solution potentially dissociates, and $C$ = molality in mol/kg $H_2O$.

Glucose has an osmotic coefficient of 1.00, whereas the $\Phi$ for sodium chloride is 0.93 at the concentrations found in serum—thus the derivation of $1.86 \times Na^+$ (mmol) in some formulas used to calculate plasma osmolality (NaCl potentially contributes two osmotically active ions times 0.93 = 1.86). Ethanol has an osmotic coefficient of 0.83. The total osmolality or osmotic pressure of a solution is equal to the sum of the osmotic pressures or osmolalities of all solute species present. The electrolytes $Na^+$, $Cl^-$, and $HCO_3^-$, which are present in relatively high concentrations, make the greatest contributions to serum osmolality. Nonelectrolytes such as glucose and urea, which are normally present at lower molal concentrations, contribute less, and serum proteins contribute less than 0.5% of the total serum osmolality because even the most abundant protein is present at millimolar concentrations.

## Determination of Plasma and Urine Osmolality

Determination of plasma and urine osmolality can be useful in the assessment of electrolyte and acid-base disorders. Comparison of plasma and urine osmolalities can determine the status of water regulation by the kidneys in settings of severe electrolyte disturbances, as might occur in diabetes insipidus or the syndrome of inappropriate antidiuretic hormone (SIADH). The major osmotic substances in plasma are $Na^+$, $Cl^-$, glucose, and urea; thus expected plasma osmolality can be calculated from the following empirical equation:

$$mOsmol/kg = 2 \times Na^+ \ (mmol/L)$$
$$+ glucose \ (mmol/L)$$
$$+ urea \ (mmol/L)$$

or

$$mOsmol/kg = 2 \times Na^+ \, (mmol/L)$$
$$+ \, glucose \, (mg/dL)/18$$
$$+ \, Urea \, (mg/dL)/2.8$$

The reference interval for plasma osmolality is 275 to 300 mOsmol/kg. Comparison of measured osmolality versus calculated osmolality can reveal the presence of an **osmolal gap,** which can be important in determining the presence of exogenous osmotic substances. Comparison of calculated and measured osmolalities can also confirm or rule out suspected pseudohyponatremia caused by the electrolyte exclusion effect. Virtually all clinical laboratories use freezing point depression osmometers for the measurement of osmolality because of its simplicity and the fact that vapor pressure osmometers will not detect volatile substances such as methanol, ethanol, or isopropanol. Furthermore, freezing point depression, unlike vapor pressure, is independent of changes in ambient temperature.

## Freezing Point Depression Osmometer

The components of a freezing point depression osmometer, often simply referred to as an osmometer (Fig. 24.2) are as follows:

1. A thermostatically controlled freezing chamber (Peltier device) maintained at −7°C.

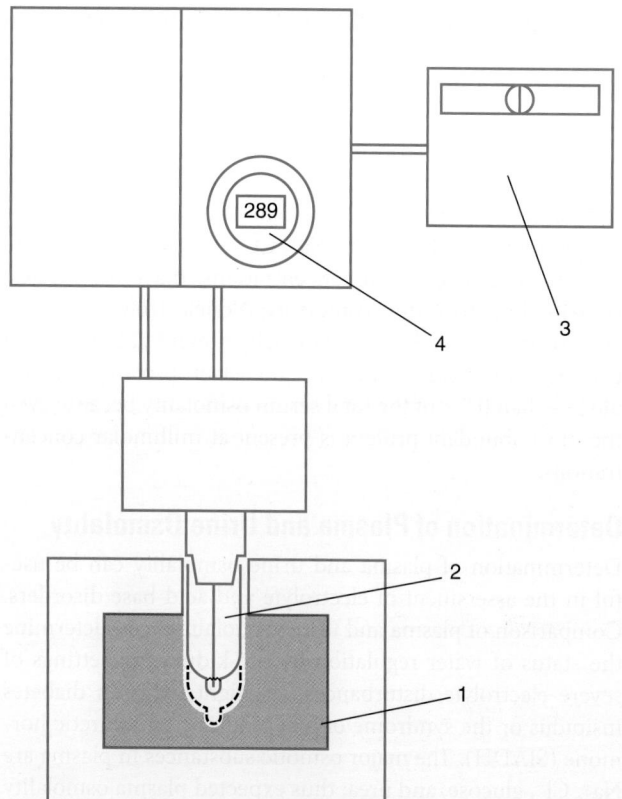

Fig. 24.2 Block diagram of a freezing point depression osmometer. The test tube is shown above the cooling block *(gray shaded area)* and inside the cooling block *(dashed line)*. 1, Cooling block (Peltier Device); 2, thermistor; 3, galvanometer; 4, potentiometer with direct readout.

2. A mechanism to agitate the sample tube to initiate (or "seed") freezing of the sample.
3. A thermistor probe connected to a circuit to measure the temperature of the sample. (The thermistor is a resistor whose resistance varies rapidly and predictably with temperature.)
4. A galvanometer that displays the freezing curve and that is used as a guide when the measuring potentiometer is used.
5. A measuring potentiometer.

In most instruments, components 4 and 5 are replaced by an automated system that provides the user with either a light-emitting diode (LED) or touchscreen display that indicates the final measured osmolality of the sample.

During analysis, the sample, in which the thermistor probe and the stirring wire are centered, is lowered into the block and is supercooled to a temperature several degrees below its freezing point (−7°C). When sufficient super cooling has occurred, the sample is agitated via a piston or other device, such as a stir rod, which initiates freezing of the supercooled solution. This freezing occurs only to the slush stage, with about 2% to 3% of the solvent solidifying. The released heat of fusion initially warms the solution, and then the temperature plateaus and remains stationary, indicating the equilibrium temperature at which both freezing and thawing of the solution occur. At the end of the equilibrium temperature plateau, the sample temperature will again decrease as the sample freezes further toward a complete solid. An example of the calculation to obtain osmolality is as follows: if the observed freezing point is −0.53°C, then:

$$mOsmol/kgH_2O = \frac{-0.53}{-1.86} \times 1000 = 285$$

where −1.86°C is the molal freezing point depression of pure water.

### POINTS TO REMEMBER

- Dissolved solutes will result in a solution with an increased osmotic pressure, lowered vapor pressure, increased boiling point, and decreased freezing point.
- Freezing point depression osmometers are the most commonly used technique to measure osmolality in the clinical laboratory.
- Comparison of plasma and urine osmolality can be useful for the assessment of water balance and disorders such as diabetes insipidus and the syndrome of inappropriate antidiuretic hormone.
- A gap between the measured and calculated osmolality can reveal the presence of unmeasured osmolytes.

## BLOOD GASES AND pH

The detection and clinical management of respiratory and metabolic disorders often depend on rapid and accurate measurements of the **partial pressures** of oxygen ($pO_2$) and carbon dioxide ($pCO_2$) in blood. Measures to support

## BOX 24.1  Conversion Factors, Prefixes, Symbols, and Descriptors Used in Discussions of Gases Measured in Blood and Expired Air[a]

**Conversion Factors**

1 mm Hg = 0.133 kPa

1 kPa = 7.5 mm Hg

  kPa: 1 kilopascal = 1000 pascal. The pascal is the SI derived unit of pressure; it equals 1 Newton/m$^2$.

**General Prefixes**

*P (or p):* partial pressure or tension

  Usage: $pO_2$, $pCO_2$, $pH_2O$

  Alternative: $pO_2$

*S:* saturation fraction

  Usage: $SO_2$

  Alternative: $sO_2$

*c:* substance concentration

  Usage: $ctO_2$ for concentration of total $O_2$

  Usage: $ctCO_2$ for concentration of total $CO_2$

  Usage: $cHCO_3^-$ for concentration of bicarbonate

*d:* dissolved gas, used with substance concentration *(c)*

*t:* total, used with substance concentration *(c)*; thus

$$ctCO_2 = cHCO_3^- + cdCO_2$$

  *Specimen origin* is indicated by lower case letters. Whole blood and plasma are distinguished by capitals.

a: arterial B: blood

v: venous P: plasma

c: capillary

  Usage: $pO_2(aB)$, for partial pressure of $O_2$ in arterial blood

**Prefixes Associated With External Respiration**

*V:* volume of air or blood (unit, L)

*V̇:* volume rate (unit, L/min)

*F:* substance fraction, also called mole fraction

*E:* expired air

*I:* inspired air

*A:* alveolar air

  Usage: *v̇(A)*, alveolar ventilation; *v̇(B)*, cardiac output; $FO_2(I)$, fraction of $O_2$ in inspired air; $pO_2(A)$, partial pressure of $O_2$ in alveolar air; and $pCO_2(E)$, partial pressure of $CO_2$ in expired air.

**Other Descriptors**

BTPS: *Body Temperature* (37°C or 310.16 K) and ambient *Pressure*, fully *Saturated* ($pH_2O$ = 47 mm Hg or 6.25 kPa)

STPD: *Standard Temperature* (0°C or 273.16 K) and standard *Pressure* (760 mm Hg or 101.08 kPa) of *Dry* gas

Amb: ambient atmosphere (unit is atm, atmosphere)

B: barometric (atmospheric)

BTPS: Usage: *P(amb)*, *P(Amb)*

SVP: *Saturated Vapor Pressure*, the vapor pressure of water. $SVP_T$ means SVP at a specified temperature (e.g., $SVP_{37}$°C = 47 mm Hg; $pH_2O$[saturated])

ATPS: *Ambient Temperature and Pressure, Saturated* with water vapor

[a]This list is not complete but is presented to facilitate interpretation of terms used in the text and to illustrate various forms that may be encountered in the literature.

From Maas AH. IFCC reference methods for measurement of pH, gases and electrolytes in blood: reference materials. *Eur J Clin Chem Clin Biochem.* 1991;29:253–261.

life in patients with cardiopulmonary impairment depend largely on assisted ventilation using mixtures of gases that are tailored in response to blood gas results. Modern blood gas analyzers are simple to operate and, with appropriate maintenance and quality control, are capable of rapid, reliable data. Details of the pathophysiology of blood gases in relation to respiration and acid-base disorders are discussed in detail in Chapter 36.

Nomenclature for this area of analysis has been recommended by the CLSI, but alternative nomenclatures exist and are in common use, as summarized in Box 24.1.

## BEHAVIOR OF GASES

Measurement of the partial pressures of $O_2$ and $CO_2$ in blood depends on the application of certain physical principles (Table 24.1). The partial pressure of a gas in a gas mixture is defined as the substance fraction of gas (mole fraction) times the total pressure. Pressure, *P* (or *p*), may mean total pressure, as in the expression *P*(Amb) for the mixture of gases in ambient air, or partial pressure of oxygen in arterial blood, as in $pO_2(aB)$.

We can determine the partial pressure of $O_2$, or $pO_2$, of room air by multiplying the atmospheric pressure by the fraction of room air that is $O_2$ (~21% or 0.21).

$$pO_2 = (pAmb - pH_2O) \times 0.21$$

where *pAmb* is the atmospheric (barometric) pressure.

In the above equation, we have added an additional variable, the partial pressure of water vapor. If the gas (air) is fully saturated with water, the $pH_2O$ cannot exceed 47 mm Hg. To calculate the $pO_2$ of room air, we also need to know the atmospheric (barometric) pressure. At sea level, the atmospheric pressure is 760 mm Hg. Using these values, we can estimate the $pO_2$ of room air to be:

$$pO_2 = (760 \text{ mm Hg} - 47 \text{ mm Hg}) \times 0.21$$

$$pO_2 = 149.7 \text{ mm Hg}$$

The $pO_2$ of the room air will vary according to the ambient atmospheric pressure and the degree of saturation with water vapor.

The SI unit of *P* is the pascal (Pa); however, millimeters of mercury (mm Hg, also called *torr*) continue to remain a popular reporting unit in some countries (see Box 24.1 for conversion factors). The use of SI units does have a practical advantage in that 1 atmosphere (atm) almost equals 100 kPa (1 atm = 101.325 kPa). Partial pressures expressed in kilopascals are therefore very close estimates of percentages of the gases in the mixture at 1 atm.

## TABLE 24.1   Physical Principles Applied in Blood Gas Measurements

| | |
|---|---|
| **Boyle's law:** The volume of an ideal gas at a constant temperature varies inversely with the pressure exerted to contain it. | $V \propto 1/P$ |
| **Charles' (Gay-Lussac's) law:** The volume of an ideal gas at a constant pressure varies directly with its absolute temperature. | $V \propto T$ |
| **Avogadro's hypothesis:** Equal volumes of different ideal gases at the same temperature and pressure contain the same number of molecules. | $n_i/V_i = n_j/V_j$ |
| **Dalton's law:** The total pressure exerted by a mixture of ideal gases is the sum of the partial pressures of each of the gases in the mixture. | $P = \Sigma P_i$ |
| **Henry's law:** The amount of a sparingly soluble gas dissolved in a liquid is proportional to the partial pressure of the gas over the liquid. | $c = \alpha \times P$ |

When assessing the partial pressure (tension) of a gas dissolved in blood, it is important to know that the partial pressure in blood is equal to the partial pressure of that gas in an imaginary ideal gas phase in equilibrium with the blood. One way to understand this concept is to imagine a blood sample exposed to room air. Over time, the partial pressures of the gases in the blood sample will equilibrate to the partial pressures of the air, and the $pO_2$ and $pCO_2$ of the blood sample will change to match the $pO_2$ and $pCO_2$ of room air. Within a whole blood sample, the partial pressure of a gas is the same in erythrocytes and plasma; consequently, the partial pressure of a gas is the same in whole blood and plasma.

Proper interpretation of blood gas results takes into consideration all of the various spaces where gases are present. This includes the gases in the ambient environment (room air), whether or not the patient is receiving supplemental $O_2$, the patient's bronchial tree, the patient's alveoli, and the measuring chamber of the blood gas instrument. In all these spaces, atmospheric (barometric) pressure, $P(Amb)$, is the prevailing pressure, which will vary with altitude and barometric pressure. The partial pressures of the gases present in these spaces must add up to the value of $P(Amb)$. Measurements of partial pressure used for clinical management are always made at *Body Temperature* (37°C), at $P(Amb)$, and in the presence of *Saturated water vapor* ($pH_2O = 47$ mm Hg). Use of this *BTPS* convention (see Box 24.1) has the following practical effects:

1. It relates laboratory data for blood gases strictly to the geographic location of the patient, so that reference intervals become altitude dependent.
2. It assumes a standard body temperature of 37°C and that the measuring device holds the sample of blood at exactly 37°C. It also implies that in circumstances such as *imposed hypothermia*, when a patient's temperature is not 37°C, blood gas values determined at 37°C might need to be

corrected to the actual body temperature to obtain an estimate of blood gas partial pressures in the patient.
3. It recognizes that partial pressures of measured gases in the blood coexist with a constant and standard saturated vapor pressure (SVP), which is identical for both the calibration conditions of the instrument and the measurement conditions of the blood sample.

Dalton's law of partial pressures governs the calibration and control of blood gas instruments. *Dalton's law* (see Table 24.1) may be written for room air as follows:

$$P(Amb) = pO_2 + pCO_2 + pN_2 + pH_2O + pX$$

where $pX$ is the partial pressure of any other gas in the air sample.

Consider a calibrator gas certified to contain 15% $O_2$ (L/L or mol/mol) and 5% $CO_2$, the remainder being $N_2$. The mole fractions (or $F$) of the gases in the dry mixture are 0.15, 0.05, and 0.80, respectively. This mixture, after saturation with water vapor at 37°C (to mimic a patient's blood or alveolar air), is introduced into a blood gas instrument's measuring chamber (held at 37°C to mimic a patient's body temperature) for the purpose of calibrating the instrument for subsequent measurements of gases in patients' samples. If the local barometric pressure, $P(Amb)$, on this occasion is 747 mm Hg, then humidified calibrator gas is present in the chamber at ambient, barometric pressure, such that

$$P(Amb) = 747 \text{ mm Hg} = pO_2 + pCO_2 + pN_2 + pH_2O$$

To set the instrument to the $pO_2$ and $pCO_2$ of the calibrator gas, the $pH_2O$ at 37°C, which is equal to the SVP of water, and 47 mm Hg must be included. Therefore,

$$747 \text{ mm Hg} - pH_2O = pO_2 + pCO_2 + pN_2$$
$$= 747 - 47$$
$$= 700 \text{ mm Hg}$$

If $P(Amb)$ corrected for $pH_2O$ represents the sum of partial pressures for the dry gases whose mole fractions we know, we can calculate the exact $pO_2$ and $pCO_2$ values for the calibrator gas, under circumstances of measurement, and enter these calibrator values into the instrument.

The law of partial pressure is also applied in defining gas mixtures used to determine $pO_2(0.5)$ or $P_{50}$ and other derived quantities, and to assess instrumentation accuracy with quality control materials.

It is important to note that $pO_2$ and $pCO_2$ are only related to the concentration of dissolved $O_2$ ($cdO_2$) and dissolved $CO_2$ ($cdCO_2$) in blood, respectively (see Henry's law; Table 24.1.) The total concentration of $O_2$ in blood ($ctO_2$) is the sum of concentrations of dissolved $O_2$ and of $O_2$ bound to hemoglobin, with $cdO_2$ being a small component of $ctO_2$ (see the later section on hemoglobin saturation). The total concentration of $CO_2$ ($ctCO_2$) is defined operationally as the sum of concentrations of dissolved $CO_2$, carbonic acid, $HCO_3^-$, undissociated bicarbonate, and carbonate ions.

*Henry's law* predicts the amount of dissolved gas in a liquid in contact with a gaseous phase (see Table 24.1). The solubility coefficient of $O_2$ in blood, $\alpha O_2$, is 0.00140 (mmol/L)/mm Hg. When arterial $pO_2$ is normal ($\approx$100 mm Hg), the $cdO_2$ in arterial blood is 0.140 mmol/L, which is a very small proportion of the $ctO_2$ of blood ($\approx$9 mmol/L), the majority of which is composed of $O_2$ bound by hemoglobin. Increasing the $O_2$ fraction of inspired air to 100% or increasing the pressure of inspired air, as in a hyperbaric chamber, forces more $O_2$ into solution.

The $cdCO_2$ can be calculated in the same way: $\alpha CO_2$ at 37°C in plasma = 0.0306 mmol/L/mm Hg. At a $pCO_2$ of 40 mm Hg, the $cdCO_2$ will be 1.224 mmol/L ($cdCO_2$ = 40 mm Hg × 0.0306 mmol× $L^{-1}$× mm $Hg^{-1}$ = 1.224 mmol/L). In the determination of blood gases, $pCO_2$ is determined along with blood pH. As will be subsequently explained, these two parameters in conjunction with the Henderson-Hasselbalch equation permit the calculation of $HCO_3^-$.

## APPLICATION OF THE HENDERSON-HASSELBALCH EQUATION IN BLOOD GAS MEASUREMENTS

Carbon dioxide and water react slowly and spontaneously to form carbonic acid, which in turn rapidly dissociates into hydrogen ions and $HCO_3^-$.

$$CO_2 + H_2O \xrightleftharpoons{K_{hydration}} H_2CO_3 \xrightleftharpoons{K_{dissociation}} H^{\oplus} + HCO_3^{\ominus}$$

Thus, the proportion of the total concentration of $CO_2$ ($ctCO_2$), that is in the form of $HCO_3^-$, versus $cdCO_2$, and the $H^+$ ion concentration ($cH^+$), are interrelated.

This relationship and its effect on pH are described by the Henderson-Hasselbalch equation below. In plasma, a small proportion of the $cdCO_2$ includes undissociated (dissolved) carbonic acid. The concentration in plasma can be expressed as $cdCO_2 = \alpha \times pCO_2$, where $\alpha$ represents the solubility coefficient of $CO_2$.

$$pH = pK' + \log\frac{cHCO_3^-}{\alpha \times pCO_2}$$

$pK'$ in the above equation is the negative log of the apparent overall (combined) dissociation constant for carbonic acid. It is *apparent* because concentrations are used rather than activities, and *overall* because both the $cdCO_2$ and the concentration of carbonic acid are used. $K'$ (and thus $pK'$) depends not only on the temperature but also on the ionic strength of the solution.

For blood at 37°C, the normal mean value of $pK'$ is 6.103, and the mean solubility coefficient for $CO_2$ gas is (0.0306 mmol) × ($L^{-1}$) × (mm $Hg^{-1}$). When $pK'$ and $\alpha$ for plasma at 37°C are inserted, the Henderson-Hasselbalch equation takes the following form:

$$pH = 6.103 + \log\frac{cHCO_3^-}{0.0306 \times pCO_2}$$

where $pCO_2$ is reported in millimeters of mercury and $cHCO_3^-$ is reported in millimoles per liter.

By measuring any two of the three parameters, $pCO_2$, pH, or $cHCO_3^-$, and by using the Henderson-Hasselbalch equation with the above values for $pK'$ and $\alpha$, the other parameter may be calculated. Although used as constants, $pK'$ and $\alpha$ must be recognized as means and are susceptible to biological variation. Changes in ionic strength of ±20% causes $pK'$ to vary between 6.08 and 6.12. Variations in $pK'$ of plasma also occur with temperature ($pK$ will decrease by 0.0026 per 1°C increase and will decrease slightly with increasing pH). For most clinical purposes, these variations of $pK'$ can be ignored. However, in cases with markedly deviant ionic strength, the change in $pK'$ may be substantial. The value of $\alpha$ is affected by the presence of increased ions or proteins in solution (value decreases) or lipids (value increases); for instance, in lipemic plasma, the value of $\alpha$ may be 0.033 or higher. Thus, parameters calculated on the assumption that $pK'$ and $\alpha$ are invariant may have error under certain pathologic circumstances. Several authors suggest caution in using calculated $HCO_3^-$ values from blood gas analyzers in extremely ill patients, as the calculated and measured $tCO_2$ values can differ by greater than 10% in adult and greater than 20% in pediatric ICU patients, respectively.

## OXYGEN IN BLOOD

The total $O_2$ content ($ctO_2$) of a blood sample is the sum of the concentrations of dissolved and hemoglobin-bound $O_2$. At a blood $ctO_2$ of 9 mmol/L, the $O_2$ associated with hemoglobin as **oxyhemoglobin** ($O_2Hb$) is 8.86 mmol/L. The $O_2Hb$ is defined as erythrocyte hemoglobin with $O_2$ reversibly bound to $Fe^{2+}$ of its heme group.

Hemoglobin A (Hb A, the adult gene product) reversibly binds $O_2$ via the heme-$Fe^{2+}$ moiety and binds biological effectors at other allosteric sites. Methemoglobin (MetHb), carboxyhemoglobin (COHb), sulfhemoglobin (SulfHb), and cyanmethemoglobin, collectively termed dyshemoglobins, are forms of hemoglobin that are not capable of reversible $O_2$ binding because of chemical alterations of the heme moiety.

In contrast to the dyshemoglobins, the *hemoglobinopathies* are the result of Hb A gene variants (commonly termed *hemoglobin variants*), these changes in gene sequence and consequent changes in amino acid sequence may alter hemoglobin's $O_2$ affinity. Greater than 900 hemoglobin variants have been described, of which only a small fraction are clinically significant (for details see Chapter 28).

Uptake of $O_2$ by blood in the lungs is governed primarily by the $pO_2$ of alveolar air and by the ability of $O_2$ to diffuse freely across the alveolar membrane into blood. At the $pO_2$ normally present in alveolar air ($\approx$102 mm Hg) with a normal erythrocyte membrane and normal hemoglobin A, greater than 95% of hemoglobin will bind $O_2$. At a $pO_2$ greater than 110 mm Hg, more than 98% of normal hemoglobin A binds $O_2$. When all hemoglobin is saturated with $O_2$, further increases in the $pO_2$ of alveolar air simply increase the concentration of dissolved $O_2$ in arterial blood. Delivery of $O_2$

by blood to tissues is governed by the large gradient between the $pO_2$ of arterial blood and that of the tissue cells, and by the dissociation of $O_2$ from $O_2Hb$ in erythrocytes at the lower $pO_2$ of the blood-tissue cell interface.

Three properties of arterial blood are essential to ensure adequate $O_2$ delivery to tissues:

1. Arterial $pO_2$ must be sufficiently high ($\approx$90 mm Hg) to create a diffusion gradient from arterial blood to the tissue cells. The $pO_2$ at the venous end of the capillaries is typically ~30 to 45 mm Hg; thus, the normal arteriovenous difference in $pO_2$ is 50 to 60 mm Hg. Low arterial $pO_2$ (*hypoxemia*) results in tissue $O_2$ starvation (*hypoxia*).
2. The $O_2$-binding capacity of blood must be normal (i.e., the concentration of hemoglobin capable of binding and releasing $O_2$ must be normal). Decreased functional Hb concentration will cause so-called **anemic hypoxia**.
3. Hemoglobin must be able to bind $O_2$ in the lungs yet release it at the tissue. In other words, the affinity of hemoglobin for $O_2$ must be normal. Too great an affinity of hemoglobin for $O_2$ may cause "affinity-based" tissue hypoxia, in which $O_2$ is not released at the capillary-tissue interface. Approximately 100 high-affinity hemoglobin variants have been described to date; however, individually, they are all rare. Hemoglobin F, while not a hemoglobin variant, has a higher affinity for oxygen than hemoglobin A.

## HEMOGLOBIN OXYGEN SATURATION

Before the factors that affect hemoglobin affinity for $O_2$ are discussed, it is important to define the concept of hemoglobin **oxygen saturation ($SO_2$)**:

$$SO_2 = \frac{\text{Oxygen Content}}{\text{Oxygen Capacity}}$$

This is the fraction (percentage) of functional hemoglobin that is saturated with oxygen and is essentially an indirect means of estimating the $pO_2$. At least three different approaches exist for determining oxygen "saturation," and although each is distinct, they are often used interchangeably to determine "oxygen saturation." These three terms—hemoglobin oxygen saturation ($SO_2$), fractional oxyhemoglobin ($FO_2Hb$, also abbreviated %$O_2Hb$), and estimated oxygen saturation ($O_2Sat$)—have distinct definitions described in CLSI C46-A2. Ambiguous use of these terms occurs because, in healthy subjects with functional hemoglobin within the reference interval, the values of all three entities are very similar. However, these assumptions can lead to erroneous conclusions in seriously ill patients and those with dyshemoglobins or hemoglobin variants.

Spectrophotometric methods are used to determine $O_2Hb$ and $HHb$, and $SO_2$ are calculated according to

$$SO_2 = \frac{cO_2Hb}{cO_2Hb + cHHb}$$

where $cO_2Hb$ is the concentration of oxyhemoglobin, $cHHb$ is the concentration of deoxyhemoglobin (aka reduced

hemoglobin), and the sum of oxyhemoglobin and deoxyhemoglobin represents all hemoglobin capable of reversibly binding $O_2$. $SO_2$ is usually expressed as a percent in the United States, but it may also be expressed as a decimal fraction of 1.00.

$SO_2$ most is often determined by simple pulse **oximetry** but may also be an available calculation on modern blood gas analyzers. It is important to note that $SO_2$ is incapable of detecting and measuring COHb, MetHb, or SulfHb concentrations. Pulse oximeters measure absorbance at 660 and 940 nm, for which $O_2Hb$ and $HHb$ have unique absorbance patterns. Use of $SO_2$ in the initial evaluation of a patient with dyshemoglobins can be very misleading. For instance, in a comatose patient with 15% COHb, the $SO_2$ by simple pulse oximetry might read 0.95, whereas the fraction of oxyhemoglobin would actually only be 0.80. It is reasonable to assess for the presence of dyshemoglobins before $SO_2$ is used for clinical purposes. Once dyshemoglobins are ruled out, pulse oximeters are appropriate for monitoring hemoglobin $O_2$ saturation, and they serve this purpose extremely well. The reference interval for $SO_2$ from healthy adults is 0.94 to 0.98 (94% to 98%).

Another expression of oxygen "saturation" is fractional oxyhemoglobin ($FO_2Hb$), which is calculated as

$$FO_2Hb = (cO_2Hb/cHHb + cCOHb + cMetHb + cSulfHb)$$

This value requires determination of all hemoglobin species and can be performed on a co-oximeter present in modern blood gas analyzers. These instruments spectrophotometrically determine the total amount of hemoglobin and the percent of each of the aforementioned species by measuring light absorbance at fixed wavelengths between 535 and 670 nm. Newer co-oximeters use a diode array and up to 128 wavelengths, and as each species of hemoglobin has its own absorbance pattern, an integrated software algorithm calculates the percent of each one. The reference interval for $FO_2Hb$ is 0.90 to 0.95 (90% to 95%).

Finally, using empirical equations, the blood gas instrument's integrated software can also estimate the oxygen saturation from the measured pH, $pO_2$, and hemoglobin. This value should be clearly referred to as *estimated oxygen saturation*, but it frequently is reported and referred to as "$O_2Sat$." If calculated values such as "$O_2Sat$" are reported, they should be interpreted with reservation because the algorithm assumes normal hemoglobin affinity for $O_2$, normal 2,3-bisphosphoglycerol (2,3-BPG) concentrations, and the absence of dyshemoglobins. The $O_2Sat$ calculated value estimates have been found to vary by as much as 6% from measured values.

The amount of $O_2$ that the blood can carry is determined by three major factors: (1) the $pO_2$, which reflects how much $O_2$ is dissolved in the blood; (2) the amount of functional hemoglobin available in erythrocytes; and (3) the affinity of available hemoglobin for $O_2$. Decreases in $pO_2$ indicate a reduced ability of $O_2$ to diffuse from alveolar air into the blood. This may be due to hypoventilation or to increased venoarterial shunting (blood passing from the right side to left side of the heart without exposure to alveolar air) that is secondary to cardiac or pulmonary insufficiency. The result of both possibilities is an increased fraction of blood that has not reached equilibrium with alveolar air. Hypoventilation and increased shunting are also characterized by an increased $pCO_2$, as the $CO_2$ dissolved in blood cannot reach equilibrium with alveolar air. Decreases in total hemoglobin concentration can result from a decreased number of erythrocytes that contain a normal concentration of hemoglobin (normochromic anemia) or a decreased mean erythrocyte concentration of hemoglobin (hypochromic anemia). Decreased concentrations of *functional* hemoglobin ($O_2Hb$ and HHb) can occur as a result of poisonings that convert hemoglobin into COHb, MetHb, or SulfHb, which cannot properly bind or exchange $O_2$.

Clinically, it is important to distinguish between arterial hypoxemia (decreased arterial $pO_2$ and decreased $FO_2Hb$ caused by decreased availability of $O_2$) and cyanosis (decreased $FO_2Hb$ caused by abnormally high concentrations of reduced hemoglobin [HHb] or high COHb, MetHb, or SulfHb). Note that in the setting of cyanosis, measurement of $SO_2$ or an estimated $SO_2$ ("$O_2Sat$") could be normal if cyanosis is due to the presence of COHb, MetHb, or SulfHb.

## Hemoglobin-Oxygen Dissociation

The degree of association or dissociation of $O_2$ with hemoglobin is determined by $pO_2$ and the affinity of hemoglobin for $O_2$. When the $SO_2$ of blood is determined over a range of $pO_2$ and is plotted against $pO_2$, a sigmoidal curve called the $O_2$ *dissociation curve* is obtained. The *shape* of the curve is affected by the increasing efficiency with which HHb molecules bind $O_2$. Hemoglobin is capable of binding four $O_2$ molecules per hemoglobin protein (one $O_2$ per $Fe^{2+}$—heme moiety), and the affinity of hemoglobin for $O_2$ increases as successive $Fe^{2+}$-heme moieties bind $O_2$ (*cooperativity*; see also Chapter 28). The *location* of the curve relative to the $pO_2$ required to achieve a particular concentration of $SO_2$ in the blood is a function of the affinity of hemoglobin for $O_2$.

The affinity of hemoglobin for $O_2$ depends on five factors: temperature, pH, $pCO_2$, 2,3-BPG concentration, and the presence of dyshemoglobins such as COHb and MetHb. Dissociation of $O_2$ in relation to 2,3-BPG concentration and abnormal hemoglobin proteins, such as fetal hemoglobin (Hb F), thalassemias, and other hemoglobinopathies, are discussed in Chapter 28.

The graph in Fig. 24.3 shows the effect of plasma pH on the $O_2$ dissociation curve (the Bohr effect). Similar graphs can be made for variations of $pCO_2$, temperature, and 2,3-BPG concentration.

## Determination of $P_{50}$

$P_{50}$ is defined as the $pO_2$ at which hemoglobin in blood is half saturated with $O_2$. The measured value of $P_{50}$ differs from the standard theoretical value of $P_{50}$ when the pH differs from 7.40, $pCO_2$ differs from 40 mm Hg, temperature differs from 37°C, and 2,3-BPG differs from 5.0 mmol/L. The value of $P_{50}$

therefore becomes a measure of change in hemoglobin affinity because of the factors that affect it.

### Clinical Significance

Increased values for $P_{50}$ indicate a shift of the $O_2$ dissociation curve to the right (i.e., decreased affinity of the hemoglobin for $O_2$). This means that hemoglobin binds $O_2$ less tightly, and $O_2$ will more readily dissociate from hemoglobin at a higher $pO_2$, facilitating dissociation of $O_2$ from hemoglobin in peripheral tissues. The decreased affinity of hemoglobin for $O_2$ at higher $pO_2$ does not, however, impair sufficient binding of adequate amounts of $O_2$ in the lungs.

The causes of a decreased affinity (shift to the right) are hyperthermia, acidemia (decreased blood pH), hypercapnia (increased $pCO_2$), high concentrations of 2,3-BPG, and the presence of a hemoglobin variant with decreased $O_2$ affinity. Low hemoglobin affinity for $O_2$ in the setting of anemia (as a result of increases in 2,3-BPG) is a desirable compensatory mechanism. The compensatory responses in healthy individuals to alter the $P_{50}$ can be remarkable. For instance, in fully acclimatized (70 days) high-altitude climbers (Mt. Everest), full cognition was maintained without supplemental oxygen at an altitude of 8400 m and an average $P(a)O_2$ of only 25 mm Hg.

Low values for $P_{50}$ signify a shift of the $O_2$ dissociation curve to the left (i.e., increased affinity of hemoglobin). The main causes are hypothermia, acute alkalemia (increased blood pH), hypocapnia (low $pCO_2$), low 2,3-BPG, and variant hemoglobin. The physiologic consequence of increased affinity of hemoglobin for $O_2$ is less efficient dissociation of $O_2$ from hemoglobin, lower delivery of $O_2$ to peripheral tissues, and lower tissue $pO_2$.

## MEASUREMENT OF $pCO_2$, $pO_2$, AND pH

### Specimens and Preanalytic Variation

Proper specimen collection and handling are critical for accurate pH, $pO_2$, and $pCO_2$ measurements.

Arterial or venous specimens are collected anaerobically with lyophilized (balanced) heparin anticoagulant in 1 to 3 mL sterile syringes. Lyophilized heparin is preferable to liquid heparin because liquid heparin, which has atmospheric $pO_2$ and $pCO_2$ values, dilutes the sample, with the effect being greatest when the syringe is not completely filled. An increasing ratio of liquid heparin to blood can have an increasingly marked effect on measured $pCO_2$ and the parameters calculated from it. Sample dilution with 10% volume of liquid heparin having an atmospheric $pCO_2$ of 0.25 mm Hg has been shown to lead to a 10 to 20 mm Hg decrease in measured blood $pCO_2$.

*Anaerobic techniques* for collection mean no exposure of blood to atmospheric air. The $pCO_2$ of air is about 0.25 mm Hg, which is much less than that of blood ($\approx$40 mm Hg). Thus, the $CO_2$ content and $pCO_2$ of blood exposed to air will decrease, and blood pH, which is a function of $pCO_2$, will rise. The $pO_2$ of atmospheric air ($\approx$155 mm Hg) is $\approx$60 mm Hg higher than that of arterial blood and $\approx$100 mm Hg higher than that of venous blood. Therefore, blood from patients breathing room air, which is exposed to atmospheric air, gains $O_2$, and blood

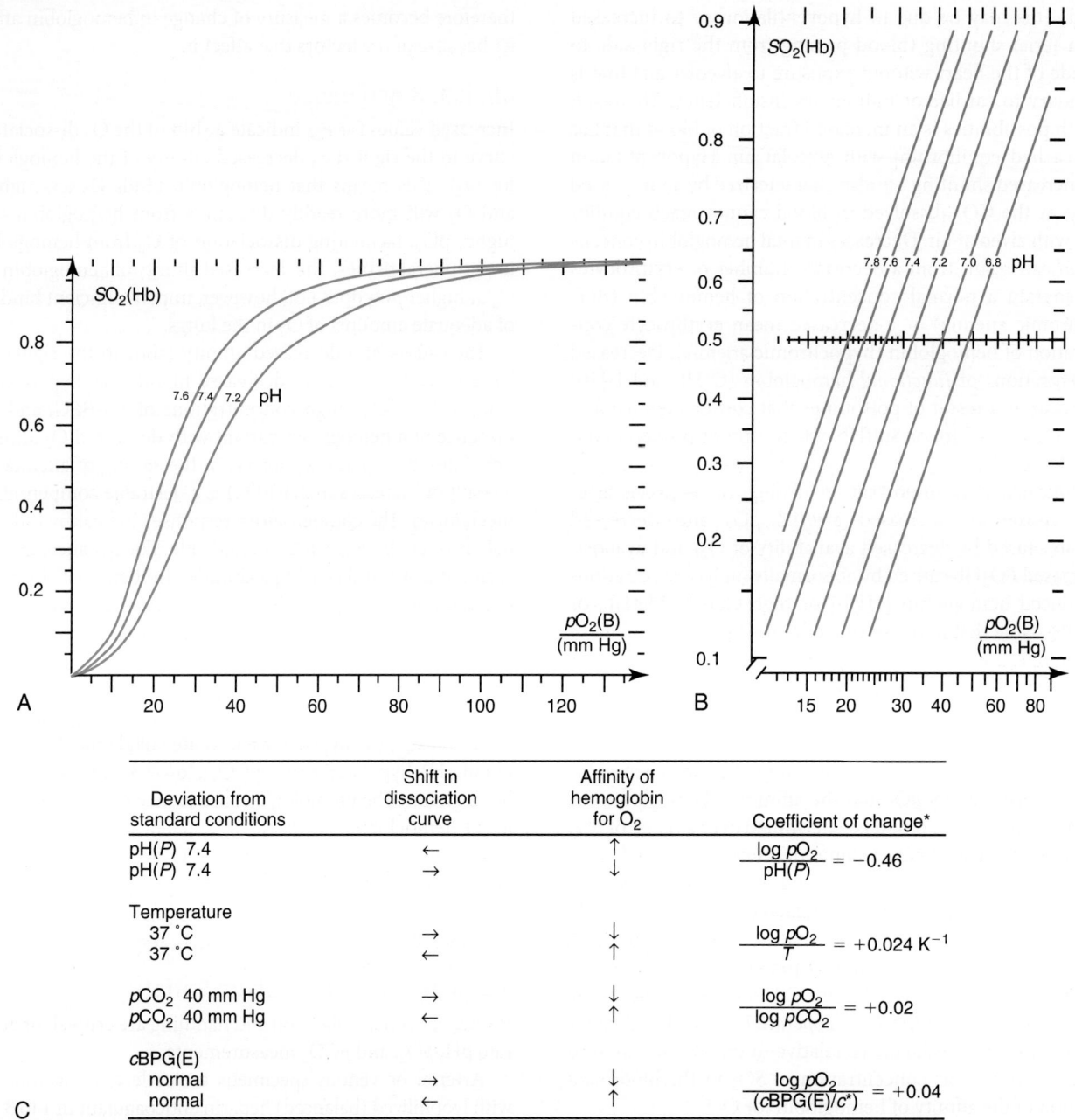

Fig. 24.3 (A) **Oxygen dissociation curves** for human blood with different plasma pH but constant $pCO_2$ of 40 mm Hg, a 2,3-diphosphoglycerol (2,3-BPG) concentration in erythrocytes of 5.0 mmol/L, and temperature at 37°C. (B) A Hill plot. Conditions are the same as in (A). The coefficients given in this chart form the basis for the correction of measured $pO_2$. (C) The effect of pH(P) to shift the dissociation curve is called the *Bohr effect*; the coefficient above for $\Delta$log $pO_2$/$\Delta$pH(P) applies to conditions when the $pCO_2$ is 40 mm Hg, and changes in pH(P) are due to changes in concentrations of noncarbonic acids and bases. If, however, the changes in pH(P) are being caused by changes in $pCO_2$, then the absolute value of the coefficient is greater (i.e., $\Delta$log $pO_2$/$\Delta$pH[P] = −0.49). The coefficients for the Bohr effect are specified for $pO_2$ of whole blood but use the pH of plasma, pH(P). The coefficient for BPG effect is based on the BPG concentration in the erythrocytes, $c$BPG(E). $c^* = 1$ mmol/L.

with a $pO_2$ greater than 150 mm Hg, as occurs in patients undergoing $O_2$ therapy, loses $O_2$. Blood can also be exposed to air simply from the air in the needle and the syringe hub's dead space. Error will be minimal if the resulting bubble is ejected immediately after drawing by holding the syringe tip up and expelling the bubble(s). The potential effect of small bubbles on blood gas results was clearly demonstrated in one study in which a 100 µL bubble of room air was added to

ten 2 mL blood samples with $pO_2$ values between 25 and 40 mm Hg. In these samples, $pO_2$ increased an average of 4 mm Hg in only 2 minutes, whereas $pCO_2$ decreased 4 mm Hg. Before analysis, mixing of the sample by vigorously rolling the syringe between the palms should be done to establish a homogeneous sample.

Sample dilution with IV fluid is another source of potential error for venous blood gas samples. Venous blood gas samples drawn from an in-dwelling catheter with heparin locks for short- and long-term intravenous therapies are common. The $pO_2$ and $pCO_2$ values of IV fluids will mirror atmospheric $pO_2$ and $pCO_2$ values (~155 mm Hg and 0.25 mm Hg, respectively). Failure to flush the catheter properly prior to sample collection will have unpredictable effects on measured quantities and is often indicated by bizarre, non-physiological results.

*Arterialized capillary blood* is sometimes an acceptable alternative to arterial blood when an arterial cannula is not available, or when repeated arterial punctures must be avoided. Freely flowing cutaneous blood originates in the arterioles and corresponds closely to arterial blood in composition. However, arterialized capillary blood is not acceptable when systolic blood pressure is less than 95 mm Hg. Capillary puncture should be preceded by warming of the selected skin puncture site for 10 minutes to achieve vasodilation and adequate blood flow. For collection from the finger of a child or an adult or from an infant's heel, warming may be accomplished by immersing the arm or leg in water warmed to 42°C. The first blood drop to appear should be wiped away, and subsequent free-forming drops should be taken up in a capillary collection tube containing lyophilized heparin. Only free-flowing blood provides a satisfactory sample, and collecting the drops as soon as they form minimizes aerobic exposure.

*Transport and analysis* of specimens should be prompt. The pH of freshly drawn blood decreases on standing at a rate of 0.04 to 0.08 pH unit/h at 37°C, 0.02 to 0.03/h at 22°C, and less than 0.01/h at 4°C. The decrease in pH is accompanied by a corresponding decrease in glucose and an equivalent increase in lactate. $pCO_2$ increases by $\approx$5 mm Hg/h at 37°C, by 1 mm Hg/h at 22°C, and by only $\approx$0.5 mm Hg/h at 2 to 4°C. The primary cause of these changes is glycolysis by leukocytes, platelets, and reticulocytes. In freshly drawn blood with a normal $pO_2$ that is maintained anaerobically, cell respiration causes $pO_2$ to decrease at a rate of $\approx$2 mm Hg/h at room temperature. Adverse effects of glycolysis and respiration on pH, $ctCO_2$, $pO_2$, and $pCO_2$ of blood can best be prevented by analysis within 30 minutes after collection. If analysis must be delayed longer than 30 minutes, the syringe should be immersed in a mixture of ice and water until analysis. Under these conditions, changes are negligible because glycolysis is inhibited. With today's blood gas instrumentation, introduction of a chilled sample carries little risk of low-temperature effect on measurements because thermal equilibration to 37°C is rapid and complete.

The aforementioned small changes in values that can be expected with delays in analysis are true *only* when the WBC count is normal or only slightly elevated. Glycolysis and the resulting effects on pH, $pO_2$, and $pCO_2$ increase dramatically with markedly elevated WBC, such as occurs in leukemia. Experiments have shown that $pO_2$ decreases by 20 mm Hg in just 2 minutes and by 40 mm Hg in only 5 minutes with WBC values greater than 100,000/µL. Indeed, for samples with these types of WBC values, it is very difficult to overcome this

effect. Even after the sample is immersed in ice, thermal equilibrium takes several minutes, allowing significant $pO_2$ loss before the contents reach 4°C. The only alternative to obtaining accurate blood gas values on such patients is immediate analysis performed at the point of care.

## Reference Intervals

Reference intervals for arterial and venous blood $pO_2$, $pCO_2$, and pH are summarized in Table 24.2. Differences in blood gas values between arterial and venous blood are most pronounced for $pO_2$. $pO_2$ is generally $\approx$40 to 60 mm Hg lower in venous blood after $O_2$ is released in the capillaries, whereas $pCO_2$ is 2 to 7 mm Hg higher in venous blood. pH is generally only 0.03 to 0.05 pH units lower in venous blood.

When assessing $pO_2$ and $pCO_2$ values, it is important to note that both will decrease with increasing altitude, but compensatory mechanisms keep pH values the same.

$pCO_2$ values decrease with altitude above sea level at a rate of 3 mm Hg/km (5 mm Hg/mile) and will vary with changes in posture; $pCO_2$ is 2 to 4 mm Hg higher for a sitting or standing person than for one in the supine position. During pregnancy, $pCO_2$ also falls gradually to a mean of about 28 mm Hg just before term.

## Instrumentation

A schematic diagram characteristic of a typical instrument is shown in Fig. 24.4. Electrochemical principles and structural features of electrodes are discussed in Chapter 10.

Operation of a traditional blood gas instrument begins with the operator presenting a blood specimen at the sample probe. The sample is taken through the probe by a peristaltic pump that loads the chamber with 60 to 150 µL of sample. The sample then resides in the chamber long enough to allow thermal equilibration and completion of measurements. On completion of measurement, the pump pushes the sample to waste.

Because electrodes are not stable over long periods of time, frequent calibration of pH, $pCO_2$, and $pO_2$ is required. The instrument (see Fig. 24.4) is designed so that a software-controlled valve (self-calibrating) admits calibrator gases, standard buffers, or a sample to a small chamber (C) maintained at 37°C ± 0.1°C. Most instruments contain a barometer so that barometric pressure P(Amb) is always known

## TABLE 24.2 Adult Reference Intervals for Arterial and Venous Blood Gas Measurements

|  | Arterial | Venous[a] |
|---|---|---|
| pH | 7.35–7.45 | 7.32–7.42 |
| $pCO_2$ | 35–45 mm Hg | Female: 36–49 mm Hg<br>Male: 39–52 mm Hg |
| $pO_2$ | 80–100 mm Hg | 44–69 mm Hg |

[a]Venous reference interval data from: Ress KL, Koerbin G, Li L, et al. Reference intervals for venous blood gas measurement in adults. *Clin Chem Lab Med.* 2021;59:947–954.

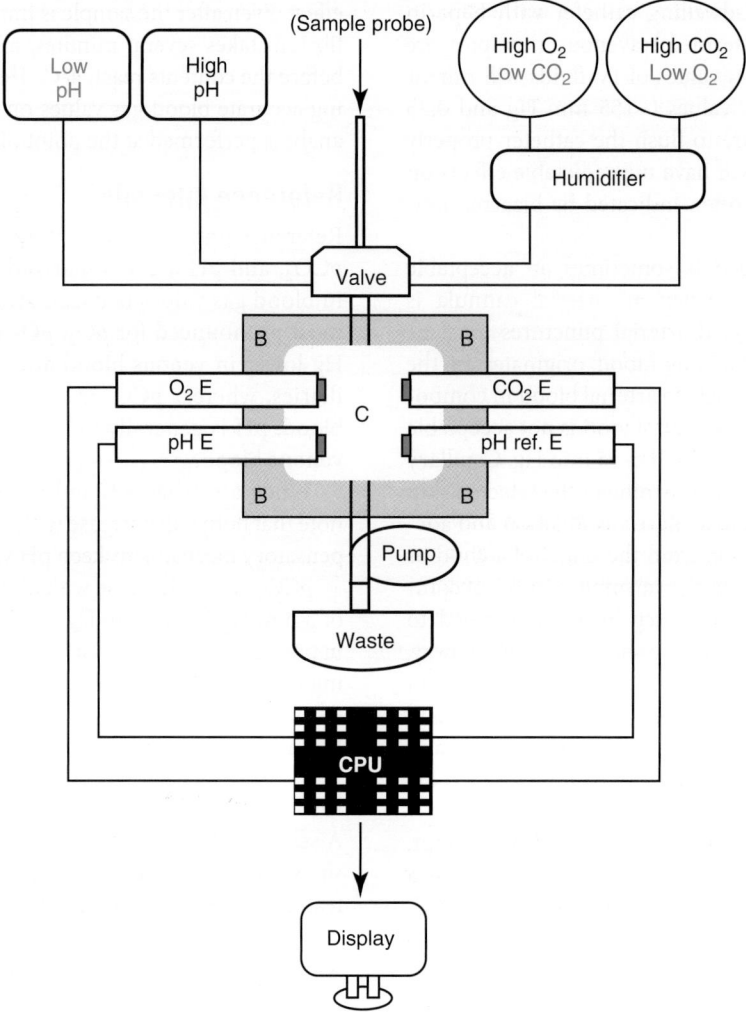

**Fig. 24.4** Diagram of blood gas instrumentation. *B,* Constant temperature block at 37°C; *C,* chamber; *CPU,* computer; *E (electrodes),* pH and gas standards are shown at top of diagram.

during calibration. Almost all manufacturers now produce small, portable, stand-alone, and easy-to-operate instruments designed for "satellite lab" operations; several handheld devices that use disposable electrodes are also available. Readers are referred to Chapter 17 for a discussion of **point-of-care testing**.

## Maintenance of Instrumentation

The software sophistication of modern equipment and availability of high-quality calibrator materials have made reliable and accurate determination of blood pH and gases primarily a matter of meticulous maintenance, adherence to the manufacturer's recommended procedures, control of the equipment, and proper collection and handling of specimens. The instrument's software programs often provide display warnings and diagnostic routines that alert the operator and assist in troubleshooting. The manufacturer's suggested maintenance schedule should be considered a minimum guideline, with reliance on experience to indicate maintenance frequency.

Cleanliness of the sample chamber and path is especially important. Automatic flushing to cleanse the sample chamber and path after each blood sample measurement is a feature of most instruments without disposable electrodes. Despite proper flushing, however, complete or partial clogging of the chamber, the path, or both may occur. Fibrin threads and small clots may be present in the specimen or may form while the sample resides in the warm chamber. If allowed to remain, they can affect subsequent measurements or calibrations by interfering with contact of blood, buffers, or gases with electrode membranes. Users of the blood gas instruments must also pay particular attention to only use the manufacturer's approved cleaning solutions on the outside of the instrument. The use of contraindicated solutions may rapidly deteriorate instrument electrodes, leading to errors and delays in testing.

## Quality Assurance and Quality Control

Elements of good quality assurance of blood gas and pH measurements include (1) proper maintenance of the instrument,

(2) use of appropriate control materials, (3) verification of electrode linearity, (4) checking of barometer accuracy, and (5) accurate measurement of temperature.

Minimum calibration and quality control (QC) frequency is mandated by federal law in the United States (Clinical Laboratory Improvement Amendments [CLIA] '88). CLIA regulations require a one-point calibration every 30 minutes (or within 30 minutes of a patient sample) and a two-point calibration every 8 hours. For QC, the minimum CLIA required frequency is one concentration of QC material every 8 hours, with the entire range of control concentrations covered in every 24-hour period. In many laboratories, however, the practical answer is to run three concentrations of QC for pH, $pO_2$, and $pCO_2$ on every instrument in use, at least once per shift, following completion of maintenance and troubleshooting procedures. Newer analyzers, particularly the smaller satellite laboratory and point-of-care instruments, frequently have an *auto quality control* (QC) feature or use *electronic QCs*. Auto QC consists of onboard QC material that is automatically sampled and analyzed by the instrument at designated intervals that fulfill regulatory requirements. Electronic QC, which is most common in devices with disposable electrode cartridges, consists of cartridges that verify the electronic response of the instruments. For further discussion of these issues, see Chapter 17 on point-of-care instrumentation.

CLIA similarly mandated external quality assurance (proficiency testing) and set criteria for satisfactory interlaboratory performance as follows: pH, target value ± 0.04; $pO_2$, target value ± 3 SD; and $pCO_2$, target value ± 8% or ± 5 mm Hg, whichever is greater.

## Blood-Based and Fluorocarbon-Based Control Materials

Commercial blood-based control material usually consists of tanned human erythrocytes suspended in buffered medium and sealed in vials with a gas mixture of known $O_2$ and $CO_2$ contents. Non-blood fluorocarbon materials with $O_2$-carrying properties similar to those of blood are also available. These products are usually made at three concentrations: pH, $pCO_2$, and $pO_2$. Unopened, these types of control materials have the advantages of a long, refrigerated shelf life.

## Aqueous Fluid Control Materials

These materials consist of a buffered medium with gas mixtures in sealed glass ampules. Immediately prior to opening the vial and introducing it into the instrument, the fluid is equilibrated with the gas by vigorous shaking by hand. The disadvantages of aqueous controls stem from their dissimilar matrix to blood. Lower viscosity and surface tension confer different washout characteristics and impair their ability to detect clogging. Greater electrical conductivity reduces their effectiveness in detecting inadequate grounding, and lower thermal coefficients make them slower to detect failures of temperature control. Nevertheless, aqueous commercial controls are the most commonly used materials for quality control purposes.

## Sources of Analytical Error

General causes of analytical error include calibration of the instrument with incorrect set points for pH buffers or calibrator gases, degraded calibration materials, failure of temperature control of the measurement chamber, and a dirty sample chamber or path. Incorrect calibration may arise from wrong entries made for buffer or gas values into the instrument software, incorrect manual calculations of $pCO_2$ and $pO_2$ values for calibrator gases, or from using gases that are dry because the humidification device is not working properly. Measurements of $pO_2$ are particularly sensitive to temperature error. To keep systematic error to 1% to 2%, the temperature control at 37°C must be within ±0.1°C. Built-in barometers can be checked by contacting nearby meteorological stations or by verifying the pressure against a NIST-certified barometer placed in the laboratory. Gases other than $O_2$ present in a blood sample may affect performance of the $pO_2$ electrode. The anesthetic gases halothane and nitrous oxide have a direct effect because both can be reduced at the polarized cathode in competition with $O_2$. Under most circumstances, however, these effects are small and can be ignored.

## TEMPERATURE CORRECTION OF MEASURED pH, $pCO_2$, AND $pO_2$

In the Henderson-Hasselbalch equation, $pK'$ and $\alpha$ are used as constants for a temperature of 37°C. The temperature-controlled sample chamber of an instrument is specified to be 37°C ± 0.1°C, and it is at that temperature that all measurements of pH and partial pressure of gases are made. The body temperature of a febrile patient may be elevated to 40°C to 41°C, or a patient may be made hypothermic for certain surgeries and have a temperature as low as 23°C. The patient's actual temperature can be entered on most blood gas instruments, from which the software can calculate and present a temperature-corrected pH and $pCO_2$ using formulas obtained from the Clinical and Laboratory Standards Institute document C46-A2. Correction of pH and $pCO_2$ to the actual temperature of the patient is usually omitted in states of hyperthermia. However, significant disagreement exists with respect to hypothermic states.

### POINTS TO REMEMBER

Blood gas instruments use the Henderson-Hasselbalch equation to calculate bicarbonate concentration and extremes of sample ionic strength; protein and lipid concentrations may alter the accuracy of this calculated value.

The presence of bubbles in blood gas syringes has the potential to dramatically change the $pO_2$ and $pCO_2$ of blood gas samples.

Hemoglobin oxygen saturation ($SO_2$), fractional oxyhemoglobin ($FO_2Hb$), and estimated oxygen saturation may produce very dissimilar values in the presence of dyshemoglobins and hemoglobin variants.

Blood gas analyzers have more stringent requirements for the frequency of calibration and quality control assessment.

## REVIEW QUESTIONS

1. The most common method for measuring sodium and potassium is:
   a. flame emission spectrophotometry.
   b. enzymatic methods.
   c. atomic absorption spectrophotometry.
   d. ion-selective electrode.

2. Which of the following will shift the $O_2$ dissociation curve to the right?
   a. Hyperthermia
   b. Acute alkalemia
   c. Hypocapnia
   d. Low 2,3-BPG

3. Which of the following present the least risk of erroneous blood gas values?
   a. 30 minutes at ambient temperature
   b. WBC >100,000/μL
   c. Air bubbles in the sample
   d. First drop from a capillary puncture

4. The vapor pressure osmometer has fallen out of popular use due to several technical drawbacks. Which of the following is false regarding this instrument?
   a. It does not include any volatile solutes in its measurement of serum osmolality.
   b. It is sensitive to changes in ambient temperature.
   c. It contains a thermistor, a galvanometer, and a measuring potentiometer.
   d. It would be able to detect an increase in osmolality attributable to increased blood glucose.

5. Solutes change the behavior of the solvent to which they are added in predictable ways, conferring colligative properties to the solution, including:
   a. decreased osmotic pressure.
   b. increased vapor pressure.
   c. decreased boiling point.
   d. decreased freezing point.
   e. increased transmittance.

6. The most common cause of falsely elevated sweat chloride testing results is:
   a. eczema.
   b. improper gauze placement.
   c. hypothyroidism.
   d. postcollection evaporation.
   e. analytic error.

7. What is the expected effect on plasma $K^+$ concentration if a freshly drawn sample is stored on the bench for 1.5 hours prior to being centrifuged?
   a. An increase in plasma $K^+$ of ~2 mmol/L
   b. A decrease in plasma $K^+$ of ~0.2 mmol/L due to transcellular shift into RBCs
   c. An insignificant increase in plasma $K^+$ of ~0.2 mmol/L
   d. A decrease in plasma $K^+$ due to increased hemolysis
   e. A decrease in plasma $K^+$ ~2 mmol/L due to transcellular shift into RBCs

8. Hemolysis of a plasma sample will most likely affect which of the following, and why?
   a. Sodium; it is present in equal amounts both intracellularly and extracellularly
   b. Glucose; it moves out of cells into plasma
   c. Insulin; it is the major intracellular anion and is present in high amounts in RBCs
   d. Potassium; it is localized mainly within cells, particularly RBCs

9. Which of the following equations is the correct Henderson-Hasselbalch equation?
   a. $pK' = pH + \log [cHCO_3]/[cH_2CO_3]$
   b. $pK' = pH + \log [cH_2CO_3]/[cHCO_3]$
   c. $pH = pK' + \log [cHCO_3]/[cH_2CO_3]$
   d. $pH = pK' + \log [cH_2CO_3]/[cHCO_3]$

10. Some methods of electrolyte analysis rely on the assumption that plasma is approximately 93% water. Conditions that alter the plasma composition, such as hyperlipidemia or hyperproteinemia, will cause which of the following?
    a. Pseudohyperkalemia
    b. Pseudonatritis
    c. Electrolyte inclusion effect
    d. Electrolyte exclusion effect

## SUGGESTED READINGS

Abraham B, Fakhar I, Tikaria A, et al. Reverse pseudohyperkalemia in a leukemic patient. *Clin Chem*. 2008;54:449–451.

Berry MN, Mazzachi RD, Pejakovic M, et al. Enzymatic determination of potassium in serum. *Clin Chem*. 1989;35:817–820.

Billman GF, Hughes AB, Dudell GG, et al. Clinical performance of an in-line, ex vivo point-of-care monitor: a multicenter study. *Clin Chem*. 2002;48:2030–2043.

Bisson J, Younker J. Correcting arterial blood gases for temperature: (when) is it clinically significant? *Nurs Crit Care*. 2006;11:232–238.

Brydon WG, Roberts LB. The effect of haemolysis on the determination of plasma constituents. *Clin Chim Acta*. 1972;41:435–438.

CLSI (Clinical and Laboratory Standards Institute). *C46–A2. Blood Gas and pH Analysis and Related Measurements*. Wayne, PA: CLSI; 2009.

Graber M, Subramani K, Corish D, et al. Thrombocytosis elevates serum potassium. *Am J Kidney Dis*. 1988;12:116–120.

Grocott MPW, Martin DS, Levett DZH, et al. Arterial blood gases and oxygen content in climbers on Mount Everest. *N Engl J Med*. 2009;360:140–149.

Hill CE, Burd EM, Kraft CS, et al. Laboratory test support for Ebola patients within a high-containment facility. *Lab Med*. 2014;45:e109–e111.

Lacher DA, Hughes JP, Carroll MD. Estimate of biological variation of laboratory analytes based on the Third National Health and Nutrition Examination Survey. *Clin Chem*. 2005;51:450–452.

Mansour MMH, Azzazy HME, Kazmierczak SC. Correction factors for estimating potassium concentrations in samples with in vitro hemolysis: a detriment to patient safety. *Arch Pathol Lab Med.* 2009;133:960–966.

Nijsten MW, de Smet BJ, Dofferhoff AS. Pseudohyperkalemia and platelet counts. *N Engl J Med.* 1991;325:1107.

Oliver Jr TK, Young GA, Bates GD, et al. Factitial hyperkalemia due to icing before analysis. *Pediatrics.* 1966;38(5):900–902.

Quiles R, Fernández-Romero JM, Fernández E, et al. Automated enzymatic determination of sodium in serum. *Clin Chem.* 1993;39:500–503.

Ress KL, Koerbin G, Li L, et al. Reference intervals for venous blood gas measurement in adults. *Clin Chem Lab Med.* 2021;59:947–954.

Zou J, Nolan DK, LaFiore AR, et al. Estimating the effects of hemolysis on potassium and LDH laboratory results. *Clin Chim Acta.* 2013;421:60–61.

# 25

# Hormones

*Timothy J. Cole*

## OBJECTIVES

1. Define the following:
   - Amino acid–derived hormone
   - Autocrine system
   - Endocrine system
   - Endocrinology
   - Hormone
   - Hormone receptor
   - Incretin hormone
   - Paracrine system
   - Protein or polypeptide hormone
   - Steroid hormone
2. Describe the three classifications of hormones; include examples of each, chemical structures, characteristics, half-life, and tissues of origin.

3. List and describe three physiological functions of hormones; include the role of hormones in each category and give examples of hormones in each category.
4. Compare the two types of receptor-hormone interactions; include examples of each type, postreceptor actions, and the specific effects that each type of interaction produces in a cell.
5. Provide examples of feedback mechanisms in the endocrine system.
6. List and describe four techniques used to assess hormones; include basic principles, specimen requirements, and an advantage of each technique.

## KEY WORDS AND DEFINITIONS

**Autocrine** A mode of hormone action in which a cell secretes a hormone that binds to autocrine receptors on that same cell, leading to changes in the cell.

**Circadian rhythms** Rhythmic repetition of certain phenomena in living organisms at about the same time each day.

**Cyclic adenosine monophosphate (cAMP)** A cyclic nucleotide that serves as an intracellular and, in some cases, extracellular "second messenger" mediating the action of many peptide or amine hormones.

**Endocrine** A mode of hormone action in which a specialized endocrine cell secretes a hormone into the bloodstream to circulate and act on another target cell of the body.

**Endocrine system** The system of glands that release their secretions (hormones) directly into the circulatory system. In addition to the endocrine glands, included are the chromaffin and the neurosecretory systems.

**Endocrinology** The scientific study of the function and pathology of the endocrine glands.

**Gonadotropin** Any hormone that stimulates the gonads.

**G-protein–coupled receptors (GPCRs)** A large superfamily of membrane receptors whose intracellular effects are mediated by G-proteins.

**G-proteins** Guanine nucleotide-binding proteins (G-proteins) are a family of intracellular proteins involved in transmitting chemical signals from outside the cell, and causing changes inside the cell. They communicate

signals from many hormones, neurotransmitters, and other signaling factors.

**Half-life** In endocrinology, the time required for a hormone to fall to half its original concentration in the specified fluid or blood.

**Homeostasis** The maintenance of equilibrium of internal body functions in response to external changes.

**Hormone** A chemical substance that has a specific regulatory effect on the activity of a certain organ or organs on cell types.

**Paracrine** A type of hormone function in which hormone synthesized in and released from endocrine cells binds to its receptor in nearby cells of a different type and affects their function.

**Phospholipase C-γ** Any esterase that catalyzes the hydrolysis of the phosphoric ester bond of a membrane phospholipid, generating a phosphorylated alcohol and diacylglycerol.

**Pituitary gland** A small oval gland attached to the base of the vertebrate brain and consisting of an anterior and a posterior lobe (also known as the hypophysis and the pituitary body).

**Receptor** A molecular structure, normally a protein, within a cell or on the surface characterized by (1) selective binding of a specific substance and (2) a specific physiological effect that accompanies the binding; examples include (1) cell surface receptors for peptide hormones, neurotransmitters, antigens, complement

fragments and immunoglobulins, and (2) cytoplasmic receptors for steroid and other lipid-derived hormones.
Second messenger  Any of several classes of intracellular signaling molecules that translate electrical or chemical messages from the environment (first messengers) into cellular responses.

Zinc finger motif  Found in nucleic acid–binding proteins that contain one or more zinc-binding domains (tandemly repeated, highly conserved stretches of 28 amino acids).

---

Endocrine hormones are chemical messengers that circulate in body fluids at variable concentrations and mediate communication between cells and tissues. They regulate development of the embryo, energy balance and integrated cellular metabolism, maintenance of homeostasis, cognition, and reproductive events throughout life. Hormones are classified into three major classes: polypeptide hormones, amino acid–derived hormones, and steroid- and other lipid-derived hormones. Each hormone is released for a specific purpose, has a defined half-life in circulation, and can negatively feedback to regulate subsequent hormone biosynthesis and release. Hormones act on target cells by activating protein receptors that are either imbedded in the cell plasma membrane or reside intracellularly. The two largest groups of cell surface receptors are the G-protein–coupled receptors (GPCRs) and the enzyme-coupled receptor (ENZCR) families of proteins. Intracellular hormone receptors comprise the nuclear receptor (NR) superfamily. Receptor activation initiates intracellular signal transduction pathways that result in hormone-directed cellular and physiological change. Accurate measurement of hormone status is critical for the clinical diagnosis of illness and disease.

## BACKGROUND

Hormones are a diverse group of chemical messengers synthesized and secreted by endocrine glands, organs, or isolated cells that have specific regulatory effects on the activity of specific target cells. As a component of the body's endocrine system, each hormone is produced at one or more sites in the body, and in general, exert their action(s) at distant target sites. Some hormones exert actions locally (paracrine), and other hormones exert their action on their cell of origin, regulating their own synthesis and secretion (autocrine). Classic endocrine hormones include insulin, thyroxine, and cortisol; neurotransmitters and neurohormones are examples of paracrine hormones, and certain growth factors that stimulate synthesis and secretion of other hormones from the same cell are examples of autocrine hormones. Table 25.1 lists hormones that are commonly measured in the clinical laboratory. Hormones are classified as either polypeptides or proteins, derivatives of amino acids, and lipophilic steroids or other lipid derivatives.

### Polypeptide or Protein Hormones

Adrenocorticotropic hormone (ACTH), insulin, and parathyroid hormone (PTH) are examples of polypeptide or protein hormones (see Table 25.1). They are water soluble and circulate freely in plasma as the secreted complete active molecule

or as active or inactive fragments. The half-life of these hormones in plasma is relatively short (≤10 to 30 minutes), and their concentrations may vary dramatically depending on specific physiological and pathological states. These hormones initiate cellular responses by binding to a vast array of cell surface membrane receptors on target cells and activate intracellular signal-transduction pathways that lead to a specific action or changes within the target cell. For example, insulin when released from pancreatic β-cells, binds to cell-surface insulin receptors at target tissues, such as the adipose and muscle, to promote the increased uptake of glucose from the bloodstream.

### Amino Acid–Derived Hormones

Thyroid hormone such as thyroxine and the catecholamines are examples of hormones that are derived from amino acids; in both of these cases they are derived from tyrosine. They are water soluble and circulate in plasma bound to specific transport proteins (thyroxine) or circulate freely (catecholamines). Thyroxine binds avidly to three specific binding proteins, transthyretin, thyroid-binding globulin, and albumin, and has a half-life of approximately 7 to 10 days; free-circulating catecholamines such as epinephrine have a short half-life of a minute or less. The catecholamines interact with a family of nine closely related cell surface adrenergic GPCRs and initiate intracellular second messenger signal-transduction systems, whereas thyroid hormones move freely across the cell membrane to activate dimers of two specific intracellular NRs, thyroid hormone receptor-α and -β.

### Steroid and Other Lipid-Derived Hormones

Endogenous lipophilic steroid hormones such as cortisol, estrogen, and testosterone are synthesized from cholesterol, are hydrophobic, and virtually insoluble in water. These hormones circulate in plasma, reversibly bound to specific transport plasma proteins (e.g., cortisol-binding globulin, sex hormone-binding globulin) with only a small fraction unbound that is freely circulating to exert physiological action. The half-life of circulating steroid hormones is 30 to 90 minutes. Free steroid hormones at their sites of action, because of their hydrophobicity, enter the cell by passive diffusion and bind with intracellular NRs in either the cytoplasm or the nucleus.

## SYNTHESIS, RELEASE, AND GENERAL ACTION OF HORMONES

The physiological functions of hormones can be broadly categorized as (1) those affecting growth, development, and

## TABLE 25.1   Representative Endocrine Hormones

| Endocrine Organ and Hormone | Hormone Type | Major Sites of Action | Principal Actions |
|---|---|---|---|
| **Brain—Hypothalamus** | | | |
| Thyrotropin-releasing hormone (TRH) | Peptide (3aa, Glu-His-Pro)* | Anterior pituitary | Release of thyroid-stimulating hormone (TSH) and prolactin (PRL) |
| Gonadotropin-releasing hormone (Gn-RH) | Peptide (10aa) | Anterior pituitary | Release of luteinizing hormone (LH) and follicle-stimulating hormone (FSH) |
| Corticotropin-releasing hormone (CRH) | Peptide (41aa) | Anterior pituitary | Release of adrenocorticotrophic hormone (ACTH) and β-lipotropic hormone (LPH) |
| Growth hormone–releasing hormone (GH-RH) | Peptides (40, 44aa) | Anterior pituitary | Release of growth hormone (GH) |
| Neuropeptide Y (NPY) | 36aa peptide released mainly from paraventricular neurons | Hypothalamus, thalamus, hippocampus, and gastrointestinal tract | Increased food intake, energy storage, reduced anxiety, and stress |
| Somatostatin (SS) or growth hormone-inhibiting hormone | Peptides (14, 28aa) | Anterior pituitary | Suppression of secretion of many hormones |
| Kisspeptin | Peptide (54aa precursor cleaved to 13 and 14aa active peptides) | Gn-RH hypothalamic neurons | Stimulation of Gn-RH release via the G-protein–coupled receptor GPR54 |
| **Anterior Pituitary Lobe** | | | |
| Thyrotropin or TSH | Glycoprotein, heterodimer‡ (α, 92aa; β, 112aa) | Thyroid gland | Stimulation of thyroid hormone formation and secretion |
| Follicle-stimulating hormone (FSH) | Glycoprotein, heterodimer‡ (α, 92aa; β, 117aa) | Ovary | Growth of follicles with LH, secretion of estrogens, and ovulation |
| | | Testis | Development of seminiferous tubules; spermatogenesis |
| Luteinizing hormone (LH) | Glycoprotein, heterodimer‡ (α, 92aa; β, 121aa) | Ovary | Ovulation; formation of corpora lutea; secretion of progesterone |
| | | Testis | Secretion of androgens |
| Prolactin (PRL) | Peptide (199aa) | Mammary gland | Proliferation of mammary gland; initiation of milk secretion; antagonist of insulin action |
| Growth hormone (GH) or somatotropin | Peptide (191aa) | Liver | Production of insulin-like growth factor (IGF-1) (promoting growth) |
| | | Liver and peripheral tissues | Anti-insulin and anabolic effects |
| Corticotropin hormone or adrenocorticotropin hormone (ACTH) | Peptide (39aa) | Adrenal cortex | Stimulation of adrenocortical steroid biosynthesis and secretion |
| **Posterior Pituitary Lobe** | | | |
| Vasopressin or antidiuretic hormone | Peptide (9aa) | Arterioles / Renal tubules | Increase of blood pressure; water reabsorption |
| Oxytocin | Peptide (9aa) | Smooth muscles (uterus, mammary gland) | Contraction; action in parturition and in sperm transport; ejection of milk |
| **Pineal Gland** | | | |
| Melatonin | Indoleamine | Hypothalamus | Suppression of gonadotropin and GH secretion; induction of sleep |
| Serotonin or 5-hydroxytryptamine (5-HT) | Indoleamine | Cardiovascular, respiratory, and gastrointestinal systems; brain | Neurotransmitter; stimulation or inhibition of various smooth muscles and nerves |

*Continued*

## TABLE 25.1 Representative Endocrine Hormones—cont'd

| Endocrine Organ and Hormone | Hormone Type | Major Sites of Action | Principal Actions |
|---|---|---|---|
| **Thyroid Gland** | | | |
| Thyroxine ($T_4$) and triiodothyronine ($T_3$) | Iodoamino acids | General body tissue | Stimulation of oxygen consumption and metabolic rate of tissue |
| Calcitonin or thyrocalcitonin | Peptide (32aa) | Skeleton | Uncertain in humans |
| **Parathyroid Gland** | | | |
| Parathyroid hormone (PTH) or parathyrin | Peptide (84aa) | Kidney | Increased calcium reabsorption, inhibited phosphate reabsorption; increased production of 1,25-dihydroxycholecalciferol |
| | | Skeleton | Increased bone resorption |
| **Adrenal Cortex** | | | |
| Aldosterone | Steroid | Kidney | Salt and water balance |
| Androstenedione | Steroid | Hormone precursor | Converted to estrogens and androgens |
| Cortisol | Steroid | Many | Metabolism of carbohydrates, proteins, and fats; anti-inflammatory effects; others |
| Dehydroepiandrosterone (DHEA) and dehydroepiandrostenedione sulfate (DHEAS) | Steroids | Hormone precursors | Converted to estrogens and testosterone |
| **Adrenal Medulla** | | | |
| Norepinephrine and epinephrine | Aromatic amines | Sympathetic receptors | Stimulation of sympathetic nervous system |
| Epinephrine | Aromatic amines | Liver and muscle, adipose tissue | Glycogenolysis Lipolysis |
| **Ovary** | | | |
| Activin A and B | Peptides¶ 2 $\beta_A$ subunits 2 $\beta_B$ subunits | Pituitary, ovarian follicle | Stimulates release of FSH; enhances FSH action; inhibits androgen production by theca cells |
| Estrogens | Phenolic steroids | Female accessory sex organs | Development of secondary sex characteristics |
| | | Bone | Control of skeletal maturation |
| Follistatin | Peptides (288aa, 315aa) | Pituitary, ovarian follicles | Inhibits FSH synthesis and secretion by binding activin |
| Inhibin A and B | Peptide ($\alpha$ subunit and $\beta_A$ or $\beta_B$ subunit) | Hypothalamus, ovarian follicle | Inhibits FSH secretion; stimulates theca cell androgen production |
| Progesterone | Steroid | Female accessory reproductive structure | Preparation of the uterus for ovum implantation, maintenance of pregnancy |
| Relaxin | Peptide# | Uterus | Inhibition of myometrial contraction |
| **Testis** | | | |
| Testosterone | Steroid | Male accessory sex organs | Development of secondary sex characteristics, maturation, and normal function |
| **Pancreas** | | | |
| Glucagon | Peptide (29aa) | Liver | Glycogenolysis |

## TABLE 25.1    Representative Endocrine Hormones—cont'd

| Endocrine Organ and Hormone | Hormone Type | Major Sites of Action | Principal Actions |
|---|---|---|---|
| Insulin | Peptide** | Liver, fat, muscle | Regulation of carbohydrate metabolism; lipogenesis |
| **Gastrointestinal Tract** | | | |
| Gastrin§ | Peptide (17aa) | Stomach | Secretion of gastric acid, gastric mucosal growth |
| Ghrelin§ | Peptide (28aa) | Anterior pituitary | Secretion of GH |
| **Kidney** | | | |
| 1,25-(OH)$_2$ cholecalciferol | Sterol | Intestine Bone | Facilitation of absorption of calcium and phosphorus; increase in bone resorption in conjunction with PTH |
| | | Kidney | Increase in reabsorption of filtered calcium |
| Erythropoietin | Peptide (165aa) | Bone marrow | Stimulation of red cell formation |
| Renin-angiotensin-aldosterone system | Peptides (renin, 297aa; Ang I, 10aa; Ang II, 8aa, produced from Ang I by angiotensin-converting enzyme) | Renin (from kidney) catalyzes hydrolysis of angiotensinogen (from liver, 485aa) to Ang I in the intravascular space | Ang II increases blood pressure and stimulates secretion of aldosterone (see adrenal) |
| **Liver** | | | |
| IGF-1, formerly called somatomedin | Peptide (70aa) | Most cells | Stimulation of cellular and linear growth |
| IGF-2 | Peptide (67aa) | Most cells | Insulin-like activity |
| **Heart** | | | |
| Atrial natriuretic peptide (atriopeptin) | Peptide with an intrachain disulfide bond (28aa) | Vascular, renal, and adrenal tissues | Regulation of blood volume and blood pressure |
| B-type natriuretic peptide | Peptide with an intrachain disulfide bond (32aa) | Vascular, renal, and adrenal tissues | Regulation of blood volume and blood pressure |
| **Adipose Tissue** | | | |
| Adiponectin | Peptide oligomers of 30 kDa subunits | Muscle Liver | Increases fatty acid oxidation Suppresses glucose formation |
| Leptin | Peptide (167aa) | Hypothalamus | Inhibition of appetite, stimulation of metabolism |
| Tissue necrosis factor-α | 157aa secreted protein | Adipose in an autocrine or paracrine fashion | Pluripotent cytokine with a wide range of actions |
| **Bone** | | | |
| Osteocalcin | 49aa | Bone, pancreas, adipose tissue | Bone mineralization and calcium homeostasis, systemic metabolism |
| Osteopontin | 314aa | Bone, pancreas, neutrophils | Bone remodeling, immune functions, chemotaxis |
| Osteonectin | 285aa | Bone, paracrine action | Bone mineralization |

*aa, Amino acid residues.

†Also produced by gastrointestinal tract and pancreas.

‡Glycoprotein hormones composed of two dissimilar peptides. The α-chains are similar in structure or identical; the β-chains differ among hormones and confer specificity.

¶Each activin and inhibin is found in multiple forms.

#Two chains linked by two disulfide bonds: α, 24aa; β, 29aa.

**Two chains linked by two disulfide bonds: α, 21aa; β, 30aa.

§Also produced in the brain.

‖Androstenedione is also produced in the ovary and testis.

A more complete list endocrine hormones can be found in *Tietz Textbook of Laboratory Medicine*, 8th ed., Chapter 38: Hormones.

maturation; (2) control of systemic homeostasis, energy balance, and integrated metabolism; and (3) regulation of reproduction.

## Synthesis and Release of Hormones

Many hormones are synthesized in specialized endocrine cells within specific endocrine glands. These include the polypeptide hormone insulin, which is synthesized in the β-cells of the pancreas; estradiol, which is synthesized in the granulosa cells of the ovary; and epinephrine (or adrenalin), which is synthesized by the medullary chromaffin cells of the adrenal gland. Some hormones require biosynthesis via complex enzymatic pathways, such as the cardiovascular hormone aldosterone, which is synthesized from precursor cholesterol in the outer zona glomerulosa cell layer of the adrenal cortex. Other hormones require simpler modification of a precursor compound such as vitamin D. All hormones attain a structural specificity that allows them to bind strongly to and activate specific receptors on target cells. In general, hormones are released from endocrine cells when they are required, either from intracellular stores or by induction of rapid biosynthesis. The biosynthetic pathways of hormones are critical to maintain homeostasis. Defects in those pathway enzymes can lead to debilitating endocrine disease, such as the genetic condition of congenital adrenal hyperplasia (CAH), which is a disease caused by mutations in the steroid biosynthetic enzymes of the adrenal cortex, which are required for production of cortisol, aldosterone, and androgen precursors from cholesterol. The loss of end-product hormone production or the inappropriate buildup of steroid precursors can lead to complex cardiovascular and reproductive development dysfunction and gender ambiguity. Examples of the three broad functional categories of hormone action are presented in the following and illustrate specific aspects on the synthesis, release, turnover, and action of endocrine hormones.

## Growth, Development, and Maturation

Normal embryonic development and postnatal growth of the whole human organism is dependent on the complex integrative function of many hormones, including growth hormone, insulin-like growth factor-1 (IGF-1), thyroxine, the gonadal steroids (estrogen and androgen), and cortisol. Several pituitary hormones, such as growth hormone, ACTH, and thyroid-stimulating hormone (TSH), are responsible specifically for the growth and development of other endocrine glands, such as the adrenal, gonads, and thyroid. For example, growth hormone is synthesized and secreted by anterior pituitary somatotroph cells and stimulates the production and release of hepatic IGF-1. Both factors then have broad somatic growth actions, particularly in bone and cartilage. Therefore, these pituitary hormones are responsible for control of synthesis and secretion of many secondary hormones. These hormones provide important negative feedback control on the secretion of the pituitary hormones. Other regulators of secretion of the pituitary hormones include **circadian rhythms** and the hypothalamic pulse generator that controls the pulsatile secretion of **gonadotropins**.

## Energy Homeostasis and Integrated Metabolism

Energy homeostasis and the activity of many metabolic pathways in cells are tightly regulated by a diverse number of systemic and locally released hormones. There is a continual change in demand for energy use and storage during states such as feeding, exercise, starvation, infection, injury and/or trauma, or emotional stress. These states initiate the release and action of many hormones to regulate energy use and nutrient metabolism, modulate energy storage, and regulate physical and behavioral responses to stress. These hormonal activated pathways in cells are complex and may involve hormones from different organs. In general, systemic nutrient uptake, appetite, energy storage, and release are under neurological control via actions of specific hypothalamic and neuroendocrine hormones (e.g., leptin and neuropeptide Y).

The following are examples to illustrate the feedback control of hormone secretion and action, which is critical to maintain homeostasis:

- Regulation of blood glucose concentrations: in response to a glucose load following a meal, insulin is promptly released from the pancreatic β-cells, which regulate the uptake of glucose into peripheral metabolic tissues (fat, muscle, liver, and brain) for the metabolism necessary to produce energy from glucose. As circulating glucose concentrations return to preload concentrations, insulin secretion slows. Several counter-regulatory hormones come into play to further regulate this process to ensure that blood glucose concentrations do not become too low. These counter-regulatory hormones include glucagon, cortisol, epinephrine, and growth hormone.
- Regulation of serum calcium (see Chapter 39): The calcium-sensing receptor (CaSR) on the parathyroid gland recognizes the ambient concentration of ionized calcium, which in turn regulates the synthesis and secretion of the hormone PTH. When ionized calcium concentrations fall (so imperceptibly that most analytical methods cannot detect the change), PTH synthesis and secretion are stimulated. Increased plasma levels of PTH will restore serum ionized calcium by enhancing renal tubular reabsorption of calcium and calcium efflux from bone. PTH also catalyzes the synthesis of the renal hormone calcitriol (1, 25-dihydroxycholecalciferol), which acts on the gut to increase intestinal absorption of calcium. These very rapid responses of PTH and calcitriol quickly restore ionized calcium to concentrations where the CaSR is no longer activated, and PTH and calcitriol synthesis and secretion return to basal levels.
- Water and electrolyte homeostasis is regulated by the steroid hormone aldosterone released from the adrenal gland, renin from the kidney, and vasopressin (antidiuretic hormone) from the posterior **pituitary gland**.

## Endocrine Control of Reproduction

The gonadotropin hormones, luteinizing hormone (LH), and follicle-stimulating hormone (FSH), are released from anterior pituitary gonadotroph cells in response to hypothalamic gonadotropin-releasing hormone to regulate the development, growth, and functions of the ovary and testis. In turn, the ovarian and testicular hormones estradiol and testosterone, respectively, initiate and regulate the following: pubertal growth; development and maintenance of secondary sex characteristics; the growth, development, and maintenance of the skeleton and muscles; and in part, the distribution of body fat.

## CELL SIGNALING MECHANISMS OF HORMONE RECEPTORS

The specific action of an endocrine hormone on its target cell or tissue is a function of the interaction between the hormone and its cognate protein receptor. Several types of hormone-receptor interactions occur with cells, and an individual cell may express and contain hundreds of different receptors that may be responding to multiple specific hormones at any given time. The hormone-receptor complex provides the strong specificity of the hormone's action, eliciting a target tissue response. Many endocrine hormones circulate in picomolar or nanomolar concentrations ($10^{-9}$ to $10^{-12}$ mol/L) but elicit specific and strong responses in specific target cells. Hormone receptors may be present on the cell surface imbedded in the plasma membrane or reside intracellularly within the cytoplasm or nucleus. Receptors at the cell surface and intracellular NRs initiate a variety of different post-receptor cellular responses by activating complex intracellular signal transduction pathways. This is shown schematically in Fig. 25.1 for three common classes of hormone receptors. Binding of the hormone or ligand to the receptor initiates activation of the receptor and initiation of downstream signaling that cause cellular changes both in the cytoplasm and the nucleus.

## Cell Surface Hormone Receptors

Polypeptide or hydrophilic hormones bind to cell surface receptors, and the conformational change or the protein–protein interactions initiated resulting from this binding activates an effector system within the cells, which is responsible for the downstream actions of the hormone (see Fig. 25.1). For many peptide and polypeptide hormones, the intracellular effector that is activated by the hormone–receptor interaction is a specific intracellular G-protein (guanyl-nucleotide–binding protein), and the cell surface receptors are called GPCRs (see Fig. 25.1). GPCRs are the largest family of cell surface receptors, with approximately 830 genes coding for human GPCRs. GPCRs are large proteins with seven membrane-spanning domains, an amino-terminal, a hormone-binding domain that is extracellular, and an intracellular carboxy-terminal tail of loop domains. The second major class of cell surface hormone receptors is the ENZCRs (see Fig. 25.1). These receptors have been divided into six subfamilies of receptors, of which the most well-characterized family is the receptor tyrosine-kinase (RTK) group of receptors, which mediate the actions of many common hormones and growth factors, such as insulin, IGF-1, epidermal growth factors, and fibroblast growth factors. These receptors are characterized by initiating intracellular kinase cascades and regulating cell growth and metabolism, and are common targets for mutation in tumor cells. A third class of cell surface receptors are the ion channel–coupled receptors that when bound and stimulated by a hormone open a channel in the cell membrane to allow the influx or efflux of a specific ion by passive diffusion. We will not discuss this receptor class any further in this chapter.

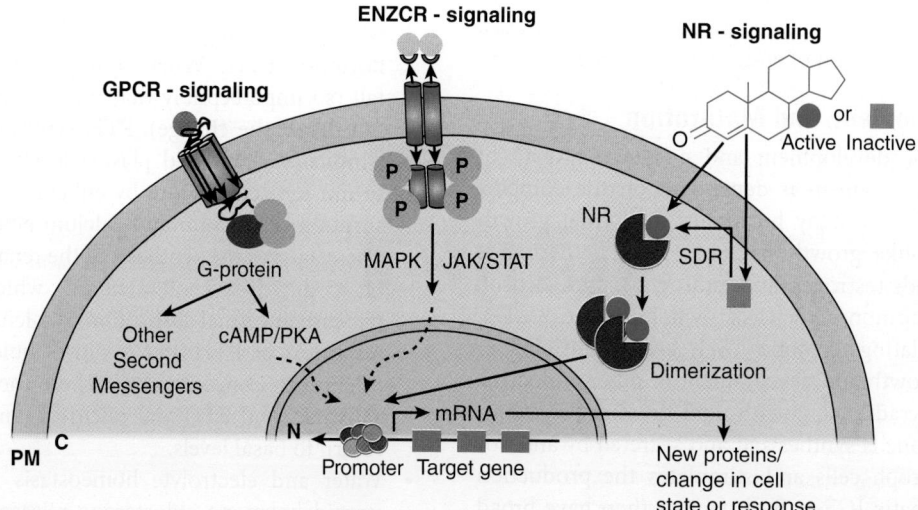

**Fig. 25.1** Endocrine cell signaling is mediated by both cell surface and intracellular hormone receptors. Cell surface receptors comprise two main classes of proteins called G-protein–coupled receptors *(GPCR)* and enzyme-coupled receptors *(ENZCR)*, whereas intracellular hormone receptors form the nuclear receptor *(NR)* superfamily of proteins. Cell surface receptors bind a circulating hormone using a specific extracellular protein domain and transduce a signal to the interior of the cell. In contrast, receptors for lipophilic hormones (e.g., a steroid hormone) reside within the cell, in many cases in the cytoplasm in an inactive complex of proteins. The activated NR is then targeted to the nucleus. *cAMP,* Cyclic adenosine monophosphate; *JAK/STAT,* Jak kinase/STAT pathway; *MAPK,* MAP kinase pathway; *N,* nucleus; *P,* phosphate; *PKA,* protein kinase A; *PM,* plasma membrane.

## SIGNAL TRANSDUCTION FROM CELL SURFACE G-PROTEIN–COUPLED RECEPTORS

GPCRs are grouped under four main classes, each of which contain receptors for specific types of hormones. The class A GPCRs contain the rhodopsin-like receptors that include receptors for olfactory compounds and melatonin; class B represents the secretin-like GPCRs (receptors for secretins, glucagon, and vasoactive intestinal polypeptide); class C, the largest by number, contains the metabotropic glutamate and/or pheromone receptors; and the class D contains the fungal mating pheromone receptors. GPCRs are seven transmembrane proteins that on hormone binding undergo a conformational change allowing direct interaction of the intracellular C-terminal tail of the activated GPCR with specific G-proteins that are organized in a trimeric complex of an α, β, and γ G-protein subunit. Activated G-protein subunits then initiate signaling cascades via activation of specific enzymes or generation of small molecules that serve as potent second messengers to mediate the hormone response within the cell. The best-known effector enzyme is adenylyl cyclase, which generates the important second messenger cyclic adenosine monophosphate (cAMP) (see Fig. 25.1). The activated G-protein α binds a molecule of GTP and is inactivated by an intrinsic GTPase activity that converts the bound GTP to GDP, thereby turning off the downstream signaling pathway.

## SIGNAL TRANSDUCTION FROM CELL SURFACE ENZYME-COUPLED RECEPTORS

The insulin receptor is a member of the second major class of cell surface hormone receptors, called the ENZCRs. These have been classified into six subfamilies of ENZCRs, with the best characterized being the large family of RTKs, a family of 90 characterized receptors. These receptors mediate the actions of many common growth factor hormones such as the epidermal, fibroblast, platelet-derived, and vascular endothelial growth factors. RTKs are single transmembrane spanning proteins that dimerize upon hormone binding, an event that initiates intracellular signaling responses (see Fig. 25.1). The receptor dimer is then auto-phosphorylated by intrinsic C-terminal tyrosine kinase catalytic domains. The phosphorylated Tyr residues act as specific binding sites for effector signaling proteins, such as phosphoinositol-3-kinase (PI-3-kinase) and phospholipase C-γ, which then transmit the signal within the cell. These effector proteins contain SH2 domains that specifically recognize phosphotyrosine residues on the activated receptor. Mitogen-activated protein (MAP)–kinase pathway activation results in subsequent downstream target gene activation, as well as cell proliferation and differentiation. These pathways do not use second messengers but involve activated enzyme cascades. RTKs and downstream signaling components are often mutated in cancer cells that then acquire a high-proliferative phenotype. Gene mutations often produce constitutively active receptors or signaling proteins such as rat sarcoma (RAS) and PI-3-Kinase.

## Intracellular Nuclear Receptors and Signal Transduction

Lipid-soluble hormones (e.g., estradiol) are primarily transported bound to plasma proteins such as albumin, with only a small fraction of the hormone circulating free or unbound. Free hormone enters the cell via passive diffusion and in most cases binds to intracellular NRs in the cytoplasm, or in some cases the nucleus (see Fig. 25.1). Some inactive lipid-derived hormones require enzymatic activation in cells via the action of one of the 71 members (in humans) of the short-chain alcohol dehydrogenase reductase (SDR) family of intracellular enzymes. Some SDR enzymes function to inactivate lipid hormones and protect the inappropriate activation of NR signaling in particular target cells. NRs are characterized by a hormone or ligand-binding domain, a central DNA-binding domain, and an amino-terminal variable domain that contributes to recruitment of nuclear proteins such as transcriptional coactivators. In general, lipid-soluble hormones bind and activate the ligand-binding domain of intracellular NRs that then signal specific changes to the nucleus (see Fig. 25.1). The human genome contains a group of 48 NR genes that encode the NR superfamily of receptors and are activated by a range of lipophilic steroid, dietary lipids, vitamins, fatty acid, and special small molecule ligands (e.g., thyroid hormone). A large number of these receptors are still classified as orphan receptors with no known hormone ligand, and little is understood of their functional role in human biology and in clinical disease. Hormone binding initiates a conformational change that enables the hormone-receptor complex to translocate to the nucleus and bind specific regulatory DNA hormone response elements (HREs) near to specific target genes. Hormone translocation of the cytoplasmic NRs to the nucleus, once activated, is mediated by a conformational change in the receptor that exposes a nuclear localization sequence normally located within the DNA-binding domain. The binding specificity of the activated NR for specific HREs near the target gene is determined by the first zinc finger in the receptor's DNA-binding domain. Binding of the hormone-receptor complex to HREs promotes recruitment of a co-activator, and sometimes, co-repressor proteins that ultimately mediate activation or repression of target gene transcription. Messenger RNA levels of target genes can be enhanced up to 1000-fold, leading to large changes in the synthesis of specific proteins that then drive cellular and physiological change. In addition to these nuclear gene expression changes, many NRs can be activated to produce rapid so-called "non-genomic" effects in the cytoplasm or at the cell membrane, although the cellular effects and mechanisms involved are less well understood.

## CLINICAL DISORDERS OF HORMONE ACTION

Although several chapters of this textbook detail a variety of endocrine disorders, a brief introduction to endocrine disorders is given here. In general, endocrine diseases may result from a deficiency or an excess of a single hormone or several hormones, or from resistance to the action of hormones in target cells. Hormone deficiency can be congenital (genetically inherited) or acquired, and hormone excess can result from endogenous overproduction (from within the body) or from exogenous overmedication. Hormone resistance can occur at several levels but can most simply be characterized as receptor-mediated, post-receptor-mediated, or at the level of the target tissue. The clinical manifestations will depend on the hormone system affected and the type of abnormality. Diabetes mellitus is an example of an endocrine metabolic disorder and is the most common endocrine disorder in Western countries. It is classified as either type 1 or type 2. Type 1 diabetes results from failure of the pancreas to secrete insulin, although the pancreas is otherwise normal. Type 2 diabetes results from end-organ resistance to the action of insulin, which, in this case, is secreted from the pancreas in abundant amounts and circulates at high concentrations. Secondary diabetes occurs when a non-endocrine disease, such as pancreatitis, destroys the pancreas, including the insulin-secreting cells. The biochemical hallmark of diabetes is hyperglycemia which can be present when there is insulin deficiency or insulin excess, and insulin excess can accompany both hyperglycemia and hypoglycemia. Steroid hormone production in the adrenal cortex is critical for post-natal life. The adrenal gland synthesizes the steroids cortisol, aldosterone, and androgen precursors using a complex series of enzymatic reactions that modify the substrate cholesterol. Deficiencies in any of these important steroid biosynthetic enzymes can lead to defects in adrenal steroid production and lead to the clinical condition of CAH. The most common genetic deficiency that affects young children is the loss of the enzyme 21-hydroxylase and is characterized by glucocorticoid (cortisol) and mineralocorticoid (aldosterone) deficiency associated with genital virilization and hyperandrogenism in females. Clinical treatment of CAH relies on replacement of cortisol and aldosterone, sodium supplements and reducing excess androgen secretion via blocking ACTH secretion.

# TECHNIQUES FOR MEASUREMENT OF HORMONES AND RELATED ANALYTES

Hormones are measured with a variety of analytical techniques, including bioassay, receptor assay, immunoassay, and instrumental techniques, such as mass spectrometry interfaced with liquid or gas chromatography. Bioassays are based on observations of physiological responses specific for the hormone being measured. In vivo bioassays usually involve the injection of test materials (such as blood or urine from a patient) into suitably prepared animals; target gland or organ responses such as growth or steroidogenesis are then measured. In vitro bioassays involve the incubation of tissue samples, membranes, dispersed cells, or permanent cell lines in a defined culture medium, with subsequent measurement of an appropriate hormone response. Bioassays tend to be imprecise and are now rarely used in clinical medicine.

Receptor-based binding assays depend on the in vitro interaction of a hormone with its biological receptor. In this type of assay, unlabeled hormone displaces trace amounts of radioactively labeled hormone from specific receptor sites. In general, receptor-binding assays are simpler to perform and have greater sensitivity than bioassays, and also have an advantage

over immunoassays in that they reflect the biological function of a hormone, namely, the capacity to combine with specific receptors. By contrast, immunoassays may measure active hormone and inactive prohormone, hormone polymer, and metabolites when all share the common antigenic determinant or set of determinants of the assay antibody. In general, receptor-binding assays are not as sensitive as immunoassays, and proteolytic enzymes in the biological specimen may sometimes degrade the receptor or destroy the labeled tracer.

Enzyme-linked immunosorbent assays or standard immunoassays that use specific antibodies are widely used to quantify hormones. Currently labeled antibody (immunometric) assays with nonisotopic labels are the method of choice for measuring concentrations of most hormones, especially peptides and proteins. Immunometric assays use saturating concentrations of two or more antibodies (often monoclonal) that are prepared against different epitopes of the protein molecule. One of the two antibodies is usually attached to a solid phase separation system and extracts the hormone from the serum specimen. The second antibody is linked to a signal molecule, which is then measured. A more recent alternate approach used to measure hormone concentrations is to use mass spectrometry coupled with gas and liquid chromatography to provide either qualitative or quantitative measurement of hormone levels. Technical advancements in mass spectrometry have resulted in the development of matrix-assisted laser desorption and/or ionization and electrospray ionization techniques that allow sequencing of peptides and mass determination of picomole quantities of analytes. Tandem mass spectrometry offers greater analytical sensitivity, accuracy, and speed, and may allow simultaneous determination of multiple hormones related to a clinical condition. For additional information on these techniques, refer to Chapters 13 and 15.

## Specimen Requirements

To prevent preanalytical variation, appropriate protocols must be followed when sending samples to the laboratory for hormone measurement (for further discussion on this topic refer to Chapter 3). Some hormones are directly affected by food (e.g., insulin) or by circadian variability (e.g., cortisol). In many clinical circumstances, the metabolic environment plays a crucial role in hormone production, and it is essential to obtain a simultaneous sample for measurement of both the hormone and the molecule(s) regulated by that hormone. An isolated measurement of plasma insulin without concurrent knowledge of the plasma glucose, or measurement of PTH independent of serum calcium, is of little, if any value. When a patient is evaluated for possible hormone deficiency or hormone excess, it is often necessary to perform a stimulation or suppression test. Most hormone assays can be performed on plasma or serum, and many can be performed on urine samples, usually a 24-hour collection. Increasingly, saliva has become a convenient body fluid for hormone analysis, particularly for hormones secreted in a diurnal rhythm (e.g., cortisol). Unlike blood sampling, which requires the patient to present to a blood drawing facility, patients can be provided with salivary collection material so they can provide specimens to the laboratory collected at multiple times during the day.

## REVIEW QUESTIONS

1. What direct effect do steroid hormones have by binding and activating specific intracellular nuclear receptors?
   a. Enzyme phosphorylation
   b. Gene expression changes
   c. cAMP formation
   d. DNA replication
2. What is the classical result that occurs when a protein hormone binds a cell membrane receptor?
   a. Phosphorylation of intracellular enzymes
   b. Inhibition of mRNA within the cell nucleus
   c. Replication of DNA and division of the cell
   d. Glycosylation of intracellular proteins
3. Select the amino acid–derived hormone:
   a. Testosterone
   b. Thyroid hormone
   c. Growth hormone
   d. Prostaglandin
4. Which of the following hormones is classified as a polypeptide?
   a. Cortisol
   b. Estrogen

   c. Adrenocorticotropic hormone
   d. Thyroid hormone
5. What type of hormone assay best reflects hormone functionality as opposed to the quantification of the hormone itself?
   a. Receptor-based assay
   b. Mass spectrometry–based assays
   c. Bioassay technique
   d. Liquid chromatography
6. For a pancreatic hormone involved in cellular energy production what type of response will be caused by its release in response to a glucose load?
   a. Modification of the response to stress
   b. Synthesis of milk proteins
   c. Promotion of bone development and growth
   d. Homeostatic control of metabolism
7. Which of these is a characteristic of steroid hormones?
   a. Account for the majority of hormones
   b. Circulate freely
   c. Water soluble
   d. Long half-life in the circulation

## SUGGESTED READINGS

Claahsen-van der Grinten HL, Speiser PW, Ahmed SF, et al. Congenital adrenal hyperplasia—current insights in pathophysiology, diagnostics, and management. *Endocrine Rev.* 2022;43(1):1–159.

Cole TJ, Short KL, Hooper SB. The science of steroids. *Semin Fetal Neonatal Med.* 2019;24(3):170–175.

Evans RM, Mangelsdorf DJ. Nuclear receptors, RXR, and the big bang. *Cell.* 2014;157(1):255–266.

Hubbard SR, Miller WT. Receptor tyrosine kinases: mechanisms of activation and signaling. *Curr Opin Cell Biol.* 2007;19:117–123.

Isberg V, Mordalski S, Munk C, et al. GPCRdb: an information system for G protein-coupled receptors. *Nucleic Acids Res.* 2016;44:D356–D364.

Jameson JL. Principles of endocrinology. In: Jameson LJ, de Kretser DM, eds. *Endocrinology Adult and Pediatric.* Philadelphia: Elsevier; 2016:3–15.

Kallberg Y, Oppermann U, Jörnvall H, et al. Short-chain dehydrogenase/reductase (SDR) relationships: a large family with eight clusters common to human, animal, and plant genomes. *Protein Sci.* 2002;11(3):636–641.

Katritch V, Cherezov V, Stevens RC. Structure-function of the G protein-coupled receptor superfamily. *Annu Rev Pharmacol Toxicol.* 2013;53:531–556.

Kelly DP. Introduction to the nuclear receptor review series. *Circ Res.* 2010;106:1557–1558.

Lefkowitz RJ, Rockman HA, Koch WJ. Catecholamines, cardiac beta-adrenergic receptors, and heart failure. *Circulation.* 2000;101:1634–1637.

Lemmon MA, Schlessinger J. Cell signaling by receptor tyrosine kinases. *Cell.* 2010;141:1117–1134.

McKenna NJ, O'Malley BW. Minireview: Nuclear receptor coactivators: an update. *Endocrinology.* 2002;143:2461–2465.

Oldham WM, Hamm HE. Heterotrimeric G protein activation by G-protein coupled receptors. *Nat Rev Mol Cell Biol.* 2008;9:60–71.

Pawson T. Specificity in signal transduction: from phosphotyrosine-SH2 domain interactions to complex cellular systems. *Cell.* 2004;116:191–203.

Qi M, Elion EA. MAP kinase pathways. *J Cell Sci.* 2005;118:3569–3572.

Seow BKL, McDougall ARA, Short KL, et al. Identification of betamethasone-regulated target genes and cell pathways in fetal rat lung mesenchymal fibroblasts. *Endocrinology.* 2019;160(8):1868–1884.

Shaw RJ, Cantley LC. Ras, PI(3)K and mTOR signaling controls tumour cell growth. *Nature.* 2006;44:424–430.

Wisler JW, Rockman HA, Lefkowitz RJ. Biased G protein-coupled receptor signaling: changing the paradigm of drug discovery. *Circulation.* 2018;137(22):2315–2317.

Yen FM, Ando S, Feng X. Thyroid hormone action at the cellular, genomic and target gene levels. *Mol Cell Endocrinol.* 2006;246:121–127.

# Catecholamines and Serotonin

*Graeme Eisenhofer and Thomas G. Rosano*

## OBJECTIVES

1. Define the following terms:
   a. 5-hydroxyindole acetic acid
   b. Carcinoid
   c. Carcinoid syndrome
   d. Catecholamine
   e. Gastroenteropancreatic neuroendocrine tumor
   f. Homovanillic acid
   g. Metanephrine
   h. Neuroblastoma
   i. Normetanephrine
   j. Paraganglioma
   k. Pheochromocytoma
   l. Serotonin
2. Discuss the following biogenic amines, including function and clinical relevance, synthesis, metabolism, and storage and release:
   a. Norepinephrine
   b. Epinephrine
   c. Dopamine
   d. Serotonin
   e. Melatonin
3. List the clinically relevant metabolites of the biogenic amines as detailed in Objective 2 above.
4. State the clinical significance and function of the catecholamines and serotonin in each of the following systems:

   a. Central nervous system
   b. Sympathetic nervous system
   c. Adrenal medullary system
   d. Peripheral dopaminergic system
   e. Enteric nervous system
5. Compare pheochromocytoma and neuroblastoma, including causes, symptoms, organ(s) and/or cell type involved, and laboratory evaluation of each; describe the clonidine suppression test and the results obtained when pheochromocytoma is present.
6. Explain the laboratory values obtained for serotonin and 5-HIAA in the assessment of a gastroenteropancreatic tumor and the carcinoid syndrome.
7. Describe the collection techniques used to obtain specimens for catecholamine, metanephrine, and serotonin analysis.
8. Describe how diet interferes with serotonin analysis; state how tricyclic antidepressants interfere in the measurement of catecholamines.
9. List the laboratory methods used to analyze metanephrines, catecholamines, serotonin, and 5-HIAA.
10. Analyze and solve case studies related to catecholamine and serotonin disorders using descriptions of symptoms and results of laboratory analyses.

## KEY WORDS AND DEFINITIONS

**Carcinoid syndrome** A syndrome due to carcinoid tumors that is characterized by attacks of severe cyanotic flushing of the skin—lasting from minutes to days—and by diarrheal watery stools, bronchoconstrictive attacks, sudden drops in blood pressure, edema, and ascites. Symptoms are caused by secretion from the tumor of serotonin, prostaglandins, and other biologically active substances.

**Carcinoid tumor** A slow-growing tumor arising from enterochromaffin cells, usually in the small intestine, appendix, stomach, or colon, and less commonly in the bronchus; sometimes used alone to refer to the gastrointestinal tumor (also called *argentaffinoma*).

**Catecholamine** One of a group of biogenic amines having a sympathomimetic action, the aromatic portion of whose molecule is catechol, and the aliphatic portion an

amine; examples include dopamine, norepinephrine, and epinephrine.

**Catecholamine metabolites** Products of catecholamine metabolism, such as dihydroxyphenylacetic acid, methoxytyramine, homovanillic acid, dihydroxyphenylglycol, methoxy-hydroxyphenylglycol, normetanephrine, metanephrine, and vanillylmandelic acid.

**Chromaffin cell** Neuroendocrine cell derived from embryonic neural crest found in the medulla of the adrenal gland and in other ganglia of the sympathetic nervous system; so-named because of the presence of cytoplasmic granules that give a brownish reaction with chromium salts.

**3,4-Dihydroxyphenylglycol (DHPG)** The metabolite produced within the peripheral sympathetic or central nervous system noradrenergic nerves by deamination of norepinephrine (can also be formed from epinephrine); *O*-methylated to methoxy-hydroxyphenylglycol in extraneuronal tissues.

**L-Dopa** An amino acid—3,4-dihydroxyphenylalanine—produced by oxidation of tyrosine by tyrosine hydroxylase; the precursor of dopamine and an intermediate product in the biosynthesis of norepinephrine and epinephrine. Can also be formed in melanocytes by the actions of tyrosinase as part of the production of melanin.

**Dopamine** A catecholamine formed in the body by the decarboxylation of dopa; an intermediate product in the synthesis of norepinephrine; acts as a neurotransmitter in the central nervous system, produced peripherally and acts on peripheral receptors.

**Epinephrine (adrenaline)** A catecholamine hormone secreted by the adrenal medulla.

**Gastroenteropancreatic neuroendocrine tumor (GEP-NET)** Encompasses neuroendocrine tumors of the digestive system and pancreas but also covers neuroendocrine pulmonary tumors and includes carcinoids.

**Homovanillic acid (HVA)** A product of dopamine metabolism; elevated urinary concentrations are used to diagnose neuroblastoma.

**5-Hydroxyindoleacetic acid (5-HIAA)** A metabolite of serotonin (5-hydroxytryptamine) that is excreted in large amounts by patients with carcinoid tumors.

**Metanephrine** A catecholamine metabolite resulting from *O*-methylation of epinephrine; formed mainly within adrenal chromaffin cells; excreted mainly in the urine as a sulfate-conjugated metabolite; measurements of the free and conjugated metabolites provide useful tests for diagnosis of pheochromocytoma.

**Methoxy-hydroxyphenylglycol (MHPG)** A metabolite of epinephrine and norepinephrine formed primarily from *O*-methylation of dihydroxyphenylglycol and in smaller amounts from deamination of normetanephrine and metanephrine; found in brain, blood, CSF, and urine, where its concentrations can be used to measure catecholamine turnover.

**Neuroblastoma** An often malignant tumor of neural crest-derived neuroblasts, usually arising in the autonomic nervous system (sympathicoblastoma) or in the adrenal medulla, that affects mostly infants and children up to 10 years of age.

**Neuroendocrine tumors (NET)** Neoplasms that arise from cells of the endocrine and peripheral nervous systems, most commonly in the digestive tract, but also found in the lung, pancreas, pituitary, thyroid, and other tissues. Include gastroenteropancreatic neuroendocrine tumors, as well as paragangliomas, neuroblastomas, neuroectodermal tumors, medulloblastomas, retinoblastomas, and pineoblastomas. Usually contain secretory granules and often produce biogenic amines and polypeptides.

**Norepinephrine (noradrenaline)** A major neurotransmitter produced by some brain neurons and peripheral sympathetic nerves that acts on α- and β1-adrenergic receptors; produced in the adrenal chromaffin cells as a precursor for epinephrine.

**Normetanephrine** An *O*-methylated metabolite of norepinephrine produced in extraneuronal cells and the adrenal medulla; excreted in the urine largely as a sulfate-conjugated metabolite; measurements of free and conjugated metabolites provide useful tests for diagnosis of pheochromocytoma.

**Paraganglioma** A tumor of neural crest derived chromaffin cells or chromaffin cell precursors associated with sympathetic paraganglia.

**Pheochromocytoma** A usually benign, well-encapsulated, lobular, vascular tumor of chromaffin tissue of the adrenal medulla.

**Serotonin (5-hydroxytryptamine)** A monoamine vasoconstrictor synthesized in the intestinal enterochromaffin cells or in central or peripheral neurons; found in high concentrations in many body tissues, including intestinal mucosa, pineal body, and central nervous system.

**Vanillylmandelic acid (VMA)** The main end product of norepinephrine and epinephrine metabolism excreted in the urine; formed primarily in the liver from oxidation of methoxy-hydroxyphenylglycol.

# BACKGROUND

Catecholamines and serotonin are biogenic amines that facilitate neuronal or hormonal signaling for a wide range of physiological processes. The naturally occurring catecholamines, dopamine and norepinephrine (noradrenaline), function as neuromodulators in the brain. Norepinephrine also functions as a neuromodulator in peripheral sympathetic nerves that innervate tissues throughout the body. Epinephrine (adrenaline) functions as a hormone released by the adrenal medulla. Catecholamines are critical in maintaining the body's homeostasis and in responding to acute and chronic stress through orchestration of cardiovascular, metabolic, glandular, and visceral organ activities (see Suggested Readings: Goldstein 2010, below). Serotonin (5-hydroxytryptamine) serves as a neuromodulator in the brain and as a modulator of vascular and gastrointestinal functions in the periphery (see Suggested Readings: Kema et al. 2000, below). Abnormal production of catecholamines or serotonin occurs in a number of neuroendocrine tumors, where clinical signs and symptoms reflect the pharmacological properties of the secreted amines. Laboratory measurement of biogenic amines or of their metabolites aids in tumor detection and monitoring, and analytical advances have produced sensitive and specific laboratory methods for clinical practice.

# CHEMISTRY, BIOSYNTHESIS, RELEASE, AND METABOLISM

## Chemistry

The **catecholamines**—dopamine, norepinephrine (noradrenaline), and epinephrine (adrenaline)—are phenylethylamines with hydroxyl groups on positions three and four of the benzene ring and an ethylamine sidechain on position one (Fig. 26.1). Hydroxyl and methyl substitutions on the ethylamine sidechain distinguish the individual catecholamines in terms of both structure and function. The catecholamines demonstrate varying degrees of alkaline instability in biological fluids, and their dihydroxybenzene or catechol structure is sensitive to oxidative formation of quinones in the presence of air and light. *Serotonin* with its indoleamine structure is distinct from the catecholamines but is an important naturally occurring biogenic amine. Melatonin is the principal indoleamine produced from serotonin by the pineal gland.

## Biosynthesis

The rate-limiting step in catecholamine biosynthesis involves conversion of tyrosine to 3,4-dihydroxyphenylalanine (L-dopa) by the enzyme, tyrosine hydroxylase (Fig. 26.2). A related enzyme, tryptophan hydroxylase, catalyzes conversion of tryptophan to 5-hydroxytryptophan in the first step of serotonin synthesis. Tissue sources of catecholamines are principally dependent on the presence of tyrosine hydroxylase, which is largely confined to dopaminergic and noradrenergic neurons of the central nervous system and to the sympathetic and adrenal medullary systems in peripheral tissues. Similarly, sources of serotonin are largely dependent on the presence of tryptophan hydroxylase in central nervous system serotonergic neurons, the pineal gland, and some peripheral endocrine tissue, particularly enterochromaffin cells of the digestive tract. Platelets also contain large amounts of serotonin derived from serotonin synthesized in enterochromaffin cells of the gastrointestinal tract.

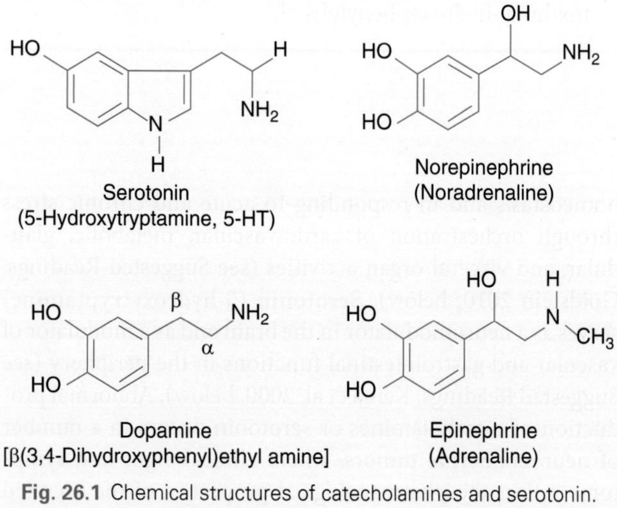

Conversion of L-dopa to dopamine and 5-hydroxytryptophan to serotonin is catalyzed by aromatic-L-amino acid decarboxylase (see Fig. 26.2), an enzyme with a wide tissue distribution and broad substrate specificity for aromatic amino acids. The dopamine and serotonin formed in the cytoplasm by aromatic-L-amino acid decarboxylase are transported into vesicular secretory granules, where the amines are concentrated and stored ready for exocytotic release as the principal neuromodulators of central nervous system dopaminergic and serotonergic neurons. The dopamine formed in noradrenergic neurons and chromaffin cells is further converted to norepinephrine by dopamine β-hydroxylase, an enzyme specifically located in secretory granules. The additional presence of phenylethanolamine N-methyltransferase in adrenal medullary chromaffin cells leads to further conversion of norepinephrine to epinephrine.

Melatonin is synthesized from serotonin in the pineal gland by two highly specific enzymes; the first step is catalyzed by serotonin-N-acetyltransferase and the second by hydroxyindole-O-methyltransferase.

## Storage and Release

Monoamines stored in secretory granules exist in a highly dynamic equilibrium with the surrounding cytoplasm, with passive outward leakage of monoamines into the cytoplasm counterbalanced by inward active transport under the control of vesicular monoamine transporters (Fig. 26.3). Monoamines share the acid environment of the secretory granule matrix with ATP, peptides, and proteins, the best known of which are the chromogranins. The chromogranins are common components of monoamine-containing secretory granules. Their widespread presence among endocrine tissues has led to their measurement in plasma as useful, albeit relatively nonspecific, markers of neuroendocrine tumors.

Monoamines are released from secretory vesicles into the extracellular space through the process of exocytosis. This event is stimulated by an influx of calcium, primarily controlled in neurons by nerve impulse-mediated membrane depolarization, and in adrenal medullary cells by acetylcholine released from innervating splanchnic nerves. Neuronal release may also occur by calcium-independent nonexocytotic processes involving increased loss of monoamines from storage vesicles into the cytoplasm and reversal of normal inward carrier-mediated transport to outward transport of monoamines into the extracellular environment. Examples of this process include the release of catecholamines induced by tyramine and amphetamine.

## Uptake and Metabolism

Because the enzymes responsible for metabolism of catecholamines have intracellular locations, the primary mechanism limiting the duration of action of catecholamines in

**Fig. 26.1** Chemical structures of catecholamines and serotonin.

**Catecholamine biosynthesis**

**Serotonin & melatonin biosynthesis**

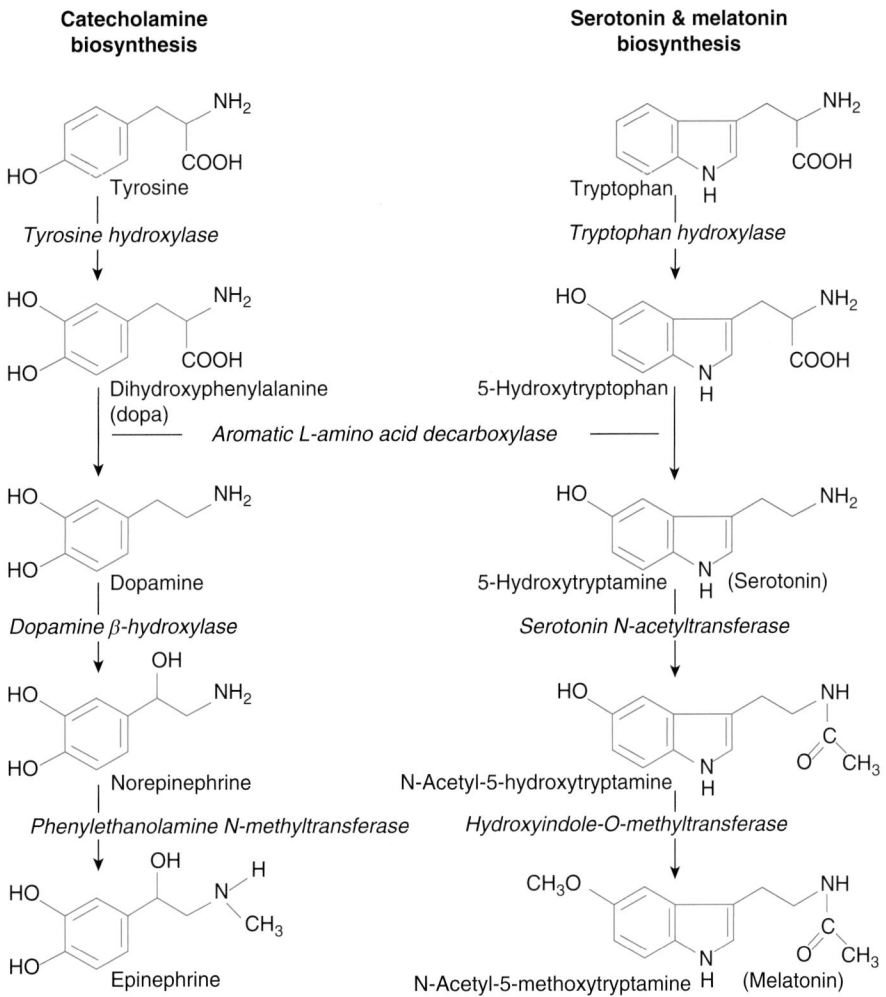

Fig. 26.2  Biosynthesis of catecholamines and serotonin, and metabolism of serotonin to melatonin.

the extracellular space is uptake by active transport (see Fig. 26.3). Uptake is facilitated by transporters that belong to two families of proteins with mainly neuronal or extraneuronal locations. Neuronal monoamine transporters provide the principal mechanism for rapid termination of the signal in neuronal transmission, whereas transporters at extraneuronal locations are more important for limiting the spread of the signal and for clearing catecholamines from the bloodstream. Of the norepinephrine released by sympathetic nerves, about 90% is removed back into nerves by neuronal uptake, 5% is removed by extraneuronal uptake, and 5% escapes these processes to enter the bloodstream. In contrast, of the epinephrine released directly into the bloodstream from the adrenals, about 90% is removed by extraneuronal monoamine uptake.

In addition to terminating the actions of released monoamines, plasma membrane monoamine transporters function in sequence with vesicular monoamine transporters to recycle catecholamines for rerelease (see Fig. 26.3). Thus, most of the norepinephrine released and recaptured by sympathetic nerves is sequestered back into secretory granules by vesicular

monoamine transporters, thereby reducing the requirements for synthesis of new transmitter. Plasma membrane monoamine transporters also function as part of metabolizing systems, requiring the additional actions of enzymes for irreversible inactivation of the released amines.

Catecholamines undergo metabolism by multiple pathways involving differing series of several enzymes with differing expression in various cells and tissues (Fig. 26.4). Most metabolism occurs within the same cells in which catecholamines are synthesized and is dependent on leakage of amines from secretory granules into the cytoplasm. In sympathetic nerves, the presence of monoamine oxidase (MAO) leads to conversion of norepinephrine to **3,4-dihydroxyphenylglycol (DHPG)**. This is then largely metabolized in extraneuronal tissues by catechol-O-methyltransferase (COMT) to **3-methoxy-4-hydroxyphenylglycol (MHPG)**. **Vanillylmandelic acid (VMA)**, the primary end product of norepinephrine and epinephrine metabolism, is produced almost exclusively in the liver. This process is dependent on the hepatic localization of alcohol dehydrogenase, an enzyme required for conversion of MHPG to VMA.

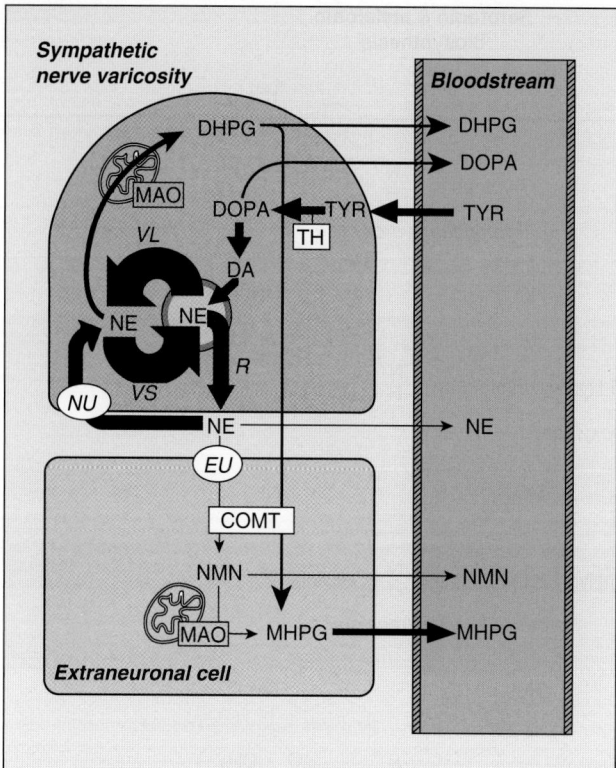

**Fig. 26.3** Schematic diagram illustrating the dynamics of synthesis, exocytotic release (*R*), neuronal reuptake (*NU*), extraneuronal uptake (*EU*), vesicular leakage (*VL*), vesicular sequestration (*VS*), and metabolism of norepinephrine (*NE*) in sympathetic nerve endings in relation to extraneuronal tissue and the bloodstream. Relative magnitudes of the various processes are reflected by the relative sizes of arrows. *COMT*, Catechol-*O*-methyltransferase; *DA*, dopamine; *DHPG*, 3,4-dihydroxyphenylglycol; *L-DOPA*, 3,4-dihydroxyphenylalanine; *MAO*, monoamine oxidase; *MHPG*, 3-methoxy-4-hydroxyphenylglycol; *NMN*, normetanephrine; *TH*, tyrosine hydroxylase; *TYR*, tyrosine.

In adrenal chromaffin cells, the additional presence of COMT leads to metabolism of norepinephrine to **normetanephrine** and of epinephrine to **metanephrine** (see Fig. 26.4). Because the intraneuronal deamination pathway far predominates over the extraneuronal *O*-methylation pathway, normetanephrine and metanephrine represent relatively minor products of catecholamine metabolism. As a consequence, the adrenal medulla represents the single largest tissue source of normetanephrine and metanephrine, accounting for 24%–40% of the former and more than 90% of the latter. The metanephrine and normetanephrine produced in the adrenal medulla or in extraneuronal tissues—the former from catecholamines leaking from secretory granules and the latter from catecholamines released from sympathoadrenal sources—may be deaminated to MHPG and then converted to VMA in the liver or may be sulfate-conjugated by a sulfotransferase enzyme expressed mainly in the gastrointestinal tissues.

Serotonin is not a substrate for COMT; it follows simpler pathways of metabolism than those for catecholamines. Serotonin is deaminated to **5-hydroxyindoleacetic acid (5-HIAA)**, the major urinary excretion product of serotonin metabolism.

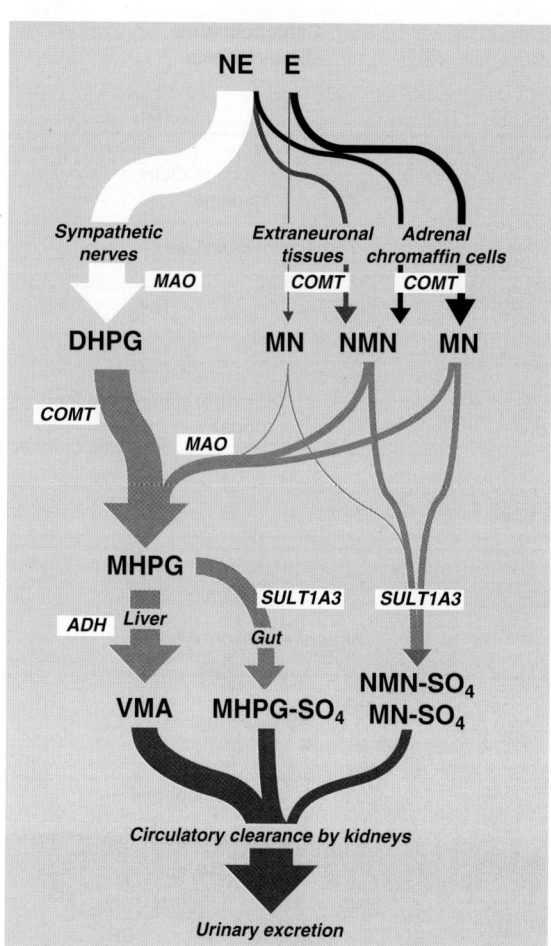

**Fig. 26.4** Schematic diagram showing the main pathways for metabolism of the norepinephrine and epinephrine derived from sympathoneuronal or adrenal medullary sources. Deamination in sympathetic nerves (*white*) is the major pathway of catecholamine metabolism and involves intraneuronal deamination of norepinephrine leaking from storage granules, or of norepinephrine recaptured after release by sympathetic nerves. Metabolism in adrenal chromaffin cells (*black*) involves *O*-methylation of catecholamines leaking from storage granules into the cytoplasm of adrenal medullary cells. The extraneuronal pathway (*light grey*) is a relatively minor pathway of metabolism of catecholamines released from sympathetic nerves or the adrenal medulla, but it is important for further processing of metabolites produced in sympathetic nerves and adrenal chromaffin cells. The free metanephrines produced in extraneuronal tissues or adrenal chromaffin cells are further metabolized by deamination or sulfate conjugation. *ADH*, Alcohol dehydrogenase; *COMT*, catechol-*O*-methyltransferase; *DHPG*, 3,4-dihydroxyphenylglycol; *E*, epinephrine; *MAO*, monoamine oxidase; *MHPG*, 3-methoxy-4-hydroxyphenylglycol; *MHPG-SO₄*, 3-methoxy-4-hydroxyphenylglycol sulfate; *MN*, metanephrine; *MN-SO₄*, metanephrine-sulfate; *NE*, norepinephrine; *NMN*, normetanephrine; *NMN-SO₄*, normetanephrine-sulfate; *SULT1A3*, phenolsulfotransferase type 1A3; *VMA*, vanillylmandelic acid.

## PHYSIOLOGY OF CATECHOLAMINE AND SEROTONIN SYSTEMS

Catecholamines and serotonin regulate physiological events at the cellular level through interaction with families of cell surface receptors. Norepinephrine and epinephrine act on two broad classes of adrenergic receptors: α- and β-adrenoceptor families. Dopamine transmits signals primarily by interaction with a large family of dopamine receptors. An even larger family of serotonergic receptor subtypes has been identified by histological and molecular techniques. The major physiological effects of catecholamines and serotonin are explained in part by these diverse receptor interactions that occur in function-specific locations throughout the vasculature and organ systems of the body.

## Central Nervous System

Norepinephrine, dopamine, and serotonin are produced primarily in regions of the brainstem by neurons with projections to other areas of the brain or spinal cord. About half of the norepinephrine in the brain is produced in norepinephrine-producing neurons in the lower brainstem that send diffuse axonal projections throughout the brain as high as the cerebral cortex. They also send descending fibers to the spinal cord, where they synapse with preganglionic sympathetic neurons that communicate with the peripheral sympathetic nervous system. The norepinephrine-producing neurons of the brainstem participate in regulating the activity of the sympathetic nervous system and the overall state of attention and vigilance.

Dopamine produced in dopaminergic neurons has functions and shows distributions that are notably different from those of norepinephrine. Dopamine in the brain influences reward-seeking behavior and is important for initiation and maintenance of movement. Disturbances in dopamine production and release in the brain are therefore involved in drug-dependency states and are central to the movement disorder that characterizes Parkinson disease. Dopamine neurotransmission is also involved in processing sensory signals and in regulating hormonal release. Dopaminergic neurons in the retina and olfactory bulb have ultrashort projections that transmit signals within these neuronal centers for vision and smell. Dopamine neurons in the hypothalamus have regulatory influences on release of several hormones of the pituitary gland.

Serotonin, similar to norepinephrine, is produced by small clusters of neurons in the brainstem. This biogenic amine serves a diverse range of behavioral and physiological functions including memory, learning, feeding behavior, sleep patterns, thermoregulation, pain modulation, cardiovascular function, and hypothalamic regulation of pituitary hormones.

## Sympathetic Nervous System

Sympathetic nerve transmission operates below the level of consciousness in controlling the physiological function of many organs and tissues of the body (Fig. 26.5). The sympathetic nervous system plays a particularly important role in regulating cardiovascular function in response to postural, exertional, thermal, and mental stress. With sympathetic activation, heart rate is increased, peripheral arterioles are constricted, skeletal arterioles are dilated, and blood pressure is elevated. Sympathetic signals work in balance with the parasympathetic component of the autonomic nervous system to maintain a stable internal environment.

Efferent or outgoing signals from the central nervous system are transmitted by preganglionic cholinergic sympathetic neurons that exit the spinal cord and converge on sympathetic ganglia along the spinal column or in visceral ganglia (see Fig. 26.5). The terminal branches of the postganglionic fibers that project from these ganglia into target organs have varicosities that form a rich ground plexus for synaptic contact with a large number of effector cells in glands and muscle fibers. Most sympathetic postganglionic nerves liberate norepinephrine as their neurotransmitter. In limited locations, sympathetic nerve endings release acetylcholine. Sympathetic fibers that release acetylcholine innervate sweat glands and the adrenal medulla, the latter stimulating release of epinephrine from chromaffin cells.

Plasma and urinary norepinephrine are derived primarily from postganglionic sympathetic neurons with little contribution from the central nervous system or from hormonal release by the adrenal medulla. Because of intervening neuronal and extraneuronal removal processes, the amount of norepinephrine that escapes into the bloodstream represents less than 10% of the total norepinephrine released by sympathetic nerves. Alterations in release and plasma concentrations of norepinephrine occur in response to physiological and pathological states, such as exercise, overeating, low salt intake, upright position, mental stress, and aging, all of which increase sympathetic outflow. Increased plasma concentrations of norepinephrine are also found in disorders such as cardiac failure, hypertension, and depression.

## Adrenal Medullary System

The human adrenal glands overlie the superior poles of the kidneys. Each gland consists of an outer cortex and a thin inner central medulla containing chromaffin cells. A characteristic feature of adrenal medullary chromaffin cells is the presence of numerous catecholamine storage granules. These granules turn brown when exposed to potassium bichromate solutions, ammoniacal silver nitrate, or osmium tetroxide because of the oxidation and polymerization of epinephrine and norepinephrine. This process is known as the *chromaffin reaction*, hence the terms *chromaffin cells* and *chromaffin granules*.

Although often considered a part of the sympathetic nervous system, the adrenal medulla produces and secretes epinephrine with different functions from the norepinephrine secreted by sympathetic nerves. The adrenal medulla and the sympathetic nerves are regulated separately, often in divergent directions in response to different forms of stress. Epinephrine is secreted from adrenal chromaffin cells directly into the bloodstream to act on cells distant from sites of release. Epinephrine and norepinephrine have overlapping but different potencies of effect on α- and β-adrenoceptors. The proximity of sites of norepinephrine and epinephrine release to adrenoceptors determines differences in adrenoceptor-mediated responses to the two catecholamines. Because of the above factors, epinephrine exerts its effects on different populations of adrenoceptors than those affected by norepinephrine. Epinephrine released from the adrenal glands is more important as a metabolic hormone

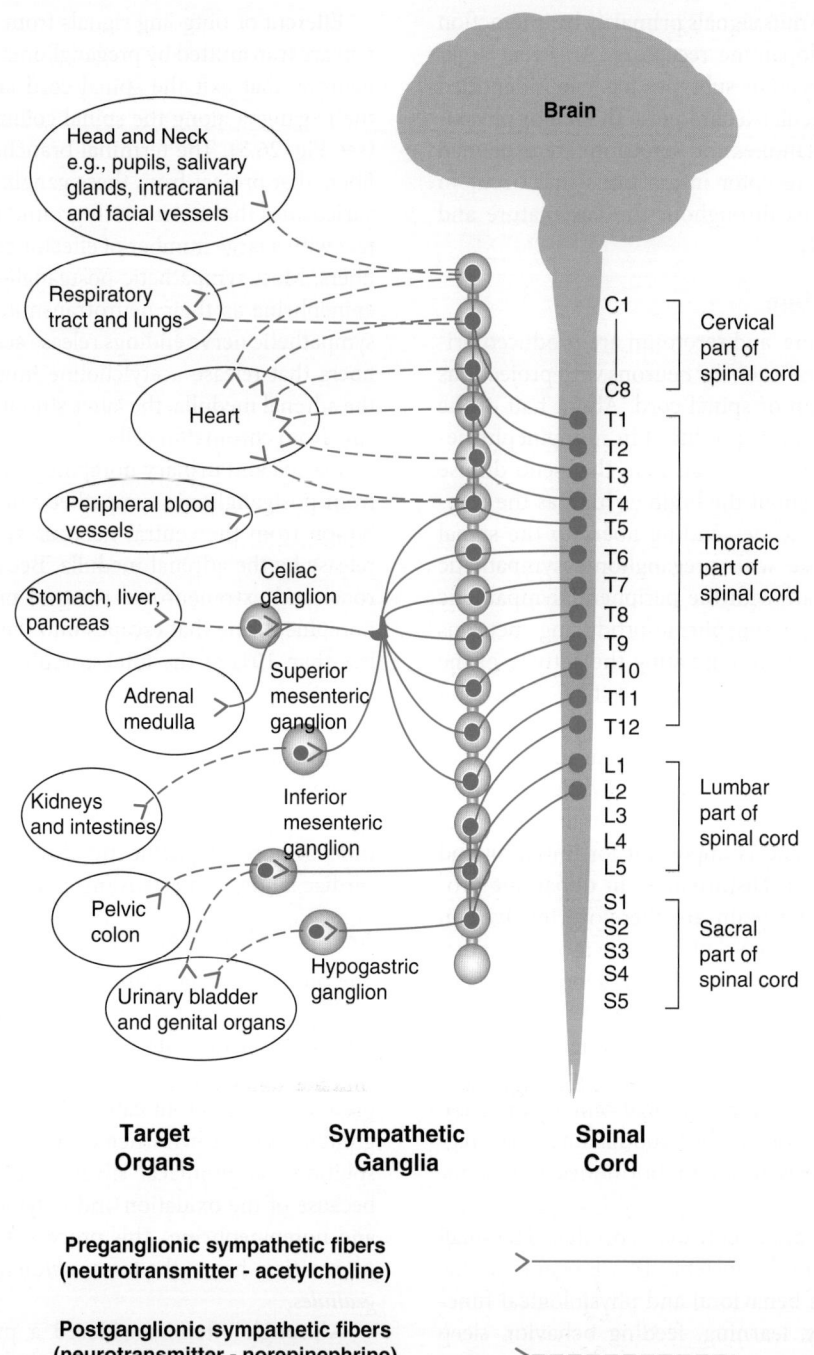

| Target Organs | Sympathetic Ganglia | Spinal Cord |
|---|---|---|

**Preganglionic sympathetic fibers**
**(neutrotransmitter - acetylcholine)**

**Postganglionic sympathetic fibers**
**(neurotransmitter - norepinephrine)**

**Fig. 26.5** Schematic diagram of sympathetic division of the autonomic nervous system. Preganglionic cholinergic fibers (*solid lines*) from the spinal cord project to the paravertebral sympathetic chain, visceral peripheral ganglia, and the adrenal medulla, whereas postganglionic noradrenergic fibers (*dashed lines*) project from sympathetic ganglia to sympathetically innervated target organs. About 5%–10% of the norepinephrine released from sympathetic nerves innervating target organs escapes neuronal and extraneuronal uptake to enter the bloodstream. This contrasts with epinephrine, which functions as a circulating hormone and is released directly from the adrenal medulla into the bloodstream. Most of the catecholamines entering the bloodstream are removed by extraneuronal uptake processes and are metabolized (e.g., in the liver), so that only small proportions are excreted in the urine.

than as a hemodynamic regulatory hormone. In particular, epinephrine stimulates lipolysis, ketogenesis, thermogenesis, and glycolysis and raises plasma glucose by stimulating glycogenolysis and gluconeogenesis. Epinephrine also has potent effects on pulmonary function, causing dilation of airways.

## Peripheral Dopaminergic System

Dopamine is usually thought of as a neuromodulator in the brain or as an intermediate in the production of norepinephrine and epinephrine in peripheral tissues. The contribution of the brain to plasma concentrations and urinary excretion of dopamine metabolites is, however, relatively minor, and

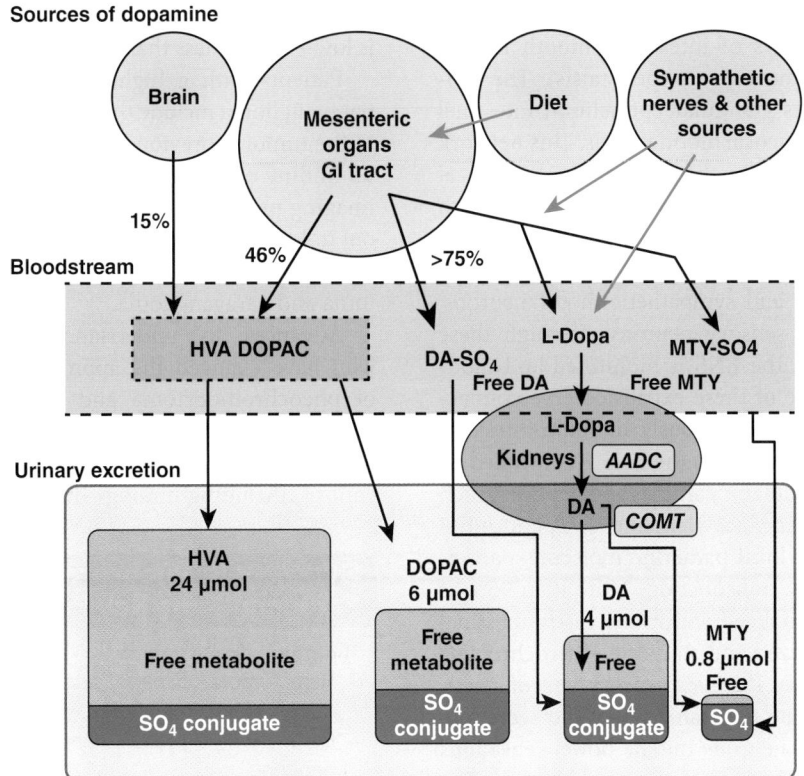

**Fig. 26.6** Schematic representation of the main sources of dopamine and the principal metabolites of dopamine in plasma and urine. The brain makes a relatively minor contribution, whereas dopamine synthesized in the gastrointestinal tract or derived from the diet contributes substantially to dopamine metabolites in the bloodstream and urine. This contrasts with the free dopamine excreted in urine, which is derived almost entirely from renal extraction of circulating L-dihydroxyphenylalanine and local decarboxylation to dopamine by L-aromatic amino acid decarboxylase. Abbreviations: *HVA*, homovanillic acid; *DOPAC*, dihydroxyphenylacetic acid; *DA*, dopamine; *DA-SO₄*, dopamine-sulfate; *L-Dopa*, L-dihydroxyphenylalanine; *MTY*, 3-methoxytyramine; *MTY-SO₄*, 3-methoxytyramine-sulfate; *AADC*, aromatic acid decarboxylase.

dopamine produced in sympathetic nerves and the adrenal medulla is mainly converted to norepinephrine. Most circulating and urinary dopamine and dopamine metabolites appear to be derived from other sources (Fig. 26.6).

In the kidneys, dopamine functions as an autocrine or paracrine effector substance contributing to the regulation of sodium excretion. Unlike neuronal catecholamine systems, production of dopamine in the kidneys is largely independent of local synthesis of L-dopa by tyrosine hydroxylase. Production of dopamine in the kidneys depends mainly on uptake of L-dopa from the circulation and conversion to dopamine by aromatic amino acid decarboxylase (see Fig. 26.6). Thus, most of the free dopamine excreted in urine derives from renal uptake and decarboxylation of circulating L-dopa.

Although the kidneys represent the major source of urinary free dopamine, this source does not account for the much larger quantities of excreted dopamine metabolites, such as homovanillic acid (HVA) and dopamine sulfate. Substantial proportions of these metabolites are produced in the gastrointestinal tract, where dopamine appears to function as an enteric neuromodulator or as a paracrine or autocrine substance. However, unlike in the kidneys, where dopamine is produced mainly from circulating L-dopa, in

the gastrointestinal tract, production of dopamine requires the presence of tyrosine hydroxylase or other sources of L-dopa.

Consumption of food increases plasma concentrations of L-dopa, dopamine, and dopamine metabolites, particularly dopamine sulfate, indicating that dietary constituents may represent an important source of peripheral dopamine (see Fig. 26.6). It is now clear that dopamine sulfate is produced mainly in the gastrointestinal tract from both dietary and locally synthesized dopamine. This is consistent with findings that the gastrointestinal tract contains high concentrations of the specific sulfotransferase enzyme responsible for sulfate conjugation of catecholamines and catecholamine metabolites.

## Enteric Nervous System

The enteric nervous system (ENS) is defined as an independent and integrated system of neurons and supporting cells located in the gastrointestinal tract, gallbladder, and pancreas. The ENS is composed of two networks or plexuses of intrinsic neurons: the myenteric plexus and the submucous plexus. Both are embedded in the wall of the gut and extend from the esophagus to the anus. These networks contain more than 100 million sensory neurons, interneurons, and motor neurons. The myenteric plexus lies between the longitudinal and circular layers of intestinal smooth muscle and controls propulsive movements (peristalsis). The submucous plexus innervates glandular epithelium, intestinal endocrine cells, and submucosal blood vessels. This network senses the environment within the lumen, regulates local blood flow, controls epithelial cell secretion, and links with the gut microbiome.

The ENS is connected to the central nervous system by extrinsic parasympathetic and sympathetic motor neurons, and by spinal and vagal sensory neurons. Through these bidirectional connections, the ENS is monitored and modified. Despite the presence of these extrinsic nerve connections, the ENS functions autonomously in some intestinal regions. Neural transmission within the ENS is controlled by a large variety of neuromodulatory amines and peptides, such as serotonin, norepinephrine, acetylcholine, ATP, and nitric oxide. Serotonin acts as a local paracrine molecule, participating in mucosal sensory transduction. More than 95% of the body's serotonin is produced within the gastrointestinal tract, and most is synthesized and stored in enterochromaffin cells in the gut mucosa. Intrinsic sensory neurons activated by serotonin stimulate peristaltic reflex and secretion, whereas extrinsic sensory neurons initiate bowel sensations such as nausea, vomiting, abdominal pain, and bloating. The paracrine actions of serotonin are terminated by uptake into epithelial cells by the same serotonin transporter used in serotonergic neurons.

## CLINICAL APPLICATIONS

Measurements of catecholamines, serotonin, and their metabolites are used in investigations of a range of pathophysiological processes, but clinical laboratory measurements of the amines and their metabolites are directed primarily at the diagnosis of neuroendocrine tumors. Catecholamine-producing neuroendocrine tumors include pheochromocytomas, paragangliomas, and neuroblastomas, whereas serotonin-producing tumors are typically carcinoids.

### Pheochromocytoma and Paraganglioma

Catecholamine-producing tumors that derive from chromaffin cells may occur within the adrenal glands, where they are referred to as pheochromocytomas, or at extra-adrenal sites, where the tumors are termed *paragangliomas*. The tumors are rare, with an annual detection rate of up to 8 per million. Autopsy studies, indicating prevalences of 0.05%–0.1%, suggest that most of the tumors remain undetected and contribute to premature death.

The presence of a pheochromocytoma or paraganglioma is usually suspected because of signs and symptoms that reflect the biological effects of catecholamines released by the tumor. Hypertension, the most common sign, can be sustained or paroxysmal. Symptoms include headache, palpitations, diaphoresis (excessive sweating), pallor, nausea, attacks of anxiety, and generalized weakness. Among patients tested because

of such signs and symptoms, the pretest prevalence of tumors is low—usually less than 1%.

Patients with a higher risk for pheochromocytoma or paraganglioma include those with a hereditary predisposition to the tumor, a previous history of the tumor, or the incidental finding of an abdominal mass during routine abdominal imaging procedures. In such patients, testing may be carried out independently of the presence of signs and symptoms. See Box 26.1 for a summary of the key points of pheochromocytoma and paraganglioma.

Advances in understanding catecholamine metabolism have changed the approach to biochemical diagnosis of pheochromocytoma and paraganglioma, concentrating now on measurements of metanephrines rather than their precursor catecholamines. This has followed several observations, including findings that adrenal medullary cells and

---

**BOX 26.1    Pheochromocytoma and Paraganglioma Key Points**

**Biology**
- Rare tumors of mainly adrenal chromaffin cells that produce, store, metabolize, and secrete catecholamines, usually with a predominance of norepinephrine over epinephrine
- Those developing from extra-adrenal sympathetic chromaffin tissue—termed *paragangliomas*—usually produce near exclusively norepinephrine and very rarely predominantly dopamine.

**Presentation**
- Tumor usually suspected because of signs and symptoms of catecholamine excess (e.g., hypertension, palpitations, headaches, excessive sweatiness), or the incidental finding of an adrenal mass during routine imaging procedures for unrelated medical conditions.
- Most pheochromocytomas are benign; 15% of adrenal tumors and 35% of extra-adrenal tumors are malignant.
- At least 30% of pheochromocytomas have a hereditary basis, resulting from mutations of 10 genes identified to date.
- Less than 1% of patients tested because of signs and symptoms have the tumor (low pretest prevalence), but the prevalence is higher among patients with identified mutations of disease-causing genes or those with an incidental adrenal mass; thus testing in these patients is recommended independently of the presence of signs and symptoms.

**Biochemical Tests**
- Diagnosis depends principally on evidence of tumoral production of catecholamines, best determined from measurements of metanephrines in urine or plasma.
- Because secretion of catecholamines by tumors is episodic, but metabolism to metanephrines within tumors is continuous, measurements of plasma or urinary fractionated metanephrines provide more reliable diagnostic tests for the tumor than measurements of catecholamines (metanephrines increased in >97% and catecholamines in 69%–92% of patients with pheochromocytomas).

pheochromocytoma tumor cells contain COMT, the enzyme that converts catecholamines to their *O*-methylated metabolites.

Normally, most norepinephrine is metabolized by deamination within sympathetic nerves, so that *O*-methylation represents a minor pathway of catecholamine metabolism. In patients with pheochromocytoma, intratumoral *O*-methylation becomes a dominant pathway of catecholamine metabolism. Consequently, the presence of the tumor leads to relatively large increases in production of *O*-methylated metabolites, compared with minor increases in deaminated metabolites. The metanephrines are produced continuously as a result of ongoing leakage of catecholamines from chromaffin granule stores into the cell cytoplasm; in contrast, catecholamines are often released episodically or in relatively low quantities compared with metanephrines.

Higher diagnostic accuracy of plasma free or urinary fractionated metanephrines compared to the parent catecholamines and other metabolites is supported by numerous studies. Consequently, current guidelines stipulate measurements of plasma or urinary fractionated metanephrines as first-line tests for diagnosis of pheochromocytoma or paraganglioma. Measurements of plasma free metanephrines are particularly sensitive so that negative results of these measurements exclude most tumors. Exceptions include small (<1 cm) tumors encountered during routine screening and tumors that do not synthesize norepinephrine and epinephrine. Among the latter, tumors that produce only dopamine may be detected by measurements of plasma or urinary methoxytyramine, the *O*-methylated metabolite of dopamine. Measurements of plasma dopamine also are useful, whereas urinary dopamine is largely derived from renal extraction and decarboxylation of L-dopa and therefore provides a relatively insensitive and nonspecific test for detection of a dopamine-producing tumor (see Fig. 26.6).

Plasma or urinary fractionated metanephrines are usually elevated sufficiently to conclusively establish the presence of most cases of pheochromocytoma. However, in about 20% of patients with the tumor, increases are smaller. Such true-positive results are difficult to distinguish from the larger proportion of false-positive results. Additional biochemical testing is then necessary. Before further biochemical testing is initiated, consideration should be given to eliminating possible causes of false-positive results. These may occur because of inappropriate sampling conditions (e.g., blood sampling without a preceding 20-min period of supine rest), medications such as tricyclic antidepressants, or clinical conditions that increase sympathetic outflow.

When biochemical testing continues to yield equivocal results, the clonidine suppression test may be useful for further confirming or excluding a pheochromocytoma. As originally introduced, this test was designed to distinguish patients with increases in plasma catecholamines caused by pheochromocytoma from those with increases caused by sympathetic activation. By activating $\alpha_2$-adrenoceptors in the brain and on sympathetic nerve endings, clonidine suppresses norepinephrine release by sympathetic nerves. Decreases in elevated plasma

norepinephrine after clonidine therefore suggest sympathetic activation, whereas lack of decrease suggests a pheochromocytoma. The test has subsequently been shown to be useful for distinguishing increases in plasma normetanephrine due to a pheochromocytoma from those due to sympathetic activation.

Up to 40% of pheochromocytoma and paraganglioma have a hereditary basis and result from mutations of at least 14 disease-causing genes identified to date. Pheochromocytomas occur at a relatively low prevalence in about 2% of patients with neurofibromatosis type 1 (NF1). Risk for the other hereditary conditions is higher. Pheochromocytomas in multiple endocrine neoplasia type 2 (MEN 2) result from mutations of the *ret* proto-oncogene, which also predisposes to medullary thyroid cancer. In von Hippel-Lindau syndrome (VHL), family-specific mutations of the VHL tumor suppressor gene determine the varied clinical presentation of tumors, which, in addition to pheochromocytomas and paragangliomas, include retinal angiomas, central nervous system hemangioblastomas, and tumors in the kidneys, pancreas, and testis. Familial paragangliomas and pheochromocytomas may occur secondary to mutations of genes for four subunits of succinate dehydrogenase (*SDHA, SDHB, SDHC,* and *SDHD*). Mutations of genes encoding transmembrane protein 127 (*TMEM127*), MYC-associated factor X (*MAX*) fumarate hydratase and malate dehydrogenase 2 represent other tumor-susceptibility genes. Somatic mutations of some of the same genes and others account for many of what have been termed sporadic cases of pheochromocytoma and paraganglioma.

Mutations of the different tumor susceptibility genes have been found to give rise to distinct catecholamine metabolite profiles (Fig. 26.7). Tumors in patients with MEN 2 and NF1 are almost always confined to the adrenals and are characterized by increases in plasma-free metanephrine, indicating epinephrine production. In contrast, tumors in patients with *VHL, SDHD,* and *SDHB* mutations, including those at adrenal locations, are characterized by increases in plasma or urinary normetanephrine without increases in metanephrine. Increases in methoxytyramine, the metabolite of dopamine, are additionally present in up to 70% of patients with mutations of *SDHD* and *SDHB* genes. In some patients, methoxytyramine represents the only metabolite increased.

The distinct mutation-dependent biochemical profiles can be useful for stratifying patients for genetic testing, when interpreting genetic test results and during routine screening of tumors. For mutations that confer a high risk of disease, such screening is generally recommended at yearly intervals and should include biochemical testing for evidence of excess catecholamine production individualized according to the expected biochemical profile of the tumor.

Although most often benign, about 10% of pheochromocytomas and 35% of paragangliomas metastasize. The risk of malignancy is particularly high in patients with *SDHB* mutations. Tumors in such patients typically produce low quantities of catecholamines and are much larger at diagnosis than tumors in other patients. This fact, along with their typically extra-adrenal location, explains their higher predisposition to malignancy.

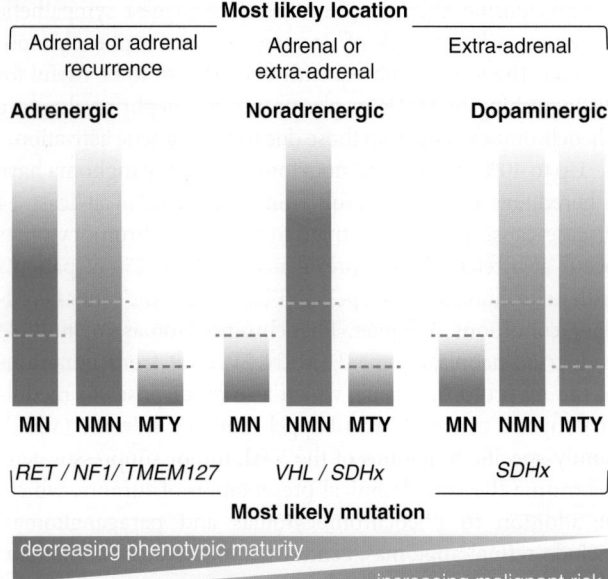

**Most likely location**

Adrenal or adrenal recurrence | Adrenal or extra-adrenal | Extra-adrenal

**Adrenergic** | **Noradrenergic** | **Dopaminergic**

MN  NMN  MTY | MN  NMN  MTY | MN  NMN  MTY

*RET / NF1/ TMEM127* | *VHL / SDHx* | *SDHx*

**Most likely mutation**

decreasing phenotypic maturity

increasing malignant risk

**Fig. 26.7** Catecholamine biochemical phenotypes among patients with mutations of *RET, NF1, TMEM127, VHL* and *SDHB, SDHD, SDHC* and *SDHA (SDHX)* genes as reflected by patterns of increases in plasma normetanephrine (NMN), metanephrine (MN) and methoxytyramine (MTY) and in relation to tumor location, phenotypic maturity, and malignant risk. (From Eisenhofer G, Peitzsch M. Laboratory evaluation of pheochromocytoma and paraganglioma. *Clin Chem.* 2014;60:1486–1499. Reproduced with permission from the American Association for Clinical Chemistry.)

Diagnosis of malignant pheochromocytoma on the basis of histopathological features is not possible and instead requires evidence of metastatic lesions in liver, lungs, bones, lymph nodes or other sites where chromaffin cells normally do occur. All patients with a previous history of tumor are at risk for recurrent or malignant disease and should undergo periodic tumor screening. Measurements of plasma methoxytyramine appear to serve as a promising biomarker for malignant pheochromocytoma and thus may be useful during biochemical testing of patients at risk due to a past history of the disease.

## Neuroblastomas

**Neuroblastomas** are neoplasms that derive from primordial neural crest cells of the sympathetic nervous system. Neuroblastomas are almost exclusively a pediatric cancer, accounting for approximately 7% of all childhood neoplasms; they are the most common malignancies in the first year of life. The incidence of neuroblastoma is approximately 10 cases per million children. A vast majority of neuroblastomas develop sporadically. Activating mutations in the tyrosine kinase domain of the anaplastic lymphoma kinase oncogene account for most cases of hereditary neuroblastoma and may occur as somatic mutations in 5%–15% of sporadic cases. Mutations of **paired-like homeobox 2b** (*PHOX2B*), also known as **neuroblastoma Phox** (*NBPhox*), account for other cases of hereditary neuroblastoma.

Most neuroblastomas are intra-abdominal, arising in the adrenal gland or in the upper abdomen. Less frequent

locations include chest, neck, and pelvis. About 60% are extra-adrenal. Metastases in disseminated neuroblastomas may involve bone marrow, bone, lymph nodes, liver, and, less frequently, skin, testis, and intracranial structures.

The biological behavior of a neuroblastoma varies from regression or maturation to an aggressive course with an unfavorable outcome. Neuroblastomas are also notable for a subset of cases with complete regression or maturation to ganglioneuroma, a benign neoplasm. Most clinically diagnosed tumors, however, are aggressive and have an unfavorable outcome. This highly variable clinical outcome underlies a need for diagnostic markers to stratify patients for therapeutic intervention. Age at diagnosis serves as a primary criterion for stratification; infants younger than 18 months have a more favorable outcome than older children. Beyond this, stratification for therapeutic intervention considers clinical stage of the disease (localized vs. disseminated), histopathological features, and consideration of v-myc myelocytomatosis viral related oncogene (*MYCN*) expression status. Unfortunately, the overall incidence of metastatic neuroblastoma at the time of diagnosis is approximately 60%, and the need for earlier detection of children with the progressive disseminating tumor remains a diagnostic challenge. See Box 26.2 for a summary of the key points of neuroblastomas.

---

### BOX 26.2 **Neuroblastoma Key Points**

**Biology**
- Tumors occurring almost exclusively in children that develop from primitive neural crest cells of the sympathoadrenal system, with about 60% derived from extra-adrenal sympathetic tissue and 40% from the adrenals
- Biological behavior of tumors is highly variable, with some tumors spontaneously regressing but most (60%) having an aggressive course with disseminated malignant disease and an unfavorable outcome.

**Presentation**
- Neuroblastomas produce variable amounts of dopamine and norepinephrine but show a poor capacity for storage and release of catecholamines. Consequently, the tumors rarely produce signs and symptoms of catecholamine excess.
- Suspicion of disease is usually based on palpation of a mass, space-occupying complications of the tumor, or effects of bone marrow involvement.
- Hereditary causes of neuroblastomas are rare; most neuroblastomas occur sporadically.

**Biochemical Tests**
- Biochemical testing is based on overproduction of dopamine and norepinephrine, but because the tumors have poorly developed machinery for catecholamine storage and release, laboratory tests mainly involve measurements of catecholamine metabolites.
- Measurements of urinary VMA and HVA represent the most widely used tests to assess catecholamine excess but are not accurate; diagnosis relies largely on histopathological analysis of biopsy specimens.

Neuroblastomas display a relative lack of the catecholamine storage vesicles common to other catecholamine-producing tumors. Consequently, intratumoral storage of catecholamines is inefficient and the catecholamines synthesized within tumor cells are largely metabolized. Although neuroblastoma tumor cells may have the capacity to synthesize dopamine and some norepinephrine, they also lack PNMT and do not produce epinephrine. Consequently, hypertension and signs and symptoms of catecholamine excess are uncommon in neuroblastoma and affected children commonly present with complications from compression effects of tumors on neighboring structures or hematological abnormalities from bone marrow involvement.

HVA and VMA, produced, respectively, from dopamine and norepinephrine, have been the most widely used biomarkers for diagnosis of a neuroblastoma, particularly before the turn of the 21st century when screening programs were in place to detect disease. Such programs, however, fell out of favor when it was clarified by several studies that outcomes were not improved by screening. In one of the largest of those studies, in which the population with negative screening results was tracked for occurrence of neuroblastoma, an elevation in VMA, HVA, or both, acid metabolites were detected in only 73% of children who developed disease. Furthermore, many of those in whom neuroblastoma was detected had disease that spontaneously regressed while those in whom disease was not detected were likely to have more aggressive forms of the disease. Diagnostic sensitivity of these measurements in screening programs was therefore shown to be limited, particularly for the children in whom it was most important to detect disease.

Currently, diagnosis of neuroblastoma depends principally on biopsy-dependent histopathology, which from molecular analyses (e.g., *MYCN* amplification status) is critical for staging, management, and therapeutic intervention. Thus, apart from indicating a functional catecholamine-producing tumor, there is minimal priority given to laboratory tests of catecholamine excess. Even after diagnosis when there may be need for therapeutic monitoring, the emphasis to assess disease burden is on imaging studies rather than biochemical measurements of catecholamine excess.

Given the limited value of urinary HVA and VMA for diagnosis of neuroblastoma, there have been some attempts to identify additional markers of catecholamine overproduction in order to improve disease detection. Plasma measurements of dopamine and L-dopa, the amino acid precursor of dopamine, have some clinical value and allow the alternate use of plasma. There is also emerging evidence that measurements of plasma normetanephrine and methoxytyramine provide improved diagnostic sensitivity for detection of neuroblastoma than urinary HVA and VMA.

The aforementioned developments are largely limited by the importance of biopsy-driven diagnostic and prognostic procedures that allow for disease staging. Nevertheless, there is some evidence to suggest that the pattern of catecholamine metabolism is associated with biological and genomic prognostic factors in neuroblastoma. An immature metabolic

pattern in neuroblastoma associated with relative deficiency in tumoral conversion of L-dopa to dopamine and to norepinephrine, is suggested to be associated with unfavorable clinical outcomes. In this way, higher ratios of HVA to VMA or plasma methoxytyramine to normetanephrine have been indicated to provide some prognostic value. Similarly, elevations of urinary methoxytyramine have been shown to be associated with poor survival and to correlate with tumoral MYC activity. There may be some remaining utility for measurements of specific catecholamine metabolic pathway constituents in the laboratory evaluation of children with neuroblastoma.

## Gastroenteropancreatic Neuroendocrine and Carcinoid Tumors

**Gastroenteropancreatic neuroendocrine tumors**, including classical **carcinoid tumors**, are derived from a variety of neuroendocrine cell types, in particular, enterochromaffin cells. These tumors are widely distributed in the body and are highly heterogeneous in their clinical presentation. The usual carcinoid tumor is solid and yellow–tan in appearance. Tumor cells exhibit a monotonous morphology, with pink granular cytoplasm and round nuclei with infrequent mitoses. Most of these neuroendocrine tumors are recognized by their reactions to silver stains and to neuroendocrine cell markers, such as chromogranin and neuron-specific enolase.

The tumors are traditionally classified according to their presumed origin from the embryonic foregut (bronchus, lung, stomach, duodenum, and pancreas), midgut (ileum, jejunum, appendix, and proximal colon), or hindgut (rectum and distal colon). The most common sites for these tumors are bronchus or lung—33%, ileum or jejunum—20%, rectum—10%, and appendix—8%. The annual detection rate of clinically significant gastroenteropancreatic tumor has been estimated at 2.5–5 cases per 100,000 persons, but has been steadily increasing presumably as a result of improved diagnostic testing. These tumors may develop in all age groups but appear most frequently in adults; a mean age of 63 has been reported for tumors of the small intestine and respiratory tract. Clinically, most patients are asymptomatic until metastases are present. Bowel obstruction and abdominal pain are the most frequent presenting symptoms.

Gastroenteropancreatic neuroendocrine tumors show aggressive malignant behavior depending on origin, depth of penetration, and size of the primary tumor. Most rectal carcinomas are found incidentally at endoscopy. They are often smaller than 1 cm and have a low rate of metastasis, even though they may show extensive local spread. Carcinoids of the appendix are seen in about 1 in every 300 appendectomies. Almost all measure smaller than 1 cm, and distant metastasis is rare. By contrast, 90% of intestinal neuroendocrine tumors that penetrate halfway through the muscle wall will have spread to lymph nodes and distant sites at the time of diagnosis. More than 70% of these tumors 1–2 cm in diameter metastasize to the liver. Fortunately, most grow slowly, and patients may live for many years. See Box 26.3 for

## BOX 26.3  Gastroenteropancreatic and Carcinoid Tumor Key Points

**Biology**
- Neuroendocrine tumors derived from enterochromaffin cells of the gastrointestinal and respiratory tracts
- Usually develop as small tumors (<2 cm) with slow growth but with propensity to metastasize
- Synthesize, store, and release a variety of peptide hormones and biogenic amines, including serotonin

**Presentation**
- Bowel obstruction and abdominal pain
- Symptoms related to secretion of vasoactive amines and peptides resulting in carcinoid syndrome (flushing, diarrhea, bronchoconstriction, and right-sided heart failure); relatively uncommon and usually occurring only after development of metastases

**Biochemical Tests**
- Biochemical tests for carcinoids include measurements of serotonin, serotonin metabolites (5-HIAA), and the serotonin precursor (5-HTP) in urine, plasma, whole blood, and platelets
- False-positive results are a common problem resulting from dietary influences.

a summary of the key points of carcinoid and gastroenteropancreatic neuroendocrine tumors.

As with normal gut endocrine cells, gastroenteropancreatic neuroendocrine tumors synthesize, store, and release a variety of hormones and biogenic amines. One of the best characterized of these substances in **carcinoid syndrome** is serotonin. These tumors also produce and secrete other biologically active substances, including histamine, kallikrein, bradykinins, tachykinins, prostaglandins, dopamine, norepinephrine, and peptide hormones. Production of these substances varies in relation to the tissue origin of the tumor. Midgut neuroendocrine tumors release large quantities of serotonin, whereas tumors derived from the foregut secrete primarily 5-hydroxytryptophan (5-HTP) (a serotonin precursor) and histamine, rather than serotonin. Primary hindgut neuroendocrine tumors usually show no secretory activity. Pancreatic neuroendocrine tumors are capable of producing gastrin, insulin, glucagon, and vasoactive intestinal peptide (VIP).

Secretion of vasoactive substances into the systemic circulation plays an important role in development of the carcinoid syndrome. The fully developed syndrome associated with humoral manifestations of these tumors is striking but uncommon, usually occurring only after metastasis to the liver and release of these substances directly into the systemic circulation. The classic clinical presentation of the carcinoid syndrome includes pronounced flushing (especially on the face and neck), diarrhea, and bronchoconstriction, and eventual right-sided valvular heart failure. Overproduction of serotonin is found in 90%–100% of patients with the carcinoid syndrome and is thought to be responsible for diarrhea through its known effects on gut motility and fluid secretion.

Clinical laboratory evaluation of the carcinoid syndrome relies on measurements of serotonin and its metabolites in body fluids and tissue. In patients with the typical carcinoid syndrome, 5-HTP is converted to serotonin and is stored in tumor secretory granules and in platelets. A small amount of serotonin remains in plasma, but most is converted to 5-HIAA, which is excreted in urine. These patients have increased blood and platelet serotonin concentrations and increased urinary 5-HIAA excretion. However, some foregut neuroendocrine tumors lack aromatic L-amino acid decarboxylase and secrete 5-HTP rather than serotonin into the bloodstream. Patients with these tumors have normal serotonin concentrations in blood and in platelets, but urinary amounts are increased because 5-HTP is converted to serotonin in the kidney; urinary 5-HIAA may be slightly elevated.

Patients with serotonin-producing carcinoid tumors usually have striking increases in urinary 5-HIAA excretion (at least 10-fold), but occasionally elevations are smaller. False-positive elevations have been known to occur if the patient ingests a wide range of serotonin-rich foods or medications. Conversely, alcohol, aspirin, and other drugs suppress 5-HIAA concentrations. Patients should avoid these agents during 24-h urine collections. Fasting plasma 5-HIAA has been proposed as a convenient replacement for urine collections.

Most physicians rely on measurement of 5-HIAA to diagnose carcinoid syndrome. But when a patient strongly suspected for carcinoid syndrome shows normal or borderline increases in urinary 5-HIAA, documentation of elevated serotonin concentrations in whole blood or platelets may help establish the diagnosis. Platelet serotonin has been reported to be more sensitive than urinary 5-HIAA for detecting carcinoids that produce small or moderate amounts of serotonin, such as foregut and hindgut carcinoids and midgut carcinoids with low tumor volume. Also, platelet serotonin concentrations are not affected by the patient's diet. Platelets can be saturated at high serotonin secretion rates, however, and 5-HIAA is often preferred for monitoring high serotonin production. Measurements of chromogranin A provide an important complement to measurements of serotonin and 5-HIAA, and are particularly useful for many gastroenteropancreatic neuroendocrine tumors that do not produce appreciable amounts of serotonin.

## ANALYTICAL METHODOLOGY

In clinical practice, laboratory determinations of catecholamines, serotonin, and their metabolites in biological fluids are performed primarily for diagnosis and follow-up of patients with catecholamine- or serotonin-producing tumors. In accordance with changes in recommended clinical procedures, most laboratories now offer measurements of urinary or plasma metanephrines (normetanephrine and metanephrine) as primary tests for diagnosis of pheochromocytoma and paraganglioma. Liquid chromatography with tandem

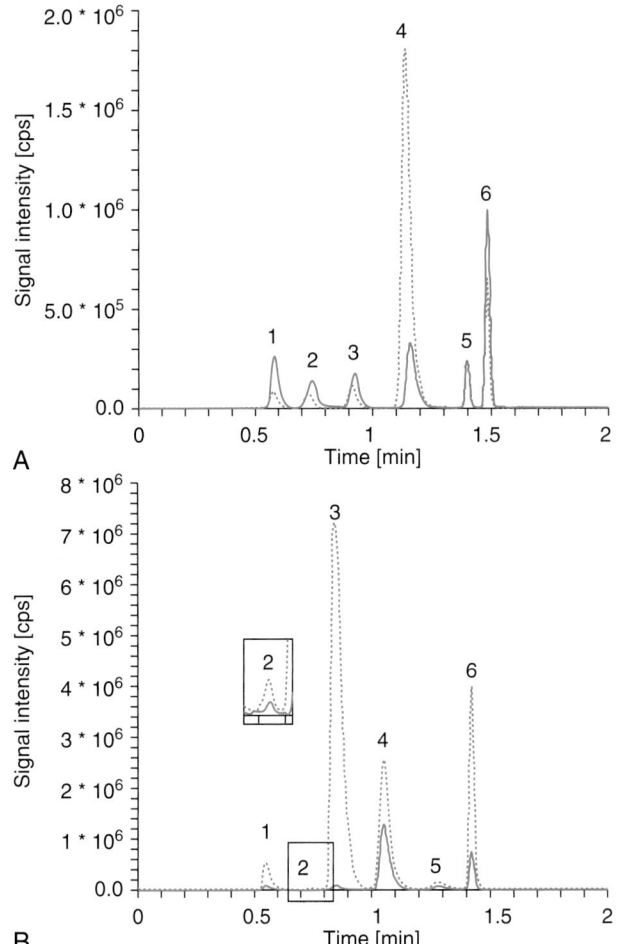

**Fig. 26.8** Chromatograms obtained by LC-MS/MS for simultaneous measurement of urinary catecholamines and their free *O*-methylated derivatives for a calibrator (**A**) and extracted urine samples of two patients (**B**). Chromatographic peaks (*) are shown for norepinephrine (1), epinephrine (2), normetanephrine (3), dopamine (4), metanephrine (5), and 3-methoxytyramine (6), with respective concentrations in the calibrator (**A**) of 59.1, 54.6, 54.6, 65.3, 50.7, and 59.8 nmol/L. For the calibrator, internal standards are shown by a *dotted line*. Patient sample-derived chromatograms (**B**) represent urinary output of catecholamines and their *O*-methylated metabolites from a patient with confirmed pheochromocytoma (*dashed line*) and a patient without pheochromocytoma. Note the much larger signal intensity (peak height) for normetanephrine (3) in the patient with, than without, pheochromocytoma.

mass spectrometry (LC-MS/MS) has increasingly become the method of choice for these measurements (Fig. 26.8). Measurements of catecholamines, usually in urine and less frequently in plasma, are also employed at some medical centers as secondary tests. Measurements of urinary VMA have shown declining importance. For assessments of catecholamine excess in children with neuroblastoma, urinary HVA and VMA remain the most commonly ordered biochemical tests in clinical practice, but other catecholamine metabolites and dopamine are also measured. Diagnostic evaluation of patients with carcinoid tumor routinely involves measurement of 5-HIAA; measurement of serotonin in platelets and urine has also been advocated.

## Collection and Storage of Samples

The conditions under which plasma or urine samples are collected is crucial to the reliability and interpretation of test results. Some clinicians prefer 24-h collections of urine to blood sampling because the former avoids the rigid sampling conditions associated with blood catecholamine collection and is more convenient for clinical staff to implement. However, 24-h urine collections are often difficult and inconvenient for patients. The reliability of the collection timing is frequently in doubt.

Although plasma metanephrines are less affected than catecholamines by various stressors, to minimize false-positive test results, it remains important to follow a number of precautions. First and foremost, it is important to take blood after at least 20 min with patients in the supine position. Emotional distress during phlebotomy-associated needlestick can increase not only plasma catecholamines, but also metanephrines in those sensitive to this procedure. Thus, blood sampling should be carried out under conditions of minimal stress and during cold weather after a suitable period of acclimation to warmer indoor temperatures. For urine collection, the influences of diet and sympathoadrenal activation associated with physical activity, cold environmental temperatures or changes in posture are not as easily controlled as they are for blood collections. First morning urine collections with correction for differences in duration of collection using urinary creatinine excretion provides an alternative to 24-h urine collection that may overcome some of these problems.

For measurements of urinary metanephrines, no preservatives are required, whereas for catecholamines, samples are best preserved with hydrochloric acid to maintain urine acid. For storage over protracted periods, aliquots are best kept frozen at −80°C to minimize auto-oxidation and deconjugation. Blood samples for both metanephrines and catecholamines are most usually collected into tubes containing heparin or ethylenediaminetetra-acetic acid (EDTA) as an anticoagulant and stored on ice before centrifugation at 4°C, with separation of plasma for further storage at −80°C.

Whole blood measurement of serotonin is popular because time-consuming isolation of platelets is not required. For whole blood serotonin, venous blood is drawn into a tube containing potassium EDTA as an anticoagulant, gently mixed and placed on ice, and transferred to a storage tube. An aliquot of blood is then removed for a platelet count. Blood serotonin samples are stored frozen at −20°C, preferably within 2 h after collection.

Platelet-rich plasma samples are prepared from whole blood by low-speed centrifugation. To prevent lowering of serotonin concentration, platelet-rich plasma is prepared within 1 h after the blood is collected and placed on ice. Plasma and pellets are stored frozen at −20°C and are analyzed within 1–2 weeks after collection.

Twenty-four-hour urine samples for serotonin and 5-HIAA are collected in 2-L brown polypropylene bottles, each of which contains 250 mg of sodium metabisulfite and

EDTA as preservatives. Samples are acidified to pH 4 with acetic acid before freezing. Most importantly, the specimen should be refrigerated during collection.

## Interferences from and Influences of Diet and Drugs

Dietary constituents or drugs may cause direct analytical interference in assays or may influence the physiological processes that determine plasma and urinary concentrations of monoamines and monoamine metabolites. In the former circumstances, interference is highly variable depending on the particular measurement method. In the latter circumstances, interference is usually of a more general nature and independent of the measurement method.

Development of new drugs, variations in assay techniques, and continuing improvements in analytical procedures make it difficult to identify which directly interfering medications should be avoided for a given analytical test. For modern mass spectrometric-based detection methods, however, such interferences are rarely a problem compared with electrochemical and spectrophotometric detection methods.

More readily identifiable and generalized sources of interference that are independent of the particular assay method tend to be associated with drugs that have primary actions on monoamine systems. Because these systems serve as important therapeutic targets, such drugs represent a relatively common source of false-positive results. Tricyclic antidepressants and other drugs that block norepinephrine reuptake are a major source of false-positive results for measurements of norepinephrine and normetanephrine. Other medications that cause significant interference, but are less commonly encountered during testing for pheochromocytoma, include L-dopa, Sinemet, α-methyldopa (Aldomet), and MAO inhibitors.

Dietary interference is sometimes particularly troublesome for measurements of serotonin metabolites, requiring detailed dietary instruction for these patients. Dietary sources of 5-hydroxyindoles such as walnuts, bananas, avocados, eggplants, pineapples, plums, and tomatoes should be restricted 3–4 days before and during urine collection. If possible, patients should abstain from all known medications that may impact plasma or urinary measurements of indoles. Measurements of methoxytyramine are subject to influences of dietary catecholamines. For plasma measurements, an overnight fast is sufficient to avoid such influences.

## Reference Intervals

Use of appropriately established reference intervals is critical for effective screening for monoamine-producing tumors. Urinary and plasma metanephrines vary with age, have different ranges in hospitalized patients compared to other populations and also differ between sexes. For plasma metanephrines, it is essential that reference intervals are established using blood samples collected supine and for methoxytyramine after an overnight fast. Age is particularly important to consider for the pediatric population but is also important in adults for plasma normetanephrine. Because of variations

in methods of analysis and subsequent analytical test results, any laboratory establishing measurements of monoamines or metabolites for diagnostic purposes should validate its own reference intervals in line with current standards in clinical practice. Nevertheless, expanding use of mass spectrometry is likely to facilitate harmonized reference intervals as a consequence of improved analytical accuracy and relative freedom from bias, as may be assessed through participation in interlaboratory comparison studies and proficiency programs.

## Urinary and Plasma Fractionated Metanephrines

The metanephrines, normetanephrine and metanephrine, and the O-methylated metabolite of dopamine, methoxytyramine, are present in plasma and urine in free and sulfate-conjugated forms. Plasma concentrations of the conjugates are 20- to 30-fold higher than those of the free metabolites, reflecting more rapid circulatory clearance of free than conjugated metabolites. Clearance of free metabolites occurs by active uptake into tissues followed by deamination or conjugation. The conjugated metabolites so produced are cleared relatively slowly by renal extraction and elimination in the urine. Metanephrines in urine are therefore routinely measured after acid hydrolysis and represent mainly conjugated metabolites, whereas metanephrines in plasma are usually measured in the free form.

Measurements of metanephrines in urine and plasma are now widely performed in many laboratories by LC-MS/MS (see Fig. 26.8). Such methods offer advantages of short chromatographic run times, high sample throughput, and elimination of drug interference that render obsolete earlier methods, which used liquid chromatography with electrochemical detection (LC-EC). A sample preparation step, usually employing ion exchange chromatography, remains a requirement; however, this is accomplished quite simply with some methods allowing on-line sample purification.

Immunoassay measurements of plasma and urine metanephrines are used by some laboratories, particularly when sample throughput is not high enough to justify the expense of LC-MS/MS instrumentation. Nevertheless, immunoassay methods suffer from poor accuracy and imprecision and are not recommended for routine clinical use.

## Urinary and Plasma Catecholamines

LC-EC methods remain commonly used for measurements of plasma catecholamines, but mass spectrometric methods are being increasingly used for measurements of urinary catecholamines and have also been developed for plasma catecholamines. Applications related to diagnosis of catecholamine-producing tumors have waning importance, but the measurements can be useful for other purposes, such as diagnosis of autonomic failure, where it can be important to assess sympathoneuronal function.

The most common extraction procedure employed for LC-EC measurements of catecholamines involves alumina extraction, sometimes combined with an additional cation-exchange step. For LC-MS/MS measurements, simpler methods of extraction can be used, such as 96-well-based ion-exchange chromatographic. Using the appropriate exchange resins, an advantage of these methods over those previously used for preparation of samples for LC-EC is that both catecholamines and metanephrines can be purified and measured together by LC-MS/MS. As outlined later, newer methods have also been developed that involve in situ derivatization that provides for stabilized derivatives of catecholamines that can be measured together with other amines as well as acid metabolites.

## Urinary Vanillylmandelic Acid and Homovanillic Acid

Vanillylmandelic acid (VMA) is the major end product of norepinephrine and epinephrine metabolism, whereas homovanillic acid (HVA) is the major end product of dopamine metabolism. Both metabolites are excreted in urine in relatively high amounts, making their analysis relatively simple. VMA in contrast to HVA is not significantly conjugated. Nevertheless, because large amounts of HVA are also present in urine in the free form, both metabolites are commonly measured without a hydrolysis step. Compared with metanephrines and catecholamines, measurements of VMA and HVA have limited value for diagnosis of pheochromocytoma or paraganglioma but are commonly used to test for neuroblastoma.

Urinary VMA and HVA are best determined by gas or liquid chromatography coupled with mass spectrometry, which are highly specific methods that also allow for additional measurement of 5-HIAA. Gas chromatography-based methods typically employ extraction of urinary analytes into an organic phase followed by derivatization of analytes in the dried down residue. Sample preparation is simpler still for LC-MS/MS methods, some of which involve only dilution of urine in a suitable injection vehicle.

## Serotonin and 5-Hydroxyindoleacetic Acid

Analyses of serotonin, its deaminated acid metabolite, and 5-HIAA and its precursor, 5-hydroxytryptophan (5-HTP), provide important biomarkers for diagnosis of carcinoid tumors. Typically, circulating serotonin is almost entirely confined to platelets, so that measurements are usually performed in whole blood, platelet-rich plasma, or isolated platelet pellets.

Measurements of urinary serotonin are of less importance because the serotonin in this matrix reflects primarily clearance of plasma-free serotonin and renal decarboxylation of circulating 5-HTP. Nevertheless, urinary measurement can be helpful in identifying tumors deficient in aromatic amino acid decarboxylase that produce substantial amounts of 5-HTP, which consequently shows up in urine as serotonin. Such tumors, however, may be more directly detected by measurement of circulating 5-HTP.

Measurements of 5-HIAA are most commonly carried out in urine. As an end product of serotonin production, 5-HIAA better reflects tumor burden than serotonin. Measurements in plasma after an overnight fast have been advocated as more reliable because they avoid the confounding influence of dietary serotonin.

Liquid chromatography with fluorometric or electrochemical detection remain the most frequently used method for measurements of serotonin and 5-HIAA. Due to higher analytical sensitivity, amperometric or coulometric detection is often favored over fluorometric detection. To enhance analytical sensitivity, some HPLC procedures incorporate precolumn derivatization with fluorescent and chemiluminescent reagents, thereby achieving detection limits in the femtomole range. Usually, these techniques have been developed for measuring serotonin and 5-HIAA separately, a consequence of differences in analyte chemistry (e.g., amine vs carboxylic acid), which define the required sample purification procedure and the purified analyte that is detected.

As with measurements of metanephrines and catecholamines, use of mass spectrometric-based methods of quantification for serotonin and 5-HIAA is increasing. With these methods, sample clean-up procedures are simpler, enabling online sample purification. An even more advanced method has been developed that involves a simple in-matrix derivatization step before further sample processing. The resulting non-polar nature of the derivatives allows for sample clean up, chromatography and mass spectrometric measurements of acid, amine, and other metabolites, so that serotonin, 5HIAA, 5HTP and tryptophan can be measured together as a single panel. The non-polar nature of derivatives not only allows for a single simple clean up step, but also offers improved chromatographic separation and heightened ionization efficiency to achieve improved analytical sensitivity. A similar method developed for simultaneous measurement of metanephrines and catecholamines allows for accurate measurement of even the low picomolar concentrations of methoxytyramine and dopamine in as little as 50 μL of plasma.

## REVIEW QUESTIONS

1. The urinary metabolite measured as an indicator of norepinephrine synthesis is:
   a. dopamine.
   b. homovanillic acid (HVA).
   c. serotonin.
   d. vanillylmandelic acid (VMA).
2. False-positive elevations of 5-hydroxyindoleacetic acid (5-HIAA) in urine can occur if:
   a. an individual is a chronic alcoholic.
   b. a patient is receiving aspirin therapy.
   c. an individual has recently eaten fruit, such as bananas, kiwis, and plums.
   d. a patient is currently using tricyclic antidepressants.
3. The two urine metabolites that are most widely used for biochemical testing for children neuroblastoma are:
   a. HVA and VMA.
   b. VMA and 5-HIAA.
   c. HVA and 5-HIAA.
   d. dopamine and epinephrine.

4. Midgut neuroendocrine tumors release which of the following substances in large quantity when compared with tumors derived from other developmental gut components?
   a. 5-Hydroxytryptophan
   b. Serotonin
   c. Epinephrine
   d. Dopamine

5. The method most frequently used for measuring 5-HIAA in urine to detect serotonin production is:
   a. nephelometry.
   b. mass spectrometry.
   c. liquid chromatography.
   d. ion exchange chromatography.

6. Although a 24-hour urine collection is often considered a better specimen for catecholamine analysis, blood samples can be used. Specimen requirements include:
   a. collection in no anticoagulant and immediate freezing of the specimen at −80°C.
   b. collection in potassium EDTA with preparation of a platelet-rich plasma sample.
   c. collection in sodium oxalate from a fasting upright individual.
   d. collection in heparin or EDTA anticoagulant from a fasting supine individual.

7. A catecholamine-producing tumor derived from the chromaffin cells of the adrenal medulla is referred to as a:
   a. neuroblastoma.
   b. pheochromocytoma.
   c. paraganglioma.
   d. gastroenteropancreatic neuroendocrine tumor.

8. True or false: More than 95% of the serotonin in the body is produced within the gastrointestinal tract.
   a. True
   b. False

9. Chromaffin cells are located in a tissue, where they are responsible for synthesis of a certain hormone. Which is it?
   a. Kidney; renin
   b. Brain; dopamine
   c. Adrenal gland; epinephrine
   d. Gut; serotonin

10. Epinephrine is also called:
   a. noradrenaline.
   b. adrenaline.
   c. metanephrine.
   d. serotonin.

## SUGGESTED READINGS

Aluri V, Dillon JS. Biochemical testing in neuroendocrine tumors. *Endocrinol Metab Clin North Am.* 2017;46:669–677.

Cheung NK, Dyer MA. Neuroblastoma: developmental biology, cancer genomics and immunotherapy. *Nat Rev Cancer.* 2013;13:397–411.

Docherty JR, Alsufyani HA. Pharmacology of drugs used as stimulants. *J Clin Pharmacol.* 2021;61(suppl 2):S53–S69.

Eisenhofer G, Klink B, Richter S, Lenders JW, Robledo M. Metabologenomics of phaeochromocytoma and paraganglioma: an integrated approach for personalised biochemical and genetic testing. *Clin Biochem Rev.* 2017;38:69–100.

Eisenhofer G, Kopin IJ, Goldstein DS. Catecholamine metabolism: A contemporary view with implications for physiology and medicine. *Pharmacol Rev.* 2004;56:331–349.

Eisenhofer G, Prejbisz A, Peitzsch M, et al. Biochemical diagnosis of chromaffin cell tumors in patients at high and low risk of disease: plasma versus urinary free or deconjugated O-methylated catecholamine metabolites. *Clin Chem.* 2018;64:1646–1656.

Goldstein DS. Catecholamines 101. *Clin Auton Res.* 2010;20:331–352.

Hofland J, Zandee WT, de Herder WW. Role of biomarker tests for diagnosis of neuroendocrine tumours. *Nat Rev Endocrinol.* 2018;14:656–669.

Kema IP, de Vries EG, Muskiet FA. Clinical chemistry of serotonin and metabolites. *J Chromatogr B Biomed Sci Appl.* 2000;747(1–2):33–48.

LaBrosse EH, Comoy E, Bohuon C, Zucker JM, Schweisguth O. Catecholamine metabolism in neuroblastoma. *J Natl Cancer Inst.* 1976;57:633–638.

Lenders JWM, Duh QY, Eisenhofer G, et al. Pheochromocytoma and paraganglioma: an endocrine society clinical practice guideline. *J Clin Endocrinol Metab.* 2014;99:1915–1942.

Lenders JWM, Kerstens MN, Amar L, et al. Genetics, diagnosis, management and future directions of research of phaeochromocytoma and paraganglioma: a position statement and consensus of the Working Group on Endocrine Hypertension of the European Society of Hypertension. *J Hypertens.* 2020;38:1443–1456.

Martin AM, Young RL, Leong L, et al. The diverse metabolic roles of peripheral serotonin. *Endocrinology.* 2017;158:1049–1063.

McCorvy JD, Roth BL. Structure and function of serotonin g protein-coupled receptors. *Pharmacol Ther.* 2015;150:129–142.

Park JR, Bagatell R, Cohn SL, et al. Revisions to the International Neuroblastoma Response Criteria: a consensus statement from the National Cancer Institute Clinical Trials Planning Meeting. *J Clin Oncol.* 2017;35:2580–2587.

Peitzsch M, Butch ER, Lovorn E, et al. Biochemical testing for neuroblastoma using plasma free 3-O-methyldopa, 3-methoxytyramine, and normetanephrine. *Pediatr Blood Cancer.* 2020;67:e28081.

Schilling FH, Spix C, Berthold F, et al. Neuroblastoma screening at one year of age. *N Engl J Med.* 2002;346:1047–1053.

Spohn SN, Mawe GM. Non-conventional features of peripheral serotonin signalling – the gut and beyond. *Nat Rev Gastroenterol Hepatol.* 2017;14:412–420.

van Faassen M, Bischoff R, Eijkelenkamp K, de Jong WHA, van der Ley CP, Kema IP. In matrix derivatization combined with LC-MS/MS results in ultrasensitive quantification of plasma free metanephrines and catecholamines. *Anal Chem.* 2020;92:9072–9078.

van Faassen M, Bouma G, de Hosson LD, et al. Quantitative profiling of platelet-rich plasma indole markers by direct-matrix derivatization combined with LC-MS/MS in patients with neuroendocrine tumors. *Clin Chem.* 2019;65:1388–1396.

Verly IRN, Matser YAH, Leen R, et al. Urinary 3-methoxytyramine is a biomarker for MYC activity in patients with neuroblastoma. *JCO Precis Oncol.* 2022;6:e2000447.

# Vitamins and Trace Elements

*Ravinder Sodi\**

## OBJECTIVES

1. Classify the vitamins discussed in this chapter according to their water or fat solubility.
2. State the chemical names of each vitamin discussed in this chapter.
3. Summarize the physiological roles of each vitamin discussed.
4. Describe the symptoms of toxicity and deficiency of each vitamin.
5. Describe methods used in the analysis of each vitamin and the factors which affect them.
6. State what is meant when an element is considered "essential."
7. Summarize the physiological functions and clinical significance of each trace element discussed.
8. Describe methods used in the analysis of trace elements and the factors which affect them.
9. Describe disorders associated with deficiency of the trace elements discussed.

## KEY WORDS AND DEFINITIONS

**Acrodermatitis enteropathica**  A hereditary disorder due to defective zinc uptake resulting in dermatitis, diarrhea, and alopecia.

**Acute-phase response (APR)**  A response of the body to inflammation that results in an increase or decrease in the plasma concentrations of a class of proteins known as acute-phase reactants.

**Apoenzyme**  A protein moiety of an enzyme that requires a coenzyme to be fully functional.

**Beriberi**  A disease caused by a deficiency of thiamine (vitamin $B_1$) and characterized by polyneuritis (dry form), cardiac pathology with edema (wet form).

**Coenzyme**  An organic molecule (sometimes derived from a vitamin) of low molecular weight that, when combined with an inactive protein called an *apoenzyme,* forms an active compound or a complete enzyme called a *holoenzyme,* which functions catalytically in an enzyme system.

**Cofactor**  A natural reactant, usually a metal ion or a coenzyme, which is required in an enzyme-catalyzed reaction.

**Hartnup disease**  An inborn error of metabolism affecting the absorption of nonpolar amino acids (particularly tryptophan) characterized by a massive aminoaciduria.

**Hemorrhagic disease of the newborn**  A self-limited hemorrhagic disorder of the first days of life, caused by a deficiency of the vitamin K–dependent blood coagulation factors II, VII, IX, and X.

**Imerslund-Grasbeck syndrome**  A rare autosomal recessive, familial form of vitamin $B_{12}$ deficiency caused by defects in the cubam receptor located in the terminal ileum, which is involved in vitamin $B_{12}$ absorption.

**Kashin–Beck disease**  A chronic, endemic disease of the bone resulting from mainly selenium and iodine deficiency.

**Keshan disease**  A fatal, congestive cardiomyopathy caused by a deficiency of essential trace elements in the diet, particularly selenium.

**Menkes syndrome**  An X-linked recessive disorder of copper metabolism caused by mutations in the *ATP7A* gene (locus Xq12–q13), which encodes a copper transporter, leading to copper deficiency. Signs and symptoms include kinky hair, hypotonia, and developmental delay.

**Nyctalopia**  Visual disturbances that occur in dim light that may be caused as a result of vitamin A deficiency among other causes. Also known as night blindness.

**Pellagra**  A clinical deficiency syndrome due to a deficiency of niacin (or failure to convert tryptophan to niacin) and characterized by dermatitis, inflammation of mucous membranes, diarrhea, and dementia.

**Pernicious anemia**  A deficiency in the production of red blood cells through a lack of vitamin $B_{12}$.

*The author acknowledges the contributions of Professor Alan Shenkin, Dr. Norman B. Roberts, and Dr. Andrew Taylor in the previous editions of this chapter.

Recommended dietary allowance (RDA)  The average daily level of intake of nutrients sufficient to meet the requirements of nearly all (97% to 98%) healthy people.

Scurvy  A condition due to a deficiency of ascorbic acid (vitamin C) in the diet.

Systemic inflammatory response syndrome (SIRS)  The systemic inflammatory response to a wide variety of severe clinical insults.

Total parenteral nutrition (TPN)  The practice of feeding a person intravenously, circumventing the gut.

Trace elements  Inorganic molecules found in human and animal tissues in milligram per kilogram amounts or less.

Vitamer  Term used to describe any of several compounds that possess a given vitamin activity.

Vitamin  An essential organic micronutrient that must be supplied exogenously and in many cases is the precursor to a metabolically derived coenzyme.

Wilson disease  A rare, progressive, autosomal recessive disease due to a defect in metabolism of copper, resulting in excessive copper accumulation in the liver, brain, eye, and other organs.

Wernicke encephalopathy  Condition arising as a result of thiamine deficiency, which presents with ophthalmoplegia, ataxia, and confusion, usually in alcoholics.

Xerophthalmia  Refers to the spectrum of ocular manifestations due to vitamin A deficiency, ranging from night blindness to conjunctival dryness to the appearance of small gray plaques with foamy surfaces (Bitot spots).

# VITAMIN AND TRACE ELEMENT STATUS

An adequate supply of vitamins and trace elements is critical in maintaining health. There is increasing public awareness that good nutrition, including supplementation with vitamins and trace elements, is necessary for improving the quality of life, but this has not necessarily been supported by randomized trials in selected groups. The general principle regarding assessment of nutritional status is to determine the extent to which the metabolic demand for nutrients has been or is currently being met by the supply. In clinical practice, this requires balancing supply and demand.

The requirements for most nutrients, including vitamins and trace elements, to maintain health have been characterized and made available in reports from the Institute of Medicine (IOM) of the National Academies (US). However, the effects of disease may increase demands. For example, hypermetabolism, as a result of trauma or infection, increases the need for protein and energy and for the vitamin and trace element cofactors necessary for related metabolism. Increased losses from the gut, kidney, and skin, or through dialysis, may also increase the overall demand for these nutrients.

An estimate of supply may be obtained from a careful dietary history, especially if performed by a dietitian, together with knowledge of any artificial nutritional supplements or therapy that may have been provided enterally or intravenously. Table 27.1 summarizes the Recommended Dietary Allowance (RDA) used in the United States and the Population Reference Intakes from the European community for vitamins and trace elements in adults. Table 27.1 also summarizes the amounts present in 2000 kcal of most tube feeds used in nutritional support and common dietary sources. For details regarding children, see the suggested readings. Table 27.2 summarizes the functions of vitamins in humans.

To improve accuracy of assessment of nutritional status, clinicians often turn to the laboratory to obtain a result that may reflect the net balance of supply and demand. Clinical laboratorians need to be aware of when such tests are useful and how to place the results of laboratory tests into the context of the clinical situation of the patient. It is important to be aware of the limitations of laboratory tests, especially in acutely ill patients. Nutritional assessment in health and disease is considered in detail by Ayling and Marshall (see Suggested Readings).

## Effect of Inflammation on Vitamins and Trace Elements

The concentration in plasma of various vitamins and trace elements can alter significantly when a systemic inflammatory response syndrome (SIRS; previously known as the acute-phase response [APR]) results from trauma or infection. This usually occurs independently of tissue stores. The associated changes may be due to alterations in the binding proteins in plasma, such as albumin or retinol-binding protein (RBP), which decrease as part of SIRS or due to protein malnutrition. Studies in patients with SIRS, as categorized based on elevated C-reactive protein (CRP) concentrations, have documented decreases in vitamins A, E, $B_2$, $B_6$, C, D, and carotenoids. One study in 1303 patients examined the effect of the magnitude of SIR on plasma micronutrient concentrations with the aim of providing guidance on the interpretation of results. The findings are shown in Table 27.3. This study concluded that the degree of inflammatory response affected the interpretation of plasma micronutrient concentrations and showed that a reliable clinical assessment could only be made if the CRP was less than 10 mg/L for vitamins A and D or less than 5 mg/L for vitamins B6 and C. There have been guidelines issued on nutrition support by national bodies such as the National Institute for Health and Care Excellence (NICE) in the United Kingdom that recommend the monitoring of micronutrient concentrations in patients receiving total parenteral nutrition (TPN); therefore, when implementing guidelines and deciding on nutritional support, it is important to take the effect of SIRS into account.

# VITAMINS

## Vitamin A

Vitamin A is the nutritional term for the group of compounds with a 20-carbon structure containing a methyl-substituted

## TABLE 27.1 Daily Oral and Intravenous Vitamin and Trace Element Intakes for Adults

| | RDA (USA) | PRI (Europe) | Some Natural Food Sources | Amount in 2000 kcal Tube Feed | IV Intake |
|---|---|---|---|---|---|
| **Vitamins** | | | | | |
| A, µg | 900 (men); 700 (women) | 700 | Liver, yellow/orange fruits, leafy vegetables, fish, milk | 1000–2160 | 1000 |
| E, mg | 15 (men and women) | 0.4/g PUFA | Fruits and vegetables, meats, vegetable oils, unprocessed cereals, nuts, seeds | 20–64 | 9.1 |
| K, µg | 120 (men); 90 (women) | 100–200 | Leafy green vegetables, especially spinach, eggs, liver | — | 150 |
| $B_1$, mg | 1.2 (men); 1.1 (women) | 1.1 | Brown rice, vegetables, potatoes, liver, eggs | 1.4–3.4 | 6 |
| $B_2$, mg | 1.3 (men); 1.1 (women) | 1.6 | Vegetables such as green beans and asparagus, bananas, dairy products | 2–6 | 3.6 |
| $B_6$, mg | 1.3 (men and women <50 years); 1.7 (men >50 years); 1.5 (women >50 years) | 1.5 | Meat, bananas, vegetables, nuts | 2–13.8 | 6 |
| $B_{12}$, µg | 2.4 | 1.4 | Meat and animal products | 3–15 | 5 |
| Folate, µg | 400 | 200 | Leafy vegetables, cereals, especially if fortified, bread, pasta, liver | 340–880 | 600 |
| C, mg | 90 (men); 75 (women) | 45 | Fruits, especially citrus fruits, and vegetables | 100–300 | 200 |
| Biotin, µg | 30[a] | 15–100 | Eggs, organ meats, yeast, milk | 100–660 | 60 |
| Niacin, mg | 16 (men); 14 (women) | 18 | Meat, fish, eggs, vegetables, mushrooms, nuts | 18–45 | 40 |
| Pantothenic acid, mg | 5[a] | 3–12[b] | Meat, vegetables like broccoli, avocados, grains | 7–20 | 15 |
| **Trace Elements** | | | | | |
| Copper, mg | 0.9 | 1.1 | Organ meats, seafood, nuts, seeds, grains, cocoa products | 2–3.4 | 0.3–1.3 |
| Selenium, µg | 55 | 55 | Organ meats, seafood, nuts, vegetables (dependent of soil selenium content) | 30–130 | 40–100 |
| Zinc, mg | 11 (men); 8 (women) | 9.5 | Red meats and some seafood | 13–36 | 2.5–6.0 |
| Iodine, µg | 150 | 150 | Milk, iodized salt | N/A | 70–170 |
| Manganese, mg | 2.3[a] (men); 1.8[a] (women) | 1–10[b] | Nuts, legumes, tea, grains | 2.4–8 | 0.06–0.1 |
| Chromium, µg | 25[a] (men); 35[a] (women) | 30–200 | Cereals, meats, fish | 10–20 | 10–15 |
| Molybdenum, µg | 45[a] | 74–240 | Legumes, grains, and nuts | 19 | 10–25 |

[a]Adequate intake.
[b]Acceptable range.
IV, Intravenous; PRI, population reference intake (Europe); PUFA, polyunsaturated fatty acids; RDA, recommended dietary allowance (US).
Reference intakes for pregnant and lactating women, infants and children vary with age and weight (see Ayling and Marshall in Suggested Readings).

cyclohexenyl ring (β-ionone ring) and an isoprenoid side chain (Fig. 27.1), with a hydroxyl group (retinol), an aldehyde group (retinal), a carboxylic acid group (retinoic acid), or an ester group (retinyl ester) at the terminal C15. Included in the vitamin A family are a subcategory known as vitamin A2 (dehydroretinal and dehydroretinol) and the dietary carotenoids (C40 polyisoprenoid compounds). The latter are also known as provitamin A because they are cleaved biologically to yield retinol. The principal dietary carotenoids are β-carotene, α-carotene, and β-cryptoxanthin.

## TABLE 27.2  Vitamins Required by Humans

| Common or Generic Name | Vitamer or Common Chemical Name | Function | Symptoms and Causes of Deficiency or Associated Diseases | Currently Used Methods | Reference Intervals |
|---|---|---|---|---|---|
| **Fat-Soluble Vitamins** | | | | | |
| Vitamin A | Retinol, retinal, retinoic acid, carotenoids | Antioxidant, role in vision, gene expression, embryonic development, immune and reproductive functions | Nyctalopia (night blindness), Bitot spot, xerophthalmia, keratomalacia; common in infants and children, especially in less developed countries; due to fat malabsorption, cystic fibrosis, and may occur due to retinol-binding protein deficiency as a result of protein malnutrition, liver disease, and zinc deficiency | HPLC, LC-MS/MS | 1–6 years: 20–40 µg/dL (0.70–1.40 µmol/L) 7–12 years: 26–49 µg/dL (0.91–1.71 µmol/L) 13–19 years: 26–72 µg/dL (0.91–2.51 µmol/L) >19 years: 30–80 µg/dL (1.05–2.80 µmol/L) |
| Vitamin E | Tocopherols, tocotrienols | Antioxidant (prevents the peroxidation of unsaturated fatty acids), role in gene transcription, immunity, inhibits platelet aggregation, recently been implicated in bone physiology | Lipid peroxidation, red blood cell fragility causing hemolytic anemia especially in premature infants; may occur due to fat malabsorption, cystic fibrosis | HPLC, LC-MS/MS | Premature neonates: 0.1–0.5 mg/dL (2.3–11.6 µmol/L) 1–12 years: 0.3–0.9 mg/dL (7–21 µmol/L) 13–19 years: 0.6–1.0 mg/dL (14–23 µmol/L) >19 years: 0.5–1.8 mg/dL (12–42 µmol/L) As a ratio of cholesterol: 3.5–9.5 µmol/mmol cholesterol |
| Vitamin K | Phylloquinones (K₁), menaquinones (K₂), menadiones (K₃) | Coagulation, bone metabolism | Increased clotting time, hemorrhagic disease of the newborn; also due to fat malabsorption, cystic fibrosis, liver disease | Prothrombin time, PIVKA, HPLC, LC-MS/MS | 0.2–2.2 nmol/mmol triglyceride |
| **Water-Soluble Vitamins** | | | | | |
| Vitamin B₁ | Thiamine, aneurin | Forms the coenzyme thiamine pyrophosphate (TPP) required for decarboxylation reactions involved in carbohydrate metabolism, and nerve function | Beriberi, Wernicke-Korsakoff syndrome in alcoholics, rare thiamine-responsive IEM | Erythrocyte transketolase, HPLC, LC-MS/MS | Erythrocyte transketolase activity: 0.75–1.30 U/g Hb (48.4–83.9 kU/mol Hb) Percent TPP effect (activation): Normal: 0%–15% Marginal: 16%–25% Deficient: >25% TPP concentration: 173–293 nmol/L or 280–590 ng/g Hb (erythrocytes); 90–140 |

| Vitamin | Function | Clinical significance / deficiency | Methods | Reference values |
|---|---|---|---|---|
| (Riboflavin, continued) | coenzymes involved in reduction-oxidation (redox) reactions in the body | photophobia, riboflavin-dependent IEM | reductase activation by FAD: reductase, HPLC, LC-MS/MS | FAD: Adequacy: 1.20 Marginal: 1.21–1.40 Deficiency: >1.41 Serum or plasma concentrations of riboflavin (median [range]): plasma FAD: 101 [57–170] nmol/L; plasma FMN: 6.3 [3.3–14.1] nmol/L; plasma riboflavin: 11 [4–34] nmol/L; erythrocyte FAD: 1.9 [0.7–3.8] pmol/g Hb; erythrocyte FMN: 0.11 [0.04–0.44] pmol/g Hb; erythrocyte riboflavin: 0.02 [0.01–0.13] pmol/g Hb |
| Vitamin $B_3$ | Niacin, nicotinic acid, nicotinamide | Coenzyme or cosubstrate in many biological redox reactions, and thus for energy metabolism | Pellagra (dermatitis, dementia, diarrhea) Seen in communities with corn-based staple diets, in carcinoid syndrome (precursor tryptophan diverted to serotonin formation), Hartnup disease (unable to absorb tryptophan), and medications such as isoniazid | HPLC & LC-MS/MS for urine metabolite, nicotinamide coenzymes | 2.4–6.4 mg/day (17.5–46.7 µmol/day) or 1.6–4.3 mg/g creatinine (11.7–31.4 µmol/g creatinine) |
| Vitamin $B_5$ | Pantothenic acid, panthenol, pante-theine | General metabolism, acetyl and acyl transfer | Burning feet syndrome | Microbiological, CPB, HPLC, LC-MS, GC-MS | Whole blood or serum: 344–583 µg/L (1.57–2.66 µmol/L) Urinary excretion: 1–15 mg/day (5–68 µmol/day) |
| Vitamin $B_6$ | Pyridoxine, pyridoxal, pyridoxamine | The active form pyridoxal phosphate is required for synthesis, catabolism of various amino acids | Epileptiform convulsions, dermatitis, anemia, medications, such as penicillamine and isoniazid, decrease it, pyridoxine-responsive IEM notably homocystinuria, and hyperhomocysteinemia (together with vitamin $B_{12}$ and folate deficiencies) | Aspartate transaminase, HPLC, LC-MS/MS | Plasma PLP: 9.5–24 ng/mL (39–98 nmol/L). Erythrocyte PLP: 250–680 pmol/g Hb |

Continued

## TABLE 27.2    Vitamins Required by Humans—cont'd

| Common or Generic Name | Vitamer or Common Chemical Name | Function | Symptoms and Causes of Deficiency or Associated Diseases | Currently Used Methods | Reference Intervals |
|---|---|---|---|---|---|
| Vitamin B$_7$ | Biotin, vitamin H | Coenzyme for carboxylation reactions involved in gluconeogenesis, lipogenesis, and catabolism of branched-chain amino acids; roles in cell signaling, epigenetic regulation of genes and chromatin structure | Dermatitis, developmental delay Seen with excessive raw egg consumption, those on parenteral nutrition, and IEM notably biotinidase deficiency | Microbiological, CPB, carboxylases, avidin binding, urinary metabolites | 0.5–2.20 nmol/L |
| Vitamin B$_9$ | Pteroylglutamic acid, folic acid, folate | Required for the interconversions of amino acids such as homocysteine to methionine and the biosynthesis of purines and pyrimidines, required for DNA synthesis | Megaloblastic anemia, neural tube defects Caused by gut sterilization, malabsorption, decreased intake, increased requirements (e.g., pregnancy), medications (e.g., methotrexate), anticonvulsants Deficiency linked to hyperhomocysteinemia, cancer and stroke | Red blood cell and serum folate, CPB, microbiological, homocysteine | >3 µg/L (7.0 nmol/L) for serum folate and <150 µg/L (340 nmol/L) for RBC folate |
| Vitamin B$_{12}$ | Cyanocobalamin, hydroxocobalamin, methylcobalamin | Required for erythropoiesis, methylation processes necessary for DNA and cell metabolism, and is a cofactor for various enzymes, notably those involved in the metabolism of methylmalonic acid and homocysteine | Pernicious and megaloblastic anemia, peripheral neuropathy Caused by decreased intake (vegetarians), short bowel syndrome (loss of distal ileum), malabsorption syndromes, medications (N$_2$O, phenytoin, methotrexate, and proton pump inhibitors), and Imerslund-Grasbeck syndrome Deficiency results in methylmalonic aciduria and homocysteinemia | CPB, immunometric, microbiolcgical, methylmalonate, homocysteine, holotranscobalamin | WHO consultation defined a serum vitamin B$_{12}$ concentration <203 ng/L (150 pmol/L) as deficient |
| Vitamin C | Ascorbic acid | Connective tissue formation, antioxidant | Scurvy, infantile scurvy (Barlow disease) Linked with osteoporosis, anemia, diabetes mellitus, cancer | Spectrophotometric-enzymatic methods, HPLC | 0.4 and 1.5 mg/dL (23–85 µmol/L) or 20–53 µg/10$^8$ leukocytes (1.14–3.01 fmol/leukocyte) |

Reference intervals are likely to vary between laboratories and are influenced by variables including the systemic inflammatory response.

*CPB,* Competitive protein binding; *FAD,* flavin adenine dinucleotide; *FMN,* flavin mononucleotide; *Hb,* hemoglobin; *HPLC,* high-performance liquid chromatography; *IEM,* inborn errors of metabolism; *LC-MS/MS,* liquid chromatography-tandem mass spectrometry; *PIVKA,* protein induced by vitamin K absence or antagonism; *RBC,* red blood cell; *RIA,* radioimmunoassay; *WHO,* World Health Organization.

## Absorption, Transport, Metabolism, and Excretion

Preformed vitamin A precursors, most often in the form of retinyl ester or carotenoids, are subject to emulsification and mixed micelle formation by the action of bile salts before they are transported into the intestinal cell. Here the retinyl esters arc moved across the mucosal membrane and hydrolyzed to retinol within the cell to be then re-esterified by cellular RBP II and packaged into chylomicra, which then enter the mesenteric lymphatic system and pass into the systemic circulation. A small amount of the ingested retinoid is converted into retinoic acid in the intestinal cell.

Carotenoids, also in micellar form, are absorbed into the duodenal mucosal cells by passive diffusion. Once inside the mucosal cell, β-carotene is principally converted to retinal by the enzyme β-carotene-15,15′-dioxygenase. Retinal is converted by retinal reductase to retinol and esterified. The newly synthesized retinyl esters, from both preformed vitamin A and carotenoids, along with exogenous lipids and nonhydrolyzed carotenoids, then pass with chylomicrons via the lymphatic system to the liver, where uptake by parenchymal cells again involves hydrolysis. In the liver, retinol is bound with RBP and transthyretin (TTR or thyroxine-binding prealbumin) in a 1:1:1 complex of sufficient size to prevent loss by glomerular filtration and is returned to the circulation or stored as esters within the stellate cells.

## Functions

The participation of retinal in vision is considered the most important physiologic function of vitamin A. All-*trans*-retinol is the predominant circulating form of vitamin A. Cells of the retina isomerize this to the 11-*cis* alcohol that is reversibly dehydrogenated to 11-*cis* retinal, which combines with proteins (e.g., opsin) to generate photosensitive pigments, such as rhodopsin. Illumination of such pigments causes photoisomerization and the release of all-*trans*-retinal and the protein, a process that couples the large conformational change with ion flux and optic nerve transmission. The all-*trans*-retinal is isomerized to the 11-*cis* isomer, which combines with the liberated protein to reconstitute the photopigment in a visual cycle, as shown in Fig. 27.2.

Other functions of vitamin A include its role in reproduction, growth, embryonic development, and immune function; many of these functions are mediated through the binding of retinoic acid to specific nuclear receptors that regulate genomic expression.

## Deficiency

Vitamin A deficiency primarily affects infants and children, and its prevalence is subject to World Health Organization

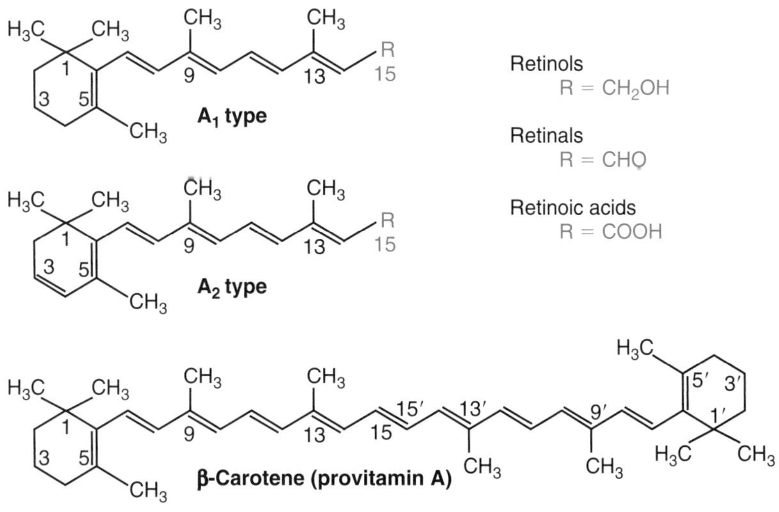

### TABLE 27.3 Median Plasma Vitamin Concentrations According to C-Reactive Protein (CRP) Concentrations

| CRP Concentration (mg/L) | Vitamin A (µmol/L) | Vitamin D (nmol/L) | Vitamin B₆ (µmol/L) | Vitamin C (µmol/L) |
|---|---|---|---|---|
| <5 | 2.0 | 34 | 48 | 23 |
| >5–10 | 2.0 | **33** | **27** | 18 |
| >10–20 | **1.8** | **31** | **32** | **17** |
| >20–40 | **1.6** | **27** | **24** | **8** |
| >40–80 | **1.4** | **23** | **18** | **6** |
| >80 | **1.0** | **20** | **15** | **5** |

Data in bold depict significant (P < .05) decrease compared to CRP category <5 mg/L.
Conversion factors for traditional units: Vitamin A—divide by 0.0349 to µg/dL; Vitamin D—divide by 2.496 to ng/mL; Vitamin B₆—divide by 4.046 to ng/mL; Vitamin C—divide by 56.78 to mg/dL.
Modified from Duncan A, Talwar D, McMillan DC, et al. Quantitative data on the magnitude of the systemic inflammatory response and its effect on micronutrient status based on plasma measurements. *Am J Clin Nutr.* 2012;95:64–71.

Fig. 27.1 Vitaminic forms of A₁, A₂, and β-carotene.

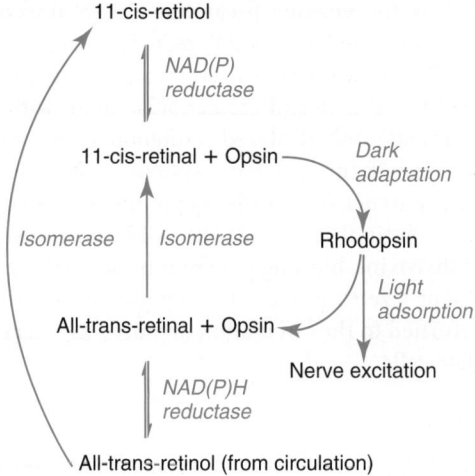

**Fig. 27.2** Participation of A vitamers in the visual cycle. *NAD,* Nicotinamide-adenine dinucleotide.

(WHO) surveillance. Risk factors include poverty, low birth weight, poor sanitation, malnutrition, infection, and parasitism. As hepatic accumulation of vitamin A occurs during the last trimester of pregnancy, preterm infants are relatively vitamin A deficient at birth.

Neonatal vitamin A supplementation has been a matter of some controversy, with trials giving mixed results dependent on the population studied. At the present time, neonatal vitamin A supplementation is not recommended as a public health intervention. Fat malabsorption, particularly caused by celiac disease or chronic pancreatitis, and protein-energy malnutrition predispose to vitamin A deficiency. Liver disease diminishes RBP synthesis, and ethanol abuse leads to both hepatic injury and competition with retinol for alcohol dehydrogenase, which is necessary for the oxidation of retinol to retinal and retinoic acid. Vitamin A deficiency may lead to anemia, although the precise mechanism is not known.

Clinical features of vitamin A deficiency include degenerative changes in eyes and skin, and poor dark adaptation or *night blindness* (nyctalopia) followed by degenerative changes in the retina. Xerophthalmia refers to the spectrum of ocular manifestations due to vitamin A deficiency, ranging from night blindness to conjunctival dryness to the appearance of small gray plaques with foamy surfaces *(Bitot spots)*. These lesions are reversible with vitamin A administration. More serious effects of deficiency are known as *keratomalacia*, and cause ulceration and necrosis of the cornea that lead to perforation, prolapse, endophthalmitis, and blindness. Usually associated skin changes include dryness, roughness, papular eruptions, and follicular hyperkeratosis.

## Toxicity

Toxic effects of hypervitaminosis A occur mainly as a result of ingestion of excess vitamin or as a side effect of inappropriate therapy. The elderly are more susceptible to

vitamin A toxicity at lower doses, as exposure to retinyl esters is longer because of delayed postprandial clearance of lipoproteins.

Symptoms of acute toxicity present as abdominal pain, nausea, vomiting, severe headaches, dizziness, sluggishness, and irritability, followed within a few days by desquamation of the skin and recovery. Chronic toxicity from moderately high doses taken for protracted periods is characterized by bone and joint pain, hair loss, dryness and fissures of the lips, anorexia, benign intracranial hypertension, weight loss, and hepatomegaly.

Epidemiologic and experimental evidence has supported the view that high vitamin A intake in humans, acting via 13-*cis*-retinoic acid, is teratogenic. A further intriguing association, supported in part by epidemiologic studies, is that observed between excessive vitamin A intake and reduction in bone mineral density (BMD). Hypervitaminosis A is also a known cause of hypercalcemia, especially in chronic kidney disease.

Carotenemia results from chronic excessive intake of carotene-rich foods, principally carrots, and is usually reported in infants and children. This condition, in which yellowing of the skin is observed, is benign because the excess carotene is deposited rather than converted to vitamin A. Carotenemia has also been linked to amenorrhea, but the mechanism behind this association remains unknown. Elevated concentrations have also been found in hypothyroid patients, in whom conversion to vitamin A is decreased, and in patients with hyperlipemia associated with diabetes mellitus.

## Laboratory Assessment of Status

Although measurement of the plasma concentration of vitamin A is the most convenient and widely used assessment of vitamin A status, it is not an ideal indicator because it does not decline until liver stores become critically depleted, which is thought to occur at a concentration of approximately 20 μg/g liver.

Vitamin A status is assessed by the measurement of retinol concentration. Retinol circulates in plasma as a 1:1:1 complex with RBP and TTR. The circulating concentration of RBP is determined by dietary protein and zinc, which are necessary for RBP synthesis. Thus, protein malnutrition, liver disease, and zinc deficiency resulting in RBP deficiency will lead to hypovitaminosis A. In contrast, renal failure resulting in decreased excretion of RBP has been reported to result in hypervitaminosis A. Another confounding factor in the assessment of vitamin A status is the effect of inflammation, as discussed earlier. Both RBP and TTR are negative acute-phase proteins; thus, inflammatory changes will result in transient falls in both proteins and plasma retinol. To distinguish inflammatory from nutritional causes of reduced plasma retinol concentrations, it may be necessary to measure CRP.

Currently high-pressure liquid chromatography (HPLC; see Chapter 12) after solvent extraction with fluorometric or spectrophotometric detection is mainly used to measure vitamin A. HPLC has brought enhanced specificity, lowered limits of detection, improved accuracy using primary standards, reference materials, and quality assurance schemes, and made acceptable reproducibility achievable (between batch coefficients of variation [CV] of <15% for both vitamin A and β-carotene). In the normal-phase HPLC, compounds to be separated are adsorbed to microparticulate silica gel and are eluted in the order of least polar to most polar. Reversed-phase HPLC is preferable for acid-sensitive compounds such as 5,6-epoxyretinoic acid. Photometric, electrochemical, and mass spectrophotometric detectors have all been used. Refer to Chapter 12 for general principles of chromatography. Dried blood spots are now being used for the assessment of vitamin A status. Vitamin A is light-sensitive, and samples should be protected from light.

## Vitamin D

Vitamin D plays an essential role as a hormone in the control of calcium and phosphorous metabolism and bone physiology. It is discussed in Chapter 39.

## Vitamin E

Vitamin E is the nutritional term for the group of tocopherols and tocotrienols that have biological activity similar to RRR-α-tocopherol (formerly D-α-tocopherol). They exist in several forms—α, β, γ, and δ—that indicate the presence or absence of methyl groups at positions 5 and 7 (Fig. 27.3). The α-tocopherol is the only form known to meet human requirements.

### Absorption, Transport, Metabolism, and Excretion

In the presence of bile, vitamin E is absorbed from the small intestine. Most forms of vitamin E are absorbed nonselectively and are secreted in chylomicron particles along with triacylglycerol and cholesterol. Some of this chylomicron-bound vitamin E is transported and delivered to the peripheral tissue (mainly adipose tissue) with the aid of lipoprotein lipase. The liver takes up the chylomicron remnants, where α-tocopherol is incorporated into very low-density lipoproteins (VLDLs) by α-tocopherol transfer protein (α-TTP), enabling further distribution of α-tocopherol throughout the body. Vitamin E is excreted via the bile and in the urine as tocopheronic acid and its β-glucuronide conjugate.

### Functions

The inhibition of free radical-mediated lipid peroxidation is the main role of vitamin E. Tocopherols and tocotrienols inhibit lipid peroxidation largely because they scavenge lipid peroxyl radicals faster than the radicals can react to adjacent fatty acid side chains or membrane proteins. The resultant tocopheryl or tocotrienyl radicals may then react with additional peroxyl radicals to produce tocopherones (nonradicals), or they may be regenerated by transfer of an electron to ascorbate to form the ascorbyl radical. Thus, vitamins E and C act synergistically to reduce lipid peroxidation (Fig. 27.4). α-Tocopherol also induces inhibition

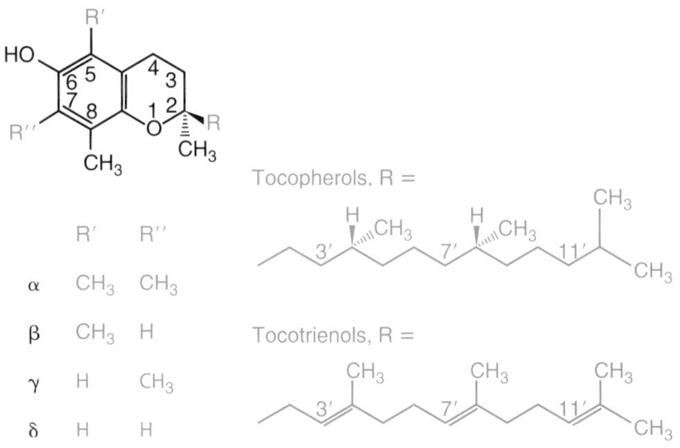

Fig. 27.3 Vitaminic forms of vitamin E.

of cell proliferation, platelet aggregation, and monocyte adhesion, which are thought to be the result of direct interaction of α-tocopherol with cell components. There is some evidence that vitamin E may have antiinflammatory properties. A recent study has shown that serum vitamin E is a determinant of bone mass by stimulating osteoclast fusion.

### Deficiency

Premature and low-birth-weight infants are particularly susceptible to the development of vitamin E deficiency because placental transfer is poor, and infants have such limited adipose tissue where much of the vitamin is normally stored. Manifestations of deficiency include peripheral neuropathy, ataxia, skeletal myopathy, retinopathy, edema, and *hemolytic anemia*. Anemia reflects the shortened life span of erythrocytes with fragile membranes; it does not respond to iron therapy, which may aggravate the condition. Although symptoms of vitamin E deficiency are rare in children and adults, deficiency can occur in some conditions, such as fat malabsorption states including cystic fibrosis and chronic cholestasis in children that in turn cause neuropathy and hemolytic anemia. The genetic disorder *abetalipoproteinemia* (vitamin E is transported on lipoproteins) can also confer vitamin E deficiency (see Chapter 23).

### Toxicity

Vitamin E toxicity is usually only ever achieved by excessive dietary supplementation. The US Food and Nutrition Board has recommended a tolerable upper limit of 1000 mg/day of vitamin E for adults 19 years and older.

### Laboratory Assessment of Status

HPLC is currently the method of choice for quantification of tocopherols in serum, as it offers the advantages of accuracy and reproducibility (between-batch CV of <5%) and the ability to quantitate multiple analytes, including vitamin A and some carotenoids, in a single analytical run. Both α- and γ-tocopherols are the principal vitamers seen, although others may be detected with minor modifications to the analytical conditions. HPLC-mass spectrometry methods have also

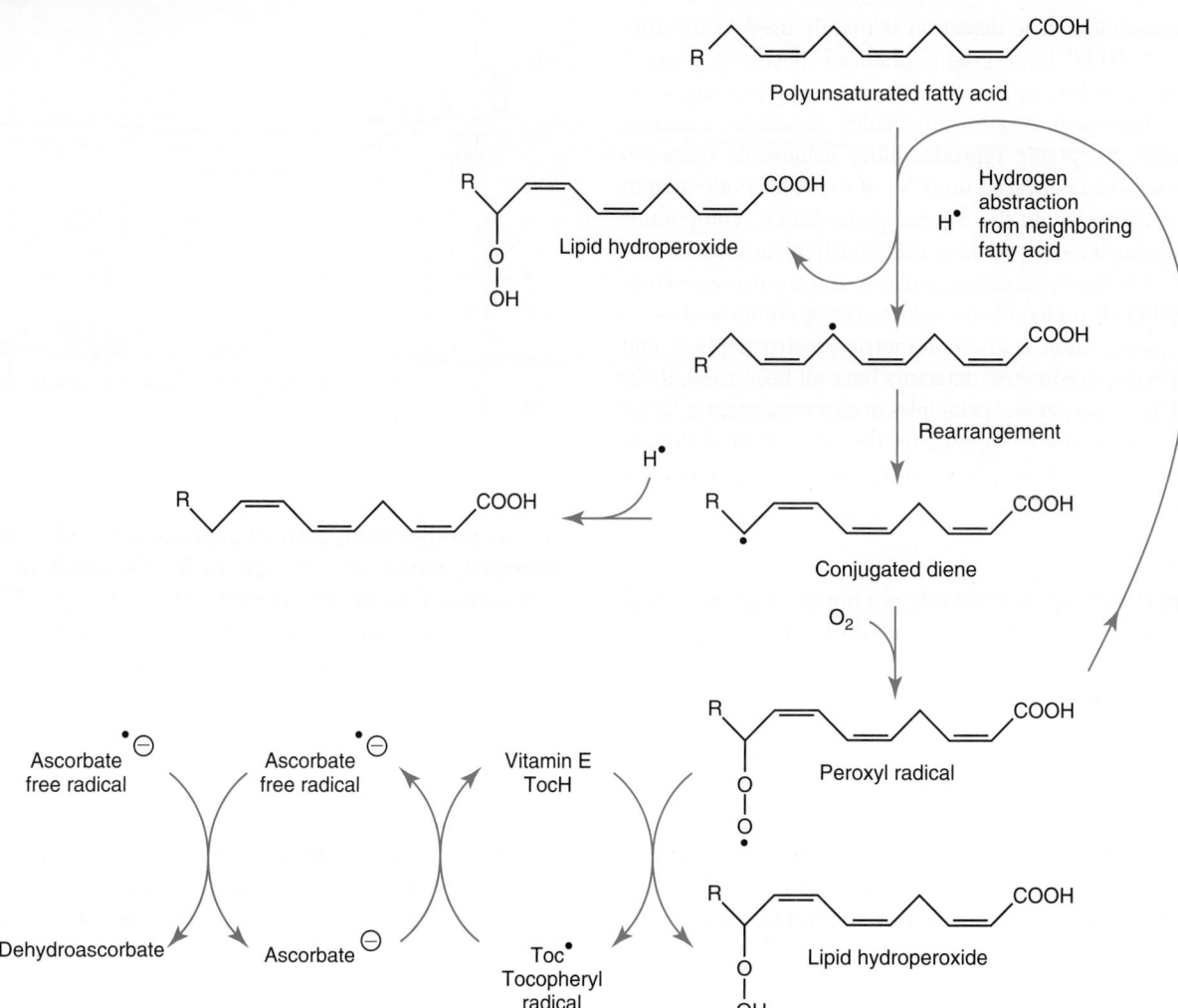

Fig. 27.4 Lipoperoxidation and synergistic action of vitamin E and vitamin C.

been developed and are increasingly being used, given the widespread adoption of this technique by clinical laboratories. Vitamin E is light-sensitive, and it is recommended that samples should be protected from light.

## Vitamin K

Vitamin K is the common generic name for a group of compounds with a methylated naphthoquinone structure (2-methyl-1,4-napthoquinones), which are substituted with side chains at carbon 3. *Phylloquinone* (K$_1$ type) synthesized in plants and *menaquinones* (K$_2$ type) of bacterial origin are the two principal natural classes of vitamin K (Fig. 27.5). Several synthetic analogs and derivatives have been used in human nutrition; most relate to or derive from *menadione* (K$_3$).

### Absorption, Transport, Metabolism, and Excretion

As for other fat-soluble vitamins, the absorption of natural vitamin K from the small intestine into the lymphatic system is facilitated by bile. Vitamins K$_1$ and K$_2$ are bound to chylomicrons for transport from mucosal cells to the liver. Menadione (K$_3$) is more rapidly and completely absorbed from the gut before entering the portal blood. In the liver, intracellular distribution is seen mostly in the microsomal

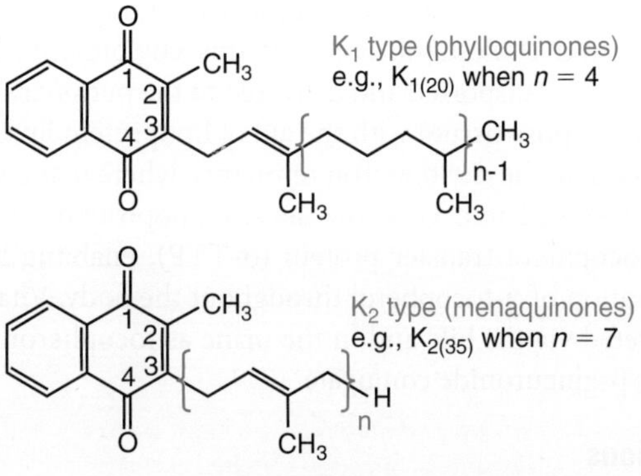

Fig. 27.5 Vitaminic forms of vitamin K.

fraction, where phenylation of menadione to form K$_2$ occurs. Release of vitamin K to the bloodstream allows association with circulating β-lipoproteins for transport to other tissue. Only traces of urinary metabolites of vitamins K$_1$ and K$_2$ appear in urine.

### Functions

The main role of vitamin K is as a cofactor to vitamin K–dependent carboxylase, an enzyme necessary for the posttranslational conversion of specific glutamyl residues in target proteins to γ-carboxyglutamyl (Gla) residues. This γ-carboxylation increases the affinity of these proteins for calcium. The antihemorrhagic function of vitamin K depends on the formation of the Gla proteins prothrombin (factor II), proconvertin (factor VII), plasma thromboplastin component (factor IX), and Stuart factor (factor X), which together with two other hemostatic vitamin K–dependent proteins, proteins C and S, and $Ca^{2+}$ initiate a process to form thrombin that then catalyzes the conversion of fibrinogen to a fibrin clot.

Proteins that contain γ-carboxyglutamyl are also abundant in bone tissue, with osteocalcin accounting for up to 80% of the total γ-carboxyglutamyl content of mature bone. Epidemiologic studies have shown an association between low vitamin K intake and hip fracture risk. Evidence indicates that vitamins K and D may act synergistically in maintaining bone density.

## Deficiency

Although vitamin K deficiency in adults is uncommon, the risk is increased with fat malabsorption states, such as (1) bile duct obstruction, (2) cystic fibrosis, and (3) chronic pancreatitis and liver disease. Risk is also increased by the use of drugs that interfere with vitamin K metabolism, such as the coumarin anticoagulants (e.g., warfarin) and antibiotics containing the N-methylthiotetrazole side chain (e.g., cephalosporin). Other at-risk groups are hospitalized patients with poor nutrient intakes or those receiving TPN, when fat-soluble vitamin supplements may not fully meet requirements. Conversely, ingestion of supraphysiologic doses of vitamins A and E has been reported to induce vitamin K deficiency, probably through competitive mechanisms. Defective blood coagulation and demonstration of abnormal noncarboxylated prothrombin are at present the only well-established signs of vitamin K deficiency.

**Vitamin K deficiency bleeding (VKDB) formerly known as** hemorrhagic disease of the newborn associated with bleeding particularly in the umbilicus, gastrointestinal tract, and nose can develop because of (1) poor placental transfer of vitamin K, (2) hepatic immaturity leading to inadequate synthesis of coagulation proteins, and (3) the low vitamin K content of early breast milk. Severe diarrhea and antibiotics used to suppress diarrhea exacerbate the situation, so prothrombin concentrations can drop significantly, resulting in bleeding. This condition is routinely prevented by the prophylactic administration of phylloquinone intramuscularly immediately after birth.

## Toxicity

The use of high doses of naturally occurring vitamin K ($K_1$ and $K_2$) appears to have no known toxic effect; however, menadione ($K_3$) treatment can lead to the formation of erythrocyte cytoplasmic inclusions known as Heinz bodies and hemolytic anemia.

## Laboratory Assessment of Status

Because of its relatively low plasma concentration, vitamin K has long presented an analytical challenge. For this reason, vitamin K status has traditionally been assessed by functional

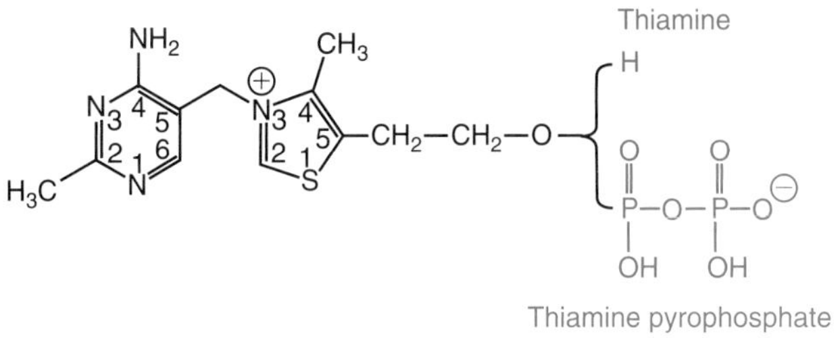

Fig. 27.6 Thiamine and the pyrophosphate coenzyme.

methods, primarily by its effect on clotting time. The *prothrombin time (PT)* is assessed by adding a portion of tissue thromboplastin to recalcified plasma and measuring the clotting time against a normal control sample. In vitamin K deficiency, the PT may rise above 30 seconds (normal, 10 to 14 seconds), and at least 2 seconds beyond the control time. Attempts at cross-laboratory standardization led to the introduction of the international normalized ratio (INR), by which PT can be expressed as a fraction of the control time.

A more sensitive assessment of vitamin K status with respect to prothrombin can be made by the immunoassay of des-γ-carboxy prothrombin, or undercarboxylated prothrombin, PIVKA-II (protein induced by vitamin K absence or antagonism). PIVKA-II has proved to be a useful marker of subclinical vitamin K deficiency. Another measurement of deficient γ-carboxylation, plasma undercarboxylated osteocalcin, has been shown to correlate individually with PIVKA-II and plasma phylloquinone concentrations and has a better correlation with plasma phylloquinone than PIVKA-II.

Direct measurement of plasma phylloquinone is probably the best indicator of vitamin K status and has been shown to correlate with intake. HPLC methods are the mainstay of vitamin K measurement. HPLC-mass spectrometry methods have also been developed.

Vitamin K is light-sensitive, and it is recommended that samples should be protected from light.

## Vitamin $B_1$

The structure of *thiamine* (3-[4-amino-2-methyl-pyrimidyl-5-methyl]-4-methyl-5-[β-hydroxyethyl]thiazole) is that of a pyrimidine ring, bearing an amino group, linked by a methylene bridge to a thiazole ring (Fig. 27.6). The thiazole has a primary alcohol side chain at C5, which can be phosphorylated in vivo to produce thiamine phosphate esters, the most common of which is thiamine pyrophosphate (TPP; also known as thiamine diphosphate [cocarboxylase]). Monophosphate and triphosphate esters also occur.

## Absorption, Transport, Metabolism, and Excretion

Thiamine absorption occurs primarily in the proximal small intestine by a saturable (thiamine transporter) process at low concentrations (1 μmol/L or lower) and by simple passive diffusion beyond that, although percentage absorption diminishes with increased dose. Absorbed thiamine undergoes intracellular phosphorylation, mainly to the pyrophosphate, but at the serosal side, 90% of transferred thiamine is present in the free form. Thiamine uptake is enhanced by thiamine deficiency and is reduced by thyroid hormone, diabetes, and ethanol ingestion. The free vitamin is present in plasma, but the coenzyme, TPP, is the primary cellular component. Approximately 30 mg is stored in the body, with 80% as pyrophosphate, 10% as triphosphate, and the rest as thiamine and its monophosphate. About half of body stores are found in skeletal muscle, with much of the remainder in heart, liver, kidneys, and nervous tissues (including the brain, which contains most of the triphosphate).

## Functions

Thiamine is required by the body as the pyrophosphate (TPP) in two general types of reactions: (1) the oxidative decarboxylation of 2-oxo acids catalyzed by dehydrogenase complexes, and (2) the formation of α-ketols (ketoses) as catalyzed by trans-ketolase and as the triphosphate (TTP) within the nervous system. TPP functions as the $Mg^{2+}$-coordinated coenzyme for active aldehyde transfers in multienzyme dehydrogenase complexes that affect decarboxylative conversion of α-keto (2-oxo) acids to acyl-coenzyme A (acyl-CoA) derivatives, such as pyruvate dehydrogenase and α-ketoglutarate dehydrogenase. These are often localized in the mitochondria, where efficient use in the Krebs tricarboxylic acid (citric acid) cycle follows.

*Transketolase* is a TPP-dependent enzyme found in the cytosol of many tissues, especially the liver and blood cells, in which principal carbohydrate pathways exist. In the pentose phosphate pathway, which additionally supplies reduced nicotinamide-adenine dinucleotide phosphate (NADPH) necessary for biosynthetic reactions, this enzyme catalyzes the reversible transfer of a glycoaldehyde moiety from the first two carbons of a donor ketose phosphate to the aldehyde carbon of an aldose phosphate. TTP is also thought to be involved in the regulation of ion channels—specifically, chloride channels of large unitary conductance, the so-called maxi-Cl channels.

## Deficiency

Causes of thiamine deficiency include inadequate intake caused by diets largely dependent on milled, nonenriched grains, such as rice and wheat, or the ingestion of raw fish containing thiaminases, which hydrolytically destroy the vitamin in the gastrointestinal tract. Tea may also contain anti-thiamine factors. Chronic alcoholism often leads to thiamine deficiency caused by reduced intake, impaired absorption, impaired use, and reduced storage, and may lead clinically to the *Wernicke-Korsakoff syndrome*. Wernicke encephalopathy classically presents with ophthalmoplegia, ataxia, and confusion. Other at-risk groups include those receiving parenteral nutrition without adequate thiamine supplementation, elderly patients taking diuretics, and patients undergoing long-term renal dialysis.

Beriberi (origin: Sinhalese, from a word meaning weakness) is the disease resulting from thiamine deficiency. Clinical signs of thiamine deficiency primarily involve the nervous and cardiovascular systems. In adults, symptoms most frequently observed include mental confusion, anorexia, muscular weakness, ataxia, peripheral paralysis, ophthalmoplegia, edema *(wet beriberi)*, muscle wasting *(dry beriberi)*, tachycardia, and an enlarged heart. In infants, symptoms appear suddenly and severely, often involving cardiac failure and cyanosis. Commonly, the distinction between wet (cardiovascular) and dry (neuritic) manifestations of beriberi relates to the duration and severity of the deficiency, the degree of physical exertion, and caloric intake. The wet or edematous beriberi results from severe physical exertion and high carbohydrate intake, whereas the dry or polyneuritic beriberi stems from relative inactivity with caloric restriction during the chronic deficiency. Nervous system involvement includes peripheral neuropathy, Wernicke encephalopathy, and the amnesic psychosis of Korsakoff syndrome. More rarely, but especially in seriously ill patients in hospitals, an acute form of cardiac failure has been described *(Shoshin beriberi)*, which may be fatal but can be successfully and rapidly reversed with high-dose intravenous thiamine.

## Toxicity

No reports have described adverse effects from consumption of excess thiamine from food and supplements.

## Laboratory Assessment of Status

The free or phosphorylated forms of thiamine can be measured directly in a suitable body fluid or tissue, or its properties as an enzymatic cofactor can be exploited in a functional assay.

The most commonly used enzyme for the functional assay is transketolase. Transketolase catalyzes two reactions in the pentose phosphate pathway. As an enzyme within the erythrocyte, transketolase is independent of nonspecific changes in the extracellular plasma. As vitamin $B_1$ deficiency becomes more severe, (1) thiamine becomes limiting in the body cells, (2) the amount of the coenzyme is depleted, and (3) transketolase activity subsequently diminishes. The *TPP effect* measures the extent of depletion of the transketolase enzyme for coenzyme by assaying enzyme activity before and after TPP addition.

Circulating thiamine concentration may be directly measured in plasma, erythrocytes, or whole blood. The plasma (or serum) concentration is thought to reflect recent intake and is mainly unphosphorylated thiamine at low concentrations (around 10 to 20 nmol/L). Because the erythrocyte contains approximately 80% of the total thiamine content of whole blood (mainly as the pyrophosphate) and erythrocyte thiamine stores deplete at a similar rate to other major organs, HPLC measurement of TPP in erythrocytes is a good indicator of body stores. Whole blood samples may be analyzed in a similar manner to washed erythrocytes and may provide the advantage of simpler sample handling, but they are subject to variable plasma dilution. However, a good correlation has been obtained between erythrocyte and whole blood TPP concentrations, particularly when whole blood TPP included a correction for hemoglobin (Hb).

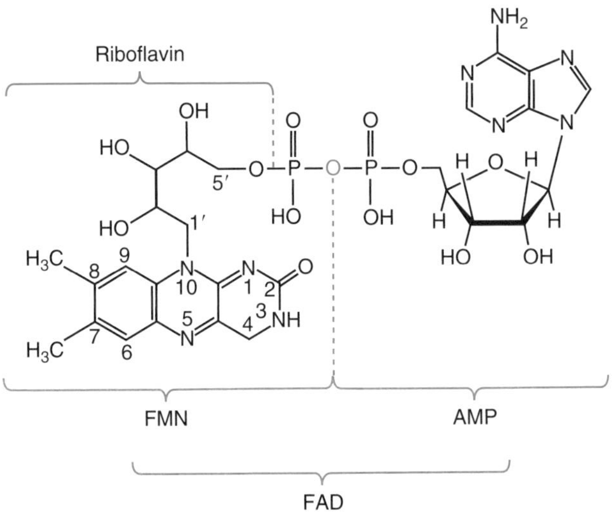

Fig. 27.7 Riboflavin and flavin mononucleotide *(FMN)* as components of flavin adenine dinucleotide *(FAD)*. *AMP,* Adenosine monophosphate.

## Vitamin B₂

Riboflavin, commonly known as vitamin $B_2$, is the precursor of all biologically important flavins, notably flavin mononucleotide, FMN (riboflavin-5′-phosphate) and flavin adenine dinucleotide, FAD (Fig. 27.7). FMN is formed from riboflavin by flavokinase-catalyzed phosphorylation, and FAD is formed from FMN and ATP by the action of FAD synthetase, also called *pyrophosphorylase*. FAD is further converted by covalent bonding to form various tissue flavoproteins.

### Absorption, Transport, Metabolism, and Excretion

Most dietary riboflavin is taken in as a complex of proteins with the coenzymes FMN and FAD. These coenzymes are released from noncovalent attachment to proteins because of gastric acidification. Nonspecific action of pyrophosphatase and phosphatase on the coenzyme occurs in the upper gut. The vitamin is primarily absorbed in the proximal small intestine by a saturable active transport system. Bile salts appear to facilitate uptake, and a modest amount of the vitamin circulates via the enterohepatic system. The transport of flavins in human blood involves loose binding to albumin and tight binding to numerous immunoglobulins. Pregnancy increases the concentration of carrier protein for riboflavin, which results in a higher rate of riboflavin uptake at the maternal surface of the placenta. Uptake of riboflavin into the cells of organs such as the liver is facilitated, possibly requiring a specific carrier at physiologic concentrations, but it can occur by diffusion at higher concentrations.

### Functions

Riboflavin and its coenzyme derivatives are involved in a large variety of chemical reactions. These derivatives are capable of one- and two-electron transfer processes and play a pivotal role in coupling the two-electron oxidation of most organic substrates to the one-electron transfer of the respiratory chain, thus being involved in energy production. They also function as electrophiles and nucleophiles, with covalent intermediates of flavin and substrate frequently involved in catalysis. Flavoproteins catalyze dehydrogenation reactions, hydroxylations, oxidative decarboxylations, deoxygenations, and reductions of oxygen to hydrogen peroxide. Other major functions of riboflavin include drug metabolism in conjunction with the cytochrome P450 enzymes and lipid metabolism. Flavins also have pro-oxidative and antioxidative functions. They are thought to contribute to oxidative stress through their ability to produce superoxide and to catalyze the production of hydrogen peroxide. As an antioxidant, FAD is a coenzyme to glutathione reductase in the regeneration of reduced glutathione from oxidized glutathione, which is necessary for the removal of lipid peroxides. Riboflavin deficiency is associated with increased lipid peroxidation. FAD is a cofactor to methylenetetrahydrofolate reductase (MTHFR) in the remethylation of homocysteine.

### Deficiency

Although riboflavin has a wide distribution in foodstuffs, many people live for long periods on low intakes; consequently, minor signs of deficiency are common in many parts of the world. In addition to poor intake, other causes of deficiency include hypothyroidism and adrenal insufficiency, which inhibit the conversion of riboflavin to its coenzyme derivatives; drugs such as chlorpromazine, imipramine, and amitriptyline, which have a similar tricyclic structure to riboflavin; the anticancer drug doxorubicin; and the antimalarial quinacrine. Excess ethanol ingestion interferes with both digestion and absorption of riboflavin.

Because flavin coenzymes are widely distributed in intermediary metabolism, the consequences of deficiency may be widespread. Riboflavin coenzymes are involved in the metabolism of vitamin $B_{12}$ and folic acid (irreversible reduction of 5,10-methylenetetrahydrofolate to 5-methyltetrahydrofolate) and therefore are a determinant of plasma homocysteine concentration; they are also involved in the metabolism of pyridoxine (PN; conversion to pyridoxal 5-phosphate [PLP]); and niacin (conversion of 5-hydroxytryptamine to tryptophan that is required for niacin synthesis). Therefore, deficiency will affect enzyme systems other than those requiring flavin coenzymes per se.

The deficiency syndrome is characterized by (1) sore throat; (2) hyperemia; (3) edema of the pharyngeal and oral mucous membranes; (4) cheilosis; (5) angular stomatitis; (6) glossitis (magenta tongue); (7) seborrheic dermatitis; and (8) normochromic, normocytic anemia associated with pure red blood cell (RBC) aplasia of the bone marrow.

### Toxicity

Probably as a result of its limited solubility and limited gastric absorption, no adverse effects have been associated with ingestion of riboflavin appreciably above RDA amounts.

### Laboratory Assessment of Status

Riboflavin status can be assessed by (1) determination of urine riboflavin excretion, (2) a functional assay measuring

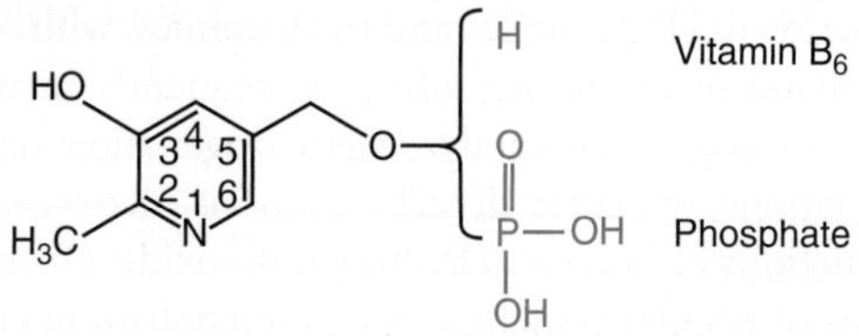

**Fig. 27.8** Free and phosphorylated forms of vitamin $B_6$. R = $CH_2OH$ for pyridoxine, $CH_2NH_2$ for pyridoxamine, and CHO for pyridoxal.

the erythrocyte glutathione reductase activity as assessed by the activation coefficient (EGRAC), which is the ratio between enzyme activity determined with and without the addition of the cofactor, FAD, or (3) direct measurement of riboflavin or its metabolites in plasma or erythrocytes. The trend is that most laboratories now utilize direct measurement rather than functional assays.

Direct measurement of riboflavin, FMN, and FAD in plasma or erythrocytes is undertaken by HPLC, usually with fluorescence detection after protein precipitation, or by capillary zone electrophoresis with laser-induced fluorescence detection (CZE-LIF). In critically ill patients, plasma FAD, which is bound to albumin, may fall as a result of the systemic inflammatory response and due to redistribution of FAD, as there is increased tissue requirement, whereas red cell FAD is unaffected. Therefore, the measurement of red cell FAD is more sensitive and recommended, especially in critically ill patients. As vitamin $B_2$ is light-sensitive, samples should be protected from light.

## Vitamin $B_6$

The vitamin $B_6$ group comprises three natural forms, *pyridoxine* (pyridoxol; *PN*), *pyridoxamine (PM)*, and *pyridoxal (PL)*, which are 4-substituted 2-methyl-3-hydroxy-5-hydroxymethyl pyridines (Fig. 27.8). During metabolic conversion, each vitamer becomes phosphorylated at the 5-hydroxymethyl substituent. PLP is the coenzyme form that participates in many $B_6$-dependent enzyme reactions.

### Absorption, Transport, Metabolism, and Excretion

The phosphorylated sources are hydrolyzed by the intraluminal action of intestinal alkaline phosphatase to enable cellular uptake. The nonphosphorylated forms are readily absorbed by the mucosal cells through a process of passive diffusion. In other cells requiring vitamin $B_6$, the unphosphorylated vitamers may be "metabolically trapped" as phosphorylated forms by cytoplasmic PL kinase, which is responsible for catalyzing the ATP-dependent phosphorylation of all three vitamin forms. Transport to the liver via the portal vein is done by the unphosphorylated form.

Release of free vitamin, mainly PL, occurs when physiologic nonsaturating concentrations of vitamin are absorbed. Here the phosphates are hydrolyzed by nonspecific alkaline phosphatase located on the plasma membrane of cells. Some PLP is released into the circulation by the liver and circulates complexed to proteins—mostly albumin. PLP is the principal tissue form of vitamin $B_6$, whereas PL constitutes much of the circulating vitamin. The main catabolite excreted in urine is

4-pyridoxic acid (4-PA), which is formed by the action of the FAD-dependent general liver aldehyde oxidase.

### Functions

As coenzyme PLP, vitamin $B_6$ functions in more than 100 reactions that embrace the metabolism of macronutrients, such as proteins, carbohydrates, and lipids. These enzymes include aminotransferases; decarboxylases that lead to the formation of various functional amines, including epinephrine and norepinephrine; phosphorylases; and cystathionine β-synthase in the trans-sulfuration pathway of homocysteine. The biosynthesis of heme depends on the early formation of 5-aminolevulinate from PLP-dependent condensation of glycine and succinyl-CoA, followed by decarboxylation. In lipid metabolism, PLP-dependent condensation of L-serine with palmitoyl-CoA forms 3-dehydrosphinganine, a precursor of sphingomyelins. Therapeutically, vitamin $B_6$ has been used for the treatment of some intractable seizures in neonates and infants and for the treatment of other vitamin $B_6$–responsive inborn errors of metabolism and the carpal tunnel syndrome.

### Deficiency

Vitamin $B_6$ deficiency in isolation is rare; it is more usual in association with deficits in other vitamins of the B-complex. Deficiency has been observed with the antituberculosis drug isoniazid (isonicotinic acid hydrazide). Penicillamine (β-dimethyl cysteine), used in the treatment of patients with Wilson disease, inactivates PLP by forming a thiazolidine derivative. Other drugs that can cause vitamin $B_6$ deficiency include the antiparkinsonian drugs benserazide and carbidopa, which react by forming hydrazones, and theophylline.

Several vitamin $B_6$–responsive inborn errors of metabolism are known, including homocystinuria, xanthurenic aciduria, primary cystathioninuria, and pyridoxine-responsive epilepsy. Low vitamin $B_6$ status (together with low vitamin $B_{12}$ and folate status) in humans has been linked to hyperhomocysteinemia and is an independent risk factor for cardiovascular disease, although clinical trials have been inconclusive.

### Toxicity

Although no adverse effects have been observed with high intakes of vitamin $B_6$ from food sources, high oral supplemental doses have been found to have neurotoxic and photosensitive effects. Based on the end point of development of sensory neuropathy, a tolerable upper intake amount of 100 mg/day for adults is recommended.

### Laboratory Assessment of Status

As with the other B vitamins that act as coenzymes, biochemical assessment of vitamin $B_6$ can be made by direct chemical analysis of the vitamer or its metabolites, or by functional means. Measurements that have been used are PLP in plasma or red cells, its metabolite 4-PA in urine or plasma, the activity and activation coefficient of the red cell aminotransferases (aspartate and alanine), and the tryptophan load metabolite excretion test. Because no single marker adequately

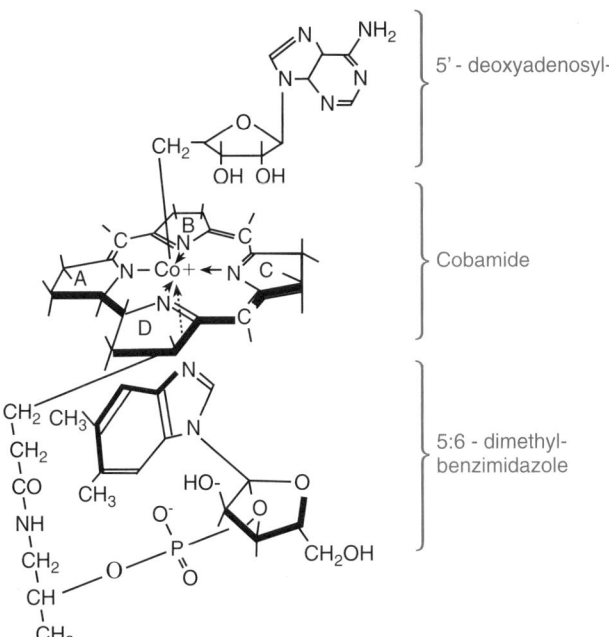

**Fig. 27.9** The structure of 5'-deoxyadenosyl cobalamin.

reflects status, a combination of these markers offers the best approach.

Plasma PLP and plasma or urine 4-PA are most commonly measured by HPLC, PLP with fluorescence detection following precolumn fluorophore formation as a semicarbazone or a pyridoxic acid phosphate, and 4-PA with its natural fluorescence. Using ion-pair reversed-phase chromatography, plasma vitamin $B_6$ vitamers (PLP, PL, PN, PMP, PM, and 4-PA) can be measured.

Functional assessment of vitamin $B_6$ status may be made by measuring the activity of red cell aspartate (or alanine) aminotransferase and its activation coefficient on incubation with PLP, although because the **apoenzyme** is highly unsaturated with PLP, the results obtained have greater variability than those derived by corresponding methods for vitamins $B_1$ and $B_2$ and thus are considered less useful.

Vitamin $B_6$ is light-sensitive; samples should be protected from light.

## Vitamin $B_{12}$

Vitamin $B_{12}$ is one of the most structurally complex small molecules produced by nature, and the only known carbon-metal bond (involving cobalt) found in a biologically active molecule. The generic term *vitamin $B_{12}$* refers to a group of physiologically active substances chemically classified as cobalamins or corrinoids. They are composed of tetrapyrrole rings surrounding central cobalt atoms and nucleotide side chains attached to the cobalt atoms. The cobalamin tetrapyrrole ring, exclusive of cobalt and other side chains, is called a *corrin*. All compounds containing this corrin nucleus are corrinoids. The cobalt-corrin complex is termed *cobamide* (Fig. 27.9). Cobalamins differ in the nature of additional side groups bound to cobalt. Examples include methyl (methylcobalamin), 5'-deoxyadenosine (deoxyadenosyl [short form,

adenosyl], cobalamin, or coenzyme $B_{12}$), hydroxyl (hydroxocobalamin), $H_2O$ (aquocobalamin, or vitamin $B_{12b}$), and cyanide (cyanocobalamin).

### Absorption, Transport, Metabolism, and Excretion

Vitamin $B_{12}$ is known to be tightly bound to proteins and must be released from food by acid and the enzyme pepsin present in the stomach. The synthetic form is free and therefore readily available for metabolism. Acid-blocking drugs such as proton pump inhibitors (e.g., omeprazole) can cause vitamin $B_{12}$ deficiency. The free vitamin $B_{12}$ molecule is bound to haptocorrin (HC, R protein) and travels with it into the duodenum, where the HC is digested by pancreatic enzymes. Liberated vitamin $B_{12}$ then binds to intrinsic factor (IF), a glycoprotein with a molecular weight of approximately 50 kDa that is produced by the gastric parietal cells in the fundus and body of the stomach. One molecule of IF binds one molecule of vitamin $B_{12}$. Gastric secretion of IF is stimulated by food, histamine, and gastrin produced by the antrum portion of the stomach; it is inhibited by vagal blockade. When the vitamin $B_{12}$–IF complex reaches the distal ileum, it is bound by specific receptors known as the cubam complex, which consists of two subunits, namely cubilin and amnionless, on the surface of mucosal epithelial cells, and it is internalized. The vitamin $B_{12}$–IF complex is dissociated within the mucosal epithelial cells by lysosomes and released into blood.

In circulation, vitamin $B_{12}$ then binds to two circulating binding proteins, HC (referred to as holohaptocorrin when bound to vitamin $B_{12}$ and previously known as transcobalamin [TC] I) and TC (holotranscobalamin when bound to vitamin $B_{12}$ and previously known as TC II); however, it is only the TC-bound fraction for which there is a receptor-mediated cellular uptake, as described earlier, and which is therefore the bioactive fraction. The function of HC that is released by granulocytes is currently unknown, and low haptocorrin concentrations, found in approximately 15% of persons with low serum cobalamin, could be one of the most common causes of low cobalamin concentrations. HC accounts for 80% to 94% of endogenous plasma vitamin $B_{12}$, whereas TC accounts for the remainder, but the latter is the more important vitamin $B_{12}$ transport protein in plasma. TC transports vitamin $B_{12}$ to receptors on cell membranes throughout the body. The TC–vitamin $B_{12}$ complex enters the cell by pinocytosis. Lysosomal proteolysis degrades TC and releases the vitamin $B_{12}$. Unbound vitamin $B_{12}$ can enter the tissue cells, but the process is very inefficient.

As discussed earlier, only vitamin $B_{12}$ bound to TC is capable of cellular uptake and as a result malabsorption of TC-bound vitamin $B_{12}$ leads to deficiency in a large proportion of cases. Almost all vitamin $B_{12}$ (bound to TC) is taken up by hepatocytes as the blood in the portal vein passes through the liver, where it is stored and released into blood to meet physiologic demands. If the quantity of vitamin $B_{12}$ exceeds the capacity of hepatocyte receptors, most of the excess is excreted by the kidneys. Normally, approximately 1 mg of vitamin $B_{12}$ is stored in the liver—a quantity equivalent to the daily metabolic requirement for 2000 days. Thus, when the dietary supply of vitamin $B_{12}$ is interrupted or mechanisms of absorption are impaired, vitamin $B_{12}$ deficiency does not become evident for several years.

Vitamin $B_{12}$ is continually secreted in the bile, but most is reabsorbed and is available for metabolic functions. If circulating vitamin $B_{12}$ concentrations exceed the binding capacity of the blood, the excess will be excreted in the urine, but in most circumstances, the highest losses of vitamin $B_{12}$ occur through the feces.

## Functions

Vitamin $B_{12}$ is a cofactor or coenzyme for various enzyme systems. In humans it is required in both adenosylcobalamin and methylcobalamin. Adenosylcobalamin is a coenzyme to L-methylmalonyl-CoA mutase in the conversion of L-methylmalonyl CoA to succinyl-CoA. The conversion of L-methylmalonyl-CoA to succinyl-CoA links propionyl-CoA, which is formed from branched-chain amino acids such as valine, isoleucine, and methionine with the tricarboxylic acid (TCA) cycle. Congenital defects of mutase synthesis or the inability to synthesize adenosylcobalamin results in life-threatening methylmalonic aciduria and metabolic ketoacidosis. Methylcobalamin is a coenzyme to methionine synthase in the conversion of homocysteine to methionine. In this reaction (Fig. 27.10), methylcobalamin serves as an intermediate in the transfer of a methyl group from 5-methyltetrahydrofolate to homocysteine for the formation of methionine. Methionine is required for protein synthesis

and as the methyl donor, S-adenosylmethionine. Congenital defects in methionine synthase or the synthesis of methylcobalamin result in severe hyperhomocysteinemia. As discussed under the section on vitamin $B_6$, defects in the enzyme cystathionine β-synthase or its cofactor vitamin $B_6$ also result in hyperhomocysteinemia.

## Deficiency

Deficiency of vitamin $B_{12}$ in humans is associated with macrocytosis, megaloblastic anemia, and neuropathy. The most common cause of vitamin $B_{12}$ deficiency is pernicious anemia, an autoimmune disease in which chronic atrophic gastritis in the fundus and body region of the stomach results from autoantibodies to gastric parietal cells directed against gastric parietal cell $H^+/K^+$-ATPase, which is responsible for secreting acid ($H^+$) in exchange for potassium ($K^+$). Loss of parietal cells also leads to decreased production of IF. In addition to IF deficiency, blocking autoantibodies that bind the vitamin $B_{12}$-binding sites of IF prevents the formation of vitamin $B_{12}$–IF complex required for recognition by the cubam complex in the distal ileum. At-risk groups include (1) those older than 65 years of age; (2) those with malabsorption; (3) vegetarians or vegans; (4) those with autoimmune disorders (pernicious anemia usually occurs as part of the autoimmune polyglandular syndrome type 3B that includes autoimmune thyroiditis); and (5) those taking prescribed medication known to interfere with vitamin absorption or metabolism, including nitrous oxide (also known as laughing gas that inactivates vitamin $B_{12}$ by oxidizing its cobalt atom), phenytoin,

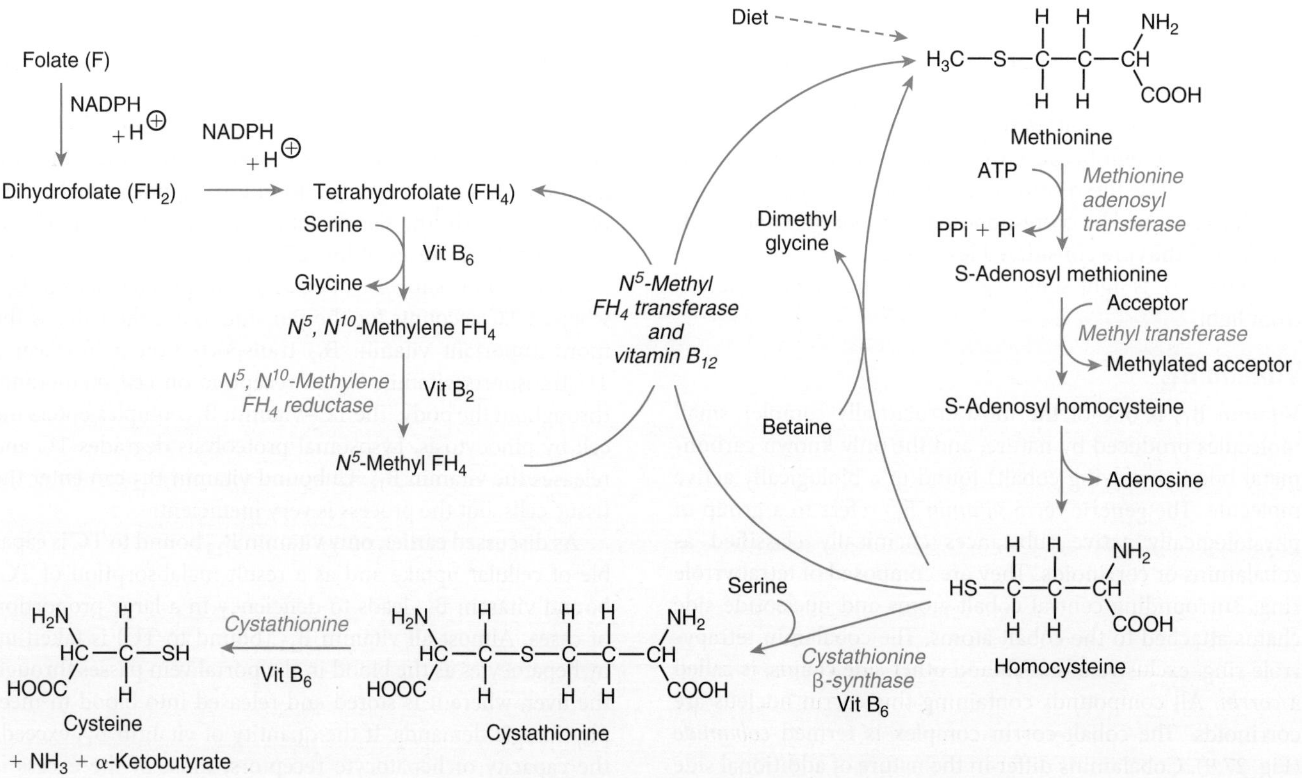

Fig. 27.10 Metabolism of homocysteine and methionine. *ATP*, Adenosine-5′-triphosphate; *NADPH*, nicotinamideadenine dinucleotide phosphate; *Pi*, inorganic phosphate; *PPi*, inorganic pyrophosphate.

dihydrofolate (DHF) reductase inhibitors, metformin, and proton pump inhibitors; as well as (6) infants with suspected metabolic disorders.

Intestinal malabsorption of vitamin $B_{12}$ may be caused by gastrectomy or ileal resection, with an inverse relationship noted between the length of ileum resected and absorption of vitamin $B_{12}$. Other causes of malabsorption include tropical sprue, inflammatory disease of the small intestine such as celiac disease, intestinal stasis with overgrowth of colonic bacteria, which consume vitamin $B_{12}$ ingested by the host, and human immunodeficiency virus (HIV) infection. Another cause of vitamin $B_{12}$ malabsorption is failure to extract cobalamin from food. This is particularly a problem in patients with compromised gastric status or early in the course of development of pernicious anemia.

Vegetarians have a lower intake of vitamin $B_{12}$ than omnivores, and although clinical signs of deficiency are uncommon, biochemical markers of status indicate functional vitamin $B_{12}$ deficiency.

A large number of disorders are associated with cobalamin deficiency in infancy or childhood. Of these, the most commonly encountered is the Imerslund-Grasbeck syndrome, a condition that is characterized by inability to absorb vitamin $B_{12}$, with or without IF, and proteinuria. It appears to be due to an inability of intestinal mucosa to absorb the vitamin $B_{12}$–IF complex as a result of mutations in cubilin or amnionless. The second most common of these is congenital deficiency of gastric secretion of IF. Very rarely, congenital deficiency of vitamin $B_{12}$ in a breast-fed infant is due to deficiency of vitamin $B_{12}$ in maternal breast milk resulting from unrecognized pernicious anemia in the mother. This is rare because most women with undiagnosed and untreated pernicious anemia are infertile. Methylmalonic acidemias (acidurias) and homocysteinemias may be due to vitamin $B_{12}$ deficiency and, depending on the underlying mutation, may or may not be responsive to supplementation with the vitamin.

The hematologic effects of vitamin $B_{12}$ deficiency are indistinguishable from those of folate deficiency. Classical morphologic changes in the blood, in approximate order of appearance, are as follows: hypersegmentation of neutrophils, macrocytosis, anemia, leukopenia, and thrombocytopenia, with megaloblastic changes in bone marrow accompanying peripheral blood changes.

In addition to hematologic changes, vitamin $B_{12}$ deficiency can lead to a demyelinating disorder of the central nervous system. Serious and often irreversible neurologic disorders can occur, such as burning pain or loss of sensation in the extremities, weakness, spasticity and paralysis, confusion, disorientation, and dementia. This condition has been termed *subacute combined degeneration of the spinal cord*. Neurologic symptoms may occur without any discernible hematologic changes in the blood. Vitamin $B_{12}$ deficiency may be associated with other mainly gastrointestinal complications, such as glossitis of the tongue, appetite and weight loss, flatulence and constipation, mental changes, and infertility.

Depending on the laboratory and the procedure used, reference intervals vary widely. A recent WHO consultation defined a serum vitamin $B_{12}$ concentration less than 203 ng/L (150 pmol/L) as deficient. Vitamin $B_{12}$ concentrations within the reference interval may not necessarily reflect adequate vitamin $B_{12}$ status because serum concentrations may be maintained at the expense of tissue stores.

## Toxicity

No adverse effects have been associated with excess vitamin $B_{12}$ intake from food or supplements in healthy people.

## Laboratory Assessment of Status

Both direct and indirect (functional) methods are available for assessment of vitamin $B_{12}$ status. Indirect tests include assays for urinary and serum concentrations of methylmalonic acid (MMA), plasma homocysteine, the deoxyuridine suppression test, and the now rarely used vitamin $B_{12}$ absorption (Schilling) test. Cytochemical staining of RBC precursors and the test for IF-blocking antibodies are other ancillary methods of assessing vitamin $B_{12}$ status.

Multiple automated and semiautomated systems are available for measuring vitamin $B_{12}$ using, for example, chemiluminescence as a signal. Most immunometric methods use solid-phase separation by immobilizing the IF antibodies on beads or magnetic particles. Spurious elevations of vitamin $B_{12}$ have been reported in patients with pernicious anemia when using automated analyzers based on the competitive binding of serum vitamin $B_{12}$ with reagents using IF. This has been attributed to the high levels of IF-blocking autoantibodies in these patients interfering in the assay. Up to 70% of patients with pernicious anemia have IF-blocking antibodies. Assay manufacturers are aware of this problem and have taken steps to inactivate the IF-blocking antibodies. However, at the present time, the scale of the problem is unknown, and alternative methods should be used if in doubt, including the measurement of IF-blocking antibodies.

Indirect tests assess the functional adequacy of vitamin $B_{12}$. Serum MMA concentration is increased when lack of adenylcobalamin causes a block in the conversion of methylmalonyl-CoA to succinyl-CoA. It is a sensitive test of status, being often the first analyte to be raised in subclinical vitamin $B_{12}$ deficiency. It has a further advantage in that it is unaffected by folate deficiency. Unfortunately, MMA is increased by renal insufficiency and in persons above the age of 65 years. Plasma total homocysteine concentration is also a sensitive indicator of vitamin $B_{12}$ status because methylcobalamin is required for the remethylation of homocysteine to methionine, but it is not specific, being elevated in deficiencies of folate, vitamin $B_{12}$, vitamin $B_2$, and vitamin $B_6$. There are several preanalytical variables affecting it: high-protein meal and venous stasis may increase it; it is decreased in the supine position as it is bound to albumin. EDTA plasma is the most widely recommended sample type and should be centrifuged within 1 hour or kept cold by collecting on ice until centrifugation.

The measurement of holotranscobalamin is potentially useful as a specific marker of biologically available vitamin $B_{12}$ because it is the only vitamin $B_{12}$ moiety that is specifically available for uptake by all cells and has been shown to have the best diagnostic accuracy for vitamin $B_{12}$ deficiency.

## Folic Acid

Vitamin $B_9$, folate, and folic acid are generic terms for a family of compounds that function as coenzymes in the processing of one-carbon units and that are derived from pteroic acid to which one or more molecules of glutamic acid are attached. Pteroic acid is composed of a pteridine ring joined to a p-aminobenzoic acid residue. When pteroic acid is conjugated with one molecule of L-glutamic acid, pteroylglutamic acid is formed; this can be reduced to dihydrofolic acid (DHF) with hydrogens in positions 7 and 8, or to tetrahydrofolate (THF) with hydrogens in positions 5, 6, 7, and 8. Only the reduced forms are biologically active. Other folate derivatives have multiple glutamic acid residues ranging from 1 to 7. As a summary, folate is converted by specific enzymes to DHF, which is then converted to THF, which is in turn converted to methylene-THF, and finally to 5-methyl-THF.

### Absorption, Transport, Metabolism, and Excretion

Folate is absorbed from dietary sources mainly as reduced methyl- and formyl-tetra-hydropteroylpolyglutamates. The bioavailability of folate from food sources is variable and is dependent on factors such as incomplete release from plant cellular structure, entrapment in food matrix during digestion, inhibition of deglutamation by other dietary constituents, and possibly the degree of polyglutamation. Polyglutamate forms of folate present in food are first converted to monoglutamates, by pteroylpolyglutamate hydrolase, in the intestinal mucosa. Absorption of monoglutamyl folates at low concentrations occurs through a saturable transport process at an acidic pH of around 5, with an additional, apparently nonsaturable absorption mechanism when intestinal folate concentrations exceed 5 to 10 µmol/L. After cellular uptake, most of the folate is reduced and methylated and enters the circulation as THF, circulating loosely bound to albumin or, to a lesser degree, to a high-affinity folate-binding protein (FBP). Uptake by certain cells (kidney, placenta, and choroid plexus) occurs by membrane-associated FBPs that act as folate receptors, and the reduced folate carrier, a member of the SLC19 family, facilitates uptake by most tissue. Once THF is demethylated and converted to the polyglutamyl form by folylpolyglutamate synthase, it is retained within the cell. For release into the circulation, the polyglutamates are reconverted to monoglutamates by polyglutamate hydrolase.

Folic acid and vitamin $B_{12}$ metabolism are linked by the reaction that transfers a methyl group from THF to cobalamin. In cases of cobalamin deficiency, folate is "trapped" as methyl-THF and is "metabolically dead." It cannot be recycled as THF back into the folate pool to serve as the main one-carbon unit acceptor for many biochemical reactions. Eventually, cellular depletion of methylene-THF ensues, causing a reduction in thymidylic acid synthesis, which, in turn, results in megaloblastic anemia and neuropathies. This concept is supported by the fact that THF corrects megaloblastic anemia in patients with congenital methylmalonic aciduria and homocystinuria, whereas it is not corrected with methyl-THF.

Protein-free plasma folate is filtered at the glomerulus, and most is reabsorbed by the proximal renal tubules. Most of the biliary excreted folate is reabsorbed in the enterohepatic circulation. Fecal losses are similar to urinary losses.

### Functions

Folate coenzymes, together with coenzymes derived from vitamins $B_{12}$, $B_6$, and $B_2$, are essential for one-carbon metabolism. Biochemically, a carbon unit from serine or glycine is transferred to THF to form methylene-THF, which is then (1) used in the synthesis of thymidine (and incorporation into DNA), (2) oxidized to formyl-THF for use in the synthesis of purines (precursors of RNA and DNA), or (3) reduced to methyl-THF, which is necessary for the methylation of homocysteine to methionine. Much of this methionine is converted to S-adenosylmethionine, a universal donor of methyl groups to DNA, RNA, hormones, neurotransmitters, membrane lipids, and proteins. Some of these reactions are illustrated in Fig. 27.11.

### Deficiency

Deficiency of folate may result from (1) absence of intestinal microorganisms (gut sterilization), (2) poor intestinal absorption (e.g., after surgical resection, in celiac disease or sprue), (3) insufficient dietary intake (including chronic alcoholism), (4) excessive demands (as in pregnancy, liver disease, and malignancies), (5) administration of antifolate drugs (e.g., methotrexate), and (6) anticonvulsant therapy (that increases folate requirements, especially during pregnancy). Inadequate folate intake leads first to decreased serum folate concentration, then to a decrease in RBC folate concentration and an increase in plasma homocysteine, and then to megaloblastic changes in the bone marrow and other tissues. Megaloblastic anemia (characterized by large, abnormally nucleated erythrocytes in the bone marrow) is the major clinical manifestation of folate deficiency, although sensory loss and neuropsychiatric changes may also occur. Deficiencies of folate and iron may coexist in malnourished people, in which case the latter may mask the expected macrocytic and megaloblastic changes.

Pregnancy brings increased demand to folate stores because of increased DNA synthesis, and one-carbon transfer reactions and low serum folate concentrations in pregnancy are associated with adverse outcomes, including preterm delivery, infant low birth weight, and fetal growth retardation. In addition, many observational studies have confirmed a reduction in risk of neural tube defects (NTDs) with periconceptual folic acid supplementation. Current suggestions are that women planning pregnancy should take at least 400 µg/day until the 12th week of pregnancy, although a daily intake of 5 mg of folic acid is recommended, especially for those with a previous history of NTD. Recent meta-analyses have strongly suggested a significant association of the variant

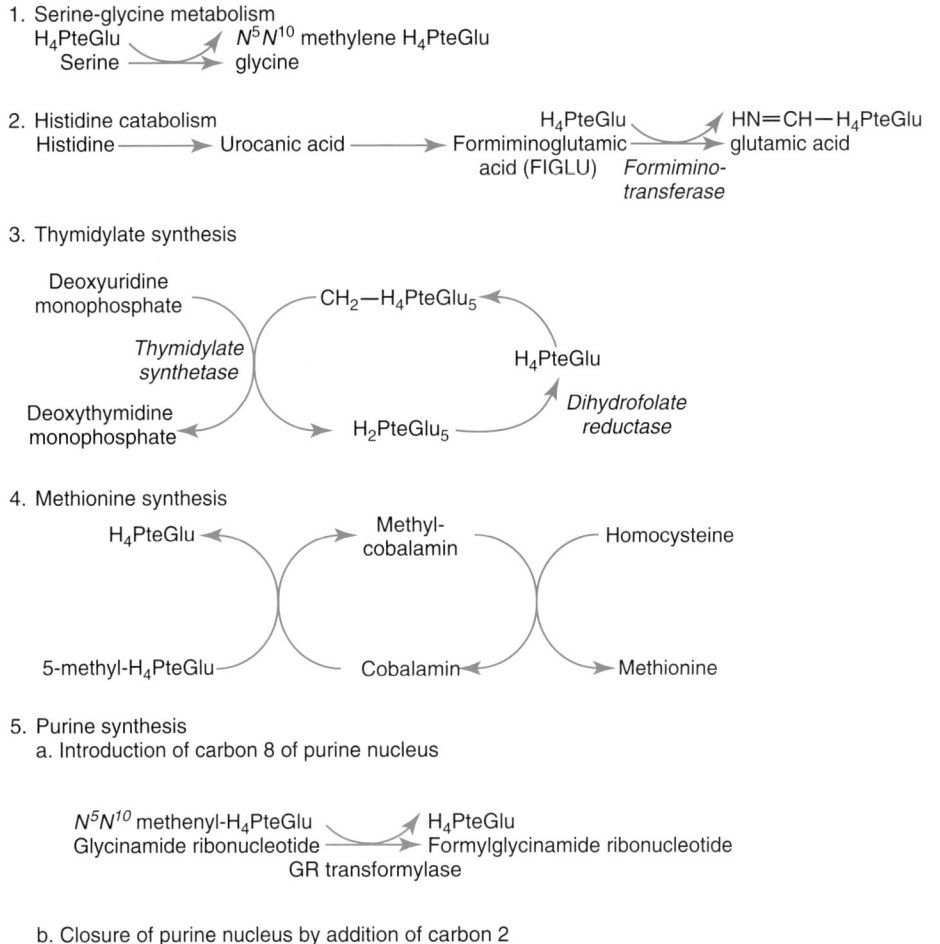

1. Serine-glycine metabolism

$H_4PteGlu$ → $N^5N^{10}$ methylene $H_4PteGlu$
Serine → glycine

2. Histidine catabolism

Histidine → Urocanic acid → Formiminoglutamic acid (FIGLU) → $H_4PteGlu$ → HN=CH—$H_4PteGlu$ glutamic acid
*Formimino-transferase*

3. Thymidylate synthesis

Deoxyuridine monophosphate → $CH_2$—$H_4PteGlu_5$
*Thymidylate synthetase*
Deoxythymidine monophosphate → $H_2PteGlu_5$
$H_4PteGlu$
*Dihydrofolate reductase*

4. Methionine synthesis

$H_4PteGlu$ ← Methyl-cobalamin — Homocysteine
5-methyl-$H_4PteGlu$ — Cobalamin — Methionine

5. Purine synthesis

a. Introduction of carbon 8 of purine nucleus

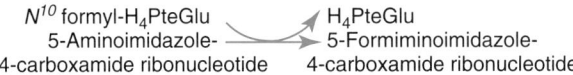

$N^5N^{10}$ methenyl-$H_4PteGlu$ → $H_4PteGlu$
Glycinamide ribonucleotide → Formylglycinamide ribonucleotide
GR transformylase

b. Closure of purine nucleus by addition of carbon 2

$N^{10}$ formyl-$H_4PteGlu$ → $H_4PteGlu$
5-Aminoimidazole-4-carboxamide ribonucleotide → 5-Formiminoimidazole-4-carboxamide ribonucleotide

Fig. 27.11 The five major metabolic functions of folate in human cells.

5,10-methyleneterahydofolate reductase (MTHFR) C677T polymorphism with increased risk of NTDs.

The increase in plasma homocysteine concentration has been postulated to be an independent risk factor for coronary artery disease and cerebrovascular disease. The involvement of folate in its coenzyme forms with homocysteine and methionine metabolism is summarized in Fig. 27.10. Folate is the principal micronutrient determinant of homocysteine status, and supplementation with folate (0.5 to 5.0 mg/day) has been used as a treatment modality to reduce circulating homocysteine concentrations. However, the most recent Cochrane meta-analyses of trials of homocysteine-lowering therapy with folate, vitamins $B_6$ or $B_{12}$ given alone or in combination have not shown a reduction in cardiovascular disease.

Folate appears to have a protective effect on colorectal cancer development, but is associated with increased risk of gastric cancer, prostate cancer, and may be associated with lung cancer. One meta-analysis of 10 randomized clinical trials (RCTs) showed a borderline significant increase in frequency of overall cancer in the folic acid-supplemented group compared with controls.

## Toxicity

No adverse effects have been reported from the consumption of folate-fortified foods; thus, any signs of toxicity are associated with supplemental folate. Most of the limited evidence suggests that excessive folate supplementation can precipitate or exacerbate neuropathy in vitamin $B_{12}$–deficient subjects, and it is this end point that has been used to set a tolerable upper intake concentration of 1 mg/day from fortified foods or supplements for adults. One recognized complication of folate supplementation is that it "masks" vitamin $B_{12}$ deficiency because the associated anemia responds to folate. This may delay treatment of any neurologic abnormalities. It has been recommended that if a low serum folate is present concomitantly with low vitamin $B_{12}$, the latter should be corrected first.

## Laboratory Assessment of Status

Folate status may be reliably assessed by direct measurement of serum and RBC or whole blood concentrations using immunometric assays, and its metabolic function as a coenzyme may be assessed by metabolite concentrations such as

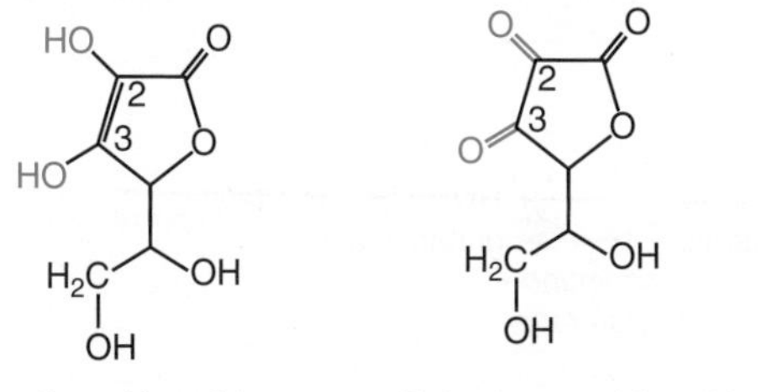

Fig. 27.12 L-Ascorbic and dehydroascorbic acids.

plasma homocysteine. Serum folate concentrations are considered indicative of recent intake and not of tissue stores, but serial measurements have been used to confirm adequate intake. Whole blood and RBC folate concentrations are more indicative of tissue stores over the lifetime of RBCs and are therefore a better indicator of longer-term folate status than serum folate. Because folate is taken up only by the developing RBC in the bone marrow and not by the mature cell, RBC concentrations reflect folate status over the 120-day life span of the cell. However, in general, serum and RBC folate provide equivalent information regarding folate status.

Plasma homocysteine is considered a sensitive indicator of folate status and is strongly correlated with serum folate concentrations in the lower range, which is below 10 nmol/L (4.5 µg/L). A homocysteine concentration above 15 µmol/L is indicative of folate deficiency. However, as the concentration of homocysteine is dependent on age, gender, renal function, genetic factors, and the status of other vitamins ($B_6$ and $B_{12}$), it is not a specific marker of folate status.

Due to the instability of folate in serum, it is therefore recommended that if delay in transportation is anticipated, serum should be separated from RBCs by centrifugation and stored frozen until analysis. As there is a significant amount of folate in RBCs, hemolysis invalidates serum folate results.

## Vitamin C

The term *vitamin C* refers to all molecules that exhibit antiscorbutic properties (derived from Latin word for scurvy, *scorbutus*) in humans and includes both ascorbic acid and its oxidized form, dehydroascorbic acid (DHA), as shown in Fig. 27.12.

### Absorption, Transport, Metabolism, and Excretion

Gastrointestinal absorption of ascorbic acid occurs throughout the ileum via a combination of sodium-dependent active transport at low concentrations and simple diffusion at high concentrations. Vitamin C is found in most tissues, including the brain, but glandular tissues, such as pituitary, adrenal cortex, corpus luteum, and thymus, have the highest amounts, and the eye lens has 20 to 30 times the plasma concentration. In plasma, vitamin C exists predominantly as the ascorbate ion. Excretion of unchanged ascorbate occurs increasingly with increased dosage, with almost all of an injected dose of more than 500 mg excreted over 24 hours.

### Functions

Ascorbic acid, working in synchrony with vitamin E, is one of the most effective antioxidants in biological fluids and is capable of scavenging physiologically important reactive oxygen species and reactive nitrogen species. Vitamin C has been shown to also exhibit pro-oxidant properties, and although pro-oxidants tend to have deleterious effects, pharmacologic doses of ascorbate may have beneficial pro-oxidant activity in the treatment of certain diseases, especially cancer. It is increasingly being recognized that the balance between antioxidant and pro-oxidant activity is important for health, and too much antioxidant might actually be harmful.

Ascorbic acid acts as a cofactor for a number of mixed function oxidases in hydroxylation processes, in which it promotes enzyme activity by maintaining metal ions in their reduced form (particularly iron and copper). Vitamin C has a functional role in the formation of collagen by acting as a cofactor for protocollagen hydroxylase, the enzyme responsible for hydroxylation of prolyl and lysyl residues within nascent peptides in connective tissue proteins. Among these are collagen and related proteins, which make up the intercellular material of cartilage, dentin, and bone.

Ascorbate is also involved in: (1) carnitine biosynthesis, serving as a cofactor to 6-*N*-trimethyl-L-lysine hydrolase; (2) γ-butyrobetaine hydrolase, which converts γ-butyrobetaine to carnitine; (3) degradation of tyrosine via 4-OH phenylpyruvate dioxygenase; (4) synthesis of adrenal hormones via dopamine β-hydroxylase; (5) biosynthesis of corticosteroids and aldosterone; (6) hydroxylation of cholesterol in the formation of bile acids; and (7) folate metabolism and leukocyte functions.

Vitamin C also has an important role in the intestinal absorption of nonheme iron by maintaining it in its reduced ferrous ($Fe^{2+}$) form. More recently identified functions include nucleic acid and histone dealkylation and proteoglycan deglycanation.

### Deficiency

Scurvy results due to deficiency of vitamin C and still occurs in developed countries, albeit rarely either as part of general malnutrition or in isolation. Those most at risk of the disease include (1) elderly men, particularly those who live alone; (2) those with alcohol dependence and smokers; (3) those taking unbalanced diets, especially populations who have limited access to fresh fruits and vegetables either due to weather conditions or disasters both natural and manmade; (4) some mentally ill patients; (5) renal failure patients undergoing peritoneal dialysis or hemodialysis; (6) those with increased requirements, such as the sick and pregnant women; and (7) some patients with cancer.

Lack of vitamin C or scurvy affects collagen, resulting in defective connective tissue, bones, and dentin formation, manifesting as swollen, tender, and often bleeding or bruised loci at joints. Bone formation is usually impaired causing poor growth and lesions. Infantile scurvy, also known as *Barlow disease*, exhibits a bayonet-rib syndrome. The gums are livid and swollen, cutaneous bleeding often begins on the lower thighs as perifollicular hemorrhages, and large spontaneous bruises (ecchymoses) may arise almost anywhere on the body. This condition may be misconstrued as child abuse. Ocular hemorrhages, drying of salivary and lacrimal glands, parotid swelling, femoral neuropathy, edema of the lower extremities, and psychologic disturbances have also been described. Some scorbutic patients may develop anemia, display radiologic changes characteristic of osteoporosis, or die suddenly from heart failure.

Vitamin C deficiency has also been linked to anemia, diabetes mellitus, various types of cancer, cataract formation, and osteoporosis, but there is no clear evidence for a causal link. A meta-analysis found that regular vitamin C supplementation did not significantly reduce the incidence of common cold in the general population.

## Toxicity

Rare adverse effects include increased oxalate excretion and kidney stone formation, increased uric acid excretion, excess iron absorption, lowered vitamin $B_{12}$ concentrations, systemic conditioning, and "rebound" scurvy. The tolerable upper intake amount for vitamin C is 2 g/day for adults older than 19 years.

## Laboratory Assessment of Status

At present, no useful functional tests of vitamin C adequacy are available; thus, laboratory assessment of status is made by direct measurement of plasma, urine, or tissue concentrations of ascorbic acid, total vitamin C, or (rarely) metabolite. Plasma ascorbate concentration is considered a reliable indicator of vitamin C intake and has been measured photometrically by oxidation with 2,4-dinitrophenylhydrazine to form the red *bis*-hydrazone, or with 2,4-dichlorophenol-indophenol, which is reduced to a colorless form. A more specific approach is to use the enzyme ascorbate oxidase to convert ascorbate to dehydroascorbate, which then is coupled with *o*-phenylene diamine to form a product that is measured fluorometrically or at 340 nm on an automated analyzer. HPLC methods offer the potential advantage of specificity but are generally time-consuming. Detection may be done by precolumn derivatization to the fluorescent quinoxaline, or by electrochemical or coulometric means. Care must be taken during the analysis to prevent oxidation of the ascorbate before detection by using dithiothreitol or homocysteine added to the sample and mobile phase.

Vitamin C in plasma or serum is known to be readily degraded by oxidation caused by high temperature, light, neutral pH, pro-oxidant material such as certain enzymes, and interaction with iron or copper. Plasma samples should be treated with a metal-chelating and protein-precipitating acid, such as metaphosphoric or sulfosalicylic acids, soon after a phlebotomy followed by prompt freezing. Dithiothreitol may also be used as a preservative.

## Biotin

*Biotin* is *cis*-tetrahydro-2-oxothieno[3,4-ᴅ]-imidazoline-4-valeric acid (Fig. 27.13). The vitamin in most organisms occurs mainly bound to protein.

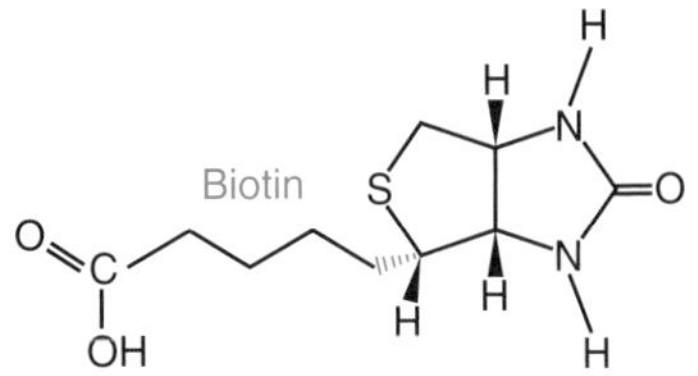

Fig. 27.13  Structure of biotin.

### Absorption, Transport, Metabolism, and Excretion

Biotin in the diet is largely linked to lysine residues on protein, and digestion of these proteins by gastrointestinal proteases and peptidases produces biocytin (ε-*N*-biotinyl lysine) and biotinyl peptides, and the latter may be further hydrolyzed by intestinal biotinidase to release biotin. Avidin, a protein found in raw egg whites, binds biotin tightly and prevents its absorption, and therefore raw egg consumption has been known to result in biotin deficiency.

A biotin carrier, the sodium-dependent multivitamin transporter (SMVT) for which pantothenic acid and lipoate compete, is located in the intestinal brush border membrane and transports biotin against a sodium ion concentration gradient. At higher biotin doses (>25 μmol/L), there is passive diffusion across cell membranes. By contrast, transport of biotin across the basolateral membrane is sodium-independent and electrogenic. The enzyme biocytinase (biotin amidohydrolase) in plasma and erythrocytes catalyzes the hydrolysis of biocytin to yield free biotin. Biotin is cleared from the circulating blood more rapidly in deficient than in normal mammals; it is taken up by such tissues as the liver, muscle, and kidney and is localized in cytosolic and mitochondrial carboxylases.

### Functions

The principal biochemical function of biotin in humans is as a cofactor for carboxylation reactions. Five carboxylases are currently found in human tissue; one of these, an acetyl-CoA carboxylase, is inactive and may act as a storage vehicle for biotin. The others are carboxylases for acetyl-CoA, propionyl-CoA, β-methylcrotonyl-CoA, and pyruvate. Recent advances have implicated biotin in the epigenetic regulation of gene expression.

### Deficiency

Biotin deficiency is uncommon but may be seen (1) with prolonged consumption of raw egg white, which contains the protein avidin that binds biotin in the intestines, preventing absorption; (2) in those on TPN without biotin supplementation; and (3) in those with inborn errors of biotin metabolism. The first two situations may be complicated by effects on gut flora that produce biotin.

Symptoms of biotin deficiency include anorexia, nausea, vomiting, glossitis, pallor, conjunctivitis, ataxia, hypotonia, depression, dry scaly dermatitis, and developmental delay in infants and children. Significantly lowered urinary excretion or circulating blood concentrations have been found in alcoholic individuals, in patients with achlorhydria, and among

urinary metabolites, $N'$-methylnicotinamide and $N'$-methyl-2-pyridone-5-carboxamide. HPLC-based methods are currently the methods of choice, although some capillary electrophoresis methods have been developed. Another approach that may prove valuable is the ratio of erythrocyte niacin coenzymes NAD to NADP. NAD concentrations respond to the niacin status, whereas NADP concentrations remain relatively constant under different conditions of niacin status. The niacin number is NAD/NADP × 100; a niacin number less than 130 is indicative of a risk of developing niacin deficiency.

## Pantothenic Acid

*Pantothenic acid*, also known as vitamin $B_5$ (name derived from Greek *pantothen* meaning "from everywhere"), is of ubiquitous occurrence in nature, where it is synthesized by most microorganisms and plants. It is the amide formed by the linkage between pantoic acid (D-2,4-dihydroxy-3,3-dimethylbutyric acid) derived from L-valine, and β-alanine derived from L-aspartate.

### Absorption, Transport, Metabolism, and Excretion

Pantothenic acid is taken in as dietary CoA compounds and 4'-phosphopantetheine and is hydrolyzed by pyrophosphatase and phosphatase in the intestinal lumen to dephospho-CoA, phosphopantetheine, and pantetheine, which are further hydrolyzed to pantothenic acid. The vitamin is primarily absorbed as pantothenic acid through a saturable process at low concentrations and through simple diffusion at higher ones. After absorption, pantothenic acid enters the circulation and is taken up by cells in a manner similar to its intestinal adsorption. Pantothenic acid is excreted in the urine after hydrolysis of CoA compounds by enzymes that cleave phosphate and the cysteamine moieties.

### Functions

Pantothenic acid has two major metabolic roles—the first as part of CoA, and the second as the prosthetic group of the acyl-carrier protein (ACP). In the former role, CoA is primarily involved in acetyl and acyl transfer reactions in catabolic processes of carbohydrate, lipid, and protein chemistry.

### Deficiency

The widespread availability of pantothenic acid in food is commensurate with its many roles and makes dietary deficiency of pantothenate unlikely in humans. Symptoms have been produced in a few volunteers who received ω-methylpantothenic acid as an antagonist and in people fed semisynthetic diets virtually free of pantothenate. Subjects became irascible and developed postural hypotension and rapid heart rate on exertion, epigastric distress with anorexia and constipation, numbness and tingling of the hands and feet, hyperactive deep tendon reflexes, and weakness of finger extensor muscles.

### Toxicity

No reports have described adverse effects, except for occasional mild diarrhea, with oral pantothenic acid given in doses as high as 20 g/day.

### Laboratory Assessment of Status

No convenient or reliable functional tests of pantothenic acid status are currently available; thus, assessment is made by direct measurement of whole blood or urine pantothenic acid concentrations. Methods that have been used to measure pantothenic acid in human samples include radioimmunoassay, liquid chromatography coupled to mass spectrometry, gas chromatography–mass spectrometry, and a stable isotope dilution assay based on liquid chromatography–mass spectrometry. CoA and ACP have been measured by enzymatic methods.

## TRACE ELEMENTS

The term trace element was originally used to describe the residual amount of inorganic analyte quantitatively determined in a sample. More sensitive methods allow accurate determination of most inorganic micronutrients present at very low concentrations in body fluids and tissue. Those present in body fluids (μg/L) and tissue (mg/kg) are, however, still widely referred to as "trace elements." The corresponding dietary requirements are quoted in mg/day or μg/day, respectively. The biological effects of deficiency disease define the essential trace elements. For example, an element is considered essential when signs and symptoms induced by a deficient diet are uniquely reversed by an adequate supply of the particular trace element under investigation.

### Dose-Effect Relationships

At low intakes of essential trace elements, deficiency disease may be seen. With increasing supply, a plateau region of optimal status is reached. Still higher intakes result in adverse effects. The concentration window separating beneficial from toxic intakes varies depending on the element in question. This is similar to the dose-effect relationship described for organic micronutrients (Fig. 27.15). Therefore, the RDA is set at amounts that are sufficient to prevent deficiency. A tolerable upper intake value that will prevent toxicity has been proposed for the

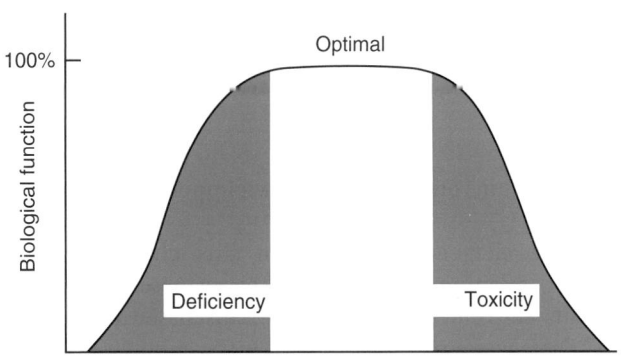

**Fig. 27.15** Model of the relationship between tissue concentration and intake of an essential nutrient and dependent biological function.

## TABLE 27.4   Reference Intervals for Trace Elements

| Trace Element | Mass Unit | SI Units |
|---|---|---|
| Chromium (serum) | 0.1–0.15 µg/L | <6 nmol/L |
| Chromium (urine) | <1–1.0 µg/24 h | 2–19 nmol/24 h |
| Cobalt (serum) | <0.6 µg/L | <10 nmol/L |
| Cobalt (urine) | <1 µg/g creatinine | <17 nmol/L |
| Copper (serum) Concentrations increase during pregnancy and oral contraception | 70–140 µg/dL | 10–22 µmol/L |
| Copper (urine) | <50 µg/24 h | <0.7 µmol/24 h |
| Wilson disease | >200 µg/24 h | |
| Wilson disease post penicillamine | >1700 µg/24 h | >3 µmol/24 h >25 µmol/24 h |
| Copper (liver) Wilson disease | 8–40 µg/g dry weight >250 µg Cu/g dry weight | |
| Iodine (urine) WHO-recommended urinary concentrations for various population groups are given in (WHO/NMH/NHD/EPG/13.1) | 76–546 µg/L | 0.60–4.30 µmol/L |
| Manganese (serum) | 0.6–2.3 µg/L | 11–42 nmol/L |
| Manganese (blood) | 5–15 µg/L | 90–270 nmol/L |
| Molybdenum (serum) | 0.4–1.2 µg/L | 4–12 nmol/L |
| Molybdenum (urine) | 14.4–119 µg/24 h | 0.15–1.24 µmol/24 h |
| Selenium (serum) | 60–125 µg/L | 0.75–1.57 µmol/L |
| Adult (UK) | 26–77 µg/L | |
| <1.5 years old | 40–88 µg/L | 0.33–0.97 µmol/L |
| 1.5–3 years old | 48–100 µg/L | 0.51–1.12 µmol/L |
| 4–18 years old | | 0.6–1.29 µmol/L |
| Zinc (serum) | 63–134 µg/dL | 9.6–20.5 µmol/L |
| Zinc (urine) | 0.2–1.3 mg/24 h | 3–21 µmol/24 h |

*WHO,* World Health Organization.

inorganic micronutrients of known importance to human health.

Trace elements discussed in this chapter include copper, selenium, zinc, iodine, manganese, chromium, cobalt, and molybdenum. Iron is discussed in Chapter 28. Dietary sources, RDAs, and intravenous intakes are shown in Table 27.1. The reference intervals are given in Table 27.4.

## LABORATORY ASSESSMENT OF TRACE ELEMENT STATUS

### Specimen Requirements

Direct determination of trace elements is done in many types of specimens—blood, plasma or serum, and urine. Less often, other sample types (e.g., leukocytes, saliva) may be analyzed. Tissue samples, obtained by needle biopsy (e.g., liver, bone) or following an autopsy, as well as hair and nail samples offer a noninvasive means of sampling tissue. Measurements of hair and nails for essential elements may be of value on a group basis during studies of severely depleted populations but are of limited value in the investigation of individual hospital patients. Problems of external contamination from environmental pollution, cosmetics, shampoos, and other sources are difficult to control.

### Preanalytical Factors

Numerous variables can affect trace element determinations before analysis of the sample and should be considered. Age, sex, ethnic origin, time of sampling in relation to food intake, time of day, medication, and other factors should be noted. In patients with infection, after injury or postsurgery, the systemic inflammatory response affects the concentration of essential elements in circulating blood, independently of nutritional status. Zinc and selenium are bound to albumin and so decrease as part of the systemic inflammatory response that results in a drop in albumin concentration, whereas copper increases owing to the upregulation of ceruloplasmin synthesis, which is a positive acute-phase reactant.

### Collection Equipment

Contamination from collection equipment can be a problem. Trace metal-free vacutainers are commercially available. To avoid contamination from the needle during venous sampling, at least the third specimen from the order of draw should be used. For some elements, collection is via plastic cannulae with the sample then placed into acid-washed containers. Urine collection bottles may be washed thoroughly with ultrapure water. For random urine samples and tissue biopsy samples, a plain plastic container with no added preservative is preferable.

### ANALYTICAL METHODS FOR MEASURING TRACE ELEMENTS

Analytical methods should provide sufficient sensitivity to reliably determine the concentrations in the limited specimen usually available. Techniques that are appropriate include atomic absorption spectrometry (AAS), inductively coupled plasma-optical emission spectrometry (ICP-OES), and inductively coupled plasma-mass spectrometry (ICP-MS). UV-vis spectrophotometry is possible for elements where concentrations are higher. Other techniques have been applied to elemental analysis. Using laser ablation, ICP-MS or x-ray fluorescence spectrometry, 2D or even 3D images of trace element distributions within biological materials can be produced. Speciation methods involve techniques to separate compounds of individual elements in a sample. A typical procedure involves HPLC coupled to ICP-MS, to separate methyl mercury from inorganic mercury. Details of these procedures are given in Chapter 13.

## Copper

### Absorption, Transport, Metabolism, and Excretion

Copper absorption occurs mainly in the small intestine, although some gastric uptake has been shown. The extent of intestinal copper absorption varies with dietary copper content and is around 50% at low intakes (<1 mg/day) but only 20% at higher intakes (>5 mg/day). Absorption is reduced by other dietary components such as zinc (which induces metallothionein that binds $Cu^{2+}$), vitamin C (which converts $Cu^{2+}$ to insoluble, nonabsorbable $Cu^+$), molybdate, and iron, and is increased by amino acids and dietary sodium.

Absorbed copper is transported to the liver in portal blood, bound to albumin, where it is incorporated by hepatocytes into cuproenzymes and other proteins, and it is then exported as ceruloplasmin via peripheral blood to tissues. Although two-thirds of the 80 to 100 mg total body content is located in the skeleton and muscle, the liver is the key organ in copper homeostasis. The ceruloplasmin molecule contains 6 to 8 atoms of copper per molecule, with 6 atoms of copper involved in the protein's ferroxidase and free radical scavenging activities.

Ceruloplasmin is a positive acute-phase reactant, and concentrations increase during infection, after tissue injury, and in pregnancy and during the use of oral contraceptives. The increase is accompanied by a rise in serum copper concentration. A smaller amount of copper in plasma (<10%) is bound to albumin by specific peptide sequences, and this copper is in equilibrium with plasma amino acids. This fraction may be important for cellular uptake.

Copper is predominantly excreted via bile into feces. Patients with cholestatic jaundice or other forms of liver dysfunction are at risk for copper accumulation caused by failure of excretion.

### Functions

Copper is a catalytic component of numerous enzymes and a structural component of other important proteins. These include the following:

*Energy Production.* Cytochrome *c* oxidase contains copper and iron. Located on the external face of mitochondrial membranes, the enzyme catalyzes four-electron reduction of molecular oxygen, establishing a high-energy proton gradient across the inner mitochondrial membrane that is necessary for ATP production.

*Connective Tissue Formation.* Protein-lysine 6-oxidase (lysyl oxidase) is a cuproenzyme essential for stabilizing extracellular matrixes by cross-linking of collagen and elastin.

*Iron Metabolism.* Copper-containing enzymes, ferroxidase I (ceruloplasmin) and ferroxidase II, and hephaestin in the enterocyte oxidize ferrous, to ferric, iron. This allows incorporation of $Fe^{3+}$ into transferrin and eventually into Hb.

*Central Nervous System.* Dopamine monooxygenase is an enzyme that requires copper as a cofactor and uses ascorbate as an electron donor. This enzyme catalyzes the conversion of dopamine to norepinephrine, an important neurotransmitter. Monoamine oxidase, one of the numerous amine oxidases, is a copper-containing enzyme that catalyzes the degradation of serotonin in the brain and is involved in the metabolism of catecholamines.

*Melanin Synthesis.* Tyrosinase is a copper-containing enzyme that is present in melanocytes and catalyzes the synthesis of the melanin biopigments pheomelanin and eumelanin.

*Antioxidant Functions.* Both intracellular and extracellular superoxide dismutases (SODs) are Cu- and Zn-containing enzymes, able to convert superoxide radicals to hydrogen peroxide, which can be removed subsequently by catalase and other antioxidant defenses.

*Regulation of Gene Expression and Intracellular Copper Handling.* Copper-dependent proteins act as transcription factors for specific genes, such as those regulating SOD and catalase. Synthesis of metallothionein, important in regulating the intracellular distribution of copper, is controlled by copper-responsive transcription factors. Additional specialized proteins act as "copper chaperones" to deliver copper to intracellular sites and prevent oxidative damage by free copper ions.

*Aceruloplasminemia* is another genetic defect resulting in failure of hepatic synthesis of ceruloplasmin leading to secondary iron overload, and insulin-dependent diabetes developing in the 4th to 5th decade of life.

### Deficiency

The main conditions resulting from or causing copper deficiency are:

*Anemia.* Copper deficiency is a rare but treatable cause of hematologic abnormalities. Usual hematologic features include anemia, leucopenia, and rarely thrombocytopenia. The mechanism is not clear.

*Zinc-Induced Hypocupremia.* Zinc intake (e.g., via dental fixatives) induces metallothionein expression in the intestinal mucosa, which sequesters copper, blocking its absorption and leading to copper deficiency.

*Menkes Syndrome.* This is a rare (1/100,000 live births), X-linked mutation disorder due to impaired intestinal transport of copper caused by a mutation in the ATP7A gene that leads to severe copper deficiency. It occurs in male infants at 2 to 3 months who present with hypotonia, seizures, failure to thrive, kinky hair (pili torti), facial changes, and neurologic abnormalities. Low concentrations of copper in plasma, liver, and brain occur because of the impaired intestinal absorption. Findings include very low plasma copper and ceruloplasmin concentrations. Deficiency of the copper enzyme dopamine monooxygenase in CSF may allow early diagnosis. Therapy with parenteral copper histidine is rarely successful, and patients usually die following aortic rupture.

*Neuropathy.* Copper deficiency–associated myeloneuropathy is an increasingly recognized disorder. Deficiency secondary to celiac disease and excessive zinc intake are among the causes suggested.

## Toxicity

Toxicity can arise from ingestion of contaminated diet or drinking water. Symptoms of acute poisoning include bloody vomiting, melena, and hypotension. Fatal renal failure has been recorded following accidental or intentional ingestion of copper sulfate. Indian childhood cirrhosis is recognized in children who may be genetically sensitive to copper in drinking water.

Wilson disease, a genetic disorder due to a mutation in the *ATP7B* gene, affects copper incorporation into ceruloplasmin and excretion into bile causing increased copper accumulation in tissues. With an incidence of 1/30,000 live births, Wilson disease is one of the more common genetic disorders. The presentation is highly variable. Primarily, it affects either the liver or the brain, but rare cases are diagnosed with renal tubular disease or hemolytic anemia. Severe liver disease typically develops in young children, while neurological signs tend to appear in teenagers and early adults, but onset and diagnosis may be made at any age. Initial investigations include plasma copper and ceruloplasmin, which will usually be low. Although the total plasma copper is decreased, the non-ceruloplasmin-bound free fraction is increased. However, methods for analysis of this fraction are not particularly reliable. Other signs and symptoms include copper deposits in the eye (Kayser-Fleischer rings), abnormal liver function tests, and increased urine copper excretion. In cases that are difficult to diagnose, analysis of liver biopsies for copper may help and a test involving an oral dose of stable[65] Cu isotope has been developed. Genetic testing is possible, but because several hundred mutations exist, this may not always be informative. Transplantation is required for cases of acute liver disease, while the chronic form of Wilson disease is treated by oral chelating agents (penicillamine) that remove excess copper from tissue and increase urinary excretion. Maintenance therapy may involve oral administration of zinc salts or ammonium molybdate that block intestinal absorption of copper.

## Laboratory Assessment of Status

Serum copper and ceruloplasmin concentrations are measured, but factors that increase the hepatic synthesis of ceruloplasmin, such as the SIR, pregnancy, or estrogen-containing contraceptive pill, will increase plasma copper independently of dietary copper intake. Urinary excretion of copper is decreased during dietary deprivation, but the change from an already low basal value is small, which makes this of limited use.

## Selenium

### Absorption, Transport, Metabolism, and Excretion

Intestinal absorption of various dietary forms of selenium is efficient and is not regulated. The inorganic salts, selenite ($Se^{IV}$) and selenate ($Se^{VI}$), used in some dietary supplements and in food fortification are almost completely absorbed, but much of the selenate ion is rapidly excreted in urine. Selenium from inorganic salts is more rapidly incorporated into glutathione peroxidase and other selenoproteins than selenium from organic sources containing selenomethionine. However, selenium-enriched yeast containing the organic forms is considered less toxic and is widely used as a dietary supplement.

Whole body selenium is about 15 mg, with higher concentrations in the kidney and liver, followed by the other organs. The concentrations of selenium in whole blood and in plasma are related to dietary intake. About 50% to 60% of total plasma selenium is present as the protein selenoprotein P, a highly basic protein having multiple histidine residues and about 10 atoms of selenium per molecule. Around 30% of plasma selenium is present as glutathione peroxidase (GSHPx-3), the remainder being incorporated into albumin as selenomethionine.

The major route of excretion is via the urine and reflects recent dietary selenium intake. The amounts excreted vary widely, ranging from less than 20 µg/L to more than 1000 µg/L.

## Functions

More than 30 biologically active selenocysteine-containing proteins have been identified and their biological function investigated. Some of these are discussed below.

*Glutathione Peroxidase (GSHPx).* This enzyme has at least eight isoforms with GSHPx-3 present in plasma. These enzymes use the reducing power of glutathione to remove an oxygen atom from hydrogen peroxide and lipid hydroperoxides.

*Iodothyronine Deiodinase.* Type I (Dio1), II (Dio2), and III (Dio3) isoforms of this enzyme are responsible for conversion of the precursor hormone $T_4$ to the active hormone $T_3$. Type 1 is located in the thyroid, liver, kidney, and muscle and is responsible for more than 90% of plasma $T_3$ production. Pituitary, brain, and brown adipose tissue contain the type II and III deiodinases.

*Thioredoxin Reductases.* Three isoforms catalyze the NADPH-dependent reduction of thioredoxin and are important in maintaining the intracellular redox state.

*Selenophosphate Synthetase.* This enzyme is required for the intracellular synthesis of selenoproteins via a monoselenium phosphate intermediate.

*Selenoprotein P.* This protein is the major selenium-containing protein in blood plasma; it may be a transport protein for the element, and it has an antioxidant function.

## Deficiency

Selenium enters the food chain mainly as selenomethionine from plants. The soil content of selenium is highly variable, and the geographic source of plant and animal foodstuffs determines the dietary intake. Soils in parts of China and New Zealand are particularly low in selenium, while wheat and other cereal products from North America, where concentrations in soil are high, are good sources.

**Keshan Disease.** Conclusive evidence of a role for selenium in human nutrition came with the results from large-scale trials in China that showed the protective effects of selenium supplementation in children and young adults suffering from an endemic cardiomyopathy. This was observed in areas of the country (Keshan region) with low soil selenium concentrations.

**Kashin–Beck Disease.** A type of severe arthritis described in parts of China and neighboring areas of Russia.

*Nutritional Depletion in Hospital Patients.* The need for selenium supplementation, with monitoring, during nutritional support is well established, and few cases of symptomatic deficiency are now reported.

*Thyroid Function.* As noted earlier, deiodinase enzymes are selenoproteins and are necessary for normal thyroid function. Children with biochemical and clinical signs of hypothyroidism were successfully treated with oral selenium. A report of a study in the United Kingdom concluded that supplementation had no effect on thyroid status.

*Immune Function.* Deficiency of selenium is accompanied by loss of immunocompetence, and this is related to the reduction of selenoproteins in the liver, spleen, and lymph nodes.

*Inflammatory Conditions.* Many conditions associated with inflammation and increased oxidative stress could be influenced by selenium status.

*Cardiovascular Disease.* A protective role for selenium against cardiovascular disease has been extensively investigated, but with no conclusive findings.

*Viral Virulence.* It is possible that an unusually virulent strain of the Coxsackie virus is part of the cause of cardiomyopathy in selenium-depleted regions of China.

*Cancer Chemoprevention.* Epidemiologic surveys suggest an association between cancer incidence and soil selenium. However, a large selenium and vitamin E study known as the Selenium and Vitamin E Cancer Prevention Trial (SELECT) concluded that selenium or vitamin E, alone or in combination at the doses and formulations used, did not prevent prostate cancer in healthy men.

## Toxicity

Clinical signs of selenosis include garlic odor on the breath, hair loss, nail damage, nervous system and skin disorders, poor dental health, and paralysis in extreme cases. The tolerable upper limit has been set at 400 µg/day for adults and less than 280 µg/day for children. Cases of toxicity and even death from self-administration or homicidal dosages have been reported. Some parts of the world, generally where there are volcanic soils, are naturally selenium-rich, and locally produced food contains high concentrations of selenium. Consumption of these foods leads to chronic selenosis typified by cases reported from Enshi City in the Hubei region of China.

## Laboratory Assessment of Status

Selenium concentrations in whole blood or plasma/serum are the usual markers of selenium status. Samples may be analyzed by electrothermal-AAS or by ICP-MS (note the interference due to the $Gd^{2+}$ ion). Urinary selenium is measured where there is occupational exposure. Measurement of glutathione peroxidase (GSHPx-3) activity in whole blood or serum is an additional biomarker of selenium status. Results are dependent on the substrate and other assay conditions so that comparisons among different studies require careful interpretation. Plasma selenoprotein P may be determined, but methods are not readily available. Plasma selenoprotein P, plasma GSPHx-3, and total plasma selenium concentration are all lowered by the APR to injury or infection. This effect should be considered when results are being interpreted. Hair and nail selenium concentrations can be useful in population studies.

## Zinc

Zinc is second to iron as the most abundant trace element in the body.

### Absorption, Transport, Metabolism, and Excretion

Intestinal absorption of zinc is controlled in the face of variable dietary zinc input and is usually from 20% to 50% of the dietary content. Uptake from the gut lumen into intestinal cells is achieved and regulated by zinc transporter proteins. Several factors, such as dietary phytate, fiber calcium, and iron, reduce intestinal absorption by forming insoluble complexes. Profound zinc deficiency in humans was first recognized in a population where geophagia (eating soil) was practiced; because zinc is bound to the soil components, deficiency resulted.

Absorbed zinc is transported to the liver by the portal circulation, where incorporation into metalloenzymes and plasma proteins occurs. Plasma contains less than 1% of the total body content of zinc and lies within a narrow concentration interval. About 80% of plasma zinc is associated with albumin, and most of the rest is tightly bound to $\alpha_2$-macroglobulin. The zinc on albumin is in equilibrium with plasma amino acids (mostly histidine and cysteine), and this small (<1%) ultrafiltrable fraction may be important in cellular uptake mechanisms (Fig. 27.16). Red cell zinc concentrations are about 10 times higher than in plasma. Fecal excretion includes both unabsorbed dietary zinc and zinc resecreted into the gut. The amount normally equals the total dietary intake and is about 10 to 15 mg/day. Urine excretion of zinc is normally about 0.5 mg/day, but this can increase markedly during catabolic illness.

### Functions

More than 300 zinc metalloenzymes have been described. Some important examples include carbonic anhydrase, alkaline phosphatase, RNA and DNA polymerases, and alcohol dehydrogenase. The key roles of zinc in protein and nucleic acid synthesis explain the failure of growth and impaired wound healing observed in individuals with zinc deficiency.

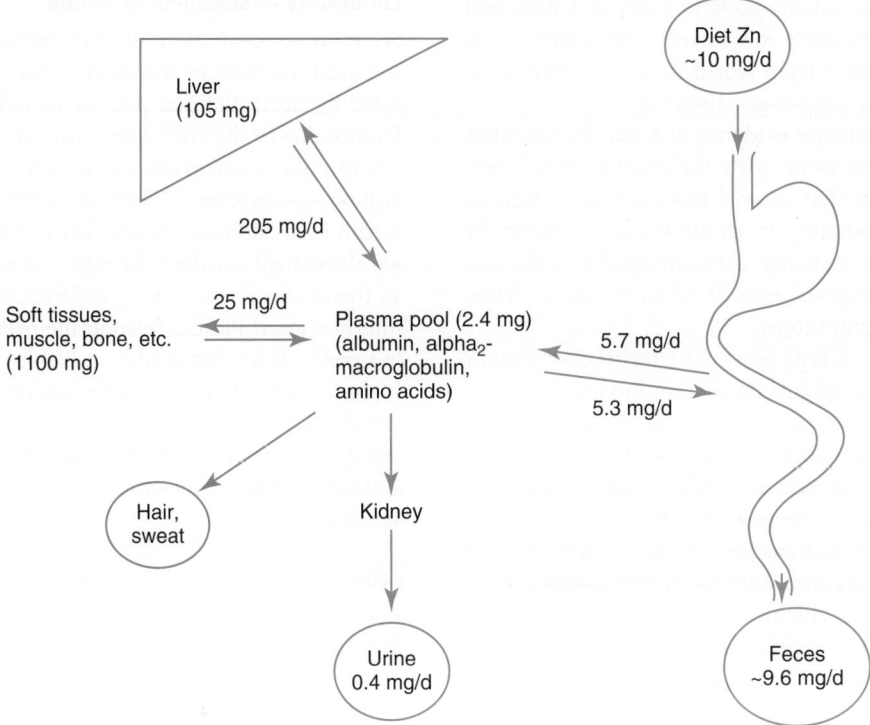

**Fig. 27.16** Zinc metabolism.

In some enzymes, such as Cu and Zn SOD, structural stability is ensured by zinc protein binding and the catalytic activity of the enzyme by the active copper site. Proteins can form domains that bind tetrahedral zinc atoms by coordination with histidine and cysteine to form folded structures known as "zinc fingers." These molecules have important roles in gene expression and hormone function.

### Deficiency

Increased amounts are required during pregnancy and lactation. Strict vegetarians may need as much as 50% more zinc per day because of increased phytic acid and fiber in their diet. As might be expected from the multiple biochemical functions of zinc, the clinical presentation of deficiency disease is varied, nonspecific, and related to the degree and duration of depletion. Signs and symptoms include depressed growth with stunting; increased incidence of infection, possibly related to alterations in immune function; diarrhea; altered cognition; defects in carbohydrate use; reproductive teratogenesis; skin lesions; alopecia; eyesight defects; and other adverse clinical outcomes.

Acrodermatitis enteropathica is an autosomal recessive disorder resulting in failure to absorb zinc, and characterized by severe periorificial and acral dermatitis, alopecia, and diarrhea. Patients with this disorder have abnormally low blood zinc concentrations (<30 μg/dL). Symptoms are reversed by oral zinc supplementation. Regular monitoring of serum concentrations is recommended.

*Immune Function.* Zinc depletion impairs immunity and has a direct effect on the gastrointestinal tract that increases the severity of enteric infections. A review of controlled trials of zinc supplementation of children in low-income countries found significant clinical benefits with substantial reduction in the incidence of severe diarrhea and respiratory infection.

*Subclinical Effects of Deficiency.* Marginal zinc deficiency, not severe enough to cause clinical signs and symptoms, may be associated with "subclinical" effects. These include susceptibility to sickle cell disease, impaired immune response, and mental well-being.

### Toxicity

Zinc toxicity is unusual and is generally associated with ingestion of zinc-contaminated food or water. Symptoms include abdominal pain, diarrhea, nausea, and vomiting. Chronic ingestion can lead to a zinc-induced deficiency of copper.

### Laboratory Assessment of Status

Although plasma zinc determination is insensitive to dietary zinc intake and is subject to a variety of influences, it remains the most widely used laboratory test to confirm severe deficiency and to monitor adequacy of zinc provision, especially when interpreted together with changes in serum albumin and the APR. A clinical and biochemical response to zinc supplementation supports a diagnosis of deficiency. It is important to recognize that a low plasma zinc concentration may not mean deficiency. Plasma albumin is a negative acute-phase reactant that redistributes, together with zinc, into interstitial space from the plasma pool during infection, after trauma, and in chronic disease. It is essential to consider plasma zinc results along with plasma albumin and a marker of the APR. Increased urine zinc is an important source of loss in the severely injured catabolic patient. Urine output increases with amino acid infusion given during TPN.

## Iodine

### Absorption, Transport, Metabolism, and Excretion

Absorption of dietary iodide is not entirely understood. The $Na^+/I^-$ symporter (NIS) on the apical surface of enterocytes of the small intestine is responsible for uptake into vesicles within the cell, but movement into the circulation is not clear. Under normal circumstances, 90% to 95% of the intake is absorbed. Subsequent transport, movement into thyroid cells (which also involves an NIS), synthesis of thyroid hormones, and release are discussed in Chapter 42. Iodine is primarily excreted in the urine.

### Functions

The essential function for iodine relates to thyroid physiology (see Chapter 42). While iodine is concentrated in thyroid tissue and hormones, around 70% of the body's iodine is distributed in many other tissues. Its role in mammary tissue relates to fetal and neonatal development, but its role in other tissues is partially unknown.

### Deficiency

Deficiency of iodine is a major health problem throughout the world, occurring in regions where the soil and groundwater are deficient in the element. Deficiency may also develop following prolonged use of special diets that may have low iodine content. The most serious adverse effect of iodine deficiency is impaired development of nervous tissue in the fetus. Thyroid hormones are required for neuronal migration and myelination of the fetal brain. Severe maternal iodine deficiency during pregnancy increases the risk of stillbirths and congenital abnormalities. A decrease in intelligence quotient (IQ) points has been shown in children who are iodine deficient.

### Toxicity

Iodine is a strong oxidizing agent and acts as an acid corrosive. Iodine vapor irritates the eyes, skin, and mucous membranes. Common causes of acute toxicity include accidental or deliberate ingestion, resulting in corrosive damage to the gastrointestinal tract, cardiovascular collapse, and renal failure; liberal use of iodine to open wounds; large injections of iodine-containing radiocontrast media; and amiodarone treatment for cardiac arrhythmias. Iodine toxicity causes a rapid decrease in release of thyroxine and 3,5,3′-triiodothyronine from thyroglobulin, decreased uptake of iodide by the thyroid gland, and hence decreased synthesis of thyroid hormones. This culminates in acute hypothyroidism.

### Laboratory Assessment of Status

Urine is the matrix of choice for suspected iodine toxicity and for the assessment of recent iodine *intake*. For epidemiological studies, such as population-based surveys, the *median* urinary iodine concentration can be used to classify that *population's* iodine status. Adequate iodine status is indicated by a population median urinary iodine concentration greater than 0.79 μmol/L (100 μg/L). However, the urine iodine test is not an appropriate test to diagnose iodine deficiency in individuals. Urine iodine levels have a low predictive value in an individual because urinary iodine concentration varies substantially between days and seasons, as well as within a day (up to threefold) as a consequence of circadian rhythm and due to differences in fluid intake. Because the thyroid gland can store large amounts of iodine (12 to 16 mg in an iodine-sufficient individual), a "low" urine iodine concentration no more indicates iodine deficiency than a low urinary concentration sodium indicates sodium deficiency. It is recommended, however, that iodine status can be reliably estimated if 10 repeat random urine samples are collected. Iodine concentration in serum or whole blood provides no useful information relevant to iodine nutritional status.

## Manganese

### Absorption, Transport, Metabolism, and Excretion

Dietary manganese is absorbed from the small intestine. Diets high in iron, calcium, magnesium, phosphates, fiber, phytic acid, oxalate, and tannins from tea can reduce the absorption. Once absorbed, manganese is transported to the liver bound to albumin; it is then exported to other tissues bound to transferrin and possibly to $\alpha_2$-macroglobulin. Excretion of manganese occurs primarily via bile into feces, with urine output being very low and not sensitive to dietary intake.

### Functions

Manganese is a constituent of many important metalloenzymes. $Mn^{2+}$ ions can be replaced by $Mg^{2+}$, $Co^{2+}$, and other cations during the activation of some enzymes. Some important manganese-dependent enzymes are discussed.

*Superoxide Dismutase (SOD).* Manganese-dependent SOD is a mitochondrial enzyme that is an important factor in limiting oxygen toxicity. The enzyme catalyzes the breakdown of the superoxide radical $O_2^-$ to $H_2O_2$, which is then removed by catalase and glutathione peroxidase.

*Pyruvate Carboxylase.* This enzyme is required to catalyze the formation of phosphoenolpyruvate (PEP), from pyruvate, a key reaction in the hepatic synthesis of glucose.

*Arginase.* Arginase is the terminal enzyme in the urea cycle, hydrolyzing L-arginine to urea and ornithine and completing the deamination of amino acids. Arginase is most concentrated in the liver but is also found in other tissues. The activity of arginase affects the production of nitric oxide by limiting the availability of L-arginine, which is required for synthesis of nitric oxide synthetase.

*Glycosyl Transferases.* These enzymes are responsible for the sequential addition of carbohydrate molecules to proteins to form proteoglycans, and ultimately connective tissue and cartilage.

## Deficiency

Overt manganese deficiency has not been documented in humans eating natural diets. Symptoms in experimentally induced manganese deficiency in animal studies include impaired growth and reproductive function, skeletal abnormalities, and impaired glucose tolerance and cholesterol synthesis.

Prolidase deficiency in infants is a rare genetic disorder that is known to be associated with abnormalities of manganese biochemistry. One study suggests there is low arginase activity due to a defect in the supply of manganese for enzyme activation.

## Toxicity

Prolonged exposure to manganese-containing dust or fumes at work is well recognized, with neurologic symptoms resembling Parkinson disease developing slowly over a period of months or years. Patients with severe liver disease may have neurologic and behavioral signs of manganese neurotoxicity resulting from failure to excrete manganese in bile. Manganese deposition in the globus pallidus results in $T_1$-weighted magnetic resonance imaging (MRI) signal hypersensitivity. By causing deficits in neurotransmitter production, manganese ions may be partially responsible for symptoms of postsystemic hepatic encephalopathy. Deposition of manganese in the brain has been demonstrated in children with biliary atresia, in adult cirrhotic patients, and in patients receiving manganese intravenously during TPN, especially those with cholestasis. A study in adults that compared the effects of increasing doses of manganese in patients receiving home parenteral nutrition showed a good correlation between blood manganese, MRI intensity, and $T_1$ values in the globus pallidus.

Increases in serum manganese to greater than 1.6 µg/L (>30 nmol/L) or in blood manganese to greater than 20 µg/L (>360 nmol/L) are indices of manganese retention.

## Laboratory Assessment of Status

Manganese status should be monitored in at-risk patients. Serum manganese, lymphocyte Mn SOD activity, and blood arginase are potentially useful when possible nutritional depletion is assessed. Blood or serum manganese in combination with brain MRI scans and neurologic assessment detect excessive exposure.

## Chromium

Chromium occurs in biology as $Cr^{3+}$ or $Cr^{6+}$, each having markedly different properties. The element has no redox or acid-base properties, but in its $Cr^{6+}$ form it is a strong oxidant that can cause tissue damage (e.g., chromic acid), although it is normally rapidly reduced to $Cr^{3+}$.

## Absorption, Transport, Metabolism, and Excretion

Absorption is increased marginally by ascorbic acid, amino acids, oxalate, and other dietary factors. After absorption, chromium binds to plasma transferrin with an affinity similar to that of iron. It then concentrates in human liver, spleen, other soft tissue, and bone. Urine chromium is the main route for excretion.

## Functions

While symptoms have been reported in severely chromium-deficient rats (impaired growth, reduced life span, corneal lesions, and alterations in carbohydrate, lipid, and protein metabolism), studies by other groups yielded inconsistent results.

## Deficiency

Chromium is proposed to play a role in impaired glucose tolerance, diabetes, and cardiovascular disease. Clinical signs attributed to chromium deficiency were described in a few patients receiving TPN for a prolonged period using fluids that did not supply sufficient chromium. All had similar presentations, with previously stable patients developing insulin-resistant glucose intolerance, weight loss, and, in some cases, neurologic deficits. Addition of substantial amounts of $Cr^{3+}$ to the intravenous fluids (150 to 200 µg/day) reversed glucose intolerance and reduced insulin requirements with eventual improvement in neurologic symptoms. These cases influenced the US Food and Nutrition Board to designate chromium as an essential trace element, although this is not universally accepted.

## Toxicity

Hexavalent chromium is a recognized carcinogen, and industrial exposure to fumes and dusts containing this metal is associated with increased incidence of lung cancer, dermatitis, skin ulcers, and hypersensitivity reactions. Chromium picolinate is a widely used dietary supplement, and this compound may cause renal and hepatic damage when used at high doses.

In addition, markedly increased concentrations (up to 1000-fold) have been observed in both plasma and urine in patients with problem hip prostheses.

## Laboratory Assessment of Status

Measurement of chromium in blood plasma or serum, the diet, in oral and intravenous nutritional support regimens requires great care to prevent contamination before and during analysis. Increased amounts of chromium in urine confirm recent occupational or environmental exposure. Monitoring urine chromium during trials that use pharmacologic dosages of chromium confirms compliance and detects potential toxicity.

## Cobalt

Cobalt (Co) is essential for humans as an integral part of vitamin $B_{12}$ (cobalamin). No other function in the human body is known. Non-vitamin $B_{12}$ cobalt does not interact with the body's vitamin $B_{12}$ pool.

Increased exposure from industrial uses, particularly with hard metal blades, leads to high mean urinary Co concentrations. Increases are also associated with hip prostheses for which concentrations can be markedly raised with no apparent clinical evidence of overt toxicity; however, there is some emerging evidence of cobalt toxicity with wear from metal-on-metal hip prostheses.

Erythropoiesis can be stimulated by inorganic cobalt ions ($Co^{2+}$), even in nonanemic subjects, and cobalt chloride was once administered at daily doses of 25 to 50 mg for use as an antianemic agent and $Co^{2+}$ therapy proved effective in stimulating erythropoiesis in both nonrenal and renal anemia. The mode of action is to stabilize hypoxia-inducible transcription factors that increase the expression of the erythropoietin gene. Because the mass of Hb is a critical factor in aerobic sports, use of cobaltous salts is tempting for athletes and horse racing trainers to stimulate erythropoiesis. But there are risks to health with severe organ damage, primarily in the heart and the sensory systems, the gastrointestinal tract, and the thyroid.

## Molybdenum
### Absorption, Transport, Metabolism, and Excretion
Molybdenum is efficiently absorbed over a wide range of dietary intakes, mainly as molybdate, although competitive inhibition of absorption by sulfate reduces intestinal uptake. Concentrations in whole blood are about 1.0 µg/L (10 nmol/L), and some 80% to 90% or more of molybdenum is bound to red cell proteins. Transport of small amounts in plasma may involve $\alpha_2$-macroglobulin. Urine output directly reflects the dietary intake of molybdenum.

### Functions
Several important mammalian enzymes, including sulfite oxidase, xanthine dehydrogenase, and aldehyde oxidase, require molybdenum as a cofactor. The organic component is a molybdopterin complex. Sulfite oxidase is probably the most important enzyme in relation to human health, catalyzing the last step in the degradation of sulfur amino acids by oxidizing sulfite to sulfate and transferring electrons to cytochrome $c$. Xanthine dehydrogenase and aldehyde oxidase hydroxylate heterocyclic substances, such as purines and pteridines.

### Deficiency
Molybdenum deficiency has not been observed in healthy people consuming a normal diet. A single case report described a patient receiving prolonged parenteral nutrition during treatment for severe Crohn disease who developed an intolerance to intravenous amino acids, especially L-methionine. Clinical signs included tachycardia, visual defects, neurologic irritability, and eventually coma. Symptoms improved on discontinuation of amino acid infusion. Biochemical abnormalities included high methionine and low uric acid concentrations in plasma. Treatment with ammonium molybdate (300 µg/day, IV) improved the clinical and biochemical abnormalities.

Very rare, usually fatal, recessive inherited diseases result from defects in the biosynthesis of molybdenum cofactor. Symptoms include failure to thrive and seizures with lens dislocations and cerebral atrophy developing later. Diagnosis is made by detection of excess sulfite in urine.

### Toxicity
Molybdenum compounds have low toxicity in humans. Reports have described increased blood uric acid in those with occupational exposure and in Armenian populations that have an abnormally high dietary intake (10 to 15 mg/day). A single report of acute toxicity from self-administration of 300 to 800 µg/day with a cumulative total of 13.5 mg over 18 days led to acute psychosis and seizures but is inconsistent with another study in healthy men who were given as much as 1500 µg/day for 24 days with no adverse effects reported. Excess molybdenum intake prevents copper absorption through formation of an insoluble thiomolybdate-copper complex. This is the basis for using ammonium molybdate in the management of Wilson disease.

### Laboratory Assessment of Status
Whole blood and serum or plasma molybdenum concentrations are too low to be reliably used to detect deficiency. However, urinary output is responsive to increases or decreases in input. Measuring urate or sulfite in the urine is the most valuable means of confirming molybdenum cofactor disorder or possible molybdenum deficiency.

## POINTS TO REMEMBER

### Vitamins

| | | |
|---|---|---|
| Vitamin A | Retinol | Antioxidant; important role in vision |
| Vitamin E | Tocopherols | Antioxidant; multiple functions including bone metabolism |
| Vitamin K | Phylloquinones | Coagulation; bone metabolism |
| Vitamin $B_1$ | Thiamine, aneurin | Coenzyme for decarboxylation and transketolation reactions; involved in carbohydrate metabolism |
| Vitamin $B_2$ | Riboflavin | Prosthetic group for oxidation-reduction reactions |
| Vitamin $B_3$ | Niacin | Hydrogen acceptors (as nicotinamide adenine dinucleotide and nicotinamide adenine dinucleotide phosphate) in many oxidation-reduction reactions |
| Vitamin $B_5$ | Pantothenic acid | Coenzyme A required for metabolism of carbohydrates, fats, and proteins |
| Vitamin $B_6$ | Pyridoxine | Coenzyme for enzymes involved in metabolism of various amino acids |

## POINTS TO REMEMBER—cont'd

| | | |
|---|---|---|
| Vitamin $B_7$ | Biotin, vitamin H | Coenzyme for carboxylation reactions involved in gluconeogenesis and lipogenesis |
| Vitamin $B_9$ | Folate | Required for the interconversions of amino acids and the biosynthesis of purines and pyrimidines |
| Vitamin $B_{12}$ | Cobalamin | Required for erythropoiesis, methylation processes necessary for DNA metabolism, and is a cofactor for various enzymes |
| Vitamin C | Ascorbic acid | Connective tissue formation; antioxidant |
| **Trace Elements** | | |
| Copper | | Catalytic component of numerous enzymes and has structural roles |
| Selenium | | Component of numerous selenocysteine-containing proteins such as glutathione peroxidase and iodothyronine deiodinase |
| Zinc | | Component of numerous metalloenzymes and proteins including transcription factors |
| Iodine | | Important role in thyroid hormone synthesis |
| Manganese | | Constituent of many important metalloenzymes such as superoxide dismutase |
| Chromium | | Implicated roles in impaired glucose tolerance, diabetes, and cardiovascular disease |
| Cobalt | | Integral component of vitamin $B_{12}$ (cobalamin) |
| Molybdenum | | Cofactor for several enzymes such as sulfite oxidase and xanthine dehydrogenase |

## REVIEW QUESTIONS

1. Which enzyme activity is decreased as a result of vitamin $B_1$ deficiency?
   a. Glutathione reductase
   b. Glutathione peroxidase
   c. Transketolase
   d. Methyltetrahydrofolate reductase
2. Which of the following statements best describes the effects of systemic inflammatory response (SIR) on vitamin status?
   a. SIR causes a decrease in the vitamins A, E, $B_2$, $B_6$, C, D, and carotenoids.
   b. SIR causes an increase in the vitamins A, E, $B_2$, $B_6$, C, D, and carotenoids.
   c. SIR does not have an appreciable effect on any vitamins in blood circulation.
   d. SIR causes a decrease in albumin and CRP that affects vitamin status.
3. Which of the following statements best accounts for vitamin A deficiency?
   a. It is dependent on renal functioning.
   b. It is not caused by liver disease.
   c. It may result due to decreased retinol binding protein (RBP) concentration in circulating blood.
   d. Circulating retinol always correlates with total body vitamin A stores.
4. Which of the following is a major cause of fat-soluble vitamin deficiency?
   a. Decreased fat intake
   b. Hemolytic disease
   c. Renal insufficiency
   d. Malabsorption syndromes
5. Which of the listed vitamin deficiencies is not associated with the disease state?
   a. Xerophthalmia—vitamin A
   b. Beriberi—vitamin $B_1$
   c. Wernicke-Korsakoff syndrome—vitamin $B_2$
   d. Hartnup disease—niacin
6. Which of the following enzymes does not require selenium for functionality?
   a. Glutathione peroxidase
   b. Selenophosphate synthetase
   c. Glutathione reductase
   d. Iodothyronine deiodinase
7. Which of the following best facilitates the diagnosis of copper dysfunction as in Wilson disease?
   a. Liver biopsy
   b. 24-hour urine copper output
   c. Urine copper post penicillamine challenge
   d. Serum copper
8. Which of the following conditions does not result in low serum copper and ceruloplasmin?
   a. Menkes syndrome
   b. Wilson disease
   c. Keshan disease
   d. Aceruloplasminemia
9. How would you investigate a patient suspected of taking excess supplements of essential trace elements such as Cu, Zn, and/or Se? By measuring:
   a. different organo-inorganic species.
   b. urine output corrected for creatinine.
   c. impact on renal and/or liver function.
   d. whole blood and plasma content of the named trace elements.

## SUGGESTED READINGS

Ayling R, Marshall WD. *Nutrition and Laboratory Medicine.* London: ACB Venture Press; 2007.

Bates CJ. Vitamin analysis. *Ann Clin Biochem.* 1997;34:599–626.

Battersby AR. How nature builds the pigments of life: the conquest of vitamin $B_{12}$. *Science.* 1994;264:1551–1557.

Gibson RS. *Principles of Nutritional Assessment.* 2nd ed. Oxford: Oxford University Press; 2005.

Roberts NB, Taylor A, Sodi R. Vitamins and trace elements. In: Nader R, Horwarth AR, Wittwer CT, eds. *Tietz Textbook of Clinical Chemistry and Molecular Diagnostics.* 6th ed. St. Louis: Elsevier; 2018:639–718.

Rosenfeld L. Vitamine—vitamin. The early years of discovery. *Clin Chem.* 1997;43:680–685.

Shenkin A. The role of vitamins and minerals. *Clin Nutr.* 2003;22(suppl 2):S29–S32.

Taylor A. Detection and monitoring of disorders of essential trace elements. *Ann Clin Biochem.* 1996;33:486–510.

# 28

# Hemoglobin and Iron

*Christina Ellervik and Dorine W. Swinkels*

## OBJECTIVES

1. Define the following:
   - Anemia of chronic disease
   - Ferritin
   - Hereditary hemochromatosis
   - Hemoglobin
   - Hemoglobinopathy
   - Soluble transferrin receptor (sTfR)
   - Thalassemia
   - Transferrin
   - Transferrin saturation
   - Transfusion-induced iron overload
2. Describe the structure and physiological role of hemoglobin.
3. State the function of hemoglobin and its significance in health and disease.
4. List four different types of hemoglobin and state the makeup of the globin chains in each.
5. List four different types of thalassemia and state the globin deficiency and genetic defect in each.
6. Compare the differences between hemoglobinopathy and thalassemia with regard to causes and laboratory values.
7. List analytical methods used to assess the presence of a hemoglobinopathy or thalassemia.
8. Describe the principle of the cyanmethemoglobin method of hemoglobin determination.
9. Describe iron food sources.
10. Describe iron uptake, transport, distribution, and storage.
11. Describe systemic and cellular iron regulation.
12. List the three major disorders of iron metabolism.
13. Describe and contrast causes, clinical and laboratory findings for iron deficiency, hereditary hemochromatosis, and iron distribution disorder (anemia of chronic disease).
14. Compare the causes of primary, secondary, and juvenile hemochromatosis.
15. State the principle of chromogenic serum iron determination and the clinical significance of the results.
16. Define total iron-binding capacity (TIBC) and state how TIBC value is determined.
17. Describe how to calculate transferrin saturation (TSAT).
18. List analytical methods used to assess serum ferritin, iron, transferrin, hepcidin, and soluble transferrin receptor.
19. Describe how biological and pre-analytical variation impact laboratory findings for serum ferritin, iron, transferrin.

## KEY WORDS AND DEFINITIONS

**Anemia of chronic disease** Anemia of inflammation.

**Beta-thalassemia major** The homozygous form of β-thalassemia, a severe condition evident from the neonatal period with complete absence of hemoglobin A.

**Beta-thalassemia minor** The heterozygous form of β-thalassemia; it is usually asymptomatic, although hemoglobin A synthesis may be retarded and there is sometimes moderate anemia and splenomegaly.

**Carboxyhemoglobin** A form of hemoglobin in which the sites usually bound to oxygen are bound to carbon monoxide.

**Complete blood count (CBC)** The determination of the quantity of each type of blood cell in a milliliter of blood, often including the amount of hemoglobin, the hematocrit, and the proportions of various white cells. In certain countries it is referred to as the "full blood count."

**Ferritin** The iron/apoferritin complex, which is one of the chief forms in which iron is stored in the body; it occurs in the (1) gastrointestinal mucosa, (2) liver, (3) spleen, (4) bone marrow, and (5) reticuloendothelial cells.

**Heme** Any quadridentate chelate of iron with the four pyrrole groups of a porphyrin, further distinguished as ferroheme or ferriheme, referring to the chelates of Fe(II) and Fe(III), respectively.

**Hemochromatosis** A rare genetic disorder caused by deposition of hemosiderin in the parenchymal cells, resulting in tissue damage and dysfunction of the liver, pancreas, heart, and pituitary. Also called iron overload disease.

**Hemoglobin (Hb)** The oxygen-carrying pigment of the erythrocytes, formed by the developing erythrocyte in bone marrow. It is a conjugated protein containing four heme groups and globin, with the property of reversible oxygenation.

**Hemoglobinopathy** Any inherited disorder caused by abnormalities of hemoglobin, resulting in conditions such as sickle cell anemia, hemolytic anemia, or thalassemia.

**Hemosiderin**  An intracellular storage form of iron; the granules consist of an ill-defined complex of ferric hydroxides, polysaccharides, and proteins having an iron content of about 33% by weight.

**Hepcidin**  Hepcidin is a peptide hormone produced by the liver that regulates systemic iron.

**Hereditary hemochromatosis**  A genetically heterogeneous group of inherited disorders of iron metabolism characterized by failure to prevent excessive amounts of iron from entering the circulatory pool and accumulating in the tissues.

**Hereditary persistence of fetal hemoglobin**  A condition characterized by continued production of fetal hemoglobin beyond the point when it is normally replaced by hemoglobin A.

**Methemoglobin**  A form of hemoglobin where its iron atom is changed from the ferrous to the ferric state.

**Myoglobin**  A heme-containing protein found in red skeletal muscle.

**Sickle cell anemia**  An autosomal dominant type of hemolytic anemia that is caused by the presence of hemoglobin S with abnormal sickle-shaped erythrocytes *(sickle cells).*

**Soluble transferrin receptor**  A circulating truncated form of the transferrin receptor used in the diagnosis of iron deficiency.

**Thalassemia**  A heterogeneous group of hereditary hemolytic anemias having a decreased rate of synthesis of one or more hemoglobin polypeptide chains and classified according to the chain involved ($\alpha,\beta, \delta$); the two major categories are $\alpha$- and $\beta$-thalassemia.

**Transferrin**  A beta globulin that carries iron in the blood.

**Transferrin saturation**  The ratio of serum iron to total iron binding capacity, expressed as a ratio or percentage.

**Transfusion-induced iron overload**  Iron overload caused by transfusion.

## HEMOGLOBIN

### Biochemistry

Hemoglobin (Hb) is a globular protein with a diameter of 6.4 nm and a molecular mass of approximately 64,500 Da. Hb consists of four globin subunits: two $\alpha$- and two non–$\alpha$-chains ($\beta$-, $\gamma$-, or $\delta$-chains). Heme is composed of porphyrin to which an iron atom is attached. The four globin chains form a thick-walled globular shell surrounding a central cavity, in which the heme portion, attached by interaction of the histidine residues of the globin chains to the iron in heme, is suspended (Fig. 28.1). The heme iron is normally in the ferrous ($^{2+}$) oxidation state.

### Globin Structure of Normal and Fetal Hemoglobin

In healthy human adults, HbA is composed of two normal $\alpha$- and two normal $\beta$-polypeptide chains and is represented symbolically as $\alpha_2\beta_2$; it represents at least 96% of the total Hb contained in a sample of whole blood. HbA$_2$ is typically approximately 2.5% to 3.0% of total Hb; it contains two $\alpha$- and two $\delta$-chains and is designated as $\alpha_2\delta_2$. HbA$_2'$ is considered a variant of HbA$_2$ and is the result of a glycine-to-arginine substitution in the 16th position of the $\delta$-chain. It rarely forms more than 3% of the total Hb. Fetal Hb (HbF) predominates during fetal life but rapidly diminishes during the first year of postnatal life. In healthy adults, less than 1% of Hb is HbF. It consists of two $\alpha$- and two $\gamma$-chains ($\alpha_2\gamma_2$).

### Modified Hemoglobins

In addition to the Hbs discussed previously, carboxyhemoglobin, methemoglobin, and sulfhemoglobin are other Hbs whose structure has been environmentally or chemically modified.

Each of the modified Hbs has a characteristic spectral pattern, as shown in Fig. 28.2. These spectral characteristics form the basis of analysis in the many co-oximeters and blood gas analyzers that provide, in a single analysis, the simultaneous quantitative measurement of carboxyhemoglobin, methemoglobin, and sulfhemoglobin. The spectral scans are performed using multidiode arrays covering a number of wavelengths, followed by patented calculations that discriminate between normal and modified Hbs.

*Carboxyhemoglobin.* Carboxyhemoglobin is formed by the preferential attachment of carbon monoxide instead of oxygen to Hb, compromising the oxygen-carrying ability of hemoglobin. Carboxyhemoglobin concentrations are increased in smokers and employees with certain environmental exposures. Carboxyhemoglobin saturation that varies from 15% to 25% may be associated with dizziness, headaches, and nausea, and greater than 50% saturation is considered life threatening. The half-life of carboxyhemoglobin is 4 to 6 hours.

*Methemoglobin.* The Fe of heme is normally in the reduced ferrous state (Fe$^{2+}$). Under alkaline conditions, the Fe is oxidized to the ferric state (Fe$^{3+}$) by toxic agents, such as nitrates (found in some well waters), aniline dyes, chlorates, drugs (e.g., quinones, phenacetin, and sulfonamides), or local anesthetics (e.g., procaine, benzocaine, and lidocaine). This oxidation converts the heme to hematin and the Hb to methemoglobin. Patients with methemoglobin are cyanotic because methemoglobin is unable to reversibly bind oxygen. Methemoglobin is normally reduced to Hb in the cell by the reduced form of the nicotinamide-adenine dinucleotide–cytochrome reductase system.

*Sulfhemoglobin.* Sulfhemoglobin is produced by the reaction of sulfur-containing compounds with heme to form an irreversible chemical alteration and oxidation of Hb by the

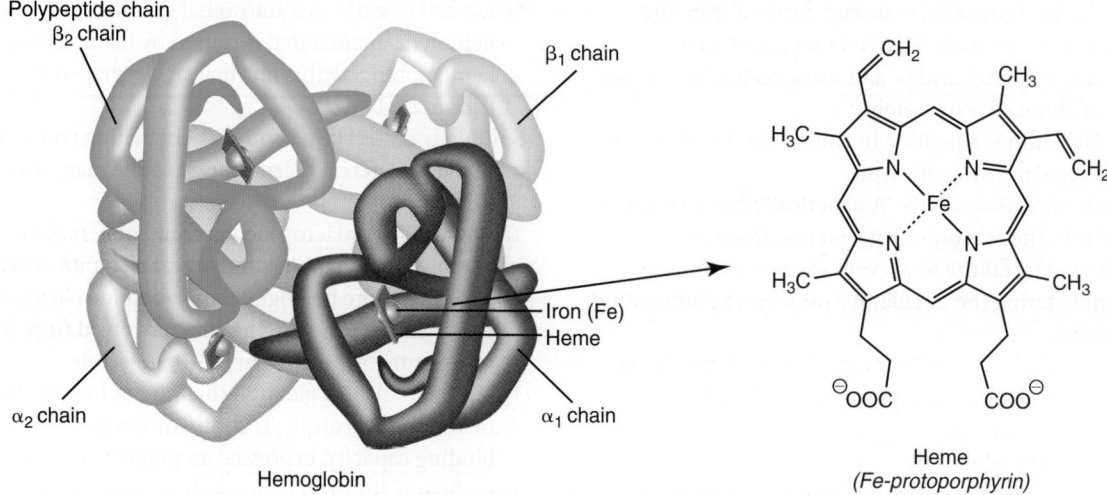

**Fig. 28.1** Model of the hemoglobin tetramer with the α-chain subunits facing the reader. Each subunit contains a molecule of heme attached to an atom of Fe.

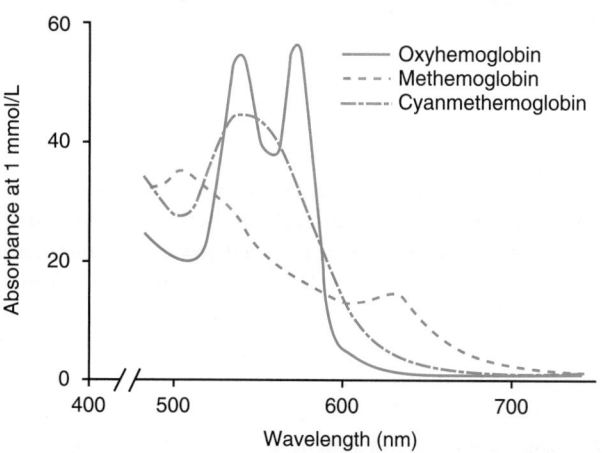

**Fig. 28.2** Spectrophotometric absorption curves for oxyhemoglobin, methemoglobin, and cyanmethemoglobin. Oxyhemoglobin and cyanmethemoglobin are used in measuring the concentration of hemoglobin *(Hb)*. The peak at 630 nm, which is distinctive for methemoglobin, is abolished by the addition of cyanide, and the resultant decrease in absorbance is directly proportional to the methemoglobin concentration. All heme proteins exhibit their maximum absorbance in the Soret band region of 400 to 440 nm. Because the absorbance of Hb in the Soret region is approximately 10 times the absorbance at 540 nm, the Soret peaks have been omitted from this diagram. The absorbance curve for methemoglobin is greatly influenced by small changes in pH. The curve given here was obtained at a pH of 6.6.

introduction of sulfur in one or more of the porphyrin rings. The most common cause of sulfhemoglobinemia is exposure to drugs, such as phenacetin and sulfonamides. Sulfhemoglobin cannot transport oxygen, and cyanosis is noted at low concentrations.

## Physiological Role

The Fe of heme is in the ferrous state ($Fe^{2+}$) and is able to combine reversibly with oxygen to act as the major oxygen-carrying moiety. The term *cooperativity* is used to describe the interaction of globin chains in such a way that oxygenation of one heme group enhances the probability of oxygenation

of the other heme group. The *Bohr effect* refers to reduction of oxygen affinity, with a decrease in pH from the physiologic range (7.35 to 7.45) to 6.0 and is another result of this cooperativity. Because the pH of the tissue decreases as a result of the presence of the end products of anaerobic metabolism, carbon dioxide ($CO_2$) and carbonic acid, the delivery of oxygen to the exercising tissue is enhanced. The oxygen dissociation curve of normal blood Hb is sigmoidal (Fig. 28.3). Physiologically, the $CO_2$ reversibly combines with the amino terminal groups of Hb to form carbamated Hb, which facilitates the removal of approximately 10% of the $CO_2$ that forms because of metabolism in the tissue to the lungs. Removal and transport of $CO_2$ from the tissue are enhanced by the preference for the attachment of more $CO_2$ by carbamated Hb.

## Clinical Significance

The **thalassemia** syndromes and **hemoglobinopathies** are clinical disorders related to Hb pathophysiology. Although they may have some similar clinical manifestations, they form two distinct disease groups of genetic origin. The thalassemias originate from insufficient or absent globin chain production due to gene deletion or nonsense mutations, which are mutations that affect the transcription or stability of messenger ribonucleic acid (mRNA) products. The name *thalassemia* is derived from the Greek word for "sea," *thalassa*, because early cases of β-thalassemia were described in children of Mediterranean origin.

Hemoglobinopathies, the most common single gene disorder in the world, are structural Hb variants arising from mutations in the globin genes, which result in substitutions or disruptions in the normal amino acid residue sequence in one or more of the globin chains of Hb.

The thalassemias and hemoglobinopathies occur worldwide and are particularly prevalent in Southeast Asia, Southern China, Mediterranean countries (particularly Greece and the Greek Cypriot part of Cyprus), India, the Middle East, Africa, and the islands of the South Pacific. With increasing migration, the thalassemias—once considered rare genetic diseases

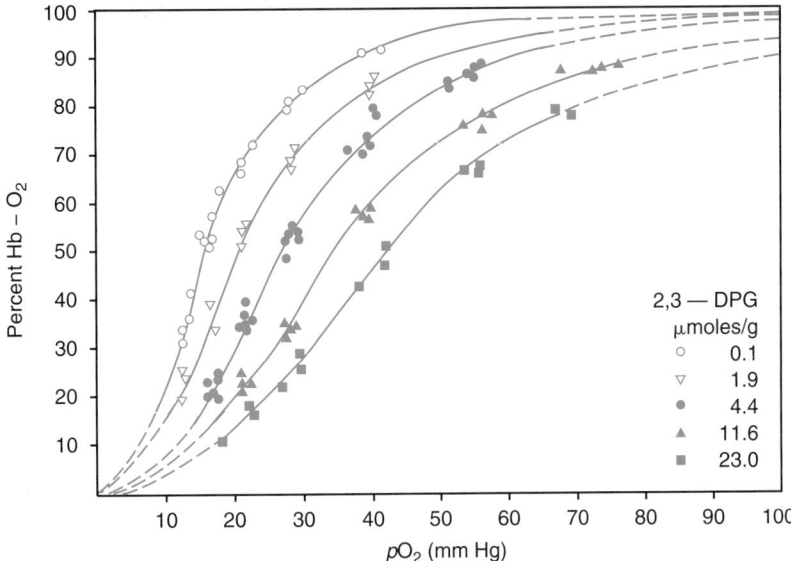

**Fig. 28.3** Normal oxygen dissociation curve of hemoglobin *(Hb)*. Changes in 2,3-diphosphoglycerate *(2,3-DPG)* concentration in the erythrocyte greatly influence the position of the curve. As the concentration of 2,3-DPG increases, the curve shifts to the right. *pO₂*, Partial pressure of oxygen. (From Duhm J. The effect of 2,3-DPG and other organic phosphates on the Donnan equilibrium and the oxygen affinity of human blood. In: Roth M, Astrup P, eds. *Oxygen Affinity of Hemoglobin and Red Cell Acid Base Status.* Copenhagen, Denmark: Alfred Benzon Foundation; 1972.)

in Northern Europe, Australia, and North America—are now becoming more common all over the world.

## Thalassemia Syndromes

Thalassemias are identified by the globin chain in which a production deficiency occurs. For example, α- and β-thalassemias result from a deficiency in α- or β-globin chain production, respectively. They are further clinically classified depending on the extent of globin chain production and the resultant severity of the anemia. All the thalassemias have a similar pattern of inheritance: in most cases the gene defects are transmitted in a Mendelian autosomal fashion. Thus, the severe symptomatic varieties result from the interaction of more than one genetic determinant. The inheritance of α-thalassemia is more complicated because it involves the products of the linked pairs of α genes (αα).

*Alpha (α)-thalassemias.* The α-thalassemias arise from deficiencies in production of the α-globin chains and are caused by deletions or (less frequently) point mutations in one or more of the four α-globin genes. There are two major classes of α-thalassemias: α⁰ in which both α genes are inactivated (−/), and α⁺ thalassemias, in which only one of the pair is defective either due to α deletion or to α mutation. The conventional nomenclature for the point mutations of an α-gene is "αᵀα," and for deletion, it is "−α." The clinical spectrum of α-thalassemias correlates well with the number of the affected α-genes (i.e., from normal to the loss of all four genes). The inheritance of a normal allele (ααα) with one of the α⁺or α⁰ results, most frequently, in an *"alpha (α)-thalassemia minor"* (− −/αα; −α/αα; −αᵀα/αα; αᵀα/−α; −α/−α) (Table 28.1). *Alpha (α)-thalassemia minor* is also called *alpha (α)-thalassemia*

*trait.* The complete blood count (CBC) in patients with alpha (α)-thalassemia minor shows a mildly reduced Hb with low mean corpuscular volume (MCV) and mean corpuscular hemoglobin (MCH). Alpha-thalassemias are common in areas where β-thalassemia is also found at a high frequency. Thus, the coinheritance of α- and β-thalassemia traits may occur and even ameliorate the hematological parameters. *Alpha-thalassemia silent* describes an α-thalassemia trait with a single α-globin chain gene deletion or mutation (−α/αα;αᵀ α/αα).

*Hemoglobin Bart's* results from deletion of all four α-globin genes, with the subsequent inability to produce any α-globin chains, leading to failure of synthesis of Hb A, F, or A₂. In the fetus, an excess number of γ-globin chains join together to form unstable tetramers known as Hb Bart's (γ⁴). Mothers who carry a fetus with Hb Bart's usually present clinically between 20 and 26 weeks' gestation with pregnancy-induced hypertension, polyhydramnios, and hydrops fetalis.

**Hemoglobin H disease.** This disorder is usually caused by a three α-globin gene deletion (−−/−α) and is characterized by a chronic anemia of variable severity.

*Beta (β)-thalassemias.* The β-thalassemias result from a reduction in the synthesis of the β-globin chain. The high frequency of β-thalassemia in the tropics is believed to reflect an advantage of heterozygotes against *Plasmodium falciparum* malaria.

The clinical classification of β-thalassemia includes beta-thalassemia major (TM; transfusion-dependent), thalassemia intermedia (TI; of intermediate severity, nontransfusion-dependent), and beta-thalassemia minor

## TABLE 28.1    The Alpha-Thalassemias

| Condition | Affected Number of Alpha-Globin Genes | Phenotype |
|---|---|---|
| Silent carrier | One | Asymptomatic or occasional low red blood cell indices |
| Alpha (α)-thalassemia trait (also called alpha-thalassemia minor) | Two | Mild microcytic and hypochromic anemia |
| Hemoglobin H disease | Three | Mild-to-moderate anemia, splenomegaly, jaundice |
| Alpha-thalassemia major/Hb Bart's hydrops | Four | Most severe form<br>Hb Bart's hydrops<br>Death in utero or at birth |

*Hb*, Hemoglobin.
Data from Vichinsky EP. Alpha thalassemia major—new mutations, intrauterine management, and outcomes. *Hematol Am Soc Hematol Educ Program*. 2009;35–41.

(asymptomatic). The severity of the clinical manifestations correlates well with the degree of imbalance of globin chains, depending on the β-globin gene defects and their interaction. The production of β-globin chains is quantitatively reduced to different degrees, whereas the synthesis of α-globin continues as normal, resulting in an accumulation of excess unmatched α-globin chains in the erythroid precursors. Clinical manifestations of β-thalassemia range from mild anemia to severe life-threatening disease that requires lifelong transfusions (Table 28.2).

**Beta-thalassemia (beta-thalassemia major; beta-TM).** Beta-TM results from mutations that interfere with translation or are involved in the initiation, elongation, or termination of globin chain synthesis. Mutations that interfere with translation account for almost 50% of all β-thalassemia mutations. Included in this are frame shift or nonsense mutations that produce premature termination codons, which result in incomplete translation of the β-globin gene and nonproduction of the β-globin chain, leading to β-thalassemia. Clinical presentation usually occurs at younger than 1 year of age, with features such as small size for age, abdominal girth expansion, and failure to thrive. Physical examination of the patient may reveal frontal bossing (an unusually prominent forehead) caused by thickening of the cranial bones, pallor, and prominence of the cheek bones, which in older children obscures the base of the nose and exposes the teeth. These features are a result of marrow expansion (up to a 30-fold increase) caused by ineffective erythropoiesis with production of highly unstable α-globin tetramers, leading to a sequence of events responsible for bone marrow expansion, anemia, hemolysis, splenomegaly, and increased Fe absorption. Typical CBC results include severe anemia with Hb concentration between 3 and 6.5 g/dL (30 and 65 g/L), MCV of 48 to 72 fL, and MCH of 23 to 32 pg, and varying size of red blood cells (RBCs) (anisocytosis).

**Beta-thalassemia intermedia (beta-TI).** Beta-TI is a clinical term used to describe patients with anemia and splenomegaly, but who do not have the full spectrum of clinical severity found in TM. Most β-TI patients are homozygotes or compound heterozygotes for mild-to-moderate

β-gene mutations (β⁺/β⁺; β/β⁺), less commonly, only a single β-globin gene is affected. Mildly affected patients are almost completely asymptomatic until adult life, experiencing only mild anemia and spontaneously maintaining Hb levels between 7 and 10 g/dL (70 to 100 g/L). In adult life, Hb is significantly reduced to values between 6 and 10 g/dL (60 to 100 g/L).

**Beta-thalassemia minor (beta-thalassemia trait).** Patients with β-thalassemia minor are often asymptomatic, except at times of hematopoietic stress, such as infection or pregnancy, when they can become more anemic. The CBC of patients with a β-thalassemia trait shows mild anemia with low normal or decreased Hb concentration and hematocrit, decreased MCV (<80 fL) and MCH (<25 pg), and variable red cell distribution widths.

**Delta-/beta-thalassemia.** The δβ-thalassemias are the result of deletions that affect various parts of the β-globin locus.

**Hereditary persistence of fetal hemoglobin.** The term **hereditary persistence of fetal hemoglobin (HPFH)** is used to describe a group of genetic conditions in which the concentration of Hb F is increased above the upper limit of the reference interval because of a reduction in β-globin synthesis and a compensatory increase in δ-globin synthesis. HPFH is divided into *deletional* and *non-deletional* HPFH.

## Hemoglobinopathies

*Nomenclature.* Hb variants are named using (1) letters (Hbs S, D, E, and so on), (2) the family name of the index case (Hb Lepore), (3) the place of discovery of the variant or place of origin of the initial identified case (the propositus; Hb Edmonton), or (4) the name of the river (Hb Saale) flowing through the city in which the propositus lived. In some cases, both a letter and a name are used, as in Hb J-Baltimore, indicating that the Hb is classified as having electrophoretic mobility similar to that of other J Hbs, but differs from them in amino acid sequence, and was originally discovered in Baltimore. The term *AS trait* (sometimes abbreviated to *S trait*) is used to describe a heterozygous state in which one of the β-globin chains is S and the other is A. In instances in which no normal β-globin chain is present (e.g., HbSD), the

## TABLE 28.2  Typical Clinical Characteristics of Beta-Thalassemia Major and Intermedia

| | Beta-Thalassemia Major | Beta-Thalassemia Intermedia |
|---|---|---|
| Age at onset, years | <2 | >2 |
| Transfusion | Dependent: lifelong, regular | Non-dependent: frequent, occasional, never |
| Organ manifestations | | |
| Endocrine | Hypothyroidism<br>Hypoparathyroidism<br>Hypogonadism<br>Diabetes | Uncommon |
| Cardiac and vascular system | Cardiac siderosis<br>Left-sided heart failure | Silent cerebral ischemia<br>Pulmonary hypertension<br>Right-sided heart failure<br>Venous thrombosis |
| Liver, biliary system | Hepatic failure<br>Viral hepatitis | Hepatic fibrosis<br>Hepatic cirrhosis<br>Hepatic cancer<br>Gallstones |
| Musculoskeletal and skin | Osteoporosis | Osteoporosis<br>Leg ulcers<br>Skeletal deformities |
| Extramedullary hematopoiesis | Rare | Common |
| Splenomegaly | Mild if optimal treatment | Common and moderate to severe |
| **Genetics** | | |
| Type of mutation | Severe | Mild/silent |
| Parents | Both are carriers of beta-thalassemia minor | One or both are carriers of beta-thalassemia minor |
| Co-inheritance of alpha-thalassemia | No | Yes |

β-globin chain present in the higher concentration is usually, although not always, placed first. A systematic nomenclature system is now used alongside the variant name to describe the affected chain and location on the chain and the amino acid substitution. For example, Hb Spanish Town [α27(β8)-$^{Glu \to Val}$], a Hb variant named after a district in Kingston, Jamaica, and found in Jamaicans of African descent, results from a substitution of valine for glutamic acid in position 27 of the α-globin chain, which is located in position 8 of the B helix of the α-chain.

*Classification of hemoglobin variants.* Hb variants are classified according to the type of mutation. Single point mutations in α-globin chains give rise to substitution of one amino acid residue. As an example, Hb San Diego [β109(G11)$^{Val \to Met}$] has a methionine residue instead of the normal valine at position 109 of the β-chain.

**Types of hemoglobin variants.** Types of Hb variants include (1) deletion, (2) insertion, (3) deletion/insertion, (4) elongation, and (5) hybrid/fusion/crossover Hbs.

**Hemoglobin S.** Hemoglobin S [β6(A3)$^{Glu \to Val}$] in the heterozygous or homozygous state is the most widespread of the Hb variants and arises from a substitution of valine for glutamic acid at position six in the A helix of the β-globin chain. Approximately 8% of African Americans are heterozygous for Hb S, and homozygous Hb S is found in one in 500 newborns in this group. The widespread distribution of the single point gene mutation responsible for the synthesis of Hb S in areas where *P. falciparum* malaria is endemic is due to the protection of Hb S heterozygotes from the worst manifestations of this malaria. The homozygous condition is described as sickle cell anemia or sickle cell disease because of the sickle-shaped RBCs that occur when a sickle cell crisis occurs (Fig. 28.4). It is sometimes written as β$^S$β$^S$.

### Analytical Methods

Thalassemias and hemoglobinopathies are diagnosed and monitored using multiple assays. The methods used are divided into those used for presumptive identification (e.g., CBC, high-performance liquid chromatography [HPLC], and electrophoresis) and those used for definitive identification (deoxyribonucleic acid [DNA] sequencing and mass spectrometry). In addition to these tests, the iron status of the patient should be ascertained. Information on the ethnicity and/or nationality of the patient also provides useful information.

Ethylenediaminetetraacetic acid (EDTA) whole blood should be collected and testing should be performed within 5 days of collection; samples should be stored at 4°C.

### Analytical Methods for Hemoglobin

Analytical techniques used to measure RBCs and their indices, Hb, and related compounds include (1) determination of complete blood count, (2) electrophoresis, (3) immunoassay, (4) separation techniques such as HPLC, capillary

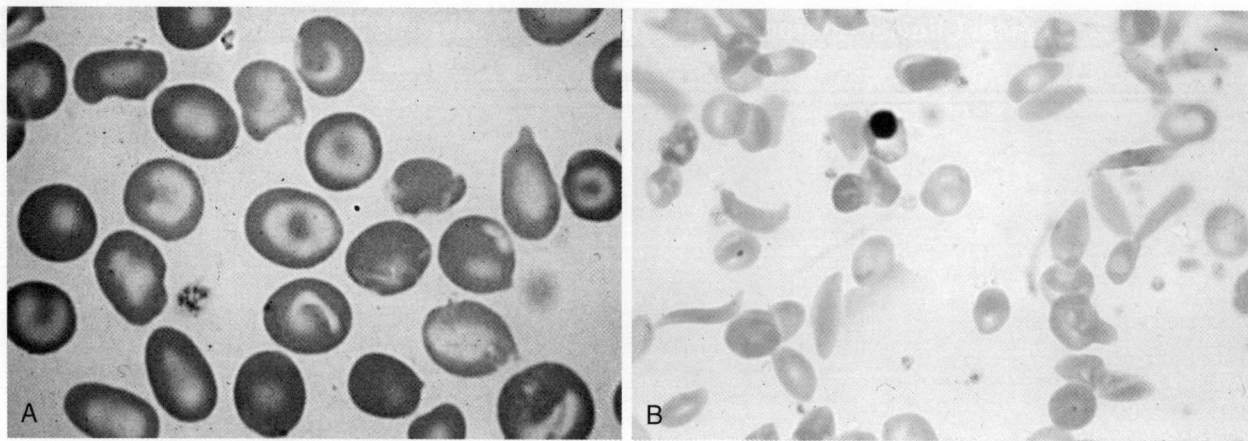

**Fig. 28.4** Peripheral blood smear from patients with (A) homozygous hemoglobin (Hb) E and (B) homozygous hemoglobin (Hb) S.

electrophoresis, and mass spectrometry, (5) molecular techniques such as DNA analysis, and (6) specific tests for specific variants.

*Routine measurement of hemoglobin.* Hemoglobin can be measured as part of the CBC on anticoagulated venous whole blood using automated hematology analyzers, on anticoagulated venous whole blood using manual methodology, and on capillary blood using point of care analyzers.

The CBC consists of (1) numbers of RBC (erythrocytes), (2) numbers of white blood cells (leukocytes), (3) numbers of platelets (thrombocytes), (4) a measure of Hb, and (5) various cell indices (Table 28.3). Measurement of hemoglobin using either manual, automated hemoglobin analyzers, or portable hemoglobinometers most often utilize a colorimetry method, in which hemoglobin is oxidized first to methemoglobin and then to cyanmethemoglobin, which is a stable color-intensive molecule that can be read photometrically.

*Electrophoresis.* Electrophoresis using agarose gel under alkaline conditions (pH 9.2) is the most common initial screening method for the detection and preliminary identification of hemoglobinopathies. Visualization of separated Hb bands is achieved by using a protein-binding stain, such as Amido Black or Ponceau S. Hb bands stain blue with Amido Black and reddish pink with Ponceau S.

At alkaline pH, Hbs migrate according to electrical charge, with HbH moving the fastest (closest to the anode). The order of migration (fastest to slowest) is HbH, HbN, HbI, HbJ, HbA, HbF, HbS, and HbC. HbD and HbG comigrate with HbS, whereas HbE, HbO, and $HbA_2$ comigrate with HbC. Hemoglobin Constant Spring migrates slightly toward the cathode. An easy way to remember the sequence is HbA goes to the anode, whereas HbC migrates to the cathode. HbF and HbS follow after HbA in alphabetical order.

Electrophoresis at pH 6.4 using a citrate buffer is performed when an abnormal band is noted on alkaline Hb electrophoresis. The same Hb variants separated on agarose electrophoresis at pH 6.4 and stained with acid violet are shown in the *right panel* of Fig. 28.5. The order of migration (cathode to anode, fastest to slowest) is HbF, HbA, HbS, and

HbC. HbD, HbG, HbI, HbJ, HbO, $HbA_2$, and HbE comigrate with HbA.

Specific types of electrophoresis that are used for Hb analysis include isoelectric focusing, conventional electrophoresis, and capillary electrophoresis.

**Isoelectric focusing electrophoresis.** Isoelectric-focusing electrophoresis (IEF) has greater resolving power than conventional electrophoresis, but it is more expensive, time-consuming, and technique-dependent to perform. Commercial IEF gels are made of cellulose acetate or polyacrylamide with the pH gradient produced by the inclusion of amphoteric materials of different pHs in bands in the gel. Locations of the Hb bands are identified using stains similar to those used in conventional electrophoresis. The bands or zones produced by IEF (Fig. 28.6) are more clearly defined than those seen with conventional electrophoresis, and reliable quantification of separated Hbs may be made at high concentrations using densitometry.

**Capillary isoelectric focusing electrophoresis.** Capillary IEF combines the detection sensitivity of capillary electrophoresis with the resolution qualities and existing extensive data on Hb variant separation by immunoelectrophoresis and the automated sampling and digital data acquisition techniques developed for chromatography. With this approach, the hemolysate is introduced into the capillary chamber using low-pressure injection and then is focused at high voltage (typically $\approx 30$ kV and 0.5 to 1.5 µA), during which it is essential to maintain adequate cooling. The separated Hbs are then eluted, using low-pressure and simultaneous voltage, past a single-wavelength spectrophotometric detector set to read at 415 nm or a dual-wavelength detector set at 415 and 450 nm.

**Capillary electrophoresis.** The introduction of commercial capillary electrophoresis instrumentation for the separation of Hbs has made this technique available to clinical laboratories. Separation in an alkaline buffer at a specific pH using high voltages is based on charge difference, electrolyte pH, and electro-osmotic flow. Hb measurement is commonly performed at a wavelength of 415 nm, and identification is based on retention time.

## TABLE 28.3 Definition of the Parameters That Constitute a Complete Blood Count

| Parameter | Definition |
|---|---|
| WBC | The number of WBCs in the blood |
| WBC differential count | The number (or percentage) of each type of WBC present in the blood: neutrophils, basophils, eosinophils, lymphocytes, monocytes |
| RBC count | The number of RBCs in the blood |
| Hct | The Hct is the proportion of blood volume that is occupied by RBCs |
| Hb | The protein molecule in RBCs that carries oxygen |
| MCV | The MCV is the average volume of RBCs |
| Mean corpuscular Hb | The average amount of Hb in the average RBC |
| Mean corpuscular Hb concentration | The average concentration of Hb in a given volume of blood |
| Red cell distribution width | A measurement of the variability of RBC size |
| Platelet count | The calculated number of platelets in a volume of blood |
| Platelet distribution width | A measurement of the variability of platelet size |
| Plateletcrit | The proportion of blood volume that is occupied by platelets |
| Mean platelet volume | The average volume of platelets |

*Hb,* Hemoglobin; *Hct,* hematocrit; *MCV,* mean corpuscular volume; *RBC,* red blood cell; *WBC,* white blood cell.

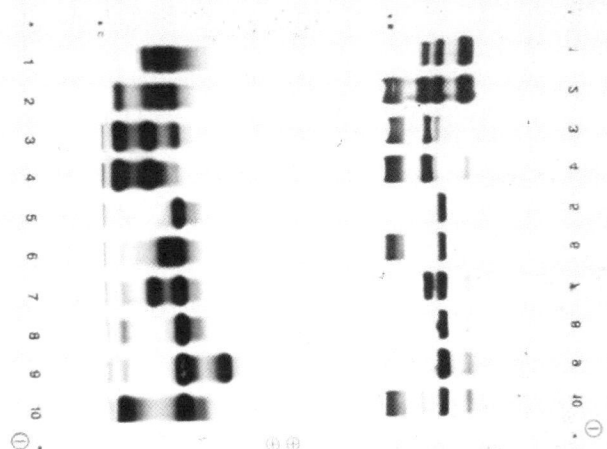

Fig. 28.5 Alkaline *(left)* and acid *(right)* electrophoresis of various hemoglobinopathies. Lane 1, hemoglobin (Hb) S, Hb FA control. Lane 2, HB S, Hb F, HbCA control. Lane 3, transfused sickle cell (SC) disease. Lane 4, SC disease. Lane 5, Hb A (normal). Lane 6, Hb Presbyterian. Lane 7, Hb S. Lane 8, raised Hb A2 (β-thalassemia trait). Lane 9, Hb J Baltimore. Lane 10, Hb C.

***High-performance liquid chromatography.*** HPLC using a column packed with cation-exchange resin provides—in a single analytical protocol—the quantification of HbF and HbA$_2$. With it, the initial identification of an Hb variant on the basis of elution time may be made. It has also been used to detect α-thalassemia phenotypes.

After injection and subsequent adsorption onto the particles of a cation-exchange resin, molecules of Hb are eluted using gradient elution. The detection of eluted Hbs is achieved by monitoring the effluent solvent stream using a dual-wavelength photometer (usually set to measure at wavelengths of 415 and 690 nm) (Fig. 28.7).

## Mass Spectroscopy

Mass spectrometry (MS) is becoming an accepted method for the characterization of Hb variants involving substitution of one or more amino acids in the globin protein chains. Tandem mass spectrometry (MS/MS) has been used for newborn screening for sickle cell disease and thalassemias.

Several MS-based approaches, sometimes using laborious preparative steps, have been described:
1. Measurement of the mass of intact globin chains and the relative proportion of β and δ globin chains. Alpha or β variants are followed up by peptide-based analysis, based on tryptic digestion of whole blood, using electrospray MS/MS in multiple reaction monitoring (MRM) mode to confirm identity.
2. Ultra-performance liquid chromatography coupled with MS/MS using predetermined tryptic peptides to screen for clinically important structural variants.
3. Mass measurement of intact globin chains without complex pre-analytical sample digestion/separation procedures followed by top-down electron transfer dissociation (ETD) fragmentation of selected globin chains for the confirmation of variants.

These techniques offer a faster and more specific detection and sequence confirmation of clinically significant Hb variants than conventional methods, but method implementation and result interpretation require special instrumentation and technical skill.

## Deoxyribonucleic Acid Analysis

DNA analysis is used in the investigation of thalassemias and hemoglobinopathies to identify specific individuals at risk and those who may benefit from genetic counseling in populations with a known high incidence of disease. For example, DNA analysis has been used to do the following:
1. Diagnose α$^0$- and α$^+$-thalassemia.

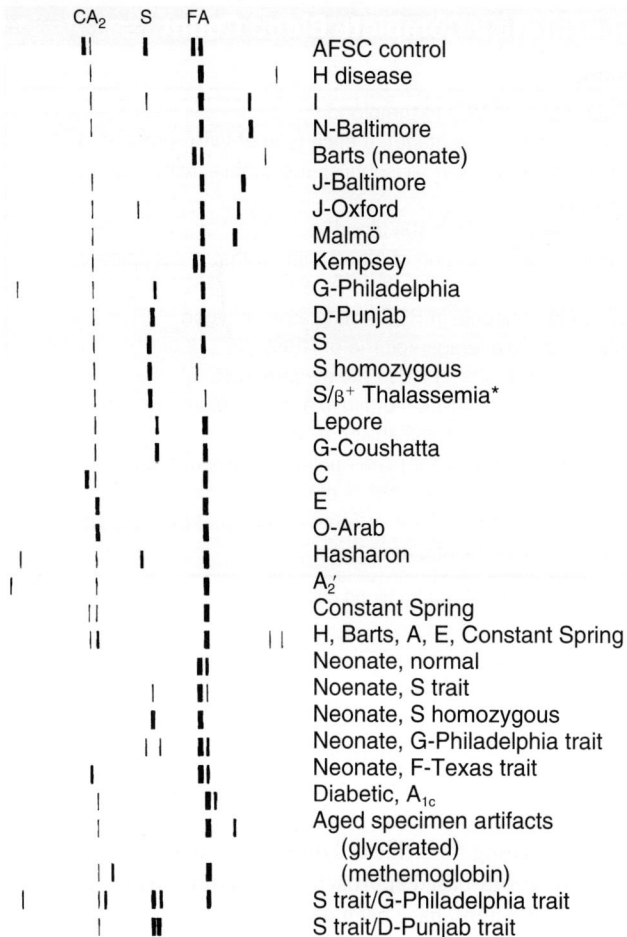

Fig. 28.6 A diagram of isoelectric focusing patterns for a variety of hemoglobin (Hb) variants. The conditions shown represent heterozygotes (traits), unless otherwise indicated. The width of the bars approximates the relative density of the bands observed. The acid anodic (pH 6) side is to the *right,* and the alkaline cathodic (pH 8) side is to the *left.* The same pattern is observed in homozygous patients with HbS disease who have received HbA by transfusion.

2. Investigate potentially life-threatening disorders of Hb synthesis in the fetus; it is performed at less than 10 weeks' gestation on chorionic villus samples.
3. Characterize the β-thalassemia genotype.
4. Screen at-risk populations for clinically significant Hb variants.
5. Distinguish between conditions that have similar laboratory and clinical presentations but are the result of different genetic conditions.

## Specific Tests

Tests that are used to measure Hbs and related analytes include those for HbH, HbS, unstable Hbs, and globin chains.

*Determining hemoglobin H.* HbH is an insoluble tetramer consisting of four β-globin chains that is produced when production of α-globin chains is decreased. If the tetramers are oxidized, precipitation occurs, and the precipitate may be viewed microscopically. In the laboratory, this oxidation

is achieved by staining unfixed cells with freshly prepared methylene blue or brilliant cresyl blue at 37°C.

*Sickling and hemoglobin S solubility tests.* Sickling tests are useful in confirming the presence of HbS in a sample after initial electrophoresis at alkaline pH. When HbS is oxygenated, it is fully soluble. When HbS is deoxygenated, polymerization occurs, forming deformed red cells with a characteristic rigid sickle shape. In the laboratory, deoxygenation and lysis of RBCs is achieved using a solution of sodium metabisulfite in a phosphate buffer. The addition of the sodium metabisulfite reagent to an HbS-containing blood sample induces the typical sickle shape of RBCs (which is the basis of the sickling test by microscopic investigation of the blood film preparation). The reaction also causes turbidity (which is the basis of the solubility test). In the HbS solubility test, turbidity is visualized by holding a lined card or a card with writing on it behind the reaction test tube (Fig. 28.8). A positive sample is not transparent, whereas a negative sample is. False negative results are obtained on anemic patients (Hb <8 g/dL; or <80 g/L) or on samples with hematocrit less than 15% (0.15). False positive results are found in samples with (1) Heinz bodies, (2) high concentrations of monoclonal protein, (3) hyperlipidemia, or (4) cold agglutinins. The test is subjective, and the combination of two identification techniques, such as HPLC and alkaline electrophoresis, may eliminate the necessity to perform this test on a routine basis.

*Tests for unstable hemoglobins.* These tests use heat (heat stability test) or isopropanol (isopropanol stability test) to precipitate the unstable Hb, and must be performed on fresh blood. A precipitate will form if unstable hemoglobins are present. More than 100 unstable Hbs are mainly the result of the interchange of nonpolar amino acid residues for polar amino acid residues in positions in the α- or β-globin chain associated with the heme cleft.

## IRON

Iron is involved in the function of all cells. It can accept and donate electrons, depending on its oxidation state: ferrous iron (Fe[II]) or ferric iron (Fe[III]). Iron is mostly locked into Fe protoporphyrin (heme) and Fe–sulfur clusters, which serve as enzyme cofactors. Hemoproteins are involved in numerous biological functions, such as oxygen binding and transport (Hbs), oxygen metabolism (catalases, peroxidases), cellular respiration, and electron transport (cytochromes). Proteins containing nonheme Fe are important for fundamental cellular processes such as DNA synthesis, cell proliferation and differentiation (ribonucleotide reductase), gene regulation, drug metabolism, and steroid synthesis. However, Fe can also cause damage, because Fe(II) catalyzes the generation of highly reactive hydroxyl radicals (·OH) from hydrogen peroxide ($H_2O_2$) ($Fe^{2+} + H_2O_2 \rightarrow Fe^{3+} + HO^- + HO\cdot$), which is called the "Fenton reaction." These hydroxyl radicals damage cellular membranes, proteins, and DNA. A large number of scavenger molecules protect cells against Fe-mediated tissue damage. Proteins sequester Fe to reduce this threat.

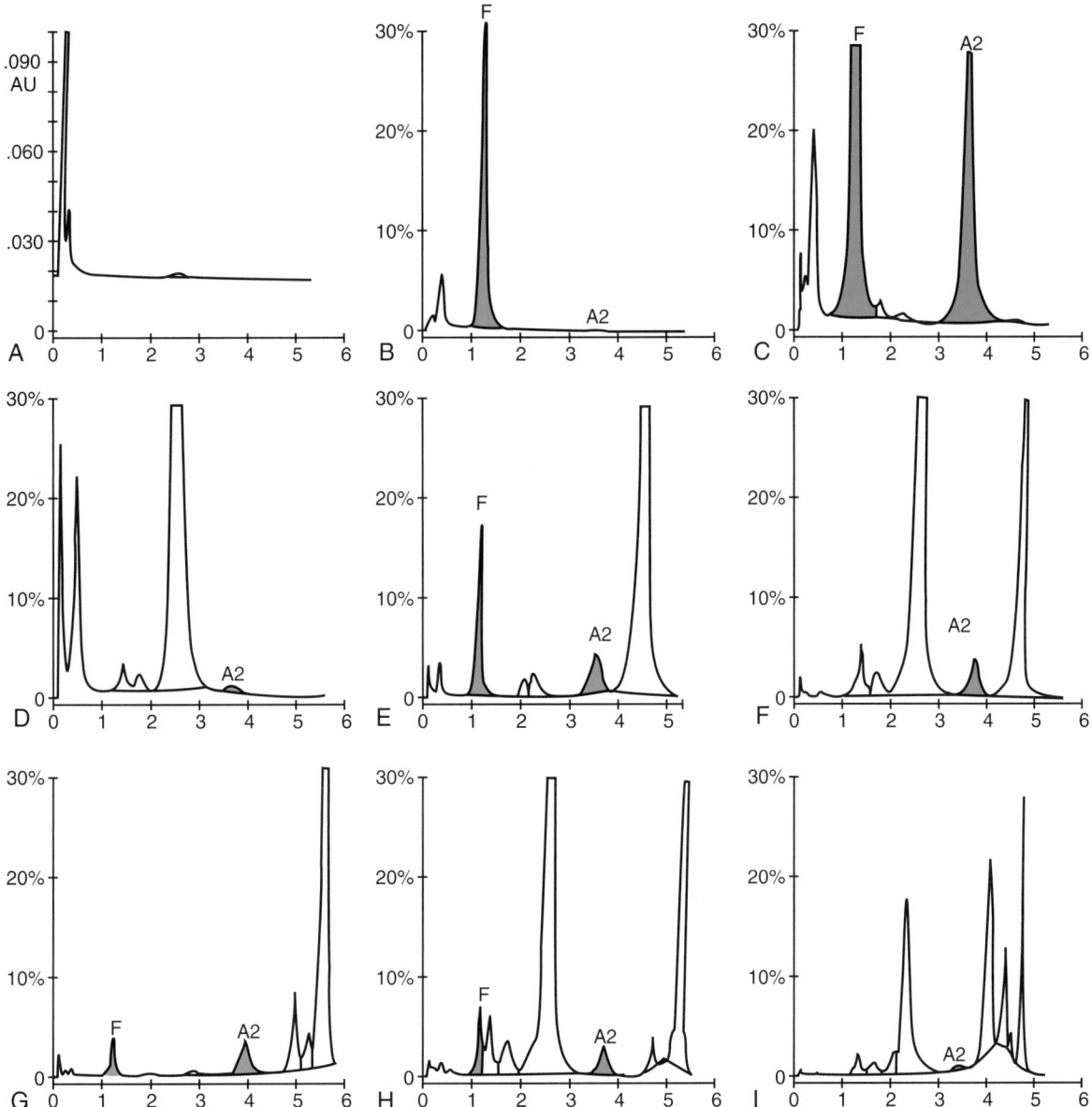

**Fig. 28.7** High-performance liquid chromatography chromatograms obtained on the Bio-Rad Variant β-thal short program for (A) hemoglobin (Hb) Bart's; (B) β⁰-thalassemia major; (C) B⁺-thalassemia homozygous E; (D) HbH; (E) homozygous S; (F) S trait; (G) homozygous C; (H) C trait; and (I) HbS-HbG Philadelphia. (From Clarke GM, Trefor N, Higgins TN. Laboratory investigation of hemoglobinopathies and thalassemias: review and update. *Clin Chem.* 2000;46:1284–1290.)

Iron circulates in a form bound to plasma transferrin, which is needed to offer the highly insoluble Fe(III) to cells via the transferrin receptor. Iron can safely be stored within cells in the form of ferritin and hemosiderin. Under normal circumstances, only small amounts of Fe exist outside this physiologic sink, although stored Fe can be mobilized for reuse. Many diseases arise from imbalances in Fe homeostasis. Too much iron accumulates in hereditary hemochromatosis (HH) and in the iron-loading anemias, which are often aggravated by multiple transfusions. In iron-deficiency anemia (IDA), insufficient amounts of iron are available for heme synthesis. In anemia of chronic disease (ACD), iron is redistributed to macrophages to promote resistance to infections.

## Iron Metabolism
### Systemic and Cellular Iron Regulation

The control of iron homeostasis acts at both the cellular and the systemic level, and involves a complex system of different cell types, transporters, and signals. To maintain systemic iron homeostasis, communication between cells that absorb Fe from the diet (duodenal enterocytes), consume Fe (mainly erythroid precursors), and store Fe (hepatocyte and tissue macrophages) must be tightly regulated. Each of these cell types plays an essential role in the homeostatic Fe cycle. Hepcidin controls Fe absorption and macrophage Fe release. Hepcidin is synthesized in the liver upon changes in body iron needs, anemia, hypoxia, and inflammation, and is secreted in

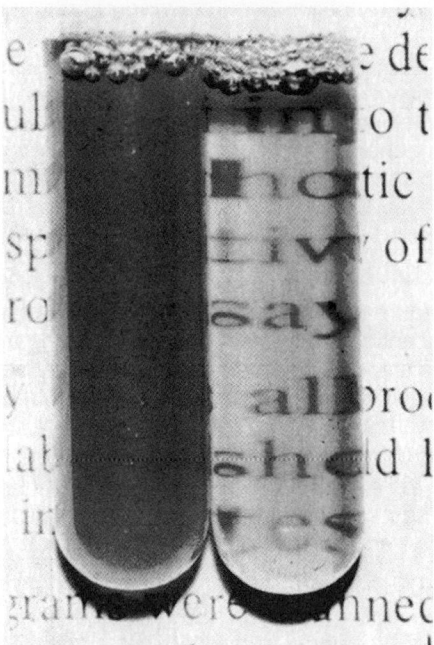

**Fig. 28.8** Solubility test for hemoglobin (Hb) S. Deoxyhemoglobin S *(left tube)* is insoluble in 2.3 mol/L phosphate buffer. In contrast, normal hemolysate *(right tube)* is sufficiently transparent that print can easily be read through it.

the circulation. It counteracts the function of ferroportin, a major cellular Fe exporter protein in the membrane of macrophages and the basolateral site of enterocytes, by inducing its internalization and degradation Fig. 28.9.

## Body Iron Distribution

See Table 28.4 for average distribution of body iron.

*Ferritin.* Ferritin is a heteropolymer of 24 subunits of two types, L (light) or H (heavy), which assemble to make a hollow spherical shell that can take up atoms of Fe stored as ferric oxyhydroxide phosphate. The ferroxidase activity of H-ferritin converts Fe(II) to Fe(III), which is necessary for Fe deposition into the nanocage. L-ferritin induces Fe nucleation. L-ferritin is predominant in iron-storing tissues (liver, reticuloendothelial), whereas H-ferritin is preferentially expressed in cells with a significant antioxidant activity (brain, heart). Ferritin occurs in nearly all body cells and stores iron in a form that is shielded from body fluids and is therefore unable to cause oxidative damage. Ferritin in hepatocytes and macrophages provides a reserve of iron that is available for synthesis of Hb and other heme proteins. In healthy men, ≈1000 mg of storage iron is present, mostly as ferritin. In healthy premenopausal women, storage iron varies up to ≈300 mg. Relative to tissues, minute quantities of relatively iron-poor ferritin are also present in serum in concentrations roughly proportional to total body iron stores. However, when elevated, serum ferritin does not always correlate with body iron content. Relatively large amounts of ferritin may be released into plasma as the result of diverse pathological conditions, among which are infections, chronic inflammatory diseases, chronic liver diseases, the metabolic syndrome, and nonalcoholic steatohepatitis (NASH).

*Hemosiderin.* Hemosiderin is formed when ferritin is aggregated and partially deproteinized in secondary lysosomes. Like ferritin, hemosiderin is found predominantly in cells of the (1) liver, (2) spleen, and (3) bone marrow. Unlike ferritin, hemosiderin is insoluble in aqueous solutions.

*Tissue iron.* Numerous cellular enzymes and coenzymes require Fe as an integral part of the molecule or as a cofactor. These include *peroxidases* and *cytochromes,* all of which are heme proteins, like Hb. Other enzymes, such as *aconitase* and *ferredoxin,* contain iron that is coordinated with sulfur in a so-called Fe–sulfur cluster. These enzymes and coenzymes occur in all nucleated cells of the body and form the *tissue Fe compartment,* normally ≈150 mg of Fe (see Table 28.4).

Myoglobin very closely resembles a single Hb subunit and contains a single heme per molecule.

*The labile iron pool.* A fraction of the circulating nontransferrin-bound iron (NTBI) is redox-active and designated labile plasma Fe. Although there are methods for measuring serum NTBI and labile plasma Fe, insufficient standardization and clinical correlation currently limit clinical use of these measurements.

*Iron transport.* Iron is transported from one organ to another in the plasma by the transport protein *apotransferrin.* The apotransferrin/Fe$^{3+}$ complex is called mono-ferric or diferric (=holo) transferrin. When transferrin binds to the *transferrin receptor* of cells, the transferrin/receptor complex is internalized into an endosome that becomes acidified, releasing the Fe(III) from transferrin. Fe(III) is then converted to Fe(II) by a ferrireductase, and transported to the cytosol via the divalent metal transporter DMT1. The apotransferrin is then transported back to the cell surface, ready to transport another transferrin molecule to the interior of the cell. This series of reactions has been designated the *transferrin cycle.*

### Regulation of iron homeostasis

**Systemic iron regulation.** The total body iron content can only be regulated by absorption from the upper intestinal tract, whereas iron loss occurs passively from sloughing of skin and mucosal cells, as well as from blood loss. Hepcidin, a peptide hormone produced by the liver, regulates systemic iron by decreasing Fe absorption from the diet as well as Fe export from macrophages. As a consequence, elevated hepcidin levels result in a decrease of plasma Fe concentration.

**Normal iron balance.** The average daily American diet contains 10 to 15 mg of Fe, much of it in the form of (1) heme proteins, (2) Hb, and (3) myoglobin in meat. Normally, ≈1 to 2 mg of Fe is absorbed each day, mostly by the duodenum. To be absorbed, inorganic Fe must be in the Fe$^{2+}$ state. Dietary heme is taken up via an unknown transport system.

**Proteins that affect iron homeostasis.** Many proteins influence iron homeostasis. Mutations in genes that encode these proteins may cause several inherited iron disorders, among which are iron overload or iron deficiency. Table 28.5 summarizes the effects of some of these proteins on iron homeostasis.

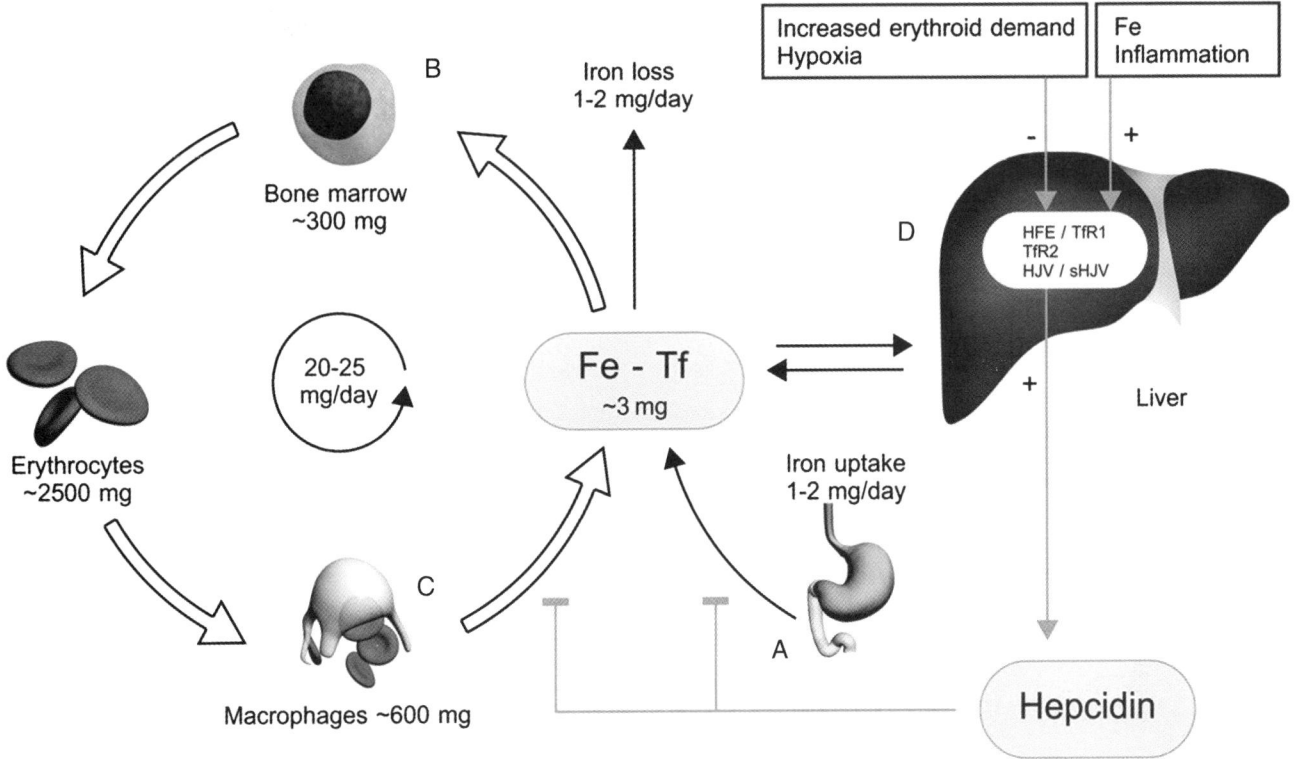

**Fig. 28.9** Systemic iron (Fe) homeostasis. The largest flux of Fe takes place in the recycling of Fe from senescent erythrocytes out of (A) macrophages to incorporation in (B) erythroid precursors in the bone marrow. Values for the different tissues and fluxes are approximate. The (D) liver and (C) reticuloendothelial macrophages function as major iron stores. Only 1 to 2 mg Fe is absorbed and lost every day. Importantly, the total amount of Fe in the body can only be regulated by absorption, whereas Fe loss occurs only passively from sloughing of skin and mucosal cells, as well as from blood loss. Hepcidin, a recently identified antimicrobial, β-defensin-like peptide secreted by the liver, decreases the plasma Fe concentration by inhibiting Fe export by ferroportin from (A) duodenal enterocytes and (C) reticuloendothelial macrophages. As a consequence, an increase in hepcidin production results in a decrease in plasma Fe concentrations. Hepcidin expression of the hepatocyte is regulated by circulating and stored Fe, inflammatory stimuli, the erythroid Fe demand, and hypoxia, by pathways involving expression of *HFE, TFR2,* hemojuvelin *(HJV),* and *TMPRSS6* genes. In HFE-, transferrin receptor (TfR)-2, and HJV-related hereditary hemochromatosis, hepcidin production is low despite increased liver Fe, which results in inappropriately increased Fe absorption. Defects in the *TMPRSS6* gene, encoding for matriptase-2, result in Fe refractory iron-deficiency anemia. The letters *A, B, C,* and *D* refer to sites with special functions in iron metabolism. (From Swinkels DW, Janssen MC, Bergmans J, et al. Hereditary hemochromatosis: genetic complexity and new diagnostic approaches. *Clin Chem.* 2006;52:950–968.)

### TABLE 28.4  Iron Content of Compartments in an Average Male

| Compartment | Iron Content (mg) |
| --- | --- |
| Hemoglobin | 2,500 |
| Storage iron[a] | 1,000 |
| Myoglobin | 130 |
| Other cellular iron-containing proteins | 150 |
| Transport (transferrin) | 3 |
| Total | 3,000–5,000 |

[a]Sum of parenchymal and reticuloendothelial iron stored in ferritin or hemosiderin.

## Clinical Significance

Iron deficiency, iron overload, and ACD are the most prevalent disorders of iron metabolism. Iron disorders may be classified according to (1) pathophysiology (see Table 28.5), (2) heritability (genetic or acquired), or (3) as being "primary" (e.g., resulting from a defect in an iron metabolism-related protein) or "secondary" (e.g., the consequences of defects in other proteins).

### Iron Deficiency

Iron deficiency and IDA—defined when anemia and iron deficiency coexist—are global health problems and common medical conditions seen in everyday clinical practice.

Iron deficiency is particularly a disorder of children and premenopausal women in low- and middle-income countries, but it can also occur in men, and in high-income countries in people of all ages. In children, iron deficiency is frequently caused by the increased physiologic needs for dietary iron for growth and development. In adults, and especially premenopausal women, iron deficiency is almost always the result of chronic blood loss or childbearing.

## TABLE 28.5    Features of Iron Metabolism Disorders

| Disorder | Gene | Inheritance | Age at Presentation | Systemic Iron Overload | Anemia | Ferritin | TSAT |
|---|---|---|---|---|---|---|---|
| **Impaired Hepcidin-Ferroportin Axis** | | | | | | | |
| HH type 1 | *HFE* | AR | Adult | Variable | No | Variable | High |
| HH type II A | *HAMP* | AR | Child | Yes | No | High | High |
| HH type II B | *HJV* | AR | Child to young adult | Yes | No | High | High |
| HH type III | *TfR2* | AR | Young adult | Yes | No | High | High |
| HH type IVA | *SLC40A1* (LOF[a]) | AD | Adult | Yes | Sporadically | High | Normal |
| HH type IV B | *SLC40A1* (GOF) | AD | Adult | Yes | No | High | High |
| **Iron Transport Disorder** | | | | | | | |
| ***Low Iron Availability for Erythropoiesis*** | | | | | | | |
| IRIDA | *TMPRSS6* | AR/AD | | No | Yes | Low–normal | Low |
| Aceruloplasminemia | *CP* | AR | | Yes | Yes | High | Normal/low |
| Anemia of chronic disease | NA | NA | Variable | No[a] | Yes | Normal–high | Low |
| ***Defect in Iron Acquisition of Erythroid Progenitor Cells*** | | | | | | | |
| Hypotransferrinemia | *Tf* | AR | | Yes | Yes | High | 100% |
| Microcytic anemia with iron loading | *DMT1* | AR | | Yes | Yes | Variable | High |
| **Erythroid Dysmaturation** | | | | | | | |
| Nontransfusion-dependent thalassemias (β-thalassemia intermedia; HbH disease) | Globin | AR | Variable | Yes | Yes | High | High |
| **Sideroblastic Anemia Congenital** | | | | | | | |
| X-linked sideroblastic anemia | *ALAS-2* | XL | Child | Variable | Mild/no anemia | Variable | Variable |
| Sideroblastic anemia | *SLC25A38* | AR | Child | Yes | Severe | High | High |
| Sideroblastic anemia | *GLRx5* | AR | Adult | Yes | Mild | High | High |
| Sideroblastic anemia with ataxia | *ABCB7* | XL | Child | No | Mild | Normal | Normal |
| Myelodysplastic syndrome (RA, RARS) | NA | NA | Adult | Variable | Variable | Variable | Variable |
| Congenital dyserythropoietic anemia Type Ia, Ib, II, III, IV | *CDAN1, C15ORF41, SEC23B, KIF23, KLF1* | Variable | Child | Variable | Yes | Variable | High |
| **Other Iron Disorders** | | | | | | | |
| Localized iron overload | | | | | | | |
| Neurodegeneration with brain iron accumulation | | | | | | | |
| Neonatal hemochromatosis | NA | NA | Neonate | Yes | No | Yes | Yes |
| Iron overload in sub-Saharan Africa | Unclear | Unclear | Adult | Yes | No | Yes | Yes |
| Hyperferritinemia-cataract syndrome | *FTL*-IRE | AD | Variable | No | No | High | Normal |
| Chronic liver disease | NA | NA | Variable | No/mild | Variable | Variable/high | Variable |
| Metabolic syndrome | | | | | | | |
| Steatohepatitis | | | | | | | |
| Cirrhosis | | | | | | | |

*Continued*

## TABLE 28.5  Features of Iron Metabolism Disorders—cont'd

| Disorder | Gene | Inheritance | Age at Presentation | Systemic Iron Overload | Anemia | Ferritin | TSAT |
|---|---|---|---|---|---|---|---|
| Parenteral iron loading/chronic erythrocyte transfusion | NA | NA | Variable | Yes | No | High | High |
| Iron deficiency (anemia) | NA | NA | Variable | No | Variable | Low | Low |

[a]Often referred to as "ferroportin disease."

*GOF*, Gain of function mutation; *HH*, hereditary hemochromatosis; *IRE*, iron response element; *IRIDA*, iron refractory iron-deficiency anemia; *LOF*, loss of function mutation; *RA*, refractory anemia; *RARS*, refractory anemia with ringed sideroblasts; *TSAT*, transferrin saturation.

Iron deficiency and IDA are associated with impaired quality of life, work productivity, aerobic exercise capacity, and fatigue, and there is also a relationship between iron status and depression and cognitive functioning. Iron deficiency also affects immune function and the susceptibility to infections. Furthermore, iron deficiency is a predictor of mortality in patients with chronic kidney disease and heart failure; treating iron deficiency in patients with heart failure improves quality of life.

IDA is generally an acquired condition due to blood losses, malabsorption, insufficient iron intake, or a combination of these. Some patients with chronic disease are especially vulnerable to develop absolute iron deficiency (e.g., patients with gastrointestinal tumors because of blood losses). Patients with advanced chronic kidney disease also have a negative Fe balance as a result of reduced dietary intake, impaired absorption from the gut, and increased Fe losses. In addition, patients with chronic kidney disease also often have a functional iron deficiency because the available circulating iron cannot keep pace with the requirements of erythropoiesis.

In patients with iron refractory iron-deficiency anemia (IRIDA), an inherited form of IDA due to a defect in the *TMPRSS6* gene encoding for the protein matriptase-2, the iron deficiency does not improve with oral Fe supplementation. This disorder is an indication for intravenous Fe treatment.

Many different measurements have been advocated for the diagnosis of iron deficiency. Overall, a low ferritin level is a sensitive and specific indicator of iron deficiency uncomplicated by other diseases. A transferrin saturation (<15% to 20%) indicates an iron supply that is insufficient to support normal erythropoiesis (Tables 28.6 and 28.7). Hb below normal combined with iron deficiency defines IDA. Soluble transferrin receptor (sTfR) is helpful in the investigation of the pathophysiology of anemia, to distinguish IDA from ACD and to detect functional iron deficiency. In the different stages of iron deficiency, the various biochemical and hematological tests efficiently complement each other and help characterize the severity in the individual patient (Fig. 28.10).

### Anemia of Chronic Disease

Anemia of chronic disease, also named anemia of inflammation, is a common disorder. It is often observed in patients with infectious and inflammatory diseases, among whom are patients with chronic kidney disease, inflammatory bowel disease, chronic heart failure, malignancy, and hepatic disease. ACD is an acquired iron distribution disorder, with relatively low circulating Fe levels, despite the presence of adequate total body Fe stores. The pathogenesis of ACD includes shortened erythrocyte survival, impaired marrow function, and disturbances of Fe metabolism. In ACD, the release of Fe from cells to the circulation is inadequate to support heme formation, and Fe is sequestered in reticuloendothelial macrophages. The ACD is typically normocytic and normochromic. Patients with ACD have anemia, low Fe, low transferrin, low transferrin saturation (TSAT), normal or moderately elevated ferritin, elevated hepcidin, and mostly normal sTfR concentrations.

### Iron Overload

Iron overload disorders are typically insidious, causing progressive and sometimes irreversible tissue damage before clinical symptoms develop. Iron overload disorders can be categorized according to whether the underlying pathophysiological defect is in the hepcidin-ferroportin axis, erythroid maturation, or in iron transport. There are also some less-common disorders that do not fit into one of these categories (see Table 28.5). Iron overload may also develop as a consequence of multiple RBC transfusions and parenteral Fe supplementation.

*Disorders of the hepcidin-ferroportin axis.* Each of the six disorders in this group has a primary form of iron overload and is a subtype of hereditary hemochromatosis (primary HH) (see Table 28.5). Five of the six different HH disorders may lead to a classical HH phenotype: normal Hb, elevated ferritin and TSAT, and tissue iron overload (see Tables 28.6 and 28.7). The pathophysiology of these five conditions is similar, with an increased Fe absorption exceeding the needs of the body, which leads to increased Fe stores due to inadequate hepcidin-mediated down-regulation of ferroportin. This leads to iron deposition in parenchymal organs (e.g., the liver and the pancreas).

Initial clinical symptoms of tissue iron overload are often nonspecific: fatigue and joint pain. In later stages, disease manifestations may include diabetes mellitus, hypogonadism and other endocrinopathies, liver cirrhosis, cardiomyopathy, skin pigmentation, and in cirrhotic patients, increased susceptibility of liver cancer. Early diagnosis and therapeutic

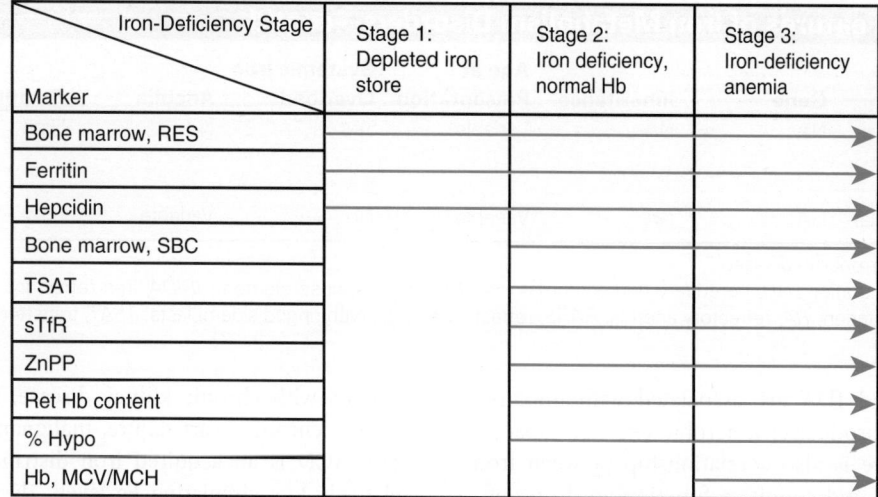

| Iron-Deficiency Stage / Marker | Stage 1: Depleted iron store | Stage 2: Iron deficiency, normal Hb | Stage 3: Iron-deficiency anemia |
|---|---|---|---|
| Bone marrow, RES | | | |
| Ferritin | | | |
| Hepcidin | | | |
| Bone marrow, SBC | | | |
| TSAT | | | |
| sTfR | | | |
| ZnPP | | | |
| Ret Hb content | | | |
| % Hypo | | | |
| Hb, MCV/MCH | | | |

Fig. 28.10 Alterations in biochemical and hematological parameters at different stages of Fe deficiency. Iron-deficiency stage 1: bone marrow hemosiderin within reticuloendothelial system *(RES)* cells and ferritin reflect the Fe stores and allow the diagnosis of Fe depletion. In this stage, hepcidin is low (mostly undetectable) to increase maximal iron uptake from the diet and release from the RES stores. Iron-deficiency stage 2: pathological values of transferrin saturation *(TSAT)*, bone marrow sideroblast count *(SBC)*, soluble transferrin receptor *(sTfR)*, zinc protoporphyrin *(ZnPP)*, reticulocyte hemoglobin *(Ret-Hb)* content, percentage of hypochromic cells *(% Hypo)* indicate that Fe-deficient erythropoiesis has already developed. Iron-deficiency stage 3: Hb below reference values defines Fe-deficiency anemia, which is accompanied by low red cell indexes. *MCH*, Mean corpuscular hemoglobin; *MCV*, mean corpuscular volume. (Modified from Hastka J, Lasserre JJ, Schwarzbeck A, et al. Laboratory tests of iron status: correlation or common sense? *Clin Chem.* 1996;42:718–724.)

phlebotomy can prevent the development of tissue damage, reduce morbidity and mortality, and provide long-term survival similar to the general population. Repeated phlebotomy is the treatment for HH.

The most common form of HH is attributed to variants in the *HFE*-gene. The best described variants in HFE-hemochromatosis are (1) the variant in the cDNA of *HFE* at position 845, a G to A nucleotide change resulting in a cysteine to tyrosine replacement (p.Cys282Tyr or C282Y); and (2) the variant at *HFE* cDNA position 187, a C to G nucleotide change resulting in a histidine to asparagine replacement in the protein (p.His63Asp or H63D). Of the White population, approximately 1 in 200 are *HFE* C282Y homozygotes, and approximately 1 in 10 carry the variant. In patients with Fe overload and of European ancestry, nearly 80% have been found to be homozygous for the C282Y variant in *HFE*. A smaller proportion (5%) are compound heterozygous for the C282Y/H63D variants. Although 38% to 76% of C282Y homozygous people develop raised serum iron, ferritin, and TSAT, disease penetrance is 2% to 38% in men and only 1% to 10% in women, who are more likely to present after menopause, presumably because menstrual blood loss and childbearing protects them from iron overload. Also, both disease severity and clinical expression correlate well with the degree of iron overload, but are heterogeneous among patients, depending not only on the age of diagnosis but also on other genetic and dietary modifiers that remain still largely unknown. Among C282Y/H63D compound heterozygotes the risk of disease progression is low, and documented iron overload

disease is rare. Furthermore, C282Y/H63D compound heterozygous hemochromatosis patients with clinical disease expression frequently have additional risk factors for iron overload or liver disease. Homozygosity for H63D is also rarely associated with hemochromatosis and is not considered a disease-associated genotype. Most patients with HFE-associated HH do not present until middle age (and in women, not until after menopause).

*Disorders of erythroid maturation.* This class of disorders represents forms of secondary iron overload, and includes the iron-loading anemias, among which are thalassemia syndromes (especially the β-thalassemias), sideroblastic anemias, and the congenital dyserythropoietic anemias. These diseases are characterized by ineffective erythropoiesis (i.e., by apoptosis of erythroid precursors), failure of erythroid maturation, and consequent expansion of the number of erythroid precursor cells in the bone marrow.

*Disorders of iron transport and iron acquisition.* The common pathophysiologic feature of these disorders is insufficient delivery and acquisition of transferrin-bound Fe to the RBC precursors in the bone marrow for heme synthesis, despite Fe stores. The resulting iron-restrictive erythropoiesis, anemia, and hypoxia all contribute to low hepcidin-induced iron overload.

*Other forms of iron overload.* Chronic erythrocyte transfusion is the most common cause of this group of disorders. Transfusion-induced iron overload is common in patients with severe β-TM and sickle cell disease. Transfusion-induced iron overload also occurs in persons with (1) severe aplastic anemia, (2) Blackfan-Diamond syndrome, (3) Fanconi

**TABLE 28.6 Laboratory Tests for Iron Status in Adults (Standard International Units)**

| Iron Status Test | Iron Deficiency | Functional Iron Deficiency | Iron-Deficiency Anemia | IRIDA | Anemia of Chronic Disease | Iron-Deficiency Anemia and Anemia of Chronic Disease | Iron Overload in Hereditary Hemochromatosis | Reference Interval |
|---|---|---|---|---|---|---|---|---|
| **Current** | | | | | | | | |
| Iron (µmol/L) | Low | Low–normal | Low | Low | Low | Low | High | 13–36[a] |
| Transferrin (g/L)/TIBC (µmol/L) | High | Normal | High | High | Low | Variable | Low | 2.0–3.6 45–78[a] |
| Transferrin saturation (%) | 15–20[a] | 15–20[a] | <15[a] | <10[b] | <15–20[a] | <15–20[a] | >45[a,c] | 15–45[a,c] |
| Ferritin (µg/L) | <12–30[a,d] | <100–200[a] | <12[a] | Variable[e] | <100[a] | <100[a] | Men: >300 Women: >200 | Men: 40–300[a,f] Women: 20–200[a,f] |
| Hb (mmol/L) | Normal | Normal | Low | Low | Low | Low | High–normal | Men: >8.1[f] Women: >7.4[f] |
| MCV (fL) | Normal | Normal | <80 | Low | Low–normal | Low | High-normal | 80–95[f] |
| MCH (fmol) | Normal | Normal | <27 | Low | Low–normal | Low | High-normal | 1.67–2.11[f] |
| **Proposed** | | | | | | | | |
| Hepcidin | Low | Low | Very low | High for TSAT[g] | High | Normal–high | Low for ferritin[h] | Varies[a] |
| sTfR (mg/L) | High | High | High | High | Low–normal | Variable | Low–normal | Varies[a] |
| sTfR/log ferritin | NA | NA | >2[a,i] | NA | <1[a,i] | >2[a,i] | NA | Varies[a] |
| ZnPP mmol/mol heme | High | High | High | High | High | High | Low–normal | <40–80[a] |
| Reticulocyte hemoglobin content (fmol) | <1.74[a,j] | <1.80[a,k] | Low | Low | Low–normal | Low | High–normal | 1.87–2.23[a,l] |
| Bone marrow iron[m] | Negative | Variable | Negative | Positive | Positive | Positive | Positive | Positive |

[a]Results vary with the methodology used.

[b]In more severe cases, less than 5%.

[c]Some guidelines propose a threshold of 50% for men.

[d]In populations exposed to infections and in patients with renal failure, inflammatory bowel disease, chronic heart failure, or other (low-grade) inflammatory diseases, threshold values indicating iron deficiency are generally considered to be higher than in those without these diseases (see the following). In these situations, levels more than 100 µg/L generally excludes absolute iron deficiency and for levels between 30 and 100 µg/L, other parameters are needed to diagnose iron deficiency.

[e]Mostly low-normal in untreated patients.

[f]Based on Camaschella C. Iron-deficiency anemia. *N Engl J Med.* 2015;372(19):1832–1843.

[g]Absolute levels vary, but in the absence of inflammation. levels are high for circulating iron levels.

[h]Absolute levels vary, but levels are low for serum ferritin levels.

[i]Value from (a) Weiss G, Goodnough LT. Anemia of chronic disease. *N Engl J Med.* 2005;352(10):1011–1023; and (b) Punnonen K, Irjala K, Rajamäki A. Serum transferrin receptor and its ratio to serum ferritin in the diagnosis of iron deficiency. *Blood.* 1997;89(3):1052–1057.

[j]For CHr, based on Mast AE, Blinder MA, Lu Q, et al. Clinical utility of the reticulocyte hemoglobin content in the diagnosis of iron deficiency. *Blood.* 2002;99(4):1489–1491.

[k]For CHr, from Thomas DW, Hinchliffe RF, Briggs C, et al. Guideline for the laboratory diagnosis of functional iron deficiency. *Br J Haematol.* 2013;161(5):639–648.

[l]For CHr, from Piva E, Brugnara C, Spolaore F, et al. Clinical utility of reticulocyte parameters. *Clin Lab Med.* 2015;35(1):133–163.

[m]By Perls staining of bone marrow for iron in reticulocytes according to Gale and colleagues.

*Hb*, Hemoglobin; *IRIDA*, iron refractory iron-deficiency anemia; *MCH*, mean corpuscular Hb; *MCV*, mean corpuscular volume; *sTfR*, soluble transferrin receptor; *TIBC*, total iron-binding capacity; *TSAT*, transferrin saturation; *ZnPP*, zinc protoporphyrin.

## TABLE 28.7 Laboratory Tests for Iron Status in Adults (Traditional Units)

| Iron Status Test | Iron Deficiency | Functional Iron Deficiency | Iron-Deficiency Anemia | IRIDA | Anemia of Chronic Disease | Iron-Deficiency Anemia and Anemia of Chronic Disease | Iron Overload in Hereditary Hemochromatosis | Reference Interval |
|---|---|---|---|---|---|---|---|---|
| **Current** | | | | | | | | |
| Iron (µg/dL) | Low | Low-normal | Low | Low | Low | Low | High | 70–200[a] |
| Transferrin (g/L) | High | Normal | High | High | Low | Variable | Low | 2.0–3.6 |
| TIBC (µg/dL) | | | | | | | | 251–436[a] |
| Transferrin saturation (%) | 15–20[a] | 15–20[a] | <15[a] | <10[b] | <15–20[a] | <15–20[a] | >45[c] | 15–45[a,c] |
| Ferritin (µg/L) | <12–30[d] | <100–200[a] | <12[a] | Variable[e] | <100[a] | <100[a] | Men: >300 / Women: >200 | Men: 40–300[a,f] / Women: 20–200[a,f] |
| Hb (g/dL) | Normal | Normal | Low | Low | Low | Low | High–normal | Men: >13[f] / Women: >12[f] |
| MCV (fL) | Normal | Normal | <80 | Low | Low–normal | Low | High–normal | 80–95[f] |
| MCH (pg) | Normal | Normal | <27 | Low | Low–normal | Low | High–normal | 27–34[f] |
| **Proposed** | | | | | | | | |
| Hepcidin | Low | Low | Very low | High for TSAT[g] | High | Normal–high | Low for ferritin[h] | Varies[a] |
| sTfR (mg/L) | High | High | High | High | Low–normal | Variable | Low–normal | Varies[a] |
| sTfR/log ferritin | NA | NA | >2[a,i] | NA | <1[a,i] | >2[a,i] | NA | Varies[a] |
| ZnPP mmol/mol heme | High | High | High | High | High | High | Low–normal | <40–80[a] |
| Reticulocyte hemoglobin content (pg) | <28[a,i] | <29[a,k] | Low | Low | Low–normal | Low | High–normal | 30.2–35.9[a,l] |
| Bone marrow iron[m] | Negative | Variable | Negative | Positive | Positive | Positive | Positive | Positive |

[a]Results vary with the methodology used.

[b]In more severe cases, less than 5%.

[c]Some guidelines propose a threshold of 50% for men.

[d]In populations exposed to infections and in patients with renal failure, inflammatory bowel disease, chronic heart failure or other (low grade) inflammatory diseases, threshold values indicating iron deficiency are generally considered to be higher than in those without these diseases (see the following). In these situations, levels more than 100 µg/L generally exclude absolute iron deficiency and for levels between 30 and 100 µg/L, other parameters are needed to diagnose iron deficiency.

[e]Mostly low-normal in untreated patients.

[f]Based on Camaschella C. Iron-deficiency anemia. *N Engl J Med*. 2015;372(19):1832–1843.

[g]Absolute levels vary, but in the absence of inflammation. levels are high for circulating iron levels.

[h]Absolute levels vary, but levels are low for serum ferritin levels.

[i]Value from (a) Weiss G, Goodnough LT. Anemia of chronic disease. *N Engl J Med*. 2005;352(10):1011–1023; and (b) Punnonen K, Irjala K, Rajamäki A. Serum transferrin receptor and its ratio to serum ferritin in the diagnosis of iron deficiency. *Blood*. 1997;89(3):1052–1057.

[j]For CHr, based on Mast AE, Blinder MA, Lu Q, et al. Clinical utility of the reticulocyte hemoglobin content in the diagnosis of iron deficiency. *Blood*. 2002;99(4):1489–1491.

[k]For CHr, from Thomas DW, Hinchliffe RF, Briggs C, et al. Guideline for the laboratory diagnosis of functional iron deficiency. *Br J Haematol*. 2013;161(5):639–648.

[l]For CHr, from Piva E, Brugnara C, Spolaore F, et al. Clinical utility of reticulocyte parameters. *Clin Lab Med*. 2015;35(1):133–163.

[m]By Perls staining of bone marrow for iron in reticulocytes according to Gale and colleagues.

*Hb*, Hemoglobin; *IRIDA*, iron refractory iron-deficiency anemia; *MCH*, mean corpuscular Hb; *MCV*, mean corpuscular volume; *sTfR*, soluble transferrin receptor; *TIBC*, total iron-binding capacity; *TSAT*, transferrin saturation; *ZnPP*, zinc protoporphyrin.

anemia, (4) acute leukemia, (5) autoimmune hemolytic anemias, and (6) myelodysplasia with refractory anemia.

Rarely, iron overload develops in persons who ingest large quantities of supplemental Fe. Iron overload also occurs in persons with renal insufficiency as a result of excessive intravenous supplements.

## Analytical Methods

Several methods are used to measure iron and related analytes. These include methods for (1) serum iron, (2) iron-binding capacity, (3) transferrin saturation, (4) serum ferritin, (5) hepcidin, (6) sTfR, and (7) red cell indices.

### Methods for Serum Iron, Total Iron-Binding Capacity, Transferrin, and Transferrin Saturation

Except when atomic absorption spectroscopy is used, hemolysis has very little effect on serum Fe assay results because Hb Fe is not released from heme by acid treatment. Markedly hemolyzed specimens should be rejected for analysis. Because Fe is ubiquitous, scrupulous care is necessary to ensure that glassware, water, and reagents do not become contaminated with extraneous Fe.

Iron is released from transferrin by decreasing the pH of the serum. It is reduced from Fe(III) to Fe(II) and then is complexed with a chromogen such as bathophenanthroline or ferrozine.

Such iron/chromogen complexes have extremely high absorbance at the applicable wavelength, which is proportional to the Fe concentration.

Transferrin can be measured directly by immunological techniques. Alternatively, transferrin is quantified in terms of the amount of Fe it will bind, a measure called total iron binding capacity (TIBC).

Serum unsaturated iron-binding capacity (UIBC) and TIBC are determined by the addition of sufficient $Fe^{3+}$ to saturate iron-binding sites on transferrin. Excess $Fe^{3+}$ is removed, e.g., by adsorption with (1) light magnesium carbonate ($MgCO_3$) powder, (2) a silica column, or (3) anion exchange resin, and the assay for iron content is then repeated. From this second measurement, the TIBC is obtained.

Many automated chemistry analyzers now measure UIBC and calculate TIBC, rather than measuring it directly. UIBC is measured by adding a known excess concentration of iron to serum. By leaving the pH near neutral, only the iron that did not bind to transferrin is measured upon the addition of an iron binding chromogen. TIBC is calculated by adding the UIBC to the serum iron level.

The combination of total serum iron and either TIBC or transferrin measurement allows the calculation of the saturation of transferrin with iron:

$$\text{Transferrin saturation}\,(\%) = (100 \times \text{serum iron})\,/\,\text{TIBC}$$

Transferrin concentration can be used to derive TIBC, and indirectly, TSAT. Because 1 mol of transferrin (average molecular mass 79,570 Da) has the capacity to bind two atoms of Fe (atomic mass 55.84 Da), the theoretically derived formulas for calculating transferrin (and TSAT) from TIBC and vice versa are:

$$\text{Transferrin}\,(g/L) = 0.007 \times \text{TIBC}\,(\mu g/L)$$
$$\text{TIBC}\,(\mu g/dL) = \text{transferrin}\,(mg/dL) \times 1.41$$
$$\text{TIBC}\,(\mu mol/L) = \text{transferrin}\,(g/L) \times 25.2$$
$$\text{TSAT}\,(\%) = (\text{Serum iron}\,(\mu g/dL))/$$
$$(\text{transferrin}\,(mg/dL)) \times 70.9$$
$$= (\text{Serum iron}\,(\mu mol/L))/$$
$$(\text{transferrin}\,(mg/dL)) \times 398$$

These mathematical derivations have some weaknesses. The results of immunological measurements of transferrin concentration correlate with those of the TIBC assay. Note that the relationship is not entirely linear as a small portion of Fe in serum is bound to proteins other than transferrin. Therefore, calculated TIBC values are slightly greater than the amount of transferrin-bound Fe. However, these small differences are of no practical or clinical consequence.

*Reference intervals.* Reference intervals for serum iron differ by as much as 35% between commercial methods. Therefore, a generic reference interval cannot be applied, and each laboratory should independently define its own reference intervals. The reference value used for TSAT also differs between laboratories. The approximate and most used reference interval is 15% to 45%. There is diurnal variation of serum iron and TSAT in many healthy people that should be considered.

*Clinical relevance.* The serum iron concentration refers to the $Fe^{3+}$ bound to serum transferrin and does not include the Fe contained in serum as free Hb and ferritin. In clinical situations, serum iron measurements are often combined with TIBC or transferrin, to calculate the TSAT that is considered more useful for clinical interpretation.

The serum iron concentration or TSAT is decreased in many, but not all, patients with IDA and with chronic inflammatory disorders (see Table 28.5). Elevated serum iron or TSAT occur (1) in iron overload such as HH, (2) in patients with aplastic anemia, (3) in children with acute iron poisoning, (4) after oral or parenteral iron use, and (5) as the result of acute liver injury.

Because only about one-third of the Fe-binding sites of transferrin are occupied by $Fe^{3+}$ in healthy individuals, serum transferrin has much reserve iron-binding capacity (UIBC). TIBC is a measurement of the maximum concentration of Fe that transferrin binds. TIBC or transferrin is increased in subjects with iron deficiency and is decreased in those with chronic inflammatory disorders, chronic liver diseases, and malnutrition. In many persons with untreated HH, TIBC is slightly decreased.

### Methods for Serum Ferritin

The most common current commercially available methods for serum ferritin include: (1) enzyme immunoassay, and (2) chemiluminescent immunoassay.

*Reference intervals.* Reference intervals for serum ferritin concentrations are summarized in Tables 28.6 and 28.7. Reference intervals and diagnostic cutoffs differ distinctly between laboratories. This can be attributed to variation in definition of reference population, variation in assay techniques, and lacking traceability to a reference measurement system.

*Clinical relevance.* Under normal conditions, serum ferritin concentrations are usually proportional to the body's iron content. The circulating protein is largely apoferritin. The plasma ferritin concentration declines very early in the development of iron deficiency—long before changes are observed in (1) blood Hb concentration, (2) RBC size, or (3) serum iron concentration. Thus, the measurement of serum ferritin concentration is used as a highly sensitive indicator of iron deficiency that is uncomplicated by other concurrent disease. On the other hand, many chronic diseases cause increased serum ferritin levels (see Table 28.5). Elevated ferritin has a low specificity for parenchymal iron overload and most subjects with elevated serum ferritin levels do not have HH or other iron overload disorders.

Since an elevated TSAT facilitates parenchymal iron deposition, the combination of high TSAT with hyperferritinemia can be observed in HH and transfusion-induced Fe overload.

In subjects with proven hemochromatosis or iron overload, serum ferritin measurements are useful gauges to the progress of phlebotomy therapy in achieving the clinically desired level of iron depletion.

## Methods for Hepcidin

Currently, several in-house and commercial immunochemical assays and laboratory-developed mass spectrometry assays provide reliable hepcidin results. Some of the MS-based assays have been thoroughly validated and are used in patient care, but most assays are labeled for "research use only."

*Reference interval.* Because hepcidin assays are not harmonized and standardized, there are no universal reference intervals or decision limits.

*Clinical relevance.* The measurement of hepcidin has provided important insights into the pathophysiology of iron disorders, among which are HH, anemia of inflammation, and IRIDA. Proof-of-concept studies highlight hepcidin as a promising tool in the diagnosis of IRIDA, and the guidance of iron supplementation therapy. The recent identification of a commutable reference material should allow for future harmonization.

## Methods for Soluble Serum Transferrin Receptor

Soluble or serum transferrin receptor (sTfR1 or sTfR)—a truncated form of the transferrin receptor—is a single polypeptide chain with a molecular mass of 84.9 kDa that can be measured by a variety of standard immunoassay techniques. The automated homogeneous immunoturbidimetric assay is characterized by a high sample throughput and excellent precision. In addition, sTfR concentrations can be assessed by immunofluorometric assays, which are based on immunoreactants labeled with fluorescent probes. The high sensitivity of fluorescence measurement combined with the sensitivity of the probe to changes in its environment offered the possibility of monitoring the concentration of sTfR directly in the reaction mixture.

*Reference intervals.* Current commercial methods for the assay of sTfR are characterized by different reference intervals.

*Clinical relevance.* Soluble TfR is useful in the investigation of the pathophysiology of anemia, to distinguish IDA from ACD and to detect functional iron deficiency. Cell membranes of developing erythroid cells, especially the erythroblasts, in bone marrow are rich in transferrin receptors (TfRs) to which the Fe-transferrin complex binds. The number of TfRs increases in the presence of high erythroid proliferation rates and low iron supplies, and decreases in bone marrow hypoplasia and suppression. These variations in the quantity of TfRs in erythropoietic tissue are also reflected in changes in sTfR.

## Red Blood Cell Indices

MCV, MCH, and MCH concentration (MCHC) are indices that are included in the CBC test. One of their uses is to characterize the RBCs of patients with anemia. Low values of MCV and MCH are indicators of IDA. MCV, MCH, and MCHC are slightly higher for untreated HH patients compared to healthy individuals.

## Bone Marrow Examination

Bone marrow examination is the gold standard assessment of body iron. The absence of stainable bone marrow iron is the most commonly accepted reference criterion of iron deficiency. One way of evaluating iron stores is by examining a bone marrow aspirate for hemosiderin within reticuloendothelial cells. In iron deficiency, marrow hemosiderin is absent; in the anemia of chronic disorders, iron is always present. Iron stores are greatly increased in β-TM and in sideroblastic anemias. However, this method for quantification of iron stores may be misleading when iron stores are not normally distributed between reticuloendothelial and parenchymal tissues as occurs in ACD. Another way of evaluating bone marrow iron includes evaluation of iron in the erythroblasts, which represents the useable and functional iron stores. Bone marrow examination for the sole purpose of assessing iron stores is rarely justifiable. It may be helpful in the diagnosis of unexplained forms of anemia and if there are concerns that a high serum ferritin value is not a true reflection of body iron stores.

## REVIEW QUESTIONS

1. Heme is a:
   a. chelate of iron with the four pyrrole groups of a porphyrin.
   b. conjugated protein and an oxygen-carrying pigment of the erythrocytes.
   c. protein found in red skeletal muscle that releases oxygen.
   d. colorless compound formed in the intestines by the reduction of bilirubin.
2. The role of hemoglobin is to:

a. transport iron between organs.

b. store iron and readily release it when body iron stores are low.

c. reversibly bind oxygen.

d. conjugate bilirubin in the liver.

3. In an individual with suspected β-thalassemia, which of the following laboratory results would correctly indicate the presence of this disease?

a. Increased hemoglobin concentration, mean corpuscular volume (MCV) and mean corpuscular hemoglobin concentration (MCHC) with the peripheral blood smear showing increased macrocytes and Howell–Jolly bodies

b. Decreased hemoglobin concentration, MCV, and MCHC with the peripheral blood smear indicating microcytosis, target cells, and polychromasia

c. Decreased hemoglobin concentration, increased MCV and MCHC, and persistence of hemoglobin F with the peripheral blood smear indicating spherocytosis and nucleated red blood cells

d. Increased hemoglobin concentration and normal MCV and MCHC with a normal peripheral blood smear

4. Which of the following is associated with low serum iron and high total iron binding capacity (TIBC) or transferrin?

a. Hemochromatosis

b. Iron-deficiency anemia

c. Iron intoxication

d. Anemia of chronic disease

5. This readily soluble iron/protein complex is the form in which iron is stored in tissues:

a. Ferritin

b. Transferrin

c. Hemosiderin

d. Hemoglobin

6. The correct formula for determining the percent of transferrin saturation % is:

a. MCV < 70 mL = increased transferrin

b. Total iron binding capacity ÷ Serum iron

c. Total iron binding capacity × 100

d. [Serum iron: TIBC] × 100

7. The major difference between thalassemia and hemoglobinopathy is that:

a. in thalassemia the globin chains of hemoglobin are structurally altered.

b. in thalassemia the serum level of conjugated bilirubin is dramatically increased.

c. in a hemoglobinopathy the globin chains of hemoglobin are structurally altered.

d. in a hemoglobinopathy the globin chains of hemoglobin are insufficiently produced.

8. Anemia of chronic disease is characterized by:

a. elevated transferrin saturation (TSAT) and elevated or normal ferritin.

b. elevated TSAT and low or normal ferritin.

c. low TSAT and low or normal ferritin.

d. low TSAT and elevated or normal ferritin.

9. Symptomatic hereditary hemochromatosis is best characterized by:

a. elevated TSAT and elevated ferritin.

b. normal TSAT and elevated ferritin.

c. elevated TSAT and normal ferritin.

d. normal TSAT and normal ferritin.

## SUGGESTED READINGS

Beguin Y. Soluble transferrin receptor for the evaluation of erythropoiesis and iron status. *Clin Chim Acta*. 2003;329:9–22.

Bhutani VK, Johnson L, Sivieri EM. Predictive ability of predischarge hour-specific serum bilirubin for subsequent significant hyperbilirubinemia in healthy term and near-term newborns. *Pediatrics*. 1999;103:6–14.

Camaschella C. Iron-deficiency anemia. *N Engl J Med*. 2015;372:1832–1843.

Doumas BT, Poon PKC, Perry BW, et al. Candidate reference method for determination of total bilirubin in serum: development and validation. *Clin Chem*. 1985;31:1779–1789.

Fleming RE, Ponka P. Iron overload in human disease. *N Engl J Med*. 2012;366:348–359.

Girelli D, Nemeth E, Swinkels DW. Hepcidin in the diagnostics of iron disorders. *Blood*. 2016;127:2809–2813.

Musallam KM, Rivella S, Vichinsky E, et al. Non-transfusion dependent thalassemia. *Haematologica*. 2013;98:833–844.

Nicolle S, Jackson N, Radi K, et al. Evaluation of mass spectrometry based approaches for the diagnosis of hemoglobinopathies. *Blood*. 2013;122:4679.

Piel FB, Weatherall DJ. The α-thalassemias. *N Engl J Med*. 2014;371:1908–1916.

Schoorl M, Schoorl M, van Pelt J, et al. Application of innovative hemocytometric parameters and algorithms for improvement of microcytic anemia discrimination. *Hematol Rep*. 2015;7:5843.

Weiss G, Goodnough LT. Anemia of chronic disease. *N Engl J Med*. 2005;352:1011–1023.

# Porphyrins and Porphyrias

*Michael N. Badminton, Caroline Schmitt, and Aasne K. Aarsand*

## OBJECTIVES

1. Define the following terms:
   - 5-Aminolevulinic acid (ALA)
   - Heme
   - Porphyrin
   - Porphobilinogen (PBG)
   - Porphyria
   - Zinc protoporphyrin
2. Summarize the biosynthetic pathway of heme, including intracellular sites of each synthetic step, rate-limiting steps and the individual enzymes.
3. List six functions of heme.
4. Compare and contrast the acute and nonacute porphyrias, including causes, symptoms, and laboratory analyses; describe the tests that differentiate between the two categories of porphyria.

5. List and categorize eight porphyrias; state the major elevated intermediates involved in each.
6. List the abnormalities of porphyrin metabolism that are unrelated to porphyria.
7. Explain the effects of lead toxicity on the heme biosynthetic pathway and on iron status.
8. List the specimen collection and storage requirements for samples undergoing porphyrin analysis.
9. Describe the laboratory methods of analysis for the following:
   - Porphobilinogen
   - 5-Aminolevulinic acid
   - Porphyrins in urine, stool, blood, and plasma
   - DNA assessments
10. Analyze and solve case studies related to abnormal porphyrin metabolism and lead toxicity.

## KEY WORDS AND DEFINITIONS

**Acute intermittent porphyria (AIP)** An autosomal dominant acute hepatic porphyria caused by a mutation in the *HMBS* gene (locus 11q23.3), which encodes hydroxymethylbilane synthase.

**Acute porphyrias** Inherited disorders of heme biosynthesis, characterized by acute attacks of neurovisceral symptoms; potentially life threatening; diagnosed by elevated urine porphobilinogen (PBG).

**5-Aminolevulinic acid (ALA)** Immediate precursor of porphobilinogen; two molecules of ALA combine to form one molecule of porphobilinogen.

**Congenital erythropoietic porphyria (CEP)** An autosomal recessive porphyria due to mutations in the *UROS* gene (locus 10q26.2), which encodes uroporphyrinogen-III synthase.

**Coproporphyrin** A porphyrin with four methyl and four propionic acid side chains attached to the tetrapyrrole backbone.

**Cutaneous porphyrias** Disorders of heme biosynthesis in which accumulations of porphyrins in the skin cause skin damage on exposure to sunlight.

**Erythropoietic protoporphyria (EPP)** An autosomal recessive disorder due to mutations in the *FECH* gene (locus 18q21.3), which encodes ferrochelatase, causing a partial deficiency of the enzyme.

**Ferrochelatase (FECH)** A mitochondrial enzyme of the lyase class that catalyzes the insertion of ferrous iron into protoporphyrin IX to form heme.

**Hereditary coproporphyria (HCP)** An autosomal dominant acute hepatic porphyria caused by a mutation in the *CPOX* gene (locus 3q11.2) that results in partial deficiency of coproporphyrinogen oxidase activity.

**Porphobilinogen (PBG)** Immediate precursor of the porphyrins; a pyrrole ring with acetyl, propionyl, and aminomethyl side chains; four molecules of PBG condense to form one molecule of 1-hydroxymethylbilane, which is then converted successively to uroporphyrinogen-III, coproporphyrinogen-III, protoporphyrinogen-IX, protoporphyrin-IX, and heme.

**Porphyrins** Any of a group of compounds containing the porphyrin structure; four pyrrole rings connected by methylene bridges in a cyclical configuration, to which different side chains are attached.

**Porphyria cutanea tarda (PCT)** The most common form of porphyria, characterized by inhibition of hepatic uroporphyrinogen decarboxylase which results in cutaneous photosensitivity.

**Porphyrias** A group of mainly inherited metabolic disorders that result from partial deficiency in one of the enzymes of heme biosynthesis or, in one disorder, increased activity of the enzyme, which cause increased accumulation and excretion of porphyrins, their precursors, or both.

**Porphyrin precursors** ALA and PBG, the biosynthetic intermediates which are metabolized to porphyrinogens and porphyrins.

**Protoporphyrin** A porphyrin with four methyl, two vinyl, and two propionic acid side chains attached to the tetrapyrrole backbone.

**Upregulation** A process by which the cell increases the quantity of a cellular component such as a specific protein or RNA.

**Uroporphyrin** A porphyrin with four acetic acid and four propionic acid side chains attached to the tetrapyrrole backbone.

**Variegate porphyria (VP)** An autosomal dominant acute hepatic porphyria due to a mutation in the *PPOX* gene (locus 1q23.3), which encodes protoporphyrinogen oxidase.

**X-linked erythropoietic protoporphyria (XLEPP)** An erythropoietic porphyria caused by a mutation in the *ALAS2* gene (locus Xp11.21), that results in increased ALA synthase 2 activity.

**Zinc protoporphyrin (ZPP)** A normal but minor by-product of heme biosynthesis found in the red blood cell; when insufficient $Fe^{2+}$ is available for heme biosynthesis, increased ZPP is formed.

---

The porphyrias are a group of eight uncommon inherited diseases resulting from either partial deficiency in one of the enzymes of heme biosynthesis or, in one disorder, increased activity of the rate-controlling enzyme of erythroid heme biosynthesis. Each disorder is associated with a specific pattern of overproduction of pathway intermediates, which are present in the blood and excreted in excessive amounts in urine, feces, or both. The clinical consequences depend on the nature of the heme precursors that accumulate. In the acute porphyrias, excess porphyrin precursors (5-aminolevulinic acid [ALA] and porphobilinogen [PBG]) are associated with potentially fatal acute neurovisceral attacks that are often provoked by various commonly prescribed drugs or hormonal factors. In the nonacute porphyrias, and in those acute porphyrias in which skin lesions occur, accumulation of porphyrins results in photosensitization of sun-exposed skin. Diagnosis depends on laboratory investigations to demonstrate the pattern of heme precursor accumulation and excretion specific for each type of porphyria through examination of appropriate specimens using adequately sensitive and specific methods. DNA analysis is rarely necessary for diagnosis of symptomatic cases, but it is the method of choice when investigating healthy, at-risk relatives. Abnormalities of porphyrin accumulation and excretion also occur in a wide variety of other disorders that are collectively more common than the porphyrias. Recognition of secondary porphyrin disorders is important to avoid diagnostic errors.

## PORPHYRIN CHEMISTRY

In this section, porphyrin structure, nomenclature, and chemical characteristics are reviewed.

### Structure and Nomenclature

The basic porphyrin structure consists of four monopyrrole rings connected by methene bridges to form a tetrapyrrole ring (Fig. 29.1). The porphyrin compounds of relevance to the porphyrias differ in the substituents occupying peripheral positions 1 through 8 (Fig. 29.2). Variation in the distribution of the same substituents around the peripheral positions of the tetrapyrrole ring gives rise to porphyrin isomers,

which are depicted by Roman numerals (e.g., I, II, III). The reduced form of a porphyrin, known as a *porphyrinogen* (see Fig. 29.1), differs by the presence of six additional hydrogens (four on the methylene bridges and two on ring nitrogens). Porphyrinogens are unstable in vitro and spontaneously oxidize to the corresponding porphyrins. Under the lower cellular oxygen tension, porphyrinogens are sufficiently stable to act as intermediates of the heme biosynthetic pathway; aromatization to protoporphyrin at the penultimate step requires protoporphyrinogen oxidase.

### Chelation of Metals

The arrangement of four nitrogen atoms in the center of the porphyrin ring enables porphyrins to chelate various metal ions. Protoporphyrin that contains iron is known as heme; ferroheme refers specifically to the $Fe^{2+}$ complex and ferriheme to $Fe^{3+}$. Ferriheme associated with a chloride counter ion is known as hemin, or hematin when the counter ion is hydroxide.

### Spectral Properties

Porphyrins, named from the Greek root for "purple" ("porphyra"), owe their color to the conjugated double-bond structure of the tetrapyrrole ring. Porphyrinogens have no conjugated double bonds and are therefore colorless. Porphyrins show particularly strong absorbance near 400 nm, often called the Soret band, and as a result of this exposure,

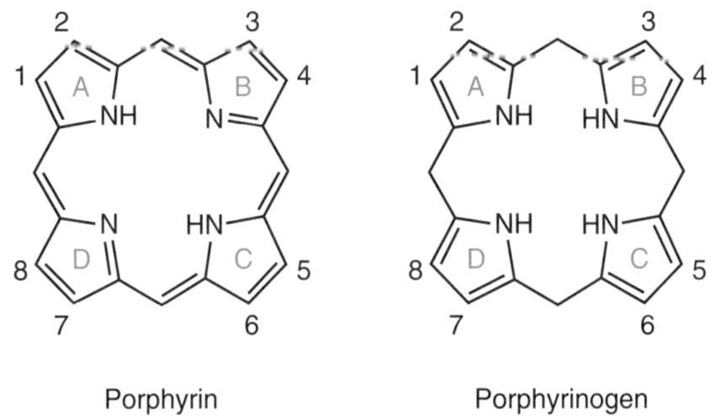

Fig. 29.1 Porphyrin and porphyrinogen structures: numbers 1 to 8 represent various substituents, the nature and order of which determine the type of porphyrin or porphyrinogen. Numbering system and ring designations are based on the Fischer system.

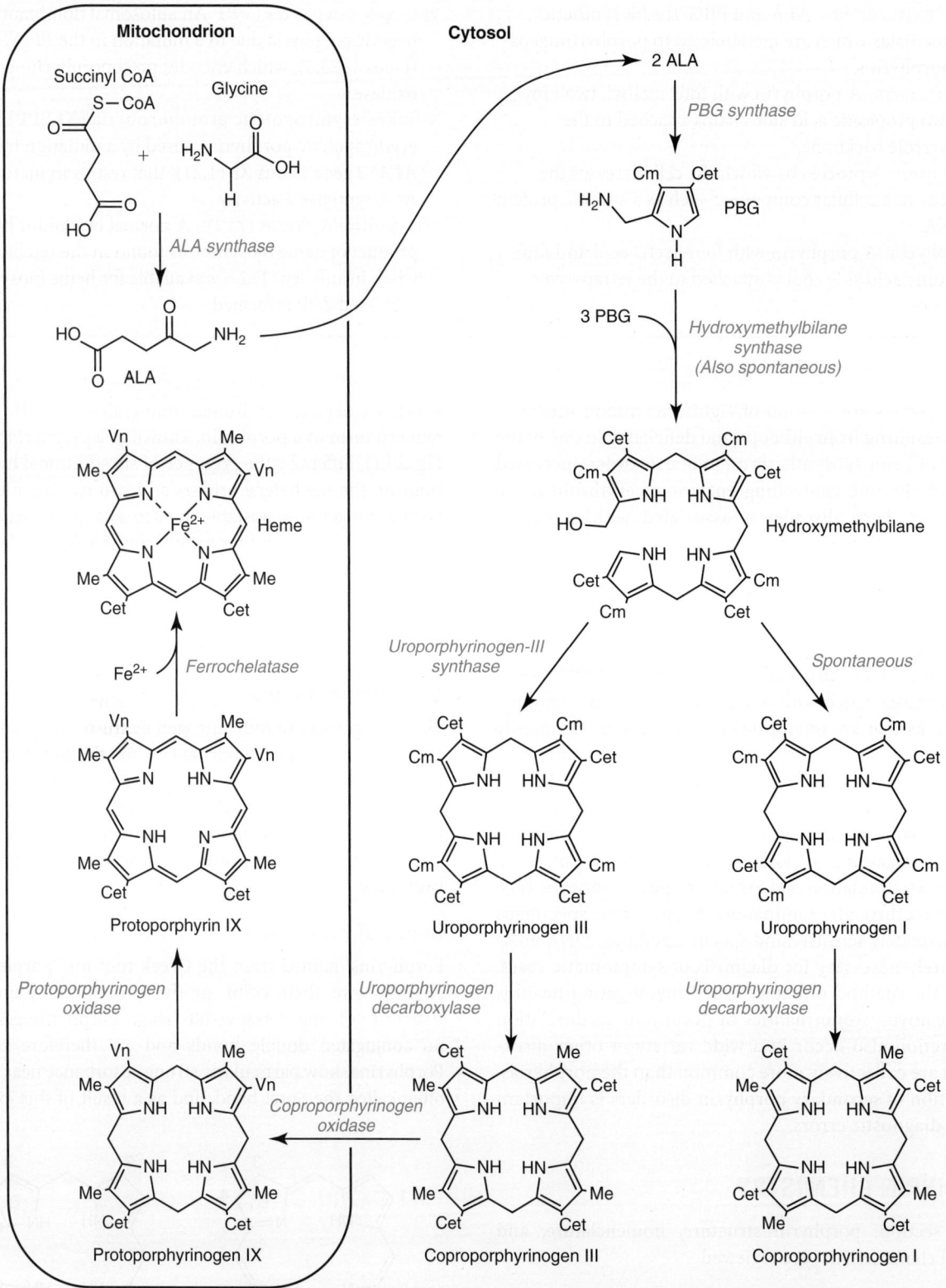

**Fig. 29.2** Biosynthetic pathway of porphyrins and heme. $C_{et}$, —$CH_2CH_2COOH$; $C_m$, —$CH_2COOH$; *Me*, —$CH_3$; *Vn*, $CH = CH_2$. *ALA*, 5-Aminolevulinic acid; *CoA*, coenzyme A; *PBG*, porphobilinogen.

display a characteristic orange–red fluorescence in the range of 550 to 650 nm. Absorbance and fluorescence are altered by substituents around the porphyrin ring and by metal binding. Zinc chelation shifts the fluorescence emission peak of protoporphyrin to shorter wavelengths and reduces the fluorescence intensity. The strong binding of iron alters the character of protoporphyrin to the extent that heme lacks significant fluorescence.

## HEME BIOSYNTHESIS

The complex tetrapyrrole ring structure of heme is built up in a stepwise fashion from precursors succinyl–coenzyme A (CoA) and glycine (see Fig. 29.2). The pathway is present in all nucleated cells, and it has been estimated that daily synthesis of heme in humans is 5 to 8 mmol/kg body weight. The pathway is compartmentalized, with some steps occurring in the mitochondrion and others in the cytoplasm.

### Enzymes of Heme Biosynthesis

The genes for all enzymes of human heme biosynthesis have been characterized (Table 29.1) and enzyme structures determined by x-ray crystallography.

### 5-Aminolevulinate Synthase (EC 2.3.1.37)

5-Aminolevulinate synthase (ALAS), the initial enzyme of the pathway is mitochondrial and has a housekeeping (ALAS1) and erythroid (ALAS2) isoenzyme. It catalyzes the formation of ALA (sometimes referred to as aminolevulinate to emphasize its ionic nature at physiological pH) from succinyl-CoA and glycine and requires a pyridoxal phosphate cofactor, which forms a Schiff base with the amino group of glycine at the enzyme surface. The carbanion of the Schiff base displaces CoA from succinyl-CoA with the formation of α-amino-β-ketoadipic acid, which is then decarboxylated to ALA. The activity of ALAS is rate limiting

as long as the catalytic capacities of other enzymes in the pathway are normal.

### 5-Aminolevulinic Acid Dehydratase (EC 4.2.1.24)

Aminolevulinic acid dehydratase (ALAD) (also known as PBG synthase) is a cytoplasmic enzyme that catalyzes the formation of the monopyrrole PBG from two molecules of ALA with the elimination of two molecules of water. The enzyme requires zinc as a cofactor and reduced sulfhydryl groups at the active site, and it is therefore susceptible to inhibition by lead.

### Hydroxymethylbilane Synthase (EC 2.5.1.61)

Hydroxymethylbilane synthase (HMBS) (also known as PBG deaminase) is a cytoplasmic enzyme that catalyzes the formation of one molecule of the linear tetrapyrrole 1-hydroxymethylbilane (HMB; also known as preuroporphyrinogen) from four molecules of PBG with the release of four molecules of ammonia. The enzyme is susceptible to allosteric inhibition by intermediates farther down the heme biosynthetic pathway, notably coproporphyrinogen-III and protoporphyrinogen-IX.

### Uroporphyrinogen-III Synthase (EC 4.2.1.75)

Uroporphyrinogen synthase (UROS) is a cytoplasmic enzyme that rearranges and cyclizes HMB to form uroporphyrinogen-III. Each pyrrole ring of HMB contains a methylcarboxylate and an ethylcarboxylate substituent, which are in the same orientation. By the rotation of zero, one, or two alternate or two adjacent pyrrole rings, it is possible to arrive at four different isomers (I to IV). Apart from closing the ring structure, the enzyme rotates the D-ring via a spirane intermediate, producing type III, the only isomer that can contribute to heme biosynthesis. HMB is unstable, and in those porphyrias in which excess HMB accumulates, cyclization occurs nonenzymatically forming the type I

## TABLE 29.1 Human Enzymes and Genes of Heme Biosynthesis

| Enzyme | Monomer Mol Mass (kDa)[a,b] | Chromosomal Location of Gene | Gene Size (kb) | Expression |
|---|---|---|---|---|
| ALAS1 | 70.6 | 3p21.2 | 17 | Ubiquitous |
| ALAS2 | 64.6 | Xp11.21 | 22 | Erythroid cells |
| ALAD | 36.3 | 9q32 | 13 | Ubiquitous and erythroid-specific mRNAs |
| HMBS | 37.0 | 11q23.3 | 10 | Ubiquitous and erythroid-specific isoforms |
| UROS | 29.5 | 10q26.2 | 34 | Ubiquitous and erythroid-specific mRNAs |
| UROD | 40.8 | 1p34.1 | 3 | Ubiquitous |
| CPOX | 40.3 | 3q11.2 | 14 | Ubiquitous |
| PPOX | 50.8 | 1q23.3 | 5 | Ubiquitous |
| FECH | 47.8 | 18q21.3 | 45 | Ubiquitous |

[a]ALAD is a homo-octamer, and HMBS and UROS are monomers; all other enzymes are homodimers.
[b]Molecular masses for ALAS1, ALAS2, CPOX, and FECH include presequences that are cleaved during mitochondrial import.
*ALAD*, Aminolevulinic acid dehydratase; *ALAS*, aminolevulinate synthase; *CPOX*, coproporphyrinogen oxidase; *FECH*, ferrochelatase; *HMBS*, hydroxymethylbilane synthase; *mRNA*, messenger ribonucleic acid; *PPOX*, protoporphyrinogen oxidase; *UROD*, uroporphyrinogen decarboxylase; *UROS*, uroporphyrinogen-III synthase.

isomer. Normally, only minimal amounts of uroporphyrinogen-I are produced.

## Uroporphyrinogen Decarboxylase (EC 4.1.1.37)

The last cytoplasmic enzyme in the pathway catalyzes the decarboxylation of all four carboxymethyl groups to form the tetracarboxylic coproporphyrinogen. The enzyme can use I and III isomers of uroporphyrinogen as substrate. Decarboxylation commences on ring D and proceeds stepwise through rings A, B, and C with the formation of heptacarboxylate, hexacarboxylate, and pentacarboxylate intermediates at a single active site. Decreased uroporphyrinogen decarboxylase (UROD) activity causes accumulation of these intermediates in addition to its substrate, uroporphyrinogen. At high substrate concentrations, decarboxylation occurs by a random mechanism.

## Coproporphyrinogen Oxidase (EC 1.3.3.3)

Coproporphyrinogen oxidase (CPOX), which is located in the mitochondrial intermembrane space, catalyzes the sequential oxidative decarboxylation of the 2- and 4-carboxyethyl groups to produce the more lipophilic protoporphyrinogen-IX, with the formation of a tricarboxylic intermediate, harderoporphyrinogen. Oxygen is required as the oxidant, and the enzyme requires sulfhydryl groups for activity, making it a target for inhibition by metals. The enzyme is specific for the type III isomer only. The product of the enzyme differs from the substrate in that replacement of two of the carboxyethyl groups by vinyl groups introduces a third substituent into the molecule. The number of possible isomeric forms is therefore increased, and conventionally the numbering system changes, so that the III isomer becomes the IX isomer. In UROD-deficient states, one of the ethylcarboxylate groups of the accumulated pentacarboxylate porphyrinogen is decarboxylated by CPOX to form the isocoproporphyrin series of porphyrins.

## Protoporphyrinogen Oxidase (EC 1.3.3.4)

Protoporphyrinogen oxidase (PPOX), a flavoprotein located in the inner mitochondrial membrane, catalyzes the removal of six hydrogens (four from methylene bridges and two from ring nitrogens) to form protoporphyrin-IX. Although nonenzymatic oxidation also occurs in vitro, under the low cellular oxygen tension, PPOX is essential for oxidation to occur. The protoporphyrin produced is the only porphyrin that functions in the heme pathway. Other porphyrins are produced by nonenzymatic oxidation and originate from porphyrinogens that have irreversibly escaped from the pathway.

## Ferrochelatase (EC 4.99.1.1)

Ferrochelatase (FECH) (also known as heme synthase) is an iron-sulfur protein located in the inner mitochondrial membrane. This enzyme inserts ferrous iron into protoporphyrin to form heme. During this process, two hydrogens are displaced from the ring nitrogens. Other metals in the divalent state also act as substrates, yielding the corresponding chelate (e.g., incorporation of $Zn^{2+}$ into protoporphyrin to yield zinc

protoporphyrin [ZPP]). In iron-deficient states, $Zn^{2+}$ successfully competes with $Fe^{2+}$ in developing red cells, so that the concentration of ZPP in erythrocytes increases. In lead poisoning, impaired iron delivery or utilization within the mitochondrion has the similar effect of increasing erythrocyte ZPP. Other dicarboxylic porphyrins also serve as substrates (e.g., mesoporphyrin).

## REGULATION OF HEME BIOSYNTHESIS

Heme supply in all tissues is controlled by the activity of mitochondrial ALAS. Two isoforms of ALAS are known. The ubiquitous isoform, ALAS1, is encoded by a gene on chromosome 3p21 and is expressed in all tissues. Because it has a half-life of approximately 1 hour, changes in its rate of synthesis produce short-term alterations in enzyme concentration and cellular ALAS activity. Synthesis of ALAS1 is under negative feedback control by heme. In the liver, ALAS1 is induced by a wide variety of drugs and chemicals that induce microsomal cytochrome P450–dependent oxidases (CYPs). This effect is thought to be mediated mainly by direct transcriptional activation of drug-responsive nuclear receptors, rather than occurring secondary to depletion of an intracellular regulatory heme pool as a consequence of use of heme for CYP assembly. The induction of ALAS1 is prevented by heme, which acts by destabilizing messenger ribonucleic acid (mRNA) for *ALAS1*, by blocking mitochondrial import of pre-ALAS1, by increased proteolysis and possibly by inhibiting transcription. In addition, ALAS1 activity is regulated by a transcriptional co-activator, PGC-1α; an effect that links the rate of hepatic heme biosynthesis with nutritional status.

The erythroid isoform, ALAS2, is encoded by a gene on chromosome Xp11.21 and is expressed only in erythroid cells. Its activity is regulated by two distinct mechanisms. Transcription is enhanced during erythroid differentiation by the action of erythroid-specific transcription factors, and mRNA concentrations are regulated by iron. Iron deficiency in erythroid cells promotes specific binding of iron regulatory proteins (IRPs) to an iron-responsive element (IRE) in the 5′ untranslated region (UTR) of *ALAS2* mRNA with consequent inhibition of translation.

### Function of Heme

Heme functions as a prosthetic group in various proteins in which, depending on the function of the protein, the iron shifts freely between the 2+ and 3+ valency states. Heme biosynthesis is ubiquitous but occurs mainly in the bone marrow (70% to 80%) and approximately a further 15% in the liver. Heme-containing proteins participate in a variety of redox reactions, including:

1. Oxygen transport (by hemoglobin in the blood) and storage (by myoglobin in muscle)
2. Mitochondrial respiration (by cytochromes $b_1$, $c_1$, and $a_3$)
3. Enzymatic destruction of peroxides (by catalase and peroxidase)
4. Drug metabolism (by microsomal cytochrome P-450 mixed-function oxidases)

## TABLE 29.2    Adult Reference Intervals

| Specimen | Analyte | Reference Interval (SI Units) | Reference Interval (Traditional Units) |
|---|---|---|---|
| Urine | Porphobilinogen | <1.5 µmol/mmol creatinine<br><10 µmol/L | <3.0 mg/g creatinine<br><0.23 mg/dL |
| | 5-Aminolevulinic acid | <3.8 µmol/mmol creatinine<br><50 µmol/L | <4.4 mg/g creatinine<br><0.66 mg/dL |
| | Total porphyrin | <35 nmol/mmol creatinine<br>20–320 nmol/L | <216 µg/g creatinine<br>14–224 µg/L |
| | Uroporphyrin | 0.8–3.1 nmol/mmol creatinine | 5.9–22.8 µg/g creatinine |
| | Heptacarboxylate porphyrin | <0.9 nmol/mmol creatinine | <6.3 µg/g creatinine |
| | Coproporphyrin-I | 1.2–5.7 nmol/mmol creatinine | 6.9–33.0 µg/g creatinine |
| | Coproporphyrin-III | 4.8–23.8 nmol/mmol creatinine | 27.8–137.7 µg/g creatinine |
| | % Coproporphyrin-III[a] | 68–86 | 68–86 |
| Feces | Total porphyrin | 10–200 nmol/g dry wt | 6–117 µg/g dry wt |
| | Coproporphyrin-I | 1.1–5.5 nmol/g feces<br>2%–33% | 0.7–3.6 µg/g feces |
| | Coproporphyrin-III | 0.2–2.5 nmol/g feces | 0.1–1.6 µg/g feces |
| | Coproporphyrin-III/I ratio | 0.3–1.4 | 0.3–1.4 |
| | Total dicarboxylate porphyrin | 0.5–12.8 nmol/g feces<br>60%–98% | 0.3–7.2 µg/g feces |
| Erythrocytes | Total porphyrin | 0.4–1.7 µmol/L erythrocytes | 25–106 µg/dL erythrocytes |

[a]Percentage of total coproporphyrin.
Laboratories should verify that these ranges are appropriate for use. Further guidance is provided in Chapter 5.
*wt*, Weight.

5. Desaturation of fatty acids (by microsomal cytochrome $b_5$)
6. Tryptophan metabolism (by tryptophan oxygenase)

Reactions of nitric oxide (NO) are often mediated by the reaction of heme with NO in control enzymes such as guanylate cyclase.

Other naturally occurring tetrapyrrole derivatives include vitamin $B_{12}$ and chlorophyll, each of which contains an atom of chelated cobalt and magnesium, respectively.

## SOLUBILITY AND EXCRETION OF HEME PRECURSORS

Typically, only minute quantities of heme precursors accumulate in the body, and the route of excretion largely depends on solubility. The porphyrin precursors ALA and PBG are water soluble and are excreted almost exclusively in urine as is uroporphyrinogen. PBG polymerizes readily, particularly at high concentrations in acid solution to form primarily the I-isomer of uroporphyrin. The last intermediate of the pathway, protoporphyrin (and also protoporphyrinogen), is insoluble in water and is excreted in the feces via the biliary tract. The other porphyrins are of intermediate solubility and appear in both urine and feces. Coproporphyrinogen-I is taken up and excreted by the liver in preference to the III isomer, so that coproporphyrinogen-I predominates in feces and coproporphyrinogen-III in urine. All porphyrinogens in the urine or feces are slowly oxidized to the corresponding porphyrins.

Once in the gut, porphyrins are susceptible to modification by gut flora. The two vinyl groups of protoporphyrin are reduced to ethyl groups, hydrated to hydroxyethyl groups, or removed, giving rise to a variety of secondary porphyrins. Gut flora can also metabolize heme (from dietary, gut cell lining, or gastrointestinal bleeding) to produce a variety of dicarboxylic porphyrins. In addition, some bacteria are capable of de novo synthesis of porphyrins.

The differing solubility of individual porphyrins is of importance not only in determining the route of excretion from the body but also in the design of analytical methods for their extraction and fractionation. At pH 7, the carboxyl groups are ionized, and the molecule has a net negative charge. Below pH 2, the pyrrole nitrogens and the carboxyl groups become protonated so that the molecule has a net positive charge. At physiologic pH, the solubility of a given porphyrin is determined by the number of substituent carboxyl groups. Uroporphyrin has eight carboxylate groups and is the most soluble porphyrin in aqueous media. Protoporphyrin has only two carboxylate groups, is insoluble in water, but dissolves readily in lipid environments, and binds readily to the hydrophobic regions of proteins such as albumin. Coproporphyrin, with four carboxylate groups, has intermediate solubility. Reference ranges for porphyrins and porphyrin precursors in blood, urine, and feces are reported in Table 29.2.

## THE PORPHYRIAS

The porphyrias are a group of metabolic disorders associated with a disturbance of heme biosynthesis (Table 29.3). All are inherited in monogenic patterns, apart from some forms of porphyria cutanea tarda (PCT) and rare erythropoietic porphyrias associated with malignant myeloid disorders. Each type of porphyria is defined by the association of characteristic clinical features with a specific pattern of accumulation

## TABLE 29.3    Main Types of Human Porphyria

| Disorder | Defective Enzyme | Prevalence[a] (Per Million) | Neurovisceral Crises | Skin Lesions | Inheritance |
|---|---|---|---|---|---|
| **Acute Porphyrias** | | | | | |
| ADP | ALAD | – | + | – | AR |
| AIP | HMBS | 5.9 | + | – | AD |
| HCP | CPOX | 0.9 | + | +[b,c] | AD |
| VP | PPOX | 3.2 | + | +[b,c] | AD |
| **Nonacute Porphyrias** | | | | | |
| CEP | UROS | 0.3 | – | +[c] | AR |
| PCT | UROD | 40 | – | +[c] | Complex (20% AD) |
| EPP | FECH | 9.2 | – | +[d] | AR |
| XLEPP | ALAS2 | 0.15 | – | +[d] | XL |

[a]Estimated prevalence of clinically overt disease.
[b]Skin lesions and neurovisceral crises may occur alone or together.
[c]Fragile skin, bullae.
[d]Acute photosensitivity without fragile skin, bullae.
AD, Autosomal dominant; ADP, ALA dehydratase deficiency porphyria; AIP; acute intermittent porphyria; ALAD, aminolevulinic acid dehydratase; ALAS, aminolevulinate synthase; AR, autosomal recessive; CEP, congenital erythropoietic porphyria; CPOX, coproporphyrinogen oxidase; EPP, erythropoietic protoporphyria; FECH, ferrochelatase; HCP, hereditary coproporphyria; HMBS, hydroxymethylbilane synthase; PCT, porphyria cutanea tarda; PPOX, protoporphyrinogen oxidase; UROD, uroporphyrinogen decarboxylase; UROS, uroporphyrinogen-III synthase; VP, variegate porphyria; XL, X-linked; XLEPP, X-linked erythropoietic protoporphyria.

of heme precursors that reflects increased formation of the substrate of the enzyme that is partially deficient or becomes secondarily rate-limiting in that type of porphyria (Table 29.4). The porphyrias are characterized clinically by two main features: skin lesions in sun-exposed areas and acute neurovisceral attacks, typically comprising of abdominal pain, peripheral neuropathy, and mental disturbance. The skin lesions are caused by porphyrin-catalyzed photodamage, of which singlet oxygen is the main mediator. Acute attacks are associated with increased formation of ALA and consequently PBG from induced activity of hepatic ALAS1 and partial hepatic heme deficiency, often in response to induction of hepatic CYPs by drugs and other factors, such as hormones. The relationship of these biochemical changes to the neuronal dysfunction that underlines all clinical features of the acute attack is uncertain. The leading hypothesis for pathophysiology is that ALA, or a product of ALA or PBG, is neurotoxic, possibly through interference with the gamma amino butyric acid (GABA) receptor pathway. As listed in Table 29.3, the porphyrias are classified as acute (in which acute neurovisceral attacks occur) or nonacute.

### Acute Porphyrias

The four acute porphyrias include ALA dehydratase deficiency porphyria (ADP), acute intermittent porphyria (AIP), variegate porphyria (VP), and hereditary coproporphyria (HCP). These disorders are autosomal dominant except for the very rare disorder, ADP, which is autosomal recessive.

The inherited defect in each of the autosomal dominant acute porphyrias (see Table 29.3) is a mutation in one copy of a gene that encodes an enzyme involved in heme synthesis, resulting in complete or near-complete enzyme deficiency from that allele. Heme supply is maintained at normal or

near-normal concentration by upregulation of ALAS1, with a consequent increase in the substrate concentration for the defective enzyme. These compensatory changes vary between tissues; they are most prominent in the liver and are undetectable in most other organs. They also vary between individuals with some showing no evidence of overproduction of heme precursors, and others having biochemically manifest disease with or without clinical symptoms.

Low clinical penetrance (the frequency of expression of an allele when it is present in the genotype) is a prominent feature of all the autosomal dominant acute porphyrias. Family studies indicate that many genetically affected individuals are asymptomatic throughout life.

All the autosomal dominant acute porphyrias show extensive allelic heterogeneity, but founder mutations are present in some populations and explain the high frequency of VP in South Africans of Dutch descent and of AIP in Sweden.

### Clinical Features

The life-threatening, acute neurovisceral attacks that occur in AIP, VP, and HCP are clinically identical. Acute attacks are very rare before puberty, usually occur first between the ages of 15 and 40 years, and are more common in women. Precipitating factors have been identified in about two-thirds of patients who present with acute attacks. The most important are drugs; alcohol, especially binge drinking; the menstrual cycle; calorie restriction; infection; and stress. Pregnancy, although associated with large hormonal changes, is usually well tolerated in most women with acute porphyria. Drugs known to provoke acute attacks include barbiturates, sulfonamides, progestogens, and some anticonvulsants, but many others have been implicated in the precipitation of acute attacks (www.drugs-porphyria.org).

## TABLE 29.4 Porphyrias: Patterns of Overproduction of Heme Precursors During Clinically Overt Phase of Disease

| Porphyria | Urine PBG/ALA | Urine Porphyrins | Fecal Porphyrins | Erythrocyte Porphyrins | Plasma Fluorescence Emission Peak |
|---|---|---|---|---|---|
| ADP | ALA | Copro-III | Not increased | ZPP | — |
| AIP | PBG > ALA | Mainly uroporphyrin from PBG | Normal or increased[a] Copro-III/I ratio normal | Not increased | 615–622 nm[b] |
| CEP | Not increased | Uro-I, Copro-I | Copro-I | ZPP, Proto, Copro-I, Uro-I | 615–620 nm |
| PCT | Not increased | Uro, Hepta[c] | Isocopro, Hepta, Penta | Not increased | 615–622 nm |
| HCP | PBG > ALA[d] | Copro-III, uroporphyrin from PBG | Copro-III, Copro-III/I ratio increased | Not increased | 615–622 nm[b] |
| VP | PBG > ALA[d] | Copro-III, uroporphyrin from PBG | Proto IX>Copro-III X-porphyrin Copro-III/I ratio increased[e] | Not increased | 624–628 nm |
| EPP | Not increased | Not increased | ±Proto[f] | Metal-free proto | 626–634 nm[g] |
| XLEPP | Not increased | Not increased | ±Proto | Metal-free proto, ZPP[h] | 626–634 nm[g] |

[a]Slight increase only unless uroporphyrin is present.
[b]Not always increased.
[c]Other methylcarboxylate-substituted porphyrins are increased to a smaller extent; uroporphyrin is a mixture of type I and III isomers; heptacarboxylate porphyrin is mainly type III.
[d]PBG and ALA may be normal when only skin lesions are present.
[e]Coproporphyrin-III/I ratio increased, but usually less than in overt HCP.
[f]Not increased in about 40% of patients.
[g]Protoporphyrin (Proto) bound to globin. If hemolysis is present the peak shifts to the left (i.e., at 626–628 nm or is quenched).
[h]Zn-protoporphyrin (ZPP) 20%–60% of total erythrocyte protoporphyrin.
*ADP*, ALA dehydratase deficiency porphyria; *AIP*; acute intermittent porphyria; *ALA*, aminolevulinic acid; *CEP*, congenital erythropoietic porphyria; *EPP*, erythropoietic protoporphyria; *HCP*, hereditary coproporphyria; *PBG*, porphobilinogen; *PCT*, porphyria cutanea tarda; *VP*, variegate porphyria; *XLEPP*, X-linked erythropoietic protoporphyria.

The main clinical features are summarized in Table 29.5. Acute attacks almost always start with abdominal pain that rapidly becomes very severe and may also be present in the back and thighs. Vomiting, constipation, tachycardia, and hypertension are frequent with convulsions as a consequence of hyponatremia or secondary to central nervous system involvement. In severe cases, a predominant motor neuropathy develops that may progress to flaccid quadriparesis. The acute phase may be accompanied by mental confusion with abrupt changes in mood, hallucinations, and other psychotic features. Persistent psychiatric illness is not a feature of the acute porphyrias, although mild anxiety or depression may be present in some patients. Abdominal pain usually resolves within 2 weeks, but recovery from neuropathy may take many months and is not always complete. Most patients have one or a few attacks followed by complete recovery and prolonged remission. About 5% have repeated acute attacks over a period of years, which in women may be premenstrual.

Skin lesions similar to those of PCT and other bullous porphyrias are present in about 80% of patients with clinically manifest VP (see Table 29.3), and about 60% of patients with VP present with skin lesions alone. The skin

## TABLE 29.5 Clinical Features of an Acute Neurovisceral Attack of Porphyria

| Symptom/Sign | Percentage of Acute Attacks |
|---|---|
| Abdominal pain | 85–90 |
| Nonabdominal pain | 25–70 |
| Vomiting and nausea | 30–90 |
| Constipation/diarrhea | 50–80 |
| Psychologic symptoms (insomnia, anxiety, depression, confusion, hallucinations) | 20–85 |
| Acute encephalopathy (headache, somnolence, seizures, altered consciousness) | 2–20 |
| Motor neuropathy (muscle weakness, pain, low/absent tendon reflexes) | 10–90 |
| Hemi/tetraparesis | 30–40 |
| Respiratory paralysis | 10–55 |
| Sensory neuropathy | 10–40 |
| Hypertension | 40–75 |
| Tachycardia (>80/min) | 30–85 |
| Hyponatremia (<135 nmol/L) | 30–60 |

Data modified from Harper P, Sardh E. Management of acute intermittent porphyria. *Expert Opin Orphan Drugs.* 2014;2(4):349–368.

is less commonly affected in HCP; skin lesions without an acute attack are uncommon and may be provoked by intercurrent cholestasis.

Treatment is initially supportive and focuses on managing the symptoms and other clinical features. Specific treatment to shorten an acute attack is based on suppressing hepatic ALAS activity by infusion of human hemin, or for recurrent attacks, administration of a novel RNA interference therapy, givosiran. Carbohydrate infusions can ameliorate an acute attack by downregulation of hepatic *ALAS1* transcription, but this treatment is less effective than intravenous hemin and care needs to be taken not to precipitate or worsen hyponatremia.

In severe cases where givosiran is not accessible, liver transplantation has been used.

Long-term complications of acute porphyrias, particularly AIP, include chronic renal failure, hypertension, and primary liver cancer.

### Management of Families

The diagnosis of autosomal dominant acute porphyria should be followed by an investigation of the patient's family to identify affected, often asymptomatic relatives, so they can be advised to avoid drugs and other factors known to provoke acute attacks and to allow for assessment related to risk of long-term complications.

### POINTS TO REMEMBER

**Acute Porphyrias**
- Present clinically after puberty.
- Low clinical penetrance means that there is usually no family history.
- AIP is associated with acute attacks, whereas VP and HCP may present with acute attacks, skin photosensitivity, or both.
- Acute attacks are due to autonomic, central, and motor neuropathy.
- Common precipitants are prescribed drugs, hormonal fluctuations, binge drinking, low carbohydrate intake, infection, and stress.
- Treatment is aimed at suppressing hepatic ALAS activity.

### Nonacute Porphyrias

The nonacute porphyrias fall into two categories depending on whether patients have bullous skin lesions (**PCT**, **congenital erythropoietic porphyria [CEP]**) or acute photosensitivity (**erythropoietic protoporphyria [EPP]**, **X-linked erythropoietic protoporphyria [XLEPP]**).

### Porphyria Cutanea Tarda

PCT is by far the most common porphyria. The disease occurs at all ages in both sexes with onset usually during the fifth and sixth decades. Lesions on sun-exposed skin, particularly the backs of the hands, the forearm, and the face, are present in all patients. These lesions are identical

to those seen in the other bullous porphyrias (see Table 29.3). Increased mechanical fragility of the skin, with trivial trauma leading to blisters (bullae) and erosions, is present in virtually all patients.

A combination of skin lesions with liver damage is strongly associated with alcohol abuse, estrogens, infection with hepatotropic viruses, particularly hepatitis C (HCV), smoking, and mutations in the hemochromatosis (*HFE*) gene. PCT may also complicate HIV infection. Hepatic iron overload, in combination with at least one of the other associated factors, is present in almost all patients.

PCT results from decreased activity of UROD in the liver, which is understood to be secondary to a UROD inhibitor, porphomethene, generated by iron-dependent partial oxidation of uroporphyrinogen. This inhibition leads to the overproduction of uroporphyrin and other carboxymethyl-substituted porphyrins, which accumulate in the liver and skin, where they act as photosensitizers. This iron dependence explains why patients with iron overload disorders, such as hemochromatosis, develop PCT. Two main types of PCT can be identified in most populations; about 80% of patients have the sporadic (type I) form of PCT, in which the enzyme defect is restricted to the liver and is a result of viral illness (e.g., HCV) or exogenous substances (e.g., hepatic iron overload, alcohol excess). The *UROD* gene appears to be normal. The rest have familial (type II) PCT, which is inherited in an autosomal dominant manner with low clinical penetrance. In this form, the mutation of one *UROD* gene leads to half-normal UROD activity in all tissues. However, the hepatic enzyme activity has to be 20% or less of normal for porphyrins to accumulate and cutaneous symptoms to appear. This further reduction in activity is dependent on the additional triggering factors associated with liver damage outlined above and explains the low clinical penetrance. PCT may also be caused by exposure to certain polyhalogenated aromatic hydrocarbons, such as hexachlorobenzene and 2,3,7,8-tetrachlorodibenzo-*p*-dioxin. Initially management is based on skin protection, sunlight avoidance, and removing exogenous triggers. Treatment aimed at lowering circulating porphyrins involves either hepatic iron depletion by venesection, or low dose chloroquine (or hydroxychloroquine) to remove porphyrins from the liver. Treatment to eradicate HCV is also curative.

### Congenital Erythropoietic Porphyria

CEP is the least common but most severe of the cutaneous porphyrias. The clinical features vary in severity from hydrops fetalis with death in utero—through the onset in infancy of severe skin lesions with transfusion-dependent hemolytic anemia—to mild skin lesions, resembling PCT.

With age, progressive scarring (particularly if erosions become infected), and atrophic changes lead to photomutilation with erosions of the terminal phalanges; destruction of ears, nose, and eyelids; and alopecia. Accumulation of porphyrin in bone is visible as erythrodontia—brownish-red teeth that fluoresce in UVA light. The skin changes are usually accompanied by hemolytic anemia and splenomegaly. Hemolysis may be fully compensated or mild, but in some patients, anemia is severe enough to require repeated transfusion. Treatment is focused on strict sunlight protection, with bone marrow transplantation reserved for the most severely affected.

CEP is an autosomal recessive disease resulting from decreased UROS activity (see Table 29.3). Patients are homoallelic or heteroallelic for mutations in the *UROS* gene or, rarely, the *GATA1* gene, which encodes an erythroid transcription factor.

## Erythropoietic Protoporphyria and X-Linked Erythropoietic Protoporphyria

The protoporphyrias are characterized by life-long acute photosensitivity caused by accumulation of protoporphyrin-IX in the skin. In EPP, overproduction of protoporphyrin-IX results from decreased activity of FECH. EPP is an autosomal recessive disease where most individuals are compound heterozygotes for a *FECH* mutation that abolishes or severely decreases FECH activity and a hypomorphic *FECH* c.315-48C allele (rs2272783). In approximately 4% of EPP families, affected individuals are heteroallelic or homoallelic for *FECH* mutations. In XLEPP, a gain-of-function mutation in *ALAS2*, usually a deletion within the C-terminal region, leads to formation and accumulation of protoporphyrin in excess of the amount required for hemoglobinization. XLEPP is inherited in an X-linked pattern with expression of disease in males and most females. In rare cases, XLEPP is associated with a mutation in *CLPX*, a modulator of erythroid heme biosynthesis. The symptoms of XLEPP are clinically indistinguishable from EPP.

Patients with either form of protoporphyria present with acute photosensitivity characterized by burning pain, which normally starts between birth and the age of 6 years. Onset after the age of 40 years is very rare; most cases are due to acquired FECH deficiency associated with myelodysplasia. Exposure to sun is followed by an intensely painful, burning, prickling, itching sensation in the skin, usually within 5 to 30 minutes, which is most frequently on the face and the back of the hands. The phototoxic reaction persists for several hours up to days, and symptoms are not relieved by shielding the skin from light. Recurrent sun exposure leads to chronic skin changes, such as shallow linear scars over the bridge of the nose and elsewhere on the face, and the skin may become thickened and waxy, especially over the knuckles. Presently, treatment options are mainly prophylactic, focusing on avoidance of sunlight, including protective clothing, use of reflectant sunscreens, narrowband ultraviolet B phototherapy, and an α-melanocyte–stimulating hormone analogue, afamelanotide, which stimulates skin pigmentation.

The most severe complication of protoporphyria is progressive hepatic failure, which is caused by the accumulation of protoporphyrin in the liver. About 15% of patients have abnormal biochemical tests of liver function, particularly increased aspartate aminotransferase; however, only about 5% of patients develop liver failure, which will require liver transplantation with or without bone marrow transplantation.

---

### POINTS TO REMEMBER

**Cutaneous Porphyrias**
- Porphyrins absorb light with wavelengths around 400 nm.
- The absorbed radiant energy either
  - Interacts with molecular oxygen to create reactive oxygen species which cause porphyrin-catalyzed photo damage.
  - Released as red fluorescent light, which is the basis of porphyrin analytical methods.
- Photosensitivity can occur in any porphyria where porphyrin ring structures accumulate, that is, all the porphyrias except AIP and ADP.
- Symptoms manifest clinically as an immediate or delayed photosensitivity dependent on the type of porphyrins that accumulate and their localization within the skin.
- Protection of the skin from sunlight is essential to reduce symptoms.

---

## Abnormalities of Porphyrin Metabolism Not Caused by Porphyria

Abnormalities of porphyrin metabolism or excretion, or both, may occur in a number of conditions other than the porphyrias and need to be considered when porphyrin results are interpreted from patients in whom porphyria is suspected. Many of these conditions are more common than the porphyrias. Relevant disorders include exposure to various toxins, for example, lead, hereditary tyrosinemia, renal and hepatobiliary disorders, hematological diseases, and situations where there is increased heme in the gastrointestinal system (diet, bleeding, bacteria). These abnormalities and their causes are detailed in Table 29.6. Conversely, there are a number of conditions that can give rise to skin lesions identical to those that characterize bullous porphyrias, but in which no abnormality in accumulation or excretion of porphyrins can be demonstrated. This is usually described as "pseudoporphyria" and is mainly associated with photosensitization from prescribed drugs, sunbeds, and in some patients undergoing hemodialysis for chronic renal failure.

## LABORATORY DIAGNOSIS OF PORPHYRIA

Laboratory investigation is essential for the diagnosis and exclusion of the porphyrias both in patients with symptoms of acute porphyria and in patients with typical cutaneous lesions because none of the clinical features are sufficiently distinctive to allow diagnosis on clinical grounds alone.

### Patients With Symptoms of Porphyria

In patients with current symptoms caused by porphyria, excessive production of heme precursors is always present. Diagnosis depends on demonstrating specific patterns of overproduction of heme precursors (see Table 29.4) and is usually straightforward, provided appropriate specimens are examined for the relevant intermediates using adequately sensitive techniques. Although the porphyrias are uncommon disorders, the variability of the associated clinical

## TABLE 29.6   Secondary Disorders of Porphyrin Metabolism

| Sample | Increased Heme Precursors | Clinical Conditions |
|---|---|---|
| Urine | Coproporphyrin | Liver dysfunction, fever, drugs, alcohol |
| | Aminolevulinic acid | Lead poisoning, hereditary tyrosinemia |
| Feces | Protoporphyrin, other dicarboxylic porphyrins | Intestinal bleed, high protein intake |
| Plasma | Uroporphyrin | Renal failure |
| | Coproporphyrin | Liver dysfunction |
| Erythrocytes | Zinc protoporphyrin | Iron deficiency anemia |
| | | Lead poisoning |

features may make it necessary to consider them as differential diagnoses in many clinical situations. It is important therefore to apply diagnostic strategies that not only allow for the diagnosis of a porphyria, but also adequately exclude the diagnosis. The diagnostic strategy of choice depends on the mode of presentation.

### Patient Presenting With Suspected Acute Attack

Failure to correctly diagnose an attack of acute porphyria not only delays appropriate life-saving treatment but may result in unnecessary surgery or administration of drugs that aggravate the attack with potentially fatal consequences. A false diagnosis of porphyria may be equally serious because of delayed vital surgery or other treatment, and may also lead to analgesic (including opiate) misuse and dependency. The essential first-line investigation is the measurement of urinary PBG by an adequately sensitive and specific method, in a morning or random urine sample. Twenty-four-hour urine collections are not recommended. Testing for ALA is often performed along with PBG. Based on the currently available evidence, PBG excretion is always increased during an acute attack of AIP, HCP, or VP, usually to a concentration that exceeds 10 times the upper reference limit. Normal PBG excretion, at a time when symptoms are present, provides very strong evidence against any type of acute porphyria as their cause, except for the very rare ADP. In ADP, PBG is normal or only slightly elevated, while ALA is markedly increased as is urinary coproporphyrin excretion. The same pattern may be observed in lead poisoning (see Tables 29.4 and 29.6).

*Differentiation between the acute porphyrias.* Management of the attack is the same regardless of the type of acute porphyria, so further investigation is not a matter of urgency. However, differentiation between the acute porphyrias is necessary for deciding which gene to examine by DNA analysis and for the selection of appropriate tests for use in family studies, as well as assessing for the risk of skin symptoms. The absence of skin lesions does not exclude VP or HCP (see Table 29.3).

Once the diagnosis of acute porphyria has been established, the most efficient diagnostic strategy uses plasma fluorescence scanning and fecal porphyrin fractionation with coproporphyrin III and I separation to differentiate between AIP, VP, and HCP (see Table 29.4).

Investigation of an asymptomatic patient with past symptoms consistent with an acute attack.

Diagnosis may be less straightforward when a patient presents for investigation after all clinical symptoms have resolved. Appropriate investigations include those described earlier.

In VP and HCP, excretion of PBG and ALA is usually normal in the absence of acute symptoms. Data indicate that ALA and PBG excretion remain increased in AIP patients for many years after an acute attack. If, however, all these tests are normal, the patient may have AIP in remission, but is most likely to have had a nonporphyric illness with symptoms mimicking those of acute porphyria. If clinical suspicion remains high, mutational analysis of *HMBS*, supplemented by assay of HMBS activity in mutation-negative patients, may help to distinguish these possibilities.

### Patients With Cutaneous Symptoms

Active skin lesions of cutaneous porphyrias require increased circulating porphyrins to reach the skin. Thus, analysis of plasma porphyrins by fluorescence emission spectroscopy is usually the first step when diagnosing cutaneous porphyrias (Fig. 29.3). The route of further investigation to identify the specific porphyria is dictated by the clinical presentation. Urine ALA and PBG have no role in the diagnosis of cutaneous porphyrias.

*Patients with acute photosensitivity without skin fragility or bullae.* When suspecting EPP/XLEPP, the essential investigation consists of the measurement of erythrocyte protoporphyrin concentration using a sensitive fluorometric method. Screening tests using solvent extraction of blood or fluorescence microscopy of erythrocytes are unreliable. If the erythrocyte (proto)porphyrin concentration is within the reference interval, EPP/XLEPP is excluded. If the concentration is increased, it is important to determine whether the increase is caused mainly by metal-free protoporphyrin, as in EPP, both free and ZPP as in XLEPP, or primarily by ZPP, as in iron deficiency and lead toxicity (Tables 29.4 and 29.6).

DNA analysis is required to confirm the diagnosis of XLEPP in patients with an increased percentage of ZPP or in patients with a family history suggestive of XLEPP.

*Patients with bullae/fragility/scarring.* Clinically indistinguishable skin lesions occur in PCT, VP, HCP, CEP (see Table 29.3), and other rare variants such as the homozygous

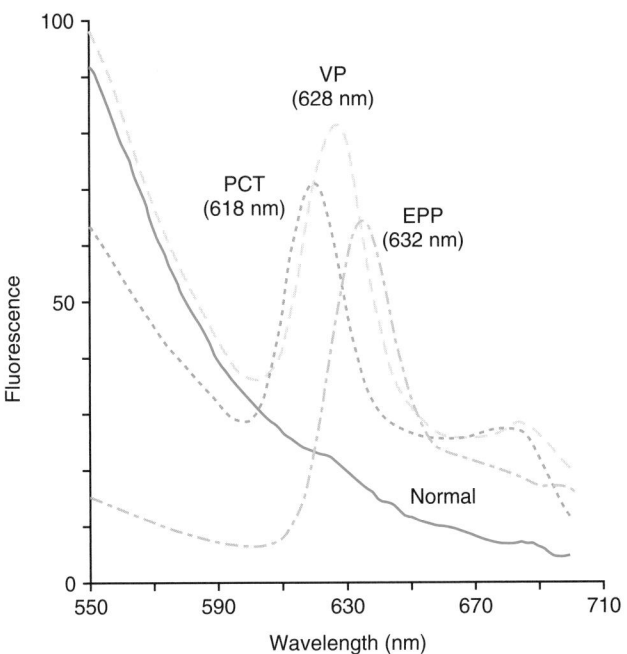

**Fig. 29.3** Fluorescence emission spectra (excitation, 405 nm) of dilutions in phosphate-buffered saline (PBS) of plasma from a normal individual and from patients with various porphyrias. *EPP*, Erythropoietic protoporphyria; *PCT*, porphyria cutanea tarda; *VP*, variegate porphyria.

or compound heterozygous forms of the autosomal dominant porphyrias. In addition, identical skin lesions characterize pseudoporphyria, in which porphyrin metabolism is normal. Initial investigations should include the fluorescence emission spectroscopy of plasma. If this is normal, then porphyria is excluded as the cause of any active bullous skin lesions.

A positive plasma porphyrin fluorescence scan with any increase in total urinary porphyrin should be further investigated by the determination of individual porphyrins in urine and feces using a technique capable of resolving all porphyrins of clinical interest, including isomers. The pattern observed in each of these porphyrias is unique (see Table 29.4).

Patients may present for investigation after their skin lesions have healed. In PCT, excretion and plasma porphyrin concentrations return to normal during remission, but the proportions of individual porphyrins in urine and feces may remain abnormal for longer than the total porphyrin concentrations, and the determination of individual porphyrins may suggest the diagnosis. The plasma fluorescence scan in VP and fecal coproporphyrin-III excretion in HCP remain abnormal during clinical remission.

## Asymptomatic Relatives of Patients With Porphyria

Depending on the type of porphyria, investigating healthy, at-risk relatives may be beneficial.

### Predictive Testing of Autosomal Dominant Acute Porphyrias

The screening of family members to identify asymptomatic individuals who have inherited AIP, VP, or HCP, and therefore

are at risk for acute attacks, is an essential part of the management of families with these disorders. Mutation detection by DNA analysis is the method of choice for family studies, unless a mutation cannot be identified in the proband, as metabolite measurements have low negative predictive value in asymptomatic individuals. Family members should be appropriately counseled prior to testing, and testing of children is clinically justifiable. Patients with a predictive diagnosis of acute porphyria should be counseled on the avoidance of agents or behaviors that can trigger acute attacks.

### Erythropoietic Protoporphyria

In EPP caused by mutations in the *FECH* gene, testing the unaffected partner for the presence of the hypomorphic *FECH* c.315-48C allele is helpful in assessing the risk that a future child will have clinically overt disease; the presence of this allele increases the risk from about 1 in 100 to 1 in 4. In XLEPP, mutational analysis of the *ALAS2* gene may be required to identify female carriers, who show phenotypic and biochemical heterogeneity, reflecting the degree of X-chromosomal inactivation of the mutant gene.

### Other Porphyrias

Family investigation has a more limited role in the clinical management of other porphyrias. In PCT, the autosomal dominant familial form has been identified by erythrocyte UROD assay or mutational analysis, but as yet little evidence suggests that family studies are necessary unless requested by anxious relatives, as the identification of a mutation does not alter the management of the patient or family.

For severe homozygous or compound heterozygous porphyrias, such as CEP, ADP, the homozygous dominant form of PCT, hepatoerythropoietic porphyria (HEP), and homozygous dominant acute porphyrias, mutation analysis may be required if prenatal diagnosis in subsequent pregnancies is indicated.

## LABORATORY ANALYSIS

The analytical methods used to diagnose and monitor porphyria are briefly described here. Full descriptions can be found in *Tietz Textbook of Laboratory Medicine*, 7th edition.

### Preanalytical Aspects
### Specimen Collection and Stability

Urinary porphyrins and precursors are best analyzed in fresh, random (10 to 20 mL) samples collected without preservative. All samples must be protected from light to avoid deterioration; as an example, urinary porphyrin concentrations have been observed to decrease by up to 50% if kept in the light for 24 hours. Samples for urine analysis must be kept refrigerated, or results must be interpreted with caution, as urinary PBG concentration rapidly decreases if stored at room temperature, whereas ALA concentration is stable. Repeated freeze-thaw cycles may also result in considerable loss of analytes, particularly PBG. Precursors and porphyrins in urine should be expressed as a ratio to creatinine concentration to correct for dilution. Very dilute urine (creatinine <2 mmol/L) is unsuitable for analysis, and it may be helpful to request an early morning urine sample to ensure it is appropriately concentrated.

Urine often is of normal color in the nonacute porphyrias, except in CEP, when it is usually red, occasionally to such an extent that it is mistaken for hematuria. During an acute attack, urine may be a reddish-brown color because of the presence of uroporphyrin and other pigments formed by the nonenzymatic polymerization of PBG. This color may be evident immediately or develop progressively during handling and storage.

About 5 to 10 g wet weight of feces is adequate for porphyrin measurements. Diagnostically, important changes in concentration are unlikely to occur within 36 hours at room temperature, and samples are stable for many months at −20°C.

Blood, anticoagulated with ethylenediaminetetraacetic acid (EDTA), shows no loss of protoporphyrin for up to 8 days at room temperature, and for at least 8 weeks at 4°C in the dark. Freeze thawing, however, can result in hemolysis, which will interfere with plasma fluorescence analysis.

## Quality Management and External Quality Assessment

Participation in external quality assessment (EQA) schemes, preferably assessing the total testing process, and the use of internal quality controls (IQCs) are important for porphyria-related analyses. IQC is available commercially for urine analytes (porphyrin, ALA, and PBG) but not for fecal, plasma, or erythrocyte porphyrins. The European Porphyria Network (EPNET) operates a clinical EQA scheme, assessing the total testing process for porphyria-related analyses in all sample types. A specialized analytical EQA scheme covering all sample types is operated by the Royal College of Pathologists of Australasia. The European Molecular Quality Network (EMQN) provides a quality scheme for the molecular testing of the porphyria genes.

## Methods for Porphyrin Precursors in Urine and for Porphyrins in Urine and Feces

The water-soluble metabolites, PBG and ALA, are excreted by the kidneys and usually are measured in the urine in the clinical laboratory.

### Porphobilinogen

Most methods for PBG are based on the reaction of Ehrlich's reagent (dimethylaminobenzaldehyde in acidic solution) with the α-methene carbon of the pyrrole ring to form a colored product variously described as "rose red" or "magenta," which has a characteristic absorption spectrum with a peak at 553 nm and a shoulder at 540 nm. Porphyrins do not contain any α-methene hydrogens and so do not react. Some other substances in urine may react with the reagent to give red products, notably urobilinogen, may inhibit the reaction, or are pigmented themselves and so mask the red chromogen. All need to be removed. This is best achieved by

ion-exchange chromatography (first described by Mauzerall and Granick), but methods for accurate quantification of PBG based on this procedure are time-consuming. A commercial method for the measurement of both PBG and ALA, based on that of Mauzerall and Granick, is available (Recipe Clinical Diagnostics, Munich, Germany). Methods based on high-performance liquid chromatography (HPLC) coupled to detection by mass spectrometry are also being used to measure urinary ALA and PBG simultaneously. These methods are not yet in widespread use due to equipment expense. However, laboratories that have access to a metabolic platform could integrate ALA and PBG measurement in the panel of amino acids. One of the advantages of these more sensitive methods is the quantitation of ALA and PBG in plasma for patients with severe kidney disease.

Several qualitative methods have been described, including the Watson-Schwartz and Hoesch tests. However, these have been criticized for poor detection limits and interferences and if used, it is essential to include appropriate controls and to confirm all positive test results using a specific quantitative method.

### 5-Aminolevulinic Acid

It is possible to measure ALA directly, but it is usually converted into an Ehrlich-reacting pyrrole through condensation with a reagent, such as acetylacetone, after separation from PBG by two-stage anion-exchange chromatography (see above).

### Analysis of Porphyrins in Urine and Feces

The methods for porphyrin fractionation are complex and time-consuming and are not available in every laboratory. Consequently, simple qualitative screening tests are often used to differentiate the majority of specimens that do not require further investigation from the few that justify fractionation of the individual porphyrins. Screening tests in which extracts of urine or feces are examined visually for typical red–pink fluorescence of porphyrins are not sensitive analytically and should not be used. Methods based on spectrophotometric scanning of acidified urine (Fig. 29.4) or fecal extracts for the presence of the Soret band (~400 nm) are recommended and yield semiquantitative information. A commercial method for the photometric determination of total porphyrins in urine is available with a preliminary extraction step by ion exchange chromatography to remove some interfering substances (Recipe Clinical Diagnostics). Quantitative fluorometric methods are also available.

All methods for the fractionation of porphyrins are based on the varying solubilities of individual porphyrins caused by their different β-substituents and, to a lesser extent, on the substituent order around the macrocycle. Methods include differential extraction with solvents, paper and thin-layer chromatography, and HPLC. Solvent extraction methods should not be used because they yield only limited and sometimes misleading information. Reversed-phase HPLC with fluorometric detection, the current method of choice, separates all porphyrins of clinical interest, including isomers

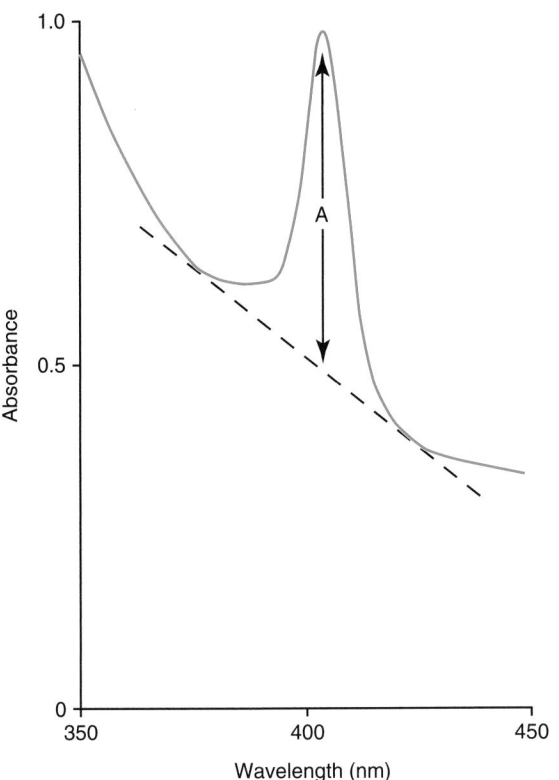

**Fig. 29.4** Absorption spectrum of acidified urine showing the procedure for measurement of corrected absorbance *(A)* of the porphyrin peak.

and metal chelates, without the need for prior methylation. Commercial methods offer fractionation and quantitation of the different urine porphyrins but do not allow the separation of uroporphyrin isomers I and III (Recipe Clinical Diagnostics; Chromsystems Instruments & Chemicals, Gräfelfing, Germany). Representative HPLC chromatograms associated with porphyrin excretion patterns in several different porphyrias are shown in Fig. 29.5.

## Analysis of Blood Porphyrins

The methods described here require a spectrofluorometer with a red-sensitive photomultiplier. If such equipment is not available locally, samples must be referred to a specialized laboratory.

The most widely used method for erythrocyte total porphyrin is based on double extraction and fluorometry. If erythrocyte (proto)porphyrin concentration is increased, it is important to differentiate between metal free protoporphyrin, as in EPP, both free and ZPP as in XLEPP, or primarily ZPP, as in iron deficiency and lead toxicity (Fig. 29.6). This requires extraction with a neutral solvent, such as ethanol or acetone, to prevent the demetalation caused by strong acids, followed by fluorescence spectroscopy or HPLC to distinguish metal-free protoporphyrin from ZPP (fluorescence emission maxima 630 nm and 587 nm, respectively).

## Analysis of Plasma Porphyrins

Plasma porphyrins may be determined by fluorescence emission spectroscopy of saline-diluted plasma or HPLC

analysis of deproteinized extracts. The fluorescence emission method offers the advantages of simplicity and inclusion of porphyrins that are bound covalently to plasma proteins and HPLC analysis cannot, from a diagnostic point of view, replace that method. Porphyrins at neutral pH fluoresce in the 610 to 640 nm region; the wavelength of maximum emission depends primarily on the porphyrin structure, but it is also influenced by the nature of the porphyrin-protein complex (see Fig. 29.3). Plasma fluorescence emission spectroscopy is an essential front-line investigation for suspected cutaneous porphyria. Fractionation of porphyrins in plasma is also available in specialist laboratories, but it provides limited information in addition to urine and fecal porphyrin fractionation.

> **POINTS TO REMEMBER**
>
> **Diagnostics**
> - Identification of individual porphyrias usually requires analysis of urine, feces, and blood samples.
> - All specimens must be protected from light.
> - Clinical information is necessary for correct interpretation of results.
> - Symptomatic porphyria is always associated with increased production of porphyrins ± porphyrin precursors.
>   - Active acute autosomal dominant porphyria can be diagnosed by demonstrating increased PBG excretion in a random urine sample.
>   - Active cutaneous porphyrias can be diagnosed as a first step by finding a positive plasma porphyrin fluorescence emission screen in a freshly separated plasma sample.
> - For EPP a blood sample for erythrocyte protoporphyrin analysis is essential and urine analysis has no role in the diagnosis.
> - Fluorescent porphyrin analysis requires a red-sensitive photomultiplier for detection.

## Enzyme Measurements

Assay of individual enzymes of the heme biosynthetic pathway is rarely required for the assessment of patients with symptoms of porphyria. However, measurement of enzyme activities may be useful for family studies when it is not possible to identify the individual mutation, or when DNA analysis is not available. Erythrocytes are a convenient source of cytoplasmic enzymes (ALAD, HMBS, UROS, and UROD); however, assay of the mitochondrial enzymes (CPOX, PPOX, and FECH) requires nucleated cells, and sampling thus requires specialized techniques.

## DNA Analysis

DNA analysis is required in the porphyrias mainly for family screening, for identifying the pattern of inheritance in families with EPP, and as an aid in assessing the prognosis in CEP. As most mutations are restricted to one or a few families, identification of a mutation in a new family almost always requires analysis of the entire gene.

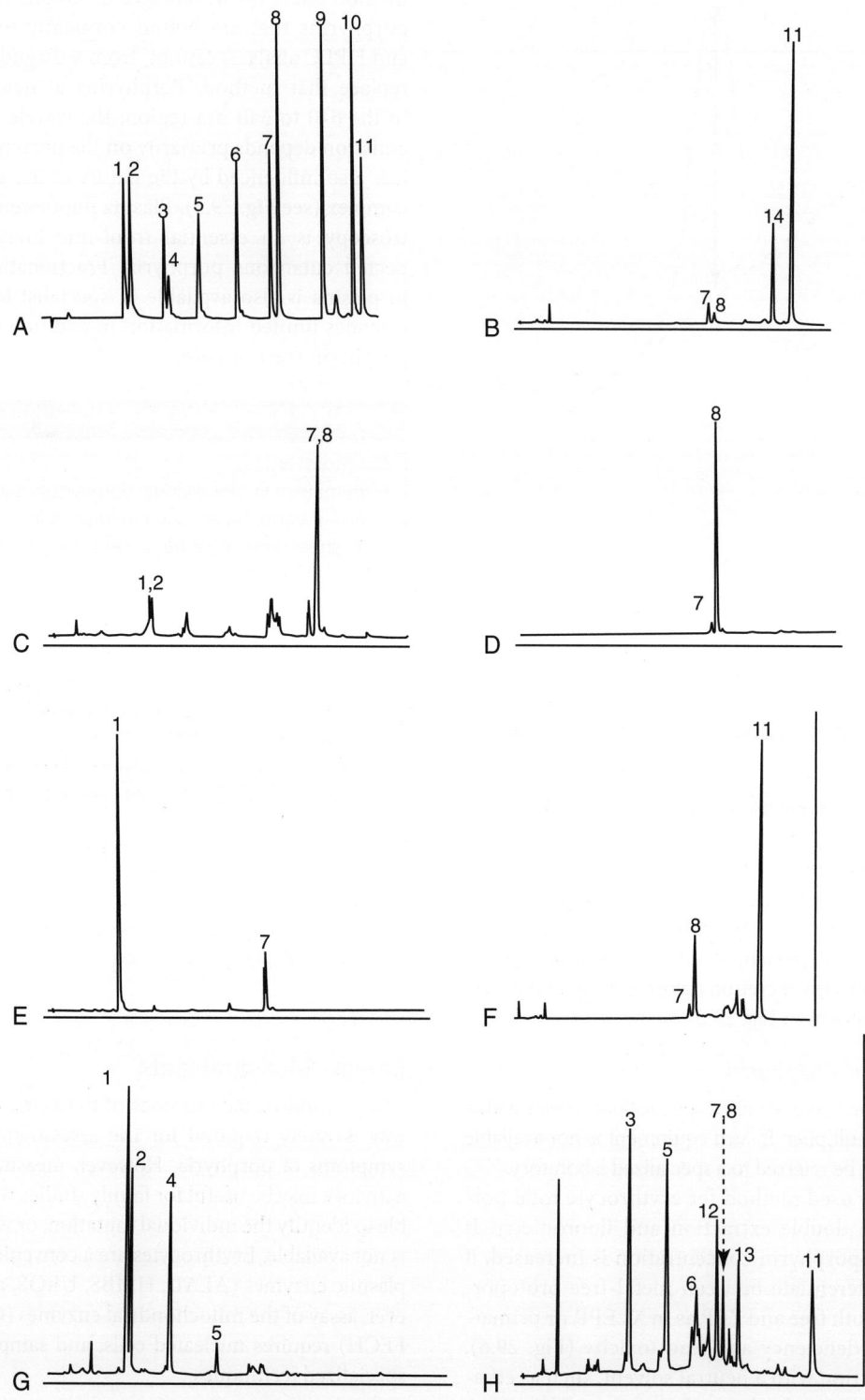

**Fig. 29.5** Representative chromatograms obtained by reverse-phase high-performance liquid chromatography for (A) working standard, (B) normal feces, (C) normal urine, (D) feces—hereditary coproporphyria, (E) urine—congenital erythropoietic porphyria, (F) feces—variegate porphyria, (G) urine—porphyria cutanea tarda, and (H) feces—porphyria cutanea tarda chromatographic conditions. Peaks are *(1)* uroporphyrin-I, *(2)* uroporphyrin-III, *(3)* heptacarboxylate porphyrin-I, *(4)* heptacarboxylate porphyrin-III, *(5)* hexacarboxylate porphyrin, *(6)* pentacarboxylate porphyrin, *(7)* coproporphyrin-I, *(8)* coproporphyrin-III, *(9)* deuteroporphyrin-IX, *(10)* mesoporphyrin-IX, *(11)* protoporphyrin-IX, *(12)* hydroxyisocoproporphyrin, *(13)* isocoproporphyrin and *(14)* pemptoporphyrin-IX.

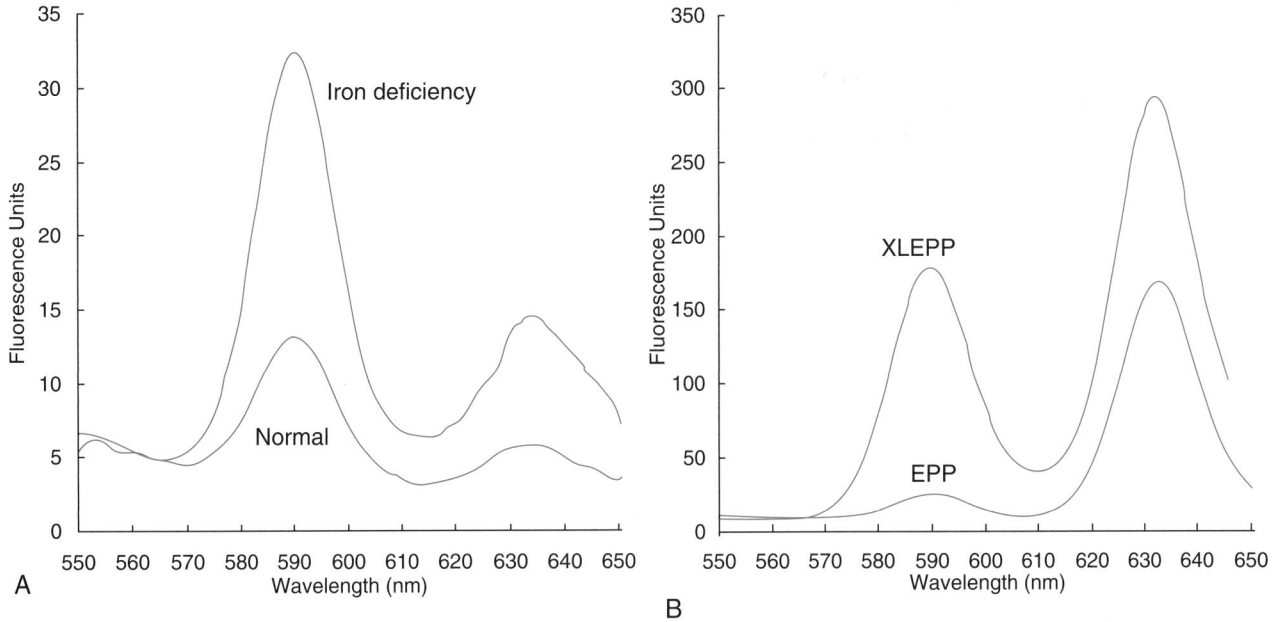

**Fig. 29.6** Fluorescence emission spectra (excitation at 405 nm) of ethanolic extracts of erythrocytes from a normal individual and with iron deficiency (A) and from patients with erythropoietic protoporphyria *(EPP)* or X-linked protoporphyria *(XLEPP)* (B). Fluorescence emission maxima are around 587 nm for ZPP and around 630 nm for metal-free protoporphyrin. Note that different scales are used.

Analysis of a gene for the presence of a mutation is most commonly carried out using direct sequencing and gene dosage analysis of genomic DNA. Unclassified variants continue to be identified in the porphyria genes, and these need to be assessed individually. Once the mutation that causes porphyria in a family has been identified, relatives are screened for its presence by direct sequencing of the region containing the mutation, or by some other mutation-specific method (see Chapter 48).

The clinical sensitivity of mutation detection in most porphyrias is above 90%, provided gene dosage analysis is included in the analysis.

## REVIEW QUESTIONS

1. The precursors of the tetrapyrrole ring structure of porphyrin are:
   a. 5-aminolevulinic acid and iron.
   b. acetyl CoA and porphyrin.
   c. succinyl CoA and glycine.
   d. zinc and porphyrinogen.

2. The indispensable test that allows the diagnosis of an acute attack of autosomal dominant porphyria to be made is:
   a. serum coproporphyrin.
   b. urine porphobilinogen (PBG).
   c. serum zinc protoporphyrin.
   d. red blood cell zinc protoporphyrin.

3. Another name for protoporphyrin that contains iron is:
   a. heme.
   b. porphobilinogen.
   c. coproporphyrin.
   d. ferrochelatase.

4. The skin lesions and photosensitivity observed in patients with nonacute cutaneous porphyrias are the result of:
   a. autonomic neuropathy.
   b. excessive production of ALA.
   c. accumulation of porphyrins in the liver.
   d. excess presence of porphyrins in skin that generate oxygen radicals.

5. In lead toxicity, what replaces iron as a substrate for ferrochelatase to be incorporated into protoporphyrin?
   a. Carbon dioxide
   b. Zinc
   c. Copper
   d. Lead

6. The most common of all the porphyria disorders is:
   a. variegate porphyria.
   b. acute intermittent porphyria.
   c. porphyria cutanea tarda.
   d. congenital erythropoietic porphyria.

7. The last two steps of heme biosynthesis occur in the:
   a. mitochondrion.
   b. cytosol.
   c. endoplasmic reticulum.
   d. cell nucleus.

8. The best specimen type for analyzing porphobilinogen is:
   a. heparinized plasma separated and frozen immediately after collection.
   b. a 24-hour urine collection collected in a dark brown container and preserved with 0.1% HCl.
   c. a fresh early morning urine specimen collected without preservative and protected from light.
   d. blood anticoagulated with EDTA and protected from light.

9. Erythropoietic protoporphyria is characterized by which of the following?
   a. Paralysis caused by the accumulation of porphobilinogen in muscle
   b. Acute photosensitivity caused by protoporphyrin-IX accumulation in skin
   c. Blisters and erosions on sun-exposed skin
   d. Severe abdominal pain and peripheral neuropathy caused by the induction of hepatic cytochromes

10. The reduced form of a porphyrin is known as a:
   a. protoporphyrin.
   b. heme molecule.
   c. pyrrole ring.
   d. porphyrinogen.

## SUGGESTED READINGS

Aarsand AK, Villanger JH, Støle E, et al. European specialist porphyria laboratories: diagnostic strategies, analytical quality, clinical interpretation, and reporting as assessed by an external quality assurance program. *Clin Chem.* 2001;57:1514–1523.

Benton CM, Couchman L, Marsden JT, et al. Direct and simultaneous quantitation of 5-aminolaevulinic acid and porphobilinogen in human serum or plasma by hydrophilic interaction liquid chromatography-atmospheric pressure chemical ionization/tandem mass spectrometry. *Biomed Chromat.* 2013;27:267–272.

Bissell DM, Anderson KE, Bonkovsky HL. Porphyria. *N Engl J Med.* 2017;377:862–872.

Danton M, Lim CK. Porphyrin profiles in blood, urine and feces by HPLC/electrospray ionization tandem mass spectrometry. *Biomedical Chromat.* 2006;20(6–7):612–621.

Elder GH. Porphyria cutanea tarda and related disorders. In: Kadish KM, Smith KM, Guilard R, eds. *The Porphyrin Handbook. Medical Aspects of Porphyrias.* Vol. 14. Amsterdam: Academic Press; 2003:67–92.

Elder G, Harper P, Badminton M, et al. The incidence of inherited porphyrias in Europe. *J Inherit Metabol Dis.* 2013;36:849–857.

Erwin AL, Desnick RJ. Congenital erythropoietic porphyria: recent advances. *Mol Genet Metabol.* 2019;128:288–297.

Ford RE, Magera MJ, Kloke KM, et al. Quantitative measurement of porphobilinogen in urine by stable-isotope dilution liquid chromatography-tandem mass spectrometry. *Clin Chem.* 2001;47:1627–1632.

Gouya L, Puy H, Robreau AM, et al. The penetrance of autosomal dominant erythropoietic protoporphyria is modulated by expression of wild type FECH. *Nat Genet.* 2002;30:23–27.

Hift RJ, Meissner PN. An analysis of 112 acute porphyric attacks in Cape Town, South Africa: evidence that acute intermittent porphyria and variegate porphyria differ in susceptibility and severity. *Medicine (Baltimore).* 2005;84:48–60.

Hindmarsh JT, Oliveras L, Greenway DC. Plasma porphyrins in the porphyrias. *Clin Chem.* 1999;45:1070–1076.

Holme SA, Anstey AV, Finlay AY, et al. Erythropoietic protoporphyria in the United Kingdom: clinical features and effect on quality of life. *Br J Dermatol.* 2006;155:574–581.

Lim CK, Peters TJ. Urine and faecal porphyrin profiles by reversed-phase high-performance liquid chromatography in the porphyrias. *Clin Chim Acta.* 1984;139:55–63.

Marsden JT, Rees DC. Urinary excretion of porphyrins, porphobilinogen and δ-aminolaevulinic acid following an attack of acute intermittent porphyria. *J Clin Pathol.* 2014;67:60–65.

Mauzerall D, Granick S. The occurrence and determination of delta-aminolevulinic acid and porphobilinogen in urine. *J Biol Chem.* 1956;21:435–446.

Meyer UA, Schuurmans MM, Lindberg RL. Acute porphyrias: pathogenesis of neurological manifestations. *Semin Liver Dis.* 1998;18:43–52.

Phillips JD, Bergonia HA, Reilly CA, et al. A porphomethene inhibitor of uroporphyrinogen decarboxylase causes porphyria cutanea tarda. *Proc Nat Acad Sci USA.* 2007;104:5079–5084.

Stein PE, Badminton MN, Rees DC. Update review of the acute porphyrias. *Br J Haematol.* 2017;176:527–538.

Whatley SD, Ducamp S, Gouya L, et al. C-terminal deletions in the ALAS2 gene lead to gain of function and cause X-linked dominant protoporphyria without anemia or iron overload. *Am J Hum Genet.* 2008;83:408–414.

Whatley SD, Mason NG, Woolf JR, et al. Diagnostic strategies for autosomal dominant acute porphyrias: retrospective analysis of 467 unrelated patients referred for mutational analysis of the HMBS, CPOX, or PPOX gene. *Clin Chem.* 2009;55:1406–1414.

Woolf J, Marsden JT, Degg T, et al. Best practice guidelines on first-line laboratory testing for porphyria. *Ann Clin Biochem.* 2017;54:188–198.

# Therapeutic Drug Monitoring

*Michael C. Milone and Leslie M. Shaw\**

## OBJECTIVES

1. Review basic principles of applied pharmacokinetics and drug monitoring.

2. Discuss the rationale for drug monitoring and some of the pitfalls of applying it in the clinical setting.

3. List drugs that are commonly monitored during their use.

## KEY WORDS AND DEFINITIONS

**Antiepileptic** A substance that prevents or alleviates seizures.

**Applied pharmacokinetics** The use of pharmacokinetic principles to guide the clinical application of therapeutic drugs.

**Beta-blocker** A drug that induces adrenergic blockade at either Pl- or P2-adrenergic receptors or at both.

**Bioavailability** The fraction of a drug absorbed into the systemic circulation relative to the same drug administered intravenously.

**Biotransformation** The chemical alteration of a xenobiotic within the body that generally enhances the xenobiotic's aqueous solubility and excretion.

**Dose-response relationship** The relationship between the dose of an administered drug and the response of the organism to the drug.

**Drug half-life** The time required for one-half of an administered drug to be lost through metabolism and elimination.

**Drug interactions** The effects of one drug on the intestinal absorption, metabolism, or action of another drug.

**Enzyme induction** Increased synthesis of an enzyme in response to an inducer or other stimulus.

**First-pass effect** Extensive metabolism of a drug with a high hepatic extraction rate by the liver before it reaches the systemic circulation.

**Generic drug** A drug not protected by a trademark. Also, the scientific name as opposed to the proprietary, brand name.

**Immunophilin** A generic term for an intracellular protein that binds immunosuppressive drugs such as cyclosporine, FK 506, or rapamycin.

**Immunosuppressant** An agent capable of suppressing immune responses.

**Pharmacodynamics** The study of the biochemical and physiological effects of drugs and the mechanisms of their actions, including the correlation of actions and effects of drugs with their chemical structure; also, such effects on the actions of a particular drug or drugs.

**Pharmacokinetics** The activity or fate of drugs in the body over a period of time, including the processes of absorption, distribution, localization in tissues, biotransformation, and excretion.

**Therapeutic drug monitoring** The process of using drug concentration or other pharmacodynamic biomarkers to guide drug dosing.

**Xenobiotics** A chemical substance foreign to the biological system.

---

The ability of medicines to both heal and hurt has been recognized since ancient times. Immortalized by the writing of the Renaissance Swiss-German physician Paracelsus over 500 years ago:

*All things are poison and nothing is without poison, only the dose makes that a thing is not a poison.*

\*The authors gratefully acknowledge the contributions by Christine L.H. Snozek, Gwendolyn A. McMillan, and Thomas P. Moyer on which this chapter is based.

The challenge in medicine is therefore to determine the optimal dose of medicine that will help a patient with limited associated harm.

Studies in the 1990s identified adverse events associated with drug therapy as ranking within the top 10 causes of death in the United States. Although many severe or fatal events may not be preventable, more than one-third appear to be preventable. In addition to the tragic life-and-death consequences of adverse drug events (ADEs), failed drug therapy also has a significant economic impact. The estimated cost of ADEs ranges from $17 to $29 billion in the United States alone. Just examining hospital-associated ADEs, the average cost of treating each preventable event is estimated to be greater than $3000 in addition to the increased length of stay. The causes of preventable drug-related adverse events vary; however, inadequate monitoring of therapy represents major sources of preventable ADEs contributing to as much as 40% of these events. Improving monitoring strategies is therefore likely to have an important impact on both health and its associated cost.

There are many ways in which drug therapy can be monitored. Clinical signs and symptoms of toxicity are often an effective way to detect toxicity or treatment failure. **Beta-blockers** represent a typical example. Blood pressure and heart rate monitoring can be used to assess the efficacy and toxicity of these drugs. Both are also easily measurable in the clinical setting and even at home. As a result, there is little need to perform monitoring beyond these straightforward clinical assessments.

The efficacy and toxicity of some drugs, however, can be much more difficult to monitor based on clinical signs and symptoms alone. The consequences of inappropriate insulin treatment are insidious, potentially life threatening, and very difficult to detect. Excessive insulin can lead to an acute decrease in blood glucose culminating in coma, brain injury, and death. Inadequate insulin dosing, although not as acutely life threatening, leads to vascular disease, end-stage renal failure, blindness, and neuropathy, which result in significant morbidity and mortality. Laboratory testing of blood glucose, a biomarker of insulin's mechanism of action, provides a means to monitor insulin therapy and prevent complications. It is so important in diabetes therapy that it has driven commercial development of point-of-care (POC) devices that patients can use to routinely monitor therapy at home. Biomarkers of drug efficacy or toxicity like blood glucose, although highly desirable, are not always available. In the absence of a useful drug effect biomarker, measuring the drug itself provides a potential surrogate.

**Therapeutic drug monitoring** (TDM) is the traditional term used for the activity of measuring drug concentrations to tailor the dose of the medication to an individual. There is an implicit assumption in TDM of a relationship between drug concentrations and efficacy or toxicity outcomes. The use of TDM and **applied pharmacokinetics** to guide drug therapy began in the 1960s, coincident with the development of robust analytical techniques. Since that time, TDM has become the standard of care for monitoring therapy with many drugs, including antiepileptic drugs (AEDs), immunosuppressive drugs (ISDs), and antibiotics. TDM is a complex process that involves pharmacists, laboratory professionals, and physicians. To justify the costs associated with TDM, it must improve clinical outcome and reduce the overall cost of drug therapy. Prospective, randomized, concentration-controlled trials (RCCTs) of TDM are limited; however, some of these RCCTs show that concentration control can improve efficacy and reduce drug therapy toxicity. The cost-effectiveness of TDM is lacking for most drugs, but TDM has been shown to improve the costs of aminoglycoside therapy.

TDM may also aid in the detection of nonadherence to drug therapy, which represents a frequent and important cause of preventable ADEs.

# FUNDAMENTAL PRINCIPLES OF APPLIED PHARMACOKINETICS

## Basic Concepts and Definitions

Pharmacology comprises that body of knowledge surrounding chemical agents and their effects on living processes. This is a broad field, and it has traditionally been confined to those drugs that are useful in the prevention, diagnosis, and treatment of disease. Pharmacotherapeutics is that part of pharmacology concerned primarily with the application or administration of drugs to patients for the purpose of prevention and treatment of disease. For this aspect of medical practice to be effective, the pharmacodynamic and pharmacokinetic properties of drugs should be understood.

### Pharmacodynamics

**Pharmacodynamics** is concerned with the interaction of pharmacologically active substances with target sites, and the biochemical and physiological consequences leading to therapeutic or adverse effects. For many drugs, the *mechanism of action* at the molecular level is poorly understood, if at all. A pharmacological effect (i.e., the therapeutic or toxic response to a drug) may be elicited either by direct interaction of the drug with the receptor that controls a specific function or by a drug-mediated alteration of the physiological process regulating the function. For most drugs, the intensity and duration of the observed pharmacological effect are proportional to the concentration of the drug at the receptor. The site at which a drug acts to initiate events leading to a specific biological effect is called the drug's *site of action*.

The *mechanism of action* of a drug is the biochemical or physical process that occurs at the *site of action*. Drug action is usually mediated through a receptor. Cellular enzymes and structural or transport proteins are important examples of drug receptors. Nonprotein macromolecules may also bind drugs, resulting in altered cellular functions controlled by membrane permeability or DNA transcription. Some drugs are chemically similar to natural endogenous substances and may compete for binding sites. In addition, some drugs may block formation, release, uptake, or transport of essential substances. Others may produce an effect by interacting with relatively small molecules to form complexes that actively bind to receptors.

Although the exact molecular interactions that give rise to the mechanism of action for many drugs remain obscure, numerous theoretical models have been developed to explain drug action. One concept postulates that a drug binds to intracellular macromolecular receptors through ionic and hydrogen bonds and van der Waals forces. This theoretical model further postulates that if the drug-receptor complex is sufficiently stable and able to modify the target system, an observable pharmacological response will occur. As Fig. 30.1 illustrates, the response is concentration dependent until a

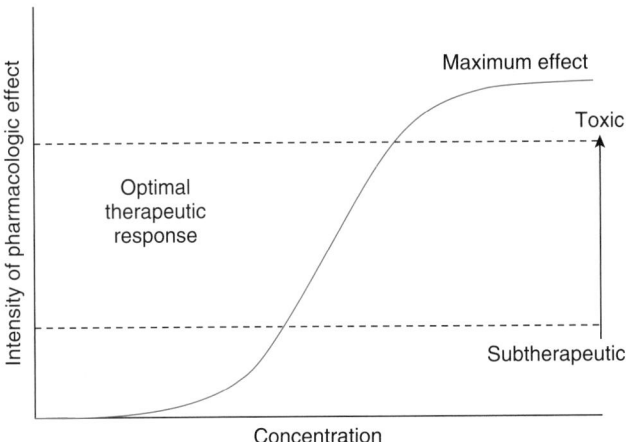

**Fig. 30.1** The dose-effect relationship. The probability of increasing pharmacologic response and risk of toxicity parallels concentration for most drugs. The plateau (maximum effect) is likely due to saturation at the receptor.

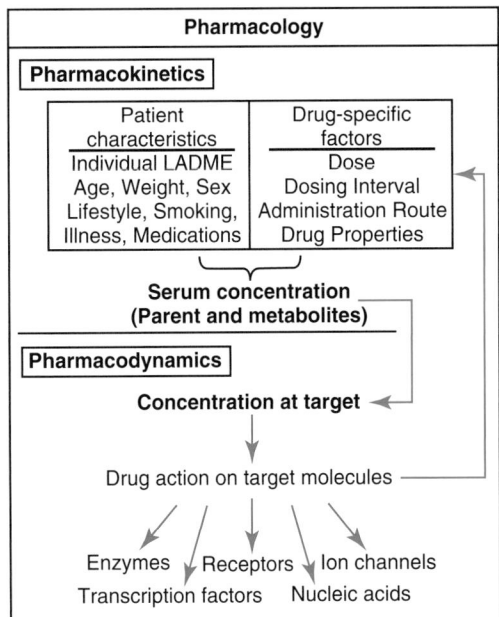

**Fig. 30.2** Conceptual relationship between pharmacodynamics and pharmacokinetics. Many drug- and patient-specific factors determine both the serum concentration of a therapeutic compound and its metabolites. Serum concentration, in turn, is related to the amount of drug present at the target site, resulting in effects on a variety of molecules (several examples shown) to induce a pharmacologic response. The efficacy and degree of response provide feedback to allow optimization of the dosing regimen for an individual patient.

maximal effect is reached. The plateau may be due to saturation at the receptor or overload of a transport process.

The utility of monitoring drug concentration is based on the premise that pharmacologic response correlates with the concentration of the drug at the site of action (receptor). Although attempts have been made to measure the concentration of drugs at the receptor site in a patient, in general, this approach is technically impractical, if not impossible for most drugs. Studies have shown that for many drugs, a strong correlation exists between the serum drug concentration and the observed pharmacological effect. In addition, years of relating blood concentrations to drug effects have demonstrated the clinical utility of drug concentration information. One must nevertheless always keep in mind that a serum drug concentration does not necessarily equal the concentration at the receptor; it merely reflects it.

## Pharmacokinetics

**Pharmacokinetics** describes the of uptake of drugs by the body, the distribution into tissue, the **biotransformations** (i.e., metabolism), and the elimination of the drugs and their metabolites from the body. Applied pharmacokinetics is the discipline that uses the principles of pharmacokinetics to enhance the safety and effectiveness of a drug in a patient. It is this aspect of pharmacology that most strongly influences the interpretation of TDM results and that is dealt with in more detail in this chapter. Fig. 30.2 illustrates the conceptual relationship between pharmacodynamics and pharmacokinetics, and the many factors affecting drug concentration and pharmacological response.

## Drugs Constantly Undergo Change in the Body

Many factors are now recognized as having a profound influence on the pharmacokinetics of drugs and consequently on a patient's pharmacological response (Box 30.1). Consideration of the patient's history, with particular emphasis on his or her pathophysiologic state and adjunct drug therapy, is essential at the initiation of drug therapy and TDM because these

factors may affect the absorption, distribution, metabolism, and excretion (ADME) of a drug.

## Absorption

Most drugs administered chronically to patients are administered extravascularly. Although intramuscular and subcutaneous routes are used, the oral route accounts for most of the extravascular doses administered. The absorption process depends on the drug dissociating from its dosing form, dissolving in gastrointestinal fluids, and then diffusing across biological membrane barriers into the bloodstream. The rate and extent of drug absorption may vary considerably depending on the nature of the drug itself (e.g., solubility, $pK_a$), on the matrix in which it is present, and on the physiological environment (e.g., pH, gastrointestinal motility, vascularity).

The fraction of a drug dose that is absorbed into the systemic circulation is referred to as its **bioavailability.** The bioavailability of a particular drug, if the drug is to be useful, must generally be great enough so that the active component can pass in sufficient amount and in a desirable time from the gut into the systemic circulation. Bioavailability of greater than 70% is desirable for drugs to be orally useful. An exception would be where the lumen of the gastrointestinal tract is the site of drug action (e.g., antibiotics used to sterilize the gut, such as oral vancomycin). Low bioavailability would then be considered advantageous.

Some drugs that are rapidly and completely absorbed nevertheless have low bioavailability to the systemic circulation. This is true of drugs with a high *hepatic extraction rate.*

## BOX 30.1    Factors That Affect Drug Distribution in Humans

**Demographic Factors**
Age
Weight
Gender
Race
Genetics (e.g., metabolic enzyme polymorphisms)

**Health-Related Factors**
Liver disease (cirrhosis, hepatitis, cholestasis)
Kidney disease
Thyroid disease (hypothyroidism or hyperthyroidism)
Cardiovascular disease (arrhythmias, congestive heart failure)
Gastrointestinal disease (e.g., sprue or other malabsorption, peptic ulcer disease)
Cancer
Surgery
Burns
Volume status (e.g., dehydration)
Nutritional status (cachetic or anorexic)
Pregnancy or other factors affecting plasma proteins or body composition

**Extracorporeal Factors**
Hemodialysis
Peritoneal dialysis
Cardiopulmonary bypass
Hypothermia or hyperthermia

**Chemical and Environmental Factors Influencing**
Absorption of drug
Food or coadministered drug affecting extent or rate of absorption
Immediate- or extended-release formulation
Distribution of drug
Coadministered drugs affecting protein binding to plasma proteins or tissue
Metabolism of drug
Food, herbs, or drugs competing for metabolism
Coadministration of drugs that induce metabolic enzymes (e.g., phenobarbital)
Coadministration of drugs that inhibit metabolic enzymes (e.g., cimetidine)
Excretion of drug
Coadministration of a drug that competes for renal tubular secretory pathways (e.g., probenecid, penicillin)
Coadministration of drugs that enhance renal tubular reabsorption

After oral administration, drugs that are absorbed in the lumen of the small intestine are carried by the portal vein directly to the liver. The liver may extensively metabolize a drug with a high hepatic extraction rate before it reaches the systemic circulation leading to low oral bioavailability. This phenomenon is called the first-pass effect.

In addition to the extent of absorption, the rate of absorption is also important. The absorption of a drug is generally considered a first-order process, and the absorption rate constant of a drug is usually much greater than its elimination rate constant. Efforts are now being made in the pharmaceutical industry to decrease the apparent rate of absorption of many drugs by manipulating their formulations to produce sustained (or extended) release products. Formulations that provide sustained release permit drugs taken orally to be taken at less frequent intervals. Conditions that may influence the extent or rate of drug absorption include abnormal gastrointestinal motility, diseases of the stomach and the small and large intestines, gastrointestinal infections, radiation, food, and interaction with other substances in the gastrointestinal tract.

## Distribution

After a drug enters the vascular compartment, it interacts with various blood constituents and is carried by various transport processes to different body organs and tissues. The overall process is referred to as *distribution*. The factors determining the distribution pattern of a drug are binding of the drug to circulating blood components, binding to fixed receptors, passage of the drug through membrane barriers, and the ability to dissolve in structural or storage lipids. Molecular weight, $pK_a$, lipid solubility, and other physical and chemical properties of the drug are important determinants of distribution.

Once a drug enters the systemic circulation, it distributes and comes to equilibrium with many of the blood components, such as plasma proteins. An equilibrium exists between *free* and *protein-bound* drug fractions. It is generally believed that only the free fraction of the drug is available for distribution and elimination. In addition, only the free drug is available to transit across cellular membranes or to interact with the drug receptor to elicit a biological response. Therefore, changes in the protein-binding characteristics of a drug can have a profound influence on the distribution and elimination of a drug as well as on the manner in which total plasma or serum steady-state concentrations are interpreted. Each drug has its own characteristic protein-binding pattern that depends on its physical and chemical properties. As a general rule, however, acidic drugs are bound primarily to albumin, and basic drugs primarily to globulins, particularly $\alpha_1$-acid glycoprotein (AAG). Some drugs bind to both albumin and globulins.

Anything that alters the concentration of free drug in the plasma ultimately alters the amount of drug available to enter the tissues and interact with specific receptor systems. Disease states can alter free drug concentrations. For example, in uremia, the composition of plasma is altered by an increase in nonprotein nitrogen compounds, by acid-base and electrolyte imbalances, and often by a decrease in albumin; free drug concentrations are frequently increased. It is important to also recognize that even though the total drug concentration may remain unchanged, displacement of a drug from its plasma protein–binding sites increases free drug concentrations and can result in clinical toxicity. For example, phenytoin is 90% bound and 10% free in healthy subjects. In uremic patients, 20% to 30% of the total plasma concentration of phenytoin may be free. If one considers a healthy patient who has a total plasma phenytoin concentration of 15 µg/mL, the free phenytoin concentration is likely to be 1.5 µg/mL. If a uremic patient has a total concentration of 15 µg/mL, the free drug concentration may be 4.5 µg/mL. A free phenytoin concentration of 4.5 µg/mL is sufficient to precipitate severe phenytoin side effects, including lethargy and increased seizure frequency. In uremic patients, it is advisable to quantitate free phenytoin concentrations and adjust the drug dose to maintain free phenytoin concentration at approximately 2.0 µg/mL.

Equilibrium dialysis represents the gold-standard method for measuring the free, unbound concentration of a drug. However, this method typically requires 16 to 18 hours of incubation to achieve equilibrium, which severely limits the turnaround time for testing. Ultrafiltration techniques are a useful alternative that can usually be accomplished in a fraction of the time. In ultrafiltration, a sample of serum or plasma is forced through a filter membrane with a low molecular weight cutoff value, typically by centrifugation, to yield a protein-free sample. Provided this process is done rapidly and under appropriate temperature control, ultrafiltration can provide a useful estimate of the free drug concentration in circulating blood.

## Metabolism

### Biotransformation

The liver is the principal organ responsible for xenobiotic metabolism. One of its major roles is to convert lipophilic nonpolar molecules to more polar water-soluble forms. The drug molecule (a xenobiotic) can be modified by phase I reactions, which alter chemical structure by oxidation, reduction, or hydrolysis; or by phase II reactions, which conjugate the drug (glucuronidation or sulfation) to water-soluble forms. Typically, both phase I and phase II reactions occur. Most drug metabolism takes place in the microsomal fraction of the hepatocytes, where many environmental chemicals and endogenous biochemicals (xenobiotics) are also processed and by the same mechanisms.

Enzymes of the hepatic microsomal system can be induced or inhibited. Microsomal enzyme induction leads to an increase in the activity of the enzymes present, most commonly through increases in the number of oxidizing enzymes. The many isoenzymes of cytochrome P450 are affected variably by different enzyme-inducing drugs. Phenobarbital and theophylline represent prototypical enzyme inducers with broad induction effects; however, they induce different cytochrome P450 isoforms leading to effects on different drugs. Because the drug-metabolizing enzymes of the liver are also relatively nonspecific and interact with a wide variety of endogenous and exogenous substances, the presence of one drug may inhibit the metabolism of a second drug that is coadministered. When patients are on a drug with a narrow therapeutic index (TI), their dosing regimen would need to be adjusted should a known enzyme-inducing or inhibiting drug be added to or deleted from their therapy.

The role of TDM becomes particularly apparent for drugs that undergo hepatic metabolism. Wide variability in the rate of metabolism of any given drug exists not only in different patients in the general population, but also in the same patient at different times and in different circumstances. This variability is due to factors such as age, weight, gender, genetics, exposure to environmental substances, diet, coadministered drugs, and disease. Furthermore, unlike kidney function, where creatinine provides a useful biomarker of function, there is no acceptable, endogenous, biochemical marker by which hepatic function, and consequently hepatic capability for drug clearance, can be routinely assessed before drug therapy is initiated.

### Excretion

Excretion of drugs or chemicals from the body can occur through biliary, intestinal, pulmonary, or renal routes. Although each of these represents a possible mechanism of drug elimination, renal excretion is a major pathway for the elimination of most water-soluble drugs or metabolites and is important in TDM. Alterations in renal function may have a profound effect on the clearance and apparent half-life of the parent compound or its active metabolite(s); decreased renal function causes increased serum drug concentrations and increases the pharmacological response.

Kidney function, in contrast to liver function, is readily evaluated by estimation of creatinine clearance. Renal clearance of creatinine at 120 mL/min approximates the glomerular filtration rate of 90 to 130 mL/min (see also Chapter 21). Therefore, measurement of creatinine clearance or estimated glomerular filtration rate (eGFR) on a routine basis provides an effective tool to evaluate kidney function. A strong correlation has been shown to exist between creatinine clearance and the total body clearance or elimination rate constant of those drugs primarily dependent on the kidneys for their elimination. Examples of drugs whose therapeutic use is adjusted to account for changes in creatinine clearance include the aminoglycoside antibiotics gentamicin, tobramycin, and amikacin.

### General Considerations for the Clinical Use of Therapeutic Drug Monitoring

There is no universal set of rules that determine whether a drug might benefit from TDM; however, numerous characteristics of a drug contribute to the need for TDM. TDM is most valuable when the drug in question is used chronically, has variable pharmacokinetics, and has a narrow TI. For drugs with a narrow TI, there is little if any window between blood concentrations associated with efficacy and those associated with toxic effects. The immunosuppressive calcineurin inhibitor drug, tacrolimus, is a narrow TI drug with wide variability in pharmacokinetics as shown in Fig. 30.3. The concentrations of tacrolimus that are associated with efficacy (i.e., freedom from graft rejection) and those associated with kidney toxicity overlap considerably. TDM helps navigate this "tightrope." By itself, however, narrow TI is not necessarily sufficient to warrant TDM. Many narrow TI drugs are routinely used without monitoring such as most cancer chemotherapy drugs. Additional factors therefore contribute to

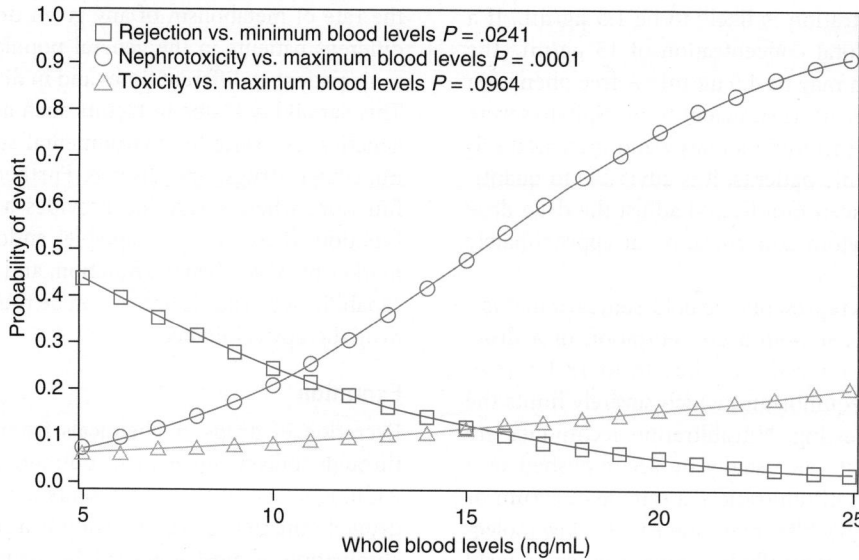

**Fig. 30.3** The pharmacodynamics of tacrolimus in renal transplantation. (Reprinted with permission from Venkataramanan R, Shaw LM, Sarkozi L, et al. Clinical utility of monitoring tacrolimus blood concentrations in liver transplant patients. *J Clin Pharmacol.* 2001; 41[5]:542–551.)

the need for TDM such as the severity of failed drug therapy (e.g., antimicrobials) or toxicity (e.g., ISDs). Difficulty in recognizing efficacy or toxicity with use of these drugs can be life threatening. Many patients, especially those with chronic disease, also require prolonged drug therapy. Poor compliance with dosing is particularly evident with patients who are characteristically free of pain or unusual discomfort as with epilepsy, asthma, hypertension, mild heart disease, and transplantation. Patients may develop a sense that their disease has been cured and they no longer need the drug. The end result of noncompliance is exacerbation of the existing disorder and treatment failure. Drug concentration values therefore provide positive feedback to physicians regarding compliance.

## Preanalytical Factors That Affect Therapeutic Drug Monitoring Results

To interpret a TDM result, it is critical that the dose of drug given to the patient is known. Dosage uniformity standards exist for US Food and Drug Administration (FDA)-approved drugs. Although most drug formulations are fairly consistent, the actual dose of a drug in a single tablet, suspension, or vial may vary. United States Pharmacopeia (USP) standards dictate that the mean dose contained in a tablet must be within ±10% of the product labeling and no tested sample may fall outside of 75% and 125% of the mean. As a result, the dose content for a single dose could theoretically vary by as much as 25% and still fall within acceptable USP content uniformity limits. This is further compounded by inaccuracies introduced by manipulation of the dose (e.g., splitting of scored tablets, failure to administer or consume the entire dose or from vomiting). Drugs may also degrade over time, which depends on storage, leading to further dose inaccuracy.

Beyond dose accuracy, pharmacokinetics is inherently time based. Accurate timing of sample collection is an important factor, especially when timed samples, such as peak or trough samples, are the primary means of monitoring. Vancomycin trough samples provide an example where collection immediately prior to the next dose is recommended due to the relatively short **half-life** of this drug (~6 to 12 hours). Premature sampling may lead to falsely increased concentrations that could alter decision making given the generally narrow therapeutic range for this drug. In contrast, drugs with slow distribution but long half-life, such as digoxin, are optimally sampled in the post distributive phase of greater than 6 hours following dosing. Sampling during the steady state (generally >4 doses) is also an important assumption made for monitoring of many drugs such as vancomycin.

Variation in collection and handling of samples for TDM can also affect the quality of concentration data. Although serum is the preferred sample for monitoring of many drugs, different collection tubes are available for generating serum that include plain glass or plastic tubes without additive (e.g., red-stoppered BD Vacutainer tubes) and specialized serum separator tubes (e.g., yellow-stoppered BD Vacutainer tubes) that contain a gel that separates serum from the cellular components following centrifugation. The latter tube may affect drug concentration due to adsorption of the drug by the gel following prolonged contact. The adsorptive effects vary across drugs and have been shown to significantly reduce the concentration of some drugs, such as phenytoin, particularly when the collection tubes are underfilled. The stability of drugs following collection may also vary, with some drugs requiring prompt serum generation followed by freezing for optimal stability (e.g., busulfan).

The importance of preanalytical factors in the accuracy and precision of TDM results should not be underestimated. It is imperative that laboratories engage and work with the many parts of the health care system, including pharmacists, nurses, and the phlebotomy team.

## Analytical Factors That Affect Results

The laboratory plays a central role in the TDM process. Analytical factors are important considerations in the interpretation of drug concentration data. Notable challenges in the analytical field include the availability of standardized reference material and the selectivity of methods for the drug of interest.

Determining whether a method gives accurate results over the long term and across laboratories is often a difficult task. This is generally accomplished by comparing the results of testing against a definitive analytical method or using a certified reference material. Definitive methods generally use time-consuming and expensive techniques to establish material purity and quantity that are not practical in most clinical laboratories. The availability of certified reference material (also frequently referred to as standardized reference material) to which methods may be compared is a critical factor in helping control systematic error (refer to Chapter 7). Early studies of method comparability for AEDs demonstrated that concentrations varied greatly across laboratories as well as within laboratories over time. These data led to the development of a standard reference material of sufficient purity and accuracy in the early 1980s by the National Institute for Standards and Technology (NIST) to allow standardization of AED monitoring methods across different laboratories and manufacturers. Unfortunately, this type of standardized reference material is unavailable for the majority of monitored drugs.

The ability of a given method to detect a compound of interest among many potential substances present in a sample (referred to as method selectivity) represents another potential source of systematic error. Selectivity is particularly important for TDM tests because many drugs are structurally related, including some endogenous compounds. Most drugs are also extensively metabolized through several different biotransformation pathways. These metabolites are often similar to the parent compound in structure, but pharmacologic activity is variable. Tacrolimus provides a useful example. Antibodies directed against tacrolimus that are used for immunoassays demonstrate similar reactivity toward tacrolimus along with two of its metabolites, 15-desmethyl-tacrolimus and 31-desmethyl-tacrolimus. Although both metabolites are detected equally, the 15-desmethyl metabolite exhibits little immunosuppressive activity, whereas the 31-desmethyl metabolite exhibits equal immunosuppressive activity when compared to that of tacrolimus. This metabolite interference with target drug detection can lead to inappropriate changes in drug dosing when not recognized. Beyond metabolites, interference can also occur from unrecognized substances within the sample matrix such as bilirubin. For immunoassay-based testing, heterophile antibodies, such as human-anti-mouse antibody (HAMA), are difficult to detect and can adversely affect testing in unpredictable ways (see Chapter 15).

### Concept of a Therapeutic Range

The relationship between serum drug concentration and clinical outcome is the basis for TDM as depicted in Fig. 30.1. One of the most common interpretative errors encountered regarding TDM is the presumption that a concentration within a reported therapeutic range will ensure treatment success in the absence of toxicity, and concentrations outside that range will not. In reality, the probability of success and toxicity are a continuum across the concentration range. These probabilities are maximized and minimized, respectively, within the therapeutic range. Nevertheless, therapeutic success can certainly occur at concentrations below the therapeutic range. More importantly, success may also be achieved by concentrations above the therapeutic range without associated toxicity in some patients. Experienced users of TDM often recognize these relationships, and they weigh the risks and potential benefits of drug concentrations in the context of the clinical situation using the therapeutic range as a guide.

Similar to a reference interval for any laboratory test, therapeutic ranges are based on population data from drug therapy trials, and in some instances, confirmed or established by RCCTs. The application of these population-based ranges to an individual therefore assumes similarity to the target population. Differences in metabolism, physiology, and/or the underlying disease process can alter these relationships, leading to unexpected and undesirable results. Phenytoin used for seizure control illustrates this limitation. A fairly good relationship between serum phenytoin concentration and seizure control exists. However, several factors have been shown to alter the dose-response relationships for phenytoin that might impact the utility of defined therapeutic ranges. The presence of concomitant liver disease significantly alters the pharmacokinetics of phenytoin due to its high degree of binding to albumin, a protein that is significantly altered with moderate–severe liver disease. As a result, individuals with liver disease are at significantly higher risk of toxicity at total serum phenytoin concentrations that are appropriate for individuals without liver disease. The recognition of this problem led to the development of methods for measuring phenytoin that is unbound to albumin in serum (also known as free phenytoin). Nevertheless, this example illustrates the need for caution in applying population-based relationships to individual patients who may not be represented by the population used for defining the therapeutic range.

# THERAPEUTIC DRUG MONITORING OF DRUGS IN COMMON CLINICAL USE

## Antiepileptic Drugs

### Phenytoin

Phenytoin (diphenylhydantoin), most commonly available as *Dilantin* but also available in generic form, is used in the treatment of primary or secondary generalized tonic-clonic seizures, partial or complex-partial seizures, and status epilepticus. The drug is not effective for absence seizures. Phenytoin likely has many targets, but the most well-described mechanism of action is the modulation of voltage-gated sodium channels through prolonged channel inactivation, which reduces the ability of the neuron to respond at high frequency. The physiological effect of this action is reduction in central synaptic transmission, which aids in control of abnormal neuronal excitability.

Phenytoin is not readily soluble in aqueous solutions. When administered by intramuscular injection, most of the dose precipitates at the site of injection and is then slowly absorbed. A prodrug called *fosphenytoin* (Cerebyx) was introduced as a therapeutic form of phenytoin to improve phenytoin's pharmacology. Fosphenytoin has increased aqueous solubility for intramuscular injection. After injection, it is rapidly converted to phenytoin. Absorption of oral phenytoin is slow and sometimes incomplete. Variations in the drug preparation have been blamed for low bioavailability. Once absorbed, the drug is tightly bound to protein (90% to 95%). As with all drugs, the pharmacological effect of phenytoin is directly related to the amount present in the free (unbound) state. Only free phenytoin is available to cross biological membranes and interact at biologically important binding sites. The degree of protein binding can be reduced by the presence of other drugs, anemia, and hypoalbuminemia, which can occur in the elderly.

The optimal total phenytoin therapeutic concentration for seizure control without side effects is 10 to 20 µg/mL (40 to 79 µmol/L). Free phenytoin concentration in the range of 1 to 2 µg/mL (1 to 8 µmol/L) is frequently considered optimal. A side effect of phenytoin not related to plasma concentration is development of gingival hyperplasia.

Phenytoin is metabolized by the liver, and it may become saturated within the therapeutic range due to its zero-order pharmacokinetics. Once metabolism is saturated, small dose increments result in large changes in blood concentration (Fig. 30.4); this phenomenon partially explains the wide variation in dosage among patients that is required to accomplish a therapeutic effect. Because of this saturation phenomenon, first-order kinetics do not generally apply to total phenytoin at blood concentrations in excess of 5 µg/mL (20 µmol/L). A number of drug interactions result in alteration of the disposition of phenytoin by enhancing metabolism (e.g., alcohol, barbiturates, and carbamazepine), competing with metabolism (e.g., chloramphenicol, cimetidine, disulfiram, isoniazid, and dicumarol), or displacing

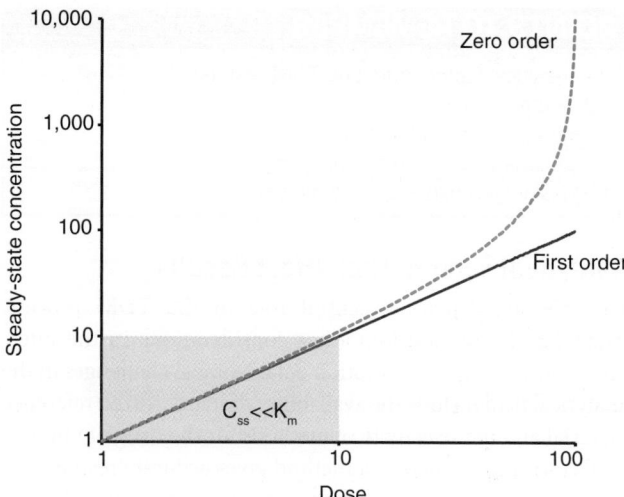

**Fig. 30.4** Nonlinear response to dose changes. Drugs with first order kinetics *(solid black line)* display serum steady-state concentrations that vary proportionately with dose. In contrast, for drugs with zero-order kinetics *(dotted blue line)*, an increase in dose may result in a disproportionate increase in serum steady-state concentrations.

phenytoin from normal binding to serum protein (e.g., salicylate and valproic acid).

### Carbamazepine

Carbamazepine, proprietary name *Tegretol*, is used in the treatment of generalized tonic-clonic, partial, and partial-complex seizures. It is also used for the treatment of pain associated with trigeminal neuralgia and as a mood-stabilizing drug in bipolar disorder. Like phenytoin, carbamazepine modulates the synaptic sodium channel, which prolongs inactivation, reducing the ability of the neuron to respond at high frequency. The physiological effect of this action is reduction in central synaptic transmission, which aids in control of abnormal neuronal excitability.

After oral administration, carbamazepine is slowly absorbed with wide individual variability. The drug is highly protein bound (80%). The elimination half-life early in therapy is approximately 24 hours. With chronic therapy, the enzymes responsible for metabolism are induced, and the elimination half-life is reduced to 15 to 20 hours. Because hepatic metabolism is the principal means by which the drug is eliminated from plasma, any reduction in liver function results in drug accumulation.

The therapeutic concentration range for optimal pharmacological effect of carbamazepine is 4 to 12 µg/mL (17 to 51 µmol/L); however, this range is dependent upon concomitant use of other AEDs. Toxicity associated with excessive carbamazepine ingestion occurs at plasma concentrations in excess of 15 µg/mL (63 µmol/L) and is characterized by symptoms of blurred vision, paresthesia, nystagmus, ataxia, drowsiness, and diplopia. Side effects unrelated to plasma concentration include development of an urticarial rash, which usually disappears on discontinuation of the drug, and hematologic depression (leukopenia, thrombocytopenia, and aplastic anemia).

The active metabolite of carbamazepine is carbamazepine–10,11–epoxide. This metabolite has been found to accumulate in children to concentrations equivalent to carbamazepine. It may contribute to symptoms of intoxication in children who have a therapeutic plasma concentration of the parent drug. Because carbamazepine is metabolized through the hepatic oxidative enzyme system, drugs that induce this system (phenytoin, phenobarbital) increase the rate of carbamazepine clearance.

Coadministration of phenobarbital, phenytoin, or valproic acid increases the rate of carbamazepine metabolism and reduces the blood concentration. Erythromycin and propoxyphene interfere with metabolism and increase carbamazepine concentrations.

Because of carbamazepine's relatively long half-life, the specimen yielding the most useful information is the one representing the trough concentration, although in the case of suspected mild intoxication, the peak value of the plasma concentration correlates more closely with toxicity. The peak specimen should be collected 4 to 8 hours after the oral dose in the setting of immediate-release formulations of carbamazepine.

## Valproic Acid

Valproic acid, brand name *Depakene* or *Depakote*, is used for treatment of absence seizures. It has also been shown to be useful against tonic-clonic and partial seizures when used in conjunction with other AEDs such as phenobarbital or phenytoin. Beyond its use in the treatment of epilepsy, valproate also has mood-stabilizing effects that make it a useful agent, and alternative, in the treatment of bipolar disorder. The drug inhibits the enzyme gamma-aminobutyric acid (GABA) transaminase, resulting in an increase in the concentration of GABA in the brain. GABA is a potent inhibitor of presynaptic and postsynaptic discharges in the central nervous system.

Valproic acid is rapidly and almost completely absorbed after oral administration. Peak concentrations occur 1 to 4 hours after an oral dose. The principal metabolite, 2-*n*-propyl-3-ketopentanoic acid, has anticonvulsant activity comparable to that of valproic acid, although this metabolite does not accumulate in plasma. The single-dose half-life is 16 hours in healthy adults, but this reduces to 12 hours on chronic therapy and may be as short as 8 hours in children. In neonates and in hepatic disease, when metabolism is reduced, the half-life becomes prolonged. Valproic acid is highly protein bound (93%). In circumstances when competition for protein binding increases, such as in uremia, cirrhosis, or concurrent drug therapy, the percent of free valproic acid increases. The minimum effective therapeutic concentration of valproic acid is 50 µg/mL (346 µmol/L). Concentrations in excess of 100 µg/mL (693 µmol/L) have been associated with hepatic toxicity and acute toxic encephalopathy.

## Ethosuximide

Ethosuximide, proprietary name *Zarontin,* is used for the treatment of absence seizures characterized by brief loss of consciousness. Ethosuximide reduces the flow of calcium through T-type calcium channels in the synapse of thalamic neurons; because thalamic neurons are the main source of 3-Hz spike-wave rhythms in absence seizures, reduction of calcium flow slows the rate of these seizure-inducing pulses.

Ethosuximide is readily absorbed from the gastrointestinal tract. The drug is cleared mainly by metabolism as either the hydroxyethyl compound or the glucuronide ester of the hydroxyethyl metabolite with a half-life of approximately 33 hours, although this may be prolonged in adults. The trough specimen yields the most useful information regarding therapeutic efficacy. The optimal therapeutic concentration of ethosuximide is 40 to 100 µg/mL (283 to 708 µmol/L). Toxicity related to an excessive blood concentration of ethosuximide is rare. Symptoms of gastrointestinal distress, lethargy, dizziness, and euphoria may be encountered early in therapy, but patients usually become tolerant to these symptoms.

## Topiramate

Topiramate, brand name *Topamax*, is a sulfamate-substituted monosaccharide anticonvulsant that is also approved for use in migraine headache therapy. The mechanisms by which topiramate exerts these effects is not clearly established. It is proposed that several effects may contribute to topiramate's pharmacologic activity including blockage of voltage-dependent sodium channels, augmentation of the neurotransmitter gamma-aminobutyrate action at some of the subtypes of the GABA-A receptor, antagonism of the AMPA/kainite subtype of glutamate receptors, and inhibition of isozymes II and IV of carbonic anhydrase.

Brand name Topamax is generally well and rapidly absorbed following oral administration with a usual $T_{max}$ between 2 and 4 hours and bioavailability of up to 95%. Coingestion of food can delay absorption by approximately 2 hours without effect on $T_{max}$. Average steady-state serum concentrations can fall by approximately 50% when either phenytoin or carbamazepine is coadministered. The metabolism of topiramate is not well understood or described, but renal clearance of unchanged drug has been reported to account for the majority of clearance in the absence of coadministered inducing drugs such as phenytoin or carbamazepine. In the presence of the latter, the contribution of hepatic clearance increases. Thus, upon introduction of one of these inducing drugs into the patient's regimen, or withdrawal, closer monitoring of serum concentrations of topiramate is warranted. In the presence of significant renal disease, lowering the dosage and judicious use of TDM are recommended. Topiramate is only weakly bound to plasma proteins, and therefore circumstances that alter drug binding in serum do not affect topiramate clearance or steady-state concentrations. Based on retrospective studies and a concentration-controlled study, the usual range of concentrations is 5 to 20 µg/mL (15 to 59 µmol/L).

## Lamotrigine

Lamotrigine, proprietary name *Lamictal,* is not a GABA analog, but binds to the GABA receptor; it is therefore considered a GABA receptor agonist. Lamotrigine acts like phenytoin and carbamazepine, and blocks repetitive nerve firings induced by depolarization of spinal cord neurons. Lamotrigine was approved by the FDA in 1994 for adjunctive therapy of partial seizures in adults. It has yet to be approved for use in children. Studies also suggest lamotrigine is effective against absence seizures.

Lamotrigine is well tolerated and completely absorbed from the gastrointestinal tract after oral administration. It is 60% bound to plasma proteins. Optimal response appears to occur with blood concentrations in the range of 2.5 to 15 µg/mL (~10 to 60 µmol/L). However, dizziness, ataxia, diplopia, blurred vision, nausea, and vomiting are signs of toxicity that may occur when the blood concentration exceeds 10 µg/mL (40 µmol/L). Half-life ranges from 15 to 35 hours with monotherapy. Elimination occurs through hepatic metabolism; the primary metabolite is the glucuronide ester. Coadministration with cytochrome $P_{450}$-inducing drugs, such as phenobarbital, phenytoin, or carbamazepine, results in reduced lamotrigine concentrations; dosage increases of approximately 30% are required to maintain optimal blood concentrations.

## Levetiracetam and Brivaracetam

Levetiracetam, marketed under the trade name *Keppra*, is an anticonvulsant drug approved in the United States for adjunctive therapy in patients with partial onset seizures. Brivaracetam (marketed as Briviact, Nubriveo or Brivajoy) is a newer AED with a similar approved indication. Levetiracetam and brivaracetam belong to the lactam class of molecules that share a 5-member pyrrolidone ring, which include piracetam and ethosuximide. The mechanism of action for these drugs, although not fully understood, appears to be via binding to the synaptic vesicle protein, SV2A, leading to a reduction in the rate of synaptic vesicle release. Brivaracetam has an ~15- to 30-fold greater affinity for SV2A compared with leviracetam, and it also exhibits more selectivity than leviracetam, which also inhibits α-amino-3-hydroxy-5-methyl-4-isoxazolepropionic acid (AMPA) receptors and high-voltage-gated calcium currents in addition to binding to SV2A.

Levetiracetam and brivaracetam are both available in oral and intravenous formulations with greater than 95% oral bioavailability. Food intake causes a modest delay in absorption with reduced peak serum concentrations; however, overall bioavailability is unaffected. Both drugs exhibit a circulating half-life of approximately 8 to 9 hours. Levetiracetam is metabolized to an inactive acetamide form by hydrolysis via amidase (~27% to 34%) with the majority of the drug excreted by the kidneys unchanged into urine. Clearance of the drug is therefore affected by kidney disease. An increase in levetiracetam clearance has been observed during the third trimester of pregnancy; however, this change in clearance is variable. Because there is no significant hepatic metabolism of levetiracetam, liver function does not affect the pharmacokinetics of this drug. In contrast, brivaracetam, while also hydrolyzed by amidase, is significantly metabolized to inactive metabolites by CYP2C9 and CYP2C19 with the vast majority of the drug (92%) excreted as metabolite in the urine. Clearance is therefore reduced in individuals with hepatic impairment necessitating dose reduction. Due to the low renal clearance of active drug, there is little impact of renal impairment on parent drug PK.

Serum concentrations of levetiracetam and brivaracetam appear to correlate linearly with dose within the typical dosing range. Although the optimal target range for serum concentration has not been fully defined for either drug, retrospective analysis of data from clinical trials suggests that serum concentrations within the range of 12 to 46 µg/mL (70 to 270 µmol/L) are associated with efficacy for leviracetam and 0.2 to 2 µg/mL (0.9 to 9 µmol/L) for brivaracetam. Due to the structural similarity of these drugs and known or potential cross-reactivity in immunoassays, caution should be used in monitoring patients undergoing a switch in drug therapy involving these drugs using these methods. If monitoring is required when there is a possibility of both drugs being present, a valid method without these interferences such as liquid chromatography with tandem mass spectrometry (LC-MS/MS) should be used. Alternatively, sufficient time should be allowed for clearance of the discontinued drug prior to monitoring.

## Felbamate

Felbamate, proprietary name *Felbatol,* was approved by the FDA in 1993 for primary or adjunctive therapy of partial seizures. Its use is limited to those patients who fail other drug treatments because felbamate carries with it a substantial risk of aplastic anemia and liver failure that is not related to blood concentration. Biweekly monitoring of complete blood count, serum aminotransferases, and bilirubin is recommended to detect early onset of these side effects. Felbamate is particularly effective in control of Lennox-Gastaut syndrome.

Felbamate is completely absorbed from the gastrointestinal tract. The drug is 30% bound to plasma proteins, and optimal blood concentrations for felbamate, although poorly defined, have been suggested to range from 30 to 60 µg/mL (126 to 252 µmol/L). It is eliminated by hepatic metabolism, with its half-life ranging from 14 to 21 hours. Felbamate saturates metabolism when the concentration exceeds 120 µg/mL (504 µmol/L); at that concentration, metabolism converts from first order to zero order. There are currently no commercially available immunoassays for felbamate. High-performance liquid chromatography (HPLC) and capillary electrophoresis have been reported for felbamate analysis.

## Phenobarbital

Phenobarbital is used in the treatment of all seizures except absence seizures, and it is known by a wide variety of proprietary names and found in combination with many other drugs. It is particularly useful for treatment of generalized tonic-clonic, partial, focal motor, temporal lobe, and febrile seizures.

Absorption of oral phenobarbital is slow but complete. The time at which peak plasma concentrations are reached is widely variable and ranges from 4 to 10 hours after the dose. Phenobarbital is 40% to 60% bound to plasma proteins. The elimination half-life is from 70 to 100 hours and is age dependent (children average 70 hours, geriatric patients 100 hours).

Because hepatic metabolism is one of the prime routes of elimination, reduced liver function results in prolonged half-life.

The optimally effective therapeutic concentration of phenobarbital is between 15 and 40 µg/mL (66 to 177 µmol/L). The predominant side effect observed in adults at blood concentrations greater than 40 µg/mL (177 µmol/L) is sedation, although tolerance to this effect develops with chronic therapy.

Phenobarbital is metabolized in the liver to *p*-hydroxyphenobarbital, which is largely excreted as glucuronide or sulfate ester. When renal and hepatic functions are decreased, patients experience decreased clearance of the drug. Elimination of phenobarbital may be decreased in the presence of valproic acid and salicylate if reduction in urinary pH occurs. During chronic administration of valproate or salicylate, the concentration of phenobarbital may increase 10% to 20%, and a dose adjustment may be necessary to avoid intoxication. Phenobarbital induces mixed-function oxidative enzymes, resulting in increased metabolism of other xenobiotics after approximately 1 to 2 weeks of therapy.

Because of the long elimination half-life of phenobarbital, the blood concentration does not change rapidly. Therefore, a serum specimen collected late in the dose interval (trough) is representative of the overall effect. Results from specimens collected 2 to 4 hours after the dose can be misleading, because they may be construed to be the peak concentration when in actuality they precede the peak. Table 30.1 summarizes pharmacokinetic data of anticonvulsant drugs.

## Primidone

Primidone, proprietary name *Mysoline,* is effective in the treatment of tonic-clonic and partial seizures. The mechanism of action of this drug is similar to that described for phenobarbital, and the therapeutic effect is due partially to the accumulation of its major metabolite, phenobarbital. A second metabolite of primidone, phenylethylmalonamide, also has some **antiepileptic** activity.

Primidone is rapidly and completely absorbed after oral administration. Once absorbed, it is not highly protein bound and it has a half-life of approximately 10 hours. Disposition of the drug is not known to be significantly altered by other disease states or other drugs.

The optimal therapeutic concentration of primidone in adults has been established as 5 to 12 µg/mL (23 to 55 µmol/L). Because phenobarbital is an active metabolite of primidone, concurrent analysis of phenobarbital is required for complete result interpretation. The previously defined therapeutic range for phenobarbital applies to adequate primidone therapy. The phenobarbital concentrations rise gradually over a period of 1 to 2 weeks after therapy is initiated. Toxicity due to accumulation of primidone occurs at serum concentrations in excess of 15 µg/mL (69 µmol/L) and is usually associated with symptoms of sedation, nausea, vomiting, diplopia, dizziness, ataxia, and a phenobarbital concentration greater than 40 µg/mL (177 µmol/L). Specimen collection is dictated by the same rules that apply for phenobarbital; the trough concentration is most useful.

Coadministration of acetazolamide with primidone results in decreased gastrointestinal absorption of primidone and subsequent diminished plasma concentrations. Primidone administered in association with phenytoin produces a modest increase in the phenobarbital/primidone ratio because phenytoin competes with the hepatic hydroxylating enzymes associated with phenobarbital's metabolism. Coadministration of valproic acid, for the same reasons outlined for phenobarbital, causes a modest increase in both primidone and phenobarbital serum concentrations.

## Zonisamide

Zonisamide is the generic name used in the United States for a widely used seizure medication whose common brand name is Zonegran. The FDA approved zonisamide for use in 2000 with the suggestion that it be used together with other anticonvulsants in the treatment of partial seizures in adults.

Orally administered zonisamide is generally well absorbed with little to no effect of concomitant food consumption, and this drug is only weakly bound to plasma proteins. Zonisamide is extensively metabolized by oxidative, acetylation, and other pathways and has essentially linear pharmacokinetics, resulting in linearity for doses ranging from 10 to 15 mg/kg/day. Concomitantly administered inducing drugs such as phenytoin or carbamazepine cause increased metabolism-based clearance and therefore a need for dose adjustment that can be aided by TDM of zonisamide. When concomitant therapy with an inducing drug is being withdrawn, adjustment of zonisamide dosing using TDM is warranted.

A target TDM range of 10 to 40 µg/mL (47 to 188 µmol/L) has been recommended, based largely on retrospective studies and, as with all other anticonvulsants, there is significant overlap of serum zonisamide concentrations between seizure-free patients and patients who do not respond to therapy with this drug, and between patients who encounter side effects and those who do not. Thus finding an optimal therapeutic concentration within the individual patient is an essential need, not simply titrating the patient to be within the target therapeutic range.

## Antibiotics

Antibiotics that require TDM include aminoglycosides, chloramphenicol, sulfonamides, vancomycin, trimethoprim, β-lactams, and tetracyclines. Pharmacokinetic details of these antibiotics are summarized in Table 30.2.

### Aminoglycosides

Aminoglycosides are polycationic agents that kill aerobic gram-negative bacteria. They act by binding to the 30S ribosomal subunit of bacterial mRNA, thereby inhibiting protein synthesis. They are inactive under anaerobic conditions because an oxygen-dependent active transport mechanism is involved in the transfer of aminoglycosides across the bacterial cell wall. The aminoglycoside class of drugs includes amikacin, gentamicin, kanamycin, neomycin, netilmicin, sisomicin, streptomycin, and tobramycin.

The aminoglycosides are a very polar group of compounds and are thus poorly absorbed from the intestinal tract. They

## TABLE 30.1   Pharmacokinetic Parameters of Antiepileptic Drugs

| Drug | RECOMMENDED THERAPEUTIC RANGE µg/mL | µmol/L | Mean Time to Steady State (days) | Observed Range of Half-Life in Adults (h) | Mean Oral Bioavailability (%) | Protein Binding (%) | Important Metabolizing Enzymes |
|---|---|---|---|---|---|---|---|
| Carbamazepine | 4–12 | 17–51 | 2–4 | 8–12 | 70 | 75 | CYP3A4 |
| Clonazepam | 0.015–0.060 | 0.048–0.190 | 3–10 | 17–56 | >90 | 85 | CYP3A4 |
| Ethosuximide | 40–100 | 283–708 | 7–10 | 30–60 | >90 | 0 | CYP3A4 |
| Felbamate | 30–60 | 126–252 | 3–4 | 14–21 | >90 | 25 | CYP3A4 |
| Gabapentin | 2–12 | 12–70 | 1–2 | 5–9 | Variable | 0 | NA |
| Lamotrigine | 2.5–15 | 10–59 | 3–6 | 20–30 | >90 | 55 | NA |
| Levetiracetam | 12–46 | 70–270 | 1–2 | 6–8 | >90 | 0 | NA |
| Phenobarbital | 10–40 | 43–172 | 12–24 | 70–140 | >90 | 50 | CYP2C19 |
| Phenytoin | 10–20 (free: 1.0–2.0) | 40–79 | 5–17 | 30–100 | 80 | 90 | CYP2C9, 2C19 |
| Primidone | 5–10 | 23–46 | 2–4 | 3–22 | >90 | 20 | CYP2C9, 2C19 |
| Topiramate | 5–20 | 15–59 | 4–5 | 20–30 | 80 | 15 | NA |
| Valproic acid | 50–100 | 346–693 | 2–4 | 11–20 | >90 | 90 | CYP2C9,2C19, 2B6, 2E1, 2A6 |
| Zonisamide | 10–40 | 47–188 | 9–12 | 50–70 | 65 | 50 | CYP2C9, 3A4 |

## TABLE 30.2   Pharmacokinetic Parameters of Commonly Monitored Antibiotics

| Drug | Therapeutic Targets[a] (µg/mL [µmol/L]) | Half-Life (h) | Oral Bioavailability (%) | Protein Binding (%) |
|---|---|---|---|---|
| **Aminoglycosides** | | | | |
| Amikacin | $C_{max}$: 25–35 (43–60) $C_{min}$: 1–8 (1.7–13.7) | 2[b] | NA | <11 |
| Gentamicin | $C_{max}$: 5–12 (10.5–25) $C_{min}$: <1 (<2) | 2[b] | NA | <30 |
| Tobramycin | $C_{max}$: 5–12 (11–25.7) $C_{min}$: <1 (<2) | 2[b] | NA | <15 |
| **Glycopeptides** | | | | |
| Vancomycin | $C_{min}$: >10–15 (>6.9–10.4) | 6–12[c] | <1[d] | 10–50 |
| **Other** | | | | |
| Chloramphenicol | $C_{max}$: 10–25 (31–77) $C_{min}$: 1–8 (3–25) | Adults: 1.5–4.1 Newborn: ≥24[f] | 70–80[e] | 60 |

[a]Target blood concentrations depend upon the infection (e.g., tissue compartment), organism and its sensitivity to the antibiotic (i.e., minimal inhibitory concentration).

[b]Clearance of aminoglycoside antibiotics is dependent upon kidney function. The half-life shown is the average elimination phase half-life in healthy individuals; however, the half-life may be significantly prolonged in individuals with renal disease.

[c]Vancomycin best conforms to a multicompartment (2- or 3-compartment) pharmacokinetic model. The half-life shown represents the terminal, elimination half-life.

[d]Absorption of vancomycin from the gastrointestinal tract leading to toxic concentrations has been observed in individuals with pseudomembranous colitis.

[e]Bioavailability of chloramphenicol depends upon the chemical form (succinate or palmitate).

[f]Chloramphenicol clearance is reduced in neonates due to limited glucuronide conjugating activity of the liver. Half-life is generally >24 hours immediately after birth and decreases to ~10 hours by 2 weeks of age.

are routinely administered intravenously or intramuscularly to achieve a high degree of bioavailability. When administered directly into the blood, they rapidly distribute to the extracellular fluid but do not cross cell membranes or bind to plasma proteins; this behavior is consistent with their unusually low volume of distribution. Most tissues and non-renal or hepatic secretions contain very small concentrations of aminoglycosides, with the exception of the renal cortex, where the drug is concentrated, and bile, because of active hepatic secretion. The drugs are mainly excreted by glomerular filtration. Elimination half-lives are short, ranging from 2 to 3 hours. Because clearance is highly dependent on renal function, any impairment of glomerular filtration causes accumulation of these drugs.

Therapy with antibiotic agents like the aminoglycosides differs from the approach used for most other drugs discussed in this chapter. The goal is to achieve a concentration in plasma such that the bacteria are killed but the host remains undamaged. Because the organisms treated are variable and can become resistant to certain drugs, treatment with specific aminoglycoside agents should always be directed by susceptibility testing. Table 30.2 identifies target maximum peak and trough serum concentrations.

Dose corrections must be made in patients with compromised renal function because these patients have prolonged half-life and slower elimination. This should then be followed up by quantification of the blood concentration and dose adjustment following the method outlined by Gilbert.

Toxicity associated with aminoglycosides manifests as delayed-onset vestibular and cochlear sensory cell destruction and acute renal tubular necrosis. The degree and severity of cell damage are variable among the different drugs, but they all cause cell damage if the concentrations are high. Unfortunately, the therapeutic concentration guidelines identified in Table 30.2 do not guarantee the avoidance of toxicity; a small number of patients experience toxic effects regardless of the concentration. Fortunately, most patients reverse the toxic effects without direct intervention if the toxicity is associated with reasonable blood concentrations. Irreparable loss of vestibular, cochlear, or renal function usually correlates with administration of one of the aminoglycosides at increased blood concentrations for periods longer than 2 weeks.

## Chloramphenicol

Chloramphenicol, proprietary name *Chloromycetin* and others, is used as a bactericidal agent. It acts by binding to the 50S ribosomal subunit of bacteria mRNA and inhibits protein synthesis in prokaryotic organisms. Use of this drug depends on its relative toxicity against the microorganism versus the host. The drug is used against gram-negative bacteria such as *Hemophilus influenzae, Neisseria meningitidis, Neisseria gonorrhoeae, Salmonella typhi,* all *Brucella* species, *Bordetella pertussis, Vibrio cholerae,* and *Shigella.* These organisms are all susceptible to a concentration of 6 µg/mL (19 µmol/L). Organisms that require higher concentrations of 12 µg/mL (37 µmol/L) are *Escherichia coli, Klebsiella pneumoniae, Pseudomonas pseudomallei, Chlamydia,* and *Mycoplasma.*

Chloramphenicol is rapidly absorbed in the gastrointestinal tract. Peak serum concentrations occur 1 to 2 hours after the oral dose. In plasma, chloramphenicol is approximately 50% protein bound and is cleared with a half-life of 2 to 3 hours. Peak serum concentrations of chloramphenicol palmitate or succinate occur 4 to 6 hours after administration. Chloramphenicol distributes to all tissues, and it concentrates in the cerebrospinal fluid. The drug is actively metabolized by the liver by *N*-acetylation and glucuronidation. Thus, chloramphenicol accumulates in cases of hepatic disease. Renal disease does not dramatically reduce clearance.

Host toxicity displayed after chloramphenicol therapy includes hematologic toxicity and cardiovascular collapse; both show a modest relationship to blood concentration. These effects are associated with serum concentrations in excess of 25 µg/mL (77 µmol/L). Development of idiosyncratic aplastic anemia has also been observed, but this complication appears unrelated to dose or blood concentration. Cardiovascular collapse, which occurs primarily in newborns, has been related to a total serum chloramphenicol concentration in excess of 40 µg/mL (155 µmol/L). An oral dose of 50 mg/kg/day results in an optimal peak serum concentration of 10 to 25 µg/mL (31 to 77 µmol/L) in a healthy adult.

Methods for chloramphenicol determination must be able to differentiate between the prodrug forms, chloramphenicol palmitate or succinate, and their active metabolite, chloramphenicol.

## Vancomycin

Vancomycin is a glycopeptide that is bactericidal against gram-positive bacteria and some gram-negative cocci. Vancomycin is used because of its activity against methicillin-resistant staphylococci and corynebacteria. It has thus become popular for treatment of endocarditis and sepsis caused by these organisms.

Although the drug is generally poorly absorbed when given orally, absorption leading to toxicity has been observed in patients with pseudomembranous colitis. It has an average elimination half-life of 5 to 6 hours. Blood concentration–related toxicity involves the auditory nerve. Concentrations less than 30 µg/mL (21 µmol/L) are rarely associated with this development. Toxicities not related to dose or blood concentrations include fever, phlebitis, and pain at the infusion site. Erythema or flushing of the face, neck, and upper torso occurring within 5 to 10 minutes following vancomycin infusion (sometimes referred to as "red man syndrome" or "red neck syndrome") has also been observed. This syndrome is due to acute, non-IgE-mediated mast cell degranulation, and is generally controlled by slow infusion and coadministration of antihistamines. In patients with impaired renal function, the serum concentration may increase to toxic concentrations because of reduced clearance.

## Antifungal Antibiotics

Over the past decade, increasing evidence has accumulated to support the use of TDM to enhance the therapeutic safety and efficacy of antifungal medicines. The azole class of antifungals has the most data supporting concentration monitoring. There are limited data supporting the monitoring of flucytosine. Studies of TDM for other classes of antifungal medicines including the echinocandins (i.e., caspofungin) and the polyenes (e.g., amphotericin B) have generated data showing no or limited value to monitoring these drugs.

A recent review of proficiency testing data that evaluated 5 years of data from 57 different laboratories around the world demonstrated that a wide variation in results, especially at low concentrations, is common leading to results that can deviate by more than 20%. New immunoassays for voriconazole and posaconazole have been described, but experience with these is limited. The availability of reliable immunoassays for these antifungals could foster more widespread experience in the effectiveness of their monitoring. Metabolism of the drugs can also affect interpretation of concentration data as discussed in more detail later.

## Antineoplastic Agents
### Methotrexate

Methotrexate has proved useful in (1) the management of acute lymphoblastic leukemia in children; (2) choriocarcinoma and related trophoblastic tumors in women; (3) carcinomas of the breast, tongue, pharynx, and testes; (4) maintenance of remission in leukemia; and (5) treatment of severe, debilitating psoriasis. High-dose methotrexate administration followed by leucovorin rescue is effective in treatment of carcinoma of the lung and osteogenic sarcoma. Intrathecal administration is effective in treating meningeal leukemia or lymphoma.

Methotrexate inhibits DNA synthesis by decreasing availability of pyrimidine nucleotides. Methotrexate competitively inhibits the enzyme dihydrofolate reductase, thus decreasing the concentrations of the tetrahydrofolate essential to the methylation of the pyrimidine nucleotides and consequently the rate of pyrimidine nucleotide synthesis. Leucovorin, a folate analog, is used to rescue host cells from methotrexate inhibition; as a synthetic substrate for dihydrofolate reductase, leucovorin administration allows resumption of tetrahydrofolate-dependent synthesis of pyrimidines and reinitiation of DNA synthesis. Methotrexate is a nonspecific cytotoxin, and prolongation of blood concentrations appropriate to killing tumor cells may lead to severe, unwanted cytotoxic effects such as myelosuppression, gastrointestinal mucositis, and hepatic cirrhosis.

Serum concentrations of methotrexate are commonly monitored during high-dose therapy (>50 mg/m²) to identify the time at which active intervention by leucovorin rescue should be initiated. Criteria for blood concentrations indicative of a potential for toxicity after single-bolus high-dose therapy are as follows:

1. Methotrexate concentration greater than 10 μmol/L 24 hours after dose
2. Methotrexate concentration greater than 1 μmol/L 48 hours after dose
3. Methotrexate concentration greater than 0.1 μmol/L 72 hours after dose

Characteristically, blood concentrations are monitored at 24, 48, and 72 hours after the single dose, and leucovorin is administered when methotrexate concentrations are inappropriately high for a post-dose phase. The route of elimination for methotrexate is primarily renal excretion. During the period of high blood concentrations, particular attention must be paid to maintaining output of a large volume of alkaline urine. The $pK_a$ of methotrexate is 5.5; thus small decreases in urine pH result in significant reduction in its solubility. Keeping urinary pH alkaline diminishes the risks of intratubular precipitation of the drug and obstructive nephropathy during the treatment period. Monitoring blood concentrations therefore provides the basis for decisions for timing of initiation and continuance of leucovorin treatment and for managing urinary pH.

## Busulfan

Busulfan is a DNA alkylating agent available in both oral and intravenous formulations. High-dose busulfan is often used as part of the myeloablative preparative regimen for hematopoietic stem cell transplantation (HSCT). Clinical use of busulfan is complicated by significant interpatient variability in pharmacokinetic behavior with reported coefficients of variation of 23% and 25% for the oral and intravenous (IV) formulations, respectively. Age, obesity, underlying disease, and organ dysfunction also exert a significant influence on observed clearance for busulfan. Children younger than 6 years typically display more than twice the average clearance of 2.5 mL/min/kg reported for adults. The observed variability in the pharmacokinetic behavior of busulfan is relevant because several studies have identified a pharmacodynamic relationship between exposure to busulfan and both its toxicity and efficacy. Exposure to busulfan is typically estimated by measurement of several plasma concentrations over a 6-hour dose interval. This exposure is generally expressed as either the area under the concentration-time curve (referred to as the AUC) or the mean steady-state concentration ($\overline{C}_{SS}$). Dosing of busulfan is usually every 6 hours or once daily over 4 days for a total of 16 or 4 doses, respectively. As a result, a study is typically performed following the first dose, and the results are promptly reported to effect a dose adjustment as early as possible in the course of the treatment regimen; however, the completion and reporting of a busulfan pharmacokinetic study are not a simple task. A variety of chromatographic methods are used for measurement of busulfan in plasma with gas chromatography–mass spectrometry (GC-MS) and LC-MS/MS generally the preferred methods. Given the complexity of the analytical methodology, onsite testing is not always available. Sample extraction and analysis also usually require several hours to complete for a single patient. Nevertheless, using the above TDM approach with dose adjustment, exposures that are within less than 10% of the target exposure are possible, and toxicity can be avoided without a compromise in efficacy.

## Immunosuppressive Drugs
### Tacrolimus

Tacrolimus, proprietary name *Prograf* and formerly called FK506, is a macrolide antibiotic isolated from a strain of *Streptomyces tsukubaensis* that has significant **immunosuppressant** properties. Tacrolimus mediates its immunosuppressive action by entering the lymphocyte, and binding to a receptor known as FK506-binding protein (FKBP). Once bound to FKBP, this drug-receptor complex interacts with, and blocks, the calcium-dependent phosphatase, calcineurin, which is critical for the translocation of the nuclear factor of activated T cells (NFAT) to the nucleus, where the latter regulates the transcription of cytokines and other genes important for T cell activation, proliferation, and function. Calcineurin inhibition therefore leads to marked suppression of T cell–mediated immune responses such as those involved in solid organ transplant rejection and graft-versus-host disease following bone marrow transplantation. NFAT plays a role in other cell types, likely contributing to the toxic effects of tacrolimus.

Tacrolimus is administered predominantly orally in capsule form (Prograf) containing 0.5 mg, 1 mg or 5 mg of the drug. A sterile solution containing the equivalent of 1 mg/mL of tacrolimus for intravenous administration and an ointment containing 0.1% or 0.03% for topical use on skin are also available. Rapid but incomplete absorption is characteristic of standard oral tacrolimus formulations, with an average time to peak concentration of 1.6 to 2.3 hours and average oral bioavailability of 17% to 22%. Recently, several prolonged release formulations of tacrolimus have been developed with the first, Advagraf, now available commercially. Extended-release formulations afford delayed maximal concentrations with improved bioavailability leading to a slight reduction in dose to achieve equivalent AUC.

There is a fairly good correlation between tacrolimus trough concentration, graft rejection, and toxicity. The target range for tacrolimus blood concentrations depends upon the concomitant use of other ISDs, the transplant type, and the time following transplantation. An example of the immunosuppressive regimens used at the authors' institution with the associated tacrolimus target ranges are shown in Table 30.3.

The steady-state trough concentration of tacrolimus per unit of dose varies widely within and between patients. The between-subject variability of dose-normalized tacrolimus has been estimated to be fivefold. Factors known to contribute to this variability are many and include hematocrit; plasma albumin concentration; patient age; genotypes of metabolizing enzyme CYP3A5; drug-drug, herb-drug, and food-drug interactions; and disease. The influence of one or more of these factors in transplant patients explains the

wide within- and between-subject variability of tacrolimus concentrations. This, taken together with the narrow TI and the requirement of contemporary practice to lower the tacrolimus dosing and target trough concentration during the first transplant year and beyond to limit nephrotoxicity, is the basis for the need for close concentration monitoring of this drug.

Due to the high binding of tacrolimus to FK506 binding proteins within cells including erythrocytes, the plasma concentration of tacrolimus is typically 1.5% to 8% of whole blood. Methods for quantitative analysis of this drug therefore generally begin with cell lysis and protein precipitation of whole blood to liberate cell-bound tacrolimus to allow measurement of the total drug present within whole blood. The lysis step is most commonly performed as a manual step using a water-miscible solvent (e.g., methanol) solution containing $ZnSO_4$ followed by centrifugation. Performance of this initial step is one of the critical points in tacrolimus analysis, and it represents an important source of potential error if not performed correctly or consistently.

Interferences in the measurement of tacrolimus include metabolites of the drug and other substances present in human blood such as antibodies that react with components of the assay (for additional discussion on interference in immunoassay, refer to Chapter 15). The former represents the more frequent and challenging interfering substance as discussed previously in the section on Analytic Factors affecting testing results.

## Cyclosporine

Cyclosporine, proprietary names *Sandimmune* (cyclosporine A, or CsA) and *Neoral,* is a cyclic peptide composed of 11 amino acids, some of novel structure, isolated from the fungus *Trichoderma polysporum.* The compound has been shown to be effective in suppressing solid organ allograft rejection

## TABLE 30.3 Immunosuppressive Regimens and Associated Tacrolimus Target Ranges Used at the Author's Institution

| Organ | Immunosuppressive Regimen | Time Posttransplant | TACROLIMUS THERAPEUTIC RANGE µg/L | nmol/L |
|---|---|---|---|---|
| Kidney | Tacrolimus + MMF | 0–3 months | 8–12 | 10.4–15.6 |
| | | 4–12 months | 6–10 | 7.8–13 |
| | | >12 months | 5–8 | 6.5–10.4 |
| Pancreas | Tacrolimus + MMF | 0–6 months | 8–12 | 10.4–15.6 |
| | | 7–12 months | 6–10 | 7.8–13.0 |
| | | >12 months | 5–8 | 6.5–10.4 |
| Heart | Tacrolimus + MMF | 0–12 months | 10–12 | 13–15.6 |
| | | 13–24 months | 8–10 | 10.4–13 |
| | | >24 months | 5–8 | 6.5–10.4 |
| Liver | Tacrolimus + steroids ± azathioprine or MMF | 0–3 months | 8–12 | 10.4–15.6 |
| | | 3–6 months | 5–8 | 5.2–10.4 |
| | | 6–12 months | 4–8 | |
| Lung | Tacrolimus + MMF + steroids | 0–12 months | 8–12 | 10.4–15.6 |
| | | >12 months | 6–8 | 7.8–10.4 |
| Bone marrow | Tacrolimus | | 5–15 | 6.5–19.5 |

*MMF,* Mycophenolate mofetil.

and graft-versus-host disease following bone marrow transplantation. CsA is approved for use in renal, cardiac, hepatic, pancreatic, and bone marrow transplants.

CsA acts by a mechanism that is very similar to tacrolimus. Following entry into the cell, CsA forms a complex with cytoplasmic receptors termed "cyclophilins" that are molecularly distinct from FKBP. These cyclosporine-cyclophilin molecular complexes interact with and inhibit the calcineurin phosphatase preventing NFAT activation that is critical for lymphocyte proliferation and function.

Absorption of CsA in the form of *Sandimmune* is highly variable, ranging from 5% to 40%. There is a poor relationship between dose and blood concentration; however, the whole-blood concentration of CsA correlates with the degree of immunosuppression and toxicity. A microemulsion form of CsA, *Neoral,* has more reproducible absorption, averaging 40%, and exhibits better correlation among dose, blood concentration, and clinical response.

Immunosuppression requires trough whole-blood concentrations of at least 100 ng/mL (83 nmol/L). Kahan and colleagues found that trough whole-blood concentrations exceeding 600 ng/mL (499 nmol/L) were associated with hepatic, renal, neurological, and infective complications.

Therapeutic trough blood concentrations of CsA for renal transplants are 100 to 300 ng/mL (83 to 250 nmol/L), whereas 200 to 350 ng/mL (166 to 291 nmol/L) is used as the target concentration for cardiac, hepatic, and pancreatic transplants; however, concomitant immunosuppression used in combination therapy, similar to combined drug therapy in other situations such as AED therapy in epilepsy, significantly affects the range of concentrations that are effective. Simultaneous immunosuppression with low-dose prednisone and either azathioprine (AZA) or mycophenolate mofetil (MMF) allows the patient to enjoy a good response to CsA at lower concentrations—some renal transplant patients obtain a satisfactory response with trough CsA concentrations of 70 ng/mL (58 nmol/L).

CsA is slowly absorbed, and peak concentrations are reached in 4 to 6 hours. Like tacrolimus, CsA is also highly (~90%) protein bound and concentrated in erythrocytes. The degree of concentration in erythrocytes is temperature dependent in vitro; thus measurement of plasma concentration requires strict attention to specimen temperature if reproducible results are to be obtained. Because of this effect, the best specimen for analysis is whole blood. CsA is also heavily metabolized, and immunoassays are generally subject to metabolite interference similar to the effects described for tacrolimus.

Several drugs alter the disposition of CsA. Ketoconazole, erythromycin, melphalan, amphotericin B, and aminoglycoside antibiotics all prolong metabolism of CsA sufficiently to increase the risk of nephrotoxicity. Coadministration of phenytoin, phenobarbital, carbamazepine, and rifampin results in induction of cytochrome $P_{450}$ enzymes, which increase the rate at which CsA is metabolized. Intravenous administration of sulfadimidine and trimethoprim decreases CsA concentrations.

Currently, nonisotopic immunoassays performed on whole blood are the most commonly used methods for measurement of CsA; however, many laboratories use HPLC and LC-MS/MS methods, which are more specific and less subject to metabolite interference. It is therefore important to ensure consistency with TDM by following individuals with the same method over time and to interpret results within the context of the method used.

## Sirolimus

Sirolimus, also known as rapamycin, is a macrocyclic antibiotic that is a fermentation product of the actinomycete *Streptomyces hygroscopicus* that was isolated from soil samples collected on Rapa Nui (Easter Island) following a search for novel antifungal agents. Structurally, sirolimus is a lipophilic macrocyclic lactone comprised of a 31-member macrolide ring. It demonstrates antifungal, antitumor, and immunosuppressive activity in animal model studies, and it is approved in the United States for the prophylaxis of acute rejection in renal transplant patients.

The complex of sirolimus and the intracellular **immunophilin,** FKBP12, modulates the immune response by combining with the specific cell-cycle regulatory protein called mTOR (the mammalian target of rapamycin) and inhibiting its activation. This inhibition results in suppression of cytokine-driven T-lymphocyte proliferation, inhibiting the progression from the $G_1$ to the S phase of the cell cycle.

The metabolism of sirolimus by the human body is driven by oxidative metabolism via CYP3A in the gastrointestinal tract and liver. There are at least seven metabolites characterized as 41-*O*- and 7-*O*-demethyl, several hydroxy, hydroxy-demethylated, and di-demethylated sirolimus. Total sirolimus metabolites accounted for 48% to 70%, and no single metabolite accounted for more than 10% of sirolimus in trough whole blood from stable renal transplant patients; however, the immunosuppressive activity of individual metabolites is reported to be lower than the parent drug.

Sirolimus is available as both an oral solution and tablet. Sirolimus is rapidly absorbed from the gastrointestinal tract with the average time to reach maximal concentration in whole blood of about 2 hours. The average bioavailability of sirolimus is low, at 15%, and attributable to extensive intestinal and hepatic metabolism by CYP3A and to counter-transport by the multidrug efflux pump P-glycoprotein in the gastrointestinal tract. This absorption barrier varies considerably within a single patient and from patient to patient. It is also the site of clinically important drug-drug and drug-food interactions.

Sirolimus distributes extensively into blood cells as reflected by the average blood-to-plasma ratio of 36:1 in renal transplant patients. Approximately 95% distributes into red blood cells, 3% in plasma, and 1% each in lymphocytes and granulocytes. The extensive and avid binding of sirolimus to the ubiquitously distributed intracellular FKBP12 accounts for the high blood-to-plasma sirolimus concentration ratio. Approximately 2.5% of the sirolimus within the plasma fraction is unbound with the remainder bound to plasma proteins.

The relationship between sirolimus whole-blood trough concentrations and efficacy and toxicity has been investigated in renal transplant patients who received concomitant full-dose CsA and corticosteroid therapy. According to these analyses, the minimum effective sirolimus concentration below which there is a significant increase in risk for acute rejection is 4 to 5 μg/L (4.4 to 5.5 nmol/L). The threshold concentration of 13 to 15 μg/L (14 to 16 nmol/L) was identified, above which the risks increase for the concentration-related side effects, thrombocytopenia (<100,000 platelets/mm$^3$), leukopenia (<4000 leukocytes/mm$^3$), and hypertriglyceridemia (>300 mg/dL or 3.4 mmol/L serum triglycerides). More studies are needed to define these relationships for other transplant populations and for different concomitant immunosuppressants.

Several chromatographic (i.e., LC-MS, LC-MS/MS, HPLC) detection methods have been validated and are in use in laboratories worldwide. A commercial, automated immunoassay has also been developed. This latter assay, while showing high precision, exhibits modest bias due to metabolite interference (~25%) when results are compared to chromatographic methods.

## Everolimus

In April 2010, everolimus, a more water-soluble analog of sirolimus, was approved for use in CsA-sparing regimens including the requirement for adjusting everolimus doses using target trough blood concentrations in renal transplant patients. The target ranges were established from earlier retrospective studies and used prospectively to demonstrate equivalent acute rejection rates compared to the combination of standard dose CsA and empiric dose MMF. More recently, the use of everolimus has expanded with approval in liver transplantation in combination with low-dose tacrolimus.

The mechanism of action and pharmacodynamic effects of everolimus are comparable to those for sirolimus. Similar to the other ISDs, wide pharmacokinetic variability of everolimus has been observed. This variability is driven by the variable metabolism via CYP3A4/5 and p-glycoprotein along with frequent drug-drug interactions that are comparable to those observed for sirolimus. Everolimus trough concentrations show a significant, linear correlation with overall drug exposure as assessed by AUC with a coefficient ($r^2$) of 0.79. Similar degrees of correlation between everolimus trough concentration and thrombocytopenia, leucopenia, hypertriglyceridemia, or hypercholesterolemia have been observed in an investigation of 54 stable renal transplant patients (18 to 68 years). Based upon the robust correlation between trough concentration and both efficacy and toxicity, a trough concentration of 3 to 8 ng/mL (3.1 to 8.3 nmol/L) has been suggested as the optimal target range.

The bioanalytical method used for measurement of everolimus concentration in the pharmacokinetic assessments and prospective TDM protocols of many clinical investigations is a validated LC-MS/MS method. In the future, we can anticipate the availability of immunoassays for everolimus, and it will be essential to understand the comparison between these methods and the current chromatographic methods.

## Mycophenolic Acid

Mycophenolic acid (MPA) is a product of the *Penicillium* species that exhibits antitumor, antiviral, antifungal, antibacterial, and immunosuppressive activity. MPA is administered as its morpholinoethyl ester, MMF. MMF, also known as RS–61433, is considered a prodrug because its immunosuppressive activity is expressed only after its hydrolysis to MPA in the body. MPA inhibits inosine monophosphate dehydrogenase, an important enzyme in the purine metabolic pathway. T lymphocytes rely on this pathway for purine synthesis, whereas other cells use the hypoxanthine–guanosine ribosyl transferase salvage pathway for purine biosynthesis. Thus MPA selectively inhibits purine synthesis, and thus transcription, in T lymphocytes. MPA is of interest clinically because it has immunosuppressive activity similar to the thiopurine, AZA, but without many of its side effects.

MMF is completely absorbed and rapidly and completely metabolized to MPA, the active metabolite. The latter is metabolized in the liver by phase II enzymes to form the major metabolite, mycophenolic acid glucuronide (MPAG). The elimination half-life of MPA averages 18 hours, the volume of distribution averages 4 L/kg, and typical serum concentrations range from a peak of 12 μg/mL (37.4 μmol/L) to a trough value of 2 μg/mL (6.24 μmol/L). Based on the available studies, the optimal immunosuppression for MPA appears to be achieved with target AUCs in the 30 to 60 mmol*min/mL range. Although poorly correlated, this is approximated by trough serum concentrations in the range of 2 to 4 μg/mL (6.24 to 12.5 μmol/L).

## Other Drugs

### Digoxin

Digoxin, proprietary name *Lanoxin,* is one of a group of cardiac glycosides obtained from digitalis plants (e.g., *Digitalis lanata*). Although used substantially less frequently than in the past due to newer drugs, digoxin is still used for treatment of supraventricular arrhythmias such as atrial fibrillation due to its activity on atrioventricular nodal conduction. Digoxin also acts as an inotropic agent that restores the force of cardiac contraction in congestive heart failure. However, this latter use has decreased substantially with the introduction of new ionotropic drugs. Digoxin has a complex mechanism of action that includes inhibiting both cellular Na$^+$ efflux and K$^+$ influx in myocardial cells, increasing calcium ion availability and improving cardiac contractility altering autonomic activity within the heart to promote parasympathetic activity.

Absorption of digoxin is variable and dependent on the drug formulation. Digoxin is concentrated in tissues, and at steady state, the concentration of digoxin in cardiac tissue is 15 to 30 times that of plasma. Accumulation of digoxin in tissue lags the plasma concentration—that is, although the peak plasma concentration is reached 2 to 3 hours after the oral dose, the peak tissue concentration occurs 6 to 10 hours after an oral dose. Although pharmacological effects and toxicity correlate with tissue concentration rather than plasma concentration, the safe therapeutic plasma concentration of digoxin has been reported to range from 0.8 to 2.0 ng/mL (1 to 2.6 nmol/L). This range is not determined at the peak plasma concentration but rather at the time of peak tissue concentration. Thus, to ensure a correlation between plasma concentration and tissue concentration, the appropriate time to collect the *specimen* is 8 hours or more after the dose, at which time serum digoxin has reached distributional equilibrium with the drug in tissues. Results from specimens collected earlier than 8 hours after the dose are misleading because high concentrations may be misinterpreted as toxic concentrations, whereas they are more likely due to incomplete distribution.

Digoxin *toxicity* is characterized by nonspecific symptoms of nausea, vomiting, anorexia, and predominance of green/yellow visual distortion. Cardiac symptoms of intoxication include multiform premature ventricular contractions, ventricular bigeminy, ventricular tachycardia, and ventricular fibrillation. Children can tolerate higher concentrations and do not usually exhibit toxicity until the digoxin concentration exceeds 4 ng/mL (5.2 nmol/L).

Currently, immunoassays remain the most widely used method for measurement of digoxin in serum and biological fluids. Use of Digibind or DigiFab digoxin-specific Fab fragments, which neutralize the drug and are used in the setting of acute toxicity, can complicate digoxin measurement by many immunoassays. Results of digoxin monitoring following administration of Digibind should therefore be interpreted with caution.

## Lithium

Lithium, whose proprietary names include *Eskalith, Lithane, Lithonate,* and others, is administered as lithium carbonate and used for the treatment of the manic phase of affective disorders, mania, and manic-depressive illness. The mechanism of action for lithium is not entirely clear. Early research suggested that it acts by enhancing re-uptake of catecholamines, thereby reducing their concentration in the neuronal junction and producing a sedating effect on the central nervous system. More recently, lithium and other mood-affecting drugs, such as valproic acid, carbamazepine, and the tricyclic antidepressants, have been shown to inhibit GSK3-β, a protein central to the Wnt/β-catenin signaling pathway that affects gene expression involved in many aspects of cellular behavior, neuronal polarity, plasticity and survival, and brain development. GSK3-β appears critical in the action of dopamine and serotonin on the brain affecting behavior. At least two mechanisms account for lithium's effects on GSK3-β. Lithium directly competes with magnesium, which is an important cation for GSK3-β activity. It also indirectly affects GSK3-β by inhibiting a critical phosphatase normally required for its activation. Although other mechanisms of action cannot be excluded, the mechanisms described above are likely to account for many of lithium's effects on mood.

Absorption of lithium from the gastrointestinal tract is complete, with peak plasma concentration reached 2 to 4 hours after an oral dose. This cation does not bind to protein.

Lithium elimination is biphasic; during the first phase, 30% to 40% of the dose of lithium is cleared, with an apparent half-life of 24 hours. During the second phase, the remainder of lithium incorporated into the cellular ion pool is cleared, exhibiting a half-life of 48 to 72 hours. Clearance is predominantly a function of the kidneys, where active reabsorption occurs. Reduced renal function causes prolonged clearance times.

The optimal therapeutic response to lithium has not been related to a specific serum concentration; however, toxicity is related to serum concentration. Serum lithium concentrations are monitored to ensure patient compliance and to avoid intoxication. It is recommended that a standardized 12-hour post-dose serum lithium concentration be used to assess adequate therapy. A concentration in excess of 1.5 mmol/L *in a specimen drawn 12 hours after the dose* indicates a significant risk of intoxication. Early symptoms of intoxication include apathy, sluggishness, drowsiness, lethargy, speech difficulties, irregular tremors, myoclonic twitching, muscle weakness, and ataxia. These symptoms, although not life threatening, are uncomfortable for patients and indicate that the onset of life-threatening seizures is imminent.

Severe intoxication, characterized by muscle rigidity, hyperactive deep tendon reflexes, and epileptic seizures, is usually associated with lithium concentrations in excess of 2.5 mmol/L.

The concentration of lithium in serum, plasma, urine, or other body fluids can be determined by several methods including flame emission photometry, atomic absorption spectrometry, ion-selective electrode or inductively coupled plasma–mass spectrometry (ICP-MS) or inductively coupled plasma–optical emission spectrometry (ICP-OES). In contemporary clinical practice, automated methods are primarily used for routine measurement of lithium in serum using a chromophore (e.g., a substituted porphyrin) that forms a colored product readily detected spectrophotometrically upon binding to lithium. The availability from NIST of a standard reference material (NIST SRM 3129a) provides manufacturers with the opportunity to prepare traceable calibrators and improve standardization of assays.

## Theophylline

Theophylline, available under many proprietary names, relaxes bronchial smooth muscles to relieve or prevent asthma. The therapeutic effect of theophylline is likely due to antagonism of adenosine receptors in smooth muscle, whereas the toxic effects are due to inhibition of cyclic nucleotide phosphodiesterase. With increased use of β–adrenergic agonists, and because of the considerable toxicity associated with it, theophylline is now considered a second-level approach used only in treatment of persistent asthma.

Theophylline is readily absorbed after oral, rectal, or parenteral administration. If the drug is taken orally without food, the blood concentration peaks within 2 hours. If it is administered with food or as a slow-release formula, peak concentrations occur 3 to 5 hours after the dose. Once absorbed, it is 50% protein bound. The drug is rapidly cleared in adolescents and in adults who smoke due to its higher rate of metabolism due to increased levels of CYP1A2. In these individuals, the half-life ranges from 3 to 4 hours. Nonsmoking adults in good health have an elimination half-life of about 9 hours. The half-life in neonates and in adults with congestive heart failure can be prolonged to 20 to 30 hours, depending on the degree of liver immaturity or loss of liver function. Coadministration of cimetidine, ciprofloxacin, and ticlopidine leads to reduced clearance of theophylline.

The optimum therapeutic effect occurs at concentrations ranging from 8 to 20 μg/mL (44 to 111 μmol/L). Suppression of exercise-induced bronchospasm in asthmatic patients occurs at concentrations exceeding 10 μg/mL (56 μmol/L) and is optimal at 15 μg/mL (83 μmol/L). Neonatal apnea treated with theophylline responds to slightly lower concentrations, ranging from 5 to 10 μg/mL (28 to 56 μmol/L). When the blood level exceeds 20 μg/mL (111 μmol/L), the secondary side effects become significant.

Symptoms of theophylline toxicity include nausea, vomiting, headache, diarrhea, irritability, and insomnia. Transient central nervous system stimulation occurring at initial administration is not directly related to blood concentration. This effect diminishes with chronic use. Serious toxicity characterized by cardiac arrhythmias and seizures is usually associated with serum concentrations in excess of 30 μg/mL (167 μmol/L). Once seizure activity begins, the final prognosis is very poor. Morbidity is reported in nearly all patients, and mortality can be as high as 50%.

## Caffeine

A minor metabolite of theophylline in adults, caffeine has been shown to accumulate to significant concentrations in neonates. Caffeine itself is an effective inhibitor of apnea, which may explain the lower therapeutic concentration required for control of neonatal apnea. Therapy with caffeine alone has also been demonstrated as effective in the treatment of neonatal apnea; it is gaining popularity because of caffeine's long half-life in neonates (>30 hours). The optimal therapeutic concentration of caffeine in this situation ranges from 8 to 14 μg/mL (41 to 72 μmol/L).

## Biologics: The New Frontier of Therapeutic Drug Monitoring

Biologic drugs (also called biopharmaceuticals) represent a varied group of therapeutic agents that are distinct from traditional small-molecule pharmaceuticals. Biologics can range from a peptide or protein to a whole cell and have origins that often require complex production methods using living cells (i.e., biotechnology). Monoclonal antibody (mAb)-based therapeutics represent a rapidly expanding area of biologic drug development. Therapeutic monitoring of mAb-based therapeutics like infliximab, in addition to potentially enhancing their efficacy and safety, may also reduce the economic impact of these revolutionary, yet expensive drugs.

The pharmacology of mAbs is quite distinct from small-molecule drugs. As proteins with a large molecular size (150 kD), mAbs cannot efficiently cross the plasma membranes of cells necessitating parenteral administration, primarily intravenous infusion. Metabolism and elimination of mAbs are also quite distinct from small molecules. Receptor-mediated endocytosis of mAb through Fc-receptors (FcRs) present throughout the reticulo-endothelial system and subsequent proteolytic degradation represents a primary mode of clearance especially when complexed with its target antigen. Host antibodies can also form against mAb, especially those derived from other species, and these anti-drug antibodies (ADAs) can further enhance clearance. However, not all FcR-mediated internalization leads to degradation. Neonatal FcR (FcRn), which was originally identified in placenta and binds IgG and albumin, is expressed across a wide range of cells including endothelium, hepatocytes, gastrointestinal epithelium, and kidney glomerular and tubular cells. FcRn mediates recycling of antibody and albumin within the endosomal compartment of cells, protecting these proteins from degradation contributing to the approximately 20-day half-life of antibody. FcRn also plays important roles in IgG transcytosis such as across the gastrointestinal epithelium, which further contributes to mAb clearance. Due to the variety of mechanisms of antibody clearance and the impact of ADAs, mAb concentrations can vary widely in relationship to dose.

TDM has been advocated for many therapeutic mAbs. Although evidence for utility for most mAb therapeutics is absent, TDM is common for the anti-TNF antibodies.

## Infliximab

Infliximab (IFX) is a chimeric monoclonal antibody with antigen binding, variable domains derived from a mouse monoclonal antibody grafted onto a human IgG1 κ antibody framework. IFX binds to tumor necrosis factor (TNF)-alpha and neutralizes the activity of this important inflammatory cytokine as its primary mechanism of action. IFX was initially approved for the treatment of Crohn's inflammatory bowel disease (IBD) where it induces significant clinical improvement in 60% to 90% of patients with initial therapy. It is now approved for the treatment of multiple moderate to severe inflammatory disorders including both adult and pediatric IBD, rheumatoid arthritis, psoriatic arthritis, plaque psoriasis, and ankylosing spondylitis.

Although many factors influence the response to IFX therapy including the variable role of TNF-α in disease, pharmacokinetics has been shown to play a significant role in response to therapy. IFX concentrations in blood are influenced by body weight, and weight-based dosing of IFX is the standard approach. Albumin concentration has also been shown to correlate with IFX clearance, perhaps due to the association with FcRn for both molecules. ADAs are thought to be the dominant factor mediating loss of therapeutic response, and these ADAs can affect response through both direct neutralization of IFX function as well as accelerating IFX clearance. Although changing therapy to another agent such as adalimumab, a fully human anti-TNFα mAb may be necessary, some ADA resistance may be overcome by changes in dosing.

Prospective as well as many retrospective studies have shown that trough concentrations of IFX above 1 mg/mL are needed to achieve an optimal response to therapy. The American Gastroenterology Association has recommended reactive TDM defined as measurement of IFX trough and anti-drug antibodies in response to new or continual active IBD during initial therapy. This group has proposed a 5 µg/mL trough threshold concentration as a guide to dose escalation in the setting of poor response. Dose escalation in response to symptoms alone without TDM may be an effective strategy for achieving maximal response. However, TDM has been shown to improve decision making and decrease cost by 15% to 30%, which is significant given the high cost of IFX.

Several methods are available for measuring IFX concentrations in blood. Immunoassays provide a simple method for IFX quantitation, representing one of the earliest methods available. These methods are subject to interference by ADAs, and it is therefore imperative that screening for ADAs is included in the testing algorithm. Alternative approaches that indirectly monitor IFX concentrations through their binding to labeled TNF-α that shift chromatographic mobility (Prometheus Anser IFX) or neutralization of TNF-α activity in a biologic assay are also commercially available. More recently, LC-MS/MS -based methods for IFX measurement have been described, which have the advantage of avoiding interference by ADAs. Nevertheless, screening for ADAs is still an essential part of IFX TDM even with LC-MS/MS methods, because the presence of ADA is important to decision making around dosing and switching to alternative therapies such as the fully human adalimumab.

## REVIEW QUESTIONS

1. Which statement regarding lithium TDM is true?
   a. Serum lithium concentration is highly correlated with therapeutic effect.
   b. Free (unbound) lithium should be measured in the setting of hypoalbuminemia.
   c. A 2-hour post-dose lithium concentration is the optimal sample for TDM.
   d. Immunoassay is a commonly used method for lithium measurement.
   e. Lithium toxicity is related to serum concentration.
2. Which of the following is associated with an increased risk for 6-mercaptopurine (6-MP) toxicity?
   a. Obesity
   b. S-methylation via thiopurine S-methyltransferase (TPMT) deficiency
   c. Concomitant use of acetaminophen
   d. Glucose-6-phosphate dehydrogenase (G6PD) deficiency
   e. Epilepsy
3. Which of the following statements best describes tacrolimus testing?
   a. Tacrolimus is typically measured in whole blood.
   b. Metabolites do not interfere with antibody-based immunoassays.
   c. Tacrolimus is routinely measured at 4 hours following a dose.
   d. Inhibition of mTOR activation is the primary mechanism of action for tacrolimus.
   e. Steady-state trough concentrations of tacrolimus show minimal variation.
4. Methotrexate is:
   a. a drug used in the treatment of generalized seizure disorders.
   b. typically combined with leucovorin treatment when used in high doses.
   c. routinely monitored by measurement of pre-dose concentrations.
   d. exhibits reduced solubility in alkaline urine that can contribute to obstructive nephropathy.
   e. an inhibitor of calcium channels.
5. Which of the following best describes valproic acid pharmacology and monitoring?
   a. Valproic acid is poorly absorbed orally necessitating intravenous administration.
   b. Valproic acid is primarily used in the treatment of schizophrenia.
   c. Inhibition of calcineurin is valproic acid's primary mechanism of action.
   d. Valproic acid is highly protein bound and its serum concentrations are affected in uremia, cirrhosis, and other drug therapy.
   e. Valproic acid pharmacokinetics is unaffected by liver function as it shows minimal hepatic metabolism.

## SUGGESTED READINGS

Atkinson AJ. *Principles of Clinical Pharmacology*. 3rd ed. San Diego: Academic Press, Elsevier; 2012.
Bauer LA. *Applied Clinical Pharmacokinetics*. 3rd ed. New York: McGraw-Hill; 2014.
Bettinger TL, Crismon ML. Lithium. In: Burton ME, ed. *Applied Pharmacokinetics & Pharmacodynamics: Principles of Therapeutic Drug Monitoring*. Philadelphia: Lippincott Williams & Wilkins; 2006:789–812.

Carruthers SG, Melmon KL. *Melmon and Morrelli's Clinical Pharmacology: Basic Principles in Therapeutics*. 4th ed. New York: McGraw-Hill; 2000.
Ferrari S, Sassoli V, Orlandi M, et al. Serum methotrexate (MTX) concentrations and prognosis in patients with osteosarcoma of the extremities treated with a multidrug neoadjuvant regimen. *J Chemother*. 1993;5(2):135–141.
Gibaldi M, Prescott LF. *Handbook of Clinical Pharmacokinetics*. New York: ADIS Health Science Press; 1983.

Goodman LS, Brunton LL, Blumenthal DK, et al. *Goodman & Gilman's the Pharmacological Basis of Therapeutics*. New York: McGraw-Hill Medical; 2011.

Hendeles L, Weinberger M. Theophylline: therapeutic use and serum concentration monitoring. In: Taylor WJ, Finn AL, eds. *Individualizing Drug Therapy: Practical Applications of Drug Monitoring*. New York: Gross, Townsend, Frank; 1981:32–65.

Jusko WJ, Thomson AW, Fung J, et al. Consensus document: therapeutic monitoring of tacrolimus (FK-506). *Ther Drug Monit*. 1995;17(6):606–614.

Keating GM, Lyseng-Williamson KA. Everolimus: a guide to its use in liver transplantation. *BioDrugs*. 2013;27(4):407–411.

MacDonald A, Scarola J, Burke JT, et al. Clinical pharmacokinetics and therapeutic drug monitoring of sirolimus. *Clin Ther*. 2000;22(suppl B):B101–B121.

Patsalos PN, Berry DJ, Bourgeois BF, et al. Antiepileptic drugs–best practice guidelines for therapeutic drug monitoring: a position paper by the Subcommission on Therapeutic Drug Monitoring, ILAE Commission on Therapeutic Strategies. *Epilepsia*. 2008;49(7):1239–1276.

Rowland M, Tozer TN, Rowland M. *Clinical Pharmacokinetics and Pharmacodynamics: Concepts and Applications*. 4th ed. Philadelphia: Lippincott William & Wilkins; 2009.

Rybak MJ, Lomaestro BM, Rotschafer JC, et al. Vancomycin therapeutic guidelines: a summary of consensus recommendations from the Infectious Diseases Society of America, the American Society of Health-System Pharmacists, and the Society of Infectious Diseases Pharmacists. *Clin Infect Dis*. 2009;49(3):325–327.

Schentag JJ. Aminoglycosides. In: Evans WE, Schentag JJ, Jusko WJ, eds. *Applied Pharmacokinetics: Principles of Therapeutic Drug Monitoring*. San Francisco: Applied Therapeutics; 1980.

Slattery JT, Clift RA, Buckner CD, et al. Marrow transplantation for chronic myeloid leukemia: the influence of plasma busulfan levels on the outcome of transplantation. *Blood*. 1997;89(8):3055–3060.

Staatz C, Tett S. Clinical pharmacokinetics and pharmacodynamics of mycophenolate in solid organ transplant recipients. *Clin Pharmacokinet*. 2007;46(1):13–58.

Terra SG, Washam JB, Dunham GD, et al. Therapeutic range of digoxin's efficacy in heart failure: what is the evidence? *Pharmacotherapy*. 1999;19(10):1123–1126.

Touw DJ, Neef C, Thomson AH, et al. Cost-effectiveness of therapeutic drug monitoring: a systematic review. *Ther Drug Monit*. 2005;27(1):10–17.

Wright JD, Boudinot FD, Ujhelyi MR. Measurement and analysis of unbound drug concentrations. *Clin Pharmacokinet*. 1996;30(6):445–462.

# 31

# Clinical Toxicology

*Loralie Langman, Laura K. Bechtel, and Christopher P. Holstege*

## OBJECTIVES

1. Define the following terms:
   Anion gap
   Confirmatory test
   Osmolal gap
   Screening test
   Spot test
   Sympathomimetic
   Toxicology
   Toxidrome
2. State and explain the formulae for calculating anion gap and osmolal gap; given appropriate information, calculate and interpret the results of these formulae and list possible interferences with these calculated measurements.
3. For each of the following cellular hypoxia causative agents, describe the agent, the toxic effects, the treatment, and the method(s) of analysis, including specimen requirements and laboratory results:
   Carbon monoxide
   Cyanide
   Methemoglobin-forming agents
4. For each of the following alcohols, describe the pharmacological action, the metabolites, the antidotes, and the method(s) of analysis, including specimen requirements and laboratory results:
   Ethanol
   Ethylene glycol
   Isopropanol
   Methanol
5. For each of the following analgesics, describe the toxic effects of overdose, the dose and time of symptom onset, the metabolizing enzyme and metabolite, the antidote, and the method(s) of analysis, including specimen requirements and laboratory results:
   Acetaminophen
   Salicylate
6. For the following cholinergic/anticholinergic toxidrome agents, describe the clinical uses if any, the mechanism of action, the metabolites, the methods of analysis, and the laboratory results for each:
   Antihistamines
   Antimuscarinics
   Antipsychotics
   Organophosphates/carbamates
   Tricyclic antidepressants
7. For the following drugs, describe the manifestations of intoxication, the metabolizing enzyme and metabolite, the pharmacological response, clinical uses if any, the antidote, and the screening tests and confirmatory methods for each:
   Amphetamines/methamphetamines
   Barbiturates
   Benzodiazepines
   Cannabinoid
   Cocaine
   Marijuana
   Opioids
   Phencyclidine
8. List and describe substances used in drug-facilitated sexual assault, including drug classification, pharmacological effects, and methods of analysis.
9. For the following specimen types, state the advantages and disadvantages of each when used for drug analysis, and list a method of analysis for each:
   Hair
   Meconium
   Saliva (oral fluid)
   Sweat
10. Discuss the strengths and weaknesses as well as the uses of screening assay compared to confirmatory assay.

## KEY WORDS AND DEFINITIONS

**Amphetamine** A sympathomimetic amine that has a stimulating effect on the central and peripheral nervous systems.

**Analgesics** Agents that relieve pain without causing loss of consciousness.

**Analyte** is a substance or chemical constituent that is of interest in an analytical procedure.

**Anticholinergic toxidrome** The signs and symptoms characteristic of poisoning due to a substance that causes inhibition of the muscarinic receptor.

**Antihistamines** Antagonists of the H1 or H2 histamine receptors that are used to treat allergic reactions or gastric hyperacidity.

**Barbiturate**  Any of a class of sedative-hypnotic agents derived from barbituric acid or thiobarbituric acid and classified into long-, intermediate-, short-, and ultrashort-acting classes.

**Benzodiazepines**  Any of a group of minor tranquilizers that have a common molecular structure and similar pharmacological activity, including antianxiety, sedative, hypnotic, amnestic, anticonvulsant, and muscle-relaxing effects.

**Cholinergic toxidrome**  The signs and symptoms characteristic of poisoning due to a substance that causes excessive muscarinic receptor agonism

**Clinical toxicology**  A subdivision of toxicology that involves clinical care of patients exposed to toxins, including the analysis of drugs, heavy metals, and other chemical agents in body fluids and tissues for the purpose of patient care.

**Chiral center**  is defined as an atom in a molecule that is bonded to four different chemical species, allowing for optical isomerism. This characteristic of a molecule makes it impossible to superimpose it on its mirror image.

**Confirmatory testing**  As used in programs that test for drugs of abuse, confirmatory tests are used to confirm a positive or sometimes negative result that had been presumptively classified as positive for a specific drug. Examples of techniques used for confirmatory testing include gas chromatography-mass spectrometry (GC-MS) and high-performance liquid chromatography-tandem mass spectrometry (LC-MS/MS).

**Enantiomer**  A molecule that exhibits stereoisomerism through the presence of one or more chiral centers (i.e., stereoisomers that are nonsuperimposable mirror images).

**Ethylene glycol**  An ethylene compound with two hydroxy groups located on adjacent carbons. It is a common ingredient in antifreeze.

**Gamma-hydroxybutyrate (GHB)**  A potent sedative, hypnotic, euphorigenic agent that is illicitly ingested for its pleasurable effects or used criminally to facilitate assaults.

**Half-life ($t_{1/2}$)**  The length of time it takes for one-half of an administered drug to decrease due to a biological process.

**Intoxication**  A state of impaired mental or physical functioning resulting from ingestion of alcohol or drug.

**Lysergic acid diethylamide (LSD)**  A derivative of an alkaloid found in certain fungi that has hallucinogenic properties.

**Medication half-life**  The time required for the plasma concentration of a drug to reach half of its original concentration.

**Miosis**  Constriction of the pupil of the eye, resulting from a normal response to an increase in light or caused by certain substances or pathological conditions.

**Opiate/opioid**  *Opiate* refers to any of a group of naturally occurring (poppy plant) or semi-synthetic narcotic alkaloids with pharmacological actions and chemical structure similar to morphine. *Opioid* is a general term that is applied to all substances with morphine-like properties, regardless of origin or chemical structure.

**Poison**  Any substance that, when relatively small amounts are ingested, inhaled, or absorbed, or when it is applied to, injected into, or developed within the body, has chemical action that may cause damage to structure or disturbance of function, producing symptoms, illness, or death.

**Screening test**  An initial test, such as that used to "screen" specimens to eliminate "negative" ones from further consideration and to identify presumptively positive specimens that then require confirmatory testing.

**Sedative-hypnotic**  A substance that depresses activity of the central nervous system and reduces anxiety and induces sleep.

**Toxidrome**  A syndrome caused by toxins in the body.

**Toxin**  A poisonous substance that is produced by living cells or organisms and is capable of causing disease when introduced into the body tissues and is often capable of inducing neutralizing antibodies or antitoxins.

# INTRODUCTION

Toxicology is a broad, multidisciplinary science whose goal is to determine the effects of chemical agents on living systems. Innumerable potential **toxins** inflict harm, including pharmaceuticals, herbals, household products, environmental agents, occupational chemicals, substances of use/misuse, drugs used in sexual assaults, and substances used by athletes for their performance-enhancing effects. Each year, millions of cases of human exposure to poisons are reported to the **poison** centers across the world. The Centers for Disease Control and Prevention has reported that poisoning is one of the top causes of injury-related death in the United States in all age groups.

This chapter provides a general overview of **clinical toxicology** and the laboratory services necessary to support the care of poisoned patients. Because a comprehensive discussion of all aspects of toxicology is beyond the scope of this chapter, the clinical significance and toxicity of only a select number of common pharmaceuticals, substances of use/misuse, and other chemicals are discussed. A more extensive review of the subject and additional references are found in Langman et al. (2022).

## Basic Information

In practice, it is neither possible nor necessary to test for the thousands of clinically significant toxins that may be encountered. In reality, only a handful of substances account for the majority of cases of intoxication treated in most emergency departments. The scope of clinical toxicology testing provided by the laboratory depends on the pattern of local substance use/misuse and on the available resources of the institution.

The value of substance testing (screening) is well established in (1) the workplace, (2) for some athletic competitions, (3) to identify substance use/misuse, (4) to evaluate substance exposure and/or withdrawal in newborns, (5) to monitor patients being prescribed controlled substances and in substance use/misuse treatment programs, and (6) to aid in the prompt diagnosis of toxicity for which a specific antidote or treatment modality is required. In many other instances of toxicity, the value of drug screening, especially on an emergency basis, is controversial.

## Clinical Considerations

To operate effectively, the laboratory should be closely associated with the health care team that is directly managing the patient. Through close and collaborative work, clinical information provided helps to guide appropriate ordering of tests and to ensure that interpretation of results is complete and accurate. For example, the team caring for the patient should provide the following information with the laboratory request:

1. The time and date of the suspected exposure along with the time and date of sample collection
2. History obtained from the patient or from witnesses that might aid in identification of the toxin
3. Assessment of the physical state of the patient at the time of presentation

Such information is useful for guiding test selection and interpretation of results.

## Analytical Considerations

Because of the wide variety of chemical substances individuals might be exposed to in society, no single analytical technique is adequate for broad-spectrum substance detection. Therefore, several analytical approaches in combination are generally required. Other critical issues include speed of analysis, turnaround time, and availability of services. An analysis that requires several hours to complete or that is not available during all hours may be of little value in a clinical emergency. Alternatively, a rapid test that may provide false information could result in erroneous diagnostic and therapeutic decisions.

## Clinical Evaluation

When a health care team initially evaluates a patient who presents with a potentially toxicologically induced problem, the final diagnosis is often determined by reviewing the history, performing a directed physical examination, using ancillary tests (e.g., electrocardiogram, radiology), and applying a rational approach to laboratory testing.

## Toxic Syndromes

Toxic syndromes (toxidromes) are clinical syndromes that are essential for the successful recognition of poisoning patterns and are a constellation of clinical signs and symptoms that

suggests a specific class of poisoning. The most commonly encountered toxidromes include anticholinergic, cholinergic, opioid, sedative-hypnotic, serotonergic, and sympathomimetic (Table 31.1). Many toxidromes have overlapping features. For example, anticholinergic findings are highly similar to sympathomimetic findings, with an exception being effects on sweat glands. In this exception, anticholinergic agents produce warm, flushed dry skin, but sympathomimetic agents produce diaphoresis. Toxidrome findings may also be affected by individual variability, comorbid conditions, and co-ingestants. For example, tachycardia associated with sympathomimetic or anticholinergic toxidromes may be absent in a patient who is concurrently taking beta-antagonist

### TABLE 31.1  Symptoms of the Important Toxidromes

| Toxidrome | Symptom |
|---|---|
| Anticholinergic | Agitation |
| | Blurred vision |
| | Decreased bowel sounds |
| | Dry skin |
| | Flushing |
| | Hallucinations |
| | Hyperthermia |
| | Ileus |
| | Lethargy/coma |
| | Mumbling speech |
| | Mydriasis |
| | Psychosis |
| | Tachycardia |
| | Urinary retention |
| Cholinergic | Diarrhea |
| | Diaphoresis |
| | Urination |
| | Miosis |
| | Bradycardia |
| | Bronchorrhea |
| | Emesis |
| | Lacrimation |
| | Salivation |
| Opioid | Bradycardia |
| | Decreased bowel sounds |
| | Hypotension |
| | Hypothermia |
| | Lethargy/coma |
| | Miosis |
| | Shallow respirations |
| | Slow respiratory rate |
| Sedative-hypnotic | Ataxia |
| | Blurred vision |
| | Confusion |
| | Diplopia |
| | Dysesthesias |
| | Hypotension |
| | Lethargy/coma |
| | Nystagmus |
| | Respiratory depression |
| | Slurred speech |

*Continued*

## TABLE 31.1 Symptoms of the Important Toxidromes—cont'd

| Toxidrome | Symptom |
|---|---|
| Sympathomimetic | Agitation |
| | Diaphoresis |
| | Excessive motor activity |
| | Excessive speech |
| | Hallucinations |
| | Hypertension |
| | Hyperthermia |
| | Insomnia |
| | Restlessness |
| | Tachycardia |
| | Tremor |
| Serotonergic | Agitation |
| | Confusion |
| | Hallucinations |
| | Rigors |
| | Diaphoresis |
| | Hyperthermia |
| | Tachycardia |
| | Diarrhea |
| | Myoclonus |
| | Hyperreflexia |
| | Clonus |
| | Tremor |
| | Nystagmus |

medications. Additionally, although toxidromes may be applied to classes of drugs, one or more toxidrome findings may be absent for some individual agents within these classes. For instance, meperidine is an opioid analgesic, but it does not induce miosis, which helps to define the "classic" opioid toxidrome. When accurately identified, the toxidrome may provide invaluable information for diagnosis and subsequent treatment.

# SCREENING PROCEDURES FOR DETECTION OF SUBSTANCES

Screening procedures are designed for the relatively rapid and generally qualitative detection of drugs or other toxic substances. Screening procedures may be designed to detect a particular drug or drug class. In general, screening tests have adequate clinical sensitivity but lack specificity. A negative result may rule out in many cases the presence of clinically significant concentrations of a particular drug, but not necessarily all drugs within a class. Because of possible interferences, a positive result should be considered "presumptive positive" and should be confirmed by an alternate procedure of greater specificity. Screening tests frequently include simple visual color tests (spot tests) and immunoassays.

## Spot Tests

Spot tests are less frequently employed now because some have been largely replaced by rapid immunoassays that may be performed at the point of care (POC) or in the central laboratory. For a more comprehensive description, refer to previous editions of this textbook.

### Electrocardiogram

Because numerous drugs cause changes in the electrocardiogram (ECG), interpretation of the ECG in the poisoned patient has been known to significantly facilitate appropriate laboratory testing, diagnosis, and management of care.

### Anion Gap

A basic metabolic panel is recommended and is an important initial screening test for all poisoned patients. When low serum bicarbonate is discovered on a metabolic panel, the clinician should determine whether an elevated anion gap exists. The formula most commonly used for the anion gap (AG) calculation is as follows:

$$AG = [Na^+] - [Cl^- + HCO_3^-]$$

The reference interval for this anion gap is accepted to be 6 to 14 mmol/L.

An increase in the anion gap, accompanied by a metabolic acidosis, represents an increase in unmeasured endogenous (e.g., lactate) or exogenous (e.g., salicylates) anions. Clinically useful mnemonics for causes of high anion gap metabolic acidosis are the classic MUDPILES (representing Methanol, Uremia, Diabetic/Starvation/Alcoholic Ketoacidosis, Propylene glycol, Iron/Isoniazid/Inhalants, Lactate, Ethylene glycol, and Salicylate) and the more recently proposed GOLD MARK (Glycols [ethylene and propylene], Oxoproline, L-lactate, D-lactate, Methanol, Aspirin, Renal failure, and Ketoacidosis).

It is imperative that clinicians who admit poisoned patients initially presenting with an increased anion gap metabolic acidosis investigate the cause of that acidosis. Many symptomatic poisoned patients may have an initial mild metabolic acidosis upon presentation caused by processes resulting in elevated serum lactate (e.g., transient hypoxia or hypovolemia). However, with adequate supportive care (e.g., oxygenation and hydration), the anion gap acidosis should steadily improve. If, despite adequate supportive care, an anion gap metabolic acidosis worsens in a poisoned patient, the clinician should consider continued absorption of exogenous acids (e.g., salicylate), formation of acidic metabolites (e.g., ethylene glycol, methanol, toluene metabolites), and cellular ischemia with worsening lactic acidosis (e.g., cyanide) as potential causes.

### Osmolal Gap

The main osmotically active constituents of serum are $Na^+, Cl^-, HCO_3^-$, glucose, and urea. Several empirical formulae based on measurement of these substances have been used to estimate serum osmolality. In practice, one has not shown itself to be superior to the others, yet each equation demonstrates significant differences in the osmolal gap reference interval. Therefore, reference intervals must be validated on appropriate patient populations. Two commonly used and easily performed formulae (in conventional and SI units) are presented here:

Conventional Units

$$OSMc \ (mOsm/kg) = 2 \ Na \ (mmol/L) \\ + \ glucose \ (mg/dL)/18 \\ + \ urea \ (mg/dL)/2.8$$

$$OSMc \ (mOsm/kg) = 1.86 \ Na \ (mmol/L) \\ + \ glucose \ (mg/dL)/18 \\ + \ urea \ (mg/dL)/2.8 + 9$$

SI Units

$$OSMc \ (mOsm/kg) = 2 \ Na \ (mmol/L) \\ + \ glucose \ (mmol/L) \\ + \ urea \ (mmol/L)$$

$$OSMc \ (mOsm/kg) = 1.86 \ Na \ (mmol/L) \\ + \ glucose \ (mmol/L) \\ + \ urea \ (mmol/L) + 9$$

The difference between the actual osmolality (OSMm), measured by freezing-point depression, and the calculated osmolality (OSMc) is referred to as delta-osmolality, or the osmolal gap (OSMg).

$$OSMg = OSMm - OSMc$$

Elevated OSMg implies the presence of unmeasured osmotically active substances. Compounds that increase serum osmolality when present in significant concentrations include volatile alcohols such as ethanol, methanol, isopropanol, acetone, and ethylene glycol. The calculation of OSMg is commonly used as a screen. However, it is important to remember that volatile alcohols are not detected when osmolality is measured with a vapor pressure osmometer. Therefore, for the purpose of determining the OSMg, only osmolality measurements based on freezing-point depression are acceptable.

It would be expected that for each 100 mg/dL (21.7 mmol/L) of ethanol (molecular weight = 46.068 g/mol) in serum it should result in an approximate increase of 21.7 mOsm/kg, however, this is not found to be the case. It has been observed that ethanol does not follow a completely predictable relationship with OSMg. In severe ethanol intoxication, OSMg increases disproportionately with increasing ethanol concentration making it appear that something is present besides the alcohol.

What constitutes a normal osmolal gap is widely debated. Large variability is seen in the normal population. But it is generally accepted that a significant residual osmolal gap (>10 mOsm/kg) after correction for ethanol, suggests the possible presence of one of the other volatile alcohols. This information, in conjunction with the presence or absence of metabolic acidosis or serum acetone, is helpful to the clinician when specific measurements of alcohols other than ethanol are not available on an emergency basis (Table 31.2). It must be realized that ketones and other substances administered to patients such as polyethylene glycol, mannitol (osmotic diuretic), and propylene glycol (solvent for diazepam and phenytoin) may increase serum osmolality.

## Immunoassay

Different types of immunoassays are useful in screening specimens for drugs. In some cases, these assays are relatively specific for a single drug (LSD), but others can detect several drugs within a class (e.g., opiates). The detection limit for various members of a class of drugs or the degree of cross-reactivity for similar drugs varies, and each manufacturer of immunoassay reagents should be consulted for specific information. These assays are easy to perform; many are available for use on automated instrumentation and may be able to provide "semiquantitative" results. For the vast majority of substances of use/misuse, immunoassays are the methods of choice for rapid initial screening. However, for more comprehensive drug screening, chromatographic procedures complement immunoassays.

## Point of Care

Numerous POC drug test devices for urine (and oral fluid) are designed for easy, rugged, and portable use by nontechnical personnel. Although these devices are relatively simple to use, proper training of non-laboratory users is important for optimal performance. These non-instrument-based immunoassay test devices are designed for use at the site of collection. Results are available within minutes and are variously configured; they can detect only one drug or many drugs simultaneously. A more detailed description of these methods is found in the package insert for each specific test kit.

## Gas Chromatography

Gas chromatography (GC) is relatively rapid, capable of resolving a broad spectrum of drugs, and widely used for qualitative and quantitative drug analysis. Common detectors for drug detection by GC are flame ionization and alkali flame ionization (nitrogen phosphorus) detectors. A GC coupled to a mass spectrometer (GC-MS) provides an analytical system with the greatest accuracy of identification. Numerous methods for general drug screening by GC-MS spectrometry have been published.

## High-Performance Liquid Chromatography

The resolving power of high-performance liquid chromatography (HPLC) in separating chemical constituents has been applied to the complex challenge of comprehensive drug

| TABLE 31.2 | Laboratory Findings Characteristic of Ingestion of Alcohols | | | |
|---|---|---|---|---|
| Alcohol | Serum Osmolal Gap | Anion Gap Metabolic Acidosis | Serum Acetone | Urine Oxalate |
| Ethanol | + | − | − | − |
| Methanol | + | + | − | − |
| Isopropanol | + | − | + | − |
| Ethylene glycol | + | + | − | + |

screening in biological fluids. Advantages of HPLC over GC include its usefulness in analyzing polar compounds without derivatization (e.g., morphine, benzoylecgonine) and thermally labile drugs (e.g., chlordiazepoxide). The advent of diode array detectors that provide a spectral scan of compounds as they elute from the column has greatly increased the discriminatory power of this technique. Analytical systems based on coupling of liquid chromatography (LC) with mass spectrometry (MS) (LC-MS or LC-MS/MS) significantly improve resolution of drugs from complex matrices.

# PHARMACOLOGY AND ANALYSIS OF SPECIFIC DRUGS AND TOXIC AGENTS

The toxic consequences of several drugs and toxins are individually discussed in this section. They have been grouped into the following categories: agents that cause cellular hypoxia, alcohols, analgesics (nonprescription), agents related to anticholinergic and cholinergic toxidrome, substances of use/misuse, and substances used in drug-facilitated crimes.

# AGENTS THAT CAUSE CELLULAR HYPOXIA

Carbon monoxide and methemoglobin-forming agents interfere with oxygen transport, resulting in cellular hypoxia. Cyanide interferes with oxygen use and therefore causes an apparent cellular hypoxia.

## Carbon Monoxide

Carbon monoxide (CO) is a colorless, odorless, tasteless gas that is a product of incomplete combustion of carbonaceous material. Small amounts of CO are produced endogenously in the metabolic conversion of heme to biliverdin.

When inhaled, CO combines tightly with the heme iron ($Fe^{2+}$) of hemoglobin to form carboxyhemoglobin. The binding affinity of hemoglobin for CO is about 250 times greater than that for oxygen. Moreover, the binding of CO to a hemoglobin subunit increases the oxygen affinity for the remaining subunits in the hemoglobin tetramer. Thus, at a given tissue $PO_2$ value, less oxygen dissociates from hemoglobin when CO is also bound, shifting the hemoglobin-oxygen dissociation curve to the left. Consequently, CO not only decreases the oxygen content of blood, but it also decreases oxygen availability to tissue. This produces a greater degree of tissue hypoxia than would result from an equivalent reduction in oxyhemoglobin due to hypoxia alone. CO may also bind to other heme proteins, such as myoglobin and mitochondrial cytochrome oxidase $a3$; this may limit oxygen use when tissue $PO_2$ is very low.

Treatment for CO poisoning involves removal of the individual from the contaminated area and administration of oxygen. The half-life ($t_{1/2}$) of carboxyhemoglobin in the body is variable. Low carboxyhemoglobin concentrations relative to the severity of poisoning may be observed if the patient was removed from the CO-contaminated environment several hours before blood sampling.

## Analytical Methods

CO may be released from hemoglobin and then measured by GC, or it may be determined indirectly as carboxyhemoglobin by spectrophotometry. GC methods are accurate and precise even for very low concentrations of CO. Spectrophotometric methods are rapid, convenient, accurate, and precise, except at very low concentrations of carboxyhemoglobin (<3%).

GC methods measure the CO content of blood and are considered to be reference procedures. When blood is treated with potassium ferricyanide, carboxyhemoglobin is converted to methemoglobin, and CO is released into the gas phase. Measurement of the released CO may be performed by GC using various methods and detectors. CO binding capacity is determined after an aliquot of the blood specimen is treated with CO to saturate the hemoglobin. The results are then expressed as percentage of carboxyhemoglobin:

$$\% \ HbCO = \frac{CO_{content}}{CO_{capacity}} \times 100$$

Spectrophotometric methods rely on the characteristic spectral absorption properties of carboxyhemoglobin. The most common are based on automated, multi-wavelength measurements of several hemoglobin species, using a co-oximeter.

Spectrophotometric methods generally compare favorably with GC procedures at carboxyhemoglobin concentrations greater than 2% to 3%, but their precision is poor below these concentrations. Therefore, they are sufficiently accurate and precise for measurement of CO after exogenous exposure, but they are too insensitive to detect the increased endogenous production of CO that occurs in hemolytic anemia.

Fetal hemoglobin and adult hemoglobin differ slightly in their spectral properties. Consequently, falsely high carboxyhemoglobin values of 4% to 7% may occur when blood from neonates is measured by some spectrophotometric methods by using fewer wavelengths. Moreover, erroneous results may occur with lipemic and icteric specimens and in the presence of methylene blue (see section below).

## Methemoglobin-Forming Agents

The heme iron in hemoglobin is normally present in the ferrous state ($Fe^{2+}$). When oxidized to the ferric state ($Fe^{3+}$), methemoglobin is formed, and this form of hemoglobin cannot bind oxygen. Congenital methemoglobinemia may result from a deficiency of NADH-methemoglobin reductase or, more rarely, from hemoglobin variants (hemoglobin M) in which heme iron is both more susceptible to oxidation and more resistant to reduction by the methemoglobin reductase system.

An acquired (toxic) methemoglobinemia may be caused by various drugs and chemicals (Table 31.3). The normal percentage of methemoglobin is less than 1.5% of total hemoglobin. All symptoms associated with methemoglobinemia are consequences of hypoxia associated both with diminished $O_2$ content of blood and with decreased $O_2$ dissociation from

## TABLE 31.3   Examples of Acquired Causes of Methemoglobinemia

| Local Anesthetics | Nitrites and Nitrates | Miscellaneous |
|---|---|---|
| Benzocaine | Ammonium nitrate | Aminophenol |
| Lidocaine | Amyl nitrite | Aniline, *p*-chloroaniline |
| Prilocaine | Butyl nitrite | Bromates |
| | Isobutyl nitrite | Chlorates |
| **Antimicrobials** | Potassium nitrate | 4-Dimethyl-amino-phenolate (4-DMAP) |
| Chloroquine | Sodium nitrate | Metoclopramide |
| Dapsone | | Nitrobenzene |
| Primaquine | **Nitrogen Oxides** | Nitroethane |
| Sulfonamides | Nitric oxide | Nitroglycerin |
| Trimethoprim | Nitrogen dioxide | Phenazopyridine |
| | | Potassium permanganate |
| **Analgesics** | | Propanil |
| Phenazopyridine | | |
| Phenacetin | | |

hemoglobin species. The $PO_2$ is normal in these patients, and therefore so is the calculated hemoglobin oxygen saturation. Thus, a normal $PO_2$ in a cyanotic patient is a significant indication of the possible presence of methemoglobinemia, therefore, measurement of methemoglobin is important in these cases. Specific therapy for toxic methemoglobinemia involves the administration of methylene blue. Methylene blue and sulfhemoglobin cause spectral interference in the measurement of methemoglobin with some co-oximeters but not with the Evelyn-Malloy method.

### Analytical Methods

Methemoglobin may be measured using the manual spectrophotometric method of Evelyn and Malloy or by performing automated multi-wavelength measurements with a co-oximeter. Methemoglobin interferes with the noninvasive pulse oximetry method, measuring the absorbance of light at 660 nm (oxyhemoglobin) and 940 nm (deoxyhemoglobin). Because methemoglobin is not stable at room temperature, specimens should be kept on ice or refrigerated, but not frozen. The stability of methemoglobin at 4°C has not been well studied. Some sources report significant decreases in methemoglobin concentration after 4 to 8 hours, whereas others describe little or no change after 24 hours. Freezing results in an increase in methemoglobin concentration.

### Cyanide

Cyanide consists of one atom of carbon triple-bonded to one atom of nitrogen (C≡N). Inorganic cyanides (also known as *cyanide salts*) contain cyanide in anion form (CN⁻) and are used in numerous industries. Organic compounds that have a cyano group bonded to an alkyl residue are called *nitriles*. Iatrogenic cyanide poisoning may occur during use of nitroprusside.

Cyanide in serum readily crosses all biological membranes and avidly binds to heme iron ($Fe^{3+}$) in the cytochrome *oxidase-$a_3$* complex within mitochondria. When bound to cytochrome oxidase-$a_3$, cyanide is a competitive inhibitor that causes decoupling of oxidative phosphorylation. Patients exposed to toxic concentrations of cyanide exhibit a wide variety of clinical effects depending on the poisoning severity. Hydroxycobalamin or the cyanide antidote kit should be administered as soon as cyanide poisoning is suspected.

### Analytical Methods

After microdiffusion, whole blood CN⁻ is measured by spectrophotometry or by headspace GC.

## ALCOHOLS OF TOXICOLOGICAL INTEREST

Several alcohols are toxic and medically important; they include ethanol, methanol, isopropanol, acetone (also a metabolite of isopropanol), and ethylene glycol.

### Ethanol

Ethanol is a widely available and often used and misused chemical substance. Consequently, measurement of ethanol is one of the more frequently performed tests in the toxicology laboratory. The principal pharmacological action of ethanol involves central nervous system (CNS) depression, and effects vary depending on the blood ethanol concentration and an individual's tolerance (Table 31.4). A blood alcohol concentration of 80 mg/dL (0.08 g/100 mL or 0.08% w/v, 17.4 mmol/L) has been established as the *per se* limit for operation of a motor vehicle in many states in the USA, but in some states it is 50 mg/dL.

When consumed with other CNS depressant drugs, ethanol exerts a potentiation or synergistic depressant effect. This occurs at relatively low alcohol concentrations, and numerous deaths have resulted from combined ethanol and drug or other substance ingestion. Ethanol is also a teratogen, and alcohol consumption during pregnancy can result in a newborn with fetal alcohol spectrum disorder (FASD). FASD is an umbrella term that describes the variety of effects that can occur in an individual whose mother consumed alcohol during pregnancy (http://www.nofas.org; last accessed March 9, 2022). These effects may include physical, mental, behavioral, and/or learning disabilities with possible lifelong implications and are 100% preventable when a woman completely abstains from alcohol during her pregnancy.

## TABLE 31.4    Stages of Acute Alcoholic Influence/Intoxication

| Blood Alcohol Concentration (%w/v) | Influence | Clinical Signs/Symptoms |
|---|---|---|
| 0.01–0.05 | Subclinical | Influence/effects not apparent or obvious |
| | | Behavior appears normal |
| | | Impairment detectable by special tests |
| | | May have loss of small-muscle control (e.g., focusing your eyes) |
| | | Some loss of judgment |
| 0.03–0.12 | Euphoria | Mild euphoria |
| | | Increased sociability, talkativeness, self-confidence |
| | | Decreased inhibitions |
| | | Muscle coordination becomes impaired (e.g., balance, speech, vision, reaction time, and hearing) |
| | | Slowed information processing |
| | | Impairment of perception and memory |
| 0.09–0.25 | Excitement | Emotional instability; loss of critical judgment comprehension |
| | | Decreased sensory response; increased reaction time |
| | | Reduced visual acuity, peripheral vision, and glare recovery |
| | | Sensorimotor incoordination; impaired balance |
| | | Drowsiness |
| 0.18–0.30 | Confusion | Disorientation, mental confusion; dizziness |
| | | Exaggerated emotional states (fear, rage, grief, etc.) |
| | | Disturbances of vision (diplopia, etc.) and of perception of color, form, motion, dimensions |
| | | Increased pain threshold |
| | | Ataxia; dysarthria, apathy, lethargy |
| 0.25–0.40 | Stupor | General inertia; approaching loss of motor functions |
| | | Markedly decreased response to stimuli |
| | | Marked muscular incoordination; inability to stand or walk |
| | | Vomiting; incontinence of urine and feces |
| | | Impaired consciousness; sleep or stupor |
| 0.35–0.50 | Coma | Unconsciousness; coma; anesthesia |
| | | Depressed or absent reflexes |
| | | Subnormal temperature |
| | | Impairment of circulation and respiration |
| | | Possible death |
| 0.45 + | Death | Possible death from respiratory arrest |

Modified from Dubowski KM. Alcohol determination in the clinical laboratory. *Am J Clin Pathol*. 1980;74:747–504.

Ethanol is metabolized principally by liver alcohol dehydrogenase (ADH) to acetaldehyde, which is subsequently oxidized to acetic acid by aldehyde dehydrogenase (Fig. 31.1). The rate of elimination of ethanol from blood approximates a zero-order process. This rate varies among individuals, averaging about 15 mg/dL/h for males and 18 mg/dL/h for females. At both low (<20 mg/dL) and high (>300 mg/dL) ethanol concentrations, elimination more closely resembles first-order kinetics. The elimination rate is also influenced by drinking practices (e.g., individuals who consume large amounts of ethanol have increased elimination rates caused by enzyme induction).

## Methanol

Methanol is used as a solvent in several commercial products, as a constituent in windshield wiper fluid, copy machine fluids, fuel additives (octane boosters), paint remover or thinner, antifreeze, canned heating sources, deicing fluid, shellacs, and varnishes.

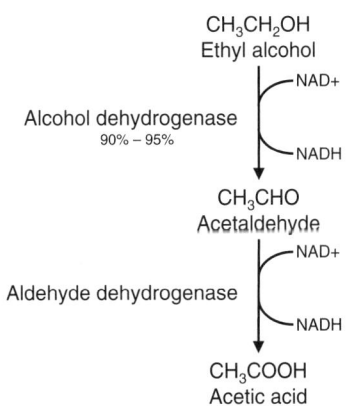

Fig. 31.1 Metabolism of ethanol.

Methanol is oxidized by liver ADH (at about one-tenth the rate of ethanol) to formaldehyde. Formaldehyde in turn is rapidly oxidized by aldehyde dehydrogenase to formic acid, which may cause serious acidosis and optic neuropathy, resulting in blindness or death. The mainstay of therapy for methanol toxicity includes the administration of fomepizole or ethanol as a competitive ADH inhibitor plus either folate or folinic acid, sodium bicarbonate, and hemodialysis when required.

## Isopropanol and Acetone

Isopropanol is readily available as a 70% aqueous solution for use as rubbing alcohol, but can also be found in cleaners, disinfectants, antifreezes, cosmetics, solvents, and inks. Isopropanol is rapidly metabolized by ADH to acetone, which is eliminated much more slowly. Therefore, concentrations of acetone in serum often exceed those of isopropanol during the elimination phase after isopropanol ingestion. Acetone has CNS depressant activity similar to that of ethanol, and because of its longer half-life, it may prolong the apparent CNS effects of isopropanol. Supportive care is the mainstay of treatment, with dialysis only in severe intoxication.

## Ethylene Glycol

Ethylene glycol is present in antifreeze products, deicing products, detergents, paints, and cosmetics. Ethylene glycol itself is relatively nontoxic; however, metabolism of ethylene glycol by ADH results in the formation of numerous acid metabolites, including oxalic acid and glycolic acid, which are responsible for much of the toxicity of ethylene glycol. It is difficult to define a serum ethylene glycol concentration associated with a high probability of death, and the determination of ethylene glycol and glycolic acid may provide useful information in cases of ethylene glycol ingestion. The mainstay of therapy for ethylene glycol toxicity includes administration of fomepizole or ethanol as a competitive ADH inhibitor, and sodium bicarbonate and hemodialysis when required.

## Analysis of Ethanol

### Serum/Plasma and Blood Ethanol

Serum, plasma, and whole blood are suitable clinical specimens for the determination of ethanol. Alcohol distributes into the aqueous compartments of blood; because the water content of serum is greater than that of whole blood, higher alcohol concentrations are obtained with serum as compared with whole blood. Experimentally, the serum-to-whole blood ethanol ratio is 1.18 (1.10 to 1.35) and varies slightly with hematocrit. Therefore, laboratories that perform alcohol determinations should make clear the choice of specimen.

Because of the volatile nature of alcohols, specimens should be kept capped to avoid evaporative loss. Blood may be stored, when properly sealed, for 14 days at room temperature or refrigerated at 4°C, with sodium fluoride/potassium oxalate (gray top) preservative.

To measure ethanol in serum/plasma, enzymatic analysis is the method of choice for many laboratories. In this method, ADH catalyzes the oxidation of ethanol to acetaldehyde and reduction of $NAD^+$ to NADH. With this reaction, the formation of NADH, measured at 340 nm, is detected and is proportional to the amount of ethanol in the specimen:

$$Ethanol + NAD \xrightarrow{ADH} Acetaldehyde + NADH$$

The current methods are very specific for ethanol, with cross-reactivity by isopropanol, acetone, methanol, and ethylene glycol typically less than 1%. However, the recommendation remains that the venipuncture site be cleansed with an alcohol-free disinfectant, such as aqueous benzalkonium chloride.

Spuriously increased results for ethanol have been described in the presence of both high concentrations of lactate dehydrogenase (LDH) and lactate. However, not all ethanol assays are known to have this interference. It is recognized that the lactate and LDH must hit some critical concentration for the interference to occur with those affected assays. Theoretically, other dehydrogenases and substrates may cause similar interferences.

### Urine Ethanol

Urine has been used as an alternative, less invasive specimen for determination of alcohol use. During the postabsorptive phase that follows alcohol ingestion, the concentration of alcohol in urine is roughly 1.3 times that in blood. However, the use of urine alcohol measurements to estimate blood concentrations is discouraged because the ratio is highly variable, and, perhaps more important, because the urine alcohol concentration may better reflect an average of the blood alcohol concentration during the period in which urine is collected in the bladder.

### Analysis of Volatile Alcohols

Flame ionization GC remains the most common method of detection and quantitation of volatile alcohols in biological samples. Not only does it distinguish between ethanol, methanol, isopropanol, and acetone, it has the capability to measure concentrations as low as 10 mg/dL (0.01%).

### Other Ethanol Markers

Ethyl glucuronide (EtG), ethyl sulfate (EtS), and phosphatidylethanols (PEth) are markers of ethanol consumption. EtG and EtS are phase II metabolites of ethanol. EtG is formed through the UDP-glucuronosyltransferase catalyzed conjugation of ethanol with glucuronic acid. EtS is formed directly by the conjugation of ethanol with a sulfate group.

EtG and EtS can be used as markers of recent ethanol intake in a variety of clinical and legal settings. It is recommended to monitor both EtG and EtS in urine.

PEth are a group of phospholipids with a common phosphoethanol head group with two fatty acid chains which differ in chain length and degree of unsaturation. PEth can be detected in blood for as long as 3 weeks after a few days of moderately heavy drinking (about four drinks per day). Therefore, PEth may be utilized in conjunction with EtG and EtS to discriminate incidental ethanol exposure from moderate to heavy "binge" alcohol drinking.

## ANALGESICS (NONPRESCRIPTION)

### Acetaminophen

Acetaminophen has analgesic and antipyretic actions. In normal doses, acetaminophen is safe and effective, but may cause severe hepatic toxicity when consumed in overdose quantities. Initial clinical findings in acetaminophen toxicity are relatively mild and nonspecific and include nausea, vomiting, and abdominal discomfort. These conditions are not predictive of impending hepatic necrosis. The measurement of serum acetaminophen concentration becomes paramount for proper assessment of the severity of overdose and for appropriate decision making for antidotal therapy with N-acetylcysteine (NAC) using the Rumack-Matthew nomogram (1975).

Acetaminophen is normally metabolized in the liver to glucuronide (52% to 57%) and sulfate (30% to 44%) conjugates and less than 5% of acetaminophen is excreted unchanged. A minor fraction is oxidized by a cytochrome P450 pathway, primarily CYP2E1, forming a highly reactive intermediate, N-acetyl-p-benzoquinone imine (NAPQI) which normally undergoes electrophilic conjugation with glutathione. However, in acetaminophen overdose, the normal conjugations pathway becomes saturated; consequently, a greater portion is metabolized by the CYP2E1 pathway resulting in increased NAPQI. When the tissue stores of glutathione become depleted, NAPQI reacts with cellular molecules leading to hepatic necrosis. Specific therapy for acetaminophen overdose is administration of NAC, which acts as a glutathione substitute. Antidotal therapy with NAC is most effective when administered before hepatic injury occurs, as signified by elevation of activities of aspartate transaminase (AST) and alanine transaminase (ALT).

Many spectrophotometric methods are available for determination of acetaminophen. In general, these methods are simple and relatively easy to perform but are subject to various interferences such as bilirubin or bilirubin byproducts absorbing at similar wavelengths. Some methods also measure the nontoxic metabolites and parent acetaminophen, and thus may produce misleading results. Therefore, only methods specific for parent acetaminophen should be used. Immunoassays are widely used clinically for this purpose, as they are rapid, easily performed, and accurate. A qualitative, one-step lateral flow immunoassay (cutoff of 25 μg/mL) may be suitable for point-of-care application, yet it has a low positive predictive value.

## Salicylate

Acetylsalicylic acid (aspirin) has analgesic, antipyretic, and anti-inflammatory properties. Salicylates directly stimulate the central respiratory center and thereby cause hyperventilation and respiratory alkalosis. Additionally, salicylates cause uncoupling of oxidative phosphorylation. As a result, heat production (hyperthermia), oxygen consumption, and metabolic rate may be increased. Salicylates also enhance anaerobic glycolysis but inhibit the Krebs cycle and transaminase enzymes, which leads to accumulation of organic acids and thus to metabolic acidosis.

Following acute salicylate overdose, patients initially may be asymptomatic, especially if that product is enteric coated. Patients may develop nausea, vomiting, abdominal pain, tinnitus, tachypnea, oliguria, and altered mental status ranging from agitation to lethargy to coma. Individuals with chronic intoxication present in a similar fashion as those with acute

exposures, yet such exposures typically are more insidious and therefore are often misdiagnosed.

Use of salicylate concentrations to guide management must be done cautiously and only in conjunction with careful evaluation of a patient's clinical status. The absorptive phase of salicylates is often unpredictable (delayed or erratic) because of bezoar formation, enteric-coated product, gastric outlet obstruction, or pylorospasm. Therefore, a specimen drawn soon after the original ingestion may not be reflective of the potential peak concentration; consequently, monitoring of serial concentrations can be very useful. Because products containing salicylates are readily available, the clinical effects of salicylate toxicity are nonspecific, and lack of metabolic acidosis does not rule out the potential for salicylate toxicity, clinicians should have a low threshold for obtaining serum salicylate concentrations.

Classic methods for measurement of salicylate in serum are based on the method of Trinder. Despite the limitations of these methods, they continue to be used to assess salicylate overdose. The Trinder method results agree very closely with those of a reference HPLC procedure. A qualitative, one-step lateral flow immunoassay (cutoff of 100 μg/mL) is commercially available for point-of-care application but has a low positive predictive value (0.47). GC and LC methods are the most specific methods for salicylate, but their general availability, especially for emergency use, is limited and probably is not necessary.

## AGENTS RELATED TO ANTICHOLINERGIC TOXIDROME

Numerous agents can induce an anticholinergic toxidrome (e.g., tricyclic antidepressants, antihistamines). These agents have divergent therapeutic applications, but in overdose often share similar anticholinergic toxidrome.

### Tricyclic Antidepressants and Related Drugs

Tricyclic antidepressants (TCAs) are so named because of their three-ring structure. They represent a class of drugs prescribed for the treatment of depression and neuropathic pain. The TCAs have been largely supplanted by the newer, less toxic selective serotonin reuptake inhibitors (SSRIs) and other atypical agents for the treatment of depression. The N-demethylated metabolites of several TCAs are pharmacologically active and contribute variably to overall pharmacodynamic activity (Table 31.5).

The therapeutic mechanism of TCAs is the blockade of neuronal reuptake of serotonin and/or norepinephrine. However, TCAs have many other pharmacological actions that contribute to adverse effects at both therapeutic and toxic doses. Cardiovascular effects are the most serious manifestation of TCA overdose, accounting for the majority of fatalities.

### Analytical Methods

TCAs are measured by chromatographic methods or by immunoassay. Immunoassays are rapid and relatively easy to perform but may be subject to interference by other drugs

## TABLE 31.5  Examples of Tricyclic Antidepressants and Their Active Metabolites

| Parent Drug | Active Metabolite(s) |
| --- | --- |
| Amitriptyline | Nortriptyline |
| Nortriptyline | |
| Imipramine | Desipramine |
| Desipramine | |
| Trimipramine | |
| Doxepin | N-desmethyldoxepin (nordoxepin) |
| Clomipramine | Desmethylclomipramine |

## TABLE 31.6  Examples of Classical and Atypical Antipsychotics

| Antipsychotics | Examples |
| --- | --- |
| **Classical Antipsychotics** | |
| Phenothiazines | Chlorpromazine |
| | Promethazine |
| | Prochlorperazine |
| | Perphenazine |
| | Fluphenazine |
| | Thioridazine |
| | Mesoridazine |
| | Trifluoperazine |
| Thioxanthenes | Flupenthixol |
| | Zuclopenthixol |
| Dibenzoxazepines | Loxapine |
| Dihydroindolones | Molindone |
| Butyrophenones | Droperidol |
| | Haloperidol |
| Diphenylbutylpiperidines | Pimozide |
| Benzamides | Sulpiride |
| **Atypical Antipsychotics** | |
| Dibenzodiazepines | Clozapine |
| | Olanzapine |
| Dibenzothiazepines | Quetiapine |
| Benzisoxazoles | Risperidone |
| Benzisothiazols | Ziprasidone |

and they cannot necessarily be used to identify which TCA is being quantitated. In cases of overdose, qualitative identification (serum or urine) is sufficient because the severity of intoxication is more reliably indicated by an increase in the QRS interval on an ECG than by the serum concentration.

## Antipsychotic Drugs

The antipsychotic drugs are generally used for primary psychiatric disorders; however, certain members of this group are used for other indications. Antipsychotic compounds are traditionally divided and subdivided according to their chemical structure (Table 31.6).

The principal manifestations of phenothiazine toxicity involve the CNS and the cardiovascular system. The presentation for most of these drugs is related to their mechanisms of action, which include dopamine blockade (CNS depression), $\alpha_1$-blockade (hypotension and miosis), anticholinergic, and K-efflux blockade (QT prolongation). Toxicity is strongly correlated with peak serum concentrations.

Neuroleptics are measured by chromatographic methods and by immunoassay.

## Antihistamines

Antihistamines are medications that are popular over the counter (OTC) treatments of allergic reactions and as sleep aids. Histamine is released from mast cells and plays an important physiological role in immediate hypersensitivity and allergic responses. Histamine functions as a neurotransmitter in the CNS and stimulates gastric acid secretion. Currently available antihistamine drugs clinically antagonize H1 and H2 histamine receptors. The principal H2 receptor response is stimulation of gastric acid secretion, whereas other actions of histamine such as smooth muscle contraction, vasodilation, increased capillary permeability, pain, and itching are primarily mediated by H1 receptors.

First-generation lipophilic antihistamines (e.g., diphenhydramine) bind H1 receptors, exhibit peripheral and CNS effects, and bind to muscarinic receptors, resulting in anticholinergic activity. Second-generation antihistamines (e.g., fexofenadine [Allegra]) are highly specific for peripheral H1 receptors and do not penetrate the CNS. Therefore, second-generation H1 receptor antagonists display minimal sedative and anticholinergic effects. Individuals overdosed with first-generation H1 antihistamines present clinically with CNS depression or stimulation and peripheral anticholinergic effects.

Commonly available antihistamines are detected using GC-MS/MS and LC-MS/MS. However, the clinical necessity of quantitative serum antihistamine concentrations is questionable, as poor correlation has been noted among patient's age, dose, blood concentration, clinical effects, and death.

Although detection of antihistamines is not typically clinically relevant for the acutely toxic patient, it is important to note that very high concentrations of first-generation antihistamines, such as promethazine and diphenhydramine, have been documented to cross-react with urine substances of use/misuse immuno-methods used for screening purposes. Therefore, physicians and medical review officers (MROs) should be aware of potential false-positive results from on-site drug testing devices, as well as immuno-screening.

## Antimuscarinic Agents

Numerous pharmaceutical agents and several plant and mushroom species contain antimuscarinic compounds (e.g., atropine, scopolamine) that cause anticholinergic symptoms when ingested. Testing for atropine and scopolamine is performed by LC-MS methods.

## AGENTS RELATED TO CHOLINERGIC TOXIDROME

Acetylcholine is an essential neurotransmitter that affects parasympathetic synapses (autonomic and CNSs), sympathetic preganglionic synapses, and the neuromuscular junction (see also prior section, "Toxic Syndromes"). The duration of acetylcholine's action is controlled by acetylcholinesterase (AChE) and plasma/serum cholinesterase (pseudocholinesterase (PChE) or butyrylcholinesterase). Acetylcholinesterase is found in erythrocytes, in the lungs, spleen, in nerve endings, and in the gray matter of the brain. It is responsible for the hydrolysis of acetylcholine released at the nerve endings to mediate transmission of the neural impulse across the synapse. PChE is found in the plasma, the liver, the pancreas, the heart, and in the white matter of the brain. Agents inducing a cholinergic toxidrome are diverse and act by either inactivation of cholinesterase enzymes or direct stimulation of acetylcholine receptors.

## Organophosphate and Carbamate Compounds

Organophosphate compounds irreversibly inactivate AChE by phosphorylating the serine hydroxyl group at the active site of the cholinesterase catalytic triad (Ser-Glu-His). Carbamates exert their effect through carbamylation rather than phosphorylation of the serine hydroxyl group. In contrast to the phosphoryl-serine bond, the carbamyl-serine bond undergoes spontaneous hydrolysis, and therefore regeneration of enzyme activity occurs.

The clinical features of organophosphate poisoning result from overstimulation of muscarinic and nicotinic receptors. Activation of muscarinic receptors causes signs and symptoms described by the mnemonics SLUDGE (Salivation, Lacrimation, Urination, Defecation, GI distress, Emesis) or DUMBBELS (Diarrhea, Urination, Miosis, Bradycardia, and Bronchorrhea-bronchoconstriction, Emesis, Lacrimation, Sweating-salivation). Stimulation of nicotinic receptors at the neuromuscular junction causes muscle fasciculations, cramping, weakness, and respiratory muscle paralysis. Stimulation of nicotinic receptors at sympathetic ganglia results in hypertension, tachycardia, pallor, and mydriasis. Thus, the patient's ultimate presenting signs and symptoms depend on the balance of muscarinic and nicotinic receptor activation.

Specific therapy for organophosphate and carbamate insecticide poisoning includes administration of atropine, to block the muscarinic (but not the nicotinic) actions of acetylcholine, and pralidoxime, to reactivate cholinesterase in organophosphate poisoning. Treatment requires immediate attention and should not rely on confirmatory testing. Therefore, cholinesterase activity is often monitored by clinicians following acute intentional and accidental exposure, and to determine response to therapy.

AChE activity present at nerve junctions is similar to that present in red blood cells and is a useful index of neurotoxicity. PChE is also inhibited by these insecticides; activity declines then return to normal more rapidly than AChE and is readily measured in clinical laboratories without isolation of red blood cells. However, AChE is more sensitive than PChE activity and often is used to confirm exposure and to predict enzyme reactivation during treatment. Both AChE and PChE enzyme activities are typically monitored using spectrophotometric methods adapted on common analyzers.

In acute poisoning, symptoms generally begin when cholinesterase activity is inhibited by about 50% of the lower limits of the reference interval, and this degree of inhibition is of diagnostic value. However, the degree of cholinesterase inhibition generally does not correlate well with the clinical severity of poisoning. Interpretation of test results is made more difficult by considerable individual variability of reference activities.

## SUBSTANCES OF USE/MISUSE

Many definitions exist for the term "substances of use/misuse." For this chapter, this term is defined as "a drug that is repeatedly and deliberately used in a way other than prescribed or socially sanctioned (i.e., a drug that is taken for nonmedicinal reasons)."

Substances of use/misuse are widespread in society, and public awareness has been heightened as to their impact on public safety and on lost productivity in industry. To resolve these issues, governmental, industrial, educational, and sports agencies increasingly require drug testing of prospective and existing employees, students, and participants in professional and amateur athletics. Moreover, substance use/misuse during pregnancy is a matter of concern, both medically and socially. Testing for substances of use/misuse may be a medical requirement for organ transplantation candidates, pain management clinics, substances of use/misuse treatment programs, and psychiatric programs. Drug testing for these purposes represents a significant activity for toxicology laboratories.

Testing for substances of use/misuse usually involves testing a single urine specimen for various drugs. It should be noted, however, that testing of a single random urine drug specimen detects only recent substance use/misuse, and it does not differentiate casual use from chronic substance use/misuse. The latter requires sequential drug testing and clinical evaluation. Moreover, urine drug testing (UDT) alone cannot determine the degree of impairment, the dose of drug taken, or the exact time of use. Because of these and other limitations of testing for drugs in urine, integrating the use of alternate biological specimens for drug testing is a matter of growing interest.

Initial screening tests for the previously listed drugs are typically immunoassays. These assays are calibrated at established cutoff concentrations. Specimens yielding responses greater than the cutoff (threshold) value are considered "presumptive positive," whereas values below the cutoff are considered negative. Immunoassays may demonstrate limited and variable specificity within certain drug classes. Similar drugs may result in a positive test, for example, pseudoephedrine, present in cold medications, may produce a positive response in immunoassays designed to detect amphetamine and methamphetamine. Therefore, it is imperative that positive screening tests be confirmed by an alternate, more definitive test. The most widely accepted methods for confirmatory testing are GC-MS or LC-MS/MS.

In the following sections, the pharmacological and analytical aspects of commonly measured drugs will be discussed.

## Amphetamine Type Stimulants

Several stimulants and hallucinogens chemically related to phenylethylamine are referred to collectively as amphetamine-type stimulants (ATSs). They are considered to be symphomimetic drugs, as they mimic or enhance endogenous transmitters in the sympathetic nervous system.

Amphetamine and methamphetamine are CNS stimulant drugs that have limited legitimate pharmacologic use, including narcolepsy, obesity, and attention-deficit hyperactivity disorders (ADHDs). They produce an initial euphoria and have a high misuse potential. These drugs have a stimulating effect on both the central and peripheral nervous systems. In the brain, a primary action is to increase the concentrations of extracellular monoamine neurotransmitters (dopamine, serotonin, norepinephrine).

Amphetamine and methamphetamine increase blood pressure, heart rate, body temperature, and motor activity, relax bronchial muscle, and depress the appetite. Misuse of these substances may lead to strong psychological dependence, marked tolerance, and mild physical dependence associated with tachycardia, increased blood pressure, restlessness, irritability, insomnia, personality changes, and a severe form of chronic intoxication psychosis similar to schizophrenia. These unpleasant responses reinforce repetitive use of the drugs to maintain the "high." Tolerance and psychological dependence develop with repeated use of amphetamines. Long-term effects may include depression and impaired memory and motor skills, probably caused by a decrease in dopamine transporters and by damage to dopaminergic and serotonergic neurons. Methamphetamine has greater CNS efficacy, most likely because of its greater ability to penetrate the CNS.

Many pharmaceutical amphetamine products are available with different proportions of isomers and biologic half-lives. The purity of dextro (d) versus levo (l) or ratio of isomers have different effects on dopaminergic and noradrenergic pathways to assist clinicians with treating attention deficit disorders and potentially reducing dependence and misuse.

In addition to hepatic metabolism, amphetamine is eliminated as an unchanged drug in urine. Elimination is dependent on urine pH. Therefore, elimination half-life (renal excretion and hepatic metabolism) varies with urine pH from 7 to 14 hours at acid pH to 18 to 34 hours at alkaline pH.

### Designer Amphetamines

The terms "designer drugs" and "club drugs" originated in the 1980s. These drugs include phenylethylamine, benzylpiperazine, phenylpiperazine, pyrrolidinophenone, and cathinone and derivatives (Table 31.7) and have gained popularity and notoriety among people who participate in all-night dance parties (raves) and who visit nightclubs. Most designer drugs produce feelings of euphoria and energy and a desire to socialize; they also promote social and physical interactions. They are used at these events to enhance energy for prolonged partying and/or dancing, and to distort or enhance visual and auditory sensations. The moniker "club drug" does not imply

that recreational use is restricted to this social environment. In this context, designer drugs mistakenly have the reputation of being safe; several experimental studies in rats and humans and epidemiologic studies have revealed risks to humans such as life-threatening serotonin syndrome, hepatotoxicity, neurotoxicity, psychopathology, and the misuse potential of such drugs.

### Ephedrine and Pseudoephedrine

Ephedrine and pseudoephedrine are diastereoisomers that possess two asymmetrical carbon atoms and exist as isomers that occur naturally in various plants of the *Ephedra* genus.

Ephedrine is both an α-adrenergic and a β-adrenergic receptor agonist. In addition, it enhances the release of norepinephrine from sympathetic neurons and is considered a mixed-acting sympathomimetic drug. Adverse effects such as hypertension, tremors, myocardial infarction, seizures, and stroke have resulted in fatalities. Because of this, the U.S. Food and Drug Administration (FDA) banned the sale of dietary supplements containing ephedra in 2004.

Pseudoephedrine is used primarily as a decongestant because of its vasoconstrictive properties (α-adrenergic action). Pseudoephedrine can be used as a precursor for the illicit synthesis of methamphetamine. Because of this, the quantity per purchase of products containing these drugs is now restricted in many places.

### Methylphenidate (Ritalin)

Methylphenidate is a psychostimulant with pharmacological properties similar to those of amphetamine. It is commonly used to treat ADHD and narcolepsy. It also exists as an isomer, as d-methylphenidate and as l-methylphenidate. The pharmacological actions of methylphenidate are almost solely performed by the D-isomer. Diversion and misuse of methylphenidate has been increasing among children and adults because of its stimulant and purported aphrodisiac properties. In overdose, the clinical effects of methylphenidate are similar to those of amphetamines.

### Analytical Methods

The initial screening test for amphetamines and related drugs is typically immunoassay. For confirmatory testing of a presumptive positive test, a quantitative drug measurement is performed using GC-MS or LC-MS/MS.

Most amphetamine immunoassays have been designed to detect amphetamine/methamphetamine; others have been designed to detect MDMA and MDA; and others to more broadly capture the ATS group, all with varying cross-reactivity. Few amphetamine immunoassays were suitable for detection of the designer amphetamine or methylphenidate, while some other chemically related compounds, such as pseudoephedrine, have been shown to produce positive results. Additionally, many psychotropic medications have been reported to interfere with immunoassays. Regarding methylphenidate, it should be noted that its detection by urine drug immunoassay is problematic, as it does not cross-react well with

## TABLE 31.7   Designer Drugs Related to Phenylethylamine, Benzylpiperazine, Phenylpiperazine, Pyrrolidinophenone, and Cathinone

| | |
|---|---|
| Phenylethylamines | 3,4-Methylenedioxymethamphetamine (MDMA; Ecstasy) |
| | 3,4-Methylenedioxyethylamphetamine (MDEA; "Eve") |
| | 3,4-Methylenedioxyamphetamine (MDA), which is also a metabolite of MDMA |
| | Paramethoxyamphetamine (PMA) |
| | Paramethoxymethamphetamine (PMMA) |
| | 2,5-Dimethoxy-4-methylamphetamine (DOM) |
| | 2,5-Dimethoxy-4-methylthioamphetamine (DOT) |
| | 4-Iodo-2,5-dimethoxyamphetamine (DOI) |
| | 2,5-Dimethoxy-4-bromo-amphetamine (DOB) |
| | 2,5-Dimethoxy-4-bromo-methamphetamine (MDOB) |
| | 3,4-(Methylenedioxyphenyl)-2-butanamine (BDB) |
| | N-Methyl-1-(3,4-methylenedioxy-phenyl)-2-butanamine (MBDB) |
| | 6-Chloro-3,4-methylenedioxymethamphetamine (Cl-MDMA) |
| | 3,4-Methylenedioxymethcathinone |
| | 4-Bromo-2,5-diemethoxy-phenylethylamine (2C-B) |
| | 2,5-Dimethoxy-4ethylthio-phenylethylamine (2C-T-2) |
| | 2,5-Dimethoxy-4 propylthio-phenylethylamine (2C-T-7) |
| Benzylpiperazines | 1-Benzylpiperazine (BZP) |
| | 1-(3,4-Methylenedioxybenzyl)-piperazine (MDBP) |
| Phenylpiperazines | 1-(3-Trifluoromethylphenyl)piperazine (TFMPP) |
| | 1-(3-Chlorophenyl)piperazine (mCPP) |
| | 1-(4-Methoxyphenyl)piperazine (MeOPP) |
| Pyrrolidinophenone | α-Pyrrolidinopropiophenone (PPP) |
| | 4-Methoxy-α-pyrrolidinopropiophenone (MOPPP) |
| | 3,4-Methylenedioxy-α-pyrrolidinopropiophenone (MDPPP) |
| | 4-Methyl-α-pyrrolidinopropiophenone (MPPP) |
| | 4-Methyl-α-pyrrolidinohexanophenone (MPHP) |
| Cathinones | Beta-keto analogs of methamphetamine |
| | • Methcathinone |
| | • Mephedrone (4-MMC) |
| | • Methylone (MDMC) |
| | • Butylone (bk-MBDB) |
| | • Ethylone |
| | • 4-Methylethcathinone (4-MEC) |
| | • 4-Fluoromethcathinone (3-FMC) |
| | • 3-Fluoromethcathinone (4-FMC) |
| | • Ethcathinone |
| | • Methedrone |
| | • Naphyrone |
| | α-Pyrrolidinophenone-derived |
| | • α-Pyrrolidinovalerophenone (α-PVP) |
| | • α-Pyrrolidinopropiophenone (PPP) |
| | • 4-Methoxy-α-pyrrolidinopropiophenone (MOPPP) |
| | • 3,4-Methylenedioxy-α-pyrrolidinopropiophenone (MDPPP) |
| | • 4-Methyl-α-pyrrolidinopropiophenone (MPPP) |
| | • 4-Methyl-α-pyrrolidinohexanophenone (MPHP) |
| | • 3,4-Methylenedioxypyrovalerone (MDPV) |

amphetamine antibodies, and is present in low concentration. Confirmation analysis using mass spectrometry methods are typically required.

All positive immunoassay results should be confirmed by a second independent method. However, if the other designer amphetamines are suspected, due to the poor cross-reactivity, a negative amphetamine immunoassay screen cannot rule out the presence of these drugs. Several GC- and LC-based methods for identification and quantitation of these drugs in biological samples have been described. **Chiral** identification can be used to differentiate "street" methamphetamine (a mixture of d and l) from the over-the-counter decongestant formulations (low dose l-methamphetamine). Clinically, this is frequently not necessary.

## TABLE 31.8  Prescription Drugs That Either Are or Are Metabolized to Amphetamine or Methamphetamine

| Drug | | Drugs Detected |
|---|---|---|
| Adderall | amphetamine | Amphetamine |
| Dexedrine | D-amphetamine | D-amphetamine |
| Deprenyl | selegiline | L-methamphetamine |
| | | L-amphetamine |
| Vyvanse | lisdexamfetamine | D-amphetamine |
| Didrex | benzphetamine | D-methamphetamine |
| | | D-amphetamine |

## TABLE 31.9  Half-life and Significant Active Metabolites of Select Barbiturates

| Drug | Active Metabolite |
|---|---|
| **Ultra-Short-Acting** | |
| Thiopental | Pentobarbital |
| Methohexital | |
| Thiamylal | |
| **Short-Acting and Intermediate-Acting** | |
| Pentobarbital | |
| Secobarbital | |
| Butalbital | |
| Aprobarbital | |
| Amobarbital | |
| Butabarbital | |
| **Long-Acting** | |
| Phenobarbital | |
| Mephobarbital | Phenobarbital |

Most published methods for analysis of members of the amphetamine class employ liquid-liquid extraction (LLE) or solid-phase extraction (SPE). ATSs are considered volatile and are lost during a dry-down or evaporation step during extraction. Also, because of their extreme volatility at the high temperatures encountered in GC-MS, and of lack of specificity of the mass spectrum, derivatization before analysis is frequently used. LC-MS and LC-MS/MS have gained in popularity. Other prescription drugs that are metabolized to amphetamine or methamphetamine are listed in Table 31.8.

## Barbiturates

The success of barbital in 1903 and phenobarbital in 1912 led to the synthesis and testing of more than 2500 barbiturate derivatives. However, because of their low therapeutic index and high potential for misuse, they have been largely replaced by safer benzodiazepines. Nevertheless, barbiturates continue to be available. The classification of barbiturates as ultra-short-acting, short-acting, intermediate-acting, and long-acting refers to the duration of effect, not to the elimination half-life (Table 31.9).

The barbiturates produce varying degrees of CNS depression, ranging from mild sedation to general anesthesia, and exert their effects by activating inhibitory GABAA receptors and inhibiting excitatory AMPA receptors that explain their CNS-depressant effects.

### Analytical Methods

Numerous commercial immunoassays for barbiturates are available, and although the degree of cross-reactivity of other barbiturates varies with each assay, most have sufficient cross-reactivity to detect the major, therapeutically used barbiturates.

Confirmatory methods for barbiturates include GC with flame ionization detection, nitrogen phosphorous detection, and MS, capillary electrophoresis-ultraviolet (UV), LC using ultraviolet (LC-UV) detection, and LC-MS.

### Benzodiazepines

The prototype benzodiazepines are diazepam and nordiazepam (N-desmethyl diazepam). Over 30 members of this group are presently used worldwide. As a class of drugs, benzodiazepines are among the most prescribed drugs in the Western hemisphere because of their efficacy, safety, low addiction potential, and minimal side effects, and because of the high public demand for sedative and anxiolytic agents. The benzodiazepines given by themselves or in combination with other drugs, particularly narcotic analgesics (opioids), are among the most widely misused drugs.

Virtually all results of the pharmacologic effects of benzodiazepines are caused by their actions on the CNS. The most prominent of these effects are sedation, hypnosis, decreased anxiety, muscle relaxation, anterograde amnesia, and anticonvulsant activity. Benzodiazepines are believed to exert most of their effects by interacting with inhibitory neurotransmitter receptors directly activated by GABA. Benzodiazepines act at GABAA but not GABAB receptors by binding directly to a specific site that is distinct from that of GABA binding. Ethanol increases both the rate of absorption of benzodiazepines and the associated CNS depression, and there are significant additive effects with other sedative or hypnotic drugs.

Benzodiazepines may be divided into three categories based on their onset time and elimination half-lives: short-acting agents, intermediate-acting agents, and long-acting agents (Table 31.10). These pharmacokinetic properties in part determine the primary clinical applications for some benzodiazepines. Benzodiazepines undergo hepatic oxidation (phase I) and conjugation (phase II), often forming metabolites with pharmacologic activity (see Table 31.10)

Treatment of benzodiazepine toxicity is primarily supportive. Flumazenil may be used in select cases as a competitive inhibitor of the benzodiazepine site on the GABA complex.

## TABLE 31.10  Half-Life of Select Benzodiazepines

| Drug | Significant Phase I Metabolites |
|------|--------------------------------|
| **Short-Acting** | |
| Midazolam | α-Hydroxy-midazolam |
| Estazolam | 3-Hydroxy-estazolam |
| Flurazepam | Hydroxy-ethyl-flurazepam |
| | N-desalkylflurazepam[a] |
| Temazepam | Oxazepam |
| Triazolam | α-Hydroxy-triazolam |
| **Intermediate-Acting** | |
| Flunitrazepam[b] | 7-Amino-flunitrazepam |
| **Long-Acting Agents** | |
| Diazepam | Nordiazepam[a] |
| | Oxazepam[a] |
| | Temazepam[a] |
| Quazepam | 3-Hydroxy-quazepam |
| | N-Desalkyl-2-oxo-quazepam |
| | 2-Oxo-3-hydroxy-quazepam |
| Alprazolam | α-Hydroxy-alprazolam |
| Chlordiazepoxide | Nordiazepam[a] |
| | Oxazepam[a] |
| Clonazepam | 7-Amino-clonazepam |
| Clorazepate[c] | Nordiazepam[a] |
| | Oxazepam[a] |
| Lorazepam | |
| Oxazepam | |

[a]Active metabolite.
[b]Not available in the United States.
[c]Converted to nordiazepam by gastric HCl.

## Analytical Methods

Benzodiazepines are measured through a variety of techniques. However, their structural diversity and wide variation in potency provide a challenge for laboratories seeking to detect all relevant members in one analytical scheme.

Several commercial immunoassay systems are available for detection and screening. Cross-reactivity in screening immunoassays of the various benzodiazepines and their metabolites varies considerably from manufacturer to manufacturer, and screening assays cannot be used to distinguish between the individual benzodiazepines. Most assays are calibrated to a common metabolite such as oxazepam, temazepam, or nordiazepam. However, the large number of different functional groups that may be present on the benzodiazepine nucleus makes it difficult to detect all drugs in this class, and some compounds may not be detected by many assays. Other factors, such as low doses and short half-lives, make the detection of some benzodiazepines especially challenging. In the absence of sufficiently sensitive or specific immunoassays, direct analysis by a confirmatory method is warranted in suspected cases.

New-generation sedative-hypnotics such as zolpidem (Ambien), eszopiclone (Lunesta), and zaleplon (Sonata)

modulate the GABAA receptor, much like the benzodiazepines, yet they are structurally different, thus not detectable by immunoassay.

Analysts need to be aware that the specimen type will dictate the target substance. Blood analyses invariably will target the parent benzodiazepine and perhaps the major active metabolite (e.g., nordiazepam for diazepam and other analogues metabolized to nordiazepam), whereas in urine, a metabolite is often the required target species.

Many benzodiazepines are analyzed without derivatization by GC. These include diazepam, nordiazepam, flurazepam, and alprazolam. Drugs that are more polar, including those with hydroxyl groups such as oxazepam, temazepam, and lorazepam or a nitro group (clonazepam, nitrazepam), display poor chromatographic characteristics and require derivatization. Some consider GC-MS as the definitive confirmatory method; however, LC with UV detection (240 nm) and LC-MS/MS can be used to detect benzodiazepines and metabolites without derivatization.

## Cannabinoids

Cannabinoids are a group of compounds found in the plant *Cannabis sativa* and have been used for centuries as medicinal and psychotropic agents. The main psychotropic effects are euphoria, distorted perceptions, relaxation, and a feeling of well-being.

Delta-9-tetrahydrocannabinol (THC) is the primary psychoactive component of the *C. sativa* plant. It binds to the endogenous cannabinoid receptors, CB1 (neuronal) and CB2 (immune cells). The distribution pattern of CB1 receptors in the CNS accounts for most of the clinical effects of THC such as those affecting mood, memory, cognition, pain, and appetite. CB2 may regulate immune and inflammatory processes.

When marijuana is smoked, THC diffuses into the plasma in seconds and is distributed into multiple phases. First, it distributes to highly vascularized tissues in minutes because of its lipophilic nature. THC then is redistributed back into the bloodstream, undergoes hepatic metabolism, and slowly accumulates into less vascularized and fatty tissues. After cessation of marijuana smoking, THC and its metabolites are slowly released from fat stores.

The main psychotropic effects after inhalation of marijuana occur within minutes and can persist for several hours. The peak plasma concentration of THC is dependent on the dose and occurs during the early acute phase (6 to 10 minutes). Numerous factors contribute to the variability in dose, such as method of consumption, depth of inhalation, exposure frequency, and cannabis potency. Onset of clinical symptoms and peak plasma concentrations after oral ingestion of THC is slower (2 to 6 hours) than after inhalation. The intensity of clinical effects described for smoked cannabis occurs during multiple phases. These phases are categorized as acute (0 to 60 minutes), post-acute (60 to 150 minutes), and residual (>150 minutes). The ratio of THC to 11-nor-delta-9-tetrahydrocannabinol-9-carboxylic acid (THC-COOH) metabolite has been used to estimate the time of exposure to marijuana. This approach may be useful in naive users but is unreliable in chronic misusers of marijuana.

THC is metabolized by CYP2D6 liver enzymes to greater than 100 metabolites. The main active metabolite, 11-hydroxy- THC, is further oxidized to the most abundant inactive metabolite, THC-COOH.

Cannabinoids have some medicinal use. For example, dronabinol (Marinol) contains synthetic THC and is used to treat anorexia and nausea in patients with acquired immunodeficiency syndrome (AIDS), nausea and vomiting associated with chemotherapy, or asthma and glaucoma.

Legitimate concern has been raised concerning positive results from "passive inhalation" of nearby users, or for use or consumption of hemp. Since 1998, the U.S. Federal Government has prohibited the importation of *C. sativa* seeds and oil containing greater than 0.3% THC to reduce human exposure to THC. These measures were successful in reducing potential positive cannabinoid drug screen results from dietary sources.

### Analytical Methods

An immunoassay method is typically used to screen for potential cannabinoids. Immunoassay screens have been designed to detect cannabis use in urine samples using antibody reagents developed against the inactive THC-COOH metabolite; these reagents cross-react with numerous other THC metabolites. A positive screening result for THC obtained by immunoassay is frequently confirmed by detection of THC-COOH by GC-MS/MS or LC-MS/MS analysis of the urine specimens.

A positive result from a urine cannabinoid screen or a positive result found by confirmatory testing does not indicate intoxication or degree of exposure. The window of detection for the urine concentration of THC-COOH varies among casual (2 to 7 days) and chronic misusers (up to 73 days) of marijuana and is dose dependent. Variables affecting the duration of detection include dose, frequency of exposure, route of exposure, body composition, fluid excretion, and method of detection. In practice, monitoring of abstinence is particularly challenging, as dilution of urine due to normal biological fluctuations (hydration) or

ingested adulterants has caused a negative result 1 day and a positive on the next. To correct for hydration fluctuations, urine concentrations of THC-COOH are normalized per milligram creatinine in monitoring individuals who are resuming cannabis use.

### Cocaine

Cocaine is an alkaloid found in *Erythroxylon coca*. In clinical medicine, it is used for local anesthesia and vasoconstriction in nasal surgery, and to dilate pupils in ophthalmology. Cocaine misuse has a long history, and cocaine is still one of the most common illicit substances of use/misuse.

Cocaine is sold on the street in two forms: a hydrochloride salt (powder) and a free-base product known as "crack." The hydrochloride salt form of cocaine is administered by nasal insufflation ("snorting") or intravenously. Crack comes as a rock crystal that is heated and its vapors inhaled. It should be noted that "crack" cocaine is not to be confused with "freebasing," which is a process in which the user purifies cocaine HCl by mixing an aqueous solution of cocaine with baking soda or ammonia and adding diethyl ether, thereby extracting the free form of the drug into the organic solvent. However, because of the extremely flammable nature of diethyl ether, and therefore the risk of igniting any remaining ether, this is no longer a common practice.

Chemically, cocaine is methylbenzoylecgonine (COC). Its metabolism is complex (Fig. 31.2) and occurs via both nonenzymatic hydrolysis and enzymatic transformation in the plasma and liver, producing both active and inactive metabolites. COC is rapidly metabolized to benzoylecgonine (BE) and ecgonine methyl ester, both of which are inactive. It should be noted that cocaethylene, produced when cocaine and ethyl alcohol are used simultaneously, possesses the same CNS stimulatory activity as cocaine in experimental animals. Norcocaine (NC) is of clinical interest because of its conversion to potentially hepatotoxic metabolites.

BE has a half-life longer than COC. It is the most commonly monitored **analyte** in urine for determination of COC use. BE is further metabolized to minor metabolites such as m-hydroxybenzoylecgonine (m-HOBE), which has been shown to be an important metabolite in the meconium

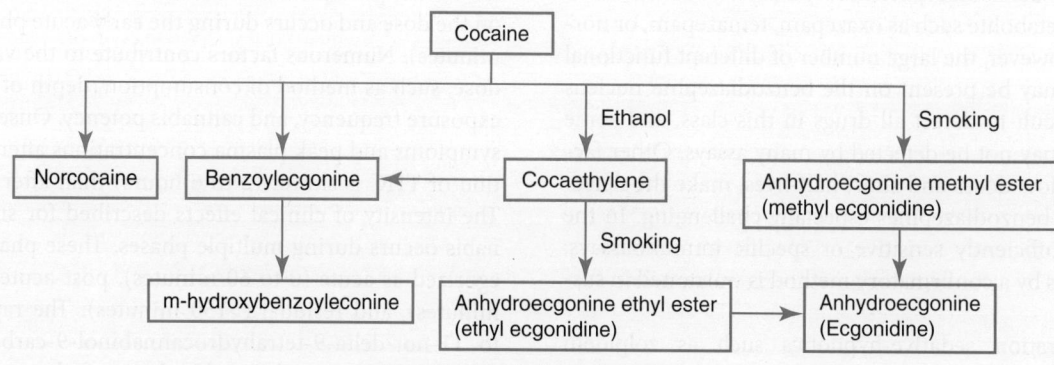

**Fig. 31.2** Metabolism of cocaine.

of cocaine-exposed babies. Anhydroecgonine methyl ester (AEME; methyl ecgonidine) has been identified as a unique COC metabolite after smoked COC ("crack") administration. Anhydroecgonine ethyl ester (AEEE; ethyl ecgonidine) has been identified in COC smokers who also use ethyl alcohol.

Cocaine is a potent CNS stimulant that elicits a state of increased alertness and euphoria with actions similar to those of amphetamine but of shorter duration. These CNS effects are thought to be largely associated with the ability of cocaine to block dopamine reuptake at nerve synapses, thereby prolonging the action of dopamine in the CNS. It is this response that leads to recreational use of cocaine. Cocaine also blocks the reuptake of norepinephrine at presynaptic nerve terminals; this produces a sympathomimetic response.

The CNS and cardiovascular effects of cocaine exhibit acute tolerance; its effects are more pronounced when the concentration of cocaine in blood is increasing than when it is at a similar but decreasing concentration (clockwise hysteresis). Thus, it is difficult to correlate isolated blood concentration values with psychomotor effects.

COC is frequently used with other drugs, most commonly ethanol. This combination produces greater euphoria and an enhanced perception of well-being relative to COC. CE appears to be equipotent to COC with regard to dopamine transporter affinity but is less potent than cocaine pharmacologically. It has been suggested that simultaneous COC and ethanol use carries an 18- to 25-fold increase in risk of toxicity than that associated with COC alone.

## Analytical Methods

The half-life of COC is 0.5 to 1.5 hours, whereas the half-life of BE is 4 to 7 hours. Thus, BE is the analyte of choice in screening for cocaine use. The initial screening test for cocaine use is the immunoassay detection directed against the primary metabolite BE.

Most confirmatory assays offer quantification of both parent drug and metabolite. Numerous methods have been described for measurement of COC and various metabolites. GC techniques for analysis of COC and its metabolites require derivatization, especially of polar metabolites. GC-MS is the method of choice for many laboratories. Liquid chromatography with tandem mass spectrometry (LC-MS/MS) methods can simultaneously assess many of the more polar secondary metabolites such as CE, NC, AEME, and AEEE. For these reasons, LC-MS/MS methods are gaining in popularity.

## Lysergic Acid Diethylamide

Lysergic acid diethylamide (LSD) is an extremely potent psychedelic ergot alkaloid derived from the fungus *Claviceps purpurea*, which grows on wheat and other grains. LSD shares structural features with serotonin (5-hydroxytryptamine), a major CNS neurotransmitter and neuromodulator. The drug LSD binds to serotonin receptors in the CNS and acts as a serotonin agonist. The principal psychological effects of LSD are perceptual distortions of color, sound, distance, and shape (synesthesia); depersonalization and loss of body image; and rapidly changing emotions from ecstasy to depression or paranoia. The most common adverse effects of LSD are panic attacks. In addition, unpredictable recurrence of hallucinations (flashbacks) may occur weeks or months after last drug use, and LSD may elicit psychotic reactions (thought disorders, hallucinations, depression, and depersonalization).

The drug is rapidly absorbed from the gastrointestinal tract, and its effects begin within 40 to 60 minutes, peak at about 2 to 4 hours, and subside by 6 to 8 hours. The elimination half-life is about 3 hours. LSD is extensively metabolized, and the metabolite 2-oxo-3-hydroxy-LSD is present in urine at concentrations 10- to 43-fold greater than those of LSD.

## Analytical Methods

Because of the very high potency of LSD and its subsequent rapid and extensive metabolism, only about 1% to 2% of the drug is excreted unchanged in urine. Thus, detection of LSD presents an especially difficult analytical challenge. Even with sensitive assays, the detection window for LSD is generally only 12 to 24 hours. The detection window may be extended, perhaps twofold to threefold, by including 2-oxo-3-hydroxy-LSD in the confirmatory test, while using sensitive techniques such as GC-MS/MS, LC-MS/MS, or LC-MS. To avoid degradation of LSD and 2-oxo-3-hydroxy-LSD or epimerization of LSD to iso-LSD, urine specimens should be protected from sunlight, bright fluorescent light, and elevated temperature at alkaline pH.

## Opiates and Opioids

The term opioid describes compounds that encompass the natural and semi-synthetic opiates that include variations on the structure of morphine and fully synthetic opioids with minimal structural homology to the natural alkaloids. The defining characteristic of this class of drugs is their morphine-like activity stemming from interaction with opioid receptors. Other compounds that are referred to as "opioids" include receptor antagonists and mixed agonist/antagonists, as well as other opium-derived alkaloids such as papaverine.

Opioids interact with the family of opioid receptors that are variably distributed throughout the body. The classical opioid receptors are divided into the mu, delta, and kappa ($\mu$, $\delta$, and $\kappa$, or MOR, DOR, and KOR, respectively) subfamilies. Opioid receptor agonists typically produce analgesia, and antagonists block this response. Most opioids have both substantial addictive capacity and potentially life-threatening side effects. Thus, the benefits of their use in non-end-stage patients must be carefully weighed against the chance of serious consequences. The development of tolerance and the risk of prescription diversion complicate even further the process of monitoring long-term opioid therapy for compliance and efficacy.

One of the more important CYP enzymes, CYP2D6, is particularly notable for its role in variable clinical response to opioids; it will be discussed in greater detail in a later section. Many additional CYP enzymes, including CYP3A and CYP2C and others, are involved in opioid metabolism. It is important to note that several of these enzymes are subject to substrate inhibition and/or induction. Substrate-dependent changes in metabolic activity are affected by other drugs, herbal supplements, and endogenous compounds that are substrates of the same enzyme. For example, methadone concentrations may be lower than expected in a patient taking St. John's Wort—a noted CYP3A4 inducer—but higher in a patient ingesting a CYP3A4 inhibitor such as grapefruit juice.

## Types of Opiates

*Natural opium alkaloids.* Opium is obtained from the unripe seed capsules of the poppy plant, *Papaver somniferum.* The milky juice is dried and powdered to make powdered opium, which contains several alkaloids. These alkaloids are divided into two distinct chemical classes: *phenanthrenes* and *benzylisoquinolines.* The principal phenanthrenes are morphine, codeine, and thebaine. The principal benzylisoquinolines are papaverine which is a smooth muscle relaxant, and noscapine.

Poppy seeds from the poppy plant *P. somniferum* contain morphine and to a lesser extent codeine. Ingestion of bakery products containing poppy seeds leads to excretion of morphine (and codeine) in urine. In practice, caution is required when the results of a positive urine test for morphine and codeine are interpreted.

**Morphine.** Morphine's major metabolites are glucuronide conjugates, including inactive morphine-3-glucuronide (M3G; ≈60%), active morphine-6-glucuronide (M6G; ≈10%), and a small amount of morphine-3,6-diglucuronide. With long-term administration, and when morphine concentrations are high, a minor fraction is converted to hydromorphone (up to 2.5% of the urine morphine concentration).

The detection time for morphine in urine is usually 48 to 72 hours, but this varies with individual differences in metabolism excretion and route and frequency of use.

**Codeine.** Because of its use as an antitussive and analgesic, codeine is frequently prescribed, and is commonly combined with non-opiate analgesic agents such as aspirin and acetaminophen. Codeine has only about one-tenth the analgesic potency of morphine and is generally considered a prodrug. The small fraction of codeine converted to morphine by CYP2D6 is considered to be responsible for the analgesic effect. During the early phase of excretion, codeine and conjugates predominate, but after this time, morphine conjugates are the major product. Approximately 3 days after codeine use, morphine and its conjugates are the only metabolites detected.

*Semi-synthetic opiates, fully synthetic and opioid antagonists, and mixed agonists/antagonists.* Examples of semisynthetic opiates include heroin, hydrocodone, hydromorphone, oxycodone, and oxymorphone and their metabolites; they are outlined in Table 31.11.

## Analytical Methods

Many different immunoassay methods are used to screen for opiates. Given their relatively rapid turnaround time and ability to detect several opiates, immunoassays are the methods of choice to screen urine samples for their opiate content. Antibodies in opiate screens commonly target morphine, and there is significant variability in cross-reactivity such that many opiates and opioids with high misuse potential such as oxycodone are often poorly detected.

The cutoff concentrations used for drugs in federally regulated tests, in particular opioids (2000 ng/mL), are too high to be of value in monitoring compliance of pain management patients or other clinical settings. For these circumstances a cutoff of 300 ng/mL morphine (or morphine equivalents) is commonly used to distinguish negative from positive urine specimens. Monitoring compliance for synthetic opioids (fentanyl, tramadol, methadone) and semisynthetic opiates (hydrocodone, oxycodone) in pain management programs should use drug-specific immunoassays because of the low cross-reactivity of these drugs in most opiate immunoassays.

It is important for drug testing laboratories to communicate relevant aspects of the metabolic interconversion of opiates to physicians responsible for these programs.

GC-MS and LC-MS/MS are techniques of choice for confirmatory testing after a positive screening result or when looking for opiates that are not well detected by immunoassay. GC-MS has historically been considered the method of choice. However, despite the long-standing role of GC in opiate analysis, LC methods are becoming more common and are often analytically advantageous. One notable example is that LC provides the ability to analyze glucuronide-conjugated metabolites, as well as parent compounds. In addition, LC methods can be used to measure polar metabolites without prior derivatization, and on-column extraction is possible with some LC systems.

## Phencyclidine and Ketamine

Phencyclidine (PCP) and ketamine are potent analgesics and general anesthetics. They are classified as dissociative anesthetics because they produce rapid-acting dissociation of perception, consciousness, movement, and memory. PCP and ketamine share similar structural features and pharmacological actions. The effects are dose dependent and vary between individuals. PCP is listed as a Schedule II drug in the U.S. Federal Controlled Substance Act and is not approved for human use. Ketamine is a Schedule III drug that is commonly used as an anesthetic. Both have been used illicitly as substances of use/misuse, as well as in cases of drug-facilitated sexual assault. At anesthetic doses it produces profound analgesia, but the individual is awake yet incapacitated, with limited voluntary limb movement. They bind and antagonize the excitatory glutaminergic system by binding to NMDA receptors. They also decrease GABA transmission, disrupt cortical activity, and increase dopamine and norepinephrine synaptic reuptake.

## TABLE 31.11    Examples of Semisynthetic Opiates Include Heroin, Hydrocodone, Hydromorphone, Oxycodone, and Oxymorphone and Their Metabolites

| Parent Drug | Primary Metabolite Active(s) | Minor Metabolite(s) |
|---|---|---|
| **Natural and Semi-synthetic Opiates** | | |
| morphine | | hydromorphone (<3%) |
| codeine | morphine | hydrocodone (<11%) |
| heroin | 6-acetylmorphine, morphine | |
| hydromorphone | | |
| hydrocodone | hydromorphone, norhydrocodone | dihydrocodeine |
| oxycodone | oxymorphone, noroxycodone | |
| oxymorphone | noroxymorphone | |
| **Fully Synthetic Opioids** | | |
| fentanyl | nor-fentanyl | |
| meperidine | normeperidine | |
| methadone | EDDP (2-ethylidene-1,5-dimethyl-3,3-diphenylpyrrolidine) | |
| tramadol | N-desmethyltramadol, O-desmethyltramadol | |
| **Opioid Antagonists and Mixed Agonists/Antagonists** | | |
| buprenorphine | | |
| naloxone | noroxymorphone (nornaloxone) | |
| naltrexone | | |

## Analytical Methods

Whether or not PCP and ketamine are included in a general urine drug screen depends on applicable regulations and on the prevalence of use in the local community. In some locations, the prevalence of PCP or ketamine use may be too low to warrant routine screening. Initial screening is typically done by immunoassay. Immunoassays for PCP are generally reliable; however, false positives have been reported because of high concentrations of dextromethorphan, diphenhydramine, and thioridazine. Immunoassay-positive specimens should be confirmed using GC-MS or LC-MS techniques. Note, these techniques will also detect norketamine and dehydronorketamine, the active metabolites of ketamine.

## Specimen Validity Testing

Several techniques are used by persons attempting to mask or adulterate drugs to avoid detection. These tactics may include the exchange of urine from a drug-free individual or dilution of the urine specimen by excessive consumption of water, use of a diuretic, or simple addition of water to the specimen to reduce drug concentrations to below cutoff limits. Also, readily available adulterants, such as detergent, bleach, salt, alkali, ammonia, tetrahydrozoline, or acid, may be added to the specimen after collection in an attempt to interfere with immunoassay screening procedures. Other more sophisticated adulterants specifically marketed to avoid drug detection include glutaraldehyde, nitrite, chromate, and a combination of peroxide and peroxidase. These adulterants also interfere with immunoassays to variable degrees, and the oxidizing agents (nitrite, chromate, and peroxide/peroxidase) may result in destruction of morphine, codeine, and the principal metabolite resulting from marijuana use, thus interfering with their GC-MS confirmation and with immunoassays.

Direct observation of urine collection is the most stringent means to guard against specimen exchange or adulteration. However, an individual's right to privacy and dignity must be weighed against the need for the highest degree of certainty of specimen integrity. Alternative measures to prevent specimen adulteration include limitations on clothing or other personal belongings allowed in the specimen collection area, addition of coloring agent to toilet water, and inactivation of the hot water tap.

## DRUG-FACILITATED CRIMES

Drug-facilitated crimes (DFCs) are defined as voluntary or surreptitious use of alcohol, drugs, and/or chemical agents to incapacitate an individual and facilitate a criminal act. These crimes include drug-facilitated sexual assault (DFSA). In addition to alcohol, the drugs that have been implicated in DFCs include such substances as choral hydrate, benzodiazepines, nonbenzodiazepine sedative-hypnotics, gamma-hydroxybutyric acid (GHB), dextromethorphan, ketamine, phencyclidine, and nonprescription medications such as antihistamines and anticholinergics. The Society of Forensic Toxicologists Drug-Facilitated Crimes Committee has recommended analytical cut-off for testing of commonly encountered compounds (http://www.soft-tox.org/files/MinPerfLimits_DFC2017.pdf, accessed April 3, 2022). Clinical effects include impaired judgment, confusion, reduced inhibitions, sedation, hypnosis, loss of muscle coordination, and sometimes anterograde amnesia. Because of the amnesic properties of these drugs, victims often may not report their sexual assault for several days. Therefore, sensitive analytical techniques are necessary to detect these drugs and their metabolites in urine or hair samples after a single dose.

## Choral Hydrate

Chloral hydrate is classified as a sedative and as a hypnotic. The CNS depressant effects of chloral hydrate are believed to be due to its active metabolite trichloroethanol. The clinical diagnosis of chloral hydrate intoxication is difficult to differentiate from alcohol or sedative-hypnotics due to their shared similar clinical effects. The exact mechanism of action of chloral hydrate has not been determined. The elimination half-life of choral hydrate is very short (4 minutes), but the half-life of its metabolite trichloroethanol is 6 to 10 hours. If co-ingested with alcohol, the metabolism of chloral hydrate is impaired. Because both ethanol and chloral hydrate are metabolized by CYP2E1 and ADH, co-ingestion not only exacerbates the clinical effects but also prolongs the duration of action.

### Analytical Methods

Chloral hydrate is not detected on routine drug screens. Chloral hydrate and its metabolite trichloroethanol (TCE) are detected with the use of LC-MS and less commonly with capillary gas chromatography with electron-capture detection (GC-ECD), or GC-flame ion detection (GC-FID).

## Benzodiazepines

Numerous benzodiazepines have been reported in sexual assault victims, including diazepam, triazolam, temazepam, clonazepam, and etizolam (see Benzodiazepine section above for more details). Flunitrazepam specifically achieved significant public awareness. It is a fast-acting sedative-hypnotic categorized as a Schedule I drug in the United States, but sexual predators are able to acquire this drug through illegal trafficking. Sexual assault predators use flunitrazepam because it is easily dissolved into a beverage, it is relatively tasteless and odorless, it quickly incapacitates their victims, and routine drug screens do not detect its presence.

### Analytical Methods

Detection of flunitrazepam is especially challenging because of the low doses and the low degree of cross-reactivity of most immunoassays with the principal urinary metabolite, 7-aminoflunitrazepam (see Benzodiazepine analytical methods above), although specific immunoassays have been developed. Direct analysis or confirmatory testing of 7-aminoflunitrazepam by GC-MS or LC-MS/MS is indicated in suspected cases.

## Nonbenzodiazepine Sedative-Hypnotics

A new generation of sedative-hypnotics are available that are structurally different from benzodiazepines. These are Schedule IV drugs which include zopiclone, eszopiclone, zolpidem, and zaleplon and are utilized as sleep aids. These drugs are readily prescribed, easily shared, and often sold illegally. The rapid onset and amnesic properties of this class of drugs result in disinhibition, passivity, and retrograde amnesia which are favorable characteristics for use in DFC.

The pharmacological effects of these agents result from their interaction with a specific subtype of GABAA receptor complex. These drugs modulate the GABAA receptor chloride channel by binding to the benzodiazepine (BZ) receptors in the brain without binding to peripheral BZ receptors.

### Analytical Methods

Although these drugs do not cross-react with most benzodiazepine immunoassays, specific reagent systems (ELISA) directed against the non-benzodiazepine hypnotics are available. But most screening and confirmatory testing are performed by GC-MS or LC-MS/MS.

## Gamma-Hydroxybutyrate, 1,4-Butanediol, and γ-Butyrolactone

Gamma-hydroxybutyrate (GHB) and its synthetic precursor compounds, 1,4-butanediol (1,4-BD) and γ-butyrolactone (GBL), are Schedule I agents in the United States, and availability is restricted in numerous other countries. GHB is an odorless and colorless liquid, or it can be obtained as an off-white powder that easily dissolves in liquids. When ingested, it has CNS depressant effects, resulting in sedation and hypnosis.

GHB is a naturally occurring substance that is produced in the brain. It is metabolized to GABA by multiple endogenous enzymes. Consumption of GHB, or the synthetic GHB precursor compound 1,4-BD or GBL, will promote GABA activity. In addition to increased metabolism to GABA, GHB has direct effects on the CNS by binding GHB-specific receptors and GABA receptors.

GHB is rapidly metabolized ($t_{1/2} \approx 30$ minutes). Onset of its effects occurs in approximately 15 to 30 minutes and the duration of response is short, typically 1 to 3 hours for a normal dose (1 to 5 g) and 2 to 4 hours with excessive doses.

### Analytical Methods

GHB is not detected on most screens but can be identified with the use of GC-FID or GC-MS. Because GHB is metabolized rapidly, timely sample collection is an important facet of GHB assay. Plasma samples should be collected within 6 to 8 hours after ingestion, and urine samples within 10 to 12 hours. Endogenous concentrations of GHB are typically 1.0 mg/L and after exogenous exposure may return to normal levels within 8 to 12 hours after ingestion. Therefore, timely presentation of the sexually assaulted victims and physician recognition of GHB symptoms are essential for prosecution of sexual offenders.

## Dextromethorphan

Dextromethorphan (DXM) is structurally related to the opioids, but it does not bind to opioid receptors at normal dose. The (L−) isomer of dextromethorphan (levomethorphan, levorphan) (not available in the United States), is a potent opioid analgesic and is an example of the stereoselective nature of opioid receptor binding. DXM lacks analgesic activity but does have antitussive activity comparable with that of codeine. DXM is present in numerous OTC cough medications, often in combination with other medications.

## Analytical Methods

Clinically approved doses of DXM are not detected by most clinical opiate immunoassays, but larger doses may cross-react. ELISA assays are available to detect DXM and its major metabolite, dextrorphan. The presence of DXM or dextrorphan in a sample is confirmed by GC-MS or LC-MS/MS. Dextrorphan is the enantiomer of levorphanol, a potent opioid agonist available in the United States (Levo-Dromoran). Unless chiral analytical techniques are used, these enantiomers are not resolved.

## PAIN MANAGEMENT

UDT is an essential tool in the field of Pain Medicine. In the late 1990s, awareness grew about the personal and economic costs of poorly controlled pain. Prominent physicians and professional organizations at local, national, and international levels supported judicious opioid use to address not only acute and cancer-related pain, but any patient presenting with pain. In short order, the negative consequences of widespread opioid use surfaced. Since 1999, the number of opioid-related deaths in the United States has more than doubled and now exceeds the number of deaths related to heroin and cocaine misuse combined.

Approximately 9.5 million people misused opioids in 2020, and approximately 1.2 million of those people initiated prescription pain reliever misuse.

Despite widespread agreement that treating chronic pain with opioids can be risky, and requires commitment to monitoring, controversy in pain medicine exists as to the type and frequency of UDT. This controversy likely stems from the paucity of high-quality research demonstrating that UDT significantly reduces the risks of misuse, and diversion. Additionally, evidence exists that inconsistent UDTs do not necessarily alter prescribing practices. Coincident are concerns about conflicts of interest and physician enticement, as UDT is now a multi-billion-dollar industry that has a history of incentivizing physicians to frequently order testing.

UDT is an important tool in clinical pain medicine. The current epidemic of prescription medication misuse underscores the need for a consistent approach to monitoring that utilizes both subjective and objective measures. While some advocate that routine UDT should include all testable substances with abusive potential, such practices are costly and likely unnecessary in many cases. High risk patients, classified by using validated clinical screening tools, require more careful and more frequent monitoring. POC and other enzyme immunoassay screening methods cannot differentiate between medications within the same drug class and may completely miss semi-synthetic and synthetic opioids. For this reason, confirmatory testing with GC or LC should be performed at least annually and on all inconsistent samples. If misuse or diversion is suspected, the physician must act in a way that promotes patient health and safety, while abiding by state and federal law. Such actions should be openly discussed and explicitly written in the opioid prescribing contract, signed at the initiation of every opioid treatment plan.

## DETECTION OF SUBSTANCES OF USE/MISUSE USING OTHER TYPES OF SPECIMENS

Blood, serum, and urine samples are typically collected for the purpose of determining exposure to various agents. However, sampling of blood is considered invasive, and collection of urine may require some invasion of privacy and loss of dignity. In addition, urine specimens are subject to adulteration or manipulation to evade detection. For these reasons, alternate biological specimens have been investigated as alternative types of samples for drug analysis.

### Meconium

The first intestinal discharge from newborns is meconium, which is a viscous, dark green substance composed of intestinal secretions, desquamated squamous cells, lanugo hair, bile pigments, and blood. Meconium also contains pancreatic enzymes, free fatty acids, porphyrins, interleukin-8, and phospholipase. Meconium begins to form during the second trimester and continues to accumulate until birth; drugs taken by the mother can be detected in the meconium of the newborn. Drug testing is necessary in infants to substantiate the clinical indication of prenatal exposure to illicit drugs.

The disposition of drug in meconium is not well understood. The proposed mechanism is that the fetus excretes drug into bile and amniotic fluid. Drug accumulates in meconium by direct deposition from bile or through swallowing of amniotic fluid. Therefore, the presence of drugs in meconium has been proposed to be indicative of in utero drug exposure potentially in the second and third trimesters—a longer historical measure than is possible by urinalysis.

Meconium testing has some limitations. For example, meconium is usually passed by full-term newborns within 1 to 2 days; however, low birth weight infants may have delayed passage (median age of 3 days). Thus, meconium collection may be missed completely, or significant delay is seen in detection of intrauterine drug exposure.

Meconium is a sticky material that is difficult to work with in the clinical laboratory. Meconium drug screening has been adapted to various analytical immunoassays, but as with any immunoassay-based drug screen, confirmatory testing by LC-MS/MS or GC-MS is necessary. Confirmatory assays for meconium are more difficult than those for urine. Recovery of drugs from meconium is low (10% to 50%). Some debate continues as to which are the most appropriate drug analytes that should be measured in meconium; Table 31.12 attempts to summarize current knowledge. Meconium drug testing is far less standardized than UDT. Assay cutoff limits and units (ng/g meconium or ng/mL extract) may vary; suitable reference or control materials are not yet available.

## TABLE 31.12    Drugs and Metabolites of Significance in Meconium

| Drug Class | Confirmation Compound |
|---|---|
| Cocaine | cocaine |
| | benzoylecgonine |
| | cocaethylene |
| | m-hydroxybenzoylecgonine |
| Opiates | morphine |
| | codeine |
| | 6-monoacetylmorphine (6-MAM) |
| | hydromorphone |
| | hydrocodone |
| | oxycodone |
| Cannabinoids | 9-carboxy-11-nor-delta-9-THC |
| | 11-hydroxy-delta-9-tetrahydrocannabinol |
| | 8,11-dihydroxy-delta-9-tetrahydrocannabinol |
| Amphetamines | amphetamine |
| | methamphetamine |
| | MDMA |
| | MDA |
| | MDEA |
| Ethanol | fatty acid ethyl esters |
| PCP | PCP |

MDEA, 3,4-Methylenedioxyethylamphetamine; MDMA, 3,4-methylenedioxymethamphetamine; MDA, 3,4-methylenedioxyamphetamine; PCP, phencyclidine; THC, delta-9-tetrahydrocannabinol.

## Oral Fluid

Oral fluid is recognized by the FDA (2020) as an alternative specimen for employment-related drug testing. Analysis of saliva for drugs was first done almost 30 years ago for the purpose of therapeutic drug monitoring. It has since been evaluated for use in forensic toxicology, with recognition of its advantages over other biological matrices. Most studies on saliva in humans use whole saliva. It should be noted that the term "oral fluid" is now preferred for the specimen collected from the mouth.

Several advantages are associated with monitoring oral fluid as contrasted with monitoring plasma or serum concentrations. For example, collection of oral fluid is considered to be a noninvasive procedure, direct observation is possible thus minimizing risk of adulteration, and some of the risks associated with drawing of blood are avoided. Furthermore, for the patient, the fear, anxiety, and discomfort that may accompany the drawing of blood are diminished. Significant disadvantages of oral fluid are (1) the window of detection is similar to blood or serum and is short compared to urine, (2) glucuronide metabolites (size and charge) may poorly distribute into oral fluid, (3) pH may affect deposition into oral fluid, (4) protein binding diminishes deposition, and (5) a small volume of sample is collected. The problem of small sample size is usually overcome by using methods that simultaneously extract multiple drug groups.

In principle, oral fluid drug concentration is related to plasma free drug concentration; therefore, oral fluid has the potential to show a relation between behavior/impairment and drug concentration, making it a possible matrix for monitoring drug intoxication or for conducting therapeutic drug management. Since disposition of drugs in oral fluid is dependent upon chemical and metabolic processes appropriate interpretation is required. In recent years, great interest has been expressed in the use of oral fluid testing for roadside drug screening, monitoring the compliance of individuals on drug maintenance programs, and workplace drug testing. Low concentrations of drugs and metabolites necessitate sensitive screening methods.

## Hair

Hair is advantageous as a biological specimen for drug analysis because it is easily obtained with less embarrassment, and it is not easily altered or manipulated to avoid drug detection. Hair also differs from other human materials used for toxicological analysis in that it has a substantially longer detection window (months to years). Once deposited in hair, drugs are very stable, and analysis can be performed even after centuries.

The exact mechanism by which chemicals are incorporated into hair is still being studied. It has been suggested, however, that passive diffusion may be augmented by binding of the drug to intracellular components of hair cells such as the hair pigment melanin. Factors that may affect how drugs are incorporated into hair are not well established but may include rate of hair growth, anatomical location of hair, hair color (melanin content), and hair texture (thick or fine, porous or not). These factors are determined by genetic factors and by the effects of various hair treatments. This may lead to biases in hair testing for substances of use/misuse.

Drugs, when deposited in hair, are generally present in relatively low concentrations; thus, sensitive analytical techniques are required for detection. Immunoassay procedures have been modified for use with hair. For confirmatory testing, GC-MS is generally the method of choice; however, various GC-MS/MS or LC-MS/MS methods have been used. External exposure to drugs causes them to be detected in hair; one of the most crucial issues facing hair analysts today is technical and false positives. The need to distinguish between passive exposure (environmental contamination) and active consumption is fundamental; consequently, decontamination procedures for hair are compulsory. These usually involve a washing step.

## Sweat

Drugs may be excreted in sweat, and analysis may provide an alternative detection technique. Sweat patch collection devices that resemble an adhesive bandage may be worn for several days to several weeks. During this time, a drug, if present, accumulates in the absorbent pad in the patch, while water vapor escapes through the semi-permeable covering. Thus, sweat drug testing offers the possibility of monitoring drug use over extended periods without the need for frequent collection of urine. Sweat drug excretion may also be an important mechanism by which drugs enter hair.

## REVIEW QUESTIONS

1. The preferred specimen type for determination of neonate exposure to drugs during the second or third trimester of pregnancy is:
   a. fetal oral fluid.
   b. meconium.
   c. fetal hair.
   d. newborn infant urine.

2. The antidotal therapy for acetaminophen overdose is:
   a. forced alkaline diuresis.
   b. inhibition of the GABA channel.
   c. pralidoxime.
   d. *N*-acetylcysteine.

3. The primary advantage of high-performance liquid chromatography (HPLC) over gas chromatography (GC) for comprehensive drug screening for a broad range of chemicals is that:
   a. HPLC does not require a derivatization step.
   b. HPLC can be performed at the individual's bedside.
   c. GC gives diverse color hues and requires considerable technical skill.
   d. GC drug testing methods are subject to many types of interference.

4. Which of the following drugs is not consistently detected in the benzodiazepine immunoassay screen?
   a. Diazepam
   b. Clonazepam
   c. Oxazepam
   d. Nordiazepam

5. To confirm heroin use, testing of which urinary metabolite is considered unique and specific for this drug?
   a. Morphine
   b. Codeine
   c. Meperidine
   d. 6-Acetylmorphine

6. For assessment of substance use/misuse, the most widely accepted laboratory method for drug *confirmation* is:
   a. immunoassay.
   b. GC-MS.
   c. HPLC-UV.
   d. TOF.

## SUGGESTED READINGS

Baselt RC. *Disposition of Toxic Drugs and Chemical in Man.* 12th ed. Seal Beach, CA: Biomedical Publications; 2020.

Brunton LL, Knollmann BC, eds. *Goodman and Gilman's The Pharmacological Basis of Therapeutics,* 14th ed. New York: McGraw Hill; 2022.

Cabezas J, Lucey MR, Bataller R. Biomarkers for monitoring alcohol use. *Clin Liver Dis (Hoboken).* 2016;8:59–63.

Cone EJ, Huestis MA. Interpretation of oral fluid tests for drugs of abuse. *Ann N Y Acad Sci.* 2007;1098:51–103.

Drummer OH. Methods for the measurement of benzodiazepines in biological samples. *J Chromatogr.* 1998;713:201–225.

Dubowski KM. Alcohol determination in the clinical laboratory. *Am J Clin Pathol.* 1980;74:747–750.

Jarvie DR, Heyworth R, Simpson D. Plasma salicylate analysis: a comparison of colorimetric, HPLC and enzymatic techniques. *Ann Clin Biochem.* 1987;24(Pt 4):364–373.

Jones G. Post-mortem toxicology. In: Moffat A, ed. *Clarke's Analysis of Drugs and Poisons.* 3rd ed. London, UK: Pharmaceutical Press; 2004:95–108.

Kadiev E, Patel V, Rad P, et al. Role of pharmacogenetics in variable response to drugs: focus on opioids. *Expert Opin Drug Metab Toxicol.* 2008;4:77–91.

Kraut JA, Madias NE. Serum anion gap: its uses and limitations in clinical medicine. *Clin J Am Soc Nephrol.* 2007;2:162–174.

Lacy TL, Nichols JH. Therapeutic drugs III: Neuroleptic (antipsychotic) drugs. In: Levine B, ed. *Principles of Forensic Toxicology.* 2nd ed. Washington, DC: AACC Press; 2003:315–325.

Langman LJ, Bechtel LK, Meier BM, et al. Chapter 43: Clinical toxicology. In: Rifai N, Chiu RWK, Young I, eds. *Tietz Textbook of Laboratory Medicine.* 7th ed. St Louis, MO: Elsevier; 2022:454.

Middleberg RA, Langman LJ. Chapter 16. Clinical aspects of alcohol testing. In: Caplan YH, Goldberger BA, eds. *Garriott's Medicolegal Aspects of Alcohol.* 6th ed. Tucson, AZ: Lawyers & Judges Publishing Company Inc; 2015:435–448.

Moore C, Negrusz A, Lewis D. Determination of drugs of abuse in meconium. *J Chromatogr.* 1998;713:137–146.

Moore KA. Amphetamines/sympathomimetic amines. In: Levine B, ed. *Principles of Forensic Toxicology.* 2nd ed. Washington, DC: AACC Press; 2003:245–264.

Juurlink N. Antipsychotics D. In: Nelson LS, Howland MA, Lewin NA, eds. *Goldfrank's Toxicologic Emergencies.* 11th ed. New York, NY: McGraw-Hill Education; 2019.

Palmer RB. A review of the use of ethyl glucuronide as a marker for ethanol consumption in forensic and clinical medicine. *Semin Diagn Pathol.* 2009;26:18–27.

Payne JP, Hill DW, Wood DG. Distribution of ethanol between plasma and erythrocytes in whole blood. *Nature.* 1968;217:963–964.

Ropper A, Samuels M. Chapter 41. Disorders of the nervous system caused by alcohol, drugs, toxins, and chemical agents. In: Ropper A, Samuels M, eds. *Adams and Victor's Principles of Neurology.* 12th ed. New York: McGraw-Hill Companies, Inc; 2023.

Rumak BH, Matthew H. Acetaminophen poisoning and toxicity. *Pediatrics.* 1975;55:871–876.

The Centers for Disease Control Guideline for Prescribing Opioids for Chronic Pain—United States, 2016. http://www.cdc.gov/mmwr/volumes/65/rr/pdfs/rr6501e1.pdf; accessed 06/29/2016. *Details the use of urine drug testing.*

# 32

# Toxic Elements

*Frederick G. Strathmann and Lee M. Blum*

## OBJECTIVES

1. Identify several elements commonly associated with toxicity.
2. Compare available specimen types for applicability in the assessment of elemental toxicity.
3. Give examples of preanalytical concerns regarding elemental testing.
4. Summarize the key information regarding clinical presentation and treatment for elemental toxicity covered in this chapter.

## KEY WORDS AND DEFINITIONS

**Antidotal treatment** The use of any chemical or physiological procedure to prevent, minimize, or terminate the adverse effects of toxicity from an exogenous substance.

**Decontamination** Neutralization or removal of toxic substances.

**Neuropathy** Damage to a nerve that may impair sensation, movement, or other aspects of health.

**Signs of toxicity** Objective evidence of toxicity to someone other than the exposed individual.

**Symptoms of toxicity** Subjective evidence of toxicity experienced by the exposed individual.

**Toxicokinetics** The study of the time course of xenobiotic absorption, distribution, metabolism, and excretion.

## PREVALENCE OF ELEMENTAL TOXICITIES

The incidence of elemental exposure across large populations attributable to arsenic, cadmium, lead, or mercury appears to be on the same scale as the more common inborn errors of metabolism, such as neonatal hypothyroidism and phenylketonuria, and is of the same order of magnitude as the incidence of adult-onset hemochromatosis. Screening for these latter diseases is indicated because they are treatable, and treatment significantly reduces long-term morbidity. The same may also be true for elemental toxicities. When identified early, disease caused by elemental exposure is readily treatable with good outcomes. Conversely, if exposure is not identified and reduced, serious and sometimes irreparable damage to the nervous, renal, and cardiovascular systems can occur. Review of the periodic table provides some insight into the determination of an element's potential toxicity (Fig. 32.1).

### POINTS TO REMEMBER

- The incidence of elemental poisoning across large populations attributable to arsenic, cadmium, lead, or mercury poisoning appears to be on the same scale as the more common inborn errors of metabolism.
- When identified early, disease caused by elemental exposure is readily treatable with good outcomes.

## DIAGNOSING TOXICITY

Confirming the diagnosis of elemental toxicity is difficult because **signs** and **symptoms** are similar to those of many non–element-dependent diseases. Diagnosis of elemental toxicity requires demonstration of all of the following factors: (1) a source of elemental exposure must be evident, (2) the patient must demonstrate signs and symptoms typical of the element, and (3) abnormal element concentration in the appropriate tissue must be evident. If one of these features is absent, a conclusive diagnosis of elemental toxicity cannot be made. The laboratory plays a key role in this process, and appropriate specimen collection coupled with accurate analysis can make a major difference in correct diagnosis.

In clinical practice, analysis of toxic elements should always be considered in the clinical workup of the patient with (1) renal disease of unexplained origin, (2) bilateral peripheral **neuropathy**, (3) acute changes in mental function, (4) acute inflammation of the nasal or laryngeal epithelium, or (5) a history of exposure. Certain elements should be considered as the active, causative, or deficient agent in specific circumstances.

## TREATMENT

The route of exposure is an important aspect in elemental toxicity that can influence treatment and clinical outcomes. The clinical approach to elemental exposure comprises one of the

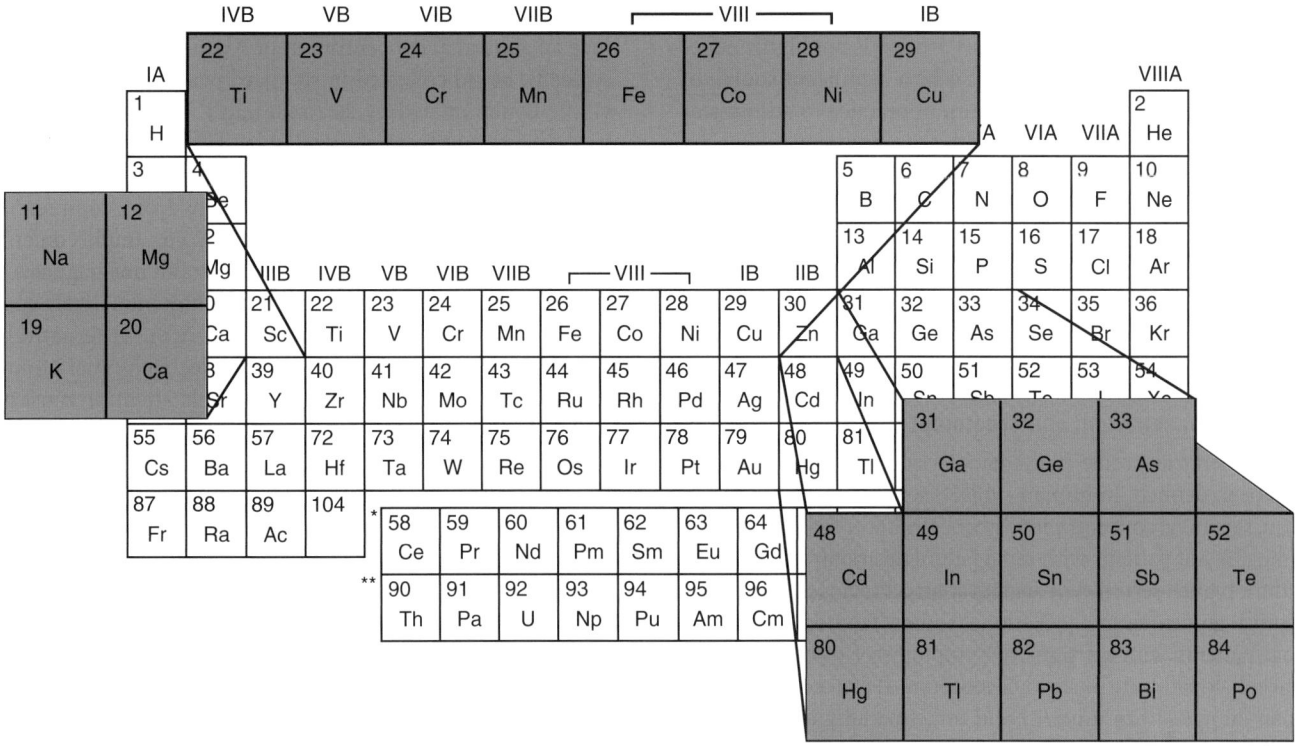

**Fig. 32.1** Periodic table, with emphasis on toxic elements.

following treatments: (1) removal from exposure if the source is known, (2) **decontamination**, (3) enhanced elimination, or (4) **antidotal treatment**.

Removal from the source of exposure can be complicated if the element responsible is unknown or the source of exposure is in question. For less extreme cases of exposure or if evidence to support more invasive treatments is lacking, removal, often in conjunction with supportive care, may be the only form of treatment available.

Decontamination strategies may include gastric lavage, activated charcoal, and supportive therapies to maintain the ABCs (airway, breathing, blood circulation), as well as attention to water, electrolyte balance, and neurologic complications. Prevention of absorption in the gastrointestinal (GI) tract is one mechanism for treating the chronic copper overload seen in patients with Wilson disease.

Enhancement of elimination can be done through diuresis, biliary excretion, hemodialysis, or exchange transfusion. Distribution of the element, once absorbed, has an impact on the utility of each of these approaches, and for several elements there is a lack of supporting data demonstrating improved outcomes after their use.

Antidotal treatments for elemental toxicities range from highly specific (e.g., deferoxamine for iron and aluminum) to considerably less specific (e.g., ethylenediaminetetraacetic acid [EDTA] for most divalent cations). The intent is to counteract the detrimental effects of the toxic element or to sequester it in a less toxic form. Although it is a highly useful method for treating elemental toxicity, the downside to chelation therapy is the potential for depletion of essential elements. The five most commonly used chelators are dimercaprol (British

anti-Lewisite [BAL]), dimercaptosuccinic acid (DMSA or succimer), dimercaptopropane sulfonate (DMPS), EDTA, and D-penicillamine.

### POINTS TO REMEMBER

**Diagnosing Elemental Toxicity**
- Confirming the diagnosis of elemental toxicity is difficult because signs and symptoms can be similar to those of many non–element-dependent diseases.
- The route of exposure is an important aspect of elemental toxicity that can influence treatment and clinical outcomes.

## SPECIFIC ELEMENTS

### Aluminum

In 1972, Alfrey and colleagues first described an encephalopathy in patients undergoing prolonged hemodialysis for renal failure. The disease was characterized by abnormal speech, myoclonic jerks, and seizures. Patients with these signs also showed a predominance of osteomalacic fractures. Subsequently, it was found that exposure of patients to (1) aluminum (Al)-laden dialysis water, (2) Al-containing oral phosphate binders, and (3) Al-laden albumin administered during dialysis were the primary causes of these signs of Al toxicity. Al is also a developmental toxicant if administered parenterally.

#### Sources of Exposure

Under normal physiologic conditions, the usual daily dietary intake of Al is 5 to 10 mg, which is primarily excreted by the kidney. Patients with renal failure lose this ability and are candidates for Al toxicity. The dialysis process is not highly effective at eliminating Al and can also be a significant source of exposure. Furthermore, it is common practice to administer Al-based gels orally to patients with renal failure to reduce the amount of phosphate absorbed from their diet to avoid excessive phosphate accumulation. A small fraction of this Al may be absorbed, and patients with renal failure can accumulate it. After dialysis, the albumin removed during dialysis may be replaced with albumin products that have high Al content resulting from the pharmaceutical purification process of passing the product through Al silicate filters.

## Clinical Presentation and Treatment

A biochemical profile that characterizes Al overload disease has been defined. In human subjects with normal renal function, serum Al concentration is typically lower than 6 µg/L (0.2 µmol/L), but patients with renal failure invariably have significantly higher serum Al concentrations. Previously published clinical guidelines by the National Kidney Foundation suggest that patients with no signs or symptoms of osteomalacia or encephalopathy are likely to have serum Al concentrations less than 20 µg/L (0.74 µmol/L) and intact parathyroid hormone (PTH) concentrations of 150 to 300 ng/L (16.5 to 33 nmol/L), which are typical for secondary hyperparathyroidism associated with renal failure. Patients with signs and symptoms of osteomalacia or encephalopathy typically have serum Al concentrations greater than 60 µg/L (2.2 µmol/L) and PTH concentrations less than 65 ng/L (7.15 nmol/L), which are indicative of Al-related bone disease. Patients with serum Al concentrations greater than 20 and less than 60 µg/L (>0.7 and <2.2 µmol/L) were identified as candidates for likely onset of Al-related bone disease. These patients required aggressive efforts to reduce their daily Al exposure, including (1) switching from Al-containing phosphate binders to calcium-containing phosphate binders, (2) ensuring that dialysis water contains less than 10 µg/L (0.4 µmol/L) of Al, and (3) ensuring that albumin used during postdialysis therapy is Al-free.

Al-related bone disease has been diagnosed and treated with deferoxamine, an avid chelator of both iron and Al. The deferoxamine infusion test is useful for the ultimate diagnosis of Al overload disease, and the drug has demonstrated utility for treating acute Al overload.

Adverse health effects in workers occupationally exposed to airborne Al compounds have included pneumoconiosis (aluminosis) and fibrosis of the lungs, and toxicity of the central nervous system, including balance disorders, difficulties with memory and concentration, impaired cognitive abilities, irritability, depression, and decreased psychomotor performances. Although rare, contact sensitization of the skin by Al is also possible.

## Preanalytical and Analytical Aspects

Preanalytical considerations related to collection of specimens for Al analysis are significant. Most of the common evacuated blood collection devices used in phlebotomy today have rubber stoppers made of Al silicate. Puncture of the rubber stopper for blood collection is sufficient to produce an abnormal concentration of Al due to contamination. Typically, blood collected in standard evacuated blood tubes will be contaminated by 20 to 60 µµg/L (0.7 to 2.2 µmol/L) of Al; this is readily demonstrated by collecting blood from a healthy volunteer into a standard evacuated phlebotomy tube. Special evacuated blood collection tubes from commercial suppliers are required for Al testing to avoid sample contamination, which leads to misinterpretation and misdiagnosis.

Analysis of Al is routinely performed by inductively coupled plasma-mass spectrometry (ICP-MS). Alternatively, atomic absorption spectrometry with electrothermal atomization may be employed, but considerable attention must be paid to matrix interferences.

## Regulatory and Occupational Exposure Aspects

Occupational exposure to Al compounds primarily occurs through inhalation of airborne particles in dust and fumes. The solubility of the Al compounds affects their **toxicokinetics** and adds to subsequent health risks. In general, inhaled soluble particles (e.g., aluminum sulfate, hydrated aluminum chloride, and aluminum nitrate) are rapidly absorbed through the lungs, whereas the less or sparsely soluble particles (e.g., aluminum metal, aluminum oxide, aluminum hydroxide, aluminum phosphate, and aluminum silicate) are retained in the lungs and then slowly released into the systemic circulation. The amount of Al absorbed by inhalation also appears to be related to particle size. Al fumes are absorbed more readily than dust particles, and ultrafine nanoparticles of aluminum oxide can penetrate cell membranes.

Biological monitoring of occupational exposure to Al can be determined by analysis of blood, serum, or urine. The concentration of Al in these specimens can be affected by both the intensity of a recent exposure and the Al body burden. Studies of aluminum welders indicate a fair correlation between Al in serum and urine; however, in workers with normal kidney function, urinary Al concentrations are a more sensitive indicator of occupational Al exposure than serum Al values. After exposures to low-level airborne Al, urinary Al concentrations are increased, whereas serum concentrations are generally within the range of control subjects. In chronically exposed welders, the Al concentration in urine collected after 1 or 2 exposure-free days is likely a good indicator for determining the magnitude of the Al stored in the body, whereas in newly exposed workers, the urinary Al concentration is probably more influenced by recent exposures than by the body burden.

## Antimony

Antimony (Sb) compounds have been known since ancient Egyptian times and were used as cosmetics by the women of that era. In the 16th century, Sb preparations were thought to be wonder drugs, and in the 19th century, they were prescribed for various conditions.

### Sources of Exposure

Pure metallic Sb is very brittle; however, alloys of Sb are used in various fields of technology. For example, the addition of

Sb to lead, tin, and copper increases the hardness of these elements when they are used for electrodes, bullets, type metal for printing, and ball bearings. Other uses include fire-resistant chemicals, pigments, and dyes.

Before the introduction of the anthelmintic drug praziquantel, several Sb-containing compounds were used in the treatment of leishmaniasis, a parasitic disease in which protozoa of the genus *Leishmania* are spread by sand flies, and of schistosomiasis, a disease carried by freshwater snails infected with one of the five species of the parasitic flatworm *Schistosoma*.

## Clinical Presentation and Treatment

Symptoms of acute exposure include a metallic taste, headache, nausea, dizziness, and, after a short interval, vomiting, diarrhea, and intestinal spasms. In chronic intoxication, adverse health effects include cardiac arrhythmias, upper respiratory tract and ocular irritation, spontaneous abortion, premature birth, and dermatitis. Lymphocytosis, eosinophilia, and a reduction in leukocyte and platelet counts may also be seen, an indication of liver and spleen damage. Evidence supports increased risk for the development of lung cancer in Sb smelter workers, but the increased risk may be multifactorial, and may be due to, among other factors, the presence of other elements in the work environment. It is important to remember that when intoxication occurs with metallic Sb, the effect may be caused not only by Sb but also by the lead, arsenic, and other elements that may accompany it.

## Preanalytical and Analytical Aspects

Careful selection of specimen tube type, even for certified trace element–free products, is important for the accurate measurement of Sb in blood. ICP-MS is typically used for Sb detection because of its increased sensitivity over that of other instrumentation. Historic methods for Sb measurements in blood have used time-consuming heated acid digestion for achieving better sensitivity, while simplified sample preparation methods have been published more recently.

## Regulatory and Occupational Exposure Aspects

For purposes of biological monitoring after exposure to Sb, urine samples are preferable over blood samples. In one study, urinary Sb concentrations in workers were correlated with the intensity of airborne exposure in nonferrous smelters producing antimony pentoxide and sodium antimonite ($r - 0.86$).

## Arsenic

Arsenic (As) is perhaps the best known of the elemental toxins, having gained notoriety from its extensive use by Renaissance nobility as an antisyphilitic agent and an antidote against acute As poisoning. Long-term administration of low As doses protects against acute poisoning by massive doses—a historic example of hepatic enzyme induction. This agent was memorably used in the well-known tale *Arsenic and Old Lace* as a means of terminating undesirable acquaintances. Arsenic is listed as the number 1 toxicant on the Agency for Toxic

Substances and Disease Registry (ATSDR) 2019 Substance Priority List of Hazardous Substances based on a combination of frequency, toxicity, and potential for human exposure. Despite their inherent toxicity, As-containing compounds are used for therapeutic reasons.

## Sources of Exposure

Nontoxic forms of As are present in many foods with arsenobetaine and arsenocholine, the two most common forms, commonly referred to as organic species. The foods that most commonly contain significant concentrations of these organic As species are shellfish and other predators in the seafood chain (e.g., cod, haddock). In a large US population study, for all participants over 6 years of age, the inorganic As metabolite dimethylarsinic acid (DMA) and arsenobetaine had the greatest contribution to the total urinary As output, with arsenobetaine being the primary contributor.

## Clinical Presentation and Treatment

The symptoms of As toxicity may be nonspecific and often overlap with symptoms of other toxicants. Acute As toxicity can be characterized by GI distress, including vomiting and diarrhea, and cardiac arrhythmias. Chronic toxicity may be characterized by renal failure, cardiac arrhythmias, liver dysfunction, and peripheral neuropathy, and As and its inorganic compounds are known carcinogens. Transverse white bands on the fingernails (Mees lines), hypopigmented macules, hyperpigmentation, and hyperkeratosis have been documented after As exposure.

Arsenic has been shown to interfere with the activity of several heme-biosynthetic enzymes, including aminolevulinate synthase, porphobilinogen deaminase, uroporphyrinogen III synthase, uroporphyrinogen decarboxylate, coproporphyrinogen oxidase, ferrochelatase, and heme oxygenase with resultant increases in COPRO/URO and COPRO I/III ratios. Interestingly, the madness of King George III, historically attributed to acute hereditary porphyria, has been hypothesized to instead be a case of arsenic-induced porphyria based on retrospective analyses of hair.

An effective antidote for treating As intoxication is BAL; the active agent in BAL is dimercaprol, a sulfhydryl-reducing agent. BAL was originally developed during World War II in response to the use of Lewisite, an As-based chemical warfare agent. Other dimercaprol derivatives are available for treatment, including DMSA (succimer) and dimercapto-1-propanesulfonic acid (DMPS), although the latter is not currently approved for As chelation therapy in the United States.

## Preanalytical and Analytical Aspects

To distinguish among toxic inorganic species, high-performance liquid chromatography (HPLC) techniques for evaluating biological fluids and tissues have been developed. In general, a 24-hour urine specimen with measurable arsenic will have 95% present as the organic, nontoxic species and less than 5% present as the inorganic toxic species. Despite the availability of HPLC-ICP-MS methods for As speciation, it is noted that the use of a screening method for total As before speciation is of outstanding utility in reducing unnecessary costs.

Hair analysis is frequently used to document the time of As exposure. Circulating in the blood, it will bind to protein by formation of a covalent complex with sulfhydryl groups of the amino acid cysteine. Because As has a high affinity for keratin, which has high cysteine content, the As concentration in hair or nails is greater than in other tissues. Several weeks after exposure, transverse white striae, called Mees lines, may appear in the fingernails, caused by denaturation of keratin by elements such as As, Cd, Pb, and Hg. Because hair grows at a rate of approximately 1 cm/month, hair collected from the nape of the neck can be used to document recent exposure. Axillary or pubic hair is used to document long-term (6 months to 1 year) exposure. Hair As greater than 1 µg/g dry weight indicates excessive exposure, though reports vary for results determined in hair due to analytical, environmental, and dietary factors. In one study, the highest hair As observed was 210 µg/g dry weight in a case of chronic exposure that was the cause of death.

The body treats As like phosphate, incorporating it wherever phosphate would be incorporated. Absorbed As is rapidly circulated and distributed into tissue storage sites. Blood is the least useful specimen for identifying As exposure, as blood As concentrations are elevated for only a short time after administration and rapidly disappear into the large body phosphate pool. Abnormal blood As concentrations are detected for only a few hours (<4 hours) after ingestion. This test is useful only to document an acute exposure when the As is likely to be greater than 20 ng/mL (0.3 µmol/L) for a short period. Typically, serum As is less than 40 ng/mL (0.5 µmol/L).

Arsenic has been accurately measured by ICP-MS. Mass response from the argon plasma is monitored for As (mass-to-charge ratio $[m/z] = 75$); however, the method must reduce the potential for interference from argon chloride ($m/z = 75$) with the use of a dynamic reaction cell or collision cell with kinetic energy discrimination. For more details on the ICP-MS technology, refer to Chapter 13. Urine is the sample of choice for As analysis because As is excreted predominantly by the kidney.

### Regulatory and Occupational Exposure Aspects

Cardiovascular diseases and cerebrovascular effects are associated with chronic exposures to inorganic As compounds in the workplace. Inhalation exposures to inorganic As compounds have been correlated with an increased incidence of lung cancer. The American Conference of Governmental Industrial Hygienists (ACGIH) classifies As and its inorganic compounds as A1 carcinogens (confirmed human carcinogens). The recommended ACGIH Biological Exposure Index (BEI) for inorganic As plus methylated metabolites is less than 35 µg/L (0.5 µmol/L) in an end-of-workweek urine sample after the exposure to As and soluble inorganic compounds (excluding gallium arsenide and arsine). After exposures to poorly soluble inorganic compounds, such as gallium arsenide, the urinary As concentration is more representative of

the amount absorbed rather than the total dose inhaled or ingested.

## Cadmium

An appreciation for the toxicity of cadmium (Cd) extends back to 1858 and the observed GI and respiratory effects after exposure to Cd-containing polishing agents. Famously, Cd toxicity was at the center of *itai-itai* disease (Japanese for "Ouch-Ouch"), a bone disease associated with fractures and severe pain that was identified after World War II in Japan. No biological function has been identified for Cd in humans; however, Cd serves as a metal cofactor of Cd-carbonic anhydrase in diatoms.

### Sources of Exposure

Cd is a by-product of zinc and lead smelting. It is used in industry in electroplating, in the production of rechargeable batteries and solar panels, as a common pigment in organic-based paints, and in tobacco products. Spray painting of organic-based paints without the use of a protective breathing apparatus is a common source of chronic exposure. Auto repair mechanics are a work group that has significant opportunity for exposure to Cd.

### Clinical Presentation and Treatment

Chronic exposure to Cd causes accumulated renal damage. Breathing the fumes of Cd vapors leads to nasal epithelial deterioration and pulmonary congestion resembling chronic emphysema. Renal dysfunction with proteinuria of slow onset (over a period of years) is the typical presentation. Normal blood Cd concentration is less than 5 ng/mL (44 nmol/L), with most concentrations in the interval of 0.5 to 2 ng/mL (4 to 18 nmol/L). Moderately increased blood Cd (3 to 7 ng/mL or 27 to 62 nmol/L) may be associated with tobacco use. Acute toxicity is observed when the blood concentration exceeds 50 ng/mL (444 nmol/L). Usual daily excretion of Cd is less than 3 µg/day (0.03 µmol/day). Cd concentrations also increase with age and may be involved with senescence.

### Preanalytical and Analytical Aspects

Collection of urine samples using a rubber catheter has been known to result in elevated results because rubber contains trace amounts of Cd that are extracted as urine passes through it. Brightly colored plastic urine collection containers should be avoided because the pigment in the plastic may be Cd-based. Cd has historically been quantified by atomic absorption spectrometry, and more recently by ICP-MS.

### Regulatory and Occupational Exposure Aspects

Inhalation is the primary route of Cd exposure in the occupational setting, and the amount absorbed from the lungs depends on the solubility of the Cd compound and particle size. Absorption through the GI tract can occur from the clearance of particles deposited in the lungs and from contaminated hands and food. After chronic low-level exposures, approximately half of the Cd body burden is stored in the liver and kidneys. Urine is the main route of elimination, and thus urinary Cd concentrations are widely used to biomonitor chronic exposures in workers. However, because of the high binding capacity for Cd in the body, a urine concentration may provide no information about exposure in someone newly exposed to Cd. The lag time needed before the urinary Cd concentration correlates with exposure depends on the intensity of the integrated exposure. Until sufficient time of chronic Cd exposure has passed before urine testing can be used appropriately (~1 year), blood testing is suggested for newly exposed workers or when changes in exposure occur, because blood values primarily reflect recent exposures.

The exposure assessment of Cd in the US Occupational Safety and Health Administration (OSHA) Cadmium Standard is part of an overall periodic environmental, medical, and biological monitoring program. Biomonitoring requires testing of urine for both Cd and $\beta_2$-microglobulin with standardization to grams of creatinine for each component ($\mu$g/g creatinine) and of blood for Cd with standardization to liters of whole blood ($\mu$g/L).

## Chromium

Chromium (Cr), from the Greek word *chroma* ("color"), makes rubies red and emeralds green. Among its many uses, it is best known for its application in making stainless steel, which is resistant to corrosion and discoloration. The requirement of Cr for sugar and lipid metabolism has resulted in considerable debate on its potential role in insulin resistance. In recent years, Cr has made headlines as one of several metal ions released with wear because of highly publicized recalls of misaligned and accelerated failure rates of specific metal-on-metal (MoM) prosthetics.

### Sources of Exposure

Occupational exposure to Cr represents a significant health hazard. Cr is used extensively (1) in the manufacture of stainless steel, (2) in chrome plating, (3) in the tanning of leather, (4) as a pigment in paints and dye for printing and textile manufacture, (5) as a cleaning solution, and (6) as an anticorrosive in cooling systems. The toxic form of Cr is hexavalent $Cr^{6+}$ (Cr[VI]), and a strong oxidizing environment is required to convert the common form trivalent $Cr^{3+}$ (Cr[III]) to $Cr^{6+}$. This can occur when $Cr^{3+}$ is exposed to high temperatures in the presence of oxygen or during high-voltage electroplating.

Considerable attention has been given to Cr toxicity after release of Cr ions during normal and abnormal wear of MoM prosthetics. However, the vast majority of Cr released from MoM prosthetics has been shown to be in the trivalent form, which is considerably less toxic than hexavalent Cr. In May 2011, the US Food and Drug Administration (FDA) issued orders for postmarketing surveillance studies to manufacturers of MoM hip replacement systems in response to increasing concern over failed implant devices reported in Europe. In the United States, no guidelines have been established for the assessment of metal ions in asymptomatic patients because of a lack of knowledge regarding the prevalence of adverse events in the US population and no clear threshold values associated with an adverse event.

### Clinical Presentation and Treatment

Symptoms associated with Cr toxicity vary based on the route of exposure, Cr species, and dose, and may include dermatitis, impairment of pulmonary function, gastroenteritis, hepatic necrosis, bleeding, and acute tubular necrosis. In the case of failing MoM prosthetics, elevated Cr in serum or blood is rarely the initial finding and instead is preceded by more telling physical symptoms such as reduced range of motion, swelling and inflammation around the joint, and general discomfort or pain. Although offered by many laboratories, measurement of Cr in joint fluid has relatively little clinical utility.

### Preanalytical and Analytical Aspects

Use of a plastic cannula for blood sampling was shown to be unnecessary in the assessment of Cr; however, sporadic contamination from stainless steel needles was observed. Quantification of total Cr in urine can be used to assess exposure to all forms of Cr. The presence of Cr in erythrocytes is suggestive of exposure to $Cr^{6+}$ within the past 120 days, because $Cr^{6+}$ crosses biological membranes but $Cr^{3+}$ does not. Increased serum Cr concentrations are observed in association with orthopedic implants made from Cr alloys. ICP-MS is the preferred technology for quantification of Cr in body fluids but suffers from considerable interference because of polyatomics. Use of dynamic reactive cell technology or a collision cell with kinetic energy discrimination is required for reproducible and accurate measurements.

### Regulatory and Occupational Exposure Aspects

Industrial Cr exposures can involve trivalent and hexavalent forms, which exhibit different toxicokinetics and toxicities in the body. Urine Cr concentrations are the most useful biomarker for assessing occupational exposure to water-soluble hexavalent Cr compounds; however, other nonoccupational sources of both trivalent and hexavalent Cr from the diet, supplements, and the environment can contribute to the total Cr concentration in urine. Furthermore, because Cr has been shown to accumulate in the body, urine Cr values can be affected by both recent and past workplace exposures. The measurement of Cr in erythrocytes has been used to gauge the intensity of exposure to hexavalent Cr; however, insufficient data are available to determine a relationship between erythrocyte Cr concentrations and the risks associated with exposures.

Occupational exposures to hexavalent Cr compounds can cause respiratory irritation and tissue damage of the nose, throat, and lungs after inhalation, and can cause irritation, burns, and ulcers on the skin with contact. Hexavalent Cr has been associated with cancers of the lungs, nose, and nasal sinuses, and is classified as a human carcinogen by the Internal Agency for Research on Cancer (IARC). Hexavalent Cr compounds are categorized as human carcinogens by the ACGIH (A1) and the German Research Foundation (DFG) in Germany (category 1). The ACGIH suggests testing total Cr in urine for workplace exposure to hexavalent Cr (water-soluble fumes).

## Cobalt

The word cobalt (Co) is derived from the German *kobalt* meaning "goblin" because of its superstitious reputation among miners. Cobalt is widely distributed in the environment, is the essential cofactor in vitamin $B_{12}$, and has been widely used throughout history for decorative accents to glass and ceramics.

### Sources of Exposure

Although relatively rare, Co is widely distributed in nature and is found in green vegetables, animal foods, and seafood. Of the Co in the body, 85% is in the form of cyanocobalamin or vitamin $B_{12}$, a Co complex similar in structure to that of porphyrins. Cobalt is used in alloys in which the presence of Co results in high melting point, strength, and resistance to oxygen. The addition of Co in MoM prosthetics adds resistance to surfaces undergoing heavy wear, and the release of Co from failed prosthetics remains of outstanding concern. Cobalt is found in rechargeable batteries and provides color to plastics, inks, glass, and paint.

### Clinical Presentation and Treatment

Cobalt is not highly toxic, but large exposures will cause pulmonary edema, allergy, nausea, vomiting, hemorrhage, and renal failure. Occupational exposure occurs during production and machining of metal alloys and has been known to result in interstitial lung disease. Cardiomyopathy and renal failure are symptomatic of acute Co exposure; this was exemplified by an incident of mass population exposure to Co when beer contaminated with cobalt salts was consumed. Chronic exposure may cause pulmonary syndrome, skin irritation, allergy, GI irritation, nausea, cardiomyopathy, hematologic disorders, and thyroid abnormalities. Cobalt exposure alone may not lead to toxicity and must be considered within the context of exposure to multiple elements.

Serum Co concentrations are increased above normal (>1 µg/L or >17 nmol/L) in patients with well-positioned and functioning orthopedic implants made from Co alloys. Considerable attention has been given to Co toxicity in the context of failed MoM prosthetics, with several case reports of severe neurologic and cardiac abnormalities described. In the case of failing MoM prosthetics, elevated Co in serum or blood is rarely the initial finding and instead is preceded by more telling physical symptoms such as reduced range of motion, swelling and inflammation around the joint, and general discomfort or pain. Although offered by several laboratories, measurement of Co in joint fluid has relatively little clinical utility.

### Preanalytical and Analytical Aspects

Quantification of active vitamin $B_{12}$ is the usual way to assess nutritional status; quantification of serum, blood, or urine Co concentration is not typical for assessing vitamin $B_{12}$ status. Cobalt deficiency has not been reported in humans. Quantification of Co in urine or biological specimens is accomplished by atomic absorption spectrometry or by ICP-MS.

### Regulatory and Occupational Exposure Aspects

Absorption of Co through the lungs from inhalation of dust and fumes is the primary route of exposure in occupational settings, but absorption from dermal contact can occur. Pulmonary absorption of the inhaled Co depends on the particle size and its solubility, with smaller particles deposited in the lower respiratory tract, where they dissolve or are phagocytized and translocated. After inhalation, Co is eliminated from the body in several phases with a relatively rapid initial phase having a half-life ranging from hours to a few days and subsequent slower phases with half-lives ranging from months to years. Cobalt concentrations in urine increase proportionally more than in the blood of workers during Co exposures; Co concentrations in urine are primarily affected by recent exposures but increase through the workweek under stable exposure conditions.

The skin and respiratory tract are the two main target organs in workers exposed to cobalt metal, cobalt salts, and cobalt-containing dust. Contact of Co with the skin can cause mild irritation and allergic reactions. Inhaled cobalt dust and fumes can cause shortness of breath. Respiratory symptoms after chronic inhalation of Co can range from cough to respiratory hypersensitivity, progressive dyspnea, decreased pulmonary function, permanent disability, and death. Pathogenic lesions in the parenchymal regions of the lungs, known as "hard metal disease", can lead to severe alveolitis that progresses to end-stage pulmonary fibrosis. In the hard metal industry, the coexposure to tungsten and Co has proved more toxic than metallic Co alone.

## Lead

Lead (Pb) has been used extensively throughout history, but its use has been drastically reduced in the last few decades as a result of a better appreciation for its toxicity, especially during early childhood development.

### Sources of Exposure

Lead was present at high concentrations (up to 35% w/w) in many paints manufactured before 1972. The Pb content of paints intended for household use was limited to less than 0.5% in 1978, but Pb is still found in paint products intended for nondomestic use and in artists' pigments. Ceramic products for use in homes available from noncommercial suppliers (e.g., local artists) have been known to contain significant amounts of Pb; Pb is leached from the products by weak acids such as vinegar and fruit juices. Leaded crystal contains up to 10% Pb, which is leached during long-term storage of fluids such as fruit juice, wine, and spirits. Lead is also found in dirt from areas adjacent to homes painted with Pb-based paints, in soil near abandoned industrial sites, and on highways where it has accumulated from the use of leaded gasoline in automobiles. Use of leaded gasoline has diminished significantly since the introduction of unleaded gasoline, which has been required in personal automobiles in the United States since 1978. Water transported through Pb or Pb-soldered pipes contains some Pb, with higher concentrations found in water that is weakly acidic. Some foods (e.g., moonshine distilled in Pb pipes) and some traditional home medicines also contain Pb. Exposure to Pb from any of these sources by ingestion, inhalation, or dermal contact has been known to cause significant toxicity.

## Clinical Presentation and Treatment

The development of Pb toxicity follows a progressive pattern. Fig. 32.2 describes this progression through a series of symptoms.

The finding that Pb contributes significantly to decreased intellectual capability in the very young is of particular concern. Young children are particularly prone to the effects of Pb because they have greater opportunity for exposure. Children tend to spend a lot of time on the floor. In older homes that have been previously treated with Pb-based paints, Pb-laden paint chips and dust accumulate on the floor, which children are likely to ingest. The Centers for Disease Control and Prevention (CDC) has continued to lower the suggested normal limit for children and is now recommending 3.5 μg/dL (0.17 μmol/L) based on the 97.5% percentile of nonexposed children. In addition, the term *blood lead level of concern* has been abandoned in favor of the viewpoint that all Pb is potentially harmful and therefore unsafe.

The World Health Organization (WHO) has previously defined blood Pb concentrations greater than 30 μg/dL (1.5 μmol/L) in adults as indicative of significant exposure. In 2021, WHO indicated that blood Pb concentrations greater than or equal to 5 μg/dL (1.5 μmol/L) should prompt identification of sources of exposure and action to reduce and terminate exposure. Pb concentrations above 60 μg/dL (2.9 μmol/L) require chelation therapy with lower thresholds recommended for women of childbearing age. Similar to the outcomes reported in children, adult blood Pb concentrations have dropped to a median value of less than 1 μg/dL (0.05 μmol/L) for individuals 20 and older with a 95th percentile of 2.8 μg/dL (0.14 μmol/L).

Avoidance of continued exposure to Pb is paramount when blood Pb concentrations exceed acceptable reference intervals. Oral dimercaprol has become a standard therapy and is being used in the outpatient setting for all except those with the most severe Pb poisoning. Although chelation therapy is effective in reducing blood Pb concentrations, a 2003 study indicated that chelation therapy given to preschool children with Pb concentrations in the range of 20 to 44 μg/dL (1 to 2.1 μmol/L) showed no beneficial effect on tests of cognition or behavior. Thus, prevention is the best therapeutic option.

## Preanalytical and Analytical Aspects

The definitive test for Pb toxicity is measurement of blood Pb. Analysis of Pb is routinely performed by ICP-MS, electrothermal atomic absorption spectrometry, or anodic stripping voltammetry. Because Pb is concentrated in the erythrocytes, EDTA-anticoagulated blood is the specimen of choice for Pb analysis. Sodium heparin may also be used; however, samples that are not analyzed within 48 hours are frequently clotted and must be rejected. Care must be taken when obtaining capillary blood. Surface contamination, insufficient collection volume, or inadequate mixing with EDTA results in frequent sample rejection. Urinalysis can also be performed; urine quantification correlates with exposure.

If ICP-MS is used to measure Pb concentrations, it is essential to sum the masses of 206, 207, and 208 *m/z* to account for the natural isotopic variation of Pb in the environment. Failure to sum masses could skew results above or below the actual concentration because the isotopic abundance of a particular mass in the calibrator might not match the sample. Interestingly, this isotopic variation has been exploited previously to determine the source of Pb exposure. By determining the relative abundances of Pb in blood and of potential sources of exposure (e.g., paint chips, soil), it may be possible to identify a matching pattern. The exposure source with the same ratio of major Pb isotopes as that of the blood should then be avoided or removed from the patient's environment.

## Regulatory and Occupational Exposure Aspects

Biomarkers of exposure and biomarkers of effect have been used in assessing occupational Pb exposures. The direct

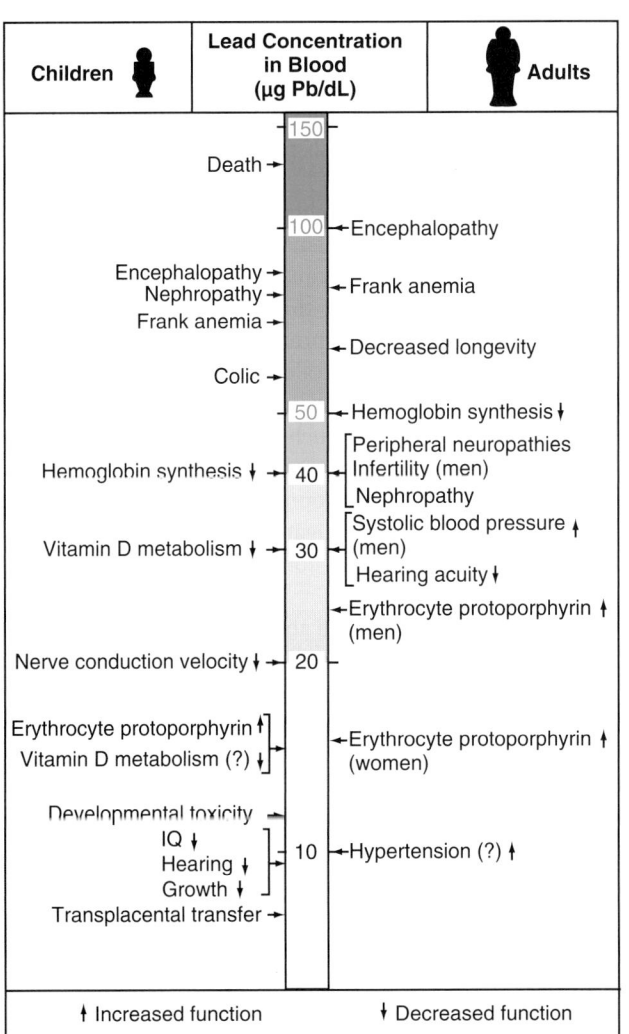

**Fig. 32.2** Effects of inorganic lead on children and adults (lowest observable adverse effect concentrations). (Reprinted with permission from Royce SE, Needleman HL, eds. *Case Studies in Environmental Medicine: Lead Toxicity*. Atlanta, GA: United States Public Health Service, Agency for Toxic Substances and Disease Registry; 1990.)

measurement of Pb in blood reflects the concentration of Pb in the soft tissues at a steady state, and therefore is an indicator of recent exposures. Most of the Pb body burden is stored in bones, so the bone Pb concentrations are a good indicator of cumulative or long-term exposures. X-ray fluorescence techniques are used to measure Pb concentrations in bone.

Exposures to Pb have been found to cause encephalopathy, peripheral neuropathy, neurologic and neurobehavioral effects, renal effects, hypertension, and reduced fertility. Because of these adverse effects, the OSHA has enacted standards to assess inorganic Pb exposure in the workplace. Workers with a single blood Pb concentration meeting the numerical criteria for medical removal must have their blood Pb values retested within 2 weeks. If a worker is medically removed, a new blood Pb concentration must be measured monthly during the removal period. Workers are permitted to return to work when their blood Pb concentration is 40 μg/dL (1.9 μmol/L) or less, according to current guidelines. However, a reported employee blood lead concentration of 25 μg/dL (1.2 μmol/L) is considered serious by OSHA and is to be handled by inspection.

According to the OSHA Lead Standards, measurement of zinc protoporphyrin (ZPP) is required on each occasion that a blood Pb measurement is made. OSHA recommends a hematocrit determination to exclude anemia whenever a confirmed ZPP of 50 μg/100 mL (0.8 μmol/L) is obtained. ZPP concentrations in excess of 100 μg/100 mL (80 μmol/L) are considered elevated. However, ZPP is an insensitive biomarker for blood Pb values less than approximately 20 μg/dL or 1 μmol/L.

## Mercury

Mercury's elemental symbol, Hg, is derived from the Greek word *hydrargyros*, meaning "water silver," and is commonly referred to as quicksilver. Mercury is one of only two elements that are liquid at standard temperature and pressure (the other is bromine). The various forms of Hg have remarkably different toxicity profiles from largely benign unless inhaled (elemental Hg), to highly toxic (Hg salts and organic forms). The phrase "mad as a hatter" was first used in reference to the Hg-induced dementia seen in workers with chronic exposure to Hg in the production of felt for hats.

### Sources of Exposure

Mercury is widely found in the environment and occurs both naturally and as the result of industrial processes, with the single largest source of Hg being its natural out-gassing from granite rock. Mercury is also found in deposits throughout the world, mostly as cinnabar (mercuric sulfide), which is the source of the red pigment vermilion.

In the past, Hg was extensively used in the manufacture of devices such as thermometers, barometers, manometers, and sphygmomanometers. However, concerns about its toxicity have resulted in the phasing out of Hg-based instruments, which have been replaced with alcohol-filled, digital, or thermistor-based versions. It is still used as a dental amalgam

and in lighting as mercury vapor lamps, although these are being replaced by sodium vapor bulbs. Mercury is used in the pulp and paper industry as a whitener, as a catalyst in the synthesis of plastics, and as a potent fungicide in antifouling and latex paints.

Chemically, it is possible to convert Hg from its elemental state to its ionized state; in industry, this is frequently accomplished by exposing $Hg^0$ to a strong oxidant, such as chlorine. Elemental Hg is also bioconverted to both $Hg^{2+}$ and alkyl Hg by microorganisms that exist in the normal human gut and in the bottom sediment of lakes and rivers. When $Hg^0$ enters bottom sediment, it is absorbed by bacteria, fungi, and related microorganisms; these organisms metabolically convert it to $Hg^{2+}$, $CH_3Hg^+$, $CH_3CH_2Hg^+$, and similar species. Consequently, the methyl mercurials are accumulated in the aquatic food chain and reach their highest concentrations in predatory fish. The normal bacterial flora present in the mouth converts a fraction of $Hg^{2+}$ to $CH_3Hg^+$; the latter has been shown to be incorporated into body tissue. As a consequence of accumulation of methylmercury in the aquatic food chain, most human exposure to Hg happens through the eating of contaminated fish, shellfish, and sea mammals. The US Environmental Protection Agency (EPA) maintains up-to-date guidance regarding the highest allowable average mercury concentration in fish per serving based on weekly fish servings.

In the late 1980s, the public became concerned about exposure to Hg from dental amalgams. However, later studies have failed to confirm a causal relationship. Basic to the initial concerns was the fact that restorative dentistry used an Hg-silver amalgam for approximately 90 years as a filling material. In 1989, Hahn and colleagues showed that a small (2 to 20 μg/day) release of $Hg^0$ from amalgam occurs when it is mechanically manipulated, such as by chewing. In addition, the habit of gum chewing can cause release of Hg from dental amalgams in even larger amounts. In 2010, the FDA issued rules that classify dental amalgam, reclassify dental mercury, and specify special controls for dental amalgam, mercury, and amalgam alloy.

Concerns have been raised about the possible relationship between Hg exposure from vaccines and autistic disorders. In the United States, the prevalence of autism has risen from 1 in approximately 2500 in the mid-1980s to 1 in approximately 300 children in the mid-1990s. Some investigators believe that this rise occurs because of the Hg that is present in vaccines as the preservative thimerosal (sodium ethyl mercury thiosulfate). However, this causality has been questioned by numerous other studies, which have not been able to confirm this relationship. In 2001, the Committee on Immunization Safety Review of the Board on Health Promotion and Disease Prevention of the Institute of Medicine initiated a study to review the connection between Hg-containing vaccines and neurodevelopmental disorders, including autism. The Committee reported that the hypothesis was biologically plausible, but that evidence was insufficient to accept or reject a causal connection. The findings of this report have been challenged, and thimerosal has been removed from most vaccines in the United States. The evidence linking Hg exposure from vaccines with autistic disorders has been highly criticized and resulted in the journal *Lancet* retracting the article linking autism to measles, mumps, and rubella (MMR) vaccines.

Historically, Hg-containing compounds have been used for therapeutic reasons. For example, Hg has been used in medications that were touted as cures for syphilis and dysentery, to treat constipation, and as diuretics. Intriguingly, the use of Hg-containing laxatives, termed "Thunder Clappers," on the Corps of Discovery Expedition with Lewis and Clark has left a discoverable trail of their movements, in more ways than one!

## Clinical Presentation and Treatment

Each form of Hg manifests differently after a toxic exposure. For elemental Hg, poor absorption in the GI system reduces toxicity but can result in GI distress with prolonged contact or deposition. With repeated injections of elemental Hg, seen in suicide attempts or psychiatric patients, the presentation was predominantly pleuritic chest pain, with other classic Hg-associated symptoms being absent. Common target organs with inorganic Hg poisoning include the GI system, kidneys, and brain.

Experience with Hg poisoning has been gained from investigation of the 1951 to 1963 industrial dumping of Hg-laden waste sludge into Minamata Bay, Japan. Fish in Minamata Bay became heavily laden with Hg through the food chain. The local human population, whose diet depended on fish from the bay, exhibited symptoms of methylmercury poisoning, including ataxia, impaired speech, visual field constriction, hearing loss, and somatosensory change, characterized histologically by cerebral cortex necrosis; this is collectively known as Minamata disease.

In adults, cases of methylmercury poisoning are characterized by the focal degeneration of neurons in regions of the brain such as the cerebral cortex and the cerebellum. Depending on the degree of in utero exposure, methylmercury may result in effects ranging from fetal death to subtle neurodevelopmental delays. Consequently, because pregnant women, women of childbearing age, and young children are particularly at risk, the EPA and FDA provide specific recommendations regarding fish consumption based on age and physical activity.

## Preanalytical and Analytical Aspects

Analysis of blood, urine, and hair for Hg concentrations is used to determine exposure. The quantity of Hg found in blood and urine correlates with the degree of toxicity, although the form of Hg can negatively affect the reliability of the relationship. Hair analysis has been used historically to document the time of peak exposure. However, it should be noted that hair analysis for elements, in general, is difficult to interpret because of contamination. Normal whole-blood Hg concentration is usually lower than 10 µg/L (49 nmol/L). Treatment with BAL or penicillamine will mobilize Hg, allowing for its excretion in the urine. Therapy is usually monitored by following urinary excretion of Hg; therapy may be terminated after the daily urine excretion rate falls below 50 µg/L (249 nmol/L).

## Regulatory and Occupational Exposure Aspects

In industry, elemental Hg is present in the air as a vapor and its inorganic salts are present as aerosols. Inhalation is the primary route of uptake from occupational exposures to Hg, although dermal absorption can also occur. Once absorbed, some elemental Hg is oxidized to the divalent form, which can bind to sulfhydryl groups in proteins such as albumin and metallothionein. Elemental Hg is mainly distributed to the kidney and brain, whereas inorganic Hg salts are mostly delivered to the kidney. Mercury is eliminated primarily through the feces and urine. Initially after exposure, more Hg may be eliminated in the feces than in the urine. This may be due to the presence of binding sites in the kidneys. The half-life of Hg in urine is approximately 40 days. Therefore, the Hg values in urine do not necessarily reflect recent exposures in newly exposed workers.

Urinary Hg concentrations are primarily used to monitor long-term exposures to elemental Hg and its inorganic salts, whereas blood Hg concentrations are mainly useful for short-term, higher-level exposures of these compounds. Urine is the preferred specimen for biological monitoring of workplace exposure to elemental Hg and its inorganic compounds, because Hg concentrations in blood can be affected by the presence of organic Hg compounds from the consumption of dietary fish. Because biological monitoring in urine reflects long-term Hg exposures, the airborne exposure values and urinary Hg concentration can be correlated, provided the exposures are relatively constant over a sufficiently long period, sample collection is standardized, and biomonitoring is initiated at least 6 months after exposure begins.

## Nickel

Found in coins since the mid-19th century, nickel (Ni) remains valuable for its corrosion resistance in plating but is often found at the center of reports involving hypersensitivity and allergic reactions to a wider range of products from cell phones to belt buckles.

## Sources of Exposure

Ni is frequently used in the production of metal alloys (which are popular for their anticorrosive and hardness properties), in Ni-based rechargeable batteries, and as a catalyst in the hydrogenation of oils. Ni alloyed with transition metals is considered nontoxic, except that it will induce inflammation at the point of contact. Nickel carbonyl ($Ni[CO]_4$), used in petroleum refining, is one of the most toxic chemicals known to humans.

In nonindustrial settings, Ni is found in a wide variety of consumer products, including utensils, jewelry, eyeglass frames, clothing buttons, braces, orthopedic implants, and some varieties of cell phones. Despite its incorporation into MoM prosthetics and increased concern with failed MoM devices (see earlier section on "Chromium"), Ni has not been implicated as a significant contributor to the associated clinical presentation.

## Clinical Presentation and Treatment

Contact dermatitis is the symptom often associated with Ni exposure in the nonoccupational setting. Ni allergy is a common contact allergen because of its ubiquitous use in jewelry and cosmetic products. Patch test studies have demonstrated a strong dose-response relationship between degree of exposure and severity of symptoms.

Patients exposed to Ni carbonyl exhibit rapid onset of pulmonary congestion and inability to oxygenate hemoglobin, followed by development of lesions of the lung, liver, kidney, adrenal glands, and spleen. Patients undergoing dialysis are exposed to Ni and accumulate Ni in their blood and other organs.

## Preanalytical and Analytical Aspects

Use of a plastic cannula for blood sampling was shown to be unnecessary in the assessment of Ni; however, sporadic contamination from stainless steel needles was observed.

## Regulatory and Occupational Exposure Aspects

Workplace exposures to various forms of Ni occur in a variety of industrial processes. Exposure to sparingly soluble Ni compounds, such as nickel sulfide, nickel oxide, nickel carbonate, and nickel sulfidic ores, generally occurs during the mining of nickel ores, the smelting and refining processes, and the grinding and welding of Ni-containing alloys. The electroplating industry is usually the main source of workplace exposures to soluble forms of Ni such as nickel acetate, nickel chloride, nickel hydroxide, and nickel sulfate. Exposure to nickel carbonyl (or nickel tetracarbonyl), an easily absorbed and highly toxic form of Ni, likely occurs in Ni refining, nickel coatings, plating glass, and as a catalyst in chemical reactions.

Occupational Ni exposure mainly occurs by inhalation of dust from sparingly soluble Ni compounds, aerosols from soluble Ni solutions, or gaseous Ni generally from nickel carbonyl. Skin contact with airborne Ni and Ni-containing solutions is also possible, as is oral ingestion in facilities with poor industrial hygiene practices and among workers who practice poor personal hygiene. The solubility of the Ni compound will affect the toxicokinetics of Ni in the body. Soluble Ni compounds are more rapidly absorbed and eliminated compared to the poorly soluble forms. Inhaled particles of sparingly soluble Ni compounds can be retained in the lung tissue and regional lymph nodes, where they can accumulate and gradually be released over time. The major elimination route for absorbed Ni is through the kidneys and into the urine.

The toxicities of most significance after occupational exposure to Ni are the allergenic and carcinogenic effects. Ni exposure can cause sensitization of the skin (e.g., contact dermatitis) and respiratory tract. Occupational exposure to Ni compounds can also increase the risk for lung and nasal cancer in workers. The IARC classifies Ni compounds as human carcinogens (group 1). Biological monitoring of Ni concentrations in body fluids after occupational Ni exposure has been extensively studied in workers, and Ni concentrations in body fluids are affected by the chemical species of the Ni to which the individual was exposed, and the time of sample collection. For example, the American Conference of Governmental Industrial Hygienists or ACGIH has different BEIs in urine for occupational exposures to nickel compounds based on the solubility of the Ni compound. However, elevated Ni concentrations in body fluids may not be directly correlated with exposure levels or risk for disease possibly because of the differences in solubility of the exposure compound and, therefore, only provide information about Ni uptake.

## Thallium

Thallium (Tl) is often referred to as the "poisoner's poison" because it is nearly tasteless and highly toxic in low doses. Isotopes of Tl are used in diagnostic imaging and were once used medicinally to treat ringworm.

### Sources of Exposure

Thallium is a by-product of zinc and lead smelting and cadmium production. Interest in Tl derives primarily from its former use as a rodenticide, with accidental exposure being the most likely reason for toxicity. Acute and often fatal poisoning has been reported after criminal use and suicide attempts. Additionally, environmental concerns are growing because Tl is a waste product of coal combustion and the manufacturing of cement. Thallium is used in photoelectric cells, lamps, semiconductors, and scintillation counters.

### Clinical Presentation and Treatment

The clinical presentation of Tl toxicity varies based on dose, age, and acute or chronic exposure. Patients exposed to high doses of Tl (>1 g) demonstrate alopecia (hair loss), peripheral neuropathy, seizures, and renal failure. Peripheral neuropathy of the feet and, less commonly, the hands occurs within 1 week after exposure, and hair loss begins at the same time and continues for several weeks. GI symptoms, including pain, diarrhea, and constipation, have been reported in acute ingestion, in addition to myalgias, pleuritic chest pain, insomnia, optic neuritis, hypertension, cardiac abnormalities, Mees lines, and liver injury.

### Preanalytical and Analytical Aspects

Typical serum concentrations in the absence of significant exposure are less than 10 ng/mL (49 nmol/L), and daily urine excretion is less than 10 µg/day (49 nmol/day). Exposed patients have been observed to have serum concentrations as high as 50 ng/mL (245 nmol/L), with urine output in excess of 500 µg/day (2446 nmol/day). Tl is routinely measured by ICP-MS in blood and urine.

### Regulatory and Occupational Exposure Aspects

Urine is the suggested specimen for biological monitoring of Tl. Although there is insufficient information available correlating occupational exposure values and urinary Tl concentrations to establish a threshold value, the biological monitoring of Tl in urine can assist in assessing the effectiveness of workplace control measures, especially because the ACGIH gives Tl and Tl compounds a "skin" notation, designating the potential for a significant contribution to the overall exposure by the cutaneous route. For exposures to Tl and inorganic Tl compounds, the Finnish Institute of Occupational Health (FIOH) has no established biomonitoring action limit but recommends testing for Tl in a post-shift urine specimen.

## REVIEW QUESTIONS

1. An individual has eaten a large meal of seafood, including shellfish and haddock, before submitting a urine specimen for analysis. What element would likely be present in a high concentration in his urine specimen?
   a. Arsenic
   b. Copper
   c. Mercury
   d. Cadmium
2. Lead inhibits _____, an enzyme that catalyzes synthesis of heme from porphyrin.
   a. ATPase
   b. RNA polymerase
   c. glutathione peroxidase
   d. aminolevulinic acid dehydratase
3. Which of the following reasons best explains why elemental toxicity is difficult to diagnose?
   a. Physicians are poorly informed about prevalence of toxic elements.
   b. Laboratories are unable to properly test for toxic elements.
   c. Signs and symptoms in elemental toxicity mirror numerous disease states.
   d. Elemental toxicity is relatively rare in developed countries.
4. Analysis of toxic elements is recommended in which of the following presentations?
   a. Renal disease due to chronic hypertension
   b. Unexplained, bilateral neuropathy
   c. Chronic inflammation of the liver
   d. No history of exposure on record
5. Which of the following correctly identifies an accepted approach to elemental exposure?
   a. Wait and see if symptoms become more severe
   b. Prospective chelation challenges with post-chelation laboratory assessments
   c. Enhanced absorption
   d. Antidotal treatment

6. The toxicity of Cd, As, Hg, and Pb is similar in regard to damage of which organ?
   a. Eye
   b. Kidney
   c. Pancreas
   d. Distal phalanges
7. Which element in its hexavalent state is toxic, while in its trivalent state it is considered largely benign?
   a. Cr
   b. Hg
   c. Pb
   d. As
8. Which element in its elemental state is largely benign unless inhaled, while its inorganic form is the basis for the phrase "mad as a hatter"?
   a. As
   b. Cr
   c. Pb
   d. Hg
9. Regarding Ni exposure, _____ Ni compounds are more rapidly absorbed and eliminated compared to the _____ forms.
   a. soluble, gaseous
   b. insoluble, soluble
   c. soluble, less soluble
   d. alloyed, pure
10. The measurement of biological samples from a worker for elements found in a workplace following occupational exposure assesses which of the following?
    a. The air concentration of the measured element
    b. The nutritional status of the worker
    c. The worker's ability to schedule time off
    d. The effectiveness of environmental control strategies used in the workplace

## SUGGESTED READINGS

Alfrey AC, Mishell JM, Burks J, et al. Syndrome of dyspraxia and multifocal seizures associated with chronic hemodialysis. *Trans Am Soc Artif Intern Organs*. 1972;18(0):25–261, 266–257.

Caldwell KL, Jones RL, Verdon CP, et al. Levels of urinary total and speciated arsenic in the US population: national health and nutrition examination survey 2003–2004. *J Expo Sci Environ Epidemiol*. 2009;19(1):59–68.

Dart RC, Sullivan JB. Mercury. In: Dart RC, ed. *Medical Toxicology*. 3rd ed. Philadelphia: Lippincott Williams & Wilkins; 2004:1437–1448.

Gerhardson L, Kazantzis G. Diagnosis and treatment of metal poisoning: general aspects. In: Nordberg GF, Fowler BA, Nordberg M, et al., eds. *Handbook on the Toxicology of Metals*. 4th ed. London: Elsevier; 2014:488–507.

Hadrup N, Lam HR. Oral toxicity of silver ions, silver nanoparticles and colloidal silver: a review. *Regul Toxicol Pharmacol*. 2014;68(1):1–7.

Haglock-Adler CJ, Strathmann FG. Simplified sample preparation in the simultaneous measurement of whole blood antimony, bismuth, manganese, and zinc by inductively coupled plasma mass spectrometry. *Clin Biochem*. 2015;48(3):135–139.

Hahn LJ, Kloiber R, Vimy MJ, et al. Dental "silver" tooth fillings: a source of mercury exposure revealed by whole-body image scan and tissue analysis. *FASEB J.* 1989;3(14):2641–2646.

Hansen G, Victor R, Engeldinger E, Schweitzer C. Evaluation of the mercury exposure of dental amalgam patients by the mercury Triple Test. *Occup Environ Med.* 2004;61(6):535–540.

Ibrahim D, Froberg B, Wolf A, Rusyniak DE. Heavy metal poisoning: clinical presentations and pathophysiology. *Clin Lab Med.* 2006;26(1):67–97, viii.

Jin T, Berlin M. Titanium. In: Nordberg G, Fowler B, Nordberg M, et al., eds. *Handbook on the Toxicology of Metals.* 4th ed. London: Academic Press; 2014: ch. 57.

Lauwerys RR, Hoet P. Biological monitoring of exposure to inorganic and organometallic substances. In: *Industrial Chemical Exposure: Guidelines for Biological Monitoring.* Boca Raton, FL: Lewis Publishers; 2001:21–181.

Lison D. Cobalt. In: Nordberg G, Fowler B, Nordberg M, et al., eds. *Handbook on the Toxicology of Metals.* 4th ed. London: Academic Press; 2014; ch. 34.

McDiarmid MA, Gaitens JM, Squibb KS. Uranium and thorium. In: Bingham E, Cohrssen B, Patty FA, eds. *Patty's Toxicology.* 6th ed. Hoboken, NJ: John Wiley & Sons; 2012:769–816.

Michalke B. Element speciation definitions, analytical methodology, and some examples. *Ecotoxicol Environ Saf.* 2003;56(1):122–139.

Michalke B, Fernsebner K. New insights into manganese toxicity and speciation. *J Trace Elem Med Biol.* 2014;28(2):106–116.

Nelson LS. Copper. In: Nelson L, Goldfrank LR, eds. *Goldfrank's Toxicologic Emergencies.* 9th ed. New York: McGraw-Hill Medical; 2011.

Newton AW, Ranganath L, Armstrong C, et al. Differential distribution of cobalt, chromium, and nickel between whole blood, plasma and urine in patients after metal-on-metal (MoM) hip arthroplasty. *J Orthop Res.* 2012;30(10):1640–1646.

Nordberg GF, Nogawa K, Nordberg M, et al. Cadmium. In: Nordberg G, Fowler B, Nordberg M, et al., eds. *Handbook on the Toxicology of Metals.* 4th ed. Academic Press; 2014: ch. 32.

Riihimäki V, Aitio A. Occupational exposure to aluminum and its biomonitoring in perspective. *Crit Rev Toxicol.* 2012;42(10):827–853.

Rogan WJ, Ware JH. Exposure to lead in children: how low is low enough? *N Engl J Med.* 2003;348(16):1515–1516.

Siddique A, Kowdley KV. Review article: the iron overload syndromes [review]. *Aliment Pharmacol Ther.* 2012;35(8):876–893.

Skerfving S, Bergdahl IA. Lead. In: Nordberg G, Fowler B, Nordberg M, et al., eds. *Handbook on the Toxicology of Metals.* 4th ed. London: Academic Press; 2014: ch. 43.

Tylenda CA, Fowler BA. Antimony. In: Nordberg G, Fowler B, Nordberg M, et al., eds. *Handbook on the Toxicology of Metals.* 4th ed. London: Academic Press; 2014: ch. 27.

# 33

# Diabetes Mellitus

*David B. Sacks*

## OBJECTIVES

1. Define the following:
   - Advanced glycation end product
   - Albuminuria
   - C-peptide
   - Diabetes mellitus
   - Epinephrine
   - Fatty acid
   - Fructosamine
   - Gestational diabetes mellitus
   - Glucagon
   - Glucose tolerance
   - Glycated albumin
   - Glycated hemoglobin
   - Hemoglobin $A_{1c}$
   - Hyperglycemia
   - Insulin
   - Insulin-like growth factor 1
   - Insulin resistance syndrome
   - Ketoacidosis
   - Ketone bodies
   - Proinsulin
2. Compare and contrast type 1 and type 2 diabetes mellitus including the following:
   - Causes
   - Symptoms
   - Insulin concentration in blood
   - Appearance of symptoms versus clinical diagnosis
   - Development of chronic complications
   - Genetic factors
3. Compare impaired glucose tolerance with impaired fasting glucose and the usefulness of these classifications as risk factors for diabetes and cardiovascular disease.
4. List three important functions of insulin.
5. Summarize how the following hormones specifically affect blood glucose concentration: insulin, glucagon, epinephrine, cortisol, somatostatin, and growth hormone.

6. Briefly describe the function of the facilitative glucose transporters, including the importance of GLUT4 in glucose uptake by skeletal muscle.
7. List five antibodies that are involved in the pathogenesis of type 1 diabetes mellitus.
8. Describe insulin resistance and the role it plays in the pathogenesis of type 2 diabetes mellitus; explain how loss of β-cell function results in development of type 2 diabetes mellitus.
9. State how diet and exercise are related to development of type 2 diabetes mellitus.
10. State the basic criteria for the diagnosis of diabetes mellitus including fasting and random plasma glucose concentration, oral glucose tolerance test, and glycated hemoglobin results.
11. Outline the procedure for and interpretation of an oral glucose tolerance test for the diagnosis of type 2 diabetes mellitus, impaired glucose tolerance, and gestational diabetes mellitus.
12. Summarize the role of the clinical laboratory in the diagnosis and short- and long-term management of diabetes mellitus.
13. Describe the assay principles of a whole blood glucose meter; calculate the difference between whole blood and plasma glucose concentrations.
14. List five variables that affect the accuracy and reproducibility of blood glucose meters; state how dehydration affects the reliability of a blood glucose meter.
15. Describe a typical implanted sensor for monitoring blood glucose including assay method, calibration, and usefulness in a person with type 1 diabetes.
16. Discuss the metabolic relationships among glucose, ketones, fatty acids, and metabolic acids including how they are altered, the effects of increased counterregulatory hormones, and the clinical significance of ketonemia and ketonuria in uncontrolled diabetes mellitus.
17. Describe the glycation of hemoglobin; state the percentage of hemoglobin $A_1$ constituted by $A_{1c}$.

597

18. Explain how measurement of glycated hemoglobin is useful in the diagnosis and monitoring of diabetes; state the cutoff value of hemoglobin $A_{1c}$ used to diagnose diabetes.
19. Specify the effects that young and old erythrocytes have on hemoglobin $A_{1c}$ values.
20. List and discuss three techniques used to determine hemoglobin $A_{1c}$ values including principles of analysis, possible interference by hemoglobin variants, and specimen requirements.
21. Describe the effects of hyperglycemia on advanced glycation end products and how these end products contribute to certain complications of diabetes.
22. State how urinary albumin excretion is useful in determining diabetic nephropathy; list the specimen collection requirements for this urine test.
23. Describe three semiquantitative analyses of urinary albumin.
24. State the healthy reference intervals used for fasting plasma glucose, oral glucose tolerance, and hemoglobin $A_{1c}$ analyses.
25. Analyze and solve case studies related to the different types of diabetes and impaired glucose tolerance using descriptions of symptoms and results of laboratory analyses.

## KEY WORDS AND DEFINITIONS

**Advanced glycation end products (AGEs)**  Proteins that have been irreversibly modified by nonenzymatic attachment of glucose; may contribute to the chronic complications of diabetes.

**Diabetes mellitus**  A group of metabolic disorders of carbohydrate metabolism in which glucose is underutilized, producing hyperglycemia.

**Gestational diabetes mellitus (GDM)**  Carbohydrate intolerance with onset during pregnancy.

**Glucose**  A six-carbon simple sugar that is the premier fuel for most organisms and an important precursor of other body constituents.

**Glycated hemoglobin**  Hemoglobin that has a sugar residue attached; HbA1c is the major fraction of glycated hemoglobin.

**Glycogen**  A polysaccharide with a formula of $(C6H10O5)$ used by muscle and liver for carbohydrate storage.

**Hyperglycemia**  Increased glucose concentrations in the blood.

**Hypoglycemia**  Decreased glucose concentrations in the blood.

**Insulin**  A protein hormone produced by β-cells of the pancreas that decreases blood glucose concentrations.

**Ketones**  Compounds that arise from free fatty acid breakdown; insulin deficiency leads to increased blood ketones, which are important contributors to the metabolic acidosis that occurs in individuals with diabetic ketoacidosis.

**Diabetes mellitus** is a group of metabolic disorders characterized by **hyperglycemia** resulting from defects in **insulin** secretion, insulin action, or both. Some patients may experience acute life-threatening hyperglycemic episodes, such as ketoacidosis or hyperosmolar coma. Acute life-threatening hypoglycemic episodes may occur as a result of therapy. As the disease progresses, patients are at increased risk for the development of specific complications, including *retinopathy* leading to blindness, *nephropathy* leading to renal failure, and *neuropathy* (nerve damage), collectively known as microvascular complications, as well as *atherosclerosis*, which is considered a *macrovascular complication*. The last may result in stroke, gangrene, or coronary artery disease.

Diabetes is a common disease, although the exact prevalence is unknown. The number of people with diabetes has increased dramatically worldwide. Estimates in 2021 indicated that ≈537 million adults have diabetes, and by 2045 this number is predicted to reach 783 million, ≈80% of whom will live in low- and middle-income countries. In the United States, the prevalence in 1999–2002 was 9.3%, 30% of whom were undiagnosed. Data from the 2011–2016 National Health and Nutritional Examination Survey (NHANES) show a prevalence of 14.6%. Similarly, the prevalence of diabetes in Asian populations has increased rapidly in recent decades, with China and India ranked first and second, respectively, among countries with the largest diabetes populations. In 2021, China was estimated to have 140.9 million adults with diabetes, while the corresponding number in India was thought to be 74.2 million. The prevalence varies widely among countries, reaching as high as 25% in the Middle East and 30% in the Western Pacific. Information about individual countries is compiled by the International Diabetes Federation (IDF) and can be found at https://diabetesatlas.org/data/en/.

Diabetes has been described as "one of the main threats to human health in the twenty-first century". It is estimated that ≈50% of individuals with diabetes worldwide remain undiagnosed. The absolute number of undiagnosed diabetes patients in the US has remained fairly stable. The prevalence of diabetes increases with age and in the US, more than 20% of the population older than 65 years have diabetes. A racial predilection has been noted; 22.1%, 20.4%, 19.1% and 12.1% of Hispanic, Black, Asian, and White people, respectively, in the US have diabetes. In 2017, diabetes was estimated to be responsible for $327 billion in health care expenditures. Worldwide diabetes generated at least $760 billion in health expenditures in 2019, though others claim costs that are twice as high, being $1.3 trillion in 2015. Acute and particularly chronic complications make diabetes the fourth most common cause of death in the developed world.

## CLASSIFICATION

Diabetes was initially diagnosed by the oral glucose tolerance test (OGTT). The 1979 classification scheme by the National Diabetes Data Group recognized two major forms of diabetes: type I (insulin-dependent) diabetes mellitus (IDDM) and type II (non-insulin-dependent) diabetes mellitus (NIDDM). The terms *juvenile-onset* and *adult-onset diabetes* were abolished. To base the classification on cause rather than on treatment, the American Diabetes Association (ADA) re-examined the classification and diagnosis of diabetes mellitus. The revised classification, published in 1997, eliminates the terms *insulin-dependent diabetes mellitus* and *non-insulin-dependent diabetes mellitus*, which now are termed *type 1* and *type 2 diabetes*, respectively (Box 33.1).

### Type 1 Diabetes Mellitus

Approximately 5% to 10% of all cases of diabetes mellitus are included in this category. Patients usually have abrupt onset of symptoms (e.g., polyuria, polydipsia, rapid weight loss) and ≈30% present with diabetic ketoacidosis. They have insulinopenia (a deficiency of insulin) caused by destruction of pancreatic islet β-cells, and are dependent on insulin to sustain life and prevent ketosis. Most patients have antibodies that identify an autoimmune process (see below). The peak incidence occurs in childhood and adolescence. Approximately 75% acquire the disease before the age of 18, but onset in the remainder may occur at any age. Age at presentation is not a criterion for classification. Three distinct stages of type 1 diabetes can be identified. Stage 1: patients are normoglycemic, but have multiple islet autoantibodies; Stage 2: patients have dysglycemia (IFG and/or IGT) with multiple islet autoantibodies; and Stage 3: hyperglycemia with clinical symptoms. In addition, there is increasing awareness of considerable disease heterogeneity in type 1 diabetes.

### Type 2 Diabetes Mellitus

This group accounts for approximately 90% of all cases of diabetes. Patients have minimal symptoms, are not prone to ketosis, and *are not dependent on insulin* to prevent ketonuria. *Insulin concentrations may be normal, decreased, or increased*, and most people with this form of diabetes have impaired insulin action. *Obesity* is commonly associated, and weight loss alone usually improves hyperglycemia in these persons. However, many individuals with type 2 diabetes may require dietary intervention, oral anti-hyperglycemic agents, insulin or other injectable drugs, to control hyperglycemia. Most patients acquire the

---

### BOX 33.1 Classification of Diabetes Mellitus

I. Type 1 diabetes
II. Type 2 diabetes
III. Gestational diabetes mellitus (GDM)
IV. Specific types of diabetes due to other causes

From the American Diabetes Association. Classification and diagnosis of diabetes. *Diabetes Care* 2017;40(Suppl 1):S11–S24.

---

disease after age 40, but it may occur in younger people. Type 2 diabetes in children and adolescents is an emerging, significant problem, especially as the prevalence of obesity in this age group rises. In Hong Kong, 90% of youth-onset diabetes is type 2, 60% in Japan and 50% in Taiwan. Some individuals cannot be classified at the time of diagnosis into type 1 or type 2 diabetes.

### Specific Types of Diabetes Mellitus Due to Other Causes

This subclass includes uncommon patients in whom hyperglycemia is due to a specific underlying disorder, such as genetic defects of β-cell function; genetic defects in insulin action; diseases of the exocrine pancreas (e.g., cystic fibrosis); endocrinopathies (e.g., Cushing's syndrome, acromegaly, glucagonoma); administration of hormones or drugs known to induce β-cell dysfunction (e.g., dilantin, pentamidine) or to impair insulin action (e.g., glucocorticoids, thiazides, β-adrenergics); infection; uncommon forms of immune-mediated diabetes; or other genetic conditions (e.g., Down syndrome, Klinefelter syndrome, porphyria). This was formerly termed *secondary diabetes.*

### Gestational Diabetes Mellitus

This was defined for many years as any degree of glucose intolerance (i.e., hyperglycemia) *with onset or first recognition during pregnancy* (i.e., women with diabetes who become pregnant are not included in this category). Estimates of the frequency of abnormal glucose tolerance during pregnancy have ranged from <1% to 28%, depending on the population studied and the diagnostic tests employed (see later in this chapter). In 2021, ≈21 million live births were estimated to be affected by hyperglycemia in pregnancy. In the United States, gestational diabetes mellitus (GDM) occurs in 6%–8% of pregnancies (≈270,000 cases annually). The prevalence of GDM is increasing, at least in part, due to the considerable increase in obesity. Women with GDM are at significantly greater risk for the subsequent development of type 2 diabetes, which ultimately occurs in 50%–60%. At 4–12 weeks postpartum, all patients who had GDM should be evaluated for diabetes using non-pregnant OGTT criteria. If diabetes is not present, patients should have lifelong screening for diabetes or prediabetes at least every 3 years.

### Categories of Increased Risk for Diabetes

People who have blood glucose concentrations above normal, but less than those required for a diagnosis of diabetes mellitus, have been recognized for many years. In 1979, this intermediate category was termed *impaired glucose tolerance (IGT)*. It was defined as a 2 h postload plasma glucose following an OGTT of 140–199 mg/dL (7.8–11.0 mmol/L). An OGTT is required to assign a patient to this class. In order to avoid an OGTT, the category of impaired fasting glucose (IFG) was added by the American Diabetes Association (ADA) in 1997 and by the WHO in 1999. IFG is diagnosed by a fasting glucose value between those of normal and diabetic individuals, namely, between 100 and 125 mg/dL (5.6 and 6.9 mmol/L). (Note that the WHO and a number of other diabetes organizations define the lower cutoff for IFG at 110 mg/mL [6.1 mmol/L]).

In 2009, hemoglobin $A_{1c}$ (Hb$A_{1c}$) was added as a criterion to diagnose type 2 diabetes. People with Hb$A_{1c}$ values below the cutoff for diabetes, i.e., 6.5% (48 mmol/mol), but above the reference interval (4%–6%; 20–42 mmol/L), are at high risk of developing diabetes. For example, the incidence of diabetes in people with Hb$A_{1c}$ of 5.5%–6.0% (37–42 mmol/mol) is 3- to 8-fold higher than the general population, while Hb$A_{1c}$ between 6.0% and <6.5% (42 and 48 mmol/mol) is more than 10 times that of people with lower concentrations.

Individuals with IFG and/or IGT and/or intermediate Hb$A_{1c}$ (5.7%–6.4%; 39–46 mmol/mol) have been referred to as having "prediabetes" as they are at high risk for progressing to diabetes. Moreover, they are at increased risk for the development of cardiovascular disease. Nevertheless, there is considerable controversy surrounding prediabetes. For example, IFG, IGT, and Hb$A_{1c}$ do not always identify the same individuals. There is also a lack of agreement on the cut-points for IFG and Hb$A_{1c}$. This is due, in large part, to the continuous nature of the risk for the development of diabetes complications and the concentration of glucose or Hb$A_{1c}$.

## HORMONES THAT REGULATE BLOOD GLUCOSE CONCENTRATION

During a brief fast, a precipitous decline in the concentration of blood glucose is prevented by breakdown of glycogen stored in the liver and synthesis of glucose in the liver. Some glucose is derived from gluconeogenesis in the kidneys. These organs contain glucose-6-phosphatase, which is necessary to convert glucose 6-phosphate (derived from gluconeogenesis or glycogenolysis) to glucose. Skeletal muscle lacks this enzyme; muscle glycogen therefore cannot contribute directly to blood glucose. With more prolonged fasting (>42 h), gluconeogenesis accounts for essentially all glucose production. In contrast, after a meal, the absorbed glucose is converted to glycogen (for storage in the liver and skeletal muscle) or fat (for storage in adipose tissue). Despite large fluctuations in the supply and demand of carbohydrates, the concentration of glucose in the blood is normally maintained within a fairly narrow range by hormones that modulate the movement of glucose into and out of the circulation. These include insulin, which decreases blood glucose, and the counterregulatory hormones (glucagon, epinephrine, cortisol, and growth hormone), which increase blood glucose concentrations (Fig. 33.1). Normal glucose disposal depends on: (1)

the ability of the pancreas to secrete insulin; (2) the ability of insulin to promote uptake of glucose into peripheral tissue; and (3) the ability of insulin to suppress hepatic glucose production. The major insulin target organs are liver, skeletal muscle, and adipose tissue. These organs exhibit some differences in their responses to insulin. For example, the hormone stimulates glucose uptake through a specific glucose transporter—GLUT4—into muscle and fat cells, but not into liver cells.

### Insulin

Insulin is a protein hormone produced by the β-cells of the islets of Langerhans in the pancreas. Insulin was the first protein hormone to be sequenced, the first substance to be measured by radioimmunoassay (RIA), and the first compound produced by recombinant DNA technology for clinical use. It is an anabolic hormone that stimulates the uptake of glucose into fat and muscle, promotes the conversion of glucose to glycogen or fat for storage, inhibits glucose production by the liver, stimulates protein synthesis, and inhibits protein breakdown. (For more details, refer to the 7th edition of *Tietz Textbook of Laboratory Medicine*.)

Human insulin (molecular weight [MW] 5808 Da) consists of 51 amino acids in two chains (A and B) joined by two disulfide bridges, with a third disulfide bridge within the A chain. Insulin from most animals is immunologically and biologically similar to human insulin, and in the past, patients were treated with insulin purified from beef or pig pancreas. Virtually all patients now use recombinant human insulins.

Preproinsulin, a protein of about 100 amino acids (MW 12,000 Da), is not detectable in the circulation under normal conditions because it is rapidly converted by cleaving enzymes to proinsulin, an 86 amino acid polypeptide. This is stored in secretory granules in the Golgi complex of the β-cells, where proteolytic cleavage to insulin and connecting peptide (C-peptide) occurs. At the cell membrane, insulin and C-peptide are released into the portal circulation in equimolar amounts. In addition, small amounts of proinsulin and intermediate cleavage forms enter the circulation.

Proinsulin, which has relatively low biological activity (approximately 10% of insulin potency), is the major storage form of insulin. Normally, only small amounts (about 3% of the amount of insulin, on a molar basis) of proinsulin enter the circulation. C-peptide was initially thought to be devoid of biological activity. Subsequent evidence reveals that C-peptide has biological activity, but its possible physiological significance remains controversial. Fasting C-peptide concentrations are fivefold to 10-fold higher than those of insulin owing to the longer half-life of C-peptide (≈35 min). The liver does not extract C-peptide, which is removed from the circulation by the kidneys and degraded, with a fraction excreted unchanged in the urine.

### Glucose Transport

One of the fundamental effects elicited by insulin is to increase glucose uptake into cells. Two families of protein modulate the transport of glucose into cells. The sodium-dependent glucose transporters (SGLTs) promote the uptake of glucose

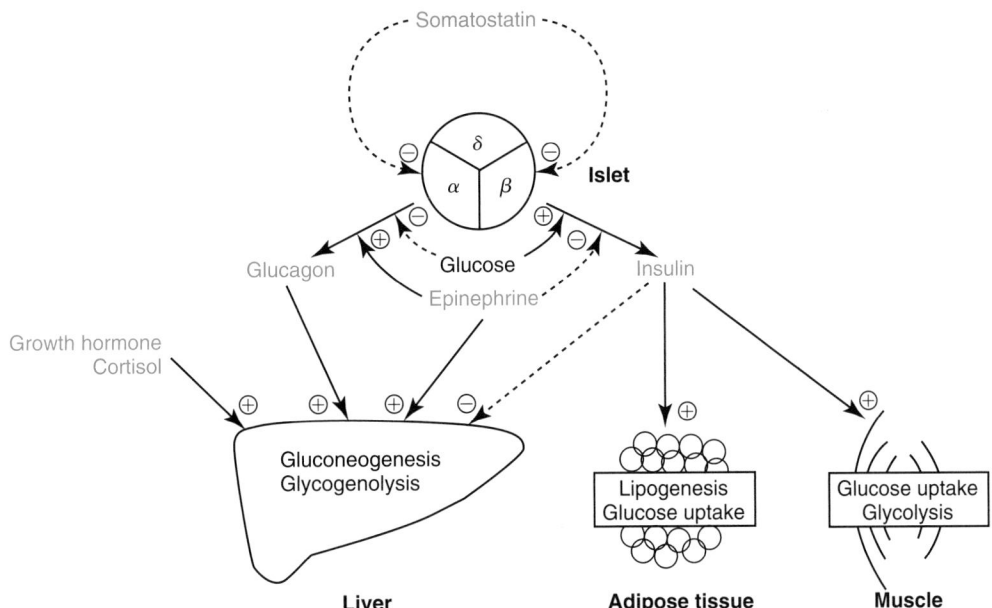

**Fig. 33.1** Hormonal regulation of blood glucose. Key: +, stimulation; −, inhibition. Cortisol, growth hormone, and epinephrine antagonize the effects of insulin.

and galactose from the lumen of the small bowel and their reabsorption from urine in the kidney. Inhibitors of SGLT2 (e.g., canagliflozin and empagliflozin) are now used to treat patients with type 2 diabetes. These drugs increase glucose excretion in the urine by suppressing glucose reabsorption in the kidney, thereby reducing blood glucose. The second family of glucose carriers, termed *facilitative glucose transporters* (GLUT) (Table 33.1), are designated GLUT1 to GLUT14, based on the order in which they were identified. Eleven have been shown to transport glucose. Many also transport other hexoses, such as galactose, fructose, mannose, and xylose. They can be divided into three classes, based on sequence similarities and characteristics. The best characterized are class I (GLUT1 to GLUT4). Less is known about those in classes II and III. GLUT1 is widely expressed and provides many cells with their basal glucose requirement. GLUT1 in the blood–brain barrier and GLUT3 in neuronal cells provide the constant high concentrations of glucose required by the brain. GLUT1 is responsible for mediating materno-placental transfer of glucose. GLUT2 is expressed in hepatocytes, β-cells of the pancreas, and basolateral membranes of intestinal and renal epithelial cells. It is a low-affinity, high-capacity transport system that allows non-rate-limiting movement of glucose into and out of these cells. GLUT2 is the major glucose transporter of hepatocytes. GLUT3 is the primary mediator of glucose transport into neurons. GLUT4 catalyzes the rate-limiting step for glucose uptake and metabolism in skeletal muscle, the major organ of glucose consumption. GLUT4 is also present in adipose tissue.

When circulating insulin concentrations are low, most of the GLUT4 is localized in intracellular compartments and is inactive. After eating, the pancreas releases insulin, which stimulates the translocation of GLUT4 to the plasma membrane, thereby promoting glucose uptake into skeletal muscle

and fat. Insulin-stimulated glucose transport into skeletal muscle is defective in type 2 diabetes mellitus, but the mechanism has not been established. Exercise also activates glucose entry into skeletal muscle, independently of insulin. Muscle contraction leads to GLUT4 translocation to the plasma membrane via a signaling pathway which differs from that stimulated by insulin.

GLUT9 is required for urate reabsorption in the kidney and appears to be associated with gout. GLUTs 6, 7, 10, 11, 12 and 14 were identified as a result of sequencing the human genome and their physiological roles remain unclear.

## Insulin-like Growth Factors

Insulin-like growth factors 1 and 2 (IGF-1 and IGF-2) are polypeptides structurally related to insulin. These hormones (previously referred to as *non-suppressible insulin-like activity* or *somatomedin*) exhibit metabolic and growth-promoting effects similar to those of insulin. Accumulating evidence implicates the IGF axis in the development of several common cancers. IGF-1 (previously known as somatomedin C) is an important mediator of growth hormone action and is one of the major regulators of cell growth and differentiation. Synthesis of IGF-1 depends on growth hormone and occurs predominantly in the liver. In addition, many other cells produce IGF-1 that does not enter the circulation but acts locally. IGF-2 is expressed mainly in early embryonic and fetal development. In adults, IGF-2 is produced in the liver and epithelial cells lining the brain. Circulating IGF-1 concentrations are approximately 1000-fold higher than insulin concentrations, and the hormone is kept inactive by binding to a family of at least six specific binding proteins. These proteins regulate IGFs by protecting the ligands in the circulation and delivering them to their target tissue. In contrast to insulin, which is unbound in the circulation, less than 10%

## TABLE 33.1   Facilitative Human Glucose Transporters

| Name | Class | Tissue | Function |
|------|-------|--------|----------|
| GLUT1 | I | Erythrocytes, brain, blood–brain barrier, fetal tissues | Basal glucose transport, particularly in erythrocytes, brain, and placenta |
| GLUT2 | I | Liver, β-cells of pancreas, small intestine, kidney, brain | Non-rate-limiting glucose transport |
| GLUT3 | I | Brain (neurons), testis | Glucose transport in neurons |
| GLUT4 | I | Skeletal muscle, cardiac muscle, adipose tissue (white and brown) | Insulin-stimulated glucose transport |
| GLUT5 | II | Small intestine, kidney | Transports fructose (not glucose) |
| GLUT6 | III | Brain, spleen, leukocytes | |
| GLUT7 | II | Small intestine, colon, testis, prostate | |
| GLUT8 | III | Testis, brain, adrenal gland, liver, spleen, brown adipose tissue, lung | |
| GLUT9 | II | Kidney, liver, small intestine, placenta, lung, leukocytes | Transports urate |
| GLUT10 | III | Heart, lung, brain, liver, pancreas, placenta, kidney | |
| GLUT11 | II | Heart, skeletal muscle | |
| GLUT12 | III | Heart, prostate, skeletal muscle, placenta | |
| HMIT (GLUT13) | III | Brain, adipose tissue | Transports myo-inositol (not glucose) |
| GLUT14 | I | Testis | |

of total serum IGF-1 is free. The biological actions of IGF are exerted through specific IGF receptors or the insulin receptor. The IGF-1 receptor is closely related to the insulin receptor in structure and biochemical properties. In contrast, the IGF-2 receptor is quite different, and its physiological relevance is not understood.

The significance of IGFs in normal carbohydrate metabolism is not known. Exogenous administration produces hypoglycemia, whereas a deficiency of IGF-1 results in dwarfism (pygmies and Laron dwarfs). IGFs, particularly IGF-2, may be produced in excess by extrapancreatic neoplasms, and patients may have fasting hypoglycemia. Clinically, IGF-1 measurement may be useful in evaluating growth hormone deficiency and excess (acromegaly), and in monitoring response to nutritional support.

## Counterregulatory Hormones

Several hormones have actions opposite to those of insulin. These counterregulatory hormones are catabolic and increase hepatic glucose production initially by enhancing the breakdown of glycogen to glucose (glycogenolysis), and later by stimulating the synthesis of glucose (gluconeogenesis). The initial response (within minutes) to low blood glucose is an increase in glucose production, stimulated by glucagon and epinephrine. Over time (3–4 h), growth hormone and cortisol increase glucose mobilization and decrease glucose use (see Fig. 33.1). Evidence also suggests that glucose production by the liver is an inverse function of ambient glucose concentration, independent of hormonal factors (glucose autoregulation). The role of other hormones or neurotransmitters is not clear but appears relatively unimportant.

## Glucagon

Glucagon is a 29 amino acid polypeptide secreted by α-cells of the pancreas. It is derived from proglucagon, which is

hydrolyzed by prohormone convertase 2 (PC2). The major target organ for glucagon is the liver, where it binds to a specific G protein-coupled receptor, which is expressed abundantly in liver and kidney, and to a lesser extent in other tissues, including heart, adipose, pancreas and brain. Glucagon stimulates the production of glucose in the liver predominantly by glycogenolysis. Gluconeogenesis is also activated and glycogenesis is inhibited. Glucagon secretion is regulated primarily by plasma glucose concentrations, with low and high plasma glucose being stimulatory and inhibitory, respectively. Long-standing diabetes mellitus impairs the glucagon response to hypoglycemia, resulting in an increased incidence of hypoglycemic episodes. Stress, exercise, and amino acids induce glucagon release. Insulin inhibits glucagon release from the pancreas and decreases glucagon gene expression, thereby attenuating its biosynthesis. Increased glucagon concentrations, secondary to insulin deficiency, contribute to the hyperglycemia and ketosis of diabetes. In addition to its effects on glycemia, glucagon directly regulates triglyceride, free fatty acid, and bile metabolism. For example, it enhances fatty acid oxidation and ketogenesis in the liver.

Proglucagon is also produced in the distal gut by enteroendocrine L cells and neurons in the nucleus of the solitary tract. In the intestinal L cells, proglucagon is cleaved by prohormone convertase 1/3 (PC1/3) to glucagon-like peptide-1 (GLP-1), GLP-2, oxyntomodulin, glicentin, and intervening peptide 2 (IP2). Food ingestion stimulates secretion of GLP-1, which acts on β-cells of the pancreas to stimulate insulin gene transcription, potentiate glucose-induced insulin secretion and inhibit glucagon secretion. GLP-1 and GIP (synthesized in and secreted from the duodenum and proximal jejunum) are incretin hormones that are responsible for up to 70% of postprandial insulin secretion. GLP-1 receptors are widely expressed, and GLP-1 also regulates glucose concentration through extrapancreatic mechanisms, including inhibiting glucose production and food intake. For these reasons, both GLP-1 receptor agonists and dipeptidyl peptidase 4 (DPP-4) inhibitors (which increase circulating GLP-1 and GIP) are used in the treatment of type 2 diabetes.

### Epinephrine

Epinephrine (also called adrenaline), a catecholamine secreted by the adrenal medulla, stimulates glucose production (glycogenolysis) and decreases glucose use, thereby increasing blood glucose concentrations. It also stimulates glucagon secretion and inhibits insulin secretion by the pancreas (see Fig. 33.1). Epinephrine appears to have a key role in glucose counterregulation when glucagon secretion is impaired (e.g., in type 1 diabetes mellitus). Physical or emotional stress increases epinephrine production, releasing glucose for energy. Tumors of the adrenal medulla, known as pheochromocytomas, secrete excess epinephrine or norepinephrine, and produce moderate hyperglycemia, as long as glycogen stores are available in the liver.

### Growth Hormone

Growth hormone is a polypeptide secreted by the anterior pituitary gland. It stimulates gluconeogenesis, enhances lipolysis, and antagonizes insulin-stimulated glucose uptake.

### Cortisol

Cortisol, secreted by the adrenal cortex in response to adrenocorticotropic hormone (ACTH), stimulates gluconeogenesis and increases the breakdown of protein and fat. Patients with Cushing's syndrome have increased cortisol production owing to tumor or hyperplasia of the adrenal cortex and may become hyperglycemic. In contrast, people with Addison's disease have adrenocortical insufficiency caused by destruction or atrophy of the adrenal cortex and may exhibit hypoglycemia.

### Other Hormones Influencing Glucose Metabolism
#### Thyroxine

Thyroxine, secreted by the thyroid gland, is not directly involved in glucose homeostasis, but it stimulates glycogenolysis and increases the rates of gastric emptying and intestinal glucose absorption. These factors may produce glucose intolerance in thyrotoxic individuals, but patients usually have a fasting plasma glucose concentration within the reference interval

#### Somatostatin

Somatostatin, also called growth hormone–inhibiting hormone, is a 14 amino acid peptide found in the gastrointestinal tract, the hypothalamus, and the δ-cells of the pancreatic islets. Although somatostatin does not appear to have a direct effect on carbohydrate metabolism, it inhibits the release of growth hormone from the pituitary. In addition, somatostatin inhibits secretion of glucagon and insulin by the pancreas, thus modulating the reciprocal relationship between these two hormones.

## CLINICAL UTILITY OF MEASURING INSULIN, PROINSULIN, C-PEPTIDE, AND GLUCAGON

Although there is interest in the possible clinical value of measurement of the concentrations of insulin and its precursors, the assays are useful primarily for research purposes. There is no role for routine testing for insulin, proinsulin, or C-peptide in most patients with diabetes. Measurement of C-peptide is sometimes necessary in the US for patients to obtain insurance coverage for continuous subcutaneous insulin infusion pumps. Occasionally, C-peptide measurements may help distinguish type 1 from type 2 diabetes in ambiguous cases (e.g., patients who have type 2 phenotype, but present with ketoacidosis). It must be emphasized that the diagnostic criteria for diabetes mellitus do not include measurements of hormones, which remain predominantly research tools.

### Insulin

The primary clinical application of insulin measurement is in the evaluation of patients with fasting hypoglycemia (discussed in more detail in Chapter 22). Measurement of circulating insulin could be helpful in evaluating insulin resistance and insulin secretion. Increased concentrations of insulin in nondiabetic individuals are an independent predictor of the development of coronary artery disease. Nevertheless, it is not clear whether the increased insulin is responsible for the risk of coronary disease, and the clinical value of measuring it in this context is questionable.

In the past, measurement of insulin was advocated by some in the evaluation and management of patients with polycystic ovary syndrome. Women with this condition have insulin resistance with androgen excess and abnormal carbohydrate metabolism that may respond to oral antihyperglycemic agents. However, it is not clear whether assessing insulin resistance by measuring insulin concentrations affords any advantage over clinical signs of insulin resistance (body mass index, acanthosis nigricans), and the American College of Obstetrics and Gynecology (ACOG) does not recommend routine measurements of insulin. Although a few investigators have advocated measuring insulin along with glucose during an OGTT as an aid to the early diagnosis of diabetes mellitus, this approach is not recommended. Insulin measurements do not add significantly to diabetes risk prediction generated with traditional clinical and laboratory measurements.

Although insulin has been assayed for over 60 years, no highly accurate, precise, and reliable procedure is available to measure the amount of insulin in a patient sample. The term *immunoreactive insulin* is used in reference to assays that may recognize, in addition to insulin, substrates that share antigenic epitopes with insulin. Examples include proinsulin, proinsulin conversion intermediates, and insulin derivatives, produced by glycation or dimerization. Antisera raised against insulin show some cross-reactivity with proinsulin but not with C-peptide. Specificity is not a problem in healthy individuals because the low proinsulin concentrations do not appreciably affect the absolute values of insulin.

In certain situations (e.g., islet cell tumors and patients with diabetes), proinsulin is present at higher concentrations, and direct assay of plasma may falsely overestimate the true insulin concentration. Because proinsulin has very low activity, incorrect conclusions regarding the availability of biologically active insulin may be reached in patients with diabetes. The magnitude of the error depends on the concentration of proinsulin and the extent of cross-reactivity of the antiserum with proinsulin.

A stable isotope dilution mass spectrometry (IDMS) assay has been developed to measure insulin, proinsulin, and C-peptide. The difference in mass between the three analytes allows specific measurement of each protein. Comparison of patient samples revealed that most, but not all, results were higher by immunoassay than by mass spectrometry. Thus, immunoassays may overestimate insulin, particularly at low concentrations. The high protein concentration in the serum requires extraction of proteins (e.g., by immunoaffinity) and purification by high-performance liquid chromatography (HPLC) before quantification by mass spectrometry. This method is not suitable for routine laboratory analysis but is the best higher-order measurement procedure available and can be used as a candidate reference measurement procedure.

Reference intervals vary among assays, and each laboratory should ideally establish its own reference intervals. After an overnight fast, insulin concentrations in healthy, normal, non-obese people vary from 12–150 pmol/L (2–25 µIU/mL). More specific assays that have minimal cross-reactivity with proinsulin reveal a fasting plasma insulin concentration of <60 pmol/L (<10 µIU/mL). Concentrations up to 1200 pmol/L (200 µIU/mL) can be reached during a glucose tolerance test. Fasting insulin values are higher in obese, non-diabetic people and lower in trained athletes.

### Insulin Antibodies

Antibodies to insulin develop in almost all patients who are treated with exogenous insulin. Note that these antibodies are distinct from insulin autoantibodies, which are present in some patients with type 1 diabetes before they receive insulin (see Pathogenesis of Type 1 Diabetes Mellitus, below). Insulin antibodies rarely produce adverse effects. On rare occasions (usually in insulin-treated patients with type 2 diabetes), high titers of insulin antibodies may cause insulin resistance; this tends to be self-limited. Patients who use inhaled insulin have significantly increased concentrations of insulin antibodies. A quantitative estimate of the concentration of circulating insulin antibody does not appear to be of significant benefit.

When there is a clinical suspicion of insulin antibodies, insulin should be measured before and after the sample is diluted. Nonlinear values are highly suggestive of assay interference. Assays to identify insulin antibodies involve the separation of free insulin from bound insulin, followed by measurement of insulin by immunoassay. Separation can be achieved by precipitation with PEG or by gel filtration chromatography, which separates molecules on the basis of molecular mass.

### Proinsulin

High proinsulin concentrations are usually noted in patients with benign or malignant β-cell tumors of the pancreas. Most patients with β-cell tumors have increased insulin, C-peptide, and proinsulin concentrations, but occasionally only proinsulin is increased because the tumors have defective conversion of proinsulin to insulin. Despite its low biological activity, proinsulin production may be adequate to produce hypoglycemia. In addition, a rare form of familial hyperproinsulinemia, produced by impaired conversion to insulin, has been described. Measurement of proinsulin can be useful to determine the amount of proinsulin-like material that cross-reacts in an insulin assay. Patients with type 2 diabetes have increased proportions of proinsulin and proinsulin conversion intermediates, high concentrations of which are associated with cardiovascular risk factors. Even relatively mild hyperglycemia produces hyperproinsulinemia, with values greater than 40% of insulin concentration in type 2 diabetes. Interestingly, published evidence reveals that almost all individuals with long-standing type 1 diabetes retain the ability to synthesize proinsulin. Increased proinsulin concentrations may also be detected in patients with chronic renal failure, cirrhosis, or hyperthyroidism.

Accurate measurement of proinsulin has been difficult for several reasons: the blood concentrations are low; antibody production is difficult; most antisera cross-react with insulin and C-peptide, which are present in much higher concentrations; the assays measure intermediate cleavage forms of proinsulin; and reference preparations of pure proinsulin were not readily available. Biosynthetic proinsulin has allowed the production of monoclonal antibodies to proinsulin and has provided reliable proinsulin calibrators and reference preparations.

Reference intervals for proinsulin are highly dependent on the method of analysis, the degree of cross-reactivity of the antisera, and the purity of proinsulin calibrators. Each laboratory should establish its own reference intervals. Reference intervals in healthy, fasting individuals reported in the literature range from 1.1–6.9 pmol/L to 2.1–12.6 pmol/L. Proinsulin is stable in EDTA at room temperature for at least 24 h.

### C-Peptide

Measurement of C-peptide has several advantages over insulin measurement. Because hepatic metabolism is negligible, C-peptide concentrations are better indicators of β-cell function than is peripheral insulin concentration. Furthermore, C-peptide assays do not measure exogenous insulin and do not cross-react with insulin antibodies, which interfere with the insulin immunoassay.

The primary indication for measuring C-peptide is to evaluate fasting hypoglycemia. Some patients with insulin-producing β-cell tumors, particularly if hyperinsulinism is intermittent, may exhibit increased C-peptide concentrations with normal insulin concentrations. When hypoglycemia is due to surreptitious insulin injection, *insulin* concentrations will be high, but C-peptide values will be low; this occurs because C-peptide is not found in commercial insulin preparations and exogenous insulin suppresses β-cell function.

Basal or stimulated (by glucagon or glucose) C-peptide concentrations provide estimates of a patient's insulin secretory capacity and rate. While useful in research, C-peptide measurement has a negligible role in the routine management of patients with diabetes. Medicare patients in the United States must have low C-peptide concentrations to be eligible for insurance coverage of insulin pumps.

Measurement of C-peptide is used to monitor patients' response to pancreatic surgery. C-peptide should be undetectable after a radical pancreatectomy and should increase after a successful pancreas or islet cell transplant. In addition, C-peptide concentration is used as an endpoint in immunomodulatory trials for the prevention of type 1 diabetes.

Measurements of urine C-peptide are useful when continuous assessment of β-cell function is desired, or when frequent blood sampling is not practical. The 24-h urine C-peptide content (in the absence of renal failure, which produces increased concentrations) correlates well with fasting serum C-peptide concentration or with the sum of C-peptide concentrations in sequential specimens after a glucose load. However, the fraction of secreted C-peptide that is excreted in the urine exhibits high intersubject and intrasubject variability, limiting the value of urine C-peptide as a measure of insulin secretion. Some have advocated C-peptide to creatinine ratio in a single urine sample to avoid the problems associated with 24-h urine collection.

Assays are not affected by anti-insulin antibodies, but methodologic problems produce large between-method variation. These difficulties include variable specificity among different antisera, variable cross-reactivity with proinsulin, and various types of C-peptide preparation used as a calibrator. The NIH formed a committee in 2002 to harmonize C-peptide measurements. Comparison of 40 serum samples using nine commercial C-peptide assay methods showed within- and between-run CVs ranging from <2% to >10%, and from <2% to >18%, respectively. Some methods had high imprecision, with between-run CVs exceeding 15%. Two IDMS methods for measuring C-peptide have been developed. Calibrating C-peptide measurements to a reference method using mass spectrometry increased comparability among laboratories.

Fasting serum concentrations of C-peptide in healthy people range from 0.78 to 1.89 ng/mL (0.25–0.6 nmol/L). After stimulation with glucose or glucagon, values range from 2.73 to 5.64 ng/mL (0.9–1.87 nmol/L), or three to five times the prestimulation value. Urinary C-peptide is usually in the range of 74 ± 26 µg/L (25 ± 8.8 µmol/L).

## Glucagon

Very high concentrations of glucagon are seen in patients with α-cell tumors of the pancreas called glucagonomas. Patients with this tumor frequently have weight loss, necrolytic migratory erythema, diabetes mellitus, stomatitis, and diarrhea. Skin lesions often occur first and are frequently overlooked. Most tumors have metastasized when finally diagnosed. Low glucagon concentrations are associated with chronic pancreatitis and long-term sulfonylurea therapy.

A competitive RIA is available for measuring glucagon. Calibrator values are assigned at the manufacturers using the WHO glucagon international standard (69/194). Immunoassays that do not use radioactivity have been developed. A comparison of 10 commercially available assays reveals that some show cross-reactivity with other peptides from proglucagon, and all lack sensitivity at low glucagon concentrations.

Fasting plasma concentrations of glucagon vary depending on the method, ranging from 0–20 ng/L up to 135 ng/L (0–5.7 pmol/L to 38.7 pmol/L). Values up to 500 times the upper reference limit may be found in patients with autonomously secreting α-cell neoplasms.

## PATHOGENESIS OF TYPE 1 DIABETES MELLITUS

Type 1 diabetes mellitus results from cellular-mediated autoimmune destruction of the insulin-secreting cells of pancreatic β-cells by a chronic mononuclear cell infiltrate, called insulitis. In the vast majority of patients, destruction is mediated by T cells. The α-, δ-, and other islet cells are preserved. The autoimmune process begins months or years before the clinical presentation, and an 80%–90% reduction in the volume of β-cells is required to induce symptomatic type 1 diabetes. The rate of islet cell destruction is variable and is usually more rapid in children than in adults.

### Antibodies

Circulating antibodies can be detected in the serum years before the onset of hyperglycemia. These are not used in the routine management of patients with diabetes. The best characterized islet autoantibodies are as follows:

1. *Islet cell cytoplasmic antibodies* (ICAs) react with a sialoglycoconjugate antigen present in the cytoplasm of all endocrine cells of the pancreatic islets. These antibodies are detected in the serum of 0.5% of normal subjects and 75%–85% of patients with newly diagnosed type 1 diabetes. The antibodies are detected by immunofluorescence microscopy on frozen sections of human pancreatic tails. The ICA assay is cumbersome, labor intensive, and difficult to standardize, and is performed in few clinical laboratories.
2. *Insulin autoantibodies* (IAAs) are present in ≈80%–90% of children who develop type 1 diabetes before age 5 years, but in <40% of individuals who develop diabetes after age 12. Their frequency in healthy people is similar to that of ICA. An important caveat is that insulin antibodies develop rapidly (<2 weeks) after initiation of insulin therapy. Therefore, IAA should not be measured in insulin-treated patients as assays do not distinguish insulin antibodies from IAA.
3. *Antibodies to the 65 kDa isoform of glutamic acid decarboxylase* (GADA) have been found up to 10 years before the

onset of clinical type 1 diabetes and are present in ≈60% of patients with newly diagnosed type 1 diabetes. GADA may be used to identify patients with apparent type 2 diabetes who will subsequently progress to type 1 diabetes.

4. *Antibodies to insulinoma-associated antigens* (IA–2A and IA–2βA), directed against two tyrosine phosphatases, have been detected in ≈40%–60% of newly diagnosed type 1 diabetes patients.

5. *Antibodies to zinc transporter ZnT8* is found in 60–80% of patients with new-onset type 1 diabetes. These are detected in ≈26% of patients with type 1 diabetes who are negative for other islet autoantibodies.

Autoantibody markers of immune destruction are present in 85%–90% of individuals with immune-mediated diabetes when fasting hyperglycemia is initially detected. Approximately 5%–10% of White adult patients who have the type 2 diabetes phenotype also have islet cell autoantibodies, particularly GADA. This condition has been termed *latent autoimmune diabetes of adulthood* (LADA) (previously termed type 1.5 diabetes or slow-onset diabetes in adults). Up to 1%–2% of healthy individuals have a single autoantibody and are at low risk of developing immune-mediated diabetes. Because the prevalence of immune-mediated diabetes is low (≈0.3% in the general population in most countries), the positive predictive value of a single autoantibody will be extremely low. The presence of multiple autoantibodies is associated with a high risk of type 1 diabetes. Screening for islet autoantibodies is controversial because no acceptable therapy has been documented to reliably prevent or delay the clinical onset of diabetes in islet autoantibody-positive individuals.

## Genetics

Susceptibility to type 1 diabetes is inherited, but the mode of inheritance is complex and has not been defined. It is a multigenic trait, and the major locus is the major histocompatibility complex on chromosome 6. At least 11 other loci on 9 chromosomes also contribute, with the regulatory region of the insulin gene *INS* on chromosome 11p15 being an important locus. The human leukocyte antigen (HLA)-DQ and -DR genetic factors are by far the most important determinants for risk of type 1 diabetes. The concordance rate between identical twins is around 30%. Approximately 95% of White patients with type 1 diabetes express HLA-DR3 or HLA-DR4 histocompatibility antigens. However, up to 40% of the nondiabetic population also express these alleles. In contrast, the HLA-DQB1*0602 allele significantly decreases the risk of type 1 diabetes. HLA typing can indicate absolute risk of diabetes. The risk of a sibling developing diabetes is 1%, 5%, and 10%–20% if the number of haplotypes shared is none, one, and two, respectively. However, only 10% of patients with type 1 diabetes have an affected first-degree relative. Overall, more than 40 non-HLA-susceptibility gene markers have been confirmed, but these have smaller effects than HLA. Non-HLA genetic factors that increase risk include the insulin gene (*INS*), cytotoxic T-lymphocyte-associated protein 4 (*CTLA4*), and protein tyrosine phosphatase non-receptor type 22 (lymphoid) (*PTPN22*). The multiplicity of

independent chromosomal regions associated with a predisposition to type 1 diabetes suggests that other susceptibility genes will be identified. Routine measurement of genetic markers is not of value at this time for the diagnosis or management of patients with type 1 diabetes.

### Environment

Environmental factors are involved in initiating diabetes. Viruses such as rubella, mumps, enterovirus, and Coxsackievirus B, have been implicated. It seems likely that autoimmunity to β-cells is initiated by a viral protein (that shares amino acid sequence with a β-cell protein) or some other environmental insult. Genetic susceptibility and other host factors (e.g., HLA type) determine the progression of the β-cell destruction. Epidemiological studies have implicated early exposure to cows' milk as a trigger of type 1 diabetes. This model is contentious and has been debated for decades. Environmental trials have failed to show a meaningful impact on the natural course of type 1 diabetes.

## PATHOGENESIS OF TYPE 2 DIABETES MELLITUS

At least two major identifiable pathological defects have been reported in patients with type 2 diabetes. One is a decreased ability of insulin to act on peripheral tissue. This is called *insulin resistance*. The other is *β-cell dysfunction*, which is an inability of the pancreas to produce sufficient insulin to compensate for the insulin resistance. Thus, a relative deficiency of insulin occurs early in the disease and absolute insulin deficiency late in the disease. The debate over whether type 2 diabetes is due primarily to a defect in β-cell secretion or to peripheral resistance to insulin, or to both, has been raging for decades. Regardless of the etiology, type 2 diabetes is an extremely heterogeneous disease, and no single cause is adequate to explain the progression from normal glucose tolerance to diabetes. The fundamental molecular defects in insulin resistance and insulin secretion result from a combination of environmental and genetic factors.

### Loss of β-Cell Function

Increased β-cell demand induced by insulin resistance is ultimately associated with progressive loss of β-cell function that is necessary for the development of fasting hyperglycemia. The major defect is a loss of glucose-induced insulin release, which is termed *selective glucose unresponsiveness*. Hyperglycemia appears to render the β-cells increasingly unresponsive to glucose (called *glucotoxicity*), and the degree of dysfunction correlates with both glucose concentration and duration of hyperglycemia. Restoration of euglycemia rapidly resolves the defect. Increased free fatty acids in serum have also been implicated in β-cell failure (termed *lipotoxicity*). Other insulin secretory abnormalities in type 2 diabetes include disruption of the normal pulsatile release of insulin and an increased ratio of plasma proinsulin to insulin. The number of β-cells is also reduced in patients with type 2 diabetes.

## Insulin Resistance

*Insulin resistance* is defined as "a decreased biological response to normal concentrations of circulating insulin"; it is found in obese, nondiabetic individuals and in patients with type 2 diabetes. The underlying pathophysiologic defect(s) has (have) not been identified, but insulin resistance is usually attributed to a defect in insulin action. Systematic inflammation, indicated by increased concentrations of pro-inflammatory cytokines (e.g., interleukin-6 and tumor necrosis factor) in the blood and inflammatory cells in adipose tissue and liver, contributes to insulin resistance. Measurement of insulin resistance in a routine clinical setting is difficult, and surrogate measures, such as fasting insulin concentration or the euglycemic insulin clamp, are used to provide an indirect assessment of insulin function. The euglycemic clamp is performed in hospital under close supervision. The subject receives a constant intravenous infusion of insulin in one arm with concurrent intravenous infusion of variable amounts of glucose in the other arm to maintain blood glucose at a normal fasting concentration. This provides a measure of sensitivity to insulin. A simpler, but indirect, approach (termed *homeostasis model assessment, HOMA*) is a calculation derived from fasting glucose and insulin concentrations. A broad clinical spectrum of insulin resistance ranges from euglycemia (with marked increase in endogenous insulin) to hyperglycemia (despite large doses of exogenous insulin). Several rare clinical syndromes are also associated with insulin resistance. The prototype is the type A insulin resistance syndrome, which is characterized by hyperinsulinemia, acanthosis nigricans, and ovarian hyperandrogenism.

The insulin resistance syndrome (also known as syndrome X or the metabolic syndrome) is a constellation of associated clinical and laboratory findings, consisting of insulin resistance, hyperinsulinemia, obesity, dyslipidemia (high triglyceride and low high-density lipoprotein [HDL] cholesterol), and hypertension. Individuals with this syndrome are at increased risk for cardiovascular disease. Several different definitions of the metabolic syndrome have been proposed by different organizations; some consensus was reached in 2009, except for waist circumference. The metabolic syndrome is diagnosed if an individual meets three or more of the following criteria:

- increased waist circumference population- and country-specific, e.g., Europe, Canada, and the United States: >35 inches (>88 cm) (women) or >40 inches (>102 cm) (men)
- triglycerides >150 mg/dL (>1.7 mmol/L)
- HDL cholesterol <51 mg/dL (<1.3 mmol/L) (women) or <39 mg/dL (<1.0 mmol/L) (men)
- blood pressure ≥130/85 mm Hg
- fasting plasma glucose ≥100 mg/dL (≥5.6 mmol/L).

The concept of the "metabolic syndrome" has been questioned by several experts, including the person who first described it, and influential clinical diabetes organizations. A WHO Expert Consultation concluded that while the metabolic syndrome may be useful as an educational concept, it has limited practical utility for diagnosis and management, and further efforts to redefine it are inappropriate.

## Environment

Environmental factors, such as diet and exercise, are important determinants in the pathogenesis of type 2 diabetes. Convincing evidence links obesity to the development of type 2 diabetes, but the association is complex. Although 60%–80% of patients with type 2 diabetes are obese, diabetes develops in <15% of obese individuals. In contrast, virtually all obese subjects, even those with normal carbohydrate tolerance, have hyperinsulinemia, and are insulin resistant. Other factors, such as family history of type 2 diabetes (genetic predisposition), the duration of obesity, and the distribution of fat are important. Nevertheless, the rising prevalence of diabetes is believed to be a consequence of the increase in obesity (defined as a body mass index ≥30 kg/m$^2$), the prevalence of which was reported to be 39.6% in US adults in 2016 and is predicted to reach 48.9% by 2030. It is important to note that intervention can delay or prevent the onset of type 2 diabetes. Several studies have documented that life-style changes (weight reduction and exercise) in individuals with IGT reduced the incidence of type 2 diabetes.

An inverse relationship has been noted between the degree of physical activity and the prevalence of type 2 diabetes. For every 500 kcal increase in daily energy expenditure, a 6% decrease in age-adjusted risk of type 2 diabetes occurs. This effect is independent of both body weight and a parental history of diabetes. The mechanism of the protective effect of exercise is thought to be increased sensitivity to insulin in skeletal muscle and adipose tissue.

## Type 2 Diabetes Susceptibility Genes

It is widely acknowledged that genetic factors contribute to the development of type 2 diabetes. For example, the concordance rate for type 2 diabetes in identical twins approaches 100%. Type 2 diabetes is 10 times more likely to occur in an obese person who has a parent with diabetes than in an equally obese person without a family history of diabetes. However, the mode of inheritance is unknown, and type 2 diabetes has been described as a "geneticist's nightmare". It is genetically complex and not inherited according to simple Mendelian rules. Multiple genetic factors interact with exogenous influences (such as environmental factors) to produce the phenotype.

Numerous factors complicate the search for susceptibility genes in type 2 diabetes. A variety of approaches have produced several genes that are associated with type 2 diabetes. Genome-wide association studies (GWAS) have substantially contributed to our understanding of the genetic architecture of type 2 diabetes, with more than 240 genetic loci and 400 genetic variants identified. Most of these genetic loci are associated with the insulin secretion pathway, rather than with insulin resistance. Despite considerable effort to identify the genetic basis of type 2 diabetes mellitus, genetic defects identified to date account for only ≈5% of patients with type 2 diabetes. Moreover, the risk alleles in these loci all have relatively small effects (odds ratios, 1.1 to 13). Combined analysis of 48 different type 2 risk loci did not significantly affect the time from diagnosis to prescription of the first drug.

## MONOGENIC DIABETES MELLITUS

Mutation of a single gene that results in β-cell dysfunction accounts for ≈2% of diabetes. At least 40 genes have been identified that cause monogenic diabetes. The ADA advocates that monogenic diabetes should be considered in diabetes diagnosed within the first 6 months of life, "atypical diabetes" (without typical features of type 1 or type 2 diabetes, especially with a strong family history of diabetes) or in children with mild hyperglycemia, especially if non-obese. Monogenic diabetes is usually separated into two categories, on the basis of age of onset of hyperglycemia.

### Neonatal Diabetes Mellitus

Persistent hyperglycemia occurring before the age of 6 months is termed *neonatal* (or *congenital*) *diabetes*. Genetic testing has identified monogenic etiology in ≈85% of these patients. The ADA recommends that all children diagnosed with diabetes in the first 6 months of life should have immediate genetic testing for neonatal diabetes. Accurate diagnosis is important as some patients require insulin while others can be managed with oral hypoglycemic agents. Some forms are transient, and insulin-requiring diabetes may resolve spontaneously between 6 and 18 months of age.

### Maturity-Onset Diabetes of the Young

Maturity-onset diabetes of the young (MODY) phenotypically resembles type 2 diabetes, but occurs in young (usually <25 years) non-obese patients who have a family history of diabetes. Inheritance is autosomal dominant, and patients have no autoantibodies for type 1 diabetes. The clinical spectrum of MODY is broad, ranging from asymptomatic hyperglycemia to an acute presentation. Thirteen genes on different chromosomes are associated with this disorder. The most common form (estimated prevalence 1 in 1000), MODY2, results from mutations in the gene that encodes glucokinase (an enzyme that catalyzes the phosphorylation of glucose in the β-cell), leading to partial deficiency of insulin secretion. Patients have mild fasting hyperglycemia and glucose lowering therapy is rarely needed. Most of the other MODYs are caused by mutations in the genes that encode transcription factors that regulate expression of genes in pancreatic β-cells, resulting in impaired insulin synthesis or secretion or a reduced β-cell mass. MODY mutations have substitution, deletion, or insertion of nucleotides in the coding regions of the genes. These mutations are detected by PCR. OGTT, islet autoantibodies and C-peptide may be helpful in differentiating MODY from type 1 or type 2 diabetes, but genetic testing, now widely available, is required to establish the diagnosis of MODY. Genetic testing for MODY should be performed in those diagnosed in childhood or early adulthood with diabetes that is not characteristic of type 1 or type 2 diabetes and occurs in successive generations.

## DIAGNOSIS OF NON-GESTATIONAL DIABETES MELLITUS

For many years the diagnosis of diabetes mellitus was dependent solely on the demonstration of hyperglycemia. For type 1 diabetes, the diagnosis is usually easy because hyperglycemia appears abruptly, is severe, and is accompanied by serious metabolic derangements. Diagnosis of type 2 diabetes may be difficult because hyperglycemia often is not severe enough for the patient to notice symptoms of diabetes. Nevertheless, the risk of complications makes it important to identify people with the disease.

### Hemoglobin A$_{1c}$

A major change in the diagnosis of diabetes was recommended in 2009. An International Expert Committee advised that HbA$_{1c}$, which reflects long-term blood glucose concentrations, could be used for the diagnosis of type 2 diabetes (Box 33.2). An HbA$_{1c}$ value ≥6.5% (≥48 mmol/mol) was selected as the decision point, based on the prevalence of retinopathy. This recommendation has been endorsed by the ADA and several other influential clinical organizations, including the WHO, the International Diabetes Federation, and the European Association for the Study of Diabetes, and has been widely (albeit not universally) accepted. HbA$_{1c}$ concentrations 5.7%–6.4% (39–46 mmol/mol) indicate subjects at high risk of developing diabetes. Note that some organizations define high risk as HbA$_{1c}$ concentrations of 5.5%–6.4% (37–46 mmol/mol), while others recommend 6.1%–6.4%

---

**BOX 33.2    Criteria for the Diagnosis of Diabetes[a]**

1. HbA$_{1c}$ ≥6.5% (48 mmol/mol)[b]
   OR
2. FPG ≥7.0 mmol/L (126 mg/dL)[c]
   OR
3. 2-h Plasma glucose ≥11.1 mmol/L (200 mg/dL) during an OGTT[d]
   OR
4. In a patient with classic symptoms of hyperglycemia or hyperglycemic crisis, a random plasma glucose ≥11.1 mmol/L (200 mg/dL)[e,f]

[a] In the absence of unequivocal hyperglycemia, diagnosis requires two abnormal test results from the same sample or in two separate test samples.
[b] The test should be performed in a laboratory using a method that is NGSP certified and standardized to the DCCT assay. Point-of-care assays should not be used for diagnosis.
[c] Fasting is defined as no caloric intake for at least 8 h.
[d] The OGTT should be performed as described by WHO, using a glucose load containing the equivalent of 75 g anhydrous glucose dissolved in water.
[e] The classic symptoms of hyperglycemia include polyuria, polydipsia, and unexplained weight loss.
[f] "Random" is any time of the day without regard to time since previous meal.
Adapted from the American Diabetes Association. 2. Classification and diagnosis of diabetes. *Diabetes Care* 2022;45(Suppl 1):S17–S38.

(43–46 mmol/mol). $HbA_{1c}$ was also recommended as an alternative to glucose for screening for diabetes. This last recommendation has also been accepted by the ADA and other clinical organizations.

## Fasting Plasma Glucose

FPG concentrations of 126 mg/dL (7.0 mmol/L) or greater on more than one occasion are diagnostic of diabetes mellitus (see Box 33.2). Some investigators believe that fasting hyperglycemia may be a relatively late development in the course of type 2 diabetes, delaying the diagnosis and leading to underestimation of the prevalence of diabetes mellitus in the population. Readers should be aware of the limitations of FPG in diabetes diagnosis, including the requirement that the patient fast ≥8 h, large biological variation (even in a single individual on different days), and the risk of glycolysis in the test tube.

## Oral Glucose Tolerance Test

Although more sensitive than FPG determinations, glucose tolerance testing is affected by multiple factors that result in *poor reproducibility* (Box 33.3). Moreover, approximately 20% of OGTTs fall into the non-diagnostic category (e.g., only one blood sample exhibits increased glucose concentration). Unless results are grossly abnormal initially, some bodies recommend that the OGTT should be performed on two separate occasions to establish the diagnosis of diabetes.

The following conditions should be met before an OGTT is performed: discontinue, when possible, medications known to affect glucose tolerance; perform in the morning after 3 days

---

### BOX 33.3 Factors Other than Diabetes that Influence the Oral Glucose Tolerance Test

**Patient preparation**
- Duration of fast
- Prior carbohydrate intake
- Medications (e.g., thiazides, oral contraceptives, corticosteroids)
- Trauma
- Intercurrent illness
- Age
- Activity
- Weight

**Administration of glucose**
- Form of glucose (anhydrous or monohydrate)
- Quantity of glucose ingested
- Volume in which administered
- Rate of ingestion

**During the test**
- Posture
- Anxiety
- Caffeine
- Smoking
- Activity
- Time of day
- Sample preservation

---

of unrestricted diet (containing at least 150 g of carbohydrate/day) and activity, and perform the test after a 10–16-h fast only in ambulatory outpatients (bed rest impairs glucose tolerance), who should remain seated during the test without smoking cigarettes. Glucose tolerance testing should not be performed on hospitalized, acutely ill, or inactive patients. The test should begin between 7:00 a.m. and 9:00 a.m. Venous plasma glucose should be measured fasting, then 2 hours after an oral glucose load. For non-pregnant adults, the recommended load is 75 g, which may not be a maximum stimulus; for children, 1.75 g/kg, up to 75 g maximum is given. The glucose should be dissolved in 300 mL of water and ingested over 5 minutes. A commercial, more palatable form of glucose may be ingested, but whether the anhydrous or monohydrate form of glucose should be used, is still in question.

An OGTT is rarely used in clinical practice for the diagnosis of diabetes in the US and many other countries owing to its lack of reproducibility and inconvenience. The sensitivity of FPG concentrations is lower than the OGTT for diagnosing diabetes, and some authors claim that the OGTT better identifies patients at risk for developing complications of diabetes. An FPG value <100 mg/dL (<5.6 mmol/L) or a random glucose concentration <140 mg/dL (<7.8 mmol/L) is sufficient to rule out the diagnosis of diabetes mellitus.

## DIAGNOSIS OF GESTATIONAL DIABETES MELLITUS

Gestational diabetes mellitus (GDM) was defined for many years as any degree of glucose intolerance with onset or first recognition during pregnancy. This can include women with pre-existing, but undiagnosed, diabetes. Due to the increasing prevalence of type 2 diabetes, the number of pregnant women with undiagnosed type 2 diabetes has increased. Therefore, several organizations (including the ADA and WHO) now recommend that women with risk factors for type 2 diabetes should be screened at the first antenatal visit using standard diagnostic criteria (see Box 33.2). Women diagnosed with diabetes by this approach should receive a diagnosis of diabetes complicating pregnancy. Other women should be rescreened for GDM at 24–28 weeks of gestation using the criteria in Table 33.2.

Normal pregnancy is associated with increased insulin resistance, especially in the late second and third trimesters. Euglycemia is maintained by increased insulin secretion, with GDM developing in those women who fail to augment insulin sufficiently. Risk factors for GDM include a family history of diabetes in a first-degree relative, obesity, advanced maternal age, glycosuria, and selected adverse outcomes in a previous pregnancy (e.g., stillbirth, macrosomia). Recommendations for screening and diagnosis remain controversial and lack consensus.

The Hyperglycemia in Pregnancy and Adverse Outcome (HAPO) study was a large (≈25,000 pregnant women), prospective, multinational study published in 2008. The study revealed strong, graded, linear associations between maternal glycemia and adverse outcomes. Based on these data, it

## TABLE 33.2  Screening for and Diagnosis of Gestational Diabetes Mellitus

**I  One-step**

1. Perform at 24–28 weeks of gestation in pregnant women not previously diagnosed with diabetes
2. Perform in the morning after an overnight fast of at least 8 h
3. Measure fasting venous plasma glucose
4. Give 75 g of glucose orally
5. Measure plasma glucose hourly for 2 h after glucose is given
6. At least one value must meet or exceed the following:

| | Glucose concentration |
|---|---|
| Fasting | 92 mg/dL (5.1 mmol/L) |
| 1 h | 180 mg/dL (10.0 mmol/L) |
| 2 h | 153 mg/dL (8.5 mmol/L) |

**II  Two-step**

**A.  Step 1 (screening)**

1. Perform at 24–28 weeks of gestation[a] in pregnant women not previously diagnosed with diabetes
2. Give 50 g oral glucose load without regard to time of day or time of last meal
3. Measure venous plasma glucose at 1 h
4. If glucose is ≥130, 135 or 140 mg/dL (7.2, 7.5 or 7.8 mmol/L)[b], proceed to step 2 and perform a 100 g glucose tolerance test

**B.  Step 2 (diagnosis)**

1. Perform in the morning after an overnight fast of at least 8 h
2. Measure fasting venous plasma glucose
3. Give 100 g of glucose orally
4. At least two[c] of the values must meet or exceed the following:

| | Glucose concentration |
|---|---|
| Fasting | 95 mg/dL (5.3 mmol/L) |
| 1 h | 180 mg/dL (10.0 mmol/L) |
| 2 h | 155 mg/dL (8.6 mmol/L) |
| 3 h | 140 mg/dL (7. 8 mmol/L) |

[a]The WHO states that this test can be performed at any time during pregnancy.
[b]The American College of Obstetricians and Gynecologists (ACOG) recommends any of the commonly used thresholds of 130, 135, or 140 mg/dL (7.2, 7.5, or 7.8 mmol/L).
[c]ACOG states that one increased value can be used for diagnosis (Committee on Practice Bulletins—Obstetrics. Practice Bulletin No. 190: Gestational Diabetes Mellitus. *Obstet Gynecol* 2018;131:e49–e64.)
Modified from the American Diabetes Association. Classification and diagnosis of diabetes: Standards of medical care in diabetes—2022. *Diabetes Care* 2022;45(Suppl 1):S17–S38.

was recommended that all pregnant women not previously known to have diabetes should be evaluated for GDM by a 75-g OGTT at 24–28 weeks' gestation. Diagnostic cutpoints for fasting, 1- and 2-hour plasma glucose concentrations have been established (see Table 33.2, one-step).

These criteria, which increase the incidence of GDM by approximately 2.5-fold, have not been accepted by all clinical organizations around the globe. The ADA accepts either the one-step strategy based on the HAPO study or the prior two-step method. ACOG endorses the two-step method, but states that only one increased value, rather than two, can be used to diagnose GDM. Universal criteria to diagnose GDM remain elusive.

The two-step is as follows:

1. Screen by a 50-g oral glucose load (the patient does not need to be fasting). A plasma glucose value greater than or equal to commonly used thresholds of 130, 135, or 140 mg/dL (7.2, 7.5, or 7.7 mmol/L, respectively) at 1 hour after glucose ingestion indicates the necessity for definitive testing. Approximately 15% of pregnant women meet this criterion and require a full OGTT. This subgroup includes approximately 80% of all women with GDM.
2. The diagnosis of GDM can be made on the basis of the result of the 100-g, 3-h OGTT. This should be performed on a different day from the 50-g OGTT.

Multiple studies have evaluated other markers to diagnose GDM. Although conceptually appealing (as neither fasting nor drinking a glucose load is necessary), markers of long-term glycemia (e.g., HbA$_{1c}$, fructosamine, or glycated albumin) have not shown adequate sensitivity or specificity. An area of considerable recent interest is GDM in early pregnancy, i.e., the first trimester (1–12 weeks). The most rapid fetal development occurs in the first trimester, more than 4 months before GDM screening is conducted. Questions that require answers include: "which analytes should be used to identify GDM in early pregnancy?"; "is diagnosis of GDM early in pregnancy of clinical value?"; and "will identification and/or treatment of GDM in early pregnancy improve outcomes for mother and baby?" Several clinical studies are underway to address these questions.

Although usually asymptomatic and not life-threatening to the mother, GDM is associated with increased neonatal mortality and morbidity, including hypocalcemia, hypoglycemia, and macrosomia. Maternal hyperglycemia causes the fetus to secrete more insulin, resulting in stimulation of fetal growth and macrosomia. Recognition is important because therapy can reduce perinatal morbidity and mortality. Maternal complications include a high rate of cesarean delivery and hypertension. In addition, mothers with GDM are at significantly increased risk of subsequent type 2 diabetes.

Distinct from GDM is pregnancy in a patient with preexisting diabetes. This is associated with an increased incidence of congenital malformation, but meticulous glycemic control during the first 8 weeks of pregnancy can significantly decrease the risk of congenital malformation. Tight control results in an increased incidence of maternal hypoglycemia, which is teratogenic in animals but does not cause malformation in humans.

Women with GDM should be screened for diabetes 6–12 weeks postpartum using non-pregnant OGTT criteria (see Box 33.2). (HbA$_{1c}$ is not recommended because of the antepartum therapy for hyperglycemia.) If glucose values are normal, glycemia should be reassessed at least every 3 years using glucose or HbA$_{1c}$.

# CHRONIC COMPLICATIONS OF DIABETES MELLITUS

Patients with type 1 or type 2 diabetes are at high risk for the development of chronic complications. Diabetes-specific microvascular pathology in the retina, renal glomeruli, and peripheral nerves produces retinopathy, nephropathy, and neuropathy, respectively. As a result, diabetes is the most frequent cause of new cases of blindness in the industrialized world in persons between 25 and 74 years of age and is the leading cause of end-stage renal disease. Diabetes is also associated with a marked increase in atherosclerotic macrovascular disease involving cardiac, cerebral, and peripheral large vessels. Therefore, patients with diabetes have a high rate of myocardial infarction (the major cause of mortality in diabetes), stroke, and limb amputation.

## Type 1 Diabetes

Although it was theorized for many years that better glycemic control would decrease rates of long-term complications of diabetes, it was not until the publication of the Diabetes Control and Complications Trial (DCCT) in 1993 that this hypothesis was verified. The DCCT was a multicenter, randomized trial that compared the effects of intensive and conventional therapy on the development and progression of complications in 1441 patients with type 1 diabetes, all of whom required insulin. During the study period, which averaged 6.5 years, intensively managed patients maintained significantly lower mean blood glucose concentrations. Compared with conventional therapy, intensive therapy reduced the risks of retinopathy, nephropathy, and neuropathy by 40% to 75%. Intensive therapy delayed the onset and slowed the progression of these complications, regardless of age, gender, or duration of diabetes. Absolute risks of retinopathy and nephropathy were proportional to the mean $HbA_{1c}$ (see later). Although intensive therapy also reduced the development of hypercholesterolemia, macrovascular complications were not significantly decreased in the initial assessment. However, analysis after 17 years of follow-up documented a 42% lower incidence of cardiovascular disease in the intensively treated group. This landmark study has had a considerable impact on therapeutic goals and comprehension of the pathogenesis of complications of diabetes.

At the conclusion of the DCCT, 95% of participants enrolled in the long-term follow-up study, the Epidemiology of Diabetes Interventions and Complications (EDIC) study. Five years after the end of the DCCT, no difference in metabolic control (as assessed by $HbA_{1c}$ measurements) was noted between the former conventional and intensively treated groups. Nevertheless, further progression of retinopathy and neuropathy was significantly lower in the former intensive group, demonstrating that the beneficial effects of intensive treatment persisted for at least 19 years beyond the period of strictest intervention.

## Type 2 Diabetes

The role of hyperglycemia in the development of complications in individuals with type 2 diabetes was established in the United Kingdom Prospective Diabetes Study (UKPDS). The UKPDS was a major, randomized, multicenter clinical study that included 5102 patients with newly diagnosed type 2 diabetes who were followed for an average of 10 years. Analogous to the findings of the DCCT, the UKPDS demonstrated that in patients with type 2 diabetes, intensive treatment diminishes the development of microvascular complications by approximately 10% to 40%. Intensive treatment also decreased the rate of occurrence of macrovascular complications. Although the reduction was not statistically significant initially, follow-up 10 years after the study ended showed a significant reduction in myocardial infarction among patients who had received intensive therapy. Analogous to the EDIC findings, long-term benefits for microvascular complications were observed with follow-up of patients in the UKPDS, despite loss of glycemic separation between intensive and standard cohorts after the study ended. An important caveat of both the DCCT and the UKPDS was that intensive therapy produced a three-fold increase in the incidence of severe hypoglycemia.

# ROLE OF THE CLINICAL LABORATORY IN DIABETES MELLITUS

The clinical laboratory has a vital role in both the diagnosis and management of diabetes (Table 33.3). The National Academy of Clinical Biochemistry (NACB)/AACC published evidence-based guidelines for laboratory analysis in diabetes in 2002, 2011, and 2023. These guidelines were reviewed and endorsed by the ADA as a Position Statement. A brief overview is presented here.

## Diagnosis

### Preclinical (Screening)

Several large clinical trials are underway to assess a variety of therapeutic strategies designed to delay or prevent the onset of type 1 diabetes. Until effective intervention becomes available and cost-effective screening strategies are developed for young children, screening for antibodies and determining HLA type is not currently warranted, except in clinical research studies. A decrease in glucose-stimulated insulin secretion is the first functional abnormality in both type 1 and type 2 diabetes. Nevertheless, tests of insulin secretion are not currently recommended for routine clinical use.

Screening asymptomatic individuals for type 2 diabetes has been the subject of much controversy. The ADA, which previously did not support screening, now advocates screening in all asymptomatic individuals over the age of 35 years. If the $HbA_{1c}$ is <5.7% (39 mmol/mol) or the FPG is <100 mg/dL (5.6 mmol/L), testing should be repeated at 3-year intervals. Due to the rising incidence of type 2 diabetes in adolescents, screening is now recommended (starting at age 10 years) for those overweight (BMI >85th centile), with one other risk factor, e.g., family history, certain ethnic group, or maternal history of GDM.

### Clinical

The laboratory diagnosis of diabetes is made exclusively by the demonstration of hyperglycemia, as evidenced by

## TABLE 33.3 Role of the Laboratory in the Management of Diabetes Mellitus

**Diagnosis**

| | |
|---|---|
| Preclinical (Screening) | Immunologic markers (autoantibodies) |
| |   ICA |
| |   IAA |
| |   GADA |
| |   Protein tyrosine phosphatase antibodies (IA-2) |
| |   Zinc transporter ZnT8 antibodies |
| | Genetic markers (e.g., human leukocyte antigen [HLA]) |
| | Insulin secretion |
| |   Fasting |
| |   Pulses |
| |   In response to a glucose challenge |
| | Blood glucose (fasting) |
| | Oral glucose tolerance test (OGTT) |
| | Hemoglobin A$_{1c}$ (HbA$_{1c}$) |
| Clinical | Blood glucose (fasting) |
| | Oral glucose tolerance test (OGTT) |
| | HbA$_{1c}$ |
| | Ketones (urine and blood) |
| | Other (e.g., insulin, C-peptide, stimulation tests) |

**Management**

| | |
|---|---|
| Acute | Glucose |
| |   Blood |
| |   Urine |
| | Ketones |
| |   Blood |
| |   Urine |
| | Acid-base status (pH ([H$^+$]), bicarbonate) |
| | Lactate |
| | Other abnormalities related to cellular dehydration or therapy (e.g., potassium, sodium, phosphate, osmolality) |
| Chronic | Glucose |
| |   Blood (fasting, random, continuous monitoring) |
| |   Urine |
| | Glycated proteins |
| |   HbA$_{1c}$ |
| |   Fructosamine |
| |   Glycated albumin |
| | 1,5-Anhydroglucitol (1,5-AG) |
| | Urine protein |
| |   Albuminuria (previously termed "microalbuminuria") |
| |   Proteinuria |
| | Evaluation of complications (e.g., creatinine, cholesterol, triglycerides) |
| | Evaluation of pancreas transplant (C-peptide, insulin) |
| | Eligibility for insulin pump (C-peptide) |

measurements of venous plasma glucose or HbA$_{1c}$. Although other tests (e.g., C-peptide, insulin analysis) have been proposed to assist in the diagnosis and classification of the disease, they do not have a role outside of research studies.

## Management

### Acute

In diabetic ketoacidosis, hyperosmolar nonketotic coma, and hypoglycemia, the clinical laboratory has an essential role in both diagnosis and monitoring of therapy. Several analytes are frequently measured to guide clinicians in treatment regimens to restore euglycemia and correct other metabolic disturbances. The metabolic abnormalities of these conditions are beyond the scope of this book, and interested readers are referred to a standard textbook of medicine. The AACC/ADA guidelines also provide information on the tests that are used.

### Chronic

The DCCT and UKPDS studies documented a correlation between blood glucose concentrations and the development of long-term complications of diabetes. Measurement of glucose and glycated proteins provides an index of short- and long-term glycemic control, respectively (see Glycated proteins, below). Detection of and monitoring for complications are achieved by assaying creatinine, urine albumin, and serum lipids. The success of newer therapies, such as islet cell or pancreas transplantation, can be monitored by measuring serum C-peptide or insulin concentrations.

## SELF-MONITORING OF BLOOD GLUCOSE

Patients with diabetes, especially those who need insulin, require careful monitoring to maintain control of blood glucose. Therapeutic regimens include multiple daily insulin injections, insulin pumps, and continuous subcutaneous insulin injections. *Testing urine for glucose is not adequate for monitoring patients on insulin therapy.* Although some evidence suggests that it may be effective for monitoring type 2 diabetes, the ADA states that limitations of urine testing make blood glucose measurements the preferred method for assessing glycemic control.

Portable meters for measurement of blood glucose concentrations are used in three major settings: in acute and chronic care facilities (at the patient's bedside and in clinics or hospitals); in physicians' offices, and by patients or their caregivers at home, work, and school. Patients measure their own blood glucose concentrations and modify their insulin doses based on the result. In 2006, the overall rate of daily self-monitoring of blood glucose (SMBG) was 63.4% among all adults with diabetes in the United States, and 86.7% among those treated with insulin.

A large number of simple test strips permit rapid glucose measurements on a drop of whole blood. At least 75 different blood glucose meters are commercially available in the US. These meters vary in size, weight, calibration method, and other features, and use the same enzyme-catalyzed reactions, predominantly glucose oxidase or glucose dehydrogenase, as described in Chapter 22 for glucose analysis. The reagents are combined in dry form on a small surface area of a test strip.

To perform the measurement, a sample of blood (usually from a fingerprick, but anticoagulated whole blood collected in ethylenediaminetetraacetic acid [EDTA] or heparin may be used) is placed on the test pad, which is attached to a plastic support. The test strip is then inserted into the meter. (In some devices, the strip is inserted into the meter before the sample is applied.) After a fixed time, the result appears on a digital display screen. These meters use reflectance photometry or electrochemistry to measure the rate of the reaction or the final concentration of the products. Reflectance photometry measures the amount of light reflected from a test pad containing reagent. In electrochemical systems, the enzymatic reaction produces a flow of electrons in an electrode incorporated on the test strip. The current, which is directly proportional to the amount of glucose in the sample, is converted to a digital readout. Large variability has been noted among meters as to the test time (5–45 seconds), the claimed reading range (30–500 mg/dL to 0–600 mg/dL: 1.7–28 mmol/L to 0–33 mmol/L) and the minimum blood volume (0.3–1.5 µL). Calibration is automatic on some devices, whereas others use lot-specific code chips or strips. All manufacturers supply control solutions. Advances in technology facilitate data analysis and sharing. Some meters have Bluetooth capabilities (enabling transmission of data to a smartphone or computer), cellular connections that automatically send data to the "cloud," USB ports, and/or communication with an insulin pump. Strict adherence to the instructions is necessary to obtain accurate results. Some meters have a porous membrane that separates erythrocytes, and analysis is performed on the resultant plasma. Whole blood glucose concentrations are approximately 10%–15% lower than plasma or serum concentrations, but meters can be calibrated to report plasma glucose values, even when the sample is whole blood. An International Federation of Clinical Chemistry and Laboratory Medicine (IFCC) working group recommended that glucose meters be harmonized using a factor of ×1.11 to report the concentration of glucose in plasma, irrespective of the sample type or technology.

## Analytical Goals

Multiple analytical goals have been proposed for the performance of glucose meters. The recommendations promulgated in 2002 by the Clinical and Laboratory Standards Institute (CLSI) (previously called the National Committee for Clinical Laboratory Standards [NCCLS]) and in 2003 by the International Organization for Standardization (ISO) are that 95% of results should fall within 20% of laboratory-measured glucose concentrations when greater than 75 mg/dL (>4.2 mmol/L) and within 15 mg/dL (0.83 mmol/L) of a laboratory glucose measurement if the glucose concentration is <75 mg/dL (<4.2 mmol/L). In both CSLI and ISO guidelines, 5% of these results can be considerably outside these limits. Note that the CLSI guideline is for meter use in acute and chronic care facilities (mainly hospitals), while the ISO guidelines pertain to meters for self-testing (i.e., SMBG). Many experts believe these acceptance criteria are too wide. The CLSI and ISO documents were revised in 2013, with tightening of acceptance criteria. The current CLSI guideline POCT12-A3 indicates that for 95% of the samples,

the difference between meter and laboratory measurement should be <12.5% when the laboratory glucose value is >100 mg/dL (≥5.6 mmol/L) and <12 mg/dL (<0.67 mmol/L) when the glucose concentration is <100 mg/dL (<5.6 mmol/L). In addition, no more than 2% of results can differ by more than 20% at >75 mg/dL (≥4.2 mmol/L) and by more than 15 mg/dL (>0.83 mmol/L) when the glucose concentration is <75 mg/dL (<4.2 mmol/L). The revised ISO goals, also issued in 2013, are that for 95% of the samples, the difference between meter and laboratory measurement should be <15% when the laboratory glucose value is >100 mg/dL (≥5.6 mmol/L) and <15 mg/dL (<0.83 mmol/L) when the glucose concentration is <100 mg/dL (<5.6 mmol/L). Moreover, 99% of results must be within zones A and B of the consensus error grid (see below). In the United States, the FDA issued guidance in 2016 for glucose meters. Two separate documents were released, one for home use (SMBG) and the other for hospitals. The analytic goals are more stringent than either the CLSI or ISO guidelines.

A different method uses an error grid to try to define clinically important errors by identifying broad target ranges. An approach using simulation modeling concluded that meters that achieve both a CV and a bias less than 5% rarely lead to major errors in insulin dosage. Lack of consensus on quality goals for glucose meters reflects the absence of agreed-upon objective criteria. When biological variation criteria are used, a goal for total error (including both bias and imprecision) of 6.1% or less has been proposed.

Glucose meters are also used to calculate insulin dose in patients without diabetes on tight glucose control protocols in intensive care units (ICUs). Evidence in 2001 showed that intensive insulin therapy significantly reduced mortality and morbidity of critically ill patients in the surgical ICU. Some subsequent studies were unable to replicate these findings. Many factors, such as hypoxia, shock, and low hematocrit, are common in these patients and can compromise glucose analysis in capillary blood samples. The use of glucose meters in these settings has been questioned by some experts. Some meters may have adequate analytical performance (as noted above), but the use of skin puncture (fingerstick) samples introduces serious error in patients who have conditions such as shock.

## Performance of Glucose Meters

The most common errors in SMBG, such as proper application, timing, and removal of excess blood, have been reduced by advances in technology, but can still occur. Additional innovations that reduce operator error include: (1) systems that abort testing if the sample volume is inadequate; (2) built-in programs that simplify quality control; and (3) increased memory that allows the instrument to store up to several hundred glucose readings that can be downloaded into a computer.

Several factors affect the accuracy and reproducibility of SMBG. These include: (1) user variability—up to 50% of values may vary by more than 20% from reference values; (2) hematocrit—the presence of anemia (false increase) or polycythemia (false depression) may result in up to 30% variability; and (3) defective reagent strips or instrument malfunction (rare). Other variables include changes in altitude, environmental temperature, or humidity; hypotension; hypoxia; and high triglyceride concentrations. In addition, *these assays are unreliable at very high and very low glucose concentrations* (<60 and >500 mg/dL; <3.3 and >28 mmol/L). Because dehydration, a common feature of diabetic ketoacidosis, greatly increases blood viscosity, inaccurately low blood glucose results may be obtained. Several drugs interfere, but not with all meters. Another important factor is the lack of correlation among meters, even from a single manufacturer, caused by different assay methods and architecture. Moreover, results from 2 meters of the same brand have been observed to differ substantially. Patient factors are also important, particularly adequate training when the meter is used for SMBG. Recurrent education at clinic visits and comparison of SMBG with concurrent laboratory glucose analysis improved the accuracy of patients' blood glucose readings. It is important to evaluate the patient's technique at regular intervals.

Meter performance varies widely. Under carefully controlled conditions in which all assays were performed by a single medical technologist, approximately 50% of analyses met the ADA criterion of less than 5% deviation from reference values. Performance of older meters was substantially worse. Note that medical technologists perform better than patients. Comparison with laboratory values of almost 22,000 measurements of capillary glucose by patients using meters revealed no significant improvement in meter performance between 1989 and 1999.

An analysis in 2012 revealed that only 18 of 34 (53%) glucose meters approved for use in Europe fulfilled the minimum accuracy requirements of the 2013 ISO standard. A 2017 study found that only 2 of 17 meters for SMBG use met the ISO standard when their performance was tested with challenging sets of samples. The imprecision of meters precludes their use from the diagnosis of diabetes and limits their usefulness in screening for diabetes.

## CONTINUOUS GLUCOSE MONITORING

Major limitations to performing SMBG are that it is painful and inconvenient. Since the 1960s, attempts have been made to develop a painless method for monitoring blood glucose concentrations. The concept underlying these methods is that the concentration of glucose in the interstitial fluid correlates with the blood glucose concentration.

Several implanted biosensors with detection systems based on enzymes, electrodes, or fluorescence have been developed. The most widely used method is an electrochemical sensor that is implanted subcutaneously. The devices—continuous glucose monitors (CGM)—use glucose oxidase to measure glucose every 5–15 min. The measurement range is 40–400 mg/dL (2.2–22.2 mmol/L) or 20–500 mg/dL (1.1–27.8 mmol/L). In addition to the

sensor, the CGM has a transmitter on the skin and a receiver for the data. The latter can be a dedicated receiver, a smart phone, or a smart watch.

CGMs can conveniently be divided into three types: (1) real-time CGM, which transmits glucose values to a receiver or smart phone in real time; (2) intermittently scanned (or flash) CGMs, which display readings only when the user swipes a reader or smart phone over the sensor; and (3) professional CGMs, which store results that are downloaded later in the physician's office. CGM systems, which became widely available in the early 2000s, have become more accurate, smaller, and easier to use. Some alert users to current or impending high or low glucose. These devices are, however, subject to some limitations. An important caveat is that changes in glucose concentration in the interstitial fluid occur 4–20 minutes later than in the blood. Implantation of a needle type of sensor into the subcutaneous tissue induces inflammatory responses in the host that alter the sensitivity of the device. Therefore, devices need to be replaced every 7–14 days. A sensor that is surgically implanted under the skin has a 90–180 day life. Until 2017, all sensors were used only as an adjunct to SMBG; meters were still required to adjust insulin dose. Newer CGMs can be used instead of meters. Another improvement is factory calibration. Older systems required calibration by the user every 12 hours with a glucose meter and were subject to the imprecision of the meter. This requirement has been eliminated from some new CGMs, which are factory calibrated.

Another strategy uses microdialysis, which measures glucose outside the body. Fluid is pumped from a storage bag through a microfiber under the skin. The solution carries the glucose sample back to a biosensor, which measures glucose every second and stores an average value every 3 minutes. This device, which is available in parts of Europe, but not in the United States, can be worn for 14 days.

Several randomized studies in adults with type 1 diabetes showed that those using real-time CGM had better long-term glycemic control than patients using intensive insulin therapy and SMBG. Newer features, such as automated suspension of insulin delivery for up to 2 hours when glucose concentrations reach a preset low threshold, significantly reduce the rate of hypoglycemia and improve HbA$_{1c}$ in patients with type 1 diabetes. CGM may be particularly useful in patients with hypoglycemic unawareness or frequent episodes of hypoglycemia. The potential use of CGM in pregnant women with diabetes is under investigation. Automated closed-loop insulin delivery systems (also termed the "artificial pancreas") are a focus of intense research. The system employs a control algorithm that modulates insulin delivery according to real-time interstitial glucose measured by a CGM. Closed-loop systems have been shown to be superior to conventional insulin pump therapy and are likely to become used more widely in the near future.

## NON-INVASIVE GLUCOSE MONITORING

Non-invasive in vivo monitoring of glucose, i.e., without implanting a probe or collecting a sample of any type, has been an area of active investigation for many years. The approaches most widely evaluated involve passing a beam of light through a vascular region and analyzing the resulting light. Near-infrared spectroscopic devices measure the absorption or the reflection of light from subcutaneous tissue. Although glucose has a specific absorption at 1035 nm, many substances interfere. A computer, individually calibrated, screens out interfering information to obtain the glucose result. Alternative approaches include Raman scattering spectroscopy and photoacoustic spectroscopy. Notwithstanding the investment of considerable resources, no noninvasive sensing technology is approved for glucose measurement in patients. Major technological hurdles must be overcome before noninvasive sensing technology will be sufficiently reliable to replace existing portable meters, implantable biosensors, or minimally invasive technologies.

# KETONE BODIES

The development of ketosis requires changes in both adipose tissue and the liver. *The primary substrates for ketone body formation are free fatty acids* from adipose stores. Normally, long-chain fatty acids are taken up by the liver, re-esterified to triglycerides, and stored in the liver or incorporated in very low-density lipoproteins and returned to the plasma. In contrast to other tissues, the brain cannot use free fatty acids for energy. When glucose is unavailable, ketone bodies supply the vast majority of the brain's energy. After a 3-day fast, ketone bodies provide 30%–40% of the body's energy requirements. In uncontrolled diabetes, the low insulin concentrations result in increased lipolysis and decreased re-esterification, thereby increasing plasma free fatty acids. In addition, the increased glucagon/insulin ratio enhances fatty acid oxidation in the liver. Increased counterregulatory hormones also augment lipolysis and ketogenesis in fat and liver, respectively. Thus, increased hepatic ketone production and decreased peripheral tissue metabolism lead to acetoacetate accumulation in the blood. A small fraction undergoes spontaneous decarboxylation to form acetone, but most of it is converted to β-hydroxybutyrate.

The relative proportions in which the three ketone bodies are present in blood vary, depending on the redox state of the cell. In healthy people, β-hydroxybutyrate and acetoacetate—which are present at approximately equimolar concentrations—constitute virtually all the serum ketones. Acetone is a minor component. In severe diabetes, the ratio of β-hydroxybutyrate to acetoacetate may increase to 6:1 because of the presence of a high concentration of nicotinamide adenine dinucleotide (NADH), which favors β-hydroxybutyrate production.

## Clinical Significance of Ketones

Excessive formation of ketone bodies results in increased blood concentrations of ketones (*ketonemia*) and increased excretion of ketones in the urine (*ketonuria*). This process is observed in conditions associated with decreased availability of carbohydrates (such as starvation or frequent vomiting) or decreased use of carbohydrates (such as diabetes mellitus, glycogen storage disease [von Gierke disease], and alkalosis). The popular high-fat, low-carbohydrate diets are ketogenic and increase ketone bodies in the circulation. Diabetes and alcohol consumption are the most common causes of ketoacidosis. Urine ketone test results are positive in more than 30% of first-morning-void specimens from pregnant women.

Diabetic ketoacidosis (DKA) is a potentially life-threatening acute complication of diabetes. Patients have hyperglycemia (glucose >200 mg/dL [11 mmol/L]), increased ketones (the concentration is not specified) and metabolic acidosis (pH <7.3 with serum bicarbonate <15 mEq/L [15 mmol/L]). Measurement of ketones by either a semiquantitative nitroprusside assay (on urine or serum) or quantification of β-hydroxybutyrate in the blood is acceptable for diagnosis of DKA. Although not always excreted in proportion to blood ketone concentrations, because of convenience and cost, urine ketones are widely used by patients with type 1 diabetes for early identification of ketosis. The ADA states that ketone testing is an important part of monitoring by patients with diabetes, particularly those with type 1 diabetes, pregnancy with pre-existing diabetes, and GDM. Patients with type 1 diabetes should test for ketones during acute illness or stress, with consistent increases in blood glucose (>300 mg/dL; >16.7 mmol/L), during pregnancy, or when symptoms of ketoacidosis are present. Patients treated with SGLT2 (sodium glucose transport) inhibitors are at increased risk of ketoacidosis and should check ketones at any sign of illness. Accumulating evidence suggests that β-hydroxybutyrate in the blood is better than urine ketones in patients with type 1 diabetes, reducing frequency of hospital admission and shortening time to recovery from DKA.

Most of the tests for ketone bodies detect or measure acetoacetate only. This may produce a paradoxical situation. When a patient initially presents in ketoacidosis, the test results for ketones may be only weakly positive. With therapy, β-hydroxybutyrate is converted to acetoacetate, and the ketosis appears to worsen.

## Measurement of Ketones in Body Fluids

None of the commonly used methods for the detection and determination of ketone bodies in serum or urine reacts with all three ketone bodies. The Gerhardt ferric chloride test reacts with acetoacetate only. Tests using nitroprusside are at least 10 times more sensitive to acetoacetate than to acetone and give no reaction at all with β-hydroxybutyrate. Traditional tests for β-hydroxybutyrate are indirect; they require brief boiling of the urine to remove acetone and acetoacetate by evaporation (acetoacetate first breaks down spontaneously to acetone), followed by gentle oxidation of β-hydroxybutyrate to acetoacetate and acetone with peroxide, ferric ions, or dichromate. The acetoacetate thus formed may be detected with the Gerhardt test or by one of the procedures in which nitroprusside is used. Quantitative enzymatic assays for β-hydroxybutyrate that can be performed directly on blood or serum are commercially available. These assays are available for high throughput instruments in the central laboratory or using hand-held devices at point of care.

The semiquantitative AimTab and Ketostix are frequently used but are insensitive to β-hydroxybutyrate. It is important to bear in mind, therefore, that a negative nitroprusside test result does not rule out ketoacidosis.

### AimTab

AimTab tablets contain a mixture of glycine, sodium nitroprusside, disodium phosphate, and lactose. Acetoacetate or acetone (to a lesser extent) in the presence of glycine forms a lavender–purple complex with nitroprusside. β-Hydroxybutyrate does not react with nitroprusside. Disodium phosphate provides an optimum pH for the reaction, and lactose enhances the color.

### Ketostix

Ketostix is a modification of the nitroprusside test, in which a reagent strip is used instead of a tablet. The Ketostix test gives a positive reaction within 15 seconds with a specimen containing at least 50 mg of acetoacetate per liter. The color chart from the manufacturer gives readings for ketone concentrations of 50, 150, 400, 800, and 1600 mg/L. Acetone also reacts, but the test is less sensitive to it.

### Determination of β-Hydroxybutyrate

In this test, β-hydroxybutyrate in the presence of $NAD^+$ is converted by β-hydroxybutyrate dehydrogenase to acetoacetate, producing reduced NAD (NADH). Diaphorase catalyzes the reduction of nitroblue tetrazolium (NBT) by NADH to produce a purple compound, and its absorbance is read at 505 nm. The assay can be performed on serum or plasma on open-channel automated chemistry analyzers and on whole blood with hand-held meters.

$$\text{β-Hydroxybutyrate} \underset{\substack{\\ NAD^{\oplus} \quad NADH + H^{\oplus}}}{\overset{\substack{\text{β-Hydroxybutyrate} \\ \text{dehydrogenase}}}{\rightleftharpoons}} \text{Acetoacetate}$$

$$NADH + NBT \overset{Diaphorase}{\rightleftharpoons} NAD^{\oplus} + \text{Reduced NBT}$$

Serum β-hydroxybutyrate values vary from 0.21 to 2.81 mg/dL (0.02–0.27 mmol/L) in healthy people after an overnight fast. Ketone bodies in the blood can reach 20 mg/dL (2 mmol/L) with prolonged exercise. Patients with diabetic ketoacidosis usually have β-hydroxybutyrate concentrations >30 mg/dL (>3 mmol/L).

### Determination of Ketone Bodies in Urine

Test strips such as AimTab, Ketostix, Ketosis Test Strips, and TRUEplus Ketone Test Strips are suitable for detecting ketone bodies in urine. The sensitivity and specificity of these tests are the same as outlined for serum.

## GLYCATED HEMOGLOBIN

Measurement of glycated proteins, primarily glycated hemoglobin (GHb), is effective in monitoring long-term glucose control in people with diabetes mellitus. It provides a retrospective index of integrated plasma glucose values over an extended period of time, and is not subject to the wide fluctuations observed when blood glucose concentrations are assayed. GHb concentrations are therefore a valuable and widely used adjunct to blood glucose determinations for monitoring long-term glycemic control. In addition, GHb is recommended for the diagnosis of diabetes and is a measure of risk for the development of microvascular complications of diabetes.

*Glycation is the nonenzymatic addition of a sugar residue to amino groups of proteins.* Human adult hemoglobin (Hb) usually consists of HbA (≈97% of the total), $HbA_2$ (2.5%), and HbF (0.5%). HbA is made up of four polypeptide chains, two α-chains and two β-chains. Chromatographic analysis of HbA identifies several minor hemoglobins, namely $HbA_{1a}$, $HbA_{1b}$, and $HbA_{1c}$, which are collectively referred to as $HbA_1$, *fast hemoglobins* (because they migrate more rapidly than HbA in an electrical field), *glycohemoglobins*, or **glycated hemoglobins**. The Joint Commission on Biochemical Nomenclature of the International Union of Pure and Applied Chemistry recommends the term *neoglycoprotein* for such derivatives and the term *glycation* to describe this process. Therefore, although *glycosylated* and *glucosylated* have been widely used in the literature, the term *glycated* is preferred. $HbA_{1c}$ is formed by the condensation of glucose with the N-terminal valine residue of each β-chain of HbA to form an unstable Schiff base (aldimine, pre-$HbA_{1c}$; Fig. 33.2). The Schiff base may dissociate or may undergo an Amadori rearrangement to form a stable ketoamine, $HbA_{1c}$. $HbA_{1a1}$ and $HbA_{1a2}$, which make up $HbA_{1a}$, have fructose-1,6-diphosphate and glucose-6-phosphate, respectively, attached to the amino terminal of the β-chain. $HbA_{1b}$ contains pyruvic acid linked to the amino terminal valine of the β-chain, probably by a ketamine bond. $HbA_{1c}$ *is the major fraction*, constituting approximately 80% of $HbA_1$.

Glycation may also occur at sites other than the end of the β-chain, such as lysine residues or the α-chain. The sum of all GHbs, referred to as total glycated hemoglobin, cannot be separated from nonglycated hemoglobin by methods based

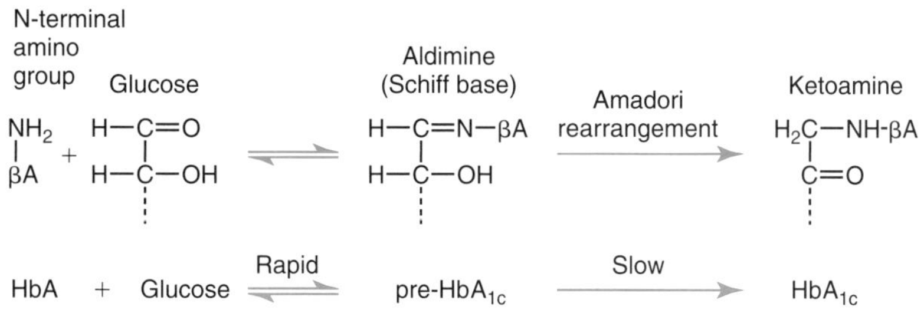

Fig. 33.2 Formation of hemoglobin (Hb)$A_{1c}$.

on charge, but are measured by boronate affinity chromatography.

Formation of GHb is essentially irreversible, and the concentration in the blood depends on both the life span of the red blood cell (RBC; average 120 days) and the blood glucose concentration. Because the rate of formation of GHb is directly proportional to the concentration of glucose in the blood, *the GHb concentration represents integrated values for glucose over the preceding 8 to 12 weeks*. This provides an additional criterion for assessing glucose control because GHb values are free of day-to-day and hour-to-hour glucose fluctuations and are unaffected by exercise or food ingestion immediately before collection of the blood sample. The contribution of the plasma glucose concentration to GHb depends on the time interval, with more recent values (such as during the preceding month) providing a larger contribution than earlier values (such as 3 months earlier). The blood glucose in the preceding 1 month determines 50% of the $HbA_{1c}$, whereas days 60–120 determine only 25%. After a sudden alteration in blood glucose concentrations, the rate of change in $HbA_{1c}$ is rapid during the initial 2 months, followed by a more gradual change approaching steady state 3 months later.

Interpretation of GHb depends on RBCs having a normal life span. Patients with hemolytic disease or other conditions with shortened RBC survival exhibit a substantial reduction in $HbA_{1c}$. $HbA_{1c}$ can still be used to monitor these patients, but values must be compared with previous values from the same patient—not with published reference intervals. Similarly, individuals with recent significant blood loss have falsely low values because of a higher fraction of young erythrocytes. High $HbA_{1c}$ concentrations have been reported in iron-deficiency anemia. The effects of hemoglobin variants (such as HbF, HbS, and HbC) depend on the specific method of analysis used (see later). Depending on the particular hemoglobinopathy and assay, results may be spuriously increased or decreased. Most manufacturers of $HbA_{1c}$ assays have modified their assays to eliminate interference from many of the common hemoglobin variants. Therefore, $HbA_{1c}$ can be accurately measured by selecting an appropriate instrument, provided the RBC life span is not altered (see https://ngsp.org for additional information). Another source of error in selected methods is *carbamylated hemoglobin*, formed by attachment of urea. It is present in large amounts in renal failure, which is common in people with diabetes. Carbamylated hemoglobin does not interfere with most modern methods. Most

interferents produce small effects and $HbA_{1c}$ can be measured accurately in the vast majority of patients with diabetes.

## Hemoglobin $A_{1c}$ in Diagnosis of Diabetes

In 2009, an International Expert Committee advised that $HbA_{1c}$ could be used for the diagnosis of diabetes (see Box 33.2). An $HbA_{1c}$ value greater than 6.5% was selected as the decision point, based on the prevalence of retinopathy. This recommendation has been endorsed by both the ADA and the WHO. $HbA_{1c}$ concentrations 5.7%–6.4% indicate individuals at high risk of developing diabetes. $HbA_{1c}$ was also recommended as an alternative to glucose for screening for diabetes. This last recommendation has been accepted by the ADA.

## Hemoglobin $A_{1c}$ in Monitoring of Diabetes

$HbA_{1c}$ is firmly established as an index of long-term blood glucose concentrations and a measure of the risk for developing microvascular complications in patients with diabetes. Absolute risks of retinopathy and nephropathy are directly proportional to the mean $HbA_{1c}$ concentration. In persons without diabetes, $HbA_{1c}$ is directly related to risk of cardiovascular disease.

## Methods for Determination of Glycated Hemoglobins

More than 250 different methods have been described for the determination of GHbs. Most methods separate GHb from nonglycated hemoglobin using techniques based on charge differences (ion-exchange chromatography, HPLC, electrophoresis, and isoelectric focusing) or structural differences (affinity chromatography and immunoassay). Electrophoresis methods have been replaced by capillary electrophoresis that specifically measures $HbA_{1c}$. An enzymatic assay for $HbA_{1c}$ is also commercially available. The $HbA_{1c}$ result is expressed as a percentage of total hemoglobin. Most laboratories in the United States use immunoassay or HPLC and report $HbA_{1c}$. The selection of method by a laboratory is influenced by several factors, including sample volume, patient population, and cost. It is advisable to consult clinicians in this process. The ADA recommends that laboratories use only $HbA_{1c}$ assays that are certified by the NGSP (previously the National Glycohemoglobin Standardization Program) as traceable to the DCCT reference. These assays are listed on the NGSP website (https://ngsp.org) and are updated several times a year.

## High-Performance Liquid Chromatography

$HbA_{1c}$ and other hemoglobin fractions are separated by HPLC, with cation exchange chromatography. Several fully automated systems are commercially available. Assays require only 5 μL of whole blood, and fingerprick samples can be collected in a capillary tube for analysis. Anticoagulated blood is diluted with a hemolysis reagent containing borate. Samples are incubated at 37°C for 30 minutes to remove the Schiff base and are inserted into the autosampler. (Some instruments have a shorter preincubation step, and others separate labile GHb chromatographically, eliminating the step to remove the Schiff base.) A step gradient using three phosphate buffers of increasing ionic strength is passed through the column. Detection is performed at 415 and 690 nm, and results are quantified by integrating the areas under the peaks. Analysis time is as short as 3 minutes. $HbA_{1c}$ by HPLC was used for analysis of all patient samples in the DCCT.

## Immunoassay

Assays for $HbA_{1c}$ have been developed using antibodies raised against the Amadori product of glucose (ketoamine linkage) plus the first few (4–8) amino acids at the N-terminal end of the β-chain of hemoglobin. A widely used assay measures $HbA_{1c}$ in whole blood by inhibition of latex agglutination. The agglutinator, a synthetic polymer containing multiple copies of the immunoreactive portion of $HbA_{1c}$, binds the anti-$HbA_{1c}$ monoclonal antibody that is attached to latex beads. This agglutination produces light scattering, measured as an increase in absorbance. $HbA_{1c}$ in the patient's sample competes for the antibody on the latex, inhibiting agglutination, thereby decreasing light scattering. Immunoassays are generally calibrated to give values that match HPLC values. The antibodies do not recognize labile intermediates or other GHbs (such as $HbA_{1a}$ or $HbA_{1b}$) because both the ketoamine with glucose and specific amino acid sequences are required for binding. Similarly, several hemoglobin variants, such as HbF, $HbA_2$, HbS, and carbamylated hemoglobin, are not detected. The procedure has been adapted for capillary blood samples using a bench-top analyzer with reagent cartridges designed for use in physicians' office laboratories.

## Affinity Chromatography

Affinity gel columns are used to separate GHb, which binds to *m*-aminophenylboronic acid on the column, from the nonglycated fraction. The boronic acid reacts with the *cis*-diol groups of glucose that are bound to hemoglobin to form a reversible five-member ring complex, thus selectively holding the GHb on the column. Nonglycated hemoglobin does not bind. Sorbitol is added to elute the GHb. Absorbance of bound and non-bound fractions, measured at 415 nm, is used to calculate the percentage of GHb.

The major advantages of affinity chromatography are as follows: no interference from nonglycated hemoglobins and negligible interference from the labile intermediate form of $HbA_{1c}$. It is unaffected by variations in temperature and has reasonably good precision. Hemoglobin variants such as HbS, HbC, HbD, or HbE produce little effect.

Affinity methods measure total GHb. This includes components other than $HbA_{1c}$ because the assay detects ketoamine structures on lysine and valine residues on both α- and β-chains of hemoglobin. Although the method detects all GHbs, most commercial systems are calibrated to report a standardized $HbA_{1c}$ value. The value is derived from an equation obtained from linear regression between total GHb and $HbA_{1c}$ analysis by HPLC. A linear relationship has been demonstrated, and standardized $HbA_{1c}$ values are thus comparable with values obtained by methods specific for $HbA_{1c}$. Columns and reagents are commercially available.

## Capillary Electrophoresis

Advantages of capillary electrophoresis include high resolving ability (due to the high voltage that can be applied) and small sample volume (see Chapter 11). Briefly, charged molecules are separated by their electrophoretic mobility in an alkaline buffer (pH 9.4), and by electrolyte pH and electroosmotic flow. Hemoglobins are detected by absorption spectroscopy at the cathodic end of the capillary. An automated liquid-flow capillary electrophoresis method to measure $HbA_{1c}$ is commercially available in several countries and is approved by the FDA in the United States .

## Enzymatic

Enzymatic assays to measure $HbA_{1c}$ have been developed based on a colorimetric method in which fructosyl peptide oxidase catalyzes the oxidative deglycation of *N*-(deoxyfructosyl)-Val-His. The procedure has been adapted for analysis on a high-throughput automated analyzer and has been approved by the FDA for use in the United States.

### Assay Standardization

Clinical laboratories measure GHb with diverse assays that use multiple methods and quantify different components. The DCCT results accentuated the need for accurate GHb measurement and provided a strong impetus for standardization of GHb assays. Committees were established under the auspices of the American Association for Clinical Chemistry (AACC) in 1993 and the IFCC in 1995 to standardize GHb assays.

The NGSP was established in 1996 to implement the protocol developed by the AACC to calibrate GHb results to DCCT-equivalent values. Employing a network of reference laboratories, the NGSP interacts with manufacturers of GHb methods to help them calibrate their methods and trace values to the DCCT. Manufacturers apply for certification by performing precision testing and report results in DCCT-equivalent $HbA_{1c}$ values. This calibration effort has markedly improved harmonization of results and has reduced imprecision. Results obtained using NGSP-certified assays can be compared directly with results of the DCCT and UKPDS, allowing alignment with clinical outcomes data. The ADA recommends that clinical laboratories in the United States use only assays certified by the NGSP and participate in proficiency testing offered by the College of American Pathologists (CAP). The CAP $HbA_{1c}$ survey uses pooled whole blood specimens at several $HbA_{1c}$ concentrations. Target values are assigned by the NGSP network. Thus, individual laboratories can directly compare their $HbA_{1c}$ results with those of the DCCT and UKPDS.

A different approach was adopted by the IFCC. A working group was established to devise a reference system for standardization based on $HbA_{1c}$. The IFCC group developed a mixture of purified $HbA_{1c}$ and $HbA_0$ as primary reference material. Two candidate reference methods, namely, electrospray ionization mass spectrometry (ESI-MS) and capillary electrophoresis, were proposed. These specifically measure the glycated N-terminal valine of the β-chain of hemoglobin. Analysis is performed by digesting the hemoglobin molecule with endoproteinase Glu-C, which cleaves the β-chain between Glu-6 and Glu-7, releasing the N-terminal hexapeptide. Glycated and nonglycated hexapeptides are separated and quantified by HPLC-ESI-MS or by HPLC and capillary electrophoresis. $HbA_{1c}$ is measured as the ratio between glycated and nonglycated N-terminal hexapeptides. The IFCC Working Group has established a network of laboratories to implement and maintain the reference system. Comparisons between IFCC and NGSP reference methods (and reference systems from Japan and Sweden) indicate a close and stable relationship and allow manufacturers to calibrate their instruments to a higher-level reference method. However, $HbA_{1c}$ results obtained using IFCC reference methods are 1.5%–2% absolute $HbA_{1c}$ units lower than those of the NGSP (and lower than other reference systems). The IFCC method is not suitable for routine analysis of patient samples.

## Test Limitations

Interpretation of $HbA_{1c}$ depends on red blood cells having a normal lifespan. Patients with hemolytic disease or other conditions with shortened red blood cell survival exhibit a substantial reduction in $HbA_{1c}$. Similarly, individuals with recent significant blood loss have falsely low values owing to a higher fraction of young erythrocytes. One study has suggested that the differences in mean red cell lifespan may explain most of the inter-individual variability in the relationship between average glucose and $HbA_{1c}$ concentrations.

The effects of hemoglobin variants (such as HbF, HbS, and HbC) depend on the specific method of analysis used. Depending on the particular hemoglobin variant and assay, results may be spuriously increased or decreased. Boronate affinity chromatographic methods are minimally affected by hemoglobin variants. Visual inspection, or an automated report, of the chromatogram from HPLC and capillary electrophoresis methods can alert the laboratory to a variant. Most manufacturers of $HbA_{1c}$ assays have modified their assays to eliminate interference from the most common hemoglobin variants. Therefore, accurate measurement of

$HbA_{1c}$ is possible by selecting an appropriate instrument, provided the erythrocyte lifespan is not altered (see https://ngsp.org for additional information).

Race influences $HbA_{1c}$ concentration. Published evidence suggests that $HbA_{1c}$ concentrations in Black, Asian, and Hispanic people are higher than in the White population. A 2017 meta-analysis in individuals without diabetes showed significantly higher $HbA_{1c}$ concentrations in Black (0.26%, 2.8 mmol/mol), Asian (0.24%, 2.6 mmol/mol), and Latino people (0.08%, 0.9 mmol/mol) than in the White population. Nevertheless, whether these differences have clinical relevance remains controversial. For example, race did not modify the association between $HbA_{1c}$ and adverse cardiovascular outcomes or death. Moreover, all measures of long-term glycemia, namely, $HbA_{1c}$, fructosamine, glycated albumin and 1,5-anhydroglucitol (1,5-AG), were higher in Black than in White people, and had similar associations with risk for nephropathy, retinopathy and cardiovascular disease in the different races. Clinical studies are ongoing to resolve this question.

Carbamylated hemoglobin is formed by the covalent attachment of isocyanic acid, which is derived from urea, to hemoglobin. Renal failure is common in diabetes patients and results in high concentrations of urea in the blood. While carbamylated hemoglobin interfered in older methods, it does not influence most modern methods of $HbA_{1c}$ analysis. High $HbA_{1c}$ concentrations have been reported in iron deficiency anemia. The mechanism is unknown, but increased glycation by malondialdehyde has been proposed. Other factors that have been reported to interfere with some methods include hyperlipidemia and selected medications. Most of the interferents produce relatively small effects, and for the vast majority of patients with diabetes, $HbA_{1c}$ can be measured accurately.

## Reporting $HbA_{1c}$

$HbA_{1c}$ is reported in the NGSP system as a percentage of total hemoglobin. These values, which are equivalent to those reported in the DCCT and the UKPDS, represent the most widely used reporting system in patient care and in the published literature, though practice varies in different countries. The IFCC method reports $HbA_{1c}$ in System International (SI) units, namely, mmol $HbA_{1c}$/mol total Hb. Comparison between the IFCC and NGSP networks produced a master equation that permits conversion between the two reference systems. For example, an $HbA_{1c}$ result of 7% (in NGSP/DCCT/UKPDS units) is equivalent to 53 mmol/mol (in IFCC units). A calculator to convert between units is available at https://ngsp.org/convert1.asp. A few countries have elected to report $HbA_{1c}$ exclusively in SI units.

In some countries, an estimated average glucose (eAG) is reported together with $HbA_{1c}$. A conversion table is available at https://ngsp.org/A1ceAG.asp. A large, prospective clinical study revealed a significant correlation between $HbA_{1c}$ and mean plasma glucose concentrations. The concept of reporting eAG with $HbA_{1c}$ is not accepted by all and is controversial.

## Performance Goals

Some expert groups have proposed goals for HbA$_{1c}$ assay accuracy and precision, and these have tightened over the years. Within-subject biological variation (CVi) of HbA$_{1c}$ is less than 1.5%. ADA guidelines recommend an intralaboratory CV of less than 2% and an interlaboratory CV of less than 1.5%. For a single method, the goal should be an interlaboratory CV of less than 2.5%.

## Specimen Collection and Storage

Patients need not be fasting. Venous blood should be collected in tubes containing EDTA, oxalate, or fluoride. Sample stability depends on the assay method used. Whole blood may be stored at 4°C for up to 1 week. Above 4°C, HbA$_{1a+b}$ increases in a time- and temperature-dependent manner, but HbA$_{1c}$ is only slightly affected. Samples are not stable at −20°C. For most methods, whole blood samples stored at −70°C or colder, are stable for at least 18 months.

## Reference Intervals

Values for GHbs are expressed as a proportion of total blood hemoglobin. HbA$_{1c}$ should be reported. The reference interval (using an NGSP-certified method) is 4%–6% (20–42 mmol/mol).

Results are not affected by acute illness. Intraindividual variability is minimal (CV ≈1%). HbA$_{1c}$ increases slightly with age and differs among racial groups (e.g., higher in the African American and Hispanic population than in the White population). It is not known whether this has clinical significance. In patients with poorly controlled diabetes, values rarely exceed 15%. HbA$_{1c}$ >15% or <4% should prompt additional studies to determine the possible presence of variant hemoglobin. Note that target values derived from DCCT and UKPDS, not the reference values, are used to evaluate metabolic control in patients with diabetes.

There is no specific value of HbA$_{1c}$ below which the risk of diabetic complications is eliminated completely. The ADA states that for most patients the goal of treatment should be to maintain HbA$_{1c}$ at <7% (53 mmol/mol). (Some organizations recommend an HbA$_{1c}$ target of <6.5% [48 mmol/mol].) These goals are applicable only if the assay method is certified as traceable to the DCCT reference. Assay precision is important because each 1% change in HbA$_{1c}$ represents an approximate 30 mg/dL (1.7 mmol/L) change in average blood glucose.

No consensus has been reached on optimum frequency of testing. The ADA recommends for patients with type 1 or type 2 diabetes that *HbA$_{1c}$ should be routinely monitored at least every 6 months in patients meeting treatment goals (and who have stable glycemic control).* Measurement should be at least every 3 months if either of these criteria is not met.

## POCT HbA$_{1c}$

Several small or hand-held devices are available to measure HbA$_{1c}$ at the point of care, as discussed above. Although many of these devices are NGSP-certified, published evaluations reveal that most POC devices for HbA$_{1c}$ do not exhibit adequate analytical performance to meet clinical needs. A meta-analysis of 13 devices in 61 studies found nine devices with negative mean bias and four with positive bias;

mean CVs were >2% at HbA$_{1c}$ <6%. Importantly, the test is waived in the US and so proficiency testing is not mandated. Therefore, minimum objective information is available concerning their performance in the hands of those who measure HbA$_{1c}$ in patient samples. For these reasons, the ADA advises that POCT devices for HbA$_{1c}$ should not be used for diagnosis or screening for diabetes. While some advocate that immediate feedback of HbA$_{1c}$ results at the time of the patient visit improves glycemic control, not all studies support this premise. Moreover, a systematic review and meta-analysis concluded that there is insufficient evidence of the effectiveness of POCT HbA$_{1c}$ in the management of diabetes.

# GLYCATED SERUM PROTEINS

In selected patients with diabetes (e.g., GDM), assays that are more sensitive than HbA$_{1c}$ to shorter-term alterations in average blood glucose concentrations may be needed. Nonenzymatic attachment of glucose to amino groups of proteins other than hemoglobin (e.g., serum proteins, membrane proteins, lens crystallins) to form ketoamines also occurs. Because serum proteins turn over more rapidly than erythrocytes (the circulating half-life for albumin is about 20 days), *the concentration of glycated serum albumin reflects glucose control over a period of 2 to 3 weeks.* Therefore, deterioration of control and improvement with therapy are evident earlier than with HbA$_{1c}$.

## Fructosamine

*Fructosamine* is the generic name for plasma protein ketoamines. The name refers to the structure of the ketoamine rearrangement product formed by the interaction of glucose with the ε-amino group on lysine residues of albumin. Analogous to HbA$_{1c}$, fructosamine may be used as an index of the average concentration of blood glucose over an extended time.

Because all glycated serum proteins are fructosamines and albumin is the most abundant serum protein, measurement of fructosamine is thought to be largely a measure of glycated albumin, but this has been questioned by some investigators. Although the fructosamine assay can be automated and is cheaper than HbA$_{1c}$, *there is a lack of consensus on its clinical utility.* An important limitation is the lack of long-term prospective studies with clinical outcomes. There is no agreed target for optimum glycemic control nor a threshold for diagnosis of diabetes.

Fructosamine may be useful in circumstances where HbA$_{1c}$ is of little value, such as in patients with hemoglobin variants that are associated with decreased erythrocyte life span. It may also have a role in conjunction with HbA$_{1c}$. Gross changes in protein concentration and half-life may have large effects on the proportion of protein that is glycated. Thus, fructosamine results may be invalid in patients with nephrotic syndrome, cirrhosis of the liver, or dysproteinemias, or after rapid changes in acute-phase reactants. *There is no role for fructosamine in the diagnosis of diabetes.*

## Determination of Fructosamine

Methods for measuring glycated proteins include: (1) affinity chromatography using immobilized phenylboronic acid (similar to the GHb assay); (2) HPLC of glycated lysine residues after hydrolysis of the glycated proteins; (3) a photometric procedure in which mild acid hydrolysis releases 5-hydroxymethylfurfural—proteins are precipitated with trichloroacetic acid and the supernatant is reacted with 2-thiobarbituric acid; and (4) other procedures using phenylhydrazine and ε-*N*-(2-furoylmethyl)-L-lysine (furosine). None of these assays is popular because they are not suitable for routine clinical laboratories. Prolonged storage at ultra-low temperatures (−96°C) prevents in vitro glycation of serum proteins.

An alternative method of measuring fructosamine is based on the principle that under alkaline conditions, fructosamine undergoes an Amadori rearrangement. The resultant compounds have reducing activity that can be differentiated from other reducing substances. In the presence of carbonate buffer, fructosamine rearranges to the eneaminol form, which reduces nitroblue tetrazolium (NBT) to a formazan. Absorbance at 530 nm is measured at two time points, and the absorbance change is proportional to the fructosamine concentration. A 10-minute preincubation period is necessary to allow fast-reacting interfering reducing substances to react. The assay is easily automated and has excellent between-batch analytical precision. Hemoglobin (>100 mg/dL; 1 g/L) and bilirubin (>4 mg/dL; ≈68 μmol/L) may interfere; therefore, moderate to grossly hemolyzed and icteric samples should not be used. Ascorbic acid concentrations greater than 5 mg/dL may cause negative interference.

### Reference Intervals for Fructosamine

Values in a nondiabetic population are 195 to 300 μmol/L using a colorimetric assay. The reference interval for the enzymatic assay is reported to be 151 to 285 μmol/L.

## Glycated Albumin

Albumin, which comprises approximately 60% of total serum protein, makes up more than 80% of total glycated serum proteins. The N-terminus and 59 lysine residues are potential glycation sites and it is not known how many of these are glycated in vivo. Analysis of human plasma by HPLC tandem mass spectrometry and [$^{13}C_6$]-glucose labeling identified 35 different glycation sites on albumin. Assays that measure only glycated albumin (GA), rather than all glycated serum proteins (i.e., fructosamine), are commercially available.

The clinical use of GA is limited by the same caveats that apply to fructosamine: limited evidence relating it to the complications of diabetes and lack of long-term prospective studies with clinical outcomes. Accumulating evidence suggests that GA may be useful for predicting diabetes and its microvascular complications. Recent data show that combining GA with HbA$_{1c}$ increased the detection of prediabetes in African immigrants to the US. Additional studies are required to more clearly define the clinical value of GA in diabetes.

### Determination of Glycated Albumin

Methods that have been used to quantify GA include: a colorimetric procedure in which mild acid hydrolysis releases 5-hydroxymethylfurfural—proteins are precipitated with trichloroacetic acid and the supernatant is reacted with 2-thiobarbituric acid; RIA using beads coated with antibody to albumin, and $^{125}$I-labeled antibody directed against glucitollysine epitopes of GA previously reduced by sodium borohydride (NaBH$_4$) to reduce the Schiff base; enzyme-linked immunosorbent assay (ELISA) in which GA binds to a monoclonal antibody coated on a plate, followed by incubation with an enzyme-linked antihuman albumin antibody; enzyme-linked boronate immunoassay where boronic acid-HRP conjugate binds to the cis-diols of GA, which is immobilized by an antihuman albumin antibody coated onto a microtiter plate; affinity chromatography using immobilized phenylboronic acid, followed by elution and measurement of albumin; boronate affinity chromatography; HPLC with anion exchange chromatography to separate albumin, followed by boronate affinity chromatography to separate glycated from nonglycated albumin; enzymatic assay using ketoamine oxidase; and mass spectrometry.

Probably the most widely used method globally is enzymatic. The assay has two steps. In the first, glycated amino acids are eliminated by oxidation with ketoamine oxidase. In the second step, GA is hydrolyzed by an albumin-specific proteinase to glycated amino acids, which are subsequently oxidized by ketoamine oxidase to glucosone, producing hydrogen peroxide. This is quantified with a chromogen by measuring absorbance at 546/700 nm. Total albumin is measured with bromocresol purple and GA is expressed as a percentage of total albumin. This assay is commercially available in a few countries and has been used in numerous published studies. It was approved in 2018 by the FDA for use in the United States.

### Reference Intervals for Glycated Albumin

Reference intervals vary considerably, depending on the method, ranging from 0.8% to 1.4% to 18% to 22%. The reference interval for the enzymatic assay, which is expressed as a percentage of total albumin, is 11.9% to 15.8%.

Concentrations in women are slightly higher than in men. There is an inverse association with BMI (body mass index); GA is lower at higher BMI. The reason for this is unknown. Values in the Black population are significantly higher than in the White population. Intraindividual variation is low (CV 2.1%), but between-subject variation is reported to be 10.6%. In patients with poorly controlled diabetes, values may increase by up to 5-fold. Factors that influence albumin metabolism have been reported to alter GA independently of glycemia. These include the nephrotic syndrome, thyroid disease, cirrhosis of the liver, smoking, hyperuricemia, and hypertriglyceridemia. Samples can be stored as long as 23 years at −70°C.

## Advanced Glycation End Products

The molecular mechanism by which hyperglycemia produces toxic effects is unknown, but glycation of tissue proteins may be important. Nonenzymatic attachment of glucose to long-lived proteins, lipids, or nucleic acids produces stable Amadori early-glycated products. These undergo a series of additional rearrangements, dehydration, and fragmentation reactions, resulting in stable advanced glycation end products (AGEs). The amounts of these products do not return to normal when hyperglycemia is corrected, and they accumulate continuously over the life span of the protein. Hyperglycemia accelerates the formation of protein-bound AGE, and patients with diabetes thus have more AGE than healthy subjects. Through effects on the functional properties of protein and the extracellular matrix, AGEs may contribute to the microvascular and macrovascular complications of diabetes.

Measurement of AGEs in the circulation has also been used as a biomarker to monitor the complications of diabetes. However, the diverse structures and composition of AGEs has resulted in assay difficulties. Analysis by ELISA has lacked standardization, yielding variable results. The development of stable isotope dilution analysis liquid chromatography-tandem mass spectrometry, in conjunction with careful pre-analytic sample preparation, shows potential to resolve these problems. Some AGE products fluoresce, which forms the basis of noninvasive measurement of skin autofluorescence with a portable reader. Some studies have revealed a positive association of skin autofluorescence with complications of diabetes, but adjustment for HbA$_{1c}$ rendered associations nonsignificant. Limitations of skin autofluorescence measurements include lack of specificity for AGE and most AGEs are not fluorescent. The clinical role of AGE is undefined.

## 1,5-ANHYDROGLUCITOL

Another marker of long-term glycemia is 1,5-anhydroglucitol (1,5-AG), which reflects glucose concentrations over the preceding 2–14 days. It is a 1-deoxy form of glucose that originates predominantly from the diet, with the vast majority (>99.9%) normally being reabsorbed from the glomerular filtrate by the SGLT4 sodium-dependent glucose transporter. When blood glucose concentrations exceed the renal threshold (usually ≈180 mg/dL [≈10.0 mmol/L]), reabsorption of 1,5-AG decreases, leading to a rapid reduction in serum 1,5-AG concentrations. Therefore, low 1,5-AG indicates hyperglycemia, correlating particularly with postprandial blood glucose concentration. An automated colorimetric assay is commercially available (and FDA approved for use in the United States). The reference interval is 10.7–32.0 μg/mL (males) and 6.9–29.3 μg/mL (females). Black people have higher 1,5-AG than White people. Several factors unrelated to glycemia may alter 1,5-AG values, including diet, medications, renal disease, and liver disease. SGLT2 inhibitors, oral agents used to treat diabetes, spuriously alter 1,5-AG as they increase glycosuria. The evidence linking it to outcomes is limited and the clinical value of measuring 1,5-AG remains to be established.

## ALBUMINURIA

### Clinical Significance

Patients with diabetes mellitus are at high risk of developing renal damage. End-stage renal disease requiring dialysis or transplantation develops in approximately one-third of patients with type 1 diabetes, and diabetes is the most common cause of end-stage renal disease in the United States and Europe. Although nephropathy is less common in patients with type 2 diabetes, approximately 60% of all cases of diabetic nephropathy occur in these patients because of the higher incidence of this form of diabetes. Persistent proteinuria detectable by routine

screening tests (equivalent to a urinary albumin excretion rate [AER] >200 μg/min or >300 mg/24 h) indicates overt diabetic nephropathy. This is usually associated with long-standing disease and is unusual less than 5 years after the onset of type 1 diabetes. Once diabetic nephropathy occurs, renal function deteriorates rapidly, and renal insufficiency evolves. Treatment at this stage can retard the rate of progression without stopping or reversing the renal damage. Preceding this stage is a period of increased AER not detected by routine dipstick methods. This range of 20–200 μg/min (or 30–300 mg/24 h) of increased AER has been called "microalbuminuria". The term microalbuminuria, although widely used, is misleading. It implies a small version of the albumin molecule rather than an excretion rate of albumin greater than normal but less than that detectable by routine methods. Current nomenclature has eliminated the terms microalbuminuria and macroalbuminuria.

The presence of increased AER denotes an increase in the transcapillary escape rate of albumin and is therefore a marker of microvascular disease. Persistent AER >20 μg/min represents a 20-fold greater risk for the development of clinically overt renal disease in patients with type 1 and type 2 diabetes. Prospective studies have demonstrated that increased urinary albumin excretion precedes and is highly predictive of diabetic nephropathy, end-stage renal disease, cardiovascular mortality, and total mortality in patients with diabetes mellitus. Intensive glucose-lowering therapy can significantly reduce the risk of development of increased AER and overt nephropathy in individuals with diabetes. In addition, increased AER identifies a group of nondiabetic subjects at increased risk for coronary artery disease. Interventions, such as control of blood glucose concentrations and blood pressure, particularly with angiotensin-converting enzyme (ACE) inhibitors, slow the rate of decline in renal function.

### Specimen Collection and Storage

Variations in urine flow rate in a person may be corrected by expressing albumin as a ratio to creatinine (i.e., ACR). AER is increased by physiological and other factors (e.g., exercise within 24 h, posture, diuresis), infection, fever, marked hyperglycemia, and marked hypertension. Samples should not be collected after exertion, in the presence of urinary tract infection, during acute illness, immediately after surgery, or after an acute fluid load. All the following urine samples are currently acceptable: 24-h collection; overnight (8–12 h, timed) collection; 1- to 2-h timed collection (in laboratory or clinic), and first morning sample for simultaneous albumin and creatinine measurement. The AER is more practical and convenient for the patient than timed specimens and is the recommended method. A first-morning-void sample is best because it has lower within-person variation than a random urine sample. At least three separate specimens, collected on different days, should be assayed because of high within-subject biological variation (CVi of 30%–50%) and diurnal variation (50%–100% higher during the day). Urine should be stored at 4°C after collection. Alternatively, 2 mL of 50 g/L sodium azide can be added per 500 mL of urine, but preservatives are not recommended for some assays. Bacterial contamination and glucose have no effect. Specimens are stable in untreated urine for 1 week at 4°C and for 5 months at −80°C. The albumin concentration decreases by 0.27%/day at −20°C.

An estimated glomerular filtration rate (eGFR) should also be calculated from serum creatinine in patients who have a positive screening test. Serum creatinine and eGFR should be performed at least annually in all adults with diabetes because some patients have decreased GFR without albuminuria.

## Semiquantitative Assays

Several semiquantitative assays are available for screening for albuminuria. These test strips, most of which are optimized to read "positive" at a predetermined albumin concentration, have been recommended for screening programs. In view of the wide variability in AER, a "normal" value does not rule out renal disease. Because these assays measure albumin concentration, dilute urine may yield a false-negative test result. Refrigerated urine samples should be allowed to reach at least 10°C before analysis. Standard dipstick methods for proteinuria lack adequate sensitivity for low urine albumin concentrations and should not be used to assess albuminuria.

## Quantitative Assays

All sensitive, specific assays for urine albumin use immunochemistry with antibodies to human albumin. Four methods are available: RIA, ELISA, radial immunodiffusion, and immunoturbidimetry. Each method has advantages and disadvantages, and the choice depends on local experience and technical support. In general, these *methods have similar imprecisions, detection limits, and reference intervals*. Details of these methods are found in an expanded version of this chapter in the 6th edition of *Tietz Textbook of Clinical Chemistry and Molecular Diagnostics*.

## REFERENCE INTERVALS

| Albuminuria | µg/min | mg/24 h | mg/g creatinine | mg/mmol creatinine |
|---|---|---|---|---|
| Normal to mildly increased | <20 | <30 | <30 | <3 |
| Moderately increased[a] | 20–199 | 30–299 | 30–299 | 3–29 |
| Severely increased[b] | ≥200 | ≥300 | ≥300 | ≥30 |

[a]Previously termed "microalbuminuria".
[b]Also termed "overt nephropathy". Previously called "clinical albuminuria".

The ADA recommends initial albuminuria measurement in patients with type 1 diabetes who have had diabetes for 5 years or longer, and in all type 2 diabetic patients. Because of the difficulty involved in dating the onset of type 2 diabetes, screening should commence at diagnosis. Analysis should be performed annually in all patients who have a negative screening result. Screening may be performed with a semiquantitative assay. If the screening result is positive, albuminuria should be evaluated by a quantitative assay. Diagnosis requires the demonstration of albuminuria in at least two of three samples measured within a 3- to 6-month period. If the confirmatory test result is positive, treatment should be initiated.

## POINTS TO REMEMBER

- HbA$_{1c}$
  - Glycated hemoglobin is formed by nonenzymatic attachment of glucose to hemoglobin.
  - HbA$_{1c}$ has glucose attached to the N-terminal valine of the β-chain of hemoglobin.
  - The concentration of HbA$_{1c}$ depends on the concentration of glucose in the blood and the erythrocyte lifespan.
  - The average erythrocyte lifespan is 120 days, and HbA$_{1c}$ therefore reflects the average blood glucose concentration over the preceding 8–12 weeks.
  - Any condition that substantially changes erythrocyte lifespan will alter HbA$_{1c}$.
  - HbA$_{1c}$ is used to diagnose diabetes, monitor glycemic control, evaluate the need to change therapy, and predict the development of microvascular complications.
- Glucose
  - Hyperglycemia results from defects in insulin secretion and/or insulin action.
  - Blood glucose homeostasis is regulated by several hormones, including insulin, glucagon, epinephrine, and cortisol.
  - Blood glucose concentrations fluctuate widely during the day, depending on food ingestion, exercise, and other factors (e.g., stress).
  - Self-monitoring of blood glucose using portable meters in patients with diabetes who require insulin has been shown to improve patient outcomes.
- Self-monitoring of blood glucose in non-insulin treated patients is not yet proven to be effective.
- The use of continuous glucose monitoring systems (CGMS), which use subcutaneously implanted glucose sensors, by patients on insulin is increasing.
- Type 2 diabetes
  - Type 2 diabetes is the most common form of diabetes, accounting for ≈90% of all cases.
  - The onset is insidious, and patients have minimal symptoms.
  - Many patients have irreversible complications at the time of diagnosis.
  - Patients exhibit both insulin resistance and inadequate insulin secretion.
  - Insulin resistance is very difficult to measure, and at diagnosis, the patient may have normal, increased, or decreased insulin concentrations.
  - The molecular defects are a consequence of both genetic and environmental factors.
  - The gene (or genes) that causes the common forms of type 2 diabetes have not been identified.
  - Obesity is linked to the development of type 2 diabetes and lifestyle changes (weight loss and exercise) can delay the onset of the disease.

## AT A GLANCE

**Diagnosis of Diabetes**

Diabetes is diagnosed if at least one of the following criteria is met:

- Fasting plasma glucose (FPG) ≥126 mg/dL (7.0 mmol/L)
- 2-hour plasma glucose ≥200 mg/dL (11.1 mmol/L) during an oral glucose tolerance test
- $HbA_{1c}$ ≥6.5% (48 mmol/mol)

The same test should be repeated on a different day to confirm the diagnosis.

Glucose should be measured in venous plasma.

Glycolysis should be minimized by collecting the blood in a tube containing a rapidly effective inhibitor of glycolysis, e.g., granulated citrate buffer. If that cannot be achieved, the tube should be placed immediately after collection in an ice-water slurry and separating plasma from cells within 30 min.

Plasma glucose and $HbA_{1c}$ should be measured in an accredited laboratory; point-of-care $HbA_{1c}$ devices are not suitable for screening or diagnosis.

$HbA_{1c}$ analysis should be performed using a method that is National Glycohemoglobin Standardization Program (NGSP)–certified and standardized to the Diabetes Control and Complications Trial (DCCT) assay.

## REVIEW QUESTIONS

1. Hemoglobin $A_{1c}$ ($HbA_{1c}$) indicates compliance of a patient with diabetes with his or her insulin-taking regimen by monitoring glucose control. $HbA_{1c}$ concentration represents the integrated glucose value in the blood over what period?
   a. 8 to 12 days
   b. 8 to 12 weeks
   c. 8 to 12 months
   d. 1 day

2. Which of the following values obtained during an oral glucose tolerance test (OGTT) is diagnostic of diabetes mellitus?
   a. 2-hour specimen = 125 mg/dL (6.9 mmol/L)
   b. Fasting glucose = 138 mg/dL (7.7 mmol/L)
   c. Fasting glucose = 110 mg/dL (6.1 mmol/L)
   d. 2-hour specimen = 80 mg/dL (4.4 mmol/L)

3. Type 2 diabetes:
   a. is associated with resistance to the action of insulin.
   b. is caused by destruction of pancreatic β-cells.
   c. is also known as insulin-dependent diabetes mellitus.
   d. occurs less frequently than type 1 diabetes.

4. All of the following results are confirmatory and diagnostic laboratory values for diabetes mellitus *except*:
   a. nonfasting blood glucose >200 mg/dL. (11.1 mmol/L).
   b. 2-hour oral glucose tolerance values >200 mg/dL (11.1 mmol/L).
   c. urine glucose >250 mg/dL. (13.9 mmol/L).
   d. fasting plasma glucose >126 mg/dL. (7.0 mmol/L).

5. Release of glucose from its storage form is referred to as:
   a. glycogenesis.
   b. glycogenolysis.
   c. glycolysis.
   d. glyconeogenesis.

6. Which of the following hormones produces *hyperglycemia*?
   a. Epinephrine
   b. Glucagon
   c. Thyroid hormone
   d. All of the above hormones produce hyperglycemia.

7. Whole blood glucose values are approximately what percent different from plasma glucose values?
   a. 20% higher
   b. 11% lower
   c. 11% higher
   d. There is no difference between whole blood glucose and plasma glucose values.

8. The development of ketosis in uncontrolled diabetes is a result of:
   a. increased lipolysis of fatty acids from adipose stores and decreased re-esterification of these fatty acids to triglycerides.
   b. increased nonenzymatic addition of glucose to proteins, lipids, and nucleic acids that form ketoamines.
   c. increased formation of advanced glycation end products that do not return to normal levels when diabetes is controlled.
   d. formation of circulating antibodies that are formed against the excess adipose tissue present in a person with diabetes.

9. Which of the following hormones promotes *decreased* blood glucose?
   a. Epinephrine
   b. Glucagon
   c. Cortisol
   d. Insulin

10. The purpose of examining urinary albumin excretion in an individual with type 1 or type 2 diabetes is to:
    a. assess the ability of the pancreas to synthesize sufficient insulin.
    b. determine the rate of formation of advanced glycation end products.
    c. assess the possibility of overt diabetic nephropathy.
    d. examine the health of the liver in its ability to synthesize albumin.

## SUGGESTED READINGS

American Diabetes Association. 2. Classification and Diagnosis of Diabetes: Standards of Medical Care in Diabetes—2022. *Diabetes Care.* 2022;45(suppl 1):S17–S38.

Atkinson MA, Eisenbarth GS, Michels AW. Type 1 diabetes. *Lancet.* 2014;383:69–82.

Beck RW, Bergenstal RM, Laffel LM, Pickup JC. Advances in technology for management of type 1 diabetes. *Lancet.* 2019;394:1265–1273.

Bry L, Chen PC, Sacks DB. Effects of hemoglobin variants and chemically modified derivatives on assays for glycohemoglobin [Review]. *Clin Chem.* 2001;47:153–163.

DCCT. The effect of intensive treatment of diabetes on the development and progression of long-term complications in insulin-dependent diabetes mellitus. *N Engl J Med.* 1993;329:977–986.

DeFronzo RA, Ferrannini E, Groop L, et al. Type 2 diabetes mellitus. *Nat Rev Dis Primers.* 2015;1:15019.

Kamel KS, Halperin ML. Acid-base problems in diabetic ketoacidosis. *N Engl J Med.* 2015;372:546–554.

Kilpatrick ES, Butler AE, Ostlundh L, Atkin SL, Sacks DB. Controversies around the measurement of blood ketones to diagnose and manage diabetic ketoacidosis. *Diabetes Care.* 2022;45:267–272.

Klonoff DC, Parkes JL, Kovatchev BP, et al. Investigation of the accuracy of 18 marketed blood glucose monitors. *Diabetes Care.* 2018;41:1681–1688.

Little RR, Rohlfing C, Sacks DB. The National Glycohemoglobin Standardization Program: Over 20 years of improving hemoglobin $A_{1c}$ measurement. *Clin Chem.* 2019;65:839–848.

Metzger BE, Lowe LP, Dyer AR, et al. Hyperglycemia and adverse pregnancy outcomes. *N Engl J Med.* 2008;358:1991–2002.

Miller WG, Bruns DE, Hortin GL, et al. Current issues in measurement and reporting of urinary albumin excretion. *Clin Chem.* 2009;55:24–38.

Rask-Madsen C, King GL. Vascular complications of diabetes: mechanisms of injury and protective factors. *Cell Metab.* 2013;17:20–33.

Sacks DB, Arnold M, Bakris GL, et al. Guidelines and recommendations for laboratory analysis in the diagnosis and management of diabetes mellitus. *Clin Chem.* 2011;57:e1–e47.

Sacks DB. A1C versus glucose testing: a comparison. *Diabetes Care.* 2011;34:518–523.

Scott MG, Bruns DE, Boyd JC, Sacks DB. Tight glucose control in the intensive care unit: are glucose meters up to the task? *Clin Chem.* 2009;55:18–20.

UK Prospective Diabetes Study (UKPDS) Group. Intensive blood-glucose control with sulphonylureas or insulin compared with conventional treatment and risk of complications in patients with type 2 diabetes (UKPDS 33). *Lancet.* 1998;352:837–853.

van den Berghe G, Wouters P, Weekers F, et al. Intensive insulin therapy in the critically ill patients. *N Engl J Med.* 2001;345:1359–1367.

Warshauer JT, Bluestone JA, Anderson MS. New frontiers in the treatment of type 1 diabetes. *Cell Metab.* 2020;31:46–61.

Welsh KJ, Kirkman MS, Sacks DB. Role of glycated proteins in the diagnosis and management of diabetes: research gaps and future directions. *Diabetes Care.* 2016;39:1299–1306.

# 34

# Cardiac Function

*Fred S. Apple, Peter A. Kavsak, and Allan S. Jaffe*

## OBJECTIVES

1. Define the following terms:
   a. Acute coronary syndrome (ACS)
   b. Acute myocardial infarction (AMI)
   c. Angina
   d. Atherosclerosis
   e. Cardiac biomarker
   f. Cardiac troponin (cTn)
   g. Congestive heart failure (CHF)
   h. Coronary artery disease (CAD)
   i. High-sensitivity cardiac troponin assay
   j. Electrocardiogram (ECG)
   k. Ischemia
   l. Myocardium
   m. Myocardial infarction
   n. Myocardial injury
   o. Natriuretic peptide (NP)
   p. Plaque
   q. Reperfusion
   r. Type 1 myocardial infarction (MI)
   s. Type 2 myocardial infarction
2. Describe the anatomy of the heart, including layers, chambers, and protein makeup of muscle.
3. List the events in the process of atherosclerotic plaque formation.
4. Describe an ideal cardiac biomarker, including necessary characteristics, analytical considerations, and persistence in blood following an AMI.
5. Compare cardiac troponin I and T, including structural differences, physiological function, localization, and usefulness in diagnosing an AMI.
6. Define the two analytical criteria required to designate a cTn assay as high sensitivity.
7. For the following cardiac biomarkers, list and describe their location within heart tissue, physiological function if known, clinical utility for diagnosing disease, tissue specificity, other pathophysiological conditions that cause increased values, and the specimen requirements needed for laboratory analysis:
   a. B-type natriuretic peptide (BNP)
   b. cTnI and cTnT
   c. N-terminal portion of proBNP (NT-proBNP)
8. List three preanalytical considerations that must be assessed by a clinical laboratory that uses natriuretic peptide assays and state what units must be used to report these analytes.
9. List three preanalytical considerations that must be assessed by a clinical laboratory that uses cTn assays; state what units must be used to report these analytes.
10. Evaluate and analyze case studies related to cardiovascular disease and the use of cardiac biomarkers in the diagnosis of cardiovascular disease.
11. Describe the role of high sensitivity cardiac troponin assays for the early rule out of AMI.

## KEY WORDS AND DEFINITIONS

**99th percentile upper reference limit (URL)** A statistically derived cTn concentration determined from a minimum number of a normal, apparently healthy reference population.

**Acute coronary syndrome (ACS)** A sudden cardiac disorder that varies from angina (chest pain on exertion with reversible tissue injury), to unstable angina (with minor myocardial injury), and to myocardial infarction (with extensive tissue necrosis, which is irreversible).

**Acute myocardial infarction (AMI)** Detection of a rise and/or fall of cardiac biomarker values (preferably cardiac troponin) with at least one value above the 99th percentile upper reference interval and with at least one of the following ischemic symptoms, ECG changes of new ischemia, development of pathologic Q waves, imaging evidence of new loss of viable myocardium, or new regional wall motion abnormality or identification of an intracoronary thrombus by angiography or autopsy.

**Angina** A condition marked by severe pain in the chest, often also spreading to the shoulders, arms, and neck, caused by an inadequate blood supply to the heart.

**Atherosclerosis** Any of a group of diseases characterized by thickening and loss of elasticity of arterial walls.

**Atherosclerotic plaque** A pearly white area within the wall of an artery that causes the intimal (interior) surface to bulge into the lumen; composed of lipid, cell debris, smooth muscle cells, collagen, and sometimes calcium; also known as an atheroma; vulnerable to rupture that causes the formation of a platelet- and fibrin-rich thrombus leading to myocardial infarction and ischemic stroke.

**Cardiac biomarker**  A biological compound whose measurement is useful in the diagnosis/detection of cardiac disease; used to (1) detect cardiac disorders, (2) detect risk of developing cardiac disorders, (3) monitor the disorder, or (4) predict the response of a disorder to a treatment.

**Congestive heart failure (CHF)**  A clinical syndrome due to heart disease, characterized by breathlessness and abnormal sodium and water retention, often resulting in edema; also called heart failure.

**Coronary arteries**  The two main arteries that provide blood to the heart, surrounding the heart like a crown, coming out of the aorta, arching down over the top of the heart, and dividing into two branches.

**Electrocardiogram (ECG)**  A graphic recording of the electrical activity produced by the heart.

**Myocardial injury**  Any mechanism of injury to the heart that results in an increase in cTnI or cTnT blood concentrations above the sex-specific 99th percentile upper reference limit.

**Myocardial ischemia**  Deficiency of blood supply to the heart muscle due to obstruction or constriction of the coronary arteries.

**Myocardium**  The middle and thickest layer of the heart wall, composed of cardiac muscle.

**Necrosis**  The sum of the morphological changes indicative of cell death and caused by the progressive degradative action of enzymes.

**Non-ST segment elevation myocardial infarction (NSTEMI)**  A myocardial infarction in which the ST segment is not elevated in one lead or several leads of the ECG.

**Risk stratification**  A statistical process used to determine detectable characteristics of a biomarker associated with an increased chance of experiencing adverse outcomes.

**ST segment elevation myocardial infarction (STEMI)**  Any type of myocardial infarction in which the ST segment is elevated in one lead or several leads of the ECG.

**Unstable angina**  Angina that occurs unpredictably or suddenly increases in severity or frequency.

**Ventricles (right and left)**  The two lower chambers of the heart, responsible, respectively, for pumping blood into the lungs via the pulmonary artery and into the systemic circulation via the aorta.

# BACKGROUND

Coronary heart disease causes over 25% of all deaths in the United States. Historically, most deaths caused by ischemic heart disease were acute, but as interventions have increased, the disease is becoming more chronic. Acute cardiac deaths result from ventricular arrhythmias or pump dysfunction and congestive heart failure (CHF) with or without cardiogenic shock. Death rates increase sharply with age, both during hospitalization and in the year after infarction.

Before the advent of coronary care units, treatment of AMI was focused on healing the infarcted area. The concept that infarctions evolve over time and that their size can be moderated updated this passive philosophy. We now know that re-establishing perfusion reduces the extent of myocardial injury and is an important prognostic determinant. Modern management of AMI suggested by most guidelines is aggressive and invasively oriented with the goal of reducing the extent of myocardial damage, which improves prognosis. Prevention is finally being recognized as a key element in the long-term treatment of patients with atherosclerosis. Recently, different types of MI have been recognized. Those not related to acute plaque rupture events deserve special consideration and less often require invasive management.

# ANATOMY AND PHYSIOLOGY OF THE HEART

The average human adult heart weighs approximately 325 g in men and 275 g in women and is 12 cm in length. It is a hollow muscular organ, shaped like a blunt cone, and is the size of a human fist. The heart has four chambers. The two upper chambers are termed the *right and left atria*, and the two lower chambers are termed the *right and left ventricles* (Fig. 34.1). Under normal circumstances, the atria are compliant structures (i.e., intracavitary pressure is low). When anatomy is normal, each atrium is connected to its ventricle through an atrioventricular (AV) valve, which opens and closes. The valve on the left side is called the *mitral valve* and the one on the right side, the *tricuspid valve*. The right ventricle is banana-shaped and pumps blood into the pulmonary artery through a trileaflet pulmonic valve. The left ventricle pumps blood into the aorta through a trileaflet aortic valve. Under normal conditions, the conduction or electrical system of the heart coordinates the sequential contraction of first the atria and then the ventricles. Given that they are connected, each side can affect the other. This sequence of activation optimizes the interaction and thus the efficiency of cardiac function.

The right and left coronary arteries originate from two of three cusps of the aortic valve and provide blood flow and thus nutritive perfusion to the heart. The largest vessels are

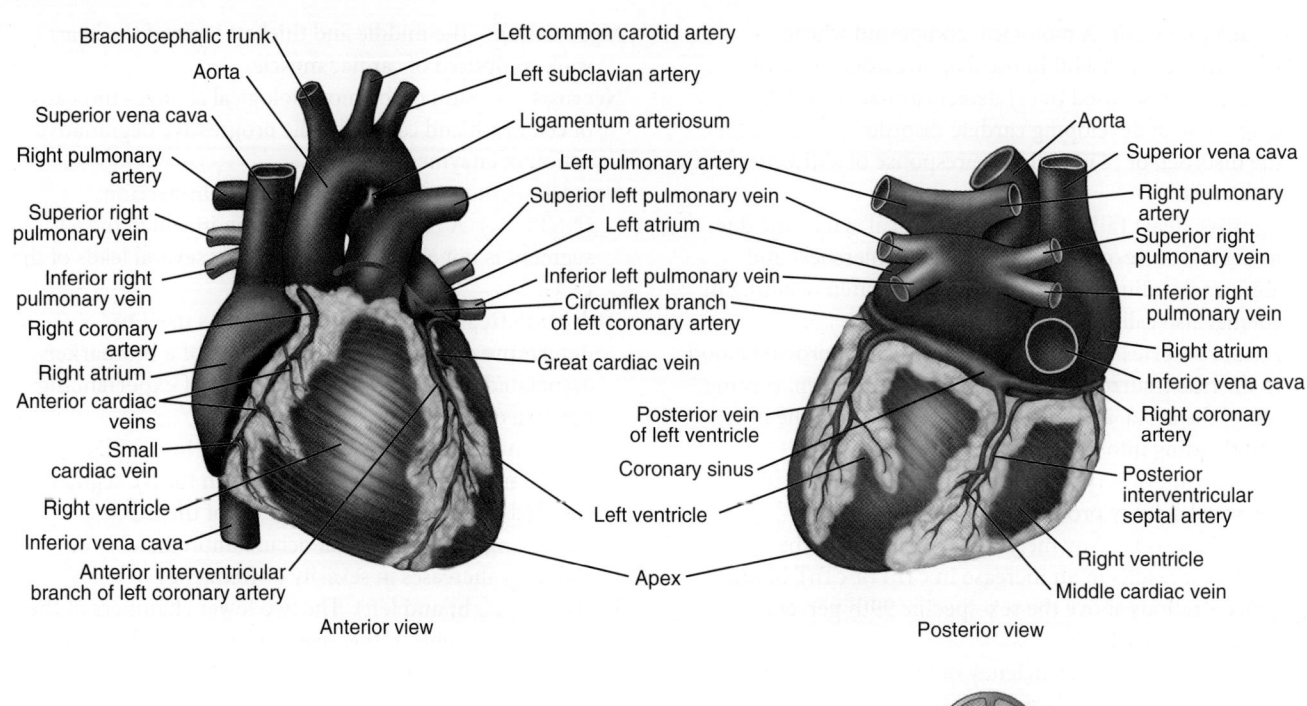

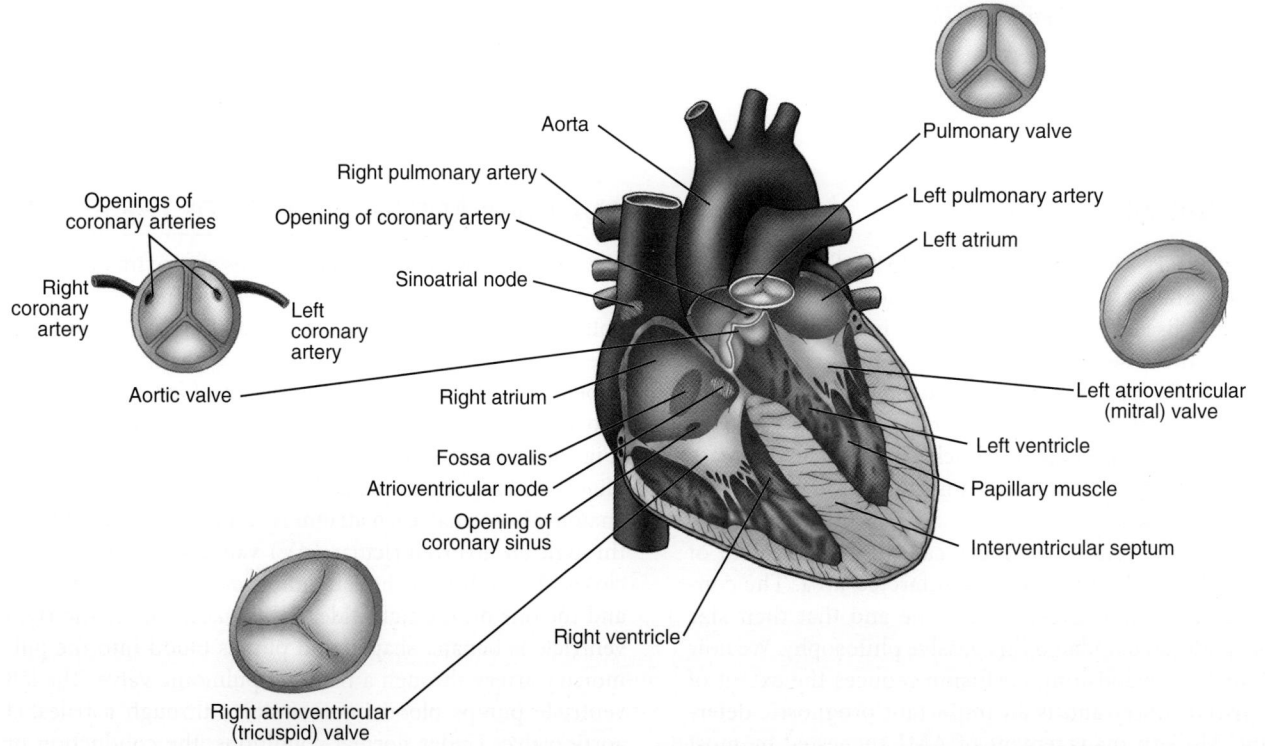

**Fig. 34.1** Anatomy of the heart. (From *Dorland's Illustrated Medical Dictionary*, 32nd ed. Philadelphia: Saunders; 2011:Panel 18.)

on the epicardium, and can be easily accessed therapeutically. Subsequent smaller branches divide, to supply the remaining **myocardium**. The endocardium is the layer most susceptible to **ischemia** because its perfusion relies on the smallest vessels.

A typical cardiac cycle consists of two intervals known as systole and diastole (Fig. 34.2). During diastole, oxygenated blood returns from the lungs to the left atrium via the pulmonary veins and deoxygenated blood returns from other parts of the body to fill the right atrium. During this period, the

AV valves are open, allowing passive filling of the ventricle. At the end of diastole, the atria contract, forcing additional blood through the AV valves and into the respective ventricles. During systole, the ventricles contract. This closes the AV valves when ventricular pressure exceeds atrial pressure. The pulmonary and aortic valves are opened when ventricular pressure exceeds pressure in the pulmonary arteries and/or the aorta, and blood flows into those conduits. During systole, a normal blood pressure in the aorta is typically

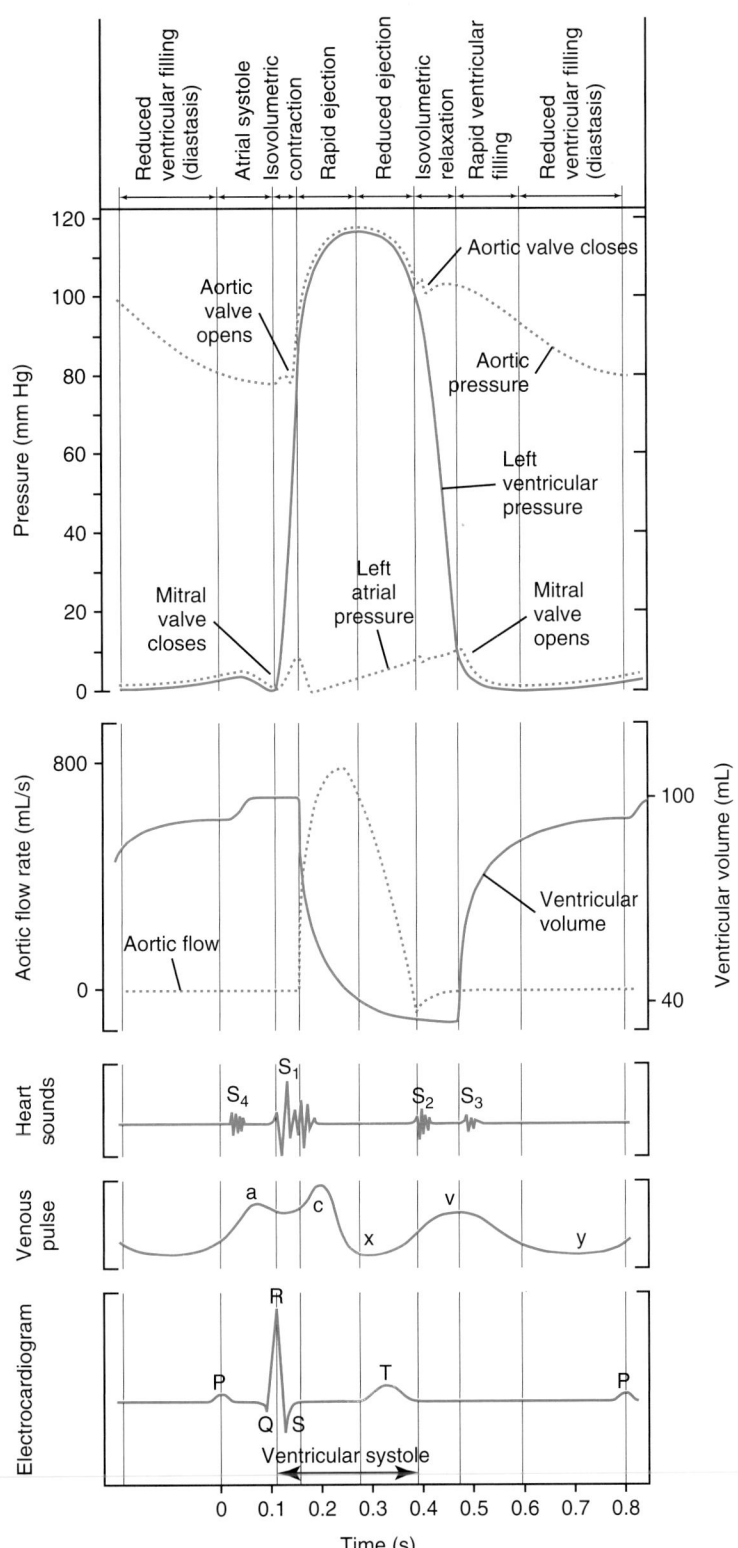

**Fig. 34.2** The cardiac cycle. (From *Dorland's illustrated Medical Dictionary*, 30th ed. Philadelphia: Saunders; 2003, with permission from the National Kidney Foundation.)

120 mm Hg; during diastole, it falls to about 70 mm Hg. At rest, the heart pumps between 60 and 80 times per minute. Measurements of cardiac output and ventricular filling pressures are the standards for assessing cardiac performance and function.

The cardiac cycle is tightly controlled by the cardiac conducting system, which initiates electrical impulses and carries them via a specialized conducting system to the myocardium. The surface **electrocardiogram (ECG)** uses leads placed on the body surface to record changes in electrical potential, and

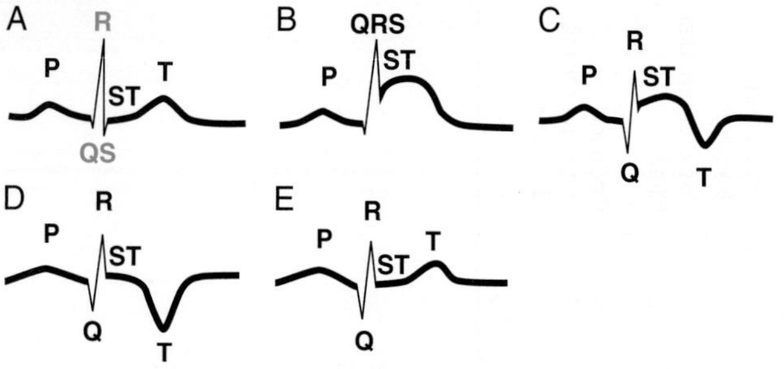

**Fig. 34.3** Electrocardiogram, serial tracing of a patient with an acute myocardial infarction. The sequence is *A*, normal; *B*, hours after infarction, the ST segment becomes elevated; *C*, hours to days later, the T wave inverts and the Q wave becomes larger; *D*, days to weeks later, the ST segment returns to near normal; and *E*, weeks to months later, the T wave becomes upright again, but the large Q wave may remain.

is a graphic tracing of the variations in electrical potential as the heart muscle excites. Clinically, the ECG is used to identify anatomic, metabolic, ionic, and hemodynamic changes in the heart. The clinical sensitivity and specificity of ECG abnormalities are influenced by a wide spectrum of clinically-variable physiologic and anatomic changes. A routine ECG is composed of 12 leads (Fig. 34.3). Each lead records the same electrical impulse but in a different position relative to the heart. Areas of abnormality on the ECG are localized by analyzing differences between the tracings in question and a normal ECG in the 12 different leads.

## CARDIAC DISEASE

### Congestive Heart Failure

CHF is a syndrome characterized by ineffective pumping of the heart, often leading to an accumulation of fluid in the lungs. There are five functional classifications of HF, resulting from the loss of function of the cardiac tissue (called *heart failure with reduced ejection fraction* (HFREF) and due to increased stiffness of the cardiac muscle (referred to as *heart failure with preserved ejection fraction* or HFPEF). Other forms of HF include those related to valvular heart disease, also called *high-output HF*; these conditions demonstrate pump insufficiency relative to systemic demand, which can be abnormally high due to other/non-cardiac disease.

### Acute Coronary Syndrome

The term **acute coronary syndrome (ACS)** encompasses clinical presentations associated with unstable ischemic heart disease. If these patients have ST segment elevation (STE), their events are called *ST elevation myocardial infarctions* (STEMI) (see Fig. 34.3). Usually, but not always, these individuals develop Q waves on their ECGs, hence the term "Q-wave MI". If patients do not have STE but have biochemical criteria for cardiac injury, they are called *non-STEMI* (NSTEMI), and most do not develop ECG Q waves. Patients who have unstable ischemia without **necrosis** are diagnosed with **unstable angina** (UA). Most UA results from an acute event in the coronary artery when circulation to a region of the heart is

obstructed. If the obstruction is high grade and persists, necrosis usually ensues. Because necrosis can take some time to develop, opening the blocked coronary artery in a timely fashion can prevent some of the death of myocardial tissue. This is clearly the case with STEMI. With NSTEMI (American Heart Association [AHA]/American College of Cardiology [ACC] guidelines), cases are usually but not always associated with chest discomfort. Because the infarct-related coronary artery is not totally occluded in NSTEMI, immediate intervention is less necessary, but intervention remains a priority.

### Clinical History

The clinical history brings substantial value to chest pain workups, as 40%–50% of patients with AMI report prior prodromal chest pain (angina pectoris). Among these patients, approximately one-third have had symptoms from 1 to 4 weeks before hospitalization; in the remaining two-thirds, symptoms predated admission by a week or less, with one-third of patients having symptoms for 24 hours or less. Most patients rate the pain of AMI as severe, but it is rarely intolerable; this pain may be prolonged, lasting up to 30 minutes.

Older individuals, patients with diabetes, and women often present atypically. Among individuals older than 80 years, less than 50% of those with AMI report chest discomfort at the time of AMI. Instead, these patients may present with shortness of breath, fatigue, or altered mental status. The pain of AMI may have disappeared by the time a physician first encounters the patient (or the patient reaches the hospital), or it may persist for several hours.

Type 1 MI events, which link to acute atherosclerosis, benefit from invasive intracoronary interventions. Type 2 MI events, which link to supply–demand mismatch, often do not require mechanical interventions even when coronary heart disease is present. In many instances, the coronary arteries may be normal or minimally diseased.

### Diagnosis of Acute Myocardial Infarction—Role of Cardiac Biomarkers

The diagnosis of **acute myocardial infarction (AMI)** established by the World Health Organization in 1986 included **biomarkers** as an integral part of the disorder and required that at least two of the following criteria be met: (1) a history of chest pain, (2) evolutionary changes on the ECG, and/or (3) elevations of serial cardiac markers to a level two times the normal value. Successive European Society of Cardiology/American College of Cardiology (ESC/ACC) consensus conferences have since led to the establishment of a Global Task Force which, in 2018, codified the role of cardiac markers—specifically, cardiac troponin I (cTnI) or T (cTnT)—as evidence of myocardial injury in the appropriate clinical situation (Box 34.1). The modern guideline recognizes the reality that neither the clinical presentation nor the ECG have adequate sensitivity and specificity to function alone in making a diagnosis of AMI. However, this guideline does not suggest that all elevations of these biomarkers should elicit a diagnosis of AMI—only those associated with appropriate clinical and ECG findings. When cardiac troponin (cTn) elevations

## BOX 34.1  Criteria for the Definition of Acute Myocardial Infarction

1. Detection of a rise and/or fall of cardiac biomarker values (preferably cardiac troponin) with at least one value above the 99th percentile upper reference interval and with at least one of the following:
   a. Ischemic symptoms
   b. ECG changes of new ischemia (new ST-T changes or new left bundle branch block)
   c. Development of pathologic Q waves in the electrocardiogram
   d. Imaging evidence of new loss of viable myocardium or new regional wall motion abnormality
   e. Identification of an intracoronary thrombus by angiography or autopsy
2. Pathologic Q waves with or without symptoms in the absence of nonischemic causes
3. Imaging evidence of a region of loss of viable myocardium that is thinned and fails to contract in the absence of a nonischemic cause
4. Pathologic findings of a prior myocardial infarction.
5. Evidence of an imbalance between myocardial oxygen supply and demand unrelated to acute atherothrombosis meets criteria for type 2 MI.

(Modified from Thygesen K, Alpert JS, Jaffe AS, et al. Fourth Universal Definition of Myocardial Infarction. *J Am Coll Cardiol.* 2018;72:2231–2264.)

are not caused by acute ischemia, the clinician is obligated to search for another cause. The guidelines classify several types of AMI, including: the spontaneous type, associated with plaque rupture or erosion; the type associated with fixed or transient coronary abnormalities but not thrombotic occlusion; fatal AMI before markers are obtained or become elevated; and MI associated with cardiac interventions, bypass surgery, and other surgical procedures.

# CARDIAC BIOMARKERS

## Cardiac Troponin I and T

The contractile proteins of the myofibril include a complex of three troponin regulatory proteins (Fig. 34.4): troponin C (the calcium-binding component), troponin I (the inhibitory component), and troponin T (the tropomyosin-binding component). Only two major isoforms of troponin C are found in human heart and skeletal muscle. These are characteristic of slow and fast twitch skeletal muscle, with the heart isoform identical to the slow-twitch skeletal muscle isoform; this precludes cTnC's use as a cardiac-specific biomarker. However, isoforms of cardiac-troponin T (cTnT) and cardiac-troponin I (cTnI) are products of unique genes, making them ideal for use as cardiac biomarkers. Troponin is localized primarily in the myofibrils (94%–97%), with a smaller cytoplasmic (loosely bound) fraction (3%–6%) that may be artifactual (due to experimental disruption of membranes during isolation and purification). Human cTnI is cardiac-specific because it has an additional 31 amino-acid residue on the amino terminal end compared with skeletal muscle TnI. cTnI

is not expressed in normal, regenerating, or diseased human or animal skeletal muscle. Similarly, cTnT is cardiac-specific because it has 11 additional amino acid amino-terminal residues compared with skeletal muscle TnT. However, during human fetal development and in diseased human skeletal muscle (e.g., in certain neuromuscular diseases), small amounts of immunoreactive cTnT are expressed. Thus, care is necessary to choose antibody pairs for the cTnT assay that do not detect these re-expressed isoforms or the immunoreactive proteins expressed in neuromuscular skeletal diseases; otherwise, cross-reactivity to the commercial (Roche) cTnT assays is possible. This may result in positive cTnT findings in the blood from noncardiac tissue (diseased skeletal muscle), falsely indicating a myocardial injury. A point-of-care (POC) hs-cTnT assay (Pylon, ET Healthcare) approved in China (by cFDA) for clinical use does not appear to have skeletal muscle interference, as their antibodies capture and detect different epitopes compared to the Roche antibodies.

After myocardial injury, multiple forms of cTn are elaborated both in tissue and in blood. These include the T-I-C ternary complex, IC binary complex, and free I; modifications of these circulating cTn forms can occur, involving oxidation, reduction, phosphorylation, and dephosphorylation, as well as both C- and N-terminal peptide degradation. It is not clear whether these processes occur solely in the myocardium, in blood, or in both. Depending on the selection of antibodies used to detect cTn, different antibody configurations can lead to a substantially different recognition pattern. Studies have shown that cTnI and cTnT forms released after MI, and the ability to measure different post-translational cTn forms, depend on the antibodies used in the immunoassay. Assays need to be developed, in which the antibodies recognize epitopes in the stable region of cTn and, ideally, demonstrate an equimolar response to the different cTn forms that circulate in the blood; however, successful standardization of cTnI and cTnT assays is unlikely .

Contemporary, POC, and high-sensitivity (hs-cTn) assays in the marketplace are well described on the IFCC Committee on the Clinical Application of Cardiac Biomarkers (C-CB) website (see Suggested Readings, below). Capture and detection antibodies in the heterogeneous assays used in clinical practice vary, and the resulting lack of standardization prevents users from switching easily from one assay to another in clinical practice or research. First, no primary reference cTn material is currently available for manufacturers to use in standardizing cTnI or cTnT assays. Second, because cTn circulates in numerous forms and the different antibodies used in assays recognize different epitopes of cTn, harmonization of assay results is not possible—even for different assays and instruments marketed by the same manufacturer. For complete standardization for cTn assays, manufacturers would need to use the same capture and detection antibodies to elicit similar cTn test specificity.

Expert consensus recommendations were published in 2018 by the American Association for Clinical Chemistry (AACC) Academy in collaboration with the International Federation of Clinical Chemistry and Laboratory Medicine

**Evidence for Cardiac Troponin Release post-MI**

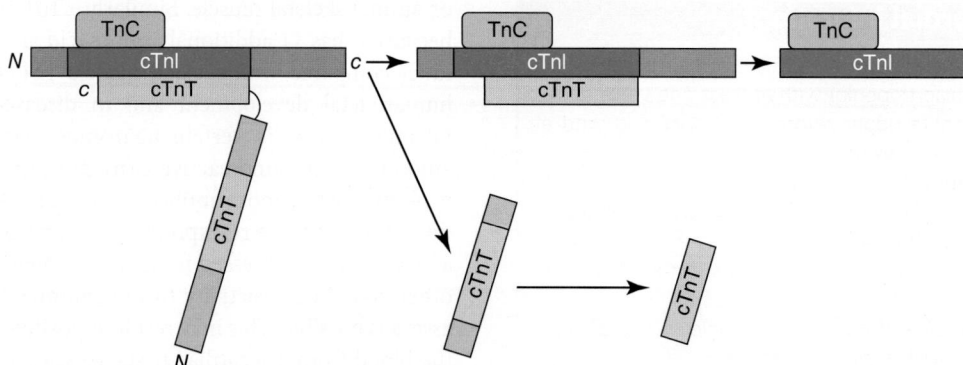

**Fig. 34.4** Schematic of troponin progression post-MI showing the amount of ITC complex decreases, with no full size cTnT or cTnI found. (From Vylegzhanina AV, Kogan AE, Katrukha IA, et al. Full size and partially truncated cardiac troponin complexes in the blood of patients with acute myocardial infarction. *Clin Chem.* 2019;65;882–892.)

Task Force on Clinical Applications of Bio-Markers (IFCC TF-CB). The document focused on clinical laboratory practice recommendations for high-sensitivity cTn (hs-cTn) assays utilizing expert opinion class of evidence to focus on the following 10 topics: (1) quality control (QC) use/approach; (2) validation of lower reportable analytical limits; (3) units used in reporting for patients and QC materials; (4) use of 99th percentile sex-specific upper reference limits vs reference intervals in testing protocols; (5) performance criteria required to define an assay as hs-cTn; (6) the laboratory's role in educating and communicating with clinicians regarding the influence of preanalytical and analytic problems that can confound hs-cTn assay results; (7) how authors need to document preanalytical and analytical variables in studies that use hs-cTn testing; (8) the role of commutable materials in efforts to harmonize and standardize hs-cTn assay results; (9) optimal result reporting time, from sample collection or sample receipt times; and (10) changes in hs-cTn concentrations over time, and the role of analytical and biological variabilities in interpreting serial hs-cTn results.

## Defining 99th Percentile Upper Reference Limits

International guidelines published by biomarker experts (cardiology, emergency medicine, laboratory medicine) and by the joint AACC Academy and IFCC C-CB agree that an increased cTn above the sex-specific **99th percentile upper reference limit (URL)** is an abnormal result. Whether a clinical laboratory defines an abnormal result >99th percentile as a critical value needs to be assessed and determined by each individual laboratory. In spite of evidence-based literature demonstrating that cTn concentrations tend to increase in individuals older than 60 years, likely because of unrecognized comorbidities, 99th percentiles are often determined across wide age ranges including patients as old as 80 years. Further frustrating the problem of selecting relevant reference subjects is the fact that clinically-defined normal individuals without known cardiovascular disease can show increased cTn concentrations and demonstrate a significantly higher risk for death. Given such problems, most laboratories: (1)

accept the manufacturer's reference interval from the package insert; (2) perform an underpowered normal study to establish a reference interval; or (3) accept a URL cutoff published in the literature, which can vary for the same assay depending on the populations studied. Implementation of the 99th percentile URL, especially by sex-specific URLs, has not been globally accepted by laboratories, most likely because of pressure from clinicians. However, the universal definition clearly states that assays are clinically usable with up to a 20% CV at the 99th percentile, and at least two serial samples are required to demonstrate the rising or falling cTn pattern indicating AMI.

One study determined overall and sex-specific 99th percentile URLs in 9 hs-cTnI and 3 hs-cTnT assays using a universal sample bank (USB) of 843 relatively diverse and apparently healthy individuals (426 men and 417 women). The overall and sex-specific 99th percentiles for all assays, before and after exclusions ($n=694$), were influenced by the statistical method used, and whether the assay had low enough analytic sensitivity to measure cTn in the specimens. Substantial differences were noted between and within both hs-cTnI and hs-cTnT assays, but men demonstrated consistently higher 99th percentiles (ng/L) than women (Fig. 34.5). However, not all assays provided a high enough percentage of measurable concentrations in women to qualify the assay as "high sensitivity," and the surrogate exclusion criteria used to define normality tended to lower the 99th percentiles.

## Guideline-Supported Recommendations

Consensus guidelines (see Suggested Readings, below) specify that, in patients who present with ischemic symptoms, a rising or falling serial pattern with at least 1 cTn concentration higher than the sex-specific 99th percentile URLs, during the first 24 hours after onset of symptoms, indicates myocardial injury owing to necrosis/cell death. Fig. 34.6 shows a representative profile of the rise and fall pattern of cTn for type 1 MI, type 2 MI, and chronic myocardial injury patients. If the elevation occurs in the clinical setting of ischemia consistent with MI, diagnosis should be made

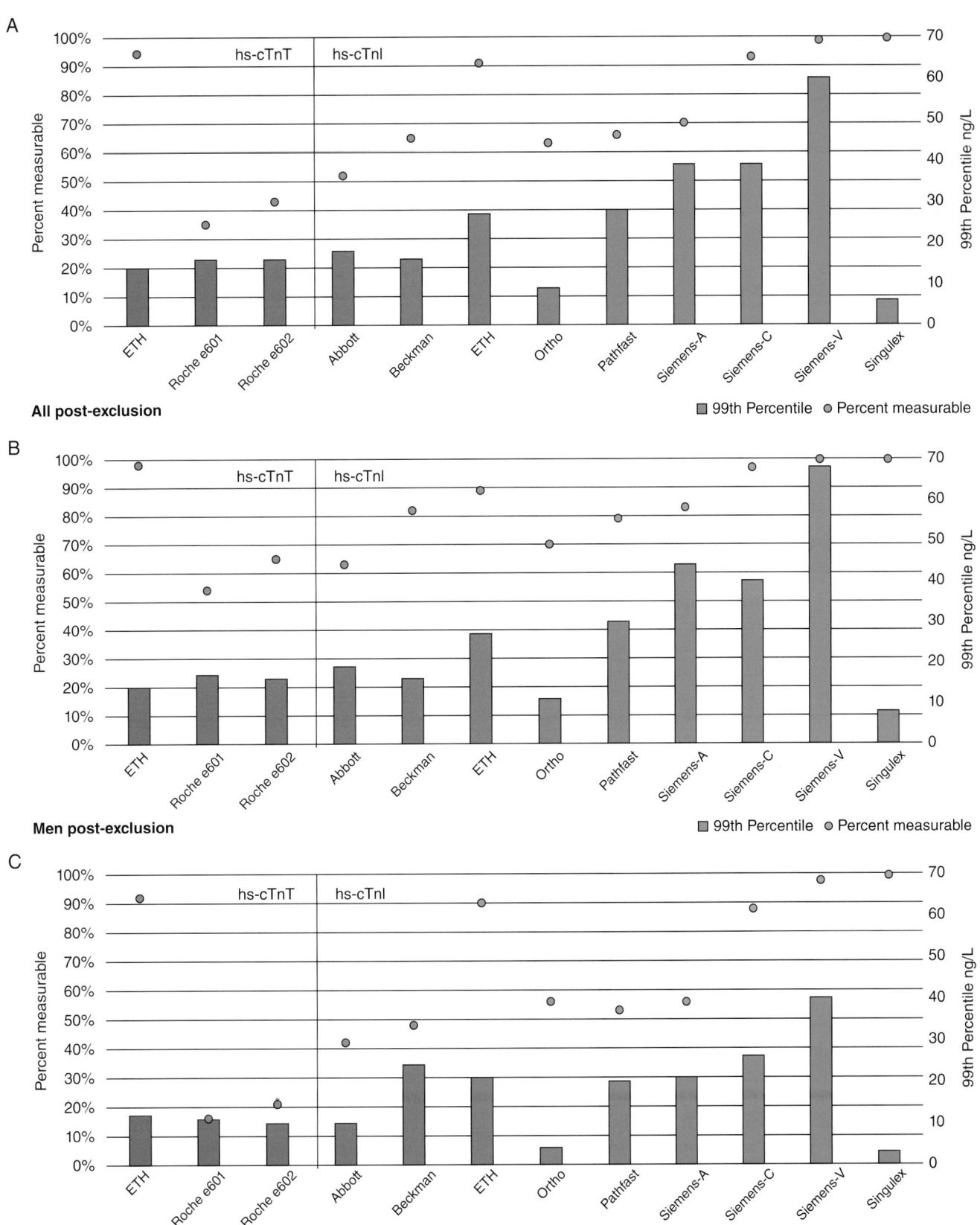

**Fig. 34.5** Comparison of both 99th percentile values (*bars*) and percent measurable concentrations (*circles*) in a presumably healthy population for high sensitivity cardiac troponin assays for (A) overall subjects, (B) men, (C) women. *ETH*, ET Healthcare; Siemens A, Atellica; *C*, Centaur: *V*, Vista. (From Apple FS, Wu AHB, Sandoval Y, et al. Sex-specific 99th percentile upper reference limits for high sensitivity cardiac troponin assays derived using a universal sample bank. *Clin Chem*. 2020;66:434–444.)

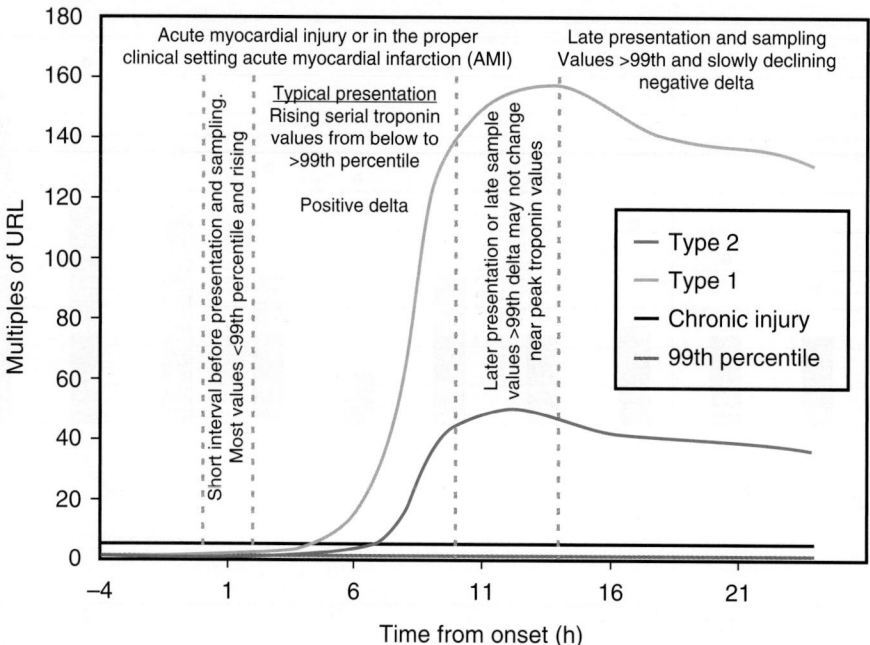

**Fig. 34.6** Kinetics for the general rise and fall pattern of cardiac troponin for type 1 myocardial infarction (MI), type 2 MI, and chronic myocardial injury. (With permission from the IFCC Task Force for Clinical Application of Cardiac Bio-Markers [TF-CB]; prepared by Paul Collinson.)

(see Box 34.1). Better imprecision at low cTn concentrations, based on high-sensitivity assays, appears to improve the value of interpreting cTn as an early rule-out/rule-in diagnostic tool and risk indicator (within 1–3 h of baseline sampling). Use of contemporary or POC cTn assays with intermediate imprecision (10%–20% CV) at the 99th percentile is deemed clinically acceptable and does not lead to patient misclassification when serial cTn results are interpreted.

HS-assays improve clinical practice for diagnostics and risk assessment, facilitating rapid (early) and improved patient management and care. Diagnostic clinical sensitivities using specimens collected serially from presentation for detection of MI have improved from 15% to 35% for the initial generations of cTn assays, to 50%–75% for current contemporary assays, and to more than 80% for HS-assays. To exclude an AMI with contemporary cTn assays, a 6-h period between draws was recommended for assessing the optimal negative predictive value (NPV) for ruling out AMI. With hs-cTn assays, the timing interval for ruling out an AMI has shortened to 2–3 hours, with >99.5% NPV and >99% clinical sensitivity from the time of baseline/first blood draw. Recent studies consistently show that in patients presenting with a low clinical likelihood of ACS, both hs-cTnI and hs-cTnT baseline concentrations below an assay's limit of detection (LoD) paired with a nonischemic ECG can be used to rule out AMI. Measurable cTn concentrations below the sex-specific 99th percentile URL or less than overall 99th percentile URL and without a significant delta (change) value (assay-dependent) 1–2 h after the baseline sample, can also provide NPV >99.5% for early rule-out in a substantial number of patients; the caveat is that this accounts for early presenters tested <2 h following onset of the index event. Using this approach can

improve triage of patients in the emergency department (ED), allowing for: (1) more rapid intervention or earlier discharge home; (2) minimal risk for adverse events; and (3) substantial financial savings to the health care system/hospital. Ongoing analytical and clinical development is underway to validate hs-POC cTn assays to further improve speed of triage.

### Analytical Considerations

Hs-cTn testing requires assays that have low limits of quantitation (LoQ; lowest concentration with 20% CV) and LoD, and low imprecision when cTn concentrations are low. Irrespective of how the testing is performed, whether in the central laboratory or at the bedside using POC assays, manufacturers need to define the imprecision profile of each assay, by displaying scatter graphs %CV vs increasing cTn concentrations from pools of human samples containing different cTn concentrations. Importantly, at least 2 cTn concentrations that cover the range between the LoD and the 99th percentile URL of the assay should be included, with one around the LoD and the other around the 99th percentile URL(s). Imprecision characteristics, including the 10% and 20% CV concentrations, the LoD, and 99th percentile data from current commercially-available assays for cTn assays, need to be addressed. As previously discussed, the absence of assay standardization limits the ability to compare results between different methods, including those produced by the same manufacturer.

### Point-of-Care Testing Considerations

Current guidelines relating to POC-based cTn testing focus mostly on administrative issues, cost-effective usage, and clinical and technical performance of cardiac biomarkers in the ED. Less sensitive POC assays have the demonstrated potential to miss a positive cTn value that would be detected as increased by more sensitive contemporary or high-sensitivity assays. Proposed elements of the POC guidelines include: (1) collective efforts by EDs, primary care physicians, cardiologists, hospital administrators, and clinical laboratory staff to develop accelerated protocols for the use of biomarkers in the evaluation of patients with possible ACS; (2) protocols should facilitate the diagnosis of MI in the ED or establish the diagnosis at other locations in the hospital; (3) quality assurance measures to reduce medical errors and improve patient treatment; (4) turnaround times for results relate to the time of presentation in the ED and, if available, to the reported time of symptom onset; (5) personnel who are knowledgeable about local reimbursement; (6) central laboratory turnaround time (TAT) goals (maximally 1 h, optimally 30 min from time of collection to time of result); (7) consideration of POC-based testing if TAT is consistently challenging; (8) similar performance specifications and characteristics for central laboratory and POC assays; (9) involvement of the central laboratory in the selection of POC assays, user training, maintenance of POC equipment, oversight of proficiency and competency of operators, and compliance with requirements of regulatory agencies; (10) POC assays should provide quantitative results; and (11) establishing quality performance specifications for new biomarkers by manufacturers. Despite manufacturers' claims, only two whole blood POC cTn assay systems are available globally that meet the criteria for classification as hs-cTn methods (see Suggested Readings, below).

For both POC and central laboratory testing, and for practical considerations, anticoagulated whole blood or plasma appears to be the optimal specimen for rapid processing. This eliminates the extra time needed for clotting and additional sample handling. Differences have been described among different plasma types (by anticoagulant used), whole blood, and serum specimens for cTnI concentrations measurement by an individual assay. Both ethylenediaminetetraacetic acid (EDTA) and heparin interfere with cTnI and cTnT antibody-binding affinity, and produce some matrix effect differences. Different sample types should not be used during an individual's work-up when serial, timed samples are being drawn to rule in or out an MI. Although clinicians and laboratorians continue to publish guidelines supporting TAT of <60 min for cTn from the time a specimen arrives in the laboratory, most studies demonstrate that TAT expectations are not being met in a large proportion of hospitals.

In medical centers where acceptable TATs are not being met, where contemporary cTn assays are still utilized, and especially in rural settings, POC-based testing may still be important whether a contemporary or high-sensitivity POC assay is used. The use of POC testing eliminates the additional time needed to transport and process specimens to, or in, the central laboratory. There remains a continued need, as requested by physicians, for laboratory services and health care providers to work together to develop better processes to meet a TAT <60 min.

## Cardiac Troponin Guidelines for the Diagnosis of Myocardial Infarction

The Fourth Universal Definition of Myocardial Infarction (2018) and the IFCC-C-CB and AACC Academy analytical guidelines provide an excellent expert consensus resource for navigating both the pathophysiology of myocardial infarction (MI) and the role of cTn monitoring. They cover: (1) differentiation of MI from myocardial injury; (2) differentiation of the types of MI; (3) the role of cardiovascular magnetic resonance and computed tomographic coronary angiography in defining etiology of myocardial injury and suspected MI.

The definition of type 1 myocardial infarction addresses the relationship of plaque disruption with coronary atherothrombosis and type 2 myocardial infarction and how oxygen demand and supply imbalance, unrelated to acute coronary atherothrombosis, are underlying factors. For types 4 and 5 myocardial infarction, there is emphasis on distinguishing procedure-related myocardial injury from procedure-related myocardial infarction.

Despite international guidance relating to when cTn testing should be requested, excessive and expensive test ordering outside guidance is common. There is substantial diversity across hospitals within the United States and internationally, relating to how cTn testing is ordered, ranging from hospital-wide serial order-sets (e.g., at presentation, and then at 3, 6, and 12 h for contemporary assays), to the 0/1 h, 0/2 h, 0/3 h and 6 h testing approaches more common for hs-cTn assays, to the offering of cTn as a single test (e.g., ordered at any time without any uniformity across a hospital/medical center). In teaching hospitals, where both attending physicians and resident physicians may place multiple orders, duplication is a possible source of excessive cTn testing.

Clinician education and monitoring of cTnI orders in the diagnosis or exclusion of MI is needed, with a clear need for electronic ordering review and/or electronic checks implemented when excessive testing is recognized. Proactive education delivered by laboratory professionals regarding cTn orders, working in concert with their clinical colleagues and information technology counterparts, should become a high priority in clinical laboratory practice to assist in health care savings.

## High-Sensitivity Cardiac Troponin Assays in Clinical Practice

With modern assays, it is clear that normal hs-cTn values are substantially lower than concentrations being reported for healthy individuals by contemporary assays, which are complicated by results less than assay LoD. Hs-cTn assays are increasingly available worldwide and have the ability to measure healthy individuals' low concentrations more accurately, making the 99th percentile URL key to reporting cTn. Any hs-cTn result value above the 99th percentile URL should be considered abnormal and indicative of myocardial injury as defined by the Fourth Universal Definition of MI (2018). Concerns about false-positive results as a result of such criteria should be minimal, assuming adequate quality assurance of the assays. Further, an increased concentration of cTn >the 99th percentile URL is required in the appropriate clinical setting along with a rising or falling pattern for the diagnosis of AMI. With the growing use of hs-cTn assays, earlier and more accurate diagnoses for ruling in and ruling out MI are being made (i.e., within 1–3 h of first blood draw compared to contemporary and POC assays; Fig. 34.7).

Fig. 34.8 shows a schematic of representative strategies to consider for early rule-in and rule-out of AMI, based on implementation of hs-cTnI testing compared to contemporary cTn assays. Many clinical situations can mimic AMI, the most common of which is myocarditis. Clinicians need to be astute and consider that an elevation in cTn—even with a rising pattern suggesting acute AMI—may not be due to ischemic heart disease. In addition, cTn testing aids diagnosis in groups that present atypically, by blending the biomarker information with the clinical.

Analytical problems in cTn testing can be caused by interferences from human anti-mouse antibodies, heterophilic antibodies, and circulating macrotroponin (troponin–antibody complexes). However, hs-cTn assays do not appear as prone to these analytical problems as the earlier generations of cTn assays. Nevertheless, a list of assay interferences involving hemolysis and biotin as potential interferents that are assay dependent, is available on the IFCC C-CB website at https://ifcc-cardiac-troponin-interference-table_v052022.pdf (insd.dk).

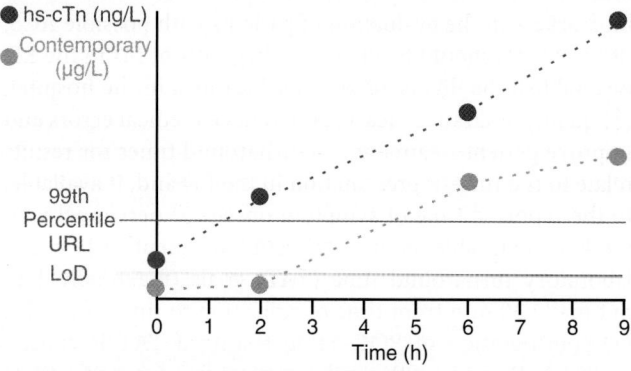

**Fig. 34.7** Cardiac troponin I kinetics comparing high-sensitivity and contemporary assays in a patient presenting within 30 minutes of an acute myocardial infarction. *Hs-cTn*, High-sensitivity cardiac troponin; *LoD*, limit of detection; *URL*, upper reference limit.

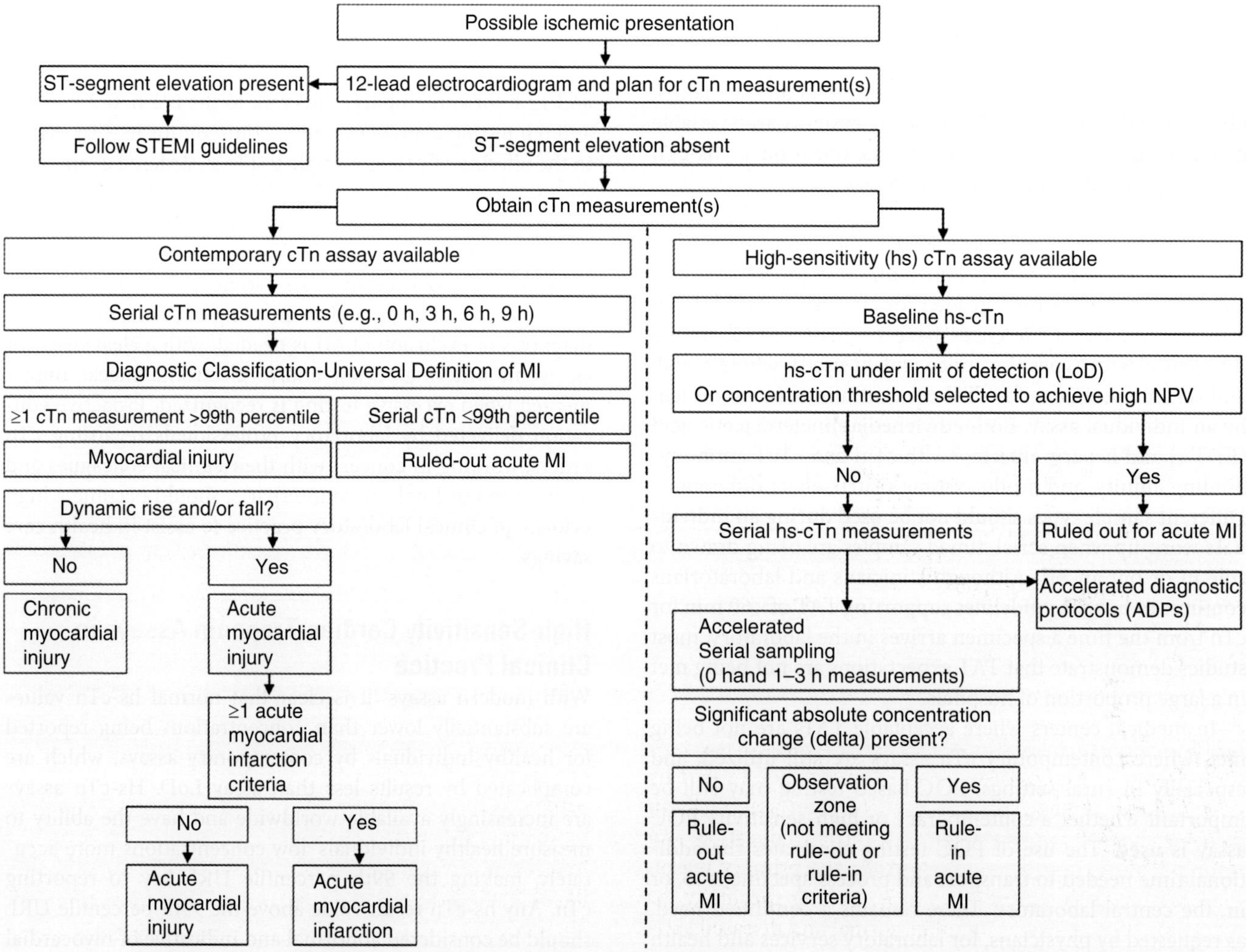

**Fig. 34.8** Schematic of representative strategies to consider for early rule-in and rule-out based on implementation of hs-cTnI testing compared to contemporary cTn assays.

Whether AMI is present is a clinical decision; thus, when cTn values are not rising, one might seriously question whether the elevations are of a more chronic nature. Care is necessary on the part of the clinician, to ensure that individuals presenting late after the onset of symptoms, whose cTn values may be near peak values, or whose values are on the long persistent tail of the time-concentration curve, may still be detected. These patients may not show a changing pattern of values because they are near the peak (range 12–48 h) of the time-concentration curve, or on the gradual down-slope. This may occur in >20% of patients.

Beyond acute rule-in and rule-out utility in diagnosing AMI, hs-cTn testing strategies have been developed to help reduce the risk of adverse events within 30 days of initial presentation. Among patients in whom MI has been excluded via testing protocols that use serial hs-cTn measurements and the assessment of absolute change criteria between baseline and later draws, the risk of adverse events during follow-up is very low (<1%, with NPV 99.5%, sensitivity of 99%). These algorithms have been studied extensively and are safe and effective in chest pain populations for both hs-cTnI and hs-cTnT assays, with the potential limitation that early presenters (<2h from symptom onset) may require additional testing for accurate detection of a rising pattern of cTn results. Conversely, in patients who present late after symptom onset, cTn concentrations may appear stable ("flat") on serial sampling over short periods of time, and also require additional testing for accurate detection of a falling pattern of cTn results.

### COVID-19/SARS-CoV-2 Virus and Cardiac Troponin

An increased cTn result (above the 99th percentile URL) is not uncommon among patients with acute respiratory infections, including SARS-CoV-2 (COVID-19), and is correlated with disease severity. Studies describing the clinical course during the pandemic have shown detectable and increased hs-cTnI and hs-cTnT concentrations in 5%–30% of patients, with significantly increased concentrations in more than half of the patients at high risk of death. Mortality rates of COVID-19 were higher in hospitalized patients with concomitant myocardial injury than those without it (50% vs 5%). In this population, the risk of death from the time of symptom onset was higher in patients with evidence of myocardial injury on admission (hazard ratio, 4.3).

### Creatine Kinase MB No Longer Clinically Useful

Creatine kinase (CK) MB is now considered an obsolete test. However, CKMB discontinuation is regularly met with resistance, in part because of the difficulty clinicians have had with understanding cTn test use. This has been fueled in part by heterogeneity in the cTn assays available, and potentially in lacking laboratory involvement in clinician education and testing protocol construction. However, the primary reason for CKMB's decline mostly lies in its lacking specificity for myocardial tissue, as it is found in normal and diseased skeletal muscle. Thus, CKMB possesses no characteristics that would make it superior to cTn.

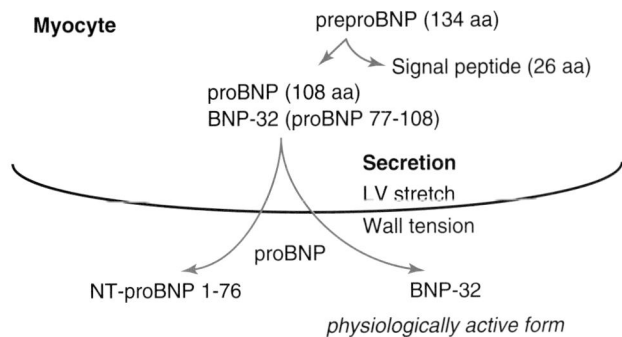

Fig. 34.9 The biotransformation and release of BNP and NT-proBNP from the myocyte into the circulation. *aa*, amino acid; *LV*, left ventricle.

## B-TYPE NATRIURETIC PEPTIDE AND CONGESTIVE HEART FAILURE

In 1981, the Canadian physiologist Adolfo J. de Bold and colleagues reported that intravenous infusion of atrial tissue extracts elicited renal excretion of sodium and water. Moreover, a rapid decrease in blood pressure and increase in blood hematocrit were observed, and the substance was named atrial natriuretic factor. This factor was purified and identified as a peptide comprising 28 amino acid residues, and re-named *atrial natriuretic peptide* (ANP). The discovery paved the way for identification of two structurally-related peptides in the porcine brain: "brain-type" natriuretic peptide (BNP) and C-type natriuretic peptide (CNP). However, BNP is mainly expressed in the heart and the name "brain" natriuretic peptide is now replaced with B-type natriuretic peptide.

### Biochemistry

BNP is a hormone that is mainly released from the myocardial ventricles. Fig 34.9 illustrates the synthesis of the preprohormone BNP and subsequent secretion of NP proteins from the cardiac myocytes; it is not known whether proBNP is split in the myocyte or later in the plasma. Corin and furin are proteases that have been identified in human heart tissue and can cleave proBNP *in vitro*. The major circulating forms of NP are NT-proBNP (function is unknown), proBNP (function is also unknown), and BNP, the physiologically active hormone. In the normal heart, the main site of BNP expression is in the atrial regions. Ventricular BNP gene expression increases drastically in heart failure that affects the ventricles. Further processing of plasma BNP involves degradation, with a loss of bioactivity through disruption of the ring structure mediated by the neutral endopeptidase, neprilysin. The circulating half-life of BNP-32 is 13–20 min. Theoretically, the half-life of proBNP 1-76 in circulation is approximately 25 min. Further, in patients with chronic HF, glycosylation (especially at amino acid 71) is more prominent and there is less active BNP available for measurement.

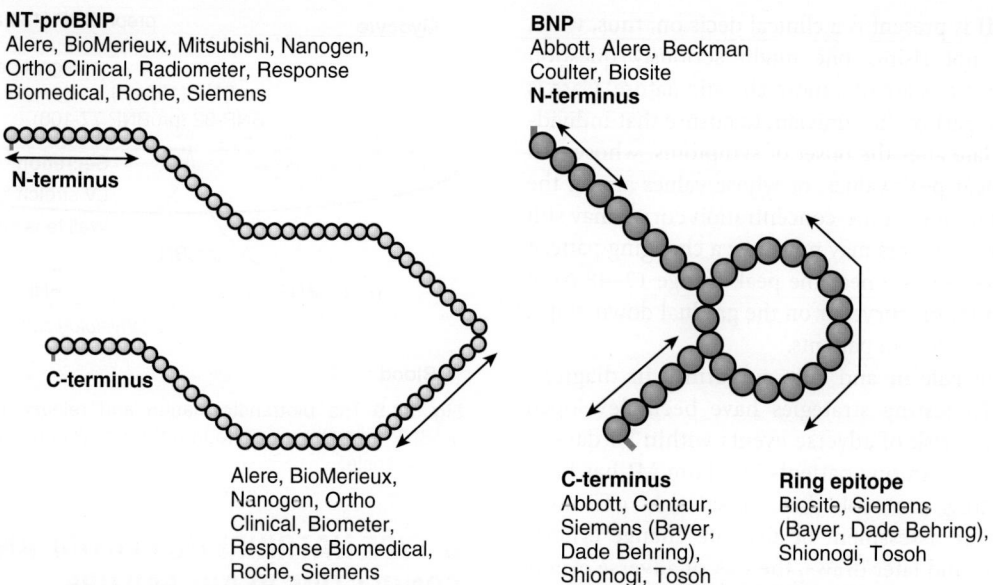

**NT-proBNP**
Alere, BioMerieux, Mitsubishi, Nanogen,
Ortho Clinical, Radiometer, Response
Biomedical, Roche, Siemens

**N-terminus**

**C-terminus**

Alere, BioMerieux,
Nanogon, Ortho
Clinical, Biometer,
Response Biomedical,
Roche, Siemens

**BNP**
Abbott, Alere, Beckman
Coulter, Biosite
**N-terminus**

**C-terminus**
Abbott, Centaur,
Siemens (Bayer,
Dade Behring),
Shionogi, Tosoh

**Ring epitope**
Biosite, Siemens
(Bayer, Dade Behring),
Shionogi, Tosoh

Fig. 34.10 Epitope locations on BNP and NT-rpoBNP used by representative commercially available assays. (From Vasile VC, Jaffe AS. Natriuretic peptides and analytical barriers. *Clin Chem.* 2017;63:50–58.)

## ANALYTICAL CONSIDERATIONS

In 2005 and 2007, IFCC committees provided recommendations on analytical and preanalytical quality specifications for natriuretic peptide (NP) assays. The updated 2019 document by the IFCC Committee on Clinical Applications of Cardiac Bio-Markers (C-CB) was an educational document, which highlighted the important biochemical, analytical, and clinical aspects pertinent to NP testing. As BNP and NT-proBNP become more integrated into clinical practice as diagnostic and prognostic biomarkers, understanding differences among individual assay characteristics is extremely important. Clinicians need to be proficient in interpreting the findings of different studies predicated on BNP or NT-proBNP concentrations monitored by different assays. The laboratory community must also work closely with *in vitro* diagnostics companies, to assist in defining assay performance characteristics. Whether BNP or NT-proBNP assays are used as biomarkers for diagnosis, therapeutic decisions, and prognosis, or used in clinical trials or studies, they should be well characterized.

A growing diversity of BNP and NT-proBNP assays are used worldwide, emphasizing the need for both analytical and clinical validation of all commercial assays to support definite clinical acceptance of these new biomarkers. At present, more companies have regulatory-approved NT-proBNP assays than BNP assays. Some assays are suitable for whole blood and thus can be used in the POC setting (examples of companies with whole blood as an acceptable sample type include Abbott i-STAT, ET Healthcare, Medience, Radiometer, Roche, and Siemens). Preliminary data from research assays for proBNP have been described, but none to-date has regulatory approval. Furthermore, Thermo-Fisher-BRAHMS has the only regulatory approved assay for mid-range (MR)-proANP, which is equivalent to BNP as a biomarker to rule out and

confirm HF. The accurate clinical performance of each NP assay, which may serve as the basis for life-and-death medical decisions, sets the stage to establish assay criteria as indispensable. Limited clinical data are available for MR-proANP.

BNP and NT-proBNP are determined by a number of different immunoassays using antibodies directed to different epitopes located on the antigen molecules (Fig. 34.10). For BNP assays, one antibody binds to the ring structure and the other antibody binds to either the carboxy- or amino-terminal end. Because degradation of BNP (amino acids [aa] 77–108) occurs by proteolytic cleavage of serine and proline residues *in vivo* and *in vitro* (Fig. 34.11), this degradation may affect antibody affinities and thus be responsible for differences in reported analyte stabilities of BNP-32 monitored by different commercial BNP assays. For NT-proBNP (a.a. 1–76) monitoring, an improved understanding of potential cross-reactivity with split products of the N-terminal portion of NT-proBNP and proBNP itself are needed. For both BNP and NT-proBNP, minimizing interferents from antibodies (e.g., heterophilic, rheumatoid factor), needs to be optimized.

Regarding specimens used in NP testing, the influence (stabilizing vs destabilizing) of anticoagulant additives, as well as the type of collection tube, have been well described. For BNP, EDTA-anticoagulated whole blood or plasma appears to be the only acceptable specimen choice. For NT-proBNP, serum, heparin plasma, and EDTA plasma appear acceptable; however, not all manufacturers and NT-proBNP assays have approvals for all three matrices, suggesting that evaluation may be needed in selecting or switching the sample type used in testing. Plastic blood collection tubes are necessary for BNP, while for NT-proBNP, either glass or plastic is acceptable.

ProBNP appears to cross-react with both BNP and NT-proBNP assays, which may have substantial implications

Early biosynthetic modifications

Endo/exoproteolytic cleavages

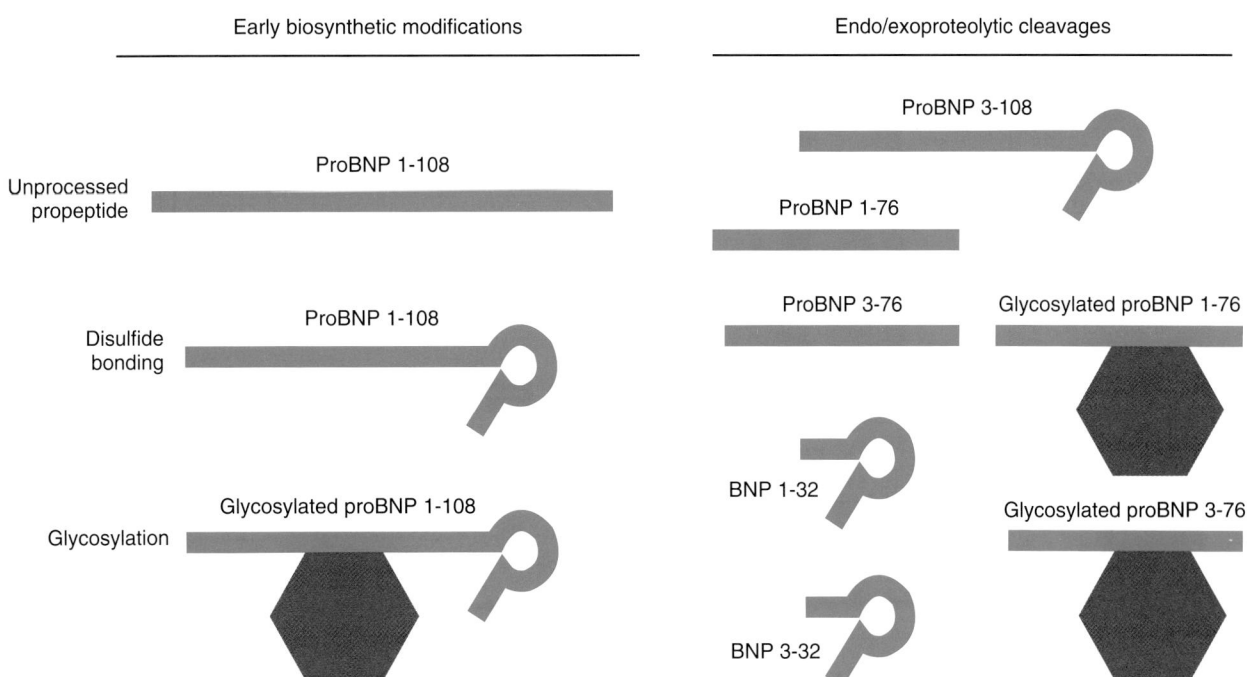

**Fig. 34.11** Schematic presentation of possible pro-brain natriuretic peptide (*proBNP*)-derived peptide products. Note that most peptides are not chemically identified but rather are suggested by biochemical methods that rely on antibody recognition. Carbohydrate is indicated by the *hexagons*. (From Rifai N. *Tietz Textbook of Clinical Chemistry and Molecular Diagnostics*, 6th ed. St. Louis: Elsevier; 2018.)

regarding clinical use (Fig. 34.12), as it is possible that most of what is measured in HF patients is proBNP. Age, gender, ethnicity, and presence of other non-HF pathologic processes can substantially influence what may otherwise be considered a normal reference concentration. Renal impairment substantially increases NT-proBNP concentrations, and BNP to a lesser extent.

For BNP, a single reference cutoff of 100 ng/L (pg/mL) has been designated for use in detecting HF; this value is likely derived from the receiver operator characteristic (ROC) curve value that was optimized for diagnostic accuracy (Fig. 34.13). However, as shown in Fig. 34.14, values in normal subjects >75 years appear to be either falsely increased or are not normal, with the 100 pg/mL cutoff detecting occult pathologic processes. For NT-proBNP, most assays use cutoffs that are age-based, i.e., for age <75 years (e.g., 125 ng/L cutoff) and age >75 years (e.g., 450 ng/L cutoff). Again, these cutoffs appear to misclassify many normal subjects, as shown in Fig. 34.14. Clinical studies (e.g., proBNP Investigation of Dyspnea in the Emergency [PRIDE]) have more appropriate age- and renal function-defined cutoffs (see Fig. 34.14). Obesity also affects measured BNP and NT-proBNP measurements, with an inverse relationship between BMI and BNP in CHF patients. Also, HF patients who received the drug nesiritide (human recombinant BNP) for therapy and management may have had confounding BNP results because nesiritide is molecularly identical to endogenous BNP; however, this compound does not appear to confound NT-proBNP measurements. Finally, a lack of

understanding of the physiologic and biologic variability of BNP and NT-proBNP in HF patients may cause clinicians to misinterpret changing (increasing or decreasing) BNP and NT-proBNP concentrations in the context of establishing the success or failure of therapy. Both BNP and NT-proBNP exhibit a within-subject biologic variability of 35%–45%. Thus, when considering what is significantly different between serial BNP or NT-proBNP values, a reference change value of 80% is necessary, although many HF trials use 30% change as a criterion for decision making. BNP or NT-proBNP monitoring may be over-used; this re-emphasizes NP's role as a confirmatory biomarker, rather than a sole marker for managing HF patients.

Data indicate low diagnostic concordance and correlation between BNP and NT-proBNP concentrations, especially among patients with chronic kidney disease using commercially available technology. In addition, the literature is scattered with reports of "home-brewed" BNP and NT-proBNP assays, which may add to the confusion when interpreting and comparing data from different studies. Whether diagnosing or ruling out HF, managing HF, screening for asymptomatic left ventricular dysfunction, or for **risk stratification** and prognostication for patients with HF, ACS, or other pathologic processes, one must consider the NP assay used, the clinical evidence available based on the individual assay, and the aim of the biomarker-based studies. No peer-reviewed literature has demonstrated that any two assays are analytically equivalent at present. Caution is suggested before the conclusions based on one particular BNP or NT-proBNP assay are translated to another assay.

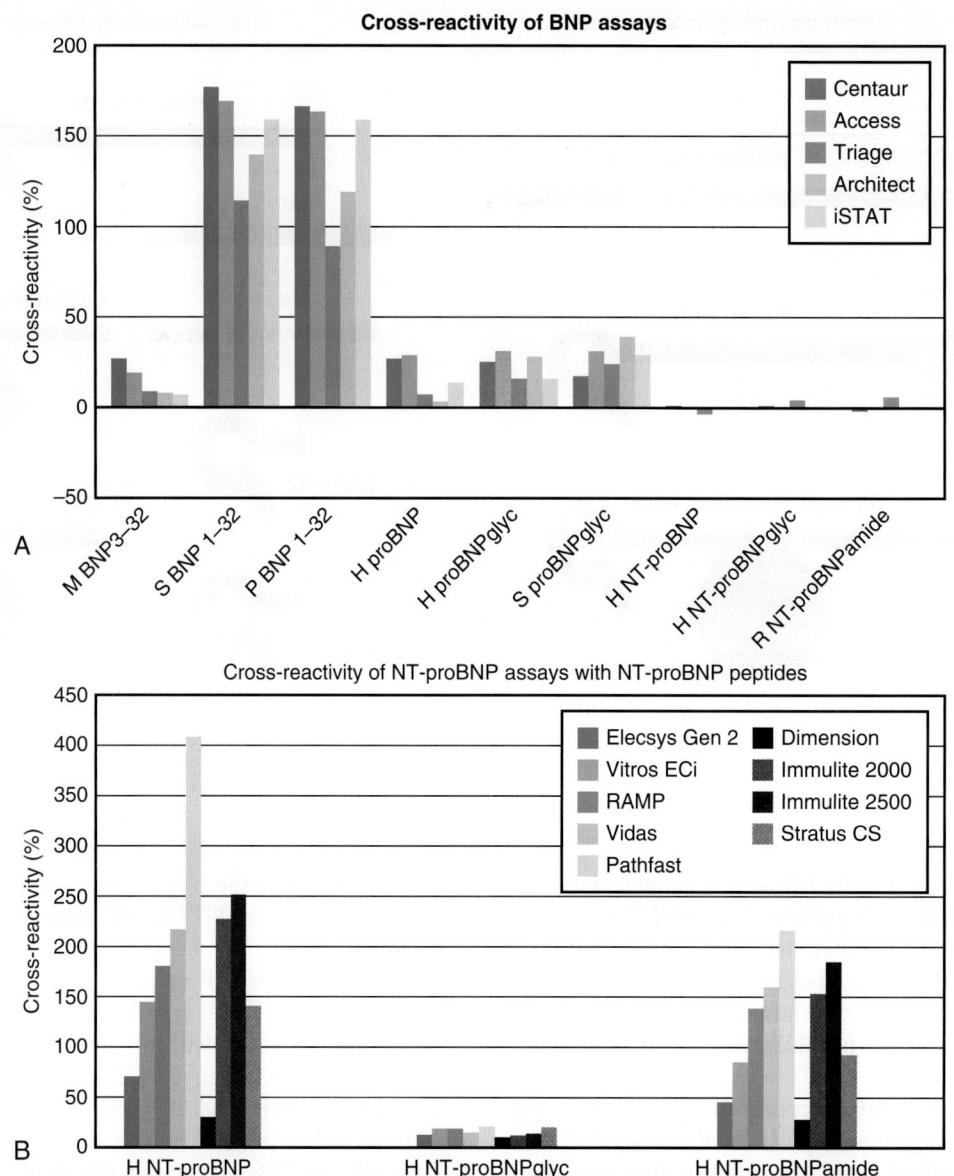

**Fig. 34.12** Cross-reactivity profiles for (A) BNP assays and (B) NT-proBNP assays, with BNP and NT-proBNP peptides, respectively. (From Saenger AK, Rodriguez-Fraga O, Ler R, et al. Specificity of B-type natriuretic peptide assays: cross-reactivity with different BNP, NT-proBNP, and proBNP peptides. *Clin Chem.* 2017;63:351–358.)

## Guidelines

Practice recommendations from the IFCC C-CB committee are provided in regards to NPs and HF, and examine: (1) the confounding nature of using different NP assays in practice, and emphasis on use of one assay, consistently; (2) the need for extensive NP assay characterization prior to clinical implementation; (3) the need for upper reference limits for NP assays to be stratified by age and sex; (4) the need for higher-order reference methods and commutable standards for BNP and NT-proBNP, to spearhead standardization efforts; (5) imprecision targets for NP assays (ideally, CV <10%); (6) diversification of populations recruited to studies of NP utility and clinical performance, to ensure better URL verification; (7) specific validation of age-stratified URLs for rule-in of acute HF; (8) the lack of a current, specific,

biomarker-guided strategy; (9) comorbidities to consider when interpreting NP test results; and (10) the long-term prognostic utility of NP tests, particularly in patients treated with NEP inhibitors.

## Clinical Utility of NP Testing

The initial validation of NP tests focused on improving the diagnosis of CHF. Rather than approaching this goal in sophisticated cardiology settings, the ED and primary care practices were key sites for NP test performance studies. The emergency setting is an extremely busy environment in which there is often a severe press for time, making cautious and careful evaluation more difficult. Also, ED physicians are generalists who must triage problems relating to almost any organ system; consequently, their ability to triage

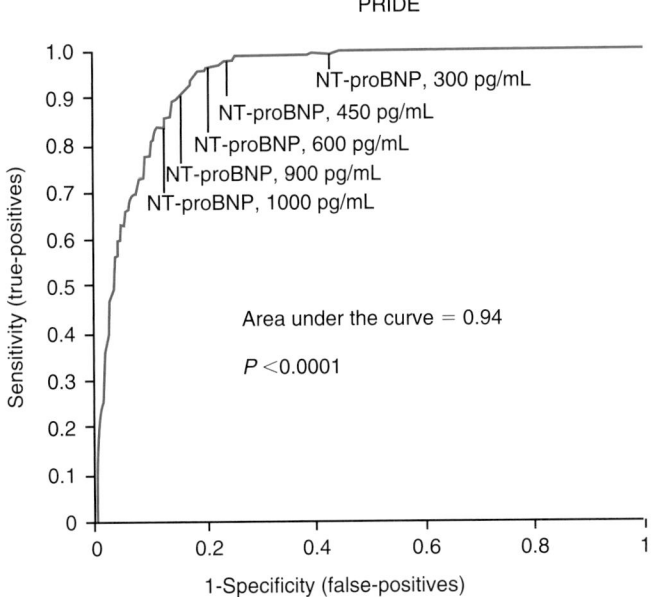

| Cut point | Sensitivity | Specificity | Positive Predictive Value | Negative Predictive Value | Accuracy |
|---|---|---|---|---|---|
| 300 pg/mL | 99% | 68% | 62% | 99% | 79% |
| 450 pg/mL | 98% | 76% | 68% | 99% | 83% |
| 600 pg/mL | 96% | 81% | 73% | 97% | 86% |
| 900 pg/mL | 90% | 85% | 76% | 94% | 87% |
| 1000 pg/mL | 87% | 86% | 78% | 91% | 87% |

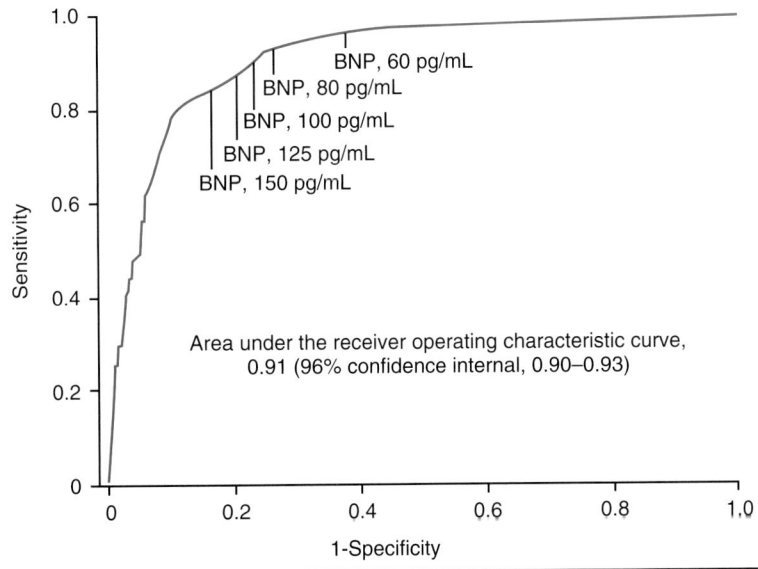

| BNP (pg/mL) | Sensitivity (%) | Specificity (%) | Positive Predictive Value (%) | Negative Predictive Value (%) | Accuracy (%) |
|---|---|---|---|---|---|
| 50 | 97 (98–98) | 62 (60–66) | 71 (68–74) | 96 (94–97) | 79 |
| 80 | 98 (91–96) | 74 (70–77) | 77 (76–80) | 92 (89–94) | 83 |
| 100 | 90 (88–92) | 76 (73–78) | 79 (78–81) | 92 (87–91) | 83 |
| 125 | 87 (86–90) | 79 (78–82) | 80 (78–83) | 87 (84–89) | 83 |
| 150 | 86 (82–88) | 83 (80–86) | 83 (80–86) | 85 (83–88) | 84 |

**Fig. 34.13** Receiver operating characteristic (ROC) analysis for brain natriuretic peptide (*BNP*) and N-terminal pro-brain natriuretic peptide (*NT-proBNP*) for the diagnosis of acute heart failure. (From Rifai N. *Tietz Textbook of Clinical Chemistry and Molecular Diagnostics*, 6th ed. St. Louis: Elsevier; 2018.)

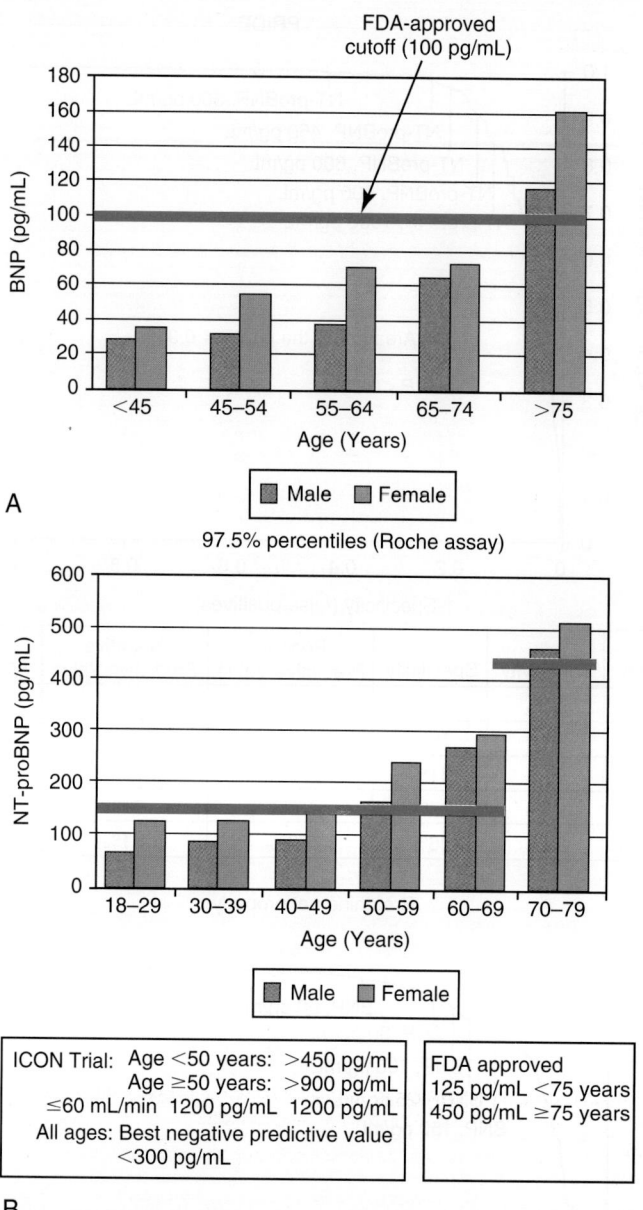

**Fig. 34.14** Representative concentration distributions in normal males and females by decade (years) with indication of the US Food and Drug Administration (*FDA*) for (A) brain natriuretic peptide (*BNP*) cleared 100 pg/mL (ng/L) cutoff value. (B) N-terminal pro-brain natriuretic peptide (*NT-proBNP*) cleared age-related cutoff values compared with those recommended by the International Collaborative on NT-proBNP ICON) trial determined by age and renal function. (From Rifai N. *Tietz Textbook of Clinical Chemistry and Molecular Diagnostics*, 6th ed. St. Louis: Elsevier; 2018.)

cardiovascular issues and assess a patient for HF is variable. Accordingly, some ED physicians have objected to the use of the ED as the primary testing ground for NP utility studies for the diagnosis of HF. General internists are in a similar position, especially in the outpatient setting where these evaluations are performed with limited resources and a heterogeneity of expertise related to this particular diagnosis. Thus, the relatively marginal improvement in diagnostic yield (74%–81% in the Breathing Not Properly [BNP] trial and 92%–96% in the PRIDE trial) is not impressive, superficially. However, in parsing the data, it is clear that the majority of the benefit of the use of NPs for HF diagnosis resides

in the triage of patients in whom clinicians are ambivalent. When patients have a very low risk for HF, it is not clear that NP testing helps at all. Similarly, when patients have a classic HF presentation, they have such a high frequency of HF, and such high pre-test probability, that NP tests are unlikely to be helpful.

However, there is a group of patients with dyspnea in whom the clinician is ambivalent, and it is this group in which NP tests are helpful. Importantly, marginal NP values often are not informative. The BNP trial suggested the use of one cutoff value at 100 ng/L, to diagnose HF (see Fig. 34.14). However, 26% of the population had values

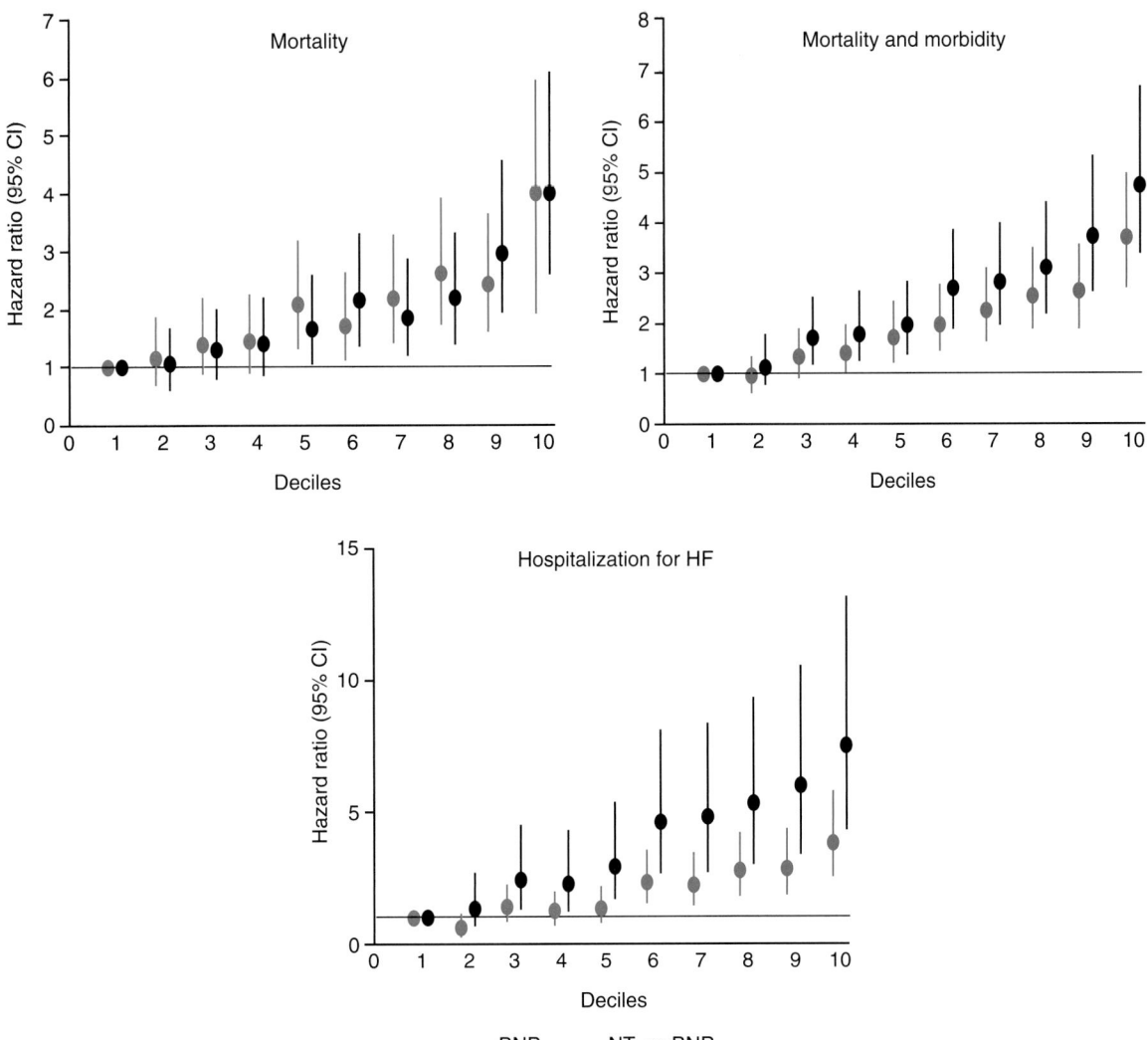

Covariates for adjustment: age, gender, NYHA class, ischemic etiology, LVEF, LVIDd, serum creatinine and bilirubin, randomized treatment, prescription of β-blockers, digitalis and diuretics, presence of AF or diabetes at study entry.

**Fig. 34.15** Relationships of brain natriuretic peptide (*BNP*) and N-terminal pro-brain natriuretic peptide (*NT-proBNP*) values and outcomes. *AF,* Atrial fibrillation; *HF,* heart failure; *LVEF,* left ventricular ejection fraction; *LVIDd,* left ventricular internal diameter end diastole; *NYHA,* New York Heart Association. (Rifai N. *Tietz Textbook of Clinical Chemistry and Molecular Diagnostics,* 6th ed. St. Louis: Elsevier; 2018.)

between 100 and 500 ng/L. One-third of this group did not have CHF according to subsequent adjudication, and two-thirds did, but unfortunately, there was no cutoff value that distinguished these groups. For this reason, a group of investigators (ICON) analyzed their data with NT-proBNP, looking to generate values that will help to both include and exclude disease. The ICON group reported that NT-proBNP <300 ng/L effectively excluded CHF, whereas values >450 ng/L in individuals who are <50 years old ruled-in HF, and values >900 ng/L diagnose HF in patients who are >50 years old. Clearly, there are gaps between these values, emphasizing that clinical judgment in addressing additional diagnostic investigation is still important and necessary in the use of NPs. It is for this reason that most guidelines groups have not suggested the routine use of NPs for diagnosis in every patient who

presents with dyspnea; instead, these groups recommend judicious use of NPs in patients in whom the diagnosis is not clear. Gender, age, and body mass index must be considered in interpreting such values. Also, it is clear that as the clinical class of the HF worsens, the NP levels rise (Fig. 34.15). Diagnosis may still be problematic, especially in patients who have other comorbidities. For example, chronic obstructive pulmonary disease and cardiovascular disease frequently overlap, and it is in these sorts of patients in whom the optimal use of NPs likely resides for HF diagnosis.

## Prognostic Considerations

Some have argued for the ubiquitous use of NPs in all patients with dyspnea. The logic for such an approach relates to the fact that individuals with higher NP values have a worse overall prognosis when compared with those with lower NP levels at presentation (either acutely or chronically). However, there is a report that extremely ill end-stage HF patients demonstrate lower NP values; while this finding could reflect exhaustion of the NP system, these observations remain to be confirmed.

One could argue that obtaining an NP value at the time of admission to hospital in a patient who has suspected CHF is valuable from the perspective of determining eventual risk. Indeed, NP values obtained in this circumstance are highly prognostic, with high risk ratios and higher NP values largely associated with worse disease. However, maximal prognostic significance is usually associated with the NP value at the time of discharge. Thus, a reasonable strategy would be to obtain one level at the time of admission and one at the time of discharge. Recent data suggest that if NP values are reduced substantially during hospitalization, patients tend to do better; however, most NP reductions reported are modest compared to the biological variability, complicating interpretation of these study data. Recent data in the outpatient setting suggest that NP result changes needed to overcome biologic variability of ≥80% are necessary to see substantive alterations in prognosis. Nonetheless, in clinical practice, there probably are differences between those individuals with more chronic disease and those with only acute disease; those with chronic disease have a chronically induced NP system that probably responds more slowly than individuals who have an acute presentation, in whom NP levels may respond more rapidly. There are no good studies defining what to do if NP levels do not respond rapidly and aggressively to change; thus, guidance for using NP to guide inpatient management could mitigate some of these problems, although sufficient information is simply not available at present.

### Considerations for Use of NPs in Therapeutic Management

Perhaps the most interesting use of NPs is in therapeutic management of the patient with HF. The logic of this approach suggests that many individuals are not as aware as they could be of their HF symptoms, and that having an objective measure may be helpful. This has recently been tested in several randomized controlled trials. The first, Systolic Heart Failure Treatment Supported by BNP (STARS-BNP) suggested benefit to such an approach, but subsequent trials have not confirmed those findings. Most recently, the Guiding Evidence Based Therapy Using Biomarker Intensified Treatment in Heart Failure (GUIDE-IT) trial was terminated early; in each arm, 37% of subjects (biomarker guided vs standard of care) reached

the primary endpoint of cardiovascular death or HF hospitalization. The negative results have been attributed to over-treatment of the control-arm (no biomarker testing) with arguments that in many of the trials, a large percentage of the patients have been elderly, and these patients may not tolerate the increased doses of therapeutic agents used in the management protocols predicated on NPs. Indeed, if subjects >75 years of age are excluded from the assessment, there is substantial benefit to this strategy.

New challenges have been posed by the development of neprilysin inhibitors, which in theory inhibit the degradation of bioactive BNP. The combination therapy of neprilysin inhibitors and angiotensin receptor blockers appears to markedly improve prognosis in patients with modest (mostly class 2) HF. In a randomized controlled trial, the therapy resulted in increased BNP values and decreased NT-proBNP values. It is likely, given the complexity of the NP system, that this view is overly simplistic, and that the agent may work on multiple proteins involved in systemic volume regulation (e.g., ANP, adrenomedullin, and possibly bradykinin, substance P, endothelin 1, and angiotensin 2). It is unclear whether the effects shown in the recent trial will impact on the use of NP measurements, but measurement of NT-proBNP may cause less diagnostic confusion early after initiation of neprilysin inhibition. A novel assay for measuring neprilysin has been developed, and the values appear to have important prognostic significance.

### Consideration of Alternative Biomarkers

ST2 (soluble interleukin 1 receptor-like 1) is an inflammatory biomarker that is being evaluated for utility in patients with HF, and perhaps acute ischemic heart disease as well. Key to this use is the understanding that the soluble form (sST2) is also released by cardiomyocyte stretch and macrophage activation that led to investigations concerning its utility in cardiovascular diseases.

Galectin-3 is an interesting marker that plays a central role in fibrosis. In response to cellular injury, the inflammatory and wound healing responses evoke the egress of macrophages into the injured area, resulting in galectin-3 release.

Another area that requires mention is multimarker testing, with the combination of NPs and other markers in a multimarker strategy to improve risk stratification, especially over the long term. Benefits may be derived from the prediction of events in older, less acutely ill individuals, using multimarker approaches. Fig. 34.16 shows additional selected cardiac biomarkers associated with prognosis in both HF and stable coronary artery disease; future studies may or may not find these promising.

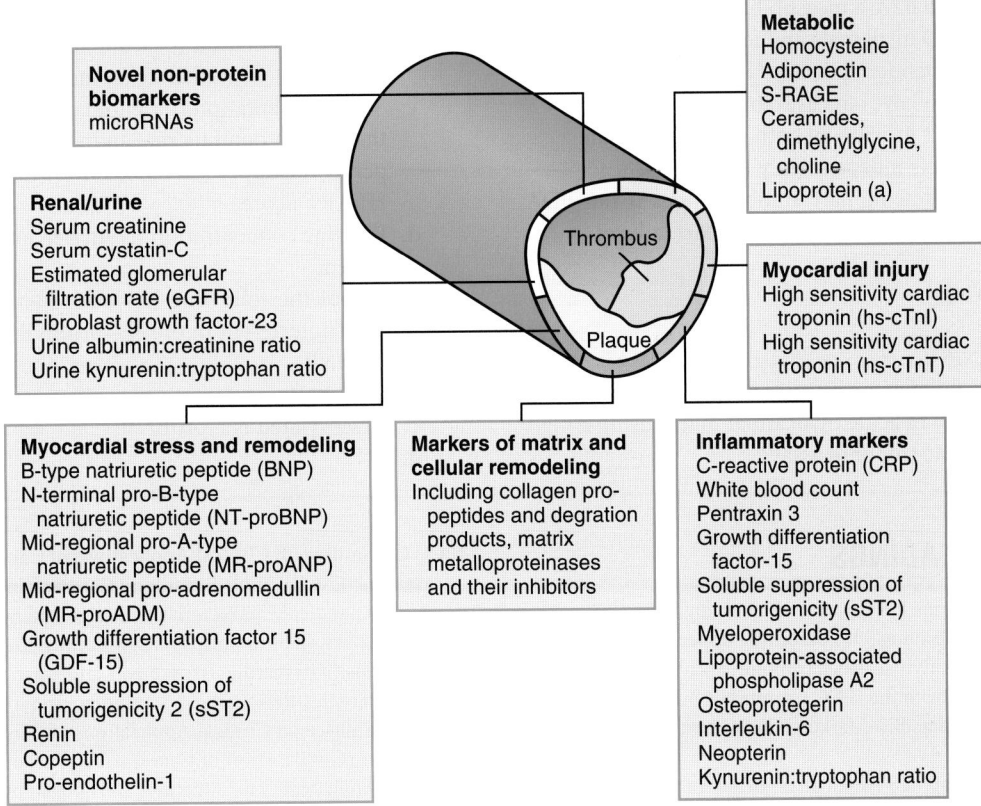

**Fig. 34.16** Selected cardiovascular biomarkers associated with prognosis in coronary artery disease. (From Omland T, White HD. State of the art: blood biomarkers for risk stratification in patients with stable ischemic heart disease. *Clin Chem.* 2017;63:165–176.)

## REVIEW QUESTIONS

1. Which of the following indicators are part of the Fourth Universal Definition of Myocardial Infarction?
   a. Ischemic symptoms
   b. Development of prolonged QT interval in the electrocardiogram
   c. Imaging evidence of new loss of viable myocardium or new regional wall motion abnormality
   d. All of the above

2. What type of myocardial injury would the following description be designated as: necrosis in which a condition other than CAD contributes to an imbalance between myocardial oxygen supply and/or demand, for example, coronary artery spasm, coronary, tachyarrhythmia, bradyarrhythmia, hypotension?
   a. Type 1 MI
   b. Type 2 MI
   c. Type 3 MI
   d. Type 4b MI

3. Which of the following should be used to set the medical decision limit for determination of acute myocardial infarction?
   a. Limit of detection (LoD)
   b. Limit of quantitation (LoQ, 20%CV)
   c. 99th percentile URL
   d. Lowest concentration that provides a 10%CV

4. Which of the following pathophysiologies is an unlikely cause of an increased blood NP concentration?
   a. Acute or chronic systolic or diastolic heart failure
   b. Systemic arterial hypertension with left ventricular hypertrophy
   c. *H. pylori* infection
   d. Endocrine disorders (e.g., Cushing syndrome)

5. Which of the following is a known predictor of adverse cardiovascular outcomes in a patient with COVID-19 disease?
   a. cTn
   b. NT-proBNP
   c. Galectin-3
   d. Soluble ST2

6. Which cardiac troponin form lacks clinical utility because it is not myocardial tissue specific?
   a. TnC
   b. TnI
   c. TnT
   d. None of the complexes

7. High sensitivity cardiac troponin assays are characterized by which of the following analytical characteristics?
   a. Have %CV <10% at LoD
   b. Have ability to have a measurable concentration above the LoD in all normal subjects

c. Have ability to have a measurable concentration above the LoD in all male and female normal subjects independently

d. Have ability to have a measurable concentration above the LoD in >50% of both male and female normal subjects independently

8. Which of the following natriuretic peptides is not FDA cleared for clinical use for ruling out heart failure?
   a. BNP
   b. MR-proANP
   c. ANP
   d. NT-proBNP

9. Which of the following strategies is the least optimal for the early rule out of acute myocardial injury using a high sensitivity cardiac troponin assay?

a. Presentation (baseline) concentration <LoD

b. Serial presentation (baseline) and 2-h concentrations that do not demonstrate an increase >4 ng/L

c. Serial presentation (baseline) and 2-h concentrations that do not demonstrate an increase above the 99th percentile upper reference limit with a normal HEART Score

d. Baseline concentration <99th percentile in low-risk patient

10. Which of the following has been identified as a cross-reactant/interferent in the NT-proBNP assay?
    a. proBNP
    b. 1–32 BNP
    c. Glycosylated NT-proBNP
    d. BNP

## SUGGESTED READINGS

Aakre K, Ordonez-Llanos J, Saenger A, et al. Analytical considerations in deriving 99th percentile upper reference limits for high-sensitivity cardiac troponin assays: educational recommendations from the IFCC Committee on Clinical Application of Cardiac Bio-Markers. *Clin Chem.* 2022;68:1022–1030.

Anand A, Lee KK, Chapman AR, et al. on behalf of the HiSTORIC Investigators. High-sensitivity cardiac troponin on presentation to rule out myocardial infarction: a stepped-wedge cluster randomized controlled trial. *Circulation.* 2021;143:2214–2224.

Apple FS, Collinson PO, Kavsak PA, et al. on behalf of the IFCC Committee Clinical Application of Cardiac Biomarkers. Getting cardiac troponin right: appraisal of the 2020 European Society of Cardiology Guidelines for the Management of Acute Coronary Syndrome in Patients Presenting Without Persistent ST-Elevation by the International Federation of Clinical Chemistry and Laboratory Medicine Committee on the Clinical Application of Cardiac Bio-Markers. *Clin Chem.* 2021;67:730–735.

Apple FS, Fantz CR, Collinson PO. Implementation of high-sensitivity and point of care cardiac troponin assays into practice: some different thoughts. *Clin Chem.* 2021;67:70–78.

Apple FS, Wu AHB, Sandoval Y, et al. Sex-specific 99th percentile upper reference limits for high sensitivity cardiac troponin assays derived using a universal sample bank. *Clin Chem.* 2020;66:434–444.

Cullen LA, Mills NL, Mahler S, et al. Early rule-out and rule-in strategies for myocardial infarction. *Clin Chem.* 2017;63:129–139.

IFCC Committee on Clinical Applications of Cardiac Bio-Markers (C-CB). BNP, NT-proBNP, and MR-proANP Assays: Analytical Characteristics Designated by Manufacturer. v052022. Available at: https://www.ifcc.org/media/479433/bnp-nt-probnp-and-mr-proanp-assays-analytical-characteristics-designated-by-manufacturer-v052022.pdf.

IFCC Committee on Clinical Applications of Cardiac Biomarkers (C-CB). Cardiac Troponin Assay Interference Table Designated by Manufacturer: Hemolysis and Biotin. v052022. Available at: https://www.ifcc.org/media/479436/ifcc-cardiac-troponin-interference-table_v052022.pdf.

IFCC Committee on Clinical Applications of Cardiac Bio-Markers (C-CB). High-Sensitivity Cardiac Troponin I and T Assay Analytical Characteristics Designated by Manufacturer. v052022. Available at: https://www.ifcc.org/media/479435/high-sensitivity-cardiac-troponin-i-and-t-assay-analytical-characteristics-designated-by-manufacturer-v052022.pdf.

IFCC Committee on Clinical Applications of Cardiac Bio-Markers (C-CB). Point of Care Cardiac Troponin I and T Assay Analytical Characteristics Designated by Manufacturer. v052022. Available at: https://www.ifcc.org/media/479438/point-of-care-cardiac-troponin-i-and-t-assay-analytical-characteristics-designated-by-manufacturer-v052022.pdf.

Kavsak PA, Hammarsten O, Worster A, et al. Cardiac troponin testing in patients with COVID-19: a strategy for testing and reporting results. *Clin Chem.* 2021;67:107–113.

Kavsak PA, Lam CSP, Saenger AK, et al. Educational recommendations on selected analytical and clinical aspects of natriuretic peptides with a focus on heart failure: A report from the IFCC Committee on Clinical Applications of Cardiac Bio-Markers. *Clin Chem.* 2019;65:1221–1227.

Libby P. The vascular biology of atherosclerosis. In: Zipes DP, Libby P, Bonow RO, Mann DL, Tomaselli GF, Braunwald E, eds. *Braunwald's Heart Disease: A Textbook of Cardiovascular Medicine.* 11th ed. Philadelphia: Elsevier; 2019:859–875.

Sandoval Y, Apple FS, Mahler SA, Body R, Collinson PO, Jaffe AS. High-sensitivity cardiac troponin and the 2021 AHA/ACC/ASE/CHEST/SAEM/SCCT/SCMR Guidelines for the Evaluation and Diagnosis of Acute Chest Pain. *Circulation.* 2022;146:569–581.

Sandoval Y, Smith SW, Sexter A, et al. Type 1 and 2 myocardial infarction and myocardial injury: clinical transition to high-sensitivity cardiac troponin I. *Am J Med.* 2017;130:1431–1439.

Sandoval Y, Smith SW, Shah ASV, et al. Rapid rule-out of acute myocardial injury using a single high-sensitivity cardiac troponin I measurement. *Clin Chem.* 2017;63:369–376.

Shah AS, Anand A, Sandoval Y, et al. for High-STEACS investigators. High-sensitivity cardiac troponin I at presentation in patients with suspected acute coronary syndrome: a cohort study. *Lancet.* 2015;386(10012):2481–2488.

Tang WH, Francis GS, Morrow DA, et al. National Academy of Clinical Biochemistry Laboratory Medicine practice guidelines: clinical utilization of cardiac biomarker testing in heart failure. *Circulation.* 2007;116:e99–109.

Thygesen K, Alpert JS, Jaffe AS, et al. on behalf of the Joint European Society of Cardiology (ESC)/American College of Cardiology (ACC)/American Heart Association (AHA)/World Heart Federation (WHF) Task Force for the Universal Definition of Myocardial Infarction. Fourth Universal Definition of Myocardial Infarction (2018). *J Am Coll Cardiol.* 2018;72:2231–2264.

Thygesen K, Alpert JS, Jaffe AS, et al. Fourth Universal Definition of Myocardial Infarction (2018). *Circulation.* 2018;138:e618–e651.

Thygesen K, Alpert JS, Jaffe AS, et al. ESC Scientific Document Group. Fourth Universal Definition of Myocardial Infarction (2018). *Eur Heart J.* 2019;40:237–269.

Wu AHB, Christenson RH, Greene DN, et al. Clinical Laboratory Practice Recommendations for the Use of Cardiac Troponin in Acute Coronary Syndrome: Expert Opinion from the Academy of the American Association for Clinical Chemistry and the Task Force on Clinical Applications of Cardiac Bio-Markers of the International Federation of Clinical Chemistry and Laboratory Medicine. *Clin Chem.* 2018;64:645–655.

# Kidney Disease

*Michael P. Delaney and Edmund J. Lamb\**

## OBJECTIVES

1. Define the following:
   Bence Jones protein
   Clearance
   Cystatin-C
   Diabetes insipidus (DI)
   Diabetic nephropathy
   Dialysis
   Diuretic
   Glomerulus
   Glomerular filtration rate (GFR)
   Juxtaglomerular apparatus
   Kidney replacement therapy (KRT)
   Micturition
   Nephrolithiasis
   Nephron
   Pyelonephritis
   Renal pelvis
   Ureter
   Urine
2. Describe the following components of the renal system, including structure, function, contribution to urine formation, and clinical significance:
   Bladder
   Bowman capsule
   Collecting tubules
   Distal convoluted tubule
   Glomerulus
   Juxtaglomerular apparatus
   Kidneys
   Loop of Henle
   Nephron
   Proximal convoluted tubule
3. State the significance of kidney blood supply in the formation of urine within the structure of the glomerulus; list the arteries that form the glomerular capillary bed.
4. List and describe the three major functions of the kidneys, including processes involved, laboratory analytes affected in each process, and how each function is controlled.
5. Describe glomerular filtration rate (GFR) and clearance in terms of clinical usefulness and effects of renal disease and age on each process.
6. Describe the renal handling of electrolytes and water, including normal physiology, hormones involved, and effect of disease on each function.
7. Discuss the following conditions, including the causes (such as drugs and toxins), symptoms, acid-base disturbances (if any), laboratory methods used to assess, and pertinent laboratory results obtained:
   Acute kidney injury (AKI)
   Acute tubular necrosis (ATN)
   Chronic kidney disease (CKD)
   Diabetes insipidus (DI)
   Glomerular disease
   Interstitial nephritis
   Kidney failure, including uremic syndrome
   Nephrotic syndrome
   Pyelonephritis
   Uremic syndrome
   Urinary tract obstruction
8. Describe two options for kidney replacement therapy (KRT), including the clinical need for the therapy and laboratory assessment of each therapy.
9. Evaluate and analyze case studies related to kidney disease and laboratory analysis of kidney disease.

## KEY WORDS AND DEFINITIONS

**Acidosis** Accumulation of acid and hydrogen ions or depletion of the alkaline reserve (bicarbonate content) in the blood and body tissues.

**Acute kidney injury (AKI)** A rapid decline in kidney function that occurs over hours and days.

**Acute nephritic syndrome** The sudden onset of hematuria, proteinuria, diminished urine production, azotemia, hypertension, and edema.

**Acute tubular necrosis (ATN)** Acute renal failure with mild to severe damage or necrosis of tubule cells.

*We are grateful for the data supplied by the United States Renal Data System (USRDS). The interpretation and reporting of these data are the responsibility of the authors and in no way should be seen as an official policy or interpretation of the US government. We are also grateful for data supplied by the United Kingdom Renal Registry. The data reported here have been supplied by the UK Renal Registry (UKRR) of the Renal Association. The interpretation and reporting of these data are the responsibility of the authors and in no way should be seen as an official policy or interpretation of the UKRR or the Renal Association. We also acknowledge the input of Professor Christopher Price to previous editions of this chapter.

**Antidiuretic hormone (ADH; vasopressin)** A nonapeptide hormone formed by the neuronal cells of the hypothalamic nuclei and stored in the posterior lobe of the pituitary gland (neurohypophysis). It has both antidiuretic and vasopressor actions.

**Azotemia** An excess of urea or other nitrogenous compounds in the blood.

**Bartter syndrome** Hypertrophy and hyperplasia of the juxtaglomerular cells, producing hypokalemic alkalosis and hyperaldosteronism.

**Bence Jones protein** An abnormal plasma or urinary protein, consisting of monoclonal immunoglobulin light chains, excreted in some neoplastic diseases. It is a characteristic protein found in the urine of most patients with multiple myeloma.

**Bowman capsule** The double-walled globular kidney structure that forms the beginning of a renal tubule and surrounds the glomerulus.

**Chronic kidney disease (CKD)** Abnormalities of kidney structure or function, present for greater than 3 months, with implications for health.

**Clearance** The volume of plasma from which a given substance is completely cleared by the kidneys per unit of time.

**Diabetic nephropathy** The nephropathy that commonly accompanies later stages of diabetes mellitus; it begins with hyperfiltration, renal hypertrophy, albuminuria, and hypertension.

**Dialysis** The removal of certain elements from the blood by virtue of the difference in the rates of their diffusion through a semipermeable membrane, for example, by means of a hemodialysis (HD) machine or filter.

**Erythropoietin** A glycoprotein hormone secreted chiefly by the kidney in the adult; it increases production of red blood cells.

**Gitelman syndrome** A syndrome of hypertrophy of juxtaglomerular cells similar to Bartter syndrome but with hypocalciuria and hypomagnesemia.

**Glomerular filtration rate (GFR)** The rate in milliliters per minute at which small molecules are filtered through the kidney's glomeruli. It is a measure of the number of functioning nephrons.

**Glomerulonephritis** Nephritis accompanied by inflammation of the capillary loops of the glomeruli of the kidney. It occurs in acute, subacute, and chronic forms.

**Glomerulus** A tuft of blood vessels found in each nephron of the kidney that is involved in the filtration of the blood.

**Hematuria** Blood in the urine.

**Hypertension** A medical condition characterized by high arterial blood pressure.

**IgA nephropathy** A common, chronic form of glomerulonephritis marked by hematuria and proteinuria and by deposits of immunoglobulin A in the mesangial areas of the renal glomeruli.

**Interstitial nephritis** Primary or secondary disease of the renal interstitial tissue.

**Juxtaglomerular apparatus (JGA)** A complex in the kidney whose function is the autoregulation of the glomerular filtration rate.

**Kidney failure** A condition where kidney function is inadequate to support life.

**Kidney replacement therapy (KRT)** Any treatment that replaces kidney function, including dialysis and transplantation.

**Liddle syndrome** A rare autosomal dominant syndrome resulting from epithelial sodium channel mutations that lead to abnormally increased channel function.

**Lithotripsy** The crushing of a calculus within the urinary system, followed at once by the washing out of the fragments; it is done either surgically or by several different noninvasive methods.

**Loop of Henle** The U-shaped part of the renal tubule, extending through the medulla from the end of the proximal convoluted tubule to the beginning of the distal convoluted tubule.

**Nephritis** Inflammation of the kidney with focal or diffuse proliferation or destructive processes that may involve the glomerulus, tubule, or interstitial renal tissue.

**Nephrolithiasis** A condition marked by the presence of renal calculi (stones).

**Nephron** The anatomical and functional unit of the kidney, consisting of the (1) renal corpuscle, (2) proximal convoluted tubule, (3) descending and ascending limbs of loop of Henle, (4) distal convoluted tubule, and (5) collecting tubule.

**Nephrotic syndrome** General name for a group of diseases involving defective kidny glomeruli, characterized by massive proteinuria with varying degrees of edema, hypoalbuminemia, and hyperlipidemia.

**Obstructive uropathy** Uropathy resulting from an obstruction in the tract.

**Oliguria** Diminished urine production and excretion.

**Peritoneal dialysis (PD)** Diffusion of solutes and convection of fluid through the peritoneal membrane. The dialyzing solution is introduced into and removed from the peritoneal cavity as either a continuous or an intermittent procedure.

**Polycystic kidney disease** The most common renal cystic condition, with deterioration of renal function.

**Polyuria** The passage of a large volume of urine in a given period.

**Proteinuria** Excessive serum proteins in the urine, such as in renal disease, after strenuous exercise, and with dehydration.

**Pseudohypoaldosteronism type 1** A hereditary disorder of infancy characterized by severe salt wasting, failure to thrive, and other signs of aldosterone deficiency.

**Pyelonephritis** An inflammation of the kidney and its pelvis as a result of infection.

**Renin** An enzyme of the hydrolase class that catalyzes cleavage of the leucine-leucine bond in angiotensinogen to generate angiotensin I.

**Uremia** An excess in the blood of urea, creatinine, and other nitrogenous end products of protein and amino acid metabolism; also referred to as azotemia.

**Uremic syndrome** The spectrum of symptoms accompanying uremia.

## INTRODUCTION

The kidneys play a central role in homeostasis, and reduced renal function strongly correlates with increasing morbidity and mortality. The basic anatomy and physiology of the kidneys are described as a foundation for understanding the pathophysiology of disease and the rationale for diagnostic and management strategies in kidney disease. Key analytical methods employed during the investigation of kidney disease are dealt with in Chapter 21.

## ANATOMY

The kidneys are a paired organ system located in the lumbar region. Their function is to (1) filter the blood and excrete the end-products of body metabolism in the form of urine; (2) regulate the concentrations of (a) hydrogen, (b) sodium, (c) potassium, (d) phosphate, and (e) other ions in the extracellular fluid; and (3) produce hormones. In an adult, each kidney is about 12 cm long and weighs about 150 g in men and 135 g in women. A kidney is of a characteristic bean shape through which pass the vessels, nerves, and ureter (Fig. 35.1).

### Nephron

The functional unit of the kidney is the **nephron**. Each kidney may contain up to 1.5 million nephrons. The nephron consists of a (1) glomerulus, (2) proximal tubule, (3) loop of Henle, (4) distal tubule, and (5) collecting duct (Fig. 35.2). The collecting ducts ultimately combine to develop into the renal calyces, where the urine collects before passing along the ureter and into the bladder. The kidney is divided into several lobes. The outer, darker region of each lobe—the cortex—consists of the glomeruli and the proximal and distal tubules. The cortex surrounds a paler inner region—the medulla—which is further divided into a number of conical areas known as the renal pyramids, the apex of which extends toward the renal pelvis, forming papillae. Medullary rays are visible striations in the renal pyramids that connect the kidney cortex with the medulla. They are composed of (1) descending (straight proximal) and (2) ascending (straight distal) thick limbs of Henle, and (3) collecting ducts and associated blood vessels (the vasa recta). The central hilus is where blood vessels, lymphatics, and the renal pelvis (containing the ureter) join the kidney.

The **glomerulus** is formed from a specialized capillary network. Each capillary develops into approximately 40 glomerular loops around 200 μm in size and consisting of a variety of different cell types supported on a specialized basement membrane. Some endothelial and epithelial cells act in concert with the specialized glomerular basement membrane (GBM) to form the glomerular filtration barrier. The glomerular capillaries are supported by a network of mesangial cells and mesangial matrix that act as connective tissue for the glomerular apparatus.

The **Bowman capsule** forms the beginning of the tightly coiled, proximal convoluted tubule *(pars convoluta)*, which on its progress toward the renal medulla becomes straightened and is then called the *pars recta*. The proximal tubule is about 15 mm long. The proximal tubule is the most metabolically active part of the nephron, facilitating the reabsorption of 60% to 80% of the glomerular filtrate volume—including 70% of the filtered load of (1) sodium and (2) chloride, most of the (3) potassium, (4) glucose, (5) bicarbonate, (6) phosphate, and (7) sulfate—and secreting 90% of the hydrogen ion excreted by the kidney.

The pars recta drains into the descending thin loop of Henle, which after passing through a hairpin loop becomes first the ascending thin limb and then the thick ascending loop. At the end of the thick ascending limb, there is a cluster of cells known as the *macula densa* (Fig. 35.3). The main role of the **loop of Henle** is to provide the ability to generate a concentrated urine, hypertonic with respect to plasma.

The cells forming the distal tubule of the nephron start at the macula densa and extend to the first fusion with other tubules to form the collecting ducts. Sodium chloride reabsorption and some potassium and hydrogen ion excretion occur at this site.

The collecting ducts are formed from approximately six distal tubules. These are successively joined by other tubules to form ducts of Bellini, which ultimately drain into a renal calyx.

### Juxtaglomerular Apparatus

Where the thick ascending limb of the loop of Henle passes very close to the glomerulus of its own nephron, the cells of the tubule and the afferent arteriole show regional specialization

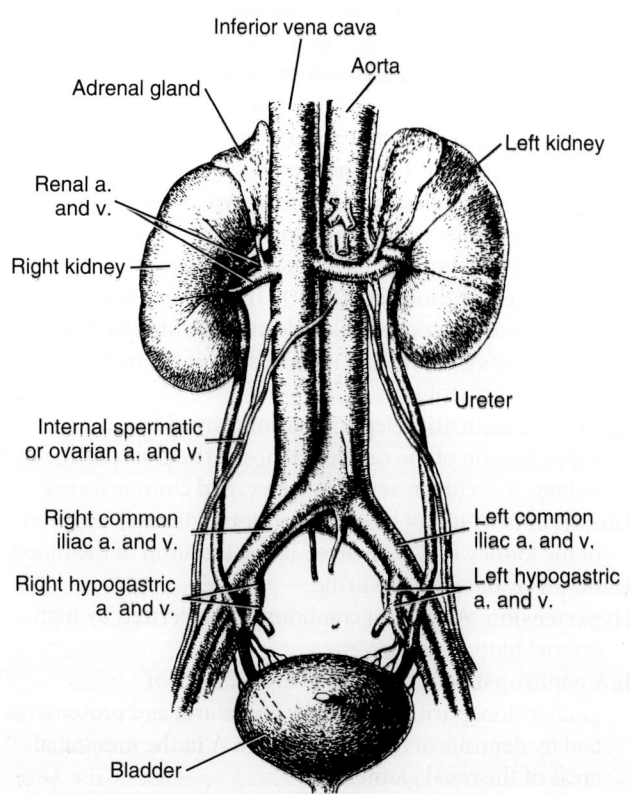

**Fig. 35.1** Vascular and anatomic relationships of the kidneys in man. (From Leaf A, Cotran RS. *Renal Pathophysiology*. 3rd ed. Oxford: Oxford University Press; 1985. Reproduced by permission of Oxford University Press.)

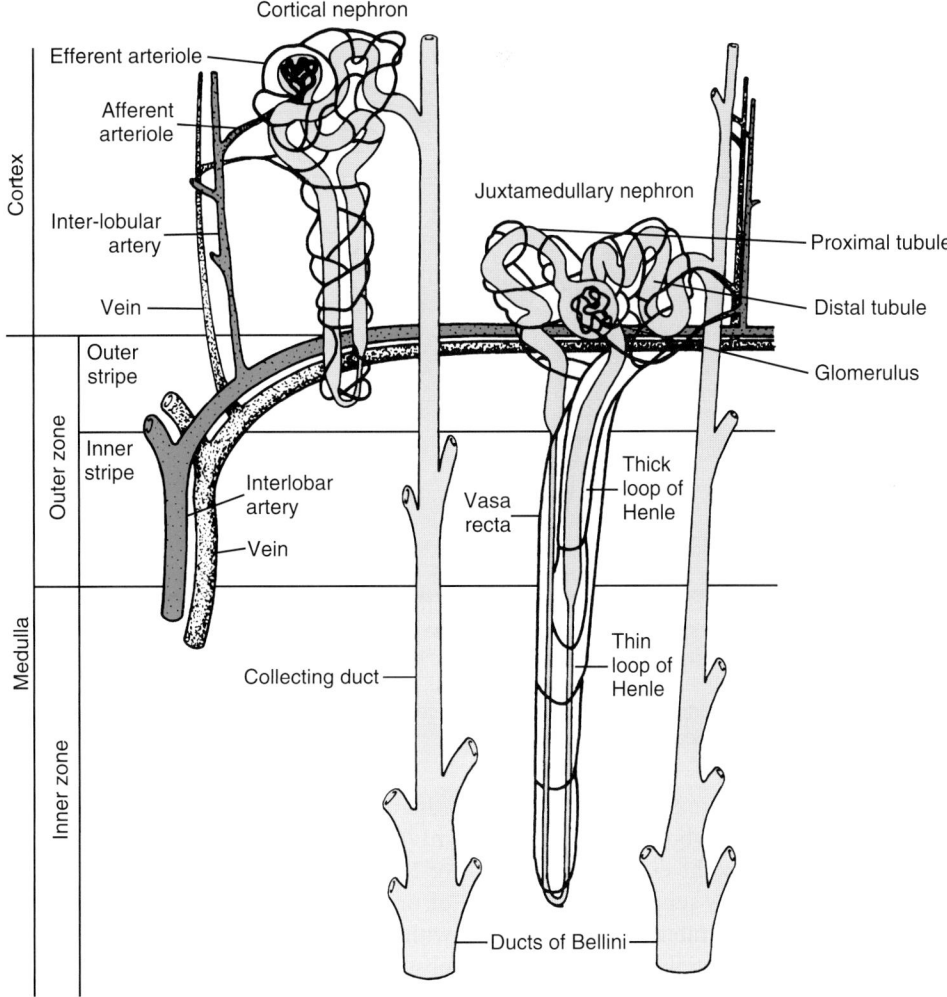

Cortical nephron

Efferent arteriole

Afferent arteriole

Cortex

Inter-lobular artery

Vein

Outer stripe

Inner stripe

Outer zone

Interlobar artery

Vein

Medulla

Inner zone

Collecting duct

Ducts of Bellini

Juxtamedullary nephron

Proximal tubule

Distal tubule

Glomerulus

Thick loop of Henle

Vasa recta

Thin loop of Henle

**Fig. 35.2** Diagrammatic representation of the nephron, the functional unit of the kidney, illustrating the anatomic and vascular arrangements. (From Pitts RF. *Physiology of the Kidney and Body Fluids.* 3rd ed. Chicago: Year Book Medical Publishers; 1974:8.)

(see Fig. 35.3). The tubule forms the macula densa; the arteriolar cells are filled with granules (containing renin or its inactive precursor, prorenin) and are innervated with sympathetic nerve fibers. This area is called the juxtaglomerular apparatus (JGA). The JGA plays an important part in maintaining systemic blood pressure through regulation of the circulating intravascular blood volume and sodium concentration. The proteolytic enzyme renin is released primarily in response to decreased afferent arteriolar pressure and decreased intraluminal sodium delivery to the macula densa. Renin release from the macula densa is also influenced by nitric oxide, renal cortical prostaglandins (predominantly PGI₂), and the sympathetic nervous system. The released renin then acts on the plasma protein angiotensinogen to generate angiotensin I. This is converted in the lungs by angiotensin converting enzyme (ACE) to the potent vasoconstrictor and stimulator of aldosterone release, angiotensin II (AII). The vasoconstriction and aldosterone release (with increased distal tubular sodium retention) act in concert with the other action of AII, to increase the release of antidiuretic hormone (ADH, vasopressin) and to increase proximal tubular sodium

reabsorption, intravascular volume, and pressure. AII also has an inhibitory effect on renin release as part of a negative feedback loop.

## Blood Supply

The renal artery divides into posterior and anterior elements, which then divide into interlobar, arcuate, interlobular, and ultimately into the afferent arterioles, which expand into the capillary bed that forms the glomerulus (see Fig. 35.2). These capillaries then rejoin to form the efferent arteriole, which then forms the capillary plexuses as well as the elongated vessels (the *vasa recta*) that pass around the remaining parts of the (1) nephron, (2) proximal and distal tubules, (3) loop of Henle, and (4) collecting duct, providing oxygen and nutrients and removing ions, molecules, and water, which are reabsorbed by the nephron. The efferent arteriole then merges with renal venules to form the renal veins, which emerge into the inferior vena cava. The complex architecture of the intrarenal vascular tree is ordered in three dimensions in a characteristic arrangement that probably serves to distribute the blood pressure and flow appropriately to the glomeruli.

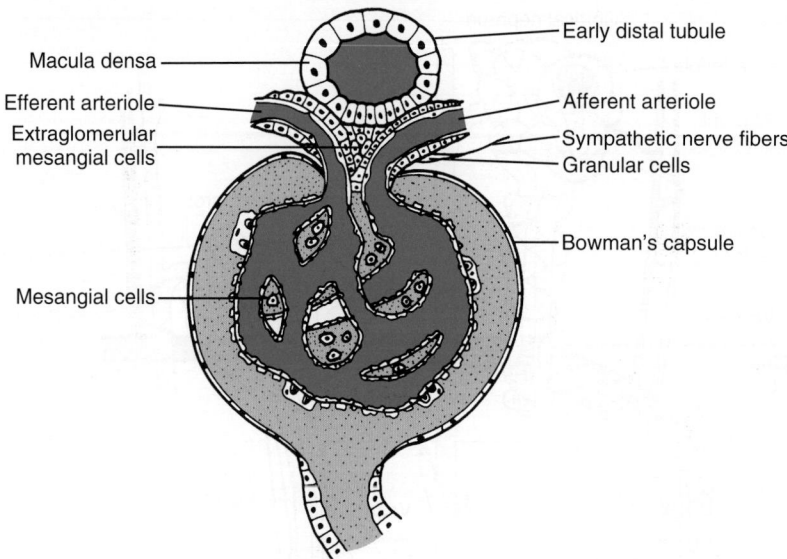

**Fig. 35.3** The juxtaglomerular apparatus. The beginning of the distal tubule (i.e., where the loop of Henle reenters the cortex) lies very close to the afferent and efferent arterioles, and the cells of both the afferent arteriole and the tubule show specialization. The cells of the afferent arteriole are thickened, granular (juxta-glomerular) cells that are innervated by sympathetic nerve fibers. The mesangial cells are irregularly shaped and contain filaments of contractile proteins. Identical cells are found just outside the glomerulus and are termed *extraglomerular mesangial cells* or *Goormaghtigh cells*. (From Lote CJ. *Principles of Renal Physiology*. 4th ed. London: Kluwer Academic Publishers; 2000.)

In the adult, the kidneys receive approximately 25% of the cardiac output; however, in the newborn infant it is 5%, only reaching adult proportions by the end of the first year of life. About 90% of this blood flow supplies the renal cortex, maintaining the highly active tubular cells. The maintenance of renal blood flow is essential to renal function, and there is a complex array of intrarenal regulatory mechanisms that ensure that it is maintained across a wide range of systemic blood pressures. The renal glomerular perfusion pressure is independent of the systemic pressure between 90 and 200 mm Hg, being maintained at a constant 45 mm Hg.

## KIDNEY FUNCTION

The main biological functions of the kidneys are (1) excretion, (2) homeostatic regulation, and (3) endocrine. The kidneys integrate these functions to maintain homeostasis and regulate the internal milieu.

### Excretory Function

*Urine* is (1) excreted by the kidneys, (2) passed through the ureters, (3) stored in the bladder, and (4) discharged through the urethra. In health, it (1) is sterile and clear, (2) is of yellow or amber color, (3) has a slightly acid pH (5.0 to 6.0), and (4) has a characteristic odor and specific gravity of about 1.024. In addition to dissolved compounds, it contains a number of cells, proteinaceous casts, and crystals (formed elements). Changes in these formed elements are studied using urine microscopy.

*Urination,* also termed *micturition* or *voiding,* is the discharge of urine. In normal adults, adequate homeostasis is maintained with a urine output of about 500 mL/day.

Alterations in urinary output are described as *anuria* (<100 mL/day), **oliguria** (<400 mL/day), or **polyuria** (>3 L/day or 50 mL/kg body weight/day). The most common disorder of urination is altered frequency, which may be associated with increased urinary volume or with partial urinary tract obstruction (e.g., in prostatic hypertrophy).

The first step in urine formation is filtration of plasma water at the glomeruli. A net filtration pressure of about 17 mm Hg in the capillary bed of the tuft drives the filtrate through the glomerular membrane. The filtrate is called an ultrafiltrate because its composition is essentially the same as that of plasma, but with a notable reduction in molecules of molecular weight exceeding 15 kDa. Each nephron produces about 100 μL of ultrafiltrate per day. Overall, approximately 170 to 200 L of ultrafiltrate passes through the glomeruli in 24 hours. In the passage of ultrafiltrate through the tubules, reabsorption of solutes and water in various regions of the tubules reduces the total urine volume, which typically ranges between 0.4 and 2 L/day.

Transport of solutes and water occurs both across and between the epithelial cells that line the renal tubules. Transport is both active (energy requiring) and passive, but many of the so-called passive transport processes are dependent upon or secondary to active transport processes, particularly those involving sodium transport. All known transport processes involve receptor or mediator molecules, many of which have now been identified and characterized using molecular biological techniques. The activity of many of these molecules is regulated by phosphorylation facilitated by protein kinase C or A. Their renal distribution has been shown to correlate with the known regional functional activities. There are inherited disorders of specific tubular transporters and a well-known generalized disorder affecting all of the transport processes, causing Fanconi syndrome.

Direct coupling of adenosine triphosphate (ATP) hydrolysis is an example of an active transport process. The most important of these in the nephron is Na$^+$,K$^+$-ATPase, which is located on the basolateral membranes of the tubuloepithelial cells. This enzymatic transporter accounts for much of renal oxygen consumption and drives more than 99% of renal sodium reabsorption.

Renal epithelial cell membranes also contain proteins that act as ion channels. For example, there is one for sodium that is closed by amiloride and modulated by hormones such as atrial natriuretic peptide (ANP). Ion channels enable much faster rates of transport than ATPases, but they are relatively fewer in number—approximately 100 sodium and chloride channels as against $10^7$ Na$^+$,K$^+$-ATPase molecules per cell.

In the tubules, the solute composition of the ultrafiltrate is altered by the processes of reabsorption and secretion, so that the urine excreted may have a very different composition from that of the original filtrate. Different regions of the tubule have been shown to specialize in certain functions. In the proximal tubule, 60% to 80% of the ultrafiltrate is reabsorbed in an obligatory fashion, along with (1) sodium, (2) chloride, (3) bicarbonate, (4) calcium, (5) phosphate, (6) sulfate, and (7) other ions. Glucose is virtually completely reabsorbed, predominantly in the proximal tubule by a passive but sodium-dependent process that is saturated at a blood glucose concentration of about 180 mg/dL (10 mmol/L). The sodium-glucose cotransporters SGLT 1 and 2 are responsible for this, and SGLT2 in particular can be subjected to inhibition with novel therapies to decrease glucose reabsorption and increase glycosuria (see below).

Uric acid is also reabsorbed in the proximal tubule by a passive sodium-dependent mechanism, but there is also an active secretory mechanism.

In the ascending limb of the loop of Henle, chloride and more sodium without water are reabsorbed, generating dilute urine. Water reabsorption in the more distal tubules and collecting ducts is then regulated by ADH. In the distal tubule, secretion (the movement of chemical substances from within tubular cells into the tubular lumen) is the prominent activity; organic ions, potassium ions, and hydrogen ions are transported from the blood in the efferent arteriole into the tubular fluid. It is also this region that secretes hydrogen ions and reabsorbs sodium and bicarbonate to aid in acid base regulation. Paracellular (between-cell) movement is driven predominantly by concentration, osmotic, or electrical gradients.

## Regulatory Function

The *regulatory function* of the kidneys has a major role in homeostasis. The mechanisms of differential reabsorption and secretion, located in the tubule of a nephron, are the effectors of regulation. The mechanisms operate under a complex system of control in which both extrarenal and intrarenal humoral factors participate.

## Electrolyte Homeostasis

The proximal convoluted tubule is predominantly concerned with reabsorption (Fig. 35.4). Water reabsorption in the proximal convoluted tubule is termed "obligatory" because its volume is related to the heavy load of solutes being returned to the blood in the efferent arteriole. The amount of bicarbonate reabsorption is related to the glomerular filtration rate (GFR) and the hydrogen ion secretory rate. The amount of phosphate reabsorption is controlled in part by plasma calcium concentration and in part by the effect of parathyroid hormone on the tubular cells. Normally, the high-threshold substances—glucose and, to a great extent, amino acids—are reabsorbed here by means of specific intracellular active transport systems. Uric acid may be either reabsorbed or secreted in the proximal convoluted tubule by a two-way carrier-mediated process.

In the ascending loop of Henle, 20% to 25% of filtered sodium is reabsorbed without concomitant reabsorption of water. This process generates dilute urine with an osmolality of 100 to 150 mOsm/kg of water and helps establish the corticomedullary osmotic gradient. The resulting hypertonicity of the interstitium is important in the pathogenesis of renal infections because the hypertonic environment interferes with leukocyte function. Subsequent water reabsorption is regulated by ADH. Although the reabsorption of Na$^+$ in the loop of Henle is complex and incompletely understood, at least one mechanism consists of an active Cl$^-$ pump with subsequent reabsorption of Na$^+$ along an electrochemical gradient. This mechanism is inhibited by loop diuretics.

The distal tubule is functionally the most active region of the nephron for the homeostatic regulation of plasma electrolytes and plasma acid-base concentrations. Here a combination of secretion and reabsorption takes place among Na$^+$, K$^+$, and H$^+$. Although excess plasma hydrogen ions are secreted all along the tubule, it is in the distal tubule that exchange of H$^+$ for Na$^+$ (which is reabsorbed) fine-tunes the balance between H$^+$ loss and retention (see Chapter 36). Potassium ions are also secreted in the distal tubule. Aldosterone is a potent modulator of Na$^+$ reabsorption in the distal tubule, particularly when the need arises to conserve Na$^+$. Production of aldosterone in the adrenal cortex is stimulated by the renin-angiotensin system and by high plasma potassium concentration. Renal secretion of renin is complex, but it is at least partly regulated by renal perfusion and plasma sodium concentration. Both inadequate perfusion and a low concentration of plasma sodium stimulate renin secretion. Organic anions, such as acetoacetate and β-hydroxybutyrate, also consume H$^+$ as they are eliminated in part in their nondissociated acid form. When H$^+$ must be conserved to maintain blood pH, distal tubule cells reduce the secretion of H$^+$, reduce NH$_4^+$ generation, reduce Na$^+$-H$^+$ exchange, and increase bicarbonate excretion. The net effect is a reduction in plasma bicarbonate and restoration of normal blood pH.

## Water Homeostasis

The production of glomerular filtrate normally amounts to about 180 L/day. The unique physiology of the kidney enables

.

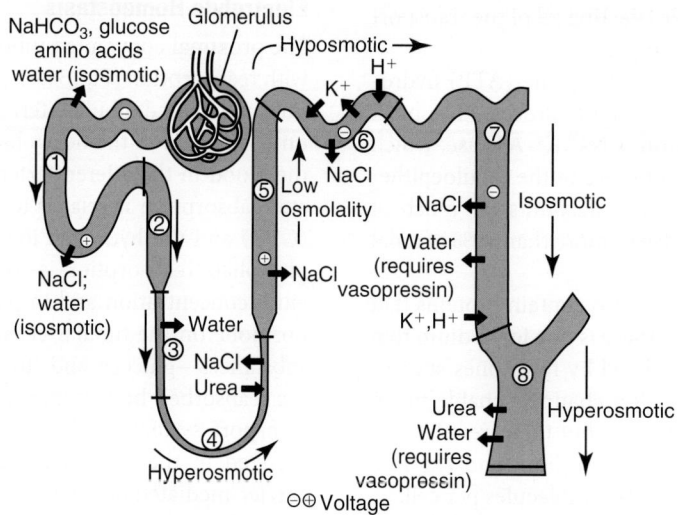

**Fig. 35.4** Countercurrent multiplication mechanism: schematic representation of the principal processes of transport in the nephron. In the convoluted portion of the proximal tubule *(1)*, salts and water are reabsorbed at high rates in isotonic proportions. Bulk reabsorption of most of the filtrate (65% to 70%) and virtually complete reabsorption of glucose, amino acids, and bicarbonate take place in this segment. In the pars recta *(2)*, organic acids are secreted, and continuous reabsorption of sodium chloride takes place. The loop of Henle comprises three segments: the thin descending *(3)* and ascending *(4)* limbs, and the thick ascending limb *(5)*. The fluid becomes hyperosmotic because of water abstraction as it flows toward the bend of the loop, and it becomes hypoosmotic because of sodium chloride reabsorption as it flows toward the distal convoluted tubule *(6)*. Active sodium reabsorption occurs in the distal convoluted tubule and in the cortical collecting tubule *(7)*. This latter segment is water impermeable in the absence of vasopressin (antidiuretic hormone, ADH), and the reabsorption of sodium in this segment is increased by aldosterone. The collecting duct *(8)* allows equilibration of water with the hyperosmotic interstitium when vasopressin is present. For additional details, see text. (From Burg MB. The nephron in transport of sodium, amino acids, and glucose. *Hosp Pract.* 1978;13:100. Modified from a drawing by A. Iselin.)

approximately 99% of this to be reabsorbed in the production of urine with variable osmolality: between 50 and 1400 mOsmol/kg $H_2O$ at extremes of water intake. Different segments of the nephron show differing permeability to water, enabling the body to both retain water and produce urine of variable concentration. Approximately 70% of the water content of the tubular fluid is reabsorbed in the proximal tubule, 5% in the loop of Henle, 10% in the distal tubule, and the remainder in the collecting ducts.

Water reabsorption occurs both isosmotically, in association with electrolyte reabsorption in the proximal tubule, and differentially, in the loop of Henle, distal tubule, and collecting duct in response to the action of the nonapeptide ADH. Absorption of water depends on the driving force for water reabsorption (predominantly active sodium transport) and the osmotic equilibration of water across the tubular epithelium. The generation of concentrated urine depends upon medullary hyperosmolality, which in turn requires low water permeability in some kidney segments (ascending limb of the loop of Henle), whereas in other kidney segments there is a requirement for high water permeability: differing permeability and the enaction of hormonal control are largely caused by the differential expression along the nephron of a family of proteins known as the aquaporins (AQP), which act as water channels.

Urinary concentration is predominantly achieved by countercurrent multiplication in the loop of Henle (see Fig. 35.4). Although the descending thin limb is very permeable

to water, the ascending limb and the collecting duct are not (the collecting ducts are also poorly permeable to urea). The fluid entering the loop of Henle is isotonic to plasma but is hypotonic on leaving it. The ascending limb has active sodium reabsorption driven by $Na^+$, $K^+$-ATPase with electroneutralizing transport of chloride, a combined process that can be inhibited by the so-called loop diuretics (e.g., furosemide). In this section of the nephron, sodium reabsorption is not accompanied by water, creating a hypertonic medullary interstitium and facilitating water reabsorption from the anatomically adjacent descending limb. The descending limb cells are permeable to sodium chloride, which is cycled from the descending limb back to the ascending limb. The continuous flow along the loop generates an osmotic gradient at the tip of the loop that can reach 1400 mOsmol/kg/$H_2O$. Approximately 5% of water is reabsorbed in the loop of Henle.

A further 10% of water reabsorption occurs in the distal tubule, with the remainder (>20 L/day) being reabsorbed in the collecting ducts. Entry of water into the collecting duct cells occurs via apical AQP2 channels under the influence of ADH. ADH also increases the permeability of collecting duct cells to urea, which is the major osmotically active component of the luminal fluid in the distal tubule. Fluid of high urea concentration therefore enters the deepest layers of the medullary interstitium, passing down its concentration gradient, contributing to medullary hyperosmolality. The regulation of ADH excretion is of vital importance to fluid homeostasis. The normal plasma osmolality is maintained very tightly between 280 and 290 mOsmol/kg $H_2O$ and is regulated by means of specific osmoreceptors found in the anterior hypothalamus. These receptors modulate the release of ADH and also affect thirst. ADH release may also be stimulated by hypotension, hypovolemia, and vomiting independently of osmoregulation. Increased free water excretion can be obtained therapeutically with highly specific inhibitors of ADH (vasopressin $V_2$ receptor antagonists).

## Endocrine Function

The *endocrine functions* of the kidneys may be regarded as (1) primary, because the kidneys are endocrine organs producing hormones, or (2) secondary, because the kidneys are a site of action for hormones produced or activated elsewhere. In addition, the kidneys are a site of degradation for hormones such as insulin and aldosterone. In their primary endocrine function, the kidneys produce (1) **erythropoietin** (EPO), (2) prostaglandins and thromboxanes, (3) renin, and (4) 1,25($OH_2$) vitamin D.

### Erythropoietin

EPO is a glycoprotein hormone secreted chiefly by the kidney in the adult and by the liver in the fetus that acts on the bone marrow cells to stimulate erythropoiesis. It is an $\alpha$-globulin having a molecular weight of 38 kDa. Physiologically the kidneys sense a reduction in $O_2$ delivery to tissue by blood and release EPO, thereby stimulating the bone marrow to make more red blood cells (RBCs). Conversely, with a surplus of $O_2$ in blood traversing the kidneys, as in some forms of polycythemia, the release of EPO into blood is diminished. The use of recombinant human EPO (rhEPO, epoetin) in the management of anemia of kidney disease is discussed below.

### Prostaglandins and Thromboxanes

Prostaglandins and thromboxanes are synthesized from arachidonic acid by the cyclooxygenase (COX) enzyme system. This system is present in many parts of the kidneys. The predominant metabolite of its vascular endothelial activity is prostacyclin ($PGI_2$). Prostaglandin $E_2$ ($PGE_2$) appears to be the major metabolite of mesangial and tubular cells. The production and activity of these biologically active compounds have an important role in regulating the physiological action of other hormones on renal vascular tone, mesangial contractility, and tubular processing of salt and water.

### Renin

Renin is produced within juxtaglomerular cells after processing and cleavage of prorenin, which is produced in the liver. Increased production of renin results in formation of AII in the lungs, which is a powerful intrarenal vasoconstrictor and also a key stimulus of aldosterone release from zona glomerulosa cells in the adrenal glands. The net effect is (1) systemic vasoconstriction, (2) intrarenal vasoconstriction, and (3) increased aldosterone release. Aldosterone controls salt and water balance in the kidney. Its effect is predominantly on the distal tubular network, affecting an increase in sodium reabsorption in exchange for potassium.

### 1,25($OH_2$) Vitamin D

The kidneys are primarily responsible for producing 1,25($OH_2$) vitamin D from 25-hydroxycholecalciferol as a result of the action of the enzyme 25-hydroxycholecalciferol 1$\alpha$-hydroxylase found in proximal tubular epithelial cells. The regulation of this system is discussed in Chapter 39.

## KIDNEY PHYSIOLOGY

The (1) GFR, (2) renal blood flow, and (3) glomerular permeability are important physiological components of renal function.

### Glomerular Filtration Rate

The GFR is considered to be the most reliable measure of the functional capacity of the kidneys and is often thought of as indicative of the number of functioning nephrons. As a physiologic measurement, it has proved to be a useful marker of changes in overall renal function.

The rate of formation of glomerular filtrate depends on the balance between hydrostatic and oncotic forces along the afferent arteriole and across the glomerular filter. The net pressure difference must be sufficient not only to drive filtration across the glomerular filtration barrier but also to drive the ultrafiltrate along the tubules against their inherent resistance to flow. In the absence of sufficient pressure, the lumina of the tubules will collapse.

A decrease in GFR precedes **kidney failure** in all forms of progressive disease. Different pathological kidney conditions have been known to progress to end-stage renal disease (ESRD) and **dialysis** dependency at rates varying from weeks to several decades. The symptoms accompanying progressive kidney disease and their correlation with falling GFR will be influenced by this rate of progression. Measuring GFR in established disease is useful in (1) targeting treatment, (2) monitoring progression, and (3) predicting when **kidney replacement therapy (KRT)** will be required. It is also used as a guide to dosage of drugs excreted by the kidneys to prevent potential drug toxicity (see Chapter 30). Measurement of GFR is discussed in Chapter 21.

### Glomerular Filtration Rate and Age

Kidney function is not constant throughout life. In utero, urine is produced by the developing fetus from about the ninth week of gestation. The GFR at birth is approximately 30 mL/min/1.73 m². It increases rapidly during the first weeks of life to reach approximately 70 mL/min/1.73 m² by age 16 days, with adult values of body surface area (BSA)-corrected GFR being achieved by 2 years of age. On average, GFR declines with age by approximately 1 mL/min/1.73 m²/year over the age of 40, and the rate of decline in GFR accelerates after age 65 years.

### Glomerular Permeability, Filtration, and Protein Loss

The glomerular permeability and filtration capabilities of the kidney control the amount of protein lost in the urine.

## Glomerular Permeability and Filtration

The glomerulus acts as a selective filter of the blood passing through its capillaries. The combination of (1) the fenestrated endothelial layer, (2) a basement membrane rich in negatively charged proteoglycans, and (3) a highly specialized terminally differentiated epithelial cell barrier produces a filter that restricts the passage of macromolecules in a (1) size-, (2) charge-, and (3) shape-dependent manner. The epithelial cells (podocytes) have foot processes that are connected to the GBM and form the final barrier to filtration via interdigitating cell foot processes connected by a slit diaphragm. Examples of the relationships between size, charge, and mass of the major urinary proteins and their glomerular handling are listed in Table 21.1. In general, proteins of molecular weights greater than albumin (66 kDa, diameter 3.5 nm) are retained by the healthy glomerulus and are termed high molecular weight proteins. However, lower molecular weight proteins are also retained to a significant extent.

## Urinary Protein Loss

Increased urinary protein loss (proteinuria) results from (1) any increase in the filtered load, (2) increased circulating concentration of low-molecular-weight proteins, or (3) decrease in reabsorptive capacity. Historically, the pattern of urinary protein loss has been used to identify the cause and to classify the proteinuria, of which there are three main types: (1) glomerular, (2) overflow, and (3) tubular proteinuria.

The normal urinary total protein loss is less than 150 mg/day. The proteins lost are made up of mostly albumin (50% to 60%) and some smaller proteins, together with proteins secreted by the tubules, of which Tamm-Horsfall glycoprotein (THG, uromodulin) is one. The normal concentrations of proteins found in urine are listed in Table 21.1. Investigation for increased urinary protein loss is mandatory in any patient with suspected kidney disease and is considered in Chapter 21.

## Consequences of Proteinuria

Many physicians believe that proteinuria is not just a consequence of, but contributes directly to, progression of kidney disease. The accumulation of proteins in abnormal amounts in the tubular lumen may trigger an inflammatory reaction, which in turn may contribute to interstitial structural damage and expansion, and progression of kidney disease. Evidence gathered from in vitro studies suggests that glomerular filtration of an abnormal amount or types of protein induces mesangial cell injury, leading to glomerulosclerosis, and that these same proteins also have adverse effects on proximal tubular cell function. Numerous studies have demonstrated that proteinuria is a potent risk marker for progression of renal disease in both nondiabetic and diabetic kidney disease. Furthermore, reducing protein excretion slows the rate of progression of proteinuric kidney disease. This has been observed in clinical trials in patients treated with ACE inhibitors and angiotensin II receptor blockers (ARBs), either alone or in combination. These drugs reduce protein loss by reducing intraglomerular filtration pressure

and possibly by stabilizing the glomerular epithelial cell slit diaphragm proteins. Similar downstream effects occur following inhibition of SGLT2. Novel medications, the SGLT2 inhibitors, are recommended in addition to ACE inhibitors and ARBs to reduce proteinuria and preserve kidney function.

## PATHOPHYSIOLOGY OF KIDNEY DISEASE

Despite the diverse initial causes of injury to the kidney, progression of kidney disease leading to loss of function and ultimately to kidney failure is a remarkably monotonous process characterized by (1) early inflammation, (2) accumulation and deposition of extracellular matrix, (3) tubulointerstitial fibrosis, (4) tubular atrophy, and (5) glomerulosclerosis (scarring). Proteinuria is thought to be one of the most important risk factors for progression of kidney diseases. The renin-angiotensin-aldosterone system (RAAS) plays a pivotal role in many of the pathophysiologic changes that cause kidney injury and is an important therapeutic target.

The kidneys have considerable ability to increase their functional capacity in response to injury. Thus a significant reduction in functioning kidney mass (50% to 60%) may occur before any major biochemical alterations appear. An increase in workload per nephron is thought to be an important cause of progressive kidney injury.

### Overview of Kidney Disease and Its Clinical Manifestations

Chronic kidney disease (CKD) is often an indolent condition with few symptoms. Most often kidney disease is detected opportunistically by measurement of blood pressure and urine and blood testing in nonsymptomatic individuals. Such testing can occur in the primary care setting or for health clearance purposes for insurance. Testing for kidney disease is recommended in those individuals considered high risk. Typical findings include isolated, invisible hematuria and isolated proteinuria. Kidney disease may also present with visible hematuria, swollen ankles, headaches, and visual disturbances due to severe hypertension, or as a manifestation of systemic disease. Symptoms suggestive of advanced kidney disease include fatigue, nausea, vomiting, poor appetite, shortness of breath, fluid retention, poor memory, loss of libido, and itching. Unfortunately, many individuals present very late in their disease and may require urgent dialysis with no previous experience with the specialist nephrology service. These patients, so-called "crash landers," have a poor prognosis compared with patients who have been cared for in a multidisciplinary specialist environment for at least 1 year. Therefore, early recognition of kidney disease is of paramount importance to outcome.

Effective management of the patient with kidney disease is dependent upon establishing a definitive diagnosis. Initial management includes a (1) detailed clinical history, (2) clinical examination, and (3) urinalysis and assessment of the urinary sediment.

**Who Should Be Tested for Chronic Kidney Disease (CKD)?[a]**

Offer testing for CKD using estimated GFR and urinary albumin to creatinine ratio (ACR) to people with any of the following risk factors:

- Diabetes mellitus
- Hypertension
- Acute kidney injury
- Cardiovascular disease (ischemic heart disease, chronic heart failure, peripheral vascular disease, or cerebral vascular disease)
- Structural renal tract disease, recurrent renal calculi, or prostatic hypertrophy
- Multisystem diseases with potential kidney involvement— for example, systemic lupus erythematosus
- Family history of kidney failure (GFR category G5) or hereditary kidney disease
- Opportunistic detection of hematuria

Do not use age, gender, or ethnicity as risk markers to test people for CKD. In the absence of metabolic syndrome, diabetes mellitus, or hypertension, do not use obesity alone as a risk marker to test people for CKD.

Monitor GFR at least annually in people prescribed drugs known to be nephrotoxic, such as calcineurin inhibitors (CNIs) (e.g., cyclosporine or tacrolimus), lithium, and nonsteroidal antiinflammatory drugs (NSAIDs).

[a] Modified from National Institute for Health and Care Excellence. Chronic Kidney Disease. Early identification and management of chronic kidney disease in adults in primary and secondary care; 2014. http://www.nice.org.uk/nicemedia/live/13712/66658/.pdf.

## Terminology of Kidney Disease

The commonly used term *acute renal failure* (ARF) has been replaced by acute kidney injury (AKI). Kidney *failure* is defined as a GFR of less than 15 mL/min/1.73 m$^2$. Not all patients with kidney failure require KRT (dialysis, or transplantation) to sustain life.

(*End-stage renal disease* [ESRD] is a US government–defined term that indicates the need for long-term chronic "renal replacement therapy" [RRT]. Each patient with ESRD is registered through the Medical Evidence form [2728] that all dialysis and transplant providers must submit. The term now includes both Medicare and non-Medicare populations. The nomenclature around "ESRD" is changing to be more relevant to patients and their caregivers. Therefore, "kidney" replaces "renal" [or nephro-])

## Classification of Chronic Kidney Disease

CKD is an important public health problem emphasizing the need for earlier identification and treatment. Historically, data obtained from epidemiologic surveys were compromised by lack of consistent surrogate markers of kidney function to identify established disease. For example, serum creatinine, calculated creatinine clearance, and measured creatinine clearance were variously used. Landmark guidelines developed by the National Kidney Foundation—Kidney Disease Outcomes Quality Initiative (NKF-K/DOQI) were

published in 2002 and were based upon categories of GFR. They have subsequently been revised and updated by Kidney Disease: Improving Global Outcomes (KDIGO) and broadly adopted by other national organizations (Table 35.1). The KDIGO 2012 guideline added a second dimension to the classification system with three identified levels of albuminuria, acknowledging the powerful additional prognostic information imparted by the presence of proteinuria (see Table 35.1).

There is a high prevalence of CKD identified with the classification system, with an estimated one in seven adults affected within the United States (United States Renal Data System Annual Data Report 2021). Most individuals with CKD do not progress to kidney failure, with prevalence rates of patients in GFR category G3 being 10 to 20 times higher than the prevalence rates of GFR categories G4 and G5. There is some concern that many individuals being identified with G3 CKD are not at increased risk; use of cystatin C to delineate risk in this population is being evaluated (for detailed description of cystatin C please refer to Chapter 21).

The major associated conditions in those patients receiving KRT are diabetes, hypertension, and cardiovascular disease. Diabetes mellitus is the largest single cause of advanced CKD and accounts for almost 50% of new dialysis patients in the United States. Hypertension is the underlying diagnosis in around 28% of new dialysis patients and is particularly prevalent among African Americans. In addition, the rate of new kidney failure in African Americans is 3.5 times higher than Whites. The myriad of kidney diseases, including (1) glomerulonephritis, (2) infection, (3) hereditary conditions, (4) systemic conditions, (5) interstitial conditions, (6) obstructive conditions, and (7) those of unknown origin account for the remainder of cases.

**Defining Chronic Kidney Disease (CKD)[a]**

CKD is defined as abnormalities of kidney structure or function, present for at least 3 months, with implications for health.

Markers of reduced kidney function or damage include:
- Reduced glomerular filtration rate (GFR <60 mL/min/1.73 m$^2$)
- Albuminuria (≥30 mg/24 h; ACR ≥30 mg/g [≥3 mg/mmol])
- Urine sediment abnormalities
- Electrolyte and other abnormalities due to tubular disorders
- Abnormalities detected by histology
- Structural abnormalities detected by imaging
- History of kidney transplantation

[a] Modified from Kidney Disease Improving Global Outcomes. Clinical practice guideline for the evaluation and management of chronic kidney disease. *Kidney Int.* 2013;3:1–150.

## Management of Chronic Kidney Disease

Irrespective of underlying cause, the rate of progression of CKD (i.e., the rate at which a patient approaches kidney failure) is dependent on both nonmodifiable factors, such as age, gender, race, and level of kidney function at diagnosis, and

**TABLE 35.1    Classification of Chronic Kidney Disease Indicating Prognosis and Secondary/Tertiary Care Referral Decision-Making by Glomerular Filtration Rate and Albuminuria Categories**

| | | | | PERSISTENT ALBUMINURIA CATEGORIES: DESCRIPTION AND RANGE | | |
| --- | --- | --- | --- | --- | --- | --- |
| | | | | A1 | A2 | A3 |
| | | | | Normal to mildly increased | Moderately increased | Severely increased |
| | | | | <30 mg/g (<3 mg/mmol) | 30–300 mg/g (3–30 mg/mmol) | >300 mg/g (>30 mg/mmol) |
| Glomerular filtration rate categories (mL/min/1.73 m$^2$): description and range | G1 | Normal or high | >90 | 55.6 | 1.9 Monitor | 0.4 Refer[a] |
| | G2 | Mildly decreased | 60–89 | 32.9 | 2.2 Monitor | 0.3 Refer[a] |
| | G3a | Mildly to moderately decreased | 45–59 | 3.6 Monitor | 0.8 Monitor | 0.2 Refer |
| | G3b | Moderately to severely decreased | 30–44 | 1.0 Monitor | 0.4 Monitor | 0.2 Refer |
| | G4 | Severely decreased | 15–29 | 0.2 Refer[a] | 0.1 Refer[a] | 0.1 Refer |
| | G5 | Kidney failure | <15 | <0.1 Refer | <0.1 Refer | 0.1 Refer |

DARK BLUE: very high risk; MIDDLE BLUE: high risk; BLUE: moderately increased risk; LIGHT BLUE: low risk (if no other markers of kidney disease, no CKD).
NOTE: Numbers in the cells show the proportion (in %) of the adult population in the United States.
[a]Referring clinicians may wish to discuss with their local nephrology service, depending on local arrangements regarding referral and monitoring.
Modified from Kidney Disease Improving Global Outcomes. Clinical practice guideline for the evaluation and management of chronic kidney disease. *Kidney Int.* 2013;3:1–150.

modifiable characteristics, including proteinuria, blood pressure control, and smoking.

Lowering blood pressure and reduction of proteinuria have been shown to decrease the progression of CKD. The Modification of Diet in Renal Disease (MDRD) Study compared the rates of decline in GFR in patients with various causes of CKD assigned to either a "usual" or "low" blood pressure goal. Outcome data suggest that the low blood pressure goal had some beneficial effect in those patients with higher concentrations of proteins in their urine. In practice, medications that inhibit parts of the RAAS are typically preferred, because these drugs have been demonstrated to reduce proteinuria and rate of progression of CKD. Major studies of SGLT2 inhibitors in patients with diabetes-related and nondiabetic albuminuric kidney disease have indicated an additional benefit of treatment in terms of preserving kidney function and reducing hard cardiovascular end points and their use, in conjunction with RAAS inhibitors, is recommended.

Protein intake is restricted spontaneously to approximately 0.6 to 0.8 g/kg/day in uremic patients not receiving dietary advice. To prevent malnutrition, patients receive professional dietary advice with diets containing an increased proportion of first-class protein and increased calorie content of up to 35 kcal/kg/day. General health measures, including cessation of cigarette smoking, are encouraged. Complications of CKD that develop before the need for KRT are numerous and include (1) cardiovascular disease, (2) bone disease, and (3) anemia. Albuminuria and proteinuria have been shown to be associated with increased risk of cardiovascular disease, cardiovascular mortality, and all-cause mortality.

## Cardiovascular Complications of Chronic Kidney Disease

The incidence of cardiovascular disease is 7- to 10-fold greater in patients with CKD than in non-CKD age- and sex-matched controls, and by the time patients develop the need for KRT, the risk increases to approximately 17 times greater.

The spectrum of cardiovascular disease in CKD includes (1) angina, (2) congestive heart failure, (3) myocardial infarction, (4) peripheral vascular disease, (5) stroke, (6) sudden cardiac death, and (7) transient ischemic attack. Structural heart diseases, such as left ventricular hypertrophy (LVH) and valvular heart disease, are very common. Up to 75% of patients commencing dialysis have echocardiographic evidence of LVH. Vascular calcification is highly prevalent in dialysis patients and is associated with reduced survival.

## Dyslipidemia in Chronic Kidney Disease

The pattern of dyslipidemia (abnormal concentration of lipids in the blood) in CKD differs from that seen in non-CKD. Although total cholesterol concentration may be normal, there is often a highly abnormal lipid subfraction profile with a predominance of atherogenic small, dense low-density lipoprotein (LDL) particles. In addition, triglyceride concentrations are high. Low cholesterol is associated with increased mortality in dialysis patients, likely reflecting coincident inflammation and malnutrition ("reverse causality"). Although there are no data to suggest that statins are of benefit in patients receiving dialysis, the Study of Heart and Renal Protection (SHARP) evaluated the use of cholesterol lowering with simvastatin and ezetimibe in 9000 patients (including 3000 dialysis patients) and demonstrated significant reductions in stroke and arterial revascularization in the treated patients followed for a median of 4.9 years.

*Disturbances in calcium and phosphorus metabolism and bone disease in chronic kidney disease.* Bone disease as a consequence of CKD has long been recognized. As GFR declines, renal activation of vitamin D decreases and plasma phosphate concentration rises, resulting in reduced ionized calcium. Consequently, the parathyroid glands increase the production of parathyroid hormone (PTH). This increased secretion of PTH stimulates resorption of calcium and phosphate from the bone, the body's major calcium reservoir. Problems develop early, typically once GFR has fallen to approximately 45 mL/min/1.73 m². Secondary hyperparathyroidism classically causes (1) bone changes, (2) so-called high turnover bone disease, and (3) increased risk of fracture.

"Adynamic," low-turnover bone disease is also highly prevalent in patients with CKD and is characterized by poor bone formation. It is more common in the elderly and those with diabetes mellitus and malnutrition. Adynamic bone is associated with (1) a low PTH concentration, (2) abnormal calcium balance, (3) hyperphosphatemia, (4) acidosis, and (5) the use of high doses of vitamin D analogues (e.g., alfacalcidol [1α-hydroxyvitamin D₃]). Vascular calcification is commonly associated with adynamic bone disease. The diagnosis of adynamic bone is ultimately made on the basis of a bone biopsy, but patients are reluctant to undergo this procedure. Unfortunately, PTH alone does not correlate with bone biopsy findings. Serum bone-specific alkaline phosphatase (ALP) measured using an immunoassay technique has good predictive value in separating high from low bone turnover, particularly in combination with PTH measurements. For example, low bone formation has been associated with bone-specific ALP concentrations less than 20 μg/L and PTH less than 200 ng/L.

High concentrations of plasma phosphate are associated with increased mortality in hemodialysis (HD) patients. Strategies to reduce phosphate concentrations are employed routinely in the treatment of patients on dialysis. Phosphate is present in many foods and is linearly associated with protein ingestion. The recommended allowance of phosphate is reduced for patients on dialysis to around 800 mg/day. Treatment with vitamin D analogs increases gut absorption of phosphate from approximately 65% to almost 85%. The use of phosphate binders, taken with meals, is almost universal in dialysis patients reducing phosphate absorption to 30% to 40%. It has been possible to normalize phosphate balance in patients treated by daily HD.

## Anemia

The World Health Organization (WHO) defines anemia as a hemoglobin concentration of less than 13 g/dL in men and less than 12 g/dL in women. In the absence of treatment, anemia is inevitable as CKD progresses. Therapies are available to correct anemia, and therefore it is mandatory to assess a patient with CKD for anemia. The National Kidney Foundation KDOQI guideline recommends that an estimated GFR of less than 60 mL/min/1.73 m² should be the cutoff value for determining the presence or absence of anemia. Detection is important since treatment may alleviate many of the symptoms of CKD and hopefully reduce risk of LVH. The pathology of anemia in CKD is multifactorial, but the predominant cause is loss of peritubular fibroblasts (specialized cells that produce collagen and other materials) within the renal cortex that synthesize EPO. Failure to produce EPO leads to decreased numbers of RBCs and concomitant decreased concentrations of hemoglobin. Other causes of anemia include (1) absolute or functional iron deficiency, (2) folic acid and vitamin B₁₂ deficiencies, and (3) chronic inflammation. RBC survival may also be reduced. Treatment with recombinant erythropoiesis-stimulating agents is recommended to correct anemia. The gene for human EPO was cloned in 1985, and rhEPO, epoetin, or erythropoietin-stimulating agents (ESAs) were introduced into clinical practice shortly afterwards. The most common side effect is hypertension, and therefore blood pressure should be well controlled before the introduction of treatment. The majority of patients respond to treatment. However, failure to respond requires thorough investigation for many potential causes, such as (1) occult blood loss, (2) hyperparathyroidism, (3) iron deficiency, (4) vitamin B₁₂ deficiency, (5) folate deficiency, and (6) inadequate dialysis. Many clinical benefits are derived from correcting anemia with ESAs, including (1) improved exercise capacity, (2) improved cognitive function, (3) better quality of life, and (4) increased libido. Later studies have, however, highlighted risks of high doses of ESA in nondialysis CKD patients with associated increase in mortality and cardiovascular morbidity. These studies have been instructive in setting the current hemoglobin target of 10.0 to 12.0 g/dL and in recommending ESA dose adjustments when hemoglobin is less than 10.5 or greater than 11.5 g/dL, to balance benefit versus safety to patients.

Treatment of anemia in CKD requires adequate iron stores. For example, in patients with CKD, a plasma ferritin less than 100 μg/L is considered to suggest iron deficiency, and a plasma ferritin of 100 to 200 μg/L in association with a transferrin saturation (TSAT) of less than 20% represents "functional" iron deficiency. Parenteral iron is the treatment of choice for absolute and functional iron deficiency since oral iron has low efficacy in CKD. Therapeutic advances in CKD-related anemia care have been developed and marketed for use. Inhibition of enzymes (prolyl-4-hydroxylase [PH] domain enzymes) that degrade hypoxia inducible factors (HIFs), a family of oxygen-sensitive proteins that regulate the cellular response to hypoxia, has been central to this paradigm shift. These orally active small molecules stimulate the body's response to hypoxia without any change to the partial pressure of oxygen in the blood or tissues. HIF-PH inhibitors can be considered as "hypoxia mimetic agents" and lead to increases in hemoglobin and enhanced utilization of iron. Several of these have been evaluated in phase III clinical trials. Roxadustat, a HIF-PH inhibitor, is being introduced into clinical practice with Marketing Authorization in the European

Union and United Kingdom for treatment of adult patients with symptomatic anemia associated with CKD.

## The Uremic Syndrome

The uremic syndrome is the group of (1) symptoms, (2) physical signs, and (3) abnormal findings on diagnostic studies that result from the failure of the kidneys to maintain adequate (1) excretory, (2) regulatory, and (3) endocrine function. It is considered the terminal clinical manifestation of kidney failure. At least 90 organic compounds have been shown to be retained in uremia.

The classic signs of uremia (azotemia) include (1) progressive weakness and easy fatigue, (2) loss of appetite followed by (3) nausea and vomiting, (4) muscle wasting, (5) tremors, (6) abnormal mental function, (7) frequent but shallow respirations, and (8) metabolic acidosis. The syndrome evolves to produce (1) stupor, (2) coma, and (3) ultimately death unless support is provided by dialysis or successful kidney transplantation. The composition of plasma is abnormally labile in response to such factors as (1) diet, (2) state of hydration, (3) gastrointestinal bleeding, (4) vomiting, (5) diarrhea, and (6) intake of therapeutic drugs. Patients with kidney failure (GFR of less than or equal to 15 mL/min/m²) will generally exhibit signs and symptoms of uremia, or a need for KRT.

The most characteristic laboratory findings are increased concentrations of nitrogenous compounds in plasma, such as urea and creatinine, as a result of reduced GFR and decreased tubular function. Retention of these compounds and of metabolic acids is followed by progressive (1) hyperphosphatemia, (2) hypocalcemia, and (3) potentially dangerous hyperkalemia. Although most patients eventually exhibit acidemia, respiratory compensation by elimination of carbon dioxide is extremely important. In addition, reduced endocrine function is manifested by inadequate synthesis of EPO and calcitriol with resulting anemia and osteomalacia. Disordered regulation of blood pressure generally leads to hypertension. Biochemical characteristics of the uremic syndrome are summarized in the Points to Remember Box.

In addition to the consequences of reduced (1) excretory, (2) regulatory, and (3) endocrine function of the kidneys, the uremic syndrome has several systemic manifestations—among them (1) pericarditis, (2) pleuritis, (3) disordered platelet and granulocyte function, and (4) encephalopathy.

Many retained metabolites have been implicated in the systemic toxicity of the uremic syndrome. Although urea was the first of these metabolites to be identified as being increased in uremia, it does not appear to be responsible for the systemic manifestations of uremia. Urea is a 60-Da water-soluble compound (see Chapter 21) that has the highest concentration of presently known uremic retention solutes in uremic plasma. Although its removal by dialysis is directly related to patient survival, the effects of urea on biological systems are not clear. Urea removal by dialysis is not necessarily representative of other molecules retained in the uremic syndrome, particularly protein-bound solutes or lower molecular weight proteins, such as PTH and cystatin C.

## POINTS TO REMEMBER

**Biochemical Characteristics of the Uremic Syndrome**
*Retained Nitrogenous Metabolites*
Urea
Cyanate
Creatinine
Guanidine compounds
Uric acid

*Fluid, Acid-Base, and Electrolyte Disturbances*
Fixed urine osmolality
Metabolic acidosis (decreased blood pH, bicarbonate)
Hyponatremia or hypernatremia
Hypokalemia or hyperkalemia
Hyperchloremia
Hypocalcemia
Hyperphosphatemia
Hypermagnesemia

*Carbohydrate Intolerance*
Insulin resistance (hypoglycemia may also occur)
Plasma insulin: normal or increased
Delayed response to carbohydrate loading
Hyperglucagonemia

*Abnormal Lipid Metabolism*
Hypertriglyceridemia
Decreased high-density lipoprotein cholesterol
Hyperlipoproteinemia

*Altered Endocrine Function*
Secondary hyperparathyroidism
Osteomalacia (secondary to abnormal vitamin D metabolism)
Hyperreninemia and hyperaldosteronism
Hyporeninemia
Hypoaldosteronism
Decreased erythropoietin production
Altered thyroxine metabolism
Gonadal dysfunction (increased prolactin and luteinizing hormone, decreased testosterone)

## Acute Kidney Injury

The definition of AKI, endorsed by KDIGO during 2012, is the occurrence of any one of the following:

1. Increase of plasma creatinine by ≥0.3 mg/dL (≥26 μmol/L) within 48 hours
2. Increase in plasma creatinine to ≥ 1.5 times baseline, which is known or presumed to have occurred within the prior 7 days
3. Reduction in urine output (documented oliguria <0.5 mL/kg/h for >6 hours)

In addition, AKI is staged 1 to 3, depending on severity. In the UK, the National Confidential Enquiry into Patient Outcome and Death: Adding Insult to Injury (http://www.ncepod.org.uk/2009report1/Downloads/AKI_summary.pdf/ accessed June 06, 2022) reported that failure (1) to identify intravascular volume depletion, (2) to withhold nephrotoxic drugs, and (3) of early diagnosis of causative conditions (such as sepsis) directly contributed to in-hospital mortality associated with AKI. Approximately 20% of postadmission AKI episodes are predictable and avoidable. Therefore, prompt administration of intravenous crystalloid solutions (such as 0.9% sodium chloride) may prevent further deterioration of AKI in many cases. Patients at risk for AKI include (1) older persons; those with (2) preexisting CKD, (3) sepsis, (4) diabetes mellitus, and (5) heart disease; and (6) patients receiving nephrotoxic drugs, particularly in the setting of hypovolemia. Clinical assessment of AKI should consider whether the precipitant is (1) prerenal, (2) intrarenal (intrinsic), or (3) postrenal. As intrinsic AKI is caused by primary vascular, glomerular, or interstitial disorders, it is important that all patients presenting with AKI undergo urinalysis to test for (1) infection, (2) hematuria, and (3) proteinuria. In most cases, the kidney lesion seen on histology is referred to as acute tubular necrosis (ATN). ATN is caused by ischemic or nephrotoxic injury to the kidney. In 50% of cases of hospital-acquired AKI, the cause is multifactorial. Urinary electrolyte measurements are seldom required or useful in the investigation of AKI. Laboratory testing of blood is crucial in the management of AKI. Blood tests also assist in establishing the underlying diagnosis, and specific investigations are requested if kidney function has not improved following volume correction. An "acute renal screen" should clearly focus on most likely diagnoses and include the tests shown in Table 35.2.

In addition to biochemical testing, there is a role for ultrasound and radiological imaging in kidney disease, and in particular, exclusion of obstruction is important. Kidney biopsy is generally reserved for cases of AKI wherein an ultrasound scan has excluded obstructed kidneys, kidney sizes are maintained, and the cause of AKI is otherwise unexplained, and an intrinsic pathology is suspected.

Metabolic acidosis is the most common acid-base disorder in patients with AKI. Reduced renal excretion of potassium and the effects of acidosis on the generation of extracellular potassium may lead to a very high concentration of potassium in the plasma. Severe hyperkalemia (plasma potassium concentration >6.5 mmol/L) is associated with life-threatening cardiac arrhythmias. Emergency treatment of hyperkalemia should be instituted as necessary. Infusion of high concentrations of glucose stimulates insulin secretion from the pancreas and uptake of potassium into the intracellular space. A fall in potassium concentration should be expected within 60 minutes. In addition, low-dose, rapid-acting insulin is sometimes administered with the glucose bolus. Additional treatment can include the use of oral, nonabsorbable potassium binders and ion exchangers that utilize the gut to increase fecal potassium losses and lower serum potassium concentration. Serum potassium concentration should be monitored hourly until risk of a life-threatening cardiac event has passed and no evidence of potassium rebound is found. Blood glucose concentration should be monitored because hypoglycemia may occur following exogenous insulin. When hyperkalemia persists despite appropriate medical measures, then dialysis should be considered. Recovery from AKI usually occurs within days or weeks following removal of the initiating

event. However, uncomplicated AKI has a mortality rate of 5% to 10%, although AKI complicating nonrenal organ system failure in the intensive care unit setting is associated with mortality rates approaching 50% to 70%.

---

### POINTS TO REMEMBER

**Causes of Acute Kidney Injury (AKI)**

Prerenal AKI:
  Hemorrhage
  Diarrhea
  Postoperative fluid and blood losses
  Sepsis
  Acute cardiac failure
Renal (intrinsic renal disease) AKI:
  Tubular
    Any of the "prerenal" causes that are severe or that are not corrected promptly leading to ATN. Other causes of ATN
    Drug nephrotoxicity
      NSAIDs, ACE inhibitors
      Aminoglycoside antibiotics
      Amphotericin
    Contrast nephropathy
    Poisoning
    TIN
      Allergic TIN associated with antibiotics and NSAIDs
      Sarcoidosis
      Pyelonephritis
  Glomerular
    ANCA-associated vasculitides, Goodpasture disease, SLE, other crescentic glomerulonephritides
    Thrombotic microangiopathies
    Cryoglobulinemia
    Atheroembolism
  Vascular
    Aortic dissection
    Renal vein thrombosis
  Miscellaneous
    Rhabdomyolysis
    Urate nephropathy
    Hepatorenal syndrome
Postrenal AKI:
  Bladder outflow obstruction
  Benign and malignant prostate disease
  Invasive bladder carcinoma
  Bilateral kidney stones or stones within a single kidney
  Retroperitoneal fibrosis

*ACE*, Angiotensin converting enzyme; *AKI*, acute kidney injury; *ANCA*, antineutrophil cytoplasmic antibody; *ATN*, acute tubular necrosis; *NSAIDs*, nonsteroidal antiinflammatory drugs; *SLE*, systemic lupus erythematosus; *TIN*, tubulointerstitial nephritis.

---

## DISEASES OF THE KIDNEY

### Diabetic Nephropathy

Diabetic nephropathy is a clinical diagnosis based on the finding of proteinuria in a patient with diabetes mellitus. Overt nephropathy is characterized by protein loss greater than 0.5 g/day, approximately equivalent to albumin loss of

## TABLE 35.2  Investigation of Acute Kidney Injury

| Test | Indication/Comments |
|---|---|
| **Urine Testing** | |
| Urine reagent strip ("dipstick") | Hematuria and proteinuria may indicate glomerular origin |
| Red cell casts on microscopy | (Not available universally; may need bedside microscope) |
| Urine microscopy and culture | Identify urinary tract infection |
| Urine protein electrophoresis and immunofixation | |
| **Blood Tests** | |
| *Baseline Studies* | |
| Urea, electrolytes, and creatinine | Check previous laboratory reports: AKI or AKI with preexisting CKD |
| Calcium, phosphate, albumin | |
| Liver function tests | Suspected multiorgan involvement or abnormal coagulation |
| Acid-base studies | Arterial blood gas or venous plasma bicarbonate concentration |
| Full blood count | Anemia, hemolysis, thrombocytopenia |
| Coagulation studies | Evidence of intravascular coagulation; need to normalize if considering kidney biopsy and central line insertion |
| *Selected Additional Investigations* | |
| Blood culture | Any infection, but especially endocarditis, severe pneumonia, or urinary tract sepsis |
| Creatine kinase | Very high in cases of muscle inflammation and necrosis (rhabdomyolysis) |
| Lactate dehydrogenase | If high, suspect renal infarction and consider hemolysis |
| Antineutrophil cytoplasmic antibodies | Vasculitides |
| Antiglomerular basement membrane antibody | Antiglomerular basement membrane disease |
| Antinuclear antibodies | SLE |
| Anti-dsDNA antibodies, extractable nuclear antigens | SLE |
| Low C3 complement | SLE, MPGN, C3 glomerulopathies |
| Low C4 complement | Systemic lupus erythematosus, atheroembolism, cryoglobulinemia, MPGN (immune complex positive) |
| Cryoglobulin | Cryoglobulinemia |
| Urate | Urate nephropathy |
| Serum protein electrophoresis | Myeloma |
| Virology studies | Hepatitis serology, human immunodeficiency virus |
| Other serology | Antistreptolysin O titer |
| **Imaging** | |
| Chest x-ray | Pulmonary edema, pneumonia, effusions, malignancy, and granulomas |
| Abdominal x-ray (kidney, ureter, and bladder) | Renal stones |
| Renal tract ultrasound scan | Identify size and symmetry of kidneys |
| | Evidence of an obstructed system |
| | Small, shrunken kidneys in advanced CKD |
| Computed tomography scan | Anatomy and perfusion |
| Magnetic resonance imaging | Angiography to identify renovascular lesions |
| Formal angiography | Critical renal artery stenosis |
| **Kidney Biopsy** | |
| | Reserved for patients with unexplained AKI in whom acute tubular necrosis is not suspected. It is anticipated that additional therapy such as steroids, cytotoxic drugs, and plasma exchange may be required |

*CKD,* Chronic kidney disease; *dsDNA,* double-stranded DNA; *MPGN,* membranoproliferative glomerulonephritis; *SLE,* systemic lupus erythematosus.

greater than 300 mg/day or category A3 albuminuria. For a variety of reasons, it is preferable to assess proteinuria as albuminuria (see Chapter 21), and albumin has long been uniformly adopted as the "criterion standard" in evaluating diabetes-related kidney damage. Patients with albuminuria exceeding 30 mg/day have pathologically increased albuminuria. Diabetic nephropathy is the most common cause of kidney failure in the United States, accounting for approximately 40% of incident patients in KRT programs. Among patients who require dialysis, those with diabetes mellitus have a 22% higher mortality at 1 year and a 15% higher mortality at 5 years than patients without diabetes. The cornerstones of treatment for diabetic nephropathy consist of (1) glycemic control; (2) blood pressure control, particularly with drugs that block the RAAS; and (3) management of cardiovascular risk. In addition, SGLT2 inhibitors are increasingly recommended for treatment to reduce cardiovascular and kidney endpoints.

## Hypertension

Hypertension is second only to diabetes mellitus as a primary diagnosis of kidney failure requiring KRT for incident patients commencing dialysis in the United States. The incidence is higher in older people and especially among the Black population in the United States. Hypertension often develops as a consequence of CKD because of alterations in salt and water metabolism and activation of the sympathetic nervous and renin-angiotensin systems. Hypertension can act as an accelerating force in the development of worsening CKD. Treatment of hypertension to predefined target blood pressure values is critical in preventing progression to kidney failure.

## Glomerular Diseases

Glomerular disease is suggested clinically by the finding of blood and protein in the urine on urine reagent strip testing. Proteinuria of greater than 1 g/day (0.88 g/g creatinine; 100 mg/mmol creatinine) in the absence of an overflow-type proteinuria, such as myoglobinuria or light chain–related disease, is invariably glomerular in origin. Although a detailed discussion of each glomerular disease is beyond the scope of this book, the most important diseases are discussed to illustrate the spectrum of disease. For further information regarding clinical guidelines, the reader is directed to the KDIGO 2021 Clinical Practice Guideline for the Management of Glomerular Diseases.

### Primary Glomerular Disease

Glomerulonephritis can be primary (affecting only the kidneys) or secondary (in which the kidneys are involved as part of a systemic process). Histopathologic classification of glomerulonephritis may appear slightly cumbersome, but it is readily simplified by consideration of the glomerular structures and cells that may be involved and the presence or absence of immune complexes. In essence, only three cell types are involved—endothelial, epithelial, and mesangial— plus the acellular GBM. The glomerular cells and the GBM have a limited range of response to injury—namely, proliferation, scarring (sclerosis), and GBM thickening. The term *focal* is used if fewer than half of the glomeruli are involved

in the disease process as seen on light microscopy, whereas *diffuse glomerulonephritis* refers to cases in which all glomeruli are involved. Immune deposits identified following immunofluorescence or immunoperoxidase staining do not define whether a disease is focal or diffuse.

***Acute nephritic syndromes.*** These disorders are characterized by rapid onset of hematuria and proteinuria, reduced GFR and salt and water retention. The urine sediment is therefore 'active', indicating an inflammatory, 'nephritic' process. Classical descriptions include reactions to infections, particularly streptococcal sore throat.

***IgA nephropathy.*** IgA nephropathy is an example of a focal glomerulonephritis with focal mesangial cell proliferation demonstrated by light microscopy. However, diffuse and global deposition of the immunoglobulin IgA can be demonstrated following immunostaining. It is the most common type of glomerulonephritis worldwide and has a particularly high prevalence around the Pacific rim. The disease tends to be slowly progressive (in terms of loss of kidney function), depending, as with most kidney diseases, on the degree of proteinuria, kidney function at time of diagnosis, and degree of interstitial fibrosis on kidney biopsy. Up to 50% of patients exhibit increased concentrations of serum IgA, although diagnosis depends on kidney biopsy findings. Clinical presentation varies considerably, from asymptomatic invisible hematuria to visible hematuria; proteinuria including nephrotic syndrome; and crescentic glomerulonephritis with kidney failure. Episodic visible hematuria is seen in some patients at the same time as an upper respiratory tract infection.

Treatment options range from tonsillectomy in patients with visible hematuria associated with respiratory infection (mainly in Japan) to no treatment in those with isolated invisible hematuria. In progressive disease, all patients are treated in a similar generic fashion as for most kidney diseases, including targeting blood pressure to less than 125/75 mm Hg and using comprehensive RAAS blockade to minimize proteinuria and consideration to SGLT2 inhibitors. In addition, selected patients may receive corticosteroids in the form of prednisone.

***Nephrotic syndrome.*** Nephrotic syndrome is defined as heavy proteinuria (>3 g/day), reduced serum albumin concentration, and edema. In comparison with nephritic syndromes, nephrotic patients may exhibit an otherwise bland urinary sediment with little hematuria. Nephrotic syndrome can occur at any age from neonate to elderly. Although the underlying kidney disease tends to vary with age, in all cases the lesion is within the glomerulus and is associated with damage to the specialized visceral epithelial cells, the podocytes. Proteinuria is a consequence of a reduction in the charge-selective properties of the filtration barrier, particularly the GBM, and of alterations in the slit diaphragms of interdigitating foot processes of adjacent podocytes.

The most common causes of nephrotic syndrome are minimal change disease (MCD), focal segmental glomerulosclerosis (FSGS), and membranous nephropathy. Detection of autoantibodies directed to M-type phospholipase $A_2$ receptor PLA$_2$R (anti-PLA$_2$R antibody) in patients with membranous nephropathy indicates primary disease rather than a secondary process and guides therapy.

Secondary causes include diabetic nephropathy, amyloidosis, and systemic lupus erythematosus (SLE). A kidney biopsy is generally undertaken in all adult patients who present with nephrotic syndrome. Nephrotic syndrome is associated with increased cardiovascular disease as a result of marked hyperlipidemia and increased risk of infection and thromboembolic disease. In addition, AKI may supervene in cases of nephrotic syndrome, and prolonged proteinuria with a poor response to treatment may lead to kidney failure.

The management of nephrotic syndrome depends on the underlying glomerular lesion, although general principles apply in all cases (Box 35.1). In addition to general measures, specific treatment targeted at inducing remission from proteinuria usually requires a combination of immunosuppressive drugs, including corticosteroids and cytotoxic drugs.

## Rapidly Progressive Glomerulonephritis

Rapidly progressive glomerulonephritis (RPGN) is a heterogeneous group of disorders characterized by a fulminant clinical course that leads to kidney failure in only weeks or months. The clinical picture of RPGN is often preceded by a systemic illness for several months.

These syndromes are often characterized by focal glomerulonephritis with glomerular ischemia, infarction, and tissue death (necrosis). Following release of inflammatory cytokines and chemokines from the necrotic capillaries, there is proliferation of the epithelial cells of the Bowman capsule. The proliferated cells lie on top of adjacent cells and form a partial circle around the inner rim of the Bowman capsule that is referred to as a *crescent*. Proliferating epithelial cells and macrophages eventually compress the glomeruli and obstruct the proximal convoluted tubules, thus severely compromising nephron function.

Anti-GBM antibodies may be present along the GBM in anti-GBM disease. Most commonly, however, there is no, or little, immunoglobulin (Ig) deposition within the glomerulus (so-called "pauci-immune"). Approximately 80% of patients with active pauci-immune necrotizing and crescentic glomerulonephritis have been shown to possess antineutrophil cytoplasmic antibodies (ANCAs), irrespective of the presence or absence of a concomitant systemic vasculitis. This strong association has allowed serologic discrimination of this type of glomerulonephritis from other types of RPGN. Two subtypes of ANCA have been described—cytoplasmic (C-ANCA) and perinuclear (P-ANCA)—reflecting the patterns observed by indirect immunofluorescence microscopy using alcohol-fixed neutrophils as a substrate. C-ANCAs are directed toward a plasma proteinase (PR3) in neutrophil primary granules, whereas the P-ANCA target antigen is usually myeloperoxidase (MPO). Immunoassays have been used to measure anti-PR3 and anti-MPO antibody titers. ANCAs appear in the plasma of almost all patients with active and generalized disease and are useful in diagnosis of the disease. However, false positives and false negatives may occur, necessitating histological diagnosis where possible.

In addition to measurement of ANCA, C-reactive protein (CRP) is helpful in assessment of the acute-phase reaction in active disease processes and response to high-intensity immunosuppressive treatment. Treatment with ongoing immunosuppression is indicated for several years, with predictable side effects contributing to the overall burden of the disease.

## Systemic Lupus Erythematosus

SLE is a chronic inflammatory disease of unknown cause that can affect the skin, joints, kidneys, lungs, nervous system, serous membranes, and/or other organs of the body. Renal involvement, termed *lupus nephritis*, occurs in up to 60% of adults with SLE. Lupus nephritis is especially common in Black and Hispanic patients in the United States. Lupus nephritis may present variably from incidental hematuria and proteinuria, nephrotic syndrome, or a fulminating RPGN. Most (75%) patients with SLE develop an abnormal urinalysis or impaired kidney function during the course of the disease. Detection of lupus nephritis involves urine testing for blood and protein and tests of kidney function. In addition, serologic testing for autoantibodies to nuclear antigens and measurement of complement components C3 and C4 are undertaken. Significant hypocomplementemia and increased anti-double-stranded deoxyribonucleic acid (anti-ds DNA) titers suggest active disease. Combined use of corticosteroids and intravenous or oral cyclophosphamide has been the conventional treatment for diffuse proliferative lupus nephritis since the 1970s. Recent data suggest that mycophenolate mofetil (MMF) and corticosteroids can be as effective as, but not superior to, intravenous cyclophosphamide for induction treatment for lupus nephritis.

## Interstitial Nephritis

A variety of chemical, bacterial, and immunologic injuries to the kidney may cause generalized or localized changes that primarily affect the tubulointerstitium rather than the glomeruli. This group of disorders is characterized by alterations in tubular function that, in advanced cases, may cause secondary vascular and glomerular damage. **Interstitial nephritis** is associated with proteinuria that is less severe than in

---

**BOX 35.1 Management of Nephrotic Syndrome**

Low-sodium diet
Protein intake of 1.0 g/kg/day
Fluid management: usually includes loop diuretics
Thromboembolism prophylaxis: may include formal anticoagulation in high-risk patients (serum albumin <20 g/L or in nephrotic syndrome due to membranous nephropathy or mesangioproliferative glomerulonephritis)
Vigilance for infections
Treatment of hyperlipidemia with 3-hydroxy-3-methylglutaryl-Co-enzyme A (HMG)-CoA-reductase inhibitors (statins)
Treatment of hypertension, primarily with RAAS blockade
Supportive treatment of AKI
Education and psychological support for patients and relatives

*AKI,* Acute kidney injury; *RAAS,* renin-angiotensin-aldosterone system.

glomerular disease. In addition to infection-related (pyelonephritis), interstitial nephritis may present in acute and chronic forms and has many causes. Acute allergic interstitial nephritis presents with AKI and marked inflammation of the interstitium. A drug hypersensitivity reaction is the most common form of acute interstitial nephritis. Urinary findings may be normal, or low-level proteinuria and eosinophils may be seen on light microscopy. More than 100 different drugs have been implicated, but NSAIDs and β-lactam antibiotics are the drugs most commonly identified. Treatment is directed at removing any causative agent. Steroids are used to promote early resolution of the clinical course, although patients can develop chronic interstitial fibrosis.

## Monoclonal Light Chains and Kidney Disease

Ig molecules are formed in secretory B cells (plasma cells) and consist of heavy chains, which denominate the antibody isotype, and either kappa (κ) or lambda (λ) light chains. The proportion of Ig containing κ versus λ is 3:2 in humans. The molecular weight of light chains is approximately 23 kDa. Excess production of light chains over heavy chains appears to be required for efficient Ig synthesis, resulting in the release of free light chains (FLCs) into the circulation. In normal individuals, the small quantity of circulating polyclonal light chains is filtered by the glomerulus, and 90% is reabsorbed in the proximal tubule and degraded by proteases.

Myeloma is a neoplastic proliferation of a clone of plasma cells that produce excessive amounts of a monoclonal (M) protein and FLCs. In multiple myeloma, complete monoclonal Igs (usually IgG or IgA) are accompanied in the plasma by variable concentrations of FLCs that appear in the urine as Bence Jones proteins (named after Henry Bence Jones, who first described these in 1848). M-proteins and FLCs can be identified in the blood and/or urine in 98% of patients with myeloma using protein electrophoresis and immunofixation. Immunoparesis, with a reduction in non-M-protein Ig, is characteristic of myeloma. The FLC immunoassay is now also used to detect monoclonal Ig. The kidneys are often affected in myeloma, with diverse clinical and pathological presentations. The three most common forms of monoclonal Ig-mediated kidney disease are cast nephropathy, monoclonal Ig deposition disease (MIDD), and AL amyloidosis. Impairment of kidney function at presentation occurs in almost 50% of patients with myeloma. Although most patients recover following treatment for other factors contributing to AKI (e.g., dehydration, hypercalcemia, infection, nephrotoxic drugs), about 10% have severe renal involvement caused by the effects of monoclonal FLCs on the kidney. Severe kidney failure may occur in myeloma following deposition of light chains within tubules—so-called "cast nephropathy" ("myeloma kidney").

## Polycystic Kidney Disease

Autosomal dominant polycystic kidney disease (ADPKD) is the second most common inherited monogenic disease (after familial hypercholesterolemia), with an estimated incidence of 1:1000. It is by far the most common inherited

kidney disease; 12.5 million people worldwide are affected. Approximately 50% of ADPKD patients develop kidney failure by age 55 years. It is therefore important to make the diagnosis in affected families and to monitor kidney function regularly. The intervals between estimations of GFR will depend on the stage of CKD, as with other progressive kidney diseases. An important clinical observation is the highly variable phenotype within families. The disease causes the development of multiple kidney cysts and extrarenal cysts occurring in the liver and pancreas. About 10% of ADPKD families have a strong family history of intracranial arterial aneurysm rupture. Hypertension is an early and frequent manifestation, and visible hematuria is a common presenting symptom. On the basis of effectiveness, cost, and safety, ultrasound is the imaging modality most commonly used to make the diagnosis.

ADPKD is caused by mutations in the genes (*PKD1* and *PKD2*) that encode polycystin 1 and 2, which are located in primary cilia. Mutations affecting *PKD1* are more prevalent than those affecting *PKD2* and tend to have a worse prognosis. Genetic testing is not used routinely as a screening tool because current techniques identify only 70% of the hundreds of different *PKD1* and *PKD2* mutations. Generic treatment should include treatment of hypertension with RAAS inhibitors and maintaining a fluid intake of 2 to 3 L/day to reduce the risk of kidney stone disease. Specific therapies are targeted at reducing cyst development and enlargement. Estimates of cyst volume can be determined using MRI techniques, and changes can be documented over a relatively short period of time. This has allowed the performance of clinical trials of novel drugs such as the vasopressin $V_2$-receptor antagonist, tolvaptan, and antiproliferative drugs such as sirolimus. Tolvaptan has been shown in the 3-year clinical study (TEMPO3:4) to slow the increase in size of the cysts, reduce pain associated with cysts, and slow the rate of change in kidney function. Adverse events, primarily thirst and polyuria, and abnormalities in liver function tests are reported, and the drug was approved for use by the US Food and Drug Administration (FDA) during 2018.

## Obstructive Uropathy

Benign prostatic hyperplasia (BPH) is one of the most common types of obstructive uropathy and is an almost universal finding in aging men. Among the most common symptoms are disorders of micturition, in particular increased frequency, and in many cases this can progress to bladder outflow obstruction. Between 10% and 40% of men with bladder outflow obstruction caused by BPH present in acute retention. Approximately 5% of this group has high-pressure chronic retention of urine, which can result in upper urinary tract obstruction and consequently CKD as a result of glomerular and tubular damage.

## Tubular Disease

Renal tubular acidosis and inherited tubulopathies are types of renal tubular disease.

### Inherited Tubulopathies

The inherited tubulopathies comprise a heterogeneous set of rare disorders, including (1) **Bartter syndrome**, (2) **Gitelman syndrome**, (3) **Liddle syndrome**, (4) pseudohypoaldosteronism type I, (5) Dent disease, and (6) X-linked dominant hypophosphatemic rickets (previously known as vitamin D–resistant rickets). Most are characterized by electrolyte disturbances. In addition to these, general reasons to suspect a tubulopathy include (1) a familial disease pattern, (2) renal impairment, (3) nephrocalcinosis, and (4) stone formation, especially if these should present at an early age. In cases in which a diuretic-sensitive channel is affected, these disorders will clearly mimic the effects of diuretic use (see discussion later in this chapter), and exclusion of covert use of diuretics is important. Although they are individually uncommon or rare, an awareness of these disorders is critical for the clinical biochemist when considering the potential differential diagnoses in patients having electrolyte imbalances.

### Diuretics

Diuretics are predominantly prescribed to treat either hypertension and/or disorders associated with fluid overload. All diuretics act by interfering with tubular reabsorption of sodium and/or chloride and therefore have accompanying effects on water retention. Different classes of diuretics act at different sites along the nephron. Classes include (1) loop, (2) thiazide, and (3) "potassium-sparing" diuretics. Many diuretics will cause hypokalemia to some degree, depending on the (1) potency, (2) dose, (3) duration of treatment, and (4) patient's underlying potassium balance.

### Kidney Stones

**Nephrolithiasis** is a condition marked by the presence of kidney stones. Such stones (also referred to as renal calculi) occur in the (1) renal pelvis, (2) ureter, and (3) bladder. Kidney stone formation is often considered to be a nutritional or environmental disease, linked to affluence, but genetic or anatomical abnormalities are also significant. Approximately 5% to 10% of the population of the Western world are thought to have formed at least one kidney stone by the age of 70 years, and the prevalence of kidney stones may be increasing. In both males and females, the average age of first stone formation is decreasing. For most stone types, there is a male preponderance. The passage of a stone is associated with severe pain called renal colic, which may last for 15 minutes to several hours and is commonly associated with nausea and vomiting.

The majority of kidney stones found in the Western world are composed of one or more of the following substances: (1) calcium oxalate with or without phosphate (frequency: 67%), (2) magnesium ammonium phosphate (12%), (3) calcium phosphate (8%), (4) urate (8%), (5) cystine (1% to 2%), and (6) complex mixtures of the above (2% to 3%). These poorly soluble substances crystallize within an organic matrix, the nature of which is not well understood. Most kidney stones are treated by **lithotripsy** that entails crushing a calculus within the urinary system, followed at once by the washing out of the fragments.

## Prostaglandins and Nonsteroidal Antiinflammatory Drugs in Kidney Disease

The prostaglandins are a series of $C_{20}$ unsaturated fatty acid derivatives of COX on cell membrane arachidonic acid (see Chapter 23). The major renal vasodilatory prostaglandin is $PGE_2$, which is synthesized predominantly in the medulla of the kidney. The major vasoconstrictor prostaglandin is thromboxane $A_2$, which is produced primarily within the renal cortex. $PGE_2$ (1) increases renal blood flow rate, (2) inhibits sodium reabsorption in the distal nephron and collecting duct, and (3) stimulates renin release. These actions promote natriuresis and diuresis. In patients with CKD, renal $PGE_2$ excretion rates are three to five times higher than those in healthy subjects, and therefore $PGE_2$ production represents a compensatory response to loss of nephron mass. Vasodilatory prostaglandins are synthesized following stimulation with renal sympathetic adrenergic and AII-dependent mechanisms to offset or modulate vasoconstriction. In the tubule, prostaglandins act as autocoids, exerting their effects locally, near the site of synthesis.

NSAIDs have analgesic, antipyretic, and antiinflammatory effects. They also block the synthesis of COX products of arachidonic acid, which have a critical role in (1) renal hemodynamics, (2) control of tubular function, and (3) renin release. Analgesic nephropathy has historically been a common cause of kidney failure in a number of countries, reaching 10% in Switzerland and Australia, but is essentially a preventable condition for which biochemical monitoring has proved useful. Older people demonstrate significant reduction of GFR within 1 week of ingestion of NSAIDs. Acute interstitial nephritis and nephrotic syndrome have been reported to occur with NSAIDs.

## KIDNEY REPLACEMENT THERAPY

KRT includes dialysis procedures such as HD, **peritoneal dialysis (PD)**, continuous hemofiltration (HF), and continuous hemodiafiltration (HDF). These techniques are used to temporarily or permanently remove toxic substances from the blood when the kidneys cannot satisfactorily remove them from the circulation. In addition, kidney transplantation has become an effective form of KRT. Extensive laboratory support is required by a KRT program (Table 35.3).

### Dialysis

Dialysis is the process of separating macromolecules from ions and low-molecular-weight compounds in solution based on the difference in their rates of diffusion through a semipermeable membrane, through which crystalloids can pass readily but colloids pass very slowly or not at all. Two distinct physical processes are involved: diffusion and ultrafiltration.

No absolute recommendation of commencement of dialysis based on GFR alone can be made. KDIGO suggest that

## TABLE 35.3  Laboratory Support for Dialysis Programs

| Clinical Condition | Laboratory Tests |
|---|---|
| **Acute Dialysis** | |
| Dialysis disequilibrium | Urea and electrolytes, bicarbonate, calcium |
| Pyrexia | C-reactive protein, white cell count, blood cultures |
| Bleeding | Clotting screen, platelets |
| | |
| **Chronic Dialysis** | |
| Anemia | Ferritin, transferrin saturation, vitamin $B_{12}$, folate |
| | Blood film, PTH, C-reactive protein |
| Sepsis | C-reactive protein, blood, urine specimens for microscopy, culture, and sensitivity |
| Nutrition | Albumin, phosphate |
| Cardiovascular disease risk | Lipid profile |
| Dialysis-related amyloid | $\beta_2$-microglobulin (not routinely measured) |
| CKD-MBD | Predialysis plasma calcium, phosphate (monthly in hemodialysis patients; every 3 months in peritoneal dialysis patients) |
| | Alkaline phosphatase |
| | PTH (at least every 3 months) |
| | Aluminum in patients receiving aluminum-based phosphate binders (every 3 months) |
| Adequacy of hemodialysis as assessed by urea clearance | Predialysis and postdialysis urea |
| Sepsis, abdominal pain in peritoneal dialysis | Microscopy and culture of peritoneal dialysate |
| Adequacy of peritoneal dialysis as assessed by weekly small solute clearance | Dialysate creatinine, urea |
| Peritoneal membrane characteristics assessed by peritoneal equilibration test (PET) | Plasma and dialysate glucose and creatinine |

*CKD,* Chronic kidney disease; *CMV,* cytomegalovirus; *CNI,* calcineurin inhibitor; *EBV,* Epstein-Barr virus; *FSGS,* focal segmental glomerulosclerosis; *GBM,* glomerular basement membrane; *MBD,* mineral and bone disease; *MPGN,* membranoproliferative glomerulonephritis; *PCP, Pneumocystis carinii* pneumonia; *PCR,* polymerase chain reaction; *PTLD,* posttransplant lymphoproliferative diseases; *SV40,* simian virus 40 (cross-reacts with BK virus).

dialysis be initiated when one or more of the following are present: symptoms or signs attributable to kidney failure (serositis, acid-base or electrolyte abnormalities, pruritus); inability to control volume status or blood pressure; a progressive deterioration in nutritional status refractory to dietary intervention; or cognitive impairment. This often but not invariably occurs in the GFR range between 5 and 10 mL/min/1.73 m². Not all individuals will be suitable for KRT, and in this setting, it is important that the multidisciplinary team facilitates care for people on the "conservative management" pathway or active symptom support.

Dialysis procedures include (1) HD and (2) PD.

## Hemodialysis

HD is the method most commonly used to treat advanced and permanent kidney failure. Clinically, it is considered the default therapy that is utilized in patients unsuitable for the alternate modalities of PD and kidney transplantation. Operationally, it involves connecting the patient to a circuit into which his or her blood flows to and from a semipermeable large surface area membrane, the hemodialyzer (Fig. 35.5). After filtration to remove wastes and extra fluid, the cleansed blood is returned to the patient. This is a complicated and inconvenient therapy requiring a coordinated effort from a health care team that includes the patient, nephrologist, dialysis nurse, dialysis technician, dietitian, and others. Patients are dialyzed in home-based or hospital-based units,

with dialysis usually performed three times a week for sessions lasting between 3 and 5 hours. This dialysis schedule is largely empirical, insofar as it reconciles adequate treatment with breaks between treatments to provide the patient with a reasonable quality of life.

HD relies on good vascular access, preferably via a surgically created upper limb arteriovenous fistula (AVF), to enable blood to be pumped around the extracorporeal circuit at a rate in excess of 300 mL/min.

Fluid management on HD is crucial for patient well-being and survival. Because conventional dialysis is based on a thrice-weekly schedule, fluid is accumulated by the patient between dialysis sessions. Many patients are anuric or at least oliguric; therefore, unrestricted fluid intake would result in fluid overload and complications of pulmonary edema and hypertension. Patients receiving HD are advised to restrict fluid intake to 1 L/day or so. This allowance is recommended to the individual patient by the dialysis nursing staff and the dietitian to ensure that adequate nutrition is maintained. Nevertheless, many patients find the fluid restriction very difficult to maintain; therefore, large weight gains between dialysis sessions are a common occurrence.

***Assessment of adequacy of hemodialysis.*** Assessment of adequacy of dialysis treatment for individual patients in the clinical setting includes consideration of the patient's well-being, cardiovascular risk, nutritional status, and degree of achievable ultrafiltration. It also includes estimates of a

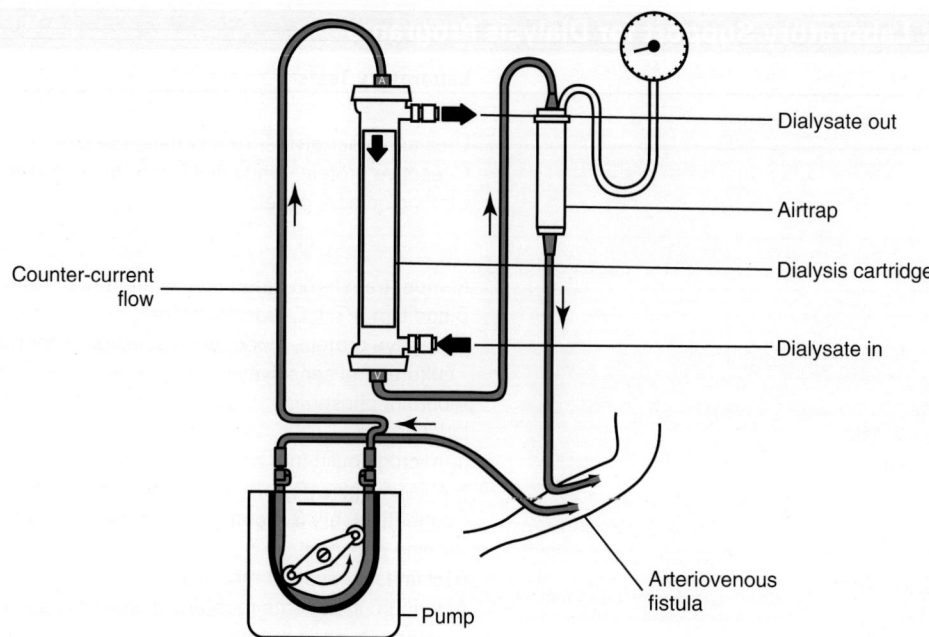

Fig. 35.5 A hemodialyzer setup.

number of laboratory parameters, such as hemoglobin, phosphate, and albumin, and clearance of the small solutes, urea, and creatinine. Although a full description of adequacy is beyond the scope of this text, in practice, a simple calculation may be performed to obtain an estimate of dialysis adequacy: the urea reduction ratio (URR). The URR is the percentage fall in plasma urea attained during a dialysis session and is measured as follows:

$$[(\text{Predialysis \{urea\}} - \text{Postdialysis \{urea\}}) / (\text{Predialysis \{urea\}})] \times 100\%$$

Observational studies in populations of dialysis patients have shown that variations in URR are associated with major differences in mortality.

## Peritoneal Dialysis

PD is a type of dialysis in which dialysate is passed into the patient's peritoneal cavity, with the peritoneum then employed as the dialysis membrane (Fig. 35.6). Use of PD varies among countries, depending on access to HD and transplantation. For example, in the United Kingdom in 2019, PD was the modality of treatment in 5.4% of the prevalent KRT population (compared to 38% receiving HD and 57% with a functioning transplant), whereas in Mexico, 90% of patients received PD during 2013, and there are worldwide initiatives to increase PD in Asia and Australasia.

Operationally, PD uses the patient's own peritoneal membrane (surface area approximately 2 m²), across which fluids and solutes are exchanged between the peritoneal capillary blood and the dialysis solution placed in the peritoneal cavity. Fluid removal (ultrafiltration) is achieved by using dialysis fluids containing high concentrations of dextrose acting as an osmotic agent; as dextrose passes across the peritoneal membrane, the concentration gradient diminishes and the rate of fluid removal decreases. Conventional therapies use four

daily exchanges of approximately 2 L of fluid, with approximately 10 L of spent dialysate generated (including ultrafiltration). Residual kidney function is critical to the success of PD because only a few milliliters per minute can contribute substantially to urea clearance and creatinine clearance ($C_{Cr}$), with each additional milliliter resulting in an extra 10 L of clearance per week. Practical reasons for opting for PD include preservation of residual kidney function and vascular access sites, a home treatment facilitating increased patient autonomy, flexibility as to where the treatment can be administered, and ease of self-treatment, with lower capital costs involved. Blood pressure control and extremes of fluid shifts are not as problematic as those that occur on conventional HD.

Automated PD is now widely available. It requires a programmable machine to regulate flow, dwell time, and drainage, and it may be performed at night. Solute clearance can be increased by leaving fluid in the peritoneum during the day and by performing an additional daytime exchange.

Peritonitis, a particular complication of PD, typically presents with a cloudy dialysate effluent and abdominal pain. Additional features such as vomiting and a high temperature suggest serious infection. Blood and dialysate samples should be taken for urgent microbiological analysis and antibiotics administered via the dialysis catheter directly into the peritoneum. If antibiotic treatment fails, then the catheter is removed and the patient is converted to HD. In the majority of cases, the episode of peritonitis responds to treatment, and PD can continue, although it is likely that repeated episodes will cause scarring and fibrosis of the peritoneal membrane, with permanent loss of ultrafiltration. Long-term, serious complications may occur, such as sclerosing encapsulating peritonitis caused by adhesions and peritoneal thickening encasing the peritoneal contents and causing bowel obstruction. This unusual condition is associated with increased frequency of peritonitis episodes and longer duration of PD.

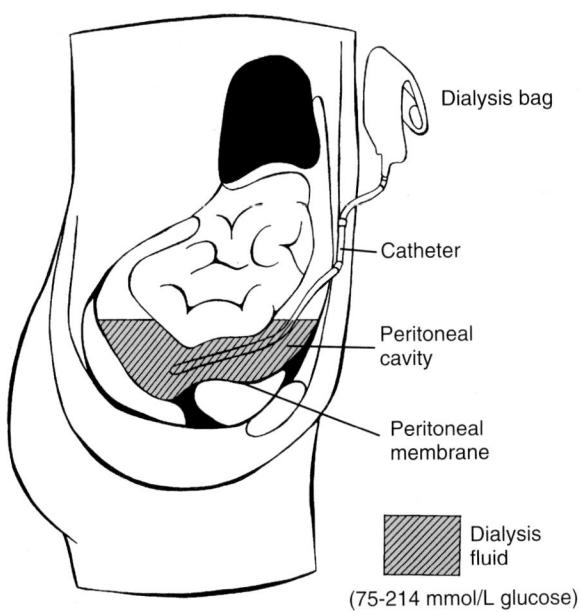

Dialysis bag

Catheter

Peritoneal cavity

Peritoneal membrane

Dialysis fluid

(75-214 mmol/L glucose)

Fig. 35.6 Diagrammatic sketch of peritoneal dialysis. To convert glucose concentration in mmol/L to mg/dL, multiply by 18. (Redrawn from Nolph KD. Peritoneal anatomy and transport physiology. In: Maher JF, ed. *Replacement of Renal Function by Dialysis*. 3rd ed. Dordrecht, The Netherlands: Kluwer Academic Publishers/Springer; 1989.)

## Malnutrition in Dialysis Patients

Dialysis patients tend to have a poor appetite. Protein metabolism is altered in the setting of chronic acidosis and low-grade inflammation. These factors in combination place patients at risk of protein and energy malnourishment. Nutritional screening is recommended in dialysis patients. Such screening may involve measurement of weight, a recent history of edema-free weight loss, the body mass index, and subjective global assessment. Serum albumin is often used as a marker of malnutrition, even though it is a relatively poor nutritional marker. However, good evidence indicates that the lower the albumin concentration, the worse the long-term prognosis.

## Kidney Transplantation

Kidney transplantation is the most effective form of KRT in terms of long-term survival and quality of life. Approximately 100,000 patients are on the waiting list for a kidney transplant, and almost 17,000 kidney transplants are performed annually in the United States. Median waiting time for a listed patient depends on his or her age, with children given priority listing. Although patients with kidney failure should have equitable access to kidney transplantation, currently fewer than one in five adult patients on dialysis in the United Kingdom are on the active deceased donor transplant waiting list. Waiting time spent on dialysis has been shown to be an important factor in determining mortality. The very best outcomes are achieved following preemptive (i.e., before dialysis has become necessary) live donor transplants. Typically, graft and patient survival at 1 year are in excess of 90%. Long-term graft survival remains a major problem, with half of transplants failing within 14 years, usually as a result of

chronic allograft injury or death with a functioning graft. Transplantation medicine provides a constant challenge to balance the immunologic risk of damage to the allograft (rejection) versus the well-being of the recipient, while avoiding excess immunosuppression that increases the likelihood of opportunistic infection and malignancy. In addition, many of the powerful immunosuppressive drugs have idiosyncratic side effect profiles.

### Preoperative Assessment

Some patients are considered unsuitable candidates for transplantation (Box 35.2). Laboratory assessment includes indicators of general operative health (e.g., electrolytes, acid-base status, clotting profile, full blood cell count, cross-matching). In addition, a full screen for infectious diseases, particularly cytomegalovirus (CMV), Epstein-Barr virus, hepatitis B and C, varicella-zoster virus, and human immunodeficiency virus (HIV) status, is undertaken; these infections can be activated by immunosuppressive therapy.

### Postoperative Assessment

During the initial postoperative phase of 1 to 2 weeks, careful monitoring of serum creatinine and urine output is required to monitor graft function. Most grafts produce measurable amounts of urine within a matter of hours, and this is a clear sign of a functioning graft; however, in a certain proportion, perhaps 5% to 10% of cases, primary nonfunction is apparent. In this subgroup, continuing dialysis support is necessary. In some patients the condition resolves without treatment, but in others a percutaneous kidney biopsy may be necessary to establish whether the graft is still viable and what form of therapy should be initiated. In otherwise uncomplicated cases, the serum creatinine concentration falls rapidly postoperatively (Fig. 35.7). Early allograft rejection episodes are suspected if the creatinine does not fall to the expected level or if there is a creatinine concentration indicating allograft dysfunction.

*Immunosuppression and therapeutic drug monitoring.* The currently used immunosuppressive drugs and regimens

**BOX 35.2 Exclusion Criteria for Consideration for a Kidney Transplant**

Serious concomitant illness (particularly if likely to shorten life expectancy or to be exacerbated by immunosuppressive treatment)
Active malignancy
Inoperable ischemic heart disease
Severe chronic lung disease
Active systemic infection (e.g., tuberculosis)
Active immunologic disease
Severe irreversible hepatic disease
Severe peripheral vascular disease
Severe obesity (body mass index >40 kg/m$^2$)
Lower urinary tract dysfunction not amenable to surgical repair
Substance abuse
Significant psychiatric disturbance

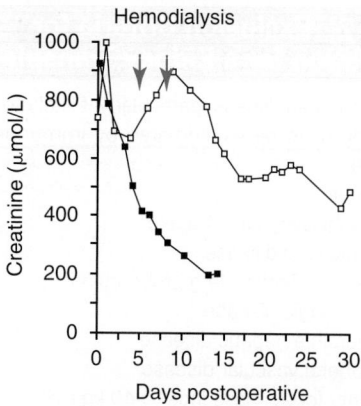

**Fig. 35.7** Posttransplantation biochemical profile. *Open squares* represent the course of a patient who experienced an early rejection episode (confirmed by biopsy, ↓) and requires initial hemodialysis support. Solid squares represent the typical profile of an uncomplicated transplant recipient. To convert creatinine concentration in μmol/L to mg/dL, multiply by 0.011.

have potentially numerous and serious side effects that are summarized in Table 35.4.

Tacrolimus and cyclosporine are both CNIs and in modern regimens tacrolimus is used in the majority of kidney transplants. The drugs have a narrow therapeutic window, and in clinical transplantation, it is important to monitor the blood concentration frequently. The most widely accepted practice is to monitor the "trough" concentration (C-0) just before the next dose. The highest concentrations are targeted during the induction phase of treatment for 2 to 3 months; subsequently, lower maintenance concentrations are desirable. Predefined target trough drug concentrations depend on a number of recipient factors and whether there is an increased risk of transplant rejection. Higher trough concentrations are required to prevent rejection in standard and high-risk cases. The CNI drugs, although central to immunosuppressive protocols can cause nephrotoxicity with acute and chronic loss of kidney function. Trough concentrations also guide sirolimus therapy (see Chapter 30).

## TABLE 35.4 Noninfectious Complications of Immunosuppressant Drugs

| Drug | Drug Dose | Target Therapeutic Range[a] | Toxicity Profile |
| --- | --- | --- | --- |
| Corticosteroids—(e.g., prednisone) | Dose depends on weight of patient and time since transplant. Typically, 20 mg daily during first week and tapering to 5 mg at 6 months and withdrawal at 12 months. | Not appropriate | Increased risk of developing diabetes mellitus<br>Deterioration in diabetes control<br>Osteopenia<br>Osteoporosis<br>Psychosis<br>Fat redistribution<br>Hypertension<br>Dyslipidemia<br>Cataracts<br>Weight gain |
| **Calcineurin Inhibitors** | | | |
| Cyclosporine | Variable<br>Depends on weight, time since transplant and achieved drug concentration. Dose given in two divided doses and predose trough concentration measured in morning blood sample | 200–300 μg/L for first 3–12 months. Thereafter, aim for 100 μg/L | Nephrotoxicity<br>Hypertension<br>Neurotoxicity<br>Hemolytic-uremic syndrome<br>Tubular electrolyte abnormalities (hypophosphatemia, hypomagnesemia, hyperkalemia)<br>Hirsutism<br>Gingival hyperplasia<br>Bone pains<br>Dyslipidemia |
| Tacrolimus | | | As for cyclosporine, except no hirsutism or gingival hyperplasia<br>Increased risk of diabetes mellitus<br>Cardiomyopathy (children)<br>Alopecia |
| Mycophenolate mofetil | Initially 2 g daily in divided doses | Not routinely measured | Abdominal pain<br>Diarrhea<br>Myelosuppression |

*Continued*

## TABLE 35.4  Noninfectious Complications of Immunosuppressant Drugs—cont'd

| Drug | Drug Dose | Target Therapeutic Range[a] | Toxicity Profile |
|---|---|---|---|
| Sirolimus | Dose depends on weight and achieved drug concentration. The drug is administered once daily. | Level depends on time since transplant. Typical early (<3 months) targets are 8–12 µg/L and thereafter 4–8 µg/L. | Lymphocele (a fluid-filled collection near to transplanted kidney)<br>Thrombocytopenia<br>Hyperlipidemia |
| Azathioprine | Usual starting dose of 2 mg/kg body weight in a single daily dose | Levels not measured. Because the enzyme thiopurine methyltransferase (TPMT) metabolizes azathioprine, the risk of myelosuppression is increased in patients with low activity of the enzyme. Enzyme activity may be determined prior to commencing treatment, and full blood counts are performed for several weeks following commencement of drug. | Myelosuppression<br>Severe interaction if used with allopurinol (treatment for gout) |
| **Selected biological agents**<br>Anti-CD25 monoclonal antibodies: basiliximab and daclizumab<br>1. Alemtuzumab (anti-CD52)<br>2. Polyclonal antithymocyte globulin (ATG) | Given at time of transplant and once thereafter<br>Used in SPK and high immunological risk settings<br>Given in response to refractory rejection episodes in selected patients | | Very well tolerated<br><br><br>Increased risk of malignancy, posttransplant lymphoproliferative disease<br>Hypersensitivity reactions |

[a]These are not recommendations but are illustrative and will vary among centers.

MMF is the morpholinoethyl ester of mycophenolic acid (MPA), a potent and reversible inhibitor of inosine monophosphate dehydrogenase isoform 2 (IMPDH), and it has become the single most used immunosuppressant in solid organ transplantation. Excellent results have been obtained with a fixed-dose regimen. IMPDH is a target for immunosuppression because lymphocytes depend on the de novo guanosine nucleotide synthesis pathway for DNA synthesis and cell division. MMF, because it is a prodrug of MPA, is rapidly absorbed following an oral dose and is deesterified to MPA, which is highly protein bound. Free MPA concentrations determine the level of immunosuppressive activity, and this can be affected by hypoalbuminemia and renal insufficiency. Therapeutic drug monitoring of MPA is possible using HPLC and immunoassay techniques. However, it has not been universally accepted in kidney transplantation programs because prospective studies have given conflicting information of its value.

In summary, long-term graft failure is a major problem, and graft loss accounts for the return of increasing numbers of patients to dialysis. The most common cause of graft loss is death with a functioning graft. Kidney failure carries a considerable burden of cardiovascular morbidity. Although some risk factors, such as volume overload and anemia, are improved following transplantation, others, including dyslipidemia and hypertension, persist. The drugs used to prevent rejection can exacerbate these. Challenges to the nephrology community are complex and include improving access to transplantation, reducing side effects of the powerful drugs used to prevent rejection, and reducing cardiovascular risk profiles for individual patients.

## Simultaneous Pancreas-Kidney Transplantation

Patients with kidney failure and diabetes mellitus, predominantly type 1, but increasingly selected patients with type 2, and limited secondary complications of diabetes may be considered for simultaneous pancreas and kidney (SPK) transplantation. Patients tend to be younger than kidney-only recipients (e.g., aged between 20 and 40 years). Patient survival now reaches over 95% at 1 year posttransplant and over 83% after 5 years. The objective of the dual transplant is to have independent kidney and pancreatic function with no requirement for dialysis nor conventional insulin therapy.

The early experience of pancreas transplantation was associated with implantation of the pancreas graft into the urinary bladder. The major fear is rejection, and a number of parameters are monitored, including plasma glucose, amylase, lipase, and 12- or 24-hour urinary amylase (for bladder-drained allografts). Historically, for patients with bladder drainage, enteric conversion may be required for refractory problems, such as dehydration, metabolic acidosis, chronic urethritis, urinary tract infection, and recurrent reflux pancreatitis. There is a long-term need for high-dose oral sodium bicarbonate supplementation in bladder-drained pancreatic transplantation because of exocrine secretory losses. Hyperamylasemia is common postoperatively and may or may not signify allograft rejection.

## REVIEW QUESTIONS

1. It is difficult to directly measure the GFR of a kidney; therefore, which one of the following is assessed to determine GFR?
   a. Renal blood flow
   b. Renal threshold
   c. Serum creatinine
   d. Urine albumin

2. Which one of the following tests evaluates renal tubular (including loop of Henle) function?
   a. Urine osmolality
   b. Inulin clearance
   c. Urine albumin
   d. Urine protein

3. The structural and functional unit of the kidney is the nephron. What structures make up a nephron?
   a. Only the structures located in the kidney cortex
   b. The glomeruli, tubules, and associated blood vessels
   c. The ureters, bladder, and urethra
   d. Only the structures located in the kidney medulla

4. Pyelonephritis is:
   a. caused by a lack of intrinsic factor.
   b. the destruction of kidney glomeruli by immune complexes.
   c. a tumor of the stomach.
   d. inflammation of both the lining of the renal pelvis and the parenchyma of the kidney especially due to bacterial infection.

5. Which one of the following hormones synthesized in cells of the JGA is involved in control of blood pressure through its action on angiotensinogen?
   a. Erythropoietin
   b. Antidiuretic hormone
   c. Renin
   d. Aldosterone

6. Regarding laboratory findings, uremia/azotemia specifically refers to:
   a. reduced kidney function.
   b. elevated nitrogenous compounds in blood.
   c. elevated serum proteins in blood.
   d. decreased urine albumin.

7. The most common glomerular disease caused by damage to the glomerular membrane from deposition of immune complexes is:
   a. IgA nephropathy.
   b. Chronic glomerulonephritis.
   c. uremic syndrome.
   d. pyelonephritis.

8. A disorder in which there is an abnormal increase in urine output, fluid intake, and often thirst and that is caused by the absence of antidiuretic hormone is:
   a. diabetes mellitus.
   b. IgA nephropathy.
   c. diabetes insipidus.
   d. nephrolithiasis.

9. Which one of the following hormones affects water reabsorption in the proximal tubule, the loop of Henle, the distal tubule, and the collecting duct of the kidney?
   a. Aldosterone
   b. Renin
   c. $1,25(OH_2)$ vitamin $D_3$
   d. Antidiuretic hormone

10. A drug prescribed to an individual to treat hypertension and/or disorders associated with fluid overload is referred to as a(n):
   a. ACE inhibitor.
   b. diuretic.
   c. cystatin C.
   d. exogenous marker.

## SUGGESTED READINGS

Bikbov B, Purcell CA, Levey AS, et al. Global, regional, and national burden of chronic kidney disease, 1990–2017: a systematic analysis for the Global Burden of Disease Study 2017. *Lancet*. 2020;395(10225):709–733.

Chapman AB, Devuyst O, Eckardt KU, et al. Autosomal-dominant polycystic kidney disease (ADPKD): executive summary from a Kidney Disease: Improving Global Outcomes (KDIGO) Controversies Conference. *Kidney Int*. 2015;88:17–27.

De Vriese AS, Glassock RJ, Nath KA, et al. A proposal for a serology-based approach to membranous nephropathy. *J Am Soc Nephrol*. 2017;28:421–430.

Devoe DJ, Wong B, James MT, et al. Patient education and peritoneal dialysis modality selection: a systematic review and meta-analysis. *Am J Kidney Dis*. 2016;68:422–433.

Haraldsson B, Nystrom J, Deen WM. Properties of the glomerular barrier and mechanisms of proteinuria. *Physiol Rev*. 2008;88:451–487.

Heerspink HJL, Stefánsson BV, Correa-Rotter R, et al. Dapagliflozin in patients with chronic kidney disease. *N Engl J Med*. 2020;383(15):1436–1446.

Kanagasundaram NS. Pathophysiology of ischaemic acute kidney injury. *Ann Clin Biochem*. 2015;52:193–205.

Kidney Disease Improving Global Outcomes. Clinical practice guideline for the evaluation and management of chronic kidney disease. *Kidney Int*. 2013;3:1–150.

Kidney Disease Improving Global Outcomes. KDIGO clinical practice guideline update for the diagnosis, evaluation, prevention, and treatment of chronic kidney disease-mineral and bone disorder (CKD-MBD). *Kidney Int. Suppl*. 2017;7:1–59.

Lamb EJ, Stevens PE, Deeks JJ. What is the best glomerular filtration marker to identify people with chronic kidney disease most likely to have poor outcomes? *BMJ.* 2015;350:g7667.

Levey AS, Eckardt KU, Dorman NM, et al. Nomenclature for kidney function and disease: report of a Kidney Disease: Improving Global Outcomes (KDIGO) Consensus Conference. *Kidney Int.* 2020;97(6):1117–1129.

Locatelli F, Fishbane S, Block GA, et al. Targeting hypoxia-inducible factors for the treatment of anemia in chronic kidney disease patients. *Am J Nephrol.* 2017;45(3):187–199.

Loudon KW, Fry AC. The renal channelopathies. *Ann Clin Biochem.* 2014;51:441–458.

National Institute for Health and Care Excellence. *Acute Kidney Injury: Prevention, Detection and Management of Acute Kidney Injury up to the Point of Renal Replacement Therapy (CG169);* 2013. https://www.nice.org.uk/.

National Kidney Foundation. Clinical practice guidelines for hemodialysis adequacy, update 2006. *Am J Kidney Dis.* 2006;48(suppl 1):S2–S90.

Parikh CR, Mansour SG. Perspective on clinical application of biomarkers in AKI. *J Am Soc Nephrol.* 2017;28:1677–1685.

Rovin BH, Adler SG, Barratt J, et al. KDIGO 2021 clinical practice guideline for the management of glomerular diseases. *Kidney Int.* 2021;100(4S):S1–S276.

UK Renal Registry. *UK Renal Registry 23rd Annual Report.* Bristol, UK: UK Renal Registry (UKRR); 2021. https://ukkidney.org/audit-research/annual-report.

United Kingdom Prospective Diabetes Study (UKPDS) Group. Intensive blood-glucose control with sulphonylureas or insulin compared with conventional treatment and risk of complications in patients with type 2 diabetes (UKPDS 33). *Lancet.* 1998;352:837–853.

Wanner C, Tonelli M. KDIGO clinical practice guideline for lipid management in CKD: summary of recommendation statements and clinical approach to the patient. *Kidney Int.* 2014;85:1303–1309.

Webster AC, Nagler EV, Morton RL, et al. Chronic kidney disease. *Lancet.* 2017;389:1238–1252.

# Physiology and Disorders of Water, Electrolyte, and Acid-Base Metabolism

*Mark A. Cervinski, Marc Berg, and Christopher McCudden*

## OBJECTIVES

1. Define the following:
   - Acid-base balance
   - Aldosterone
   - Anion gap
   - Antidiuretic hormone
   - Compensation
   - Depletional hyponatremia
   - Dilutional hyponatremia
   - Hyper- and hypovolemia
   - Interstitial fluid
   - Solute diuresis
2. State the significance of and describe the total body water (TBW) distribution between compartments, including approximate volume and composition of each compartment, electrolyte distribution, and active/passive transport for ion exchange; list the hormonal regulators of water and sodium.
3. For each of the following electrolytes, state and describe regulatory mechanisms, disorders, and causes/effects of these disorders:
   - Chloride
   - Potassium
   - Sodium

4. State the Henderson-Hasselbalch equation, and explain each of its components; explain its relation to compensatory mechanisms in acid-base disturbances.
5. Categorize the physiological buffer systems relative to their specific roles in the regulation of blood pH.
6. Explain the specific respiratory and renal mechanisms important in the regulation of acid-base balance.
7. For each of the acid-base imbalances listed below, list the causes and state the primary deficit, compensatory mechanisms, and laboratory values obtained with each:
   - Metabolic acidosis
   - Metabolic alkalosis
   - Respiratory acidosis
   - Respiratory alkalosis
8. State the formula for and calculate the anion gap; discuss the clinical usefulness of anion gap, including eight causes of an increased anion gap and four causes of normal anion gap acidosis.
9. Compare chloride-responsive, chloride-resistant, and exogenous base metabolic alkalosis, including causes and laboratory values.

## KEY WORDS AND DEFINITIONS

**Acid-base balance** The homeostatic maintenance of acids and bases within the body to achieve a physiological pH (approximately 7.40).

**Acidemia** An arterial blood pH less than 7.35.

**Alkalemia** An arterial blood pH greater than 7.45.

**Anion gap (AG)** The difference between the serum sodium concentration and the sum of the serum chloride and bicarbonate concentrations; the anion gap is high in some forms of metabolic acidosis.

**Chronic obstructive pulmonary disease (COPD)** Any disorder characterized by persistent or recurring obstruction of bronchial airflow, such as chronic bronchitis, asthma, or pulmonary emphysema.

**Compensation mechanisms for metabolic acidosis** A state of acidosis in which the pH of the blood has been returned toward normal by compensatory mechanisms.

**Depletional hyponatremia** A condition characterized by low plasma concentration of sodium associated with low

total body sodium and normal blood volume; also called euvolemic hyponatremia.

**Diabetes insipidus** A condition associated with increased thirst, polyuria, and large volume of dilute urine, exceeding 3 L/day, and causing dehydration.

**Dilutional hyponatremia** A condition characterized by low plasma concentration of sodium resulting from loss of sodium from the body with nonosmotic retention of water.

**Extracellular fluid (ECF)** A general term for all the body fluids outside the cells, including the interstitial fluid, plasma, lymph, and cerebrospinal fluid (CSF).

**Henderson-Hasselbalch equation** An equation that defines the relationship between pH, bicarbonate, and the partial pressure of dissolved carbon dioxide gas.

**Hyperkalemia** A concentration of serum potassium above 5.0 mmol/L.

**Hypernatremia** A concentration of serum sodium above 145 mmol/L.

**Hypervolemia** Abnormal increase in the volume of circulating fluid (plasma) in the body.

**Hypokalemia** A concentration of serum potassium below 3.5 mmol/L.

**Hyponatremia** A concentration of serum sodium below 135 mmol/L.

**Hypovolemia** Abnormally decreased volume of circulating fluid (plasma) in the body.

**Intracellular fluid (ICF)** The portion of the total body water (TBW) with its dissolved solutes that is within cell membranes.

**Ketoacidosis** A condition characterized as acidosis accompanied by the accumulation of ketone bodies (ketosis) in the body tissues and fluids.

**Metabolic acidosis** A pathological process that leads to the accumulation of acid that lowers bicarbonate concentration and decreases pH.

**Metabolic alkalosis** A pathological process that leads to the accumulation of base that raises bicarbonate concentration and increases pH.

**Respiratory acidosis** A pathological process that leads to the accumulation of carbon dioxide that raises $PCO_2$ and decreases pH; caused by COPD (emphysema or chronic bronchitis) or hypoventilation.

**Respiratory alkalosis** A pathological process that leads to the excessive elimination of carbon dioxide, which lowers $PCO_2$ and increases pH; caused by hyperventilation.

**Sodium–hydrogen exchanger ($Na^+$–$H^+$ exchanger)** A membrane protein that is primarily responsible for maintaining the balance of sodium; also called the sodium–hydrogen antiporter.

**Total body water (TBW)** Any of various estimates of the water content of the human body, taking into consideration the person's height, weight, and age.

# INTRODUCTION

Fluid and electrolyte homeostasis requires the interaction of multiple organ systems, chemical buffers, and highly specialized mechanisms. These systems include the lungs and kidneys, which work together to regulate water, electrolytes, and pH between and within intracellular and extracellular compartments.

Water accounts for 60% of body weight in adolescents and adult males and ≈55% for adult females. As depicted in Fig. 36.1, approximately two-thirds of total body water (TBW) is distributed into the intracellular fluid (ICF) compartment, and one-third exists in the extracellular fluid (ECF) compartment. The ECF may be further subdivided by the capillary endothelium into interstitial (≈75% of ECF) and intravascular (≈25% of ECF) compartments. The average adult has ≈5 L of blood volume (intravascular compartment) and a plasma volume of ≈35 L when the hematocrit is 40%. Although fluid from other clinically relevant ECF compartments (e.g., cerebrospinal fluid [CSF], urine) are analyzed in the clinical laboratory, most laboratory tests used to determine hydration status and electrolyte and acid-base status (e.g., electrolytes and $HCO_3^-$) are performed on samples from the *intravascular* compartment.

The minimum daily requirement for water can be estimated from urine (1200 to 1500 mL) and evaporative losses (≈400 to 700 mL from the skin and respiratory tract). Physical activity, environmental conditions, and disease all have dramatic effects on daily water (and electrolyte) requirements. On average, an adult must take in ≈1.5 to 2.0 L of water daily to maintain fluid balance. Table 36.1 lists common causes and signs and symptoms of expansion and contraction of the ECF compartment.

## WATER AND ELECTROLYTES—COMPOSITION OF BODY FLUIDS

The primary positively charged electrolytes (cations) are sodium ($Na^+$), potassium ($K^+$), calcium ($Ca^{2+}$), and magnesium ($Mg^{2+}$), whereas the negatively charged electrolytes (anions) include chloride ($Cl^-$), bicarbonate ($HCO_3^-$), phosphate ($HPO_4^{-2}$, $H_2PO_4^-$), sulfate ($SO_4^{2-}$), organic ions such as lactate, and negatively charged proteins (e.g. albumin). Electrolyte concentrations of the body fluid compartments are shown in Table 36.2. Plasma or serum $Na^+$, $K^+$, $Cl^-$, and $HCO_3^-$ concentrations, commonly analyzed in an *electrolyte profile*, provide the most relevant information about the osmotic, hydration, and acid-base status of the body. Although hydrogen ($H^+$) is a cation, its concentration is approximately 1 million-fold lower in plasma than the major electrolytes listed in Table 36.2 ($10^{-9}$ vs. $10^{-3}$ mol/L) and is negligible in terms of osmotic activity.

To maintain electroneutrality, any increase in the concentration of one anion is accompanied by a corresponding decrease in other anions, by an increase in one or more cations, or a combination of both. The converse is true for any decrease in anion concentration. In the case of polyvalent ions (e.g., $Ca^{2+}$, $Mg^{2+}$), it is important to distinguish between the substance concentration of the ion itself and the concentration of the ion charge. Thus, although the concentration of total calcium ions in normal plasma is ≈2.5 mmol/L, the concentration of the total calcium ion *charge* is 5.0 mmol/L (also called 5 milliequivalents per liter [mEq/L]).

## EXTRACELLULAR AND INTRACELLULAR COMPARTMENTS

### Plasma

Plasma generally has a volume of 1300 to 1800 mL/m² of body surface and constitutes approximately 5% of the body volume (≈3.5 L for a 66 kg subject). Total body volume is derived from body mass by using an estimated body density of 1.06 kg/L. Table 36.2 describes the electrolyte composition of plasma. Note: the mass concentration of water in normal plasma is approximately 0.933 kg/L, depending on the protein and lipid content (see "Electrolyte Exclusion Effect" in Chapter 24).

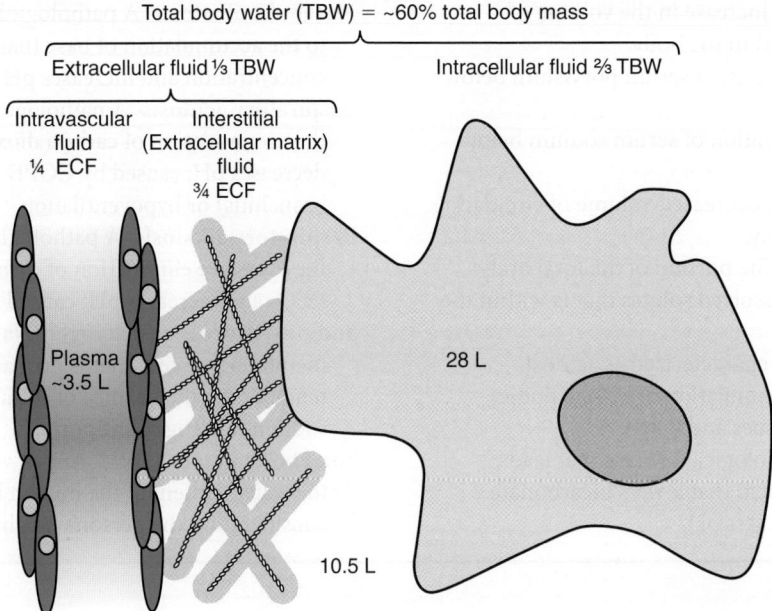

**Fig. 36.1** Volume and distribution of total body water (TBW). The intracellular and extracellular fluid compartments (ICF and ECF, respectively) are separated by cellular plasma membranes, and within the ECF, interstitial and intravascular fluids are separated by the capillary endothelium (*blue* cells). The volumes indicated represent water and not total volume. *blue*, Endothelial cells; *gray*, interstitial cell; *black cables*, collagen matrix fibers.

### TABLE 36.1    Causes and Clinical Manifestations of Changes in Extracellular Fluid Volume

|  | Clinical Manifestations | Causes |
|---|---|---|
| ECF loss | Thirst, anorexia, nausea, light-headedness, orthostatic hypotension, fainting, tachycardia, oliguria, decreased skin turgor and "sunken eyes," shock, coma, death | Trauma (and other causes of acute blood loss), "third-spacing" of fluid (e.g., burns, pancreatitis, peritonitis), vomiting, diarrhea, diuretics, renal or adrenal (i.e., sodium wasting) disease |
| ECF gain | Weight gain, edema, dyspnea (secondary to pulmonary edema), tachycardia, jugular venous distention, portal hypertension (ascites), esophageal varices | Heart failure, cirrhosis, nephrotic syndrome, iatrogenic (intravenous fluid overload) |

*ECF*, Extracellular fluid.

### TABLE 36.2    Electrolyte and Water Composition of Body Fluid Compartments

| Component | Plasma | Interstitial Fluid | Intracellular Fluid[a] |
|---|---|---|---|
| Volume, $H_2O$ (TBW = 42 L) | 3.5 L | 10.5 L | 28 L |
| $Na^+$ | 140 | 145 | 12 |
| $K^+$ | 4 | 4 | 156 |
| $Ca^{2+}$ | 2.4 | 2–3 | 0.3 |
| $Mg^{2+}$ | 1 | 0.5–1 | 13 |
| $Cl^-$ | 103 | 114 | 4 |
| $HCO_3^-$ | 27 | 31 | 12 |
| $HPO_4^{2-}$ | 1 | - | — |
| $SO_4^{2-}$ | 0.5 | - | — |

[a]These values are derived from skeletal muscle.
Except, values are expressed in millimoles per liter of *fluid*. Because the $H_2O$ content of plasma is ≈93% by volume, the corresponding electrolyte concentrations in plasma water are ≈10% higher.
*TBW*, Total body water.

## Interstitial Fluid

Interstitial fluid is essentially an ultrafiltrate of blood plasma, which surrounds tissue cells. When all extracellular spaces except plasma are included, the volume accounts for about 25% (10.5 L) of the total body volume (see Fig. 36.1). Plasma is separated from interstitial fluid by the capillary endothelial lining, which acts as a semipermeable membrane and allows passage of water and diffusible solutes but not compounds of high molecular mass such as proteins. The capillary endothelial lining is not completely impermeable to proteins, and in some pathologic conditions causing shock, such as bacterial sepsis, the permeability of the vascular endothelium increases dramatically, resulting in leakage of albumin from the vascular space, a reduction in the effective circulating volume, and hypotension.

## Intracellular Fluid

The exact composition of ICF is difficult to measure and varies by tissue type. Data for ICF (see Table 36.2), therefore, are considered only approximations. The ICF constitutes approximately two-thirds of the total body volume (see Fig. 36.1).

## Reasons for Differences in Composition of Body Fluids

The composition of the intracellular and extracellular fluids differ substantially from each other because of their separation by the cell membrane and as a consequence of both the Gibbs-Donnan equilibrium and the passive and active transport of ions and larger molecules.

## Gibbs-Donnan Equilibrium

Two solutions separated by a semipermeable membrane will establish an equilibrium, so that all ions are equally distributed in both compartments, so long as the solutes can freely pass through the membrane. At equilibrium, the total ion concentration and total concentration of osmotically active particles are equal on both sides of the membrane.

If the solutions separated by a membrane contain differing concentrations of ions that cannot freely move through the membrane (e.g., proteins), the distribution of diffusible ions (e.g., electrolytes) at the steady state will be unequal. The sum of the ion concentrations in one compartment however will be equal to the sum of ion concentrations in the other compartment (Fig. 36.2). This is referred to as Gibbs-Donnan equilibrium. Importantly, the law of electrical neutrality must also be obeyed for both compartments.

An example of the Gibbs-Donnan equilibrium and the law of electrical neutrality is the difference between $Cl^-$ concentration between plasma and CSF. As compared to plasma, CSF has a low protein concentration (nondiffusible ions), to balance both the osmotic and electrical equilibrium, the $Cl^-$ concentration in CSF is $\approx$15% higher than plasma. Osmotic pressure is normally identical inside and outside the cells because the cell membrane can correct concentration differences by excluding some small ions through active, energy-requiring transport processes. If these processes stop, the cell will swell and eventually will burst (osmotic lysis).

## Distribution of Ions by Active and Passive Transport

The electrolyte compositions of blood plasma and interstitial fluid are similar (both are ECFs) and differ markedly from that of ICF (see Table 36.2). The major ECF ions are $Na^+$, $Cl^-$, and $HCO_3^-$, but in ICF, the main ions are $K^+$, $Mg^{2+}$, organic phosphates, and protein. These unequal distributions of ions are the consequence of active and passive transport of ions and larger molecules. The difference in $Na^+$ concentration, for instance, is due to active transport of $Na^+$ from inside to outside the cell against its electrochemical gradient. This gradient is maintained predominantly by an active sodium pump deriving its energy from glycolysis-generated adenosine

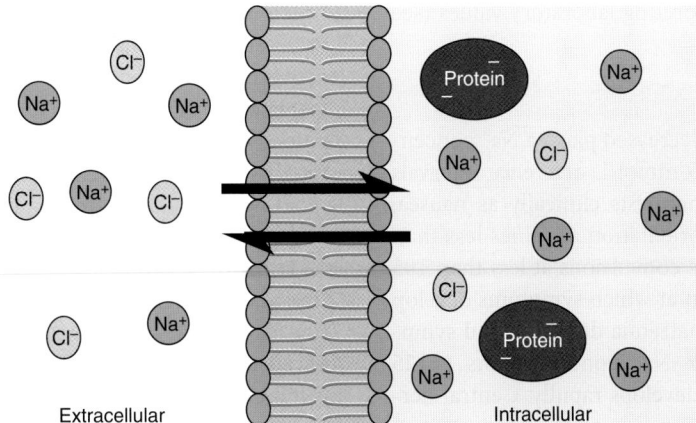

**Fig. 36.2** Diagram illustrating Gibbs-Donnan equilibrium across a cell membrane. The membrane is impermeable to negatively charged proteins but permeable to electrolytes (in this case sodium and chloride). To maintain electrical neutrality, the cations (sodium) move inside the cell, while the anions (chloride) move outside of the cell. This creates an uneven distribution of sodium and chloride across a permeable membrane, but electrical neutrality is maintained (total sum of ions on each side is the same). (From Berg M, El-Khoury JM, Cervinski MA. Disorders of water, electrolytes, and acid-base metabolism. In: Rifai N, ed. *Tietz Textbook of Laboratory Medicine*. 7th ed. St. Louis: Elsevier; 2022.)

triphosphate (ATP). A Na$^+$/K$^+$-ATPase frequently couples the active transport of Na$^+$ out of the ICF with transport of K$^+$ into the cell against the K$^+$ concentration gradient.

## ELECTROLYTES

Disorders of Na$^+$, K$^+$, Cl$^-$, and HCO$_3^-$ will now be separately considered, even though disorders of electrolyte and water homeostasis are directly connected and require systematic evaluation rather than an individual review of each ion. In all cases, it is useful to consider ion loss, gain, and processing steps, which collectively define the concentration.

## SODIUM

Disorders of Na$^+$ homeostasis can occur because of excessive loss, gain, or retention of Na$^+$, or that of H$_2$O. It is difficult to separate disorders of Na$^+$ and H$_2$O balance because of their close relationship in establishing normal osmolality in all body water compartments. As described in detail in Chapter 35, the primary organ for regulating body water and extracellular Na$^+$ is the kidney.

The kidney is responsible for maintaining electrolyte homeostasis across a wide range of gains and losses. It is important to recall that ~99% of filtered Na$^+$ is reabsorbed by the kidney, either in conjunction with Cl$^-$ and H$_2$O following passively, or in exchange for K$^+$ or H$^+$ to maintain electrical neutrality and osmotic equivalence.

The body's only nonrenal mechanism for restoring Na$^+$/H$_2$O homeostasis is ingestion of H$_2$O. Thirst is stimulated by decreased blood volume or hyperosmolality. Baroreceptors that influence renal handling of Na$^+$ and H$_2$O, and thirst, sense changes only in the intravascular blood volume and not the total ECF, while osmoreceptors in the brain sense the osmolality of the ECF surrounding the cells. Laboratory assessment of water and electrolyte disorders is made primarily from plasma; the clinician must assess the status of TBW and blood volume before interpreting laboratory values (see Table 36.1).

### Hyponatremia

**Hyponatremia** is defined as a decreased plasma Na$^+$ concentration (defined as <130 to 135 mmol/L; reference intervals vary by lab). Hyponatremia manifests clinically as nausea, generalized weakness, and disorientation at values less than 120 mmol/L, and delirium plus convulsions at less than 105 mmol/L. The Na$^+$ concentration at which symptoms develop depends on how quickly hyponatremia develops, and symptoms may manifest at higher Na$^+$ concentrations ($\approx$125 mmol/L) when hyponatremia develops rapidly. Central nervous system (CNS) symptoms are due to the movement of H$_2$O into cells to maintain osmotic balance and subsequent swelling of CNS cells. These symptoms can occur more rapidly in children, so there is a need to be particularly vigilant in the pediatric population.

Hyponatremia can be hypo-osmotic, hyperosmotic, or iso-osmotic. Thus measurement of plasma osmolality is an important initial step in the assessment of hyponatremia. Of these, the most common form is hypo-osmotic hyponatremia due to the large role that Na$^+$ plays in maintaining osmolality. Fig. 36.3 describes an algorithm for laboratory measurements and physical examination findings in the differential diagnosis of plasma Na$^+$ less than 135 mmol/L.

### Hypo-osmotic Hyponatremia

Typically when plasma Na$^+$ concentration is low, osmolality (calculated or measured) will also be low. This type of hyponatremia can be due to excess loss of Na$^+$ (**depletional hyponatremia**) or increased ECF volume (**dilutional hyponatremia**). Differentiating these initially requires clinical assessment of TBW and ECF volume by history and physical examination.

Depletional hyponatremia results from a loss of Na$^+$ from the ECF space that exceeds the concomitant loss of water. The net loss of Na$^+$ from the ECF space stimulates thirst and production of antidiuretic hormone (ADH), both of which contribute to the maintenance of hyponatremia. **Hypovolemia** is apparent in the physical examination (orthostatic hypotension, tachycardia, decreased skin turgor). If urine Na$^+$ is low (<10 mmol/L), the kidneys are properly retaining filtered Na$^+$ and the loss is extrarenal (not occurring as a result of kidney disease), most commonly from the gastrointestinal (GI) tract or skin (see Fig. 36.3). Preventing ongoing loss and restoring ECF volume with isotonic fluid is sufficient to correct hyponatremia in these situations. Alternatively, if urine Na$^+$ is increased in this setting (generally >20 mmol/L), renal loss of Na$^+$ is likely. Renal loss of Na$^+$ occurs with (1) osmotic diuresis, (2) use of diuretics (which inhibit reabsorption of Cl$^-$ and Na$^+$ in the ascending loop), (3) adrenal insufficiency (lack of aldosterone or cortisol prevents distal tubule reabsorption of Na$^+$), or (4) salt wasting nephropathies, as can occur with interstitial nephritis and tubular recovery after acute tubular necrosis or obstructive nephropathy. Renal loss of Na$^+$ in excess of H$_2$O can also occur in metabolic alkalosis from prolonged vomiting because increased renal HCO$_3^-$ excretion is accompanied by Na$^+$ ions. In this case, urine sodium is increased (>20 mmol/L), but urine chloride remains low. In proximal renal tubular acidosis (RTA) type 2, bicarbonate is lost because of a defect in HCO$_3^-$ reabsorption and is accompanied by Na$^+$ to maintain electrical neutrality. As with extrarenal Na$^+$ loss, management of hyponatremia attributable to renal Na$^+$ loss is centered on reversing the underlying cause and restoration of ECF volume.

**Dilutional hyponatremia** is a result of excess H$_2$O retention and often can be detected during the physical examination as edema. In advanced renal failure, water is retained because of decreased filtration and H$_2$O excretion. When ECF is increased but the circulating blood volume is decreased, as occurs in hepatic cirrhosis or nephrotic syndrome, a vicious cycle is established. The decreased blood volume is sensed by baroreceptors and results in increased aldosterone and ADH, even though ECF volume is excessive. The kidneys reabsorb Na$^+$ and H$_2$O in response to increased aldosterone and ADH to restore the blood volume, resulting in further increases in ECF and further dilution of Na$^+$.

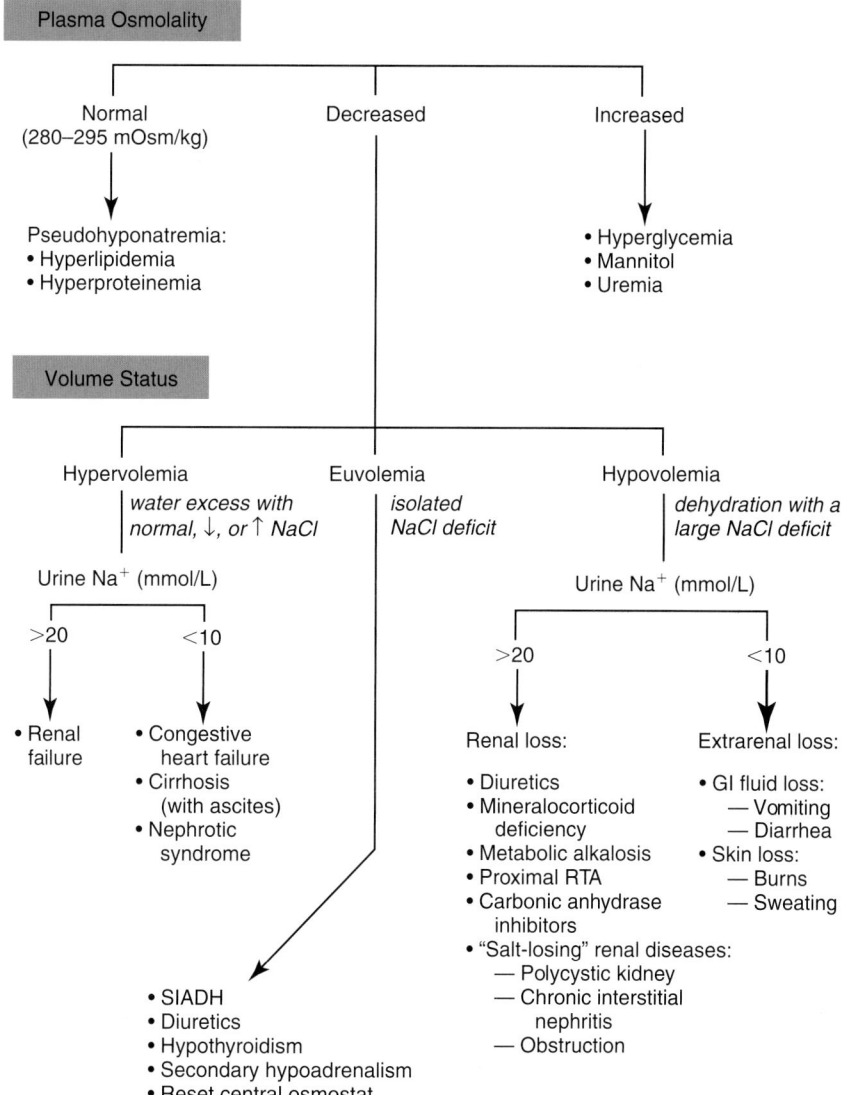

**Fig. 36.3** Algorithm for the differential diagnosis of hyponatremia. *GI*, Gastrointestinal; *RTA*, renal tubular acidosis; *SIADH*, syndrome of inappropriate secretion of antidiuretic hormone. (Modified from Kirkpatrick W, Kreisberg R. Acid-base and electrolyte disorders. In: Liu P, ed. *Blue Book of Diagnostic Tests.* Philadelphia: WB Saunders; 1986.)

In **hypo-osmotic hyponatremia** with a normal or euvolemic volume status, the most common causes are syndrome of inappropriate ADH (SIADH), primary polydipsia, and endocrine disorders such as secondary adrenal insufficiency and severe hypothyroidism (see Fig. 36.3). SIADH describes hyponatremia attributable to "inappropriate" ADH release, which stimulates excessive $H_2O$ retention and increased urine osmolality. In secondary adrenal insufficiency, due to lack of adrenocorticotropic hormone (ACTH), glucocorticoid secretion is impaired. In the absence of cortisol and ACTH, increased corticotropin-releasing hormone (CRH) secretion stimulates ADH release and causes hyponatremia. Severe hypothyroidism impairs free $H_2O$ excretion due to reduced cardiac output and glomerular filtration rate (GFR). Finally, euvolemic hyponatremia can also be found in primary polydipsia when water intake is greater than the renal capacity to excrete excess $H_2O$.

## Hyperosmotic Hyponatremia

Hyponatremia in the presence of increased quantities of other solutes in the ECF is the result of an extracellular shift of water or an intracellular shift of $Na^+$ to maintain osmotic balance between ECF and ICF compartments. The most common cause of this type of hyponatremia is severe hyperglycemia but may also occur in the setting of mannitol diuresis (see Fig. 36.3). As a rule, $Na^+$ is decreased by ≈1.6 to 2.0 mmol/L for every 100 mg/dL (5.6 mmol/L) increase in glucose above 100 mg/dL (5.6 mmol/L).

## Isosmotic Hyponatremia

If the measured $Na^+$ concentration in plasma is decreased, but measured plasma osmolality, glucose, and urea are normal, the most likely explanation is pseudohyponatremia caused by the *electrolyte exclusion effect* (see Chapter 24, Electrolytes and Blood Gases). This occurs when $Na^+$ is measured by an

## Hypernatremia

**Hypernatremia** (plasma $Na^+$ >150 mmol/L) is always hyperosmolar. Symptoms of hypernatremia are primarily neurologic (because of neuronal cell loss of $H_2O$ to the ECF) and include tremors, irritability, ataxia, confusion, and coma. As with hyponatremia, the speed at which hypernatremia develops determines the plasma $Na^+$ concentration at which symptoms occur. Acute development may cause symptoms at 160 mmol/L, whereas in chronic hypernatremia, symptoms may not occur until $Na^+$ exceeds 175 mmol/L.

In many cases, the symptoms of hypernatremia may be masked by underlying conditions. Hypernatremia rarely occurs in an alert patient with a normal thirst response and access to water. Most cases are observed in patients with altered mental status or infants, both of whom may not be capable of rehydrating themselves.

Hypernatremia arises in the setting of (1) hypovolemia (excessive water loss or failure to replace normal water losses), (2) **hypervolemia** (a net $Na^+$ gain in excess of water gain), or (3) normovolemia. Again, assessment of TBW status by physical examination and measurement of urine $Na^+$ and osmolality are important steps in establishing a diagnosis (Fig. 36.4).

### Hypovolemic Hypernatremia

Hypernatremia in the setting of decreased ECF is caused by renal or extrarenal loss of hypo-osmotic fluid, leading to dehydration. Once hypovolemia is established by physical examination, measurement of urine $Na^+$ and osmolality is used to determine the source of fluid loss. Patients with large extrarenal fluid losses will have concentrated urine (often >800 mOsmol/L) with low urine $Na^+$ (<20 mmol/L), reflecting a proper renal response to conserve $Na^+$ and water to restore ECF volume. Extrarenal causes include diarrhea, skin losses (burns, fever, or excessive sweating), and respiratory losses coupled with failure to replace the water (see Fig. 36.4). When extrarenal loss is excluded, and the patient has normal mental status and access to $H_2O$, a hypothalamic disorder (tumor or granuloma) inducing **diabetes insipidus** (DI) should be suspected. An additional consideration in the setting of poorly controlled diabetes mellitus is osmotic diuresis due to plasma glucose values greater than 600 mg/dL (33.3 mmol/L). This condition, referred to as hyperosmolar hyperglycemic nonketotic syndrome, occurs most commonly in elderly subjects with type 2 diabetes mellitus.

### Normovolemic Hypernatremia

Hypernatremia in the presence of normal ECF volume typically arises due to insensible losses through the lungs or skin and is often characterized by concentrated urine as the kidneys conserve water. Normovolemic hypernatremia arising from insensible losses is frequently a prelude to hypovolemic hypernatremia. Water or solute diuresis resulting in polyuria (generally defined as >3 L urine output/day) may also result in normovolemic hypernatremia (see Fig. 36.4). Solute diuresis is exemplified by the osmotic diuresis of diabetes mellitus and

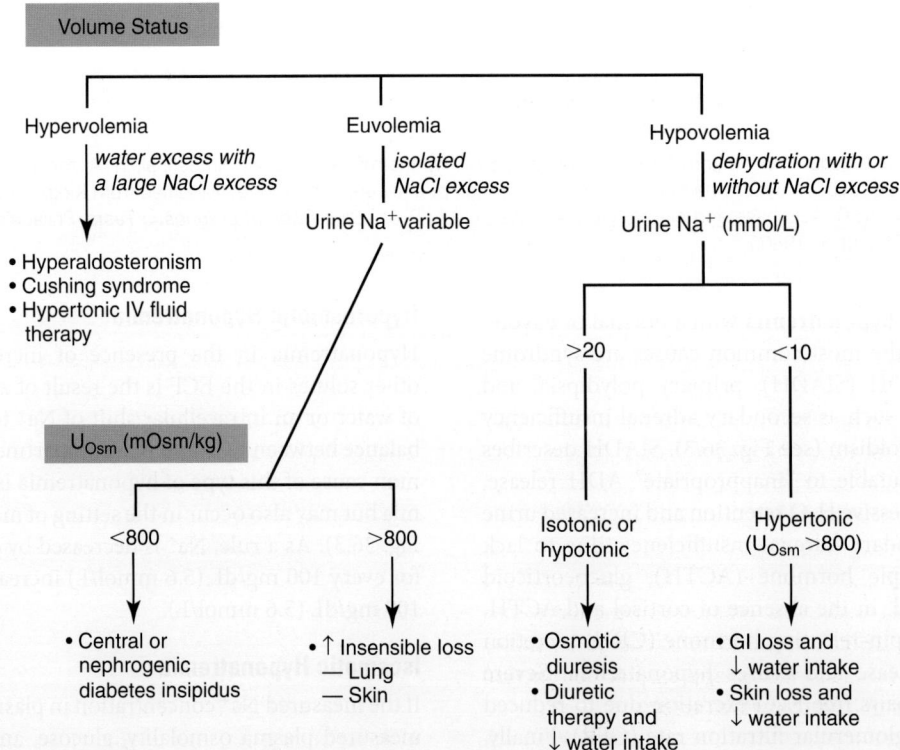

Fig. 36.4 Algorithm for the differential diagnosis of hypernatremia. (Modified from Kirkpatrick W, Kreisberg R. Acid-base and electrolyte disorders. In: Liu P, ed. *Blue Book of Diagnostic Tests*. Philadelphia: WB Saunders; 1986.)

generally is characterized by urine osmolality greater than 300 mOsmol/L and hyponatremia (see previous discussion in this chapter). Water diuresis, a manifestation of DI, is characterized by dilute urine (osmolality <250 mOsmol/L) and hypernatremia. DI can be central or nephrogenic. Central DI is due to decreased or absent ADH secretion resulting from head trauma, hypophysectomy, pituitary tumor, or granulomatous disease. Nephrogenic DI is due to renal resistance to ADH as a result of drugs (e.g., lithium, demeclocycline, amphotericin); electrolyte disorders (e.g., hypercalcemia, hypokalemia); sickle cell anemia; or Sjögren syndrome. When thirst and access to water are uncompromised, many patients with DI will remain normonatremic since their free water losses are offset by intake. Such patients only display symptoms of polyuria and polydipsia. However, overt hypernatremia can develop with the progression of underlying causes, impaired thirst, or restricted access to water. Administration of ADH (in the form of desmopressin) can be used to treat central DI, although patients with nephrogenic DI may be resistant to it.

### Hypervolemic Hypernatremia

The presence of excess TBW and hypernatremia indicates a net gain of water and Na$^+$, with Na$^+$ gain in excess of water (see Fig. 36.4). This rare condition is observed most commonly in hospitalized patients receiving hypertonic saline or sodium bicarbonate.

## POTASSIUM

Potassium (K$^+$) is the major intracellular cation, where it is found at a concentration of ~150 mmol/L. In contrast, only ~2% of total body K$^+$ is present in the ECF/plasma at a concentration of ~4 mmol/L. Despite this concentration differential, plasma K$^+$ is largely a good indicator of total K$^+$ stores. Disturbance of K$^+$ homeostasis has serious consequences ranging from muscle weakness and confusion to arrhythmias and cardiac arrest. Because of the physiological importance of K$^+$, the laboratory needs to recognize situations that may yield misleading K$^+$ results, such as hemolysis (falsely high K$^+$ concentration), and pseudohypokalemia (falsely low K$^+$ concentration).

### Hypokalemia

Causes of hypokalemia (plasma K$^+$ <3.5 mmol/L) are classified as redistribution of extracellular K$^+$ into ICF, or true K$^+$ deficits, caused by decreased intake or loss of potassium-rich body fluids (Fig. 36.5). A decrease in extracellular K$^+$ (hypokalemia) is characterized by muscle weakness, irritability, and paralysis. Severe hypokalemia (plasma K$^+$ concentrations <3.0 mmol/L) is often associated with neuromuscular symptoms and indicates a critical degree of intracellular depletion. At lower concentrations, tachycardia and cardiac conduction defects develop and can lead to cardiac arrest.

### Redistribution

Intracellular redistribution of K$^+$ is exemplified by a fall in plasma K$^+$ following insulin therapy for diabetic

hyperglycemia. Insulin plays a crucial role in maintaining the intracellular distribution of K$^+$ through active cellular transport as well as glucose control. Redistribution hypokalemia is also a feature of alkalosis, in which K$^+$ moves from ECF into cells in exchange for H$^+$ efflux and renal conservation of H$^+$ at the expense of urinary K$^+$ loss. Other causes of intracellular redistribution are listed in Fig. 36.5. Clinically, redistributive hypokalemia is generally a transient phenomenon that is reversed once underlying conditions are corrected. Hypokalemia is highly prevalent in cancer patients but must be differentiated from pseudohypokalemia. Pseudohypokalemia can occur in settings of very high white blood cell or platelet counts and is caused by high concentrations of metabolically active cells taking up K$^+$ *after* blood is collected. This may be seen in some patients within a leukemic blast crisis where there can be a time-dependent transport of K$^+$ into the leukemic cells. In these settings, it is important to process the samples as quickly as possible.

### True Potassium Deficit

Hypokalemia reflecting true total body deficits of K$^+$ can be classified into renal and nonrenal losses (see Fig. 36.5). If urine excretion of K$^+$ is less than 30 mmol/day, it can be concluded that the kidneys are properly functioning and are reabsorbing K$^+$. The cause may be decreased K$^+$ intake or extrarenal loss of K$^+$-rich fluid. Causes of decreased intake include chronic starvation and postoperative intravenous fluid therapy with K$^+$-poor solutions. GI loss of K$^+$ occurs most commonly with diarrhea and loss of gastric fluid through vomiting.

Urine excretion exceeding 30 mmol/day in a hypokalemic setting is inappropriate and indicates that the kidneys are the primary source of K$^+$ loss. Renal losses of K$^+$ may occur during the diuretic (recovery) phase of acute tubular necrosis and during states of excess mineralocorticoid (primary or secondary aldosteronism) or glucocorticoid (Cushing syndrome). Excess mineralocorticoids (aldosterone) or glucocorticoids (cortisol) cause increased distal tubular Na$^+$ reabsorption and K$^+$ excretion (see Chapter 41, Adrenal Cortex). Renal loss of K$^+$ is also caused by thiazide and loop diuretics. In addition to the redistribution of K$^+$ into cells in an alkalotic setting, K$^+$ can be lost from the kidneys in exchange for reclaimed H$^+$ ions. This cause of true hypokalemia is associated with low urine Cl$^-$ and alkaline urine. Simplistically, Na$^+$ and H$^+$ move in the opposite direction of K$^+$, and urine K$^+$ provides clues as to the underlying cause of abnormalities. True potassium deficit requires replacement of potassium. Although there are many dietary sources of potassium, such as potatoes, broccoli, bananas, salmon, and legumes, significant K$^+$ losses may require oral or intravenous supplementation with potassium chloride.

### Hyperkalemia

Hyperkalemia (plasma K$^+$ >5.0 mmol/L) is a result of (singly or in combination) (1) redistribution, (2) increased intake, or (3) increased retention. High extracellular K$^+$ (hyperkalemia) concentrations may produce symptoms of disorientation, weakness, tingling, flaccid paralysis of the extremities,

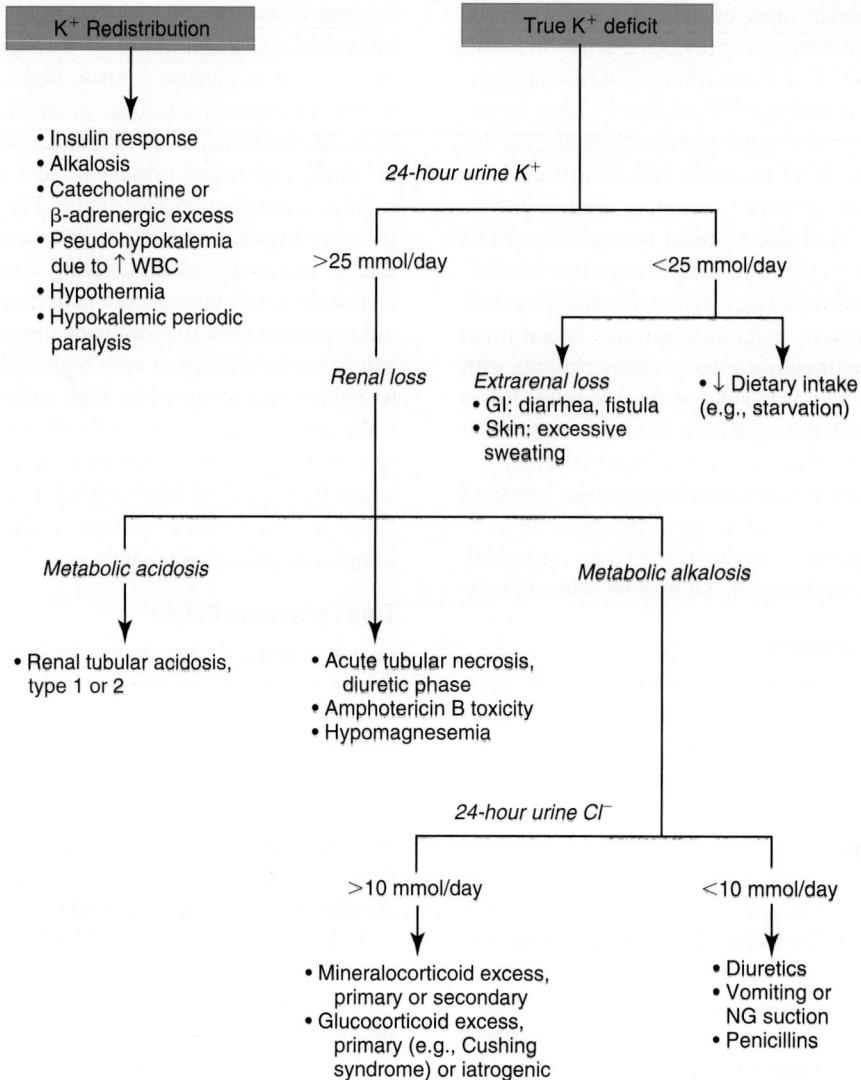

**Fig. 36.5** Algorithm for the differential diagnosis of hypokalemia. *GI,* Gastrointestinal; *NG,* nasogastric; *WBC,* white blood cell. (Modified from Kirkpatrick W, Kreisberg R. Acid-base and electrolyte disorders. In: Liu P, ed. *Blue Book of Diagnostic Tests.* Philadelphia: WB Saunders; 1986.)

weakness of the respiratory muscles, bradycardia, and cardiac conduction defects. Prolonged, severe hyperkalemia (plasma $K^+$ concentrations >7.0 mmol/L) can lead to peripheral vascular collapse and cardiac arrest. Symptoms or electrocardiogram (EKG) abnormalities are usually present at $K^+$ concentrations greater than 6.5 mmol/L. Potassium concentrations greater than 10.0 mmol/L in most cases are fatal, although fatalities can occur at significantly lower values.

In addition, preanalytical conditions—such as hemolysis, thrombocytosis (>106/μL), and leukocytosis (>105/μL) together with delayed sample analysis—have been known to cause marked pseudohyperkalemia, as described in detail in Chapter 24 (Electrolytes and Blood Gases). Collection of blood in a tube containing the wrong anticoagulant ($K_2EDTA/K_3EDTA$) can also falsely increase $K^+$. Some useful clues that indicate $K^+$ concentrations are falsely elevated include very high potassium in asymptomatic outpatients, pink/red plasma (reflecting hemolysis), and in the case of

$K_2EDTA$ contamination, extreme hypocalcemia due to chelation of serum calcium by EDTA.

### Redistribution

The transfer of intracellular $K^+$ into ECF invariably occurs in acidemia as $K^+$ shifts outward as the result of pH-induced changes in $Na^+/K^+$-ATPase activity. When acidemia is corrected, normokalemia will be restored rapidly. Extracellular redistribution of $K^+$ may also occur in (1) tissue hypoxia; (2) insulin deficiency (e.g., diabetic ketoacidosis); (3) massive intravascular hemolysis; (4) severe burns; (5) intense and sustained muscular activity, as in status epilepticus; (6) rhabdomyolysis; (7) tumor lysis syndrome, as well as (8) iatrogenic causes. Redistributive hyperkalemia can be corrected by reversing the aberrations that cause $K^+$ to shift out of cells. Insulin and sodium bicarbonate are commonly used and have a quick onset of action, particularly in the diabetic or acidemic setting.

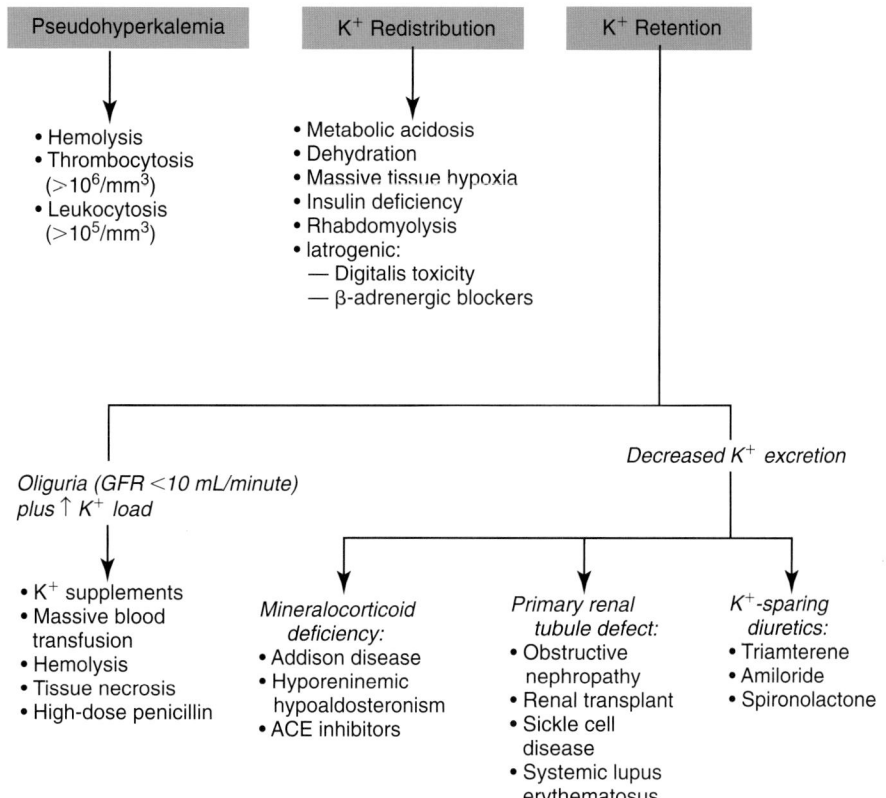

**Fig. 36.6** Algorithm for the differential diagnosis of hyperkalemia. *ACE,* Angiotensin-converting enzyme. (Modified from Kirkpatrick W, Kreisberg R. Acid-base and electrolyte disorders. In: Liu P, ed. *Blue Book of Diagnostic Tests.* Philadelphia: WB Saunders; 1986.)

## Potassium Retention

When glomerular filtration or renal tubular function is decreased, hyperkalemia will often occur due to impaired ability to excrete excess potassium. With mild renal failure, hyperkalemia may not develop, and if it does it is seldom prolonged. Decreased excretion of $K^+$ in moderate and acute renal disease and end-stage renal failure (with oliguria or anuria) are the most common causes of prolonged hyperkalemia (Fig. 36.6). Hyperkalemia occurs along with $Na^+$ depletion in adrenocortical insufficiency (e.g., Addison disease, Chapter 41) because diminished $Na^+$ reabsorption results in decreased tubular $K^+$ secretion. Drugs that block the production of aldosterone, such as inhibitors of angiotensin-converting enzyme (ACE inhibitors; e.g., lisinopril), nonsteroidal antiinflammatory drugs, and angiotensin II receptor blockers, may also cause hyperkalemia. Excess administration of potassium-sparing diuretics that block distal tubular $K^+$ secretion (e.g., triamterene, spironolactone) may also cause hyperkalemia.

## CHLORIDE

In the absence of acid-base disturbances, $Cl^-$ concentrations in plasma generally will follow those of $Na^+$. However, determination of plasma $Cl^-$ concentration is useful in the differential diagnosis of acid-base disturbances and is essential for calculating the anion gap. Fluctuations in serum or plasma

$Cl^-$ have little clinical consequence but do serve as signs of an underlying disturbance in fluid or acid-base homeostasis. The specific replacement of chloride is rarely targeted at chloride deficit independently, but it is a cornerstone of management for metabolic alkalosis.

### Hypochloremia

In general, causes of hypochloremia parallel causes of hyponatremia. Persistent gastric secretion and prolonged vomiting result in significant loss of $Cl^-$. Ultimately this results in hypochloremic alkalosis (low $Cl^-$ with excess base in the form of $HCO_3^-$) due to retention of $HCO_3^-$ by the nephron to maintain electroneutrality in conjunction with reabsorption of the filtered $Na^+$ load. Respiratory acidosis, which is accompanied by increased $HCO_3^-$, is another common cause of decreased $Cl^-$ with normal $Na^+$. This again results from the need to maintain electroneutrality where the compensatory increase in $HCO_3^-$ is balanced with $Cl^-$ excretion in urine and shifts of $Cl^-$ into cells.

### Hyperchloremia

Increased plasma $Cl^-$ concentration, like increased $Na^+$ concentration, occurs with dehydration, prolonged diarrhea with loss of sodium bicarbonate, DI, and overtreatment with normal saline solutions, which have a $Cl^-$ content of 150 mmol/L. A rise in $Cl^-$ concentration may also be seen in respiratory alkalosis because of renal compensation for excreting $HCO_3^-$.

## ACID-BASE PHYSIOLOGY

Normal metabolic processes result in the production of large amounts of metabolic acids. These products of metabolism are transported to the lungs and kidneys via the ECF and blood with no appreciable change in the ECF pH and with only a minimal difference between arterial (pH 7.35 to 7.45) and venous (pH 7.32 to 7.42) blood. This is accomplished by the buffering capacity of blood and by respiratory and renal regulatory mechanisms.

## ACID-BASE BALANCE AND ACID-BASE STATUS

Interpretation of the acid-base balance in physiology involves an accounting of the carbonic ($H_2CO_3$, $HCO_3^-$, $CO_3^{2-}$, and $CO_2$) and noncarbonic acids and conjugate bases in terms of input (intake plus metabolic production) and output (excretion plus metabolic conversion) over a given time interval. For example, during a 24-hour period, a 70 kg person exhales approximately 20 moles of $CO_2$ (volatile form of carbonic acid) through the lungs, and excretes about 70 to 100 mmol (or ≈1 mmol/kg) of nonvolatile acids (mainly sulfuric and phosphoric acids) through the kidneys.

### Acid-Base Parameters—Definitions and Abbreviations

*Acids* are chemical substances that can donate protons ($H^+$ ions) in solution, and *bases* are substances that accept protons. Strong acids readily give up $H^+$, whereas strong bases readily accept $H^+$. Thus the conjugate base of a strong acid is a weak base and vice versa.

Acidemia is defined as an arterial blood pH less than 7.35, and alkalemia indicates an arterial blood pH greater than 7.45. *Acidosis* and *alkalosis* refer to pathologic states that often lead to acidemia or alkalemia.

#### pH and pK

The pH of a solution is defined as the negative logarithm of the hydrogen ion activity (pH = −log $aH^+$). A decrease in 1 pH unit represents a 10-fold increase in $H^+$ activity. pH is measured using potentiometry (see Chapter 24) and is an assessment of $H^+$ ion activity. In the setting of pH assessment, an assumption is made that $H^+$ activity is equivalent to

concentration. The $H^+$ concentration of blood is thus equal to 40 nmol/L at pH 7.4.

The pK (also known as pK′ and pKa) is the pH at which an acid is half-dissociated, existing as equal proportions of acid and conjugate base. Acids have pK values less than 7.0, whereas bases have pK values greater than 7.0. The lower the pK, the stronger the acid, and the higher the pK, the stronger the conjugate base.

The pH of plasma is the function of two independent variables:
1. $PCO_2$, which is regulated by the lungs and represents the acid component of the carbonic acid/bicarbonate buffer system
2. The concentration of titratable base (base excess or deficit, which is defined later), which is regulated by the kidneys

### Bicarbonate and Dissolved Carbon Dioxide

Bicarbonate is the second largest fraction (behind $Cl^-$) of plasma anions. Conventionally, it is defined to include (1) plasma bicarbonate ion ($HCO_3^-$), (2) carbonate ion ($CO_3^{2-}$), and (3) $CO_2$ bound in plasma carbamino compounds (R-C-NH-COOH). Actual bicarbonate ion concentration is not measured in clinical laboratories. The analyte usually measured in plasma is total $CO_2$, which includes bicarbonate and dissolved $CO_2$ ($dCO_2$) but is often referred to as "serum bicarb".

### Henderson-Hasselbalch Equation

The Henderson-Hasselbalch equation is described in detail in Chapter 24. However, it is important to review here because it enhances understanding of pH regulation of body fluids as it relates to compensatory mechanisms in acid-base disturbances. The equation described in Chapter 24 can be written as follows:

$$pH = 6.1 + \log \frac{cHCO_3^-}{cdCO_2}$$

where $cdCO_2$ is the concentration of dissolved $CO_2$ and is equal to α (0.0306 mmol/L per mm Hg) × $pCO_2$ and 6.1 is the pK′ for the carbonic acid/bicarbonate system.

The average normal ratio of the concentrations of bicarbonate and $dCO_2$ in plasma is 25 (mmol/L)/1.25 (mmol/L) = 20/1. It follows then that any change in the concentration of bicarbonate or $dCO_2$ relative to each other must be accompanied by a change in pH. Such changes in this important ratio can occur through a change in $c$ $HCO_3^-$ (the renal component) or in $PCO_2$ (the respiratory component). Clinical conditions characterized as *metabolic* disturbances of acid-base balance are classified as primary disturbances in $cHCO_3^-$. Those characterized as *respiratory* disturbances are classified as primary disturbances in $cdCO_2$ ($PCO_2$). Various compensatory mechanisms attempting to reestablish the normal ratio of $cHCO_3^-/cdCO_2$ may result in changes in bicarbonate concentration, $dCO_2$ concentration, or both. Applications of the Henderson-Hasselbalch equation to human acid-base physiology are illustrated in Fig. 36.7.

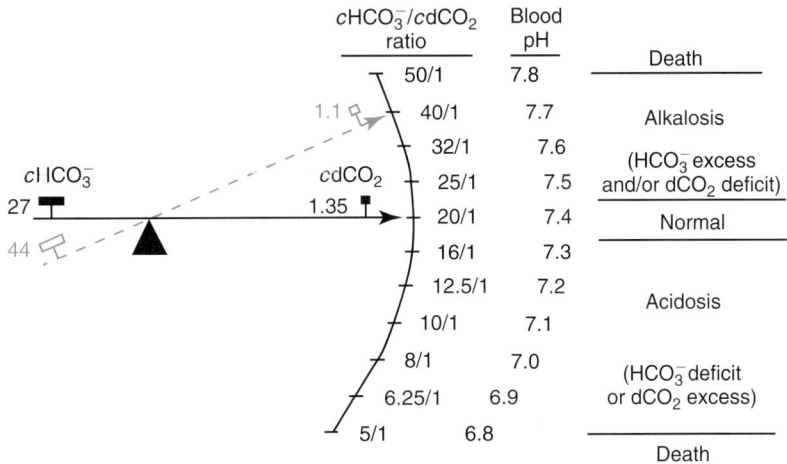

**Fig. 36.7** Diagram demonstrating the relation between pH and the ratio of bicarbonate concentration to the concentration of dissolved $CO_2$. If the ratio in blood is 20:1 ($cHCO_3^-$ = 27 mmol/L/$cdCO_2$ = 1.35 mmol/L), the resultant pH will be 7.4, as demonstrated by the *solid beam*. The *dotted line* shows a case of uncompensated alkalosis (bicarbonate excess) with $cHCO_3^-$ of 44 mmol/L and a $cdCO_2$ of 1.1 mmol/L. The ratio, therefore, is 40:1, and the resultant pH is 7.7. In a case of uncompensated acidosis, the pointer of the balance would point to a pH between 6.8 and 7.35, depending on the $cHCO_3^-/cdCO_2$ ratio. (From Weisberg HF. A better understanding of anion-cation ["acid-base"] balance. *Surg Oncol Clin North Am.* 1959;39:93–120.)

## BUFFER SYSTEMS AND THEIR ROLE IN REGULATING THE pH OF BODY FLUIDS

A buffer is a mixture of a weak acid and a salt of its conjugate base that resists changes in pH when a strong acid or base is added to the solution. If concentrations of the acid and base components of a buffer are equal, the pH will equal the p$K$. Generally, buffers work best at resisting pH changes in the interval of ±1 pH unit of its p$K$ and are more effective at higher molar concentrations. The action of buffers in the regulation of body pH can be demonstrated by using the bicarbonate buffer system as an example. If a strong acid is added to a solution containing $HCO_3^-$, and $H_2CO_3$, the $H^+$ will react with $HCO_3^-$ to form more $H_2CO_3$, and subsequently $CO_2$ and $H_2O$. The $H^+$ ions are thereby bound, and the increase in the $H^+$ concentration will be minimal.

$$H^+ + HCO_3^- \rightleftharpoons H_2CO_3 \rightleftharpoons CO_2 + H_2O$$

### Bicarbonate and Carbonic Acid Buffer System

The most important buffer of plasma is the bicarbonate/carbonic acid pair even though its p$K$ is 6.1, and normal plasma pH is 7.4. The normal bicarbonate/d$CO_2$ ratio is 20:1, which is outside the 10:1 or 1:10 ratio at which buffers work best. However, the effectiveness of the bicarbonate buffer is based on the fact that the lungs can readily dispose of or retain $CO_2$, and is present at higher concentrations than other buffers with the exception of Hb. In addition, the renal tubules can regulate bicarbonate through increased or decreased reclamation (see Chapter 35).

### Phosphate Buffer System

At a plasma pH of 7.4, the ratio $cHPO_4^{2-}/cH_2PO_4^-$ is 4 : 1 (p$K'$ = 6.8). The total concentration of this buffer in both erythrocytes and plasma accounts for about 5% of the nonbicarbonate buffer value of plasma. Organic phosphate, in the form of 2,3-diphosphoglycerate (present in erythrocytes in a concentration of approximately 4.5 mmol/L), accounts for about 16% of the nonbicarbonate buffer value of erythrocytes and plays a vital role in the titration and excretion of acids in urine.

### Plasma Protein and Hemoglobin Buffer System

Proteins, especially albumin, account for the greatest portion (>90%) of the nonbicarbonate buffer value of plasma. The imidazole groups of histidine (p$K$ ~7.3) are the most important components of proteins in the physiological pH range encountered in plasma. For example, albumin contains 16 histidine residues per molecule.

The hemoglobin within erythrocytes also plays a significant role in the physiologic buffering system of whole blood through the diffusion of $CO_2$ produced by cellular respiration in peripheral tissues into the erythrocyte and its conversion to $HCO_3^-$ and $H^+$ through the action of carbonic anhydrase. The $H^+$ initially decreases the erythrocyte fluid pH; however, this decrease in pH is rapidly compensated by the release of oxygen to the tissues from $O_2Hb$, which involves the conversion of stronger acid ($O_2Hb$) into weaker acid (HHb) that readily accepts the $H^+$. The reduced hemoglobin (HHb) also contributes to the buffering capacity of whole blood by binding $CO_2$ in the form of carbamino-$CO_2$. The $HCO_3^-$ produced by the action of carbonic anhydrase is shunted out of

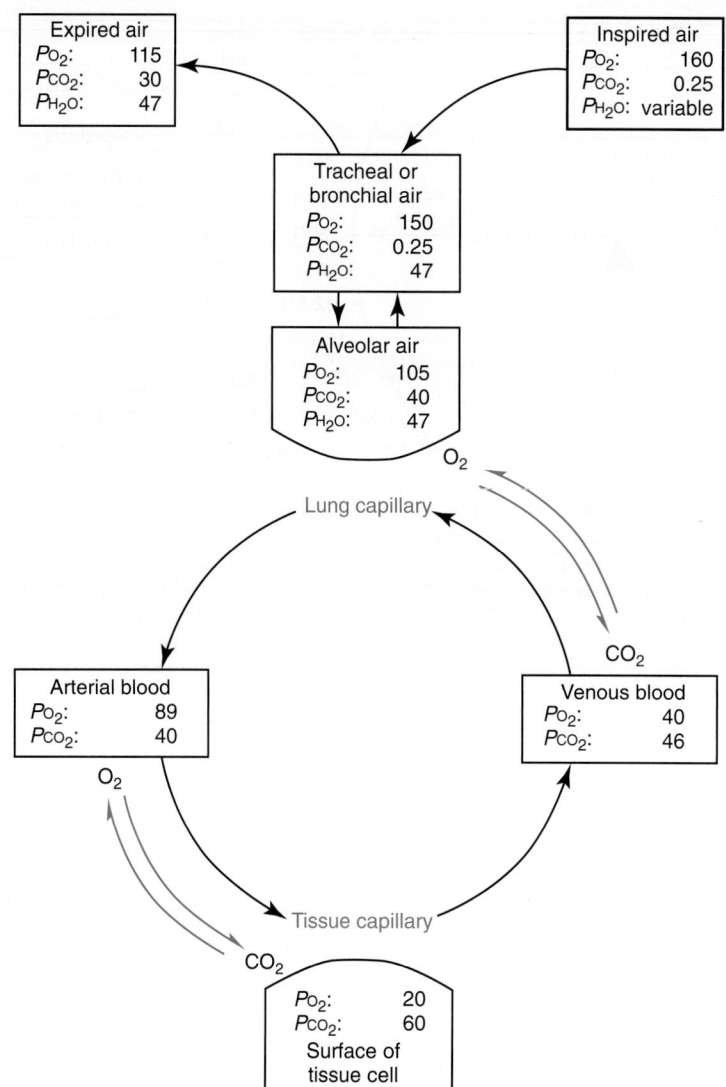

**Fig. 36.8** Partial pressures of oxygen and carbon dioxide in air, blood, and tissue. Values shown are approximations in mm Hg and are calculated assuming a 5% shunt. *Blue arrows* show directions of gradients. (Modified from Tietz NW. *Fundamentals of Clinical Chemistry*. 3rd ed. Philadelphia: WB Saunders; 1987.)

the erythrocyte in exchange for plasma $Cl^-$ to maintain electroneutrality referred to as the *chloride shift*. In the alveoli, the low $PCO_2$ and high $PO_2$ cause a reversal of reactions detailed briefly above to remove $CO_2$ (and thus acid) from circulation.

## RESPIRATORY MECHANISM IN THE REGULATION OF ACID-BASE BALANCE

In addition to supplying $O_2$ to tissue cells for normal metabolism, the respiratory mechanism contributes to maintenance of normal body pH through elimination or retention of $CO_2$ in metabolic acidosis and alkalosis, respectively.

### Exchange of Gases in the Lungs and Peripheral Tissues

Diffusion of $O_2$ and $CO_2$ across alveolar and cell membranes is governed by gradients in the partial pressure of each gas (Fig. 36.8). Dry air inspired at a pressure of 1 atm (760 mm Hg) consists of 21% $O_2$ ($PO_2 \approx 160$ mm Hg), 0.03% $CO_2$ ($PCO_2$

$\approx 0.25$ mm Hg), 78% nitrogen, and $\approx 0.1\%$ other inert gases. As inspired air passes over the mucous membranes of the upper respiratory tract, it is warmed to 37°C, becomes saturated with water vapor, and mixes with air in the respiratory tree and alveoli, resulting in partial pressures at the alveolar membrane of $\approx 105$ mm Hg for $O_2$, $\approx 40$ mm Hg for $CO_2$, and $\approx 47$ mm Hg for $H_2O$. Venous blood on the opposite side of the alveolar membrane has $PO_2 \approx 40$ mm Hg and $PCO_2 \approx 46$ mm Hg. Thus the gradient for $O_2$ is inward, toward the blood, and for $CO_2$, it is outward, toward the alveoli. $CO_2$ removal is so efficient that the $PCO_2$ in expired air is more than 100 times the $PCO_2$ in inspired air (see Fig. 36.8). In arterial blood, the $PO_2$ is slightly lower than in alveolar air (90 to 100 vs. 105 mm Hg) as the result of shunting of about 5% of blood that does not equilibrate.

At the arterial end of capillaries in peripheral tissues, the $PO_2$ of 83 to 110 mm Hg is substantially higher than the average $PO_2$ at the surface of tissue cells (20 mm Hg), and the $PCO_2$ at 40 mm Hg is substantially lower than that in the cells

(50 to 70 mm Hg). Thus, in the tissue capillary, the gradient for $O_2$ is inward to the cell; for $CO_2$, it is outward to the capillary blood.

# RENAL MECHANISMS IN THE REGULATION OF ACID-BASE BALANCE

The average pH of plasma and of the glomerular filtrate is $\approx 7.4$, whereas the average urinary pH is $\approx 6.0$, reflecting renal excretion of nonvolatile acids. Various functions of the kidneys respond to different alterations in acid-base status. In the case of acidosis, excretion of acids is increased and base is conserved; in alkalosis, the opposite occurs. The pH of the urine changes correspondingly and may vary in *random* specimens from pH 4.5 to 8.0. The ability to excrete variable amounts of acid or base makes the kidney the final defense mechanism against changes in body pH. Renal excretion of acid and conservation of $HCO_3^-$ occur through several mechanisms, including (1) $Na^+$-$H^+$ exchange, (2) production of ammonia and excretion of $NH_4^+$, and (3) reclamation of $HCO_3^-$.

## Na⁺-H⁺ Exchange

Nearly all mammalian cells contain a plasma membrane ATP-hydrolyzing protein capable of exchanging sodium ions for protons—the so-called $Na^+$-$H^+$ exchanger. In the renal tubules, the $Na^+$-$H^+$ exchangers extrude $H^+$ ions into the tubular fluid in exchange for $Na^+$ ions, and their activity is enhanced in states of acidosis and is inhibited in alkalosis.

The proximal tubules, however, cannot maintain an $H^+$ gradient of more than $\approx 1$ pH unit, whereas the distal tubules cannot maintain more than $\approx 3$ pH units. Thus maximum urine acidity is reached at $\approx$pH 4.4.

Potassium ions compete with $H^+$ at the $Na^+$-$H^+$ exchangers in the renal tubule. If intracellular $K^+$ concentration of renal tubular cells is high, more $K^+$ and less $H^+$ are exchanged for $Na^+$. As a result, urine is less acidic, and body fluid pH decreases. If $K^+$ is depleted, more $H^+$ ions are exchanged for $Na^+$; urine becomes more acidic and body fluids more alkaline. In essence, hyperkalemia contributes to acidosis and hypokalemia to alkalosis.

## Renal Production of Ammonia and Excretion of Ammonium Ions

Renal tubular cells are able to generate ammonia from glutamine and other amino acids derived from muscle and liver cells according to the following reaction:

The ammonium ion produced dissociates into ammonia and hydrogen ions to a degree dependent on the pH. Hydrogen ions secreted into the tubular lumen through the $Na^+$-$H^+$ exchangers lower the pH of tubular fluid, and at the acidic pH of urine, the equilibrium between $NH_4^+$ and $NH_3$ shifts markedly to the left, strongly favoring the formation of $NH_4^+$. Due to its positive charge, the $NH_4^+$ formed in the tubular lumen cannot readily cross cell membranes and is trapped in the tubule to be excreted in urine with phosphate, chloride, or sulfate anions.

## Excretion of H⁺ as H₂PO₄⁻

Hydrogen ions secreted into the tubular lumen by the $Na^+$-$H^+$ exchanger may also react with $HPO_4^{2-}$ to form $H_2PO_4^-$. Acidemia increases phosphate excretion and thus provides an additional buffer for reaction with $H^+$. A decrease in the GFR results in a decrease in $H_2PO_4^-$ excretion.

## Reclamation of Filtered Bicarbonate

The unmodified glomerular filtrate has the same concentration of $HCO_3^-$ as plasma; however, with increasing acidification of proximal tubule fluid, the $HCO_3^-$ concentration is decreased. The $H^+$ excreted into the proximal tubule by the $Na^+$-$H^+$ exchanger is buffered by $HCO_3^-$ and converted to $H_2CO_3$ by carbonic anhydrase, which then dissociates to form $CO_2$ and $H_2O$. The increased $CO_2$ in the tubular fluid freely diffuses into tubular cells, where it reacts with $H_2O$ through the action of cytoplasmic carbonic anhydrase forming $H_2CO_3$ and ultimately $HCO_3^-$ and $H^+$. The $HCO_3^-$ formed in this process is used to restore or maintain normal plasma pH.

Normally, $\approx 90\%$ of filtered $HCO_3^-$ (or about 4500 mmol/day) is reclaimed in the proximal tubule. When plasma $HCO_3^-$ concentration increases above $\approx 28$ mmol/L, the capacity of the proximal and distal tubules to reclaim $HCO_3^-$ is exceeded and $HCO_3^-$ is excreted in the urine. Type II RTA is caused by a decreased ability to reabsorb $HCO_3^-$ in the proximal tubules, leading to a decrease in blood pH.

# CONDITIONS ASSOCIATED WITH ABNORMAL ACID-BASE STATUS AND ABNORMAL ELECTROLYTE COMPOSITION OF BLOOD

Blood acid-base abnormalities are accompanied by characteristic changes in plasma electrolyte concentrations. Hydrogen ions cannot accumulate without concomitant accumulation of anions, such as $Cl^-$ or lactate, or without exchange for cations, such as $K^+$ or $Na^+$. Consequently, plasma electrolyte composition is often determined with measurements of blood gases and pH to assess acid-base disturbances.

Acid-base disturbances are traditionally classified as (1) metabolic acidosis, (2) metabolic alkalosis, (3) respiratory acidosis, or (4) respiratory alkalosis with renal and respiratory compensatory responses (Table 36.3).

An acidosis can only occur as the result of one (or a combination) of three mechanisms: (1) increased addition of acid, (2) decreased elimination of acid, and (3) increased loss of

## TABLE 36.3    Classification and Characteristics of Simple Acid-Base Disorders

| | Primary Change | Compensatory Response | Expected Compensation |
|---|---|---|---|
| **Metabolic** | | | |
| Acidosis | ↓ $cHCO_3^-$ | ↓ $PCO_2$ | $PCO_2 = 1.5\ (cHCO_3^-) + 8 \pm 2$ <br> $PCO_2$ falls by 1–1.3 mm Hg for each mmol/L fall in $cHCO_3^-$ <br> Last two digits of pH = $PCO_2$ (e.g., if $PCO_2$ = 28, pH = 7.28) <br> $cHCO_3^-$ + 15 = last two digits of pH ($cHCO_3^-$ = 15, pH = 7.30) |
| Alkalosis | ↑ $cHCO_3^-$ | ↑ $PCO_2$ | $PCO_2$ increases 6 mm Hg for each 10-mmol/L rise in $cHCO_3^-$  $cHCO_3^-$ + 15 = last two digits of pH ($cHCO_3^-$ = 35, pH = 7.50) |
| **Respiratory** | | | |
| *Acidosis* | | | |
| Acute | ↑ $PCO_2$ | ↑ $cHCO_3^-$ | $cHCO_3^-$ increases by 1 mmol/L for each 10 mm Hg rise in $PCO_2$ |
| Chronic | ↑ $PCO_2$ | ↑ $cHCO_3^-$ | $cHCO_3^-$ increases by 3.5 mmol/L for each 10 mm Hg rise in $PCO_2$ |
| *Alkalosis* | | | |
| Acute | ↓ $PCO_2$ | ↑ $cHCO_3^-$ | $cHCO_3^-$ falls by 2 mmol/L for each 10 mm Hg fall in $PCO_2$ |
| Chronic | ↓ $PCO_2$ | ↑ $cHCO_3^-$ | $cHCO_3^-$ falls by 5 mmol/L for each 10 mm Hg fall in $PCO_2$ |

From Narins RG, Gardner LB. Simple acid-base disturbances. *Med Clin North Am.* 1981;65:321–346.

base. Similarly, alkalosis occurs only by (1) an addition of base, (2) decreased elimination of base, and (3) increased loss of acid. This concept can be illustrated by depicting the body as a two-tank vat, one of acid and one of base, with inputs and outputs for each vat (Fig. 36.9).

## Metabolic Acidosis (Primary Bicarbonate Deficit)

The primary perturbation in metabolic acidosis is decreased plasma bicarbonate. Bicarbonate is "lost" in buffering acid created through increased production (such as the generation of acetoacetic acid in diabetic ketoacidosis) or decreased elimination of acid (seen in renal failure or some types of RTA). Serum bicarbonate can fall with resultant metabolic acidosis if there is a net loss of bicarbonate in the urine (secondary to decreased tubular reabsorption) or in the GI tract (e.g., duodenal/pancreatic fluid loss in severe diarrhea).

The resulting drop in pH from decreased $HCO_3^-$ stimulates respiratory compensation via hyperventilation, resulting in a lower $PCO_2$ and increased pH.

## Increased Anion Gap Acidosis (Organic Acidosis)

Metabolic acidoses are classified as those with an increased anion gap or a normal anion gap (Box 36.1). The concept of the anion gap was originally devised as a quality control rule when it was noted that if the sum of $Cl^-$ and $HCO_3^-$ values was subtracted from the $Na^+$ values ($Na^+ - [Cl^- + HCO_3^-]$), the difference, or "gap," averaged 12 mmol/L in healthy subjects. This *apparent* gap is due to unmeasured anions (e.g., proteins, $SO_4^{2-}$, $H_2PO_4^{2-}$) that are present in plasma. In reality, unmeasured cations (calcium, magnesium, organic cations) should

be included in the equation with sodium (and occasionally potassium), but their plasma molar concentrations are relatively small compared with circulating sodium concentration. The anion gap should be assessed in the electrolyte profiles of all patients as it is increased and is often the first indication of a metabolic acidosis (Fig. 36.10).

All anion gap metabolic acidosis, excluding inborn errors of metabolism, can be explained by one (or a combination) of eight underlying mechanisms included in the mnemonic device GOLD MARK (see Box 36.1) or the older MUDPILES (Box 36.2).

## Glycols (Ethylene and Propylene)

Ethylene glycol produces a high anion gap metabolic acidosis via its metabolism primarily to glycolic and oxalic acids. Ethylene glycol ingestion also induces the production of lactic acid by converting $NAD^+$ to NADH, which favors the production of lactic acid from pyruvate in glycolysis, preventing pyruvate from entering the tricyclic acid cycle. Precipitation of calcium oxalate and hippurate crystals in the urinary tract may lead to acute renal failure, worsening the acidosis. Ingestion of ethylene glycol will also generate a plasma osmolar gap, which can help determine the cause of an anion gap acidosis.

Propylene glycol is a common food and pharmaceutical additive, and it is commonly used in intravenous medications as a carrier for active compounds such as the benzodiazepine lorazepam. Propylene glycol is metabolized to acetate, as well as D- and L-lactate. While generally considered nontoxic, ingestion of large volumes of "non-toxic" antifreeze

## BOX 36.1   Conditions of Metabolic Acidoses With High and Normal Anion Gaps

| Cause | Retained Acid(s) | Other Laboratory Findings & Notes |
|---|---|---|
| **High Anion Gap (GOLD MARK)** | | |
| **G**lycols (ethylene and propylene) | Hippurate, glycolate, oxalate | ↑ Osmolal gap (>15 mOsmol/kg), Ethylene glycol assoc. with urine oxalate crystals |
| | | Propylene glycol associated with D-lactic acid |
| **O**xoproline | 5-oxoproline (pyroglutamic acid) from chronic acetaminophen/paracetamol use | ↑ Lactate associated with liver failure |
| **L**-Lactic acid | | |
| **D**-Lactic acid | | D-lactate from bacterial fermentation, associated with "short-bowel syndrome" |
| | | D-lactate also a metabolite of propylene glycol |
| **M**ethanol | Formate | ↑ Osmolal gap (>15 mOsmol/kg) |
| **A**spirin | Salicylate | Respiratory alkalosis |
| **R**enal failure | Sulfuric, phosphoric, and organic acids | ↑ serum creatinine and urea conc. |
| **K**etoacidosis | Acetoacetate and beta-hydroxybutyrate | ↑ serum glucose in diabetic ketoacidosis |
| **Normal Anion Gap** | | |
| Gastrointestinal fluid loss/ diarrhea | Primary loss of bicarbonate | Hypokalemia |
| Acetazolamide (carbonic anhydrase inhibitor/diuretic) | Renal bicarbonate loss | |
| ***Renal Tubular Acidosis*** | | |
| Type 1 | Decreased renal H+ secretion | Hypokalemia |
| Type 2 | Renal bicarbonate loss | Hypokalemia |
| Type 4 | Aldosterone deficiency or resistance | Hyperkalemia |
| ***Pancreatitis*** | | |
| Pancreatic fistula (external) | Loss of bicarbonate-rich fluid | |

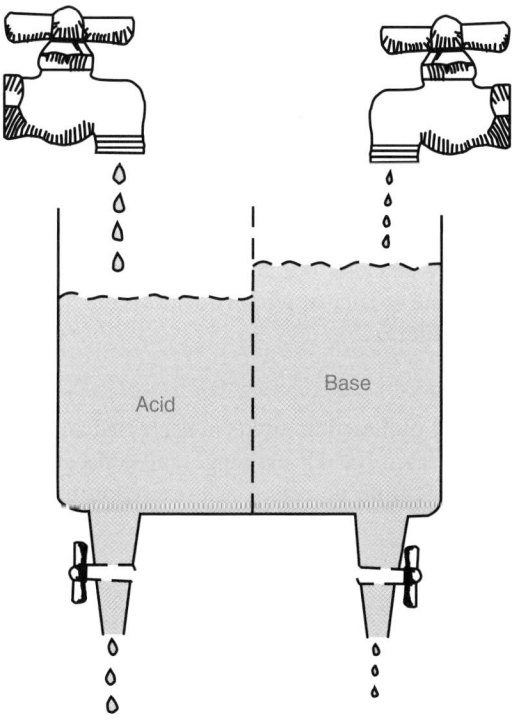

Fig. 36.9 Simple depiction of the body as a two-vat system of acid and base. At equilibrium, input and output from each vat are equal. (From Dufour DR. Acid-base disorders. In: Dufour DR, Christenson RH, eds. *Professional Practice in Clinical Chemistry: A Review*. Washington, DC: AACC Press; 1995.)

## BOX 36.2   An Older Mnemonic for High Anion Gap Acidosis (MUDPILES)

**M** Methanol
**U** Uremia (kidney failure)
**D** Diabetic ketoacidosis
**P** Paraldehyde, Paracetamol (acetaminophen)
**I** Isoniazid, Iron, or Ischemia
**L** Lactic acidosis
**E** Ethylene glycol
**S** Salicylate

containing propylene glycol (rather than the more common toxic ethylene glycol) or intravenous infusions can produce a lactic acidosis. As with ethylene glycol, propylene glycol will also produce a large osmolar gap. Differentiation between these two glycols via specific chromatographic methods is important for appropriate treatment.

### Oxoproline (Pyroglutamic Acid)

Chronic acetaminophen (paracetamol) use by patients with decreased glutathione stores can lead to an accumulation of 5-oxoproline (pyroglutamic acid) that results in an anion gap. An anion gap acidosis usually only develops in chronic acetaminophen/paracetamol users that have other comorbidities such as malnutrition, chronic renal failure, or liver disease.

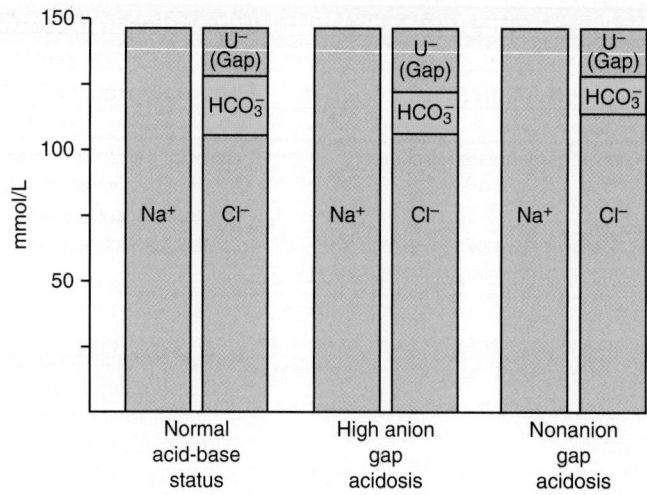

**Fig. 36.10** Simple "Gambelgram" depiction of normal gap, anion gap acidosis, and normal anion gap acidosis. Cations, $Na^+$ (and $K^+$, not shown here), are in *left bar* for each condition, whereas measured ($Cl^-$ and $HCO_3^-$) and unmeasured ($U^-$) anions are in *right bar* for each condition. (From Berg M, El-Khoury JM, Cervinski MA. Disorders of water, electrolytes, and acid-base metabolism. In: Rifai N, ed. *Tietz Textbook of Laboratory Medicine.* 7th ed. St. Louis: Elsevier; 2022.)

## L-lactate

Lactic acid, present in blood as the lactate ion, is an intermediate of carbohydrate metabolism derived mainly from muscle cells and erythrocytes (see Chapter 22). It represents the end product of anaerobic metabolism and is normally metabolized by the liver. Blood lactate concentration is affected by the rates of production and metabolism, both of which are dependent on adequate delivery of oxygenated blood to tissues.

Lactic acidosis caused by tissue hypoxia is seen most commonly in the setting of shock but can also be seen in sepsis, severe anemia, cardiopulmonary insufficiency, and due to toxins such as methanol, that disrupt mitochondrial oxidative phosphorylation. Severe tissue oxygen deprivation blocks aerobic oxidation of pyruvic acid in the tricarboxylic acid cycle, resulting in the reduction of pyruvate to lactate. Even in vigorous exercise, an aerobic threshold may be met (depending on multiple factors) and anaerobic metabolism may develop resulting in a lactic acidosis, with lactate concentrations increasing substantially to $\approx 12$ mmol/L. If the lactate-generating condition can be corrected, lactate is rapidly metabolized to $CO_2$, which then is exhaled.

## D-lactate

D-lactate is a special subset of lactic acidosis that arises from the fermentation of carbohydrates to D-lactate by intestinal bacteria. D-lactic acidosis is a rare cause of an anion gap acidosis and should only be considered in patients with "short-bowel" syndromes or following other GI surgeries resulting in "blind loops" that allow bacterial overgrowth. Most lactate measurement methods do not detect D-lactate (for more detail, see Chapter 22). D-lactate is also a metabolite of propylene glycol, however in the case of propylene glycol exposure, the concentration of D-lactate rarely sufficiently accumulates.

## Methanol

Although nontoxic itself, methanol is metabolized by the liver to formaldehyde and formic acid, the accumulation of which results in a high anion gap acidosis. Ocular symptoms include optic papillitis, retinal edema, and blindness due to optic nerve atrophy. Coma may result as well. Methanol will increase plasma osmolality, a fact that can be used for a toxicology diagnosis (see Chapter 31).

## Aspirin (Salicylates)

Acidosis from aspirin (salicylate) intoxication is complex and multifactorial. Salicylate itself is an unmeasured anion leading to an increased anion gap, but its effect on the body results in more profound acidosis through the alternation of peripheral metabolism and the production of various organic acids. Salicylate toxicity can be complex, with a number of superimposed acid-base disturbances occurring simultaneously, such as respiratory alkalosis due to salicylate-induced increased respiration rate or later respiratory acidosis due to coma and respiratory failure.

## Renal Failure

Renal tubular dysfunction results in decreased ammonia formation, decreased $Na^+$-$H^+$ exchange, and consequently metabolic acidosis from decreased acid excretion in urine (see Chapter 35).

## Ketoacidosis

The pathogenesis of ketoacidosis is discussed in detail in Chapter 33. Ketoacids such as β-hydroxybutyrate accumulate during diabetic ketoacidosis, as well as in starvation and alcoholic malnutrition. Ketoacids represented unmeasured anions and their accumulation causes a decrease in $HCO_3^-$ and a high anion gap. Treatment is directed at the process generating the ketoacids—most commonly insulin deficiency or starvation.

## Normal Anion Gap Acidosis (Inorganic Acidosis)

In contrast to high anion gap acidoses, in which bicarbonate is consumed from buffering excess $H^+$, the cause of a normal anion gap acidosis is the loss of bicarbonate-rich fluid from the kidney or the GI tract (see Box 36.1). As bicarbonate is lost, more $Cl^-$ ions are reabsorbed with $Na^+$ or $K^+$ to maintain electrical neutrality, resulting in hyperchloremia. Normal anion gap acidosis can be divided into *hypokalemic, normokalemic,* and *hyperkalemic* acidoses, which can be helpful in the differential diagnosis of this type of disorder.

### Gastrointestinal Losses

Diarrhea may cause acidosis as a result of loss of $Na^+$, $K^+$, and $HCO_3^-$. One of the primary exocrine functions of the pancreas is production of $HCO_3^-$ to neutralize gastric contents on entry into the duodenum. If the water, $K^+$, and $HCO_3^-$ in the intestine are not reabsorbed, a hypokalemic, normal anion gap metabolic acidosis will develop. The resulting hyperchloremia is due to replacement of lost bicarbonate with $Cl^-$ to maintain electrical balance.

### Renal Tubular Acidoses

These syndromes are characterized by loss of bicarbonate due to decreased tubular secretion of $H^+$ (distal or type I RTA) or decreased reabsorption of $HCO_3^-$ (proximal or type II RTA), resulting in bicarbonate "wasting" in the urine. Because the major urine-acidifying power of the kidneys rests in the distal tubules, proximal and distal RTAs may be differentiated by measurement of urine pH. In proximal RTA, urine pH becomes less than 5.5, whereas in distal RTA, the distal tubules are compromised and urine pH is greater than 5.5. Type IV RTA is due to decreased aldosterone concentration or aldosterone resistance, leading to decreased $Na^+$ reabsorption and thus decreased $H^+$ and $K^+$ secretion. A full discussion of the renal tubular acidoses and the differentiation between the types is beyond the scope of this chapter.

### Compensatory Mechanisms in Metabolic Acidosis

The buffer systems of blood (mainly the bicarbonate/carbonic acid buffer) minimize pH changes. The compensation mechanisms for metabolic acidosis seek to return arterial blood pH to 7.40. Compensation will not exceed an arterial blood pH of 7.40.

### Respiratory Compensatory Mechanism

Respiratory compensation to metabolic acidosis occurs immediately in response to a decrease in pH by increasing both the rate and depth of respiration to increase $CO_2$ elimination, decreasing $pCO_2$ and $cdCO_2$, and raising arterial pH. The maximal respiratory response may take several hours to develop. Table 36.3 depicts expected compensation in various cases of acidoses and alkaloses, and corresponding laboratory values.

### Renal Compensatory Mechanism

If possible, the kidneys respond to restore pH to 7.40 through increased acid excretion and preservation of base (increased rate of $Na^+$-$H^+$ exchange, increased ammonia formation, and increased reabsorption of bicarbonate). When the renal compensating mechanisms are functioning, urine acidity and ammonia are increased.

The renal compensatory mechanism is slower than respiratory compensation and may take several days for maximal effect.

## METABOLIC ALKALOSIS (PRIMARY BICARBONATE EXCESS)

Alkalosis occurs when excess base is added to the system, base elimination is decreased, or acid-rich fluids are lost (see the box "At a Glance"). Measurement of urine $Cl^-$ can be helpful in the evaluation of alkalosis, as metabolic alkalosis falls into $Cl^-$ responsive, $Cl^-$ resistant, and exogenous base categories (see the box "At a Glance" and Fig. 36.5).

**AT A GLANCE**

**Conditions Leading to Metabolic Alkalosis**
*Chloride Responsive (Urine $Cl^-$ Less Than 10 mmol/L)*
- Contraction alkaloses
  - Prolonged vomiting or nasogastric suction
  - Pyloric or upper duodenal obstruction
  - Prolonged or abusive diuretic therapy (loop diuretics)
  - Dehydration
- Post-hypercapnic state
- Cystic fibrosis (systemic ineffective reabsorption of $Cl^-$)

*Chloride-Resistant (Urine $Cl^-$ Greater Than 20 mmol/L)*
- Mineralocorticoid excess
  - Primary hyperaldosteronism (adrenal adenoma or, rarely, carcinoma)
  - Bilateral adrenal hyperplasia
  - Secondary hyperaldosteronism
  - Congenital adrenal hyperplasia (resulting from adrenal enzyme deficiencies in cortisol production [11β- or 17α-hydroxylase])
- Glucocorticoid excess
  - Primary adrenal adenoma (Cushing syndrome)
  - Pituitary adenoma secreting adrenocorticotropic hormone (Cushing disease)
  - Exogenous cortisol therapy
  - Excessive licorice ingestion
- Bartter syndrome (defective renal $Cl^-$ reabsorption)

*Exogenous Base*
- Iatrogenic
  - Bicarbonate-containing intravenous fluid therapy
  - Massive blood transfusion (sodium citrate overload)
  - Antacids and cation-exchange resins in dialysis patients
  - High-dose carbenicillin or penicillin (associated with hypokalemia)
- Milk-alkali syndrome

Most causes of $Cl^-$ responsive metabolic alkalosis occur as a result of *hypovolemia* (see the box "At a Glance"). The loss of acidic gastric secretions via prolonged vomiting or nasogastric suction, or the use of certain diuretics, can severely deplete the ECF and result in an acid-base disorder referred to as contraction alkalosis. The underlying mechanism of contraction alkalosis is depletion of $Cl^-$. Hydrochloric acid loss from the stomach is a particularly important cause, as both hypovolemia *and* hypochloremia can quickly develop. In the setting of hypovolemia and hypochloremia, the kidneys preferentially reabsorb $Na^+$ to restore volume, and excess $HCO_3^-$ is reabsorbed in the absence of sufficient $Cl^-$ to maintain electrical neutrality. Alkalosis may also be exacerbated by renal loss of $H^+$ (and $K^+$) in exchange for $Na^+$ reabsorption. Urine $Cl^-$ will be less than 10 mmol/L in $Cl^-$ responsive metabolic alkalosis (see Fig. 36.5) and treatment consists of correcting TBW deficit and chloride replacement, usually as NaCl. Replenishment of $Cl^-$ allows the kidney to reabsorb $Cl^-$ and excrete excess $HCO_3^-$.

## $Cl^-$ Resistant Metabolic Alkalosis

Chloride-resistant metabolic alkalosis is far less common than $Cl^-$ responsive metabolic alkalosis and is typically associated with an underlying disease (e.g., primary hyperaldosteronism, Cushing syndrome, Bartter syndrome) or with addition of an exogenous base. In these conditions, urine $Cl^-$ will usually be greater than 20 mmol/L.

In states of adrenocortical excess, $K^+$ and $H^+$ are "wasted" and $Na^+$ is reabsorbed by the kidney due to the effect of aldosterone or cortisol. The resultant hypokalemia produces an alkalosis through enhanced renal excretion of $H^+$ (in the form of $NH_4^+$) and increased $HCO_3^-$ reabsorption. The decreased tubular $K^+$ concentration observed in diseases in which endogenous mineralocorticoids, glucocorticoids, or both are increased include primary and secondary hyperaldosteronism, bilateral adrenal hyperplasia, pituitary ACTH-producing adenoma (Cushing disease), and primary adrenal adenomas producing glucocorticoids (Cushing syndrome) or aldosterone.

## Exogenous Base

Excess exogenous base states can include citrate toxicity, often following massive blood transfusion (citrate is metabolized to $HCO_3^-$ as part of the tricyclic acid cycle), aggressive intravenous therapy with bicarbonate solutions, and ingestion of large quantities of antacids in the treatment of gastritis or peptic ulcer *(milk-alkali syndrome)*.

## Compensatory Mechanisms in Metabolic Alkalosis

The compensatory mechanisms for metabolic alkalosis include both respiratory and renal compensation. Increased pH depresses the respiratory center, which decreases the respiratory rate (hypoventilation), which will increase retention of $PCO_2$ as less $CO_2$ is lost with exhalation. Respiratory compensation is, however, limited by the resultant hypoxia, preventing $PCO_2$ from increasing above 55 mm Hg. Above

pH 7.55, tetany may develop, even in the presence of a normal serum total calcium concentration, as the ionized calcium concentration decreases due to increased binding of calcium by albumin. The kidneys respond to the alkalosis by decreased $Na^+$-$H^+$ exchange, decreased formation of ammonia (and thus $NH_4^+$), and decreased reclamation of bicarbonate. However, this response is blunted in the presence of hypokalemia and hypovolemia.

## RESPIRATORY ACIDOSIS

Respiratory acidosis is only produced by conditions that decrease pulmonary elimination of $CO_2$, resulting in an increased $PCO_2$ (hypercapnia) and $dCO_2$ (and thus $H_2CO_3$, which dissociates to $H^+$ and $HCO_3^-$). This, in turn, causes a decrease in the $cHCO_3^-/cdCO_2$ ratio. Causes of decreased $CO_2$ elimination (see the box "At a Glance") are classified as acute or chronic.

---

### AT A GLANCE

**Conditions Leading to Respiratory Acidosis**
*Factors That Directly Depress the Respiratory Center*
- Opioids and barbiturates
- CNS trauma, tumors, and degenerative disorders
- Infections of the CNS such as encephalitis and meningitis
- Comatose states such as cerebrovascular accident secondary to intracranial hemorrhage
- Primary central hypoventilation

*Conditions That Affect the Respiratory Apparatus*
- Chronic Obstructive Pulmonary Disease (COPD—most common cause)
- Severe pulmonary fibrosis
- Status asthmaticus (severe asthma attack)
- Disease of the upper airways such as laryngospasm or tumor
- Pulmonary infection (severe)
- Impaired lung motion secondary to pleural effusion or pneumothorax (collapsed lung)
- Acute respiratory distress syndrome
- Chest wall disease and chest wall deformity
- Neurologic disorders affecting the muscles of respiration

*Others*
- Abdominal distention, as in peritonitis and ascites
- Extreme obesity (Pickwickian syndrome)
- Sleep disorders such as sleep apnea

---

## Compensatory Mechanisms in Respiratory Acidosis

Compensation for respiratory acidosis occurs immediately via buffer systems in blood, over time via the kidneys and, if possible, the lungs. Excess $H^+$ present in blood is buffered to a great extent by hemoglobin and protein buffer systems. The kidneys respond to respiratory acidosis in a manner similar to the way that they respond to metabolic acidosis—namely, with (1) increased $Na^+$-$H^+$ exchange, (2) increased ammonia formation (and thus $NH_4^+$ formation in the nephron), and (3) increased reclamation of bicarbonate. Renal compensation is slow to engage and is not effective before 6 to 12 hours and is not maximal for 2 to 3 days. In chronic respiratory acidosis, such as in patients with chronic obstructive pulmonary disease (COPD), full renal compensation may be seen even in patients with very high $PCO_2$ (>60 mm Hg).

The increased $PCO_2$, and resultant decrease in pH, stimulates the CNS respiratory center, resulting in an increased rate and depth of respiration, provided that the primary defect is not CNS disease. Pulmonary elimination of $CO_2$ results in a decrease in $cdCO_2$; thus the ratio of $cHCO_3^-/cdCO_2$ and pH approach normal.

## RESPIRATORY ALKALOSIS

A decrease in $PCO_2$ (hypocapnia) and the resulting primary deficit in $cdCO_2$ (respiratory alkalosis) are caused by an increased rate and/or depth of respiration. Excessive pulmonary elimination of $CO_2$ reduces $PCO_2$ and causes an increase in pH and $cHCO_3^-/cdCO_2$ ratio. This shift also results in a decrease in $cHCO_3^-$, which partially ameliorates the increase in pH. Causes of respiratory alkalosis can be classified as those with a direct stimulatory effect on the respiratory center and those due to effects on the pulmonary system (see the box "At a Glance".)

### POINTS TO REMEMBER

- Respiratory acidosis results in an increased $PCO_2$ secondary to the inability of the lungs to eliminate $CO_2$.
- Respiratory alkalosis is the result of excess elimination of $CO_2$ via hyperventilation.
- Respiratory compensatory mechanisms in primary metabolic acidosis or alkalosis settings should not be interpreted as respiratory disorders.

### AT A GLANCE

**Factors Causing Respiratory Alkalosis**
*Nonpulmonary Stimulation of Respiratory Center*
- Anxiety, panic attack
- Febrile state
- Gram-negative septicemia
- Metabolic encephalopathy (e.g., secondary to liver disease)
- CNS infections such as meningitis and encephalitis
- Cerebrovascular accident/stroke
- Intracranial surgery
- Hypoxia (e.g., severe anemia, low air pressure associated with high altitude)
- Drugs such as salicylates, epinephrine (acute treatment of anaphylaxis)
- Pregnancy, mainly third trimester
- Hyperthyroidism

*Pulmonary Disorders*
- Pneumonia
- Pulmonary emboli (blood clot)
- Interstitial lung disease
- Large right-to-left shunt ($PCO_2$ <50 mm Hg)
- Congestive heart failure
- Respiratory compensation after correction of metabolic acidosis

*Others*
- Ventilator-induced hyperventilation

## Compensatory Mechanisms in Respiratory Alkalosis

The compensatory mechanisms respond to respiratory alkalosis in two stages. In the first stage, red blood cells and tissue buffers provide $H^+$ ions that consume a small amount of $HCO_3^-$. The second stage becomes operational in prolonged respiratory alkalosis and depends on renal compensation as described for metabolic alkalosis (decreased reuptake of bicarbonate from nephron lumen).

## REVIEW QUESTIONS

1. Total body water (TBW) makes up approximately 60% of adult body weight. The majority of TBW is located in which one of the following compartments?
   a. Extracellular fluid (ECF)
   b. Intracellular fluid (ICF)
   c. Interstitial fluid
   d. Plasma
2. The anion gap, an estimate of anions not directly measured in serum, is correctly calculated by which one of the following formulae?
   a. $(Na^+) + (Cl^- + HCO_3^-)$
   b. $(Na^+) - (Cl^- + HCO_3^-)$
   c. $(Cl^-) + (HCO_3 + Na^-)$
   d. $(HCO_3^- - Na^+) - (Cl^-)$
3. Hypernatremia commonly occurs in:
   a. decreased production of antidiuretic hormone (ADH).
   b. decreased aldosterone.
   c. the syndrome of inappropriate ADH (SIADH) secretion.
   d. decreased cortisol.
4. A decrease in $PCO_2$ and a resulting primary deficit in $cdCO_2$ is referred to as
   a. metabolic acidosis.
   b. metabolic alkalosis.
   c. respiratory acidosis.
   d. respiratory alkalosis.
5. The use of spironolactone in addition to an *increased* dietary intake of this particular electrolyte can lead to

this disorder characterized by mental confusion, bradycardia, and possible eventual cardiac arrest.
   a. Sodium; hypernatremia
   b. Sodium; hyponatremia
   c. Potassium; hyperkalemia
   d. Potassium; hypokalemia
6. Which one of the following is the primary cause of respiratory acidosis?
   a. Hyperventilation
   b. Overdose of antacids
   c. Chronic obstructive pulmonary disease (COPD)
   d. Uncontrolled diabetes mellitus
7. Respiratory compensation of a metabolic alkalosis
   involves hypoventilation to increase $PCO_2$. Which of the
   following is the maximum $PCO_2$ achievable, and what
   limits $PCO_2$ from increasing beyond that threshold?
   a. 55 mm Hg, hypoxia

   b. 65 mm Hg, $CO_2$ solubility
   c. 80 mm Hg, diffusion
   d. 15 mm Hg, tetany/seizures
8. In the absence of an acid/base disorder, the normal ratio
   of bicarbonate to dissolved carbon dioxide in whole
   blood is approximately
   a. 10:1
   b. 1:20
   c. 20:1
   d. 1:10
9. Of the following causes of metabolic acidosis, which will
   present with an anion gap within the reference interval?
   a. Uremia of kidney failure
   b. Renal tubular acidosis type II
   c. D-Lactic acidosis
   d. Acetaminophen ingestion

## SUGGESTED READINGS

Adrogué HJ, Madias NE. Hypernatremia. *N Engl J Med.* 2000;342:1493–1499.

Dufour DR. Acid-base disorders. In: Dufour R, Christenson RH, eds. *Professional Practice in Clinical Chemistry: A Review.* Washington, DC: AACC Press; 1995:604–635.

Farese Jr RV, Biglieri EG, Shackleton CH, et al. Licorice-induced hypermineralocorticoidism. *N Engl J Med.* 1991;325:1223–1227.

Gandhi MJ. Refractory hyponatremia with lung cancer. In: *Tietz's Applied Laboratory Medicine.* 2nd ed. 2007:79–87.

Hoye A, Clark A. Iatrogenic hyperkalaemia. *Lancet.* 2003;361:2124.

Kadakia SC. D-lactic acidosis in a patient with jejunoileal bypass. *J Clin Gastroenterol.* 1995;20:154–156.

Lyon AW, Baskin LB. Pseudohyponatremia in a myeloma patient: direct electrode potentiometry is a method worth its salt. *Lab Med.* 2003;5:357–360.

Mehta AN, Emmett JB, Emmett M. GOLD MARK: an anion gap mnemonic for the 21st century. *Lancet.* 2008;372:892.

Mendu DA, Fleisher M, McCash SI, et al. D-lactic acidosis mediated neuronal encephalopathy in acute lymphoblastic leukemia patient: an under diagnosis. *Clin Chim Acta.* 2015;441:90–99.

Spasovski G, Vanholder R, Allolio B, et al. Clinical practice guideline on diagnosis and treatment of hyponatremia. *Eur J Endocrinol.* 2014;170:G1–G47.

# Liver Disease

*William Rosenberg, Tony Badrick, Sudeep Tanwar, and Stanley Lo*

## OBJECTIVES

1. Define the following:
   - Acinus
   - Ascites
   - Bilirubin
   - Cholestasis
   - Cirrhosis
   - Gallbladder
   - Hepatic lobule
   - Hepatitis
   - Hepcidin
   - Jaundice
   - Model for end-stage liver disease (MELD) score
   - Portal hypertension
   - Portal triad
2. Describe the microscopic and macroscopic anatomy of the hepatic system, including functional units, lobules, hepatobiliary ducts, blood supply, intrinsic cell types, and functional organization.
3. Detail the major functions of the liver, including the mechanisms of bilirubin excretion, substances synthesized and their functions, and substances metabolized and their sources.
4. List the causes and consequences of each of the following clinical manifestations of liver disease:
   - Disordered hemostasis
   - Liver enzyme release
   - Jaundice
   - Portal hypertension

5. List the enzymes synthesized in the liver, their subcellular location, tissue specificity, and mechanisms of enzyme release and clearance.
6. Compare and contrast acute liver injury with chronic liver injury, including manifestations of injury, target cells involved, specific means of cell death, and laboratory analyses used to distinguish between them.
7. List and describe five types of viral hepatitis, including type of virus, mode of transmission, involvement in liver cancer, methods of prevention, and laboratory tests used to diagnose the presence of the virus.
8. Describe the following types of liver disease, including causes, clinical presentation, and laboratory findings:
   - Acute alcoholic hepatitis
   - Alcohol related liver disease
   - Autoimmune hepatitis
   - Cholestatic hepatitis
   - Cholestatic liver diseases
   - Cirrhosis
   - Drug-induced liver injury (DILI)
   - Ischemic hepatitis
   - Primary biliary cholangitis (PBC)
   - Primary sclerosing cholangitis (PSC)
   - Toxic hepatitis
9. Describe hepatocellular carcinoma (HCC) including prevalence, risk factors, screening tests, and laboratory findings.

## KEY WORDS AND DEFINITIONS

**Alcoholic hepatitis** An acute or chronic degenerative and inflammatory lesion of the liver in patients with acute or chronic excessive alcohol use. It is potentially progressive though sometimes reversible.

**Alcohol-related liver disease** Liver injury caused by chronic excessive alcohol ingestion.

**Apoptosis** Programmed cell death as signaled by the nuclei in normally functioning human and animal cells when age or state of cell health and condition dictates.

**Ascites** Serous fluid that accumulates in the abdominal cavity.

**Autoimmune hepatitis (AIH)** A form of hepatitis, usually with hypergammaglobulinemia and serum autoantibodies.

**Bile** A greenish-yellow fluid secreted by the liver and stored in the gallbladder.

**Cholestasis** Suppression of the normal flow of bile.

**Chronic hepatitis** A collective term for a clinical and pathologic syndrome that has several causes and is characterized by varying degrees of hepatocellular necrosis and inflammation for at least 6 months.

**Cirrhosis** Liver disease characterized histologically by loss of the normal microscopic lobular architecture with fibrosis and nodular regeneration.

**Drug-induced liver injury (DILI)** A disease of the liver that is caused by prescribed medications, over-the-counter medications, vitamins, hormones, herbs, illicit drugs, and environmental toxins.

**Fulminant hepatic failure** A condition characterized by the development of severe liver injury with impaired synthetic capacity and encephalopathy in patients with previous normal liver or at least well-compensated liver disease.

**Fulminant hepatitis**    A rare and frequently fatal form of acute hepatitis B in which the patient's condition rapidly deteriorates with hepatic encephalopathy, necrosis of the hepatic parenchyma, coagulopathy, renal failure, and coma.

**Gallstones**    Solid formations in the gallbladder, most commonly composed of cholesterol and bile salts.

**Hemochromatosis**    A rare genetic disorder, due to abnormalities in genes that regulate iron metabolism.

**Hepatic failure**    A condition of severe liver dysfunction that is accompanied by a loss of normal liver functions.

**Hepatitis**    Inflammation of the liver. Typically divided into acute (duration of weeks to months) and chronic (lasting for more than 6 months).

**Hepatocellular carcinoma (HCC)**    A cancer arising from hepatocytes.

**Hepatocyte**    An epithelial liver cell that performs most of the synthetic and metabolic functions of the liver.

**Hepcidin**    A hormone produced by liver cells, in response to signals from a complex pathway, that decreases iron mobilization across intestinal and macrophage membranes, preventing excess iron in the blood (see also Chapter 28).

**Jaundice**    A clinical finding characterized by hyperbilirubinemia and deposition of pigment in the skin, mucous membranes, and sclera with resulting yellow appearance; also called icterus.

**Kernicterus**    A clinical syndrome of the neonate resulting from high concentrations of unconjugated bilirubin that passes the immature blood-brain barrier of the newborn and causes degeneration of cells of the basal ganglia and hippocampus.

**Model for End-Stage Liver Disease (MELD) Score**    A scoring system for assessing the severity of chronic liver disease.

**Necrosis**    The sum of the morphologic changes indicative of cell death and caused by the progressive degradative action of enzymes; it may affect groups of cells or part of a structure or an organ.

**Nonalcoholic fatty liver disease (NAFLD)**    A condition characterized by the buildup of extra fat in liver cells that is not caused by alcohol.

**Nonalcoholic steatohepatitis (NASH)**    An inflammatory disease of the liver of uncertain pathogenesis that is not caused by alcohol.

**Portal hypertension**    Any increase in the pressure in the portal vein (which carries venous blood from the intestines and spleen to the liver) due to anatomic or functional obstruction (e.g., cirrhosis) to blood flow in the portal venous system.

**Primary biliary cholangitis (PBC)**    A rare form of liver disease, formerly called primary biliary cirrhosis, that results in the irreversible destruction of the small bile ducts within the liver.

**Primary sclerosing cholangitis (PSC)**    A chronic, nonbacterial inflammatory narrowing of the bile ducts (usually the larger ducts outside of the liver).

**Reye syndrome**    A sudden, sometimes fatal, disease of the brain (encephalopathy) caused by specific forms of acute injury to the liver.

**Sjögren syndrome**    A systemic autoimmune disease in which immune cells attack and destroy the glands that produce tears and saliva.

**Varices**    Enlarged and tortuous veins, most commonly found in the esophagus (termed esophageal varices).

**Viral hepatitis**    Liver inflammation caused by viruses. Specific hepatitis viruses have been labeled A, B, C, D, and E.

**Viral load**    The measurement of the amount of virus in the blood. It is expressed as the amount of virus nucleic acid per milliliter of body fluid and used to guide treatment decisions and monitor response to treatment.

**Wilson disease**    An autosomal recessive disorder associated with excessive quantities of copper in the tissue, particularly the liver and central nervous system.

## ANATOMY OF THE LIVER

The adult liver weighs approximately 1.2 to 1.5 kg. It is located beneath the diaphragm in the right upper quadrant of the abdomen and is protected by the ribs and held in place by ligamentous attachments.

### Gross Anatomy

The liver is divided into left and right anatomic lobes by the falciform ligament (Fig. 37.1). It has a dual blood supply. The portal vein carries blood from the spleen and nutrient-enriched blood from the gastrointestinal (GI) tract, supplying approximately 70% of the blood supply; the hepatic artery, a branch of the celiac axis, provides oxygen-enriched arterial blood. These two blood supplies merge and flow into the sinusoids that course between individual hepatocytes. Venous drainage from the liver ultimately converges into the right and left hepatic veins, which exit on the posterior surface of the liver and join the inferior vena cava near its entry into the right atrium.

Biliary drainage originates at the bile canaliculi that merge to form ductules that drain into the intrahepatic bile ducts, which ultimately join to form the right and left hepatic bile ducts to exit the liver at the porta hepatis, forming the common hepatic duct. The hepatic duct is joined by the cystic duct that drains the gallbladder, to form the common bile duct which then enters the duodenum (usually with the pancreatic duct) at the ampulla of Vater. The gallbladder, which

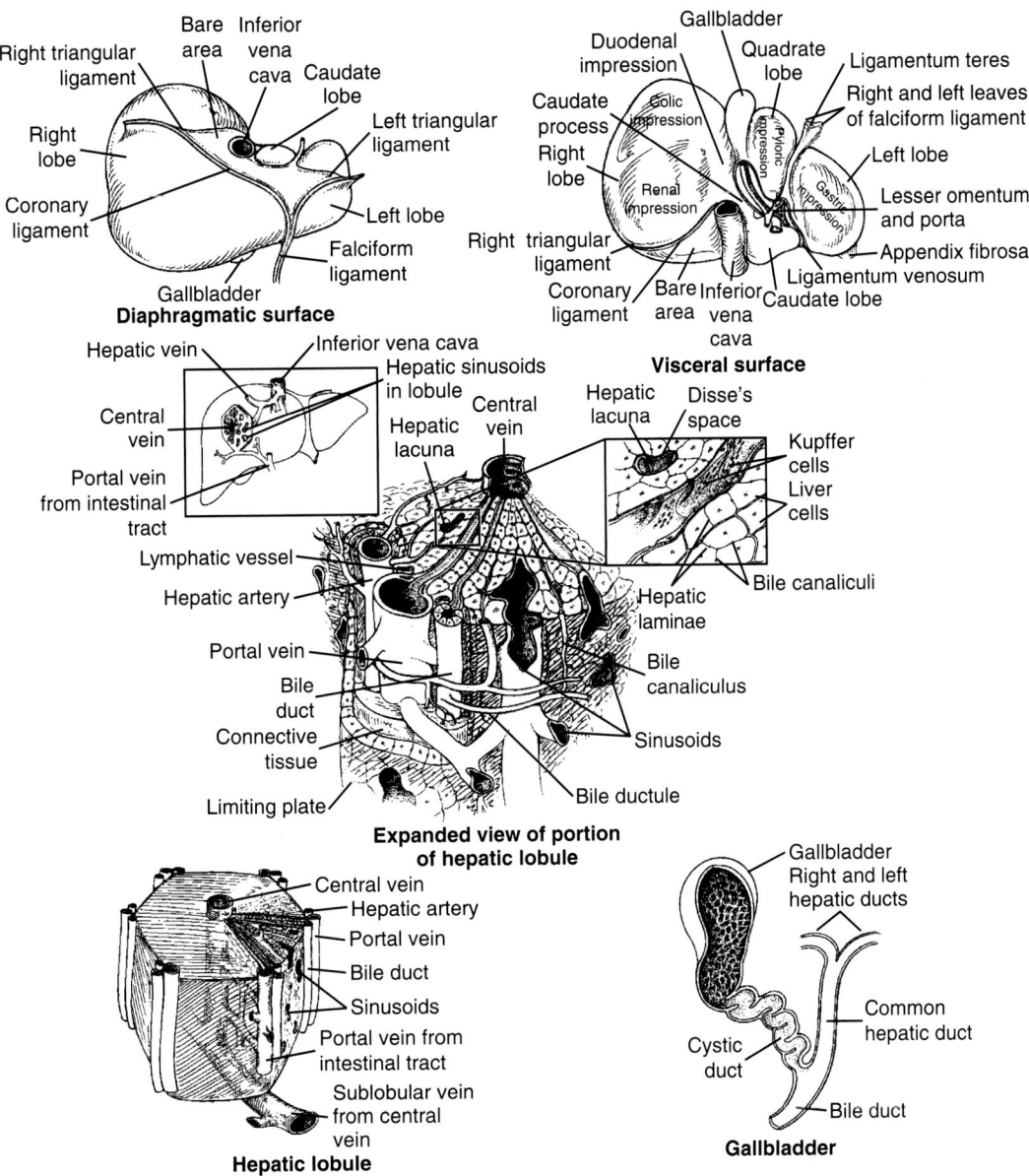

**Fig. 37.1** Structure of the liver. (From Dorland WAN. *Dorland's Illustrated Medical Dictionary.* 30th ed. Philadelphia: Saunders; 2003 [plate 26].)

is located on the undersurface of the right lobe of the liver, stores and concentrates 30 to 50 mL of bile.

## Microscopic Anatomy

The functional anatomic unit of the liver is the acinus, adjacent to the portal triad (which consists of a branch of each of the portal vein, hepatic artery, and bile duct). Each acinus is supplied by a terminal branch of the portal vein and of the hepatic artery and is drained by a terminal branch of the bile duct. The blood vessels radiate toward the periphery, forming sinusoids, which perfuse the liver and ultimately drain into the central (terminal) hepatic vein (Fig. 37.2). The sinusoids are lined by fenestrated endothelial cells (which allow free filtration of blood) and phagocytic Kupffer cells derived from blood monocytes.

Hepatocytes are the major functioning cells in the liver and are responsible for approximately 70% of liver mass. They perform most of the metabolic and synthetic functions of the liver. Hepatic stellate cells are located between the endothelial lining of the sinusoids, and the hepatocytes are within a small cleft referred to as the space of Disse. In their normal, quiescent state, stellate cells serve as a site of storage for fat-soluble vitamins, particularly vitamin A. When stimulated, stellate cells are morphologically and functionally transformed. They synthesize collagen and are the cells responsible for fibrosis and, eventually, cirrhosis. They also synthesize nitric oxide, which helps to regulate intrahepatic blood flow.

The blood supply to each acinus is zonal (Fig. 37.3). Zone 1, the area immediately adjacent to the portal tract, is

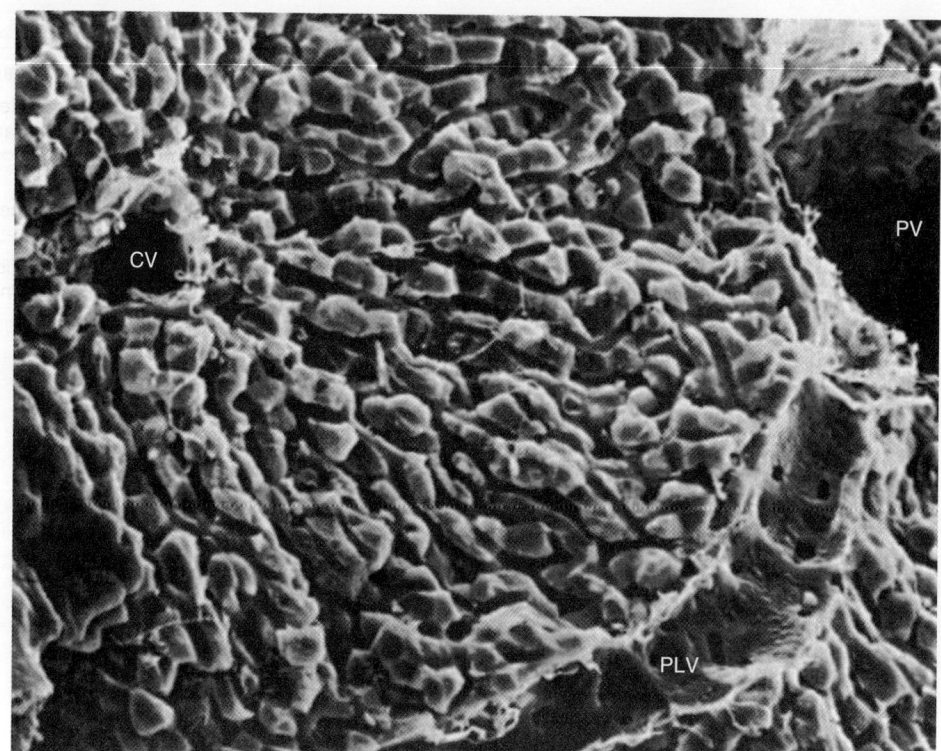

**Fig. 37.2** A low-magnification scanning electron micrograph depicting a portion of a liver lobule from a rat liver. *CV*, Central vein; *PLV*, perilobular venules; *PV*, portal vein. (From Zakim O, Boyer TD. *Hepatology: A Textbook of Liver Disease.* 3rd ed. Philadelphia: WB Saunders; 1996.)

enriched with lysosomes and mitochondria and forms a base for hepatic regeneration. Zone 2 predominantly contains hepatocytes that perform the major metabolic functions of the liver. The periphery of the acinus, zone 3, is enriched with the endoplasmic reticulum, is active metabolically, and has relatively low oxygen tension. Zone 1 is more susceptible to injury from viral hepatitis, autoimmune hepatitis (AIH), primary biliary cirrhosis (PBC), and some drugs.

### Ultrastructure of the Hepatocyte

Hepatocytes contain a well-developed organelle substructure (Fig. 37.4). Mitochondria, which constitute approximately 18% of hepatocyte volume, are the sites of oxidative phosphorylation and energy production. The smooth endoplasmic reticulum contains microsomes that are involved in bilirubin conjugation; detoxification (cytochrome $P_{450}$–dependent isoenzymes), and synthesis of steroids, cholesterol, and bile acids. Several microsomal enzymes, including $\gamma$-glutamyltransferase (GGT), are induced by many drugs and inhibited by others. This is the site of most drug metabolism and many important drug interactions.

Peroxisomes are found near the smooth endoplasmic reticulum and contain oxidases that use molecular oxygen to modify a variety of substrates, leading to the production of hydrogen peroxide. They also contain catalase, which decomposes hydrogen peroxide. Peroxisomes catalyze the $\beta$-oxidation of fatty acids that have 7 to 18 chain lengths. Approximately 5% to 20% of the metabolism of ethanol also occurs in the peroxisomes. Lysosomes are dense

organelles that contain hydrolytic enzymes that act as scavengers. Deposition of iron, lipofuscin, bile pigments, and copper occurs in the lysosomes. The Golgi apparatus lies near the canaliculus and is involved in the secretion of various substances, including bile acids and albumin.

## BIOCHEMICAL FUNCTIONS OF THE LIVER

The liver is involved in various excretory, synthetic, and metabolic functions. Clinical laboratories perform numerous tests that are useful in the biochemical assessment of these functions.

### Hepatic Excretory Function

Organic compounds of both endogenous and exogenous origin are extracted from the sinusoidal blood, biotransformed, and excreted into the bile or urine. Assessment of this excretory function provides valuable clinical information. The most frequently used tests involve the measurement of plasma concentrations of endogenously produced compounds, such as bilirubin and bile acids. In specialist centers, these tests may be augmented by the determination of the rate of clearance of exogenous compounds, such as aminopyrine, lidocaine, and caffeine.

#### Bilirubin

Bilirubin derived from heme is mainly a product of red blood cell turnover. It is extracted and biotransformed in the liver and excreted in bile and urine.

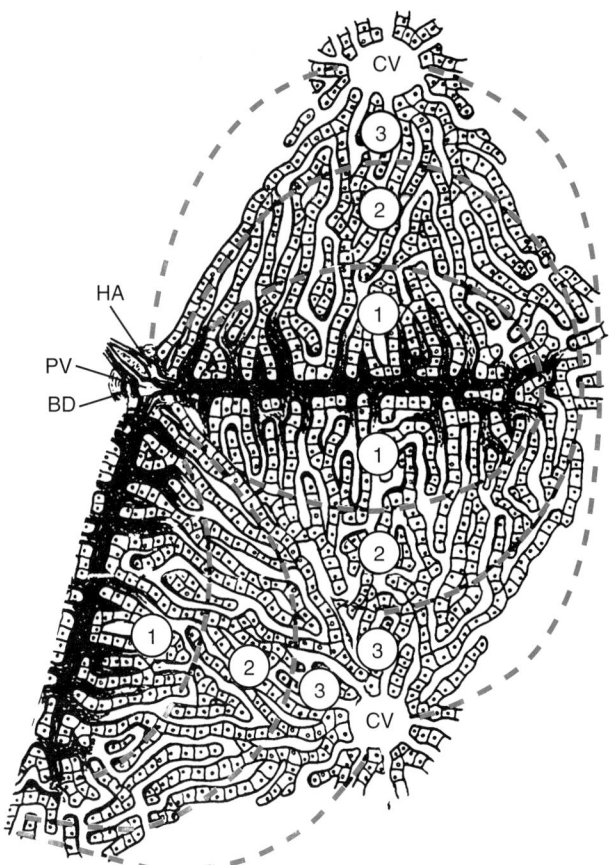

Fig. 37.3 Blood supply of the simple liver acinus. Zones 1, 2, and 3 indicate corresponding volumes in a portion of an adjacent acinar unit. Oxygen tension and the nutrient level in the blood in sinusoids decrease from zone 1 through zone 3. *BD*, Bile duct; *CV*, central vein; *HA*, hepatic artery; *PV*, portal vein. (From Zakim O, Boyer TD. *Hepatology: A Textbook of Liver Disease.* 3rd ed. Philadelphia: WB Saunders; 1996.)

Bilirubin is transported from sites of production (mainly the spleen) and is loosely bound to albumin in its native, unconjugated form. Bilirubin is transported across the hepatocyte membrane and is rapidly conjugated with glucuronic acid to produce bilirubin glucuronides, which are then excreted into bile by an energy-dependent process.

The measurement of unconjugated (indirect) and conjugated (direct) bilirubin fractions can be used to classify the likely cause of hyperbilirubinemia into prehepatic, hepatic, and posthepatic causes.

## Bile Acids

Regulation of bile acid metabolism is a major function of the liver. Cholesterol homeostasis is in large part maintained by the conversion of cholesterol to bile acids and subsequent regulation of bile acid metabolism. Bile acids facilitate both hepatic excretion of cholesterol and solubilization of lipids for intestinal absorption.

## Hepatic Synthetic Function

The liver has extensive synthetic capacity and plays a major role in the regulation of protein, carbohydrate, and lipid metabolism (see Chapters 18, 22, and 23). The liver is vital to the regulation of blood glucose and to the synthesis of proteins, triglycerides, fatty acids, cholesterol, and bile acids.

## Protein Synthesis

The liver is the primary site of the synthesis of most plasma proteins (see Chapter 18) in the rough endoplasmic reticulum of hepatocytes, followed by release into the hepatic sinusoids. Many factors may affect plasma protein concentrations. Because there are extensive functional reserves and relatively long half-lives of proteins such as albumin, the reduction in plasma proteins is indicative of extensive liver damage. For this reason and others, the sensitivity and specificity of plasma protein concentrations for the diagnosis of liver disease are far from ideal. Short-lived hepatic proteins (such as transthyretin and prothrombin) fall quickly, whereas those proteins with longer half-lives are normal or minimally changed. Serial determination of plasma proteins provides prognostic information; for example, worsening of prothrombin time (PT) during acute hepatitis suggests a poor prognosis.

### Plasma proteins

**Albumin.** This is one of the most commonly measured plasma proteins; it is synthesized exclusively by the liver. With liver disease, hypoalbuminemia is noted primarily in cirrhosis, AIH, and alcoholic hepatitis. One important consideration in measurement of albumin is the inaccuracy of dye-binding methods in patients with liver disease. Although bromocresol green measurements tend to overestimate albumin concentration at low concentrations, bromocresol purple methods give falsely low values in patients with jaundice because of the interference of bilirubin at the site of binding.

**Transthyretin (pre-albumin).** This protein has a short half-life of 24 to 48 hours, making it a sensitive indicator of current synthetic ability. Transthyretin is typically decreased in cirrhosis (among other conditions) as a result of decreased synthesis. It is commonly used as a measurement of nutritional status.

**Immunoglobulins.** Plasma immunoglobulin (Ig) concentrations are commonly increased in cirrhosis, AIH, and PBC, but they are normal in most other types of liver disease. IgG is increased in AIH and cirrhosis; IgM is increased in PBC. IgA tends to be increased in all types of cirrhosis. None of these findings are specific, and they are seldom used in the diagnosis of liver disease, but serial measurement of IgG levels can be used to monitor disease activity in AIH.

**Ceruloplasmin.** The concentration of this protein is decreased in Wilson disease, cirrhosis, and many causes of chronic hepatitis, but it may be increased by inflammation, cholestasis, hemochromatosis, pregnancy, and estrogen therapy (see section on Wilson Disease).

**Alpha$_1$-antitrypsin.** Concentrations of this protein, which is the major serine protease inhibitor (serpin) in plasma, is decreased in homozygous deficiency and cirrhosis and is increased by acute inflammation. It is discussed in greater detail later in the section on alpha$_1$-antitrypsin (AAT) deficiency.

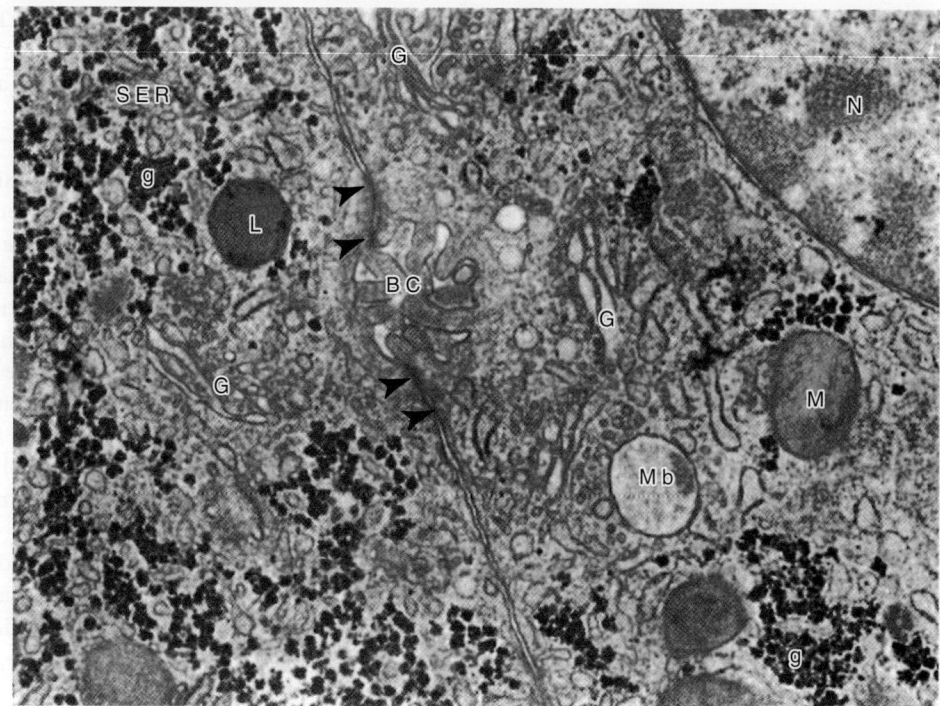

**Fig. 37.4** Portions of two human liver cells showing the relationship of the organelles and a typical bile canaliculus *(BC). Arrowheads* indicate light junctions. *g,* Glycogen; *G,* Golgi; *L,* lysosome; *M,* mitochondria; *Mb,* microbody; *N,* nucleus; *SER,* smooth endoplasmic reticulum. (From Zakim O, Boyer TD. *Hepatology: A Textbook of Liver Disease.* 3rd ed. Philadelphia: WB Saunders; 1996.)

**Alpha-fetoprotein.** The concentration of this protein, a normal component of fetal blood, falls to adult values by 1 year of age. Mild increases are seen in patients with acute and chronic hepatitis and indicate hepatocellular regeneration. It is present at higher concentrations in hepatocellular carcinoma (HCC).

*Coagulation proteins.* The coagulation proteins, inhibitors of the coagulation system, including antithrombin, protein C, and protein S, are synthesized in the liver. Some of the coagulation factors (II, VII, IX, and X) or coagulation inhibitors (protein C and S) require vitamin K for posttranslational carboxylation within the hepatocyte. Activated protein C in plasma inhibits coagulation by inactivating factors V and VIII. Parenchymal liver disease of sufficient severity to impair protein synthesis or obstructive liver disease, sufficient to impair intestinal absorption of vitamin K, is therefore a potential cause of bleeding disorders. Because of the great functional reserve of the liver, failure of hemostasis usually does not occur except in severe or long-standing liver disease.

*Lipid and lipoprotein synthesis.* The liver plays a key role in the metabolism of lipids and lipoproteins (see Chapter 23). On a daily basis, approximately 33% of the fatty acids originating from adipose tissue enter the liver, where they undergo esterification into triglycerides or are oxidized. Oxidation is favored in the fasting state and esterification is favored in the nonfasting state. Excessive esterification results in fatty liver, a disorder in which excess triglycerides are deposited in large vacuoles that displace other cellular components. Most cholesterol is synthesized endogenously, in the liver. Hepatic cholesterol and cholesterol of dietary origin enter the hepatic pool, where they are converted to bile acids, incorporated into lipoproteins, or used in the synthesis of liver cell membranes. The relative rates of secretion of bile acids, cholesterol, and lecithin are important factors in the pathogenesis of cholesterol gallstones.

*Urea synthesis.* Patients with end-stage liver disease may have low concentrations of urea in plasma (see Chapter 35). The rate of urea excretion in urine is lower in these patients than that in healthy individuals. In addition, plasma concentrations of urea precursors—ammonia and amino acids—are elevated. Lower specific activities of enzymes involved in urea synthesis are also seen. These findings suggest that patients with liver disease have an impaired ability to metabolize protein nitrogen and to synthesize urea. The rate of hepatic urea synthesis also depends on exogenous intake of nitrogen and on endogenous protein catabolism.

## Hepatic Metabolic Function

A recurring theme is the central importance of the liver in metabolic and regulatory pathways. The functional expression of the complex, integrated organelle structure includes the metabolism of drugs (activation and detoxification) and the disposal of exogenous and endogenous substances, such as galactose and ammonia. In addition, metabolic abnormalities due to specific inherited enzyme deficiencies can affect the liver. A classic example is galactosemia. In this condition, congenital absence of galactose 1-phosphate uridyltransferase allows accumulation of the toxic metabolite

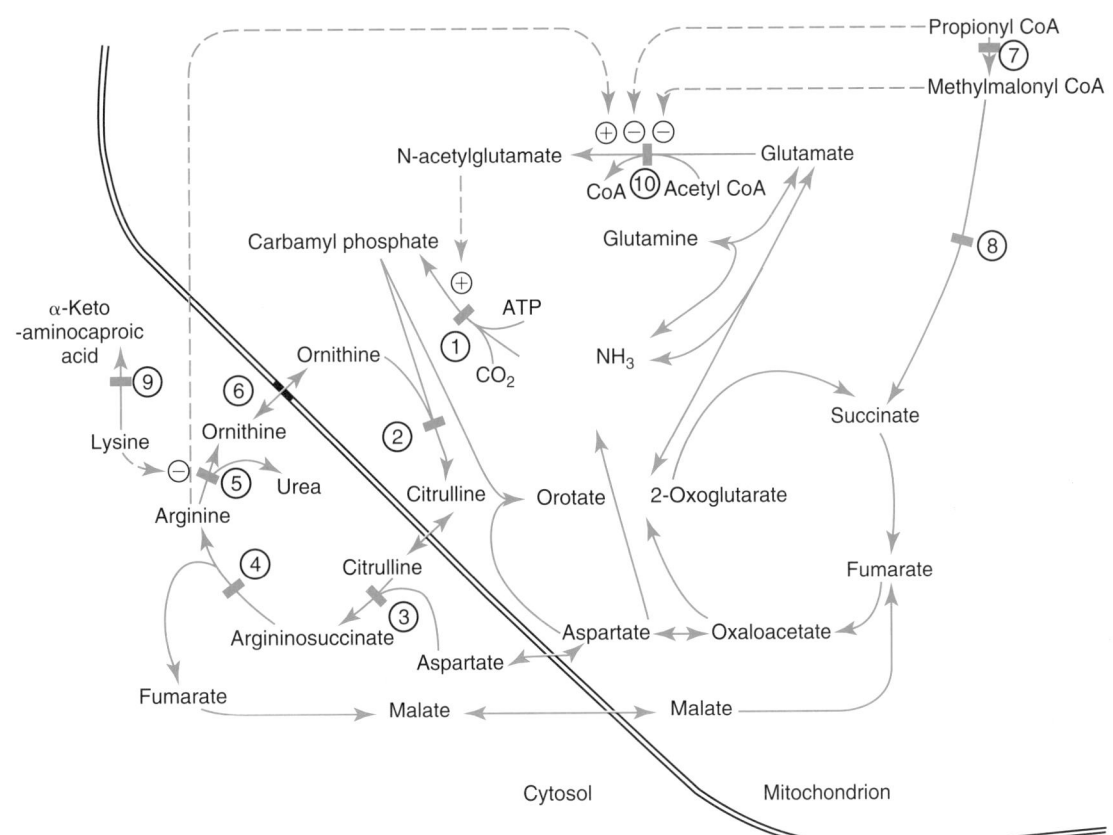

Fig. 37.5 Major metabolic pathways for the use of ammonia by the hepatocyte. *Solid bars* indicate the sites of primary enzyme defects in various metabolic disorders associated with hyperammonemia. *(1)* Carbamyl phosphate synthetase 1, *(2)* ornithine transcarbamylase, *(3)* argininosuccinate synthetase, *(4)* argininosuccinate lyase, *(5)* arginase, *(6)* mitochondrial ornithine transport, *(7)* propionyl coenzyme-A *(CoA)* carboxylase, *(8)* methylmalonyl CoA mutase, *(9)* L-lysine dehydrogenase, and *(10)* N-acetyl glutamine synthetase. *Dotted lines* indicate the site of pathway activation (+) or inhibition (−). (From Flannery OB, Hsia YE, Wolf B. Current status of hyperammonemia syndromes. *Hepatology.* 1982;2:495–506.)

galactose 1-phosphate, which causes injury to the liver, brain, and kidneys.

## Ammonia Metabolism

The major source of circulating ammonia is the GI tract. Plasma ammonia concentration in the hepatic portal vein is typically 5- to 10-fold higher than that in the systemic circulation. It is derived from the action of bacterial proteases, ureases, and amine oxidases on the contents of the colon and from the hydrolysis of glutamine in both the small and large intestines. Under normal circumstances, most of the portal vein ammonia load is metabolized to urea in hepatocytes through the Krebs-Henseleit (urea) cycle during the first pass through the liver; this process includes intramitochondrial and cytosolic enzyme-catalyzed steps (Fig. 37.5).

Ammonia enters the tissue of the central nervous system by passive diffusion. The rate of entry increases in proportion to the plasma concentration and is dependent on pH. Ammonia crosses the blood-brain barrier more readily than the ammonium ion. Fasting venous plasma ammonia concentration is useful in the differential diagnosis of encephalopathy to determine if it is hepatic in origin. In acute liver failure, ammonia concentrations in excess of 200 µmol/L are associated with cerebral edema and a poor prognosis.

*Bilirubin metabolism.* The proposed structure of bilirubin is shown in the upper portion of Fig. 37.6. However, the insolubility of the bilirubin molecule in water and its solubility in a variety of nonpolar, lipid solvents are not predicted from this linear tetrapyrrole structure. X-ray crystallography shows bilirubin assuming a ridge-tiled configuration, stabilized by six intramolecular hydrogen bonds. This Z-Z *(trans)* conformation (see Fig. 37.6) prevents the interaction of bilirubin with polar groups in aqueous media. When exposed to light, the Z-Z configuration is converted by rupture of the intramolecular double bonds to the E-E *(cis)* conformation, which is more water-soluble than the Z-Z conformation. Thus light-exposed forms of bilirubin are more water soluble and are readily excreted in the bile. This is the rationale for irradiating jaundiced newborns with 450 nm light.

Bilirubin IXα is produced from the catabolism of heme. For each mole of heme, one mole each of carbon monoxide, bilirubin, and ferric iron is produced. Daily bilirubin production from all sources averages from 250 to 300 mg.

Approximately 85% of the total bilirubin produced is derived from the heme moiety of hemoglobin released from senescent erythrocytes that are destroyed in the reticuloendothelial system. The remaining 15% is produced from RBC precursors destroyed in the bone marrow and from the catabolism of other heme-containing proteins.

In blood, bilirubin is bound to albumin and is transported to the liver. It dissociates from albumin at the membrane of the hepatocyte and is transported across the membrane into the liver (Fig. 37.7). Inside the liver cells, bilirubin is reversibly bound to soluble proteins known as ligandins or *protein Y*. Inside the hepatocytes, bilirubin is rapidly conjugated with glucuronic acid to produce bilirubin monoglucuronide and diglucuronide, which then are excreted into bile (see Fig. 37.7). The microsomal enzyme bilirubin uridine diphosphate (UDP)–glucuronyltransferase (EC 2.4.1.17) catalyzes the formation of bilirubin monoglucuronide. In adults, virtually all bilirubin excreted in bile is in the form of glycosidic conjugates.

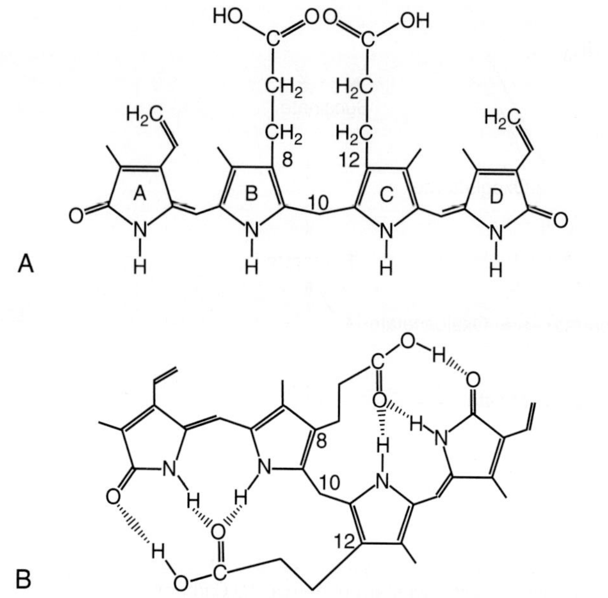

In the intestine, bilirubin glucuronides are hydrolyzed by the catalytic action of β-glucuronidase from the (1) liver, (2) intestinal epithelial cells, and (3) bacteria. The unconjugated bilirubin is then reduced by anaerobic intestinal microbial flora to form a group of three colorless tetrapyrroles collectively called urobilinogen. In the lower intestinal tract, the three urobilinogen are spontaneously oxidized to produce the bile pigments, which are orange-brown and the major pigments of stool.

## Carbohydrate Metabolism

Because the liver is a major processor of dietary and endogenous carbohydrates, liver disease affects carbohydrate metabolism in a variety of ways (see Chapters 22 and 33). However, none of the conventional modes of evaluating carbohydrate metabolism have value in the diagnosis of liver disease. Because the liver is the major site of both glycogen storage and gluconeogenesis, hypoglycemia is a common complication in certain liver diseases, particularly **Reye syndrome, fulminant hepatic failure,** advanced cirrhosis, and HCC.

**Fig. 37.6** Bilirubin IXα structure. (A) A linear molecular representation of unconjugated bilirubin. (B) The preferred structure of unconjugated bilirubin IXα, Z-Z configuration. The structure is stabilized by hydrogen bonding. The "ridge" involves carbon atoms 8 through 12.

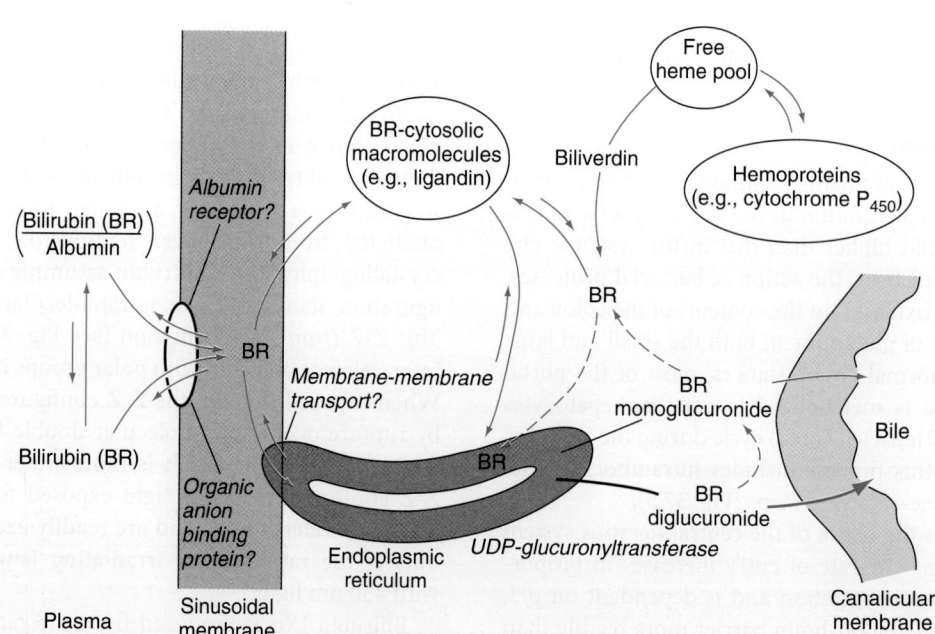

**Fig. 37.7** At a glance. Bilirubin uptake, metabolism, and transport in the hepatocyte. (From Gollan JL, Schmid R. Bilirubin update: formation, transport, and metabolism. In: Popper H, Schaffner F, eds. *Progress in Liver Diseases.* Philadelphia: WB Saunders 1982.)

## Hepatic Storage Function

The liver serves as a major site for storage of energy-rich carbohydrate substrates. Hepatic glycogen is released to other tissues when the need exists.

## Nutritional and Metabolic Abnormalities

Severe metabolic and nutritional derangements have been observed in cirrhotic patients, including alterations in glucose metabolism caused by insulin resistance, and hypokalemia caused by secondary hyperaldosteronism. In addition, hypoalbuminemia is frequently present because of decreased production and sinusoidal leakage of albumin in patients with portal hypertension. In patients with chronic cholestasis, impaired delivery of bile salts to the duodenum may result in malabsorption of lipids and fat-soluble vitamins, leading to deficiencies in vitamins A, D, E, and K (see Chapters 23 and 27).

## Disordered Hemostasis in Liver Disease

The liver manufactures most of the soluble clotting factors (except for factor VIII and von Willebrand factor) and a number of inhibitors of clotting (proteins C and S, antithrombin III). The liver also clears activated clotting factors from the circulation. Bile acids are necessary for vitamin K absorption and are needed to produce the active forms of several clotting factors, as well as proteins C and S. Disorders of fibrinogen also occur in liver disease.

## Enzymes Released From Diseased Liver Tissue

Because hepatic function is often normal in many patients with liver disease, the plasma activities of several cytosolic, mitochondrial, and membrane-associated enzymes are measured because they are increased in many forms of liver disease.

## DISEASES OF THE LIVER

The liver has a limited number of ways of responding to injury. Acute injury to the liver may be asymptomatic but often presents as jaundice. The major acute liver disorders are acute hepatitis and cholestasis. Chronic liver injury generally takes the clinical form of chronic hepatitis; its long-term complications include cirrhosis and HCC.

## Mechanisms and Patterns of Injury

Cell death occurs by necrosis (death of cell), apoptosis (programmed cell death), or both. The target cell determines the pattern of injury, with hepatocyte injury leading to hepatocellular disease and biliary cell injury leading to cholestasis. All cellular injury induces fibrosis as an adaptive or healing response, with the duration of injury and genetic factors determining whether cirrhosis and ultimately carcinoma occur (Fig. 37.8).

In general, the aminotransferase enzymes and alkaline phosphatase (ALP) are used to distinguish the pattern (see the following "At a Glance" box), the plasma albumin determines the chronicity, and the PT or factor V concentration determines the severity. Classically, liver fibrosis has been assessed using liver biopsy, but in recent years several noninvasive methods of assessment of liver fibrosis have been described and evaluated. Although liver biopsy yields incomparable information about the nature, severity, and chronicity of liver disease, noninvasive tests may provide more accurate assessment of liver fibrosis, and in particular, disease severity and prognosis.

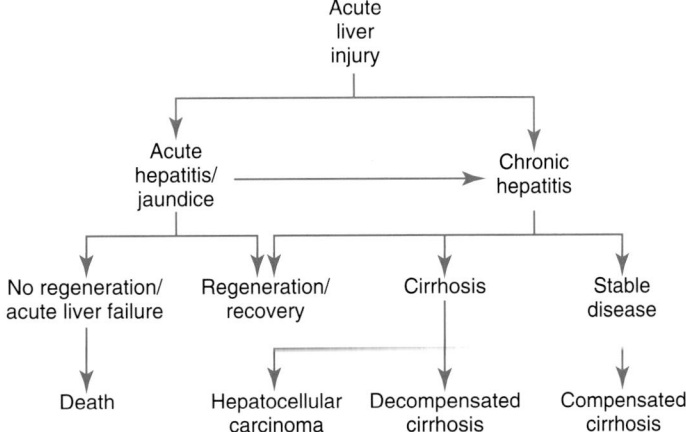

**Fig. 37.8** Natural history of liver disease. With acute injury to the liver, several outcomes are possible. In many individuals, damage is clinically inapparent and recovery occurs with clearance of the causative agent. In some, clinical acute hepatitis occurs. In most of these, clearance of the causative agent results in complete recovery; in a small minority, damage is so severe that acute liver failure (fulminant hepatitis) develops, which is usually fatal without liver transplantation. A variable percentage of persons with acute liver injury (dependent on the cause) progress to chronic hepatitis. In some, recovery eventually occurs naturally or following treatment of the underlying cause. Among those in whom chronic hepatitis persists, many will never progress to cirrhosis. Most of those who do will remain well for many years, but approximately 3% per year develop decompensated cirrhosis (bleeding varices, ascites, hepatic encephalopathy) or hepatocellular carcinoma. These are the most common causes of death from liver disease.

## AT A GLANCE

Algorithm for using abnormal liver function tests to classify and diagnose various types of liver disease.

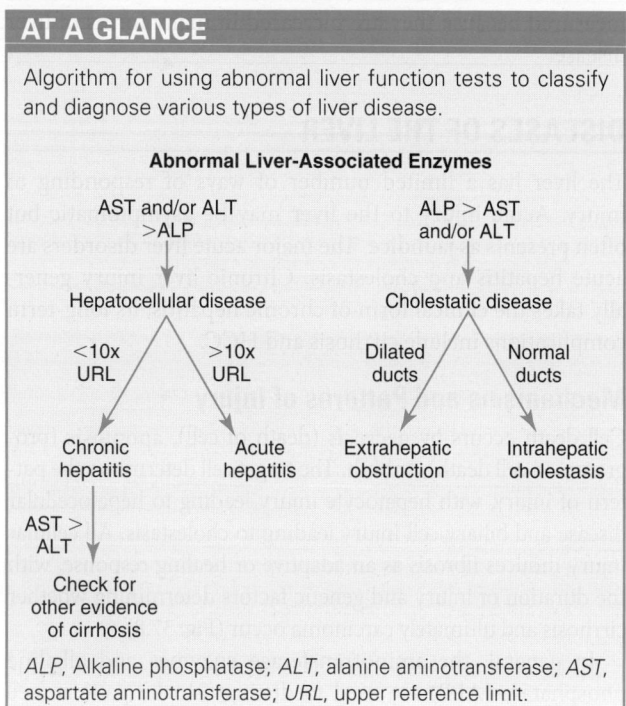

**Abnormal Liver-Associated Enzymes**

AST and/or ALT >ALP → Hepatocellular disease

ALP > AST and/or ALT → Cholestatic disease

Hepatocellular disease:
- <10x URL → Chronic hepatitis
- >10x URL → Acute hepatitis

Cholestatic disease:
- Dilated ducts → Extrahepatic obstruction
- Normal ducts → Intrahepatic cholestasis

Chronic hepatitis → AST > ALT → Check for other evidence of cirrhosis

*ALP,* Alkaline phosphatase; *ALT,* alanine aminotransferase; *AST,* aspartate aminotransferase; *URL,* upper reference limit.

---

Initial evaluation is best accomplished by examining the pattern of liver-associated enzymes. If elevation primarily affects one of the aminotransferases, then hepatocellular disease is likely; an increase primarily in *ALP* suggests a cholestatic disorder. If only ALP is elevated, then it is appropriate to consider nonhepatic sources before further investigation (using measurement of other canalicular enzymes such as *GGT* or ALP isoenzymes). If the liver is the source of elevated ALP, then an imaging study to evaluate the ducts is the next test performed; dilated ducts establish a mechanical cause of obstruction, and normal ducts indicate intrahepatic cholestasis requiring further evaluation, as discussed in the text. Predominant increases in aminotransferases suggest hepatocellular injury; values more than 10 times the upper reference limit *(URL)* usually indicate acute hepatitis and lower values are typical of chronic hepatitis. If aspartate aminotransferase *(AST)* is higher than alanine aminotransferase *(ALT),* common causes include early hepatic injury, nonhepatic injury (such as muscle injury), and with mildly increased values, cirrhosis.

### Disorders of Bilirubin Metabolism

**Jaundice** is a condition characterized by hyperbilirubinemia and deposition of bile pigment in the (1) skin, (2) mucous membranes, and (3) sclera, with a resulting yellow appearance of the patient; it is also called icterus. Defects in bilirubin metabolism resulting in jaundice occur at each step of the metabolic pathway (see Fig. 37.7). Bilirubin disorders are characterized by elevations in conjugated or unconjugated bilirubin in the absence of other abnormal liver tests.

Disorders that cause jaundice in the neonate are classified as unconjugated or conjugated hyperbilirubinemia.

*Neonatal unconjugated hyperbilirubinemia.* Unconjugated hyperbilirubinemia poses a risk for development of **kernicterus** (acute bilirubin encephalopathy), especially in low-birth-weight infants. It is possible to prevent this syndrome by phototherapy and exchange transfusion in infants with elevated unconjugated bilirubin concentrations. Causes of unconjugated hyperbilirubinemia in the neonate are (1) physiological jaundice of the newborn, (2) hemolytic disease owing to Rhesus (Rh) or ABO incompatibility, and (3) breast milk hyperbilirubinemia.

Babies frequently become jaundiced within a few days of birth; this condition is known as *physiological jaundice of the newborn.* Unconjugated bilirubin concentrations reach a peak within 3 to 5 days of birth and remain elevated for less than 2 weeks. Factors contributing to physiological jaundice include (1) increased bilirubin load in the newborn caused by the shortened life span of RBCs; (2) decreased conjugation of bilirubin resulting from relative lack of glucuronyltransferase (conjugating enzyme) in the first few days after birth; and (3) exposure of breast-feeding infants to pregnanediol, nonesterified fatty acids, and other inhibitors of bilirubin conjugation present in breast milk.

Physiological jaundice of the newborn is treated with phototherapy; exposure to light of approximately 450 nm disrupts intramolecular hydrogen bonds in the bilirubin molecule and yields several photoisomers that are more water soluble than the Z-Z-isomer and thus are excreted in the bile. Exchange transfusions are rarely necessary.

Guidelines for managing newborns with hyperbilirubinemia were introduced in 2004. These guidelines were developed to assess the newborn's risk for hyperbilirubinemia prior to their discharge. The increase in bilirubin concentration from the time of birth prior to discharge from the hospital is monitored using a nomogram. In this nomogram, the total bilirubin concentration is plotted versus the age of the newborn (hours) to determine the newborn's risk for hyperbilirubinemia.

*Neonatal conjugated hyperbilirubinemias.* Biliary atresia is a condition in which the bile ducts either fail to develop or develop abnormally. It occurs in one in 10,000 births, and females are more frequently affected. Having no exit to the intestine, bile accumulates inside the liver and eventually escapes into the blood, causing mixed hyperbilirubinemia. Etiologies include (1) certain viral infections, (2) AAT deficiency, and (3) trisomy 17 or 18.

*Extrahepatic biliary atresia,* which is more common than the intrahepatic type, may involve all or part of the extrahepatic biliary tree. If jaundice persists beyond 14 days of age, a direct or conjugated bilirubin measurement must be performed to exclude biliary atresia. If bilirubin is elevated, the urine should be tested for bile. Early identification of this condition is essential if these infants are to benefit from the operation of portoenterostomy, which should be performed no later than 60 days after birth. If portoenterostomy is not successful, liver transplantation is the treatment of choice. Children rarely live beyond 3 years unless the lesion is surgically correctable.

## Hepatic Viral Infection

Five viruses (hepatitis A, B, C, D, and E) have been identified as causes of infections that primarily target the liver. In addition, certain other viruses may infect the liver as part of a more generalized infection, of which the more important causes include cytomegalovirus (CMV), Epstein-Barr virus (EBV), and herpes simplex virus (HSV). Several other viruses have been proposed as causes of liver injury; these include hepatitis G virus (HGV), transfusion-transmitted virus, and the closely related SEN virus. Although all three are blood-borne chronic viral infections, and in the case of transfusion-transmitted virus and SEN have been known to replicate in the liver, none of these viruses appear to cause acute or chronic liver injury. The various hepatitis viruses are outlined in Table 37.1.

### Hepatitis A Virus

The incidence of hepatitis A virus (HAV) has fallen over the past four decades due to the introduction of effective vaccination. Hepatitis A is most common in young adult men, particularly in people exposed to sewage, those who eat raw seafood or inject drugs, and in men who have sex with men. It tends to be most virulent in middle-aged and older people. Epidemics have been associated with waterborne and food-borne contamination. It is estimated 50% to 70% of infected adults develop jaundice (more than hepatitis B virus [HBV] or hepatitis C virus [HCV]), and mortality is almost 2% with infection in those older than 60 years of age. HAV infection in children is rarely associated with jaundice and so is usually not detected clinically. Hepatitis A may cause severe hepatitis and death in those who have chronic hepatitis, particularly hepatitis B or C.

HAV is not cytopathic but causes liver injury by stimulating both cellular and humoral immune responses. The incubation period of hepatitis A is 15 to 50 days. The clinical course of acute hepatitis A is usually that of a mild flu-like illness that lasts for a few days to a few weeks. There is no chronic form of hepatitis A, but cholestasis (manifested by several weeks of jaundice and pruritus) may occur in some adults. Relapse has been known to happen 1 to 3 months after the acute illness in up to 5% of patients.

Diagnosis of hepatitis A is based primarily on serologic tests for antibodies to HAV. Total anti-HAV is believed to be protective and occurs with natural exposure to HAV and to the HAV vaccine. With natural exposure, HAV antibodies appear to persist for life. IgM antibodies to HAV are always present at the time of diagnosis of acute hepatitis A and generally remain present for 3 to 6 months, although they may persist for longer in approximately 14% of individuals. False-positive results can be identified through reference to the clinical context.

Three types of effective vaccines are available. A monovalent vaccine against HAV, a combined HAV and HBV vaccine, and a combined HAV and typhoid vaccine. Vaccination followed by a booster at 12 months will provide immunity for up to 20 years.

### Hepatitis B Virus

HBV is the commonest cause of acute hepatitis and the most common chronic viral infection worldwide. It is estimated 350 million individuals are chronically infected with HBV, and several times as many individuals have been exposed to HBV. The prevalence of chronic HBV infection varies worldwide, being highest in Central and Southeast Asia, Central

| TABLE 37.1 | **Types of Viral Hepatitis** | | | | | |
|---|---|---|---|---|---|---|
| | **A** | **B** | **C** | **D** | **E** | **G** |
| Type | RNA | DNA | RNA | Partial | RNA | RNA |
| Incubation period, days | 45–50 | 30–150 | 15–160 | 30–150 | 20–40 | Unknown |
| **Transmission** | | | | | | |
| Fecal-oral | Yes | No | Min | No | Yes | No |
| Household | Yes | Min | Min | Yes | Yes | No |
| Vertical | No | Yes | Min | Yes | No | Yes |
| Blood | Rare | Yes | Yes | Yes | Unknown | Yes |
| Sexual | No | Yes | Min | Yes | Unknown | Yes |
| Diagnosis | Anti-HAV IgM | HBsAg, PCR, anti-HBc IgM | Anti-HCV, PCR | Anti-HDV | Anti-HEV | Anti-HGV |
| Carrier state | No | Yes | Yes | Yes | Yes | Yes |
| Risk of chronic hepatitis | No | Depends on age, immune status | 50%–70% | Yes | Rare[a] | No |
| Risk of liver cancer | No | Yes | Yes | No | No | No |
| **Prevention** | | | | | | |
| Vaccine | Yes | Yes | No | Yes[b] | No | No |
| Immunoglobulin | Yes | Yes | No | Yes[b] | No | No |
| Response to interferon | Not used | 30% | 40%–80% | Yes | Not used | Yes |

[a]Only with severe immunosuppression.

[b]Vaccination and passive immunization against HBV protects against HDV infection.

*HAV,* Hepatitis A virus; *HBc,* hepatitis B core antigen; *HBsAg,* hepatitis B surface antigen; *HCV,* hepatitis C virus; *HDV,* hepatitis D virus; *HEV,* hepatitis E virus; *HGV,* hepatitis G virus; *IgM,* immunoglobulin M; *Min,* minimal; *PCR,* polymerase chain reaction.

Africa, and Southern Europe (prevalence >8% of the population) and intermediate (2% to 8%) in most of the rest of Asia, Africa, and South America. In endemic areas, the incidence of new infection has decreased markedly where HBV vaccination is practiced. HBV is transmitted through body fluids, primarily by parenteral or sexual contact; it can be transmitted from mother to child, usually at or after delivery (termed vertical transmission). In parts of the world with high rates of chronic infection, much of the transmission is vertical. The residual risk from transfusion is estimated to be 1 in 600,000.

Hepatitis B is caused by a 42-nm DNA virus of the Hepadnavirus family. The S gene codes for several different length variants of surface protein; the smallest form, hepatitis B surface antigen (HBsAg), is produced independently of and in excess of the amount needed for viral replication; the largest form (S1) makes up the surface coat of circulating viral particles. The C gene encodes the hepatitis B core antigen (HBcAg), which is part of the infectious core of the virus. The X gene codes for a transactivating factor that may be involved with viral replication and the development of malignancy. The precore and basal core promoter regions code for production of hepatitis B e antigen (HBeAg), a protein found only in those with circulating viral particles. The final major viral protein is a polymerase, which has several different enzymatically active sites and functions including reverse transcription. This error-prone reproductive strategy and an extremely high replication rate result in a high frequency of mutation in HBV.

*Hepatitis B e antigen and hepatitis B e antigen mutants.* The most common HBV mutations involve the regions that code for production of HBeAg. These mutants are associated with undetectable HBeAg and are usually found in patients with detectable levels of anti-HBe. They may be present at the time of infection or may develop during the course of disease. Infection with these mutant strains is associated with a higher risk of development of HCC, and the risk is stronger for the mutations in the basal core promoter region.

*Polymerase mutants.* Treatment with antiviral agents that inhibit the reverse transcriptase domain of HBV polymerase is currently the most widely used therapy for chronic HBV.

*Hepatitis B surface antigen mutants.* Mutations in the "a" determinant of HBsAg are rare but important HBsAg mutants because antibodies to HBsAg, which are developed by natural exposure or by the HBV vaccine, are primarily directed against the "a" determinant. Mutations in HBsAg can lead to failure of detection by antibodies used in HBsAg assays. Use of assays with antibodies to multiple epitopes improves detection of such mutant strains.

*Diagnostic tests for hepatitis B.* The diagnostic evaluation of HBV infection requires the integration of results from biochemical, immunologic, and molecular tests (see the following "At a Glance" box).

HBsAg, the most widely used marker for detecting current hepatitis B infection, is detected by kits using an antibody to HBsAg. False-positive results occur rarely, particularly during pregnancy; a neutralization assay is available. False-negative results can occur with mutants in the surface antigen, and

they occur more commonly in early HBV infection. Most assays are qualitative. Increasingly quantitative measurement of HBsAg is being used to guide treatment.

Antibodies to the HBcAg (anti-HBc) are the most commonly detected antibodies against HBV. Two assays are usually used: IgM and total anti-HBc. IgM anti-HBc assays typically use a large dilution of plasma (1:100) before analysis to reduce the likelihood of positivity in individuals with chronic HBV. The total antibody assay measures both IgM and IgG antibodies. Anti-HBc appears to last longer than anti-HBs in natural infection and is still present in 97% of previously infected individuals more than 30 years after exposure. Isolated anti-HBc is a relatively common finding. Although this may represent a false-positive result, particularly as a transient phenomenon after influenza vaccination, current guidelines on hepatitis B recommend consideration of individuals with isolated anti-HBc as having been exposed to HBV.

Antibodies to the HBsAg (anti-HBs) are considered evidence of immunity to hepatitis B and are the only marker found in those who have received the hepatitis B vaccine. The World Health Organization (WHO) has developed reference material that contains 10 IU/mL of anti-HBs. Current guidelines suggest that immunocompetent individuals who achieve anti-HBs of ≥10 IU/mL have effective immunity to hepatitis B.

The HBeAg and antibodies to the e antigen (anti-HBe) are typically used only in the setting of chronic HBV infection. HBeAg typically appears at approximately the same time as HBsAg in acute hepatitis. In chronic infection, HBeAg has historically been used as a marker of persistence of infectious virus; its clearance and the appearance of anti-HBe have been used as indicators of conversion to the nonreplicating state and remain goals of antiviral treatment. With widespread availability of HBV DNA assays with low detection limits, the discordance between HBeAg and the presence of infectious viral particles has become apparent. Although most untreated patients with HBV who are HBeAg positive have high viral loads (usually >$10^6$ IU/mL), detectable HBV DNA is also found (usually with lower viral load) in approximately 70% of those who are HBeAg negative, some of whom may have hepatitis that may be associated with elevated transaminases. When HBeAg-positive individuals are treated with polymerase inhibitors, loss of HBV DNA occurs in the majority. Loss of HBeAg during treatment, with development of anti-HBe, indicates a high likelihood that viral suppression will be maintained after discontinuation of treatment. In contrast, in those with HBV viremia who were HBeAg negative (and anti-HBe positive) before treatment, discontinuation of treatment usually leads to recurrence of viremia except in those with HBsAg levels less than 1000 IU/mL. Thus, HBeAg remains an important marker for monitoring therapy but must be assessed in conjunction with HBV DNA for detection of those who harbor the infectious virus.

Hepatitis B viral DNA is now routinely measured using amplification techniques. The WHO has established an international reference material for HBV DNA and results are typically reported in international units per milliliter; conversion from copies per milliliter differs on the basis of viral load and is different for various assays. An approximate conversion factor is 5 copies/mL = 1 IU/mL. Data has shown that risk of progression to cirrhosis or HCC increases at viral loads at more than 10,000 copies/mL (2000 IU/mL). Current treatment guidelines suggest that this number should be used as one criterion in treatment decision making.

Hepatitis B mutants and genotypes are usually determined by direct sequencing or with the use of line probes.

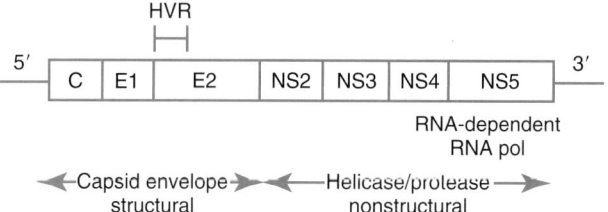

Fig. 37.9 Structure of the hepatitis C genome. *HVR,* Highly variable region.

## AT A GLANCE

### Course of acute type B hepatitis with recovery

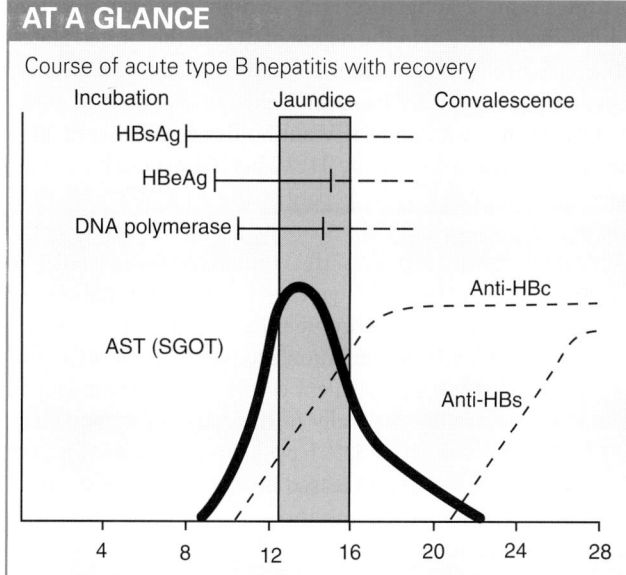

(1) Onset of hepatitis with jaundice 3 months after exposure; (2) detection of hepatitis B surface antigen *(HBsAg)* 2–8 weeks after exposure, followed by appearance of its antibody *(anti-HBs)* 2–4 weeks after HBsAg is no longer detectable; (3) detection of hepatitis B e antigen *(HBeAg)* shortly after HBsAg disappears (this is usually followed by the appearance of antibody to HbeAg *[anti-HBe]*, which persists); (4) detection of hepatitis B core antibody *(anti-HBc)* at the time of onset of disease 2–3 months after exposure. Anti-HBc immunoglobulin M will be detectable in high levels for approximately 5 months.

From Balistreri WF. Viral hepatitis: unique aspects of infection during childhood. *Consultant.* 1984;24:131–153.
*AST,* Aspartate aminotransferase; *SGOT,* serum glutamic-oxaloacetic transaminase.

***Hepatitis C virus.*** The HCV is the cause of most cases previously known as non-A, non-B hepatitis. It was recognized in 1989 and fully characterized 2 years later. It is the commonest cause of chronic **viral hepatitis** in North America, Europe, and Japan and is estimated to infect approximately 170 million individuals worldwide. HCV infection primarily occurs through plasma; major risk factors are injection drug use and transfusion. Because of its mode of spread, HCV infection is rare in children. Vertical transmission may occur from an infected mother (estimated to occur in ≈5% of infected women). Unsterile medical and dental procedures and ritual practices continue to account for new infections.

HCV is a single-stranded enveloped RNA virus of the flavivirus family, which includes other hepatitis viruses (yellow fever virus) and viruses that cause unrelated disease (such as West Nile virus). HCV RNA contains one reading frame (Fig. 37.9). The resulting polypeptide is cleaved to core and envelope antigens, and a number of nonstructural proteins, including a polymerase and a protease. As an RNA virus, HCV is subject to a high rate of spontaneous mutation, giving rise to large numbers of variants. According to various global reviews, genotype 1 (G1) is the most common (46%; affecting ≈83 million cases, one-third of which are in East Asia), followed by G3 (22% to 31%; ≈54 million), G2 (13%; ≈22 million), and G4 (13%; ≈22 million).

Chronic HCV infection is associated with evidence of chronic liver injury in most cases. Elevations in aminotransferases are usually mild and fluctuate in most infected individuals. In 15% to 20% of cases, cirrhosis becomes evident within 30 years. HCC may develop once cirrhosis is present, at an average rate of 1.5% to 3% of cases per year. In North America, Europe, and Japan, HCV is the most common risk factor in the development of HCC. Various extrahepatic manifestations of chronic HCV infection may be noted; the most common are cryoglobulinemia and porphyria cutanea tarda (see Chapter 29). Epidemiologic evidence has linked HCV to increased risk of lymphoma and type 2 diabetes mellitus.

***Diagnostic tests for hepatitis C.*** Measurement of the antibody to HCV (anti-HCV) is the principal screening test for HCV exposure. Current widely used assays incorporate enzyme-linked immunosorbent assays (ELISAs) using antigens from four different regions of the HCV genome. Tests become positive 9 to 12 weeks after exposure.

Reverse immunoblot assays (RIBAs) use a similar principle to Western blotting. HCV antigens are blotted onto a membrane and reactivity is detected after incubation with serum. Results are interpreted as negative if there is less than 1+ reactivity with any of the four antigens, indeterminate if there is 1+ or greater reactivity to only a single antigen (or to more than one antigen along with the nonspecific yeast marker superoxide dismutase), and positive with 1+ or greater reactivity to multiple antigens.

HCV RNA measurement, typically performed using polymerase chain reaction (PCR) amplification, has become the most widely used test to detect current HCV infection. Separation of serum from cells by centrifugation and refrigeration preserves the integrity of HCV RNA, and samples can be kept indefinitely if frozen. Samples collected in EDTA are stable for 24 hours, even if plasma is not separated from red cells. HCV RNA assays have been standardized against international reference material for quantification of HCV RNA in international units per milliliter.

Hepatitis C core antigen (HCV Ag) is produced by the most constant part of the HCV genome and has a similar time course to that of HCV RNA in both acute and chronic HCV infection; the currently available assay for HCV Ag becomes reliably positive when HCV RNA is 20,000 IU/mL or greater which is observed in 95% of untreated HCV RNA–positive individuals. In contrast to HCV RNA, HCV Ag is stable in storage. Currently, no commercial HCV Ag assays are available in North America.

Hepatitis C genotype shows regional diversity and is currently important for determining the selection of antiviral therapy, although pan-genotypic treatments are emerging. Several methods are currently used to determine the infecting genotype. Serologic assays are available but their correlation with direct tests is approximately 90%, and a significant minority of infected individuals have antibodies to more than one genotype. The most reliable method involves direct sequencing of regions of the genome that show characteristic patterns with specific genotypes and subtypes. Commercial assays using the 5′-untranslated region are the most widely used, although assays using the NS5b region are now available. Available assays show good agreement on genotype, but they differ in their detection limits. Sequencing methods have the advantage that they can be used to identify treatment resistance-associated variants that may develop under selection pressure from the new directly acting antiviral agents. Line probe assays are also widely used and show good agreement with direct sequencing assays.

### Hepatitis D Virus (Delta Agent)

Hepatitis D virus (HDV) is an incomplete, 36-nm single-stranded antisense RNA virus that cannot replicate on its own. It is coated with HBsAg and is dependent on HBV for its activation. It is thus a satellite virus similar to that seen in plants. It is very infectious and strongly associated with intravenous drug use; approximately 10 million individuals have been infected worldwide, although the incidence is declining with the fall in incidence of HBV infection. It occurs as a simultaneous infection with hepatitis B (coinfection) or as a superimposed infection in someone with chronic hepatitis B (superinfection). Coinfection usually runs the same time course as acute hepatitis B, and HDV is spontaneously cleared as the hepatitis B resolves, but the risk of fulminant hepatitis is higher than in HBV infection alone, and mortality is higher. Superinfection typically results in chronic HDV infection, suppression of HBV DNA replication, and more rapid progression to cirrhosis (estimated 4%/year) and HCC (estimated 3%/year). It should be assessed in all patients with HBV infection, due to its seriousness, and suspected in patients with HBV infection whose condition worsens.

Although it is traditionally diagnosed serologically by detection of anti-HDV (total or IgM) and/or HDV Ag, HDV RNA measurements are often used as evidence of current infection.

### Hepatitis E Virus

Hepatitis E virus (HEV) is a 34-nm, single-stranded, unenveloped RNA virus. It accounts for sporadic and epidemic hepatitis in tropical and semitropical countries and in people returning from these areas. HEV RNA is frequently isolated from city sewage treatment plants in nonendemic areas. It is enterically transmitted and viral RNA has been detected in plasma and in stools. The specificity of antibody tests for open reading frame 2 antigen of HEV is high. The prevalence of antibodies to HEV is in the region of 21% in the United States. HEV has been isolated from a number of animals, notably rats and pigs, and HEV has been linked to ingestion of pork.

Detection of IgM anti-HEV antibodies is considered diagnostic of acute infection by HEV, but false-positive results have been reported with hepatitis due to CMV and EBV. Molecular tests for HEV RNA can be used to diagnose infection and monitor clearance. The clinical course is similar to that of HAV infection. HEV typically has a self-limited course, but increasingly cases of chronic infection are reported, particularly in organ transplantation recipients. A peculiar feature of this disease is its virulent course in late pregnancy in India, with mortality generally in the range of 20% to 25%, although rates as high as 50% have been reported. Mortality during pregnancy is not increased in other parts of the world. Mortality is increased among the elderly and in those with chronic liver disease.

### Hepatitis G Virus

HGV, also known as GBV-C, is an RNA virus of the flaviviruses family and is closely related to HCV. It is most commonly transmitted by plasma but vertical transmission (i.e., from mother to offspring) has also been reported. HGV infection appears to have no adverse consequences, and, although it has been called a hepatitis virus, viral RNA cannot be isolated from the liver in chronic infection.

## Acute Hepatitis

Acute hepatitis refers to an acute injury directed against the hepatocytes. The injury may be mediated directly, which occurs with certain drugs, such as acetaminophen or with ischemia, or indirectly, which occurs with immunologically mediated injury from most of the hepatitis viruses and most drugs, including ethanol. Direct injury typically causes a rapid rise in cytosolic enzymes, such as AST, ALT, and lactate dehydrogenase (LDH), followed by a rapid fall, with rates of decline similar to known half-lives of the enzymes. Immunologic injury typically causes a gradual rise in cytosolic enzymes, followed by a plateau phase and gradual resolution of enzyme elevation. Although jaundice is a key clinical finding in acute hepatitis, it is often absent. An increase in AST activity to greater than 200 U/L or in ALT activity to greater than 300 U/L has sensitivity and specificity greater than 90% for acute hepatitis.

ALP usually is mildly elevated and is less than three times the URL in 90% of cases of acute hepatitis. Increased plasma concentration of bilirubin, when present, is predominantly due to direct reacting bilirubin. The distribution of direct bilirubin percentage is identical in acute hepatitis and bile duct obstruction. The features helpful in the differential diagnosis of acute hepatitis are summarized in Table 37.2.

The outcome of acute hepatitis is variable. In most cases, complete recovery occurs, and liver regeneration leads to normal structure and function. In a small percentage of cases, massive destruction of the liver leads to acute (fulminant) hepatic failure, which is associated with high mortality unless liver transplantation is performed.

## Acute Viral Hepatitis

All forms of acute viral hepatitis have similar pathology and a similar clinical course. They are all diagnosed on the basis of marked elevations in serum aminotransferase activities, usually to between 8 and 50 times the upper reference intervals, with only slight elevations in ALP and little or no effect on hepatic synthetic function. ALT is typically higher than AST because of slower clearance. Enzyme elevations typically peak before peak bilirubin occurs and remain increased for an average of 4 to 5 weeks (longer for ALT than AST because of its longer half-life). Bilirubin elevation is variable. The incidence, prevalence, and management of acute viral hepatitis are covered in the practice guideline of the World Gastroenterology Organisation.

## Toxic Hepatitis

Toxic hepatitis refers to direct damage of hepatocytes by a toxin or toxic metabolite. Toxic reactions are usually predictable and are directly related to the dose of the agent ingested. In North America and Europe, the most common cause of toxic hepatitis (and the most common cause of acute liver failure) is acetaminophen. The metabolism of acetaminophen is affected by dose, induction of metabolic enzymes, and concentrations of glutathione (Fig. 37.10). When a large dose of acetaminophen is ingested (the average lethal dose is a single ingestion of 15 g), the metabolic pathways are overwhelmed, glutathione is depleted, and toxic intermediates accumulate, causing liver damage. In glutathione depletion due to starvation or metabolic enzyme induction (such

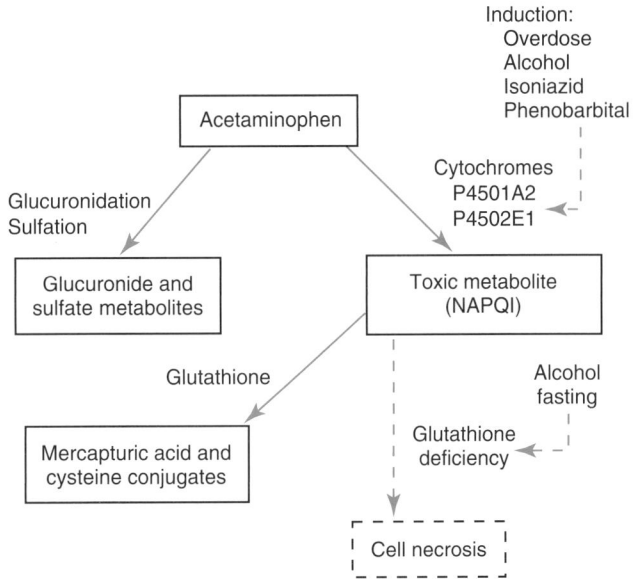

Fig. 37.10 Metabolism of acetaminophen by the liver.

## TABLE 37.2  Laboratory Features of Different Forms of Acute Hepatitis

| Type | AST/ALT | ALP | Bilirubin | PT (s) | Serology | Other |
|---|---|---|---|---|---|---|
| Viral | 8–50× URL | <3× URL | 5–15 mg/dL (86–256 µmol/L) | <15 | Positive | |
| HAV | | | | | IgM anti-HAV | |
| HBV | | | | | HBsAg, IgM anti-HBc | |
| HCV | | | | | HCV RNA ± anti-HCV | |
| Alcoholic | <8× URL | >3× URL in 25% | 5–15 mg/dL (85–256 µmol/L) | <15 | Negative | AST > ALT |
| Toxic | >50× URL | Normal | <5 mg/dL (<85 µmol/L) | >15 | Negative | Toxin usually detectable; acute renal failure common |
| Ischemic | >50× URL | Normal | <5 mg/dL (<85 µmol/L) | >15 | Negative | Acute renal failure common |
| Drug induced | 8–50× URL | >3× URL in 50% | 5–15 mg/dL (85–256 µmol/L) | <15 | Negative | Eosinophilia, skin rash common |
| Autoimmune | 8–50× URL | <3× URL | 5–15 mg/dL (85–256 µmol/L) | <15 | Positive ANA or ASMA | Low albumin, high globulins |
| Wilson | 8–50× URL | Low normal or decreased | 5–15 mg/dL (85–256 µmol/L) | <15 | Negative | Hemolytic anemia, renal failure, low ALP common; low ceruloplasmin often absent |

*ALP*, Alkaline phosphatase; *ALT*, alanine aminotransferase; *ANA*, antinuclear antibody; *ASMA*, anti–smooth muscle (or antiactin) antibody; *AST*, aspartate aminotransferase; *HAV*, hepatitis A virus; *HBc*, hepatitis B core antigen; *HBsAg*, hepatitis B surface antigen; *HBV*, hepatitis B virus; *HCV*, hepatitis C virus; *IgM*, immunoglobulin M; *PT*, prothrombin time; *URL*, upper reference limit.

as by ethanol), toxicity can occur with relatively small doses of acetaminophen (total doses of 2 to 4 g). Toxicity can also occur with excessive cumulative doses of acetaminophen. Diagnosis is often based on history and increased acetaminophen concentrations. In late presentation or when a history cannot be obtained, measurement of acetaminophen-protein adducts allows diagnosis. The first laboratory abnormality to appear is an increase in PT, followed by increased activity of cytosolic enzymes, with AST tending to be higher than ALT. Peak activities (typically >100 times the URLs) usually occur by 24 to 48 hours, followed by rapid clearance at rates approximating the known half-lives of the enzymes. PT elevations are typical and are more than 4 seconds greater than the control value in most cases. Prognosis is related most closely to the prolongation of PT; persistent elevation of PT 4 days after ingestion is associated with a poor prognosis. Other markers of risk include development of acute renal failure and the presence of lactic acidosis, particularly if the pH is less than 7.30 ([H+] >50 nmol/L).

## Ischemic Hepatitis (Shock Liver)

Hepatic hypoperfusion (ischemic hepatitis) is one of the most common causes of elevated cytosolic enzymes, which may exceed 10,000 IU/L; in hospital patients, it is the cause of most cases of acute hepatitis. Ischemic hepatitis may follow any cause of shock; the most common causes are septic and cardiogenic shock. Bilirubin elevations typically are minimal, and they usually peak several days after enzyme activity reaches its greatest point. Laboratory findings are similar to those seen in toxic hepatitis, and acute renal failure is a common complicating factor. Prognosis is primarily related to the underlying cause of hypotension. Individuals with prolonged elevation of bilirubin appear to have a poor prognosis.

### AT A GLANCE

**Assessment of Viral Hepatitis**

- In all cases of viral hepatitis, it is prudent to test patients for each of the major bloodborne viruses: HBV, HCV, and human immunodeficiency virus.
- In viremic patients, testing should include measurement of viral nucleic acid (HBV DNA and HCV RNA).
- Hepatic inflammation is indicated by the extent of elevation of aminotransferases, but these are neither sensitive nor specific.
- The staging of severity of chronic viral hepatitis is determined by the severity of liver fibrosis. Liver fibrosis can be assessed using noninvasive blood tests, fibroelastography, imaging or liver biopsy, or any combination of these tests.

## DIAGNOSTIC ALGORITHM OF VIRAL HEPATITIS

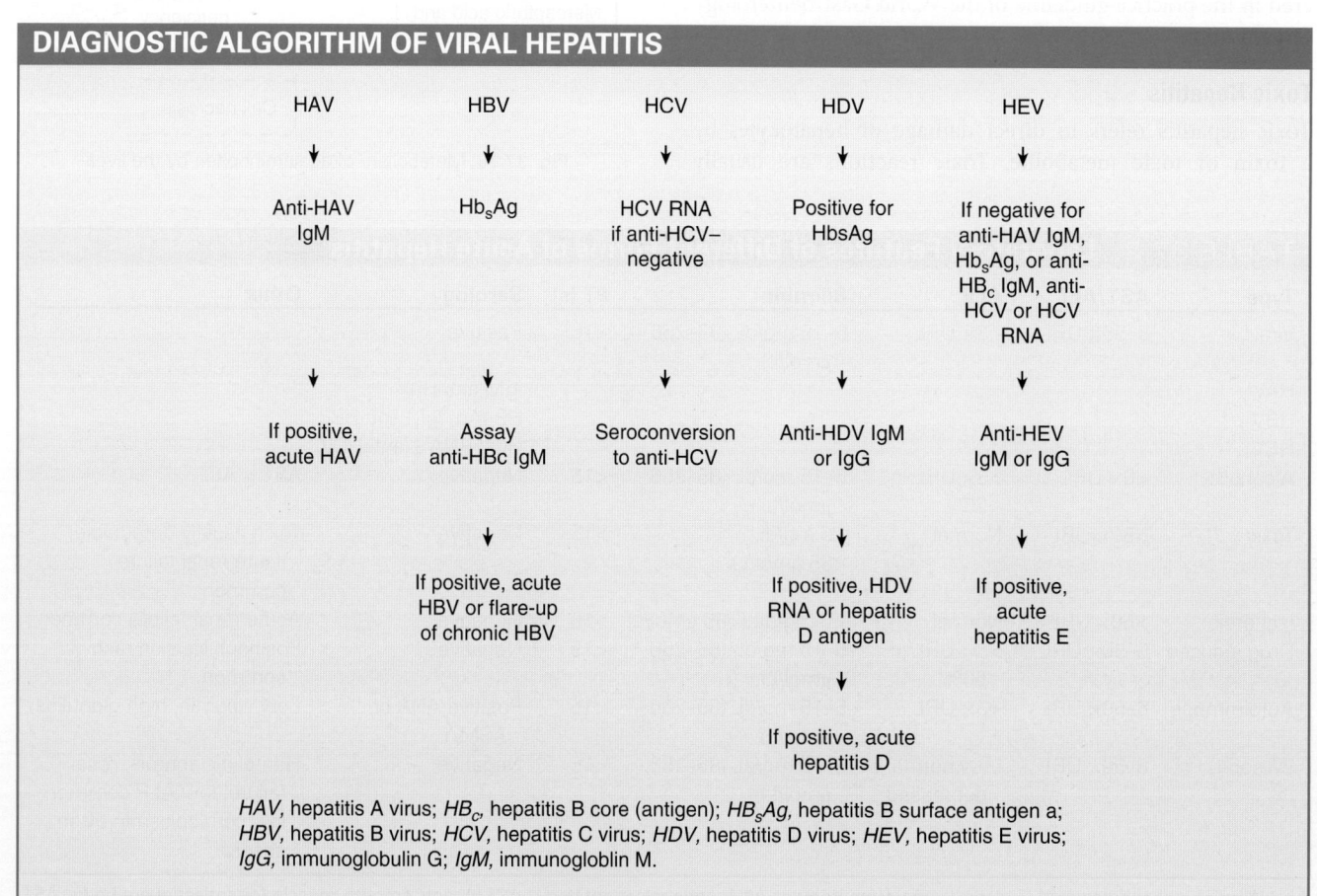

HAV, hepatitis A virus; HB_c, hepatitis B core (antigen); HB_sAg, hepatitis B surface antigen a; HBV, hepatitis B virus; HCV, hepatitis C virus; HDV, hepatitis D virus; HEV, hepatitis E virus; IgG, immunoglobulin G; IgM, immunogloblin M.

From the World Gastroenterology Organization Practice Guidelines–Management of Acute Viral Hepatitis; 2003. http://www.worldgastroenterology.org/guidelines/global-guidelines/management-of-acute-viral-hepatitis/acute-viral-hepatitis-english.

## Chronic Hepatitis

Chronic hepatitis is defined as chronic inflammation of the liver that persists for at least 6 months or signs and symptoms of chronic liver disease in the presence of elevated cytosolic enzymes. Common causes of chronic hepatitis and tests used to make a specific etiologic diagnosis are listed in Table 37.3.

The clinical features of chronic hepatitis are highly variable. Most patients are asymptomatic, but nonspecific features, such as fatigue, lack of concentration, and weakness may be present. Most patients are diagnosed because of an unexplained abnormality in aminotransferase activities or detection of positive results on a screening test for a cause of chronic hepatitis. Moderate elevations in plasma aminotransferase activities are characteristic (an average of approximately twofold, and in most cases, less than fivefold). Normal aminotransferase activities do not exclude chronic hepatitis, especially in the presence of chronic viral hepatitis or nonalcoholic fatty liver disease (NAFLD). Characteristically, ALT is elevated to a greater degree than AST. Reversal of the AST/ALT activity ratio to more than one suggests coexisting alcohol abuse or cirrhosis. Although ALT is relatively specific for the liver, skeletal muscle sources for AST and ALT should always be considered, especially in physically active young individuals. Persistent elevation of aminotransferase activity should lead to an evaluation for chronic hepatitis using the tests outlined in Table 37.3. A liver biopsy may be helpful in determining the cause and in assessing disease severity. A specific etiologic diagnosis is essential to determine prognosis and treatment. The most common causes of chronic hepatitis are chronic HBV, HCV, and NAFLD, but a variety of other disease processes may cause chronic hepatitis.

### Chronic Hepatitis B

Worldwide, HBV infection is the most important cause of chronic hepatitis. According to the WHO, approximately 350 million individuals worldwide have chronic HBV infection; most cases are found in Asia, Africa, and Southern Europe.

HBV is not cytopathic, rather injury results from an immune-mediated inflammatory attack against hepatocytes. Chronic hepatitis results when the virus is not eliminated from infected cells resulting in a continuing cycle of viral replication, reinfection of regenerating hepatocytes, and immune damage to newly infected cells that is inadequate to clear the infection.

The clinical presentation may be complicated by various extrahepatic complications (which occur in 1% to 10% of those with HBV), including polyarteritis, glomerulonephritis, polymyalgia rheumatica, cryoglobulinemia, myocarditis, and Guillain-Barré syndrome. These conditions are associated with circulating immune complexes containing HBsAg. Immunocompromised persons, such as HBV/HIV coinfected individuals, typically have higher replication markers, less hepatic inflammation, and poorer survival than those with HIV alone. The natural history of chronic hepatitis B (defined by the persistence of HBsAg) varies. Features of the different stages of chronic HBV are given in Table 37.4. The evolution of HBV infection is best defined by the nature of the host immune response and inflammatory activity. The stages of chronic HBV infection can only be classified with reference to eAg and eAb status, HBV DNA concentrations, along with ALT activities and histology. HBV DNA levels are commonly very high (exceeding $10^6$ IU/mL) during the immune-tolerant phase of infection. In the immune active and immune control phases of HBV infection, viral DNA levels exceeding 2000 IU/mL are considered to be indicative of levels of replication

### TABLE 37.3  Causes of Chronic Hepatitis and Diagnostic Strategies

| Cause | Diagnosis |
|---|---|
| Hepatitis B | History, HBsAg, anti-HBs, anti-HBc, HBV DNA |
| Hepatitis C | Anti-HCV, HCV RNA by PCR |
| Autoimmune type 1 | ANA, anti–smooth muscle antibody |
| Autoimmune type 2 | SLA, anti-LKM1 |
| Wilson disease | Ceruloplasmin |
| Drugs | History |
| AAT deficiency | AAT phenotype |
| Nonalcoholic fatty liver disease | Metabolic syndrome, liver ultrasound, liver biopsy |
| Idiopathic | Liver biopsy, absence of markers |

*AAT*, Alpha₁-antitrypsin; *ANA*, antinuclear antibody; *HBc*, hepatitis B core antigen; *HBsAg*, hepatitis B surface antigen; *HBV*, hepatitis B virus; *HCV*, hepatitis C virus; *LKM1*, liver-kidney microsomal antigen type 1; *PCR*, polymerase chain reaction; *SLA*, soluble liver antigen.

### TABLE 37.4  Patterns of Chronic Hepatitis B Virus Infection

| Type | AST/ALT | HBsAg | HBeAg | Anti-HBc | HBV DNA |
|---|---|---|---|---|---|
| Occult | Normal | Negative | Negative | Positive | Negative[a] |
| Immune control | Normal | Positive | Negative | Positive | Negative[a] |
| Immune tolerant | Normal | Positive | Positive/negative | Positive | Positive |
| Immune active | Increased | Positive | Positive/Negative | Positive | Positive, viral load >2000 IU/mL |
| HBeAg-negative chronic hepatitis | Increased | Positive | Negative | Positive | Positive, viral load usually >2000 IU/mL but <10⁶ IU/mL |

[a]May have very low level (usually <10² IU/mL) in serum.
*ALT*, Alanine aminotransferase; *AST*, aspartate aminotransferase; *HBc*, hepatitis B core antigen; *HBeAg*, hepatitis B e antigen; *HBsAg*, hepatitis B surface antigen; *HBV*, hepatitis B virus.

associated with liver damage. All phases of chronic HBV are associated with the presence of HBsAg in serum. Occult HBV infection is not associated with inflammation in the liver or elevated aminotransferases.

In general, chronic HBV passes through stages in untreated persons. For those infected early in life, the immune tolerant phase is usually followed by an immune active phase that may vary in duration and may cause significant liver damage. This phase usually gives way to a protracted period of immune control, with HBsAg positivity or occult infection if HBsAg is cleared. For those infected individuals who go on to have chronic infection as older children or adults, the immune toler-ant phase may be a short period or absent, leading straight into the immune active phase. Approximately 8% to 10% of persons per year will transition from the immune active to the immune control phase of chronic HBV. A variable, but low, proportion of those in the immune control phase will revert to the immune active phase that is manifest by levels of HBV DNA greater than 2000 IU/mL and elevated transaminases. Approximately 0.5% to 1% of persons per year will convert from HBsAg positive to HBsAg negative, entering the occult phase of infection (or, in a minority, resolved HBV). Each of these transitions can be associated with an acute rise in aminotransferase activities and a clinical picture that mimics acute viral hepatitis.

Individuals who have chronic replicating infection are at risk of developing cirrhosis and HCC. An estimated 20% to 30% of individuals with chronic hepatitis B will develop cirrhosis over a 20-year follow-up period; the risk is directly related to the amount of HBV DNA, with risk progressively increasing at viral loads of more than 2000 IU/mL (10,000 copies/mL). Once cirrhosis has developed, the annual risk of HCC is 1.5% to 5%. Although the risk of HCC is lower in individuals with HBV infection who do not have cirrho-sis, risk is directly related to viral load and rises at quantities greater than 2000 IU/mL. Even a person in the nonreplicat-ing stage of infection have a 10-fold higher risk of HCC than unexposed individuals. Worldwide, hepatitis B infection is the most common cause of liver cancer.

Efficacy of treatment is typically measured by response of ALT and/or AST and HBV DNA; goals of treatment include normalization of ALT and suppression of HBV DNA to less than the limits of detection of assays, ideally using assays with detection limits of approximately 20 to 50 IU/mL. With poly-merase inhibitors, approximately 70% to 80% of patients will achieve these goals within 1 year of treatment. Duration of treatment is largely dependent on HBeAg status before the start of therapy. For those who are HBeAg positive before treatment, loss of HBeAg and development of anti-HBe indi-cate a high likelihood of maintenance of HBV DNA control and normalization of ALT once treatment is stopped (after 6 to 12 months of further treatment once anti-HBe appears). For those who are HBeAg negative prior to treatment, sup-pression of HBV DNA for more than 3 years with HBsAg levels less than 1000 IU/mL is associated with good control after stopping treatment. Treatment should be maintained indefinitely in patients who do not achieve these goals. With interferon (IFN) therapy, response rates to 1 year of treatment

are somewhat lower than with polymerase inhibitors, but treatment requires only 6 to 12 months. Loss of HBsAg is uncommon; with most agents, the likelihood of loss of HBsAg usually is not higher than that in untreated persons, although it may be higher with IFN and tenofovir.

## Chronic Hepatitis C

Approximately 170 million individuals worldwide have been diagnosed with chronic HCV infection; most cases are found in North America, Northern Europe, and Japan. Chronic HCV infection develops in 75% to 85% of cases of acute hep-atitis C. Clearance of acute HCV infection does not appear to confer lasting immunity. Once viremia becomes estab-lished beyond 6 months after initial exposure, infection never resolves spontaneously. It is estimated that approximately 20% to 30% of patients with hepatitis C will progress to cir-rhosis over a period of 20 years. The frequency of progression appears to be increased by age older than 40 years at the time of infection, male sex, alcohol abuse, and immunosuppres-sion, but it is less than 5% after 20 years of infection in those infected during the first 20 to 30 years of life. In those who develop recurrent HCV after liver transplantation, the rate of progression to cirrhosis is faster than in primary infection. The likelihood of progression to HCC is between 1.5% and 5% per year in those with cirrhosis.

Infection with HCV is characterized by fluctuating ALT activities over time. Only approximately one-third of those with chronic HCV have continually increased ALT, and many of these individuals show variation in ALT activity. A signifi-cant minority of individuals with chronic hepatitis C and nor-mal transaminases have advanced fibrosis or cirrhosis.

Dramatic advances in the treatment of chronic hepatitis C have revolutionized outcomes for patients and changed the requirements for laboratory testing in the management of patients on treatment. Directly acting antiviral agents that target essential HCV proteins have been shown to cure infection in most patients. The critical tests required for the evaluation and monitoring of HCV infection are HCV gen-otype and viral load measurement, both of which depend on molecular tests. Although this remains a rapidly evolving field, it is highly likely that it will be possible to cure infec-tion in almost all cases within the next decade in any patient capable of adhering to a full course of treatment. The assess-ment of HCV genotype, the presence of resistance-associated sequences, and viral load may influence the choice of treat-ment and so access to molecular tests of HCV is mandatory in the treatment of hepatitis C. The extent to which liver fibrosis reverses in patients who attain clearance of HCV still needs to be established, but studies of patients who have been cured using INF-based therapies suggest that the long-term risks of liver cancer and bleeding varices are reduced even in cir-rhotic patients who attain clearance of HCV.

## Nonalcoholic Fatty Liver Disease and Nonalcoholic Steatohepatitis

NAFLD is now a major cause of chronic liver disease and is increasing in prevalence. NAFLD encompasses a range of pathology from simple steatosis to nonalcoholic steatohepatitis (NASH) characterized by an inflammatory response to hepatic fat. Fibrosis is a feature of NAFLD that is triggered by NASH and may culminate in cirrhosis. The histologic features of NASH are identical to those of alcoholic hepatitis (including hepatocyte ballooning, presence of Mallory hyaline, and neutrophil infiltration) but can be attributed to fatty liver disease in those who have no history of heavy alcohol intake. Many individuals with NAFLD have features of the metabolic syndrome (obesity, hypertension, and dyslipidemia). As many as 20% to 30% of the population in North America and Europe have NAFLD, making it far and away the most common form of liver disease and an extremely common condition in the developed world. Approximately 10% of those with NAFLD have NASH. Almost half of individuals who meet the criteria for metabolic syndrome have NAFLD. The frequency in obese or diabetic individuals is much higher, with NAFLD in 60% to 75% and NASH in 20% to 25%. Prospective studies of patients with liver disease have confirmed that NASH is a common cause of elevated liver enzymes in an unselected population of patients referred to gastroenterologists or seen in primary care settings. The frequency of cirrhosis in NASH is not well established, but it has been suggested that NASH may be a major cause of cryptogenic cirrhosis. Because weight loss develops with chronic illness, fat may disappear from the liver, leaving only fibrosis.

Current evidence suggests that accumulation of fat in NAFLD is a consequence of insulin resistance. However, the pathogenesis is likely to be more complicated because a variety of other factors lead to increased fat accumulation in the liver, including increased carbohydrate intake, certain drugs, and mutations in lipid synthesis, but they have not been associated with the development of NASH. Laboratory abnormalities may include raised ferritin levels, signs of diabetes, and dyslipidemia.

## Autoimmune Hepatitis

AIH represents a rapidly progressive form of chronic hepatitis, with up to 40% 6-month mortality in untreated individuals; it is associated with the presence of autoimmune markers. It is relatively uncommon, with an annual incidence of 1.9 cases per 100,000 population in the United States, but it is responsible for 3% to 6% of all liver transplantations; the disease recurs in approximately 30% of patients after transplantation. As with most autoimmune diseases, there is a strong female predominance. Forms of AIH have been found in individuals of all ages, with no racial or ethnic predilection. It has been associated with specific human leukocyte antigen (HLA) haplotypes, notably DR3 and DR4, as is true for many other autoimmune diseases. For details on autoimmune chronic hepatitis, refer to the AASLD (American Association for the Study of Liver Diseases) practice guidelines.

AIH is associated with the presence of liver and non-liver autoantibodies in plasma. These are helpful in diagnosis but are not likely to be the cause of liver injury. The most important antibodies for diagnosis include antinuclear antibody (ANA), anti-smooth muscle (or anti-actin) antibody (ASMA), anti-liver–kidney microsomal antigen type 1, and anti-soluble liver antigen (SLA), which is insensitive but highly specific. A summary of the most common autoantibodies, their associations, and their molecular targets (when known) is given in Table 37.5. Individuals who are negative

## TABLE 37.5  Serologic Markers of Autoimmune Liver Disease

| Antibody Name | Antigen Target | Associations |
| --- | --- | --- |
| Antiactin | Actin | AIH type 1; more specific than ASMA, poor response to corticosteroids, early age of onset |
| Anti-asialoglycoprotein receptor | Transmembrane antigen-binding protein | AIH, correlate with activity, disappear with successful treatment |
| Anti-LKM1 | Cytochrome P450 2D6 | AIH type 2; seen in only 4% of US cases; usually in children |
| Anti–liver-specific cytosol | Enzyme (possibly formiminotransferase cyclodeaminase or argininosuccinate lyase) | AIH in younger patients, often with anti-LKM1, primary sclerosing cholangitis; vary with activity of disease |
| Antimitochondrial antibody | Dihydrolipoamide acyltransferase | Primary biliary cholangitis |
| Antineutrophil cytoplasmic antibodies | Bactericidal/permeability protein, cathepsin G, lactoferrin | PSC (50%–70%), ulcerative colitis (50%–70%), AIH; nonspecific |
| Antinuclear antibody | Multiple targets (centromere, ribonucleoproteins); may not be detected by ELISA | AIH type 1, some PSC cases |
| ASMA | Actin, tubulin, vimentin, desmin, keratin | AIH type 1, seen in other autoimmune diseases in lower titers |
| Antisoluble liver antigen/liver pancreas | UGA tRNA suppressor–associated transfer protein | AIH type 3; specific for AIH, correlate with relapse after corticosteroid withdrawal |

*AIH,* Autoimmune hepatitis; *ASMA,* anti–smooth muscle antigen; *ELISA,* enzyme-linked immunosorbent assay; *LKM1,* liver-kidney microsome; *PSC,* primary sclerosing cholangitis.

for common autoantibodies, but who otherwise meet the criteria for diagnosis, have a similar prognosis and response to treatment.

## Inherited Liver Disease Presenting as Chronic Hepatitis

Inherited liver diseases that present as chronic hepatitis are relatively uncommon but important to recognize and include hemochromatosis, Wilson disease, and AAT deficiency.

**Hereditary hemochromatosis** (HH) is an autosomal recessive disorder of iron metabolism that results in excessive iron absorption and accumulation in tissues, specifically in the parenchymal cells of the liver, heart, pancreas, and other organs. HH is caused by mutations in the *HFE* gene that affect any of the proteins that control the entry of iron into the circulation. These proteins include hepcidin, HFE, transferrin receptor 2 (Tfr2), hemojuvelin (HJV) (these proteins all sense iron accumulation that hepcidin acts to correct) and the protein ferroportin (Fpn), which is a cellular transporter of iron downregulated by hepcidin (for more detail refer to Chapter 28).

HH is primarily a disease in men and postmenopausal women with common clinical features, including lethargy and weakness, arthralgia, loss of libido, upper abdominal discomfort, hepatomegaly, grey/bronze skin pigmentation, testicular atrophy, and joint swelling and/or tenderness. Untreated, HH can lead to serious complications, including liver fibrosis and cirrhosis with HCC in approximately 30% of patients with cirrhosis, diabetes mellitus, cardiomyopathy, and arrhythmias.

Liver disease due to hemochromatosis becomes more common after the age of 30 years. Liver function tests are frequently normal in asymptomatic patients. The most useful tests are fasting transferrin saturation and serum ferritin. A transferrin saturation value more than 45% is the most sensitive marker of early iron overload, but neither a raised fasting transferrin saturation nor ferritin concentration is diagnostic of HH. Ferritin is also an acute-phase reactant and can be raised nonspecifically in the presence of alcohol consumption, NAFLD, other liver disease and any systemic inflammatory condition. Serum ferritin is considered to be abnormal when it is more than 250 µg/L in premenopausal women and more than 300 µg/L in men and postmenopausal women. *HFE* gene testing can be used to confirm the diagnosis of HH and to evaluate familial risks. Cirrhosis is unlikely if the ferritin is less than 1000 µg/L, plasma AST activities are normal, and there is no hepatomegaly. Cirrhotic patients rarely regress to normal and have a lifelong risk of HCC.

Wilson disease. This is an autosomal recessive disorder of copper metabolism. It has a gene frequency of 1 in 200 and a disease frequency of 1 in 30,000. It is due to mutations in a gene on chromosome 13 that codes for a copper-transporting adenosine triphosphatase (ATP7B) found mainly in the liver and involved in movement of copper into bile; deficiency leads to accumulation of copper in the liver and eventually in other tissues.

Wilson disease usually manifests at age younger than 30 years. Patients usually present either with the hepatic or the neuropsychiatric form of the disease. Hepatic involvement tends to predominate in children, whereas in adolescents and adults, the neuropsychiatric form becomes more common. Patients presenting with neuropsychiatric manifestations commonly have advanced liver disease at presentation, whereas those presenting with liver disease may have little in the way of neurologic damage. An important presentation to recognize is antibody-negative hemolytic anemia resulting from hepatic release of copper into the circulation. Several laboratory tests are available for the diagnosis of Wilson disease; ceruloplasmin (see Chapter 18) and copper measurement (see Chapter 27). Classic findings of Wilson's disease include decreased plasma ceruloplasmin, decreased total plasma copper, increased plasma-free (or non-ceruloplasmin) copper, increased urine copper excretion, and increased hepatic copper content. Ceruloplasmin is a ferroxidase that typically is measured by enzymatic activity or by immunoassay. Controversy is ongoing over which assay format is preferable, and guidelines have not specified one type. Molecular diagnosis is complicated by the numerous gene mutations known to cause Wilson disease.

*Alpha₁-antitrypsin deficiency.* AAT is the most important of the serine protease inhibitors (collectively termed serpins; see also Chapter 18). AAT inhibits trypsin and other proteolytic enzymes, including neutrophil-derived elastase, cathepsin G, and proteinase 3. The gene for AAT (*SERPINA1*) is located on chromosome 14. Several genetic variants of AAT (differing by a single amino acid) have been classified on the basis of their electrophoretic mobility; the slowest migrating of these was termed the Z variant. The most severe forms of disease have been associated with homozygosity for the Z variant, which is found in 1 in 1000 to 2000 individuals in Europe and North America. However, it is estimated that only approximately 10% of those with AAT deficiency develop clinical disease.

The effects of AAT deficiency on the liver are controversial. In neonates, AAT deficiency is often associated with hepatitis, with up to 25% 1-year mortality. However, in those who survive the first year, evidence of liver injury diminishes and usually resolves by age 12 years.

AAT is estimated by protein electrophoresis, in which it constitutes most of the α₁-globulin band. It can also be quantified by a variety of other techniques. Determination of phenotype was typically accomplished by isoelectric focusing and had been recommended as the diagnostic test of choice in one guideline, but phenotyping cannot distinguish true homozygotes from heterozygotes who have a null genotype on the other *SERPINA1* gene. Molecular tests are now available to determine *SERPINA1* genotype.

## Drug-Induced Liver Injury

As discussed earlier, most cases of drug-induced liver injury (DILI) present as acute hepatitis. Less commonly, drugs have produced chronic liver injury in a pattern that mimics chronic hepatitis or other chronic liver injury (chronic cholestasis and hepatic granulomas). The drugs most commonly linked to chronic hepatitis are nitrofurantoin, methyldopa, and hydroxy-3-methylglutaryl-coenzyme-A (CoA) reductase inhibitors; however, a large number of drugs have been associated with liver injury, and herbal medications have been linked to chronic hepatitis. In individuals with increased activities of aminotransferases and no obvious cause, prescription drug use was significantly more likely to be present than in those with a known cause for elevated enzyme activities. As with acute drug reactions, establishing drugs as the cause of chronic hepatitis is difficult; temporal relationships to drug ingestion are not as clear as with acute hepatitis, and reactions can be seen first in those who have been taking the medication for many months. Most chronic drug reactions resolve when administration of the drug is discontinued.

## POINTS TO REMEMBER

**Most Common Causes of Chronic Liver Disease**
Alcohol
Fatty liver disease
Chronic viral hepatitis B or hepatitis C

## AT A GLANCE

**Causes of Chronic Liver Disease**
Often the cause of chronic liver disease is not immediately obvious. In this situation, a systematic approach to differential diagnosis should be taken, gathering history, and the findings of clinical examination, and blood and urine tests, as well as imaging and biopsy.
 The following etiologies of chronic liver disease should be considered:
Toxins: alcohol, drugs
Viruses: HBV, HCV
Metabolic liver diseases: fatty liver disease, hemochromatosis, AAT deficiency, Wilson disease
Immune-mediated liver diseases: AIH, PBC, primary sclerosing cholangitis
Infiltration of the liver
Tumors: benign and malignant (primary, secondary)

## Cirrhosis

Cirrhosis, which is defined anatomically as diffuse fibrosis with nodular regeneration, represents the end stage of scar formation and regeneration in chronic liver injury. Fibrosis is the common response to all forms of liver injury. Common causes of cirrhosis and their therapies are listed in Table 37.6. Virtually all chronic liver diseases are known to lead to cirrhosis (see Fig. 37.8).

In the early stages of cirrhosis when the functions of the damaged liver are sufficiently well preserved (termed compensated cirrhosis), no signs or symptoms of liver damage may be present. Laboratory abnormalities usually appear before clinical findings, such as ascites, gynecomastia, palmar erythema, and portal hypertension develop. The earliest laboratory abnormalities to develop in cirrhosis are a fall in platelet count, an increase in PT, a decrease in the plasma albumin-to-globulin concentration ratio to less than 1, and

### TABLE 37.6 Causes and Treatment of Cirrhosis

| Cause | Treatment |
|---|---|
| **Viral** | |
| Hepatitis B | Administration of nucleoside or nucleotide HBV DNA polymerase inhibitors or pegylated α-interferon |
| Hepatitis C | Directly acting antiviral inhibitors of HCV |
| **Toxic** | |
| Alcohol | Abstinence, liver transplantation |
| **Metabolic** | |
| Hemochromatosis | Phlebotomy |
| Wilson disease | Penicillamine, zinc trientine |
| α₁-antitrypsin deficiency | Gene therapy, protein administration |
| Nonalcoholic fatty liver disease | Diet, exercise, insulin sensitizers |
| **Biliary** | |
| Primary biliary cholangitis | Ursodeoxycholic acid, obeticholic acid |
| Primary sclerosing cholangitis | Liver transplantation |
| Autoimmune hepatitis | Corticosteroids, azathioprine, other immunosuppressants |
| Idiopathic | Consider immunosuppression |
| Advanced cirrhosis, irrespective of cause | Liver transplantation |

*HBV*, Hepatitis B virus; *HCV*, hepatitis C virus.

an increase in the AST/ALT activity ratio to more than 1. In general, cirrhosis progresses to decompensation slowly, at a rate of approximately 3% per year; 10-year survival with compensated cirrhosis is 90%. Once decompensation occurs, 10-year survival is only approximately 20%. However, prognosis varies with etiology and may be influenced dramatically by response to treatment (as is the case in viral hepatitis B and C) or by abstinence from alcohol in alcoholic liver disease. Jaundice is a late finding in decompensated cirrhosis. Plasma activities of aminotransferases are variable in cirrhosis and reflect underlying necroinflammatory activity. Clinical scales for assessing cirrhosis in widespread use include the Child-Pugh system. Current thinking advocates the concept of "acute on chronic" liver failure in which acute exacerbations of liver disease due to any one of a variety of causes may cause acute worsening of liver function in cirrhosis. Tests commonly used for the assessment of hepatic function are summarized in Table 37.7.

### Biomarkers of Fibrosis

Due to the limitations of liver biopsy, several noninvasive methods have been developed to detect progressive liver fibrosis and stage liver disease. Over the past two decades, numerous serum markers or biomarkers have been identified

## TABLE 37.7    Tests of Hepatic Function and Injury

| Test | Utility |
| --- | --- |
| Bilirubin | Diagnosing jaundice, modest correlation with severity |
| Alkaline phosphatase | Diagnosing disorders of metabolism and disorders of the newborn |
| Bilirubin fractionation | Diagnosing cholestasis and space-occupying lesions |
| Aspartate transaminase (AST) | Sensitive test of hepatocellular disease; AST > ALT in alcoholic disease |
| Alanine aminotransferase (ALT) | Sensitive and more specific test of hepatocellular disease |
| γ-glutamyltransferase (GGT) | Prognostic indicator for increased cardiovascular and all-cause mortality |
| Albumin | Indicator of chronicity and severity |
| Prothrombin time | Indicator of severity of cholestasis |

and described. In contrast to a liver biopsy, biomarkers are less invasive, with minimal associated procedural morbidity. Serum biomarkers of fibrosis can be categorized into direct serum markers (measuring parameters directly related to both the fibrinolytic and fibrogenic processes involved in liver matrix turnover) and indirect serum markers (combinations of serum parameters that are related to liver function, including AST and ALT).

*Direct biomarkers.* Direct biomarkers exhibit biologic plausibility because they represent alterations of extracellular matrix (ECM) composition that occur during hepatic fibrosis. Combinations of direct biomarkers can result in superior diagnostic performance for the detection of fibrosis compared with their constituent components. The enhanced liver fibrosis (ELF) test is a combination of hyaluronic acid (HA), tissue inhibitor of matrix metalloproteinase 1, and the amino-terminal fragment of procollagen III that has been validated for the detection of fibrosis in a variety of liver diseases, including viral hepatitis B and C, NAFLD in children and adults, and PBC and primary sclerosing cholangitis (PSC).

*Indirect biomarkers.* By contrast, indirect biomarkers reflect parameters that are altered because of changes in hepatic function that arise in the context of a particular stage of liver fibrosis. Indirect biomarkers include biochemical or hematologic variables that are synthesized or regulated by the liver (e.g., clotting factors, cholesterol, and bilirubin), or indicate inflammation (e.g., aminotransferases). Hitherto, the AST-to-platelet ratio index (APRI) has been one of the most studied indirect biomarkers of liver fibrosis. The AST-to-platelet ratio is calculated by dividing AST by the URL of AST (for the sex of the patient) and the platelet count and multiplying by 100. Another indirect biomarker is Fib-4, which is a combination of AST, ALT, age, and platelet count.

*Hybrid biomarkers.* Indirect biomarkers can also be combined with direct biomarkers to form combination or hybrid biomarkers. Fibrometer is a hybrid biomarker that uses age, platelets, prothrombin index, AST, $\alpha_2$-macroglobulin, HA, and urea. Hepascore is a combination of bilirubin, GGT, HA, $\alpha_2$-macroglobulin, age, and sex. Fibrotest is a combination of GGT, bilirubin, haptoglobin, $\alpha_2$-macroglobulin, apolipoprotein A1, age, and sex.

## Hepatic Glycogenoses

The glycogenoses are a group of rare inherited disorders that are characterized by excessive and/or aberrant glycogen storage in various tissues. All are transmitted as autosomal recessive traits, except for type IV, which is sex-linked. The hepatic glycogen storage diseases and their enzyme defects are discussed in more detail in Chapter 22.

## Cholestatic Liver Disease

Cholestasis (stoppage or suppression of the flow of bile) is characterized by retention of bile within the excretory system. The term obstruction is often used inappropriately, because cholestasis frequently occurs without mechanical obstruction to the biliary tract, as with many drug reactions. Mechanical obstruction must always be excluded with imaging in the first instance before other causes are considered. The major cholestatic diseases include mechanical obstruction of the bile ducts, PBC, and PSC. There are specific types of cholestasis that can occur in pregnancy; these are discussed in Chapter 44.

### Mechanical Bile Duct Obstruction

The most common cause of cholestasis is biliary tract obstruction by space-occupying lesions. Extrahepatic bile duct obstruction occurs most commonly as the result of gallstones in the common bile duct or because of tumors in the head of the pancreas or duodenum. Other causes of extrahepatic obstruction include (1) bile duct strictures, (2) extrinsic compression of the bile ducts by enlarged lymph nodes, (3) congenital biliary atresia, and (4) PSC. Extrahepatic obstruction is commonly associated with jaundice, especially when obstruction is complete. Transient increases in aminotransferases are more common with choledocholithiasis than with other causes of extrahepatic obstruction. Transient increases in carbohydrate antigen (CA) 19-9 occur with bile duct obstruction; this is an important consideration because CA 19-9 is often used as a diagnostic test for pancreatic and bile duct carcinoma (for more details see Chapter 20 on tumor markers).

Intrahepatic cholestasis caused by mechanical obstruction is also common but is rarely associated with jaundice or with visibly dilated ducts on imaging studies, although it may be associated with increased direct bilirubin. The commonest cause is drug-induced cholestasis, but viral infections can also cause intrahepatic cholestasis. Obstructive intrahepatic cholestasis leads to jaundice with lesions that are large or are located near the porta hepatis, where they may obstruct both hepatic ducts. Common causes of intrahepatic obstruction include tumors (particularly metastases), granulomatous diseases (such as sarcoidosis and tuberculosis), and infiltrative processes (such as lymphoma, leukemia, and extramedullary hematopoiesis).

## Primary Biliary Cholangitis (Formerly Primary Biliary Cirrhosis)

Primary biliary cholangitis (PBC) or nonsuppurative destructive cholangitis, is an uncommon autoimmune disorder that targets intrahepatic bile ducts. Its prevalence is approximately 2 to 8 per 100,000 population in the industrialized world but is much lower in lower-income countries. The median age at onset is 50 years, and the female-to-male ratio is approximately 6:1. An association with HLA class II antigen DR8 has been noted in some populations. A family history of PBC is seen in 1% to 4% of cases. In up to 80% of cases, the condition is associated with other autoimmune processes, most commonly Sjögren syndrome and hypothyroidism (which often develops before the onset of PBC).

The pathogenesis of PBC is not well understood. However, it is known that destruction of the bile duct is mediated by T cells in the presence of upregulation of HLA class I antigens on hepatocytes and HLA class II antigens on biliary epithelial cells. At least 95% of patients have antimitochondrial antibodies that react against the dihydrolipoamide acyltransferase component of the pyruvate decarboxylase complex. Part of this complex is found on the apical surface of biliary epithelial cells, suggesting a role for this antigen as an immune target. In individuals with coexisting Sjögren syndrome, the antigen is also expressed on the surface of salivary gland cells.

Biochemical tests and direct markers of liver fibrosis have been studied as surrogate markers of disease severity and prognostic markers of survival in PBC.

## Primary Sclerosing Cholangitis

PSC is a chronic inflammatory disease of the biliary tree that most commonly affects the extrahepatic bile ducts; involvement of intrahepatic ducts, with extrahepatic involvement or as an isolated finding, is also possible. In contrast to PBC, PSC has a male predominance (60% to 70%) and a younger median age at onset (30 years). In 70% to 90% of patients, PSC is associated with ulcerative colitis, which usually (but not always) precedes onset of PSC; conversely, only approximately 2% to 4% of patients with ulcerative colitis develop PSC. This has led to speculation that bacterial antigens in portal blood might be involved in the pathogenesis of PSC. An autoimmune component is likely because 97% of patients with PSC have one or more autoantibodies present in their plasma. The prevalence of PSC is similar to that of PBC, but it is most common in Northern Europe, where PSC is the most common indication for liver transplantation. PSC susceptibility is associated with the HLA antigens B8, DRw52a, DR8, and DR3.

## Drug-Induced Cholestasis

Drugs are a common cause of cholestasis, causing approximately 15% of cases. Drug reactions are especially common in older individuals, among whom up to 50% of individuals have

increased enzymes because of medications. Nonmedicinal drugs are also increasingly recognized as a cause of cholestasis. Drugs can cause a cholestatic picture by two major mechanisms. In some cases, only conjugated bilirubin is increased, whereas canalicular enzymes are not elevated. This picture, which is often seen with estrogen and anabolic steroids, appears to be due to inhibition of production of the multidrug resistance protein-2, an ATP-binding cassette (ABC) transporter that transports drug-conjugates and divalent bile salt conjugates into bile. More commonly, drugs induce a cholestatic hepatitis, as discussed earlier. The National Institutes of Health website, http://livertox.nih.gov, and reviews provide further information and excellent support in the investigation of suspected drug-induced liver toxicity.

## Gallstones

Gallstones are solid formations in the gallbladder that are composed of cholesterol and bile salts. Although they vary in chemical composition, they generally contain a mixture of cholesterol, bilirubin, calcium, and mucoproteins. In the United States, 70% to 85% of all gallstones are predominantly cholesterol, and more than 10% of the adult population is affected.

Three major types of gallstones are cholesterol, pigmented, and, the most common, mixed. These stones form whenever bile is supersaturated with cholesterol or unconjugated bilirubin. Whenever an increase in cholesterol or a decrease in bile acids or lecithin occurs, bile becomes lithogenic and cholesterol may precipitate. Factors that predispose to cholesterol hypersecretion include obesity, aging, certain drugs such as fibrates and nicotine, and certain hormones such as estrogen. Factors that decrease bile acid secretion include terminal ileal disease and cholestatic diseases, such as PBC, PSC, and cystic fibrosis. Genetic factors also appear to be involved. Within racial groups, women are more frequently affected than men. Diet may play a role because it appears that people who ingest diets high in polyunsaturated fats have a higher incidence, whereas those with a diet high in fiber have a decreased incidence.

Pigmented gallstones are associated with conditions in which the bilirubin concentration is increased, such as hemolytic anemia, or when bilirubin becomes insoluble (i.e., deconjugated), such as occurs in cholestasis or chronic biliary infection.

## Hepatic Tumors

The liver is host to a wide variety of benign and malignant primary tumors. It is the second most common site of metastases; metastatic tumors account for 90% to 95% of all hepatic malignancies. Primary tumors may arise from many cell lines in the liver, but they arise most commonly from parenchymal and biliary epithelial cells and from mesenchymal cells. The two most important primary liver tumors are HCC and cholangiocarcinoma.

## Hepatocellular Carcinoma

HCC is the fifth most common cancer worldwide and a leading cause of cancer death; more than 500,000 cases occur annually, with a similar number of deaths. Wide geographic and ethnic variations are noted in the incidence, suggesting that both host and environmental factors are involved in its origin. Seventy-five percent of HCC cases occur in Asia, with an annual incidence of HCC in China of approximately 30 cases per 100,000 males. Worldwide, the incidence is two- to threefold higher among men than among women. The incidence of HCC has been increasing in the United States and much of Europe because of the increasing frequency of cirrhosis caused by HCV; however, incidence has declined in many parts of the world because of the success in prevention of infection by HBV. Although cirrhosis is present in most patients with HCC, it is absent in approximately 25% to 30% of cases, often in association with HBV. More importantly, the presence of cirrhosis had been recognized before diagnosis of HCC in only one-third of cases. The incidence of HCC in cirrhosis varies greatly with the cause of cirrhosis, but viral hepatitis B and/or C is the commonest cause worldwide.

The tumor marker most widely used for screening purposes is alpha-fetoprotein (AFP); it is typically quantified using assays that measure its total concentration. Although it appears to be relatively sensitive, elevation of AFP is common in individuals with chronic hepatitis and cirrhosis; this is the same group that has the highest risk for HCC.

## LIVER TRANSPLANTATION

Clinical biochemistry, as part of the multidisciplinary transplant team, plays an important role in the management of patients before and after transplantation. Algorithms incorporating biochemical and other clinical parameters have been developed for the assessment of the need for transplantation in patients with acute and chronic liver disease. These include the Child-Pugh-Turcotte, Model for End-Stage Liver Disease (MELD) Score, and United Kingdom End-stage Liver Disease Score classifications. Post transplantation, the main focus of management is on detecting graft failure, organ rejection, and monitoring the efficacy of immunosuppression. Laboratories are closely involved in monitoring liver enzymes, tests of hepatic synthetic function, therapeutic drug monitoring, and monitoring for viruses, including recurrence of HBV or HCV and CMV, which may complicate the course of recovery in immune-suppressed patients.

### Analytical Methods for Bilirubin

Serum bilirubin is measured in body fluids by spectrophotometric or chromatographic methods.

#### Diazo Methods

The reaction of bilirubin with diazotized sulfanilic acid, known as the *diazo reaction,* is the basis of the most widely used methods for measuring bilirubin. The observation that the reaction was slow in sera from jaundiced infants and required an accelerator (ethanol) to proceed, and that it was rapid in bile and in adult sera with the addition of ethanol led to the terms indirect bilirubin and direct bilirubin, respectively.

The reaction of the coupling of bilirubin with a diazo compound is shown in Fig. 37.11. In this example, diazotized sulfanilic acid reacts with bilirubin to produce two azodipyrroles, which are reddish purple at neutral pH and blue at low or high pH values. Numerous variations of this method have been developed. All use one of a variety of "accelerators," which facilitate the reaction of unconjugated (indirect) bilirubin with the diazo reagent. The most commonly used accelerators are (1) caffeine, (2) dyphylline, and (3) several surface-active agents (surfactants).

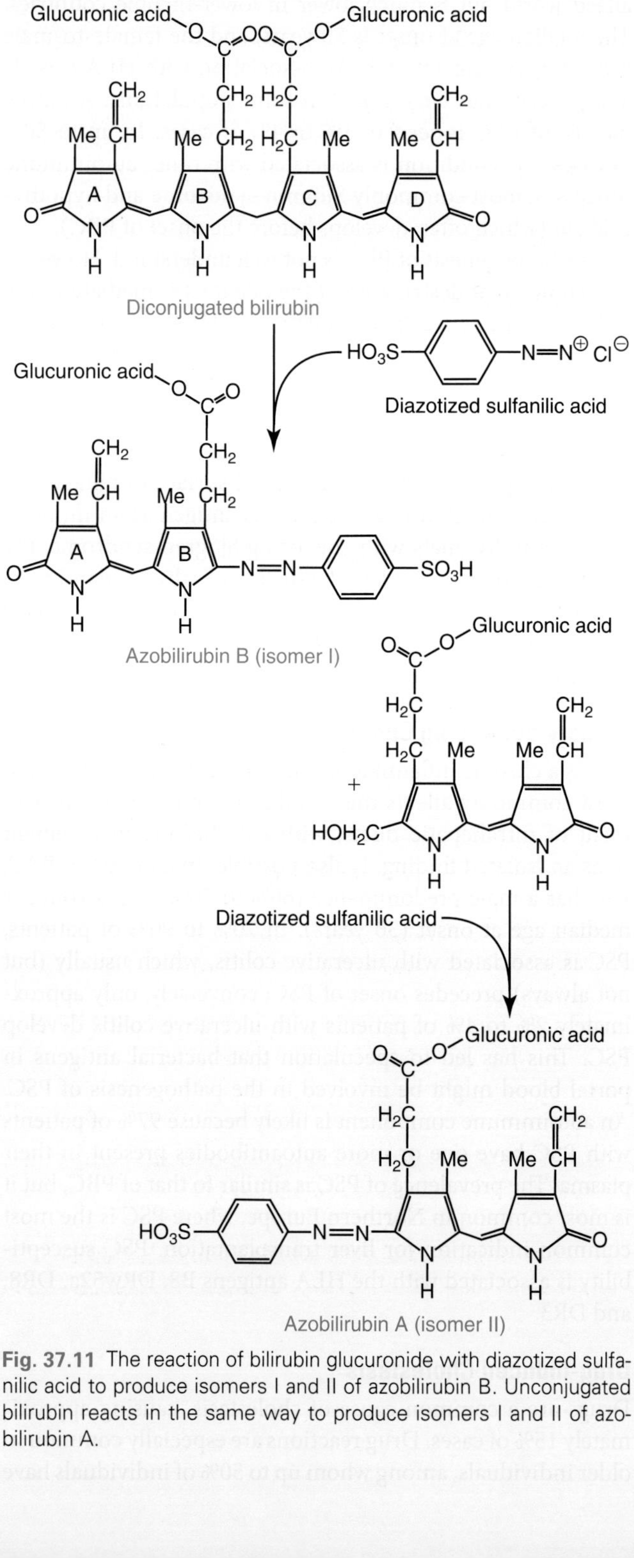

Fig. 37.11 The reaction of bilirubin glucuronide with diazotized sulfanilic acid to produce isomers I and II of azobilirubin B. Unconjugated bilirubin reacts in the same way to produce isomers I and II of azobilirubin A.

## Total Bilirubin

The Doumas-modified Jendrassik-Grof method to quantitate total bilirubin in serum is the most commonly used method in the clinical laboratory. In this procedure, serum is added to an aqueous solution of caffeine and sodium benzoate (accelerator), which displaces unconjugated bilirubin from its association sites on albumin. Formation of hydrogen bonds with caffeine renders the bilirubin water soluble and facilitates its reaction with diazotized sulfanilic acid. After a 10-minute incubation period at room temperature, alkaline tartrate is added, and absorbance of the alkaline azobilirubin is measured at 598 nm. This method is currently the reference measurement procedure for measuring total bilirubin in serum.

*Direct bilirubin.* Bilirubin monoconjugates and diconjugates (mainly glucuronides), and delta-bilirubin, because they are water-soluble, react with the diazo reagents in the absence of accelerators. A reliable method for direct bilirubin should not measure any unconjugated bilirubin. To prevent the unconjugated bilirubin from reacting, it is necessary to keep the pH of the reaction mixture near 1.0. A preferred manual method for direct bilirubin is available. Ditaurobilirubin (bilirubin conjugated with taurine and available as the disodium salt)—a water-soluble synthetic material—is used by instrument manufacturers for calibrating direct bilirubin methods; it is also present in quality control and proficiency-testing materials.

## REVIEW QUESTIONS

1. In the liver, bilirubin is conjugated to:
   a. vinyl groups.
   b. methyl groups.
   c. hydroxyl groups.
   d. glucuronide.

2. Functions of the liver include the synthesis of all of the following *except*:
   a. albumin.
   b. immunoglobulins.
   c. glycogen.
   d. coagulation factors.

3. In the liver, the small grooves between adjacent hepatocytes that carry bile to the gallbladder are the:
   a. cords.
   b. canaliculi.
   c. lobules.
   d. sinusoids.

4. Hepatocellular carcinoma (HCC) can be directly related to:
   a. an acute viral hepatitis infection.
   b. cholestasis.
   c. a chronic hepatitis B infection.
   d. the synthetic function of the liver.

5. Which type of viral hepatitis is usually spread parenterally by transfusion, shared needles, or dialysis and is considered the most common chronic viral infection in North America?
   a. Hepatitis B
   b. Hepatitis C
   c. Hepatitis A
   d. Cirrhosis

6. Laboratory tests that are initially run to determine the presence of any liver disease include:
   a. liver enzymes only.
   b. viral antigens and antibodies, serum cholesterol.
   c. hepatitis antigens and antibodies, coagulation times, and serum proteins.
   d. bilirubin, liver enzymes, prothrombin time (PT), and albumin.

7. Blockage of the bile ducts or blockage of bile flow from within the liver due to inflammation will stop normal bile flow. This is referred to as:
   a. hepatitis.
   b. hepatocellular carcinoma (HCC).
   c. cholestasis.
   d. cirrhosis.

8. A genetic disorder that is associated with elevated amounts of copper in the liver and other tissues and leads to decreased ceruloplasmin concentration in blood is:
   a. Wilson disease.
   b. Reye syndrome.
   c. cholestasis.
   d. autoimmune hepatitis.

9. A woman visits her physician with symptoms of jaundice, hepatic pain, and chalky-appearing stools. Lab values indicate elevated conjugated bilirubin, alkaline phosphatase (ALP) and γ–glutamyltransferase (GGT). These findings are most likely due to:
   a. hemolytic anemia.
   b. ineffective erythropoiesis.
   c. cholestasis due to gallstones.
   d. Reye syndrome.

10. The type of portal hypertension seen in the majority of cases is sinusoidal hypertension, which is most commonly caused by:
    a. blockage of the portal veins.
    b. hepatic vein occlusion.
    c. congestive heart failure.
    d. cirrhosis.

## SUGGESTED READINGS

Bhutani VK, Johnson L, Sivieri EM. Predictive ability of predischarge hour-specific serum bilirubin for subsequent significant hyperbilirubinemia in healthy term and near-term newborns. *Pediatrics.* 1991;103:6–14.

Choo QL, Kuo G, Weiner A, et al. Isolation of a cDNA clone derived from a blood-borne non-A, non-B viral hepatitis genome. *Science.* 1989;244:359–362.

Day CP. Non-alcoholic fatty liver disease: a massive problem. *Clin Med.* 2011;11:176–178.

Doumas BT, Poon PKC, Perry BW, et al. Candidate reference method for determination of total bilirubin in serum: development and validation. *Clin Chem.* 1985;31:1779–1789.

Dufour DR, Lott JA, Nolte FS, et al. Diagnosis and monitoring of hepatic injury. I. Performance characteristics of laboratory tests. *Clin Chem.* 2000;46:2027–2049.

European Association for the Study of the Liver. EASL Clinical practice guidelines: Management of chronic hepatitis B virus infection. *J Hepatol.* 2012;1:167–185.

Fontan R, Lok A. Noninvasive monitoring of patients with chronic hepatitis C. *Hepatology.* 2002;36:S57–S64.

Friedman SL. Evolving challenges in hepatic fibrosis. *Nat Rev Gastroenterol Hepatol.* 2010;7:425–436.

Gow PJ, Smallwood RA, Angus PW, et al. Diagnosis of Wilson's disease: an experience over three decades. *Gut.* 2000;46:415–419.

Guha IN, Parkes J, Roderick P, et al. Non-invasive markers of fibrosis in nonalcoholic fatty liver disease: validating the European Liver Fibrosis panel and exploring simple markers. *Hepatology.* 2008;47:455–460.

Hennes EM, Zeniya M, Czaja AJ, et al. Simplified criteria for the diagnosis of autoimmune hepatitis. *Hepatology.* 2008;48:169–176.

Kamath PS, Wiesner RH, Malinchoc B, et al. A model to predict survival in patients with end-stage liver disease. *Hepatology.* 2001;33:464–470.

Lam BP, Jeffers T, Younoszai Z, et al. The changing landscape of hepatitis C virus therapy: focus on interferon-free treatment. *Therap Adv Gastroenterol.* 2015;8:298–312.

Lee WM. Acetaminophen-related acute liver failure in the United States. *Hepatol Res.* 2008;38:S3–S8.

Lindor KD, Gershwin ME, Poupon R, et al. Primary biliary cirrhosis. *Hepatology.* 2009;50:291–308.

Lucey MR, Mathurin P, Morgan TR. Alcoholic hepatitis. *N Engl J Med.* 2009;360:2758–2769.

McMahon BJ. The natural history of chronic hepatitis B virus infection. *Hepatology.* 2009;49:S45–S55.

Pietrangelo A. Hereditary hemochromatosis: pathogenesis, diagnosis and treatment. *Gastroenterology.* 2010;139:393–408.

Rosenberg WMC, Voelker M, Thiel R, et al. Serum markers detect the presence of liver fibrosis: a cohort study. *Gastroenterology.* 2004;127:1704–1713.

Zimmerman HJ. Drug-induced liver disease. *Clin Liver Dis.* 2000;4:73–96.

# Gastric, Intestinal, and Pancreatic Function

*Roy A. Sherwood and Natalie E. Walsham*

## OBJECTIVES

1. Define the following terms:
   - Digestion
   - Absorption
   - *Helicobacter pylori*
   - Celiac disease
   - Steatorrhea
   - Diarrhea
2. List and describe the three phases of digestion.
3. Describe the structure and function of the stomach, intestinal tract, and pancreas.
4. List the main enzymes involved in the digestion of carbohydrates, fats, and proteins.
5. List the tests used to investigate possible celiac disease, lactase deficiency, and bacterial overgrowth and describe the test principles.
6. State the use of the following tests:
   - Serum gastrin
   - Fecal elastase
   - Antibodies against tissue transglutaminase
   - Fecal calprotectin

## KEY WORDS AND DEFINITIONS

**Acute pancreatitis** An acute episode of destruction of the pancreas due to the release of active pancreatic enzymes into pancreatic tissue.

**Breath tests** Tests that detect products of bacterial metabolism in the gut or products of human metabolism by measuring compounds in breath.

**Celiac disease** A disease caused by the destructive interaction of gluten with intestinal mucosa causing malabsorption.

**Chronic pancreatitis** An inflammatory disease characterized by persistent and progressive destruction of the pancreas.

**Crohn disease** A chronic inflammatory bowel disease that may affect any part of the digestive tract.

**Cystic fibrosis** An inherited disease caused by genetic alteration of a transmembrane conductance regulator protein (CFTR) that can lead to chronic pancreatitis and pulmonary disease.

**Diarrhea** The passage of liquid stools more than three times daily and/or a stool weight greater than 200 g/day.

**Digestion** The conversion of food in the intestines into compounds capable of being absorbed.

**Gastrin** A group of peptide hormones secreted by gastrointestinal mucosal cells that stimulate the production of acid.

**Gastritis** Inflammation of the mucosa of the stomach.

**Helicobacter pylori** A bacterium found in the stomach that can be associated with inflammation.

**Lactose intolerance** A condition due to lactase deficiency leading to the malabsorption of lactose resulting in symptoms following consumption of foods containing lactose.

**Malabsorption** An abnormality in the absorption of nutrients.

**Maldigestion** An abnormality of the digestive process due to dysfunction of the pancreas or small intestine.

**Steatorrhea** A condition of excessive fat in feces.

**Ulcerative colitis** An inflammatory bowel disease predominantly localized to the large intestine.

## INTRODUCTION TO THE ANATOMY AND PHYSIOLOGY OF THE GASTROINTESTINAL TRACT

The major organs of the gastrointestinal (GI) tract include the esophagus, stomach, small and large intestines, pancreas, liver (see Chapter 37), and gallbladder, all of which are involved in the digestive processes that commence with the ingestion of food and water and culminate with the excretion of waste products as feces.

### Anatomy

The GI tract is a hollow tube approximately 8 m in length beginning with the mouth and ending with the anus. The esophagus, which is approximately 25 cm in length, is a muscular tube connecting the pharynx to the stomach. The laboratory has little role in the investigation of disorders of the esophagus.

#### Stomach

The stomach consists of three major zones: the cardiac zone, the body, and the pyloric zone (Fig. 38.1). The upper cardiac

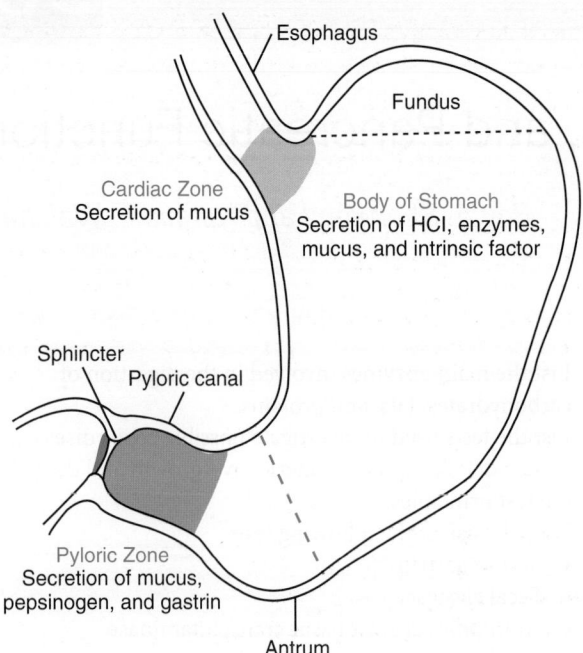

Fig. 38.1 Schematic drawing of the stomach with major zones.

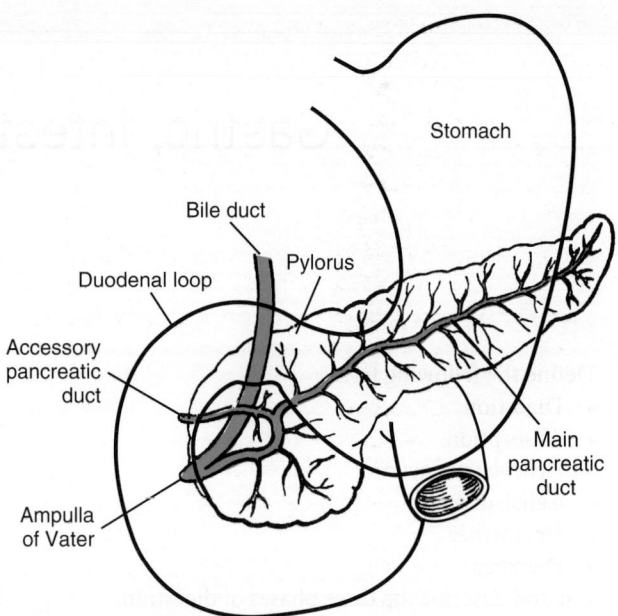

Fig. 38.2 Cross-section through the pancreas.

zone includes the fundus and contains mucus and pepsinogen II–secreting surface epithelial cells and endocrine-secreting cells. The body of the stomach contains cells of many different types: surface epithelial cells that secrete mucus, parietal cells that secrete hydrochloric acid and intrinsic factor, chief cells that secrete group I and II pepsinogens, enterochromaffin cells that secrete serotonin, and other endocrine cells. The pyloric zone is subdivided into the antrum (approximately the distal third of the stomach), the pyloric canal, and the sphincter. The cells of the pyloric zone secrete mucus, group II pepsinogens, serotonin, and **gastrin**, but not hydrochloric acid. In the stomach, food is converted into a semifluid, homogeneous material (chyme) that passes through the pyloric sphincter into the small intestine.

### Small Intestine

The small intestine consists of three parts: the duodenum, jejunum, and ileum. In adults, the small intestine is approximately 6 m in length and its cross section decreases as it proceeds distally. The duodenum is approximately 25 cm long and is the shortest part of the small intestine. The jejunum and ileum make up the remainder of the small intestine, with the ileum constituting the distal 3.5 m.

The wall of the small intestine consists of four layers: mucosa, submucosa, muscularis propria, and serosa/adventitia. The internal surface of the upper part of the small intestine contains valve-like circular folds (valvulae conniventes or plicae circulares) that project 3 to 10 mm into the lumen. Covering the entire mucous surface are small (1-mm) finger-like projections (villi). The luminal surface of each epithelial cell consists of some 1700 microvilli projecting approximately 1 μm from the cell. The folds, villi, and microvilli increase the absorptive surface area 600-fold to approximately 250 m², comparable to the area of a doubles lawn tennis court.

### Large Intestine

The large intestine is approximately 1.5 m in length, extending from the ileum to the anus and including the cecum, appendix, colon, rectum, and anal canal. The cecum is a blind pouch that begins the large intestine; it is connected to the terminal ileum via the ileocecal sphincter (or valve). The colon is approximately 1 m long and is divided into ascending, transverse, descending, and sigmoid sections. The sigmoid colon connects to the rectum, which is approximately 15 cm long, and connects to the anal canal.

### Pancreas

The pancreas is 12 to 15 cm long and lies across the posterior wall of the abdominal cavity. The head is located in the duodenal curve, with the body and tail extending to the spleen (Fig. 38.2). The pancreas secretes a juice containing digestive enzymes and bicarbonate; this enters the duodenum through the ampulla of Vater and the sphincter of Oddi to mix with the bolus of food coming from the stomach.

## Phases of Digestion

The processes of **digestion** can be divided into neurogenic, gastric, and intestinal phases.

### Neurogenic Phase

The neurogenic, or cephalic, phase is initiated by the intake of food into the mouth; the sight, smell, and taste of food stimulate the cerebral cortex and subsequently the vagal nuclei.

### Gastric Phase

When food enters the stomach, the resulting distention initiates the gastric phase of digestion, which is mediated by local and vagal reflexes. Hydrochloric acid release is caused by direct vagal stimulation of the parietal cells, local distention of the antrum, and vagal stimulation of antral cells to secrete gastrin. Gastrin also stimulates antral motility, secretion of pepsinogens and of pancreatic fluid rich in enzymes, and release of hormones such as secretin, insulin, acetylcholine, somatostatin, and pancreatic polypeptide. As a result of the acid environment, pepsinogen is rapidly converted to the active proteolytic enzyme pepsin. Food is mixed by contractions of the stomach and is partially degraded into chyme by the chemical secretions of the stomach. The pylorus plays a role in emptying chyme into the duodenum by virtue of its strong musculature.

### Intestinal Phase

The intestinal phase of digestion begins when the weakly acidic digestive products of proteins enter the duodenum. Many hormones and other regulatory peptides are released by both neural and local stimulation and act within the GI tract to regulate digestion and absorption. Digestion, absorption, and storage functions are stimulated or inhibited by different hormones. This results in a control system that regulates the action of intestinal hormones and induces the secretion of bile acids, bicarbonate, and numerous enzymes involved in the digestion of food.

During the intestinal phase, carbohydrates, proteins, and fats are degraded and absorbed. Most nutrients, including vitamins and minerals, will have been absorbed by the time the food passes from the jejunum and ileum into the large intestine. In the large intestine, water is actively absorbed, electrolyte balance is regulated, and further bacterial degradation of residual food occurs. These processes result in the formation of feces.

### Processes of Digestion and Absorption

The total quantity of fluid absorbed each day by the gut is estimated to be approximately 9 L, which is composed of 2 L oral intake, 1.5 L saliva, 2.5 L gastric juice, 0.5 L bile, 1.5 L pancreatic juice, and 1 L intestinal secretions. More than 90% of this fluid is absorbed in the small intestine. The maximal absorptive capacity for fluid is probably at least 20 L. Typically several hundred grams of carbohydrates, 100 g of fat, and 50 to 100 g of amino acids are absorbed daily in the small intestine, but the maximal absorptive capacity may be 10 times higher. This considerable reserve capacity may explain the lack of symptoms from mild disease processes. The efficiency of absorption is due to the unique features of the absorptive surface of the bowel and the relationship of the epithelial cells to the underlying rich vascular plexus and lymphatic vessels.

Digestion of food starts in the mouth through the action of salivary amylase and lingual lipase, but it principally takes place both within the lumen of the small intestine and at the mucosal (brush-border) surface. Defects of digestion may occur at one or more stages of this process. The terms **maldigestion** and **malabsorption** refer to different functional abnormalities. *Maldigestion* is a dysfunction of the digestive process that may occur at various sites in the GI tract. For example, a reduction in the acidity in the stomach will reduce peptic digestion of protein, whereas hyperacidity of the duodenum can inactivate pancreatic enzymes. Loss of brush-border enzymes in the small intestine can prevent oligosaccharides and disaccharides from being further hydrolyzed. Pancreatic insufficiency will reduce intraluminal enzyme activity in the small gut, causing maldigestion of fats and proteins. Inherited disorders of the exocrine pancreas can cause pancreatic insufficiency secondary to chronic pancreatic inflammation and ultimately lead to maldigestion. In contrast, *malabsorption* is strictly a dysfunction of the absorptive process in the small gut resulting from a reduction in the size of the absorptive surface caused by responses to factors including gluten, inflammation, infection, surgical resection, and infiltration. Various genetic defects also lead to malabsorption of specific substances (e.g., glucose-galactose malabsorption, zinc deficiency in the congenital disorder acrodermatitis enteropathica). In clinical practice, however, the term *malabsorption* is often used to encompass all aspects of impaired digestion and absorption.

In the following sections, the digestion and absorption of carbohydrates, fats, and proteins are discussed separately. It must be remembered, however, that a complex interplay takes place among nutrients, regulatory peptides, enzymes, gallbladder, and pancreatic function, the microbiota of the gut and bowel motility, leading to an integrated absorptive process that commences with the ingestion of food, and culminates in the excretion of feces.

### Digestion and Absorption of Carbohydrates

After the salivary and pancreatic α-amylases have acted on dietary starch and glycogen, the carbohydrate content of the small intestine consists of ingested monosaccharides; dietary disaccharides such as lactose, sucrose, maltose, and trehalose; oligosaccharides such as dextrins and maltotriose and indigestible oligosaccharides and polysaccharides such as cellulose, agar, and other dietary fibers.

The brush-border enzymes with disaccharidase and oligosaccharidase activity are listed in Table 38.1. The sucrase-isomaltase complex comprises most (80%) of the sucrase, isomaltase, and maltase activity of the small intestine. It hydrolyzes sucrose to its constituent monosaccharides, cleaves glucose from α-limit dextrins with 1,6 bonds, and hydrolyzes maltose. The activity of the complex is four- to fivefold greater in the jejunum than the ileum. Changes in diet have a marked effect on the expression of the complex; starvation leads to a rapid decline in activity that is quickly restored on refeeding. Secretion of all small intestinal saccharidases may decrease with infection or inflammation of the small bowel to the extent that carbohydrate malabsorption occurs, leading to **diarrhea**, flatulence, and weight loss.

The lactase–phlorizin hydrolase complex is the only brush-border enzyme able to hydrolyze lactose and is therefore essential for the survival of mammals early in life. Infectious and inflammatory diseases greatly reduce lactase–phlorizin hydrolase activity, leading to symptomatic intolerance to milk (bloating, abdominal pain, diarrhea, and flatulence).

## TABLE 38.1   Brush-Border Oligosaccharidases

| Enzyme | Principal Substrate | Products |
|---|---|---|
| Lactase (EC 3.2.1.23) | Lactose | Glucose + galactose |
| Sucrase (EC 3.2.1.48) | Maltose/sucrose | Glucose or fructose + glucose |
| Isomaltase (EC 3.2.1.10) | 1,6-α-linkages in Isomaltose and α-dextrins | Glucose |
|  | Maltose | Glucose |
| Trehalase (EC 3.2.1.28) | Trehalose | Glucose |
| Glucoamylase complex (EC 3.2.1.20) | | |

The developmental regulation of lactase is discussed later, in the section on disaccharidase deficiencies. Also present in the brush-border is the α-glucosidase maltase-glucoamylase, which removes individual glucose molecules from the nonreducing end of α(1,4)-oligosaccharides and disaccharides. This enzyme accounts for approximately 20% of the total maltase activity of the small intestine. Trehalase is also found in the brush-border of the small intestine and hydrolyzes trehalose, an α(1,1)-disaccharide of glucose found in yeast and mushrooms. The developmental pattern of trehalase appears to follow that of sucrase-isomaltase.

In addition to their actions on disaccharides, the brush-border enzymes further hydrolyze the products of amylase action, including maltose, maltotriose, and α-limit dextrins. The brush-border enzymes appear to act in an integrated manner in that a flow of substrate occurs from glucoamylase and isomaltase to sucrose, producing the monosaccharides glucose, galactose, and fructose. These monosaccharides are transported into enterocytes by the sodium-dependent glucose (and galactose) transporter (SGLT1) and the GLUT5 transporter, which transports fructose across the apical membrane of the enterocyte. Absorbed glucose and fructose are transported across the basolateral membrane, out of the enterocyte, and into the portal system by the GLUT2 transporter.

Carbohydrate digestion in the small intestine is not always complete. Up to 10% of ingested starch and sucrose can pass undigested and unabsorbed into the colon. It has been estimated that colonic bacteria require 70 g of carbohydrates per day. Much of this is derived from endogenous sources, such as glycoproteins from GI secretions, with the remainder coming from unabsorbed dietary carbohydrates and dietary fiber. Bacterial action creates short-chain fatty acids that are rapidly absorbed by the colonic mucosa and are thought to provide fuel for the colonocytes. Starch and oligosaccharides are osmotically active; they draw water into the gut and retain luminal fluidity. The colon, however, can absorb up to four times the normal colonic water load; for this reason, diarrhea is not always present in oligosaccharide malabsorption.

### Digestion and Absorption of Lipids

The recommended daily fat intake in Europe and North America is 70 to 85 g. Less than 5 g/24 h is recoverable in feces, indicating the overall efficiency of the normal processes of fat digestion and absorption. Most dietary fat is in the form of long-chain triacylglycerols (triglycerides). Pancreatic lipase is quantitatively the most important hydrolytic enzyme, but the contribution of gastric lipase to overall hydrolysis should not be underestimated. Gastric lipase is secreted by the gastric mucosa and normally accounts for up to 17.5% of fatty acids released from triglycerides following a meal. Lipase has a wide pH optimum and is active in both the stomach and duodenum. This nonpancreatic lipase may have a significant role in lipid digestion when pancreatic function is impaired and in the neonatal period before pancreatic lipase activity is fully developed. A lingual lipase is also produced but is thought to be of little significance in humans.

Fats are first emulsified in the stomach by its churning action and are stabilized by interaction with luminal lecithin and protein fragments. The lingual and gastric lipases do not require bile salts or cofactors for their action; they have a pH optimum of 3 to 6, and their action produces 1,2-diacylglycerols and fatty acids. These products further stabilize the surface of the triglyceride emulsion and in the duodenum promote the binding of pancreatic colipase. In addition, the liberated fatty acids stimulate the release of cholecystokinin (CCK) from the duodenal mucosa.

In the presence of bile salts and colipase, pancreatic lipase acts at the oil-water interface of the triglyceride emulsion to produce fatty acids and 2-monoacylglycerols. Colipase is secreted by the pancreas as an inactive proenzyme and is then activated by trypsin. Other significant enzymes involved in the breakdown of fats are cholesterol ester hydrolase, phospholipase A2, and a nonspecific bile salt–activated lipase.

Only a small proportion of ingested triacylglycerol is completely hydrolyzed to glycerol and fatty acids. These products form micelles with bile salts and lysophosphoglycerides; the micelles convey the nonpolar lipid molecules from the lumen to the epithelial cell surface and dissociate there to produce a high concentration of monoglycerols, lysophosphoglycerides, and fatty acids, which partition into the mucosal cell. Absorption involves both passive and active transport processes and is facilitated by a fatty acid–binding protein in the cytosol of the cell that has a high affinity for fatty acids. Within the cell, triacylglycerols are resynthesized from the absorbed 2-monoacylglycerols and fatty acids. The triacylglycerols—together with phospholipids, cholesterol and its ester, fat-soluble vitamins, and apolipoprotein B-48—are formed into chylomicrons that are then released by exocytosis into the lymphatic system of the small bowel. The absorption of long-chain fatty acids is facilitated by a number of transmembrane fatty acid transport proteins.

From the lymphatic system, chylomicrons enter the bloodstream via the thoracic duct and are distributed to the liver, adipose tissue, and other organs. Medium- and short-chain fatty acids (chain length <12 carbon atoms) in mixed triglycerides are preferentially split by lipases and pass into the aqueous phase, from which they are rapidly absorbed. Medium-chain triglycerides can be absorbed without complete lipolysis and in the absence of bile. They do not require micellar solubilization and are transported from the intestinal epithelial cells predominantly via the hepatic portal vein. Fig. 38.3 summarizes the processes involved in fat absorption and conditions that compromise the efficiency of one or more stages in these processes that can result in fat malabsorption.

## Digestion and Absorption of Proteins

The average daily intake of protein in developed countries is approximately 100 g, compared with an estimated requirement for adults of 50 to 70 g. Another 50 to 60 g of protein enters the intestinal tract daily in GI secretions and from desquamated mucosal cells. Normal daily fecal loss of protein is about 10 g.

Protein digestion is initiated in the stomach by the action of pepsin in a highly acidic medium. The acidity also helps denature dietary proteins, unfolding the polypeptide chains for better access by the gastric, pancreatic, and intestinal proteolytic enzymes. The polypeptides and amino acids produced in the stomach by the action of pepsin are potent secretagogues for hormones that stimulate the pancreas and intestine. Stimulated pancreatic secretion contains proenzyme forms of the proteolytic enzymes trypsin, chymotrypsin, elastase, exopeptidases, and carboxypeptidases. Stimulation of the intestine by GI hormones liberates several proteolytic enzymes from the brush-border. One of them, enterokinase, selectively cleaves a hexapeptide from the N-terminus of trypsinogen to form trypsin. Trypsin then activates more trypsin (autocatalysis) and also converts other pancreatic proenzymes into their active forms. Proteolytic enzymes may be endopeptidases (e.g., pepsin, trypsin, chymotrypsin, elastase), which hydrolyze peptide bonds within the polypeptide chain, or exopeptidases, which hydrolyze peptide bonds of the terminal amino acids (e.g., carboxypeptidase, aminopeptidase). The action of the pancreatic enzymes on partially digested proteins within the lumen produces peptides that are 2 to 6 amino acid residues in length as well as single amino acids. The peptides are largely hydrolyzed to single amino acids by the aminopeptidases and dipeptidases of the brush-border before absorption, although some dipeptides and tripeptides are absorbed and hydrolyzed to amino acids by cytosolic peptidases within the enterocytes. Multiple carrier systems with overlapping specificities for the 20 essential amino acids are involved in the transport of amino acids into cells. Absorption of amino acids by these transport systems is faster in the jejunum than the ileum. The amino acids pass across the enterocyte basolateral membrane by passive diffusion as well as by active transport systems, which are distinct from those at the brush-border membrane. The rich vascular plexus is drained by the portal circulation, and it is by this route that absorbed amino acids reach the liver and then the systemic circulation.

Mucosal diseases may affect protein assimilation through a number of mechanisms. Reduction in the number of mucosal cells decreases peptidase activity in the intestine and the absorptive capacity for amino acids. Disease may increase the turnover of intestinal cells and their rate of desquamation. This cell loss, together with increased losses of plasma proteins from the damaged intestinal surface, can cause a negative nitrogen balance.

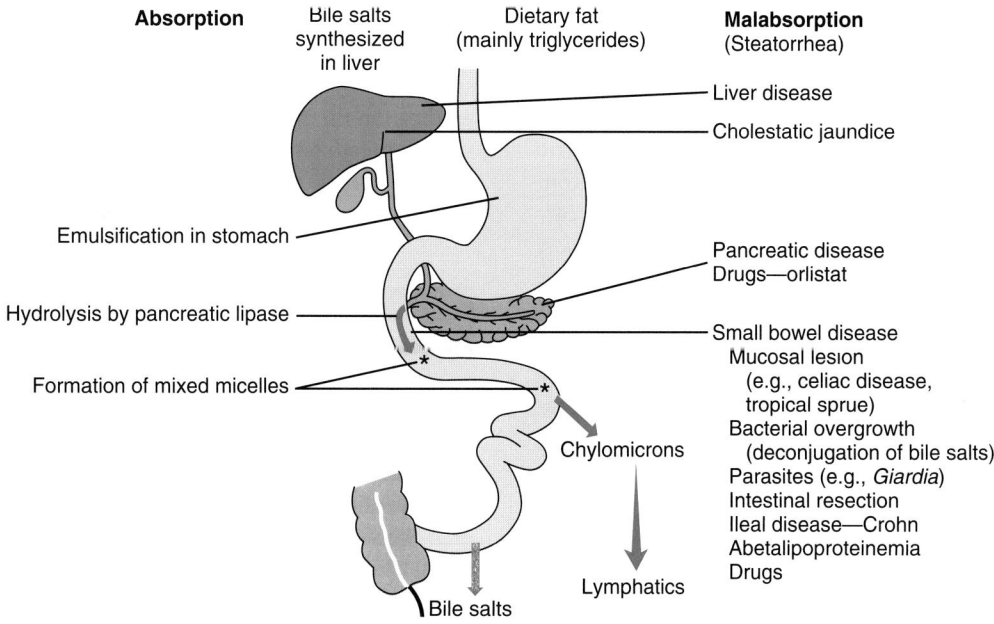

**Fig. 38.3** Summary of the processes involved in fat absorption and malabsorption. (From Clark ML, Silk DB. Gastrointestinal disease. In: Kumar P, Clark M, eds. *Clinical Medicine.* 6th ed. Edinburgh: Saunders; 2005.)

Surgical resection of the intestine not only reduces the total absorptive surface area but may also remove a segment of the gut that is specialized for the absorption of certain nutrients (resection of the distal ileum removes the active transport system for vitamin $B_{12}$–intrinsic factor complex). Resection may also alter intestinal motility, leading to stasis and bacterial overgrowth, which can intensify a negative nitrogen balance. Also, rare hereditary defects in amino acid transporters (e.g., Hartnup disease) may produce distinct syndromes.

# STOMACH: DISEASES AND LABORATORY INVESTIGATIONS

Growth in endoscopic procedures, with direct visualization of the interior of the stomach, has largely removed the need for the laboratory to carry out investigation of gastric contents. Situations remain, however, in which the laboratory continues to play a role in diagnosing gastric diseases and in monitoring the effectiveness of treatment.

## *Helicobacter pylori*

In 1985, an association was made between the presence of a spiral-shaped bacterium, **Helicobacter pylori**, and peptic ulcer diseases. *H. pylori* is now accepted to be the predominant cause of gastric and duodenal ulcers, the remainder being associated with the long-term use of nonsteroidal anti-inflammatory drugs (NSAIDs) and, rarely, gastrinomas. Most estimates suggest that *H. pylori* is present in the mucus layer of the stomach in half the world's population. In Europe, 30% to 50% of adults and at least 20% of adults in the United States are infected with the bacterium. Chronic infection produces an inflammatory response (gastritis) and increases the risk for developing a peptic ulcer (3- to 10-fold) and/or adenocarcinoma (2- to 10-fold). Up to 90% of gastric cancer patients are infected with *H. pylori*, compared with 40% to 60% of age-matched controls. *H. pylori* may cause dyspepsia in the absence of an ulcer, and current recommendations suggest a low threshold for testing for *H. pylori*; some advocate treatment without testing. Gastric cancer is the second most common cause of death from cancer worldwide. A large number of studies have been carried out that have shown an association between *H. pylori* and gastric cancer. In 1994, the International Agency for Research on Cancer declared *H. pylori* to be a causal factor for gastric cancer.

The mode of transmission of *H. pylori* is unclear. In many cases, the infection appears to originate in childhood, presumably by the fecal-oral route, because the prevalence is higher in developing countries and is inversely related to food hygiene. Almost all individuals infected with *H. pylori* develop chronic gastritis, but only 10% of cases manifest as peptic ulcers. *H. pylori* infection predominantly affects the gastric mucosa, with the antrum usually the most densely infected. At least 95% of patients with duodenal ulcers have *H. pylori* infection, and eradication of the organism results in healing of the ulcer and a reduction in relapse rates.

*H. pylori* produces urease, and hydrolysis of this endogenously produced urea to bicarbonate and ammonia may create a more hospitable environment for the survival of the organism in the stomach. This ability of *H. pylori* to hydrolyze urea forms the basis of urea breath tests and direct urease tests on gastric biopsy samples.

### Diagnostic Tests for *Helicobacter pylori*

In theory, all patients with symptoms that could be associated with *H. pylori* infection could undergo endoscopy. However, in the real world, this is neither practical nor acceptable to patients. Numerous invasive and noninvasive diagnostic tests for *H. pylori* have been described (Box 38.1) and many have been reviewed.

At gastroscopy, biopsies can be taken from the gastric mucosa from which the organism can be visually detected or cultured. The antrum is the preferred site, but multiple biopsies from the anterior and posterior walls of the antrum and the body of the stomach are recommended to avoid false-negative results in patients with patchy infection. False-negative results may also occur when biopsies are taken during treatment with proton pump inhibitors (PPIs) or within 2 weeks of stopping PPI therapy because these drugs alter the intragastric distribution of *H. pylori* and suppress its activity. PPIs can also lead to false-negative urea breath test results. Histamine ($H_2$)-receptor antagonists should be stopped at least 24 hours before a breath test. Antacids do not affect the test results. Commercially available kits can be used to identify *H. pylori* in gastric biopsy samples. These are based on a gel that incorporates urea and an indicator that changes color at an alkaline pH. The action of urease present in *H. pylori* cleaves the urea to bicarbonate and ammonia, raising the pH and inducing a color change in the indicator.

Tests for *H. pylori* are required for the diagnosis of infection and in some situations to ascertain whether eradication therapy has been successful. High sensitivity is required to ensure that positive findings are not missed; similarly, high specificity is essential to prevent the inappropriate use of eradication therapy. A common strategy is to "test and treat", using a breath test or stool antigen test, in adults with appropriate dyspeptic symptoms who are younger than 45 years of age. The age limit may vary depending on local prevalence

---

**BOX 38.1   Diagnostic Tests for *Helicobacter pylori***

**Invasive Tests: Using Gastric Mucosal Biopsy Samples**
- Histology: microscopy after Giemsa or silver staining
- Histology: microscopy after immunohistochemical staining
- Direct urease test: biopsy included in urea/indicator solution—visual endpoint
- Culture: incubation in suitable media for 4–10 days

**Noninvasive Tests: Using Breath, Blood, Saliva, or Feces**
- Breath tests: rise in $^{14}CO_2$ or $^{13}CO_2$ after ingestion of $^{14}C$- or $^{13}C$-labeled urea
- Serum, saliva, or feces tests for *Helicobacter pylori* antigen

and the age distribution of gastric cancer. Successful eradication of *H. pylori* should be confirmed with the urea breath test or by a monoclonal antibody–based stool antigen test if urea breath tests are not available. Testing to confirm eradication should be done at least 4 weeks after completion of the course of treatment.

The urea breath test for *H. pylori* is currently the most widely used method for the noninvasive diagnosis of infection. Urea labeled with carbon-13 is given orally as a drink or a capsule. *H. pylori* rapidly hydrolyzes the urea to produce labeled bicarbonate, which is absorbed into the bloodstream and broken down to be exhaled as $^{13}CO_2$. In the absence of urease, the urea is absorbed intact and excreted by the kidney. Breath samples are collected before and 45 to 60 minutes after drinking the labeled urea. The detection of labeled carbon, which is not radioactive, is usually carried out by mass spectrometry or using infrared spectroscopy. The breath test has sensitivity and specificity for *H. pylori* in excess of 95% and can be used both for diagnosis and to assess the success of eradication therapy.

Serologic methods are available to detect specific antibodies (immunoglobulin G [IgG] or IgA) against *H. pylori* in serum. However, they have some drawbacks compared with the urea breath test. The systemic antibody response is variable, with equivocal results often occurring in subjects above 50 years of age. The sensitivity (92%) and specificity (83%) are also lower than those for the breath test. Serologic tests cannot be used to confirm eradication of the bacterium because of the persistence of the antibodies for variable periods after completion of treatment and, for this reason, are no longer considered clinically useful. Point-of-care devices exist to detect *H. pylori* antibodies, but current evidence is that these perform poorly in terms of both sensitivity and specificity and cannot be recommended. These tests may be useful in specific situations, such as when PPI therapy cannot be withheld because of ulcers that are bleeding.

*H. pylori* is excreted in feces where it can be detected by several tests. Polyclonal or monoclonal antibodies to *H. pylori* can be configured into various immunoassay formats, although sensitivity and specificity are lower than for breath tests. Commercial kits are available that use the polymerase chain reaction to amplify nuclear sequences specific for *H. pylori* in feces (or saliva); they have a sensitivity and specificity of 95% and 94%, respectively, but are seldom routinely available. In time, stool tests for *H. pylori* may replace the urea breath test, particularly in assessing whether eradication has been successful.

### POINTS TO REMEMBER

**Helicobacter pylori**
- *H. pylori* is the predominant cause of gastric and duodenal ulcers.
- There is an increased risk for gastric cancer with *H. pylori* infection.
- The urea breath test is useful in the diagnosis of *H. pylori* infection.

## Gastric Acid Secretion and Gastrinomas

Before the discovery of the role of *H. pylori,* patients with gastric or duodenal ulcers were often tested for hyperacidity of the stomach, either in the basal state or after stimulation. Patients with duodenal ulcers are typically hypersecretors of acid, whereas those with peptic ulcers are more often normal or low secretors, but there was significant overlap between the two groups of patients. Collection of gastric juice and analysis of acid output was at one time extensively carried out in the investigation of possible gastrinomas. This invasive technique has now been replaced by the greater availability of plasma gastrin measurements, endoscopy, and imaging modalities, including computed tomography (CT), magnetic resonance imaging (MRI), positron emission tomography (PET), and octreotide scanning.

### Gastrin

Three molecular forms of gastrin occur in blood and tissues: G-34, G-17, and G-14. Gastrins originate from the cleavage of a single precursor, preprogastrin—a peptide consisting of 101 amino acids. The smallest peptide sequence of gastrin possessing biologic activity is the carboxy-terminal tetrapeptide (G-4), but it is only 10% to 20% as potent as G-17. A synthetic pentapeptide (pentagastrin) was used in the past to stimulate acid secretion for collection and analysis, but it is rarely used now.

Gastrin is produced and stored mainly by endocrine cells (G cells) of the antral mucosa and to a lesser extent by G cells of the proximal duodenum and Δ cells of the pancreatic islets. After secretion, gastrin is transported by the blood through the liver to the parietal cells of the fundus of the stomach, where it stimulates the secretion of gastric acid. Gastrin also stimulates secretion of gastric pepsinogens and intrinsic factor by the gastric mucosa, release of secretin from the small intestinal mucosa, and secretion of pancreatic bicarbonate and enzymes and hepatic bile; it increases gastric and intestinal motility, mucosal growth, and blood flow to the stomach. It is secreted in response to antral distention from food and by the presence of amino acids, peptides, and polypeptides in the stomach from partially digested proteins. Other stimuli of gastrin include alcohol, caffeine, insulin-induced hypoglycemia, and calcium.

Maximal secretion of gastrin occurs at an antral pH of 5 to 7. At pH 2.5, the secretion of gastrin is reduced by approximately 80%, with maximal suppression occurring at pH 1. Secretion is inhibited by the direct action of acid on the G cells. This negative feedback prevents excess acid production regardless of the stimulant.

### Gastrinoma and the Zollinger-Ellison Syndrome

In 1955, Zollinger and Ellison described a syndrome consisting of multiple peptic ulcers, gastric hypersecretion, and non–β islet cell tumors of the pancreas secreting gastrin. Gastrinomas are a rare cause (<0.5%) of gastroduodenal ulcers. The persistently high circulating gastrin concentrations lead to the hypersecretion of gastric acid and increased parietal cell mass, as the hormone is trophic to parietal cells. Most cases occur between the ages of 30 and 50 years, although the condition has been reported in patients as young as 7 and as old as 90 years of age. It is more common in men (60% of cases) than in women.

Symptoms may be those of *H. pylori* peptic ulcer disease, but they can also include diarrhea (secondary to inactivation of pancreatic enzymes in the acidic environment). Duodenal ulceration and ulcers resistant to standard therapies must be considered suspicious. Gastrinomas are most often sporadic, but they may also be associated with multiple endocrine neoplasia type 1 (MEN1, Wermer syndrome), a syndrome characterized by the presence of two or more tumors sited in the pituitary, parathyroid glands, or pancreas.

Gastrinomas are commonly located in the pancreas, but they can arise from the stomach, duodenum, or other tissues. They are more often (60%) malignant than benign, with metastases frequently present at the time of diagnosis. Measurement of plasma gastrin in a fasting sample is the initial step in aiding the differential diagnosis. A mildly elevated plasma gastrin concentration may be observed in long-term PPI therapy, hypochlorhydria, pernicious anemia, and G-cell hyperplasia. *H. pylori* infection can also lead to increased plasma gastrin and in some cases atrophic gastritis. Increases in plasma gastrin in chronic renal failure appear to be related to the severity of renal impairment.

Fasting plasma gastrin concentrations in the Zollinger-Ellison syndrome are usually markedly increased, and a concentration of more than 10 times the upper reference limit in the presence of gastric acid hypersecretion is virtually diagnostic of a gastrinoma. No correlation has been observed between the severity of symptoms and the extent of plasma gastrin elevation. However, the fasting plasma gastrin concentration at presentation in sporadic gastrinomas is related to the extent of tumor burden and the presence of hepatic metastases; it is therefore of prognostic value.

### Measurement of Plasma Gastrin

In plasma from healthy subjects, the predominant forms of gastrin are amidated G-34 and G-17. In patients with gastrinomas, the gastrins found in the circulation display unpredictable heterogeneity with a shift toward larger peptides. For the detection of gastrinomas, the assay should detect all secreted forms of gastrin to prevent false-negative findings. Gastrin is unstable in serum and plasma, and samples may lose up to 50% of their immunoreactivity over 48 hours at 2°C to 8°C because of the action of proteolytic enzymes. Blood samples should be collected in tubes containing an anticoagulant and a protease inhibitor (e.g., aprotinin) to prevent degradation.

## INTESTINAL DISORDERS AND THEIR LABORATORY INVESTIGATION

This section includes discussion of celiac disease, disaccharidase deficiency, bacterial overgrowth, bile salt malabsorption, inflammatory bowel disease (IBD), and protein-losing enteropathy and the main laboratory investigations associated with the diagnosis and monitoring of these disorders.

## Celiac Disease
### Pathophysiology of Celiac Disease

Celiac disease occurs in genetically predisposed subjects as a consequence of an inappropriate T cell-mediated immune response to ingestion of gluten from wheat and to similar proteins in barley and rye. The external trigger to the development of celiac disease in genetically susceptible individuals is found in gluten, which is the complex group of proteins found in wheat and other grains.

The identification in 1997 of small bowel tissue transglutaminase as the autoantigen of celiac disease has led to a greater understanding of the pathogenesis of the condition. The tissue transglutaminases are a family of calcium-dependent enzymes released from cells during wound healing. They catalyze the cross-linking or deamidation of proteins leading to stabilization of the wound area. Deamidation of gliadin peptides enhances their binding to human leucocyte antigen (HLA) DQ2/DQ8 and increases recognition of these peptides by gut-derived T cells from subjects with celiac disease. The characteristic enteropathy is then induced by the release of interferon-γ and other proinflammatory cytokines.

A 33–amino acid peptide of gluten appears to be the primary initiator of the inflammatory response. It is resistant to breakdown by all gastric, pancreatic, and brush-border membrane proteases, thus allowing it to reach the small intestine intact. The peptide can be detoxified by exposure to a bacterial prolyl endopeptidase, suggesting a therapeutic strategy for celiac disease.

Increased intestinal permeability in untreated celiac disease that is reversible on withdrawal of gluten from the diet has been recognized since the early 1980s. Evidence suggests that this increase in paracellular permeability may be mediated by increased expression of zonulin, a protein that opens small intestinal tight junctions, or by decreased expression of intercellular epithelial cell adhesion molecules such as Z0-1, catenin, and cadherin. The zonulin pathway is now thought to play a significant role in the entry of allergens into cells and hence in the autoimmune response.

### Clinical Considerations

Celiac disease is a common disorder in Northern European populations with a prevalence of approximately 1%, but it also occurs in Northern Indian and North African populations. It is rare among people of East Asian, and African Caribbean descent.

A wide spectrum of clinical manifestations of celiac disease is seen, with most diagnoses being made in adult life. Classic celiac disease—manifesting in infancy with failure to thrive, abdominal distention, and diarrhea—is now uncommon in developed countries. Most adults present with nonspecific symptoms; the condition may be picked up during the investigation of patients suspected of having irritable bowel syndrome (IBS). Mild iron deficiency is common. The patient at initial presentation may be seen by a wide range of clinical specialties (Table 38.2). A strong association with other autoimmune diseases, especially type 1 diabetes and autoimmune thyroid disease, has been reported. In type 1 diabetes, the prevalence of celiac disease is approximately 5%, and serologic screening to detect these cases has been advocated.

## Tests for Celiac Disease

Appropriately standardized serologic tests have high clinical sensitivity and specificity for diagnosis and monitoring of compliance with a gluten-free diet. Table 38.3 compares the sensitivity and specificity of the serologic tests commonly used for the diagnosis of celiac disease.

Historically serologic testing for celiac disease involved testing for antigliadin antibodies and antiendomysial antibodies by indirect immunofluorescence. The sensitivity and specificity of these tests were poor; they have largely been superseded by the measurement of antibodies against tissue transglutaminase (TTG) and deaminated gliadin peptide (DGP). Both IgG and IgA antibodies are detected by specific quantitative enzyme-linked immunosorbent assays (ELISAs). The diagnostic accuracy of DGP-IgA is similar to that of TTG-IgA, with sensitivities of 85% to 90% and a specificity of approximately 95%. Sensitivity for DGP-IgG is not as good as that for DGP-IgA but has a specificity approaching 99%. Patients with selective IgA deficiency (plasma IgA concentration less than 0.05 g/L, incidence ~1 in 600) are at greater risk for celiac disease. The tests directed at the IgA antibodies to TTG and DGP may produce false-negative results in patients with IgA deficiency; total IgA measurement should be considered in requesting serologic tests for celiac disease. When IgA deficiency is identified, the IgG-based tests should be used to confirm or exclude a diagnosis of celiac disease. No current recommendations suggest that DGP-based tests should replace tests based on TTG antibodies, but support has been increasing for their use in both adult and pediatric populations. The response to gluten withdrawal can be assessed clinically, by serologic tests, or by endoscopic or wireless capsule techniques. Endoscopic biopsies are considered the gold standard but are invasive and expensive, and they are now less frequently used for this purpose.

Strict adherence to a gluten-free diet leads to mucosal healing in celiac disease and reduces the risk for bowel malignancy (i.e., enteropathy-associated T-cell lymphoma [EATL]). TTG can be used as a marker for monitoring dietary adherence in addition to its diagnostic role. Failure of symptoms to respond to a prescribed gluten-free diet may indicate nonadherence to the diet, other coexisting conditions such as small bowel overgrowth, lactose intolerance, microscopic colitis, or the presence of refractory celiac disease. The latter is characterized by persistent villous atrophy with an increase in intraepithelial lymphocytes in the small bowel while the patient is on a strict long-term gluten-free diet. In both responsive and refractory celiac disease, antibody titers are typically decreased with dietary therapy and remain within reference intervals unless individuals are reexposed to gluten.

## Disaccharidase Deficiencies

The presence of the brush-border disaccharidases is essential for carbohydrate absorption; a reduction in their activity leads to carbohydrate malabsorption and intolerance. Carbohydrate malabsorption can result in osmotic diarrhea with abdominal pain and distention and flatulence resembling the symptoms of IBS. Inherited disorders of sucrase-isomaltase and of transport proteins causing glucose-galactose malabsorption and fructose malabsorption have been described but are rare. Adult lactase deficiency is common in many populations.

### Lactase Deficiency

Lactase activity has its highest prevalence in the earliest months of life and declines after weaning. The prevalence of lactase deficiency varies widely with ethnic origin; although only 5% to 15% of northern Europeans are lactase-deficient, hypolactasia or alactasia can be found in more than 70% of individuals of African and Asian origin (Table 38.4). Lactase non-persistence after infancy is mediated by a C/T nucleotide polymorphism at a position 13,910 nucleotides upstream of the lactase gene (*LCT*). Congenital lactase deficiency is a very rare disorder that becomes apparent once the infant has been exposed to milk feeds. It is an autosomal recessive disorder that if present in either homozygote or compound heterozygote form can lead to congenital lactase deficiency. Stools have a low pH and contain large amounts of lactose and

**TABLE 38.2  Examples of Clinical Specialties to Which a Child or Adult With Celiac Disease May Present**

| Clinical Specialty | Symptoms/Manifestations |
| --- | --- |
| General medicine | Tired all the time |
| Gastroenterology | Diarrhea, flatulence, weight loss |
| Hematology | Anemia |
| Obstetrics/gynecology | Infertility |
| Orthopedics | Fracture, osteopenia |
| Dermatology | Dermatitis herpetiformis, hyperkeratosis |
| Neurology | Peripheral neuropathy |
| Rheumatology | Arthropathy |
| Endocrinology | Short stature, thyroid disease |
| Diabetes | Diarrhea, anemia |

**TABLE 38.3 Comparison of Serologic Tests for Celiac Disease**

| Antibody | Method | Sensitivity (%) | Specificity (%) |
|---|---|---|---|
| IgA-endomysial antibody | Immunofluorescence on monkey esophagus or human umbilical cord | 80–100 | >99 |
| IgA-antigliadin antibody | Quantitative ELISA | 75–95 | 95 |
| IgA-antitissue transglutaminase antibody | Quantitative ELISA | >90 | >99 |
| IgA-deamidated gliadin peptide antibody | Quantitative ELISA | 90 | 90 |

*ELISA,* Enzyme-linked immunosorbent assay; *IgA,* immunoglobulin A.

**TABLE 38.4 Prevalence of Lactase Deficiency in Adults**

| Ancestral Group | Prevalence (%) |
|---|---|
| Chinese | >90 |
| African Americans | 54–81 |
| Asians | 60–90 |
| Greeks | 60–78 |
| North Europeans | 5–30 |

glucose, the latter being produced by bacterial degradation of undigested lactose. Secondary lactase deficiency is common in celiac disease owing to villous atrophy but also may occur in non-specific GI tract disorders much more frequently than previously thought.

### Tests for Lactase Deficiency

Many methods have been proposed for making the diagnosis of lactase deficiency (Box 38.2). Disaccharidase activities can be measured in duodenal or jejunal biopsies, although this is rarely done in routine practice. The xylose absorption test was first introduced as a test for carbohydrate malabsorption in the 1930s. In humans, D-xylose, a pentose sugar of plant origin, is absorbed by a passive mechanism in the jejunum. After an oral dose of D-xylose, it can be measured in blood or urine samples. It is now accepted that the amount of xylose excreted is affected not just by reduced absorption in the gut but also by renal, hepatic, and cardiac disease, and the test has largely been superseded by the hydrogen breath test. Oral lactose tolerance tests, measuring the increase in plasma glucose after ingestion of lactose, have been used to diagnose lactase deficiency. The usual dose of lactose is 50 g, but lower doses should be used in children (2 g/kg up to a maximum of 50 g). Blood samples are taken over a 2-hour period and the peak increment in glucose is recorded; a rise greater than

1.1 mmol/L (20 mg/dL) for capillary samples or greater than 1.4 mmol/L (>25 mg/dL) for venous plasma excludes lactase deficiency.

### Hydrogen Breath Tests

Hydrogen is not a normal end product of mammalian metabolism, and hydrogen in breath is derived from bacterial metabolism in the intestinal tract. After lactose ingestion, the disaccharide is normally broken down into its constituent monosaccharides, which are absorbed. In the presence of lactase deficiency, unabsorbed disaccharide passes into the large bowel, where bacteria act on it to produce hydrogen that is absorbed into the systemic circulation and subsequently exhaled. Breath hydrogen can be measured by a variety of techniques based on the electrochemical detection of hydrogen; both laboratory and handheld point-of-care devices are available. Fasting breath hydrogen is normally less than 5 ppm (5 μL/L), and concentrations greater than 20 ppm (20 μL/L) at 2 hours after oral administration of 50 g lactose in adults (2 g/kg up to a maximum of 50 g in children) are suggestive of malabsorption or bacterial overgrowth. A lower cutoff of 10 ppm (10 μL/L) has been suggested that can improve diagnostic sensitivity without altering specificity. In some individuals (estimated at 2% to 13%), the large bowel bacteria do not produce hydrogen and fasting breath hydrogen will be low; in such individuals, a normal result cannot exclude lactase deficiency. A positive breath hydrogen result after ingestion of lactose also may occur in glucose-galactose malabsorption; this can be confirmed or excluded by repeating the test substituting 25 g each of glucose and galactose for the lactose. An increase in breath hydrogen confirms the diagnosis. Lactose intolerance or malabsorption has become a very topical issue with clinicians as well as dieticians and nutritionists. Many of these have abandoned any measurements to confirm

**BOX 38.2 Methods for Detecting Lactase Deficiency**

- Lactase in mucosal biopsy
- Oral lactose tolerance
  - Measure increase in plasma glucose or galactose
  - Measure increase in breath $H_2$ or $^{13}CO_2$
  - Measure urinary excretion of lactose after oral load

malabsorption-maldigestion and simply rely on exacerbation of symptoms with the ingestion of a pint of milk. Alternatively, the diagnosis is based on symptomatic improvement when patients are placed on a dairy-free diet.

## Bacterial Overgrowth

The proximal small intestine (duodenum and jejunum) normally contains few bacteria (less than 1000 cfu/mL). Most ingested bacteria do not survive the acidic environment of the stomach; therefore few live organisms enter the small bowel. The motility of the jejunum prevents fecal-type organisms from progressing up into the jejunum from the cecum. The ileum normally contains some fecal-type bacteria. Colonization of the upper small bowel is described as bacterial overgrowth and usually occurs as a consequence of other abnormalities (structural or motility disorders) of the small intestine. Gastric hypochlorhydria (associated with the use of PPIs) may contribute to bacterial overgrowth. Abnormalities in the systemic immune system (isolated IgA deficiency, hypogammaglobulinemia, combined immunodeficiency, infection with the human immunodeficiency virus [HIV]) can result in bacterial overgrowth. Impaired motility, pancreatic insufficiency, intrinsic small bowel disease, or surgically induced blind loops are often associated with bacterial overgrowth.

Small bowel bacterial overgrowth can be asymptomatic or associated with nonspecific symptoms that include abdominal distention, flatulence, and diarrhea resembling IBS. Bacteria colonizing the small bowel (e.g., *Escherichia coli* and *Bacteroides* species) deconjugate and dehydroxylate bile salts, resulting in conjugated bile salt deficiency and mild fat malabsorption. Bacterial metabolism of vitamin $B_{12}$ can occur, leading to deficiency, whereas plasma folate concentration may be increased owing to production by the bacteria.

The gold standard diagnostic procedure is microbiologic examination of small bowel contents, but this is seldom practical. Noninvasive procedures based on oral administration of substances metabolized by bacteria to yield products that can be detected in breath are now the most common tests for bacterial overgrowth, but there is controversy as to which test to use and their sensitivity/specificity.

The $^{14}C$-glycocholate breath test was one of the first tests to be used for noninvasive diagnosis of bacterial overgrowth, but it has been superseded by tests that avoid the use of radioactive isotopes. Small bowel bacterial breath tests in routine use involve test substances labeled with $^{13}C$ and the breath hydrogen tests. Lactulose is not normally absorbed from the small bowel and is therefore available for metabolism by bacteria throughout the gut; alternatively, labeled glucose can be used. In a normal subject, breath hydrogen does not increase until the substrate reaches the large intestine; the time from ingestion to a rise in breath hydrogen is an indicator of small bowel transit time. In bacterial overgrowth, an early rise in breath hydrogen of at least 20 ppm (20 µL/L) is observed within 30 minutes of ingestion. The early increase is diagnostic when it can be distinguished clearly from the later colonic phase. Frequent measurements are essential (at 5-minute intervals) for the first 30 minutes. The finding of an increased breath hydrogen output has high specificity for bacterial overgrowth but poor sensitivity. Variations in gastric emptying rate and small bowel transit times limit the diagnostic accuracy of the breath tests.

## Bile Acid Malabsorption

Bile acids are synthesized in the liver and pass into the lumen of the small bowel via the gallbladder. Bile acids are present in bile as taurine or glycine conjugates; because the pH of bile is slightly alkaline and contains significant amounts of sodium and potassium, most of the bile acids and their conjugates exist as salts (bile salts). In practice, the terms *bile acids* and *bile salts* are frequently used synonymously. Their major function is to act as surface-active agents, forming micelles and facilitating the digestion of triglycerides and the absorption of cholesterol and fat-soluble vitamins. Little reabsorption of bile acids occurs in the proximal small bowel, but normally more than 90% is reabsorbed in the terminal ileum. The bile acids return to the liver via the portal circulation and can be resecreted into bile (enterohepatic circulation). Less than 10% of secreted bile acid is lost in the feces (~0.2 to 0.6 g/24 h).

Bile acid malabsorption leading to chronic diarrhea occurs when ileal disease is present or after resection of the terminal ileum; it may also occur after cholecystectomy and is present in some patients with IBS. Malabsorption of bile salts produces diarrhea by two different mechanisms. When significant bile salt depletion occurs, the deficiency of intraluminal bile salts leads to fat malabsorption and steatorrhea. More commonly, malabsorption of bile salts in the ileum leads to increased concentrations of bile salts in the colon, where they alter water and electrolyte absorption. This leads to net secretion of water into the lumen and diarrhea.

The most widely used test for bile acid malabsorption involves oral administration of the synthetic radiolabeled bile acid selenohomocholyltaurine (SeHCAT). Whole-body gamma counting is used to determine the basal level at 1 hour and then repeated at 7 days when in normal subjects more than 15% of the dose is retained. Retention of less than 10% of SeHCAT at 7 days can predict a good response to bile acid sequestrants.

Two blood tests have been proposed as alternatives to SeHCAT to avoid administration of a radioactive substance: fibroblast growth factor-19 (FGF-19) and 7α-hydroxy-4-cholesten-3-one (C4). C4 is the intermediary step between cholesterol and taurocholic acid and reflects the activity of hepatic cholesterol 7α-hydroxylase and therefore because this is the rate-limiting enzyme, the rate of bile acid synthesis Bile acid malabsorption is associated with increased plasma concentrations of C4 as hepatic synthesis is upregulated to maintain the pool of circulating bile acids. The presence of bile acids in the ileum has been shown to stimulate the production of FGF-19. Good correlation has been demonstrated between both serum C4 and FGF-19 and SeHCAT. These tests, however, are not yet routinely available.

With growing awareness of the role of bile salt malabsorption in chronic diarrhea in a proportion of patients with IBS or IBD and the therapeutic effectiveness of cholestyramine, measurement of C4 and/or FGF-19 may become routine.

# Inflammatory Bowel Disease and Irritable Bowel Syndrome

Intestinal symptoms including abdominal pain or discomfort with diarrhea or constipation are common to both IBD and IBS. IBD includes ulcerative colitis (UC) and Crohn disease (CD). IBS is a functional bowel disorder for which there is no identifiable pathologic process or known cause. Although IBS may produce symptoms that are sufficient to interfere with daily life, it is seldom associated with serious morbidity. IBS may affect up to 10% to 20% of the adult population in the developed world, with a typical age at presentation of 20 to 30 years and a female preponderance. The prevalence of UC is approximately 100 to 200 per 100,000 people and of CD approximately 50 to 100 per 100,000 people, with no significant difference between genders. There is, however, a difference in prevalence with ethnic origin, with IBD being more common among individuals of European ancestry than those of Asian or African origin. Up to 20% of cases of IBD manifest in childhood, although the most common age at presentation is between 15 and 30 years of age. Both UC and CD are chronic conditions that tend to follow a remitting and relapsing course. The prognosis of patients with CD tends to be worse than that of those with UC, although in the latter it is estimated that up to 10% of patients will require surgical intervention within 10 years of diagnosis.

The cause of IBD is not fully understood, but both genetic and environmental factors have been implicated. Genome-wide association studies have identified over 160 susceptibility loci/genes that are significantly associated with IBD. Studies in monozygotic twins, however, have shown a lower-than-expected concordance rate (15% to 19% for UC, 27% to 50% for CD) if IBD were an inherited disorder. It is thought that individuals with a genetic predisposition to IBD need to be exposed to a range of environmental triggers that affect the host's immunity. Tissue damage is a consequence of neutrophil activation and the production of proinflammatory cytokines/chemokines. The success of treatments based on immunosuppressive agents or tumor necrosis factor-alpha (TNF-α) inhibitors appears to support an immune basis for the development of IBD. Environmental factors implicated in triggering the development of active disease include a protective effect of breast-feeding and an increased risk in patients who have recurrent GI infections or exposure to drug therapy (antibiotics, oral contraceptives, NSAIDs) along with socioeconomic factors, stress, smoking, and diet.

In the past 20 years, several fecal markers have been proposed that can aid in differentiating IBD from IBS and in monitoring disease activity or response to treatment.

## Calprotectin

Calprotectin is a member of the S100 family of zinc- and calcium-binding proteins and is a heterodimer of S100A8/9. First discovered in 1980, it accounts for approximately 60% of cytosolic protein in neutrophils. It is also present in monocytes and macrophages at lower concentrations than in neutrophils and may have antimicrobial properties. Any disruption to the mucosal architecture of the GI tract allows neutrophils that accumulate at sites of active inflammation to be released into the lumen and subsequently shed in feces. The fecal concentration of calprotectin has been shown to correlate well with the gold standard indium-111–labeled granulocyte test and is directly related to the extent of inflammation. Calprotectin appears to be evenly distributed in fecal samples and has reasonable stability at room temperature.

The initial studies of fecal calprotectin were on its ability to differentiate between IBS and IBD. In a study of 602 consecutive referrals from primary care to gastroenterology clinics at King's College Hospital (London, UK) patients had fecal calprotectin measured and were assessed for IBS using the Rome questionnaire. The sensitivity and specificity for calprotectin for the detection of organic disease were 89% and 79%, respectively. Combining calprotectin with the Rome questionnaire had a predictive value approaching 100%.

In the past decade, there have been many studies of the value of fecal calprotectin for distinguishing IBD from IBS in adults and children and these have been the subject of several meta-analyses. A review of these meta-analyses was published in 2019 that found a range of sensitivities from 83% to 99% and specificities of 53% to 96%. Although a range of cut-off values were evaluated, most found a value between 50 and 60 µg/g of stool to give optimal results; this value is recommended by most of the manufacturers of commercial methods in current usage. The studies included in these meta-analyses included only patients already in secondary or tertiary care and may have been biased by preselection of patients in primary care before referral. A retrospective analysis of data from 946 patients from 48 primary care practices found a sensitivity of 82% and a specificity of 77%. Nevertheless, the (UK) National Institute for Health and Care Excellence (NICE) has recommended the widespread use of calprotectin in general practice to select patients at high risk for having IBD for referral to gastroenterologists, with the vast majority of the rest with IBS (normal calprotectin) remaining in primary care and treated appropriately. The cost savings of this approach are substantial.

Calprotectin has been found to differentiate between active and inactive IBD. The aim of treatment of IBD is currently to secure and maintain remission, with the ultimate aim of achieving mucosal healing. Assessment of treatment efficacy until recently has been based on clinical scores, including the Crohn's Disease Activity Index (CDAI) and the Ulcerative Colitis Disease Activity Index (UCDAI), and by changes in erythrocyte sedimentation rate (ESR) and C-reactive protein (CRP). However, many patients in clinical remission have increased fecal calprotectin concentrations, and it is perhaps these patients who would benefit from escalation of treatment to achieve mucosal healing. Several studies have demonstrated that a fall in the fecal calprotectin concentration indicates a good response to treatment and that this can precede any clinical response. It has been recommended that fecal calprotectin should be included in the range of tests utilized before consideration of initiating or changing IBD therapy. Various studies have provided data on the use of fecal calprotectin in predicting relapse or recurrence of IBD, and these have been reviewed. Treating the inflammatory component of IBD regardless of symptoms promises to alter the natural history of the disease in a way similar to that seen in rheumatoid arthritis.

Fecal calprotectin is not, however, specific to IBD and is increased in patients with colorectal carcinoma, chronic use of NSAIDs, bacterial infections, and diverticular disease. Other fecal markers that are undergoing active research include M2-PK, lactoferrin, S100A12, and cationic eosinophilic protein.

## Therapeutic Drug Monitoring in Patients With Inflammatory Bowel Disease

The increasing use of thiopurine analogs (azathioprine [AZA] and mercaptopurine [MP]) and the introduction of the anti-tissue necrosis factor (anti-TNF) drugs infliximab (IFX) and adalimumab (ADA) have led to the introduction of the concept of therapeutic drug monitoring (TDM) to gastroenterology. The metabolism of AZA (a prodrug) is complex, involving a number of enzymatic pathways that result in active, inactive, and potentially toxic metabolites. Measurement of red cell thiopurine methyltransferase (TPMT) activity has become a prerequisite before starting patients on AZA therapy because the presence of the low metabolic activity phenotype is a relative contraindication to the use of thiopurine analogs, and those who are heterozygous require a reduced dose. An alternative method, although less commonly available, is to the genotype for the *TPMT* gene by molecular testing. Measurement of the plasma concentration of 6-thioguanine (6-TG) can be used to assess adherence or the adequacy of dosage.

## ALGORITHM FOR THE USE OF FECAL CALPROTECTIN IN DIFFERENTIATING IRRITABLE BOWEL SYNDROME AND INFLAMMATORY BOWEL DISEASE

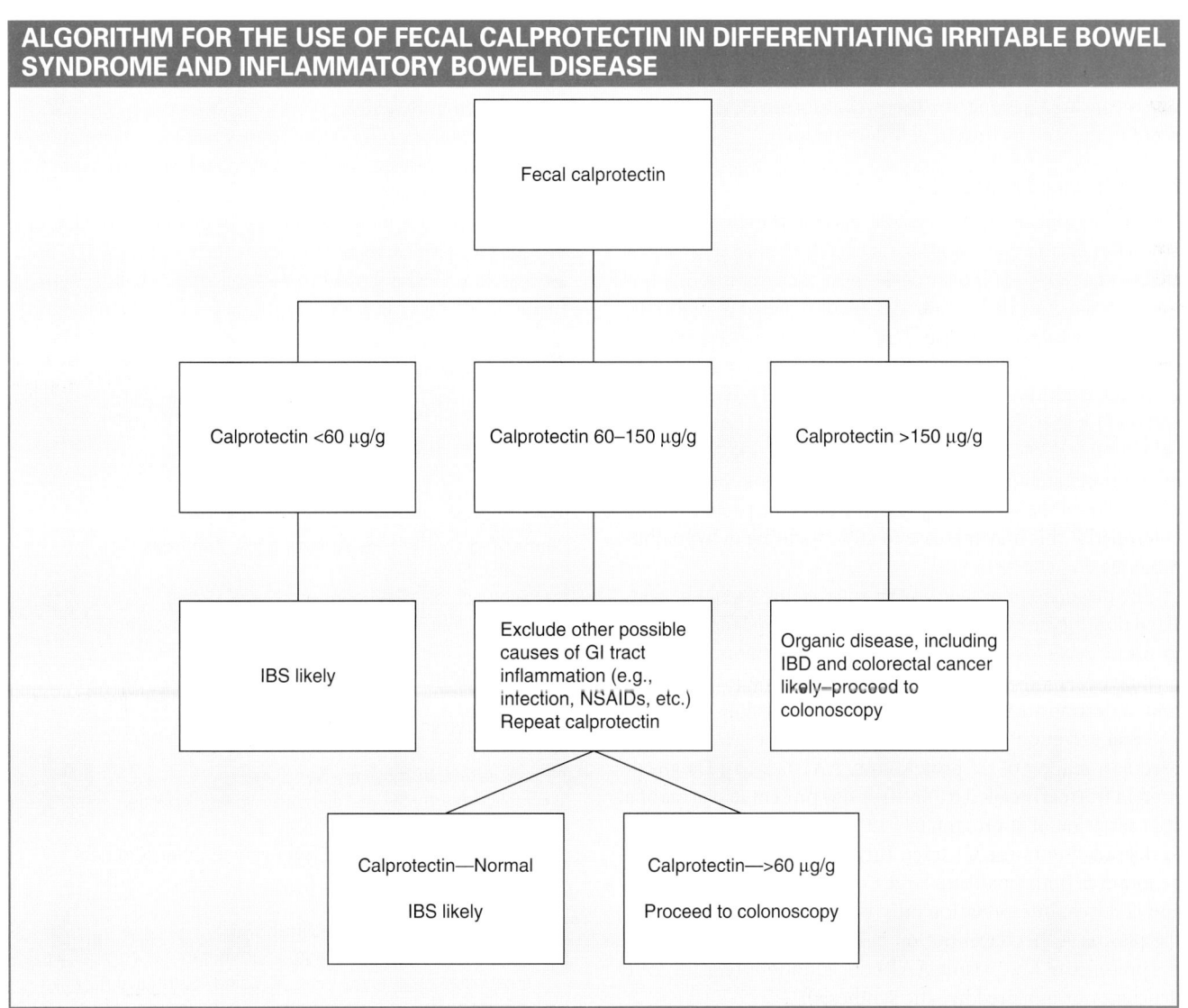

The anti-TNF drugs, particularly IFX and ADA, have proved effective in inducing and maintaining remission in patients with IBD. However, because these drugs are themselves humanized antibodies against TNF, many patients develop antibodies against them. Simultaneous measurement of the plasma drug concentrations and the antibodies against these drugs has meant that a failure to sustain a beneficial response to anti-TNF therapy can be correctly ascribed to either subtherapeutic drug concentrations or the presence of antidrug antibodies and alternative therapies can be devised and initiated. ELISA methods are commercially available for the measurement of both IFX and ADA and their corresponding antibodies. IFX and ADA can also be measured using mass spectrometry.

### Assessment of Functional Small Bowel Length

The amino acid citrulline, which is involved in the urea cycle, is predominantly synthesized in the enterocytes of the small intestine. The short bowel syndrome can be present after major surgical resection of the gut in the treatment of Crohn disease or necrosis. The remaining small bowel length can be estimated at surgery, but this is unreliable at lengths over 50 to 80 cm. Plasma citrulline concentrations have been shown to correlate well with small bowel length and absorption of xylose ($P < 0.001$), but not with CRP, CDAI, or ESR. Plasma citrulline measurements, therefore, appear to be a noninvasive means of assessing small bowel absorptive capacity that is not influenced by intestinal inflammation.

### Protein-Losing Enteropathy

Loss of significant quantities of plasma proteins into the bowel lumen and their subsequent excretion in feces is associated with a range of GI disorders. These include IBD, diseases in which the intestinal lymphatics are obstructed (lymphoma, Whipple disease), and disorders of immune status such as systemic lupus erythematosus and some food allergies.

In the healthy bowel, fecal protein is largely derived from enterocytes shed from the mucosal surface and from intestinal secretions. The normal GI loss of albumin is less than 10% of albumin catabolism, representing a daily loss of less than 1% to 2% of the circulating protein pool. In protein-losing enteropathy, this may increase to 40%, resulting in hypoalbuminemia and edema.

The diagnosis of protein-losing enteropathy should be considered in the investigation of patients with hypoalbuminemia in whom renal loss, liver disease, and malnutrition have been excluded. Methods using the administration of radioactive albumin or dextran are the gold standards but are seldom used now.

Fecal excretion of $\alpha_1$-antiprotease inhibitor (AAT) can be used as a marker of GI protein loss. AAT is a 54-kDa glycoprotein (formerly called $\alpha_1$-antitrypsin) present in plasma at a concentration of approximately 1.0 to 2.0 g/L that is resistant to degradation in the GI tract. Increased AAT excretion can be found in both small and large bowel disease both in adults and children. Interpretation must be made with knowledge of the plasma AAT concentration because the test is invalid in the presence of low plasma AAT concentrations (e.g., in AAT deficiency or impaired hepatic synthesis).

## PANCREAS: DISEASE AND ASSESSMENT OF EXOCRINE PANCREATIC FUNCTION

The pancreas plays a central role in the absorptive process for carbohydrates, fats, and proteins. Disorders of the exocrine pancreas, therefore, are frequently associated with symptoms of malabsorption such as diarrhea or steatorrhea. In this section, pediatric and adult exocrine pancreatic disorders are briefly discussed and tests that can be used to assess exocrine pancreatic function are described. Information on neuroendocrine tumors of the pancreas is also provided.

### Pediatric Disorders of the Exocrine Pancreas

Pancreatic disorders of childhood have been reviewed and are summarized in Box 38.3.

Cystic fibrosis (CF) is the most common severe autosomal recessive disease, with an estimated gene frequency in Western Europe and the United States of between 1:25 and 1:35 and a disease incidence of approximately 1 in 2500 to 1 in 3200 (see also Chapter 24). Pancreatic insufficiency is present in the neonatal period in 65% of infants with CF, and a further 15% develop it during infancy and early childhood.

**BOX 38.3    Spectrum of Pancreatic Disease in Childhood**

**Disorders of Morphogenesis**
- Annular pancreas, pancreas divisum, pancreatic hypoplasia and agenesis, heterotopic pancreas

**Inherited Syndromes Affecting the Pancreas**
- Cystic fibrosis
- Schwachman-Diamond syndrome, Johnson-Blizzard syndrome, Pearson bone marrow pancreas syndrome

**Gene Mutations Leading to Pancreatic Disease**
- Hereditary pancreatitis, cationic trypsinogen gene mutations, trypsin inhibitor gene mutations

**Pancreatic Insufficiency Syndrome**
- Isolated enzyme deficiencies: lipase, colipase, enterokinase
- Pancreatic insufficiency secondary to other disorders
- Celiac disease

**Acquired Pancreatitis in Childhood**
- Idiopathic, traumatic, drugs, viral, metabolic, collagen vascular disease, autoimmune, fibrosing, nutritional (trophic)

The 20% who do not develop pancreatic insufficiency have a better prognosis and develop fewer complications.

Measurement of pancreatic elastase-1 in feces (see the following section on noninvasive tests of exocrine function) is considered to be a reliable test for pancreatic insufficiency in infants over the age of 2 weeks with CF and in older children at the time of diagnosis. This test can also be used to detect the onset of pancreatic insufficiency in those previously sufficient.

Recurrent bouts of acute pancreatitis in childhood should arouse a suspicion of a hereditary cause. Two gene defects have been shown to be associated with pancreatitis manifesting in childhood: the cationic trypsinogen gene *(PRSS1)* and the serine protease inhibitor Kazal type 1 *(SPINK1)* gene. The majority of patients with *PRSS1*-related hereditary pancreatitis have a pathogenic mutation in exons 2 or 3 of the *PRSS1* gene. Duplication or triplication of the *PRSS1* gene has been reported to cause hereditary pancreatitis. The mechanism is assumed to be inappropriate activation of trypsin with consequent proteolytic action causing cell damage. Approximately 22% of patients with idiopathic pancreatitis have been reported to have at least one copy of the c.101A>G (p.Asn34Ser) mutation in the *SPINK1* gene, compared with approximately 2.5% of the general population. This protease inhibitor is believed to be the principal inhibitor of trypsin and chymotrypsin within the pancreas, and the mutation results in a loss of its inhibitory capacity.

## Adult Disorders of the Exocrine Pancreas

The major exocrine pancreatic disorders manifesting in adult life are acute pancreatitis, chronic pancreatitis, and carcinoma of the pancreas. The use of enzyme tests in the diagnosis of acute pancreatitis is discussed in Chapter 19. The causes of pancreatitis are given in Box 38.4.

Chronic pancreatitis is defined by irreversible pancreatic damage, with histologic evidence of inflammation and fibrosis leading to destruction of cells and loss of endocrine and exocrine function. In developed nations, the most common cause is alcohol (60% to 90% of all cases of chronic pancreatitis), although because only 5% to 15% of heavy drinkers develop the disease, other predisposing factors must be present (smoking, diet high in fat and protein).

## Tests of Exocrine Function of the Pancreas

The predominant exocrine function of the pancreas is the production and secretion of pancreatic juice, which is rich in enzymes and bicarbonate. Normal pancreatic juice is colorless and odorless; it has a pH of 8.0 to 8.3 and a specific gravity of 1.007 to 1.042. The total 24-hour volume secreted may be as high as 3000 mL.

Laboratory tests used to assess exocrine pancreatic function can be divided into invasive and noninvasive categories. Invasive tests require GI tract intubation to allow the collection of pancreatic secretions. Noninvasive tests were developed to avoid the need for intubation, which is uncomfortable for the patient, time-consuming, and therefore expensive.

---

### BOX 38.4   Causes of Pancreatitis in Adults

**Acute**
- Gallstones
- Alcohol
- Infection (e.g., mumps, Coxsackie B)
- Pancreatic tumors
- Drugs (e.g., azathioprine, estrogens, corticosteroids, didanosine)
- Iatrogenic (e.g., postsurgical, endoscopic retrograde cholangiopancreatography)
- Hyperlipidemias
- Miscellaneous (e.g., trauma, scorpion bite, cardiac surgery)
- Idiopathic

**Chronic**
- Alcohol
- Tropical (nutritional)
- Hereditary (trypsinogen and inhibitory gene defects, cystic fibrosis)
- Idiopathic
- Trauma
- Hypercalcemia

From Burroughs AK, Westaby, D. Liver, biliary tract disease and pancreatic disease. In: Kumar P, Clark M, eds. *Clinical Medicine*. 7th ed. Edinburgh: Saunders; 2009:319–385.

---

Noninvasive ("tubeless") tests are simpler to perform but in general lack the sensitivity and specificity of invasive tests, particularly for the diagnosis of mild pancreatic insufficiency.

### Invasive Tests of Exocrine Pancreatic Function

In these tests, the total volume of pancreatic juice, the concentration of bicarbonate, and activities of the pancreatic enzymes amylase, lipase, and trypsin are measured in duodenal fluid.

The secretin-cholecystokinin test is based on the principle that secretion of pancreatic juice and bicarbonate output are related to the functional mass of the pancreas. After an overnight fast, a tube is sited in the duodenum to permit the collection of pancreatic juices. Secretin (1 U/kg body weight) is given intravenously, and the duodenal fluid is collected at 15-minute intervals for at least 1 hour. Secretin stimulates the secretion of pancreatic juice and bicarbonate. CCK (or the synthetic equivalent, ceruletide, the C-terminal octapeptide sequence of the intact hormone, where the functional activity resides, Fig. 38.4) can then be given to stimulate the secretion of pancreatic enzymes, allowing a more complete assessment of pancreatic reserve than can be obtained with secretin alone. The secretin-cholecystokinin and secretin-ceruletide tests are considered the gold standard for assessing pancreatic exocrine function. Although seldom used in adults, these tests are still used in infants with pancreatic insufficiency to distinguish between CF and Schwachman-Diamond syndrome (pancreatic α-cell aplasia). In the former, mucous plugs reduce pancreatic secretion, but the enzyme concentrations increase in a normal physiologic response to cholecystokinin, whereas in the latter enzyme secretion is absent or minimal.

$$\text{CCK-8} \quad \text{Asp—Tyr—Met—Gly—Trp—Met—Asp—Phe—NH}_2$$

with SO$_3$H on the Tyr.

$$\text{Ceruletide} \quad \text{Pyr—Gln—Asp—Tyr—Thr—Gly—Trp—Met—Asp—Phe—NH}_2$$

with SO$_3$H on the Tyr.

**Fig. 38.4** Comparison of the amino acid sequences of cholecystokinin *(CCK)*-8 and ceruletide.

## Noninvasive Tests of Exocrine Pancreatic Function

A range of tubeless tests has been proposed, but none has adequate sensitivity for reliably detecting early pancreatic disease. When malabsorption is present, such tests are of value in confirming or excluding pancreatic disease. Considerable overlap often occurs between results observed in normal individuals and those found in patients with pancreatic disease; this is due mainly to the large functional reserve of the pancreas. It has been estimated that pancreatic insufficiency cannot clearly be demonstrated until at least 50% of the acinar cells have been destroyed. Clinical signs of pancreatic insufficiency often do not appear until 90% of acinar tissue has been destroyed.

The noninvasive tests are based on the reduction in secretion of pancreatic enzymes with measurement of the enzymes in feces (chymotrypsin or elastase) or detection of products of their catalytic reactions after oral administration of synthetic substrates in urine (*N*-benzoyl-L-tyrosine-*p*-aminobenzoic acid [NBT-PABA] or pancreolauryl test) or in breath ($^{13}$C mixed-chain triglyceride breath test). The NBT-PABA and pancreolauryl substrates are no longer commercially available.

Pancreatic chymotrypsin is almost completely digested in its passage through the gut in adults, but the residual activity of the enzyme in feces is stable for several days at room temperature. Its output in stool correlates poorly with chymotrypsin secretion in duodenal contents when both are measured after stimulation with secretin-CCK. In patients without pancreatic disease, the incidence of falsely low results is approximately 10% to 15% and may be due to voluminous stools (>300 g/24 h), thus less enzyme per gram of feces; inadequate food intake; partial gastrectomy or mucosal disease (e.g., celiac disease), which causes inadequate stimulation of pancreatic secretion; or obstruction of the common bile duct. Falsely normal results in patients with mild pancreatic insufficiency may be as high as 50%. In a collaborative study in children, both fecal chymotrypsin and elastase showed 100% sensitivity for detecting pancreatic insufficiency in CF; but the specificity of chymotrypsin was lower than that of elastase in a control group of children with small intestinal disease.

Pancreatic elastase-1 is a pancreas-specific protease present in pancreatic juice. It is not degraded during passage through the gut, and concentrations in feces are five- to sixfold greater than those in pancreatic juice. Elastase-1 can be measured by ELISA with two monoclonal antibodies specific to the human enzyme. Treatment of patients with pancreatic enzyme supplements, therefore, does not interfere with the test. Fecal elastase-1 has been evaluated extensively in both CF and adult pancreatic insufficiency, and its use is recommended in both groups. Fecal elastase is often undetectable (<15 µg/g) in children with CF, and values below 200 µg/g after 4 weeks of age are indicative of pancreatic insufficiency.

The test has been evaluated in adults against the secretin-CCK test and in patients whose diagnosis of chronic pancreatitis has been made on the basis of anatomic and morphologic changes detected by ultrasound and endoscopic retrograde pancreatography or CT. In a meta-analysis of 14 studies that included 428 cases of exocrine pancreatic insufficiency and 673 controls, a sensitivity for elastase of 77% and specificity of 88% was achieved when compared to the secretin test; whilst in six studies comparing elastase to fecal fat, a sensitivity of 86% and specificity of 88% was obtained. The test is routinely carried out on a small random fecal sample; thus it might be expected to give inferior diagnostic accuracy compared to evaluations carried out on portions of 24- or 72-hour fecal collections. However, with random fecal samples, specificities of 98% and 100% have been reported in healthy controls and specificities of 90% to 97% in patients with nonpancreatic GI disease. Positive results (<200 µg/g) have been reported in patients with clinical or laboratory evidence of malnutrition who also have IBD or chronic diarrhea (nonpancreatic).

Measurement of pancreatic elastase-1 in feces has a high sensitivity for the detection of severe and moderate chronic pancreatitis in adults. It has better sensitivity than other tests for detecting mild chronic pancreatitis and high sensitivity and high negative predictive value for discriminating between diarrhea of pancreatic and nonpancreatic origin. The test is not specific for pancreatitis and detects moderate to severe impairment of pancreatic exocrine secretion from any cause. It is considered to be the most suitable test to confirm pancreatic insufficiency in CF infants older than 2 weeks. A negative test does not exclude mild disease and false-positive results in some nonpancreatic diseases and in very watery samples limit its diagnostic accuracy.

---

**POINTS TO REMEMBER**

**Pancreatic Insufficiency**
- Fat malabsorption is associated with exocrine pancreatic insufficiency.
- Fecal elastase is a useful test for exocrine pancreatic insufficiency.

## Acute Pancreatitis

Acute pancreatitis is an inflammatory condition of the pancreas that may have a self-limiting short course but can be fatal. Almost all patients with acute pancreatitis have severe epigastric pain, usually of sudden onset and often radiating to the back. In more severe cases, there is nausea and vomiting, fever, hypotension, shock, and multiorgan failure that may lead to death. Biochemical features of acute pancreatitis include uremia, hypoalbuminemia, hypokalemia, hyperglycemia, metabolic acidosis, hypoxemia, and abnormal liver tests. None of these are invariably present or diagnostic for pancreatitis. In acute necrotizing pancreatitis, methemalbuminemia may be detectable. The use of enzyme measurements in the diagnosis of acute pancreatitis is explained in Chapter 19.

### AT A GLANCE

**Causes of Acute Pancreatitis**
- Gallstones
- Alcohol excess
- Drugs
- Hypertriglyceridemia
- Hypercalcemia
- Trauma
- Infections
- Rare causes including tumors

## Investigation of Maldigestion and Malabsorption

This section summarizes the causes of malabsorption and suggests a general laboratory approach to these disorders. Table 38.5 summarizes the main causes of malabsorption under the three categories of intraluminal disorders and malabsorption secondary to disorders of either transport into enterocytes or transport out of enterocytes.

The clinical presentation of a patient with malabsorption or maldigestion classically includes the following features:
*Evidence of general ill health.* Anorexia, weight loss, fatigue after minor effort, and dyspnea may be seen. Edema (due to hypoalbuminemia), tetany (low plasma calcium concentration), and dehydration secondary to electrolyte imbalance and water loss may be present. In exocrine pancreatic insufficiency, however, hyperphagia is the rule: patients may often report a very high (5000 kcal/day, 21,000 kJ/day) food intake without weight gain.
*Isolated nutrient deficiencies.* Iron, folate, or vitamin $B_{12}$ deficiency may manifest as anemia, which may be mild; vitamin K deficiency as a bleeding tendency; and vitamin D deficiency as bone disease (see Chapter 27 for more details on vitamins). They are reflected by a variety of signs and symptoms (glossitis, pallor, dermatitis, petechiae, bruising, hematuria, muscle or bone pain, or neurologic abnormalities).
*Abdominal symptoms.* These include discomfort, distention, flatulence, and borborygmi (rumbling and gurgling sounds resulting from movement of gas in the intestine).
*Watery diarrhea and possible steatorrhea.* In severe cases of steatorrhea, the stool is typically loose, bulky, offensive, greasy, light-colored, and difficult to flush away. Alternatively, the stools may appear normal but may be more bulky or be passed more frequently.

Early manifestation of malabsorption will, however, be more subtle than this list might indicate. The alteration in volume or consistency of the stool may be slight, and only mild symptoms may be attributable to the GI tract. The patient may report only anorexia, fatigue, and lack of interest in daily activities. It is in these cases that the astute physician who suspects malabsorption on clinical grounds will rely on the laboratory to assist in the diagnosis. Initial laboratory investigations consist of routine tests, with abnormalities that may indicate the possibility of malabsorption (e.g., blood hemoglobin concentration, mean red cell volume, serum concentrations of folate, ferritin, calcium, albumin, liver enzyme activities, and tests for antibodies in celiac disease).

### TABLE 38.5 Summary of Disorders Leading to Malabsorption

| **Disorders of Intraluminal Digestion** | |
|---|---|
| 1. Altered gastric function | Postgastrectomy syndrome, Zollinger-Ellison syndrome |
| 2. Pancreatic insufficiency | Chronic pancreatitis, cystic fibrosis, pancreatic cancer |
| 3. Bile acid deficiency | Disease/resection of terminal ileum, small bowel overgrowth |
| **Disorders of Transport Into Enterocytes** | |
| 1. Generalized disorders due to reduction in absorptive surface area | Celiac disease, tropical sprue |
| 2. Specific disorders | Hypolactasia, vitamin $B_{12}$ in pernicious anemia, zinc in acrodermatitis enteropathica |
| **Disorders of Transport Out of Enterocytes** | |
| 1. Blockage of the lymphatics | Primary lymphangiectasia<br>Abdominal lymphoma |
| 2. Inherited disorders | Abetalipoproteinemia |

## Evaluation of Fat Absorption

The evaluation of fat absorption or malabsorption is required in only a small minority of patients undergoing investigation for GI disorders because a firm diagnosis can often be made on clinical grounds alone.

Historically the assessment of fat malabsorption was carried out by measurement of fecal fat excretion in a timed (2 to 3 days) fecal collection. This had many limitations and is seldom performed today. A range of alternative tests have been proposed, but most had similar limitations to those for fecal fat measurement in either their sensitivity and specificity or analytic constraints. Currently, investigation of fat malabsorption is limited to the measurement of fecal elastase and the $^{13}C$ mixed-chain triglyceride breath test to identify exocrine pancreatic insufficiency with a consequent reduction in the secretion of lipase.

The $^{13}C$ mixed-chain triglyceride breath test uses $^{13}C$-labeled medium- and long-chain fatty acids as a means of assessing intraluminal pancreatic lipase activity. The labeled substrate is administered orally with a standard meal of toast and butter. Breath samples are collected over a 5-hour period and exhaled $^{13}CO_2$ is expressed as a percentage of the administered dose, with normal excretion in the range of 25% to 40%. The sensitivity and specificity of the test for identifying pancreatic insufficiency has been reported as 89% and 81%, respectively. Similar results have been reported for the $^{14}C$-triolein test using a variety of fat loads and procedures. The disadvantage of this test is the need to measure the $^{14}C$-labeled $CO_2$ immediately, which requires the availability of a scintillation counter and facilities for the administration of radioisotopes.

## Investigation of Chronic Diarrhea

Although diarrhea is a common problem, no clear definition has existed to distinguish it from the range of stool weight, frequency, consistency, or volume that occurs in the normal population. A 2003 proposal that sought to encompass these different elements suggests that for a Western diet, diarrhea may be defined as "the abnormal passage of loose or liquid stools more than three times daily and/or a volume of stool greater than 200 g/day." Guidelines suggest that diarrhea may be defined as chronic when it has continued for 4 weeks or more; such persistence indicates the likelihood of a noninfectious cause requiring further investigation.

Several quite different mechanisms can lead to diarrhea. In carbohydrate malabsorption, the presence of unabsorbed solutes in the bowel causes osmotic diarrhea as water enters the bowel from tissue. By contrast, the diarrhea in most cases of laxative abuse or VIPomas is due to the active secretion of water and electrolytes into the bowel, which is described as secondary diarrhea. IBD causes diarrhea as a consequence of the inflammatory process.

Many diseases more commonly thought to cause "diarrhea" in fact lead to more frequent passage of stools but not usually to an increased stool weight (or volume). Such disorders (e.g., IBS) generally fall outside the scope of the definition of chronic diarrhea. Guidelines for the management

### BOX 38.5   Causes of Chronic Diarrhea

**Colonic**
- Ulcerative colitis
- Crohn disease
- Microscopic colitis

**Small Bowel**
- Irritable bowel syndrome
- Celiac disease
- Small bowel enteropathies (e.g., Crohn disease)
- Bile salt malabsorption
- Disaccharidase deficiency
- GI tract infections including small bowel bacterial overgrowth

**Endocrine**
- Hyperthyroidism
- Neuroendocrine tumors (e.g., VIPoma, carcinoid tumors)
- Hypoparathyroidism
- Addison disease

of IBS are available, and the best results are achieved with an integrated approach to the problem, involving clinicians with a special interest, dietitians, a psychiatric-psychologic approach, etc.

Box 38.5 describes the many causes of chronic diarrhea; most are due to disease of the colon, in which laboratory diagnostic tests are of little value with the exception of fecal calprotectin for the differentiation of IBS from IBD.

### Laxative Abuse

Surreptitious laxative abuse is an important cause of diarrhea that is often overlooked. It may be as common as 20% of cases in secondary or tertiary referral centers. In Munchausen syndrome by proxy, adults have administered laxatives surreptitiously to young children. A clinical diagnosis rarely can be made; no single clinical feature reliably predicts a positive test. When there is a high index of clinical suspicion, urine screens for laxatives may be helpful.

### The Acute Abdomen

The acute abdomen is defined as undiagnosed intense abdominal pain lasting less than 1 week. Many of the diseases that present in this way have a high mortality if not treated surgically, but others may have high morbidity and mortality if surgical intervention is carried out. The clinical diagnosis is based primarily on the nature of the pain. Common causes of the acute abdomen are detailed in Box 38.6. Nonabdominal conditions may simulate an acute abdomen. History and examination often yield a likely diagnosis, but laboratory investigations may help in establishing this (e.g., pregnancy test in suspected ectopic pregnancy, serum amylase, or lipase in acute pancreatitis). A full blood count may reveal a raised neutrophil count suggestive of infection or anemia secondary to blood loss from the GI tract. Knowledge of renal function and acid-base status is important if surgery is being considered.

## BOX 38.6 Causes of the Acute Abdomen

**Common Causes**
- Acute appendicitis
- Acute cholecystitis, ascending cholangitis
- Small and large bowel obstruction
- Intussusception, volvulus, and strangulated hernias
- Renal/ureteric colic
- Perforated peptic/duodenal ulcer
- Acute pancreatitis
- Acute diverticulitis
- Gynecologic conditions (e.g., ectopic pregnancy, salpingitis)
- Ruptured aortic aneurysm
- Mesenteric lymphadenitis

**Less Common Causes**
- Gastroenteritis including *Salmonella, Shigella, Yersinia,* measles virus, etc.
- Crohn disease
- Pyelonephritis
- Meckel diverticulitis
- Acute intermittent porphyria

**Conditions That May Simulate the Acute Abdomen**
- Myocardial infarction or myocarditis

## Gastrointestinal Regulatory Peptides

The gut is the largest endocrine organ in the body but is also a major target for many hormones released locally or from other organs. GI regulatory peptides are released from the pancreatic islets (e.g., somatostatin) or from endocrine cells spread throughout the gut mucosa and collectively known as the diffuse endocrine system. Many of these peptides (such as vasoactive inhibitory peptide [VIP] and somatostatin) are present in the enteric nerves. They are also found in the central nervous system (CNS) and have important roles in the neuroendocrine control of the gut. Although many of them fulfill the classic criteria for a hormone by acting on distant cells, others function as neurotransmitters or have local (paracrine) effects on adjacent cells. Collectively they influence motility, secretion, digestion, and absorption in the gut. They regulate bile flow and the secretion of pancreatic hormones and affect the tonicity of the vascular walls, blood pressure, and cardiac output.

Table 38.6 summarizes the basic chemical characteristics of four of the major GI regulatory peptides and indicates their site of origin and main functions. More detailed descriptions of these peptides are given in the following paragraphs. A list of other regulatory peptides of the GI tract is presented in Table 38.7.

## TABLE 38.6 Characteristics of Prominent Forms of Principal Gut Regulatory Peptides

| Hormone/ Peptide | Molecular Weight (Da) | No. of Amino Acids | Main Gut Localization | Principal Physiologic Action |
|---|---|---|---|---|
| **Gastrin Family** | | | | |
| Cholecystokinin | 3918 | 33 | Duodenum and jejunum | Stimulates gallbladder contraction and intestinal motility; stimulates secretion of pancreatic enzymes, insulin, glucagon, and pancreatic polypeptides; has a role in indicating satiety; the C-terminal 8–amino acid peptide (CCK-8) retains full activity |
| Gastrin-17 | 2098 | 17 | Gastric antrum and duodenum | Stimulates the secretion of gastric acid pepsinogen, intrinsic factor, and secretin; stimulates intestinal mucosal growth; increase gastric and intestinal motility |
| Gastrin | 3839 | 34 | | |
| **Secretin-Glucagon Family** | | | | |
| Secretin | 3056 | 27 | Duodenum | Stimulates pancreatic and jejunal secretion of bicarbonate, enzymes, and insulin; reduces gastric and intestinal motility, inhibits gastrin release and gastric acid secretion |
| VIP | 3326 | 28 | Enteric nerves | Relaxes smooth muscle of gut, blood, and genitourinary system; increases water and electrolyte secretion from the pancreas and gut; releases hormones from the pancreas, gut, and hypothalamus |
| GIP | 4976 | 42 | Duodenum and jejunum | Stimulates insulin release; reduces gastric and intestinal motility; increases fluid and electrolyte secretion from the small intestine |

*GIP,* Glucose-dependent insulinotropic peptide; *VIP,* vasoactive intestinal polypeptide.

## TABLE 38.7    Brief Description of Other Gastrointestinal Regulatory Peptides

| Hormone/Peptide | Major Tissue Location | Principal Known Actions |
| --- | --- | --- |
| Bombesin | Throughout the gut and pancreas | Stimulates release of CCK and gastrin |
| Calcitonin gene–related peptide | Enteric nerves | Unclear |
| Chromogranin A | Neuroendocrine cells | Secretory protein |
| Enkephalins | Stomach, duodenum | Opiate-like actions |
| Enteroglucagon | Small intestine, pancreas | Inhibits insulin secretion |
| Ghrelin | Stomach | Stimulates appetite, increases gastric emptying |
| GLP-1 | Pancreas, ileum | Increases insulin secretion |
| GLP-2 | Ileum, colon | Enterocyte-specific growth hormone |
| Leptin | Stomach | Appetite control |
| Motilin | Throughout the gut | Increases gastric emptying and small bowel motility |
| Neuropeptide Y | Enteric nerves | Regulation of intestinal blood flow |
| Neurotensin | Ileum | Affects gut motility; increases jejunal and ileal fluid secretion |
| Pancreastatin | Pancreas | Inhibits pancreatic endocrine and exocrine secretion |
| Pancreatic polypeptide | Pancreas | Inhibits pancreatic and biliary secretion |
| PYY | Colon | Inhibits food intake |
| Somatostatin | Stomach, pancreas | Inhibits secretion and action of many hormones |

*CCK,* Cholecystokinin; *GLP,* glucagon-like peptide; *PYY,* peptide tyrosine tyrosine.

## Gastrointestinal Neuroendocrine Tumors and Tumor Markers

GI neuroendocrine tumors may be endocrine pancreatic tumors or neuroendocrine tumors arising from enterochromaffin cells that occur throughout the GI tract. Neuroendocrine tumors are described in Chapter 26. Approximately two-thirds of patients with tumors arising from pancreatic islet cells present with excessive hormone production. This group of tumors includes insulinomas, gastrinomas, VIPomas, glucagonomas, and somatostatinomas. Insulinomas and glucagonomas are not usually associated with GI symptoms. Gastrinomas were discussed earlier. The somatostatinoma syndrome is associated with steatorrhea, gallstones, and hyperglycemia.

The watery diarrhea hypokalemic achlorhydria syndrome (WDHA syndrome, Werner-Morrison syndrome) is a consequence of a tumor producing excessive amounts of VIP. The WDHA syndrome may be suspected in a patient who produces large volumes (>1 L/24 h) of secretory diarrhea with dehydration and hypokalemia. The diagnosis is confirmed by the finding of high plasma VIP concentrations and demonstration of somatostatin-receptor uptake on imaging.

The remaining one-third of patients with neuroendocrine tumors have no specific clinical symptoms associated with the tumors, which are described as nonfunctional.

The pattern of hormonal and precursor production by neuroendocrine tumors is complex. Most secrete several tumor markers. Chromogranin A, a member of a family of secretory proteins, has a diagnostic sensitivity of more than 90% for neuroendocrine tumors. Plasma chromogranin A concentration is elevated in most tumors and is an alternative to more specific markers in monitoring the effectiveness of therapy. Although chromogranin A has high sensitivity, false-positive findings have been observed in several nonendocrine tumors, including prostate cancer.

Chromogranin A has been reported to be slightly increased in IBD and also in other malignancies, including lung, prostate, breast, and uterine. It is increased by the use of PPIs and hydrogen receptor blockers, which can be problematic because many patients suspected of having a neuroendocrine tumor may have started on these in primary care. Chromogranin A is renally excreted, so significant renal dysfunction increases the concentration. For these reasons, chromogranin A is usually considered to be a marker of prognosis and for monitoring response to therapy rather than a diagnostic tool.

## REVIEW QUESTIONS

1. Gastrin:
   a. is secreted by the liver and stomach.
   b. is secreted when stomach pH is low.
   c. stimulates gastric acid secretion.
   d. inhibits secretion of intrinsic factor.

2. The hydrogen breath test using glucose or lactulose as a substrate assesses:
   a. intestinal bacterial overgrowth.
   b. celiac disease.
   c. the presence of *H. pylori.*
   d. bile acid malabsorption.

3. A peptide neurotransmitter that relaxes smooth muscle in the gut and increases water and electrolyte secretion is:
   a. cholecystokinin (CCK).
   b. secretin.
   c. vasoactive intestinal polypeptide (VIP).
   d. gastric inhibitory polypeptide.
4. The three phases of the digestive process include the neurogenic, gastric, and the intestinal phases. The intestinal phase is initiated:
   a. by distention of the stomach.
   b. by the sight, smell, and taste of food.
   c. upon stimulation of the cerebral cortex in the brain.
   d. when weakly acidic digestive products of proteins and lipids enter the duodenum.
5. An example of an invasive test for detection of *H. pylori* in peptic ulcer disease would be:
   a. breath testing following ingestion of $^{14}$C-labeled urea.
   b. microbiologic culture of a gastric biopsy sample.
   c. lab measurement of a specific IgG antibody.
   d. detection of a specific fecal antigen.
6. Which one of the following is considered to be a disease of the intestine?
   a. Zollinger-Ellison syndrome
   b. Peptic ulcer disease
   c. Celiac disease
   d. Cystic fibrosis (CF)
7. In Western countries, the most common cause of chronic pancreatitis in adults is:
   a. gallstones.
   b. infections.
   c. pancreatic tumors.
   d. alcohol consumption.
8. Which one of the following peptides stimulates increased pancreatic secretion of bicarbonate?
   a. Glucose-dependent insulinotropic peptide (GIP)
   b. Gluten
   c. Secretin
   d. Vasoactive intestinal polypeptide (VIP)
9. A tumor of the pancreatic islet cells that produces in part massive gastric hypersecretion, diarrhea, and steatorrhea causes:
   a. the Zollinger-Ellison syndrome.
   b. celiac disease.
   c. lactose intolerance.
   d. cystic fibrosis (CF).

## SUGGESTED READINGS

Basuroy R, Srirajaskanthan R, Prachalias A, et al. Review article: the investigation and management of neuroendocrine tumours. *Aliment Pharmacol Ther.* 2014;39:1071–1084.

Caio G, Volta U, Sapone A, et al. Celiac disease: a comprehensive current review. *BMC Med.* 2019;17:142.

Duncan A. Screening for surreptitious laxative abuse. *Ann Clin Biochem.* 2000;37:1–8.

Hofland J, Zandee WT, de Herder WW. Role of biomarker tests for diagnosis of neuroendocrine tumours. *Nat Rev Endocrinol.* 2018;14:656–669.

Kumar PJ, Clark ML. Malabsorption and weight loss. In: Bloom S, ed. *Practical Gastroenterology.* London: Martin Dunitz; 2002:371–382.

Lerner A. Serological testing of celiac disease—moving beyond the tip of the iceberg. *Int J Celiac Dis.* 2014;2:64–66.

Leus J, Van Biervliet S, Robberecht E. Detection and follow up of exocrine pancreatic insufficiency in cystic fibrosis: a review. *Eur J Pediatr.* 2000;159:563–568.

Lindsay J, Langmead L, Preston SL. Gastrointestinal disease. In: Kumar P, Clark M, eds. *Clinical Medicine.* 8th ed. Edinburgh: Saunders; 2012:229–302.

Malfertheiner P, Megraud F, O'Morain CA, et al. Management of *Helicobacter pylori* infection—the Maastricht V/Florence Consensus Report. *Gut.* 2017;66:6–30.

Masoero G, Zaffino C, Laudi C, et al. Fecal pancreatic elastase 1 in the work up of patients with chronic diarrhea. *Int J Pancreatol.* 2000;28:175–179.

Mottacki N, Simren M, Bajor A. Review article: bile acid diarrhoea—pathogenesis, diagnosis and management. *Aliment Pharmacol Ther.* 2016;43:884–898.

Papadia C, Sherwood RA, Kalantzis C, et al. Plasma citrulline concentration: a reliable marker of small bowel absorptive capacity independent of intestinal inflammation. *Am J Gastroenterol.* 2007;102:1–9.

Ponder A, Long MD. A clinical review of recent findings in the epidemiology of inflammatory bowel disease. *Clin Epidemiol.* 2013;5:237–247.

Raphael KL, Willingham FF. Hereditary pancreatitis: current perspectives. *Clin Exp Gastroenterol.* 2016;9:197–207.

Sherwood RA. Faecal markers. *J Clin Pathol.* 2012;65:981–985.

Thomas PD, Forbes A, Green J, et al. Guidelines for the investigation of chronic diarrhoea. *Gut.* 2003;52(suppl. 5):v1–v15.

Walsham NE, Sherwood RA. Fecal calprotectin in inflammatory bowel disease. *Clin Exp Gastroenterol.* 2016;9:1–9.

Yarur AJ, Abreu MT, Deshpande AR, et al. Therapeutic drug monitoring in patients with inflammatory bowel disease. *World J Gastroenterol.* 2014;20:3475–3484.

# Bone and Mineral Metabolism

*David N. Alter*

## OBJECTIVES

1. Define the following:
   a. Bone marker
   b. Matrix
   c. Osteoblast
   d. Osteoclast
   e. Osteomalacia
   f. Osteopenia
   g. Osteoporosis
   h. Rickets
   i. Type I collagen
2. Describe the structure and function of bone.
3. Detail the physiology and regulation of calcium and phosphate.
4. List causes, symptoms, and laboratory analyses used in the differential diagnosis of the following:
   a. Hypercalcemia
   b. Hypermagnesemia
   c. Hyperphosphatemia
   d. Hypocalcemia
   e. Hypomagnesemia
   f. Hypophosphatemia
5. List and describe commonly used methods in the measurement of the following analytes:
   a. Bone alkaline phosphatase (bone ALP)
   b. Parathyroid-related protein
   c. Phosphate
   d. Magnesium
   e. PTH
   f. Total/free calcium
   g. Vitamin D and metabolites
6. State the effect each of the following disorders has on total and free calcium, phosphate, albumin, and PTH:
   a. Primary and secondary hyperparathyroidism
   b. Primary and secondary hypoparathyroidism
   c. Pseudohypoparathyroidism
7. Discuss 1,25-dihydroxyvitamin D, including its metabolism, physiology, and roles in bone health, mineral metabolism, and disease.
8. List and describe five markers of bone formation and resorption.
9. For the following disorders, state the cause(s), symptoms, laboratory analyses, and lab results used to diagnose:
   a. Osteoporosis
   b. Paget disease of bone
   c. Rickets

## KEY WORDS AND DEFINITIONS

**Adynamic bone disease (ABD)** A type of renal osteodystrophy characterized by reduced osteoblasts and osteoclasts, and low bone turnover.

**Bone alkaline phosphatase** An isoenzyme of alkaline phosphatase and a biochemical marker of bone formation.

**Calcitonin** A 32-amino-acid polypeptide hormone elaborated by the parafollicular cells of the thyroid gland in response to hypercalcemia.

**CTX** An antigen produced when type I collagen is digested by the proteinase cathepsin K yielding crosslinked carboxy-terminal telopeptide of type I collagen; a plasma marker for bone resorption.

**Deoxypyridinoline (DPD)** A crosslink of type I collagen present in bone that is excreted, free or protein-bound, in serum or urine and serves as a marker of bone resorption.

**Humoral hypercalcemia of malignancy (HHM)** A malignancy caused by bone resorption mediated by circulating factors released from distant tumor cells.

**Hypercalcemia** Increased concentration of calcium in plasma; manifestations include fatigability, muscle weakness, depression, anorexia, nausea, and constipation; most commonly caused by primary hyperparathyroidism or malignancy.

**Hypercalcemia of malignancy (HCM)** Hypercalcemia caused by the presence of malignancy.

**Hypermagnesemia** A condition characterized by abnormally high concentrations of magnesium in plasma.

**Hyperphosphatemia** A condition characterized by abnormally high concentrations of phosphates in plasma.

**Hypocalcemia** A condition characterized by a low concentration of calcium in plasma.

**Hypomagnesemia** A condition characterized by a low concentration of magnesium in plasma.

**Hypoparathyroidism** The condition produced by greatly reduced function of the parathyroid glands.

**Hypophosphatemia** A condition characterized by a low concentration of phosphate in plasma.

**Mineralization**  The process by which the body uses minerals to build bone structure.

**N-telopeptide (NTX)**  A biochemical marker of bone resorption.

**Osteitis fibrosa**  A complication of hyperparathyroidism in which the bones are soft and often deformed; also called osteitis fibrosa cystica.

**Osteoblasts**  Cells responsible for formation of bone, including synthesis of type I collagen and noncollagenous proteins and mineralization of osteoid.

**Osteocalcin (OC)**  A protein found in the extracellular matrix of bone and dentin and involved in regulating mineralization in the bones and teeth.

**Osteoclasts**  Large, multinuclear cells responsible for resorption of bone.

**Osteomalacia**  Inadequate or delayed mineralization of osteoid; the adult equivalent of rickets (interruption in the development and mineralization of the growth plate in children).

**Osteopenia**  A condition characterized by decreased bone mineral density. Often a predecessor to osteoporosis. It is diagnosed with a radiologic test (Dual-Energy X-ray Absorptiometry; DEXA Scan) that is designed to assess bone mineral density.

**Osteoporosis**  A condition characterized by reduction in bone mass, leading to fractures with minimal trauma; postmenopausal osteoporosis occurs in women after menopause; senile osteoporosis occurs in both men and women later in life.

**Paget disease of bone**  A localized, bone disease characterized by osteoclastic bone resorption followed by replacement of bone in a chaotic fashion. Prevalence varies markedly between countries.

**Parathyroid hormone (PTH)**  A peptide hormone secreted by parathyroid glands in response to decreased free calcium that increases calcium in blood by increasing bone resorption, increasing renal reabsorption of calcium, and increasing the synthesis of 1,25-hydroxyvitamin D [25(OH)D]; the latter increases intestinal absorption of calcium and phosphate.

**Parathyroid hormone-related protein (PTHrP)**  A protein that mimics many actions of PTH, but is a product of a different gene that is expressed in many normal tissues and overexpressed by some tumors in cases of humoral hypercalcemia of malignancy (HHM).

**Procollagen type I carboxy-terminal propeptide (PICP)**  A biochemical marker of bone formation.

**Procollagen type I N-terminal propeptide (PINP)**  A biochemical marker of bone formation.

**Pyridinium crosslinks**  A family of molecules that links collagen molecules to each other; the breakdown products of collagen are excreted into blood then urine with attached crosslinks including pyridinoline (PYD) and deoxypyridinoline (DPD).

**Renal osteodystrophy**  Bone diseases associated with chronic renal failure, including high turnover (osteitis fibrosa or secondary hyperparathyroidism) and low turnover (osteomalacia and adynamic bone) diseases.

**Rickets**  A disorder in children caused by a lack of vitamin D, calcium, or phosphate that leads to softening and weakening of the bones. In adults it is known as osteomalacia.

**Tartrate-resistant acid phosphatase 5b (TRACP5b)**  An enzyme derived from osteoclasts; it is a marker of bone resorption.

**Vitamin D**  A fat soluble pro-hormone that is key in calcium regulation and produced in skin upon exposure to sunlight (vitamin D3, also called *cholecalciferol*) or absorbed from foods that contain it (vitamin D2 or *ergocalciferol*). A deficiency of vitamin D can result in rickets in children and osteomalacia in adults. Related tests with clinical utility include assays for 25(OH)D (calcidiol) and 1,25-dihydroxyvitamin D (calcitriol).

## OVERVIEW OF SKELETAL METABOLISM

Bone is composed primarily of an extracellular mineralized matrix with a smaller cellular fraction. It is a dynamic tissue under continuous turnover or *remodeling*. Osteoclasts and osteoblasts are located on bone surfaces and are responsible for bone resorption and formation. Osteocytes, the most abundant cells in mature bone, are located in lacunae within the bone matrix. Osteoclasts resorb bone, osteoblasts lay down new bone at a site of previous bone resorption, and osteocytes nourish the skeleton and regulate bone cell activity (Fig. 39.1). The remodeling cycle can be divided into activation, resorption, reversal, formation, and termination/resting phases.

Giant multinucleate osteoclasts resorb bone by producing hydrogen ions to mobilize minerals and lysosomal enzymes to digest the organic matrix. Osteoblasts form bone by synthesizing the organic matrix, including type I collagen, and participating in the mineralization of newly synthesized matrix. The development of the osteoblast phenotype has been divided into three phases (Fig. 39.2).

The organic matrix of bone is 90% type I collagen combined with a large number of noncollagenous proteins. The organic matrix is mineralized by the deposition of inorganic calcium and phosphate in small crystals with carbonate, magnesium, sodium, and potassium. Bone contains 99% of the body's calcium, most of the phosphate (85%), and much of the magnesium (55%).

### Bone Remodeling

From 10% to 30% of the skeleton is remodeled yearly. Bone growth and turnover is influenced by a regulatory dance of calcium, phosphate, magnesium, PTH, and 1,25-dihydroxyvitamin D (1,25(OH)$_2$D); which, in turn, is affected by thyroid hormones, estrogens, androgens, cortisol,

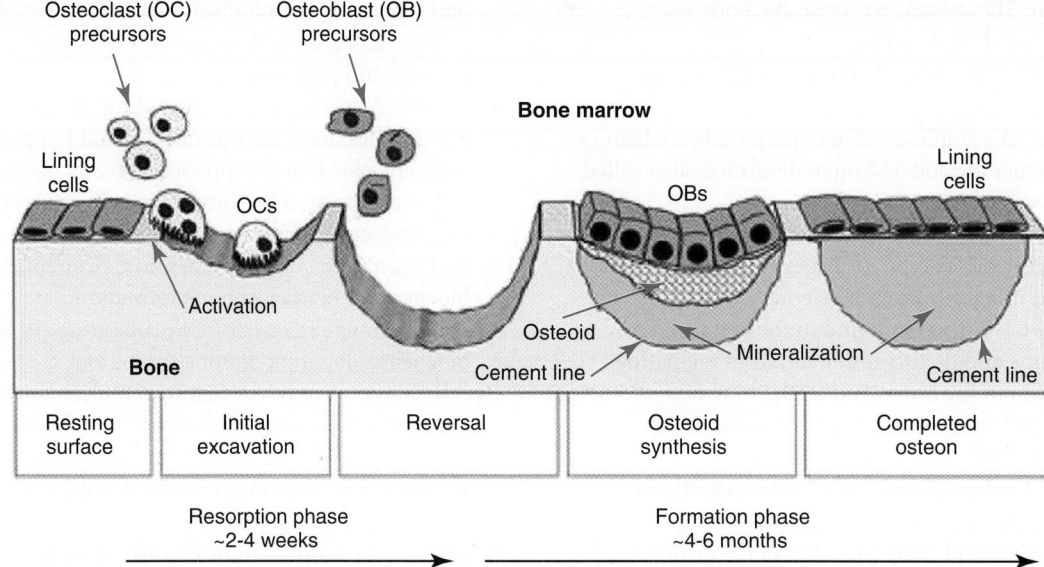

**Fig. 39.1** Bone remodeling is shown in two dimensions, *in vivo*. It occurs in three dimensions, with osteoclasts continuing to enlarge the cavity at one end and osteoblasts beginning to fill in at the other end. (From Riggs BL, Parfitt AM. Drugs used to treat osteoporosis: the critical need for a uniform nomenclature based on their action on bone remodeling. *J Bone Miner Res.* 2005;20:177–184.)

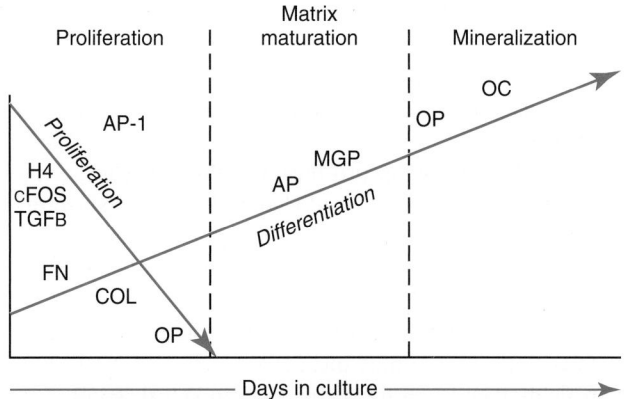

**Fig. 39.2** Development of the osteoblast phenotype. The reciprocal relationship between cell growth and differentiation is shown, *arrows* depict expression of cell cycle and cell growth-related genes (*proliferation arrow*) and that of genes related to maturation of the osteoblast phenotype and production of the extracellular matrix (*differentiation arrow*). The three principal periods in the developmental sequence are designated by *vertical broken lines*. *AP*, Alkaline phosphate; *COL*, type I collagen; *MGP*, matrix Gla protein; *OC*, osteocalcin; *OP*, osteopontin. (Modified from Lian JB, Stein GS. Development of the osteoblast phenotype: molecular mechanisms mediating osteoblast growth and differentiation. *Iowa Orthop J.* 1995;15:118–140.)

insulin, growth hormone, insulin-like growth factors (IGF-I and IGF-II), transforming growth factor-β (TGF-β), fibroblast growth factor 23 (FGF23), and platelet-derived growth factor (PDGF). In addition, numerous cytokines alter bone remodeling by stimulating resorption; these include interleukins (IL)-1, -4, -6, and -11; macrophage and granulocyte/macrophage colony-stimulating factors (MCSF, GCSF), and TNF-α.

During childhood and adolescence, bone formation markedly exceeds bone resorption (bone modeling)—a process that ends with epiphyseal closure at the end of puberty and is followed, in women, by a period of consolidation for the next 5–10 years, when the bone becomes fully mineralized. In healthy individuals, resorption and formation remain in balance for several decades. After menopause, declines in estrogen level trigger an increase in bone resorption exceeding formation resulting in a decrease in bone mass. Males do not experience this phase of rapid bone loss unless they develop altered physiology, such as hypogonadism, but they do experience longer-term age-related loss at a rate similar to that in women. This remodeling imbalance is referred to as **osteoporosis**.

## BIOCHEMICAL MEASUREMENTS IN METABOLIC BONE DISEASE

### Calcium

#### Biochemistry

Calcium is the fifth most common element in the body and the most prevalent cation. An average human (70 kg) contains 1 kg, or 25 mol, of calcium, predominantly as extracellular crystals in hydroxyapatite ($Ca_{10}(PO_4)_6(OH)_2$). Most (99%) of the total body calcium resides within the bony skeleton with 1% in soft tissues and just 0.2% in extracellular fluid (mostly blood) (Table 39.1). Calcium has many physiologically crucial roles in both intracellular and extracellular compartments. Intracellularly, calcium is a key cofactor in muscle contraction, hormone secretion, glycogen metabolism, and cell division. Most extra-skeletal calcium is extracellular with a 20,000-fold greater concentration than intracellularly (approximately 0.1 μmol/L). At the extracellular level, calcium is necessary for bone mineralization as well as being a critical cofactor in blood coagulation, and maintenance of plasma membrane potential. Calcium also stabilizes plasma membranes and influences their permeability and

**TABLE 39.1  Distribution and Physicochemical States of Calcium, Phosphate, and Magnesium in Human Plasma**

|  | Calcium | Phosphate | Magnesium |
|---|---|---|---|
| Skeleton | 99% | 85% | 55% |
| Soft tissues | 1% | 15% | 45% |
| Extracellular fluid | <0.2% | <0.2% | 1% |
| Total body | 1000 g | 600 g | 25 g |
|  | (25 mol) | (19.4 mol) | (1 mol) |
| Free (ionized) | 50% | 55% | 55% |
| Protein-bound | 40% | 10% | 30% |
| Complexed | 10% | 35% | 15% |
| Total, mg/dL | 8.6–10.3 | 2.5–4.5 | 1.7–2.4 |
| Total mmol/L | 2.15–2.57 | 0.81–1.45 | 0.70–0.99 |

Modified from Fraser WD. Bone and mineral metabolism. In: Rifai N, Horvath AR, Wittwer CT eds. *Tietz Textbook of Clinical Chemistry and Molecular Diagnostics*, 6th ed. St. Louis: Elsevier Saunders 2018:1422–1491.

excitability e.g., a decrease in blood calcium concentration causes increased neuromuscular excitability and can lead to tetany. Extracellularly, virtually all calcium is found in the blood, which has a calcium concentration ranging from 8.6 to 10.3 mg/dL (2.15–2.57 mmol/L). In blood, it exists in three physicochemical states "ionized" (free), protein-bound and complexed (see Table 39.1). Total blood calcium reflects both bound and free calcium.

Protein-bound calcium is just that; free calcium bound to proteins (mostly albumin) with its binding dependent on pH and having no biologic activity itself. Bound calcium consists of 40% of the extracellular calcium with 80% of it bound to albumin and the remainder to globulins. Calcium binds to the negatively charged sites on proteins with its binding directly related to pH, such that as pH increases, calcium binding increases and free Ca levels decline. Therefore, pH is inversely associated with free Ca levels. For every 0.1 unit decrease in pH, a 0.2 mg/dL (0.05 mmol/L) increase occurs in free calcium. Complexed calcium is also biologically active at the cellular level representing about 10% of total calcium and refers to calcium complexed with anions such as bicarbonate, phosphate, sulfate, and citrate. Free calcium, also known as "ionized calcium", refers to unbound calcium ions (cations) freely existing in plasma. It is the bioactive component of total calcium; responsible for calcium homeostasis as well as a majority of cellular and intracellular processes. Ionized calcium is more aptly referred to as free calcium as all blood calcium is ionized.

### Regulation

Calcium blood level is regulated by the parathyroid gland via its secretion of **parathyroid hormone (PTH)** in response to changes in free calcium blood level. PTH is constantly being secreted with decreased levels of free calcium triggering parathyroid gland chief cell calcium sensing receptors (CaSR) to increase PTH's rate of release. Conversely, increased levels of iCa will decrease its release. PTH has both direct and indirect roles in calcium regulation. PTH's direct role in hypocalcemic conditions is multifactorial: (1) it promotes bone resorption increasing blood calcium

and phosphate levels; (2) it promotes conversion of storage **vitamin D** (25OH Vitamin D; 25OHD) to the active form of Vitamin D (1,25-dihydroxyvitamin D, $(1,25(OH)_2D)$); and (3) it promotes calcium reabsorption in the distal tubules of the kidneys. Indirectly, PTH affects calcium homeostasis via the actions of $1,25(OH)_2D$, which plays a direct role by increasing intestinal absorption and renal tubular reabsorption of calcium and phosphate. It is reported that high levels of $1,25(OH)_2D$ will also result in bony resorption (Fig. 39.3). With respect to renal regulation of calcium, independent of hormonal control, up to 70% of filtered calcium is passively reabsorbed in the proximal tubule with the remainder (except that which is excreted) reabsorbed via co-transporters in thick ascending loop and distal tubules.

### Physiologic Variation in Calcium

Plasma calcium concentration is dynamically maintained via the previously described processes and varies with age (declines in the elderly), gender, and season. During pregnancy, total calcium levels will decline in parallel with plasma albumin leaving free calcium unchanged. In addition, fetal circulation is relatively hypercalcemic, with higher total and free calcium in cord blood than in maternal plasma. Calcium concentrations decline after birth in healthy term neonates during the first few days, but soon increase to concentrations slightly greater than in adults.

*Hypocalcemia.* Hypocalcemia may be due to a reduction in bound calcium, free calcium, or both. Typically, it reflects both but discordant (low total, normal free calcium or normal total, low free calcium) values are possible. When in doubt, it is critical to check the free calcium level. Clinically, hypocalcemia primarily manifests with both neuromuscular (e.g., paresthesias, muscle twitching, seizures, Trousseau's and Chvostek's signs) and cardiac (prolonged QT interval, hypotension, and arrhythmias) manifestations. Trousseau's sign is a carpopedal spasm induced with the use of a blood pressure cuff and Chvostek's sign is a contraction of facial muscles induced by tapping on the facial nerve (anterior to the ear). The severity and presence of these findings is directly related to the degree of hypocalcemia.

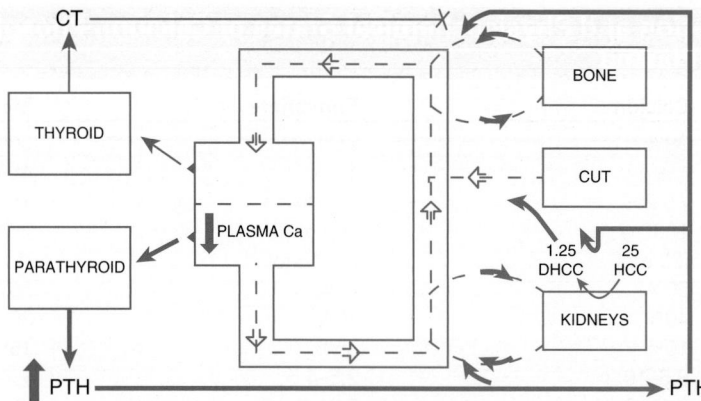

**Fig. 39.3** Regulation of calcium via parathyroid hormone (*PTH*) secretion and its direct and indirect action at the kidneys, intestine, and bone. (Modified from Fraser WD. Hyperparathyroidism. *Lancet.* 2009;374:145–158.)

Hypoalbuminemia is the most common cause of apparent hypocalcemia, particularly in hospitalized patients. Low plasma albumin is seen in chronic liver disease, nephrotic syndrome, congestive heart failure, malignancy, malnutrition, and post-surgical volume replacement with saline or colloidal fluid. Other endogenous causes of hypocalcemia include: chronic kidney disease (CKD), malignancies, drugs, and **hypoparathyroidism**. In pseudohypoparathyroidism, there exists an inherited resistance to PTH such that there are, paradoxically, increased levels of circulating PTH.

Pre-analytic variables can also result in an apparent hypocalcemia, such as with EDTA or citrate contamination seen with an order of draw error or in association with a recent blood transfusion. In the latter situation, transfusion of citrated blood can result in citrate complex formation, leading to a lower free calcium concentration without decreasing the total calcium. Hyperventilation (rapid decrease in $pCO_2$) will result in respiratory alkalosis (increased pH) causing protein binding of free calcium leading to hypocalcemia.

Treatment of symptomatic hypocalcemia may require intravenous calcium; if due to hypoparathyroidism or pseudo-hypoparathyroidism, vitamin D, or vitamin D analogs plus oral calcium are administered. PTH therapy by intramuscular injection is also available to treat hypoparathyroidism. In hypomagnesemic hypoparathyroidism, intravenous magnesium will normalize magnesium, which restores control over PTH synthesis and secretion and results in normocalcemia with calcium supplementation.

*Hypercalcemia.* Hypercalcemia results when the influx of calcium into the extracellular fluid compartment from the skeleton (increased resorption), intestine (increased absorption), or kidney (decreased excretion) is greater than its efflux. The most common signs and symptoms are remembered with the mnemonic "*STONES*", "*BONES*", "*ABDOMINAL GROANS*" and *MENTAL MOANS*". Respectively, these refer to the following sequelae: renal (stone formation); musculoskeletal (bone pain and muscle weakness); gastrointestinal tract (anorexia, nausea, constipation, and vomiting); and nervous system (confusion, fatigue, and stupor). Cardiovascular impacts are also seen with shortened QT interval and bradycardia.

Hypercalcemia is typically divided into PTH-related and non-PTH-related etiologies. Among the PTH-related group, primary hyperparathyroidism (PHPT) is the most common cause in outpatients; whereas, malignancy (**hypercalcemia of malignancy, HCM**) is the most common in hospitalized patients. Vitamin D or analog therapy has also been noted as a common cause of hypercalcemia. These three account for the majority (up to 95%) of hypercalcemia cases.

The most common cause of PHPT is parathyroid adenoma (85%), followed by parathyroid hyperplasia (12%) and then parathyroid carcinoma (1%–2%). Non-parathyroid causes of hypercalcemia are associated with very low or suppressed PTH and include hypercalcemia of malignancy, vitamin D intoxication, and medications. There are many etiologies of hypercalcemia; however, two are worthy of highlighting: (1) granulomatous disorders and (2) milk alkali syndrome. In the former, many granuloma forming disorders produce 1,25(OH)₂D independent of normal homeostatic controls but with all of its calcium increasing properties. Milk alkali syndrome occurs in the setting of calcium supplement overuse.

HCM occurs in 5%–30% of individuals with cancer. It has two primary causes: **humoral hypercalcemia of malignancy (HHM, 80%)** and osteolytic metastatic disease (20%). In cases of HHM, solid tissue malignancies, particularly squamous cell carcinomas, produce **parathyroid hormone-related protein (PTHrP)**, which stimulates bone resorption. In HHM, samples must be obtained prior to initiating treatment as lowering the calcium in HHM will stimulate PTH secretion and can cause diagnostic confusion (hypercalcemia with detectable PTH). Bony metastatic disease will cause local release of cytokines including osteoclast activating factor leading to osteolysis and subsequent release of calcium.

Treatment is directed at decreasing the plasma calcium by either saline diuresis, or medications (bisphosphonates, denosumab, calcitonin) that decrease osteoclastic resorption with emphasis on addressing the underlying disorder.

### Measurement of total calcium

**Photometric.** Spectrophotometric methods measure total calcium using metallochromic indicators or dyes. Of the metallochromic indicators that change color on selectively binding calcium; *o*-cresolphthalein complexone (CPC)

[3′,3″-bis({bis-[carboxymethyl]amino}-methyl)-5′,5″-di-methylphenolphthalein] and arsenazo III are most widely used. In alkaline solutions, the metal-complexing dye CPC forms a red chromophore with calcium; the color is measured between 570 nm and 580 nm. The sample is diluted with acid to release protein-bound and complexed calcium. Organic base, most often diethylamine, 2-amino-2-methyl-1-propanol, or 2-ethylaminoethanol, is then added to buffer the reaction and to produce an alkaline pH. Interference by magnesium is reduced by adding 8-hydroxyquinoline, by buffering the reaction mixture to near pH 12, and by measuring the absorbance near 580 nm. Urea reduces the turbidity of lipemic specimens and enhances complex formation. Adding ethanol or other organic solvents reduces blank absorbance. Calcium forms 1:1 and 2:1 complexes with CPC, the former predominating at lower concentrations. The calibration curves are nonlinear at low concentrations. Multipoint calibration has been recommended. Sodium acetate may improve linearity.

Arsenazo III [1,8-dihydroxynaphthalene-3,6-disulfonic acid-2,7-bis(azo-2)-phenylarsonic acid], at mildly acidic pH, has a higher affinity for calcium than magnesium and produces an intense, purple complex. A reaction pH of 6 is used using imidazole as a buffer as the spectral properties of arsenazo III are dependent on pH. Interference from most biological pigments is reduced by measuring the calcium–dye complex near 650 nm. Citrate can cause negative interference, particularly with dry-slide techniques. Clinically significant interference may be noted in patients receiving citrated blood or blood products. Unlike CPC, which has limited stability, the arsenazo III reagent is stable.

**Atomic absorption spectrometry methods.** The Clinical Laboratory and Standards Institute (CLSI) and the Joint Committee on Traceability in Laboratory has approved an atomic absorption spectrophotometry (AAS) method as a reference method for measuring total serum calcium. The reference method is reported to have an accuracy of 100 ± 2%, compared with 100 ± 0.2% for isotope dilution–mass spectrometry (ID–MS) the definitive method developed by the National Institute of Standards and Technology.

**Specimen requirements.** Serum and heparinized plasma are the preferred specimens. Citrate, oxalate, and EDTA anticoagulants should not be used for spectrophotometric methods as they form complexes with calcium. Acidification of urine is recommended to ensure complete dissociation of calcium from complexes that can be formed at high pH seen in some samples.

**Interferences.** Hemolysis, icterus, lipemia, paraproteins, and magnesium have been reported to interfere with photometric methods. Many methods use bichromatic analysis, multi-wavelength corrections, or blanking to reduce interference. Lipemic specimens should be ultracentrifuged before analysis, or treated to remove the lipid fraction. Although hemolysis can cause a negative error because red cells contain lower concentrations of calcium than plasma, more significant errors may be caused by the spectral interference of hemoglobin. If hemolyzed specimens must be analyzed, blanking with ethylene glycol-*O,O′*-bis(2-aminoethyl)-*N,N,N′,N′*-tetraacetic

---

## BOX 39.1  Preanalytical Factors Affecting Measurement of Serum Total or Free Calcium

**In Vivo**
- Tourniquet use and venous occlusion
- Changes in posture: 10%–12% increase in total calcium and 5%–6% increase in free calcium on standing
- Exercise
- Hyperventilation
- Fist clenching
- Alimentary status
- Alterations in protein binding
- Alterations in complex formation

**In Vitro**
- Inappropriate anticoagulants
- Dilution with liquid heparin
- Interfering levels of heparin
- Contamination with calcium
- Bungs, glassware, tubes
- Specimen handling
- Alterations in pH (free calcium)
- Adsorption or precipitation of calcium
- Spectrophotometric interference
- Hemolysis, icterus, lipemia

---

acid (EGTA) is recommended. Individual instruments and methods should be evaluated for their susceptibility to effects of interferents. Care should be taken to prevent sample contamination with calcium. How the patient is prepared and how the specimen is obtained can have a significant effect on both free and total calcium measurements (see Chapter 3 and Box 39.1).

Hypoalbuminemia provides a caveat to the measurement and reporting of total calcium. In cases of severe hypoalbuminemia, total calcium levels can be artificially depressed (total calcium approximately decreases 0.8 mg/dL for every 1 g/dL drop in albumin concentration). To adjust for this source of error, several equations have been proposed to correct reported calcium levels in situations of hypoalbuminemia. Adjusted calcium is calculated from total calcium and albumin by calculating a correction factor by multiplying the deviation of plasma albumin from the mean of its reference interval by the slope of the regression of total calcium against albumin. Two equations are frequently used with results expressed as mg/dL and mmol/L:

$$\text{Adjusted total calcium (mg/dL)} = \text{Total calcium (mg/dL)} + 0.8\,[4 - \text{Albumin (g/dL)}]$$

$$\text{Adjusted total calcium (mmol/L)} = \text{Total calcium (mmol/L)} + 0.02\,[40 - \text{Albumin (g/dL)}]$$

Many factors affect the distribution of calcium among the fractions (Box 39.2). The reliability of adjustment for serum albumin deteriorates in patients with very low or high albumin concentrations and in patients with severe disease and multiple

## BOX 39.2   Factors Altering the Distribution Between Protein-Bound, Complexed, and Free Calcium, and Compounding the Interpretation of Total Calcium

**Factors Altering Protein Binding of Calcium**
- Altered concentration of albumin or globulins
- Abnormal proteins
- Heparin
- pH
- Free fatty acids
- Bilirubin
- Drugs
- Temperature

**Factors Altering Complex Formation**
- Citrate
- Bicarbonate
- Lactate
- Phosphate
- Pyruvate and α-hydroxybutyrate
- Sulfate
- Anion gap

organ failure as seen in intensive care units. Direct determination of free calcium by ISE is preferable to adjusted calcium but it should be remembered that ISE methods are also subject to effects due to prevailing albumin concentrations.

*Measurement of free calcium.* Blood gas analyzers, using ion specific electrodes (ISEs), provide rapid whole blood determinations of plasma free calcium and electrolytes, as well as blood gases. (See also Chapters 10 and 24.)

Sensitive potentiometers measure the voltage difference between the calcium or pH and reference electrodes for calibrating solutions or samples. A microprocessor calibrates the system and calculates calcium concentration and pH. Most instruments simultaneously measure free calcium and pH at 37°C. Calcium ISEs contain a calcium-selective membrane, which encloses an inner reference solution of calcium chloride often containing saturated AgCl, physiologic concentrations of NaCl, KCl, and an internal reference electrode. The reference electrode, usually Ag/AgCl, is immersed in this inner reference solution. Modern calcium ISEs use liquid membranes containing the ion-selective calcium sensor dissolved in an organic liquid trapped in a polymeric matrix with an external reference (Ag/AgCl or calomel) electrode in contact with the specimen through a liquid/liquid junction or a salt bridge of potassium chloride or sodium formate. The potential difference across the cell is logarithmically related to the activity of free calcium ions in the sample by the Nernst equation. By convention, free calcium is converted from activity to concentration using its activity coefficient, which is itself dependent on strength. Most free calcium analyzers adjust and maintain samples at 37°C, thereby ensuring that results are physiologically relevant.

**Interferences.** Because ISEs measure ion activity, they are affected by the ionic strength of a specimen. Modern

electrodes (see Chapter 10) have high selectivity for calcium over $Na^+$, $K^+$, $Mg2^+$, $H^+$, and $Li^+$ ions. At normal concentrations, these cations have little effect on the accuracy of free calcium measurements. Wide variations in the concentration of $Na^+$ and high concentrations of $Mg2^+$ and $Li^+$ may influence the concentration of free calcium. Electrodes are insensitive to $H^+$, with insignificant interference noted between pH 5 and 9. In addition, many anions including protein, phosphate, citrate, lactate, sulfate, and oxalate form complexes with calcium ions. Although these anions reduce the concentration of free calcium by complex formation, they do not directly interfere with measurement of free calcium. Protein deposits on the electrode may act as a divalent cation exchanger, resulting in positive interference with high concentrations of $Mg2^+$ ions. Newer electrodes use a dialysis membrane or a neutral carrier to reduce or eliminate this protein effect, which typically is less than +0.02 mmol/L (0.08 mg/dL) for 1 g/dL (10 g/L) of protein. The type of dialysis technology or protein exclusion technology can result in different effects of protein concentration on free calcium measurement, especially at extremes of albumin concentration.

**Effect of pH.** Albumin, with up to 30 binding sites for calcium, accounts for 80% of the protein-bound calcium. Increasing the pH of a specimen in vitro increases the ionization and negative charge on albumin leading to an increase in protein-bound calcium and decrease in free calcium. Decreasing pH decreases ionization and negative charge, decreasing protein-bound calcium and increasing free calcium. Free calcium changes by 5% for each 0.1 unit change in pH (Fig. 39.4). Because of this inverse relationship between free calcium and pH, specimens must be analyzed at the patient's pH.

**Specimen requirements.** Specimens for free calcium must be collected and handled to minimize alterations in pH and free calcium caused by loss of $CO_2$ and blood cell metabolism. Free calcium may be measured in heparinized whole blood, heparinized plasma, or serum. Where specimens are analyzed rapidly, heparinized whole blood is preferred because it reduces processing time, uses smaller specimen volume, and avoids alteration in pH associated with centrifugation. All syringes and evacuated tubes should be filled completely, kept tightly sealed, and handled anaerobically to prevent loss of $CO_2$ and the increase in pH that may occur when specimens are exposed to air. It is best that the sample for free calcium is collected in a separate container to minimize the likelihood that the specimen may be analyzed aerobically.

Whole blood specimens should be analyzed within 15–30 min of sampling. Free calcium is reported to be stable in whole blood for at least 1 h at room temperature and for 4 h at 4°C. If specimens cannot be analyzed promptly, they can be collected in an ice-water slurry to minimize metabolism. For delayed analysis, serum may be the optimal sample type because of elimination of the anticoagulant and reduction in the occurrence of microclots. Once centrifuged, specimens are stable for hours at 25°C and for days at 4°C in a sealed tube. The use of aerobic specimens for the measurement of free calcium with correction to pH 7.4 has been criticized and

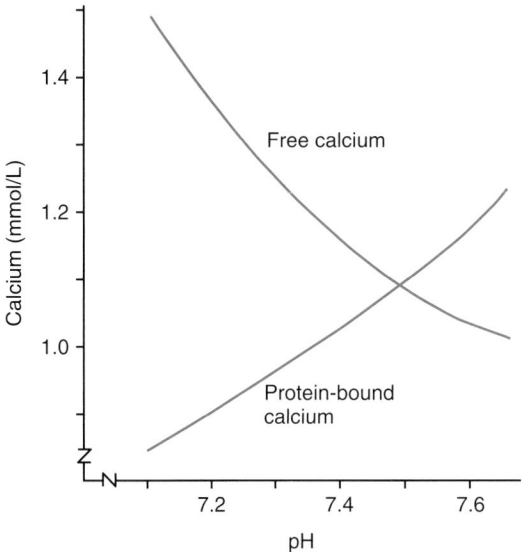

Fig. 39.4 Effect of pH on free and protein-bound calcium.

is not recommended. Free calcium at pH 7.4 may be misleading in patients with respiratory and metabolic alkalosis or acidosis.

**Effects of anticoagulants.** Heparin is the only acceptable anticoagulant for free calcium determinations; however, heparin by itself, which is historically found in conventional blood gas syringes, can significantly lower free calcium. Since the 1990s, commercial syringes containing heparin formulations that are "electrolyte balanced containing calcium" to minimize calcium binding have been in use. Most evacuated collection tubes, when filled completely, contain concentrations of heparin (15 U/mL) that only slightly decrease free calcium. It is important that all syringes and tubes be filled completely to minimize dilution and/or heparin effects.

**Calibrators and quality controls.** Various calibration solutions are used for free calcium analyzers. The buffers in which these calibrators are prepared may affect the liquid junction potential and calcium binding; this is usually corrected by the instrument software. Aqueous quality control materials are available for free calcium. Because simple aqueous controls may not reliably detect changes in performance with patient specimens, the use of serum-based quality control materials is recommended.

## Patient Preparation and Sources of Preanalytical Error

Patient preparation and the manner of specimen collection can significantly affect the results of total and free calcium determinations (see Box 39.1).

Fist clenching or other forearm exercise should be avoided before phlebotomy as either will cause a decrease in pH and an increase in free calcium. Use of tourniquet and postural changes cause fluid shifts within 2 min and 10 min, respectively, altering the concentrations of cells and large molecules such as albumin. These changes cause hemoconcentration secondary due to decreased intravascular water leading to an increased total calcium concentration by 0.2–0.8 mg/dL (0.05–0.20 mmol/L). Errors of 0.5–1.0 mg/dL (0.12–0.25

mmol/L) in total calcium may result from the increase in protein-bound calcium caused by the vascular efflux of water during stasis.

Conversely, lying recumbent has the opposite effect with lower total calcium results.

### Reference Intervals for Total and Free Calcium in Serum and Plasma

*Total calcium.* The reference intervals for serum/plasma calcium are usually defined by an upper limit of 10.1–10.5 mg/dL (2.52–2.62 mmol/L) and a lower limit between 8.5 and 8.8 mg/dL (2.12–2.20 mmol/L). Pediatric reference intervals have been established as part of the CALIPER study (see Appendix).

As an analytical goal for between-day imprecision, the coefficient of variation (CV) is ≤0.9% based on within-person biological variation. Current methods achieve between-day CVs of ≤1.5% within laboratories.

*Free calcium.* The reference interval of free calcium (in adults) is 4.6–5.3 mg/dL (1.15–1.33 mmol/L). Whole blood specimens develop a liquid junction potential different from that of serum or plasma because of the presence of erythrocytes. A positive bias that is directly proportional to the hematocrit has been reported. Free calcium values differ among capillary blood, venous blood, and serum samples because of pH differences. Reference intervals should be determined using the local instrument, specimen type, and collection protocol, and reference individuals representative of the population served.

### Interpretation of Total and Free Calcium Results

For several reasons, calcium status is best determined by measuring free calcium. Total serum calcium is complicated by its association with protein, leading to disagreement between free and total calcium values in up to 18%–31% of patients.

As a result, free calcium is more useful than total calcium determination in hospital patients who have received "interfering" substances, such as citrated blood products, bicarbonate, intravenous solutions, or calcium. Additionally, free calcium measurement is valuable for many inpatients as they may either be hypoalbuminemic or receiving medications that alter protein binding.

Abnormally low free calcium is also frequently found in critically ill patients. The calcium metabolism of patients with renal disease is best evaluated by the determination of free calcium because of alterations in protein, pH, protein binding of calcium, and calcium complexes with organic and inorganic anions. Free calcium may also be useful in the diagnosis of hypercalcemia. Patients with surgically proven PHPT often have increases in free calcium greater than total calcium. Free calcium is more sensitive than total calcium in detecting HCM, as patients frequently have decreased plasma albumin concentrations. Less commonly, paraproteins produced in myeloma may bind calcium, complicating the interpretation of total or adjusted calcium measurements.

*Urinary calcium.* Urinary calcium excretion reflects calcium intake, intestinal absorption, skeletal resorption, renal tubular filtration, and reabsorption. Healthy men and women excrete up to 300 mg (7.5 mmol) of calcium per day on a diet with unrestricted calcium content, and up to 200 mg (5 mmol) per day on a calcium-restricted diet (500 mg or 12.5 mmol calcium/day or less). Under fasting conditions, the intestinal and renal components are relatively fixed, and calcium excretion (mg/100 mL of GF) in the fasting state is used to assess the skeletal component. A value >0.16 mg/100 mL (>0.04 mmol/L) of GF implies an increase in osteoclastic bone resorption. Urine calcium testing has the utility for evaluation of kidney stone risk, osteomalacia, or osteoporosis. It is also recommended to be used in certain situations as part of a hypercalcemia workup, such as distinguishing PHPT from familial hypocalciuric hypercalcemia (FHH). In this scenario, both present with hypercalcemia and (possibly FHH) elevated levels of PTH; however, FHH will have low/normal urine calcium levels.

Specimens may be collected in a container containing acid to prevent calcium salt precipitation. HCl (6 mol/L) is commonly used. Specimens collected without acid should be acidified and allowed to stand for 1 h before thorough remixing and aliquoting. The ability of post collection acidification to redissolve all calcium salts has been questioned.

The reference interval for urinary calcium for spot fasting or timed specimens collected after an overnight fast is <0.16 mg/100 mL (<0.04 mmol/L) of glomerular filtrate (GF), as calculated by the equation:

$$\frac{UCa\,(mg/100mL\,GF)}{} = \frac{[UCa\,(mg/dL)] \times [Serum\,creatinine\,(mg/dL)]}{Urinary\,creatinine\,(mg/dL)}$$

## POINTS TO REMEMBER

**Calcium**
- The free calcium is the physiologically important ion and is tightly regulated.
- The skeleton is the major store of calcium.
- PTH and vitamin D metabolites combine to regulate calcium via the kidney, intestine, and bone.
- Calcium adjusted for albumin can supply important information regarding an individual's calcium status.
- A calcium sensing receptor is present on the chief cells of the parathyroid gland that is responsive to changes in circulating free calcium.

## Phosphate
### Biochemistry and Physiology
An adult has 600 g or approximately 20 mol of phosphorus in inorganic and organic phosphates, 85% is in the skeleton, and the rest is in soft tissue. As inorganic phosphorous is measured, the appropriate nomenclature is "phosphate" not phosphorous. In soft tissue, organic phosphate is ubiquitous in terms of location and function, with respect to intracellular processes (metabolism, gene transcription and cell growth) and compounds such as, but not limited to, nucleic acids,

phospholipids, phosphoproteins, and high-energy compounds, e.g., adenosine triphosphate (ATP). The latter are involved in many energy-intensive processes, such as muscle contractility, neurologic function, and electrolyte transport. In addition, it is important for enzyme activity across many compounds e.g., 2,3-diphosphoglycerate, the key compound regulating oxygen affinity of hemoglobin.

Inorganic phosphate exists as both monovalent ($H_2PO_4^-$) and divalent ($HPO_4^{2-}$) phosphate anions. The ratio of $H_2PO_4^-$ to $HPO_4^{2-}$ is pH dependent and varies from 1:1 in acidosis to 1:4 at pH 7.4 and 1:9 in alkalosis. Inorganic phosphate is a major component of hydroxyapatite in bone; playing an important role in the structural support of the body and providing phosphate for the extracellular and intracellular pool. Only 10% of phosphate in blood is protein-bound; 35% is complexed with sodium, calcium, and magnesium; the remainder, 55%, is free. Phosphate blood levels in adults are maintained between 0.7 and 1.4 mmol/L regulated by the following organs (in order of importance): kidneys, intestine, and skeleton, in conjunction with a combination of the circadian rhythm, and diet. It demonstrates a diurnal variation with a significant increase after the evening meal to a peak in the early hours of the morning, decreasing to a nadir later in the morning. The circadian rhythm is blunted by fasting.

Hormonal regulation of phosphate concentration has not been fully ascertained; however, it involves interactions between phosphate blood levels, parathyroid hormone (PTH), fibroblast growth factor 23 (FGF23) and 1,25(OH)$_2$D, apparently (at this point) primarily choreographed by free calcium levels with phosphate's specific role still to be ascertained. Phosphate blood levels actively increase secondary to homeostatic hypocalcemic responses, which also trigger compensatory mechanisms to prevent hyperphosphatemia. The role of PTH in this dance is to promote renal phosphate reabsorption, bone resorption (releasing phosphate and calcium); as well as conversion of 25OHD to 1,25(OH)$_2$D, which promotes intestinal absorption of phosphate and calcium. At the kidneys, FGF23 and PTH act independently of each other to decrease phosphate reabsorption in the proximal tubules leading to increased phosphaturia. It is postulated that phosphate levels might be the stimulus for osteocyte secretion of FGF23; however, that has not been yet clarified. FGF23 also serves to decrease phosphate levels by inhibition of 1α-hydroxylase activity; thereby, decreasing 25OHD conversion to 1,25(OH)$_2$D. These key effects lead to decreasing phosphate blood concentrations elevated secondary to hypocalcemic responses.

*Hypophosphatemia.* Major causes of hypophosphatemia and phosphate depletion include intracellular shift, such as seen with alcoholism; carbohydrate-induced insulin secretion; vomiting; diarrhea; inadequate intestinal phosphate absorption, such as in patients taking aluminum- or magnesium-containing antacids; renal phosphate wasting; ketoacidosis; genetic causes; and certain drugs such as anticonvulsants and diuretics. Phosphate depletion ultimately leads to membrane disorders and decreased ATP for cellular activities. Clinically, this presents as muscle weakness, respiratory difficulties, and cardiac issues, such as hypotension, decreased contractility, and arrhythmias. At very low levels metabolic encephalopathy can occur. Very low levels can affect 2,3 diphosphoglycerate (2,3-DPG) levels, which will impair oxygen release from hemoglobin, resulting in tissue hypoxia.

Treatment of hypophosphatemia depends on phosphate concentrations and on symptoms. Patients with moderate hypophosphatemia often require only treatment of the underlying disorder and, possibly, oral phosphate. In patients with marked symptoms of hypophosphatemia, particularly if respiratory muscle weakness is present, parenteral administration of phosphate is indicated.

*Hyperphosphatemia.* Hyperphosphatemia is most commonly due to, and is a major clinical issue associated with, renal failure (chronic kidney disease (CKD); see Chapter 35). In acute kidney injury and CKD, a decrease in glomerular filtration rate (GFR) reduces the renal excretion of phosphate, resulting in hyperphosphatemia. Moderate increases in phosphate levels occur in individuals with low PTH, PTH resistance, or acromegaly. In renal failure, FGF23 increases in a compensatory mechanism to counter increasing plasma phosphate; however, as kidney function deteriorates, responsiveness to FGF23 declines reducing FGF23's ability to lower phosphate levels. The clinical manifestations of hyperphosphatemia are similar to hypocalcemia and depend on the rate of onset. Signs and symptoms include the following: altered mental status, convulsions, tetany, seizures, hypotension, Chvostek's, and Trousseau's signs. Therapy for hyperphosphatemia is directed toward correcting the cause. In renal failure and in hypoparathyroidism, dietary restriction of phosphate and agents that bind phosphate in the intestine are useful in lowering phosphate.

## Measurement of Phosphate

*Photometric.* Most methods used to measure serum inorganic phosphate are based on the reaction of phosphate ions with ammonium molybdate forming a phosphomolybdate complex measured by a spectrophotometer:

$$7H_3PO_4 + 12(NH_4)_6Mo_3O_{24} + 4H_2O \rightarrow$$
$$7(NH_4)_3 \left[ PO_4(MoO_3)_{13} \right] + 51NH^{+4} + 51OH^- + 33H_2O]$$

The colorless phosphomolybdate complex may be measured directly by ultraviolet (UV) absorption (340 nm) or reduced to molybdenum blue and measured at 600–700 nm. An acidic pH is necessary for the formation of complexes. A higher pH can result in spontaneous reduction of molybdate. Solubilizing agents such as Tween 80 prevent protein precipitation. Measurement of unreduced complexes has several advantages, including simplicity, speed, and reagent stability. Disadvantages include greater interference by hemolysis, icterus, and lipemia when the 340 nm wavelength is used.

*Specimen requirements.* Serum and heparinized plasma are preferred specimens. Phosphate concentrations are 0.2–0.3 mg/dL (0.06–0.10 mmol/L) lower in heparinized plasma than in serum. Anticoagulants, such as citrate, oxalate, and EDTA, interfere with formation of the phosphomolybdate complex. Phosphate concentrations in plasma or serum are increased by prolonged storage at room temperature or 37°C. Hemolyzed specimens are unacceptable as erythrocytes contain high concentrations of organic phosphate esters. Inorganic phosphate increases by 4–5 mg/dL (1.29–1.61 mmol/L) per 24 h in hemolyzed specimens at 4°C, and more rapidly at 37°C.

Phosphate is stable in separated serum for several days at 4°C and for months when frozen, provided evaporation and lyophilization are prevented.

*Interferences.* Positive or negative interference has been noted with hemolyzed, icteric, and lipemic specimens. Mannitol, fluoride, and monoclonal immunoglobulins are reported to interfere.

*Reference intervals.* In adults, the reference interval for serum phosphate is 2.5–4.5 mg/dL (0.81–1.45 mmol/L). In children, it is 4.0–7.0 mg/dL (1.29–2.26 mmol/L). Serum phosphate concentrations are about 50% higher in infants than in adults and decline throughout childhood. Detailed pediatric reference intervals were established in the CALIPER study (see Appendix).

Urinary phosphate excretion varies with age, muscle mass, renal function, PTH, and time of day. Urinary excretion of phosphate is essentially equivalent to dietary intake. On a nonrestricted diet, the reference interval for urinary phosphate is 0.4–1.3 g/24 h (12.9–42.0 mmol/24 h).

Urine should be collected in 6 mol/L HCl, to avoid precipitation of phosphate complexes. Simultaneous measurement of phosphate and creatinine in serum and urine with fasting morning spot or 1- to 2-hour timed collections permits calculation of the renal phosphate threshold (TmPO4/GFR). The clearance of phosphate divided by creatinine clearance can be plotted on a nomogram, and the TmPO4/GFR determined.

---

### POINTS TO REMEMBER

**Phosphate**
- Phosphate is the proper term instead of "phosphorus."
- Phosphate can be stored in bone combined with calcium as hydroxyapatite.
- Abnormalities of phosphate metabolism can lead to significant bone disorders including rickets.
- Phosphate metabolism is under the regulation of PTH, vitamin D metabolites, and FGF23.
- Phosphate in serum is subject to significant fluctuation throughout the day influenced by nutritional intake.
- CKD results in significant increases in serum phosphate.

---

## Magnesium
### Biochemistry and Physiology

Magnesium is the fourth most abundant cation in the body and the second most prevalent intracellular cation. The total body magnesium content is 25 g ($\approx$1 mol), of which 55% resides in the skeleton. One-third of skeletal magnesium is exchangeable and is thought to serve as a reservoir for maintaining the extracellular magnesium. Some 45% of magnesium is intracellular. Within cells, most of the magnesium is bound to proteins and negatively charged molecules; 80%–90% of cytosolic magnesium is bound to ATP, and MgATP is the substrate for numerous enzymes. Of the total cellular magnesium 0.5%–5.0% is free. The transport of magnesium across the cellular membrane is regulated by a magnesium transport system.

Extracellular magnesium accounts for 1% of the total body magnesium content. Of the magnesium in plasma 55% is free, 30% is associated with proteins (primarily albumin), and 15% is complexed with phosphate, citrate, and other anions (see Table 39.1).

Magnesium is a cofactor for 300+ enzymes, and is essential for physiologic processes such as oxidative phosphorylation, glycolysis, cell replication, nucleotide metabolism, and protein biosynthesis. Magnesium also influences neurotransmitter release at neuromuscular junctions with clinical sequelae of extremes (hypo- and hyper-) related to this function. Reduction in plasma magnesium lowers the threshold of axonal stimulation increasing nerve conduction velocity resulting in increased neuromuscular excitability.

The Institute of Medicine recommends a daily magnesium intake of 310–420 mg. The small bowel absorbs 20%–80% of dietary magnesium; absorption is proportional to the amount in the diet. The kidneys play a major role in regulating magnesium balance. There is 70%–80% of magnesium that is ultrafilterable with 5%–15% being reabsorbed passively in the proximal tubules. In the thick ascending limb of the loop of Henle, 65%–75% is absorbed paracellularly.

*Hypomagnesemia.* **Hypomagnesemia** is common in hospital patients. Ten percent of patients admitted to hospital and 65% of patients in the intensive care unit (ICU) may be hypomagnesemic. Moderate or severe magnesium deficiency is usually due to loss of magnesium from the gastrointestinal tract (GI) or kidneys. Vomiting, diarrhea, and nasogastric suction lower, and may deplete, body magnesium. Excessive urinary losses of magnesium from the kidneys are important causes of magnesium deficiency; other causes include alcohol, diabetes mellitus, and aminoglycoside antibiotics. Magnesium deficiency is usually secondary to another disease or a therapeutic agent. Features of the primary disease may complicate or mask magnesium deficiency. Neuromuscular hyperexcitability with tetany and seizures may be present. Cardiac arrhythmia is a more serious outcome of deficiency. Determination of blood magnesium levels is the most widely used test to assess magnesium status; however, as extracellular magnesium accounts for only 1% of total body magnesium, it correlates poorly with total body magnesium. Intracellular magnesium depletion and magnesium deficiency may exist despite a normal plasma magnesium. Hypocalcemia, hypokalemia, neuromuscular hyperirritability, and cardiac arrhythmias should be an alert to the possible presence of magnesium deficiency. Acute symptomatic magnesium deficiency is treated with parenteral magnesium; mild depletion is treated with oral magnesium.

*Hypermagnesemia.* Magnesium intoxication is rarely encountered although a mild to moderate increase in magnesium concentration is observed in 12% of hospital patients. Symptomatic **hypermagnesemia** is almost always caused by excessive intake, resulting from administration of antacids, enemas, and parenteral fluids containing magnesium. Many patients have concomitant renal failure, limiting the ability to excrete magnesium. Depression of the neuromuscular system and cardiac arrhythmias are common and directly correlate with blood levels; 4–6 mEq/L (4.8–7.2 mg/dL), decreased deep tendon reflexes, lethargy; 6–10 mEq/L (7.2–12 mg/dL), absence of deep tendon reflexes, somnolence, hypotension and ECG changes; >10 mEq/L (12 mg/dL), paralysis, heart block, and respiratory failure. Calcium acutely antagonizes the toxic effects of magnesium and can promote kidney excretion; patients with severe magnesium intoxication may require intravenous calcium. Peritoneal dialysis or hemodialysis against a low-magnesium dialysis bath effectively lowers magnesium.

## Measurement of Total Magnesium

*Photometric methods.* Several metallochromic indicators or dyes change color on selectively binding magnesium. Calmagite [1-(1-hydroxy-4-methyl-2-phenylazo)-2-naphthol-4-sulfonic acid], a metallochromic indicator, forms a colored complex with magnesium in alkaline solution, measured at 530–550 nm with EGTA is added to reduce calcium interference. Methylthymol blue forms a blue complex with magnesium, measured around 600 nm.

*Atomic absorption spectrometry.* As with calcium, AAS methods provide greater accuracy and precision for magnesium measurements than do photometric methods.

*Enzymatic methods.* Enzymatic methods have been developed with hexokinase using $Mg^{2+}$-ATP as a substrate. The rate of the enzyme-catalyzed reaction is dependent on magnesium concentration. When hexokinase is used with glucose 6-phosphate dehydrogenase, the rate of the dehydrogenase reaction is monitored by measuring the formation of NADPH at 340 nm.

## Measurement of Free (Ionized) Magnesium

Free magnesium measurements in whole blood, plasma, or serum use ISEs with neutral carrier ionophores. Current ionophores or electrodes have insufficient selectivity for magnesium over calcium. It is necessary to determine both ions simultaneously and to correct for $Ca^{2+}$. pH should be measured simultaneously, as protein binding of magnesium in plasma is pH-dependent.

Discordance between total and free magnesium measurements has been reported in selected populations—cardiovascular disorders, diabetes mellitus, alcoholism, migraine headaches, asthma, renal transplant, head trauma, and pregnant women. Interferences in measurements of total magnesium, such as thiocyanate in smokers, may explain some discrepancies.

However, the clinical utility of free magnesium vs total magnesium levels is uncertain with limited discussion in the literature. In fact, as of publication, there is only one instrument that offers free magnesium testing.

## Specimen Requirements for Total and Free Magnesium

Serum and heparinized plasma are preferred specimens for measuring free and total magnesium. Zinc heparin, lithium-zinc heparin, and some newer heparins, developed for free calcium determination, should be avoided because they increase free magnesium. Anticoagulants, such as citrate, oxalate, and EDTA, are not acceptable because they form complexes with magnesium. Storage of serum for days at 4°C and for months frozen, does not affect the measured concentrations of total magnesium. Serum or plasma must be separated as soon as possible to prevent an increase in magnesium due to cell leakage. Hemolyzed specimens are unacceptable. Interference by icterus or lipemia depends on the method and can be decreased by bichromatic analysis or blanking with EDTA.

Factors that affect free calcium also alter free magnesium concentrations. Specimens should be handled anaerobically to prevent loss of carbon dioxide and analyzed without delay to prevent changes in pH. Certain silicones or other tube additives as well as thiocyanate (smokers and diet) interfere with free magnesium. Magnesium is primarily an intracellular ion, so depletion is not necessarily reflected in decreased plasma concentrations.

Urine specimens should be collected in acid to prevent precipitation of magnesium complexes. If acid must be added after collection, the entire specimen must be acidified, warmed, and mixed thoroughly before analysis.

## Reference Intervals for Total and Free (Ionized) Magnesium

Adult reference intervals for total serum magnesium are 1.7–2.4 mg/dL (0.66 to 1.07 mmol/L). The reference interval is a matter of debate, as low concentrations within the interval are associated with cardiovascular risk. Conversion factors for the units used to express magnesium concentration are given:

$$mmol/L = mEq/L \times 0.5 = mg/dL \times 0.41$$

$$mEq/L = mmol/L \times 2 = mg/dL \times 0.82$$

$$mg/dL = mEq/L \times 1.22 = mmol/L \times 2.43$$

Reference intervals for total magnesium in infants, children, and adolescents have been published; they do not differ significantly from those of adults. Pediatric reference intervals have been established as part of the CALIPER study (see Appendix).

## Hormones Regulating Bone and Mineral Metabolism

PTH and 1,25(OH)₂D are the primary hormones regulating calcium and phosphate balance, whereas FGF23 is primarily involved in phosphate homeostasis. Pharmacologic calcitonin has also been implicated in lowering plasma calcium levels but the role of physiologic calcitonin (secreted by the thyroid) as a physiologic calcium mediator has not yet been confirmed. Parathyroid hormone-related protein (PTHrP) is the mediator of humoral hypercalcemia of malignancy (HHM), but it also has physiologic functions in fetuses, and in pregnancy and lactation. Sclerostin inhibits the Wnt signaling pathway that plays a major role in osteoblast development and function, and results in decreased bone formation and turnover.

### Parathyroid Hormone

Parathyroid hormone (PTH) is synthesized and secreted by the parathyroid gland; a four lobed gland (two superior and two inferior), located bilaterally on or near the thyroid gland capsule. The chief cells of the parathyroid are responsible for synthesizing, storing, and secreting PTH; with its rate of secretion determined by free calcium concentration. Its metabolism and clearance are dependent on the liver and kidney, respectively.

*Synthesis and secretion.* Parathyroid cells have relatively few secretory granules for PTH storage, and it is synthesized as needed for secretion at the transcriptional level based on free calcium blood levels. PTH production consists of a stepwise post-transcriptional modification of an initially produced preproparathyroid hormone molecule (115 amino acids) to a final intact PTH (1-84 amino acids) hormone. Together with intact PTH, carboxyl (COOH)-terminal (C-terminal) and N-terminal fragments of the hormone are also secreted. The proportion of active hormone varies with degree of calcemia; ranging from 33% (hypo), 20% (normo) to 4% (hyper); the remainder is C-terminal with a small percentage of N-terminal fragments. The heterogeneity of the PTH fragments in blood is due to the secretion of C-terminal fragments, liver/kidney metabolism of intact hormone to C-terminal fragments and renal clearance of intact hormone. Biologically active intact PTH (amino acids 1–84) is rapidly cleared from plasma in normal subjects (half-life <5 min) by the liver (60%–70%) and the kidneys (20%–30%). The biologic significance (if any) of C and N terminal fragments is unclear; however, their concentrations vary in disease states, especially renal failure and can analytically interfere with existing PTH assays.

*Regulation.* The concentration of free calcium in blood or extracellular fluid is the primary acute physiologic regulator of PTH synthesis, metabolism, and secretion. An inverse sigmoid relationship exists between PTH secretion and free extracellular calcium, such that maximal secretion and suppression are attained with hypocalcemia and hypercalcemia, respectively. 1,25(OH)₂D, phosphate, and magnesium have roles in relation to the synthesis and secretion of PTH; however, these are secondary to the role of free calcium. Of note, elevated levels of 1,25(OH)₂D interact with vitamin D receptors in the parathyroid glands to decrease PTH secretion.

Phosphate blood levels also have a role in relation to PTH synthesis and secretion. In CKD, hyperphosphatemia leads to parathyroid hyperplasia and hyperparathyroidism. Chronic severe hypomagnesemia, such as in alcoholism, has been associated with impaired PTH secretion and acute hypomagnesemia may stimulate secretion. Chronic hypomagnesemia can cause resistance to the effects of PTH. PTH demonstrates a circadian rhythm throughout 24 hours. Variation in phosphate is important in controlling the circadian secretion of PTH.

*Biological actions.* PTH influences calcium and phosphate homeostasis directly through its actions on bone and kidneys and indirectly through actions on the intestine via the actions of $1,25(OH)_2D$ (see Fig. 39.3). PTH exerts its actions by interacting with type 1 PTH receptors located in the plasma membranes of target cells. In the kidneys PTH induces $1\alpha$-hydroxylase, increasing the conversion of 25OHD to $1,25(OH)_2D$, increases calcium reabsorption in the distal tubules and decreases phosphate reabsorption in the proximal tubules.

The effects of PTH on bone are complex, as evidenced by its stimulation of bone resorption or bone formation, depending on the concentration of PTH, the duration of exposure and the PTH signaling profile. For example, chronic exposure to high concentrations of PTH leads to increased bone resorption; whereas variable doses of PTH result in an anabolic effect on bone that may be mediated by inhibition of sclerostin expression in osteocytes. PTH increases osteoblasts and enhances their differentiation from stromal cells.

*Clinical significance.* Determination of PTH is useful in the differential diagnosis of both hypercalcemia and hypocalcemia, for assessing parathyroid function in renal failure, and for evaluating parathyroid function in bone and mineral disorders.

*Measurement of parathyroid hormone.* Circulating PTH is composed of both "inactive" fragments and intact hormone. Fragments consisting of the middle and carboxyl regions of the molecule (e.g., amino acids 34–84, 36–84) are devoid of the N-terminal region (where classic PTH activity resides) and are considered inactive degradation products. PTH assays have struggled over time because of this physiologic heterogeneity of circulating PTH-related antigens, complicated by the fact that renal failure (which is often associated with hypercalcemia) is associated with an increase in N-term fragments. Over time, PTH methodologies have progressed from "1st, 2nd , and 3rd generation" assays, with each subsequent progression an improvement on PTH specificity. In the newest PTH assays ("3rd generation"), the epitope of the N-terminally binding antibody consists of the first four to six amino acids of the PTH molecule. Such assays have been variously termed *true intact* PTH assays, *whole* PTH assays, or *cyclase-activating* PTH assays. Despite theoretical improvement, in clinical practice, they have not shown advantages over the earlier assay, "intact PTH" or "2nd generation".

PTH assays developed to measure the intact molecule of PTH(1–84) only ("2nd generation"), are called *intact assays.* These assays incorporated the use of a noncompetitive immunometric assay (IMMA) (see Chapter 15 for immunoassay discussion format using two antibodies: (1) a solid-phase capture antibody against the C-terminus, and (2) a labeled detection antibody against the N-terminus, or vice versa).

It has become clear that intact assays can overestimate the severity of PTH-related bone disease because they detect several molecular species of PTH. Blood contains N-terminally truncated PTH fragments that are long enough to react in the intact PTH assays but do not bind the PTH receptor. The term *intact* as applied to these immunometric PTH assays is a misnomer because C terminal PTH fragments are detected along with PTH(1–84).

**N-terminal-truncated parathyroid hormone and chronic kidney disease.** The N-terminal-truncated fragment(s) [non-(1–84)PTH and PTH(7–84)], containing all but a few of the N-terminal amino acids, account on average for 20%–50% of intact PTH concentrations measured by intact PTH assays in healthy subjects and CKD. The relative concentration of N-terminal-truncated PTH increases with hypercalcemia and decreases with hypocalcemia. N-terminal-truncated PTH originates from both secretion by the parathyroids and peripheral metabolism of intact hormone. The newest intact PTH assay utilizes antibodies against PTH(1–4) and requires the presence of the most N-terminal amino acid, evidenced by its failure to recognize PTH(2–34) (Fig. 39.5). The inability of some intact PTH methods to accurately measure biologically active intact hormone may explain why such intact PTH assays are not a reliable indicator of bone turnover in dialysis patients and fail to distinguish patients with low-, normal-, and high-turnover bone disease. The newest intact PTH assays (whole PTH) are not totally specific for intact PTH. Several studies highlight the lack of comparability of current PTH assays, especially in patients with CKD or those receiving hemodialysis. This has raised concerns regarding the standardization of PTH assays; therefore, production and implementation of a recognized commutable international standard material is required.

**Specimen requirements.** EDTA plasma is often preferred, although some assays require serum and results vary with sample type. Plasma should be analyzed within 72 h if stored at 4°C. Lower concentrations of PTH are observed in serum incubated at room temperature for longer than a few hours, or after one to several days at 4°C. There is no consensus on the effects of storing samples in a freezer (−20°C or −80°C) before analysis. PTH can stick to some plastic tubes and result in decreased values obtained with storage.

*Reference intervals.* Reference intervals for PTH vary with the method used and can be affected by vitamin D status of the population studied.

Typical reference intervals are:

Intact PTH : $10 - 65$ pg/mL or $1.1 - 6.8$ pmol/L

PTH $(1 - 84)$ : $6 - 40$ pg/mL or $0.6 - 42$ pmol/L

Interpretation of PTH concentrations must take account of the patient's circulating calcium at the time of sampling. Lower intervals have been established by excluding individuals with vitamin D insufficiency. Intact PTH increases with age; is low or normal during pregnancy; is lower in fetuses and umbilical cord blood; and increases during the first few

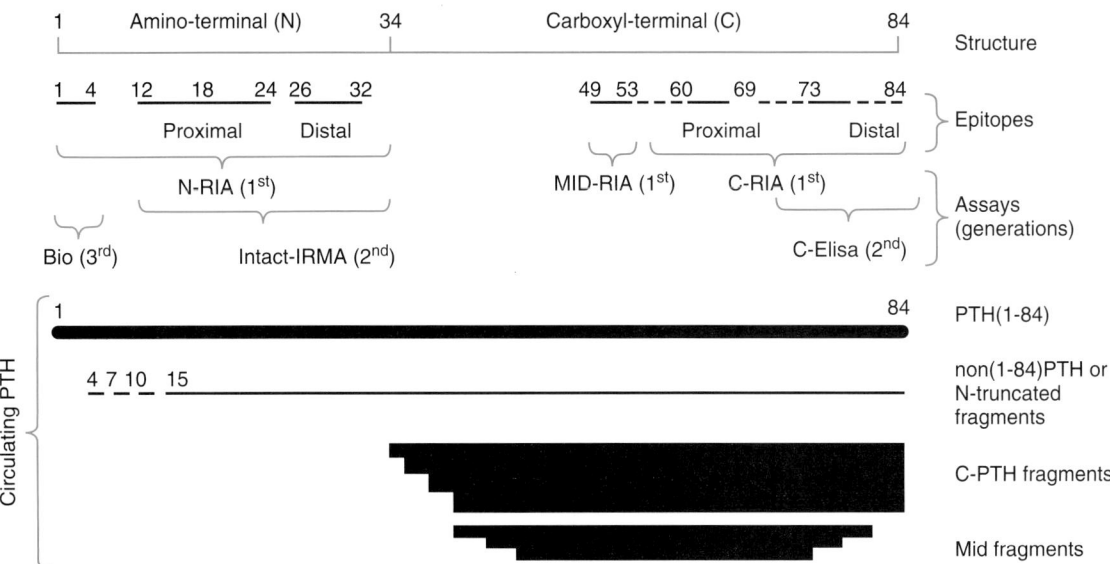

**Fig. 39.5** Relationship between parathyroid hormone (*PTH*) assays, PTH assay epitopes, and PTH molecular forms detected in circulation. The *upper panel* depicts the structure of human PTH and epitopes detected by various PTH assays. Early PTH assays detect full-length PTH(1–84) in addition to PTH fragments. These assays include RIAs that use antisera specific for the amino-terminal (N-RIA), middle (MID-RIA), or carboxyl-terminal (C-RIA) region of PTH. "Intact PTH" assays detect full-length PTH(1–84) and non-(1–84)PTH fragments. PTH assays (*Bio*) detect the full-length PTH(1–84). The *lower panel* depicts the PTH molecular forms present in the circulation. (Modified from Henrich LM, Rogol AD, D'Amour P, Levine MA, Hanks JB, Bruns DE. Persistent hypercalcemia after parathyroidectomy in an adolescent and effect of treatment with cinacalcet HCl. *Clin Chem*. 2006;52:2286–2293.)

days of life. Concentrations in children and adolescents are similar to adults.

*Interpretation of parathyroid hormone results.* PTH is the most important test for the differential diagnosis of hypercalcemia. Intact PTH is increased in most patients with PHPT (Fig. 39.6) and is below normal or close to the lower limit of the reference interval in most patients with non-parathyroid hypercalcemia. In stable hypercalcemia, increased or inappropriately detectable PTH in patients with hypercalcemia and malignancy suggests coexisting PHPT and malignancy as ectopic PTH production by tumors is extremely rare. Measurements of urinary calcium excretion are necessary to confirm hypocalciuria in cases of suspected familial benign hypocalciuric hypercalcemia (FBHH).

The short half-life of PTH (≤5 min) allows intraoperative determination of intact PTH to assess the completeness of parathyroidectomy and facilitates minimally invasive parathyroidectomy. Preoperative or intraoperative PTH may be useful for localizing hyperfunctioning parathyroid tissue by sampling multiple veins from the cervical and mediastinal regions. Postoperative PTH concentrations after thyroidectomy may be predictive of development of hypocalcemia due to a large influx of calcium into bone (hungry bone syndrome).

Subnormal or low–normal PTH is observed in most patients with hypoparathyroidism (see Fig. 39.6). The apparently detectable concentrations in patients with hypoparathyroidism or non-parathyroid hypercalcemia may be a result of imprecision of methods at low concentrations, a nonspecific serum (ligand-free matrix) effect, and/or

measurement of N-terminal-truncated PTH. In secondary hyperparathyroidism (2° HPT), PTH is increased before total or free calcium becomes abnormally low—a consequence of homeostatic mechanisms for the maintenance of serum calcium. As discussed, the most common cause of hypoparathyroidism is surgical status post adjacent neck surgery.

In patients with end-stage renal disease (ESRD), the measurement of PTH is helpful in assessing parathyroid function, in estimating bone turnover, and in improving management. Parathyroid status is usually determined by measuring PTH on predialysis specimens because factors, including changes in plasma calcium and the type of dialysis membrane, affect PTH secretion and clearance.

## POINTS TO REMEMBER

**Parathyroid Hormone**

- Measurement of intact PTH is pivotal in the differential diagnosis of calcium disorders.
- Surgical removal of the parathyroid glands is the commonest cause of hypoparathyroidism.
- Several assays exist for the measurement of PTH. Cross reactivity with PTH metabolites and standardization remains a current problem resulting in significant variation in values obtained particularly in CKD.
- Hypomagnesemia can result in failure of the chief cells to release PTH resulting in hypoparathyroidism. In such cases, patients will not normalize their circulating calcium until there is adequate magnesium replacement.

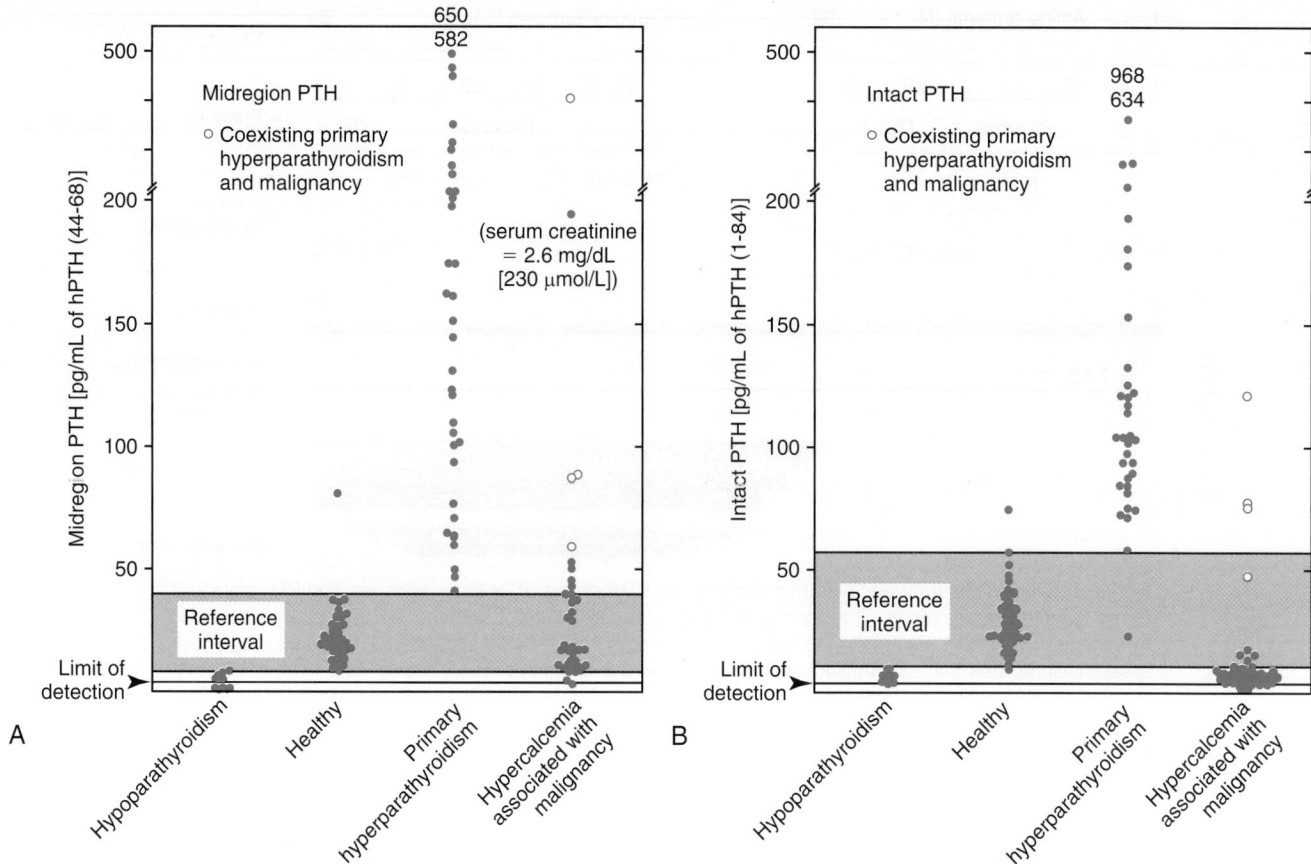

**Fig. 39.6** Parathyroid hormone (*PTH*) in healthy individuals and patients with primary hyperparathyroidism, hypercalcemia-associated malignancy, and hypoparathyroidism. PTH was measured with immunoassay for its midregion PTH (A) and for intact PTH (B). (Modified from Endres DB, Villanueva R, Sharp CF Jr., Singer FR. Measurement of parathyroid hormone. *Endocrinol Metab Clin North Am.* 1989;18:611–629.)

## Vitamin D

Vitamin D3 is produced endogenously through exposure of skin to sunlight (cholecalciferol, D3) and is absorbed from foods containing or supplemented with vitamin D (ergocalciferol, D2). Regardless of source, vitamin D is metabolized to its storage form 25OHD, which is converted to its biologically active form, $1,25(OH)_2D_3/D_2$ in hypocalcemic states. Deficiency of vitamin D results in impaired formation of bone, producing **rickets** in children and **osteomalacia** in adults.

Vitamin D and its metabolites may be categorized as cholecalciferols or ergocalciferols (Fig. 39.7). Cholecalciferol (vitamin D3) is the parent compound and is produced in skin from 7-dehydrocholesterol on exposure to UV B from sunlight. Latitude, season, aging, sunscreen use, and skin pigmentation influence the production of vitamin D3 by skin. Vitamin D2 is manufactured by irradiation of ergosterol produced by yeasts. Total vitamin D refers to vitamin D or metabolites regardless of its source.

A total of 90% of vitamin D is produced by synthesis in the skin. In North America, a significant fraction of vitamin D is acquired by ingestion of fortified foods (cereals, bread, and milk) or supplements. The recommended daily allowance is 400 IU (10 µg). In some European countries, the

recommendation for people older than 60 years is 800 IU (20 µg). There is debate about the doses of vitamin D that are considered optimal for bone health and that can improve vitamin D status sufficiently to result in increases in bone mineral density (BMD) and reduce risk of fracture. Prospective randomized trials of high-dose vitamin D supplementation have increased BMD and muscle function in women, but in some cases a detrimental effect has been observed resulting in increased falls and fractures.

***Metabolism, regulation, and transport.*** Vitamin D2 and vitamin D3 are metabolized to $25(OH)D_{2/3}$ (storage form of vitamin D) in the liver by vitamin D 25-hydroxylase (see Fig. 39.7). The concentration and half-life of 25(OH)D in blood is listed in Table 39.2. In the kidneys, 25OHD is converted to 1,25-dihydroxyvitamin D, the biologically active hormone, by 1α-hydroxylase (see Fig. 39.7). Circulating $1,25(OH)_2D$ is tightly regulated, by PTH, calcium, FGF23 and $1,25(OH)_2D$. Hypocalcemia stimulates PTH secretion and PTH increases 1α-hydroxylase activity. In opposition to hypocalcemic regulation, elevated levels of calcium, phosphate, FGF23, and $1,25(OH)_2D$ reduce 1α-hydroxylase activity putting a break on its calcium raising impact. $1,25(OH)_2D$ also induces 25(OH)D 24-hydroxylase, producing $24,25(OH)_2D$ (inactive metabolite of 25(OH)D), another break on its effects. Normal

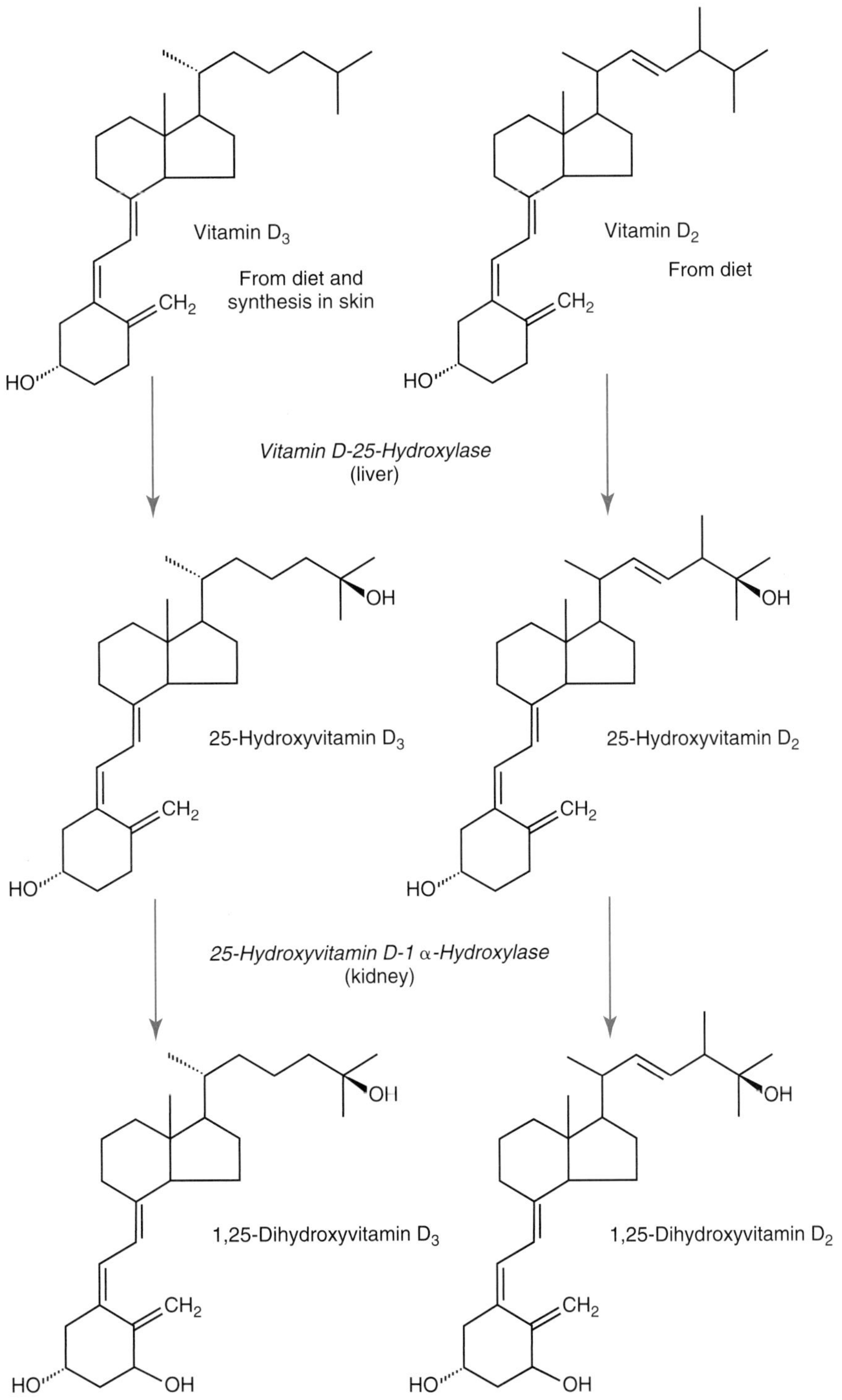

Fig. 39.7 Metabolism of vitamin D. Vitamin D2 and vitamin D3 are enzymatically hydroxylated to 25-hydroxyvitamin D in the liver and to 1,25-dihydroxyvitamin D by the kidneys.

concentrations and the half-life of 24,25(OH)₂D are listed in Table 39.2.

Vitamin D, 25(OH)D, and 1,25(OH)₂D are bound to vitamin D binding protein (DBP), a specific, high-affinity transport protein also known as *group-specific component of serum* or *Gc-globulin*. DBP is constitutively synthesized by the liver and circulates in excess (400 mg/L), with <5% of the vitamin D binding sites occupied. Only 0.03% of 25(OH)D and 0.4% of 1,25(OH)₂D are free in plasma (see Table 39.2). DBP

concentrations are increased in pregnancy and estrogen therapy and are decreased in nephrotic syndrome.

***Biological actions of 25-hydroxyvitamin D and 1,25-dihydroxyvitamin D.*** The major circulating and storage form of vitamin D is 25OHD. It has no biologic role; however, it is the vitamin D metabolite assessed for vitamin D sufficiency. 1,25(OH)₂D maintains calcium and phosphate concentrations in blood through its actions on intestine, bone, kidney, and the parathyroids. In the small intestine,

## TABLE 39.2  Vitamin D and Its Metabolites in Plasma

| Compound | Concentration | Free (%) | Half-Life |
|---|---|---|---|
| Vitamin D | <0.2–20 ng/mL | — | 1–2 days |
| | <0.5–52 nmol/L | | |
| 25-Hydroxyvitamin D | 10–65 ng/mL | 0.03 | 2–3 weeks |
| 1,25-Dihydroxyvitamin D | 25–162 nmol/L | | |
| | 15–60 pg/mL | 0.4 | 4–6 h |
| | 36–144 pmol/L | | |
| 24,25-Dihydroxyvitamin D | 0.8–2.8 ng/mL | Not established | NA |
| | 2.0–7.2 nmol/L | | |

$1,25(OH)_2D$ stimulates calcium absorption, primarily in the duodenum, and phosphate absorption by the jejunum and ileum. At high concentrations, $1,25(OH)_2D$ increases bone resorption by inducing monocytic stem cells to differentiate into osteoclasts and by stimulating osteoblasts to produce cytokine production influencing osteoclast activity. By stimulating osteoblasts, $1,25(OH)_2D$ increases ALP and osteocalcin (OC). $1,25(OH)_2D$ acts directly on the parathyroids to inhibit the synthesis and secretion of PTH.

*Clinical significance.* Determination of 25(OH)D may be useful in the differential diagnosis of hypocalcemia, hypercalcemia, or hypercalciuria and is the means for evaluation of vitamin D status in health and in bone and mineral disorders. The (UK) National Kidney Foundation guidelines have emphasized that vitamin D nutrition is assessed by measurements of 25(OH)D, not $1,25(OH)_2D$. Vitamin D nutritional status is best determined by measurement of 25(OH)D, because it is the main circulating form of vitamin D (see Table 39.2), has a long half-life and is less affected by day-to-day variation, exposure to sunlight, or food intake. Groups at higher risk for developing nutritional vitamin D deficiency include breast-fed infants, strict vegetarians who abstain from eggs and milk, strict vegans, and the elderly.

Concentrations of 25(OH)D may be decreased by reduced availability of vitamin D, inadequate conversion of vitamin D to 25(OH)D, accelerated metabolism of 25(OH)D, and urinary loss of DBP and 25(OH)D. Reduced availability of vitamin D may occur with inadequate exposure to sunlight, dietary deficiency, malabsorption syndromes, and following gastric or small bowel resection. Severe hepatocellular disease has been associated with inadequate conversion of vitamin D to 25(OH)D. Drugs such as phenytoin and phenobarbital induce drug-metabolizing enzymes that accelerate the metabolism of vitamin D and its metabolites. 25(OH)D concentrations may be reduced in patients with nephrotic syndrome because of the urinary loss of DBP and 25(OH)D. A significant proportion of adults in Europe and North America have poor vitamin D status. It has been difficult to harmonize reference intervals for 25(OH)D; this may be related to differences of opinion regarding the definition of subclinical vitamin D insufficiency.

In hypercalcemia, 25(OH)D measurement has limited value. It can confirm intoxication after ingestion of large amounts of vitamin D or 25(OH)D.

The measurement of $1,25(OH)_2D$ is diagnostic in vitamin D-dependent rickets types 1 and 2 and is helpful in disease states associated with the overproduction of $1,25(OH)_2D$, such as granuloma-forming disorders, fungal infection, Hodgkin disease, and other lymphomas. $1,25(OH)_2D$ gives confirmatory information in the evaluation of hypercalcemia, hypercalciuria, hypocalcemia, and bone and mineral disorders. $1,25(OH)_2D$ concentrations are increased in vitamin D-dependent rickets type 2, in $1,25(OH)_2D$ intoxication, and in PHPT. Reduced $1,25(OH)_2D$ can be observed in renal failure, hypercalcemia of malignancy, hyperphosphatemia, hypoparathyroidism, pseudohypoparathyroidism, type 1 vitamin D-dependent rickets, hypomagnesemia, nephrotic syndrome, and severe hepatocellular disease.

$24,25(OH)_2D$ measurements have some clinical utility. The absence of $24,25(OH)_2D$ can result in childhood hypercalcemia and stone formation. Some reports of hypercalcemia in pregnancy have described low $24,25(OH)_2D$ contributing to the pathology. Higher 25(OH)D concentrations have a strong positive correlation with $24,25(OH)_2D$ and increasing vitamin D supplementation results in proportionally greater increases in $24,25(OH)_2D$ than $1,25(OH)_2D$.

*Measurement of vitamin D metabolites.* Specific and sensitive assays exist for measuring vitamin D, 25(OH)D, $1,25(OH)_2D$, and $24,25(OH)_2D$. All assays should measure D2 and D3 metabolites equally (equimolar reactivity), because both D2 and D3 are metabolized to produce biologically active $1,25(OH)_2D$. Separate measurement of the D2 and D3 does not necessarily distinguish between dietary and endogenous sources of vitamin D, as food can be supplemented with D3 or D2.

**Measurement of 25-hydroxyvitamin D.** The metabolite is measured by competitive protein binding assay (CPBA), competitive or noncompetitive immunoassay (radioimmunoassay [RIA]), enteroinsular axis enzyme assay [EIA], immunochemiluminometric assay [ICMA], UV absorption after separation by high-performance liquid chromatography (HPLC), or by mass spectrometry after separation by chromatography (see Chapters 12 and 13). The 25(OH) D2 and D3 metabolites can be quantified separately by liquid chromatography-mass spectrometry (LC-MS)/MS. It is important to report the sum of the two concentrations $[25(OH)D_2 + 25(OH)D_3]$ because vitamin D status depends on the total concentration. Determination by HPLC with UV absorption or mass spectrometry requires appropriate equipment (see Chapter 13), specialized training, and a larger sample. Commercial enzyme immuno-assays are available in use for measurement of 25OH vitamin D on high throughput automated autoanalyzers; however, the gold standard method for 25OH vitamin D remains LC-MS. Unlike autoanalyzers, LC-MS methods have the ability to discriminate between D2 and D3 molecules.

**Measurement of 1,25-dihydroxyvitamin D.** $1,25(OH)_2D$ circulates at 1/1000 of the concentration of $25(OH)D$ and at lower concentrations than other dihydroxylated metabolites (see Table 39.2). Together with the extreme hydrophobicity and instability of the compound this greatly complicates its determination in serum.

**Measurement of 24,25 dihydroxyvitamin D.** No immunoassays have sufficient antibody specificity that enable measurement of $24,25(OH)_2D$. The methods currently in use are LC-MS/MS assays.

*Specimen requirements.* Serum is preferred for measuring vitamin D metabolites, although plasma is acceptable for assays using extraction and chromatography. Once separated from the clot, serum is stable at both room temperature and 4°C; specimens should be frozen if the analysis is delayed. Vitamin D metabolites in serum or plasma are not sensitive to light and do not require special handling.

*Reference intervals.* The Institute of Medicine published a recommendation that the lower limit for vitamin D sufficiency be lowered from 30 to 20 ng/mL (75 to 50 nmol/L) and that concentrations greater than 50 ng/mL (>125 nmol/L) be considered as cause for concern. Vitamin D insufficiency [$25(OH)D$ <20 ng/mL (50 nmol/L)] was common during the winter in adults (>30 years), White men (15%), and women (30%) living in the southern United States.

$25(OH)D$ is increased by exposure to sunlight and shows seasonal variation, with the highest concentrations in summer or fall and the lowest in winter or spring. It is recommended that testing be done at the end of winter; if results are above the cutoff, the subject is likely to have adequate concentrations throughout the year.

Vitamin D metabolite concentrations vary with age and are increased in pregnancy. Concentrations of $1,25(OH)_2D$ are higher in children than in adults and are highest during periods of greatest growth. Although $25(OH)D$ and $1,25(OH)_2D$ decrease with age, this decline may be a consequence of poor nutrition, reduced exposure to sunlight, and declining health. Concentrations of metabolites were unchanged with age in studies limited to healthy, active subjects. $24,25(OH)_2D$ concentrations are method-dependent.

## Fibroblast Growth Factor 23

*Biochemistry and physiology.* Fibroblast growth factor 23 (FGF23) promotes phosphate excretion in urine. FGF23 consists of 251 amino acids, is present in embryonic and adult tissues, and has high expression in osteoblasts and osteocytes.

*Biological actions and clinical significance.* FGF23 acts directly on the proximal tubules of the kidney in conjunction with a tubular membrane protein "Klotho" to decrease renal phosphate reabsorption, i.e., promoting phosphaturia. It also inhibits 1α-hydroxylase in the kidney resulting in a decrease

---

**POINTS TO REMEMBER**

**Vitamin D**
- Measurement of 25 hydroxyvitamin D (25OHD) is accepted as the best reflection of vitamin D status.
- Tandem mass spectrometric methods are considered the best way of measuring 25OHD; however, comparable immunoassays currently exist.
- A high percentage of the world's population are vitamin D deficient.
- Prolonged deficiency of vitamin D results in rickets in children and osteomalacia in adults.
- Care is required with high-dose vitamin D treatment as it can result in significant morbidity, increasing falls, and fractures in elderly women.

---

in the circulating concentration of 1,25-dihydroxyvitamin D. Its mechanism of release has not been fully worked out, but it appears to be secreted by osteocytes in response to blood phosphate levels. FGF23 is increased in plasma in CKD and a variety of other conditions including X-linked hypophosphatemia (XLH). FGF23 may be the best measurement at predicting deterioration in CKD and is markedly increased in CKD. The mechanism regulating FGF23 production in CKD remains unclear.

*Measurement of FGF23.* A single step IMMA incorporates an antibody to the C-terminal peptide fragments of FGF23 (cFGF23) that also reacts with the intact molecule (iFGF23) is available. This assay provides a combined estimate of both cFGF23 and iFGF23. Multiple other immunoassays for the measurement of the intact molecule are available. These assays can give different results in the same populations and so care is required when interpreting the results obtained. Reference intervals are considerably different for each assay. Pre-analytical factors are of importance and the sample type differs between assays. Users are advised to follow instructions provided by manufacturers.

*Reference intervals.* There is significant variability in the reference intervals reflecting a degree of assay variation; at the time of chapter writing, ≤59 pg/mL has been noted on several commercial laboratory's test menu websites.

*Interpretation.* Very high FGF23 concentrations can be obtained in XLH and CKD. An FGF23 concentration in the upper quartile of the reference interval may be inappropriate for a prevailing low phosphate and may require further investigation.

## Calcitonin

The release of calcitonin from the parafollicular or C cells of the thyroid gland is stimulated by circulating calcium. Calcitonin has been used pharmacologically as an inhibitor of bone resorption, but the physiologic role of endogenous calcitonin is uncertain. Calcitonin measurements have a role in the diagnosis and follow-up of medullary thyroid carcinoma (MTC), a malignant tumor of the C cells.

*Biochemistry and physiology.* Calcitonin is a 32 amino acid peptide, molecular mass 3418 Da that interacts with a specific G-protein-coupled receptor found on fully differentiated osteoclasts to inhibit their calcium uptake promoting calcium deposition on bone. During the biosynthesis of calcitonin, the original product is a larger precursor form known as procalcitonin. The structures necessary for biological function are the C-terminal portion of the molecule. Pharmacological doses of calcitonin decrease plasma calcium and phosphate primarily by inhibiting osteoclastic bone resorption. Higher concentrations of calcitonin are observed in young children, and during pregnancy and lactation. The hormone may protect the skeleton during periods of calcium stress. Multiple forms of calcitonin can be observed both in healthy individuals and in patients with MTC or nonthyroidal malignancies. Much of the immunoreactive calcitonin in the circulation is larger than the monomeric hormone.

*Clinical significance.* MTC occurs as a sporadic disease and as part of the multiple endocrine syndromes MEN2A, MEN2B, and familial MTC. These account for 5%–10% of thyroid malignancies, with sporadic MTC accounting for about 80%. After thyroidectomy in MTC patients, calcitonin can serve as a tumor marker. The use of calcitonin measurements in oncology is discussed in Chapter 20. Calcitonin is also increased in various nonthyroidal cancers, and other nonmalignant conditions including acute and chronic renal failure, hypercalcemia, hypergastrinemia, pulmonary disease, and severe illness.

*Measurement of calcitonin.* Calcitonin is measured by immunoassay; interpretation can be complicated both by the heterogeneity of the circulating antigen and by the varying characteristics of the assays. Some assays may give results that are erroneously low at high concentrations (hook effect).

*Reference intervals.* Reference intervals for calcitonin are method dependent. They should be determined for healthy and athyroidal individuals, by gender, for basal and stimulated (calcium and pentagastrin provocation tests) conditions. An upper limit for the reference interval for basal calcitonin concentration in adults is 10 pg/mL (2.9 pmol/L) the mean concentrations are lower in women, 5.8 pg/mL (1.7 pmol/L), and higher 8.8 pg/mL (2.6 pmol/L) in men. Age, growth, pregnancy, and lactation—in addition to gender—have been reported to influence circulating calcitonin.

## Parathyroid Hormone-Related Protein

PTHrP was discovered as a molecule responsible for causing HHM. It later proved to be an autocrine/paracrine factor with a multitude of functions in several organ systems. Among these are its effects on chondrocyte biology and endochondral bone formation, as well as on calcium metabolism in the fetus, and during pregnancy and lactation.

*Biochemistry and physiology.* PTHrP is derived from a gene on chromosome 12 that is distinct from the *PTH* gene on chromosome 11. The N-terminal shows close homology to PTH, and its PTH-like activity is contained within the N-terminal. Like PTH, PTHrP causes hypercalcemia and hypophosphatemia, and increases urinary cyclic adenosine monophosphate.

PTHrP exerts endocrine effects on skeletal development and calcium homeostasis during fetal life and lactation. Breast milk contains high PTHrP as does amniotic fluid. PTHrP regulates transepithelial calcium transport; it is a potent smooth muscle relaxant, and it regulates growth, differentiation, and development.

*Clinical significance.* HCM is the third most frequent cause of hypercalcemia in hospitalized patients and is caused by HHM and local osteolysis. HHM is present in approximately 75%–80% of patients with HCM. HHM is common in patients with squamous (lung, head and neck, esophagus, cervix, vulva, and skin), renal, bladder, and ovarian carcinomas. PTHrP is rarely required for diagnosis because HHM nearly always occurs in advanced disease when the diagnosis is clear. The need for PTHrP determination is greater when it becomes important in prognosis, selection of therapy, or monitoring.

*Measurement of parathyroid hormone-related protein.* Enzyme immunoassays are available for the measurement of PTHrP.

*Specimen requirements.* PTHrP is unstable in serum and plasma at 4°C and at room temperature unless collected in the presence of protease inhibitors and kept on ice. EDTA plasma should be promptly separated, and frozen as red cell enzymes degrade PTHrP.

*Reference intervals.* PTHrP concentrations are dependent on the assay and collection, varying from undetectable up to 5 pmol/L.

*Interpretation.* PTHrP is increased in 50%–90% of patients with HCM (Fig. 39.8). In addition to squamous cell carcinoma of the lung, head and neck, esophagus, cervix, and skin, increased concentrations have been found in a wide variety of other malignancies.

## Sclerostin

Sclerostin is secreted by osteocytes and articular chondrocytes, and absence favors bone formation.

*Biochemistry and physiology.* Sclerostin expression by osteocytes is regulated by mechanical forces. Immobilization increases sclerostin positive osteocytes and circulating sclerostin.

*Clinical significance.* Sclerostin is increased in hypoparathyroidism, type 2 diabetes, cancer-induced bone disease and **Paget disease of bone** (PDB). Sclerostin is decreased in 1HPT and ankylosing spondylitis.

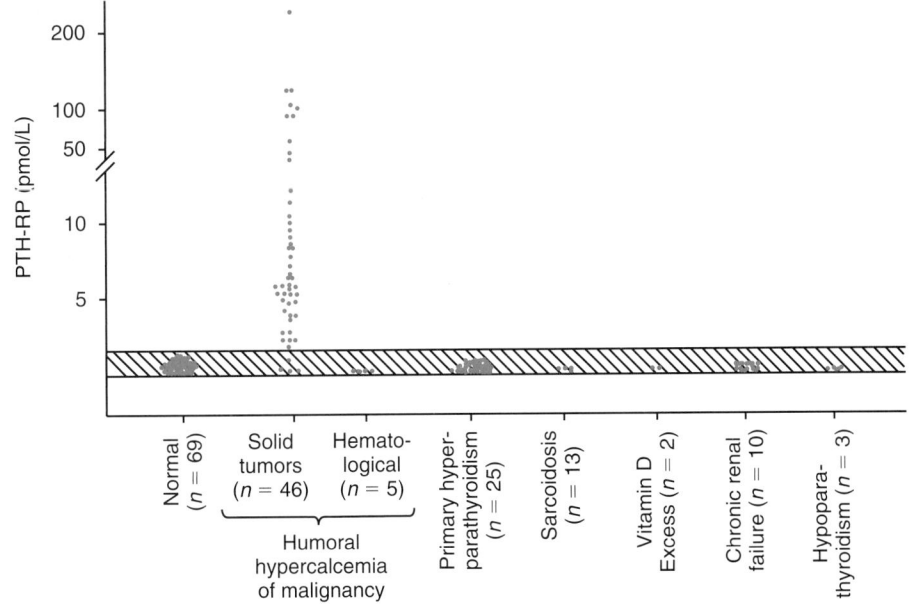

**Fig. 39.8** Parathyroid hormone-related protein (*PTH-RP*) in healthy individuals, patients with malignancies and other disorders. The *hatched area* indicates the reference interval. (Modified from Pandian MR, Morgan CH, Carlton E, Segre GV. Modified immunoradiometric assay of parathyroid hormone-related protein: clinical application in the differential diagnosis of hypercalcemia. *Clin Chem*. 1992;38:282–288.)

*Measurement of sclerostin.* Several assays are available. EDTA-plasma and serum are the recommended sample types. Significant differences exist between commercial assays.

*Reference intervals.* Using the Biomedica assay in normal adults, the mean concentrations are:

- Serum 0.8 pmol/L; plasma (EDTA) 1.3 pmol/L, plasma (heparin) 1.2 pmol/L, plasma (citrate 1.4 pmol/L).

## Biochemical Markers of Bone Turnover

Bone turnover markers are divided up into two classes: "Formation" and "Resorption". Common markers of bone formation include products of the osteoblast, the amino- or carboxy-terminal propeptides of type I collagen, **procollagen type I N-terminal propeptide (PINP)**, and **procollagen type I carboxy-terminal propeptide (PICP)**, **bone alkaline phosphatase (bALP)**, and **osteocalcin**. Common markers of bone resorption are breakdown products of type I collagen and include the amino-terminal and carboxy-terminal cross-linked telopeptide parts of collagen (**N-telopeptide [NTX]** and **C-telopeptide [CTX]**. **TRACP5b** , an enzyme released from resorbing osteoclasts is also one of the common markers of bone resorption. Less common markers are **pyridinium crosslinks** (pyridinoline [PYD] and **deoxypyridinoline [DPD]**).

### Markers of Bone Formation

Bone formation markers can be divided into three families, each reflecting a specific phase in development of the osteoblast. During each remodeling cycle, osteoblasts pass through the phases of proliferation, matrix maturation, and mineralization (see Fig. 39.2). Markers can give discordant results if bone formation is affected by a disease that targets a particular developmental phase of the osteoblast.

*PINP, PICP.* Type I collagen accounts for 90% of the bone organic matrix and provides it with tensile strength. The type I collagen, a triple helix of two identical $\alpha1(I)$ chains and an $\alpha2(I)$ chain, is synthesized as a precursor type I procollagen that contains large additional domains at both ends of the rod-like collagen molecule (Fig. 39.9). Cleavage of the C-terminal propeptide (PICP) is necessary before collagen molecules can be assembled into collagen fibers, whereas the N-terminal propeptide (PINP) may remain longer. PINP is released before bone mineralization, but in soft tissues, type I collagen may still contain the N-terminal propeptide. The concentrations of procollagen propeptides reflect the rate of collagen synthesis.

Plasma PINP in health is present mainly in intact, trimeric form. In certain situations (CKD with hemodialysis, bedridden geriatric patients), smaller forms of PINP are detected in plasma. PINP assays differ with respect to whether they measure the trimeric form (intact PINP) or both forms (total PINP). Intact propeptides are degraded by the endothelial cells of the liver. Renal clearance also occurs for the smaller circulating propeptides.

**Clinical significance.** In principle, measurement of either propeptide should give the same information. This is the case when PICP and PINP concentrations are compared in situ. In children, circulating propeptides closely reflect the somatic growth rate, and the peak of PICP and PINP concentrations occurs earlier in girls than in boys. During puberty, the increase is larger in boys than in girls.

The measurement of response to treatment for osteoporosis therapies is a major use of bone formation markers. The concentration of PINP is increased more during active bone growth than is the concentration of PICP.

**Specimen requirements.** The preferred sample for measuring procollagen propeptides is serum. The antigens are

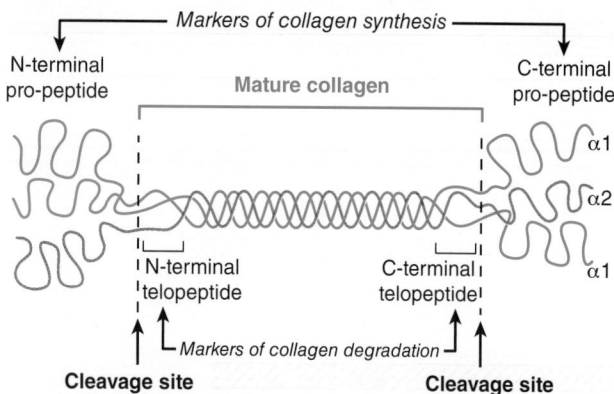

Fig. 39.9 Structure of collagen molecule. Pro-collagen is comprised of two alpha-I chains and one alpha-2 chain intertwined into a triple helix. Pro-peptide domains at the carboxy-terminals and amino-terminals are cleaved, resulting in formation of mature collagen. When collagen is degraded, during physiological turnover or pathological adverse remodeling, telopeptides (from the amino-terminals or carboxy-terminals) are cleaved and released into the plasma. (Modified from Fan D, Takawale A, Lee J, et al. Cardiac fibroblasts, fibrosis and extracellular matrix remodeling in heart disease. *Fibrogenesis Tissue Repair* 2012;5(1):15. Figure 3. *Available via license: Creative Commons Attribution 2.0 Generic*)

very stable in serum or plasma. Storage of serum at room temperature for 1 week does not decrease concentrations.

**Assays.** Automated enzyme immunoassays are available for both PINP and PICP.

**Reference intervals.** Reference intervals for PICP are 38–202 µg/L in men and 50–170 µg/L in women. For intact PINP, the reference intervals in men are 20–78 µg/L, and in women 19–84 µg/L. The reference interval for total PINP in young healthy premenopausal women (30–39 years) is 16.3–72.2 µg/L. The reference interval for total PINP in men is 13.9–85.5 µg/L. For all of the bone turnover markers, reference intervals may vary from analyzer to analyzer; please consult with your lab for the local reference intervals. Data is limited on pediatric reference intervals; however overall, children have higher concentrations immediately after birth and later during growth spurts.

*Bone alkaline phosphatase.* ALP are membrane-bound ectoenzymes that catalyze the hydrolysis of monophosphates from ester linkage under alkaline conditions (pH 8–10). Four different gene codes are known for the tissue: nonspecific, intestinal, placental, and germ cell (placental-like) isoenzymes. These isoforms are N-glycosylated, and only the liver ALP does not contain O-linked glycans. Bone ALP can be separated by anion-exchange HPLC or isoelectric focusing into four isoforms differing in their sialic acid content. During mineralization of bone, the main function of bone ALP is to hydrolyze inorganic pyrophosphate (PPi) to generate phosphate (Pi). The balance between Pi and PPi is thought to be critical for mineralization because PPi inhibits the formation of hydroxyapatite. Bone ALP is produced by osteoblasts during the matrix maturation phase (see Fig. 39.2) when the newly formed collagenous matrix is prepared for the deposition of mineral. Because ALP is firmly bound to cell membranes,

release to plasma can be delayed, and increase in plasma activity takes time.

**Clinical significance.** Total ALP or bone ALP provides the highest clinical sensitivity and specificity in the diagnosis and monitoring of PDB. Bone ALP is more sensitive than total ALP in mild (monostotic) disease. ALP is increased in PDB and reflects increased bone formation. Bone ALP is increased in osteoporosis, osteomalacia and rickets, hyperparathyroidism, renal osteodystrophy, thyrotoxicosis, acromegaly, and bone metastases. ALP and bone ALP are stable in serum *in vitro* and do not require special specimen handling. Bone ALP is more useful than osteocalcin in individuals with impaired renal function because it is not cleared by glomerular filtration.

**Measurement of bone alkaline phosphatase.** Measurement of the enzymatic activities of total and bone ALP is described in Chapter 19. Although internal standards for ALP isoenzymes have been used to increase assay precision for bone ALP activity, they tend to be technically complicated, labor intensive, imprecise, insensitive, and inaccurate. Immunoassays are currently used for bone ALP. None of the monoclonal antibodies used is completely specific for bone ALP. Current immunoassays exhibit 7%–17% cross-reactivity with liver ALP.

**Reference intervals.** Plasma concentrations of bone ALP are influenced by age and gender. Concentrations are higher in men and increase with age in men and women. Reference ranges vary with instrument, for example an immunosorbent method lists 15.0–41.3 µg/L for men and 11.6–29.6 µg/L for premenopausal women; whereas an automated chemiluminescent immunoenzymatic method, the 95th percentile limit is 14.3 µg/L for men and 20.1 µg/L for premenopausal women.

*Osteocalcin.* OC is the most abundant noncollagenous protein of human bone; it is a small protein of 49 amino acids and contains three glutamyl residues at amino acid positions 17, 21, and 24, which can be converted to γ-carboxyglutamyl residues by a post-translational, vitamin K-dependent enzymatic carboxylation. These unique carboxylated amino acids bind calcium ions and are found in proteins involved in blood coagulation and in calcium transport, deposition, and homeostasis. OC binds calcium and hydroxyapatite, suggesting a physiologic role in bone mineralization.

Osteocalcin is present in the plasma in carboxylated and undercarboxylated forms; it is the undercarboxylated form of OC that acts as a hormone. The undercarboxylated fraction represents 16%–21% of total OC. It is cleared by the kidneys and has a half-life of 5 min. Levels are increased in CKD and exhibit a diurnal variation with a nocturnal peak, decreasing by as much as 50% to a morning nadir. Circulating OC is heterogeneous; in addition to the intact molecule, several fragments also exist. Intact OC has been estimated to account for 35% of total OC, N-terminal/mid-region for 30%, and other fragments for much less in the circulation.

**Clinical significance.** The concentration of OC changes rapidly in situations that affect bone turnover. Plasma OC is increased in metabolic bone disease with increased bone formation, hyperparathyroidism, renal osteodystrophy, thyrotoxicosis, post-fractures, acromegaly, and bone metastases. OC is decreased in hypoparathyroidism, hypothyroidism, growth hormone deficiency, during estrogen therapy, treatment with glucocorticoids, bisphosphonates, and calcitonin. OC concentrations may be misleading in several situations; such as an increase in impaired renal function without a similar increase in bone formation or it may be increased during bed rest without an increase in bone formation. About 10%–30% of OC synthesized by the osteoblast is released into the circulation. OC fragments are released from the bone matrix during bone resorption and may contribute to circulating OC. Serum osteocalcin may be considered a marker of bone turnover rather than just bone formation.

**Measurement of osteocalcin.** Many immunoassays have been developed for OC since the first reported in 1980. Those assays measuring both intact OC plus the N-terminal/mid-region (1–43) fragment, are of particular interest. These assays do not measure smaller fragments of OC that are produced during bone resorption. OC concentrations are more stable when measured with assays that recognize both intact hormone (1–49) and the N-terminal/mid-region (1–43). Specificities with respect to carboxylated and undercarboxylated forms of OC are often not known.

An immunoassay for the undercarboxylated form of OC has been developed. This assay uses recombinant human undercarboxylated OC for calibration and two monoclonal antibodies, one of these specifically recognizes the 14–30 sequence, in which the three glutamic acid residues are not carboxylated.

**Specimen requirements.** OC is rapidly degraded in blood samples at room temperature or 4°C. Serum OC concentrations are more stable when assessed with methods measuring both intact OC and the N-terminal/mid-region fragment (1–43); concentrations are unchanged after 3 h at room temperature and after 24 h at 4°C.

**Reference intervals.** OC concentrations are influenced by age, gender, and diurnal variation. Men have higher OC than women. OC concentrations are increased during menopause. In one OC ELISA, the reference interval was 9.6–40.8 µg/L in men, 8.4–33.9 µg/L in premenopausal women, and 12.8–55.0 µg/L in postmenopausal women. Concentrations are higher in children—the highest of which are observed during periods of rapid growth. Pediatric reference intervals for osteocalcin and the telopeptides are not present in the CALIPER database and published studies are limited.

## Biochemical Markers of Bone Resorption

Most markers of bone resorption reflect degradation of type I collagen. These markers were initially measured in urine, but serum-based methods have been developed. An osteoclast-derived enzyme, serum TRAP5b, has been used to assess bone resorption.

*Telopeptides: NTX, CTX.* Extracellularly, type I collagen molecules are assembled into immature fibrils with limited tensile strength, which then are modified by formation of intramolecular and intermolecular covalent bonds

or crosslinks. Intermolecular crosslinking sites are located in short non-triple-helical domains at each end of the type I collagen molecule, called *telopeptides.* The activities of two enzymes—intracellular lysyl hydroxylase 2b and extracellular lysyl oxidase—regulate which variant structures of crosslinks are formed. Cathepsin K is the main enzyme that degrades bone collagen. Its activity alone is sufficient to completely dissolve insoluble collagen of adult cortical bone. Crosslinked telopeptides are released from type I collagen during bone resorption because crosslinks resist proteolysis of adjacent polypeptide chains. This may lead to the generation of the amino-terminal and carboxyl-terminal collagen crosslinks (NTX and CTX, respectively). Both of which can be detected by immunoassay.

*Collagen crosslinks: deoxypyridinoline and pyridinoline.* PYD and DPD are stable even to acid hydrolysis, whereas the pyrrole variants are quite unstable. Trivalent crosslinks are found in soft tissues and in collagen types other than type I (type II, III). PYDs were the first mature crosslinks to be identified, but their quantity in bone is relatively low, one per three to five collagen molecules, compared with the quantity of their divalent precursors, 1 per collagen molecule. The pyrrole crosslinks are concentrated at the N-terminal end of human bone collagen. Both telopeptides have a sequence including an aspartic acid residue, which can undergo racemization and α-isomerization. Immunoassays detect only one form of these structures.

**Clinical significance of telopeptides and crosslinks.** Increased urinary CTX, NTX, and DPD have been reported in osteoporosis, PDB, PHPT, and 2° HPT, hyperthyroidism, carcinoma metastases, and multiple myeloma. Inhibition of bone resorption with pharmacologic agents (bisphosphonates, denosumab) leads to a decrease in serum/plasma or urinary CTX, NTX, and DPD; this is the most common use of these markers in clinical practice.

*N-telopeptide NTX assay.* Enzyme immunoassays for NTX in urine and serum have been developed and are in use. The use of serum can significantly reduce within-subject day-to-day variation.

*C-telopeptide CTX assay.* EDTA plasma is the preferred sample. Serum can be used if rapidly separated prior to storing frozen at a minimum of −20°C. The most widely used methods recognize the α-isomer. In healthy human bone, 70%–80% of C-telopeptides have α-isomerization, but in PDB, it accounts for only 50 to 60. α-Isomerization and racemization may vary between individuals. All CTX methods require the C-terminal amino acid to be a free arginine. Serum/plasma CTX assays are available by several enzyme immunoassay types.

*Deoxypyridinoline and pyridinoline.* DPD and PYD were originally measured by HPLC. Today, DPD is measured primarily by immunoassay using automated analyzers or manual ELISA. Unlike most HPLC methods, which can measure total DPD and PYD, the immunoassays for DPD or DPD/PYD measure primarily free, but not peptide-bound, forms.

**Specimen requirements.** Serum or plasma is best collected after overnight fasting. A second morning void urine, collected by 10:00 a.m., is recommended. For treatment monitoring, specimens should be collected at the same time as the baseline specimen. Peak urinary excretion of PYDs occurs at 5:00 to 8:00 a.m., reflecting the nocturnal peak in bone turnover. Urinary PYDs reach a nadir between 2:00 and 11:00 p.m. PYDs and telopeptides are relatively stable in urine. Exposure to UV light decreases DPD and PYD.

**Comparison of urine and serum analyses.** Urine was the sample of choice for measuring bone collagen degradation. Urinary hydroxyproline analysis was replaced by more sensitive and specific crosslinks (DPD, PYD) and telopeptide (CTX, NTX) assays. Urinary measurements need to be corrected for creatinine excretion to adjust for effects of urinary concentration or dilution. Including a second analyte, with its analytical variation, adds to the uncertainty of the result. Serum and urine telopeptide assays have been compared in several studies; correlation coefficients varied from 0.6 to 0.9. Kidneys are involved in degradation of crosslinked peptides; as a result, 40% of total crosslinks in the urine are free. The mean fractional excretion of NTX (0.22) is lower than that of CTX (0.44), indicating renal degradation is greater for the former.

During antiresorptive treatment, urinary telopeptides may overestimate the decrease in bone resorption because the renal metabolism of these peptides can change. The response to antiresorptive therapy is generally greatest when measured with telopeptide assays, intermediate with total DPD, and lowest with free DPD. Serum or plasma assays have replaced urine assays in many countries.

**Reference intervals.** Concentrations of collagen crosslinks are influenced by age and gender. Concentrations are markedly higher in children, with highest concentrations observed during early infancy and adolescence, which are periods of rapid bone growth. In adults, concentrations of collagen crosslinks are relatively constant between 30 and 45 years, increasing significantly after menopause. Age-related increases have been reported in men.

*Tartrate-resistant acid phosphatase 5b (TRACP5b).* Osteoclasts secrete **tartrate-resistant acid phosphatase 5b (TRACP5b)** (see Fig. 39.2) during bone resorption and it is used to assess osteoclast number. Osteoclast number can be increased in bone disorders and is decreased by antiresorptive treatment. Early methods failed to distinguish between two isoforms: TRACP5b produced by the osteoclasts, and TRACP5a produced by inflammatory macrophages and dendritic cells. Isoform 5b is a dimer, 5a is a monomer; 10% of TRACP circulates in an enzymatically active form, the remaining 90% present as inactive fragments.

In a kinetic method, TRACP5b activity is estimated by subtracting tartrate-resistant fluoride-resistant acid phosphatase activity from total activity. Immunoassays are available for TRACP5b but not be available in the United States.

**Specimen requirements.** The preferred sample is serum. Diurnal variation is minor, indicating that the half-life of TRACP5b is longer than those of the other markers of bone resorption. TRACP5b is unstable on storage; it can be stored for up to 8 h at room temperature and up to 3 days at 4°C.

Long-term samples must be stored at −80°C. Six months' storage at −20°C reduces activity by 40%.

**Clinical significance.** In response to alendronate, TRACP5b decreased by a mean (SE) of 39% (4%), compared with 49% (4%) to 69% (5%) for urinary telopeptides (CTX and NTX), and 75% (8%) for serum/plasma CTX. Boys aged 13–17 years have higher concentrations than girls in the same age group.

**Reference interval.** An immunoassay for TRACP5b has upper limits of reference intervals of 4.2 U/L for women and 4.8 U/L for men.

## Preanalytical and Analytical Variables of Bone Turnover Marker

Controllable sources of preanalytical variability include sampling time, sample preservation, and food intake. Most bone markers have a diurnal rhythm with a peak in the early morning hours (4:00 to 8:00 a.m.) and nadir in the afternoon/evening (1:00 to 11:00 p.m.). The amplitude of this variation is greatest for resorption markers, with nadir values averaging 70% of peak values. Specimens should be collected at a standardized time of day to minimize the impact of diurnal variability. For urinary markers, collection of the second morning void is recommended.

Urinary resorption markers are usually normalized by dividing by the urinary creatinine concentration. Variability (within- and between-method) in creatinine measurements, within-subject variability in urinary creatinine, and its dependence on muscle mass contribute to the variability of urinary markers. Within-individual variability of urine markers is higher (15%–60%) than that of plasma markers (5%–10%). Bone ALP and TRACP5b do not demonstrate much diurnal variation because of their long half-lives. Food intake affects CTX concentration. The diurnal variation of plasma CTX is ±40% around the 24 h mean; fasting reduces circadian variation. Exercise can acutely increase the concentration of CTX. With other bone markers, the clinical impact of feeding versus fasting is small. The collection of samples in the fasting and resting state is standard practice.

## Metabolic Bone Diseases

Metabolic bone disease results from a partial uncoupling or imbalance between bone resorption and formation. Decreased bone mass, or **osteopenia**, is more common than increases in bone mass. The most prevalent metabolic bone diseases are osteoporosis, osteomalacia/rickets, and renal osteodystrophy. Osteoporosis is characterized by loss of bone mass, microarchitectural deterioration of bone tissue and increased risk of fracture. Rickets and osteomalacia are characterized by the defective mineralization of the bone matrix. Renal osteodystrophy is a complex condition that develops in response to abnormalities of the endocrine and excretory functions of the kidneys.

## Osteoporosis

Osteoporosis results in over 1.5 million fractures each year. It is associated with increased risk for vertebral, hip, and distal forearm fractures. At age 50, women have a lifetime fracture risk (at any of these sites) of 40%. Men have a lifetime fracture risk one-third that of women. Trabecular bone turns over at five to seven times the rate of cortical bone and so fractures of bones that are predominantly trabecular (vertebrae and distal forearm) occur earlier in life. One-third of women older than 65 years suffer vertebral crush fracture, which can occur acutely and result in disabling pain and discomfort. Long-term complications include immobility and loss of height, protuberant abdomen, hiatus hernia, chronic constipation, urinary incontinence, and loss of self-esteem. Up to 50% of vertebral fractures may be clinically silent when they occur, only to manifest later as an incidental finding on x-ray.

Fractures of cortical bone (proximal femur or hip) occur later in life. For women, the lifetime risk of hip fracture is 15% and for men 3%. The mortality rate accompanying hip fracture may be as high as 20% in the 6 months following fracture. Mortality is higher in men than women; it increases with age and is higher for those with coexisting illness and poor pre-fracture functional status. Twenty-five percent of survivors are confined to long-term care in nursing homes.

Peak bone mass is attained by 30 years and decreases slowly after 40 years in both men and women. Bone mass attained during growth is an important determinant of osteoporosis. Exercise and adequate nutrition play important roles in attaining and maintaining skeletal mass. During early adult life, bone formation is coupled with bone resorption so that bone mass remains stable. Aging is a major risk factor for bone loss. After 40 years, bone resorption exceeds bone formation, so that 0.5% of the skeletal mass is lost per year. In women, the decrease in sex steroids at menopause accelerates bone loss to 2% to 3% per year. Osteoporosis is commonly encountered in postmenopausal women. Advanced age, female gender, sex steroid deficiency, a family history of osteoporosis, alcohol abuse, smoking, and chronic disease are all risk factors. After decreased bone mass is documented by bone mass measurements, the diagnostic workup is directed at determining the cause, which could be due to endocrine or inflammatory conditions, malabsorption, and drugs, among others.

Bone markers can assess bone turnover in patients with osteoporosis, the rate of bone turnover is considered an important determinant of bone fragility in postmenopausal women. Markers for both bone resorption and bone formation can be useful in monitoring effects of antiresorptive therapy. The International Osteoporosis Foundation, National Bone Health Alliance and the International Federation of Clinical Chemistry and Laboratory Medicine recommend one formation marker (serum PINP) and one resorption marker (plasma CTX) be used as reference markers. High calcium intake (1000–1500 mg/day), adequate vitamin D (400–800 IU/day), sufficient protein intake, and a regular exercise program are helpful in maintaining bone mass and preventing osteoporosis. In secondary osteoporosis, treatment is directed at the underlying condition. Most therapies for postmenopausal osteoporosis are directed at decreasing osteoclast bone resorption.

## Osteomalacia and Rickets

Osteomalacia in adults and rickets in children are caused by a mineralization defect that occurs during bone formation, resulting in an increase in osteoid. Osteomalacia or rickets are due to either vitamin D deficiency or phosphate depletion.

Despite supplementation in some countries, of milk, bread, and some cereals with vitamin D, vitamin D insufficiency is common in North America and Europe. Breastfed infants, the elderly, strict vegetarians, and individuals with darker skin pigmentation are at increased risk. Clinical osteomalacia is uncommon. Mild to moderate vitamin D deficiency may be associated with reduced muscle strength, impaired physical performance, and falls—all of which are factors that contribute to osteoporotic fracture. Vitamin D deficiency may develop in cases of malabsorption.

Vitamin D-dependent rickets type I is an inherited defect in 25(OH)D-1$\alpha$-hydroxylase that causes impaired formation of 1,25(OH)$_2$D. The disease is manifested in infancy and can be treated with 1,25(OH)$_2$D. Vitamin D-dependent rickets type II is an inherited disorder that is characterized by high plasma concentrations of 1,25(OH)$_2$D caused by resistance to 1,25(OH)$_2$D, secondary to defects in the 1,25(OH)$_2$D receptor.

Osteomalacia and rickets may occur as the result of phosphate depletion. In developing countries, dietary calcium deprivation may lead to rickets, without vitamin D or phosphate deficiency. Clinical manifestations of rickets and osteomalacia are a consequence of the defect in mineralization. In adults, bone pain is the most common symptom, stress fractures and frank skeletal fractures occur.

Vitamin D deficiency is diagnosed by measuring serum 25(OH)D (see Table 39.2). Other findings in rickets and osteomalacia include increased ALP due to increased osteoblast activity associated with producing unmineralized osteoid. Treatment of rickets and osteomalacia is dictated by the cause. Nutritional rickets and osteomalacia are healed by treatment with physiologic doses of vitamin D, whereas higher doses may be required in malabsorption.

## Disorders of Bone and Mineral in Chronic Kidney Disease (Renal Osteodystrophy)

CKD is associated with a multitude of disorders of bone and mineral metabolism. Renal bone diseases include both high-turnover bone disease (osteitis fibrosa or 2° HPT) and low-turnover bone disease (osteomalacia and adynamic bone disease [ABD]). Quantitative histomorphometric analysis of bone biopsies, measurement of bone formation by double tetracycline labeling, and special stains are often necessary for correct diagnosis of patients with osteitis fibrosa, osteomalacia, ABD, and mixed bone disease of renal osteodystrophy.

Osteitis fibrosa (hyperparathyroid bone disease) is the most common high-turnover disease. This disorder is caused by high concentrations of serum PTH, which is a consequence of the hypocalcemia associated with hyperphosphatemia and 1,25(OH)$_2$D deficiency. Low-turnover bone diseases include osteomalacia and adynamic (*aplastic*) bone disease. Osteomalacia and ABD are distinguished by the extent of unmineralized bone matrix. Osteomalacia in chronic renal failure may reflect vitamin D deficiency caused by decreased renal synthesis of $1,25(OH)_2D$.

Bone pain is the most common complaint of patients with renal osteodystrophy. The weight-bearing bones are the sites of greatest discomfort, with leg, hip, and back pain being common. The central role of PTH in guiding therapy requires that the PTH assay used can be relied on to measure only the active hormone. This is not true for any of the assays available, and kidney disease leads to accumulation of inactive PTH fragments above concentrations seen in healthy individuals. Treatment guidelines take this into account, but inconsistencies among assays can lead to situations in which opposite therapeutic decisions could be made for a single patient, depending on the assay used.

Biochemical findings in CKD include hyperphosphatemia and hypocalcemia (see Chapter 35) with an increased immunoreactive PTH and a decreased $1,25(OH)_2D$. ALP is increased in patients with hyperparathyroidism or osteomalacia. Because magnesium is cleared by the kidney, modest increases in plasma concentration (2–4 mg/dL [0.08–0.16 mmol/L]) are common.

Early management of CKD calls for dietary restriction of phosphate and administration of phosphate-binding agents. Calcium supplements are also used. Administration of $1,25(OH)_2D$ or other active forms of vitamin D enhances intestinal calcium absorption and may act directly on the parathyroid glands to reduce PTH secretion. Ultimately dialysis or renal transplantation may be necessary.

### Paget Disease of Bone

Paget disease of bone (PDB) is a localized disease of bone characterized by osteoclastic bone resorption, followed by replacement of bone in a chaotic fashion. It is most common in Northern Europe, North America, Australia, and New Zealand in persons of Anglo-Saxon descent; prevalence may be up to 5% among people older than 40 years. It is uncommon in Asia, Africa, and Scandinavia. A family history of PDB is reported by 20%–50% of patients. Environmental factors, especially a possible paramyxovirus infection (measles, canine distemper, respiratory syncytial), may play a role in causation. PDB may affect one bone (monostotic) or several bones (polyostotic). Signs and symptoms depend on which skeletal site is affected; the skull, femur, pelvis, and vertebrae are common sites. The disease is often diagnosed from radiographs or laboratory tests (total ALP) performed for another reason. Advanced disease can produce deformities such as skull enlargement and anterior bowing of the weight-bearing bones (femur and tibia).

Increases in biochemical markers of bone resorption reflect the osteoclastic nature of the disease. Therapy is directed at decreasing osteoclastic bone resorption. Patients may require surgery for skeletal deformity that limits mobility, or for arthritic changes, fractures, or nerve compression.

### Osteogenesis Imperfecta

Osteogenesis imperfecta (OI), often termed "brittle bone disease," is a heterogeneous group of inherited connective tissue disorders that share similar skeletal abnormalities resulting in low bone mass, minimal trauma fractures, and subsequent bone deformity. In its most severe form, it can be lethal in fetal life and in neonates. Biochemical and molecular studies have identified that milder forms of OI are caused by quantitative defects in type 1 collagen and that more severe types are caused by structural defects in either of the two chains that form the heterotrimer. There is a spectrum of signs and symptoms including frontal bossing of the skull, bluish sclera, yellowish teeth, barrel chest/pectus excavatum, joint laxity, vertebral compression, and growth retardation. Recurrent fractures with minimal trauma may lead to suspicion of child abuse. When a diagnosis is in doubt, biochemical studies of collagen expressed by cultured cells, DNA sequencing of type 1 collagen, and genetic expression plus gene sequencing studies may be of value in confirming the diagnosis.

### Involvement of Bone in Malignancies

Bone metastases are the most common skeletal complication of malignancy, occurring in up to 70% of patients with advanced breast or prostate cancer, and in 15%–30% of patients with carcinoma of lung, colon, stomach, bladder, uterus, rectum, thyroid, or kidney. Metastases can have a markedly osteolytic or osteoblastic character, but often they are mixed. Patients with breast cancer have predominantly osteolytic lesions, but 5%–20% of metastases have an osteoblastic nature. Metastases of prostate cancer are mainly osteoblastic. In most carcinoma metastases, both bone degradation and formation take place and both biochemical markers of bone formation and resorption are valuable in assessing the presence of bone metastasis.

## REVIEW QUESTIONS

1. Which of the following cells is the main producer of RANKL in bone?
   a. Osteoclast
   b. Osteoblast
   c. Osteocyte
   d. Bone lining cell
   e. Chondrocyte

2. Where is the major site of regulation of magnesium excretion in the kidney?
   a. Glomerulus
   b. Proximal convoluted tubule (PCT)
   c. Cortical collecting duct (CCD)
   d. Distal convoluted tubule (DCT)
   e. Thick ascending limb of the Loop of Henle

3. When is measurement of parathyroid hormone-related peptide of greatest clinical value?
   a. In the differential diagnosis of hypocalcemia
   b. In pregnancy
   c. In patients with hypercalcemia thought to be caused by a tumor but with no obvious clear diagnosis of malignancy
   d. In chronic kidney disease
   e. In patients suspected to have primary hyperparathyroidism

4. Which of the following is the most appropriate use of a bone turnover marker?
   a. Monitoring a metabolic bone disease treatment response
   b. Diagnosis of osteoporosis
   c. Diagnosis of osteomalacia
   d. Assessment for calcium supplementation

   e. Indications for parathyroidectomy

5. Which of the following biochemical tests are of diagnostic value in Paget disease of bone?
   a. Parathyroid hormone
   b. Fibroblast growth factor 23
   c. Alkaline phosphatase
   d. 25 hydroxyvitamin D
   e. Acid phosphatase

6. What can cause a falsely high 25-hydroxyvitamin D measurement in many immunoassays?
   a. Hypercalcemia
   b. Li heparin contamination
   c. Ingestion of magnesium sulfate
   d. High concentration of the 3-epimer of 25OHD in the sample
   e. High concentration of 24,25-dihydroxyvitamin D in the sample

## SUGGESTED READINGS

Bauer DC. Clinical use of bone turnover markers. *JAMA*. 2019;322:569–570.

Bilezikian JP, Brandi ML, Eastell R, et al. Guidelines for the management of asymptomatic primary hyperparathyroidism: summary statement from the Fourth International Workshop. *J Clin Endocrinol Metab*. 2014;99:3561–3569.

Compston J, Cooper A, Cooper C, et al. UK clinical guideline for the prevention and treatment of osteoporosis. *Arch Osteoporos*. 2017;12:43.

Compton JT, Lee FY. A review of osteocyte function and the emerging importance of sclerostin. *J Bone Joint Surg Am*. 2014;96:1659–1668.

Cundy T. Paget's disease of bone. *Metabolism*. 2018;80:5–14.

Eastell R, Pigott T, Gossiel F, Naylor KE, Walsh JS, Peel NFA. Diagnosis of endocrine disease: bone turnover markers: are they clinically useful? *Eur J Endocrinol*. 2018;178:R19–R31.

Fraser WD. Bone and mineral metabolism. In: Rifai N, Horvath AR, Wittwer CT, eds. *Tietz Textbook of Clinical Chemistry and Molecular Diagnostics*. 6th ed. St. Louis: Elsevier Saunders; 2018:1422–1491.

Fraser WD. Hyperparathyroidism. *Lancet*. 2009;374:145–158.

Fukumoto S. FGF23 and bone and mineral metabolism. *Handb Exp Pharmacol*. 2020;262:281–308.

Glendenning P, Chubb SAP, Vasikaran S. Clinical utility of bone turnover markers in the management of common metabolic bone diseases in adults. *Clin Chim Acta*. 2018;481:161–170.

Goltzman D. Physiology of parathyroid hormone. *Endocrinol Metab Clin North Am*. 2018;47:743–758.

Gonciulea AR, Jan De Beur SM. Fibroblast growth factor 23-mediated bone disease. *Endocrinol Metab Clin North Am*. 2017;46:19–39.

KDIGO Clinical Practice Guideline for the Diagnosis, Evaluation, Prevention, and Treatment of Chronic Kidney Disease: Mineral and Bone Disorder (CKD-MBD). Kidney disease: Improving global outcomes (KDIGO) CKD-MBD Work Group. *Kidney Int*. 2009;113:S1–S130.

Ketteler M, Block GA, Evenepoel P, et al. Executive summary of the 2017 KDIGO Chronic Kidney Disease-Mineral and Bone Disorder (CKD-MBD) Guideline Update: what's changed and why it matters. *Kidney Int*. 2017;92:26–36.

Marini JC, Forlino A, Bächinger HP, et al. Osteogenesis imperfecta. *Nat Rev Dis Primers*. 2017;18:17052.

Pludowski P, Holick MF, Grant WB, et al. Vitamin D supplementation guidelines. *J Steroid Biochem Mol Biol*. 2018;175:125–135.

Song L. Calcium and bone metabolism indices. *Adv Clin Chem*. 2017;82:1–46.

Sturgeon CM, Sprague S, Almond A, et al. Perspective and priorities for improvement of parathyroid hormone (PTH) measurement. A view from the IFCC Working Group for PTH. *Clin Chim Acta*. 2017;467:42–47.

Szulc P, Naylor K, Hoyle NR, Eastell R, Leary ET. Use of CTX-I and PINP as bone turnover markers: National Bone Health Alliance recommendations to standardize sample handling and patient preparation to reduce pre-analytical variability. National Bone Health Alliance Bone Turnover Marker Project. *Osteoporos Int*. 2017;28:2541–2556.

Thode J, Juul-Jorgensen B, Bhatia HM, et al. Comparison of serum total calcium, albumin-corrected total calcium, and ionized calcium in 1213 patients with suspected calcium disorders. *Scand J Clin Lab Invest*. 1989;49:217–223.

# Disorders of the Pituitary Gland

*Daniel T. Holmes and Roger L. Bertholf**

## OBJECTIVES

1. Describe the anterior pituitary hormones and their releasing/inhibiting factors.
2. Discuss the levels of control of the anterior pituitary hormones including the long and short feedback loops.
3. Be familiar with the critical role of pulsatility in the release of hypothalamic-releasing hormones.
4. Discuss the factors that contribute to variations in reference intervals for anterior pituitary hormones.
5. Describe the physiologic effects of hormones secreted by the anterior pituitary gland.
6. Understand the complex interplay between growth hormone and insulin-like growth factor 1 (IGF-1).
7. List the main causes of hyperprolactinemia.
8. Be aware of macroprolactinemia as a common cause of elevated plasma prolactin.
9. Describe the role of luteinizing hormone (LH) and follicle-stimulating hormone (FSH) in gonadal steroid synthesis and ovulation.
10. State the effects of increased and decreased anterior pituitary hormone secretion and list the laboratory tests used to assess hypersecretion and hypopituitarism.
11. With respect to the posterior pituitary, understand the role of antidiuretic hormone (ADH) and its physiologic control.
12. Discuss the pathophysiology of diabetes insipidus and the syndrome of inappropriate antidiuretic hormone (SIADH).

## KEY WORDS AND DEFINITIONS

**Acid-labile subunit (ALS)** IGF-1 and IGF-2 circulate together with insulin-like growth factor binding protein-3 (IGFBP-3) and the acid-labile subunit (ALS) to form a 150-kDa trimeric protein complex.

**Acromegaly** A chronic disease of adults caused by hypersecretion of pituitary growth hormone, characterized by a constellation of endocrine, soft-tissue, and bony pathologies.

**Adrenocorticotropic hormone (ACTH)** A 39-amino-acid peptide hormone secreted by the anterior pituitary that stimulates the adrenal cortex to secrete cortisol.

**Antidiuretic hormone (ADH)** A 9-amino-acid peptide hormone synthesized in the hypothalamus but stored and released from the posterior pituitary lobe; also known as vasopressin.

**Corticotropin-releasing hormone (CRH)** A 41-amino-acid neuropeptide released by the hypothalamus that stimulates the release of ACTH by the anterior pituitary.

**Diabetes insipidus** Failure of the kidney tubules to reabsorb sufficient water; is caused by either a deficiency of ADH or defective receptor action.

**Follicle-stimulating hormone (FSH)** A glycoprotein hormone secreted by the anterior pituitary. In women, FSH stimulates the growth and maturation of ovarian follicles (eggs), stimulates estrogen secretion, and promotes endometrial changes. In males, FSH stimulates the Sertoli cells; in this way, spermatogenesis is supported.

**Gigantism** Excessive growth is caused by hypersecretion of pituitary growth hormone before the bony epiphyses have fused.

**Growth hormone (GH)** A polypeptide of 191 amino acids produced by the anterior pituitary affecting carbohydrate, lipid, and protein metabolism. GH regulates the secretion of insulin-like growth factor I (IGF-1).

**Insulin-like growth factors (IGFs)** These are members of the insulin-related peptide family; they include insulin and relaxin. Proinsulin, IGF-1, IGF-2, and relaxin are all composed of two domains joined by a connecting domain. In children, IGF-1 secretion is a major determinant of normal linear growth.

**Insulin-like growth factor binding proteins (IGFBPs)** IGFBPs have a very high affinity for IGFs and function as inhibitors of IGF action. IGFBPs have a higher affinity for IGFs than do the IGF receptors.

**Luteinizing hormone (LH)** A glycoprotein gonadotropic hormone secreted by the anterior pituitary that acts with FSH to promote ovulation and progesterone production. In males, LH stimulates testosterone secretion.

**Oxytocin** A nonapeptide hormone is synthesized in the hypothalamus and stored in the posterior lobe of the pituitary. It induces smooth muscle contraction in the uterus and mammary glands.

**Polydipsia** Chronic excessive intake of water, as seen in diabetes mellitus or diabetes insipidus.

*The authors gratefully acknowledge the contributions of Neil S. Harris, William E. Winter, and Ann McCormack to previous versions of this chapter.

**Polyuria** The passage of a large volume of urine in a given period of time, characteristic of diabetes mellitus and diabetes insipidus.

**Pro-opiomelanocortin (POMC)** This is the precursor 267-amino-acid precursor of ACTH as well as the melanocyte-stimulating hormones and beta-endorphin.

**Prolactin (PRL)** A lactogenic hormone synthesized by the anterior pituitary.

**Syndrome of inappropriate antidiuretic hormone (SIADH)** A condition where inappropriately excessive ADH secretion produces dilutional hyponatremia with an elevated urine osmolality.

**Thyroid-stimulating hormone (TSH)** A glycoprotein hormone synthesized by the anterior pituitary that sustains, stimulates, and promotes the growth and hormonal secretion of the thyroid gland; also called thyrotropin.

**Thyrotropin-releasing hormone (TRH)** A tripeptide produced by the hypothalamus that stimulates the release of TSH from the anterior pituitary.

**Vasopressin** See ADH or antidiuretic hormone.

## BACKGROUND

The anterior and posterior lobes of the pituitary gland control processes vital for survival of the individual and the species.

## CONTENT

This chapter focuses on disorders of the anterior and posterior pituitary that produce deficient or excess hormone activity.

The hypophysis is composed of the adenohypophysis (the anterior lobe of the pituitary; ≈75% of the mass of the pituitary) and the neurohypophysis (the posterior lobe of the pituitary, ≈25% of the mass of the pituitary) (Fig. 40.1).

The biology of the adenohypophysis is distinctly different from that of the neurohypophysis; the adenohypophysis is controlled by the hypothalamus via releasing or inhibiting hormones, whereas the cell bodies of the neurohypophysis are anatomically located in hypothalamic nuclei, with **oxytocin** or antidiuretic hormone (ADH) reaching the neurohypophysis through nerve axons.

The roles of the various hormones secreted by the pituitary are exceedingly diverse and include regulation of (1) the body's response to stress (**adrenocorticotropic hormone [ACTH]** and **growth hormone [GH]**), (2) the metabolic rate (**thyroid-stimulating hormone [TSH]**), (3) growth (TSH and GH), (4) reproduction (**luteinizing hormone [LH]** and **follicle-stimulating hormone [FSH]**), (5) nourishment for the newborn and infant (prolactin), (6) parturition and milk letdown during breastfeeding (oxytocin), and (7) fluid balance and blood pressure regulation in states of stress (antidiuretic hormone [ADH] and cortisol).

## ANATOMY

The pituitary is located at the base of the brain and is protected by the bony sella turcica. Direct delivery of hypothalamic regulatory hormones to the adenohypophysis occurs through the hypothalamic-pituitary portal system. Anterior and superior to the pituitary is the optic chiasm. These relations are clinically important because pituitary neoplasms can compress or invade these structures.

### Regulation of Function of the Adenohypophysis

The synthesis and release of the following anterior pituitary hormones are stimulated by hypothalamic-releasing hormones: ACTH, TSH, GH, LH, and FSH. **Prolactin** is the sole anterior pituitary hormone whose release is predominantly regulated through suppression. Corticotrophs secrete ACTH, thyrotrophs secrete TSH, somatotrophs secrete GH, gonadotrophs secrete both LH and FSH, and lactotrophs secrete prolactin. Except for LH and FSH, each hormone is normally produced by a unique cell type. The molecular composition of the anterior pituitary hormones is summarized in Table 40.1.

Multiple levels of control of the hypothalamic-pituitary-end organ-hormone axis are known (Fig. 40.2). Except for prolactin and LH at the midpoint of the menstrual cycle, negative feedback controls secretion of the adenohypophyseal hormones. The long feedback loop involves suppression of the hypothalamic-releasing hormones and the anterior pituitary trophic hormones by the hormonal

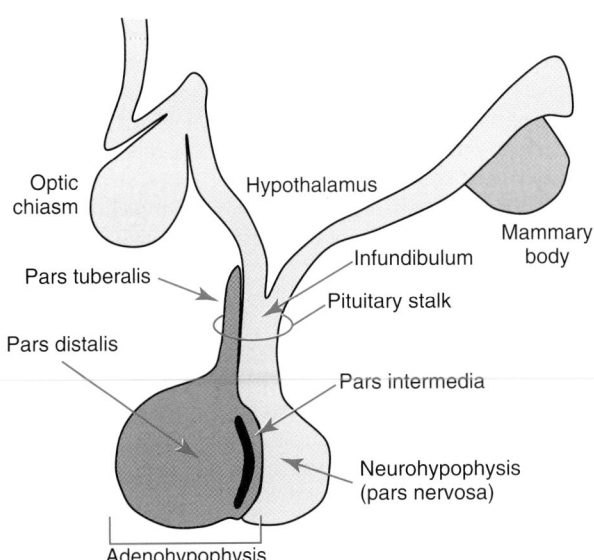

**Fig. 40.1** The hypophysis (pituitary gland) is composed of the adenohypophysis (the anterior lobe of the pituitary) and the neurohypophysis (the posterior lobe of the pituitary; pars nervosa). The adenohypophysis has three parts: the pars distalis, where most of the hormone-producing cells are located; the pars tuberalis, which is part of the pituitary stalk; and the pars intermedia.

## TABLE 40.1  Hypothalamic-Releasing or Hypothalamic-Inhibiting Hormones, Their Target Cells, and the Hormone That Is Regulated

| Hypothalamic Hormone/ Abbreviation | Amino Acids | Anterior Pituitary Target Cell | Hormone Regulated | Amino Acids | MW (kDa) |
|---|---|---|---|---|---|
| Corticotropin-releasing hormone | 41 | Corticotroph | ACTH | 39 | 4.5 |
| Thyrotropin-releasing hormone | 3 | Thyrotroph | TSH[a] | α: 92 | 28 |
| | | | | β: 118 | |
| Growth hormone–releasing hormone | 44 | Somatotroph | GH[c] | 191 | 22 |
| Somatotropin release–inhibiting hormone[b] (SRIH) | 14 | Somatotroph | GH[c] | 191 | 22 |
| Gonadotropin-releasing hormone | 10 | Gonadotroph | LH[a] | α: 92 | 32 |
| | | | | β: 121 | |
| | | | FSH[a] | α: 92 | 30 |
| | | | | β: 111 | |
| Prolactin release–inhibiting hormone | NA[d] | Lactotroph | Prolactin | 199 | 22 |

[a]All α-glycoprotein chains are identical, including the α-chain of human chorionic gonadotropin.
[b]Also known as somatostatin.
[c]Note: The 20 kDa form of GH is not shown in the table but is secreted together with the 22 kDa form of GH.
[d]Note: PRIH (dopamine) is not an amino acid per se but is a derivative of tyrosine.
*ACTH*, Adrenocorticotropic hormone; *FSH*, follicle-stimulating hormone; *GH*, growth hormone; *LH*, luteinizing hormone; *MW*, molecular weight; *TSH*, thyroid-stimulating hormone.

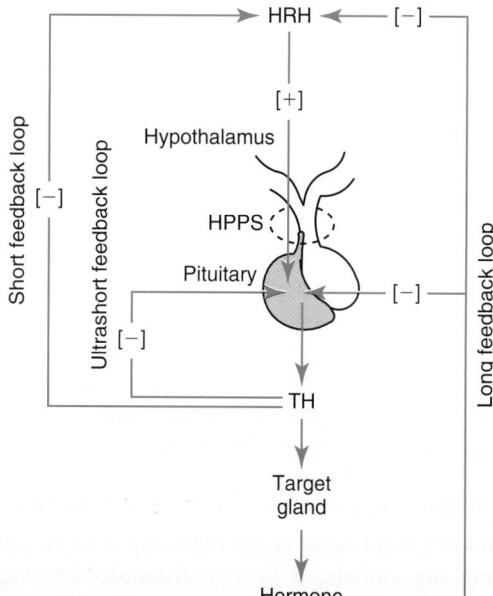

Fig. 40.2 Many anterior pituitary trophic hormones (e.g., adrenocorticotropic hormone, thyroid-stimulating hormone, growth hormone, luteinizing hormone, follicle-stimulating hormone) are regulated by hypothalamic releasing hormones *(HRHs)*. Releasing hormones secreted by the hypothalamus reach the pituitary via the hypothalamic-pituitary portal system *(HPPS)*. Long feedback loops involve negative feedback of the target cell hormone at the pituitary gland and hypothalamus. The short feedback loop involves the anterior pituitary trophic hormone feeding back at the hypothalamus, whereas the ultrashort feedback loop involves the anterior pituitary hormone feeding back at the anterior pituitary. *[+]*, Stimulation; *[–]*, suppression; *TH*, trophic hormone.

product of the target tissue. The major site of negative feedback for cortisol (regulated by ACTH), insulin-like growth factor-I (IGF-1; regulated by GH), and sex steroids and inhibins (regulated by LH and FSH) is the hypothalamus.

In contrast, for thyroid hormone (regulated by TSH), the major site of negative feedback is the anterior pituitary. Retrograde flow from the pituitary to the hypothalamus via the portal system permits the existence of short negative feedback loops in which pituitary hormones suppress the secretion of hypothalamic-releasing hormones. Ultrashort feedback loops also exist in which pituitary hormones inhibit their own secretion.

### AT A GLANCE

1. The pituitary is a master gland for many vital endocrine functions regulating growth (GH), thyroid function (thyrotropin), reproduction (LH, FSH, and prolactin), stress responses (ACTH), parturition (oxytocin), and water balance (antidiuretic hormone [ADH]).
2. The hypothalamus regulates pituitary hormone release or is the site of synthesis of the posterior pituitary hormones.

### POINTS TO REMEMBER

1. Most anterior pituitary hormones are predominantly regulated by stimulatory hypothalamic hormones. The exception is prolactin, which is regulated by suppression.
2. The pulsatility of release of hypothalamic-releasing hormones can regulate the release of anterior pituitary hormones such as LH and FSH.
3. Reference intervals may depend on the time of the day at which a measurement is obtained, the sex of the subject, their age and/or Tanner stage, and in the case of gonadotropin and sex steroid concentrations in reproductive-age women, the stage of the menstrual cycle.

## TABLE 40.2  Hypothalamic-Pituitary-End Organ Physiology

| Hypothalamic Hormone | Anterior Pituitary Hormone | Target Organ/Tissue | Target Hormone |
| --- | --- | --- | --- |
| CRH | ACTH | Adrenal cortex: zona fasciculata and zona reticularis | Cortisol |
| TRH | TSH | Thyroid follicular cell | Thyroxine ($T_4$) and 3,5,3′-triiodothyronine ($T_3$) |
| GHRH and SRIH | GH | Liver and many tissues of the body | IGF-1, IGFBP-3, and ALS |
| GnRH | LH, FSH | Gonad | Sex steroids and inhibins |
| PRIH | Prolactin | Breast | Not applicable |

*ACTH*, Adrenocorticotropic hormone; *ALS*, acid-labile subunit; *CRH*, corticotropin-releasing hormone; *FSH*, follicle-stimulating hormone; *GH*, growth hormone; *GHRH*, growth hormone–releasing hormone; *GnRH*, gonadotropin-releasing hormone; *IGFBP-3*, IGF binding protein-3; *IGF-1*, insulin-like growth factor-1; *LH*, luteinizing hormone; *MW*, molecular weight; *PRIH*, prolactin release–inhibiting hormone; *SRIH*, somatotropin release–inhibiting hormone; *TRH*, thyrotropin-releasing hormone; *TSH*, thyroid-stimulating hormone.

## HYPOTHALAMIC REGULATION

Hormones released by the hypothalamus regulating the anterior pituitary hormones are listed in Table 40.2. The secretion of corticotropin-releasing hormone (CRH) is stimulated by systemic physiologic stress. Physiologically, stress, inflammation, and hypoglycemia stimulate ACTH release. The energy state and temperature of the organism influence the secretion of thyrotropin-releasing hormone (TRH). Acute inflammatory cytokines such as interleukin (IL)-1β, IL-6, and tumor necrosis factor (TNF)-α stimulate ACTH release. Stimulators of GH–releasing hormone (GHRH) release include dopamine- and galanin-secreting neurons and brain stem neurons with catecholaminergic inputs. Physiologically, amino acids (arginine, lysine, and ornithine) and hypoglycemia stimulate GH release. In turn, the secretion of IGF-1 in response to GH is influenced by nutrition, sex steroids, thyroid hormone, and the presence or absence of chronic disease. Malnutrition, sex hormone deficiency in adolescents and adults, hypothyroidism, and chronic disease all produce GH resistance to varying extents. The regulation of gonadotropin-releasing hormone (GnRH) is complicated by the fact that GnRH must differentially control the secretion of LH and FSH, which varies greatly during the menstrual cycle. GnRH pulsatility is essential to gonadotroph responsiveness. Tonic release of GnRH will downregulate GnRH receptors on gonadotrophs, which leads to hypogonadism. The rate of pulsatility may influence the relative secretion of LH and FSH.

### Anterior Pituitary

In the anterior pituitary, (1) CRH receptors are expressed on corticotrophs, (2) TRH receptors are expressed on thyrotrophs, (3) GHRH receptors are expressed on somatotrophs, (4) GnRH receptors are expressed on gonadotrophs, and (5) prolactin-release inhibiting hormone (PRIH) receptors are expressed on lactotrophs. At pathologically high concentrations, TRH stimulates the release of LH and prolactin. Corticotrophs are stimulated by high concentrations of proinflammatory cytokines, such as IL-1, IL-6, and TNF-α.

The hormonal products of each anterior pituitary target cell (if applicable) are listed in Table 40.1 together with a summary of each system. Deficiency of an individual pituitary hormone is typically called hypopituitarism, whereas deficiency of all anterior pituitary hormones is termed panhypopituitarism.

### Growth Hormone and Insulin-Like Growth Factors

Linear growth is the consequence of (1) genetic potential, (2) nutrition, (3) the presence or absence of disease, and (4) hormonal effects. Many hormones influence growth, but the most important are GH, thyroid hormone, and sex steroids. Excess glucocorticoids can impair growth in children. GH deficiency produces morbidity in adults; thus GH is essential for health throughout life.

#### Growth Hormone

Two circulating forms of GH are present: a 22-kDa form that represents 85% to 90% of circulating GH and a 20-kDa GH that results from alternative splicing of the GH mRNA transcript. Circulating GH also exists as aggregates and oligomers. "Big GH" is a dimer of GH monomers, and "Big, big GH" is GH associated with its binding protein (GHBP). GHBP is the external domain of the GH receptor (GHR), which binds GH with high affinity and is produced by cleavage of the GHR (Fig. 40.3).

GH has both indirect and direct activity. The indirect activity of GH is mediated by IGF-1. To initiate its direct and indirect activity, GH binds to receptors (GHR) that appear to be expressed by all tissues.

#### Insulin-Like Growth Factors

Proinsulin, insulin-like growth factor (IGF)-1, IGF-2, and relaxin are all composed of two domains (A and B) joined by a connecting domain. Less than 1% of the total IGF-1 is free (the biologically active form).

Most of the circulating IGF-1 is produced by hepatocytes, but it is also produced locally throughout the body and thus acts as a paracrine and an autocrine hormone.

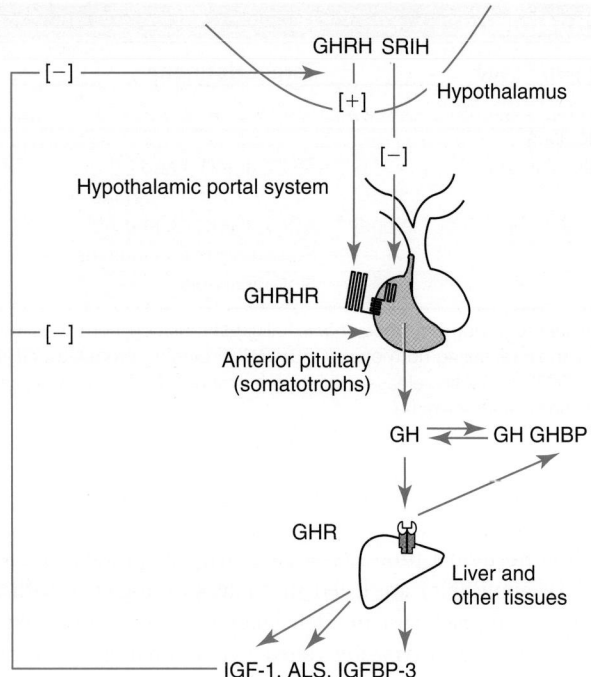

**Fig. 40.3** The hypothalamus secretes growth hormone–releasing hormone *(GHRH)* and somatotropin release–inhibiting hormone *(SRIH;* somatostatin), which regulate growth hormone *(GH)* release. The receptor for GHRH *(GHRHR)* is illustrated because mutations in this receptor can cause some forms of inherited GH deficiency. GH circulates unbound and bound to its binding protein *(GHBP)*. GHBP is the extracellular domain of the GHR, which is cleaved from the GHR and circulates in the plasma. GH releases IGF-1, IGF binding protein-3 *(IGFBP-3)*, and the **acid-labile subunit (ALS)**. IGF-1 negatively feeds back at the anterior pituitary somatotrophs and at the hypothalamus. Because transection of the pituitary stalk leads to GH deficiency, the predominant hypothalamic control of GH is stimulatory via GHRH.

Like IGF-1, IGF-2 does not normally induce hypoglycemia. However, certain tumors of mesenchymal or hepatic origin may secrete a high molecular weight and incompletely processed form of IGF-2 called "Big IGF-2" which may cause hypoglycemia. This condition is referred to as "Non-Islet-Tumor Hypoglycemia" (see Chapter 22).

### Receptors for Insulin-Like Growth Factors

Two types of receptors for IGFs have been identified: type I and type II. Structurally, the type I IGF receptor has a homology with the insulin receptor.

The type I IGF receptor binds IGF-1 with a higher affinity than IGF-2, and the affinity for insulin is lower than the affinity of the receptor for IGF-1 or IGF-2. The affinities of the insulin receptor are the opposite: insulin >>IGF-2 >IGF-1. The type II IGF receptor is structurally dissimilar from the type I IGF receptor and the insulin receptor. The type II IGF receptor is monomeric and similar to the epidermal growth factor (EGF) receptor.

### Regulation of Growth Hormone Secretion

GH ultimately stimulates the release of IGF-1, which negatively feeds back to regulate GH release via two hypothalamic

hormones: somatotropin release–inhibiting hormone (SRIH) (or somatostatin) and GH-releasing hormone (GHRH) (see Fig 40.3). Somatotrophs of the anterior pituitary gland have receptors for both hormones. Somatostatin inhibits GH release, whereas GHRH promotes the release of GH. In addition to its hypothalamic negative feedback effects, IGF-1 directly suppresses the pituitary release of GH.

Physiologically, GH secretion is episodic and pulsatile. Consequently, random measurements cannot exclude GH deficiency or confirm GH excess; between pulses, GH concentrations can be quite low and do not distinguish GH insufficiency from normal GH production. During daytime hours, the plasma concentration of GH in healthy adults remains stable and relatively low (<2 ng/mL; <2 μg/L), with several secretory spikes occurring approximately 3 hours after meals (particularly meals high in protein and arginine) and after exercise. In contrast, during the evening hours, adults and children show a marked rise in GH concentrations approximately 90 minutes after the onset of sleep, reaching a peak during the period of deepest sleep. GH is also increased by stress and hypoglycemia. Normal GH secretion requires thyroxine and age-appropriate concentrations of testosterone or estrogen.

GH is suppressed by increased blood glucose. One of the tests for GH excess measures GH after an oral glucose load (e.g., 75 g in adults and 1.75 g/kg in children); the normal response is a GH of less than 0.4 ng/mL (0.4 μg/L), using modern chemiluminescent sandwich assays for GH (Box 40.1). GH also declines with increases in free fatty acid concentrations and aging. In the presence of abnormally high concentrations of glucocorticoids, GH secretion is suppressed.

### Physiologic Actions

GH *directly* raises blood glucose by stimulating gluconeogenesis and reducing insulin sensitivity. Also, GH causes adipose tissue lipolysis, and the resulting free fatty acids provide an alternative energy source. Therefore, when glucose and free fatty acid concentrations are raised with stress—in partnership with epinephrine, glucagon, and cortisol—fuels for the fight-or-flight response are provided. GH directly stimulates the production of IGF-1, **insulin-like growth factor binding protein** (IGFBP)-3, and the ALS.

*Indirect* effects of GH are mediated through IGF-1 production, which, together with GH, is necessary for linear growth in childhood and promotes growth in soft tissue, cartilage, and bone. IGF-1 is mitogenic and antiapoptotic. GH, through IGF-1 and insulin, induces growth in a similar manner because both have protein anabolic effects and stimulate the transport of amino acids into peripheral cells. However, the respective effects of IGF-1 and insulin on glucose homeostasis oppose each other.

IGF-1 concentrations vary somewhat with gender but very strongly with age. IGF-1 rises during childhood and puberty and then shows a gradual decline throughout the remainder of life.

GH is not the only determinant of IGF-1 concentration in circulation. Therefore, a decreased IGF-1 concentration is not always synonymous with GH deficiency.

## BOX 40.1 Protocol for Glucose Suppression of Growth Hormone Test

### Rationale
Normal subjects show suppression of serum growth hormone (GH) concentrations after oral administration of glucose. Subjects with acromegaly fail to exhibit appropriate GH suppression.

### Procedure
The test should be performed after an overnight fast with the patient maintained at bed rest. After a baseline blood specimen is collected for GH and glucose measurement, a solution of 75 g of glucose is given orally (in children, 1.75 g/kg to a maximum dose of 75 g). Glucose and serum GH are measured again on specimens collected 30, 60, 90, and 120 min later.

### Interpretation
Serum GH concentrations in normal individuals fall to less than 0.4 ng/mL (0.4 µg/L) (i.e., below the lower limit of detection of the GH assay used). Subjects with acromegaly fail to show this suppression and sometimes show a paradoxical increase in GH concentration. Patients with liver disease, uremia, or heroin addiction may have false-positive results with this test (failure to suppress serum GH concentrations after oral glucose load).

## Clinical Significance

Clinically important states of GH excess or deficiency are uncommon and are often difficult to diagnose. As it pertains to GH excess, one of the diagnostic challenges is related to the pulsatility of GH release from the pituitary gland. Even when there is a net excess of GH production, at any given moment, the concentration of GH in the blood may not exceed the reference value. Conversely, when there is a net deficiency of GH, it is difficult to prove this with an isolated measurement because, even in normal subjects, GH levels are frequently undetectable. For these reasons, GH measurements are best determined as part of dynamic testing: physiologic or pharmacologic provocative stimuli are used to diagnose GH deficiency, whereas the absence of GH suppression following glucose administration is used to diagnose GH excess.

Due to its long half-life, a single measurement of IGF-1 (which can be drawn at any stage of the diagnostic process) better reflects GH IGF-1 production than random GH measurements performed outside the context of dynamic function testing. For this reason, IGF-1 is a good initial screening test for both growth hormone excess and deficiency.

## Growth Hormone Excess

Growth hormone excess results in acromegaly in adults. Much less common is pituitary gigantism, which results from GH excess in childhood. The clinical features of acromegaly involve overgrowth of the skeleton and soft tissue, producing (1) acral (extremity) enlargement, (2) organomegaly (enlarged heart and/or liver), (3) coarsening of facial features,

(4) intestinal polyposis, (5) premature cardiovascular disease, (6) increased sweating, (7) skin tags, (8) joint disease, (9) myopathy with weakness, (10) insulin resistance, (11) carpal tunnel syndrome, and other peripheral neuropathies, and often (12) diabetes mellitus. Premature cardiovascular disease is the most common cause of death from acromegaly. Gigantism is characterized by extremely tall stature in addition to the clinical features of acromegaly as pathologic GH excess occurs before epiphyseal fusion is complete.

More than 95% of cases of acromegaly result from anterior pituitary GH-secreting tumors (somatotropinomas) with the remainder of cases accounted for by pathological GHRH production from the hypothalamus or from neuroendocrine tumors arising from other organs (e.g., lung or pancreas). Somatotropinomas are usually macroadenomas (>10 mm in diameter) by the time they come to clinical attention. Approximately 5% of GH-secreting tumors are familial and caused by disorders such as multiple endocrine neoplasia type 1 syndrome, familial acromegaly, Carney syndrome, McCune-Albright syndrome, and familial isolated pituitary adenoma.

In severe or advanced cases of GH excess, the diagnosis may be established based on physical appearance alone. In less severe or early cases, the physical changes may be subtle and gradual, so a high degree of clinical suspicion is needed. In these cases, it is useful to compare the patient's current appearance to prior photographs. The reversibility of tissue changes depends largely on the duration of the disease. In addition to soft tissue changes, acromegaly may cause severe disability or death from cardiac, pulmonary, or neurologic sequelae. The most important requirement for the diagnosis of acromegaly is the demonstration of inappropriate and excessive GH secretion.

Essentially all patients with acromegaly have an abnormal GH response to oral glucose load (see Box 40.1). Patients with acromegaly typically show no change in their basal GH level or demonstrate a paradoxical increase in GH; in contrast, normal individuals show suppression of GH to less than 0.4 ng/mL (0.4 µg/L) after a 75-g oral glucose load. Serum IGF-1 is also elevated above the age-dependent reference interval in acromegaly.

## Growth Hormone Deficiency and Growth Retardation

GH deficiency is an uncommon cause of short stature with a low growth velocity. Approximately 50% of children evaluated for growth retardation have no specific organic cause; approximately 15% have an endocrine disorder, of which approximately half have GH deficiency. Children with significantly reduced height and low growth velocities with no clear explanation should be screened for GH deficiency after other endocrine disorders have been excluded.

GH deficiency in children is characterized by (1) short stature, (2) low growth velocity, (3) immature facial appearance, (4) retarded bone age on radiologic examination, and (5) increased adiposity. In cases of congenital GH deficiency, size at birth is usually normal because in utero IGF-1 does not appear to be under GH control. GH replacement therapy forms an important part of the clinical care of GH-deficient children.

The diagnosis of adult GH deficiency is difficult because of the subtle clinical presentation. However, it can occur in the setting of panhypopituitarism of any cause. Adults with GH deficiency may experience (1) reduced muscle mass, (2) increased central adiposity, (3) osteoporosis with decreased bone density, (4) an increase in fractures, (5) decreased quality of life, (6) dyslipidemia, and (7) increased risk for cardiovascular disease. Whether GH therapy is required in GH-deficient adults is controversial because of the associated expense and modest clinical benefit.

GH insufficiency can be a consequence of (1) hypothalamic disease, (2) disruption of the portal system between hypothalamic nuclei and the anterior pituitary, (3) GHRHR loss-of-function mutations, or (4) somatotroph disease. GH deficiency can occur in isolation or together with other pituitary deficiencies. Patients with isolated GH deficiency should be followed clinically for the development of other pituitary hormone deficiencies because multiple pituitary hormone deficiencies can evolve over time. In most affected children, the cause of GH deficiency is unknown (idiopathic GH deficiency). Approximately one in four children with proven GH deficiency has an organic cause of GH deficiency; half of these children will be diagnosed with a central nervous system (CNS) tumor. Biochemical stimulation testing is necessary to establish the diagnosis of GH deficiency, GH resistance, or multiple pituitary hormone deficiencies.

### Investigation of growth hormone deficiency

**Children.** A staged approach for the evaluation of GH deficiency in children is advised. Initial screening can involve one of the following tests: (1) measurement of IGF-1 (with or without IGFBP-3), or (2) GH measurement after exercise or pharmacologic stimulation. If a GH screening test is abnormal (e.g., the GH and/or IGF-1 concentration is reduced), definitive testing should be pursued. All forms of GH testing should be performed after the subject has fasted overnight.

Exercise physiologically enhances GH release. A baseline GH measurement is not required. The child exercises vigorously for approximately 20 minutes and GH is then measured. GH is also measured 20 minutes later to capture delayed GH release. Screening for GH deficiency can also be performed by measuring GH 60 to 90 minutes following clonidine, arginine, glucagon, or L-dopa administration.

If IGF-1 is within its reference interval for age and sex in children, GH deficiency is excluded. If IGF-1 is low, definitive GH testing is required. Because IGF-1 concentrations can be depressed in states other than GH deficiency, a low IGF-1 concentration does not confirm GH deficiency. IGFBP-3 is an alternative screening test for GH deficiency in children but is measured with less frequency.

GH responses to insulin-induced hypoglycemia (insulin tolerance test [ITT]) and GH responses to centrally acting pharmacologic or biologic agents are considered definitive tests. The insulin tolerance test is generally reserved for children nearing the age of adulthood because of the risks associated with the procedure and the emotional fortitude required of the patient. The stimuli are usually administered

sequentially or, less commonly, on different days. The classic diagnosis of pediatric GH deficiency requires that GH responses to two different stimuli be deficient. Stimulated GH concentrations less than 4 to 7 ng/mL (4 to 7μg/L) define GH deficiency in children. The cutoff defining GH deficiency is method-dependent and subject to interpretation by clinicians.

Of children with appropriate stature for age, approximately 80% will have a normal GH response to one stimulus and 95% will have normal GH responses to one or both of the two stimuli.

**Adults.** A history of childhood GH deficiency, CNS disease, trauma, or irradiation is an indication to test adults for GH deficiency because not all adults with childhood GH deficiency remain GH-deficient as adults. In adults, a single deficient GH response to a stimulus is diagnostic of GH deficiency if the deficiency is congenital or genetic or if multiple pituitary hormone deficiencies are due to organic disease. In adults, GH deficiency is present when stimulated GH is generally less than 3 to 5 ng/mL (3 to 5 μg/L) depending on the method of stimulation and the guidance document employed.

IGF-1 measurements in adults are often not diagnostically helpful. For reasons that are unclear, IGF-1 concentrations can be normal in GH-deficient adults. If the IGF-1 concentration is low and suspicion for GH deficiency is high, some experts would diagnose GH deficiency in the absence of GH testing in adults.

## Growth Hormone Resistance

In children with short stature and low growth velocity, if (1) IGF-1 is below the reference interval for the child's bone age, sex, and Tanner stage, (2) the random GH concentration is normal or elevated, and (3) non–GH-dependent causes of IGF-1 deficiency have been excluded, GH resistance should be considered. GH resistance is rare.

GH resistance can be congenital, resulting from loss-of-function GHR mutations or GHR signaling defects (e.g., STAT5b mutations) or from defects in the production of IGF-1 itself. Most cases of GHR deficiency display low or absent concentrations of GHBP. In acquired GH resistance, which is far more common, the IGF-1 is low (despite sufficient GH secretion) because of malnutrition, malabsorption, chronic disease, hypothyroidism, or sex hormone deficiency.

---

### POINTS TO REMEMBER

1. Secretion of GH by the pituitary gland is episodic and pulsatile, and transient elevations have been observed in normal healthy subjects.
2. A single basal or random concentration of GH provides limited diagnostic information.
3. The diagnosis of GH deficiency usually requires the use of one of a number of stimulation tests.

GH excess is typically first identified by an elevated IGF-1 level and biochemically confirmed by the failure of GH suppression after an oral glucose load.

## Prolactin

Prolactin is secreted by lactotrophs. Prolactin stimulates and sustains lactation in postpartum mammals after the mammary glands have been prepared by other hormones, including estrogens, progesterone, GH, corticosteroids, and insulin.

### Biochemistry

The hypothalamic PRIH is dopamine. Occasionally and independent of the presence or absence of disease, biologically inactive high molecular weight forms of prolactin usually caused by IgG autoantibodies bound to prolactin (termed "macroprolactin"), can cause elevations in measured prolactin concentration. Macroprolactin elevates the total prolactin concentration as a result of lower clearance. Failure to recognize macroprolactin can lead to the inappropriate diagnosis of hyperprolactinemia.

### Physiology

Prolactin is necessary for lactation after the delivery of the newborn. Prolactin is stimulated by breastfeeding, a large list of medications including a number of anti-psychotics and anti-emetics, chest wall disease, and stress. Prolactin secretion by lactotrophs is controlled predominantly through suppression by PRIH.

It is unclear if prolactin has a physiologic function in men. Postpartum, a positive feedback loop occurs between suckling and milk production. Transmitted via nerve fibers from the nipple to the CNS, suckling reduces PRIH, which increases prolactin release. The positive feedback loop of suckling, prolactin secretion, and milk production is a "stimulus secretion" reflex. However, with continued breastfeeding, prolactin concentrations decline.

### Hyperprolactinemia

Hyperprolactinemia is the most common hypothalamic-pituitary disorder encountered in clinical endocrinology. Prolactin may be elevated in women who have only subtle alterations in fertility, such as (1) anovulation with or without menstrual irregularity, (2) amenorrhea and galactorrhea, or (3) galactorrhea alone. In men, prolactin excess usually manifests as a result of low serum testosterone, with reduced libido and central weight gain. Hyperprolactinemia can also cause galactorrhea in men.

An irregular menstrual period may reveal a microadenoma (≤10 mm in diameter) in women. Elevated prolactin concentrations are observed in as many as 30% of women with the polycystic ovarian syndrome and in patients with non-functioning pituitary adenomas, which impinge on the pituitary stalk suppressing the delivery of PRIH ("stalk effect"). If a borderline elevation of prolactin is found, it is advisable to repeat the measurement on at least two other occasions, taking care to obtain a morning specimen under conditions of minimal stress to the patient Ideally, the patient should not be on any medication that could stimulate prolactin release (see later in this section). The differential diagnosis of hyperprolactinemia is extensive (Table 40.3).

### TABLE 40.3    Differential Diagnosis of Hyperprolactinemia

| | |
|---|---|
| Prolactin-producing adenoma of the pituitary | Prolactinoma<br>Combined growth hormone and prolactin-producing adenoma |
| PRIH (dopamine) deficiency | Hypothalamic disease<br>Interruption in the hypothalamic-pituitary portal system (trauma, "stalk effect" from pituitary adenoma) |
| Drugs | Antipsychotics, antiemetics, and gastroprokinetic agents having dopamine antagonist activity<br>Certain antihypertensives (verapamil, methyldopa, reserpine)<br>Antidepressants: selective serotonin reuptake inhibitors, tricyclic antidepressants, and monoamine oxidase inhibitors.<br>Opiates |
| Hormones | Estrogen, pregnancy |
| Neurogenic | Nursing (nipple stimulation)<br>Chest wall disease<br>Spinal cord injury |
| Other diseases | Hypothyroidism (pathologically elevated TRH can release prolactin)<br>Chronic renal disease<br>Cirrhosis |

*PRIH,* Prolactin release–inhibiting hormone; *TRH,* thyrotropin-releasing hormone.

The higher the prolactin concentration, the greater the likelihood that hyperprolactinemia is the result of prolactinoma. Idiopathic hyperprolactinemia is a diagnosis of exclusion. Early diagnosis of a prolactinoma is critical because therapy with oral dopamine agonists, such as bromocriptine, can reduce tumor size and control tumor progression. Surgical excision of a prolactinoma is usually considered if there is tumor growth or dopamine agonist therapy fails (the "dopamine-resistant prolactinoma"), if there is failure to quickly reverse the associated visual loss, or if the patient is intolerant to dopamine agonists.

A diagnostic challenge in the investigation of hyperprolactinemia is the presence of a pituitary incidentaloma (a radiologic image consistent with a mass that is not necessarily pathologic) in a patient with elevated prolactin that could potentially lead to inappropriate medical or surgical treatment. Unless a pituitary tumor can be demonstrated by magnetic resonance imaging (MRI), prolactin-secreting microadenoma (≤10 mm in diameter) is diagnosed by exclusion. Because half of all prolactin-secreting microadenomas are too small to be detected by imaging methods, differentiating between a small pituitary tumor, prolactin-cell hyperplasia, and idiopathic hyperprolactinemia may not be possible.

Medications that stimulate prolactin release (through PRIH suppression) are the most common cause of hyperprolactinemia in otherwise healthy individuals. When a significant elevation of prolactin is confirmed, a careful history should rule out the possibility that medications are the cause. A pregnancy test should be performed in women of reproductive age because pregnancy is a cause of hyperprolactinemia.

## Prolactin Deficiency

Prolactin is of great clinical importance in the postpartum period because it is required for lactation. However, other than the necessity of breastfeeding, prolactin deficiency in humans may not have adverse consequences.

### POINTS TO REMEMBER

1. In contrast to the measurement of other anterior pituitary hormones, prolactin can be measured in the absence of stimulation or suppression.
2. There are many causes of hyperprolactinemia that should be considered in the evaluation of hyperprolactinemia.
3. Elevations of prolactin in the absence of obvious causes or symptoms should trigger a biochemical investigation for macroprolactin.
4. The first line of treatment for prolactinomas is medical therapy through the administration of dopamine agonists.

## Adrenocorticotropic Hormone and Related Peptides

ACTH is secreted by the adenohypophysis as a derivative of pro-opiomelanocortin (POMC). ACTH acts on the adrenal cortex, stimulating its growth and the secretion of corticosteroids (specifically cortisol). ACTH production is increased during physiologic or psychologic stress.

Many variables affect the secretion of ACTH, which is both pulsatile and circadian in nature. Cortisol is the major negative feedback hormone for the inhibition of CRH and ACTH secretion. Regulation of ACTH—and a discussion of adrenal disorders including disorders of ACTH secretion—is found in Chapter 41.

## Gonadotropins (Follicle-Stimulating Hormone, Luteinizing Hormone)

LH and FSH are synthesized by gonadotrophs. Their actions have already been described. LH and FSH control the functional activity of the gonads. In males and females, gonadotropin secretion is regulated via GnRH. For more details on FSH and LH action and regulation, refer to Chapter 43.

### POINTS TO REMEMBER

1. LH and FSH are secreted from pituitary gonadotrophs in response to pulsatile GnRH.
2. FSH stimulates the growth of ovarian follicles and the secretion of estrogen (estradiol) in females and spermatogenesis in males.
3. LH in females assists in the formation of the corpus luteum and together with FSH promotes progesterone secretion; in males, LH stimulates Leydig cells to produce testosterone.

## Thyroid-Stimulating Hormone

TSH, which is synthesized in pituitary thyrotrophs, promotes the growth of thyroid follicular cells and sustains and stimulates the hormonal secretion of thyroid gland hormones 3,5,3,5′ tetraiodothyronine (thyroxine; T4) and 3,5,3-triiodothyronine (T3).

TSH binds to TSH receptors (TSHRs) located on the surfaces of thyroid follicular cells. TSH (1) stimulates the growth and vascularity of the thyroid gland, (2) stimulates the growth of thyroid follicular cells, (3) promotes thyroid hormone synthesis by increasing the uptake of iodine (via the sodium-iodide transporter), (4) promotes the organification (reduction) of iodine, (5) promotes the coupling of tyrosines, and (6) promotes the proteolytic release of stored thyroid hormone from thyroglobulin. TSH release is stimulated by TRH and suppressed by thyroid hormone (principally circulating free T4). TRH is a modified tripeptide produced by the hypothalamus. Details concerning the regulation and clinical significance of these hormones are discussed in detail in Chapter 42.

## Antidiuretic Hormone

Disorders of ADH involve excess hormone (syndrome of inappropriate ADH [SIADH]) or deficient ADH action (diabetes insipidus [DI]). DI can result from ADH deficiency, ADH resistance, or renal tubular disease; the latter two conditions are termed nephrogenic DI. Disorders of oxytocin secretion have not been described; therefore oxytocin is not discussed further in this chapter.

## Biochemistry

ADH is a nonapeptide consisting of a cyclic hexapeptide and a three-amino-acid side chain. The ADH receptor in the renal collecting ducts is termed the arginine vasopressin receptor 2 (V2 receptor). The action of ADH is to stimulate the movement of aquaporin-2 from the cytoplasm to the apical plasma membrane (Fig. 40.4). In this way ADH allows the reabsorption of water from the collecting duct. As electrolyte is not also reabsorbed, the action of ADH can be described as increasing "free water" reabsorption.

## Regulation of Antidiuretic Hormone Secretion

ADH secretion is controlled predominantly by plasma osmolality, which is sensed by osmoreceptors in the hypothalamus. Increased osmolality results in ADH release. Plasma osmolality above 280 mOsm/kg (mmol/kg) is thought to be the osmotic threshold for triggering ADH release.

In addition to the osmoreceptor mechanism of vasopressin release, physiologic regulation of ADH secretion involves a pressure–volume mechanism that is distinct from the osmotic sensor. High-pressure arterial baroreceptors of the aortic arch and carotid sinus and low-pressure volume receptors in the pulmonary venous system and atria also regulate ADH release. Therefore, ADH is secreted in response to decreased circulating blood volume or decreased blood pressure.

The thirst center is regulated by many of the same factors that determine ADH release. This center has a higher set point than the osmoreceptors and responds to osmolalities

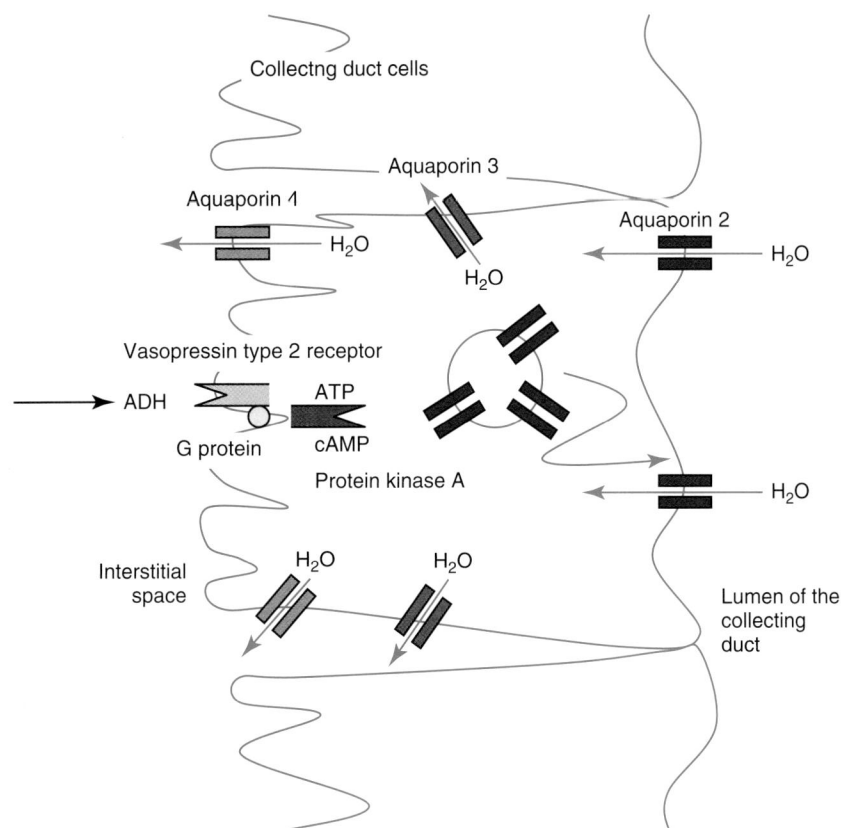

**Fig. 40.4** Vasopressin type 2 receptors on collecting duct cells bind antidiuretic hormone *(ADH)*. Through a G-protein system, adenosine triphosphate *(ATP)* is converted to cyclic adenosine 3′,5′-monophosphate *(cAMP)* via adenylate cyclase with protein kinase A activation. This leads to the translocation of aquaporin-2 water channels from an intracellular pool to the apical plasma membrane, allowing free water uptake by cells of the collecting duct. Via the basolateral plasma membrane aquaporin-3 and aquaporin-4 water channels, free water then leaves these cells.

above 290 mOsm/kg. Responses involving ADH, thirst, and renal reabsorption of sodium and water are coordinated in a complex scheme that maintains plasma osmolality in healthy individuals within a narrow interval (~285 to ~295 mOsm/kg [mmol/kg]).

## Physiologic Activity

The actions of ADH are to conserve free water (via V2 receptors) and stimulate vasoconstriction (via V1a receptors). These effects combine to maintain proper osmolality of the extracellular space (the major action of ADH) and blood pressure through the maintenance of circulating blood volume and prevention of dehydration and excessive loss of water.

ADH increases the permeability of renal collecting ducts to water, thereby increasing water reabsorption and concentrating the urine to a higher specific gravity.

## Clinical Significance

Disorders of ADH activity have been divided into hypofunction (DI) and hyperfunction (SIADH) (Fig. 40.5).

*Polyuric states and diabetes insipidus.* Exclusive of diabetes mellitus, polyuric states are divided into two main categories: (1) deficient ADH action, producing DI

(sometimes called "water diabetes"), and (2) excessive oral water intake (psychogenic polydipsia). Osmotic diuresis (e.g., secondary to hyperglycemia) may also produce polyuria and polydipsia.

In DI, polyuria results from excessive loss of water into the urine. Under normal circumstances, urine output is predominantly dependent on fluid intake. When urine output is greater than 2.5 L/day, an investigation is usually indicated. In the absence of ADH, urine output may approach 1 L/h. Increased osmolality normally stimulates thirst. Therefore, if a patient with DI has an intact thirst mechanism and access to water, excessive urinary loss of water should be matched by excessive intake of fluids. The major laboratory finding in DI is urine of low osmolality and serum sodium within the upper half of the reference interval, with a corresponding high-normal serum osmolality. If water is not available or the individual with DI is physically impaired or lacks a normal thirst mechanism, serum sodium, and osmolality rise, while urine osmolality remains relatively low, and polyuria persists. With dehydration, weight loss is acute (because of fluid loss) and patients develop progressive hypovolemic hypernatremia with attendant hypotension, tachycardia, hypovolemia/shock, and acute kidney injury; they will also deteriorate neurologically manifesting confusion, seizures, and coma.

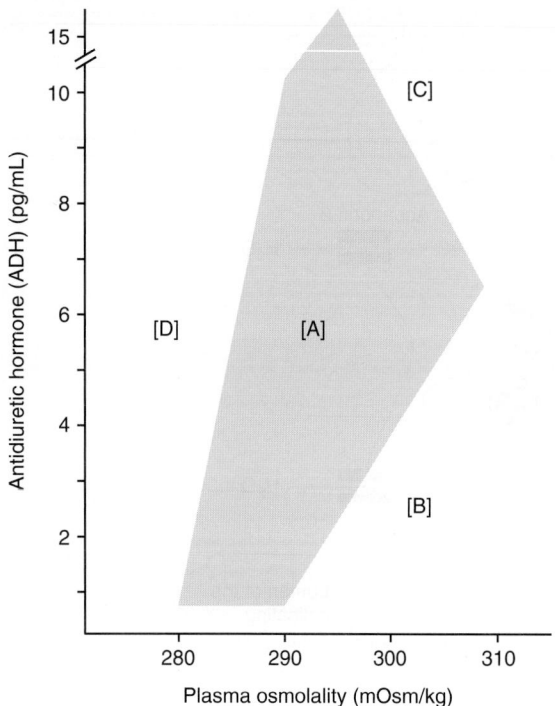

Fig. 40.5 Antidiuretic hormone (ADH) concentration versus plasma osmolality is plotted. The shaded area [A] depicts the normal physiologic relationship between ADH and plasma osmolality. Area B illustrates cases of diabetes insipidus with ADH deficiency. Area C encompasses cases of ADH resistance. Area D includes cases of syndrome of inappropriate ADH secretion (SIADH).

| TABLE 40.4 | Causes of Central Diabetes Insipidus |
|---|---|
| Congenital | Midline malformations: septo-optic dysplasia, holoprosencephaly, single central incisor, cleft lip and/or palate |
| | Malformation of the pituitary (ectopia or hypogenesis) |
| | Diabetes insipidus–diabetes mellitus–optic atrophy syndrome (Wolfram syndrome) |
| | Familial diabetes insipidus (autosomal dominant and recessive forms) |
| Acquired | Tumors (craniopharyngioma, germinoma, pinealoma, optic glioma, pituitary adenoma, metastatic tumor, leukemia) |
| | Trauma (e.g., stalk section) |
| | Infarction (e.g., septic shock, Sheehan syndrome, hypoxic injury) |
| | Infiltrative disease (sarcoidosis, hypophysitis, histiocytosis) |
| | Cysts and aneurysms |
| | Drugs (opiates, alcohol, phenytoin, alpha-adrenergic agents, etc.) |
| | Infection |
| | Increased metabolism of ADH (vasopressinase in pregnancy) |

ADH, Antidiuretic hormone.

Central DI can result from any destructive hypothalamic lesion or infundibular lesion (Table 40.4). DI resulting from such lesions can equally be termed hypothalamic, neurogenic, central, or cranial DI. When the thirst center is also abnormal, severe dehydration can occur.

In 30% of patients, central DI occurs without apparent cause. The remaining cases are associated with (1) neoplastic disease, (2) neurologic surgery, (3) head trauma, (4) ischemic or hypoxic disorders, (5) granulomatous disease, (6) infection, or (7) autoimmune disorders. DI can result from acquired or genetic tubular diseases that affect the responsiveness of renal tubules to ADH (nephrogenic DI). In the broadest sense, any form of tubular injury with impaired water reabsorption, including (1) polycystic kidney disease, (2) medullary cystic kidney, (3) chronic pyelonephritis, (4) acute tubular necrosis, (5) obstructive uropathy, (6) sickle cell nephropathy, and (7) renal amyloidosis can cause nephrogenic DI. Many drugs can cause nephrogenic DI, including (1) lithium, (2) various antimicrobials, and (3) several antineoplastic drugs. In psychogenic polydipsia (primary polydipsia), excessive water intake eventually impairs the concentrating ability of the kidney.

*Investigation of polyuria.* Assuming that diabetes mellitus is excluded, the examination of polyuric states is undertaken with measurements of plasma and urine osmolality and, if the findings are equivocal, plasma ADH concentrations. A screening test for ADH sufficiency is the measurement of the urine specific gravity in the first morning-voided urine sample where the specific gravity should be 1.010 or greater.

Failure to demonstrate an appropriate urine-specific gravity and response in a subject with a history of polyuria and polydipsia should trigger assessment of a basic metabolic panel, urinalysis, serum osmolality, and urine osmolality.

Urine osmolality less than 300 mOsm/kg (mmol/kg) combined with serum osmolality greater than 300 mOsm/kg (mmol/kg) (or with hypernatremia) is diagnostic of DI. If urine osmolality is above 600 mOsm/kg (mmol/kg), and serum osmolality is below 270 mOsm/kg (mmol/kg), DI is unlikely.

If the diagnosis of DI is unclear, a water deprivation test should be performed. Water deprivation testing should not be carried out if the subject is dehydrated at baseline or has renal insufficiency. The overnight water deprivation test is always conducted in a hospital setting because of the immediate concerns of profound hypotension and possible mortality. The water deprivation test is usually begun on the morning after an overnight fast unless the history describes large volumes of water ingested and urine produced, in which case the test should begin after breakfast. The subject remains fasting throughout the entire test. A heparin lock is inserted intravenously so that serial blood samples are obtained easily. Baseline laboratory tests include (1) sodium, (2) potassium, (3) chloride, (4) serum carbon dioxide ($CO_2$), (5) urea (blood urea nitrogen [BUN]), (6) creatinine, (7) glucose, (8) calcium, and (9) serum osmolality. Potassium and calcium are measured to exclude hypokalemia and hypercalcemia as causes of nephrogenic DI (see later).

Measurements of serum or plasma sodium, chloride, $CO_2$, and urine pH provide an assessment of the patient's renal tubular acid-base function. Renal function and hydration status are evaluated with creatinine and urea (BUN) measurements. A urine specimen is obtained for measurement of urine sodium, urine osmolality, and urine specific gravity. Body weight and vital signs at baseline are recorded. Thereafter, each hour, serum and urine tests are repeated with measurement of hourly urine output, body weight, and urine volume. If ADH measurements are requested, they can be performed at the beginning, middle, and completion of the test; however, ADH measurements are not required for making the diagnosis of DI. More recently, copeptin, a co-secreted peptide fragment produced from the proteolytic cleavage of pre-pro AVP, has been identified as a reliable surrogate for the measurement of ADH. From an analytical standpoint, copeptin has the advantage of better in vitro stability than ADH. The water deprivation test is continued for 8 to 10 hours unless the diagnosis of DI is confirmed before the full time period has elapsed.

During the water deprivation test, if urine osmolality exceeds 600 mOsm/kg (mmol/kg) on two samples 1 hour apart or a single urine sample exceeds 1000 mOsm/kg (mmol/kg), DI is ruled out and the test can be concluded. If urine osmolality is less than 600 mOsm/kg (mmol/kg), and serum osmolality is more than 300 mOsm/kg (mmol/kg), DI is diagnosed and the water deprivation test can be concluded and the patient can proceed to a vasopressin or desmopressin challenge (see below). If serum osmolality does not exceed 300 mOsm/kg (mmol/kg), the water deprivation should be continued. If mental status changes or hypotension occurs or weight loss exceeds 3%, the test should be terminated.

If DI is diagnosed during a water deprivation test or the full 8-hour test is completed without the serum and urine osmolalities failing to exceed 300 and 600 mOsm/kg, respectively, aqueous vasopressin is injected subcutaneously (1 U/ m² or, according to some sources, 5 U total), or desmopressin (des-amino-D-arginine vasopressin) is given intranasally (20 µg), intravenously or intramuscularly (2 µg). A decline in urine volume with the doubling of urine osmolality over the next 1 to 2 hours identifies the DI as central in origin with the patient being ADH deficient. Failure to respond to exogenous ADH defines nephrogenic DI. Most patients with psychogenic polydipsia are able to concentrate their urine (>600 mOsm/kg) after water deprivation, but some fail to produce concentrated urine unless the water deprivation is prolonged.

*Syndrome of inappropriate antidiuretic hormone secretion.* SIADH is a common cause of hyponatremia in hospitalized patients. The autonomous sustained production of ADH in the absence of recognized and appropriate stimuli (such as hyperosmolality) is termed SIADH. In this syndrome, plasma ADH concentrations are "inappropriately" elevated relative to decreased plasma osmolality and to normal or increased plasma volume.

SIADH may be the result of one of several factors (Table 40.5), including (1) the production of ADH by a malignancy (e.g., neuroendocrine tumors such as small cell carcinoma of the lung), (2) the presence of acute or chronic disease of the

## TABLE 40.5 Causes of the Syndrome of Inappropriate Antidiuretic Hormone

| | |
|---|---|
| CNS disease | Brain tumor |
| | Infection (e.g., meningitis, encephalitis, abscess) |
| | Prolonged seizure |
| | Psychiatric disease |
| | Stress (e.g., prolonged nausea) |
| Paraneoplastic syndrome | Small cell carcinoma (especially lung), neuroblastoma, leukemia. |
| Pulmonary disease | Hypoxia (e.g., neonatal) |
| | Infection (e.g., pneumonia, emphysema) |
| Nonpulmonary infection | HIV infection |
| Drugs | Drugs with CNS effects (anticonvulsants, anti-Parkinson drugs, antipsychotics, antipyretics, antidepressants) |
| | Angiotensin-converting enzyme inhibitors |
| | Antineoplastic agents |
| | Chlorpropamide |
| | Methylenedioxymethamphetamine ("Ecstasy") |

*HIV,* Human immunodeficiency virus; *CNS,* central nervous system.

CNS, (3) pulmonary disorders, or (4) as a side effect of certain drug therapies.

In SIADH, primary excess of ADH coupled with unrestricted fluid intake promotes increased reabsorption of water by the kidney. The consequences are decreased urine volume and increased urine osmolality. The increase in intravascular volume causes hemodilution accompanied by dilutional hyponatremia and low plasma osmolality. It is important to recognize that although osmoregulation is tightly controlled, volume regulation always takes precedence over osmoregulation. Via suppression of the renin-angiotensin-aldosterone axis, volume expansion also decreases renal sodium reabsorption; thus, the urine sodium concentration is typically only diluted to 20 to 40 mEq/L (mmol/L), indicating ongoing sodium excretion, despite dilutional hyponatremia in the blood. This hypervolemia-induced urinary sodium excretion is mediated by natriuretic peptides and is, by necessity, accompanied by some water loss that cannot be overcome by ADH. This balance of opposing factors explains why patients with SIADH are euvolemic and not edematous.

Clinical manifestations of hyponatremia are nonspecific and include nausea, weakness, and apathy in mild cases and CNS changes such as lethargy, coma, and seizures in more severe cases. No signs or symptoms are specific to SIADH. History, physical examination, and routine laboratory test results often suggest that hyponatremia is dilutional (decreased urea, hemoglobin, or albumin) or depletional (increased urea, hemoglobin, or albumin). Measurements of sodium and osmolality in blood and urine combined with clinical assessment of volume status usually permit the

## TABLE 40.6    Disorders of Overproduction and Underproduction of Pituitary Hormones

| Pituitary Hormone | Consequences of Hormone Excess | Consequences of Hormone Deficiency |
|---|---|---|
| ACTH | Cushing disease | Cortisol deficiency |
| TSH | Central hyperthyroidism | Central hypothyroidism |
| GH | Children: gigantism | Children: short stature |
|  | Adults: acromegaly | Adults: adult GH deficiency |
| LH, FSH | Alpha-chain overproduction | Hypogonadism |
| Prolactin | Galactorrhea, hypogonadism | Inadequate lactation or lactation failure in mothers after delivery |
| ADH | SIADH | DI |

*ACTH,* Adrenocorticotropic hormone; *ADH,* antidiuretic hormone; *DI,* diabetes insipidus; *FSH,* follicle-stimulating hormone; *GH,* growth hormone; *LH,* luteinizing hormone; *SIADH,* syndrome of inappropriate ADH; *TSH,* thyroid-stimulating hormone.

appropriate differential diagnosis of hyponatremic conditions.

### Diagnostic Studies

Serum osmolality can be estimated from serum sodium, glucose, and urea (BUN) but is more reliably measured directly. Various formulas are available for estimating serum osmolality (see Chapter 24 for detail).

### POINTS TO REMEMBER

1. ADH and oxytocin-synthesizing cells are located in the hypothalamus.
2. ADH deficiency or resistance causes DI with the excess loss of free water.
3. ADH excess causes the SIADH, which results in the excess retention of free water.

## SUMMARY OF PITUITARY-RELATED DISORDERS

Disorders that result from the over- or underproduction of pituitary hormones are tremendously diverse (Table 40.6). Pituitary adenomas may be secretory or nonsecretory. Corticotropinomas secrete ACTH, somatotropinomas secrete GH, and prolactinomas secrete prolactin. Gonadotropinomas are rare and usually do not secrete intact LH and/or FSH but may secrete free α subunits. TSH-omas are likewise rare, causing high free thyroxine concentration with high or inappropriately normal (i.e., unsuppressed) TSH levels. Pituitary adenomas, whether functional or not, can lead to deficiencies of other pituitary hormones through the compression and destruction of the adjacent pituitary cells. These topics are reviewed in depth in many chapters of this textbook.

## REVIEW QUESTIONS

1. Which one of the following anterior pituitary hormones is regulated through suppression via the secretion of a hypothalamic hormone?
   a. ACTH
   b. Prolactin
   c. Growth hormone
   d. LH, FSH
   e. IGF-1
2. Which one of the following hormones exerts a predominant negative feedback via the anterior pituitary? The other hormones predominantly feedback at the level of the hypothalamus.
   a. IGF-1
   b. Sex steroids
   c. Inhibins
   d. Cortisol
   e. Thyroid hormone
3. Which one of the following statements is correct?
   a. IGF-1 and IGF-2 circulate bound to albumin.
   b. IGF-1 and IGFBP-3 levels are independent of one another.

   c. IGF-1 and IGF-2 circulate together bound to IGFBP-3 and the acid-labile subunit (ALS).
   d. The acid-stable subunit binds to IGF-1.
   e. IGF-1 and insulin form a complex.
4. Which of the following statements is correct regarding growth hormone (GH)?
   a. Physiologically, GH secretion is episodic and pulsatile.
   b. GH concentrations reach very low levels during the period of deepest sleep.
   c. GH actions are mediated through cortisol.
   d. GH secretion is stable throughout the day.
   e. A single measurement of GH is sufficient for diagnostic purposes.
5. Which one of the following statements is true?
   a. GH lowers blood glucose and can cause hypoglycemia.
   b. GH raises blood glucose by stimulating gluconeogenesis and reducing insulin sensitivity.
   c. GH is suppressed by hypoglycemia.
   d. GH inhibits lipolysis.

**e.** GH is the only determinant of IGF-1 concentrations.

6. What is the most common cause of acromegaly?
   **a.** IGF-1–secreting tumors
   **b.** Macro GH
   **c.** Anterior pituitary GH-secreting tumors (somatotropinomas)
   **d.** Multiple endocrine neoplasia type 1 syndrome
   **e.** Gonadotropin-secreting tumors

7. Which one of the following statements is true regarding macroprolactin?
   **a.** This is often caused by a complex between prolactin and immunoglobulin.
   **b.** This is a very high-molecular-weight form of prolactin due to alternative splicing.
   **c.** Macroprolactin lowers the plasma prolactin concentration.
   **d.** Macroprolactin heralds a dangerous pituitary tumor.
   **e.** Macroprolactin cannot be detected in the laboratory.

8. Which one of the following statements is true?
   **a.** In men, FSH stimulates testosterone production by Leydig cells. LH directs Sertoli cells to nourish developing sperm during spermatogenesis.
   **b.** LH and FSH are secreted by separate and distinct pituitary cells.
   **c.** LH and FSH secretion is stimulated by steady high concentrations of GnRH.
   **d.** LH and FSH are single-chain polypeptides.
   **e.** LH and FSH are secreted episodically.

9. Which one of the following statements is true?
   **a.** Cortisol is directly regulated by CRH.
   **b.** The major site of cortisol feedback is the anterior pituitary gland.
   **c.** ACTH directly regulates CRH.
   **d.** Increased ACTH increases cortisol secretion.
   **e.** ACTH is a glycoprotein hormone made up of alpha and beta subunits.

10. Which of the following suggests diabetes insipidus (DI)?
    **a.** Urine osmolality greater than 600 mOsm/kg (mmol/kg)
    **b.** Serum osmolality less than 270 mOsm/kg (mmol/kg)
    **c.** Urine osmolality less than 300 mOsm/kg (mmol/kg) plus serum osmolality greater than 300 mOsm/kg
    **d.** Edema and hypertension
    **e.** Very high urine sodium

## SUGGESTED READINGS

Alter D. Disorders of the adrenal cortex and medulla. In: Clarke WA, Marzinke MA, eds. *Contemporary Practice in Clinical Chemistry*. Washington, DC: AACC Press; 2020:725–742.

Amar AP, Weiss MH. Pituitary anatomy and physiology. *Neurosurg Clin N Am*. 2003;14:11–23 v.

Ball SG. Vasopressin and disorders of water balance: the physiology and pathophysiology of vasopressin. *Ann Clin Biochem*. 2007;44:417–431.

Bernard V, Young J, Chanson P, et al. New insights in prolactin: pathological implications. *Nat Rev Endocrinol*. 2015;11:265–275.

Ciccone NA, Kaiser UB. The biology of gonadotroph regulation. *Curr Opin Endocrinol Diabetes Obes*. 2009;16:321–327.

Ellervik C, Halsall DJ, Nygaard B. Thyroid disorders. In: *Tietz Textbook of Laboratory Medicine*. 7th ed. Elsevier; 2022:806–845.

Guillemin R. Hypothalamic hormones a.k.a. hypothalamic releasing factors. *J Endocrinol*. 2005;184:11–28.

Hiers PS, Winter WE. Disorders of growth. In: Wong EC, Dietzen DJ, Bennett MJ, et al., eds. *Biochemical Basis of Pediatric Disease*. 5th ed. Association for the Aid of Crippled Children Press; 2021:327–370.

Higham CE, Johannsson G, Shalet SM. Hypopituitarism. *Lancet*. 2016;388:2403–2415.

Holmes DT, Winter WE, McCormack A, et al. Pituitary function and pathophysiology. In: Rifai N, ed. *Tietz Textbook of Laboratory Medicine*. 7th ed. Elsevier; 2022:767–804.

LeRoith D. Clinical relevance of systemic and local IGF-I: lessons from animal models. *Pediatr Endocrinol Rev*. 2008;5(suppl. 2):739–743.

Molitch ME. Diagnosis and treatment of pituitary adenomas: a review. *JAMA*. 2017;317:516–524.

Mullis PE. Genetics of isolated growth hormone deficiency. *J Clin Res Pediatr Endocrinol*. 2010;2:52–62.

Rogol AD, Hayden GF. Etiologies and early diagnosis of short stature and growth failure in children and adolescents. *J Pediatr*. 2014;164:S1–S14.

Rosenbloom AL, Connor EL. Hypopituitarism and other disorders of the growth hormone-insulin-like growth factor-I axis. In: Lifshitz F, ed. *Pediatric Endocrinology*. Informa Healthcare; 2007:65–99.

Richmond EJ, Rogol AD. Growth hormone deficiency in children. *Pituitary*. 2008;11:115–120.

Toogood AA, Stewart PM. Hypopituitarism: clinical features, diagnosis, and management. *Endocrinol Metab Clin North Am*. 2008;37:235–261.

Tomycz ND, Horowitz MB. Inferior petrosal sinus sampling in the diagnosis of sellar neuropathology. *Neurosurg Clin North Am*. 2009;20:361–367.

Yuen KC, Biller BM, Radovick S, et al. American Association of Clinical Endocrinologists and American College of Endocrinology guidelines for management of growth hormone deficiency in adults and patients transitioning from pediatric to adult care. *Endocr Pract*. 2019;25:1191–1232.

# 41

# Adrenal Cortex

*Roger L. Bertholf*

**Cortisol**  The major adrenal glucocorticoid, which is synthesized in the zona fasciculata (and, to a lesser extent, the zona reticularis) of the adrenal cortex.

**Cushing syndrome**  A condition characterized by an increased concentration of adrenal glucocorticoid hormone in the bloodstream and its effects on the body.

**Dehydroepiandrosterone (DHEA)**  A weakly androgenic steroid secreted by the adrenal cortex. It is the major androgen precursor in females.

**Glucocorticoids**  Any of the group of 21-carbon steroids (principally cortisol) produced by the adrenal cortex that regulate carbohydrate, fat, and protein metabolism.

**Hyperaldosteronism**  Abnormally elevated synthesis and secretion of aldosterone by the adrenal gland (also called *aldosteronism*).

**Mineralocorticoids**  Any of the group of 21-carbon corticosteroids (principally aldosterone) that contribute to the regulation of water, pH, and electrolyte balance.

**Renin**  A hydrolase enzyme that catalyzes cleavage of the leucine-leucine bond in angiotensinogen to release angiotensin I.

**Steroidogenic acute regulatory protein (StAR)**  A transport protein that functions to regulate cholesterol transfer within the mitochondria.

**Waterhouse-Friderichsen syndrome**  Adrenal failure caused by bleeding into the adrenal gland. It is a fulminating complication of bacterial infections, notably meningococcemia, characterized by a sudden onset and short course, cyanosis with petechial hemorrhages of the skin and mucous membranes, fever, and hypotension, which can lead to shock and coma.

**Zona fasciculata**  The thick middle layer of the adrenal cortex that contains large lipid-laden cells. It is the major source of glucocorticoids and, to a lesser extent, adrenal androgens.

**Zona glomerulosa**  The thin outer layer of the adrenal cortex. It is the source of mineralocorticoids.

**Zona reticularis**  The inner layer of the adrenal cortex. Its cells resemble those of the zona fasciculata except that they contain less lipid. The zona reticularis is the major source of adrenal androgens and a minor source of glucocorticoids.

## INTRODUCTION

The adrenal cortex, gonads, and placenta are the exclusive anatomic sites for synthesis and secretion of steroid hormones, a class of bioregulatory molecules derived from cholesterol. Three classes of steroid hormones are produced in the adrenal cortex: mineralocorticoids, glucocorticoids, and androgenic steroids. Aldosterone is the primary mineralocorticoid produced in the adrenal cortex, and it functions to increase blood volume by promoting sodium reabsorption from the renal tubules. Cortisol is the primary glucocorticoid produced in the adrenal cortex, and it has a variety of essential regulatory functions affecting glucose metabolism, inflammation, lipolysis, hemoglobin synthesis, calcium excretion, fetal development, and neurological activity, among other effects. The primary adrenal androgens are dehydroepiandrosterone and its sulfated derivative, and androstenedione, which are minor sources of androgenic activity in males but are responsible for the growth of axillary and pubic hair in females. In males and females, the gonads are the primary source of masculinizing and feminizing hormones, respectively.

The adrenal medulla is anatomically and biochemically distinct from the adrenal cortex and produces catecholamines, which are the subject of Chapter 26.

## ADRENAL ANATOMY AND PHYSIOLOGY

### Gross Anatomy

The adrenal[a] glands are pyramidal-shaped, 2 to 3 cm wide, 4 to 6 cm long, and about 1 cm thick. Arterial blood is supplied to the adrenal gland by (1) the superior adrenal (or suprarenal) artery from the inferior phrenic artery (a branch of the aorta); (2) the middle adrenal artery, which is directly from the aorta; and (3) the inferior adrenal artery, a branch of the renal artery. Venous access to the adrenal gland, which is important for diagnostic studies, is obtained through the right adrenal vein that enters into the vena cava at an acute angle, or the left adrenal vein that enters into the left renal vein.

Embryologically, the adrenal gland develops from two different primary germ layers: the adrenal cortex is derived from the intermediate mesoderm, whereas the adrenal medulla develops from the ectodermal neural crest. The fetal adrenal cortex is proportionately larger than adrenal glands observed later in life. The fetal adrenal layer is situated between the definitive cortex and the medulla and contains large steroid-secreting cells arranged in a reticular pattern. At birth, the adrenal gland exceeds the weight of an adult adrenal gland (8 to 12 g) and is several times the size of the postnatal kidney. The large size of the fetal adrenal gland (approximately 250 mg/100 g body weight) probably explains why it occasionally is traumatized during delivery. Between 3 and 18 months of age, the adrenal glands involute to approximately half their size at birth. Later in life, the adrenal glands are less susceptible to trauma and represent less than 50 mg/100 g of body weight. Adult adrenal glands weigh 4 to 6 g each. The mature adrenal cortex is morphologically divided into three layers, or zones: the glomerulosa (10% to 15% of the cortex), the fasciculata (up to 75% of the cortex), and the reticularis (5% to 10% of the cortex) (see Fig. 41.1). Each layer of the adrenal cortex has a specific function: the zona glomerulosa produces mineralocorticoids

---

[a]Also called "suprarenal" glands, the name "adrenal" is derived from the Latin prefix *ad-*, meaning "near" and *renes*, the Latin word for "kidney."

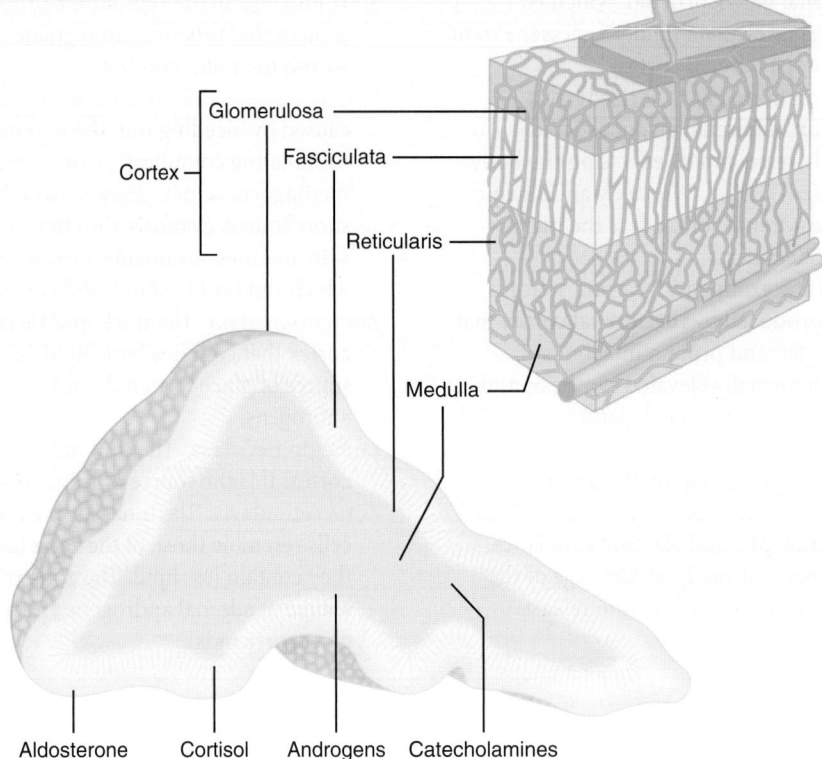

**Fig. 41.1** The adrenal gland is anatomically divided into four layers: zona glomerulosa, zona fasciculata, zona reticularis, and the medulla. The outer three layers produce steroid hormones, and the inner medulla produces catecholamines. Mineralocorticoids are produced in the zona glomerulosa; glucocorticoids are produced in the zona fasciculata, and androgens are produced in the zona reticularis. (From Bertholf RL, Cooper M, Winter WE. Adrenal cortex. In: Rifai N, ed. *Tietz Textbook of Laboratory Medicine.* 7th ed. St. Louis: Elsevier; 2022.)

(primarily aldosterone), the zona fasciculata produces glucocorticoids (primarily cortisol), and the zona reticularis produces androgens (primarily androstenedione and dehydroepiandrosterone).

### POINTS TO REMEMBER

| Adrenal Layer | Hormones | Hormonal Action |
|---|---|---|
| Zona glomerulosa | Aldosterone | Mineralocorticoid |
| Zona fasciculata | Cortisol | Glucocorticoid |
| Zona reticularis | Androstenedione Dehydroepiandrosterone | Androgenic |
| Medulla | Catecholamines | Neuromodulation |

The adrenal cortex and the gonads share several metabolic pathways for synthesis of steroid hormones because both tissues are derived from mesodermal anlagen. Two important transcription factors control the development of the adrenal cortex: steroidogenic factor-1 (SF-1), regulated by the dosage-sensitive sex reversal adrenal hypoplasia critical region on chromosome X, gene 1 (DAX-1). A complete list of adrenal proteins and enzymes mentioned in this chapter and their chromosomal loci appears in Table 41.1. Although

the three layers within the adrenal cortex are morphologically distinct, there is some degree of functional redundancy. For example, adrenocorticotropic hormone (ACTH, or corticotropin) receptors are expressed in some zona glomerulosa cells, and the enzyme that converts 11-deoxycortisol to cortisol is expressed in both the zona fasciculata and the zona reticularis.

## Zona Glomerulosa

The outermost functional layer of the adrenal cortex is the zona glomerulosa, lying just beneath the capsule. Histologically, the cells of the zona glomerulosa appear ovoid and in rosette-like clusters, from which the name glomerulosa[b] is derived. There is heterogeneity in cells of the glomerulosa and not all glomerulosa cells express the entire suite of enzymes necessary to produce aldosterone. Unique to the zona glomerulosa, however, is the enzyme aldosterone synthase, which catalyzes the final three steps in the production of aldosterone from 11-deoxycorticosterone by way of corticosterone and 18-hydroxy intermediates. Aldosterone production and secretion by the zona glomerulosa is activated through several biochemical signals. A major regulator of aldosterone secretion is angiotensin II, which binds to the angiotensin II receptor type 1 ($AT_1$), a $G_{q/11}$-coupled

---

[b]From the Latin *glomus,* meaning "ball"; it is also the root for "glomerulus."

## TABLE 41.1   Enzymes and Proteins Related to Adrenocortical Steroids

| Common Names and Abbreviations | Gene | Cytogenetic Band |
|---|---|---|
| **Enzymes** | | |
| 3β-Hydroxysteroid dehydrogenase (3BHSD) | HSD3B2 | 1p12 |
| 11β-Hydroxysteroid dehydrogenase 2 (HSD2) | HSD11B2 | 16q22.1 |
| 11β-Hydroxylase-1 (11B1H) | CYP11B1 | 8q24.3 |
| 17α-Hydroxylase (17AH) | CYP17A1 | 10q24.32 |
| 17β-Hydroxysteroid dehydrogenase type 1 (17BHSD1) | HSD17B1 | 17q21.2 |
| 17β-Hydroxysteroid dehydrogenase type 3 (17BHSD3) | HSD17B3 | 9q22.32 |
| 21-Hydroxylase (21H) | CYP21A2 | 6p21.33 |
| Aldosterone synthase (AS) | CYP11B2 | 8q24.3 |
| Aromatase (AR) | CYP19A1 | 15q21.2 |
| Cholesterol side-chain cleavage enzyme (CSCE) | CYP11A1 | 15q24.1 |
| Dehydroepiandrosterone sulfotransferase (DS) | SULT2A1 | 19q13.33 |
| **Proteins** | | |
| Angiotensin II receptor type 1 ($AT_1$) | AGTR1 | 3q24 |
| Angiotensin II receptor type 2 ($AT_2$) | AGTR2 | Xq23 |
| Corticosteroid-binding globulin (CBG) | SERPINA6 | 14q32.13 |
| Dosage-sensitive sex reversal adrenal hypoplasia critical region on chromosome X (DAX-1) | NR0B1 | Xp21.2 |
| Glucocorticoid receptor (GR) | NR3C1 | 5q31.3 |
| Melanocortin receptor-2 (MC2) | MC2R | 18p11.21 |
| Melanocortin receptor-5 (MC5) | MC5R | 18p11.21 |
| Melanocortin 2 receptor accessory protein (MRAP) | MRAP | 21q22.11 |
| Melanocortin 2 receptor accessory protein 2 (MRAP2) | MRAP2 | 6q14.2 |
| Mineralocorticoid receptor (MR) | NR3C2 | 4q31.23 |
| Pro-opiomelanocortin (POMC) | POMC | 2p23.3 |
| Sex hormone-binding globulin (SHBG) | SHBG | 17p13.1 |
| Steroidogenic acute regulatory protein (StAR) | STAR | 8p11.23 |
| Steroidogenic factor-1 (SF-1) | NR5A1 | 9q33.3 |

protein expressed on the surface of glomerulosa cells. An angiotensin II receptor type 2 ($AT_2$) is also expressed in glomerulosa cells, but its function in aldosterone regulation is less clear. It is believed that angiotensin II binding to $AT_2$ receptors opposes the vasoconstrictive and inflammatory effects of $AT_1$ activation. Angiotensin II has a variety of physiological effects; binding of angiotensin II to $AT_1$ activates phospholipase C, inducing $Ca^{2+}$ influx and stimulation of protein kinase C. In the adrenal gland, the effect is to promote aldosterone synthesis and secretion. Potassium acts synergistically with angiotensin II in the regulation of aldosterone secretion, and these are the two most important aldosterone secretagogues.

ACTH is a minor regulator of aldosterone production, although the minimum dose of ACTH required to stimulate aldosterone release is lower than the dose required to stimulate either cortisol or dehydroepiandrosterone (DHEA). The responsiveness of zona glomerulosa cells to ACTH is primarily due to the MC5 melanocortin receptor, a member of the melanocortin receptor superfamily of G protein-coupled receptors, which is expressed in all three adrenocortical layers but predominantly in the zona glomerulosa. Zona glomerulosa cells express MC2, the primary melanocortin receptor in the zona fasciculata, to a much lesser extent.

## Zona Fasciculata

The middle and largest of the three functional adrenocortical layers is the zona fasciculata,[c] which accounts for about 80% of the entire adrenocortical volume and is histologically characterized by polyhedral cells arranged radially in straight cords, or columns, toward the medulla. Lipid droplets within their cytoplasm give the parenchymal cells a foamy appearance and their descriptive name, spongiocytes.

The primary hormonal products of the zona fasciculata are glucocorticoids, which are a class of corticosteroids that bind to the glucocorticoid receptor (GR), a member of nuclear receptor subfamily 3. Cortisol, a 17α-hydroxy-C21 steroid synthesized in the zona fasciculata from 17-hydroxypregnenolone, is the principal glucocorticoid in humans, although smaller amounts of corticosterone and its 11-deoxy metabolite, which also have glucocorticoid activity, are also secreted by the adrenal gland. Cortisol synthesis and secretion is under the regulatory control of ACTH, a melanocortin produced in the anterior pituitary gland. ACTH binds to MC2, expressed by the zona fasciculata cells. The MC2 receptor is highly specific

[c]From the Latin *"fascis,"* meaning "bundle"; also the root of "fascia," "fascicle" and "fasciitis."

for ACTH, but requires the presence of a protein, melanocortin 2 receptor accessory protein (MRAP), to modulate ACTH binding.

## Zona Reticularis

The innermost layer of the adrenal cortex is the zona reticularis, histologically characterized by small, irregularly shaped, sparsely vacuolated cells arranged in randomly-oriented overlapping cords that give it the appearance of a net.[d] During fetal development, the adrenal gland consists primarily of cells that secrete the adrenal androgens DHEA and dehydroepiandrosterone sulfate (DHEAS), from what has been called the "fetal zone" of the developing adrenal gland. It is only after birth that the gland begins to differentiate into the three zones that characterize an adult adrenal gland. The zona reticularis is the last of the three adrenocortical layers to develop, emerging at the time of adrenarche. Therefore, DHEA and DHEAS production peaks during fetal development, then wanes about 1 year after birth, reappearing around age 8 to 10 years, as adrenarche approaches and expression of the sulfotransferase enzyme responsible for converting DHEA to DHEAS increases.

Hormonal regulation of adrenal androgen production and secretion is not as well understood as the control of mineralocorticoids and glucocorticoids. Reticular cells express the ACTH-specific receptor MC2, and therefore ACTH appears to be a major regulator of adrenal androgens. However, the production of adrenal androgens does not mirror cortisol production in the way that would be predicted if there were a single common mediator. Therefore, it has been suggested that additional factors modulate the adrenal androgen response. Cells of the zona reticularis and zona fasciculata express a 17α-hydroxylase enzyme that converts pregnenolone and progesterone to their respective 17-hydroxy derivatives. These C21 derivatives are further converted by the same enzyme to the C19 androgens, DHEA, and androstenedione. DHEA, DHEAS, and androstenedione have weak androgenic activity, but provide a circulating pool of precursors to more potent androgens such as testosterone and dihydrotestosterone, and estrogens such as estradiol and estriol, synthesized in the gonads. Recent evidence suggests that a minor by-product of steroid synthesis in the zona fasciculata and zona reticularis, 11-ketotestosterone (11-KT), may be responsible for most of the androgenic activity of the adrenal sex steroids; 11-KT binds to the human androgen receptor with an affinity comparable to testosterone.

## ADRENAL STEROID BIOCHEMISTRY

### Cholesterol

Steroids are characterized by a 17-carbon tetracyclic nucleus of four aliphatic rings biosynthesized by the cyclization of

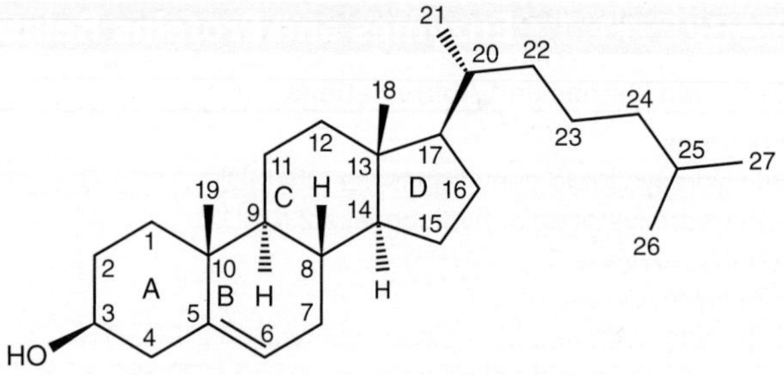

Fig. 41.2 The structure of cholesterol, the 27-carbon sterol precursor for all the adrenocortical steroids. Numbers identify individual carbon atoms, and letters identify the four ring structures. (From Bertholf RL, Cooper M, Winter WE. Adrenal cortex. In: Rifai N, ed. *Tietz Textbook of Laboratory Medicine*. 7th ed. St. Louis: Elsevier; 2022.)

squalene, a triterpene produced by the mevalonate pathway.[e] The steroid backbone consists of one pentacyclic and three hexacyclic carbon rings, designated A, B, C, and D. The conventional carbon numbering system for cholesterol is illustrated in Fig. 41.2. Sterols such as cholesterol are hydroxylated at position 3 on the A ring. Cholesterol has a double bond between carbons 5 and 6 and an eight-carbon aliphatic side group at position 17. Dietary or biosynthesized cholesterol is the precursor to all human steroid hormones.

Although cells in the adrenal cortex have the capacity to synthesize cholesterol, most of the steroid (approximately 80% of the total) is taken up by low-density lipoprotein (LDL) receptors in the adrenal cortex. Cytosolic cholesterol esterase hydrolyzes cholesterol esters to release free cholesterol, an important step that must precede transport of cholesterol into the mitochondria. In the rate-limiting step of steroid hormone biosynthesis, cholesterol gains access to the inner mitochondrial membrane with the help of steroidogenic acute regulatory (StAR) protein. In the adrenal gland, StAR expression is regulated by ACTH, but several other regulatory factors appear to be involved, as well, including gonadotropins, epidermal growth factor, insulin-like growth factor, prolactin, gonadotropin-releasing hormone, and macrophage-derived factors. Once cholesterol is transported to the inner surface of the mitochondrial membrane, cholesterol side-chain cleavage enzyme (CSCE) hydrolytically cleaves a 4-methylpentanal group from the side chain on carbon 17, leaving the C19 steroid pregnenolone, which is the precursor of all the adrenal steroids.

---

[d]Latin "*reticularis*," meaning "little net."

[e]Also called the HMG-CoA reductase, or isoprenoid pathway. β-Hydroxy β-methylglutaryl-CoA (HMG-CoA) is synthesized from acetyl CoA and acetoacetyl CoA, and then reduced to mevalonate, which is twice phosphorylated and then decarboxylated to generate isopentenylpyrophosphate (IPP). IPP isomerizes to dimethylallyl pyrophosphate (DMAPP), and then to the diphosphorylated sesquiterpene farnesyl pyrophosphate, which is the substrate for squalene synthase. Oxidosqualene cyclase cyclizes squalene to form lanosterol, which ultimately is converted to cholesterol in 19 additional biosynthetic steps.

## Adrenal Steroid Biosynthesis

The biosynthetic pathways from pregnenolone to aldosterone, cortisol, DHEA, and androstenedione are illustrated in Fig. 41.3.

In the zona glomerulosa, pregnenolone is oxidized to progesterone by 3β-hydroxysteroid dehydrogenase-2.[f] A hydroxyl group is added to the methyl group at position 21 (on the side chain) by the action of 21-hydroxylase enzyme, generating 11-deoxycorticosterone, which is subsequently converted to corticosterone by addition of a hydroxyl group at position 11, catalyzed by aldosterone synthase. Both of the final two steps in the biosynthesis of aldosterone are also catalyzed by aldosterone synthase. In the first step, 18-hydroxycorticosterone is generated by hydroxylation of the methyl group at position 18 of corticosterone, and in the second step, the newly added hydroxyl group is oxidized to an aldehyde, producing aldosterone.

In the zona fasciculata, 17α-hydroxylase adds a hydroxyl group at position 17 on pregnenolone or progesterone to generate 17-hydroxypregnenolone and 17-hydroxyprogesterone, respectively. 17-OH pregnenolone can be converted to 17-OH progesterone in the zona fasciculata by 3β-hydroxysteroid dehydrogenase-2, the same as pregnenolone is converted to progesterone in the zona glomerulosa. Carbon 21 of 17-OH progesterone is hydroxylated by 21-hydroxylase to produce 11-deoxycortisol, which is then hydroxylated at position 11 by 11β-hydroxylase-1 to generate cortisol.

In the zona reticularis, 17α-hydroxylase converts 17-OH pregnenolone and 17-OH progesterone to the C19 steroids DHEA and androstenedione, respectively, by removing the hydroxyl group from carbon 17. Androstenedione can also be produced from DHEA by $\Delta^{5-4}$ isomerization and oxidation of the C-3 hydroxyl group, catalyzed by 3β-hydroxysteroid dehydrogenase. DHEA is esterified with sulfate by DHEA sulfotransferase to form DHEAS, which is hormonally inert but can be converted back to DHEA, which has weak androgenic and estrogenic activity; therefore, DHEAS can be considered a prohormone. Primarily in the ovaries, but in other tissues as well, aromatase removes the C-19 methyl group of androstenedione to produce estrone, which is followed by aromatization of the A ring to produce estradiol.

## Adrenal Steroid Activity and Metabolism

Aldosterone binds to the mineralocorticoid receptor (MR), which is expressed throughout the body but most importantly in distal tubular epithelial tissue, where it regulates the $Na^+/K^+$ pump (epithelial sodium channel; ENaC) to influence sodium and water reabsorption and potassium excretion. The MR has equal affinity for aldosterone and cortisol, but in the distal nephron, 11β-hydroxysteroid dehydrogenase type 2

(HSD2) is co-expressed with the MR and converts cortisol to cortisone, which does not bind to the receptor.[g] Normal circulating concentrations of cortisol (10 to 20 μg/dL; 275 to 550 nmol/L) are more than 1000 times higher than aldosterone concentrations (2 to 9 ng/dL; 55 to 250 pmol/L), so in tissues where the MR is expressed without the HSD2 enzyme, its principal ligand is cortisol unless aldosterone is significantly elevated.

Hepatic UDP-glucuronosyltransferase enzymes convert aldosterone to the tetrahydroglucuronide metabolite by 18β-glucuronidation. Aldosterone has a plasma half-life of less than 20 minutes.

The GR[h] is expressed in nearly all vertebrate cells. A variety of endogenous (cortisol, corticosterone) and synthetic (dexamethasone, prednisolone) glucocorticoids bind to the GR, initiating a cascade of molecular events resulting in the up- or down-regulation of thousands of genes associated with metabolism, stress response, inflammation, and a host of other organismal functions.

Circulating cortisol is metabolized to dihydrocortisol and tetrahydrocortisol, which are conjugated to glucuronide by hepatic UDP-glucuronosyl transferase enzymes. Ten percent of cortisol is converted to the 17-ketosteroid metabolite, which is then conjugated to sulfate before being excreted in the urine. The plasma half-life of cortisol is just over 60 minutes but can be longer when cortisol concentrations are very high, presumably due to saturation of these metabolic pathways.

## Corticosteroid-Binding Proteins

Steroids are poorly soluble in water and therefore require a soluble protein for effective transport in circulation. Corticosteroid-binding globulin (CBG; also called transcortin) binds up to 90% of circulating cortisol, and a small amount of cortisol is bound to albumin, leaving only about 4% of circulating cortisol in the free, active state. Protein binding plays an important role in the regulation of hormonal activity, sequestering large fractions of circulating hormone in an inactive (bound) form and thereby modulating the concentration of the free, active hormone. This is much the same way the anion of a weak acid sequesters hydrogen ions in a chemically buffered solution, preventing rapid changes in the pH.

---

[f]Also known as $\Delta^{5-4}$-isomerase, because in addition to oxidizing the hydroxyl group on carbon 3, the enzyme also translocates the double bond from carbons 5–6 to carbons 4–5. Two isoforms of the enzyme exist, HSD3B1 and HSD3B2. The former is expressed in the placenta and peripheral tissues, and the latter is expressed in the adrenal gland and gonads. Both are coded on chromosome 1p12.

[g]There are two isoenzymes of 11β-hydroxysteroid dehydrogenase: type 1 and type 2. Both isoenzymes have 11β-dehydrogenase activity to convert cortisol to cortisone, but only type 1 isoenzyme has 11-oxoreductase activity, which converts cortisone back to cortisol. The type 2 isoenzyme is not able to catalyze the reverse reaction, so it prevents cortisol from binding to the MR.

[h]The glucocorticoid receptor (NR3C1) is closely related to paralogues NR3C2 (mineralocorticoid receptor), NR3C3 (progesterone receptor), and NR3C4 (androgen receptor). All four receptors share a 4-domain structure consisting of an amino-terminal domain, a zinc-finger DNA-binding domain, a hinge region, and a C-terminal ligand-binding domain.

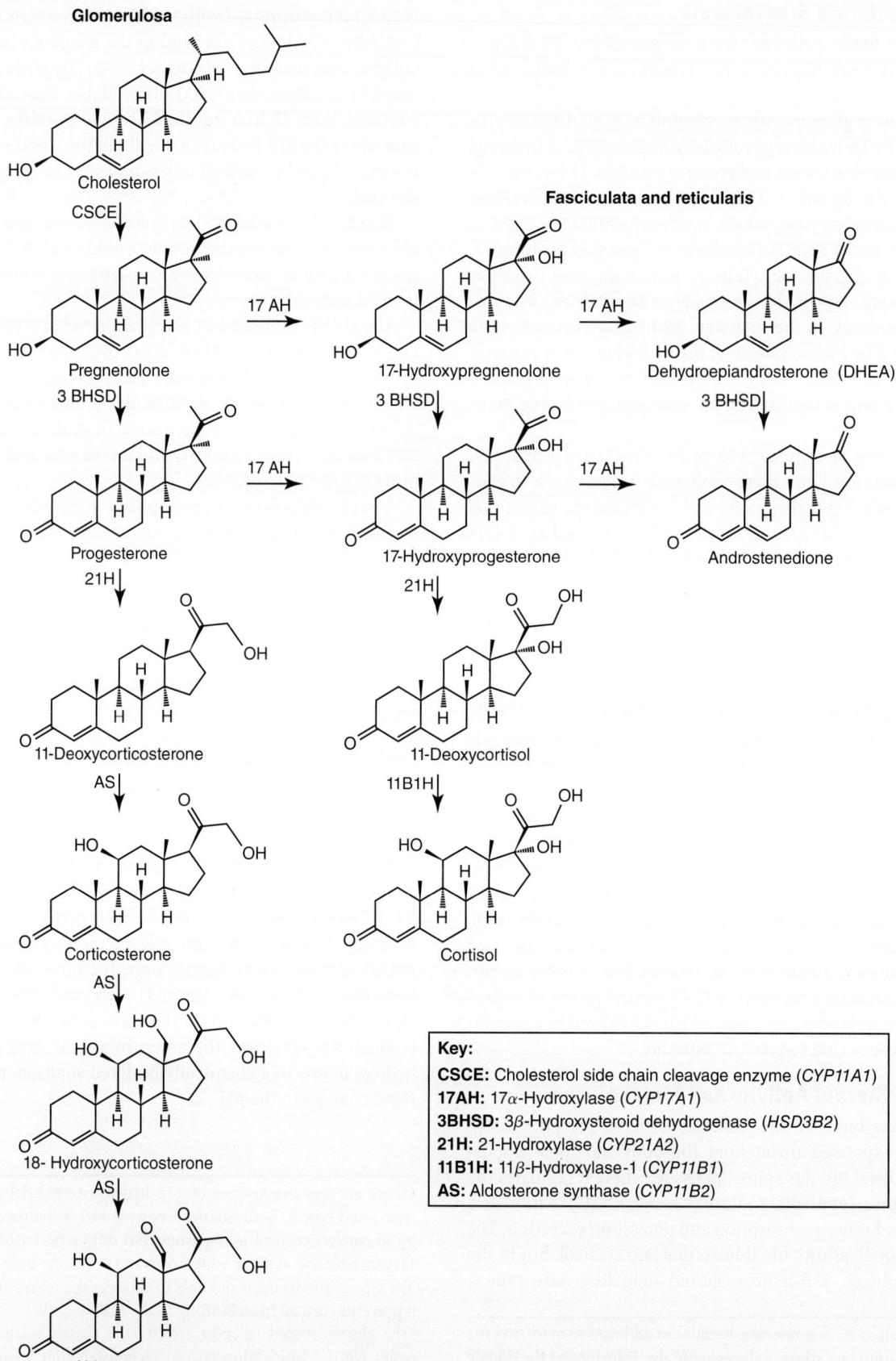

**Fig. 41.3** Adrenocortical biosynthesis of aldosterone, cortisol, androstenedione, and dehydroepiandrosterone from cholesterol. (From Bertholf RL, Cooper M, Winter WE. Adrenal cortex. In: Rifai N, ed. *Tietz Textbook of Laboratory Medicine.* 7th ed. St. Louis: Elsevier; 2022.)

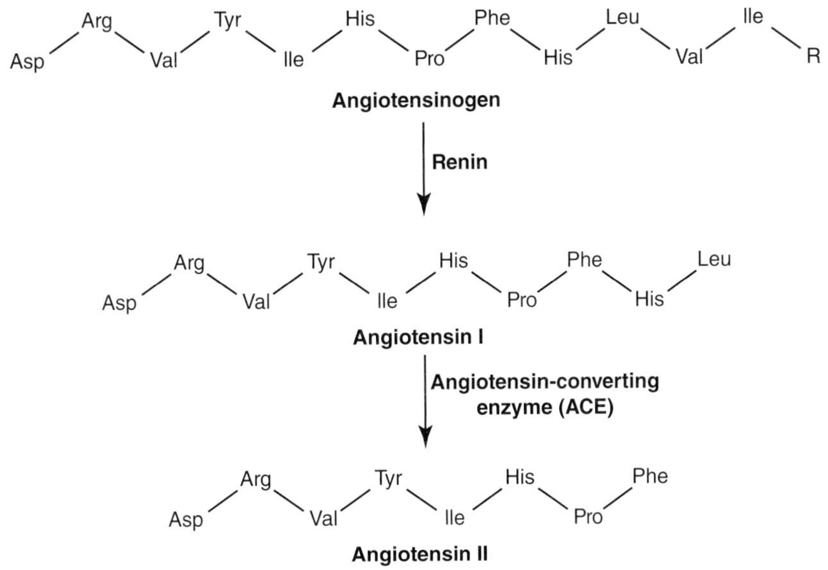

**Fig. 41.4** Production of angiotensin II from angiotensinogen and angiotensin I. Angiotensinogen is produced in the liver; renin is secreted by the kidneys; angiotensin-converting enzyme (ACE) is expressed in many tissues, but primarily the pulmonary epithelium. (From Bertholf RL, Cooper M, Winter WE. Adrenal cortex. In: Rifai N, ed. *Tietz Textbook of Laboratory Medicine.* 7th ed. St. Louis: Elsevier; 2022.)

In contrast to cortisol, aldosterone is only weakly bound to CBG and albumin; the free aldosterone concentration is about 36% of the total concentration, and most of the bound fraction is associated with albumin.

Adrenal androgens are approximately 90% bound to albumin, and about 3% bound to sex hormone-binding globulin (SHBG, also called sex steroid-binding protein), an 88 kDa homodimeric glycoprotein that serves primarily as a transport protein for testosterone and estradiol. DHEA binds weakly to SHBG, but DHEAS and androstenedione do not bind to the protein at all.

# REGULATION OF ADRENOCORTICAL HORMONES

## Mineralocorticoids

Aldosterone secretion by the zona glomerulosa of the adrenal cortex is primarily regulated by two chemical stimuli: angiotensin II and potassium. The combined action of increased angiotensin II and potassium, in addition to the minor influence of ACTH, increase the production and release of aldosterone, which in turn promotes sodium reabsorption and potassium secretion from the renal tubules. The overall physiological effect of aldosterone is to increase blood volume and pressure.

### The Renin-Angiotensin-Aldosterone System

Renin is a 36 kDa aspartyl protease enzyme produced by specialized cells in the juxtaglomerular apparatus (or complex) in the nephron. Three types of juxtaglomerular cells exist, and they produce and secrete renin in response to specific stimuli. An increase in distal tubular sodium and chloride concentration is detected by the *macula densa*; a decrease in renal perfusion is detected by baroreceptors in the granular cells, and

the juxtaglomerular cells are also sensitive to beta-1 adrenergic stimulation. The only known substrate for renin is angiotensinogen, a 62 kDa α-globulin produced in the liver. Renin cleaves the 10 N-terminal amino acids to form the hormonally inert decapeptide, angiotensin I. Angiotensin-converting enzyme (ACE), a zinc-dependent dicarboxypeptidase found primarily in the lungs but also widely distributed in endothelial and epithelial tissues, removes the two C-terminal residues from angiotensin I to produce the octapeptide angiotensin II, which is the most active form of the hormone (see Fig. 41.4). In humans, angiotensinogen is normally in excess, so the production of angiotensin I and II is rate-limited by the concentration of renin. Several angiotensin II receptors have been identified, but $AT_1$ is the best characterized and is expressed in the glomerulosa cells of the adrenal cortex and in vascular endothelium. Plasma potassium also stimulates aldosterone production through a calcium-mediated signaling pathway.

The presence of a direct feedback loop for the renin-angiotensin-aldosterone system has not been conclusively demonstrated. Some have suggested that angiotensin II inhibits renin secretion by its interaction with $AT_1$ receptors on juxtaglomerular cells, constituting a "short-loop" feedback mechanism, but this has not been proven. Indirect regulators of the system include greater perfusion of the kidneys and decreased sodium and chloride concentration in the distal tubules.

### Adrenocorticotropic Hormone

Although less important than angiotensin II and potassium in the regulation of aldosterone, ACTH also stimulates aldosterone release, and the magnitude of this stimulus is likely related to the degree of expression of the MC2 receptors in the zona glomerulosa cells. In healthy individuals, ACTH is not responsible for the diurnal rhythmicity of aldosterone release, although aldosterone regulation is influenced by ACTH in primary aldosteronism (discussed later).

---

**POINTS TO REMEMBER**

**Regulation of Mineralocorticoids**
- Renin is released by the juxtaglomerular apparatus in response to:
  - Low plasma sodium
  - Low arterial blood pressure
  - β-1 adrenergic activity
- Renin cleaves angiotensinogen to produce angiotensin I
- ACE converts angiotensin I to angiotensin II
- Angiotensin II (and K+) stimulate adrenal secretion of aldosterone
- Aldosterone promotes renal tubule reabsorption of sodium and water and excretion of potassium and protons

---

## Glucocorticoids

ACTH is the primary regulator for the adrenal production and secretion of glucocorticoids, the most active of which is cortisol. ACTH is produced by corticotropic cells in the anterior pituitary gland from its precursor, proopiomelanocortin (POMC). In the corticotrophs, a serine endoprotease cleaves POMC into two fragments, the ACTH precursor fragment (pro-ACTH) and β-lipotropin. A receptor for β-lipotropin has not been identified, therefore its function is not known. The 39 amino acid peptide hormone ACTH is released from the pro-ACTH fragment of POMC. ACTH is not further modified in corticotrophs.

ACTH synthesis and release are regulated by corticotropin-releasing hormone (CRH), a 41 amino acid peptide synthesized in the parvocellular neuroendocrine cells within the hypothalamus and released into the hypothalamo-hypophyseal portal system, where it is carried to the anterior pituitary.

ACTH circulates systemically and binds to MC2 receptors located on adrenocortical cells, leading to steroidogenesis, increased size and number of adrenocortical cells, and increased size and functional complexity of cellular organelles, resulting in cortisol synthesis and release.

Cortisol inhibits hypothalamic and pituitary release of CRH and ACTH, respectively, in a classic hypothalamic/pituitary/end hormone negative feedback loop. Other regulatory mechanisms for ACTH include a short feedback loop in which ACTH suppresses hypothalamic CRH and an ultra-short feedback loop whereby ACTH suppresses its own release. There is diurnal variation in the secretion of cortisol; highest concentrations occur approximately 2 hours before awakening, and lowest concentrations shortly after falling asleep.

## Adrenal Androgens

In comparison to mineralocorticoids and glucocorticoids, the physiological regulation of adrenal androgens is relatively poorly understood. In the fetal and adult adrenal gland,

ACTH appears to be the primary stimulus for androgen production, but other possible regulators include the mitogen-activated protein kinase (MAPK) pathway, protein kinase C and D signaling, growth factors such as insulin-like growth factor-1 and epidermal growth factor, steroidogenic-inducing protein, macrophage-derived factors, and chloride or calcium channel messengers. In addition, several endocrine signals have been shown to influence adrenal androgen secretion, including prolactin, estrogen, prostaglandins, angiotensin, growth hormone, gonadotropins, and β-endorphin.

---

**POINTS TO REMEMBER**

**Regulation of Glucocorticoids**
- Hypothalamic CRH stimulates the anterior pituitary gland to secrete ACTH
- ACTH is the primary stimulus for adrenal production of glucocorticoids
- Cortisol suppresses the release of both CRH and ACTH
- When adrenal production of glucocorticoids is insufficient, ACTH is elevated
- Dysregulation usually occurs when a tumor is producing one or more of the hormones

---

# ADRENOCORTICAL INSUFFICIENCY

The adrenal glands have considerable functional reserve; symptoms of adrenocortical insufficiency may not be evident until at least 90% of the adrenal cortex is lost or nonfunctional. Adrenocortical insufficiency can manifest with inadequate glucocorticoid activity, inadequate mineralocorticoid activity, or both. Deficiency of adrenal androgens ordinarily has few clinical consequences in males, but there is some evidence that DHEA replacement therapy is beneficial in females with adrenocortical insufficiency. When adrenocortical insufficiency is the result of destruction or dysgenesis of the adrenal gland or impairment of steroidogenesis, it is termed primary adrenocortical failure, also known as **Addison disease** (AD).[i] Glucocorticoid and mineralocorticoid deficiencies can also occur due to adrenocortical resistance to hormones that stimulate synthesis and secretion of adrenocortical steroids, when the pituitary fails to produce sufficient ACTH (secondary adrenal failure), or more rarely from CRH deficiency (tertiary adrenal failure). In addition, there are rare genetic conditions that result in impaired response to adrenocortical hormones due to mutations in the mineralocorticoid and glucocorticoid receptors (GRs).

## Addison Disease

AD refers to disorders characterized by a nonfunctioning adrenal cortex, causing glucocorticoid and mineralocorticoid deficiency. AD is relatively rare, affecting only about 1

---

[i]Thomas Addison (1793 to 1860), English physician and scientist, described a case of adrenal insufficiency in 1855. Addison was most interested in the changes in skin pigmentation associated with the disease, which are due to melanocyte-stimulating hormone activity of corticotropin (ACTH), which is elevated in adrenal insufficiency.

in 10,000 individuals in developed countries. Symptoms of AD usually include fatigue, muscle weakness, weight loss, hyperpigmentation, hypotension, lightheadedness on standing, psychosis, nausea/vomiting, and diarrhea. Laboratory investigations may reveal hypoglycemia, hyponatremia, hyperkalemia, hypercalcemia, elevated ACTH, low cortisol and aldosterone, and impaired response to stimulation tests, although not all of these abnormalities are likely to be observed in every case. In particular, hypoglycemia and hyponatremia are uncommon complications of AD. Stress from infection or trauma can exacerbate symptoms and precipitate Addisonian crisis, a life-threatening medical emergency requiring immediate supportive care.

## Causes

Although over half of the original 11 cases of *melasma suprarenale*[j] described by Thomas Addison in 1855 were associated with tuberculosis, in today's developed countries the most common cause of AD is autoimmune adrenalitis. Tuberculosis remains the most common cause of AD worldwide. In children, most AD cases (>80%) are genetic. In addition to autoimmune, infectious disease, and genetic causes, adrenal insufficiency can be precipitated by neoplastic invasion, vascular disease, various drugs, trauma, and surgery. Table 41.2 lists many of the factors that may contribute to the development of adrenal insufficiency.

Autoimmune Addison disease (AAD) can develop at any age but is most common between ages 30 and 50 years. Although AAD sometimes occurs in isolation of other autoimmune diseases (~10% of cases), most cases are associated with an autoimmune polyendocrine syndrome (APS). Four types of APS have been described; AAD is most commonly associated with APS type 2 (~70% of cases). The molecular target of autoantibodies in autoimmune adrenalitis appears to be 21-hydroxylase; autoantibodies to this enzyme can be detected in up to 95% of AAD cases.

Mycobacterium tuberculosis (TB) is the most common infection causing AD, although AD has been associated with a host of other bacterial, fungal, parasitic, and viral infections, as well (see Table 41.2). Autopsy findings indicate that adrenal gland involvement occurs in about 6% of patients with active TB. Because of adrenal functional reserve, however, TB-infected patients do not develop AD until approximately 90% of the adrenal gland is destroyed, so most cases of adrenal TB are asymptomatic. Septicemia from *Neisseria meningitides, Pseudomonas aeruginosa, Haemophilus influenza, Pasteurella multocida, Staphylococcus aureus*, and *Streptococcus* group A infections can lead to Waterhouse–Friderichsen syndrome, a hemorrhagic disorder resulting in endotoxin-induced adrenal infarction.

A variety of other factors may compromise adrenal function. Naturally, bilateral adrenalectomy, which may be used to treat bilateral pheochromocytoma, uncontrolled Cushing disease, or adrenal nodular disease, cause AD that requires glucocorticoid and mineralocorticoid replacement therapy.

Ketoconazole, fluconazole, posaconazole, etomidate, rifampicin, and several anticancer agents inhibit adrenocortical steroidogenesis. Infiltration of the adrenal gland by metastatic disease, amyloidosis, or hemochromatosis are other causes of adrenal insufficiency. Vascular complications and coagulopathies of thrombocytopenia, systemic lupus erythematosus (SLE), polyarteritis nodosa, and antiphospholipid syndrome are associated with adrenal gland destruction and AD. Heparin-induced thrombocytopenia has been associated with adrenal hemorrhage and insufficiency.

### Mineralocorticoid Deficiency

Insufficient production of aldosterone leads to hyponatremia, hyperkalemia, acidosis, and hemodynamic instability. Aldosterone deficiency may be the result of impaired synthesis, inadequate stimulation of aldosterone production and release, or resistance to the effects of aldosterone. In cases of AD, aldosterone synthesis is most often impaired by autoimmune destruction of the adrenal gland. In the development of AD, glucocorticoid deficiency usually precedes mineralocorticoid deficiency, complicating diagnosis of the disease because symptoms of glucocorticoid deficiency are mostly non-specific, and AD may not be suspected until late in the course of the disease when the patient presents in Addisonian crisis. Addisonian crisis is a potentially fatal condition characterized by circulatory collapse and shock, caused by the combined deficiencies of glucocorticoids and mineralocorticoids.

Hypoaldosteronism can result from failure of the renin-angiotensin-aldosterone regulatory system, a disorder that can be either congenital or acquired. Hyporeninemic hypoaldosteronism is the most common cause of isolated aldosterone deficiency and is usually associated with diabetes mellitus. Many nephropathies can cause a deficiency in renin production, including glomerulonephritis, pyelonephritis, nephrolithiasis, renal amyloidosis, IgA nephropathy, and nephropathy associated with multiple myeloma or SLE. In cases of hyporeninemic hypoaldosteronism, urinary aldosterone secretion and plasma renin are low and do not respond to provocation by sodium restriction, upright posture, or diuretics. Hypervolemia suppresses renin, so chronic hypertension may produce an apparent hypoaldosteronism. It has also been suggested that diabetic neuropathy may stunt the adrenergic response to postural changes, inhibiting renin release. Defects in the conversion of pro-renin to renin have also been proposed.

Congenital hypoaldosteronism is a rare autosomal recessive disorder caused by a deficiency in aldosterone synthase, the enzyme that converts 11-deoxycorticosterone to aldosterone through two intermediates, corticosterone, and 18-hydroxycorticosterone. Aldosterone synthase deficiency (ASD) is classified into two phenotypes: type 1 ASD is characterized by low or undetectable plasma aldosterone concentrations, but type 2 ASD patients may have normal plasma aldosterone levels.

Hypoaldosteronism may also result from mutations in the MR or in the proteins required for the proper function of the ENaC, which facilitates sodium reabsorption in the renal tubules. It is misleading to refer to these cases as "hypoaldosteronism,"

---

[j]*Melasma*, from a Greek word for "black spot" or "blacken" and *suprarenale*, Latin for "above the kidney."

## TABLE 41.2    Causes of Primary Adrenal Failure (Addison Disease)

| Category | Causes |
|---|---|
| Autoimmune | Sporadic<br>APS type 1 (with candidiasis and/or hypothyroidism)<br>APS type 2 (with autoimmune thyroid disease and/or type 1 diabetes)<br>APS type 4 (with other autoimmune diseases) |
| Infection | Tuberculosis: *Mycobacterium hominis, Mycobacterium avium*<br>Other bacterial: *Neisseria meningitides, Pseudomonas aeruginosa, Haemophilus influenza, Pasteurella multtocida, Streptococci, Treponema pallidum, Eschericha coli*<br>Fungal: *Pneumocystis carinii, Histoplasma capsulatum, Blastomyces dermatitidis, Paracoccidioides brasiliensis, Coccidiodes immitis, Cryptococcus neoformans, Candida albicans*<br>Parasitic: *Toxoplasma gondii*, African trypanosomiasis<br>Viral: HIV, CMV, HSV, Echovirus type 11 and 12 |
| Inborn errors | Congenital adrenal hyperplasia (mostly *CYP21A2* or *CYP11B1* mutations, but other mutations in steroidogenic enzymes occur rarely)<br>X-linked adrenal hypoplasia congenita (*DAX-1* mutation)<br>Congenital lipoid adrenal hyperplasia (*STAR* mutation)<br>Steroid factor-1 deficiency (*NR5A1* mutation)<br>Other adrenal dysgenesis (*CDKNIC, SAMD9, GL13, MKS1, DOK7, RAPSN, HYLS1, WDR73* mutations, pseudotrisomy 13) |
| Drugs | Adenolytics: mitotane, aminoglutethimide, trilostane<br>Anticancer agents: tyrosine kinase inhibitors (sunitinib, imatinib); immune checkpoint inhibitors (ipilimumab, tremelimumab, nivolumab, pembrolizumab)<br>Other: ketoconazole, fluconazole, etomidate, rifampicin, ciproterone acetate |
| Vascular | Trauma<br>Polyarteritis nodosa<br>Systemic lupus erythematosus<br>Primary antiphospholipid syndrome<br>Waterhouse-Friderichsen syndrome (intra-adrenal hemorrhage)<br>Thrombocytopenia<br>Anticoagulant therapy |
| Neoplastic | Primary: lymphomas<br>Metastatic: lung, breast, and colon cancers; melanoma |
| Surgical | Bilateral adrenalectomy for Cushing disease, pheochromocytoma, macronodular adrenal hyperplasia, or primary pigmented nodular adrenocortical disease |

*APS*, Autoimmune polyendocrine syndrome; *CMV*, cytomegalovirus; *HIV*, human immunodeficiency virus; *HSV*, herpes simplex virus.

since aldosterone production and secretion by the adrenal gland is normal. Terms used for this disorder include "mineralocorticoid resistance" and "pseudohypoaldosteronism," the latter of which is abbreviated PHA and has three phenotypes: PHA1A, an autosomal dominant form with sodium wasting; PHA1B, an autosomal recessive form with sodium wasting; and PHA2,[k] which does not involve salt wasting.

### Glucocorticoid Deficiency

Impaired production of cortisol, the primary glucocorticoid, is essential for the diagnosis of AD. A secondary cause of glucocorticoid deficiency is inadequate production and secretion of ACTH, the hormone primarily responsible for stimulating adrenocortical production of cortisol. ACTH deficiency can occur when the ability of the anterior pituitary to produce ACTH is impaired, or more rarely, if CRH production or delivery to the pituitary gland is impaired, often called tertiary glucocorticoid deficiency.

[k]Also known as familial hyperkalemic hypertension, or Gordon syndrome.

The physiological activities of glucocorticoids are summarized in Table 41.3. Growth and development, metabolism, lipid homeostasis, inflammation, gluconeogenesis and glycogenolysis, and response to stress are all regulated to some degree by glucocorticoids. Cortisol, and to a lesser extent corticosterone and cortisone, diffuse through cellular membranes and bind to the cytosolic GR, which is expressed in virtually all mammalian cells with highest expression in brain, liver, muscle, bone marrow, and lymphoid tissues. Stimulation of the GR induces a conformational change that exposes nuclear localization sequences, which interact with glucocorticoid-responsive elements in the promoter region of target genes or through other transcriptional factors. In addition, glucocorticoids exert non-genomic effects mediated through MAPK, phosphatidylinositol 3-phosphate, $Ca^{++}$/calmodulin-dependent protein kinase II, and phospholipase C signaling pathways. Loss of function mutations in the GR produce glucocorticoid resistance.

Glucocorticoid deficiency is clinically characterized by anorexia, depression, and weight loss. The primary biochemical effect of glucocorticoid deficiency is hypoglycemia.

## TABLE 41.3 Glucocorticoid Activity

| Target | ADVERSE OUTCOME | |
| --- | --- | --- |
| | Deficiency | Excess |
| Central nervous system | Anorexia | Polyphagia |
| | Depression | Depression and/or psychoses |
| **Endocrine system** | | |
| Carbohydrate metabolism | Hypoglycemia | Hyperglycemia |
| Glycogen synthesis | Decreased | Increased |
| Gluconeogenesis | Decreased | Increased |
| Insulin resistance | Decreased | Increased |
| Fatty acids and triglycerides | NSE | Increased |
| Body weight | Decreased | Increased |
| Fat distribution | NSE | Centripetal |
| Pituitary hormones | NSE | Increased thyrotropin (TSH) |
| **Musculoskeletal and connective tissue** | | |
| Muscle | NSE | Atrophy (catabolism) |
| Skin | NSE | Thinning (catabolism) |
| Bone | NSE | Osteoporosis |
| Immune system | NSE | Immunosuppression |

*NSE,* No specific effect.

Because cortisol inhibits its own secretion through a feedback mechanism that involves inhibition of CRH and ACTH, cortisol deficiency due to primary adrenocortical insufficiency is characterized by high ACTH. In contrast, secondary (pituitary) and tertiary (hypothalamic) cortisol deficiency is characterized by low ACTH. Glucocorticoid deficiency is treatable with oral glucocorticoids such as hydrocortisone (cortisol in pharmaceutical form), cortisone, or long-acting synthetic glucocorticoids like prednisolone and dexamethasone.

### Adrenal Androgen Deficiency

Except during fetal development, a deficiency in adrenal androgens may be asymptomatic. This is especially true in males, where the primary source of androgens is the testes. Adrenal androgens contribute less than 5% of the total androgenic activity in males. DHEAS produced by the fetal adrenal gland fuels placental estrogen production. In adult females, adrenal androgens provide the metabolic precursors for about half of testosterone production, varying with the menstrual cycle, but clinical symptoms associated with a deficiency of adrenal androgens in females are not well defined.

### AT A GLANCE

**Addison Disease**
- Primary adrenocortical insufficiency
- Most common causes:
  - Autoimmune destruction of the adrenal gland
  - Infectious disease
  - Adrenal hemorrhage
  - Congenital adrenal hyperplasia
- Symptoms of glucocorticoid deficiency usually appear first
- Severe mineralocorticoid deficiency can result in "Addisonian crisis"

### Proximal Causes of Adrenal Insufficiency

Adrenal insufficiency is often associated with other diseases that have a proximal influence on adrenal function. Whereas AD customarily refers to primary adrenal insufficiency, it is a rare disease and deficiency of adrenal hormones can be observed in a host of disorders in which destruction of the adrenal gland itself is not the principal cause.

### Adrenoleukodystrophy

Adrenoleukodystrophy (ALD) is an X-linked autosomal recessive disorder affecting an ATP-binding cassette protein that transports very long chain fatty acids (VLCFA) to peroxisomes for degradation. ALD presents in several phenotypes, including childhood and neonatal forms, along with adult presentations. ALD is associated with neuroinflammation, adrenomyeloneuropathy, cerebral demyelination, and adrenal steroid dysgenesis. Neurological degeneration results from demyelination due to impaired β-oxidation of saturated VLCFA, therefore ALD is diagnosed by elevated plasma concentrations of VLCFA. Approximately 90% of males with ALD develop adrenal insufficiency, whereas adrenal involvement is rare in females with heterozygous ALD. Newborn screening for ALD has been instituted in about half of the states in the US.

### Zellweger Spectrum Disorder

Zellweger spectrum disorder (ZSD)[1] is one of a group of autosomal recessive disorders that involve defects in the

[1]Zellweger spectrum disorder (Hans Ulrich Zellweger; Swiss-American pediatrician: 1909 to 1990) has also been referred to as cerebrohepatorenal syndrome; neonatal adrenoleukodystrophy (NALD), and infantile Refsum disease (Sigvald Bernhard Refsum; Norwegian neurologist: 1907 to 1991).

production of peroxisomes, which are membrane-bound organelles found in virtually all eukaryotic cells. Peroxisomes contain enzymes that are essential for cellular metabolism of lipids, along with numerous other cellular functions. Peroxisome biogenesis disorders are caused by mutations in peroxins, which are proteins necessary for the biosynthesis and assembly of peroxisomes. ZSD can have variable clinical presentations, but adrenal insufficiency is a relatively common finding in these patients. ALD is also considered a peroxisome biogenesis disorder since peroxisomal function is compromised by inadequate or absent VLCFA transport protein, but it is not classified among ZSDs.

## Steroidogenic Factor-1 Mutations

SF-1 is a member of the nuclear receptor subfamily of transcription factors that regulate gene expression. SF-1 is essential for development of adrenal and reproductive function. A phospholipid appears to be the signaling ligand for SF-1, and binding the ligand activates promoters for several genes associated with adrenal and gonadal development. Adrenal insufficiency is rare in SF-1 mutations, which most commonly present as a 46XY disorder of sex development with gonadal dysgenesis, ambiguous genitalia, and the absence of Müllerian structures.

## DAX-1 Mutations

DAX-1[m] is a nuclear receptor protein. Loss of function of this protein causes congenital adrenal hypoplasia (or adrenal hypoplasia congenita, AHC[n]). DAX-1 is considered an "orphan" nuclear receptor because its ligand has not been identified. Moreover, the exact function of the protein is not clear, although studies have suggested that DAX-1 inhibits the function of the sex-determining region on the Y chromosome (SRY). AHC is an X-linked recessive disorder characterized by hypogonadotropic hypogonadism and adrenal hypoplasia or agenesis.

Because AHC is X-linked, it occurs primarily in males. The classic form of AHC often presents within 2 months after birth and includes adrenal insufficiency, hypogonadotropic hypogonadism, and ultimately infertility. AHC may also develop later in childhood and may first be detected when the child presents in Addisonian crisis. A late-onset form of the disease also exists, usually presenting in young adulthood.

## Wolman Disease

A deficiency in lysosomal acid lipase (LAL) causes lysosomal storage disease, a large group of disorders characterized by impaired ability to hydrolyze cholesterol esters in lysosomes. Hydrolysis of the esterified cholesterol is an essential step in the biosynthesis of adrenocortical steroid hormones. Wolman disease[o] (WD) is the severest form of lysosomal storage disease, involving complete loss of LAL activity. In contrast,

patients with the similar disorder, cholesteryl ester storage disease (CESD), also caused by a mutation in the gene coding for LAL, may have up to 12% of residual enzyme activity, and their clinical course is correspondingly milder. Patients with WD typically present within the first few weeks of life with liver fibrosis and elevated aspartate and alanine transaminase enzymes, cirrhosis, hepatomegaly, vomiting, diarrhea, abdominal distention, and failure to thrive. Radiography reveals enlarged, calcified adrenal glands, a feature that is rarely seen in CESD. The distinction between WD and CESD can be made by measuring LAL activity, which is absent in WD but measurable in CESD.

## Kearns-Sayre Syndrome

Kearns-Sayre syndrome[p] (KSS) is a mitochondrial disorder that results from a 1.1 to 10 kilobase deletion from the mitochondrial genome, which normally contains ~16,600 base pairs that encode 37 genes. The most common form of KSS involves deletion of ~5000 base pairs and 12 genes. Since oxidative phosphorylation occurs in the mitochondria, loss of this function affects cellular energy production and is particularly evident in tissues and organs that have high energy requirements, such as the nervous system, skeletal and cardiac muscle, and the endocrine system. The key features of KSS are ophthalmoplegia (paralysis of the eye muscles), retinal pigmentation, and defects in cardiac conduction. Disruption of endocrine function occurs in two-thirds of KSS patients.

## Smith-Lemli-Opitz syndrome

Smith-Lemli-Opitz syndrome[q] (SLOS) is an inherited autosomal recessive disorder caused by a mutation in the gene that codes for 7-dehydrocholesterol reductase (7-DCR; also known as δ-7-dehydrocholesterol reductase, or sterol δ-7-reductase). 7-DCR catalyzes the final step in the biosynthesis of cholesterol, and a deficiency in this enzyme results in the accumulation of its substrate, 7-dehydrocholesterol and its isomer, 8-dehydrocholesterol. The clinical features of SLOS include growth retardation, intellectual disability, behavioral problems, and multiple anatomic malformations such as syndactyly, polydactyly, and microcephaly. Metabolic abnormalities in SLOS include adrenal insufficiency and undervirilization in males due to dihydrotestosterone deficiency in utero.

## Congenital Adrenal Hyperplasia

Congenital adrenal hyperplasia (CAH) is a rare autosomal recessive genetic disorder that affects the production of adrenocortical steroids. In nearly all cases of CAH, there is a deficiency in one of two enzymes: 21-hydroxylase (21H; 95% of cases), and 11β-hydroxylase (11B1H; most of the remaining cases).

---

[m]Abbreviation for "dosage-sensitive sex reversal-adrenal hypoplasia congenita critical region on the X chromosome 1."
[n]CAH customarily refers to congenital adrenal *hyper*plasia.
[o]Moshe Wolman, Israeli neuropathologist: 1914 to 2009.

[p]Thomas P. Kearns (1922 to 2011), George Pomeroy Sayre (1911 to 1992).
[q]David Weyhe Smith (1926 to 1981), Luc Lemli (1935–), and John Marius Opitz (1935–).

## 21-Hydroxylase Deficiency

Referring to Fig. 41.3, 21H converts progesterone to 11-deoxycorticosterone (11-DOC), and 17-hydroxyprogesterone (17-OHP) to 11-deoxycortisol (11-DC). A deficiency in 21H activity, therefore, results in the accumulation of progesterone and 17-OHP, creating an imbalance in adrenocortical steroid products tilted in favor of the adrenal androgens. This imbalance is particularly evident during fetal development when an excess of adrenal androgens can result in virilization of the female fetus and ambiguous genitalia at birth. In a male, 21H deficiency may not be apparent until he undergoes precocious puberty, since the testes are the principal source of androgenic hormones in males.

Expression of 21H deficiency can be variable; the most severe form, "salt-wasting 21H deficiency," results in deficient glucocorticoid and mineralocorticoid activity, and accounts for about half of 21H deficiency cases. These patients are at greatest risk for Addisonian crisis, which typically occurs within the first 2 weeks after birth. The salt-wasting form of CAH usually involves more extensive virilization of both females and males. At the other end of the spectrum, mild ("simple virilizing") 21H deficiency typically produces virilization of females, but mineralocorticoid activity remains sufficient.

CAH due to 21H deficiency is usually diagnosed by measuring 17-OHP, which typically is greater than 1000 ng/dL (30 nmol/L) in these cases (normal newborn 17-OHP: 7 to 77 ng/dL); androstenedione levels in these patients are 5 to 10 times normal. In most developed countries, neonatal screening programs include measurement of 17-OHP.

## 11β-Hydroxylase Deficiency

The second-most common cause of CAH is 11B1H deficiency, comprising approximately 5% of cases. As shown in Fig. 41.3, deficiency in 11B1H affects the conversion of 11-DC to cortisol, resulting in glucocorticoid deficiency. Children and adolescents with 11B1H deficiency often develop hypokalemic hypertension, presumably due to the mineralocorticoid activity of 11-DOC, which is elevated in the disorder. Unlike 21H deficiency, 11B1H CAH usually presents in late childhood or adolescence, although it sometimes presents as ambiguous genitalia and clitoromegaly in female infants.

## Other Causes of Congenital Adrenal Hyperplasia

Very rare causes of CAH include deficiencies in 17α-hydroxylase (17AH), 3β-hydroxysteroid dehydrogenase type 2 (3BHSD), P450 oxidoreductase, and cholesterol side chain cleavage enzyme, all of which are essential for synthesis of adrenocortical steroids. Of these, 17AH deficiency is the most common, accounting for about 1% of CAH. In 17AH deficiency, 17-OHP is decreased, unlike 21H and 11B1H deficiencies, where 17-OHP is elevated. Deoxycortisol is also decreased. Cortisol is low but the patient may be asymptomatic due to the overproduction of corticosterone, which has weak glucocorticoid activity. Since 17AH converts progesterone to 17OHP, a high ratio of progesterone to 17OHP suggests 17AH deficiency.

In the adrenal gland, 3BHSD converts pregnenolone, 17-hydroxypregnenolone, and dehydroepiandrosterone to progesterone, 17-hydroxyprogesterone, and androstenedione, respectively. In 3BHSD deficiency, adrenocortical production of aldosterone, cortisol, and adrenal androgens all are impaired. The prevalence of 3BHSD deficiency is estimated at 1 per million births. Based on the degree to which the enzyme activity is impaired, 3BHSD deficiency has been categorized into three phenotypes: salt-wasting, non-salt-wasting, and non-classic. The salt-wasting phenotype is usually detected shortly after birth, due to hyponatremia, dehydration, and poor feeding. Non-salt-wasting and non-classical phenotypes present with milder symptoms and adequate sodium uptake. Males with 3BHSD deficiency may have hypospadias or ambiguous genitalia because the enzyme is also expressed in the gonads, where it converts androstanediol to testosterone. The non-salt-wasting or non-classical phenotypes in females may go undetected until puberty, when irregular menstruation, premature pubic hair growth, and hirsutism occur; infertility is common. The disorder is characterized by low progesterone, 17-hydroxyprogesterone, and androstenedione.

Most of the enzymes involved in adrenocortical steroid synthesis belong to the cytochrome P450[r] superfamily, so a mutation in the P450 protein affects numerous enzymes. Patients with cytochrome P450 deficiency typically display the features of combined 21-hydroxylase and 17α-hydroxylase deficiency, along with multiple skeletal malformations.

CSCE catalyzes a series of three monooxygenase reactions that convert cholesterol to pregnenolone, the precursor to all steroid hormones. A deficiency in CSCE has a similar presentation to StAR deficiency since both disorders impair the ability to produce pregnenolone, and both cause lipoid CAH, a rare and severe form of CAH. Males with CSCE deficiency present with apparently female external genitalia and may be assigned the female gender at birth. Adrenal failure in these patients occurs within several months after birth.

## Disorders Producing Excess Adrenocortical Hormones

Several disorders exist that are characterized by excess mineralocorticoid or glucocorticoid activity. Some of these disorders involve hormone-secreting tumors, whereas others may be the result of genetic mutations in enzymes that metabolize steroid hormones or the receptors that respond to their activity. In many cases of glucocorticoid excess, the disorder is epiphenomenal to various unrelated physiological factors.

### Mineralocorticoid Excess

*Primary hyperaldosteronism.* Between 10% and 15% of patients with hypertension fulfill the biochemical criteria for primary aldosteronism (PA), characterized by autonomous adrenal overproduction of aldosterone. Aldosterone is regulated by the renin-angiotensin-aldosterone mechanism, so aldosterone excess can occur either from autonomous

---

[r]"P450" refers to the spectrophotometric peak absorption at 450 nm of the enzyme in its reduced state.

over-secretion by the adrenal gland or from overstimulation by renin. Most cases of **hyperaldosteronism** are caused by autonomous secretion of aldosterone by the adrenal cortex. When hyperaldosteronism is caused by excess renin or angiotensin II, it is considered "secondary" hyperaldosteronism. Autonomous hypersecretion of aldosterone may be due to a benign adrenal adenoma, adrenal hyperplasia, or carcinoma. Masses within the adrenal gland are relatively common, and often are an incidental radiographic finding, giving rise to the term "incidentaloma;" these proliferations of adrenocortical tissue have been shown to express aldosterone synthase, and therefore have the capacity to produce aldosterone. However, the exact mechanism by which adrenal tumors acquire the ability to produce aldosterone independently from renin, angiotensin II, or ACTH is not well understood. The clinical symptoms associated with autonomous aldosterone hypersecretion are given the name **Conn syndrome,**[s] which may be used synonymously with "primary aldosteronism," or simply "aldosteronism." In PA, excess mineralocorticoid activity results in sodium retention, volume expansion, hypertension, hypokalemia, and metabolic alkalosis due to renal loss of hydrogen ions.

*Glucocorticoid-remediable aldosteronism.* Expression of aldosterone synthase is normally limited to the zona glomerulosa, thereby restricting aldosterone production to the outermost layer of the adrenal cortex. However, an autosomal dominant trait involving chimeric gene duplication results in the expression of aldosterone synthase in the zona fasciculata, which normally produces only glucocorticoids and adrenal androgens. As a result, AS expression and activity become ACTH-dependent in the zona fasciculata. Glucocorticoid-remediable aldosteronism (GRA) is the most common monogenic cause of hypertension and is characterized by elevated plasma aldosterone in the presence of normal ACTH levels, leading to early onset hypertension and hypokalemia. Treatment involves suppression of ACTH by exogenous glucocorticoid therapy, which can normalize plasma aldosterone levels and resolve hypertension. Suppression of aldosterone by dexamethasone supports the diagnosis of GRA.

*Apparent mineralocorticoid excess.* Normal plasma concentrations of cortisol are 10 to 20 μg/dL (275 to 550 nmol/L), whereas normal plasma aldosterone concentrations are 7 to 30 ng/dL (200 to 800 pmol/L). In addition to being in much higher concentration than aldosterone, cortisol also binds to the MR with affinity equal to aldosterone. As previously noted, aldosterone-sensitive tissues also express 11β-hydroxysteroid dehydrogenase type 2 (HSD2) to convert cortisol to cortisone, which does not bind to the MR. HSD2 deficiency results in overstimulation of the MR by cortisol, producing a clinical picture of hyperaldosteronism, but with low plasma aldosterone concentrations. The classical triad of hypertension, hypokalemia, and suppressed aldosterone and renin usually establishes the diagnosis.

## Glucocorticoid Excess

Excess glucocorticoid production results in **Cushing**[t] **syndrome** (CS), characterized by hypertension, centripetal obesity, striae, "moon-shaped" facies, thoracic kyphosis, acne, hypertrichosis, supraclavicular fat accumulation, weakness, menstrual irregularities and sexual dysfunction, fatigue, headaches, hyperglycemia, and occasionally psychosis. The diagnosis of CS is complicated by the fact that only a few of these signs may be present, and all the signs can be associated with other disorders. Laboratory findings in CS may also produce a confusing diagnostic picture, as some of the hormones involved are secreted episodically. If the syndrome is caused by excess ACTH (secondary hypercortisolism), darkening of the skin can occur due to the melanotropic activity of ACTH. Excess cortisol production can also produce symptoms of mineralocorticoid excess (hypokalemia, metabolic alkalosis, and hypertension) due to activity of cortisol at the MR, which is normally suppressed by HSD2 conversion of cortisol to cortisone but can be saturated by excess cortisol. Prolonged elevations in cortisol can result in immunosuppression, protein catabolism, central redistribution of fat, and insulin resistance, all of which are also characteristic of metabolic syndrome.

*Classification of disorders producing glucocorticoid excess.* Glucocorticoid excess may be primary, due to autonomous production of cortisol by the adrenal cortex or cortisol-secreting tumor, or secondary, caused by overstimulation of the adrenal cortex by excess ACTH. These two disorders are also called "ACTH-independent hypercortisolism" and "ACTH-dependent hypercortisolism," respectively. A distinction can also be made between "exogenous" (or "iatrogenic") and "endogenous" CS, based on whether the source of excess hormone is pharmaceutical or adrenal. The most common cause of CS is treatment with corticosteroids for their anti-inflammatory and immunosuppressive effects. Therapeutic use of corticosteroids is relatively common, so exogenous CS should be ruled out before considering adrenal abnormalities.

Endogenous CS is a rare disorder, with an incidence of just a few dozen cases per million per year. ACTH-dependent CS accounts for over 80% of cases, and approximately 80% of those are due to an ACTH-secreting pituitary adenoma, properly referred to as "Cushing disease" (CD). Cushing disease produces the clinical picture of CS, but CS has causes other than Cushing disease. Most of the remaining cases of endogenous ACTH-dependent CS are caused by nonpituitary (ectopic) ACTH-producing tumors, and rarely by CRH-producing tumors. ACTH-independent CS is most often caused by a unilateral adrenal tumor, of which 80% are adenomas and the remainder are adrenocortical carcinomas.

*Pseudo-Cushing syndrome.* Whether ACTH-dependent or ACTH-independent, endogenous CS is a neoplastic disorder, its various causes differing only in the type and location of the functioning tumor. However, there are many physiological stimuli for cortisol secretion. The Cushing-like

[s]Jerome W. Conn (1907 to 1994), an American endocrinologist, first described primary hyperaldosteronism in 1955.

[t]Harvey Williams Cushing (1869 to 1939), American neurosurgeon and pathologist.

symptoms produced in the absence of a neoplastic source of hormone are variously called "pseudo-Cushing syndrome," "non-neoplastic hypercortisolism," or "physiologic hypercortisolism." Common non-neoplastic causes of hypercortisolism include ethanol abuse, depression, obesity, type 2 diabetes, polycystic ovary syndrome, chronic kidney disease, anorexia nervosa, intense chronic exercise, and multiple sclerosis. The presence of pseudo-CS can complicate the diagnosis of true ACTH-dependent CS since mild disease can present with laboratory findings similar to metabolic syndrome.

*Cushing disease.* An ACTH-secreting pituitary corticotroph adenoma is the clinical definition of CD, causing endogenous ACTH-dependent (secondary) hypercortisolism and CS. Cushing disease is the most common endogenous cause of CS and women are nine times more likely than men to have the disease. Corticotrophic adenomas comprise about 10% of all pituitary adenomas (prolactinomas are the most common pituitary adenoma). About half of CD cases involve a pituitary microadenoma smaller than 5 mm in diameter, which may be too small to detect with imaging studies. Therefore, diagnosis of CD often relies on biochemical evidence. Constant stimulation by excess ACTH results in bilateral adrenocortical hyperplasia. Ordinarily, hypercortisolism suppresses ACTH secretion, but CD is characterized by inappropriately high ACTH in the presence of elevated plasma cortisol. Cushing disease can be treated surgically, with radiotherapy, or chemically with steroidogenesis inhibitors, GR antagonists, or tumor suppressor agents.

*Ectopic adrenocorticotropic hormone syndrome.* In about 20% of endogenous ACTH-dependent CS cases, the source of excess ACTH is not the pituitary, but instead comes from a nonpituitary tumor, producing "ectopic ATCH syndrome," or EAS. The most common tumors causing EAS are small cell carcinomas of the lung or pulmonary carcinoid tumors, but EAS has also been associated with pancreatic and thymic neuroendocrine tumors, gastrinomas, medullary thyroid cancer, and pheochromocytoma.

*Secondary hypercortisolism due to corticotropin-releasing hormone excess.* Endogenous ACTH-dependent CS due to excess CRH is extremely rare and usually arises from lung, thymic, pancreatic, or medullary thyroid carcinomas. Most CRH-secreting ectopic tumors also secrete ACTH.

*Primary endogenous hypercortisolism.* Primary endogenous hypercortisolism, or ACTH-independent CS, is most often caused by a cortisol-secreting tumor in the adrenal cortex. The most common adrenal tumor is adenoma; cortisol-secreting and aldosterone-secreting adenomas are indistinguishable grossly and microscopically. In primary endogenous hypercortisolism, CRH and ACTH are suppressed by autonomously produced cortisol.

*Primary pigmented nodular adrenocortical disease.* A rare cause of ACTH-independent CS results from mutations in several genes associated with cAMP-PKA signaling and is characterized by multiple pigmented adrenocortical micronodules less than 10 mm in diameter. Primary pigmented nodular adrenocortical disease (PPNAD) is most often

associated with Carney syndrome,[u] an autosomal dominant mutation in a tumor suppressor gene that predisposes affected individuals to development of adrenal tumors. Patients with PPNAD have elevated cortisol levels that are not suppressed by dexamethasone.

*Primary bilateral macronodular hyperplasia.* At least 2% of endogenous ACTH-independent CS is associated with primary bilateral macronodular hyperplasia (PBMAH), which presents with multiple benign adrenal nodules up to 4 cm in diameter. Several gene mutations have been identified in PBMAH patients. PBMAH is characterized by abnormal expression of G-protein-coupled receptors in certain adrenocortical cells, imparting sensitivity to multiple hormones, including vasopressin, luteinizing hormone, serotonin, and gastric inhibitory peptide.

---

**AT A GLANCE**

**Cushing Syndrome**
- Symptoms and physical characteristics that result from overexposure to glucocorticoids
- Most common cause is exogenous (pharmaceutical) glucocorticoids
- Endogenous CS is caused by a hormone-secreting tumor
- Cushing disease is an ACTH-secreting pituitary adenoma
- CS can be difficult to diagnose because many of its symptoms are nonspecific

---

## LABORATORY INVESTIGATION OF ADRENOCORTICAL DYSFUNCTION

Determining the cause of endocrine disorders is often challenging because multiple pathologies can produce similar clinical and biochemical results. For example, glucocorticoid deficiency may occur due to the inability of the adrenal cortex to produce cortisol, failure of the anterior pituitary to produce ACTH, inadequate CRH release by the hypothalamus, or peripheral GRs that do not respond properly to cortisol. Likewise, deficient mineralocorticoid activity may be the result of impaired aldosterone synthesis, insufficient renin response to hypotension, or MR resistance to aldosterone.

An additional complication in diagnosing adrenal disorders is that the concentrations of various adrenal hormones are dynamic, so the timing of the blood collection is important. Also, long-term exposure to elevated adrenal hormone concentrations may result in decreased sensitivity to hormonal stimulation—that is, a "blunted" response—which can produce normal test results in the presence of adrenal dysfunction.

This section will describe various laboratory tests used to diagnose adrenal disorders, which will be divided into two broad categories: adrenal insufficiency, and adrenal

---

[u]J. Aidan Carney (1934-), Irish pathologist. He also described "Carney's triad," a different phenomenon related to the coexistence of three types of tumors, primarily in women.

hyperactivity. Some of the laboratory tests are used in one or the other clinical scenario, whereas a few of the tests might be used in both insufficiency and hyperactivity scenarios. Overall, the diagnostic strategy should systematically eliminate potential causes of endocrine dysfunction until the exact pathologic defect is identified. To investigate disturbances in adrenocortical hormones, multiple diagnostic tests are often required.

## Investigation of Adrenal Insufficiency (Addison Disease)

### Plasma Cortisol

Normally, cortisol is produced by the zona fasciculata in a diurnal circadian pulsatile rhythm,[v] with highest concentrations upon waking (in the morning, if the sleep-wake cycle is traditional), and lowest concentrations in the late evening. Cortisol also varies throughout the day, so random plasma cortisol levels are not useful. A morning plasma cortisol concentration less than 5 µg/dL (<140 nmol/L) is considered presumptive evidence of cortisol deficiency. Since cortisol production is a normal response to stress, a plasma cortisol of less than 5 µg/dL (<140 nmol/L) at a time of stress is also considered presumptive for cortisol deficiency regardless of the time of day. Conversely, plasma cortisol levels greater than 18 to 20 µg/dL (500 to 550 nmol/L) at any time essentially rule out glucocorticoid deficiency.

In circulation, about 70% of cortisol is bound to CBG, and another 20% is bound to albumin, so the total concentration of cortisol in plasma can vary with the CBG and albumin concentrations. Therefore, disorders that affect plasma proteins, such as impaired liver function, malnutrition, or nephrotic syndrome will influence the total cortisol level in plasma. An alternative is to measure the free concentration of cortisol, which directly reflects glucocorticoid activity since the bound fraction is hormonally inert. Two approaches to measuring the free cortisol fraction have been used: urine cortisol and saliva cortisol.

### Adrenocorticotropic Hormone

In theory, measuring plasma ACTH should distinguish between primary and secondary adrenal failure, based on whether the hormone concentration is increased or decreased, respectively. In practice, however, plasma ACTH levels are usually non-diagnostic, primarily because the hormone is labile and plasma concentrations vary throughout the day due to the diurnal pulsatility of the hypothalamic-pituitary-adrenal axis. ACTH is most often measured in conjunction with various stimulation tests, described below.

### Cosyntropin Stimulation Tests

To determine whether the adrenal cortex is able to respond appropriately to ACTH stimulation, a synthetic derivative of the hormone is administered, and the cortisol response is monitored. ACTH is a 39 amino acid oligopeptide, but the active domain is in the N-terminal 24 amino acid sequence which, when synthesized, is known by the generic names tetracosactide (or tetracosactrin) or cosyntropin, and has the trade names Cortrosyn and Synacthen (not available in the United States). In the literature and elsewhere, all these names are used to identify the synthetic ACTH analog; for simplicity, this chapter will always refer to it as cosyntropin.

In one variation of the cosyntropin stimulation test, 250 µg of cosyntropin is administered either intramuscularly or intravenously, and blood is collected 30 and 60 minutes after injection, along with a baseline blood specimen collected before injection of cosyntropin. Peak plasma cortisol less than 18 µg/dL (500 nmol/L), and/or a change from baseline plasma cortisol of less than 7 to 10 µg/dL (100 to 275 nmol/L) is consistent with primary adrenocortical failure. This approach is sometimes called the "short (or 1 hour) high-dose cosyntropin stimulation test."

A criticism of the high-dose cosyntropin stimulation test is that the dose of cosyntropin is supra-pharmacologic. Exposure to high levels of ACTH as simulated in the high-dose cosyntropin test may stimulate the adrenal cortex to produce cortisol when, at physiologic ACTH concentrations, the response remains inadequate; therefore, the test lacks sensitivity for impaired adrenocortical function. A low-dose modification of the cosyntropin stimulation tests involves administration of 1 µg of cosyntropin to more closely mimic physiological ACTH concentrations. This approach has greater sensitivity for mild adrenal insufficiency. Studies comparing the two approaches to cosyntropin stimulation have determined, however, that there is little difference in their diagnostic accuracies.

Another variation of the cosyntropin stimulation test prolongs the duration of stimulation to 8 hours, 2 days, or even 3 to 5 days. Based on the possibility that chronic deficiency in ACTH stimulation results in adrenocortical atrophy requiring sustained ACTH stimulation to reverse, the long-term cosyntropin stimulation tests maintain cosyntropin infusion over a period of hours to days, and cortisol production is assessed by measuring plasma cortisol levels and, in the case of 2, 3, or 5 day stimulation, 24 hour urine collections. Failure of plasma cortisol to exceed 18 to 20 µg/dL (500 to 550 nmol/L), or a three-fold increase in the urinary free cortisol excretion, confirms primary adrenal insufficiency.

### Corticotropin-Releasing Hormone Stimulation Test

Inadequate production and release of ACTH can be the result of anterior pituitary failure, or due to insufficient CRH production by the hypothalamus (tertiary adrenal insufficiency). The most common cause of CRH deficiency is chronic corticosteroid therapy, which suppresses the entire hypothalamic-pituitary-adrenal axis. Rapid withdrawal of exogenous glucocorticoids without a gradual taper that facilitates a

[v]A "circadian" rhythm refers to pulsatile patterns that recur on a 24-hour cycle; "diurnal" means "of or during the day." Hence a pulsatile pattern that is diurnal, is not necessarily circadian. For cortisol, it has been shown that the 24-hour cycle is superimposed on an ultradian rhythm of approximately 90 minutes.

corresponding increase in endogenous synthesis results in transient glucocorticoid deficiency. Tumors or infiltrative disease that occlude the infundibular stalk also cause tertiary adrenal insufficiency by preventing hypothalamic CRH from reaching the pituitary. Isolated CRH deficiency is very rare. In the CRH stimulation test, after collecting a baseline plasma specimen, 1 μg/kg of ovine CRH is administered intravenously and blood is collected at 15, 30, and 60 (and sometimes 120) minutes after CRH administration. An increase in plasma ACTH suggests CRH deficiency.

### Insulin-Induced Hypoglycemia Test

Hypoglycemia is a powerful stimulus for cortisol release, and therefore producing a hypoglycemic state by administering insulin is a sensitive test to assess the adequacy of the hypothalamic-pituitary-adrenal axis in a patient suspected of having CS. Specific protocols vary, but one published method involves administration of 0.15 units of insulin per kg body weight and measuring plasma ACTH and cortisol at 5- to 15-minute intervals. Plasma glucose was suppressed to less than 29 mg/dL (1.6 mmol/L). ACTH concentrations peaked at an average of 323 pg/mL (71 pmol/L), and the average peak cortisol concentration was 21 μg/dL (584 nmol/L).

Although the insulin-induced hypoglycemia test is considered the gold standard for diagnosis of secondary adrenal insufficiency, the procedure involves risk of severe hypoglycemia, and should only be performed in a hospital setting where the patient's condition can be continuously monitored and intravenous glucose can be administered immediately if the patient's condition deteriorates.

### Metyrapone Stimulation Test

A safer alternative to the insulin-induced hypoglycemia test involves administration of metyrapone, which blocks cortisol production by inhibiting 11B1H. Response to an overnight metyrapone challenge is assessed by measuring plasma 11-deoxycortisol, the substrate for 11B1H. If the hypocortisolism caused by metyrapone inhibition of 11B1H induces the appropriate hypothalamic and pituitary response, 11-deoxycortisol will be produced in excess.

Metyrapone is occasionally used to treat CS.

### Investigation of Adrenal Hyperactivity (Cushing Syndrome/Conn Syndrome)
#### 24-Hour Urine Cortisol

The most accurate measure of cortisol status is a 24-hour urine cortisol (sometimes called urinary free cortisol). The 24 hour urine cortisol has two advantages: (1) it measures the cortisol released over a 24 hour period, so circadian and ultradian variations are averaged over the entire 24 hour period, and (2) only the free cortisol is measured (assuming normal renal function) because the bound fraction is not filtered in the glomerulus; variations in CBG and/or albumin are of no consequence. Normal 24-hour urinary free cortisol is 20 to 90 μg/24 h (55 to 248 nmol/24 h). The drawbacks to 24-hour urine collections are an inconvenience to the patient and imprecision in the duration of urine collection.

### Salivary Cortisol

Measuring cortisol in saliva has gained popularity as a means for evaluating cortisol status. This approach has two advantages: (1) cortisol in the saliva mostly reflects the unbound cortisol in blood, and (2) devices are available that the patient can take home to collect saliva at a specific time, such as upon waking in the morning or before bedtime at night, when plasma cortisol is at its peak or nadir, respectively. Normal salivary cortisol is 1.4 to 10.1 μg/dL (40 to 280 nmol/L) at 7 a.m., and 0.7 to 2.2 μg/dL (20 to 60 nmol/L) at 10 p.m.

There are methods available to measure free cortisol in plasma, either by filtration or equilibrium dialysis, but these methods are uncommon.

### Dexamethasone Suppression Test

Dexamethasone is a synthetic fluorinated cortisol derivative that has 50 to 150 times the glucocorticoid activity of cortisol and is used therapeutically to treat inflammatory and autoimmune disorders. Non-therapeutic administration of dexamethasone as a diagnostic test (dexamethasone suppression test, DST) is intended to mimic the action of cortisol, to determine whether the hypothalamus and pituitary respond appropriately to increased glucocorticoid activity by suppressing CRH, ACTH, and ultimately cortisol secretion. Dexamethasone is used rather than cortisol because only very small doses are required due to its high glucocorticoid activity, and the endogenous cortisol response can be measured because immunoassays for cortisol do not cross-react with dexamethasone. An appropriate response to dexamethasone suppression is low cortisol, whereas failure to suppress cortisol is consistent with CS.

In the standard protocol, 1 mg of dexamethasone (or 0.3 mg/m² body surface area in children) is administered orally at 10 p.m. At 8 a.m. the following morning, a blood specimen is collected for plasma cortisol; a result less than 1.8 μg/dL (<50 nmol/L) is a normal response, indicating appropriate suppression of cortisol by the exogenous glucocorticoid. Plasma cortisol after overnight dexamethasone suppression greater than 1.8 μg/dL (>50 nmol/L) is consistent with CS. False-positive results of the standard overnight DST (failure to suppress a.m. cortisol) are uncommon but can result from failure to take the dexamethasone, enhanced dexamethasone metabolism,[w] or episodic variations in ACTH secretion. False-negative results may occur if dexamethasone metabolism is inhibited. A "low-dose" variation of the overnight DST uses 0.25 mg of dexamethasone rather than the standard 1 mg dose. Another variation of the DST involves administration of dexamethasone (0.5 mg orally) every 6 hours for 2 or 3 days, followed by stimulation with CRH.

Patients whose 8 a.m. cortisol is not suppressed following overnight dexamethasone administration are candidates for the high-dose suppression test to determine the mechanism

---

[w]Dexamethasone is metabolized by the cytochrome P450 oxidase, which is involved in the oxidative metabolism of many drugs and can be induced by certain drugs. Therefore, interferences with dexamethasone metabolism are common.

responsible for cortisol excess. Following collection of a baseline 24-hour urine specimen for UFC measurement on day 1 in the absence of dexamethasone suppression, patients are administered 2 mg dexamethasone every 6 hours for 48 hours on days 2 and 3 and 24-hour urine specimens are collected for measurement of UFC on both days. Decreased 24-hour UFC on days 2 and 3 (high-dose dexamethasone) indicates an ACTH-producing pituitary adenoma (Cushing disease) as the likely cause of cortisol excess, while a failure to suppress indicates either an ectopic ACTH-producing tumor or an adrenal cortisol-producing tumor.

### Desmopressin Stimulation Test

Vasopressin (or antidiuretic hormone, ADH) binds to several types of arginine vasopressin receptors (AVR) distributed widely throughout the body. A synthetic analogue of vasopressin, desmopressin,[x] is a vasopressin analogue that does not normally stimulate ACTH secretion. However, corticotroph adenomas are often responsive to desmopressin, and it, therefore, stimulates ACTH and cortisol secretion in most Cushing disease patients.

In a typical desmopressin stimulation test, 10 μg of the drug is administered intravenously, and plasma ACTH and cortisol are measured at several intervals up to 60 minutes. A peak plasma ACTH concentration in response to desmopressin stimulation greater than 27 pg/mL (6 pmol/L) is 75-87% sensitive, and 90% to 91% specific for Cushing disease.

### Bilateral Inferior Petrosal Sampling

A modification of CRH stimulation involves bilateral inferior petrosal venous sinus sampling (BIPSS) and is used to confirm a radiographically undetectable pituitary adenoma. In the BIPSS procedure, bilateral femoral vein catheters are inserted and terminate in each of the inferior petrosal sinuses; a third catheter is used to sample peripheral blood from the inferior vena cava. Stimulation with 100 μg of intravenous CRH should result in prompt release of ACTH into the petrosal sinuses by the pituitary, whereas peripheral ACTH will remain relatively unchanged. A petrosal sinus to peripheral ACTH ratio of greater than three following stimulation is diagnostic for a pituitary microadenoma. An ectopic ACTH-producing tumor, on the other hand, suppresses pituitary ACTH, and the response to CRH is therefore muted. The BIPSS procedure has the advantage of localizing the lateral location of the tumor, providing some guidance to surgical excision.

### Aldosterone and Renin

Since PA is a relatively common cause of hypertension, patients with hypertension (particularly those with drug-resistant hypertension) should be screened for PA, which is characterized by autonomous aldosterone production. Aldosterone has a half-life of 20 minutes, so random plasma aldosterone measurements are of little diagnostic value. Renin stimulates aldosterone secretion and has a similarly short half-life. However, since renin stimulates aldosterone production, changes in renin and aldosterone concentrations in plasma should reflect each other. Therefore, aldosterone is usually measured and reported as its ratio to renin concentration or activity. The upper threshold for a normal plasma aldosterone to renin ratio (ARR) is usually set somewhere between 20 and 40, depending on the assays used. Perhaps because of the rapid changes in both aldosterone and renin concentrations, the ARR suffers from a high rate of false positive results, although it is quite sensitive for PA. Therefore, ARR should be considered only a screening test for PA. Several confirmatory tests for PA are available, mostly involving measurement of the aldosterone/renin response to salt loading, either oral or by saline infusion, or fludrocortisone suppression, discussed below.

### Fludrocortisone Suppression Test

Fludrocortisone is a pharmaceutical corticosteroid used to treat salt-wasting adrenal insufficiency due to its potent mineralocorticoid activity; it also has significant glucocorticoid activity, but not clinically relevant in the doses given. In subjects with normal adrenal function, fludrocortisone suppresses plasma aldosterone. In patients with PA, aldosterone is not suppressed. Usually considered the most reliable confirmatory test for PA, fludrocortisone suppression has been compared to saline infusion and captopril challenge tests in several studies, and the finding was that all three tests have similar diagnostic accuracy.

### Saline Loading Tests

Subjects with normal adrenal function respond to increased sodium by suppressing aldosterone secretion. To assess a patient's response to increased sodium, salt can be administered either orally (oral sodium loading test) or intravenously (saline infusion test). In both cases, following the sodium challenge, plasma or urinary aldosterone is measured to determine the adrenal response to hypernatremia. The concentration (or daily excretion) thresholds for a positive result vary from one protocol to another.

### Captopril Challenge Test

Captopril inhibits ACE, reducing the ability of the enzyme to convert inactive angiotensin I to its active form, angiotensin II. Angiotensin II is the primary stimulus for aldosterone secretion, so administration of captopril normally reduces plasma or urine aldosterone. Patients with PA produce aldosterone autonomously, so their aldosterone production and secretion are unaffected by **ACE inhibitors**. Losartan, an angiotensin II receptor blocker also used to treat hypertension, has been suggested as an alternative to captopril in a protocol to assess aldosterone response to a pharmaceutical block in the renin-angiotensin-aldosterone pathway, with sensitivity and specificity comparable to the captopril challenge test.

---

[x]Desmopressin is a modified form of vasopressin (Cys-Tyr-Phe-Gln-Asn-Cys-Pro-Arg-Gly-NH$_2$), in which the C-terminal Cys is deaminated and the $d$-Arg is substituted for $l$-Arg in position 8, and is marketed under the trade name DDAVP. Pharmaceutically, desmopressin is used to treat diabetes insipidus and nighttime bedwetting in children.

## Furosemide Stimulation Test

Furosemide inhibits the sodium-potassium-chloride cotransporter in the thick ascending loop of Henle, resulting in urinary excretion of the three ions, thereby promoting diuresis, or excessive urine production.[y] Diuretics are used to treat hypertension by decreasing blood volume. Therefore, a normal response to diuresis is the release of renin from the juxtaglomerular apparatus leading to aldosterone secretion and sodium and water reabsorption. In the furosemide stimulation test, the patient is in the supine position for 30 minutes prior to the test. Following collection of a baseline blood specimen, 40 to 80 mg of furosemide is administered intravenously, and the patient maintains upright posture for 2 hours, after which blood is collected again, and the plasma renin activity (PRA) (or concentration) is measured in baseline and post-challenge specimens. The threshold for a positive result depends on the specific protocol, but typically a PRA of greater than 2 ng/mL/h is consistent with PA, because of renin suppression by chronically high aldosterone levels.

## Adrenal Vein Sampling

Adrenal tumors are rarely malignant, and the majority are non-secreting and unilateral. Aldosterone-secreting bilateral adrenal tumors can be treated pharmacologically with MR antagonists, but for unilateral aldosterone-secreting adrenal tumors, surgical adrenalectomy is the most effective treatment. When the adrenal tumor is small, radiological detection and localization is not always reliable to determine which of the adrenal glands is affected. Also, radiography cannot detect secretory activity in any sized tumor. Adrenal vein sampling (AVS) is a diagnostic procedure to determine which adrenal gland is hypersecreting aldosterone.

In the AVS procedure, catheters are introduced into the femoral veins, and under fluoroscopic guidance, are positioned in the left and right adrenal veins.[z] A third cannula is placed in a peripheral vein for reference. Blood specimens are collected from all three sites before, and 30 minutes after a bolus of 0.25 mg cosyntropin is administered, to stimulate adrenal production of aldosterone. Typically, the aldosterone to cortisol ratio is measured in each specimen; dissymmetry between the left and right adrenal vein specimens helps determine the location of the active tumor. The AVS procedure lacks standardization, and therefore it is difficult to compare the predictive value of results from one center to another.

## Analytical Methods

Assessment of adrenal function requires measurement of adrenocortical hormones, such as cortisol, aldosterone, androstenedione, and DHEAS, along with several intermediates in

their synthetic pathways. In addition, non-adrenal hormones, such as ACTH, CRH, and renin measurements can help isolate the cause of adrenal insufficiency or excess. Measurement of corticotropin-binding globulin (transcortin) occasionally is useful. Analytical methods for all these analytes have been available for decades, but many of the methods are slowly making a transition from primarily immunochemical assays to more sensitive and specific mass spectrometric assays.

### Immunoassay

All the major in vitro diagnostics manufacturers offer immunoassays for cortisol, aldosterone, DHEAS, and ACTH, which are the most commonly measured hormones associated with adrenal function. Androstenedione, 17-hydroxyprogesterone, and testosterone methods are also available on many automated immunoassay platforms. However, there are two principal limitations of immunoassays: (1) antibody specificity is not absolute and therefore the potential exists for cross-reactivity with other components in the specimen, and (2) immunoassays are quite susceptible to non-antigenic (or non-competitive) interferences.

Regarding the first limitation, adrenal steroids are particularly vulnerable because so many adrenal steroid hormones and intermediates differ from one another only by minor chemical modifications. Even if the degree of cross-reactivity is minimal, the magnitude of interference may be significant if the concentration of the interfering steroid greatly exceeds the concentration of the steroid being measured. Designing and producing immunoassays for adrenal steroids that do not cross-react with unintended antigens is technically challenging.

Non-competitive sources of immunoassay interference include heterophilic antibodies, endogenous enzyme inhibitors (which may interfere with measurement of enzyme labels), compounds that interfere with spectrophotometric measurements, or constituents that interfere with linkage proteins used to capture antibody-antigen complexes.

*Adrenal steroids.* Immunoassays are available for measuring cortisol on most automated chemistry analyzers. Automated assays for measuring plasma aldosterone are also available, although less common. Many cortisol immunoassays can measure the hormone in plasma, urine, or saliva. Interferences in various cortisol immunoassays have been reported from EDTA, biotin, hypergammaglobulinemia, heterophilic antibodies, and cortisol metabolites such as cortisone. Potential interferences in aldosterone immunoassays include the carbon-3 glucuronidated metabolite of aldosterone, which is elevated in renal failure. Interference from the glucuronidated metabolite can be eliminated by solvent extraction into dichloromethane since the glucuronidated metabolite is hydrophilic.

*Renin.* Renin is an aspartic protease produced by the pericytes in the afferent arterioles of the juxtaglomerular apparatus in the kidney from a precursor protein, prorenin. Circulating concentrations of prorenin can be 100-fold greater than the concentration of renin, although a 10:1 ratio of prorenin to renin is more common. As a result, even minimal cross-reactivity of prorenin with renin antibodies used

---

[y]This should not be confused with the furosemide stress test, which is used to evaluate acute kidney injury. The furosemide stimulation (or upright) test is recommended by the Japan Hypertension Society, and its use worldwide is limited.

[z]The right and left adrenal veins are not anatomically symmetric; the right adrenal vein is shorter and smaller than the left adrenal vein and is therefore much more difficult to locate and cannulate.

in immunoassays to measure renin can be significant. Assays that determine renin activity (usually abbreviated PRA, for plasma renin activity) by measuring the amount of angiotensin I it produces from angiotensinogen have been available for decades. More recently, immunoassays to measure the absolute amount of renin in plasma have been introduced. Each approach has advantages and disadvantages.

PRA measurements provide an indication of the biologically active fraction of renin in the specimen. However, PRA methods are difficult to standardize. Two basic approaches have been used to measure renin activity. In the classic PRA method, inhibitors of angiotensinase and ACE are first added to prevent the conversion of angiotensin I to angiotensin II (some methods "trap" angiotensin I with an antibody to prevent its conversion to angiotensin II), and then the specimen is incubated at 37°C, and the concentration of angiotensin I is measured. The rate of the reaction is influenced by pH, incubation time, and, importantly, the endogenous angiotensinogen concentration in the specimen, which can be increased in pregnancy, glucocorticoid excess, and estrogen administration. Because the angiotensinogen concentration in blood does not ordinarily exceed the $K_m$ for the renin-angiotensinogen complex, its concentration is rate limiting. Therefore, the classic PRA method produces results that vary significantly depending on the concentration of angiotensinogen. A second approach to measuring PRA uses exogenous angiotensinogen as substrate and thereby avoids the variability associated with endogenous angiotensinogen. These PRA methods add sheep-derived angiotensinogen to the specimen at a concentration that is several times the $K_m$ for the renin-angiotensinogen complex, ensuring the reaction rate is limited by renin activity alone. The advantage of using a consistent source of angiotensinogen is that the activity assays can be calibrated against renin reference materials.

An additional variable in PRA methods occurs because, in plasma, prorenin exists in two forms, depending on whether the 46 amino acid "pro" segment is in an open or closed conformation. In the open conformation, the active site of the enzyme is exposed, so this form is enzymatically active. Only about 2% of circulating prorenin is in the open conformation, but assay conditions such as cooling and low pH can cause the closed conformation of prorenin to open, which results in an overestimate of physiologic renin activity. Incubation of plasma at 22°C for 24 hours reversibly activates (unfolds) approximately 5% of prorenin, although incubation at 37°C promotes refolding of the "pro" segment to its closed form. In some assays, the closed prorenin is deliberately opened by acidification to pH 3.3 or incubation with trypsin, which removes the "pro" segment from prorenin altogether. These assays measure total renin and prorenin activity by activating all the prorenin, followed by a standard PRA assay. PRA assays are also susceptible to interference from antihypertensive drugs that inhibit renin activity.

Immunoassays for measuring the plasma renin concentration (PRC, sometimes called a "direct plasma renin test") have been available since the mid-1980s, but many of the earlier methods cross-reacted with closed and/or open prorenin. Modern renin immunoassays usually use two antibodies and chemiluminescent labels, and these assays have greater specificity for renin. One such assay involves a biotinylated capture antibody (which recognizes both renin and prorenin) immobilized to streptavidin-coated magnetic particles, and an acridinium ester–labeled signal antibody that recognizes only renin. Results of PRC immunoassays, expressed in mIU/L, correlate well with PRA results expressed in ng/mL/h, but PRC assays tend to display better inter-laboratory agreement compared to PRA methods.

Since renin indirectly stimulates aldosterone production, the ARR is typically reported so the aldosterone concentration can be interpreted in the context of renin activity or concentration.

*Adrenocorticotropic hormone.* In specimens collected at 8 a.m., normal plasma concentrations of ACTH are between 10 and 60 pg/mL (2.2 to 13.3 pmol/L). There are several commercially available immunoassays for measuring ACTH; most are two-site methods with chemiluminescent detection. ACTH is produced from a pro-hormone, pro-opiomelanocortin, which contains the entire ACTH amino acid sequence and therefore is likely to be recognized by anti-ACTH antibodies. Mass spectrometry-based analytical methods for measuring ACTH offer superior specificity.

## Mass Spectrometry

*Adrenal steroids.* LC/MS-MS methods have been described for measuring all the relevant adrenocortical steroids. Unlike immunoassays, which are designed to detect one specific adrenal androgen, LC/MS-MS can measure multiple steroids in a single analytical run because the steroids are chromatographically separated prior to measurement by tandem mass spectrometry. LC/MS-MS methods have superior precision and sensitivity when compared to immunoassays, although LC/MS-MS quantitative results may not agree with the results of immunoassays due to cross-reactivity that occurs in the latter.

*Renin and angiotensin.* Mass spectrometric measurement of proteins often requires specially adapted instruments to volatilize the large protein molecules,[aa] but oligopeptides are within the capabilities of conventional LC/MS-MS technology. Therefore, PRC is usually measured with immunoassay, but PRA methods may use mass spectrometry to measure the angiotensin products of renin activity.

*Adrenocorticotropic hormone.* Although ACTH is a 39-residue polypeptide with a molecular weight of 4540 daltons, which is quite large for LC/MS-MS applications, methods are available to measure the active form of ACTH by LC/MS-MS. Mass spectrometry has been used to resolve discrepancies between the ACTH concentrations measured by various immunoassays.

---

[aa]Matrix-assisted laser desorption ionization/time-of-flight (MALDI-TOF) mass spectrometry is commonly adapted to measure proteins.

## SUMMARY

The adrenal cortex is the source of steroid hormones classified as mineralocorticoids, glucocorticoids, and adrenal androgens. Diseases of adrenocortical origin can result in excess or deficiency of any of the steroids. Deficiencies of adrenocortical steroids are usually the result of autoimmune processes, infectious disease, or neoplastic destruction of the adrenal gland but genetic mutations that affect the activity of enzymes involved in synthesis of the adrenocortical steroids also cause adrenal insufficiency. Adrenocortical hormone excess usually is the result of functional neoplasms that may arise in the adrenal cortex, the pituitary, or ectopic locations. Because adrenal steroid hormones are under physiological regulation that is often multifactorial, laboratory diagnosis of adrenal diseases can be complex, involving stimulation or suppression of various components in the regulatory mechanism, to determine whether the adrenal response is appropriate. Historically, immunoassays have been most widely used to quantitate steroid hormones, but these are being replaced by analytical methods based on liquid chromatography and tandem mass spectrometry, which offers the advantages of higher specificity, lower detection limits, and greater flexibility to measure multiple hormones in a single process.

## LIST OF ABBREVIATIONS

7-DCR: 7-Dehydrocholesterol reductase
11-DOC: 11-Deoxycortisol
11-KT: 11-Ketotestosterone
17-OHP: 17-Hydroxyprogesterone
AAD: Autoimmune Addison disease
ACA: Adrenal cortex autoantibodies
ACTH: Adrenocorticotropic hormone (corticotropin)
AD: Addison disease
ADH: Antidiuretic hormone
AHC: Adrenal hypoplasia congenita
AITD: Autoimmune thyroid disease
ALD: Adrenoleukodystrophy
ALDP: Adrenoleukodystrophy protein
AMN: Adrenomyeloneuropathy

APS: Autoimmune polyendocrine syndrome
ARR: Aldosterone-renin ratio
BIPSS: Bilateral inferior petrosal sinus sampling
CAH: Congenital adrenal hyperplasia
CBG: Cortisol-binding globulin
CD: Cushing disease
CESD: Cholesterol ester storage disease
CRH: Corticotropin-releasing hormone
CS: Cushing syndrome
DAX-1: Dosage-sensitive sex reversal, adrenal hypoplasia critical region, on chromosome X, gene 1
DHEA: Dehydroepiandrosterone
DHEAS: Dehydroepiandrosterone sulfate
DOC: Deoxycorticosterone
DST: Dexamethasone suppression test
EAS: Ectopic ACTH syndrome
GIP: Gastric inhibitory peptide
GR: Glucocorticoid receptor
GRA: Glucocorticoid-remediable aldosteronism
GRS: Glucocorticoid resistance syndrome
KSS: Kearns-Sayre syndrome
LAL: Lysosomal acid lipase
LC-MS/MS: Liquid chromatography-tandem mass spectrometry
MAPK: Mitogen-activated protein kinase
MEN: Multiple endocrine neoplasia
MRAP: Melanocortin receptor accessory protein
MSH: Melanocyte-stimulating hormone
PBMAH: Primary bilateral macronodular adrenal hyperplasia
PHA: Pseudohypoaldosteronism
PPNAD: Primary pigmented nodular adrenocortical disease
PRA: Plasma renin activity
SF-1: Steroidogenic factor 1
SHBG: Sex hormone binding globulin
SLE: Systemic lupus erythematosus
SLOS: Smith-Lemli-Opitz syndrome
StAR: Steroidogenic acute regulatory protein
UFC: Urinary free cortisol
VLCFA: Very long-chain fatty acids
WD: Wolman disease
ZSD: Zellweger spectrum disorder

## REVIEW QUESTIONS

1. Measurement of urinary free cortisol (UFC) is typically used as a screening test for which adrenal disorder?
   a. Hyperaldosteronism
   b. Cortisol hypersecretion
   c. Adrenal insufficiency
   d. Congenital adrenal hyperplasia
2. Glucocorticoids _____ blood glucose concentrations by altering synthesis of gluconeogenic enzymes.
   a. increase
   b. decrease
   c. do not affect
3. What is the primary adrenal mineralocorticoid?
   a. Cortisol
   b. Dehydroepiandrosterone (DHEA)

   c. 11-deoxycortisol
   d. Aldosterone
4. Steroid hormone metabolism that involves the P450 enzyme system occurs in which organ?
   a. Liver
   b. Kidney
   c. Gastrointestinal tract
   d. Lungs
5. Which stimulation test is used to assess the ability of the adrenal glands to synthesize cortisol?
   a. Dexamethasone test
   b. Metapyrone test
   c. Cosyntropin test
   d. Salt-loading test

6. Which disorder is due to *primary* adrenal insufficiency?
   a. Cushing syndrome
   b. Addison disease
   c. Conn syndrome
   d. Congenital adrenal hyperplasia (CAH)
7. Which adrenal disorder is caused by loss-of-function mutations in specific adrenocortical enzymes responsible for the synthesis of cortisol?
   a. Cushing syndrome
   b. Addison disease
   c. Conn syndrome
   d. Congenital adrenal hyperplasia (CAH)
8. Which anterior pituitary hormone causes adrenocortical cells to increase in size and number, and stimulates cortisol synthesis?
   a. Corticotropin
   b. Growth hormone
   c. Corticotropin-releasing hormone (CRH)
   d. Aldosterone
9. What is one of the main functions of the mineralocorticoids?
   a. Increasing blood glucose.
   b. Increased fat breakdown.
   c. Sodium retention.
   d. Glycogen synthesis.
10. Which one of the following disorders is the result of autonomous excessive production of cortisol?
   a. Cushing syndrome
   b. Addison disease
   c. Conn syndrome
   d. Congenital adrenal hyperplasia (CAH)

## SUGGESTED READINGS

Bertholf RL. Disorders of the adrenal gland. In: Winter WE, Holmquist B, Sokoll LJ, Bertholf RL, eds. *Handbook of Diagnostic Endocrinology*. 3rd ed. London: Elsevier Academic Press; 2021:103–148.

Betterle C, Presotto F, Furmaniak J. Epidemiology, pathogenesis, and diagnosis of Addison's disease in adults. *J Endocrinol Invest*. 2019;42(12):1407–1433.

Blocki F, Zierold C, Olson G, Seeman J, Cummings S, Bonelli F. In defense of aldosterone measurement by immunoassay: a broader perspective. *Clin Chem Lab Med*. 2017;55(4):e87–e89.

Boolani A, Channaveerappa D, Dupree EJ, et al. Trends in analysis of cortisol and its derivatives. *Adv Exp Med Biol*. 2019;1140:649–664.

Buliman A, Tataranu LG, Paun DL, et al. Cushing's disease: a multidisciplinary overview of the clinical features, diagnosis, and treatment. *J Med Life*. 2016;9(1):12–18.

El Ghorayeb N, Bourdeau I, Lacroix A. Role of ACTH and other hormones in the regulation of aldosterone production in primary aldosteronism. *Front Endocrinol (Lausanne)*. 2016;7:72.

Fassnacht M, Arlt W, Bancos I, et al. Management of adrenal incidentalomas: European Society of Endocrinology Clinical Practice Guideline in collaboration with the European Network for the Study of Adrenal Tumors. *Eur J Endocrinol*. 2016;175(2):G1–G34.

Findling JW, Raff H. Diagnosis of endocrine disease: differentiation of pathologic/neoplastic hypercortisolism (Cushing's syndrome) from physiologic/non-neoplastic hypercortisolism (formerly known as pseudo-Cushing's syndrome). *Eur J Endocrinol*. 2017;176(5):R205–R216.

Fleseriu M, Castinetti F. Updates on the role of adrenal steroidogenesis inhibitors in Cushing's syndrome: a focus on novel therapies. *Pituitary*. 2016;19(6):643–653.

Hinz L, Pacaud D, Kline G. Congenital adrenal hyperplasia causing hypertension: an illustrative review. *J Hum Hypertens*. 2018;32(2):150–157.

Li N, Li J, Ding Y, et al. Novel mutations in the CYP11B2 gene causing aldosterone synthase deficiency. *Mol Med Rep*. 2016;13(4):3127–3132.

Morera J, Reznik Y. Management of endocrine disease: the role of confirmatory tests in the diagnosis of primary aldosteronism. *Eur J Endocrinol*. 2019;180(2):R45–R58.

Nieman LK. Diagnosis of Cushing's syndrome in the modern era. *Endocrinol Metab Clin North Am*. 2018;47(2):259–273.

Rege J, Rainey WE. The steroid metabolome of adrenarche. *J Endocrinol*. 2012;214(2):133–143.

Spat A, Hunyady L, Szanda G. Signaling interactions in the adrenal cortex. *Front Endocrinol (Lausanne)*. 2016;7:17.

Turcu AF, Nanba AT, Auchus RJ. The rise, fall, and resurrection of 11-oxygenated androgens in human physiology and disease. *Horm Res Paediatr*. 2018;89(5):284–291.

Vaidya A, Mulatero P, Baudrand R, et al. The expanding spectrum of primary aldosteronism: implications for diagnosis, pathogenesis, and treatment. *Endocr Rev*. 2018;39(6):1057–1088.

Vinson GP. Functional zonation of the adult mammalian adrenal cortex. *Front Neurosci*. 2016;10:238.

Vitellius G, Trabado S, Bouligand J, et al. Pathophysiology of glucocorticoid signaling. *Ann Endocrinol (Paris)*. 2018;79(3):98–106.

Yang T, He M, Hu C. Regulation of aldosterone production by ion channels: from basal secretion to primary aldosteronism. *Biochim Biophys Acta Mol Basis Dis*. 2018;1864(3):871–881.

42

# Thyroid Disorders

*Christina Ellervik, David John Halsall, and Birte Nygaard*

## OBJECTIVES

1. Define the following:
   - Central hypothyroidism
   - Colloid
   - Congenital iodine deficiency syndrome
   - Euthyroid
   - Goiter
   - Hashimoto thyroiditis
   - Iodide
   - Reverse T3 (rT3)
   - Thyroglobulin (Tg)
   - Thyroid follicle
   - Thyroid storm
   - Thyrotoxicosis
   - Thyrotropin-releasing hormone (TRH)
2. Describe the structure and function of the thyroid gland, including cell types, internal location of key hormone precursors and proteins, regulation of the thyroid gland, and functions of the hormones synthesized and secreted.
3. Describe the metabolism of thyroid hormones, including synthesis, peripheral deiodination, specific effects on target tissues, and catabolism; state the full names of the thyroid hormones.

4. State the effects of increased and decreased thyroid hormones on thyroid-stimulating hormone (TSH), TRH, and target tissues.
5. For the following disorders, state the cause(s), symptoms, laboratory analyses, and lab results used to diagnose:
   - Autoimmune thyroid disease
   - Graves disease
   - Hashimoto thyroiditis
   - Myxedema
   - Nonthyroidal illness
   - Primary and secondary hyperthyroidism
   - Primary and secondary hypothyroidism
   - T3 thyrotoxicosis
6. Name and describe the thyroid autoantibodies associated with thyroid disease, including mechanism of action, specificity of autoantibody to each disease, methods of detection, and interferences.
7. State the methods, specimen requirements, and problems with methods used to assess total and free thyroid hormones, thyroxine-binding globulin (TBG), Tg, and TSH.
8. Analyze and solve case studies related to thyroid disease and laboratory analysis of these conditions.

## KEY WORDS AND DEFINITIONS

**Autoimmune thyroid disease (AITD)** Diseases in which the immune system attacks or stimulates the body's own thyroid gland.

**Central hypothyroidism** Refers to thyroid hormone deficiency due to a disorder of the (1) pituitary, (2) hypothalamus, or (3) hypothalamic-pituitary portal circulation.

**Colloid** An amorphous material found in the follicular lumen of the thyroid gland. A critical component is thyroglobulin (Tg).

**Congenital hypothyroidism** A pathological condition resulting from severe thyroid insufficiency during prenatal development and early infancy, which may lead to severe physical and mental retardation.

**Congenital iodine deficiency syndrome** (previously known as cretinism) A pathological condition from severe iodine deficiency during prenatal development and infancy, which may lead to short stature, developmental delay, dystrophy of the bones, and low basal metabolism.

**Euthyroid** Having normal thyroid function.

**Goiter** An enlargement of the thyroid gland that causes a swelling in the front part of the neck.

**Graves disease** A disorder of the thyroid of autoimmune etiology that causes hyperthyroidism. Characterized by having at least two of the following conditions hyperthyroidism, goiter, and exophthalmos. It is also known in Europe as *Basedow disease*.

**Hashimoto thyroiditis** An autoimmune disorder in which the thyroid gland is attacked by a cell-mediated autoimmune process. Also known as *Hashimoto disease* and *chronic lymphocytic thyroiditis*, it is marked by (1) goiter, (2) chronic inflammation of the thyroid (*thyroiditis*), and (3) often hypothyroidism.

**Hyperthyroidism** A condition caused by excessive production of iodinated thyroid hormones. Symptoms and signs include increased basal metabolic rate, enlargement of the thyroid gland, rapid heart rate, high systolic blood pressure, and a number of secondary symptoms.

**Hypothyroidism** A condition of deficient thyroid gland activity leading to lethargy, muscle weakness, and intolerance to cold.

**Myxedema** A severe form of hypothyroidism in which there is an accumulation of mucopolysaccharides in the skin and other tissue, leading to a thickening of facial features and a doughy induration of the skin.

**Nonthyroidal illness (sick euthyroid syndrome)** Abnormalities of T4, FT4, T3, and TSH concentrations that are seen in people with severe illness. In general, treatment with replacement thyroid hormone is not indicated.

**Organification** A process in the thyroid gland whereby iodide is oxidized and incorporated into tyrosyl residues (tyrosine) of thyroglobulin (Tg). Organification is catalyzed by the enzyme thyroperoxidase (TPO).

**Primary hypothyroidism** A condition that develops when the thyroid gland fails to produce or secrete as much thyroxine (T4) as the body needs.

**Reverse T3 (rT3)** A biologically inert metabolite of thyroxine (T4) with three iodine molecules attached in a configuration (l-3,3′,5′-triiodothyronine) different from that of the active thyroid hormone triiodothyronine (T3).

**Subclinical hyperthyroidism** A biochemical condition with normal concentrations of serum thyroid hormones when the serum TSH concentration is repeatedly low in the absence of hypothalamic or pituitary disease.

**T3 thyrotoxicosis** A hyperthyroid condition in which T3, but not T4, is elevated.

**Thyroglobulin (Tg)** An iodine-containing glycoprotein of high molecular weight (663 kDa) which is present in the colloid of the follicles of the thyroid gland.

**Thyroid follicle** The secretory unit of the thyroid gland consisting of an outer layer of epithelial cells that enclose an amorphous material called colloid.

**Thyroid-stimulating hormone (TSH)** A polypeptide hormone synthesized by the anterior pituitary gland that promotes the growth of the thyroid gland and stimulates the synthesis and release of thyroid hormones by the thyroid gland. Also called *thyrotropin*.

**Thyroid storm** A life-threatening condition that develops in a minority of cases of untreated thyrotoxicosis (hyperthyroidism, or overactive thyroid).

**Thyroiditis** A condition characterized by inflammation of the thyroid gland.

**Thyrotoxicosis** A toxic condition resulting from excessive amounts of thyroid hormones in the body.

**Thyrotropin-releasing hormone (TRH)** A tripeptide, produced in the hypothalamus that stimulates the synthesis and release of TSH from the anterior pituitary.

**Thyroxine (T4)** The major hormone synthesized and released by the thyroid gland that contains four iodine molecules (l-3,5,3′,5′-tetraiodothyronine).

**Thyroxine-binding globulin (TBG)** One of three major plasma thyroid hormone binding proteins.

**Toxic multinodular goiter** A condition in which the thyroid gland contains multiple lumps (nodules) that are overactive and that produce excess thyroid hormones. Also known as *Parry disease* and *Plummer disease*.

**Transthyretin (TTR)** A protein found in serum and cerebrospinal fluid that binds to and transports thyroxine (T4). TTR complexes with retinol-binding protein (RBP) to prevent its loss through the glomerulus by filtration. It was once called prealbumin because it travels faster than albumin on electrophoresis gels.

**Triiodothyronine (T3)** The biologically active form of thyroid hormone is formed primarily outside of the thyroid gland by the peripheral deiodination of thyroxine (T4). It has three iodine molecules attached to its molecular structure (l-3,5,3′-triiodothyronine).

## ANATOMY

The thyroid consists of two lobes connected by an isthmus and has a butterfly shape with the right lobe being slightly larger than the left. It is located in the front of the neck just above the trachea. The gland synthesizes thyroid hormones and calcitonin through two distinct cell types: the epithelial (follicular) cells and the parafollicular (or C) cells, respectively. The normal adult thyroid gland weighs 15 to 25 g, but in specific disease states, it can attain a weight of several hundred grams.

The thyroid gland is composed of follicles or acini (Fig. 42.1). In the center of the **follicle** is the lacuna, which contains **colloids** composed predominantly of **thyroglobulin** (Tg). The parafollicular (or C) cells produce the polypeptide hormone *calcitonin*.

### Thyroid Dysgenesis

Thyroid dysgenesis is a collective designation for thyroid agenesis (or athyreosis; i.e., the complete lack of thyroid tissue), hypoplasia, hemiagenesis (lacking one lobe), and thyroid ectopia (the aberrant location of thyroid tissue along its embryological descent). The developmental defects have considerable phenotypic variations. Ectopic tissue may coexist with a normally positioned gland. It is important to localize ectopic thyroid tissue before thyroidectomy.

## THYROID HORMONES

The thyroid gland secretes two hormones, **thyroxine** (3,5,3′,5′-l-tetraiodothyronine) and **triiodothyronine** (3,5,3′-l-triiodothyronine), which are commonly known as T4 and T3, respectively (Table 42.1). In addition, the thyroid gland secretes very small amounts of biologically inactive 3,3′,5′-l-triiodothyronine (**reverse T3 [rT3]**) and minute quantities of monoiodotyrosine (MIT) and diiodotyrosine (DIT), which are precursors of T3 and T4. The structures of these compounds are shown in Fig. 42.2.

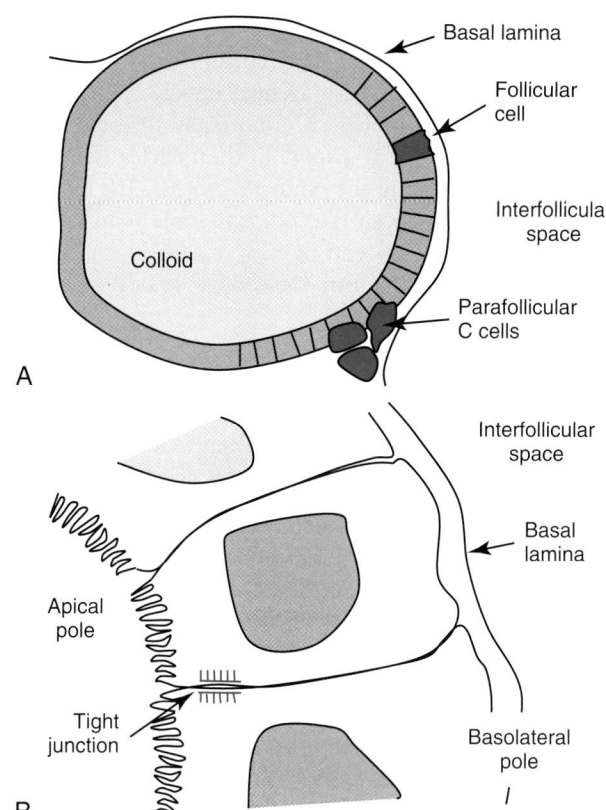

**Fig. 42.1** (A) Basic unit of the thyroid gland. The follicle is the basic unit of the thyroid gland. It is composed of thyroid follicular cells surrounding the colloid. Outside the follicular cells is a basal lamina. (B) Apical and basolateral poles of the follicular cells and tight junctions between the follicular cells. Parafollicular (C cells) that secrete calcitonin can be found beneath or outside the basal lamina. Not pictured between the follicles are capillaries and fibroblasts.

## Biological Function

The functions of thyroid hormones include (1) control of the basal metabolic rate and calorigenesis, (2) enhancement of mitochondrial metabolism, (3) stimulation of neural development and normal growth, (4) promotion of sexual maturation, (5) stimulation of adrenergic activity with increased heart rate and myocardial contractility, (6) stimulation of protein synthesis and carbohydrate metabolism, (7) increasing the synthesis and degradation of cholesterol and triglycerides, (8) increasing the requirement for vitamins, (9) increasing calcium and phosphorus metabolism, and (10) enhancing the sensitivity of adrenergic receptors to catecholamines. These effects are typically magnified in patients with either an overactive thyroid gland (e.g., in hyperthyroidism) or reduced in patients with reduced thyroid function (e.g., hypothyroidism).

## Biochemistry

Approximately 40% of secreted T4 is deiodinated in peripheral tissues by enzyme deiodinases to yield T3, and about 45% is deiodinated to yield rT3, a biologically inactive metabolite.

Therefore, with normal T4 production of 100 nmol (80 µg) daily, approximately 40 nmol (26 µg) of T3 and 45 nmol (29 µg) of rT3 are produced by peripheral deiodination.

### TABLE 42.1 Nomenclature and Abbreviations for Thyroid Tests

| Name | Abbreviation |
|---|---|
| **Hormones** | |
| Total thyroxine | T4 |
| Total triiodothyronine (3,5,3'-triiodothyronine) | T3 |
| Free thyroxine | FT4 |
| Free triiodothyronine | FT3 |
| Thyrotropin (thyroid-stimulating hormone) | TSH |
| Reverse T3 (3,3',5'-triiodothyronine) | rT3 |
| **Thyroid Hormone Binding Proteins (TBP)** | |
| Thyroxine-binding globulin | TBG |
| Transthyretin (thyroxine-binding prealbumin) | TTR |
| Albumin | Alb |
| **Tests for Autoimmune Thyroid Disease** | |
| Autoimmune thyroid disease | AITD |
| Thyroglobulin autoantibodies | Anti-Tg |
| Thyroperoxidase autoantibodies | Anti-TPO |
| TSH receptor autoantibodies | Anti-TSHR |
| TSH receptor antibodies | TRAb |
| TSH receptor-blocking antibodies | Anti-TSHRB |
| TSH receptor-stimulating antibodies | Anti-TSHRS |
| **Other Hormones, Thyroid-Related Proteins, and Conditions** | |
| Thyroid peroxidase | TPO |
| Thyrotropin-releasing hormone | TRH |
| Thyroglobulin | Tg |
| Thyroid hormone receptor | THR |
| Deiodinase 1,2,3 | D1, D2, D3 |
| Iodotyrosine dehalogenase 1 | DEHAL |
| Sodium-iodide symporter | NIS |
| TSH receptor | TSHR |
| Dual oxidase 1 and 2 | DUOX1 and DUOX2 |
| Thyroid hormone receptor-α | THRα |
| Thyroid hormone receptor-β | THRβ |

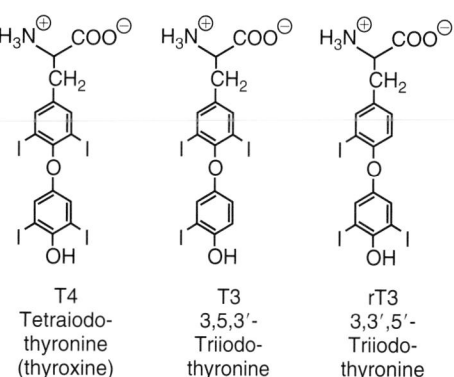

**Fig. 42.2** Chemical structures of thyroxine *(T4)*, triiodothyronine *(T3)*, and reverse T3 *(rT3)*.

From the estimated daily production rates for T3 (30 µg) and rT3 (30 µg) in a normal (**euthyroid**) state, at least 85% of T3 production and essentially all rT3 production are accounted for by peripheral deiodination of T4 rather than by direct secretion from the thyroid gland. T3 is at least four to five times more potent in biological systems than T4. Because one-third of all T4 is converted to T3 during the course of its metabolism, T4 may be considered to be a prohormone for T3. The biosynthesis of thyroid hormones occurs by a process termed **organification**. It involves the (1) trapping of circulating iodide by the thyroid gland, (2) incorporation of iodine into Tg tyrosines producing monoiodinated tyrosines and di-iodinated tyrosines, and (3) coupling of two iodinated tyrosyl residues to form the thyronines (T4 and T3) within the protein backbone of the Tg protein in the follicular lumen

(Fig. 42.3). Endocytosis followed by proteolytic cleavage of Tg releases the iodothyronines into circulation.

Dietary iodine is the basic element involved in the synthesis of thyroid hormones. It is normally ingested in the form of iodide. Iodide transport to the follicles is the first and rate-limiting step in the synthetic process. The follicular cells of the thyroid concentrate iodide to some 30 to 40 times the normal plasma concentration by means of an energy-dependent pump mechanism, the sodium-iodide symporter (NIS/SLCA5).

The synthesis of MIT and DIT (Fig. 42.4), T4 (Fig. 42.5), and T3 (Fig. 42.6), occurs mainly at the follicular cell–colloid interface but also within the colloid (see Fig. 42.3).

Tg is present in the highest concentrations within the colloid, where it is stored. The follicular cells engulf colloid

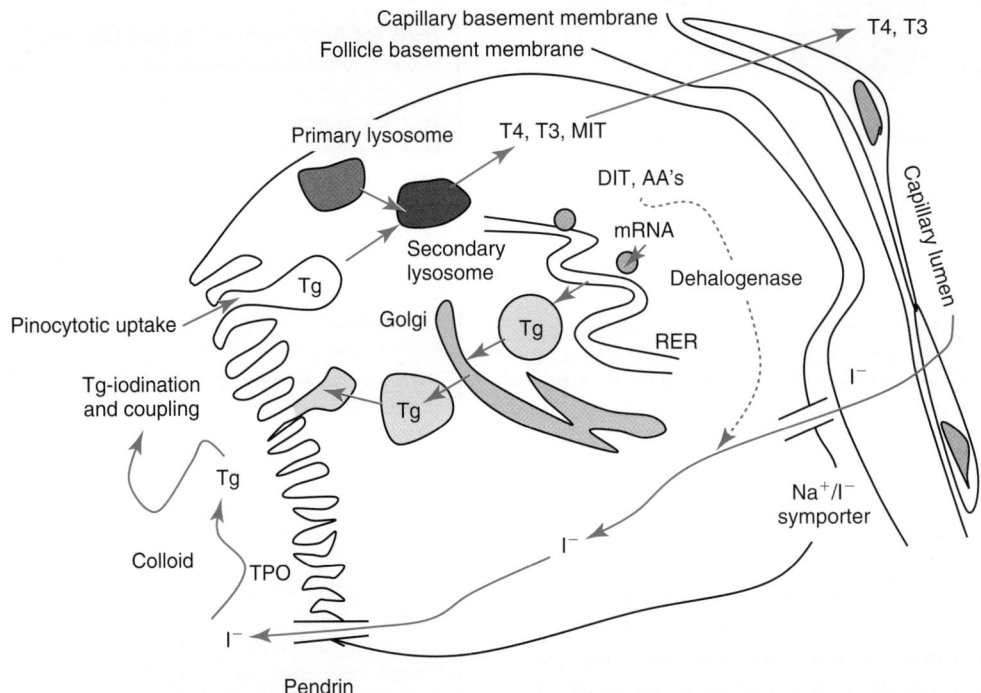

**Fig. 42.3** Synthesis of thyroid hormones begins with the absorption of iodide by the thyroid follicular cell and the Na+/I− symporter. From the cytoplasm, iodide moves into the lacunae via pendrin. Within the lacunae, thyroperoxidase *(TPO)* and the dual oxidases (DUOX [not depicted]) convert iodide to iodine, leading to iodination of tyrosine residues on thyroglobulin *(Tg)*. Tg is synthesized in the cell and exported to the lacunae. TPO is responsible for the coupling of monoiodotyrosine *(MIT)* and di-iodotyrosine *(DIT)* to form T3, and di-iodotyrosine and di-iodotyrosine to form T4. Upon the uptake of iodinated Tg (containing T4 and T3) and the fusion of this phagosome-like vesicle with a primary lysosome, Tg is degraded in a secondary lysosome, releasing T4 and T3 into the circulation, and MIT and DIT undergo deiodination via a dehalogenase to recycle the iodine for new thyroid hormone synthesis. *RER,* Rough endoplasmic reticulum.

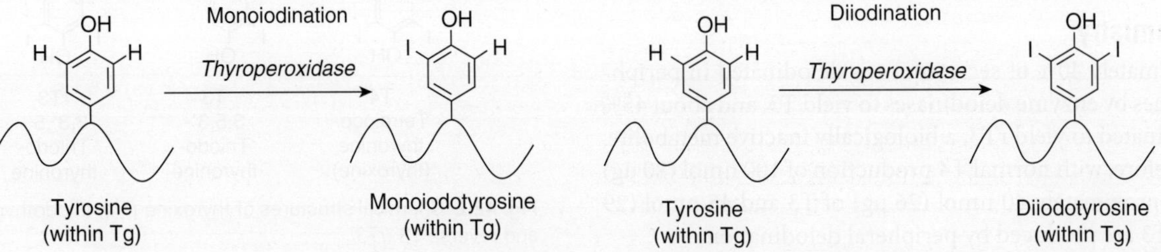

**Fig. 42.4** Monoiodination and diiodination of tyrosine. *Tg,* Thyroglobulin.

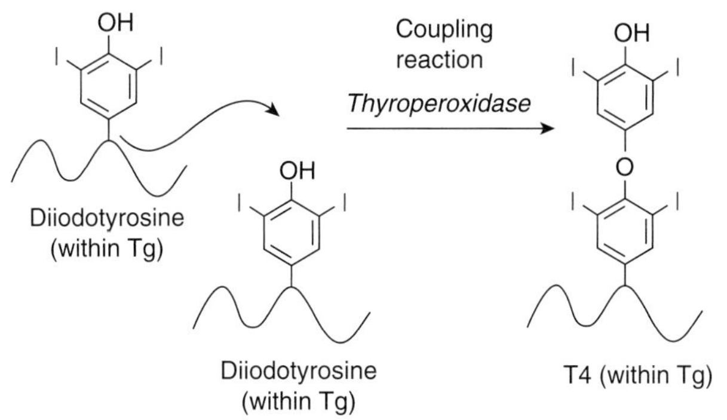


Fig. 42.5 Chemical coupling of two molecules of diiodotyrosines to produce a molecule of thyroxine (T4). The reaction is catalyzed by thyroperoxidase. *Tg*, Thyroglobulin.

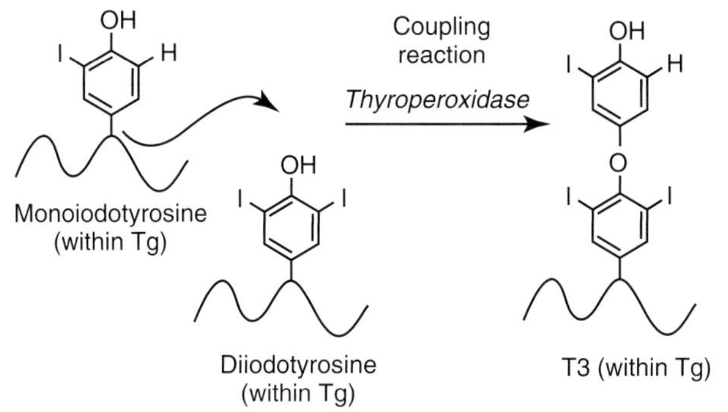


Fig. 42.6 Chemical coupling of one molecule of monoiodotyrosine and one molecule of diiodotyrosine to produce one molecule of T3. The reaction is catalyzed by thyroperoxidase. *Tg*, Thyroglobulin.

globules by endocytosis; these globules then merge with lysosomes in the follicular cell. Lysosomal proteases break the peptide bonds between iodinated residues of Tg, and MIT, DIT, T4, and T3, are released into the cytoplasm of the follicular cell. T4 and T3 diffuse into the systemic circulation after their liberation from Tg. DIT and MIT are deiodinated by an intracellular microsomal iodotyrosine dehalogenase (IYD). The freed iodide is then reused for thyroid hormone synthesis.

Each step in the synthesis of thyroid hormones is regulated by pituitary **thyroid-stimulating hormone (TSH)**. TSH (also known as *thyrotropin*) stimulates (1) the "iodide pump," (2) Tg synthesis, and (3) colloidal uptake by follicular cells. TSH also regulates the rate of proteolysis of Tg for the liberation of T4 and T3. In addition, TSH induces an increase in the size and number of the thyroid follicular cells. Prolonged TSH stimulation leads to increased vascularity and eventual hypertrophic enlargement of the thyroid gland (**goiter**). Thyroid hormones cross plasma membranes using specific transporters. One important thyroid hormone transporter is monocarboxylate transporter 8 (MCT8). MCT10 transports iodothyronines and aromatic amino acids across membranes, and MCT10 is likely more preferential than MCT8 in transporting T3 over T4 across plasma membranes. Organic anion transporting polypeptide 1C1 (OATP1C1) also has a high affinity for thyroid hormone and may be an important component of the transport of T3 and T4.

**BOX 42.1 Alterations in the Concentration or Affinity of Thyroid Hormone-Binding Proteins**

A. TBG concentration (or affinity)
   1. Genetic (inherited) causes
   2. Nonthyroidal illness
   3. Normal physiology (pregnancy, newborn)
   4. Drug use
      1. Increase (oral contraceptives, estrogens, tamoxifen, methadone)
      2. Decrease (androgens, anabolic steroids, large doses of glucocorticoids)
B. TBG-binding capacity (drugs bound to TBG, such as salicylates and phenytoin)
C. Prealbumin binding (familial euthyroid thyroxine excess)
D. Albumin binding (familial dysalbuminemic hyperthyroxinemia)
E. Thyroxine binding by autoantibodies (autoimmune thyroid disease, hepatocellular carcinoma)

*TBG*, Thyroxine-binding globulin.

## Metabolism

Free (unbound) T4 (FT4) is the primary secretory product of the normal thyroid gland. T4 undergoes peripheral deiodination of the outer ring at the 5′ position to yield T3. This deiodination occurs in a number of tissues but primarily in the liver. rT3, produced by the removal of one iodine from the inner ring of T4, is metabolically inactive and is an end-product of T4 metabolism. Peripheral deiodination is a rapidly responsive mechanism of control for thyroid hormone balance. Acute or chronic stress or illness causes a shift in the direction of this deiodination, favoring the formation of rT3 rather than T3. Various medications also shift peripheral deiodination toward the inactive product rT3.

T4 and T3 in the circulation are bound reversibly and almost completely to carrier proteins. These carrier proteins are (1) **thyroxine-binding globulin** (TBG), (2) thyroxine-binding prealbumin (TBPA; **transthyretin** [TTR]), and (3) albumin. Collectively, these proteins bind 99.97% of total T4 and 99.7% of total T3. Thus, only a very small fraction of each of these hormones is unbound and free for biological activity. Because a wide variation exists in the concentration of thyroid hormone-binding proteins, even under normal circumstances, a wide variation also exists in T4 concentrations among euthyroid individuals. Total T3 concentrations also vary with alterations in binding proteins, although usually to a lesser degree than T4 concentrations. Circumstances in which thyroid hormone-binding protein concentrations are increased or decreased are shown in Box 42.1.

## Regulation and Control

The hypothalamic-pituitary-thyroid axis is a classic endocrine negative feedback loop (Fig. 42.7). **Thyrotropin-releasing hormone (TRH)**, which is produced in the paraventricular neurons

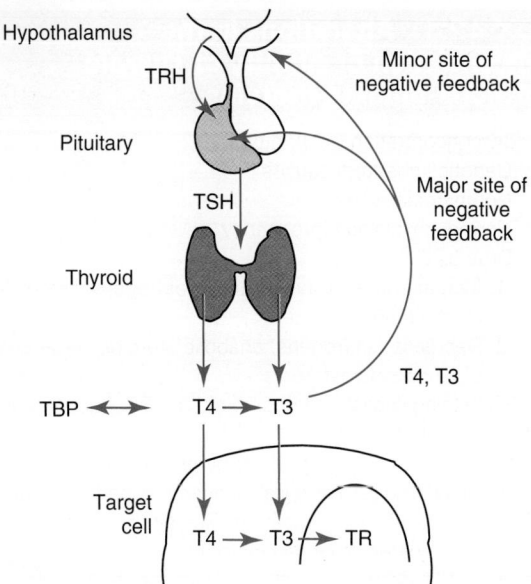

**Fig. 42.7** Metabolic control of thyroid hormones. **Thyrotropin-releasing hormone** *(TRH)* from the hypothalamus enters the hypothalamic-pituitary portal system to release thyroid-stimulating hormone *(TSH;* thyrotropin) from anterior pituitary thyrotrophs. TSH stimulates the release of **thyroxine (T4)** and triiodothyronine (T3) from the thyroid gland, although most T3 (~80%) comes from peripheral monodeiodination of T4 to T3. More than 99% of T4 and T3 are bound to various thyroid hormone-binding proteins *(TBP)*. T4 and T3 negatively feedback on the hypothalamus and, more powerfully, the pituitary. T4 and T3 enter into target tissues, where T4 is converted to T3 with T3 binding to the thyroid hormone receptor *(THR)*.

on the hypothalamus, stimulates the release of thyrotropin (also called thyroid stimulating hormone, TSH), from the anterior pituitary cells known as *thyrotrophs*. TRH is delivered to the anterior pituitary gland via the hypothalamic-pituitary portal system. TSH is the principal regulator of thyroid hormone synthesis and secretion by the thyroid gland. TSH binding to the TSH receptor (TSHR) stimulates the thyroid gland to produce thyroid hormones. TRH and TSH are inhibited by the negative feedback from thyroid hormones, although the effect on TRH in the hypothalamus is minor compared with the suppression of TSH in the pituitary. The negative feedback is such that TRH and TSH concentrations rise in thyroid hormone deficiency and decline when thyroid hormone is in excess.

### Biochemistry

TRH is the modified tripeptide l-pyroglutamyl-l-histidyl-l-prolinamide secreted by the paraventricular nuclei (PVN) in the hypothalamus (Fig. 42.8). Its concentrations rise in thyroid hormone deficiency with TRH declining when thyroid hormone is in excess. In relative terms, TRH has a greater effect on TSH glycosylation than hormone release. However, glycosylation of TSH is necessary for normal TSH bioactivity. When TRH is deficient, TSH may lack potency as the result of insufficient glycosylation, yet nonglycosylated TSH may retain much of its immunoreactivity. Chemically, TSH is a 30 kDa heterodimeric glycoprotein that shares the 14.7 kDa alpha subunit with (1) luteinizing hormone (LH), (2) follicle-stimulating hormone (FSH), and (3) human chorionic

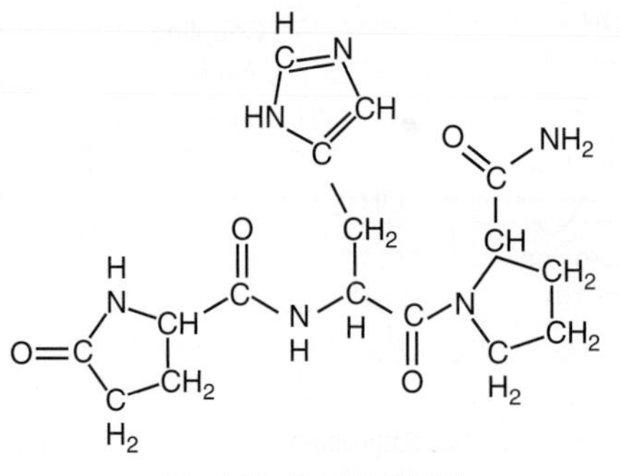

**(pyro)Glu-His-Pro(NH₂)**

**Fig. 42.8** Chemical structure of thyrotropin-releasing hormone *(TRH)*. Note that TRH is a tripeptide (L-pyroglutamyl-L-histidyl-L-prolinamide).

gonadotropin (hCG), whereas each hormone has a unique but structurally related beta subunit.

### Function

The effects of TSH on the thyroid follicular cell are mediated through the TSH receptor, a 100 kDa glycoprotein of 743 amino acids. TSH binding to the receptor activates the second messenger system involving $G_S$ proteins, adenylate cyclase, and the formation of cyclic adenosine monophosphate and stimulates the activity of the sodium-iodine symporter, the synthesis of Tg and thyroperoxidase (TPO)-mediated release of T4 and T3. TSH stimulation also increases the size and number of thyroid follicular cells.

## IODINE AND THYROID DISORDERS

Iodine (or iodide [I⁻] in its ionized form) is a trace element and an essential nutrient (see Chapter 27). Iodine is an indispensable component of the thyroid hormones T3 and T4, respectively. These hormones, together with thyronamines, are the only iodine-containing hormones in vertebrates. Without iodine, there is no biosynthesis of thyroid hormones. Thus, thyroid function requires an adequate supply of iodine to the thyroid gland.

### Geography and Iodine Supply

Iodide ions in seawater and coastal seaweed beds are oxidized to elemental iodine, which then volatilizes into the atmosphere and is returned to the soil by rain. This process (the iodine cycle) is slow and incomplete in many regions, thus leaving soils and drinking water iodine depleted.

Most iodine is found in the oceans. The major source of iodine in industrialized countries is iodized salt, and if that is not available, then dairy products.

### Iodine-Containing Products and Goitrogens

Exposure to iodine also can occur from iodine-containing products, such as disinfectants, amiodarone, radiology contrast agents, and topical antiseptics (e.g., the surgical scrub povidone–iodine). The iodine content of these agents is several thousand-fold higher than iodine appearing in naturally occurring foods. Iodine deficiency is the major cause of endemic goiter, but naturally occurring compounds and environmental pollutants may also be goitrogenic. Goitrogens can be either agents acting directly on the thyroid gland or causing a goiter by indirect action. Interestingly, cigarette smoking is associated with high plasma concentrations of thiocyanate, which can compete with iodine for uptake into the thyroid.

## Biochemistry

Dietary iodine controls its own absorption through post-transcriptional regulation of the intestinal $Na^+/I^-$ symporter (NIS). The thyroid gland has autoregulatory mechanisms to handle excess iodine intake involving the sodium iodide symporter. Excess iodine has an inhibitory effect on thyroxine synthesis in intact thyroids. In conditions of adequate dietary iodine supply, the healthy thyroid usually takes up less than 20% of absorbed iodine. However, in chronic iodine deficiency, this fraction can be more than 80%. The thyroid is thus able to adapt to low intakes of dietary iodine by marked modification of its activity. The metabolism of circulating thyroid hormones in peripheral tissues releases iodine that enters the plasma iodine pool, which in turn can be taken up by the thyroid or excreted by the kidney. Approximately 90% of ingested iodine is excreted in the urine and approximately 10% in feces.

## Iodine Deficiency

Both deficient and excessive intakes of iodine can impair thyroid function. The clinical presentations of iodine deficiency are largely age dependent. Pregnant and lactating women have higher demands for iodine because of an increase in maternal T4 production to maintain maternal euthyroidism and the transfer of thyroid hormone to the fetus early in the first trimester. In fetuses, deficiency may cause abortion, stillbirth, and congenital anomalies. In neonates, deficiency may cause congenital iodine deficiency syndrome and infant mortality. In children and adolescents, deficiency may cause impaired mental function, delayed physical development, and low IQ. In adults, deficiency may cause impaired cognitive function, reduced work productivity, thyroid autoimmunity, toxic nodular goiter, and hypothyroidism. In all ages, goiter is the most visible sign of iodine deficiency but is not specific to it.

## Iodine Excess

Thyroid dysfunction may occur in vulnerable patients if exposed to excess iodine. These patients include those with preexisting thyroid disease, older adults, pregnant and lactating women, fetuses, and neonates. Iodine excess can result in adverse thyroidal effects after only a single exposure to iodine-containing substances. Excess dietary iodine intake in pregnant and lactating women in iodine-replete areas may lead to an increase in plasma TSH concentrations and thus to subclinical hypothyroidism (SCH).

## EXTRATHYROIDAL FACTORS THAT AFFECT THYROID FUNCTION

### Epidemiologic Factors

Concentrations of thyrotropin, thyroid hormones, thyroid antibodies, and thyroid-binding proteins are to varying degrees determined genetically and by epidemiologic factors such as age, gender, ethnicity, body mass index, smoking, pregnancy, nutritional iodine, season, nonthyroidal disease, radiation, and medication.

### Drugs

Many drugs, other than those used for the treatment of thyroid disorders, interfere with thyroid hormone homeostasis. Drugs may interfere with (1) endogenous thyroid function through actions on thyroid hormone synthesis, secretion, transport, metabolism, and absorption (Table 42.2), (2) pharmacokinetics of thyroid therapy (liberation, absorption, distribution, metabolism, and excretion of drug), and (3) laboratory testing of thyroid hormones (which is described later in this chapter).

### Lithium

Lithium, which is still a widely used drug for the treatment of the bipolar disorder, is associated with subclinical and overt hypothyroidism in up to 34% and 15% of patients, respectively. These may develop even after many years of treatment. Patients should have regular thyroid function tests, at least once or twice per annum. Lithium primarily inhibits thyroid hormone secretion, although it appears also to have effects on iodine trapping, release, and coupling.

### Amiodarone

Amiodarone is an antiarrhythmic drug that comprises 37% iodine by weight and has structural similarities with thyroid hormones. The drug has a long half-life, large distribution volume, and wide tissue distribution. The mechanisms of amiodarone injury are multifactorial and involve the accumulation of iodine, the formation of free radicals, and immunologic damage. The effects of amiodarone can be divided into effects occurring in everyone treated with amiodarone, resulting in changes in thyroid function tests ("obligatory effects"), and effects only occurring in some people treated with amiodarone ("facultative effects"), resulting in clinically overt thyrotoxicosis or hypothyroidism. It may take several months for normalization of thyroid function tests after discontinuation of amiodarone treatment.

Amiodarone-induced thyrotoxicosis (AIT) is particularly prevalent (10%) in iodine-deficient regions, in men, and in patients with underlying thyroid disease (e.g., nodular goiter or Graves disease). Amiodarone-induced hypothyroidism occurs primarily in iodine-sufficient regions and in women with preexisting anti-TPO antibodies.

## NONTHYROIDAL ILLNESS

Many disorders are associated with variations in the concentration of thyroid hormones in the absence of definable thyroid disease (Table 42.3). For example, (1) significant nutritional deprivation, (2) acute severe illness, or (3) chronic illness often results in changes in thyroid function. Collectively they are characterized as *nonthyroidal illnesses* (NTI; but also called sick euthyroid syndrome). A progressive spectrum of thyroid test result anomalies often accompanies nonthyroidal illnesses in euthyroid patients. The

## TABLE 42.2  Effects of Some Drugs on Tests of Thyroid Function

| Cause | Drug | Effect |
|---|---|---|
| Inhibit TSH secretion | Dopamine<br>L-dopa<br>Glucocorticoids<br>Somatostatin | ↓ T4; ↓ T3;<br>↓ TSH |
| Inhibit thyroid hormone synthesis or release | Iodine<br>Lithium | ↓ T4; ↓ T3;<br>↑ TSH |
| Inhibit conversion of T4 to T3 | Amiodarone<br>Glucocorticoids<br>Propranolol<br>Propylthiouracil<br>Radiographic contrast agents | ↓ T3; ↑ rT3;<br>↓, ≒, ↑ T4 and FT4;<br>≒, ↑ TSH |
| Inhibit binding of T4/T3 to serum proteins | Salicylates<br>Phenytoin<br>Carbamazepine<br>Furosemide<br>NSAIDs<br>Heparin (in vitro effect) | ↓ T4; ↓ T3;<br>≒, ↑ FT4;<br>≒TSH |
| Stimulate metabolism of iodothyronines | Phenobarbital<br>Phenytoin<br>Carbamazepine<br>Rifampicin | ↓ T4; ↓ FT4;<br>≒TSH |
| Inhibit absorption of ingested T4 | Aluminum hydroxide<br>Ferrous sulfate<br>Cholestyramine<br>Colestipol<br>Iron sucralfate<br>Soybean preparations<br>Kayexalate | ↓ T4; ↓ FT4;<br>↑ TSH |
| Increase in concentration of T4-binding proteins | Estrogen<br>Clofibrate<br>Opiates (heroin, methadone)<br>5-Fluorouracil<br>Perphenazine | ↑ T4; ↑ T3;<br>≒FT4;<br>≒TSH |
| Decrease in concentration of T4-binding proteins | Androgens<br>Glucocorticoids | ↓ T4; ↓ T3;<br>=FT4;<br>≒TSH |

↓, Reduced serum concentration; ↑, increased serum concentration; ≒ no change; *FT4*, free thyroxine; *NSAID*, nonsteroidal antiinflammatory drug; *rT3*, reverse triiodothyronine; *T3*, triiodothyronine; *T4*, thyroxine; *TSH*, thyroid-stimulating hormone.
Data obtained from Smallridge RD. Thyroid function tests. In: Becker KL, ed. *Principles and Practice of Endocrinology and Metabolism.* 7th ed. Philadelphia: JB Lippincott; 1995.

earliest and most common changes that occur are a reduction in the serum concentrations of total and free T3, sometimes to extremely low concentrations, and an elevation in the serum concentration of rT3. These changes have been ascribed to a block in the 5'-deiodinases that convert T4 to T3 in peripheral tissue.

Serum TSH concentrations are usually normal in euthyroid sick patients but may be mild to moderately depressed with moderate to severe NTI or slightly elevated during recovery from a severe illness (Fig. 42.9). The causes of these transient abnormal TSH concentrations are not fully understood but may relate to the effects of endogenous or exogenous hormones, such as glucocorticoids or dopamine, which independently suppress the secretion of pituitary TSH concentrations. Other possible causes include altered nutrition or altered biological activity of immunoreactive TSH. Decreased total T4 levels may result from T4 displacement from thyroid hormone-binding proteins but with a slight increase in FT4. As patients recover from NTIs, many of the thyroid test abnormalities revert to normal. T4 concentrations will be corrected first, followed by a rise in the concentration of T3. Serum TSH may also transiently rebound to high concentrations for several days or weeks before returning to normal.

## EVALUATION OF THYROID FUNCTION

In clinical practice, thyroid function tests are routinely measured to diagnose disorders of the thyroid. For example, in combination with information obtained from (1) patient history, (2) physical examination, and (3) laboratory results, patients are classified as (1) hypothyroid, (2) hyperthyroid, or (3) euthyroid (Fig. 42.10). Almost all laboratory tests for thyroid function are commercially available on automated immunoassay instruments. The following is a brief description of tests that are commonly used for the evaluation of thyroid status. Reference intervals for the analytes discussed below are not harmonized and vary with population and analytical method.

### Measurement of Thyroid-Stimulating Hormone

Most clinical laboratories use immunometric assays to measure TSH in serum, typically with chemiluminescent probes and solid phase capture antibodies, as this format gives the required limit of detection. The limit of detection of TSH assays is a major issue because it is necessary to measure well below the population reference interval to differentiate primary hyperthyroidism from other causes of low serum TSH concentration. The previously used "generational" concept for TSH assays is now largely redundant because clinical guidelines now specify the appropriate limit of detection for TSH assays. All assays in clinical practice should be "third generation," that is the functional sensitivity (20% inter-assay coefficient of variation) should be at a concentration of 0.01 to 0.02 mIU/L. It is beholden to the clinical chemist to be aware of and monitor this aspect of the assay.

The specificity of TSH assays is largely of historical concern because modern assays show little cross-reactivity with the other highly homologous pituitary glycoprotein hormones despite sharing the common α-subunit. Although the clinical performance of TSH assays is impressive, further challenges for the clinical chemist remain. This is because of the heterogeneity of the TSH molecule. The protein is 25% by mass

## TABLE 42.3  Nonthyroidal Illness

| Hormone | Initial | Midcourse | Prolonged | Resolution |
|---------|---------|-----------|-----------|------------|
| TSH | Normal | Normal to decreased | Decreased | Increases |
| T4 | Normal | Normal to decreased | Decreased | Increases |
| T3 | Decreased (−) | Decreased (−−) | Decreased (−−−) | Increases |
| rT3 | Increased (+) | Increased (++) | Increased (+) | Decreases |

Note: The severity of decreased T3 is proportional to the number of (−) signs. The degree of increase in rT3 is proportional to the number of (+) signs.

*T3*, Triiodothyronine; *rT3*, reverse T3; *T4*, thyroxine; *TSH*, thyroid-stimulating hormone.

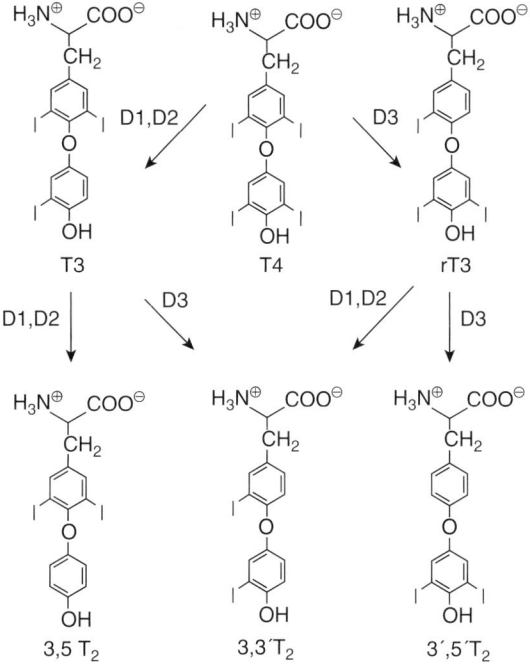

Fig. 42.9 Effects of altered deiodination. In states of nonthyroidal illness (e.g., the sick euthyroid syndrome), thyroid hormone deiodination patterns are altered with reduced T3 concentrations and elevated concentrations of reverse T3 *(rT3)*.

glycosylated and the pituitary secretes a range of glycoforms that differ with thyroid status. This makes TSH assays difficult to standardize because a homogenous reference preparation will not accurately reflect all isoforms and the glycosylation state is likely to affect the relationship between TSH immunoreactivity and biologic activity. This is of particular concern in the diagnosis of secondary (pituitary) hypothyroidism as the pituitary can produce immunoreactive but biologically inactive TSH in this setting. However, work by the IFCC has shown that clinically used TSH assays can be substantially harmonized using common calibrants despite the lack of an established reference method procedure; this may allow common reference intervals to be established.

Both serum and plasma are acceptable substrates for TSH immunoassay. TSH is stable in serum for at least 5 days at 4°C, and at least 29 years at −25°C. The unit of measurement is mIU/L.

Because TSH is used as the primary marker of thyroid function, serum TSH concentrations must be interpreted against relevant reference intervals. Within individuals, TSH concentrations are remarkably constant with the intraindividual variation being at least less than half of the reference interval.

Secretion of TSH is circadian with peak concentrations of TSH occurring between 0200 and 0400 hours, and the lowest between 1700 and 1800 hours. Low-amplitude oscillations occur throughout the day.

### Measurement of Total Thyroxine and Triiodothyronine

Circulating T4 is highly (>99.9%) protein bound, and the fraction that is bound to protein is biologically inactive. Total thyroid hormone measurements are now largely used to confirm the results of FT4 measurements when they are in doubt. Because total thyroid hormone is present in the serum in nanomolar concentrations, it is less of an analytical challenge than the measurement of free hormone. Mass spectrometric measurements are now the method of choice for total thyroid hormone analysis given the sensitivity and selectivity of modern mass spectrometers. However competitive immunoassay methods are still used widely. These methods include a displacing agent such as 8-anilino-1-napthalenesulfonic acid to release thyroid hormone from high-affinity serum binding sites. The efficiency of this process for T4 methods may contribute to relatively poor method comparisons both between immunoassay methods and between immunoassay and mass spectrometric methods.

T3 is the principal active thyroid hormone with approximately 20% of circulating T3 secreted by the thyroid gland, and the remainder is produced by the deiodination of T4 in the peripheral tissues. Like T4, T3 is highly bound to protein with less than 1% of the total concentration as a free active hormone. However, compared with T4, it is less tightly bound to serum proteins by about an order of magnitude. Consequently, the displacement of bound T3 from proteins is essentially complete in the presence of conventional blocking agents. Also, T3 does not ordinarily displace T4 from thyroid hormone-binding proteins.

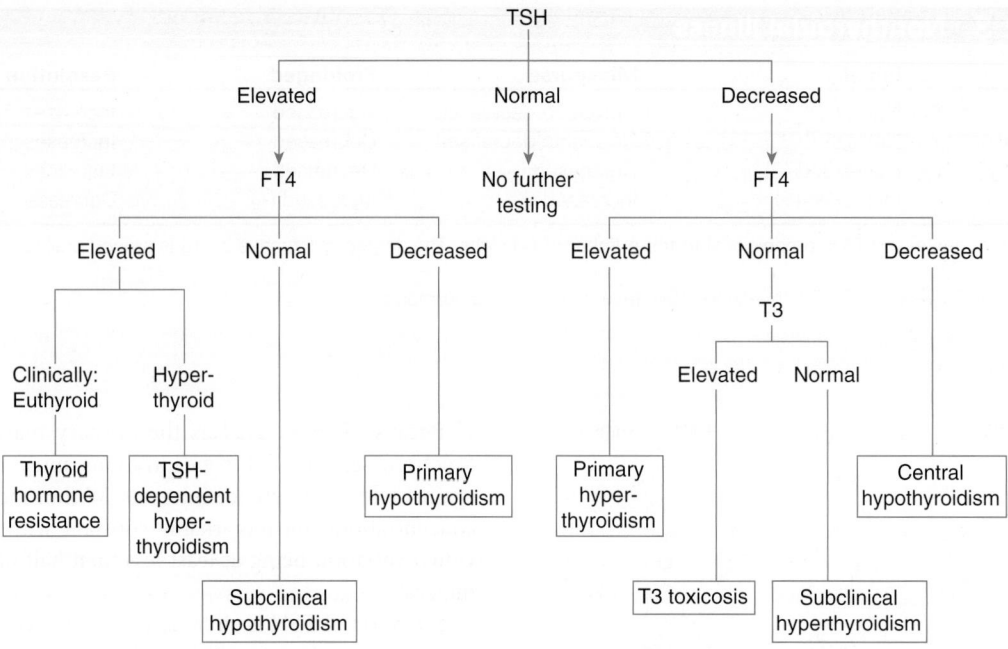

**Fig. 42.10** Suggested algorithm for the laboratory evaluation of thyroid function. *TSH,* Thyroid-stimulating hormone.

## Measurement of Reverse Triiodothyronine

Mass spectrometric assays are the preferred method for measuring circulating rT3 due to the increased selectivity of these methods. These supersede previous radioimmunoassay (RIA) methods. Unlike T4 and T3, rT3 assays have not been adapted to automated platforms due to limited diagnostic value and clinical utility.

## Measurement of Free T4

Most authorities now subscribe to the "free hormone hypothesis," that is, that the measurement of non–protein-bound T4 in circulation (FT4) is a more accurate reflection of thyroid status than the total amount of T4 (free plus bound T4). This is because T4 concentrations are clearly influenced by changes in thyroid-binding proteins as well as HPT axis regulation. However, the measurement of FT4 presents both theoretical and practical challenges, which compromises the clinical utility of this assay. Unbound FT4 is present in picomolar concentration in plasma and represents only about 0.03% of the total. FT4 must be measured despite this vast excess of bound hormone and in the presence of other iodothyronines such as T3. All current methods represent varying degrees of compromise because it is difficult to separate bound from free hormone without perturbing the equilibrium between the two species. Several assay designs have been established that have been given confusing and often nonstandard nomenclature. Pragmatically, competitive immunoassays for FT4 have gained widespread popularity and clinical use, but an awareness of the limitations of these assays is required to prevent misdiagnosis.

The first level of assay hierarchy is between "direct" methods, which use a physical separation of bound from free T4, such as equilibrium dialysis or ultrafiltration, and indirect methods that estimate FT4 in the presence of T4 binding proteins.

Direct methods are conceptually easier to understand; FT4 is separated from protein-bound T4 using a physical method such as dialysis or ultrafiltration followed by a mass spectrometric analysis of T4 in the protein-depleted fraction. Although direct methods have been proposed for routine clinical use, the complexity and expense of these methods compared with the easily automatable indirect immunoassay methods have prevented the wide-scale implementation of direct FT4 assays. Dialysis has been proposed as the international conventional reference measurement procedure for FT4 analysis. However, even dialysis methods are not infallible and need to be used with caution as the conditions that determine the equilibrium between free and bound T4 in vivo must be carefully maintained during dialysis.

Indirect immunoassays are almost universally used in clinical chemistry laboratories and are further divided into one- and two-step methods depending on whether a wash step is included to remove serum constituents before the addition of the T4 immunoassay tracer. Modern immunoassay methods are also "analog" because chemically modified T4 probes are used rather than historic radiolabeled hormones. Indirect immunoassay methods assume that the FT4:T4 equilibrium is maintained during immunoassay to such an extent that a clinically relevant estimation of FT4 can be returned. One-step methods incubate the assay antibody and tracer in the presence of all serum constituents. Two-step or "back-titration" methods allow T4 to equilibrate with the assay antibody in the presence of all serum components but wash away uncaptured components before back titrating with a tracer. Although both methods sequester a significant amount of T4 from the serum pool during the assay, the FT4:T4 equilibrium is maintained sufficiently to provide a reliable estimate of FT4 under most conditions, however, given the variety of methods used, comparability can be poor. Both one- and two-step methods will fail when the nature or concentration of T4 binding proteins is significantly different in the analytical sample compared to the serum-based calibrator used. This is apparent in samples from patients with genetic variants of thyroid-hormone binding proteins such as albumin (familial dysalbuminemic hyperthyroxinemia [FDH]) or TTR. These effects are assay dependent, with some assay designs more susceptible than others. Patients with autoantibodies generated against T4 are well described; these antibodies are particularly problematic for one-step assays because they can sequester the immunoassay tracer, giving false positive results. Two-step assays are more resistant to this class of interference because the autoantibody is removed before the immunoassay tracer is added. Both labeled tracer and labeled antibody methods are currently used in clinical practice. Although labeled antibody methods have theoretical advantages in terms of limit of detection, susceptibility to anti-T4 antibodies and binding protein abnormalities remain an issue. Harmonization initiatives by the IFCC aim to establish calibration traceability, particularly for free thyroid hormones have demonstrated that the comparability of FT4 assays in current practice could be dramatically improved.

## Measurement of Free T3

As with T4, the concentration of FT3 is thought better to correlate with biological activity than tT3. However, analysis of FT3 by immunoassay is more challenging than FT4 as it is present in serum at lower concentrations and is more easily displaced from its binding proteins. Competition immunoassay methods for FT3 are in widespread use but assays from different providers are poorly comparable; a situation that could be improved by better calibrant traceability. Advances in mass-spectrometric methods allow the measurement of FT3 by direct methods such as equilibrium dialysis or ultrafiltration followed by tandem mass-spectrometry however, unlike FT4, a reference measurement procedure has not been established. Whilst impractical for use in the routine clinical lab, the use of direct mass spectrometric methods has brought into question the reliability of competition immunoassay methods for FT3. Some authorities recommend the immunoassay of (total) T3 rather the FT3 for this reason. FT3 immunoassay methods, like FT4 methods, are also susceptible to alterations in thyroid hormone binding proteins such as familial dysalbuminemic hyperthyroxinemia, albeit to a lesser extent.

## Thyroid Hormone Metabolite Panels

Given the rapid improvement in the performance and the availability of high-resolution mass spectrometers, it is now possible to measure profiles of thyroid hormone metabolites including T3 and reverse T3 but also other iodothyronine metabolites. The clinical utility of these measurements is yet to be proven.

## Measurement of Thyroxine-Binding Globulin

Commercial immunoassays are available for the quantitation of circulating TBG in several formats including competitive immunoassays and immunoturbidimetric methods.

## Measurement of Thyroglobulin

Thyroglobulin (Tg) is detectable in the plasma and as such acts as a marker for the presence of active thyroid tissue. Tg concentrations are determined by thyroid mass, TSH stimulation, and thyroid manipulation including surgery, fine-needle aspiration, or thyroid injury. The primary use of serum Tg measurement is as a tumor marker in patients with differentiated thyroid cancer (DTC) who have undergone thyroidectomy. It is difficult to measure Tg owing to the heterogeneity of the molecule, largely because of different glycoforms, and to the prevalence of endogenous anti-Tg or anti-reagent antibodies that interfere with the immunoassay. Current practice for thyroidectomized thyroid cancer patients is to withdraw thyroxine replacement to stimulate endogenous TSH secretion or to use recombinant human TSH to stimulate any residual or neoplastic thyroid tissue. This can be inconvenient, unpleasant, and expensive. Consequently, a Tg assay with the sensitivity to detect Tg in the absence of TSH stimulation (i.e., suppressed) is desirable.

Two analytical methods are in current use, each with its advantages and limitations. Immunometric assays are very sensitive (0.1 ng/mL or lower), and amenable to automation, but prone to antibody interference. Immunometric Tg assays should be reported together with anti-Tg results. If Tg-Ab is present (≥1.8 IU/mL), the Tg value can be falsely low and the Tg value measured by immunometric assay cannot be used as a tumor marker. Instead, Tg should be assayed by mass spectrometry which can be sensitive down to 0.2 ng/mL. Mass spectrometry is robust to antibody interference.

## Measurement of Thyroid Autoantibodies

The most common causes of both hyper- and hypothyroidism are autoimmune in nature. Consequently, the detection of autoantibodies directed against the thyroid during autoimmune destruction of the gland in Hashimoto thyroiditis or activating antibodies directed against the TSH receptor in Graves disease can be useful diagnostic markers (Table 12.1).

### Thyroid Peroxidase Antibodies (TPOAb)

Anti-TPO assays are in widespread use as a marker of autoimmune hypothyroidism because their presence is widely accepted as a risk factor for developing autoimmune hypothyroidism. Immunometric methods are in widespread use, but despite the availability of an international reference preparation, methods do not agree well. Consequently, results from different assays cannot be compared. Anti-TPO assay is a very sensitive (~95%), but less specific, marker for Hashimoto thyroiditis, and it has been implicated in the disease process. The

### TABLE 42.4　Thyroid Autoantibodies

| Autoantibody | Antigen | Prevalence in Autoimmune Hypothyroidism | Prevalence in Graves Disease | Action of Antibody | Principal Clinical Use |
|---|---|---|---|---|---|
| Anti-TPO | Thyroid peroxidase | >95% | >80% | ? Cytotoxic | Diagnosis and risk of developing autoimmune hypothyroidism |
| Anti-Thyroglobulin | Thyroglobulin | 60%–80% | 50%–60% | Passive | Detection of possible antibody interference in thyroglobulin immunoassays |
| Anti-TSHR | TSH receptor | 0%–20% | 98% | Stimulatory, inhibitory, or apoptotic | Diagnosis of Graves disease |

specificity of the assay is dependent on the type of assay used and the population studied, being affected by age, gender, ethnicity, and iodine status. Anti-TPO antibodies are also typically raised in Graves disease (>80% sensitivity), but anti-TPO antibodies have been superseded by anti-TSHR antibodies for this application. Serial measurement of anti-TPO is of little value because the treatment is aimed at correcting thyroid dysfunction rather than the autoimmune process itself.

### Anti-Thyroglobulin Antibodies

Antithyroglobulin antibodies are also raised in Hashimoto hypothyroidism (sensitivity 60% to 85%) but are most frequently measured to raise awareness of the possibility of interference in Tg assays.

### Anti–Thyroid-Stimulating Hormone Receptor Antibodies

T4 secretion from the thyroid is stimulated by TSH binding to the thyroidal TSH receptor (TSHR). This receptor can also be stimulated or blocked by autoantibodies directed against the TSH receptor (TRAbs). The nomenclature to describe TRAbs is complex and is based on either the detection method used or the action of the antibody; also, a "generational" system based on the limit of detection is in use. The original TRAb assays utilized detergent-solubilized TSH receptor preparations to capture competing radiolabeled TSH or TRAb from patient serum. As such, these assays were also called Thyroid Binding Inhibitory Immunoglobulin assays (TBII). These "first generation" assays had detection limits around 2 IU/L. To reduce the limit of detection and simplify assay protocols "second generation" assays using immobilized TSHR and chemiluminescent labeled TSH were developed which halved the limit of detection and allowed the development of automated TRAb assays. "Third generation" assays use a high-affinity monoclonal TRAb (M22) instead of TSH which further reduced the limit of detection to around 0.4 IU/L. Sensitivity and specificity for third-generation TRAb assays are high. Despite high diagnostic efficiency high levels of TRAb have been described in some patients with transient hyperthyroidism, however, typical features of Graves disease were absent in these patients, necessitating a degree of caution when interpreting TRAb in this context. Whilst TRAb assays are extremely effective for the diagnosis of Graves

disease they cannot distinguish between thyroid stimulatory antibodies, blocking antibodies, and "neutral" TRAb species. There are some clinical scenarios when this can be restrictive. These include:

- The transplacental passage of TRAb: As either stimulatory or blocking antibodies can be transferred to the fetus, knowledge of the antibody class can predict fetal response and direct appropriate therapy,
- "Class switching": Production of antibodies in patients with autoimmune thyroid disease can switch between stimulating and blocking antibodies. An awareness of antibody type can anticipate the need to modify therapeutic interventions.
- Differential diagnosis of Hashimoto hypothyroidism: A significant proportion of autoimmune hypothyroid patients (8%) have TSH-blocking antibodies; this may represent a second etiology for autoimmune hypothyroidism or may precede the development of the T-cell mediated cell destruction that defines Hashimoto thyroiditis. As to whether alternate therapies can be used based on the detection of blocking antibodies is the subject of further research.

More complex cell-based assays have been designed to discriminate stimulatory and blocking antibodies; these are based on the generation of cellular cAMP as the second messenger for TSH signaling. As well as discriminating antibody type these assays have low limits of detection. Unfortunately, these assays are complex and unsuited to the routine clinical chemistry laboratory. Recently more accessible cell-based assays that incorporate a luciferase reporter construct have been developed; these assays exceed the performance of TRAbs and have been recently FDA-approved for clinical use. Given the complexity of the bioassays, attempts have been made to redesign the TSHR to be more specific for stimulating rather than blocking assays for use in the simpler competition immunoassay format. This assay utilizes a genetically modified TSH/ LH receptor fusion to replace C terminal elements in the receptor thought to be predominantly targeted by blocking antibodies. The assay uses "bridging" technology which detects TRAb by its ability to link the chimeric receptor to a reporter construct. Whilst effective as a TRAb assay, the specificity of the assay for thyroid-stimulating immunoglobulins alone (rather than blocking antibodies) is contested. TRAbs may affect other functions of TSHR apart from stimulation of T4 secretion such as thyrotroph differentiation and apoptosis, the potential impact of this effect on the diagnosis and treatment of autoimmune thyroid disease is a topic that warrants further study.

## Measurement of Urinary Iodine Concentration

Because most of the body's iodine is excreted in the urine, urinary iodine concentration (UIC) is considered a reliable and valid biomarker of the iodine intake and iodine deficiency of the population. Unfortunately, as urinary iodine is dependent on the intake of iodine and varies from day to day a single measurement of urinary iodine is not a reliable marker of iodine status in routine clinical practice.

Secondary measurements for estimating iodine deficiency are thyroid size, TSH concentration, and thyroid hormones.

## Assay Interference

Despite improvement in immunoassay design, the potential for interference, which may affect patient management, remains an ongoing challenge for the clinical chemist. Situations where the immunoreactivity of the analyte under assay conditions does not reflect its biological activity are a major cause of the diagnostic error. Several classes of interference have been described (Fig. 42.11).

## Interference Specific to Assay Design

The design of some clinical assays leaves them prone to interference from exogenous compounds such as therapeutics. Biotin supplementation disrupts the biotin-streptavidin linkage that is utilized by many immunoassay manufacturers to immobilize antibody reagents. If biotin is present at a high enough concentration in the patient sample, then immobilization of the reagent antibody can be impaired which can lead to false negative results in immunometric assays or false positive results in competitive designs. This can lead to an unfortunately plausible constellation of results for thyroid function tests giving a false negative TSH result with false positive results for thyroid hormone and thyroid stimulatory antibody tests leading to the erroneous diagnosis of Graves disease. High-concentration biotin is an established treatment for multiple sclerosis and biotin–thiamine–responsive basal ganglia disease, but biotin can also be present in over-the-counter medications at sufficient concentration to cause this effect. This presents a considerable challenge to the clinical chemist and physician as neither may be aware of the presence of the potential interferent. Whilst assay manufacturers

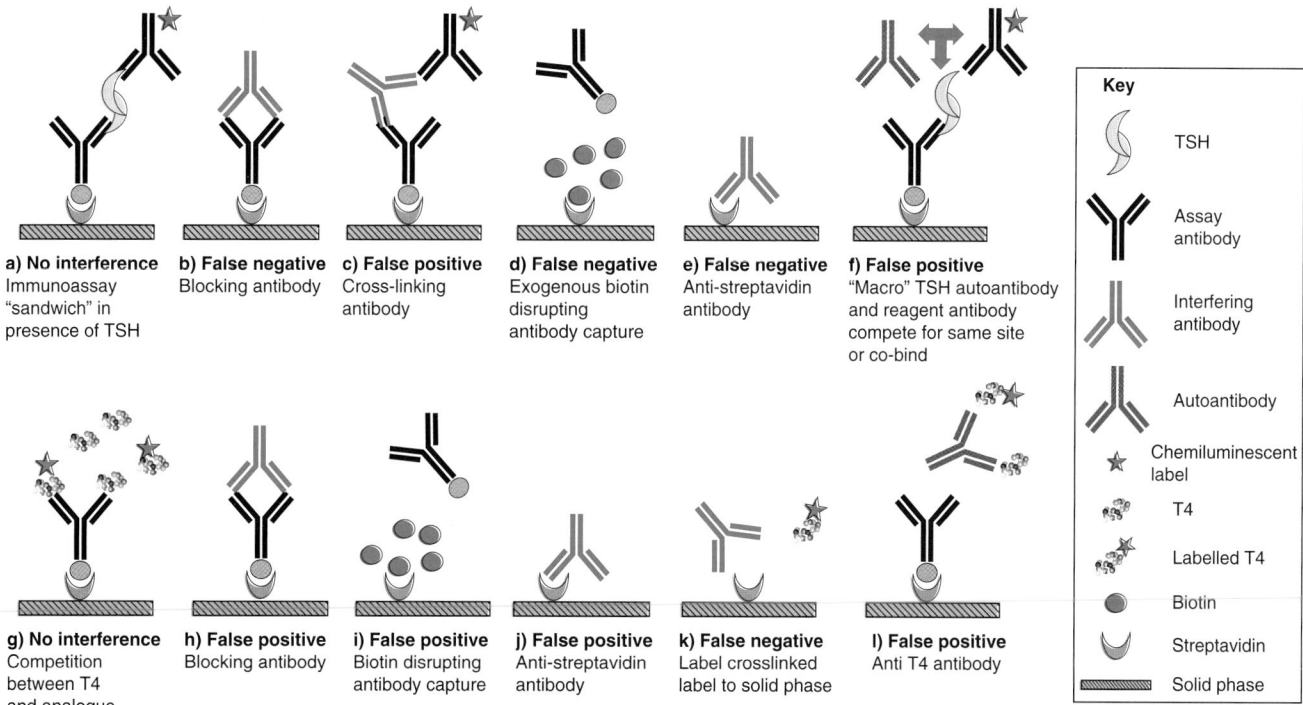

**Fig. 42.11** Mechanisms of Antibody Interference in Thyroid Immunoassay. Schematic to show how anti-reagent antibodies and autoimmune antibodies can interfere with immunoassay. With immunometric designs (a–f) a positive signal occurs when the chemiluminescent signal is immobilized to the solid phase, in the competitive designs (g–l) a positive signal occurs when the chemiluminescent signal is displaced from the solid phase. With autoantibodies, false positive interference is caused by the presence of an immunoreactive but biologically ineffective hormone species. Anti-T4 antibodies can sequester the T4 analog. Macro TSH antibodies are likely to compete with reagent antibodies but may bind simultaneously. (From Ellervik C, Halsall DJ, Bygaard B. Thyroid disorders. In: Rifai N, ed. *Tietz Textbook of Laboratory Medicine.* 7th ed. St. Louis: Elsevier; 2022.)

are attempting to eliminate this class of interference by changing assay configurations, awareness of which assay designs are susceptible to this class of interference is key to managing this potential risk of misdiagnosis. Either rechecking samples using a biotin-resistant method or re-sampling after the cessation of biotin therapy for 48 hours can eliminate this effect.

### Antibody Interference—Anti-Analyte Antibodies

Antibodies directed against T4 are well described and are common during the destructive phase of Hashimoto thyroiditis. As described above, one-step FT4 assays are prone to this class of interference, as anti-T4 antibodies present in patient serum can bind the T4 analog tracer and cause false positive results. The incidence of T4 autoantibodies has been reported at 1.8%, but the incidence of significant analytical interference is likely to be lower.

Autoantibodies directed against TSH have also been described. The TSH:Ig complex is commonly referred to as "macro-TSH" given the increase in apparent molecular mass of the TSH when analyzed by size exclusion chromatography. In the presence of anti-TSH autoantibodies the relation between biologically active TSH and the immunoassay result is complex and method dependent, as the relevant epitopes affected and the relative affinity of the autoantibody and immunoassay antibodies during assay conditions both affect the amount of detectable TSH. Gel filtration methods, which separate the TSH immunoreactive species by size, have been proposed as the gold standard methodology for quantifying macro-hormone complexes; but these methods are also flawed due to sample dilution during assay and the limitations of immunoassay as a detection method in the presence of anti-TSH antibodies. The prevalence of macroTSH may be as high as 0.8%, and as anti-TSH antibodies can be transferred trans-placentally, can be a cause of false positive **congenital hypothyroidism** screening tests.

### Anti-Assay Component Antibodies

Antibodies can also be directed against assay components; these can be specific anti-animal antibodies or weak polyspecific antibodies usually referred to as heterophile. When directed against the assay antibodies they can either block or cross-link antibodies depending on the assay design. Antibodies against assay components such as streptavidin which is often used to attach capture antibodies to solid phase components via the streptavidin-biotin linkage have also been described.

Most clinical free hormone assays are done using indirect competitive immunoassays. These assays assume that the equilibrium between free and bound hormones is maintained during assay conditions. As these assays are invariably calibrated against serum with "wild-type" binding proteins at expected physiological concentrations and in the absence of drugs that may compete with the thyroid hormone binding sites, perturbation of this equilibrium is inevitable and a source of error to which all immunoassays in current clinical use are susceptible. "Gold standard" direct methods such as

equilibrium dialysis are not necessarily immune to this class of interference either as these methods invariably incur some sample dilution, so diluents must not show a differential effect between "normal" and "abnormal" binding proteins. Familial dysalbuminemic hyperthyroxinemia is perhaps the best described binding protein abnormality that affects FT4 and to a lesser extent FT3 assays. A gain-of-function mutation in albumin (most often at codon 218) causes increased affinity for T4. This effect is clinically benign but typically generates falsely high FT4 results in most assays. The frequency of FDH is estimated at 1:10,000 but varies with ethnicity. Genetic variations in TBG and TTR that affect commonly used FT4 assays have also been described but at a lower frequency.

As the T4 binding sites on albumin are not specific, T4 can be displaced by other endogenous metabolites or drugs. Two effects are commonly seen. Best described are the effects of the older antiepileptic agents, which often generate artefactually low FT4 results as well as induce the enzymatic clearance of thyroid hormone.

### Laboratory Approaches for the Detection and Elimination of Assay Interference

Whilst most thyroid function tests accurately reflect thyroid status a small minority can give misleading information. The laboratory is faced with two challenges: when to suspect assay interference and how to confirm its presence. Several methods have been proposed for the detection of immunoassay interference but unfortunately, no single method can detect all types of interference. Consequently, the clinical laboratory has a major role to play in raising awareness of the possibility of assay interference when clinical presentation and thyroid function test results are at odds. Method comparison using a suitably orthologous method is a practical and effective method, and the availability of mass-spectrometric methods for free thyroid hormones and thyroglobulin has greatly facilitated this. For analytes where mass-spectrometric methods are currently unavailable as an alternative to immunoassay, methods that use different assay architecture (i.e., biotin resistant), antibodies from different species, or simple immunosubtraction methods such as PEG precipitation can be used with good effect.

## THYROID DISEASE

### Thyroiditis

Thyroiditis means inflammation of the thyroid. It encompasses many thyroid disorders, some of which have an autoimmune etiology, including Hashimoto thyroiditis, painless sporadic thyroiditis, and painless postpartum thyroiditis. The prevalence of individuals with high serum concentrations of thyroid antibodies varies with gender, age, and ethnicity; the prevalence is higher in women, people older than 60 years of age, and whites. It has been suggested that dietary iodine deficiency may be protective against certain types of thyroiditis because of the geographical variations in incidence seen in these conditions.

The different types of thyroiditis may cause thyrotoxicosis, hypothyroidism, or both. All types of thyroiditis may eventually progress to permanent hypothyroidism, and the risk is higher in patients with high serum thyroid antibody concentrations. As thyroid function declines, TSH secretion increases, resulting in SCH (elevated TSH, normal T4, and T3), later in overt hypothyroidism with clearly elevated TSH and a preferential expression of T3 but low T4, and finally, in thyroid failure, also low T3.

## Autoimmune Thyroid Disease

**Autoimmune thyroid disease (AITD)** comprises two main diseases, Hashimoto thyroiditis, and Graves disease. The prevalence is estimated to be 5%, but the prevalence of thyroid antibodies in the general population is 10% to 20%. AITD is a T-cell-mediated disorder leading to an immune attack of the thyroid in an individual with genetic susceptibility accompanied by environmental factors. Examples of factors that increase the risk of AITD include ethnicity, pollutants (smoking, radioiodine), dietary (iodine excess, selenium deficiency), endocrine (female gender, parity, postpartum, oral contraceptives), infections, drugs, and trauma. Pathologically, AITD is characterized by lymphocyte infiltrates within the thyroid. AITD is associated with other autoimmune diseases, either organ-specific (autoimmune polyglandular syndromes) or systemic (type 1 diabetes, rheumatoid arthritis, systemic lupus erythematosus, Sjögren syndrome, systemic sclerosis, cryoglobulinemia, sarcoidosis, psoriatic arthritis); these associations reflect common genetic susceptibilities and common pathogenic mechanisms. AITD is also associated with papillary thyroid cancer.

## Hypothyroidism

Hypothyroidism is defined as a deficiency in thyroid hormone production or secretion producing a variety of clinical signs and symptoms of hypometabolism. The term **myxedema** is used in severe or complicated cases but strictly refers only to the appearance of the skin as it becomes infiltrated with glycosaminoglycans. Hypothyroidism is a common endocrine disorder that is often overlooked but often may present serious signs and symptoms. Thyroid hormones affect the function of most of the organs and tissues of the body (Box 42.2). The clinical features of thyroid hormone deficiency are therefore quite diverse and may involve multiple systems. The thyroid gland itself may be enlarged as a goiter; either firm or granular in texture; tender or nontender, or normal, small, or impalpable, depending on the etiology of the hypothyroidism.

### Epidemiology

Worldwide, the most common cause of hypothyroidism is still iodine deficiency. However, in developed countries where iodine fortification is widespread, the most common cause of **primary hypothyroidism** is Hashimoto thyroiditis. Hypothyroidism is more common in women than men

increases with age and is higher in Whites than in Blacks or Hispanics.

### Etiology

Primary hypothyroidism is caused by the destruction of the thyroid gland because of autoimmunity (the most common cause), thyroiditis, or medical intervention such as surgery, radioiodine, and radiation (Box 42.3). Secondary hypothyroidism is caused by insufficient stimulation by TSH of an otherwise normal thyroid gland often caused by damage to the pituitary gland or hypothalamus (Box 42.4). Congenital hypothyroidism is discussed in a separate section.

> **BOX 42.2 Clinical Manifestations of Hypothyroidism**
>
> **Symptoms**
> Fatigue
> Lethargy
> Sleepiness
> Mental impairment
> Depression
> Cold intolerance
> Hoarseness
> Dry skin
> Hair loss
> Decreased perspiration
> Weight gain
> Decreased appetite
> Constipation
> Menstrual disturbances (typically menorrhagia) and infertility
> Arthralgia
> Paresthesia
>
> **Signs**
> Goiter (may be present)
> Slow movements
> Slow speech
> Hoarseness
> Bradycardia
> Dry skin
> Loss of outer lateral eyebrow
> Nonpitting edema (myxedema) (caused by the accumulation of glycosaminoglycans in subcutaneous and other interstitial tissue)
> Carpal tunnel syndrome
> Psychosis
> Galactorrhea
> Hyporeflexia
> Delayed relaxation of reflexes
> Myopathy
> Congestive cardiac failure (severe hypothyroidism)
> Coma (severe hypothyroidism)
> Growth failure and mental retardation (undetected congenital hypothyroidism)
> Prolonged jaundice (neonatal hypothyroidism) (as a result of the immaturity of uridine diphosphate glucuronyltransferase)

## BOX 42.3   Causes of Hypothyroidism

**Primary Hypothyroidism**
Thyroid dysgenesis
Destruction of thyroid tissue
Chronic autoimmune thyroiditis: atrophic and goitrous forms
Thyroid ablation
Subtotal and total thyroidectomy
Infiltrative diseases of the thyroid (amyloidosis, sarcoid, lymphoma, hemochromatosis, scleroderma)
Defective thyroid hormone biosynthesis
Congenital defects in thyroid hormonal biosynthesis
Iodine deficiency
    Drugs with antithyroid actions: lithium, iodine, and iodine-containing drugs, radiographic contrast agents

**Central Hypothyroidism**
Pituitary disease
Hypothalamic disease

**Transient Hypothyroidism**
Silent (painless) thyroiditis including postpartum thyroiditis
Subacute thyroiditis (De Quervain syndrome)

## BOX 42.4   Possible Causes of Central Hypothyroidism

**Tumors:** pituitary macroadenomas, craniopharyngiomas, meningiomas, gliomas, Rathke cleft cysts, metastases
**Iatrogenic:** cranial surgery or irradiation, drugs
**Injury:** head traumas, traumatic delivery
**Vascular:** postpartum necrosis (Sheehan syndrome), pituitary apoplexy, carotid aneurysms
**Infiltrative diseases:** sarcoidosis, hemochromatosis
**Infectious disease:** tuberculosis, syphilis, mycoses
**Genetic:** *TSHB* mutations
**Malformations:** Empty sella syndrome
**Idiopathic:** Other unknown causes

*TRHR,* Thyrotropin-releasing hormone (TRH) receptor (TRHR) gene; *TSHB,* thyroid-stimulating hormone-beta (TSHB) gene.

## Primary Hypothyroidism

Hashimoto thyroiditis is autoimmune thyroiditis. It was first described in 1912 by Hakaru Hashimoto, a Japanese physician. Also known as chronic lymphocytic thyroiditis, Hashimoto thyroiditis is the most common type of thyroiditis, and in iodine-sufficient areas, it is also the most frequent cause of hypothyroidism and goiter. It leads to the destruction of thyroid follicular cells through a T-cell–mediated autoimmune process. Histologically, the gland is infiltrated with lymphocytes and plasma cells, which can lead to the development of secondary lymphoid follicles within the gland, which are similar to the secondary follicles observed in normal lymph nodes. The initial finding is usually a firm, symmetric goiter, but over time, the gland can atrophy, reflecting the destruction of the gland. The gland may often be lobulated, which sometimes makes it difficult to distinguish from multinodular goiter. Although atrophy may occur in Hashimoto

thyroiditis, atrophic thyroiditis may also occur when autoantibodies against the TSHR bind to the receptor and block the action of endogenous TSH. TSHR-blocking autoantibodies can cross the placenta during pregnancy, causing transient hyperthyrotropinemia in infants (elevated TSH with a normal T4) or even transient congenital hypothyroidism. There is a strong association between Hashimoto thyroiditis and primary B-cell lymphoma of the thyroid, although this is a rare condition. It is thought that prolonged stimulation of the intrathyroidal B cells results in the emergence of a malignant clone. In addition, the frequency of papillary carcinoma may be increased in chronic autoimmune thyroiditis, particularly in women. Pain may indicate the presence of lymphoma. Fine-needle aspiration (FNA) biopsy or surgical biopsy may be required to distinguish between these conditions.

Patients with severe hypothyroidism may present with myxedematous (hypothyroid) coma, a syndrome of decreased consciousness, hypothermia, and other features of hypothyroidism. This condition has high mortality and requires aggressive treatment in a critical care facility with facilities for mechanical ventilation if required.

Serum TSH is the first-line measurement for the assessment of thyroid function with an age-dependent reference interval usually between 0.4 and 4.5 mIU/L. *Overt hypothyroidism* is defined as increased TSH and low FT4 (Table 42.5). SCH is defined by a high serum TSH (but usually <10 mIU/L) and a serum FT4 within the reference interval. In patients whose initial testing indicates hypothyroidism, TPO autoantibodies should also be measured, indicating an autoimmune etiology. Patients diagnosed with SCH should be followed up with repeat measurements together with the measurement of TPO antibodies preferably after a 2- to 3-month interval. The presence of antibodies indicates an increased risk of progression to overt hypothyroidism. The prevalence of SCH increases with age and is higher in women than in men.

Other conditions in which TSH is elevated but FT4 is normal encompass the recent institution of thyroid hormone replacement therapy (FT4 returns to normal before TSH declines), poor compliance with treatment in primary hypothyroidism, recovery from nonthyroidal illness, TSH assay antibody interference and rarely TSH resistance due to genetic variation in the TSH receptor.

Ninety percent of patients with Hashimoto thyroiditis have anti-TPO at presentation making these autoantibodies sensitive markers for this condition. Furthermore, 20% to 50% of patients with Hashimoto have anti-Tg autoantibodies. However, some people in the general population may also have anti-TPO and anti-Tg without Hashimoto, therefore the positive predictive value of antibody testing is low and antibody testing should not be used as a screening tool.

If overt hypothyroidism is present, patients should be treated with levothyroxine to normalize TSH. TSH-suppressing doses can be used short term to reduce goiter size. TSH should be used for monitoring. Serum thyroid antibody concentrations do not decrease with treatment but may decrease or disappear over a longer timescale.

## TABLE 42.5  Patterns of Thyroid Dysfunction

| | TSH | FT4 | Comments |
|---|---|---|---|
| Primary hypothyroidism | Increased | Decreased | — |
| Subclinical primary hypothyroidism | Increased | Normal | — |
| Primary hyperthyroidism | Decreased | Increased | T3: increased |
| T3 toxicosis | Decreased | Normal | T3: increased |
| Subclinical primary hyperthyroidism | Decreased | Normal | T3: normal |
| Thyroid hormone resistance due to defects in the thyroid hormone receptor | Normal to increased | Increased | T3: increased; rT3: increased |
| Thyroid hormone resistance due to defects in thyroid hormone metabolism of T4 converted to T3 | Mildly increased | Increased | T3: decreased; rT3: increased |
| Thyroid hormone resistance due to defects in thyroid hormone transport into cells | Normal to increased | Normal to decreased | T3: increased; rT3: decreased |

*T3,* Triiodothyronine; *rT3,* reverse T3; *FT4,* free T4; *T4,* thyroxine; *TSH,* thyroid-stimulating hormone.

## Central Hypothyroidism

Central hypothyroidism is caused by insufficient stimulation by TSH of an otherwise normal thyroid gland. The prevalence is estimated to be 1 in 20,000 to 1 in 80,000 in the general population, accounting for 1 in 1000 hypothyroid patients. Neonatal screening programs have shown a prevalence of congenital hypothyroidism of central origin of 1 in 160,000. In the Netherlands, the neonatal screening program using a combined TBG, TSH, and T4 strategy has shown that central hypothyroidism is diagnosed earlier with milder forms with an incidence of 1 in 16,000.

Central hypothyroidism may arise from pituitary disorders (secondary) or hypothalamic (tertiary) disorders including the pituitary stalk (see Box 42.4). Tertiary hypothyroidism is a result of hypothalamic defects or damage leading to insufficient stimulation of pituitary TSH production.

Central hypothyroidism can be classified into invasive or compressive lesions, iatrogenic factors (e.g., cranial surgery or irradiation), injuries (e.g., head traumas), vascular accidents (e.g., pituitary apoplexia, postpartum pituitary [Sheehan] syndrome), autoimmune disease (e.g., polyglandular autoimmune diseases), infiltrative lesions (e.g., iron overload, sarcoidosis), inherited diseases, and infectious diseases (e.g., tuberculosis). Invasive or compressive lesions include pituitary macroadenomas, craniopharyngiomas, meningiomas or gliomas, Rathke cleft cysts, metastases, empty sella syndrome, and carotid aneurysms. The inherited forms are rare and may include TSHβ mutations or TRH receptor mutations or pituitary transcription factor defects.

Transient or reversible forms of central hypothyroidism can be observed with drugs affecting the neuroendocrine TSH regulation, such as somatostatin analogs, glucocorticoids, or dopaminergic compounds acutely inhibiting TSH secretion. Transient or reversible forms may also occur during recovery from prolonged thyrotoxicosis or severe chronic diseases.

The clinical manifestations of central hypothyroidism (caused by either pituitary or hypothalamic disease) are similar to those of primary hypothyroidism but tend to be less severe (unless diagnosed in infancy). If a mass is taking up space in the cranium, headache, visual field disturbances, and hypopituitarism may develop. Nonthyroidal illness may have a similar picture as central hypothyroidism because of suppression of the hypothalamic–pituitary axis. Undiagnosed central hypothyroidism in infancy leads to severe physical and mental retardation.

The laboratory diagnosis is based on the demonstration of low, normal, or slightly elevated TSH concentrations combined with low T4 or FT4 concentrations. In neonatal screening programs, measurement of both TSH and T4 is required to differentiate between primary and secondary hypothyroidism.

## Thyrotoxicosis

The term thyrotoxicosis refers to a condition with excess thyroid hormone. The term *hyperthyroidism* refers to a sustained increase in thyroid hormone biosynthesis and secretion by the thyroid gland. The term *thyrotoxicosis* relates to its clinical manifestations: a syndrome of hypermetabolism and hyperactivity resulting from an elevation of plasma T4 or T3 concentration (most usually both). The terms *thyrotoxicosis* and *hyperthyroidism* are not entirely synonymous. For example, thyrotoxicosis can occur as a result of excessive hormone release from the thyroid in the absence of increased synthesis, as may occur in thyroiditis. Excessive intake of thyroid hormones can also cause thyrotoxicosis but not hyperthyroidism. Box 42.5 summarizes the clinical manifestations of thyrotoxicosis.

Thyrotoxicosis can affect any physiological system in the body with the frequency and severity of signs and symptoms varying considerably among patients. Some of the causes produce characteristic clinical signs; for example, orbital and cutaneous manifestations, which is unique to Graves disease. The age of the patient and the presence of concomitant disturbances may have an impact on the clinical features of hyperthyroidism, either exaggerating or diminishing them. For example, older patients may have less marked evidence of sympathetic activation, such as anxiety, hyperactivity, or

## BOX 42.5   Clinical Manifestations of Thyrotoxicosis

**Symptoms**

Nervousness, stroke, agitation, or irritability
Fatigue, lethargy
Weakness
Increased perspiration
Heat intolerance
Tremor
Hyperactivity
Palpitation
Appetite change (usually increase)
Weight change (usually weight loss)
Increased bowel movement
Menstrual disturbances

**Signs**

Hyperactivity
Tachycardia or atrial arrhythmia
Systolic hypertension
Warm, moist, smooth skin
Stare and eyelid retraction
Tremor
Hyperreflexia
Muscle weakness
Goiter
Thyroid bruits (with Graves disease, exophthalmos, pretibial
    myxedema, onycholysis, thyroid acropachy)
Digital clubbing, swelling of digits and toes
Periosteal reaction at extremities of bones

tremor, and less weight loss but marked features of cardiovascular dysfunction such as congestive cardiac failure and atrial fibrillation.

Graves disease—the most common cause of hyperthyroidism—affects approximately 0.4% of the US population and occurs more often in women than in men (5:1). It is frequently associated with other autoimmune disorders. There is a genetic susceptibility to Graves disease, as shown by a sibling occurrence risk of 11.6% and a heritability of 75% in twin studies; the rest is environmental, with smoking being a significant risk factor.

The causes of thyrotoxicosis are listed in the "Points to Remember" section. Thyrotoxicosis is usually associated with hyperthyroidism but not always. Common causes for thyrotoxicosis *not* associated with hyperthyroidism include (1) *thyroiditis* (silent painless thyroiditis, postpartum thyroiditis, subacute thyroiditis), and (2) *excess exogenous thyroid hormone* (iatrogenic or factitious).

The prevalence of the causes varies with iodine intake, such that in iodine-sufficient areas, Graves disease is the most common cause of thyrotoxicosis, accounting for 60% to 90% of cases. But in iodine-deficient areas, thyroidal autonomy is more common. Thyroiditis accounts for about 10% of all causes of thyrotoxicosis. Iodine fortification induces a temporary, modest increase in the incidence of hyperthyroidism in mild to moderate iodine-deficient regions.

## Thyroid (Thyrotoxic) Storm

A thyroid storm (also known as a thyrotoxic crisis) is a rare, severe, exaggerated, and life-threatening condition of thyrotoxicosis, which is triggered by precipitating factors (e.g., intercurrent illness or surgery). Thyroid storm is most often seen in the context of underlying Graves hyperthyroidism but can complicate thyrotoxicosis of any etiology.

## Graves Disease

Graves disease results from an autoantibody that binds to and activates the TSHR, producing the excessive release of thyroid hormone and clinical hyperthyroidism. In patients with Graves disease, the thyroid gland is no longer under the control of pituitary TSH but is constantly stimulated by the circulating antibodies with TSH-like activity. Both B and T lymphocytes are known to be directed at three well-characterized thyroid autoantigens, namely Tg, TPO, and TSHR. However, most of the evidence suggests that TSHR is the primary autoantigen of Graves disease and that the immune response to the other two thyroid antigens is caused by the resulting thyroiditis.

Graves ophthalmopathy has an autoimmune pathogenesis, with important genetic and environmental influences, particularly smoking. Orbital muscle, connective tissue, and adipose tissue are infiltrated by lymphocytes and macrophages. The extracellular compartment of extraocular muscles and orbital fibroadipose tissue becomes edematous, secondary to the deposition of hydrophilic glycosaminoglycans.

The diagnosis of Graves disease is based on laboratory demonstration of thyrotoxicosis with elevated FT4 (and FT3) and low TSH, clinical features (particularly Graves disease-specific extrathyroidal manifestations, including ophthalmopathy and dermopathy), and the presence of moderate, diffuse, and soft goiter over which a vascular bruit may be detectable.

Treatment of Graves disease includes antithyroid drugs (thionamides), radioiodine therapy, and thyroidectomy.

## Toxic Adenomas and Toxic Multinodular Goiter

Toxic adenomas and toxic multinodular goiter are conditions in which thyrocytes function and produce thyroid hormones independently of thyrotropin (TSH) and TSHR-stimulating antibodies. This autonomous secretion of thyroid hormones leads to TSH suppression and ultimately results in thyrotoxicosis. Such thyroid autonomy is a common finding in iodine-deficient areas, where it accounts for up to 60% of cases of thyrotoxicosis. However, thyroid autonomy is rare in regions with sufficient iodine supply (3% to 10% of cases with thyrotoxicosis).

## Gain-of-Function Mutations of the Thyroid-Stimulating Hormone Receptor

A familial autosomal dominant form of hyperthyroidism has been described that is caused by gain-of-function mutations in the TSH receptor. The gain-of-function mutation causes activation of TSHR in the absence of a ligand. In infants homozygous for such mutations, neonatal thyrotoxicosis, so severe as to require emergency thyroidectomy, has been observed. Certain heterozygous mutations have been reported to cause infantile hyperthyroidism.

## Central Hyperthyroidism

Central hyperthyroidism is rare but is most frequently caused by nearly always benign thyroid-stimulating hormone-secreting pituitary adenomas. A total of 75% of the tumors are macroadenomas, having a diameter larger than 10 mm at the time of diagnosis, but microadenomas (diameter <10 mm) are increasingly recognized owing to earlier diagnosis with improved imaging techniques. Patients with TSH-secreting tumors present with signs and symptoms of thyrotoxicosis, but extrathyroidal manifestations (i.e., ophthalmopathy, pretibial myxedema, and acropachy) are absent. Goiter is a common finding as a consequence of chronic TSH hyperstimulation. Patients may also have symptoms related to the mass effect of the pituitary adenoma such as visual field defects, headache, or loss of other anterior pituitary functions (menstrual disorders, galactorrhea, acromegaly).

The laboratory diagnosis is based on a non-suppressed TSH in the presence of high levels of free thyroid hormones (FT3 and FT4). Other diagnostic criteria include evidence of a pituitary mass on computed tomography or magnetic resonance imaging. There are both clinical situations (in particular) and possible laboratory artifacts that may cause a biochemical profile that is characteristic of patients with TSH-secreting tumors; these include thyroid hormone resistance, binding protein abnormalities, falsely high FT4 results, and falsely high TSH concentrations. Dynamic function tests such as T3 suppression or TRH stimulation are often required to make the differential diagnosis. The molar ratio of α-subunit to TSH may serve as a specific but insensitive marker for TSH-secreting tumors, with the ratio being increased in macroadenoma, but often within the reference interval in microadenoma and with thyroid hormone resistance.

## Subclinical Hyperthyroidism

The laboratory diagnosis of subclinical hyperthyroidism is defined by a low plasma TSH with normal concentrations of T4 and T3. The condition is classified as mild if TSH is in the range of 0.1 to 0.4 mIU/L.

Persistent subclinical hyperthyroidism may be caused by an exogenous iatrogenic overdose of levothyroxine or by endogenous causes as in primary hyperthyroidism such as Graves disease, toxic multinodular goiter, or solitary autonomous nodule. Exogenous subclinical hyperthyroidism is the most common and is reversible by reduction of levothyroxine dose, however, it is well recognized that many patients on T4 replacement may need to run FT4 just outside the reference interval to normalize TSH. In this situation, an FT3 result within the reference interval can be reassuring.

Transitory subclinical hyperthyroidism may be caused by treatment with radioiodine or antithyroid drugs in patients previously with overt hyperthyroidism or as part of thyroiditis.

## Diagnosis and Differential Diagnosis of Thyrotoxicosis

The diagnosis of Graves disease may be obvious if the patient has other clinical signs, such as exophthalmos. The laboratory diagnosis of thyrotoxicosis is based on a suppressed TSH and increased FT4 or increased FT3 or total T3. TSH is the most sensitive biomarker. A total of 2% to 4% of patients with hyperthyroidism have increased concentration of FT3 or total T3 but a normal concentration of FT4 (T3 thyrotoxicosis). Low TSH may also be drug-induced (glucocorticoids and dopamine) or caused by nonthyroidal illness.

In pituitary adenoma (secondary hyperthyroidism), TSH can be inappropriately normal or high for an elevated concentration of peripheral thyroid hormones.

If the etiology of thyrotoxicosis is uncertain, a radioactive iodine uptake test should be performed; iodine uptake of the thyroid gland is low in thyroiditis and high in Graves disease and autonomous nodules (single or multiple).

The presence of TSHR-stimulating antibodies effectively confirms a diagnosis of Graves disease. A total of 75% of patients with Graves disease have TPO antibodies, an observation that may help differentiate this disease from toxic nodular hyperthyroidism if necessary.

Due to the side effects of antithyroid drugs, patients with Graves disease should have a baseline complete blood count, including a white blood cell (WBC) count with differential, and a liver profile, including bilirubin and transaminases, before antithyroid drug therapy is initiated.

---

**POINTS TO REMEMBER: CAUSES OF HYPERTHYROIDISM**

**Endogenous Thyroid Disorders**
Autoimmune thyroid disease
Graves disease
Hashitoxicosis
Postpartum thyroiditis
Toxic multinodular goiter
Toxic adenoma
Struma ovarii
hCG-induced hyperthyroidism
    Gestational hyperthyroidism
    hCG-secreting tumors (trophoblastic tumors)
Atopic thyroid tissue
Secondary hyperthyroidism (pituitary tumor secreting TSH)

**Exogenous Disorders**
Thyroid destruction from viral or bacterial thyroiditis (e.g., de Quervain)
Iodine-induced hyperthyroidism (e.g., amiodarone)
Thyroid hormone ingestion (thyrotoxicosis factitia)

*hCG,* Human chorionic gonadotropin; *TSH,* thyroid-stimulating hormone.

# THYROID DISORDERS IN PREGNANCY AND POSTPARTUM

It is estimated that approximately 4% of pregnant women have a history of thyroid disease, develop thyroid disease during pregnancy, or are diagnosed for the first time with thyroid disease 5 years after pregnancy.

## Physiological Changes

In the first trimester of pregnancy, TSH concentrations decline as hCG stimulates the maternal thyroid gland to produce thyroid hormone, sometimes leading to a TSH concentration that is below the lower reference limit. Placental hCG shares the same α subunit with TSH but has a unique β subunit and acts in early pregnancy as a TSH agonist by binding to TSH receptors on the thyroid gland. The physiological consequences of the mild hCG stimulation of the thyroid in early pregnancy lead to a physiological rise in T4 and T3, which, by the hypothalamic-pituitary-thyroid (HPT) axis feedback mechanism, inhibits TSH secretion, which causes TSH to fall. Serum TSH decreases in the first trimester and then resets during the second and third trimesters in response to falling hCG concentrations. Concentrations of hCG are higher in a twin pregnancy, which causes a more pronounced transient TSH suppression in the first trimester relative to a singleton pregnancy.

Plasma T3 and T4 concentrations increase during pregnancy owing to an increase in TBG concentration. This increase is caused by enhanced hepatic synthesis and reduced metabolism (a result of increased estrogen levels) early in pregnancy, resulting in a 1.5-fold increase in TBG by 6 to 8 weeks of gestation. TBG remains elevated throughout pregnancy. There is a transient rise in FT4 during the first trimester owing to the relatively high circulating concentration of hCG, and FT4 gradually falls in the second and third trimesters. Changes in FT3 concentrations broadly parallel those of FT4.

Given these changes, thyroid function tests should be interpreted in the context of trimester-specific reference intervals.

## Hypothyroidism in Pregnancy

A total of 2% to 3% of all iodine-sufficient pregnant women have undiagnosed hypothyroidism, mostly SCH. Overt hypothyroidism is estimated to occur in 0.5% of all pregnant women. Worldwide, the most common cause is endemic iodine deficiency. The main cause of hypothyroidism in iodine-sufficient populations is chronic autoimmune thyroiditis. Two percent have isolated hypothyroxinemia (e.g., low thyroid hormone without plasma TSH elevation and without the presence of autoantibodies). About 10% to 20% of women in the childbearing years have detectable autoantibodies (TPO or Tg autoantibodies).

The diagnosis of hypothyroidism in pregnancy is based, as in nonpregnant subjects, on the finding of an elevated serum TSH concentration with low concentrations of FT4, using trimester-specific reference intervals (see Appendix). Untreated overt maternal hypothyroidism is associated with adverse maternal and fetal outcomes. There is an increased risk of miscarriage, preterm delivery, and preeclampsia in the mother. In the newborn, there is an increased risk of neonatal mortality caused by preterm delivery, the risk of low-for-gestational-age birth weight, and decreased IQ. The complications are similar in SCH but occur at a lower frequency. Also, in euthyroid pregnant women, positive for thyroid peroxidase and Tg antibodies, the risks of miscarriage, preterm delivery, and postpartum thyroiditis are increased.

## Thyrotoxicosis in Pregnancy

The causes of thyrotoxicosis in pregnancy are the same as for thyrotoxicosis generally; however, gestational transient hyperthyroidism is pregnancy-specific. Thyrotoxicosis may be present before pregnancy or be diagnosed in pregnancy or postpartum.

The diagnosis of thyrotoxicosis in pregnancy is made by finding a low plasma TSH concentration and elevated concentrations of FT3 and/or FT4, compared to trimester-specific reference intervals. Subclinical hyperthyroidism in pregnancy is defined as a low plasma TSH concentration with normal concentrations of FT4 or FT3.

## Graves Disease in Pregnancy

Graves disease occurs in 0.1% to 1% of all pregnancies. Uncontrolled, untreated Graves disease is associated with adverse pregnancy outcomes during and following pregnancy. Risks for the mother include fetal loss, preeclampsia, miscarriage, premature labor, thyroid storm, and congestive heart failure. Risks for the fetus and neonate include hyperthyroidism caused by TRAb crossing the placenta (fetal tachycardia, accelerated bone maturation, fetal goiter, intrauterine growth restriction, and signs of congestive heart failure, low birthweight for gestational age, poor Apgar scores, and respiratory distress syndrome), risk of hypothyroidism caused by treatment with antithyroid drugs, and congenital abnormalities caused by hyperthyroidism and the teratogenic effects of antithyroid drugs. Neonatal hyperthyroidism is infrequent and occurs in 1 in 50,000 neonates born to mothers with Graves disease. However, if it is not recognized and treated properly, the mortality rate can be as high as 30%. In pregnant patients with Graves disease, TSH and thyroid hormones should be measured every 4 to 6 weeks. The measurement of TRAb should be reserved for patients with Graves disease who become pregnant or if Graves disease is suspected during pregnancy. In the former, TRAb should be measured at diagnosis and 24 to 28 weeks gestation because these antibodies can cross the placenta, starting in the late second trimester. Testing for other thyroid autoantibodies is not required, although these are typically present in high titers.

## Gestational Transient Hyperthyroidism and Hyperemesis Gravidarum

Gestational transient hyperthyroidism usually occurs in the first trimester with a prevalence of 2% to 3% in Europeans. Gestational transient thyrotoxicosis is a nonautoimmune hyperthyroidism occurring in pregnant women with a spectrum ranging from no emesis to emesis, to hyperemesis gravidarum (when dehydration could be so severe that intravenous fluid replacement may be required). Gestational transient thyrotoxicosis occurs in 2% to 3% of all pregnancies and results from the activation of TSH receptors by hCG. Serum hCG concentrations are positively correlated with the severity of nausea and vomiting. The thyrotoxicosis of hyperemesis gravidarum usually resolves spontaneously within several weeks as the vomiting disappears. The degree of hyperthyroidism is typically mild.

## Postpartum Thyroiditis

Postpartum thyroiditis may be difficult to differentiate from Graves disease. The differences between the two include the presence of goiter, ophthalmopathy, and TRAb in Graves disease; these are usually not present in thyroiditis. Approximately 4% to 9% of unselected postpartum women develop postpartum thyroiditis, although the incidence varies with geographical location. Postpartum thyroiditis often recurs in subsequent pregnancies, and 50% of affected women eventually develop hypothyroidism. Anti-TPO positivity increases the likelihood of developing postpartum thyroiditis.

## Thyroid Function Testing in Pregnancy

TSH is a reliable indicator of thyroid function during pregnancy in most cases. Trimester-specific reference intervals for TSH and thyroid hormones should be applied. International guidelines recommend that trimester- and assay-specific reference intervals should be established or verified in each laboratory. If that is not possible, then reference intervals from the American Thyroid Association (ATA) should be applied.

The use of immunoassay for free thyroid hormones in pregnancy remains controversial as thyroid hormone-binding proteins change significantly during gestation (TBG increases and albumin falls). Direct mass spectrometric assays have been proposed for use in pregnancy for this reason. However, given the improvement in competition immunoassays for free thyroid hormones, provided method and gestational age-specific reference intervals are applied, immunoassay methods may also be used.

# THYROID NEOPLASIA

The prevalence of palpable thyroid nodules in adults is about 5%, the prevalence of nodules found on ultrasonography is 13% to 30%, and the prevalence of nodules found on autopsy is 49% to 57%. The prevalence of cancer in single nodules has been estimated to be 5% and may be less frequent in multinodular goiter. Cancer risk depends on age, sex, radiation exposure, history, family history, and other factors.

There are four main types of thyroid cancer (listed from the most common to the least common): DTC, including (1) papillary, and (2) follicular thyroid cancer, accounting for more than 90% of thyroid cancers in the United States; (3) medullary thyroid cancer (MTC) (<5%); and (4) anaplastic thyroid cancer, accounting for about 2%.

The main role of the clinical biochemist is the monitoring of TSH suppression therapy, the determination of cancer ablation by tumor makers (Tg for differentiated cancer and

Calcitonin for medullary cancer), the detection of recurrence in patients given definitive treatment, such as thyroidectomy, and prognostication.

## Differentiated Thyroid Cancer

Patients with DTC have a favorable prognosis. Tg is not a diagnostic marker, but it is a useful marker for disease recurrence in thyroidectomized patients because it should be undetectable. Immunoassays should not be used to measure Tg in patients with anti-Tg antibodies owing to measurement interference. Mass spectrometry-based methods are acceptable for use in these patients as they are not subject to interference caused by anti-Tg antibodies. Thyroid stimulation either by temporarily ceasing thyroid hormone replacement or by the administration of recombinant TSH greatly increases the sensitivity of Tg measurement, but this may not be necessary using more sensitive Tg assays. The optimal cut-off for Tg for predicting recurrence is not known. There is a general agreement that a stimulated Tg less than 1 ng/mL, with no other radiologic or clinical evidence of disease and in the absence of autoantibodies, suggests no evidence of disease, although recurrence has been described below this cut point. Newer Tg assays have a functional sensitivity of 0.1 ng/mL or less (compared to older assays with 1 ng/mL); this allows for earlier identification of recurrence and helps avoid the use of TSH stimulation.

## Medullary Thyroid Cancer

Parafollicular or C cells secrete calcitonin and give rise to MTC, with an intermediate prognosis. About 80% of MTC is sporadic (i.e., not genetically inherited and occurs randomly), and the rest is hereditary. Calcitonin is a 32-amino-acid monomeric peptide—the result of cleavage and the posttranslational processing of procalcitonin, which is itself a product of preprocalcitonin. Serum calcitonin can be used as a screening test in patients with a family history of MTC, who are at risk of developing the disease. The use of calcitonin as a screening marker in patients with nodular goiter and with no family history is debatable. Calcitonin also is used diagnostically as an immunohistochemical marker. Basal serum calcitonin and carcinoembryonic antigen (CEA) should be measured concurrently. CEA is not a specific biomarker for MTC and is not useful in the early diagnosis of MTC. However, CEA is useful for evaluating disease progression in patients with clinically evident MTC and for monitoring patients after thyroidectomy. All patients diagnosed with MTC should be tested for the genetic mutations associated with hereditary forms of the disease. To predict outcomes and plan long-term follow-up in patients treated by thyroidectomy for MTC, tumor, node, metastasis classification, the number of lymph node metastases, and postoperative serum calcitonin and CEA should be used. The genetic status also determines the prognosis in patients with hereditary MTC.

Measurements of calcitonin also may be used to monitor for persistent or recurrent disease after surgery because the concentrations correlate with tumor burden. The MTC growth rate can be determined by measuring serum levels of calcitonin or CEA over multiple time points to determine the rate at which each marker's value doubles. Furthermore, serum TSH and serum calcium should be measured postoperatively. The goals are to achieve euthyroid status and to prevent hypocalcemia.

Blood samples should be drawn in the fasting state. Calcitonin has a low stability in serum at room temperature, so the sample must be immediately separated and then frozen and transported on ice to the laboratory. Commercial chemiluminescent immunometric assays are available for calcitonin measurement. Because of inter-method differences, concentrations pre- and post-thyroidectomy and during treatment should be measured using the same assay and instrument in the same laboratory. Calcitonin values are higher in men than in women, which is likely because of a higher C-cell mass. Calcitonin may also be high during the first week of life and in low-birthweight children and premature infants. Besides gender and age, pregnancy, lactation, and growth in children may also influence circulating concentrations of calcitonin. Calcitonin may be increased in nonthyroidal cancer, inflammation and sepsis, acute and chronic renal failure, hypercalcemia, pulmonary disease, and hypergastrinemia.

## THYROID DISEASE IN CHILDREN

Fetuses are dependent on thyroid hormones for normal growth and organ development, especially brain development and maturation. TSH surges immediately after birth, reaching a peak of 25 to 160 mIU/L within 30 minutes and declining back to cord blood concentrations by postpartum day 3. TSH concentrations stabilize to near adult concentrations (reference interval generally near 0.4 to 4.5 mIU/L) within the first few weeks of life. Thyroid disease can occur at any age; however, some characteristics in newborns, children, and adolescents are worth mentioning. The consequences of a hypofunctioning thyroid in developing and maturing children may be long-lasting if not diagnosed and treated early. Neonatal hyperthyroidism may be caused by the transplacental passage of thyroid-stimulating maternal immunoglobulins (due to active maternal Graves disease) or by activating TSH receptor mutations. In older children and adolescents, the most common cause of hyperthyroidism is Graves disease, and the most common cause of hypothyroidism in iodine-replete areas is Hashimoto thyroiditis.

### Congenital Hypothyroidism

Before the introduction of newborn screening programs, the incidence of congenital hypothyroidism was estimated to be 1 in 7000 newborns. However, recent surveys estimate the incidence to be 1 in 2000 to 1 in 4000 newborns; the incidence is higher in Asians and Hispanics than in Whites and Blacks. The incidence is higher in older compared with younger mothers and in preterm infants versus term infants. Incidence rates are dependent on TSH screening cut-offs.

Permanent congenital hypothyroidism (75% to 86%) needs lifelong replacement treatment, but transient forms resolve within weeks to months after birth. Permanent

primary congenital hypothyroidism may be caused by defects in thyroid development, thyroid dysgenesis (85%), or dyshormonogenesis (15%)—a biosynthesis defect of thyroid hormone production in a structurally normal gland. Thyroid dysgenesis may consist of either thyroid agenesis, failure of the gland to descend normally during embryologic development with or without ectopy, or hypoplasia of a normal localized gland. Central hypothyroidism occurs in 1 in 25,000 to 1 in 50,000 newborns.

Transient congenital hypothyroidism is most commonly caused by inadequate maternal iodine intake in areas of endemic iodine deficiency. It may also be caused by maternal antithyroid medication during pregnancy, transfer of maternal blocking antibodies, maternal iodine exposure (e.g., amiodarone), liver hemangiomas causing increased production of deiodinase 3, and genetic defects.

Unless born with thyroid agenesis, most newborns with congenital hypothyroidism have residual thyroid function. Many newborns, even those with thyroid agenesis, do not present with classic symptoms and signs of hypothyroidism owing to the transplacental passage of maternal thyroid hormones. Early symptoms and signs of congenital hypothyroidism include a lethargic infant with increased sleep, prolonged jaundice, myxedematous facies, large fontanels, macroglossia, distended abdomen, hypothermia, and hypotonia. Later symptoms and signs include poor sucking effort leading to feeding difficulties, constipation, developmental delay with cognitive and growth retardation, myxedema, umbilical hernia, and decreased activity. Ten percent of children born with congenital hypothyroidism have other congenital birth defects, and 50% of them have congenital heart defects.

Levothyroxine is the treatment of choice with treatment goals to raise serum FT4 and normalize serum TSH. Levothyroxine treatment can prevent mental retardation in the majority of children (>90%) if commenced within the first 2 weeks of life.

### Laboratory Diagnosis of Congenital Hypothyroidism

Newborn screening for congenital hypothyroidism on dried blood spots is a successful public health program for the secondary prevention of mental retardation. Worldwide it is estimated that 25% of the newborn population undergoes screening for congenital hypothyroidism.

Screening strategies based on blood spots to differentiate between primary and secondary causes of congenital hypothyroidism differ between countries. The strategies include (a) measuring TSH initially with a reflex total T4 if TSH is abnormal, (b) measuring total T4 initially with a reflex TSH if total T4 is abnormal, and (c) measuring a combination of TSH and total T4. The initial screening occurs on the second to the fifth day of life; children discharged from the hospital on the first day of life may have a sample taken at this time. Some programs routinely obtain a second specimen at 2 to 6 weeks of age. Filter cards are mailed to a central laboratory. Each program has its own cut-offs for test results. Thyroid hormone levels and TSH are higher in the first days of life but have usually fallen to concentrations typically seen in infancy within 2 to 4 weeks.

An abnormal result on screening should lead to a confirmatory test in a serum sample, but this should not delay treatment. Confirmatory testing includes TSH and free or total T4 and should be compared with appropriate age-dependent reference intervals (see Appendix for reference intervals). Further diagnostic tests may include radionuclide thyroid uptake and scanning, thyroid sonography, and serum Tg to determine the subtype of congenital hypothyroidism, but again these investigations should not delay the initiation of treatment.

False-positive elevations in TSH within the first 2 days of life may be revealed after repeated confirmatory testing. Transplacental transfer of heterophile antibodies is well described as a false-positive interference in blood spot TSH, and maternal thyroid function tests need to be checked in this context. Preterm infants with an immature HPT axis and acutely ill term infants may have a late rise in TSH and may not show elevated TSH on the first screening test; many programs have a second screening test for these babies. Dopamine used in the treatment of ill premature neonates can also attenuate TSH release. Seasonal variations in TSH occur with an increased false-positive rate of congenital hypothyroidism in the winter (0.9%) compared with the summer (0.6%); this is in accordance with globally conducted previous studies that have identified an increased prevalence of suspected and confirmed cases of congenital hypothyroidism in the winter months.

## GENETICS

Evidence from twin studies has shown that about 65% of baseline TSH and thyroid hormone concentrations are genetically determined, with about 20% of the variability coming from common genetic variations at the population level. This suggests a genetic basis for narrow intraindividual variation in these hormone concentrations. Several loci have been identified in genome-wide association studies (GWAS) for the circulating concentrations of TSH, thyroid hormones, thyroid autoantibodies, and deiodinases.

Autoimmune susceptibility against the thyroid gland is estimated to affect 5% of the general population, and about 80% of this susceptibility can be explained by genetic factors.

### Genetics in Congenital Hypothyroidism

Thyroid dyshormonogenesis is inherited in an autosomal recessive pattern. Thyroid dysgenesis, on the other hand, is inherited in only approximately 2% of cases; the rest are considered to be sporadic.

### Thyroid-Stimulating Receptor Mutations and Resistance to Thyroid-Stimulating Hormone

Cases of familial thyrotoxicosis with no evidence of autoimmunity and children with persistent isolated neonatal hyperthyroidism should be evaluated for familial nonautoimmune autosomal dominant hyperthyroidism (FNAH) and persistent sporadic congenital nonautoimmune hyperthyroidism (PSNAH) caused by rare germline mutations in the TSHR gene.

### Thyroid Hormone Receptor Mutations and Resistance to Thyroid Hormone

Thyroid hormone resistance syndromes are caused by mutations in the two thyroid hormone receptors α (THRα) and β (THRβ). The resultant phenotypes reflect the tissue distribution of the two different forms. Best described are mutations in the THRβ gene. As THRβ is expressed in the pituitary this syndrome is characterized by raised levels of thyroid hormone with normal or slightly elevated levels of TSH. Clinical features such as hyperactivity and tachycardia reflect hyperstimulation of tissues with the unaffected THRβ receptor

Only a few patients with resistance to thyroid hormone α (RTHα) have been described. As THRβ is not expressed in the pituitary thyroid function tests are only subtly affected but clinical features of hypothyroidism such as growth retardation, constipation, and intellectual deficit are consistent with impaired expression of the THRβ form in relevant tissues.

## REVIEW QUESTIONS

1. What is the most common type of laboratory assay that is widely used to assess thyroid hormone concentrations?
   a. Ultrafiltration
   b. Immunoassay
   c. Potentiometry
   d. Estimation from using a formula
2. What stimulates the uptake of iodide by the thyroid gland for thyroid hormone synthesis?
   a. Thyroid-stimulating hormone (TSH)
   b. Thyroxine (T4)
   c. Tyrosine
   d. Thyroiditis
3. What causes primary hypothyroidism?
   a. The absence or dysfunction of the thyroid gland
   b. Increased TSH

   c. A pituitary disorder
   d. A hypothalamic disorder
4. Hyperthyroidism is also referred to as:
   a. Athyreosis
   b. Myxedema
   c. Thyrotoxicosis
   d. Exophthalmos
5. What is the function of thyroid hormones?
   a. Inhibit the secretion of growth hormone
   b. Solely regulate reproductive processes in males and females
   c. Maintain water homeostasis
   d. Regulate carbohydrate, lipid, and protein metabolism within cells

6. *Primary* hypothyroidism is indicated by which of the following sets of lab results?
   a. Increased FT4, and decreased TSH
   b. Increased FT4, and increased TSH
   c. Decreased FT4, and increased TSH
   d. Decreased FT4, and decreased TSH
7. Which of the following hormones is *not* produced by the thyroid gland?
   a. TSH
   b. Calcitonin
   c. Thyroxine (T4)
   d. Triiodothyronine (T3)
8. What is the amino acid precursor of T4?
   a. Threonine
   b. Tyrosine
   c. Thyronine
   d. Alanine
9. What is the tumor marker for differentiated thyroid cancer?
   a. Thyroid peroxidase antibodies
   b. Calcitonin
   c. Thyroglobulin antibodies
   d. Thyroglobulin
10. What is the tumor marker for medullary thyroid cancer?
   a. Thyroid peroxidase antibodies
   b. Calcitonin
   c. Thyroglobulin antibodies
   d. Thyroglobulin

## SUGGESTED READINGS

Bailey D, Colantonio D, Kyriakopoulou L, et al. Marked biological variance in endocrine and biochemical markers in childhood: establishment of pediatric reference intervals using healthy community children from the CALIPER cohort. *Clin Chem.* 2013;59:1393–1405.

Cooper DS, Biondi B. Subclinical thyroid disease. *Lancet.* 2012;379:1142–1154.

Cooper DS, Laurberg P. Hyperthyroidism in pregnancy. *Lancet Diabetes Endocrinol.* 2013;1:238–249.

Elmlinger MW, Kuhnel W, Lambrecht HG, et al. Reference intervals from birth to adulthood for serum thyroxine (T4), triiodothyronine (T3), free T3, free T4, thyroxine binding globulin (TBG) and thyrotropin (TSH). *Clin Chem Lab Med.* 2001;39:973–979.

Franklyn JA, Boelaert K. Thyrotoxicosis. *Lancet.* 2012;379:1155–1166.

Gruters A, Krude H. Detection and treatment of congenital hypothyroidism. *Nat Rev Endocrinol.* 8:104–113.

Hoofnagle AN, Becker JO, Wener MH, et al. Quantification of thyroglobulin, a low-abundance serum protein, by immunoaffinity peptide enrichment and tandem mass spectrometry. *Clin Chem.* 54;1796–1804.

Midgley JE. Direct and indirect free thyroxine assay methods: theory and practice. *Clin Chem.* 2001;47:1353–1363.

Pearce EN, Farwell AP, Braverman LE. Thyroiditis. *N Eng J Med.* 2003;348:2646–2655.

Roberts CG, Ladenson PW. Hypothyroidism. *Lancet.* 2004;363:793–803.

Stagnaro-Green A, Pearce E. Thyroid disorders in pregnancy. *Nat Rev Endocrinol.* 2012;8:650–658.

Taylor PN, Porcu E, Chew S, et al. Whole-genome sequence-based analysis of thyroid function. *Nat Commun.* 2015;6:5681.

Thienpont LM, Van Uytfanghe K, Van Houcke S, et al. A progress report of the IFCC committee for standardization of thyroid function tests. *Eur Thyroid J.* 2014;3:109–116.

Thienpont LM, Van Uytfanghe K, Beastall G, et al. Report of the IFCC working group for standardization of thyroid function tests; part 1: thyroid-stimulating hormone. *Clin Chem.* 2010;56:902–911.

Thienpont LM, Van Uytfanghe K, Beastall G, et al. Report of the IFCC Working Group for Standardization of Thyroid Function Tests; part 3: total thyroxine and total triiodothyronine. *Clin Chem.* 2010;56:921–929.

Thienpont LM, Van Uytfanghe K, Van Houcke S. Tests IWGfSoTF. Standardization activities in the field of thyroid function tests: a status report. *Clin Chem Lab Med.* 2010;48:1577–1583.

Vestergaard P, Rejnmark L, Weeke J, et al. Smoking as a risk factor for Graves' disease, toxic nodular goiter, and autoimmune hypothyroidism. *Thyroid.* 2002;12:69–75.

Zimmermann MB, Boelaert K. Iodine deficiency and thyroid disorders. *Lancet Diabet Endocrinol.* 2015;3:286–295.

# Reproductive Endocrinology and Related Disorders

*Robert D. Nerenz and Andrew R. Crawford*

## OBJECTIVES

1. Identify hormonal factors that determine male and female reproductive function.
2. Describe clinical symptoms associated with states of reproductive dysfunction.
3. Explain pathologic mechanisms responsible for infertility.
4. Describe laboratory tests used in the evaluation of reproductive disorders.

## KEY WORDS AND DEFINITIONS

**Amenorrhea** The absence of menstruation.

**Dehydroepiandrosterone (DHEA)** The most abundant adrenal androgen.

**Estradiol** The predominant female sex steroid.

**Follicle** A pouch-like sac on the surface of the ovary that contains the maturing ovum (egg).

**Follicle-stimulating hormone (FSH)** A heterodimeric glycoprotein secreted by the pituitary gland that stimulates ovarian follicle maturation and sperm production.

**Gonad** A gamete-producing gland.

**Gonadotropin-releasing hormone (GnRH)** A hypothalamic polypeptide hormone that stimulates LH and FSH release by the pituitary gland.

**Hypothalamus** The portion of the brain just above the pituitary gland that regulates its endocrine functions.

**Luteinizing hormone (LH)** A heterodimeric glycoprotein secreted by the pituitary gland that stimulates gonadal sex steroid production and triggers ovulation.

**Menopause** Cessation of menstruation, which usually occurs around the age of 50.

**Menses** The monthly flow of blood from the female genital tract.

**Pituitary** The master regulatory endocrine gland located at the base of the brain.

**Polycystic ovary syndrome (PCOS)** A female condition that is characterized by multiple ovarian follicles, ovulatory dysfunction, and increased androgen production.

**Progesterone** A steroid hormone secreted by the corpus luteum and placenta with a primary role in maintaining pregnancy.

**Ovary** Female gonad.

**Ovulation** The process of ovarian egg release.

**Sex hormone-binding globulin** A circulating plasma protein that binds estradiol, testosterone, and dihydrotestosterone.

**Testis (pl. Testes)** Male gonad.

**Testosterone** The predominant male sex steroid.

**Virilization** The induction or development of male secondary sex characteristics; especially the induction of such changes in females.

## BACKGROUND

The field of reproductive endocrinology encompasses the hormones of the hypothalamic–pituitary–gonadal axis and the adrenal glands; these hormones are crucial for reproductive function. Hypothalamic gonadotropin-releasing hormone (GnRH) directs the pituitary to synthesize and release follicle-stimulating hormone (FSH) and luteinizing hormone (LH), which in turn stimulate gonadal synthesis of the sex steroids that govern the development and maintenance of secondary sex characteristics. In states of reproductive health, serum concentrations of these hormones rise and fall in a tightly regulated and well-characterized pattern. In states of reproductive dysfunction, measurement of these hormones in the clinical laboratory often provides the necessary information to identify the underlying abnormality and guide appropriate treatment.

## MALE REPRODUCTIVE BIOLOGY

The mature testes synthesize both sperm and androgens. The testes contain a structured network of tightly packed seminiferous tubules, the lumina of which are lined by maturing germ cells and Sertoli cells. Sertoli cells play a crucial role in sperm maturation and secrete *inhibin*, a 32-kDa glycoprotein that inhibits the pituitary secretion of FSH. Surrounding the seminiferous tubules are the interstitial Leydig cells, the primary site of androgen production. The principal androgen in humans is testosterone, which serves a central role in reproductive physiology. Testosterone is required for sexual differentiation, spermatogenesis, and the promotion and maintenance of sexual maturity at puberty. At the cellular level, these effects are mediated by binding of testosterone or its more potent metabolite dihydrotestosterone (DHT) to the androgen receptor or via aromatization to estradiol and subsequent binding to the estrogen receptor. Testicular function is under the control of the hypothalamic–pituitary–gonadal axis.

## Hypothalamic–Pituitary–Gonadal Axis

GnRH is a decapeptide synthesized in the hypothalamus and transported to the anterior pituitary gland, where it stimulates the release of both FSH and LH.

In adult males, GnRH and thus LH and FSH are secreted in pulsatile patterns, with more rapid pulses favoring LH release and slower pulses favoring FSH release. In males, GnRH pulse frequency appears to be relatively constant throughout adult life. A circadian rhythm is present, with higher concentrations found in the early-morning hours and lower concentrations in the late evening. LH acts on Leydig cells to stimulate the conversion of cholesterol to pregnenolone. FSH acts on Sertoli cells and spermatocytes and is central to the initiation (in puberty) and maintenance (in adulthood) of spermatogenesis. Sex steroids and inhibin provide negative feedback control of LH and FSH secretion, respectively.

## Androgens

Androgens are a group of C-19 steroids (Fig. 43.1) responsible for masculinization of the genital tract and development and maintenance of male secondary sex characteristics. Testosterone is the principal androgen secreted in males.

### Biosynthesis of Testosterone

Testosterone is synthesized primarily by the Leydig cells of the testes (95%) and, to a lesser extent (≈5%), via peripheral conversion from the precursors dehydroepiandrosterone (DHEA) and androstenedione, which are synthesized in the zona reticularis of the adrenal glands (see Fig. 43.1).

### Androgen Transport in Blood

Testosterone and DHT circulate in plasma freely (≈2%–3%) or bound to plasma proteins. Binding proteins include the specific sex hormone-binding globulin (SHBG) and non-specific proteins such as albumin. SHBG is an α-globulin that has low capacity for steroids but binds with very high affinity ($K_a = 1 \times 10^8$ to $1 \times 10^9$), whereas albumin has high capacity but low affinity ($K_a = 1 \times 10^4$ to $1 \times 10^6$). SHBG has the highest affinity for DHT and the lowest for estradiol.

The biologically active fraction includes free testosterone; albumin-bound testosterone may also be available for tissue uptake. Therefore, bioavailable testosterone (free + albumin-bound) composes approximately 35% of total circulating testosterone.

Testosterone and SHBG exhibit rhythmic variation in their circulating concentrations. Testosterone concentrations peak at approximately 4:00 a.m. to 8:00 a.m. and reach nadir between 4:00 p.m. and 8:00 p.m. Daily variations in SHBG concentrations are similar to those of other proteins and albumin in serum, with major changes related to posture. Concentrations of SHBG are suppressed by testosterone administration and hypothyroidism and elevated in hypogonadal and hyperthyroid males.

### Metabolism of Testosterone

Circulating testosterone serves as a precursor for the formation of two additional active metabolites: DHT and estradiol. In one pathway, 5α-reductase converts 6%–8% of testosterone to DHT. Both testosterone and DHT bind the androgen receptor, but DHT binds with higher affinity. In an alternative pathway, testosterone and androstenedione are converted to estrogens (≈0.3%) through aromatase (CYP19). DHT is formed in androgen target tissues such as the skin and prostate, whereas aromatization occurs in many tissues, especially the liver and adipose tissue. Peripheral aromatization occurs primarily in adipose tissue (of both males and females), which contains high concentrations of aromatase. The rate of extraglandular aromatization therefore increases with body fat.

The main excretory metabolites of androstenedione, testosterone, and DHEA are shown in Fig. 43.2. Except for epitestosterone, these catabolites constitute a group of steroids known as *17-ketosteroids* (17-KS); they are excreted primarily in the urine.

### Testosterone Concentrations

Testosterone is required for proper sexual development and function throughout all stages of life: fetal, pubertal, and adult (Fig. 43.3). Fetal testes produce testosterone around the 7th week of gestation, with peak fetal serum concentrations of approximately 250 ng/dL (8.7 nmol/L) observed at the beginning of the second trimester, and with concentrations gradually returning to baseline by birth. Shortly after birth, the concentration of testosterone begins to increase, peaking again at approximately 250 ng/dL (8.7 nmol/L) at 2–3 months of age, and then falling to baseline again by 6–12 months. The concentration of testosterone remains low (<50 ng/dL, 1.7 nmol/L) until puberty, when the concentration of testosterone rises to 500–700 ng/dL (17.3–24.3 nmol/L) and remains elevated until 30–40 years of age, at which point circulating testosterone decreases by 0.5%–2% per year. This decline in testosterone is thought to be due to: (1) a decrease in Leydig cell numbers; (2) decreased GnRH pulse amplitude; and (3) increases in SHBG. Decreases in circulating concentrations of testosterone were previously viewed as a normal part of the aging process. Now, however, these decreases, when accompanied by symptoms of decreased libido, sexual dysfunction, decreased energy levels, and decreased muscle mass, are regarded as a syndrome with a variety of names, such as androgen deficiency in the aging male (ADAM), partial androgen deficiency of the aging male (PADAM), late-onset hypogonadism (LOH), and, erroneously, andropause. The name *andropause* is inaccurate and misleading, given that in contrast to menopause in women, concentrations of sex steroids in males do not decrease sharply with secondary cessation of reproductive function. A name put forward

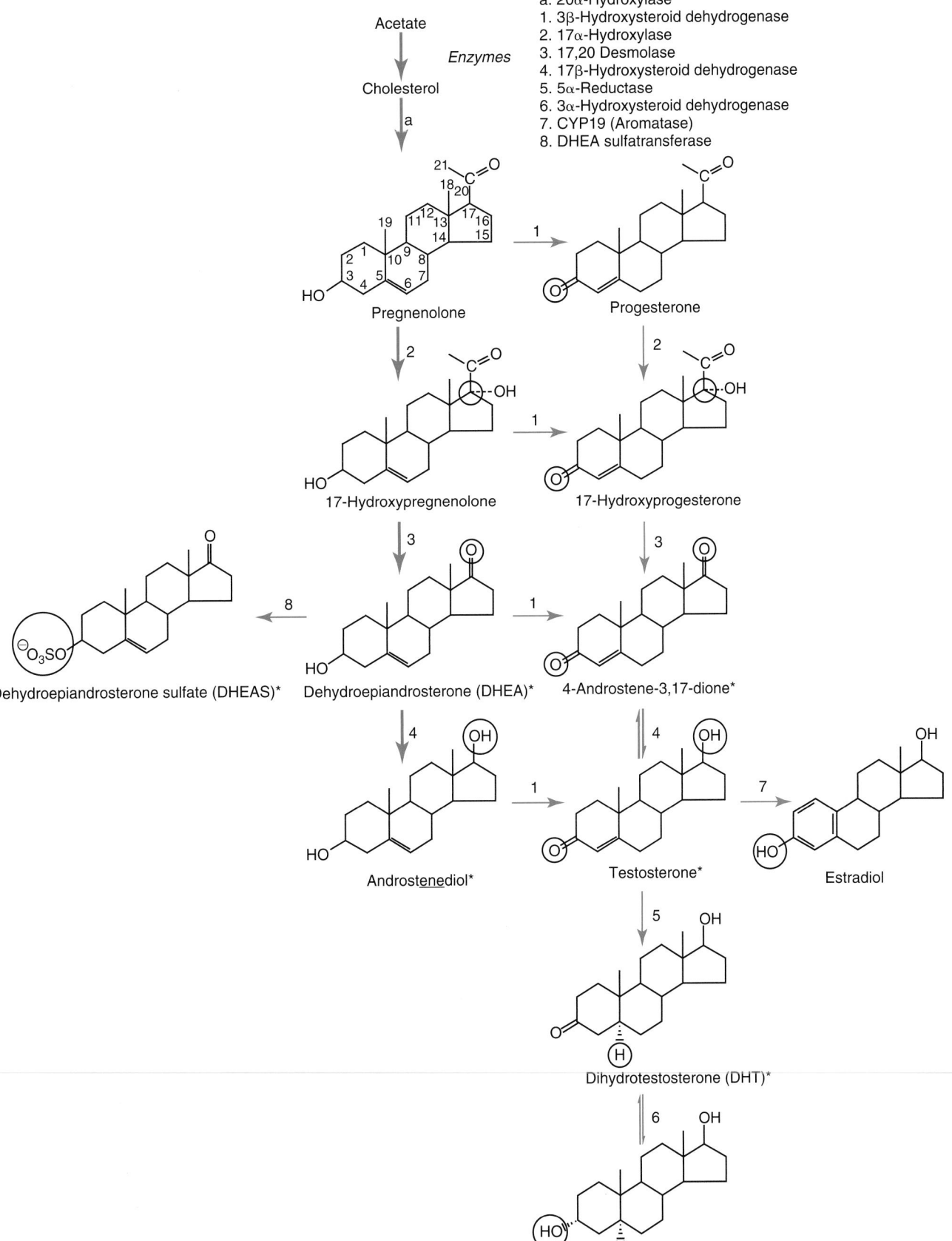

**Fig. 43.1** Biosynthesis of androgens (adrenal glands and testis). The *heavy arrows* indicate the preferred pathway. The *circled areas* represent the site of chemical change. *Denotes androgens.

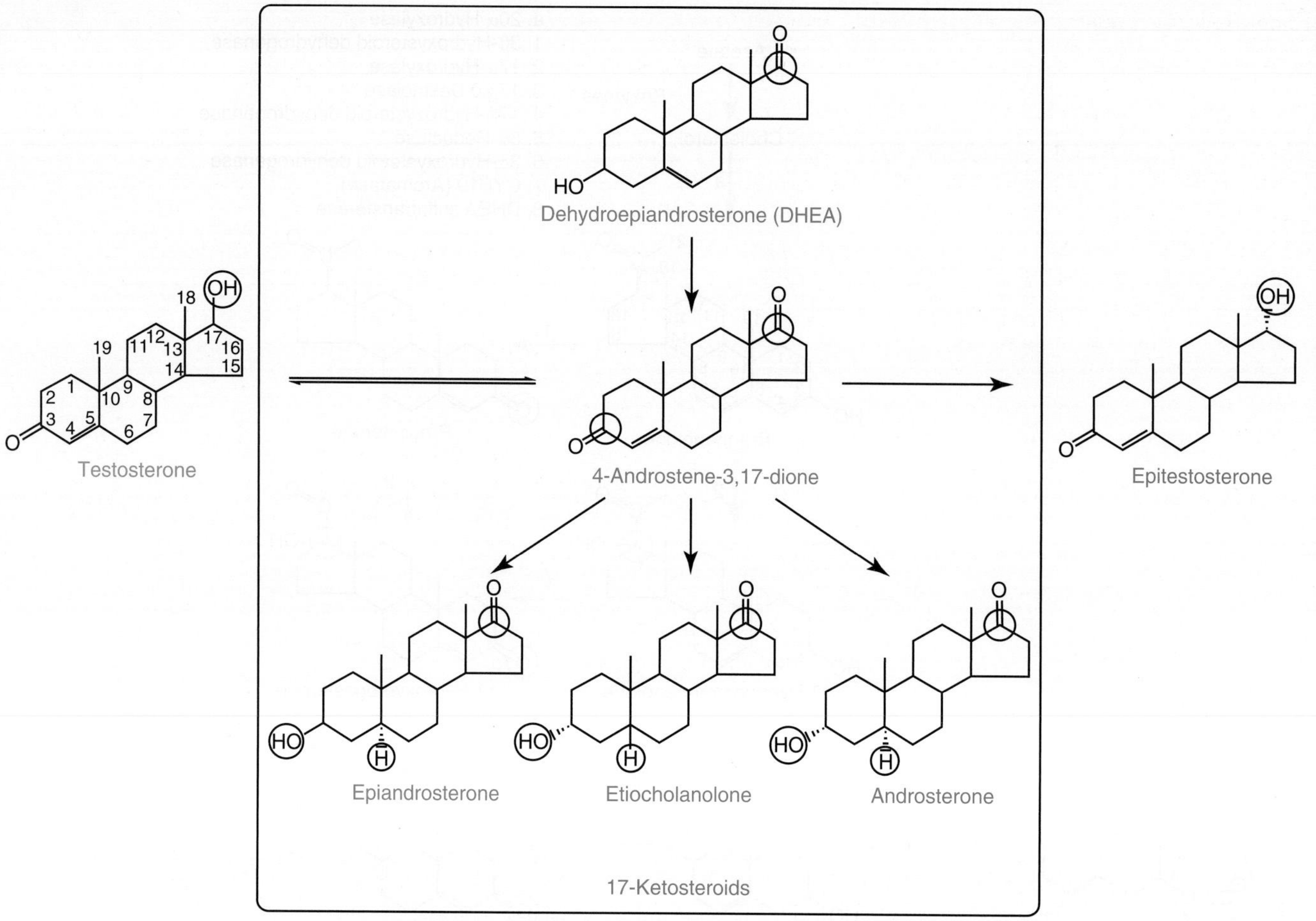

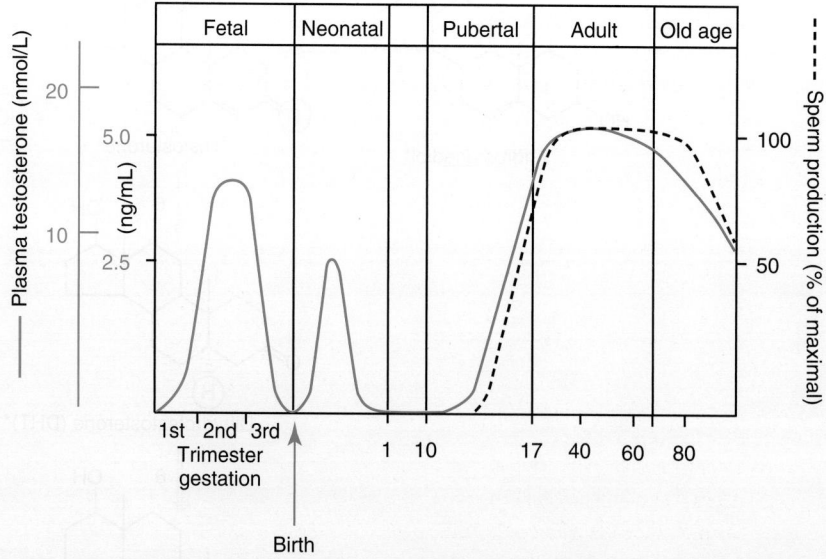

**Fig. 43.2** Catabolism of C19O2 androgens. The *circled areas* represent the site of chemical change.

**Fig. 43.3** Schematic diagram of different phases of male sexual function during life as indicated by mean plasma testosterone concentration and sperm production at different ages. (From Griffin JE, Wilson JD. The testis. In: Bondy PK, Rosenberg LE, eds. *Metabolic Control and Disease*, 8th ed. Philadelphia: WB Saunders; 1980.)

more recently is *testosterone deficiency syndrome (TDS)*, highlighting a specific deficit in testosterone as part of the clinical picture.

Diagnosis of LOH (TDS) should be based on both clinical and laboratory assessment. Clinically, patients should exhibit symptoms suggestive of testosterone deficiency described above. Patients should exhibit one to three of these symptoms with a concomitant low serum testosterone concentration to fit various diagnostic criteria. Total serum testosterone is the most widely used biochemical parameter for assessment of hypogonadism, but measurement of free or bioavailable testosterone should be considered when total testosterone is not diagnostic despite the clinical presentation of hypogonadism. To accurately diagnose male hypogonadism, unequivocally low testosterone should be demonstrated on at least two fasting early morning blood samples.

## Male Reproductive Abnormalities

A wide variety of abnormalities can affect the male reproductive system before birth, in childhood, or in adulthood. For the purposes of this chapter, they have been divided into categories of: (1) hypogonadotropic hypogonadism; (2) hypergonadotropic hypogonadism; (3) defects in androgen action (Box 43.1); (4) erectile dysfunction; and (5) gynecomastia.

## Hypogonadotropic Hypogonadism

Hypogonadotropic hypogonadism occurs when defects in the hypothalamus or pituitary prevent normal gonadal stimulation. Causative factors include congenital or acquired panhypopituitarism, hypothalamic syndromes, GnRH deficiency, hyperprolactinemia, malnutrition or anorexia, and iatrogenic causes. All of these abnormalities are associated with decreased testosterone and gonadotropin concentrations.

*Kallmann syndrome*, the most common form of congenital hypogonadotropic hypogonadism, results from a deficiency of GnRH in the hypothalamus during embryonic development. It is characterized by hypogonadism and anosmia (absent sense of smell) in male or female patients, and is inherited as an autosomal dominant trait with variable penetrance.

## Hypergonadotropic Hypogonadism

Hypergonadotropic hypogonadism results from a primary gonadal disorder. Patients with primary testicular failure have increased concentrations of LH and FSH and decreased concentrations of testosterone. Causes of primary hypogonadism are categorized as: (1) acquired causes (irradiation, castration, testicular torsion, mumps orchitis, or cytotoxic drugs); (2) chromosomal defects (Klinefelter syndrome); (3) testicular agenesis; (4) seminiferous tubular disease; (5) congenital deficiencies in enzymes involved in androgen synthesis; and (6) other miscellaneous causes.

## Defects in Androgen Action

The most common and severe defect in androgen action is *androgen insensitivity syndrome* (AIS), a disorder arising from mutations in the androgen receptor gene (*AR*). AIS may

---

### BOX 43.1 Male Reproductive Abnormalities

**Hypogonadotropic Hypogonadism**
- Panhypopituitarism (congenital or acquired)
- Hypothalamic syndrome (congenital or acquired)
  - Structural defects (neoplastic, inflammatory, and infiltrative)
  - Prader–Willi syndrome
  - Laurence–Moon–Biedl syndrome
  - GnRH deficiency (Kallmann syndrome)
  - Hyperprolactinemia (prolactinoma or drugs)
  - Malnutrition and anorexia nervosa
  - Drug-induced suppression of luteinizing hormone (androgens, estrogens, tranquilizers, antidepressants, antihypertensives, barbiturates, cimetidine, GnRH analogs, and opiates)

**Hypergonadotropic Hypogonadism**
- Acquired
  - Irradiation
  - Mumps orchitis
  - Castration
  - Cytotoxic drugs
- Chromosome defects
  - Klinefelter syndrome (47,XXY) and mosaics
  - Autosomal and sex chromosomes, polyploidies
  - Ovotesticular disorder of sex development (previously known as true hermaphroditism)
  - Defective androgen biosynthesis
  - 20α-Hydroxylase (cholesterol 20,22-desmolase) deficiency
  - 17,20-Lyase deficiency
  - 3β-Hydroxysteroid dehydrogenase deficiency
  - 17α-Hydroxylase deficiency
  - 17β-Hydroxysteroid dehydrogenase deficiency
- Testicular agenesis
- Selective seminiferous tubular disease
- Miscellaneous
  - Noonan syndrome (short stature, pulmonary valve stenosis, hypertelorism, and ptosis)
  - Streak gonads
  - Myotonia dystrophica
- Acute and chronic disease

**Defects in Androgen Action**
- Complete androgen insensitivity (*testicular feminization*)
- Partial androgen sensitivity
  - 5α-Reductase deficiency

*GnRH, Gonadotropin-releasing hormone.*

---

be classified as complete (CAIS) or partial (PAIS), depending on the amount of residual receptor function. Individuals with complete AIS (formerly known as testicular feminization) have a male karyotype (46,XY) with female external genitalia (labia, clitoris, and vaginal opening). The testes are present intra-abdominally, and because they produce anti-Müllerian hormone (AMH), no uterus, fallopian tubules, or proximal vagina is present. The circulating concentration of testosterone in these patients is greater than or equal to that of a healthy male. Concentrations of LH are increased, presumably because of resistance of the hypothalamic-pituitary system to androgen inhibition.

Males with *5α-reductase deficiency* (5-ARD) do not convert testosterone to the more potent DHT. Because DHT leads to masculinization of external genitalia in utero, males are born with ambiguous genitalia. High ratios of the circulating concentrations of testosterone to DHT are indicative of 5-ARD. Moreover, evidence indicates that DHT formation is deficient in the tissues of the urogenital tract in these patients.

In patients with cryptorchidism or ambiguous genitalia, identification of abdominal **gonads** is essential for proper diagnosis and treatment. The presence of testicular tissue has traditionally been detected by the measurement of Leydig cell testosterone production after stimulation with human chorionic gonadotropin (hCG). However, circulating inhibin and AMH concentrations reflect Sertoli cell function and may offer a noninvasive evaluation of the integrity of the seminiferous tubules.

### Erectile Dysfunction

Erectile dysfunction (formerly referred to as *impotence*) is the persistent inability to develop or maintain a penile erection that is sufficient for intercourse and ejaculation in 50% or more of attempts. A wide variety of organic and psychologic abnormalities may cause changes in sexual drive and in the ability to have an erection or to ejaculate. Psychogenic erectile dysfunction is the most common diagnosis. Other causes include vascular disease, diabetes mellitus, hypertension, uremia, neurologic disease, hypogonadism, hyperthyroidism and hypothyroidism, neoplasms, and drugs. If no obvious explanation for erectile dysfunction can be found, measurement of morning serum testosterone, LH, and thyroid-stimulating hormone (TSH) concentrations has been suggested. Elevated gonadotropin concentrations indicate primary hypogonadism.

### Gynecomastia

Gynecomastia, the benign growth of glandular breast tissue in males, is a common finding among males of various ages. This condition, which is related to an increase in the estrogen/androgen ratio, is commonly associated with three distinct periods of life. First, transient gynecomastia can be found in 60%–90% of all newborns because of the high estrogen concentrations that cross the placenta. The second peak occurs during puberty in 50%–70% of normal males. It is usually self-limited and may be due to low serum testosterone, low DHT, or a high estrogen/androgen ratio. The last peak is found in the adult population, most frequently among males aged 50–80 years. Gynecomastia may be due to testicular failure, resulting in an increased estrogen/androgen ratio, or to increased body fat, resulting in increased peripheral aromatization of testosterone to estradiol. Pathologic gynecomastia can be caused by hyperthyroidism, hyperprolactinemia, hCG-secreting tumors and states of excessive estradiol secretion (estrogen-secreting tumors) or reduced estrogen clearance such as hepatic cirrhosis and medications which have estrogen-like activity, increase the estrogen/androgen ratio, or block androgen action (such

as spironolactone). It is important to note that prolactin plays an important role in *galactorrhea* (milk production) but only an indirect role in gynecomastia.

> **POINTS TO REMEMBER**
> - GnRH stimulates LH and FSH release, which increase testosterone and sperm production, respectively.
> - LH secretion is inhibited by testosterone and FSH secretion is inhibited by inhibin.
> - Testosterone is transported in blood tightly bound to SHBG and loosely bound to albumin.
> - Free testosterone is biologically active and represents 2%–3% of total testosterone.
> - Pituitary or hypothalamic defects result in hypogonadotropic hypogonadism.
> - Primary gonadal defects result in hypergonadotropic hypogonadism.

## FEMALE REPRODUCTIVE BIOLOGY

The ovaries produce ova and secrete the sex hormones **progesterone** and estrogen. Every healthy female neonate possesses approximately 400,000 primordial follicles, each containing an immature ovum. During the reproductive life span of an adult woman, 300–400 follicles will reach maturity. A single mature **follicle** is typically produced during each normal menstrual cycle at approximately day 14. Surrounding the oocyte of the mature follicle are three distinct cell layers: *theca externa, theca interna,* and *granulosa cells*. The theca interna cells are the primary source of androgens, which are transported to adjacent granulosa cells, where they are aromatized to estrogens.

The mature follicle undergoes **ovulation** by the process of rupture (facilitated by theca externa), thereby releasing the oocyte into the proximity of the fallopian tubes. The follicle then fills with blood to form the corpus hemorrhagicum. The granulosa and theca cells of the follicle lining quickly proliferate to form lipid-rich luteal cells, replacing the clotted blood and forming the *corpus luteum* (yellow body). The resulting luteal cells produce estrogen and progesterone. If fertilization and pregnancy occur, the corpus luteum persists and continues to produce estrogen and progesterone. If no pregnancy occurs, the corpus luteum regresses, and the next menstrual cycle begins.

The uterine cavity is lined by the endometrium. The endometrium undergoes cyclic changes in preparation for implantation and pregnancy in response to cyclic changes in estrogen and progesterone. During the follicular phase, the endometrial lining increases in thickness and vascularity in response to increasing circulating concentrations of estrogen; after regression of the corpus luteum, menstruation begins as the endometrium is shed in response to the withdrawal of progesterone.

### Hypothalamic–Pituitary–Gonadal Axis

In adult females, a tightly coordinated feedback system exists between the hypothalamus, anterior pituitary, and ovaries to orchestrate menstruation. FSH serves to stimulate follicular growth, and LH stimulates ovulation and progesterone secretion from the developing corpus luteum.

## Estrogens

Estrogens are responsible for the development and maintenance of female sex organs and female secondary sex characteristics. In conjunction with progesterone, they participate in regulation of the menstrual cycle and of breast and uterine growth as well as in the maintenance of pregnancy.

Estrogens affect calcium homeostasis and have a beneficial effect on bone mass. They decrease bone resorption and accelerate linear bone growth in prepubertal females, resulting in epiphyseal closure. Long-term estrogen depletion is associated with loss of bone mineral content, an increase in stress fractures, and postmenopausal osteoporosis.

Estrogens also have well-established effects on plasma proteins that influence endocrine testing. They increase circulating concentrations of SHBG, corticosteroid-binding globulin, and thyroxine-binding globulin. Hence, prepubertal males and females have comparable concentrations of SHBG, but adult males have SHBG concentrations approximately half those of adult females. Concentrations of plasma proteins that bind copper and iron are also elevated in response to estrogen, as are those of high-density and very high-density lipoproteins. In addition, estrogens may have a preventive role in coronary heart disease.

### Chemistry

The three most biologically active estrogens in order of potency are estradiol ($E_2$), estrone ($E_1$), and estriol ($E_3$) (Fig. 43.4).

### Biosynthesis

The biochemical pathway illustrating aromatization of testosterone to estradiol and androstenedione to estrone is shown in Fig. 43.5.

Estrogens are secreted primarily in non-pregnant females by the ovarian follicles and the corpus luteum, and during pregnancy by the placenta. The adrenal glands and testes (in males) may also secrete minute quantities of estrogens. The ovary synthesizes estrogens via aromatization of androgens. Synthesis of estrogens begins in the theca interna cells with

the enzymatic synthesis of androstenedione from cholesterol. Androstenedione is then transported to the granulosa cells, where it is further metabolized directly to estrone (androstenedione → estrone), or first to testosterone and then to estradiol (androstenedione → testosterone → estradiol) by the enzyme aromatase. While the healthy human ovary produces all three classes of sex steroids (estrogens, progestins, and androgens), estradiol and progesterone are its primary secretory products. The most potent estrogen secreted by the ovary is 17β-estradiol. Because it is derived almost exclusively from the ovaries, its measurement is often considered sufficient for the evaluation of ovarian function.

Estrogens are also produced by the peripheral aromatization of androgens, primarily androstenedione. In healthy adult males and females, approximately 1% of secreted androstenedione is converted to estrone. Although the ovaries of postmenopausal females do not secrete estrogens, peripheral conversion of adrenal androstenedione results in significant blood concentrations of estrone. Because a major site of this conversion is adipose tissue, estrone is increased in postmenopausal females with obesity, sometimes yielding enough estrogen to produce bleeding.

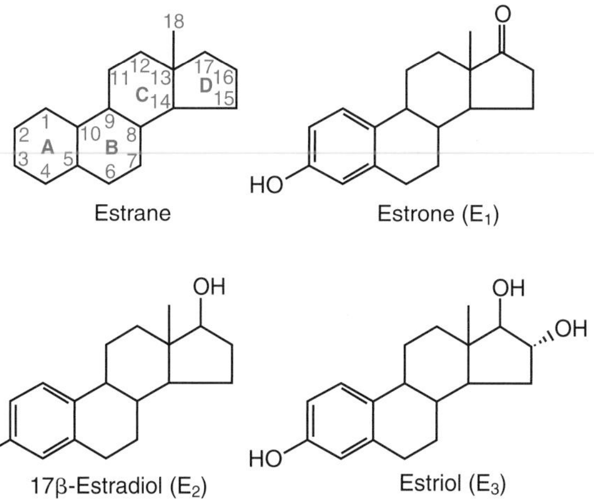

### Biosynthesis During Pregnancy

Estrogen biosynthesis differs qualitatively and quantitatively in pregnant females compared with non-pregnant ones. In pregnant females the major source of estrogens is the placenta, whereas in non-pregnant females the ovaries are the main site of synthesis. In contrast to the microgram quantities secreted by non-pregnant females, the quantity of estrogens secreted during pregnancy increases to milligram amounts. The major estrogen secreted by the ovary is estradiol ($E_2$), whereas the major product secreted by the placenta is estriol ($E_3$). Estriol is formed in the placenta by sequential desulfation and aromatization of plasma dehydroepiandrosterone sulfate (DHEA-S). Except during prenatal trisomy screening, measurements of $E_3$ have little clinical value.

### Transport in Blood

More than 97% of circulating $E_2$ is bound to plasma proteins. It is bound specifically and with high affinity to SHBG and nonspecifically to albumin. SHBG concentrations are increased by estrogens, hyperthyroidism, and administration of certain antiepileptic drugs (e.g., phenytoin/Dilantin). SHBG concentrations may decrease in hypothyroidism, obesity, or androgen excess. Only 2%–3% of total $E_2$ circulates in free form. In contrast, $E_1$ and $E_1$ sulfate circulate bound almost exclusively to albumin. As with testosterone, both free and albumin-bound fractions of $E_2$ are considered bioavailable, but measurement of this fraction has no demonstrated clinical utility.

### Metabolism

The metabolism of $E_2$ is chiefly an oxidative process dominated by three pathways, of which the fastest is oxidation of the β-hydroxy group at C-17 to a ketone (estradiol → estrone). This process is reversible; however, equilibrium favors the estrone species (Fig. 43.6).

Fig. 43.4 Biologically active estrogens.

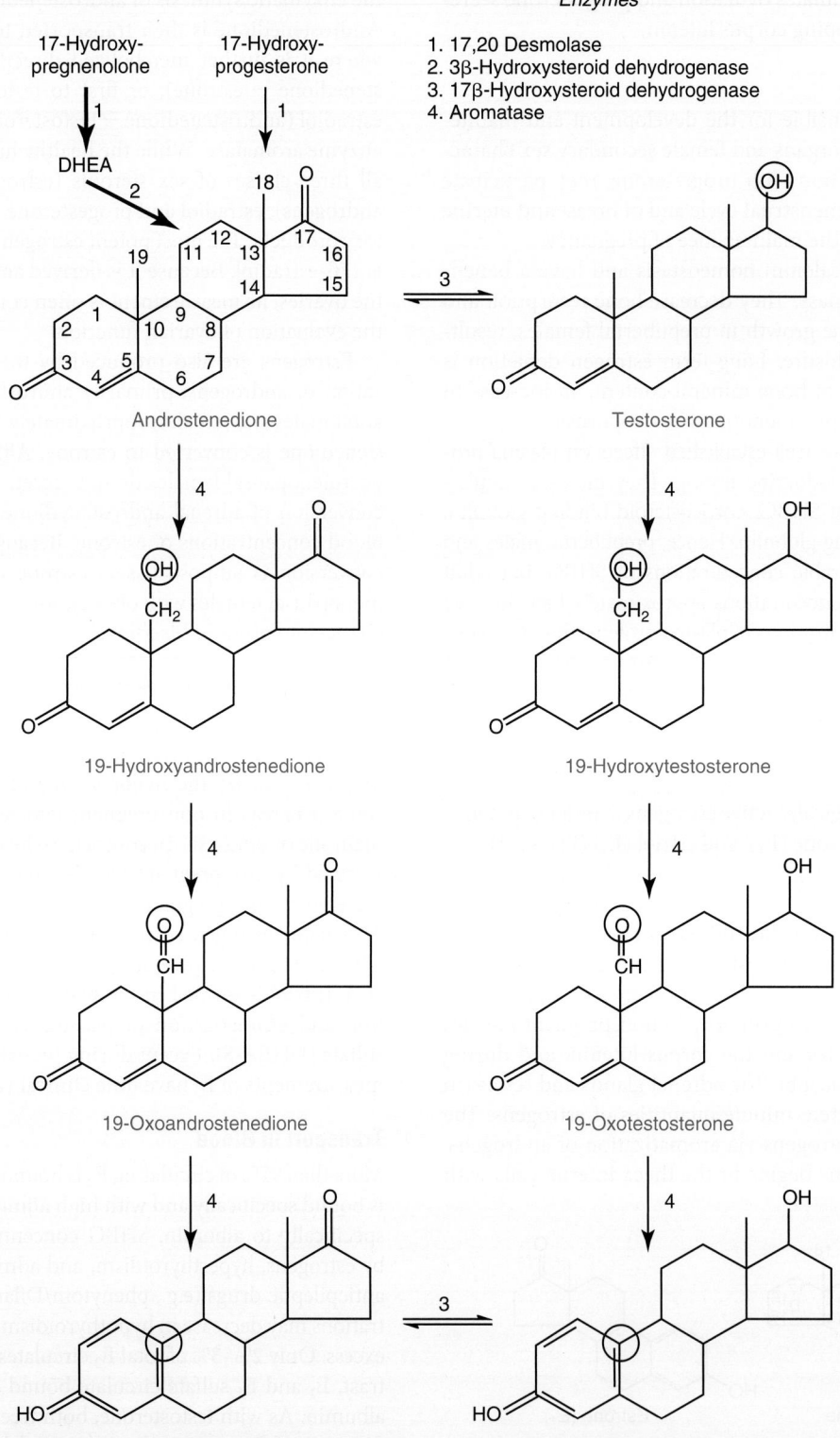

**Enzymes**

1. 17,20 Desmolase
2. 3β-Hydroxysteroid dehydrogenase
3. 17β-Hydroxysteroid dehydrogenase
4. Aromatase

**Fig. 43.5** Biosynthesis of estrogens. *Heavy arrows* indicate the Δ5–3β-hydroxy pathway. The *circled areas* represent the site of chemical change. (See Fig. 43.1 for early synthetic steps.)

## Progesterone

Progesterone, similar to the estrogens, is a female sex hormone (Fig. 43.7). In conjunction with estrogens, it helps to regulate the accessory organs during the menstrual cycle.

This hormone is especially important in preparing the uterus for implantation of the blastocyst and in maintaining pregnancy. In non-pregnant females, progesterone is secreted mainly by the corpus luteum. During pregnancy, the placenta

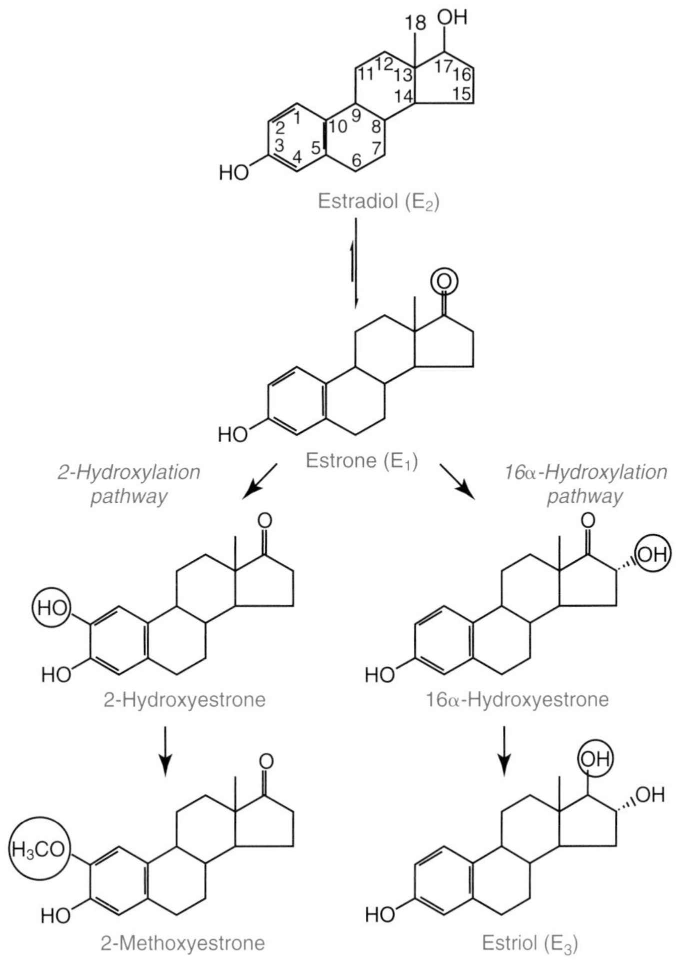

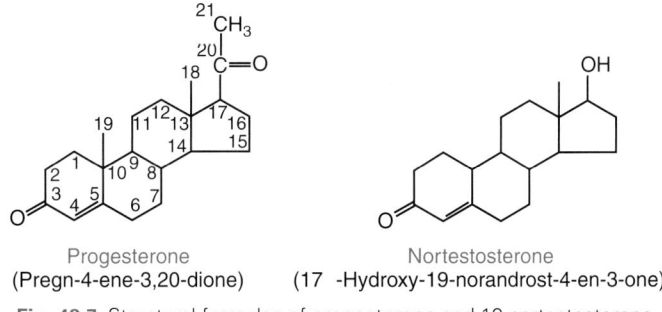

Fig. 43.6 Main pathways of estradiol metabolism in humans. The *circled areas* represent the site of chemical change.

Progesterone
(Pregn-4-ene-3,20-dione)

Nortestosterone
(17 -Hydroxy-19-norandrost-4-en-3-one)

Fig. 43.7 Structural formulas of progesterone and 19-nortestosterone.

becomes the major source of this hormone. Minor sources are the adrenal cortex in both sexes and the testes in males.

## Biosynthesis

Biosynthesis of progesterone in ovarian tissues follows the same path, from acetate to cholesterol through pregnenolone, as it does in the adrenal cortex (see Fig. 43.1). In luteal tissue, however, low-density lipoprotein cholesterol is thought to serve as the preferred precursor despite the potential of the corpus luteum to synthesize progesterone de novo from acetate. Initiation and control of luteal secretion of progesterone are regulated by LH and FSH.

## Transport in Blood

Progesterone does not have a specific plasma-binding protein but is primarily bound to albumin with a smaller fraction bound to corticosteroid-binding globulin. Reported concentrations for plasma free progesterone vary from 2% to 10% of total concentration, and the percentage of unbound progesterone remains constant throughout the normal menstrual cycle. The production rate of progesterone during the luteal phase reaches as high as 30 mg/day (95 μmol/day), whereas the production rate of progesterone by the placenta during the third trimester of pregnancy is approximately 300 mg/day (950 μmol/day).

## Metabolism

The important metabolic events leading to inactivation of progesterone are reduction and conjugation. The main metabolic pathway for the metabolism of progesterone is outlined in Fig. 43.8. Reduced metabolites are eventually conjugated with glucuronic acid and excreted as water-soluble glucuronides.

## Female Reproductive Development

Reproductive development begins with anatomy during the fetal period, followed by a postnatal period of adaptation to reduced maternal sex steroids, and finishes with sexual maturation during puberty. Healthy females remain fertile and menstruating until menopause.

### Fetal

In the genotypic female, lack of testosterone and AMH causes regression of the Wolffian ducts and maintenance of the Müllerian ducts, thus forming the female reproductive

tract. Gonadotropin activity in utero is suppressed because of high concentrations of circulating estrogens derived from the mother.

### Postnatal

When the placenta separates, concentrations of fetal sex steroids drop abruptly. Serum $E_2$ in neonates is decreased to basal concentrations within 5–7 days after birth, and persists at this concentration until puberty. The negative feedback action of steroids is thus removed, and gonadotropins are released. Postnatal peaks of LH and FSH are measurable for a few months after birth, peaking at 2–5 months and then dropping to basal concentrations. During childhood, circulating concentrations of sex steroids and gonadotropins are low and are similar for both sexes. However, in patients with primary hypogonadism (Turner syndrome), LH and FSH concentrations are higher than in unaffected children.

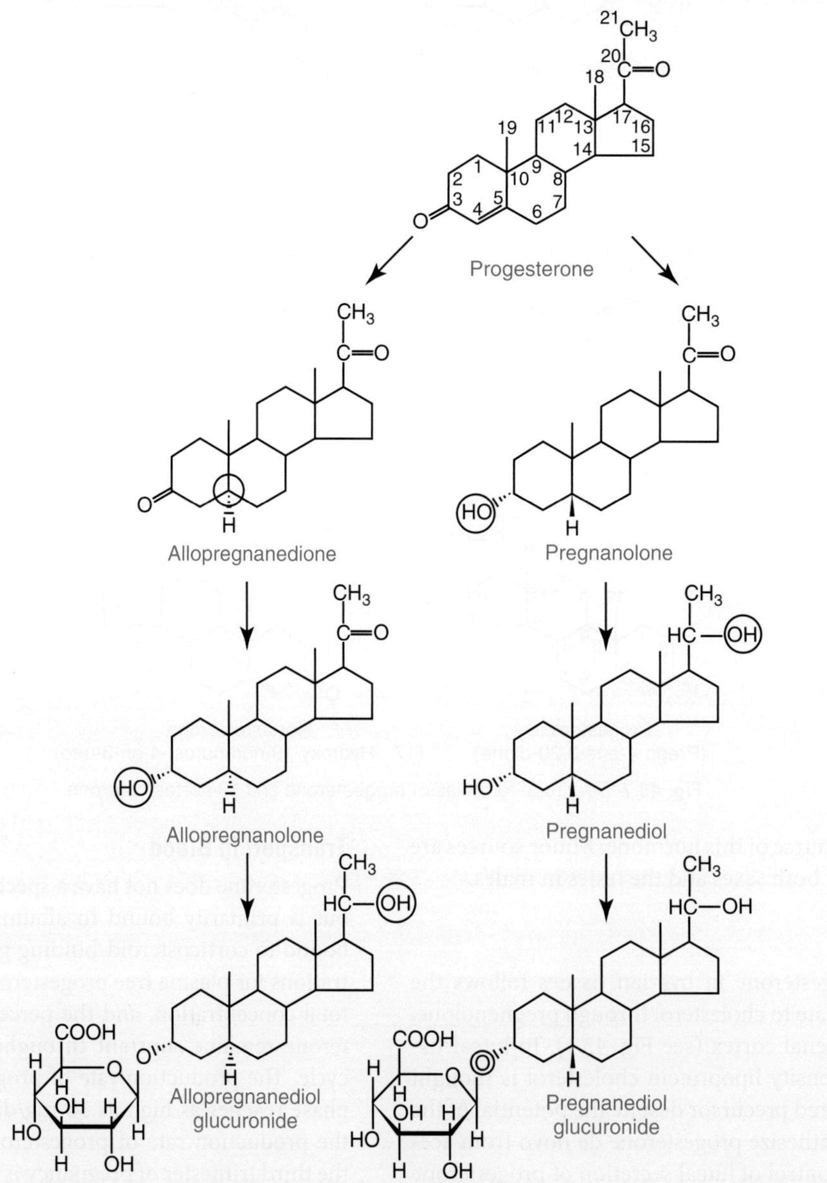

**Fig. 43.8** Metabolism of progesterone. The *circled areas* represent the site of chemical change.

## Puberty

The transition from sexual immaturity appears to begin with diminished sensitivity of the pituitary gland, hypothalamus, or both to the negative feedback effect of sex steroids. The mechanism for this change is unclear. As puberty approaches, nocturnal secretion of gonadotropins occurs. Concentrations of LH, FSH, and gonadal steroids rise gradually over several years before stabilizing at adult concentrations when full sexual maturity is reached. In females, puberty is considered precocious if the onset of pubertal development (secondary sex characteristics) occurs before age 8 years and is considered delayed if no development has occurred by age 13 years or menarche has not occurred by age 16.5 years.

Adrenarche precedes puberty by a few years. In females, the rise in adrenal androgen concentrations (DHEA, DHEA-S, and androstenedione) begins at age 6–7 years. This rise lasts until late puberty. In females, puberty is associated with elevations in estrogen secretion by the ovary in response to gonadotropin concentrations that increase in response to GnRH. Estrogen secretion by the ovary increases, causing enlargement of the uterus and breasts. In the breast, estrogen enhances the growth of ducts; progesterone augments this effect. As the breast develops, estrogen increases adipose tissue around the lactiferous duct system, contributing to the further enlargement of breast tissue. These physiologic and physical processes associated with puberty in females culminate not only in the development of secondary sexual characteristics as described, but also trigger *menarche*—the beginning of menstrual function and the first menstrual period.

### Normal Menstrual Cycle

During a normal menstrual cycle, a closely coordinated interplay of feedback effects occurs between the hypothalamus, anterior lobe of the pituitary gland, and ovaries. In addition, cyclic hormonal changes lead to functional and structural changes in the ovaries (follicle maturation, ovulation, and corpus luteum development), uterus (preparation of the endometrium for possible implantation of the fertilized ovum), cervix (to permit transport of sperm), and vagina (Fig. 43.9).

*Phases.* The menstrual cycle is measured beginning on day 1 as the first day of menstrual bleeding. Each cycle consists of a follicular phase, followed by ovulation, and then a luteal phase.

**Follicular phase.** The *follicular phase*—that is, the selection and growth of the dominant follicle—begins during the last few days of the previous luteal phase and terminates at ovulation (see Fig. 43.9). During the early part of the follicular phase, concentrations of FSH rise and then decline until ovulation (see Fig. 43.9). LH secretion begins to increase around the middle of the follicular phase. Just before ovulation, estrogen secretion by the follicle increases dramatically;

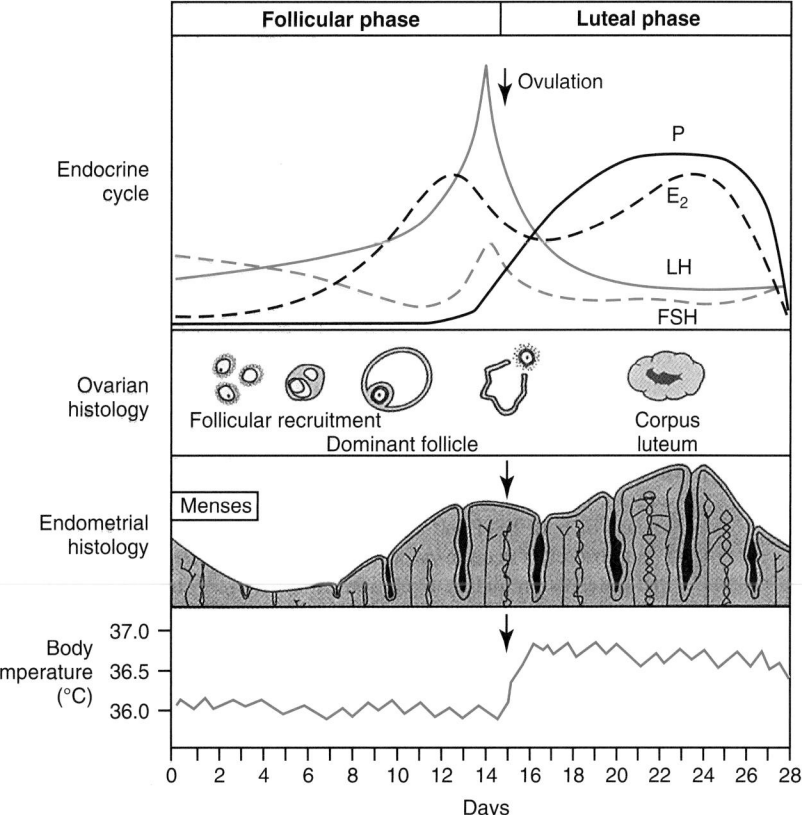

Fig. 43.9 Hormonal, ovarian, endometrial, and basal body temperature changes throughout the normal menstrual cycle. *E₂*, Estradiol; *FSH*, follicle-stimulating hormone; *LH*, luteinizing hormone. (From Carr BR, Bradshaw KD. Disorders of the ovary and female reproductive tract. In: Braunwald E, Fauci A, Kasper D, et al., eds. *Harrison's Principles of Internal Medicine*, 15th ed. New York: McGraw-Hill; 2001; used with permission.)

this stimulates the hypothalamus and triggers the LH surge, which is a reliable predictor of ovulation. Onset of the LH surge for 90% of premenopausal females occurs 16–58 hours before ovulation and peaks 3–36 hours before ovulation. Ovulation occurs around day 14 in a 28-day menstrual cycle.

**Luteal phase.** The *luteal phase*, the last half of the cycle, is characterized by the increasing production of progesterone and estrogen from the corpus luteum and gradual lowering of LH and FSH concentrations. Progesterone peaks at about 8 days' post-ovulation. If ovulation does not occur, the corpus luteum fails to form and the cyclic rise in progesterone is subnormal. If ovulation and pregnancy occur, hCG maintains the corpus luteum and progesterone continues to rise. In the absence of conception, the corpus luteum resolves, resulting in a decrease in estrogen and progesterone concentrations and a breakdown of the endometrium. The average duration of menstrual flow is 4–6 days and average menstrual blood loss is 30 mL.

**Cyclic variation.** Healthy females display considerable variation in cycle length, ranging from 26 to 34 days (28 days on average). Much of the cyclic variation can be attributed to variation in the length of the follicular phase, while the length of the luteal phase remains relatively constant.

**Gonadotropin-releasing hormone.** GnRH triggers the surge of LH that precedes ovulation. There appear to be two separate feedback centers in the hypothalamus: a tonic negative feedback center in the basal medial hypothalamus and a cyclic positive feedback center in the anterior regions of the hypothalamus. Low concentrations of $E_2$, such as those that are present during the follicular phase, affect the negative feedback center, whereas high concentrations of $E_2$, such as those seen just before the midcycle LH peak, trigger the positive feedback center. Progesterone in combination with estrogen affects the negative feedback center in the luteal phase. GnRH is released in a pulsatile fashion and has a self-priming effect; the first pulse potentiates the effects of subsequent pulses. A higher GnRH pulse frequency favors the release of LH while slower pulses favor FSH release. The magnitude of the LH response to GnRH increases steadily through the follicular phase and is greatest during the preovulatory LH surge, after which it declines again.

**Follicle-stimulating hormone.** A few days before day 1 of the cycle, FSH begins to rise (see Fig. 43.9), probably triggered by a fall in $E_2$ concentration that briefly eliminates the negative feedback effect. This rise in FSH initiates the growth of a cohort of ovarian follicles. LH and FSH release is pulsatile throughout the cycle; therefore the values shown in Fig. 43.9 represent integrated concentrations. As estrogen is released from the growing follicles, FSH concentrations fall again and remain low through the follicular phase. By days 5–7, a single dominant follicle is selected for further growth and maturation. During the luteal phase, FSH is suppressed by negative feedback from $E_2$ until a lesser FSH peak, occurring near the end of the cycle, starts off the follicular recruitment for the next cycle.

**Luteinizing hormone.** LH secretion is suppressed in the follicular phase by negative feedback from $E_2$. As $E_2$ production by the developing follicle increases, the effect of $E_2$ on the positive feedback center becomes important. Increasing release of GnRH from the hypothalamus and increasing sensitivity of the anterior lobe of the pituitary gland to GnRH lead to the preovulatory LH surge. Ovarian follicle receptors for LH, sensitized by FSH and $E_2$, transmit the stimulus to enhance differentiation of the theca cells and production of progesterone by the developing corpus luteum. During the luteal phase, LH production is suppressed by negative feedback from progesterone combined with $E_2$, but a low concentration of LH is probably necessary to prolong corpus luteum function.

**Estradiol.** Estradiol production by the ovary decreases near the end of a cycle but begins to increase again under the influence of FSH (see Fig. 43.9). Estradiol enhances the FSH effect on a maturing follicle through changes in FSH receptors of the follicular cells, but it suppresses pituitary FSH and LH release during the follicular phase through negative feedback. Before the mid-follicular phase, estrogen concentrations are less than 50 pg/mL (183.5 pmol/L), but they increase rapidly as the follicle matures, reaching a midcycle peak at between 250 and 500 pg/mL (917.5–1835 pmol/L). Estradiol concentrations decrease abruptly after ovulation but increase again as the corpus luteum is formed, reaching concentrations of approximately 125 pg/mL (458.8 pmol/L) during the luteal phase. Progesterone produced by the corpus luteum combined with $E_2$ provide negative feedback to the hypothalamus and the anterior lobe of the pituitary gland. As a result, the secretion of LH and FSH is again suppressed during the luteal phase. Estradiol is essential for the development of proliferative endometrium and is synergistic with progesterone for the development of changes in the endometrium that initiate shedding; the decrease in negative feedback from $E_2$ on the anterior lobe of the pituitary gland triggers the FSH surge that begins the development of an ovarian follicle for the next cycle.

**Progesterone.** Progesterone is not produced in significant amounts until the preovulatory LH surge and resulting ovulation. LH enhances theca cell differentiation and progesterone production, which increases by a factor of 10–20, and peaks about 8 days after the midcycle peak of LH. Progesterone is thought to stimulate the ovulatory peak of FSH and promote the growth of secretory endometrium, which is necessary for implantation of the fertilized ovum.

*Ovulation.* An intricate interplay of endocrine events contributes to follicular maturation. Growth of ovarian follicles appears to be continuous. How an individual follicle is selected for a single menstrual cycle is not known; however, the late-cycle peak in FSH concentration is likely important in this process. Once a follicle has been stimulated, $E_2$ production enhances the follicle's response to the effects of FSH. The high concentration of $E_2$ just before midcycle is responsible for triggering positive feedback in the hypothalamus, which leads to the preovulatory LH surge. After ovulation, LH is suppressed by progesterone and $E_2$, but the relatively low concentrations of LH are sufficient to maintain the corpus luteum until hCG produced by trophoblastic cells of the developing embryo binds and stimulates LH receptors. In the absence of hCG, the corpus luteum regresses and estradiol and progesterone concentrations decline; the net result of these changes is a de-repression of the pituitary and the late-cycle FSH peak that starts the next cycle.

## Menopause

Menopause is defined as the permanent cessation of menstruation resulting from loss of ovarian follicular activity. It begins with the ovaries failing to produce adequate amounts of estrogen and inhibin; as a result, gonadotropin production is increased in a continued attempt to stimulate the ovary (Fig. 43.10). The mean age of menopause in the United States is 51 years, but it varies considerably. Ovarian insufficiency may occur at any age, but menopause before age 40 years is considered premature.

Hormonal changes begin about 5 years before the actual menopause as the response of the ovary to gonadotropins begins to decrease and menstrual cycles become increasingly irregular. At this time, cyclic changes in hormone concentrations are still observed but FSH concentrations increase and $E_2$ concentrations decrease, whereas LH and progesterone concentrations remain unchanged, indicating that menstrual cycles remain ovulatory. The decrease in estrogen concentrations gives rise to vasomotor instability and "hot flashes."

After menopause, the ovary continues to produce androgens, particularly testosterone and androstenedione, as a result of increased LH release. In addition, the adrenal gland continues to secrete androgens. The resulting decrease in the estrogen/androgen ratio is the cause of the hirsutism seen in some postmenopausal females. In general, menopause may be diagnosed in females over the age of 45 on the basis of menstrual history and age without relying on laboratory test results, although serum FSH values may be helpful. In females below age 40 with menopausal symptoms and irregular

menses, other causes of menstrual irregularities should be ruled out prior to making the diagnosis of primary ovarian insufficiency (POI).

It is important to note that perimenopausal and postmenopausal females may secrete pituitary hCG. Serum concentrations are generally low (<13 IU/L), but positive hCG results often cause confusion and can delay important diagnostic tests or treatments. Pituitary versus placental hCG can be confirmed by measuring serum FSH (concentrations of FSH >45 IU/L are consistent with menopause and make pregnancy unlikely) or by 2 weeks of hormone replacement therapy (hormone replacement therapy should decrease LH, FSH, and hCG concentrations).

## Female Disorders of Sex Development

In female disorders of sex development, the gonadal sex varies from the genetic sex. Individuals with these conditions are genetically female (XX) but have phenotypic characteristics that are, to varying degrees, male. In neonates with a 46,XX karyotype and ambiguous genitalia, *congenital adrenal hyperplasia* (CAH) should be considered. In genetically XX fetuses, exposure to androgens before the 12th week of gestation causes ambiguous genitalia; after 13 weeks, it results in clitoral enlargement. Because androgen excess occurs before the 12th week of gestation in those with CAH, ambiguous genitalia are almost always present. Only deficiencies of 21-hydroxylase and 11β-hydroxylase are predominantly virilizing disorders. Deficiency of 3β-hydroxysteroid dehydrogenase is rare, but when it occurs, affected genotypically XX individuals may exhibit **virilization**. For further discussion of CAH, the reader is directed to Chapter 41.

## Precocious Puberty

Precocious puberty is the development of secondary sexual characteristics in females younger than 8 years old and

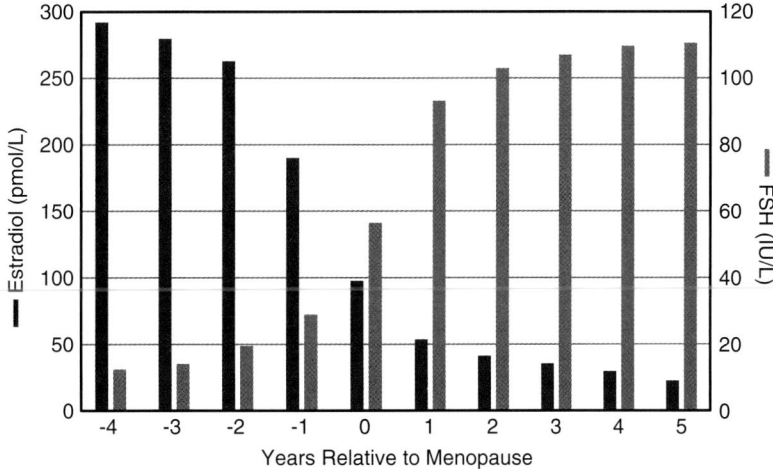

Fig. 43.10 Geometric means for follicle-stimulating hormone (*FSH*) and estradiol in relation to the final menstrual period (FMP). The horizontal axis represents time (years) with respect to the FMP (0); negative (positive) numbers represent time before (after) the FMP. (Modified from Burger HG, Dudley EC, Hopper JL, et al. Prospectively measured levels of serum follicle-stimulating hormone, estradiol, and the dimeric inhibins during the menopausal transition in a population-based cohort of women. *J Clin Endocrinol Metab.* 1999;84:4025–4030.)

males younger than 9 years old. Early puberty is manifested by the appearance of secondary sexual characteristics such as premature thelarche (breast development) for females or premature testicular enlargement for males. When presented as isolated cases, these secondary sexual characteristics are not necessarily considered to be pathologic. However, if a child demonstrates progressive development of the characteristics and/or increased rates of bone growth and maturation, causes of true precocious puberty must be considered.

GnRH-dependent precocious puberty (also called *central precocious puberty*) is due to early activation of the hypothalamic–pituitary–gonadal axis. In females, the cause is most commonly idiopathic (90%). In males, idiopathic cases account for between 26% and 60%. Central nervous system tumors have also been known to cause central precocious puberty, the most common being hypothalamic hamartoma. Neurofibromatosis can also lead to GnRH-dependent precocious puberty.

GnRH-independent precocious puberty (also called *peripheral precocity* or *pseudoprecocious puberty*) refers to precocious sex steroid secretion that is independent of pituitary gonadotropin release. CAH is a common cause of pseudoprecocious puberty. Classic forms of CAH present with virilization, growth acceleration, and accelerated bone maturation. Non-classic or late-onset forms usually present in childhood or adolescence with premature adrenarche and acne. In fact, 5%–10% of children who present with premature adrenarche have late-onset adrenal hyperplasia. Tumors of the adrenal gland, ovaries, and testes that secrete androgens or estrogens or exposure to exogenous estrogen or androgens may result in GnRH-independent precocious puberty.

Diagnosis of precocious puberty is based on clinical presentation, a thorough pubertal history, bone age determinations, and laboratory tests performed to assess gonadotropin concentrations and response to exogenous GnRH. In GnRH-dependent precocious puberty, basal LH concentrations are elevated and show an increased response to GnRH stimulation. Conversely, in GnRH-independent precocious puberty, basal LH concentrations are typically low and do not increase following GnRH stimulation.

## Irregular Menses

Amenorrhea, the absence of menstrual bleeding, is traditionally categorized as primary (women who have never menstruated) or secondary (women in whom menstruation is present for a variable time and then ceases). Amenorrhea is a relatively common disorder, with an estimated prevalence of 5% in the general population and as high as 8.5% in an unselected adolescent post-pubescent population.

*Primary amenorrhea.* Primary amenorrhea is defined as failure to establish spontaneous periodic menstruation by the age of 15 years regardless of whether secondary sex characteristics have developed. About 40% of phenotypic females who have primary amenorrhea (nearly always associated with absence of development of secondary sex characteristics) have *Turner syndrome* (45,X karyotype) or *pure gonadal*

dysgenesis (46,XX or XY karyotype). *Müllerian duct agenesis* or *dysgenesis* with absence of the vagina or uterus is the second most common manifestation, and the third most common is *androgen insensitivity syndrome* (androgen receptor deficiency and normal or elevated plasma testosterone concentrations if the patient is past puberty and is karyotype XY but has female sex characteristics).

**Evaluation of primary amenorrhea.** When puberty is delayed in a female, serum gonadotropins should be measured. Inappropriately low concentrations will be seen in inherited or acquired conditions that either directly affect GnRH release from the hypothalamus or FSH/LH release from the pituitary. Gonadotropin concentrations elevated into the postmenopausal range indicate definite gonadal failure.

*Secondary amenorrhea.* Secondary amenorrhea is defined as absence of periodic menstruation for at least 6 months in women who have previously experienced menses. *Oligomenorrhea* is infrequent menstruation that occurs fewer than nine times per year. With few exceptions, the causes of primary and secondary amenorrhea overlap (Box 43.2). Pregnancy, the most common cause of secondary amenorrhea, must be considered first and ruled out. Elevated concentrations of prolactin—iatrogenic or induced by a prolactin-secreting tumor—can result in oligomenorrhea or amenorrhea. About one-third of women with no obvious cause of amenorrhea have elevated prolactin concentrations; hyperprolactinemia may interfere with GnRH pulsatility, resulting in impaired release of LH and FSH.

Disorders of the ovary, such as Primary Ovarian Insufficiency (POI) and loss of ovarian function, can cause amenorrhea. POI has been defined as failure of ovarian estrogen production occurring in the context of a hypergonadotropic state at any age between menarche and 40 years. If the patient is younger than 25 years or shorter than 5 feet tall, karyotyping or chromosomal microarray should be performed to rule out the presence of a variety of chromosomal abnormalities involving duplications or absence of the X chromosome or the presence of a Y chromosome. Screening for the fragile X premutation (*FMR1*) should also be performed. Autoimmune disorders have been associated with 20% to 40% of cases of POI that result in amenorrhea due to destruction of the ovary. Other causes for POI include oophorectomy, cystic degeneration, trauma, infection, galactosemia, ischemia, pelvic radiotherapy, and treatment with cytotoxic chemotherapy. In rare patients, ovarian resistance to gonadotropins may be evident.

Secondary amenorrhea may also result from a uterine outflow tract abnormality, marked by the absence of menstruation despite typical cyclical hormonal changes. Endometrial damage may occur in response to a dilatation and curettage or to an infection of the endometrium. Pituitary dysfunction will also cause secondary amenorrhea. This is most often due to intrinsic pituitary tumors. However, pituitary infarction following peripartum hemorrhage (Sheehan syndrome) and pituitary apoplexy can result in panhypopituitarism. Empty sella syndrome has been reported in 4%–16% of patients with amenorrhea and galactorrhea.

## BOX 43.2    Causes of Amenorrhea

**Primary Amenorrhea**
- Lower tract defects
  - Vaginal aplasia
  - Imperforate hymen
  - Congenital vaginal atresia
- Uterine disorders
  - Congenital absence of the uterus
  - Endometritis
  - Müllerian agenesis (Mayer–Rokitansky–Kuster–Hauser syndrome)
- Ovarian disorders
  - XO gonadal and X dysgenesis and variants (Turner syndrome)
  - XX gonadal dysgenesis
  - 17-Hydroxylase deficiency of the ovaries and adrenal glands
  - Autoimmune oophoritis
  - Polycystic ovary syndrome
- Adrenal disorders (congenital adrenal hyperplasia)
- Thyroid disorders (hypothyroidism)
- Pituitary-hypothalamic disorders
  - Hypopituitarism
  - Constitutional delay in the onset of menses (physiologic)
  - Nutritional disorders
  - Kallmann syndrome

**Secondary Amenorrhea**
- Pregnancy/lactation
- Uterine disorders
  - Posttraumatic uterine synechiae (Asherman syndrome)
  - Progestational agents
- Ovarian disorders

- Polycystic ovary syndrome (hypothalamic)
- Ovarian tumor
- Primary ovarian insufficiency
- Resistant ovary syndrome
- Antimetabolite therapy
- Adrenal disorders
  - Late-onset adrenal hyperplasia
  - Cushing syndrome
  - Virilizing adrenal tumors
  - Adrenocorticoid insufficiency
- Thyroid disorders
  - Hypothyroidism
  - Hyperthyroidism
- Pituitary disorders
  - Acquired hypopituitarism
  - Physiologic or pathologic hyperprolactinemia
- Hypothalamic disorders
  - Tumor and infiltrative disease
  - Nutritional disorders
  - Excessive exercise
  - Stress
- Iatrogenic
  - Antipsychotics (phenothiazines, haloperidol, clozapine, pimozide)
  - Antidepressants (tricyclics, monoamine oxidase inhibitors)
  - Antihypertensives (calcium channel blockers, methyldopa, reserpine)
  - Drugs with estrogenic activity (digitalis, flavonoids, marijuana, oral contraceptives)
  - Drugs with ovarian toxicity (busulfan, chlorambucil, cisplatin, cyclophosphamide, fluorouracil)

**Evaluation of secondary amenorrhea.** Evaluation of women with secondary amenorrhea should begin with a careful history that includes a complete description of menstrual patterns. In addition, the patient should be evaluated for galactorrhea, hot flashes, symptoms of hypothyroidism, hirsutism, prior abdominal surgery, pelvic or uterine trauma, medications taken, nutritional history, patterns of exercise, previous contraceptive use, weight changes, stress, and chronic disease. Serum or urine β-hCG should be measured to rule out pregnancy (Table 43.1). Because both hypothyroidism and hyperprolactinemia cause amenorrhea, they are easily excluded by measuring serum TSH and prolactin.

In patients with history/physical exam suspicious for Cushing syndrome, a screening test such as 24-hour urine free cortisol, late night salivary cortisol, or low dose overnight dexamethasone suppression test, should be performed. On the basis of the preliminary assessment, magnetic resonance imaging (MRI) of the sella turcica should be performed in patients with evidence of pituitary or hypothalamic disease.

*Progesterone challenge for evaluating amenorrhea.* When the cause of amenorrhea is unclear after the initial assessment, relative estrogen status should be determined. Serum $E_2$ can be measured, but results must be interpreted with caution because serum $E_2$ fluctuates throughout the menstrual cycle. A *progesterone challenge* may be performed as a functional assessment of relative estrogen status. Women with an estrogen-primed uterus have withdrawal vaginal bleeding after treatment with oral progestin such as medroxyprogesterone acetate (Provera). If estrogen concentrations are adequate and the outflow tract is intact, menstrual bleeding should occur within a week of treatment. In patients with withdrawal bleeding, the plasma $E_2$ concentration is usually greater than 40 pg/mL (146.8 pmol/L). However, the progesterone challenge test is subject to false-positives because up to 20% of normoestrogenic women with oligomenorrhea do not experience withdrawal bleeding. It is also subject to false-negatives because up to 40% of women with oligomenorrhea and reduced plasma $E_2$ experience withdrawal bleeding.

*Androgen excess.* Amenorrhea due to androgen excess can stem from adult-onset CAH, corticotropin-dependent Cushing syndrome, or polycystic ovary syndrome (PCOS). Patients with androgen excess will often present with acne, obesity, and variable degrees of excess hair on

## TABLE 43.1  Differential Diagnosis of Secondary Amenorrhea

| CAUSES | FSH | LH | E₂ | Uterine Bleeding after Progesterone |
|---|---|---|---|---|
| **Hypothalamic** | | | | |
| CNS—hypothalamic dysfunction | | | | |
|   Idiopathic | ↓ or N | ↓ or N | ↓ or N | ± |
|   Secondary to medications | ↓ or N | ↓ or N | ↓ or N | ± |
|   Secondary to stress | ↓ or N | ↓ or N | ↓ or N | ± |
| CNS—hypothalamic dysfunction or failure due to exercise | ↓ or N | ↓ or N | ↓ or N | ± |
| CNS—hypothalamic dysfunction or failure due to weight loss | | | | |
|   Simple weight loss | ↓ or N | ↓ or N | ↓ or N | ± |
|   Anorexia nervosa | ↓ or N | ↓ or N | ↓ or N | — |
| CNS—hypothalamic failure | | | | |
|   Lesions | ↓ | ↓ | ↓ | — |
|   Idiopathic | ↓ | ↓ | ↓ | — |
| CNS—hypothalamic-adreno-ovarian dysfunction (polycystic ovary syndrome) or hyperandrogenic chronic anovulation | N | ↑* | N | + |
| **Pituitary** | | | | |
| Destructive lesions (Sheehan syndrome) | ↓ | ↓ | ↓ | — |
| Tumor | ↓ | ↓ | ↓ | — |
| **Ovarian** | | | | |
| Premature ovarian failure | ↑ | ↑ | ↓ | — |
| Loss of ovarian function (oophorectomy, infection, cystic degeneration, chemotherapy, radiation) | ↑ | ↑ | ↓ | — |
| **Uterine** | | | | |
| Uterine synechiae (Asherman syndrome) | N | N | N | — |

CNS, Central nervous system; $E_2$, estrogen; FSH, follicle-stimulating hormone; LH, luteinizing hormone; N, value within normal reference interval; ↓, value below normal reference interval; ↑, value above normal reference interval; ↑*, >25 IU/L, less than menopausal concentration; ±, positive or negative bleeding response to progesterone.
From Davajan V, Kletzky OA. Amenorrhea. In: Mishell DR, Davajan V, Lobo RA, eds. *Infertility, Contraception and Reproductive Endocrinology*, 3rd ed. Boston: Blackwell Scientific Publications; 1991.

the face, chest, abdomen, and thighs. Some individuals with 21-hydroxylase deficiency do not manifest any developmental abnormalities or salt wasting but present with signs of androgen excess. This clinical syndrome, referred to as *nonclassic adult-onset* or *late-onset CAH*, may be clinically indistinguishable from PCOS.

PCOS is characterized by infertility, hirsutism, obesity (in approximately half of those affected), and various menstrual disturbances ranging from amenorrhea to irregular vaginal bleeding (Table 43.2). Women with PCOS have an increased prevalence of diabetes, along with increased risk for coronary heart disease and endometrial cancer. PCOS patients have substantial estrogen production because of the peripheral conversion of androgens to estrogens. Abnormal bleeding patterns seen in PCOS are due to chronic anovulation and lack of progesterone stimulation and withdrawal. Chronic estrogen exposure without progesterone predisposes patients to endometrial cancer. Although this syndrome is associated with polycystic ovaries, the name is actually a misnomer in that the ovaries are covered with immature follicles rather than cysts.

## TABLE 43.2  Clinical Features of the Polycystic Ovary Syndrome[a]

| Clinical Feature | Frequency (%) |
|---|---|
| Hirsutism | 65 |
| Acne | 25 |
| Obesity | 35 |
| Infertility | 50 |
| Amenorrhea | 35 |
| Oligomenorrhea | 40 |
| Regular menstrual cycle | 20 |

[a]Data were compiled from three studies. Two used ultrasonography as the primary method of diagnosis; one used ovarian histology. Total N = 1935.
Modified from Franks S. Polycystic ovary syndrome. *N Engl J Med*. 1995;333:853.

PCOS occurs in 4%–10% of premenopausal women, and the prevalence varies depending on the diagnostic criteria used. The Rotterdam Consensus Criteria are the most widely accepted. They define hyperandrogenism, oligomenorrhea or amenorrhea, and polycystic ovaries by ultrasound as the characteristic signs and symptoms and require the presence of two of the three for diagnosis of PCOS.

Because the pathophysiologic mechanism is unknown, PCOS remains a diagnosis of exclusion, clinically defined by hyperandrogenism in women with chronic anovulation and no other cause. Relatively low FSH and disproportionately high LH concentrations are common in PCOS, although this ratio should not be used in a routine PCOS workup. Studies have reported higher serum AMH concentrations in women with PCOS relative to unaffected women, and ongoing work is evaluating the potential utility of including AMH measurement in PCOS diagnostic criteria.

*Ovarian hyperthecosis*, a non-neoplastic lesion of the ovary characterized by the presence of islands of luteinized thecal cells in the ovarian stroma, is sometimes confused with PCOS. Features that distinguish it from PCOS include higher concentrations of testosterone, androstenedione, and DHT derived from ovarian secretion.

*Hirsutism and virilization.* Hirsutism is defined as excessive growth of terminal hair in women and children in a distribution similar to that occurring in postpubertal men. It is important to distinguish true hirsutism, which is androgen responsive, from hypertrichosis, which consists of excessive growth of vellus, or non-androgen-responsive hair. Women with androgen-dependent hirsutism may have exposure to excess androgens or may have heightened sensitivity to normal circulating concentrations of androgen (Box 43.3).

Virilization is characterized by clitoral hypertrophy, deepening of the voice, temporal hair recession, baldness, increased libido, decreased body fat, and menstrual irregularities or amenorrhea. Hirsutism is usually associated with normal or slightly elevated serum androgens, whereas virilization is associated with marked increases in ovarian or adrenal androgen production and is an indication for more intensive investigation.

**Laboratory evaluation of hirsutism/virilization.** The two most important screening tests used in the evaluation of women for hirsutism and virilization are serum total or free testosterone and DHEA-S. A significant elevation in the DHEA-S concentration suggests an adrenal origin of androgens, whereas elevations in testosterone indicate an adrenal or ovarian source. Neoplastic disease is unlikely if the serum testosterone concentration is less than 200 ng/dL (6.9 nmol/L), the DHEA-S concentration is less than 700 µg/dL (19 µmol/L), or 17-KS concentrations are less than 30 mg/dL (1 mmol/L).

*Other factors.* Hypothalamic dysfunction consists of those disorders that disrupt the frequency or amplitude of GnRH release. Rarely is this due to a lesion or tumor. However, most commonly, disruption occurs in response to psychologic stress, depression, severe weight loss, anorexia nervosa, or strenuous exercise. A syndrome known as the *female athletic triad* has been described. This syndrome is prevalent in women who exercise vigorously, and it is associated with amenorrhea, disordered eating, and osteoporosis. Competitive long-distance runners, gymnasts, and professional ballet dancers appear to be at highest risk. Although the mechanism for the disturbance is unclear, symptoms and laboratory profiles are similar to those of other forms of hypothalamic amenorrhea. LH and FSH concentrations are normal or low, and $E_2$ concentrations are low.

Several hormone-producing tumors of the ovary, pituitary gland, and adrenal glands occur in combination with amenorrhea. This amenorrhea may be confused with pregnancy if the tumors produce hCG. Choriocarcinoma of the uterus or ovary may produce large amounts of hCG, which cause hyperthyroidism because of the slight thyrotropic action of hCG. Granulosa-theca cell tumors are usually associated with estrogen secretion resulting in amenorrhea and irregular menses and, rarely, excessive androgen with associated virilization.

Many drugs—particularly, antipsychotic medications—produce amenorrhea (see Box 43.2) through dopamine suppression. Dopamine exerts a tonic inhibitory effect upon prolactin; consequently, dopamine suppression leads to hyperprolactinemia. Excessive prolactin release then suppresses GnRH and FSH/LH secretion, leading to amenorrhea.

---

**BOX 43.3  Causes of Hirsutism**

- Ovarian
  - Severe insulin resistance
  - Hyperthecosis, hilus cell or stromal cell hyperplasia
  - Androgen-producing ovarian tumor
  - Menopause
- Adrenal
  - Classic congenital hyperplasia
  - 21-Hydroxylase deficiency
  - 11-Hydroxylase deficiency
  - 3β-Hydroxysteroid dehydrogenase deficiency
  - Adult or attenuated adrenal hyperplasia (nonclassical adrenal hyperplasia)
  - Androgen-producing adrenal tumor
- Familial hirsutism
- Endocrine disorders
  - Polycystic ovary syndrome
  - Hyperprolactinemia
  - Acromegaly
  - Cushing syndrome
- Idiopathic hirsutism (includes increased skin sensitivity to androgens)
- Iatrogenic
  - Androgens
  - Phenytoin
  - Diazoxide
  - Minoxidil
  - Streptomycin
  - Cyclosporine
  - Danazol
  - Metyrapone
  - Phenothiazides
  - Progestagens (19-non-steroid derivatives)

## POINTS TO REMEMBER

- Pulsatile secretion of GnRH stimulates LH and FSH release, which control oocyte maturation and ovulation and increase estradiol and progesterone production.
- Estradiol is transported in blood tightly bound to SHBG and loosely bound to albumin, whereas progesterone is bound to corticosteroid-binding globulin.
- Estradiol and progesterone both inhibit and stimulate LH and FSH release, with the type of regulation dependent on the

stage of the menstrual cycle and the serum steroid hormone concentration.
- PCOS is defined by hyperandrogenism and oligo/anovulation and remains a diagnosis of exclusion based primarily on clinical evaluation.
- Pituitary secretion of hCG is often seen in postmenopausal women, and the pituitary origin can be confirmed by the presence of concurrently elevated serum FSH.

## INFERTILITY

*Infertility* is defined as the inability to conceive after 1 year of unprotected intercourse. It has been estimated that 93% of healthy couples practicing unprotected intercourse should expect to conceive within 1 year. A specific cause of infertility is identified in approximately 80% of couples: one-third are due to female factors alone, one-third to male factors alone, and one-third to a combination of problems.

Primary infertility refers to couples or patients who have had no previous successful pregnancies. Secondary infertility encompasses patients who have previously conceived but are currently unable to conceive. These types of infertility generally share common causes.

Infertility problems often arise as a result of hormonal dysfunction of the hypothalamic–pituitary–gonadal axis.

### Male Infertility

A list of the most common male infertility factors is given in Box 43.4 and an algorithm for the evaluation of male infertility is shown in the At a Glance box—Evaluating Male Infertility. Initial evaluation of male infertility should include a detailed history and physical examination. The physical examination should pay particular attention to: (1) the external genitalia—for evidence of proper androgenization; (2) hair pattern—degree of virilization; (3) breast abnormalities—gynecomastia and/or discharge; and (4) neurologic findings—sense of smell and visual impairments. An assessment should be made for the presence of a condition predisposing to obstructive azoospermia such as enlargement of the testicular venous plexus (varicocele). The history must include: (1) reproductive history, including living children and any pregnancies that resulted

## AT A GLANCE

**Evaluating Male Infertility**
Algorithm for the evaluation of male infertility.

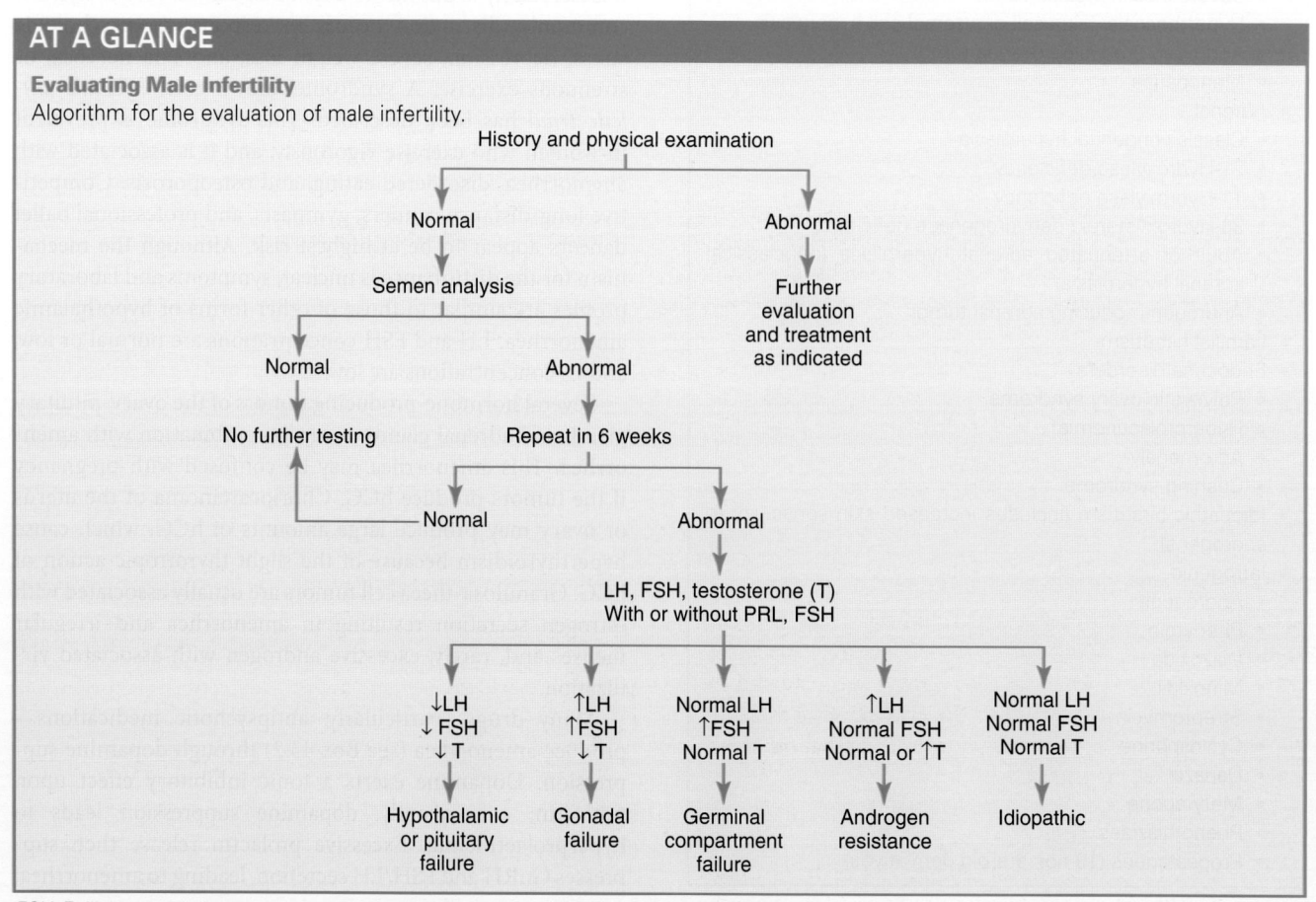

*FSH*, Follicle-stimulating hormone; *LH*, luteinizing hormone; *PRL*, prolactin; *T*, testosterone.

## BOX 43.4 Male Infertility Factors

**Endocrine Disorders**
- Hypothalamic dysfunction (Kallmann syndrome)
- Pituitary failure (tumor, radiation, surgery)
- Hyperprolactinemia (drug, tumor)
- Androgen insensitivity syndrome (AIS)
- Exogenous androgens
- Thyroid disorders
- Adrenal hyperplasia
- Testicular failure

**Anatomic**
- Congenital absence of vas deferens
- Obstructed vas deferens
- Congenital abnormalities of ejaculatory system
- Varicocele
- Retrograde ejaculation

**Abnormal Spermatogenesis**
- Unexplained azoospermia
- Chromosomal abnormalities
- Mumps orchitis
- Cryptorchidism
- Chemical or radiation exposure

**Abnormal Sperm Motility**
- Absent cilia (Kartagener syndrome)
- Antibody formation

**Psychosocial**
- Unexplained impotence
- Decreased libido

Modified from Morell V. Basic infertility assessment. *Primary Care.* 1997;24:195–204.

## TABLE 43.3 Normal Seminal Fluid Values

| Parameter | Value |
|---|---|
| Ejaculate volume | >1.5 mL (1.4–1.7)[a] |
| Sperm density | >15 million/mL (12–16)[a] |
| Total sperm count | >39 million/ejaculate (33–46)[a] |
| Motility | >32% progressive motility (31–34); >40% total (38–42)[a] |
| Morphology | >4.0% normal (3–4)[a] |
| pH | 7.2–8.0[a] |
| Color | Gray-white-yellow |
| Liquefaction | Within 40 min |
| Fructose | >1200 µg/mL |
| Acid phosphatase | 100–300 µg/mL |
| Citric acid | >3 mg/mL |
| Inositol | >1 mg/mL |
| Zinc | >75 µg/mL |
| Magnesium | >70 µg/mL |
| Prostaglandins (PGE$_1$ + PGE$_2$) | 30–200 µg/mL |
| Glycerylphosphorylcholine | >650 µg/mL |
| Carnitine | >250 µg/mL |
| Glucosidase | >20 mU per ejaculate |

[a]Values from the World Health Organization. Cooper TG, Noonan E, von Eckardstein S, et al. World Health Organization reference values for human semen characteristics. *Hum Reprod Update.* 2010;3:231.

volume of ejaculate. An appropriate increase in serum testosterone without change in the ejaculate volume may indicate mechanical blockage. Absence of, or a decrease in, specific biochemical markers such as acid phosphatase and citric acid (from prostate), fructose, and prostaglandins (from seminal vesicles) can assist in determining the location of blockage. A urine sample after the semen collection can assess for the presence of retrograde ejaculation.

### Evaluation of Endocrine Parameters

If severe oligospermia or azoospermia is found, measurement of serum testosterone, LH, and FSH concentrations is warranted, with or without measurement of prolactin and TSH. Hyperprolactinemia is a cause of secondary testicular dysfunction. Prolactin excess likely causes hypogonadism by impairing GnRH release. It also leads to under-androgenization and erectile dysfunction (see Erectile Dysfunction, above). If hyperprolactinemia is found, it is imperative to check for hypothyroidism because elevated TRH concentrations can result in hyperprolactinemia.

As testosterone is essential for normal sperm development, any disorder that results in hypogonadism (and thus low testosterone concentrations) results in infertility. In men with normal gonadotropins and testosterone and a nonpalpable vas deferens on physical exam, genetic testing of *Cystic Fibrosis Transmembrane Receptor (CFTR)* should be performed to assess for the presence of cystic fibrosis.

*Hypergonadotropic hypogonadism.* Measurement of the concentration of FSH is indicated in men with a sperm count lower than 5–10 million/mL, elevated concentrations of FSH indicate Sertoli cell dysfunction and, in azoospermic men, primary germinal cell failure, Sertoli cell-only syndrome, or

in miscarriage; (2) medications taken; (3) use of recreational and performance-enhancing drugs and alcohol; (4) systemic illness; and (5) potential toxin exposure. Sexual history should include frequency of intercourse and use of any lubricants. Issues of potency must be distinguished from those of infertility or subfertility. Testosterone should be measured, especially when the history or physical examination suggests deficient development of secondary sex characteristics. Laboratory evaluation of male infertility should begin with evaluation of the semen (Table 43.3), which should be followed by evaluation of endocrine parameters.

### Evaluation of Semen

Semen analysis measures ejaculate volume, pH, sperm count, motility, forward progression, and morphology. Although semen analysis is not a test for infertility, it is considered the most important laboratory test in the evaluation of male fertility. If semen analysis is normal, it is unlikely that other laboratory testing will be useful.

### Evaluation of Obstruction

Testosterone produced after administration of hCG causes the seminal vesicles, epididymis, and prostate to increase the genetic conditions such as Klinefelter syndrome. Radiotherapy and gonadotoxic chemotherapy can also lead to testicular failure with azoospermia. Elevated FSH (>120 IU/L) in the setting of decreased testosterone (<200 ng/dL, 7 nmol/L) and oligospermia indicate primary testicular failure.

*Hypogonadotropic hypogonadism.* Decreased concentrations of testosterone (<200 ng/dL, 7 nmol/L) and decreased concentrations of FSH (<10 IU/L) are suggestive of hypogonadotropic hypogonadism. The administration of GnRH may help to distinguish between gonadal insufficiencies caused by pituitary versus hypothalamic failure when the etiology is not clear. Because the pituitary is sensitive to sex steroids for appropriate gonadotropin secretion, patients with long-standing hypogonadism should be given exogenous testosterone for 1 week before the GnRH stimulation test is administered.

### Y-chromosome Microdeletions

Deletions in either of the azoospermia factor regions (*AZF1* and *AZF2*) on the long arm of the Y chromosome are associated with an inability to make sperm. In addition, genes such as *SRY* (sex-determining region Y) are on the short arm of chromosome Y. Deletion of these regions is associated with azoospermia or, less frequently, oligospermia. The incidence of Y microdeletions in idiopathic nonobstructive azoospermic men is 8%–18%. Testing for Y-chromosome microdeletions is performed to determine whether sperm might be retrieved on a testicular sperm extraction procedure.

## Female Infertility

Evaluating female infertility is more complex than evaluating infertility in the male. A list of the most common female infertility factors is given in Box 43.5. An algorithm for the evaluation of female infertility is shown in the At a Glance box—Evaluating Female Infertility.

### Initial Evaluation of Female Infertility

The initial evaluation of female infertility should include a detailed history and physical examination. The physical examination should include evaluation of: (1) the external genitalia and hair pattern (for signs of androgen excess, including clitoromegaly, hirsutism, and virilization); (2) the pelvis (for masses, nodularity, or tenderness); (3) the breasts (for signs of galactorrhea); (4) neurologic findings (sense of smell and visual impairments); (5) the thyroid (for enlargement or nodules); and (6) body mass index. All abnormalities in the history and physical examination should be pursued. A thorough medical and surgical history is also necessary, including an assessment of the patient's gravidity and parity, coital frequency, duration of infertility, and prior workup and treatment for infertility. History of sexually transmitted infections, assessment of previous cervical cytologic and human papillomavirus (HPV) testing and treatment, and a menstrual history should also be obtained. Concentrations of TSH, testosterone, and prolactin should be measured if menstrual cycles are absent or irregular or if signs of galactorrhea or thyroid abnormalities are present.

---

## AT A GLANCE

**Evaluating Female Infertility**
Algorithm for the evaluation of female infertility.

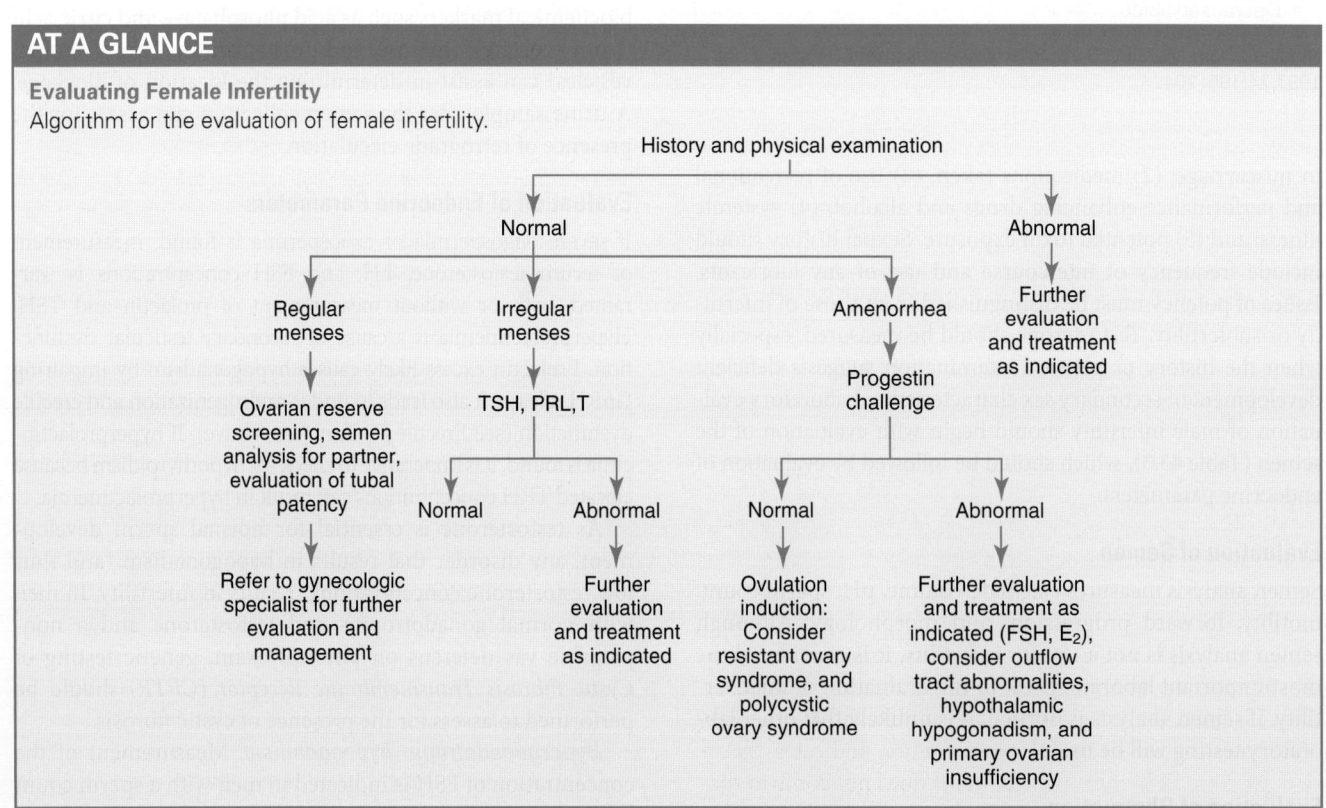

$E_2$, Estradiol; *FSH*, follicle-stimulating hormone; *LH*, luteinizing hormone; *PRL*, prolactin; *T*, testosterone; *TSH*, thyroid-stimulating hormone.

## BOX 43.5   Female Infertility Factors

**Ovarian or Hormonal Factors**
- Metabolic disease
  - Thyroid
  - Liver
  - Obesity
  - Androgen excess
  - Polycystic ovarian syndrome
- Hypergonadotropic hypogonadism
  - Menopause
  - Luteal phase deficiency
  - Gonadal dysgenesis
  - Primary ovarian insufficiency
  - Resistant ovary syndrome
- Hypogonadotropic hypogonadism
  - Hyperprolactinemia (tumor, drugs)
  - Hypothalamic insufficiency (Kallmann syndrome)
  - Pituitary insufficiency

**Tubal Factors**
- Occlusion or scarring
- Salpingitis isthmica nodosa
- Infectious salpingitis

**Cervical Factors**
- Stenosis
- Inflammation or infection
- Abnormal mucous viscosity

**Uterine Factors**
- Leiomyomata
- Congenital malformation
- Adhesions
- Endometritis or abnormal endometrium

**Psychosocial Factors**
- Decreased libido
- Anorgasmia
- Iatrogenic
- Immunologic (antisperm antibodies)

Modified from Morell V. Basic infertility assessment. *Primary Care.* 1997;24:195–204.

*Evaluation of ovulation.* In the menstruating woman, the next step is to determine whether ovulation occurs. No current laboratory tests will confirm ovum release. However, measurement of midluteal plasma progesterone does indicate that a corpus luteum has been formed. Other methods, such as measurement of the LH surge (to predict ovulation) and basal body temperature (to detect a midcycle rise in progesterone), have been used to assess ovulation.

*Progesterone measurement.* Measurement of the concentration of serum progesterone is the primary assay used for the evaluation of ovulation. It is important to note that an increase in progesterone concentration indicates that a corpus luteum has been formed, but it does not confirm that the oocyte was actually released. Beginning immediately after ovulation, serum progesterone concentrations rise (see Fig. 43.9) and peak within 5–9 days during the midluteal phase

(days 21–23). If ovulation does not occur, the corpus luteum fails to form and the expected cyclic rise in progesterone concentration is subnormal. If pregnancy occurs, hCG maintains the corpus luteum, and progesterone production continues to rise. Midluteal progesterone concentrations greater than 300 ng/dL (9.5 nmol/L) indicate that ovulation has taken place.

*Basal body temperature.* Basal body temperature charts have long been accepted as simple, cost-effective indicators of ovulation. Ovulation is associated with a rapid rise in body temperature (by 0.2°F–0.5°F, or 0.1°C–0.3°C), which persists through the luteal phase. The rise in temperature is due to increased progesterone concentration. However, similar to progesterone, the rise in body temperature is evident only retrospectively and therefore does not predict imminent ovulation in a way helpful for timing intercourse.

*Measurement of the luteinizing hormone surge.* LH appears in the urine just after the serum LH surge, 24–36 hours before ovulation (see Fig. 43.9). Measurement of LH does not confirm ovulation or provide insight into the cause of anovulation, but rather indicates when ovulation should occur and provides a guide with which to time intercourse.

### Evaluation of Endocrine Parameters

Disorders of the hypothalamus, pituitary, and ovary are endocrine causes of infertility.

*Hypergonadotropic hypogonadism.* POI is indicated by repeatedly elevated basal FSH concentrations (>30 IU/L) or a single elevation greater than 40 IU/L in a woman younger than 40 years. These patients are often hypoestrogenic ($E_2$ <20 pg/mL, 73 pmol/L) and do not respond to a progestin challenge because their endometrium is atrophic. A pelvic ultrasound will reveal a thin endometrium. Basal serum FSH has been used as an indicator of relative ovarian reserve.

*Assessing ovarian reserve.* Women in their mid-to-late 30s and early 40s with infertility constitute the largest portion of the total infertility population. These women are also at increased risk for miscarriage. This reflects a diminished ovarian reserve as a result of follicular depletion and a decline in oocyte quality. As women age, serum FSH concentrations in the early follicular phase begin to increase; this may be due to a decline in the number of small follicles secreting inhibin B.

The concomitant measurement of follicular phase serum FSH and $E_2$ is a popular screening test for assessing ovarian reserve. In general, day 3 FSH concentrations >20–25 IU/L are considered elevated and associated with a poor reproductive outcome. Concomitant measurement of serum $E_2$ concentration adds to the predictive power of an isolated FSH determination. Early follicular phase $E_2$ concentrations >75–80 pg/mL (275–294 pmol/L) may be associated with a poor response to ovarian stimulation and pregnancy outcome, although this interpretation is complicated by the slightly elevated $E_2$ concentrations observed in women with PCOS.

More recently, AMH has emerged as a helpful indicator of ovarian reserve. AMH regulates follicle development and maturation as well as $E_2$ production. AMH is produced by small, growing follicles, but is not produced during

FSH-dependent follicular growth or in atretic follicles. Serum AMH remains relatively constant throughout the menstrual cycle and decreases with age, leading to its promotion as a marker of ovarian reserve and reproductive capacity.

Current literature suggests that the most beneficial application of AMH measurement is not in AMH's ability to predict the chance of pregnancy but rather in predicting response to controlled ovarian stimulation used in assisted reproductive techniques. Patients with elevated serum AMH concentrations are often "high responders" and at risk of ovarian hyperstimulation syndrome (OHSS) if a standard ovarian stimulation protocol is used. As a result, these women may undergo a modified stimulation protocol to minimize the risk of OHSS. Conversely, women with low serum AMH concentrations are considered "low responders" and often require greater ovarian stimulation to ensure successful oocyte collection.

*Hypogonadotropic hypogonadism.* In hypogonadotropic hypogonadism, serum $E_2$ concentrations are <40 pg/mL (147 pmol/L); therefore, there is no withdrawal bleeding with a progestin challenge because the endometrium is thin. Decreased LH (<10 IU/L) and decreased FSH (<10 IU/L) are also observed. Hyperprolactinemia can cause hypogonadotropic hypogonadic infertility. TSH should be measured to exclude hypothyroidism as a cause of elevated prolactin. Prolactin concentrations can be elevated in patients with PCOS or chronic stress, and those taking medications such as antidepressants, cimetidine, and methyldopa. Prolactin concentrations can be elevated if drawn later in the day or after a meal, so they should be drawn fasting, early in the day. In cases where hyperprolactinemia is noted, MRI imaging of the brain is indicated to rule out pituitary or hypothalamic pathology.

*Ovulatory factors.* Ovulatory dysfunction is difficult to diagnose because it will manifest in the presence or absence of normal menses. Metabolic diseases of many types affect ovulatory function, including those that result in androgen excess. PCOS, which results in androgen excess, is the most common cause of anovulation. In women with hirsutism, CAH should be considered.

## Assisted Reproduction

Couples with a multitude of infertility problems, including unidentified causes and persistent infertility despite standard treatments, may benefit from assisted reproductive techniques (ART). If no definable cause is identified, standard initial therapy consists of ovulation induction with intrauterine insemination for three cycles before progression to more aggressive techniques such as controlled ovarian hyperstimulation (COH) with inseminations or in vitro fertilization (IVF) with or without intracytoplasmic sperm injection (ICSI).

The laboratory plays an important role in the process of COH. The principle involves the administration of gonadotropins to stimulate follicular growth, followed by hCG to stimulate follicular maturation and ovulation. Clinical, laboratory, and ultrasound monitoring of the treatment cycle is necessary to: (1) identify the dose and length of therapy;

(2) determine when or whether to administer hCG; and (3) obtain an adequate ovulatory response while avoiding hyperstimulation.

## Transgender Medicine

In transgender persons, the gender assigned at birth is discordant with the gender identity. The existence of primary and secondary sex characteristics that are not consistent with gender identity (*gender incongruence*) has the potential to lead to psychological distress (termed *gender dysphoria*). It is important to recognize that transgender persons each have specific goals as to measures that will lead to gender affirmation and thus limit or eliminate gender dysphoria; these measures may or may not include gender-affirming hormone therapy and/or gender-affirming surgical treatments. In adolescents meeting criteria for gender dysphoria/gender incongruence, GnRH agonists can be used after the first signs of puberty to limit the development of incongruent secondary sex characteristics. The use of GnRH agonists at this stage has the advantage of reversibility: if an individual determines that they no longer wish to pursue gender-affirming pharmacotherapy the GnRH agonist can be discontinued, leading to progression of puberty.

### Transgender Women

Treatment with $E_2$ or conjugated estrogens (oral) is necessary to allow for the development of feminizing secondary sex characteristics. $E_2$ comes in multiple formulations including transdermal, oral, or injectable. In transgender women, treatment with an anti-androgen is often necessary. Spironolactone, a mineralocorticoid receptor antagonist, also antagonizes the action of androgens at androgen receptors and can be used for this purpose. GnRH agonists such as leuprolide or goserelin acetate, or selective antagonist of the androgen receptor (bicalutamide) can also be used to block the synthesis of testicular androgens or block the effects of androgens, respectively.

### Transgender Men

In transgender men, goals of gender-affirming pharmacotherapy treatment usually include suppression of menstruation and development of male secondary sex characteristics such as voice deepening and male-pattern hair growth. Testosterone treatment is typically sufficient to suppress menstruation by reducing FSH and LH release from the pituitary. This can be accomplished by treatment with testosterone which comes in multiple formulations including transdermal, injectable, oral, or intranasal.

### Laboratory Monitoring

In individuals undergoing gender-affirming hormone therapy, the clinical response is the most important consideration. However, laboratory monitoring is essential to limit the risk of side effects and guide dosing. Transgender women who undergo treatment with $E_2$ require regular monitoring to ensure that $E_2$ concentrations do not exceed the female upper reference limit to avoid risks of venous thromboembolism, hypertension, and liver dysfunction. Testosterone should also be monitored to ensure that it is suppressed: the Endocrine Society recommends a target value of <50 ng/dL. Potassium should be monitored in patients taking spironolactone. Prolactin should be periodically assessed given the rare risk of prolactinoma with high-dose $E_2$ treatment.

In transgender men who choose testosterone therapy, testosterone should be within the male reference interval. Hematocrit and lipids should also be monitored regularly, given the risk of erythrocytosis and dyslipidemia with testosterone therapy.

## ANALYTIC METHODS FOR REPRODUCTIVE HORMONES

A variety of methods are available for measuring sex steroids in body fluids. Currently, the most common method is non-isotopic immunoassay. However, the use of mass spectrometry to measure sex steroids is increasing.

### Measurement of Sex Steroids by Mass Spectrometry

Although immunoassays are the predominant method for the detection and measurement of sex steroids ($E_2$, testosterone, progesterone, etc.), they are associated with considerable analytic problems. For example, automated testosterone immunoassays (nonisotopic) perform well in healthy adult males and $E_2$ immunoassays perform well in healthy premenopausal females, but they are unacceptable for use in children or adult patients with low hormone concentrations due to accuracy and imprecision problems at the low end of the measuring range.

Tandem mass spectrometry (MS/MS) coupled with high-performance liquid chromatography (HPLC) offers several advantages over traditional immunoassays, including lower limits of detection, enhanced analytic specificity, small sample size, decreased lot-to-lot variability, and the possibility of simultaneous measurement of multiple steroids. Because of these advantages, the Endocrine Society has suggested using extraction and chromatography followed by mass spectrometry (MS) or MS/MS as a potential gold standard for the measurement of testosterone. However, this technology has some disadvantages, including the requirement for highly trained personnel, high costs of equipment and maintenance, and lack of standardization.

Differences in assay performance are attributed to differences in assay accuracy, specificity, imprecision, and calibration that are most pronounced in steroid hormone immunoassays, but MS assays also require standardization. Lack of standardization makes it difficult to translate findings between institutions that utilize different assay methods, although this limitation is being addressed by the CDC hormone standardization (HoSt) program.

### Methods for Determining Total Testosterone in Blood

As described earlier, circulating testosterone comprises three different forms or pools: a non-protein-bound or "free" form,

a weakly bound form, and a tightly bound form. Testosterone bound to SHBG is not biologically active, whereas the free and bioavailable forms are available for target cells.

### Methods

Direct (no extraction required) immunoassay methods have been developed for the determination of testosterone in serum or plasma. In these methods, the steroid must be displaced from its binding proteins (albumin and SHBG), and results of the assay depend on the effectiveness of the displacement. However, most routine immunoassays are not sensitive enough to measure very low testosterone concentrations, such as those found in women, children, or hypogonadal men.

*Specimen collection and storage.* Serum and plasma (with EDTA or heparin as anticoagulant) have been used to measure total testosterone. Specimens should be centrifuged and separated within 24 hours. Testosterone is subject to diurnal variation, reaching a peak concentration between 4:00 a.m. and 8:00 a.m.; consequently, morning specimens are preferred. DHEA supplementation should be avoided before testing.

### Methods for Determining Free and Bioavailable Testosterone in Blood

In cases where SHBG concentrations are altered, measurements of free or bioavailable testosterone reflect androgen status more accurately than total testosterone. The three methods deemed acceptable for clinical practice include the following:
1. Estimation of the free testosterone fraction by equilibrium dialysis or ultrafiltration;
2. Calculation of free and weakly bound testosterone concentrations by mathematical modeling; and
3. Estimation of combined free and weakly bound (bioavailable) testosterone fractions by selective precipitation of the tightly bound form.

Methods not recommended for use in clinical practice include the following:
1. Estimation of free hormone using a direct radioimmunoassay using an analog tracer
2. Calculation of the androgen index using indices that reflect the ratios of testosterone pools.

### Equilibrium Dialysis/Ultrafiltration

Only a small fraction (1%–2%) of unconjugated testosterone exists in the free state (non-protein-bound) in serum or plasma. None of the conventional assay methods, including radioimmunoassay (RIA), is sufficiently sensitive to quantify free steroid directly in a protein-free ultrafiltrate of plasma. Instead, free steroid is estimated in plasma by adding a known amount of radiolabeled compound to the sample and allowing labeled and unlabeled compounds to reach equilibrium in their competition for the same binding sites on proteins. Bound and free radiolabeled fractions are then separated, and the ratio of free labeled to total labeled compound is determined. At equilibrium, this ratio is taken as a measure of the free testosterone fraction. An estimate of serum free testosterone can be calculated by multiplying the free testosterone fraction by the total testosterone concentration. Because of the labor-intensive nature of both equilibrium dialysis and ultrafiltration, these methods are used almost exclusively at reference laboratories.

## Selective Precipitation

Selective precipitation of SHBG with ammonium sulfate is also used in bioavailable testosterone methods. With this technique, aliquots of serum or plasma are first incubated with radiolabeled testosterone. Testosterone bound to SHBG is then precipitated with 50% ammonium sulfate. The samples are centrifuged, and aliquots of the supernatant containing free and albumin-bound testosterone (also known as *non-SHBG-bound testosterone*) are radioactively counted. The percentage of labeled testosterone not bound to SHBG is subsequently multiplied by the total testosterone concentration to obtain the bioavailable testosterone. Similar to equilibrium dialysis and ultrafiltration methods, performance of selective precipitation is generally limited to reference laboratories.

## Calculated Free Testosterone

Methods based on mathematical modeling use algorithms to derive non-SHBG-bound testosterone. These algorithms assume that when concentrations of total testosterone, SHBG, and albumin, and the constants for binding of testosterone to SHBG and albumin are known, free testosterone and bioavailable testosterone can be calculated. These calculations are based on a proper estimation of the association constant for the binding of testosterone to SHBG and albumin. However, various association constants for SHBG have been reported, and conditions resulting in abnormal plasma protein concentrations—such as nephrotic syndrome, cirrhosis, and pregnancy—require adjustments in the assumption for albumin concentration.

## Direct Radioimmunoassay Using Analog Tracer

RIA procedures are no longer used for the direct estimation of free testosterone. These assays used a labeled derivative (analog) of testosterone that, in theory, retains the ability to react with exogenous antitestosterone antibodies but is restricted from interacting with testosterone-binding proteins in the serum sample. Development of an analog that met these criteria was difficult to achieve and, as a result, direct RIAs have been replaced by calculation methods based on total testosterone, SHBG, and albumin concentrations or equilibrium dialysis followed by liquid chromatography-tandem mass spectrometry (LC-MS/MS).

## Androgen Index

The free androgen index is a ratio of testosterone to SHBG multiplied by 100. The free androgen index is no longer used to assess testosterone status because of the inherent variability of SHBG concentrations, pand the potential to over-estimate free testosterone in specimens with low SHBG.

## Methods for Determining Testosterone Precursors and Metabolites in Blood

Several biosynthetic precursors and metabolites of testosterone are measured using specific immunoassays (directly or after sample extraction), chromatography, or LC-MS/MS.

## Methods for Determining Dehydroepiandrosterone and its Sulfate

Measurements of DHEA or its sulfated conjugate, DHEA-S, in serum and plasma are important for investigations of adrenal androgen production, such as assessment of adrenal hyperplasia, adrenal tumors, adrenarche, delayed puberty, or hirsutism. DHEA is secreted almost entirely by the adrenal glands, and thus DHEA-S in circulation originates primarily from the adrenal source, with sulfation occurring in the liver or adrenal gland. Only small amounts of DHEA are produced in the ovaries and testes.

DHEA concentrations exhibit a circadian rhythm that reflects the secretion of adrenocorticotropic hormone (ACTH); these concentrations vary during the menstrual cycle. DHEA-S concentrations, however, do not exhibit a circadian rhythm because of their longer circulating half-life.

DHEA-S measurement is performed using nonisotopic immunoassays, competitive protein-binding assays, and MS-based methods. Immunoassays for DHEA-S demonstrate significant cross-reactivity with DHEA, androstenedione, and androsterone, yet the relatively low concentrations of these steroids have a minimal effect on assay performance.

## Specimen Collection and Storage

Serum or plasma (EDTA or heparin as anticoagulant) is suitable for DHEA or DHEA-S measurement. Early-morning collection, before 10:30 a.m., is preferred for DHEA. DHEA-S specimens are stable for at least 1 day at room temperature.

## Methods for Determining Estradiol in Blood

Both MS-based and immunoassay-based methods are used to measure estrogens in blood. MS-based methods utilizing isotope dilution provide the most accurate and reliable measurement of $E_2$. The main steps in these reference methods include solvent extraction, chromatographic fractionation, and chemical derivatization before analysis.

Several immunoassays for $E_2$ have been developed and adapted for use on fully automated immunoassay systems. All are heterogeneous assays (i.e., a separation step is needed), but most are direct assays and do not require preliminary extraction. Most procedures offer the convenience of solid-phase separation methods. For routine clinical applications, the greatest experience is with enzyme immunoassays.

To measure $E_2$ directly without extraction and chromatography, the steroid must be displaced from its binding proteins. The displacing agents used in commercial methods are usually proprietary, but in some systems, effective displacement is achieved by adding 8-anilino-1-naphthalene sulfonic acid (ANS) or a large excess of a competing steroid such as DHT to the sample.

Caution should be exercised in assaying samples from subjects who are receiving oral contraceptives or estrogen replacement therapy, because cross-reacting steroids may cause elevated results.

## Specimen Collection and Storage

Serum and plasma (with EDTA or heparin as anticoagulant) have been used. Specimens should be centrifuged and separated within 24 hours.

## Methods for Determining Estriol in Blood

Except for purposes of fetal aneuploidy screening, measurement of $E_3$ has little clinical value because in non-pregnant women, $E_3$ is derived almost exclusively from $E_2$. Automated enzymatic immunoassay methods account for all unconjugated $E_3$ measurements.

## Methods for Determining Estrone in Blood

Estrone determinations have limited clinical utility. Normally, blood $E_1$ concentrations parallel $E_2$ concentrations throughout the menstrual cycle, but at slightly lower concentrations. Some have proposed $E_1$ measurement in transgender women but as $E_2$ is the recommended gender-affirming hormone treatment, the Endocrine Society recommends measurement of $E_2$ rather than $E_1$.

## Methods for Determining Progesterone in Blood

Enzyme immunoassays constitute the predominant method used for progesterone measurement. Initial immunoassays for serum progesterone measurement used organic solvents to remove the steroid from endogenous binding proteins such as corticosteroid-binding globulin and albumin. Direct (non-extraction) measurement of progesterone in serum or plasma is considered the method of choice for routine applications.

Several immunoassays are available on fully automated systems. All are heterogeneous assays that require separation of free and antibody-bound fractions, although these assays do not have adequate functional sensitivity for the measurement of low progesterone concentrations in men, postmenopausal women, and children.

To overcome this limitation, MS-based methods are available at reference laboratories and other specialized medical centers.

## Specimen Collection and Storage

Serum or plasma (with heparin or EDTA as anticoagulant) is used and should be separated within 24 hours. The patient need not be fasting, and no special handling procedures are necessary.

## Measurement of Salivary Sex Steroids

Measurement of steroid concentrations in saliva has the potential to serve as a noninvasive and convenient procedure for the assessment of "serum free" steroid concentrations. However, primarily because of rapid fluctuations in salivary concentration necessitating the collection of multiple samples, salivary testing for sex steroids is not commonplace.

---

### POINTS TO REMEMBER

- Measurement of total serum steroid hormone concentrations requires displacement of hormone from its binding proteins.
- Immunoassay remains the most common method of steroid hormone measurement, but mass spectrometry is becoming more widely used.
- Automated testosterone and estradiol immunoassays are acceptable for use in healthy adult men and women, respectively, but most lack sufficient accuracy and precision for use in children and adults with low steroid hormone concentrations.
- Mass spectrometry-based methods offer improved accuracy and a lower limit of detection but require highly trained personnel and increased equipment costs.
- Free testosterone is most accurately measured by equilibrium dialysis or ultrafiltration in a reference laboratory. Direct immunoassay measurement of free testosterone is not recommended.

---

## REVIEW QUESTIONS

1. An elevated serum concentration of which of the following hormones is most useful in distinguishing between a pituitary versus placental source of hCG?
   a. FSH
   b. TSH
   c. Estradiol
   d. Progesterone
   e. ACTH
2. Which of the following best describes the application of mass spectrometry to steroid hormone measurement?
   a. Mass spectrometry is easily automated and does not require highly trained technologists.
   b. All mass spectrometry-based methods generate equivalent results.

   c. Mass spectrometry-based methods are usually more sensitive and specific than immunoassays.
   d. Mass spectrometry-based assays require fewer steps to validate than immunoassays.
   e. Mass spectrometry-based methods should not be used in women with low estradiol concentrations.
3. Which of the following laboratory tests would be most appropriate to assess anovulation?
   a. FSH on cycle day 4
   b. Estradiol on cycle day 10
   c. LH on cycle day 28
   d. Progesterone on cycle day 21
   e. Estrone on cycle day 14

4. Which of the following accurately describes free testosterone?
   a. Free testosterone represents the majority of circulating testosterone.
   b. Free testosterone provides an accurate reflection of androgen status in patients with altered SHBG concentrations.
   c. Measurement of free testosterone using a direct immunoassay generates the most accurate results.
   d. Free testosterone is not biologically active.
   e. Fluctuations in circulating SHBG do not affect free testosterone concentrations.

5. Which of the following is a likely diagnosis in a female patient experiencing primary amenorrhea characterized by delayed puberty with low serum FSH and LH concentrations?
   a. Gonadal dysgenesis
   b. 17α-hydroxylase deficiency
   c. Pituitary failure
   d. Uterine outflow abnormality
   e. FSH insensitivity

6. What is the most common cause of secondary amenorrhea?
   a. Prolactinoma
   b. Fragile-X primary ovarian insufficiency
   c. Autoimmune adrenal insufficiency
   d. Hypothyroidism
   e. Pregnancy

7. Which of the following correctly describes polycystic ovary syndrome (PCOS)?
   a. Females with PCOS have otherwise unexplained hyperandrogenism and anovulation.
   b. Females with PCOS have undetectable serum estrogen concentrations.
   c. Females with PCOS have a decreased risk of developing diabetes.
   d. Females with PCOS have a decreased risk of developing coronary heart disease.
   e. Females with PCOS can be diagnosed with a single definitive laboratory test.

## SUGGESTED READINGS

Bhasin S, Brito JP, Cunningham GR, et al. Testosterone therapy in men with hypogonadism: an Endocrine Society clinical practice guideline. *J Clin Endocrinol Metab.* 2018;103(5):1715–1744.

Bulun S. Physiology and pathology of the female reproductive axis. In: Melmed S, Auchus RJ, Goldfine AB, et al., eds. *Williams Textbook of Endocrinology.* 14th ed. Philadelphia: Elsevier; 2020:574–641.

Delot EC, Vilain E. Disorders of sexual development. In: Strauss J, Barbieri RL, eds. *Yen & Jaffe's Reproductive Endocrinology: Physiology, Pathophysiology, and Clinical Management.* 8th ed. Philadelphia: Elsevier; 2019:365–393.

Demers LM. Testosterone and estradiol assays: current and future trends. *Steroids.* 2008;73:1333–1338.

Dewailly D, Andersen CY, Balen A, et al. The physiology and clinical utility of anti-Mullerian hormone in women. *Human Reprod Update.* 2014;20:370–385.

Gronowski AM, Fantz CR, Parvin CA, et al. Use of serum FSH to identify perimenopausal women with pituitary HCG. *Clin Chem.* 2008;54:652–656.

Hall JE. Neuroendocrine control of the menstrual cycle. In: Strauss J, Barbieri RL, eds. *Yen & Jaffe's Reproductive Endocrinology: Physiology, Pathophysiology, and Clinical Management.* 8th ed. Philadelphia: Elsevier; 2019:149–166.

Hembree WC, Cohen-Kettenis PT, et al. Endocrine treatment of gender-dysphoric/gender-incongruent persons: an endocrine society clinical practice guideline. *J Clin Endocrinol Metab.* 2017;102(11):3869–3903.

La Marca A, Giulini S, Tirelli A, et al. Anti-Müllerian hormone measurement on any day of the menstrual cycle strongly predicts ovarian response in assisted reproductive technology. *Human Reprod.* 2007;22:766–771.

Layton JB, Li D, Meier CR, et al. Testosterone lab testing and initiation in the United Kingdom and the United States, 2000 to 2011. *J Clin Endocrinol Metab.* 2014;99:835–842.

Legro RS, Arslanian SA, Ehrmann DA, et al. Diagnosis and treatment of polycystic ovary syndrome: an Endocrine Society clinical practice guideline. *J Clin Endocrinol Metab.* 2013;98:4565–4592.

Montag M, Toth B, Strowitzki T. New approaches to embryo selection. *Reprod Biomed Online.* 2013;27:539–546.

Morley JE, Patrick P, Perry 3rd HM. Evaluation of assays available to measure free testosterone. *Metabolism.* 2002;51:554–549.

Nelson SM. Biomarkers of ovarian response: current and future applications. *Fert Steril.* 2013;99:963–969.

Practice Committee of American Society for Reproductive Medicine. Current evaluation of amenorrhea. *Fert Steril.* 2008;90:S219–S225.

Practice Committee of American Society for Reproductive Medicine. Multiple gestation associated with infertility therapy: an American Society for Reproductive Medicine Practice Committee opinion. *Fert Steril.* 2012;97:825–834.

Rosner W, Auchus RJ, Azziz R, et al. Position statement: utility, limitations, and pitfalls in measuring testosterone: an Endocrine Society position statement. *J Clin Endocrinol Metab.* 2007;92:405–413.

Santen RJ, Allred DC, Ardoin SP, et al. Postmenopausal hormone therapy: an Endocrine Society scientific statement. *J Clin Endocrinol Metab.* 2010;95:s1–s66.

Vigen R, O'Donnell CI, Baron AE, et al. Association of testosterone therapy with mortality, myocardial infarction, and stroke in men with low testosterone levels. *JAMA.* 2013;310:1829–1836.

# Pregnancy and Prenatal Testing

*Robert D. Nerenz and Julie A. Braga\**

## OBJECTIVES

1. Define the following:
   a. Alpha fetoprotein (AFP)
   b. Amnion
   c. Amniotic fluid
   d. Chorion
   e. Ectopic pregnancy
   f. Embryo
   g. Gestation
   h. Meconium
   i. Placenta
   j. Human placental lactogen (hPL), or placental lactogen (PL)
   k. Preeclampsia
   l. Prenatal screening
   m. Surfactant
2. Outline the events in the normal development of a fetus, beginning with conception and ending with birth.
3. Describe the structure and functions of the following, including hormones synthesized (if any), effect on maternal/fetal health if dysfunctional, and laboratory analyses and results used to determine health or disease:
   a. Amnion/amniotic fluid
   b. Blastocyst
   c. Chorionic villus
   d. Corpus luteum
   e. Ovaries
   f. Placenta
4. List the components of amniotic fluid and state their specific functions and what laboratory analyses are used to examine amniotic fluid.
5. Describe the major biochemical changes that take place during a normal pregnancy in maternal physiological systems, including renal, hemostatic, and endocrine changes.
6. State the clinical significance of the following laboratory analytes in the assessment of maternal and fetal health:
   a. Alpha fetoprotein (AFP)
   b. Human chorionic gonadotropin (hCG), or chorionic gonadotropin (CG)
   c. Inhibin A (inhA)
   d. Placental alpha macroglobulin-1 (PAMG-1)
   e. Pregnancy-associated plasma protein A (PAPP-A)
   f. Unconjugated estriol (uE3)
7. Describe the fetal renal, gastrointestinal, hepatic, pulmonary systems, including functions, development, and maturation, and how and why these systems are assessed by the laboratory.
8. For the following disorders, list the causes and symptoms, and state the laboratory analytical procedures, specimen requirements, and laboratory results used to assess and diagnose:
   a. Anencephaly
   b. Down syndrome
   c. Eclampsia
   d. Ectopic pregnancy
   e. HELLP syndrome
   f. Hemolytic disease of the newborn (HDN)
   g. Hyperemesis gravidarum
   h. Preeclampsia
   i. Respiratory distress syndrome (RDS)
   j. Spina bifida
9. In regard to maternal serum screening for fetal defects, describe the composition, timing during pregnancy and utility of the quadruple and integrated tests.

## KEY WORDS AND DEFINITIONS

**Acute fatty liver of pregnancy** A rare, life-threatening complication of pregnancy that occurs in the third trimester or the immediate period after delivery, characterized by fatty infiltration of hepatocytes with little inflammation or necrosis.

**Alpha fetoprotein (AFP)** A protein produced in the fetal liver that is measured in maternal serum for predicting risk of anencephaly, spina bifida, and Down syndrome in the fetus.

**Amniotic fluid** Substance derived mostly from fetal urine that protects the developing fetus.

**Anencephaly** A birth defect characterized by an underdeveloped brain, skull, and scalp.

**Assisted reproductive technologies (ART)** Procedures involving the manipulation of eggs or sperm to establish pregnancy in the treatment of infertility.

*The authors gratefully acknowledge the original contributions of Melanie Yarbrough, Ann Gronowski, David Grenache, and Geralyn Lambert-Messerlian, upon which portions of this chapter are based.

**Blastocyst** A thin-walled hollow structure in early embryonic development that contains a cluster of cells called the *inner cell mass* from which the embryo arises.

**Cholestasis of pregnancy** A condition during pregnancy characterized by impaired bile flow allowing bile salts to be deposited in the skin and the placenta.

**Chorionic villi** One of the minute vascular projections of the fetal chorion that combines with maternal uterine tissue to form the placenta.

**Conception** The union of the sperm and the ovum. Synonymous with fertilization.

**Down syndrome** A birth defect characterized by having three copies of chromosome 21. Also known as *trisomy 21*.

**Eclampsia** Convulsions and coma occurring in a pregnant woman or a woman who recently gave birth.

**Ectopic pregnancy** A pregnancy that occurs outside of the uterine cavity, most commonly in the fallopian tube.

**Embryo** A developing infant that has not yet finished organ development (before 10 weeks' gestation).

**Endometrium** The glandular mucous membrane that lines the uterus.

**Erythroblastosis fetalis** A severe hemolytic disease of a fetus or newborn infant caused by the production of maternal antibodies against the fetal red blood cells, usually involving rhesus (Rh) blood group incompatibility between the mother and fetus.

**Expected date of confinement (EDC)** The date at which an infant is expected to be born, calculated from the date of the last menstrual period (LMP). Also called *due date*.

**Fetal fibronectin (fFN)** A protein produced during pregnancy that is thought to function as a "glue" attaching the fetal sac to the uterine lining.

**Fetal lung maturity (FLM)** A parameter that determines the likelihood a neonate will develop respiratory distress syndrome. No longer routinely assessed in clinical practice.

**Fetus** A developing infant that has finished organ development (following 10 weeks' gestation).

**Gestation** The process, state, or period of carrying an embryo or fetus from conception until birth; by convention, the time is measured clinically from the first day of the last menstrual period (LMP) and reported in weeks.

**HELLP syndrome** A life-threatening pregnancy complication considered to be a variant of preeclampsia that typically occurs between 23 and 39 weeks' gestation. The name is an acronym for the diagnostic features: H, hemolysis; EL, elevated liver enzymes; LP, low platelets.

**Hemolytic disease of the newborn (HDN)** A disease of the fetus and newborn caused by maternal antibody-mediated fetal erythrocyte destruction.

**Human chorionic gonadotropin (hCG)** A placental glycoprotein hormone that stimulates the ovary to produce progesterone.

**Human placental lactogen (hPL)** A placental hormone, similar in structure and function to growth hormone, that disappears from the blood immediately after delivery.

**Hydramnios (or polyhydramnios)** An abnormality of pregnancy characterized by an accumulation of excess amniotic fluid.

**Hydrops fetalis** A condition in which a fetus or newborn baby accumulates fluids, causing swollen arms and legs and impaired breathing.

**Hyperemesis gravidarum** Extreme, excessive, and persistent vomiting in early pregnancy that may lead to dehydration and malnutrition.

**In vitro fertilization (IVF)** A procedure in which (1) eggs (ova) from a woman's ovary are removed, (2) the removed eggs are fertilized with sperm in a laboratory procedure, and (3) the fertilized egg (embryo) is returned to the woman's uterus.

**Lamellar bodies** Packages of phospholipids that are produced by type II alveolar cells and represent the storage form of surfactant. They are similar in size to platelets and are present in amniotic fluid.

**Meconium** A dark green fecal material that accumulates in the fetal intestines and is discharged at or near the time of birth.

**Molar pregnancy** A type of pregnancy caused by a chromosomal aberration, characterized by abnormal proliferation of placental tissue in the uterus. Also known as a *hydatidiform mole*.

**Multiple of the median (MoM)** In clinical screening, the statistic used to normalize analyte values.

**Neural tube defect (NTD)** A major birth defect resulting from the abnormal development of the neural tube that gives rise to the central nervous system; the two most common NTDs are *spina bifida* and anencephaly.

**Nuchal translucency (NT) test** A measurement of the size of the translucent space behind the neck of the fetus; made using ultrasound between 10 and 14 weeks of pregnancy.

**Oligohydramnios** A condition in pregnancy characterized by a deficiency of amniotic fluid.

**Omphalocele** A birth defect in which the infant's intestine or other abdominal organs protrude from the navel.

**Ovulation** The release of the egg (ovum) from the ovary.

**Placenta** A membranous vascular organ that develops in female mammals during pregnancy, lining the uterine wall and supporting the fetus, to which it is attached by the umbilical cord. Following birth, the placenta is expelled.

**Placental alpha microglobulin-1 (PAMG-1)** A protein present in blood and the amniotic fluid and cervico-vaginal discharge of pregnant women.

**Polyhydramnios (or hydramnios)** The presence of excess amniotic fluid in the uterus.

**Preeclampsia** A disorder of widespread vascular endothelial malfunction and vasospasm that occurs after 20 weeks' gestation and can present as late as 4–6 weeks postpartum. It is clinically defined by hypertension and proteinuria, with or without pathologic edema.

**Pregnancy** The period from conception to birth. It usually lasts 40 weeks, beginning from the first day of the woman's last menstrual period (LMP), and is divided into three trimesters, each lasting 3 months.

**Pregnancy-associated plasma protein-A (PAPP-A)** A protein used in screening tests for Down syndrome.

**Premature rupture of membranes (PROM)** Breakage of the sac containing the developing fetus and the amniotic fluid prior to the start of labor; rupture before the 37th week of gestation is called *preterm PROM* (*PPROM*).

**Preterm delivery** The birth of an infant before 37 weeks' gestation.

**Prolactin** A pituitary hormone that stimulates and maintains the secretion of milk.

**Puerperium** The approximate 6-week period lasting from childbirth to the return of normal uterine size.

**Pulmonary surfactant** A fluid secreted by the cells of the alveoli that serves to reduce the surface tension of pulmonary fluids.

**Respiratory distress syndrome (RDS)** A disease of premature infants caused by a deficiency of lung surfactant.

**Spina bifida** A congenital disorder caused by the incomplete closure of the embryonic neural tube (see *neural tube defect*); the most common form is meningomyelocele (also called *myelomeningocele*).

**Triploidy** A condition characterized by the individual having three times the haploid number of chromosomes in the cell nucleus.

**Trisomy 18 (Edwards syndrome)** A genetic disorder caused by the presence of all or part of an extra 18th chromosome (trisomy three chromosomes).

**Trophoblasts** The outermost layer of cells of the blastocyst that attaches the fertilized ovum to the uterine wall and serves as a nutritive pathway for the embryo.

**Umbilical cord** A flexible cordlike structure containing blood vessels that attaches a human or other mammalian fetus to the placenta during gestation.

**Yolk sac** A membranous sac attached to an embryo that provides early nourishment in the form of yolk in many animals, including humans, where it functions as the circulatory system before internal circulation begins.

**Zygote** The fertilized ovum or diploid cell resulting from the fusion of two haploid gametes.

## BACKGROUND

The clinical laboratory has an important role in monitoring pregnancy. In contrast to most clinical situations, clinicians must simultaneously care for more than one patient. Reference intervals derived from non-pregnant women for many clinical measurements no longer apply during pregnancy, further complicating the management of the patient. This chapter reviews the biology of pregnancy and discusses laboratory tests used to detect, evaluate, and monitor both normal and abnormal pregnancies.

## HUMAN PREGNANCY

To appreciate the role of laboratory tests in pregnancy, it is necessary to understand fundamental topics, such as: (1) conception, embryo development, and fetal growth; (2) the role of the placenta; (3) the importance and composition of amniotic fluid; (4) maternal physiologic adaptations to pregnancy; and (5) functional maturation of the fetus.

### Conception, Embryo, and Fetus

Normal human pregnancy (i.e., gestation) lasts approximately 40 weeks, as measured from the first day of the last normal menstrual period (LMP or LNMP). The anticipated date of birth of an infant is commonly referred to as the expected date of confinement (EDC). Physicians customarily divide pregnancy into four time intervals. The first three time intervals are called *trimesters*, each of which is ≈13 weeks. The last time interval, 37–42 weeks, is coined *term*. By convention, the first trimester, 0–13 weeks, begins on the first day of the last menses.

Ovulation occurs on approximately the 14th day of the menstrual cycle. If conception occurs, the ovum is fertilized, usually in the fallopian tube, and becomes a zygote, which is then carried down the tube into the uterus. The zygote divides, becoming a morula. After 50–60 cells are present, the morula develops a cavity, the primitive yolk sac, and thus becomes a blastocyst, which implants into the uterine wall about 5 days after fertilization. The cells on the exterior wall of the blastocyst, trophoblasts, synergistically invade the uterine endometrium and develop into chorionic villi, creating the placenta.

At this stage, the product of conception is referred to as an embryo. A cavity called the *amnion* forms and enlarges with the accumulation of amniotic fluid. Nourished by the placenta and protected by the amniotic fluid, an embryo undergoes rapid cell division, differentiation, and growth. From combinations of three primary cell types—ectoderm, mesoderm, and endoderm—organs begin to form through a process called *organogenesis*. At 10 weeks, an embryo has developed most major structures and is now referred to as a fetus. At 13 weeks, the fetus weighs approximately 13 g and is ≈8 cm long.

Rapid fetal growth occurs during the 13–26 weeks of the second trimester. By the end of the second trimester, the fetus weighs approximately 700 g and is 30 cm long. In the third trimester, fetal growth and maturation continue, and toward the end of the third trimester there is a slight deceleration in the rate of fetal growth. By the end of the third trimester, the fetus weighs approximately 3200 g and is about 50 cm long. Term pregnancy is defined as ≥37 weeks. Recently, the definition of *term pregnancy* was subdivided into: early term (37 0/7–38 6/7 weeks); full term (39 0/7–40 6/7); and late term (41 0/7–41 6/7). Normal labor, defined as rhythmic uterine contractions causing cervical dilation and eventually delivery of the fetus and placenta, normally occurs during this period.

## Placenta

The **placenta** and the **umbilical cord** form the primary link between fetus and mother. The placenta grows throughout pregnancy and is normally delivered through the birth canal immediately after the birth of the infant.

### Function

The placenta: (1) keeps the maternal and fetal circulation systems separate; (2) nourishes the fetus; (3) eliminates fetal wastes; and (4) produces hormones vital to pregnancy. It is composed of large collections of fetal vessels called *villi*. These villi are finger-like projections that insert into the *intervillous space*, which contains maternal blood that bathes the fetal villi and facilitates bidirectional exchange between mother and fetus. For substances to move from maternal circulation to fetal circulation, they must cross through the trophoblasts and several membranes. The transfer of any substance depends largely on the: (1) concentration gradient between the maternal and fetal circulatory systems; (2) presence or absence of circulating binding proteins; (3) lipid solubility of the substance; and (4) presence of facilitated transport, such as ion pumps or receptor-mediated endocytosis. The placenta is an effective barrier to the movement of large proteins and hydrophobic compounds bound to plasma proteins. Maternal immunoglobulin (Ig)G crosses the placenta via receptor-mediated endocytosis. Because of its long half-life, maternally produced IgG protects a newborn through passive immunity for the first 6 months of life. Antibody assays with low limits of detection may be positive in infants up to age 18 months, because of the persistence of maternal antibodies.

### Placental Hormones

The placenta produces several protein and steroid hormones. The major protein hormones are **human chorionic gonadotropin (hCG)** and **human placental lactogen (hPL)**. Steroid hormones including progesterone, estradiol, estriol, and estrone are synthesized in complex joint pathways involving maternal, placental, and fetal contributions. In general, hormone production by the placenta increases in proportion to the increase in placental mass (e.g., the increase in maternal serum hPL concentration with advancing gestational age is directly correlated with the increasing mass of placental tissue). hCG, which peaks at the end of the first trimester, is an exception.

### Chorionic Gonadotropin

One of the most important placental hormones is hCG. It stimulates the ovary to produce progesterone by maintaining the corpus luteum that, in turn, prevents menstruation, thereby protecting the pregnancy. Chemistry, biochemistry, and methods for measuring hCG are discussed later in this chapter.

### Placental Lactogen

Placental lactogen, also known as hPL and human chorionic somatomammotropin (hCS), is a single polypeptide chain of 191 amino acids with two intramolecular disulfide bridges. The structure of hPL is exceptionally homologous (96%) with growth hormone (GH) and less so with **prolactin** (67%). The placental secretion near term is 1–2 g/day, the largest of any known human hormone. hPL has many biological activities, including: (1) lactogenic, (2) metabolic, (3) somatotropic, (4) erythropoietic, and (5) aldosterone-stimulating effects.

### Placental Steroids

The placenta produces a wide variety of steroid hormones, including estrogen and progesterone, with large amounts of estrogens produced at term. Maternal cholesterol is the main precursor for placental progesterone production. Biosynthesis of estrogens by the placenta differs from that of the ovaries because the placenta has no 17α-hydroxylase. Thus, each of the estrogens—estrone (E1), estradiol (E2), and estriol (E3)— must be synthesized from C-19 intermediates that already have a hydroxyl group at position 17. In non-pregnant women, the ovaries secrete 100–600 μg/day of estradiol, of which about 10% is metabolized to estriol. During late pregnancy, the placenta produces 50–150 mg/day of estriol and 15–20 mg/day of estradiol and estrone. Secretion of estrogens and progesterone throughout pregnancy ensures: (1) appropriate development of the endometrium, (2) uterine growth, (3) adequate uterine blood supply, and (4) preparation of the uterus for labor.

### Amniotic Fluid

Throughout intrauterine life, the fetus lives within a fluid-filled compartment. The **amniotic fluid** provides a medium in which a fetus readily moves. It cushions a fetus against possible injury, helps maintain a constant temperature, and is inhaled and swallowed by the fetus during normal fetal lung development. This fluid is a dynamic medium whose volume and chemical composition are controlled within relatively narrow limits.

### Volume and Dynamics

The volume of amniotic fluid increases progressively until 34 weeks' gestation, when it decreases slightly through the 40th week and then more sharply declines until the 42nd week. The volume is 200–300 mL at 16 weeks; 400–1400 mL at 26 weeks; 300–2000 mL at 34 weeks; and 300–1400 mL at 40 weeks. Pathological decreases and increases in amniotic fluid volume are encountered frequently in clinical practice.

**TABLE 44.1  Composition of Amniotic Fluid (Mean Values**

| Component | Gestational Age (Weeks) | | |
| --- | --- | --- | --- |
| | 15 | 25 | 40 |
| Sodium, mmol/L | 136 | 138 | 126 |
| Potassium, mmol/L | 3.9 | 4.0 | 4.3 |
| Chloride, mmol/L | 111 | 109 | 103 |
| Bicarbonate, mmol/L | 16 | 18 | 16 |
| Urea nitrogen, mg/dL (mmol urea/L) | 11 (3.9) | 11 (3.9) | 18 (6.4) |
| Creatinine, mg/dL (μmol/L) | 0.8 (71) | 0.9 (80) | 2.2 (194) |
| Glucose, mg/dL (mmol/L) | 47 (2.6) | 39 (2.2) | 32 (1.8) |
| Uric acid, mg/dL (mmol/L) | 4.0 (0.24) | 5.7 (0.34) | 10.4 (0.61) |
| Total protein, g/dL (g/L) | 0.5 (5) | 0.8 (8) | 0.3 (3) |
| Bilirubin, mg/dL (μmol/L) | 0.13 (2.2) | 0.14 (2.4) | 0.04 (0.7) |
| Osmolality, mOsm/kg H$_2$O | 272 | 272 | 255 |

(From Benzie RJ, Doran TA, Harkins JL, Owen VM, Porter CJ. Composition of the amniotic fluid and maternal serum in pregnancy. *Am J Obstet Gynecol.* 1974;119:798–810.)

Intrauterine growth restriction and anomalies of the fetal urinary tract, such as bilateral renal agenesis or obstruction of the urethra, are associated with oligohydramnios, an abnormally low amniotic fluid volume. Increased fluid volume is known as hydramnios (also termed polyhydramnios). Conditions associated with hydramnios include: (1) maternal diabetes mellitus, (2) severe Rh isoimmune disease, (3) fetal esophageal atresia, (4) multifetal pregnancy, (5) anencephaly, and (6) spina bifida.

## Composition

Early in gestation, the composition of the amniotic fluid resembles a complex dialysate of the maternal serum. As a fetus grows, the amniotic fluid changes in several ways (Table 44.1). Most notably, the sodium concentration and osmolality decrease and concentrations of urea, creatinine, and uric acid increase. The activities of many enzymes in amniotic fluid have been studied with respect to both gestational age and fetal status but have not been found to be clinically useful. The major lipids of interest are the phospholipids (PL), whose type and concentrations reflect fetal lung maturity (FLM). Numerous steroid and protein hormones are also present in amniotic fluid. The rare syndrome of congenital adrenal hyperplasia (CAH) had been diagnosed antenatally by measuring 17-hydroxyprogesterone and pregnanetriol in the amniotic fluid near term, although this has largely been replaced by molecular genetic analysis of DNA obtained from amniocentesis or chorionic villus sampling.

Early in pregnancy, little or no particulate matter is found in the amniotic fluid. By 16 weeks' gestation, large numbers of cells are present, having been shed from the surfaces of the amnion, skin, and tracheobronchial tree. These cells are of great utility in antenatal diagnosis and are the cellular source for DNA used for karyotype analysis after amniocentesis. As pregnancy continues to progress, scalp hair and lanugo (fine hair on the body of the fetus) are shed into the fluid and contribute to its turbidity. Production of surfactant particles in the lung, termed lamellar bodies, greatly increases the haziness of the fluid. At term, amniotic fluid contains gross particles of vernix caseosa, the oily substance composed of sebum and desquamated epithelial cells covering the fetal skin.

Normal fetuses do not defecate during pregnancy. If severely stressed, a fetus may pass stool that is called meconium. This heterogeneous material contains many bile pigments and therefore stains the amniotic fluid green. Meconium-stained amniotic fluid is a sign of fetal stress.

### POINTS TO REMEMBER

**Placenta**
- A major function of the placenta is production of several protein and steroid hormones.
- hCG is a protein hormone that maintains the corpus luteum and promotes continued production of progesterone, which protects the pregnancy by preventing menstruation. After the luteo-placental shift, progesterone is synthesized by the placenta.
- hPL is a protein hormone that regulates maternal and fetal metabolism to facilitate growth and development of the fetus.
- Major steroid hormones, including progesterone and estriol, are synthesized by the fetoplacental unit.

**Amniotic Fluid**
- Amniotic fluid provides a medium to cushion and protect the fetus.
- Early in gestation, the composition of the amniotic fluid resembles a complex dialysate of the maternal serum.
- Toward the end of the first trimester, the fetal kidneys begin to produce urine, which becomes the main component of amniotic fluid.
- Fetal cells shed in amniotic fluid are a source of DNA for karyotype analysis for suspected aneuploidy.
- Decreases and increases in amniotic fluid volume can be indicative of potential pathophysiological changes in pregnancy, although many times are idiopathic.

## MATERNAL ADAPTATION

During pregnancy, a woman undergoes dramatic physiologic and hormonal changes. The large quantities of estrogens, progesterone, PL, and corticosteroids produced during pregnancy affect various metabolic, physiologic, and endocrine systems. In addition, the woman experiences: (1) an increase in resistance to angiotensin; (2) a predominance of lipid metabolism over glucose use; and (3) increased synthesis by the liver of thyroid- and steroid-binding proteins, fibrinogen, and other proteins characteristic of pregnancy. As a result of such changes, many of the laboratory reference intervals for non-pregnant patients are not appropriate for pregnant patients. Reference intervals for >70 analytes in normal pregnancy have been developed. Mean values for selected tests expressed as a percentage of control means are presented in Table 44.2. It should be noted that these reference intervals will vary depending on testing method.

### Hematologic Changes

Maternal blood volume increases during pregnancy by an average of 45%. Plasma volume increases more than red blood cell mass; therefore, despite augmented erythropoiesis, hemoglobin concentration, erythrocyte count, and hematocrit decrease during normal pregnancy, producing the so-called physiologic anemia of pregnancy. Hemoglobin concentrations at term average 12.6 g/dL (126 g/L), compared with 13.3 g/dL (133 g/L) for the non-pregnant state. The leukocyte count varies considerably during pregnancy, from 4000 to 13,000/μL. During labor and puerperium (the interval immediately after delivery), leukocyte counts may be markedly increased.

The concentrations of several blood coagulation factors are increased during pregnancy. For example, plasma fibrinogen increases by approximately 65%, from 275 to 450 mg/dL (8.1–13.2 μmol/L); this increase contributes to the increase in sedimentation rate. Other clotting factors also increase, including factors VII, VIII, IX, and X. Prothrombin and factors V and XII do not change, whereas factors XI and XIII decrease slightly. Even though the platelet count remains unchanged in most women and the prothrombin time and activated partial thromboplastin time shorten slightly (see Table 44.2), pregnancy increases the risk of thromboembolism up to five times that of non-pregnant women.

### Biochemical Changes

During pregnancy, electrolytes show little change, but an approximately 40% increase in serum triglycerides, cholesterol, PL, and free fatty acids is seen. Plasma albumin is decreased to an average of 3.4 g/dL (34 g/L) in late pregnancy; plasma globulin concentrations increase slightly. Several of the plasma transport proteins, including thyroxine-binding globulin (TBG), cortisol-binding globulin (CBG), and sex hormone-binding globulin (SHBG), increase markedly. Serum cholinesterase activity is reduced, whereas alkaline phosphatase activity in serum is tripled, mainly as the result of an increase in very heat-stable alkaline phosphatase of placental origin. In addition, creatine kinase can markedly increase upon delivery.

### Renal Function

Pregnancy increases the glomerular filtration rate (GFR) to about 170 mL/min per 1.73 m$^2$ by 20 weeks, and therefore increases the clearance of urea, creatinine, and uric acid. Concentrations of these three analytes are slightly decreased in serum for much of pregnancy. As term approaches, GFR begins to return to the non-pregnant rate. Urea and creatinine concentrations rise slightly during the last 4 weeks. During this time, tubular reabsorption of uric acid increases dramatically, which increases serum uric acid compared with the non-pregnant state. Glucosuria up to 1000 mg/day (5.55 mmol/day) may be present, owing to increased GFR, which presents more fluid to the tubules and therefore lowers the renal glucose threshold. Protein loss in the urine can increase to up to 300 mg/day.

### Endocrine Changes

The action of progesterone prevents menses and thus allows pregnancy to continue. In early pregnancy, progesterone is produced by the corpus luteum of the maternal ovary in response to hCG. In later stages the placenta directly produces enough progesterone to maintain pregnancy.

Throughout pregnancy, plasma parathyroid hormone (PTH) is increased by approximately 40%, with almost no change in the plasma free ionized calcium fraction, thus suggesting a new set point for the secretion of PTH. Calcitonin does not increase predictably during pregnancy, whereas 1,25-dihydroxyvitamin D is increased during pregnancy and promotes increased intestinal calcium absorption to support the calcium requirements for fetal skeletal development.

Increased estrogen concentration stimulates increased hepatic production of CBG. The hepatic clearance of cortisol decreases. Thus, the absolute plasma concentrations of both total and free cortisol are several times higher during pregnancy. The diurnal rhythm of cortisol, higher in the morning and lower in the evening, is maintained. Increased plasma aldosterone and deoxycorticosterone concentrations are observed.

Increasing estrogen concentrations throughout pregnancy increase the secretion of prolactin up to 10-fold. Conversely, high estrogen concentrations during pregnancy suppress the secretion of luteinizing hormone (LH) and follicle-stimulating hormone (FSH) below the detection limit and the GH response to provocative stimuli is blunted (see Table 44.2).

Although normal pregnancy is a euthyroid state, many changes occur in thyroid function. High concentrations of TBG raise the concentration of total thyroxine (T4) and triiodothyronine (T3), but a slight decrease in free T4 concentration occurs during the second and third trimesters. Increasing hCG concentrations in the second half of the first trimester cause a corresponding decrease in TSH, which then returns to non-pregnant concentrations when hCG declines in the second trimester. Thyroglobulin is significantly

## TABLE 44.2   Mean Serum and Plasma Laboratory Values During Normal Pregnancies Expressed as a Percentage of the Non-pregnant Mean (*n* = 29)

| Analyte | TIME OF GESTATION | | |
| --- | --- | --- | --- |
| | 12 Weeks | 32 Weeks | Term |
| Sodium | 97 | 98 | 97 |
| Potassium | 95 | 95 | 100 |
| Bicarbonate | 85 | 85 | 81 |
| Chloride | 98 | 100 | 99 |
| Urea nitrogen | 77 | 63 | 77 |
| Creatinine | 71 | 74 | 81 |
| Fasting glucose | 98 | 94 | 94 |
| Bilirubin, unconjugated | 56 | 67 | 78 |
| Albumin | 93 | 78 | 78 |
| Protein | 92 | 83 | 83 |
| Uric acid | 68 | 92 | 120 |
| Calcium | 98 | 94 | 97 |
| Free ionized calcium | 99 | 101 | 102 |
| Parathyroid hormone, intact | — | — | 140 |
| 1,25-Dihydroxyvitamin D | — | — | 400 |
| Phosphate | 108 | 97 | 96 |
| Magnesium | 92 | 87 | 87 |
| Alkaline phosphatase | 90 | 203 | 347 |
| Creatine kinase | 87 | 86 | 135 |
| α1-Antitrypsin | 129 | 174 | 191 |
| Transferrin | 105 | 160 | 170 |
| Cholesterol | 100 | 144 | 156 |
| HDL-cholesterol | 121 | 119 | 130 |
| LDL-cholesterol | 80 | 118 | 146 |
| Fasting triglycerides | 141 | 300 | 349 |
| Iron | 112 | 94 | 94 |
| Iron-binding capacity | 95 | 139 | 144 |
| Transferrin saturation | 136 | 68 | 64 |
| Zinc protoporphyrin | 107 | 109 | 144 |
| Ferritin | 81 | 33 | 59 |
| Thyroxine | 103 | 107 | 100 |
| Triiodothyronine | 100 | 121 | 121 |
| Free thyroxine | 98 | 72 | 74 |
| Thyroxine-binding globulin | 114 | 155 | 182 |
| Thyroid-stimulating hormone | 111 | 122 | 139 |
| Cortisol | 111 | 301 | 309 |
| Aldosterone | — | — | 1500 |
| Prolactin | — | — | 800 |
| Hemoglobin | 95 | 90 | 96 |
| Hematocrit | 94 | 91 | 97 |
| Leukocyte count | 144 | 167 | 240 |
| Prothrombin time | 99 | 97 | 97 |
| Activated partial thromboplastin time | 95 | 91 | 93 |
| Platelet count | 98 | 96 | 100 |
| Fibrinogen | 119 | 154 | 165 |

*HDL*, High-density lipoprotein; *LDL*, low-density lipoprotein.
Data from Lockitch G, ed. *Handbook of Diagnostic Biochemistry and Hematology in Normal Pregnancy.* Boca Raton: CRC Press; 1993.

increased, especially in the third trimester. Very few (<0.2%) pregnant individuals develop hyperthyroidism, and hypothyroidism is very rare. Postpartum thyroid dysfunction is common and is frequently unrecognized and misdiagnosed as routine postpartum symptoms of fatigue and weight changes. The fetal thyroid-pituitary axis functions independently from the mother's axis by the end of the first trimester. However, if the mother has preexisting Graves' disease (hyperthyroidism caused by autoantibodies that stimulate the thyroid), those antibodies can cross the placenta, causing hyperthyroidism in the fetus. If the mother has anti-TSH autoantibodies, the infant can develop transient hypothyroidism.

# FUNCTIONAL DEVELOPMENT OF THE FETUS

Fetal organs mature during the third trimester but not at the same rate. This section reviews the lung, liver, kidneys, and blood maturation in the fetus.

## Lungs and Pulmonary Surfactant

In normal air-breathing lungs, a substance called **pulmonary surfactant** coats the alveolar epithelium and responds to alveolar volume changes by reducing surface tension in the alveolar wall during expiration. Surfactant is needed because the surface tension is an inverse function of the radius of the airway. Thus, small alveoli have a higher collapsing force than larger alveoli. Surfactant opposes the force and keeps the small alveoli from collapsing. Specialized alveolar cells synthesize pulmonary surfactant and package it into laminated storage granules called *lamellar bodies*. These storage granules are 1–5 μm in diameter and contain PL, cholesterol, and protein. Pulmonary surfactant production starts as early as 20 weeks' gestation, but adequate amounts do not accumulate until about 36 weeks. Exudation of pulmonary fluid (via the trachea) and fetal breathing movements transport lamellar bodies into the amniotic fluid.

Pulmonary surfactant is a complex mixture of lipids and proteins; <5% is composed of carbohydrates. The principal phospholipids present in surfactant are lecithin (phosphatidylcholine) and phosphatidylglycerol (PG), while phosphatidylinositol and sphingomyelin are present in much lower abundance. The protein fraction of lamellar bodies is approximately 4% and is composed of four surfactant-specific proteins: SP-A, SP-B, SP-C, and SP-D.

## Liver

Hematopoiesis occurs in the liver during the first two trimesters and is transferred to the fetal bone marrow during the third trimester. The liver is also responsible for production of specific proteins (such as albumin and clotting factors), metabolism and detoxification of many compounds, and secretion of substances such as bilirubin. A clinically useful protein produced by the liver is **alpha fetoprotein (AFP)**. Bilirubin secretion and detoxification mechanisms are immature until late in pregnancy and even in the first few months after birth. Thus, premature infants often have high serum bilirubin concentrations and metabolize drugs poorly.

## Kidneys

Toward the end of the first trimester, the fetal kidneys begin to produce urine, which becomes the main component of amniotic fluid. Early nephrons cannot produce concentrated urine, and pH regulation is also limited. Complete maturation occurs after birth. Although kidneys are not required for fetal survival, amniotic fluid is required for normal lung development. Without fluid to breathe, the fetal lungs fail to properly develop. Thus, newborns without kidneys die of pulmonary failure.

## Fetal Blood Development

Fetal blood is produced first by the embryonic yolk sac, then by the liver, and finally by the fetal bone marrow. With the switch of erythropoiesis to the fetal liver and spleen, fetal hemoglobin (HbF) production begins. HbF consists of two α- and two γ-chains (α2γ2). Small amounts of adult hemoglobin, HbA (α2β2), are also produced, but HbF predominates during the remainder of fetal life.

As the fetal bone marrow begins red cell production, HbA production increases. At birth, fetal blood contains 75% HbF and 25% HbA. HbF production rapidly diminishes during the first year of postnatal life. In normal adults, <1% of hemoglobin is HbF. The difference between fetal and adult hemoglobin is very significant, as HbF has a higher affinity for oxygen than HbA. Thus, in the placenta, oxygen is released from the maternal HbA, diffuses into the chorionic villi, and preferentially binds to the fetal HbF. In addition, 2,3-diphosphoglycerate (2,3-DPG) does not bind HbF and therefore cannot decrease its affinity for oxygen.

# MATERNAL AND FETAL HEALTH ASSESSMENT

For optimal care during pregnancy, a woman should consult her physician, preferably before conception. Preconception evaluation should include a medical, reproductive, and family history; physical examination; and laboratory testing.

## Laboratory Testing

The following laboratory tests are recommended as part of a preconception evaluation: (1) hematocrit; (2) blood type and Rh compatibility; (3) erythrocyte antibody screen; (4) Papanicolaou smear (or human papillomavirus [HPV] test) if indicated; (5) rubella titer; (6) cystic fibrosis carrier status; (7) spinal muscular atrophy carrier testing. Infectious disease testing should also be considered, including: (1) rapid plasma reagin/syphilis IgG; (2) gonorrhea and chlamydia testing; (3) human immunodeficiency virus (HIV) antigen and antibody screen; (4) hepatitis B surface antigen; and (5) hepatitis C antibody. Depending on demographic risks, genetic testing for disorders such as Tay–Sachs disease, thalassemia, and sickle cell disease should be offered. A careful diet history is warranted. Folic acid supplementation should be recommended to reduce the risk of **neural tube defects (NTDs)**. Women at high risk for diabetes mellitus should be screened for this disorder (see Chapter 33).

Many laboratory tests are useful for managing normal and abnormal pregnancies (see "At a Glance: Laboratory Evaluation of Maternal Health", below). Screening for fetal NTDs and aneuploidy should be offered to all pregnant patients. Depending on diabetes risk, glucose tolerance testing should be performed immediately or at 24–28 weeks. Maternal observation and recording of fetal movements, ultrasound examination (biophysical profile), and fetal heart rate patterns (nonstress test and contraction stress tests) are the currently accepted methods for monitoring fetal well-being.

## Diagnosis and Dating of Pregnancy

It is important for maternal and fetal health to accurately detect early pregnancy and establish an accurate estimate of

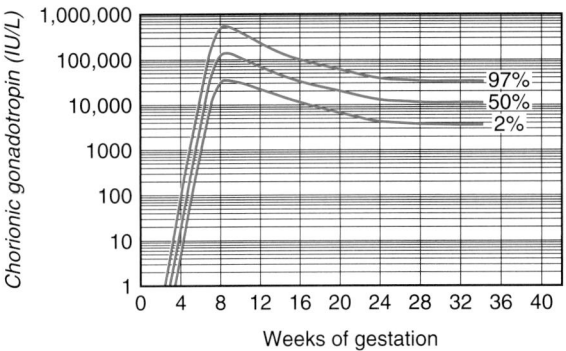

Fig. 44.1 Concentration of chorionic gonadotropin (hCG) in maternal serum as a function of gestational age. *Lines* represent the 2nd, 50th, and 97th percentiles. The maternal serum values from 14 to 25 weeks are medians calculated from 24,229 pregnancies from testing performed at ARUP Laboratories, Inc., from January to October 1997. (From Ashwood ER. Evaluating health and maturation of the unborn: the role of the clinical laboratory. *Clin Chem.* 1992;38:1523–1529, with permission.)

gestational age. The most useful test for detecting pregnancy is the hCG test.

Qualitative tests for hCG in blood or urine are used to screen for pregnancy. In the first 8 weeks of pregnancy, the hCG concentration in maternal serum rises geometrically (Fig. 44.1). Detectable amounts (>5 IU/L) are present in the serum 8–11 days after conception. hCG usually becomes detectable in the urine 1–3 days later, although this interval is highly variable. For women aged 13–40 years, serum hCG concentrations of ≥5 IU/L are consistent with pregnancy. Modestly elevated hCG values are infrequently seen in menopausal women and are thought to be secreted by the pituitary following removal of feedback inhibition by ovarian steroids. Concentrations in approximately half of pregnant women reach 25 IU/L on the first day of their missed period. The peak concentration occurs at about 8–10 weeks and is hugely variable, ranging from 30,000–500,000 IU/L. Subsequently, hCG concentrations start to decline in serum and urine, and by the end of the second trimester, a 90% reduction from peak concentration has usually occurred. The presence of twins approximately doubles hCG concentrations.

## AT A GLANCE

**Laboratory Evaluation of Maternal Health**
*First Prenatal Visit*
- Complete blood count (CBC)
- Rh(D) typing and antibody screen
- Pap smear
- Urine culture
- Rubella immunity
- Varicella immunity
- Hepatitis B screening
- Hepatitis C screening
- HIV antigen/antibody test
- Sexually transmitted infection (STI) testing
  - Syphilis
  - Chlamydia
  - Gonorrhea

Women at increased risk may also receive testing for the following:
- Genetic testing for inherited disease
- Hemoglobinopathies
- Gonorrhea
- Tuberculosis
- Toxoplasma
- Hepatitis C

Additional testing that may be offered during pregnancy:
- Carrier screening for cystic fibrosis and spinal muscular atrophy
- Detection of fetal anomalies
  - Maternal serum screening (first and second trimester)
  - Cell free DNA screening (at 10 weeks' gestation or later)
- Oral glucose tolerance testing (between 24 and 28 weeks' gestation)
- Group B *Streptococcus* screening cultures (between 35 and 37 weeks' gestation)

## COMPLICATIONS OF PREGNANCY

Although most pregnancies progress without problems, complications can arise in the mother, placenta, or fetus.

### Abnormal Pregnancies

Conditions arising primarily in the mother include: (1) ectopic pregnancy, (2) hyperemesis gravidarum, (3) preeclampsia, (4) HELLP syndrome, (5) liver disease, and (6) hemolytic disease of the newborn. The clinician must distinguish abnormal changes in laboratory tests from normal physiologic changes induced by pregnancy (see Table 44.2).

### Ectopic Pregnancy and Threatened Abortion

When a fertilized egg implants in a location other than the body of the uterus, the condition is called an ectopic pregnancy. Most abnormal implantations occur in the fallopian tube; they can also occur in the abdomen, although this is rare. Common symptoms of ectopic pregnancy include abdominal pain, vaginal bleeding, and adnexal mass. Tubal rupture from the expanding non-distensible fallopian tube can cause a life-threatening hemorrhage and is a common cause of maternal death from ectopic pregnancy. Management of ectopic pregnancy can be surgical or medical (with methotrexate). Early detection and proper management of ectopic pregnancy are the most effective means of preventing maternal morbidity and mortality.

Ultrasound examination is used to evaluate women with symptoms. When ultrasound is non-diagnostic, serial quantitative measurements of serum hCG are used to identify women with ectopic pregnancy or abnormal intrauterine pregnancy. These conditions frequently produce abnormally low hCG concentrations and slow rates of increase (longer doubling time).

### Trophoblastic Disease

Serum hCG determinations are very useful for monitoring patients with germ cell-derived neoplasms or other hCG-producing tumors, such as lung carcinoma. The use of hCG in these diseases is discussed in Chapter 20.

## Preeclampsia and Eclampsia

**Preeclampsia** is a pregnancy condition characterized by hypertension and other end organ involvement, including proteinuria, cerebral vasospasm, hematologic abnormalities such as hemolysis and thrombocytopenia, and elevated transaminases. The 2020 diagnostic criteria established by the American College of Obstetricians and Gynecologists require the presence of new onset hypertension and proteinuria or, in the absence of proteinuria, new onset thrombocytopenia, renal insufficiency, impaired liver function, pulmonary edema or headache that does not respond to medication.

It can occur any time after 20 weeks (although there are cases of preeclampsia occurring at less than 20 weeks in abnormal pregnancies, such as **molar pregnancies**). It affects 3%–5% of pregnancies and continues to be a major cause of maternal and perinatal mortality. If the mother develops generalized seizures, the condition is called **eclampsia**. Most maternal deaths are due to central nervous system complications, but ischemic liver damage may also occur. The only cure for preeclampsia is delivery of the placenta.

## HELLP Syndrome

The **HELLP syndrome** (hemolysis, elevated liver enzymes, and low platelet counts in association with preeclampsia) is a life-threatening obstetric complication that occurs in 0.1% of pregnancies. Its most prominent features are thrombocytopenia and disseminated intravascular coagulation. Most cases occur between 27 and 36 weeks' gestation, but the syndrome also may occur postpartum. Women typically present with epigastric or right upper quadrant pain, malaise, nausea, vomiting, and headache. Lactate dehydrogenase (LD) values may be very high reflecting high levels of red blood cell hemolysis, and alanine aminotransferase (ALT) and aspartate aminotransferase (AST) are usually 2–10 times their upper reference limits. Treatment for HELLP is delivery of the fetus.

## Liver Disease

Several liver disorders are unique to pregnancy. These include: (1) hyperemesis gravidarum, (2) **cholestasis of pregnancy**, and (3) fatty liver of pregnancy. These disorders must be distinguished from the normal physiological changes of pregnancy (see Table 44.2). Significant changes normally seen in pregnancy include a dilutional decrease in serum albumin and an increase of alkaline phosphatase (from the placenta). Notably, total bilirubin, 5′-nucleotidase, gamma-glutamyl transferase (GGT), ALT, and AST are unchanged in mothers with a normal pregnancy. Changes in these analytes reflect hepatobiliary disease. Also discussed in this section are non-pregnancy-related liver disease in pregnancy and the effect of pregnancy on preexisting liver disease.

### Hyperemesis Gravidarum

**Hyperemesis gravidarum** is characterized by nausea and vomiting and, in severe cases, dehydration and malnutrition.

It typically occurs in the first trimester. When hyperemesis is severe enough to cause dehydration, abnormal liver enzyme values—usually less than four times the upper reference limit—are seen in approximately 50% of patients. Mild hyperbilirubinemia may occur. However, significant liver disease does not occur, and liver biopsy results are normal. Low birth weight babies are common, especially for women who develop malnutrition.

### Cholestasis of Pregnancy

Pregnancy does not preclude the acquisition or aggravation of non-pregnancy-related liver disease. Thus, cholestasis during pregnancy may reflect the presence of: (1) hepatotoxicity from drugs, (2) primary biliary cholangitis (formerly primary biliary cirrhosis), (3) Dubin–Johnson syndrome, or (4) cholelithiasis. Abdominal ultrasound, endoscopic retrograde cholangiography, or liver biopsy may be necessary to exclude these conditions.

The onset of cholestasis during pregnancy usually occurs in the third trimester and is manifested clinically by diffuse pruritus and, in 10% of patients, jaundice. The typical features of cholestasis, including pale stools and dark urine, are present and last until delivery. Women who experience cholestasis while taking oral contraceptives usually develop cholestasis of pregnancy. Diagnosis is made based on symptoms in combination with total bile acids levels of 10 nmol/mL or higher. Serum bilirubin rarely exceeds 5 mg/dL (85.5 μmol/L). Alkaline phosphatase is typically 2–4 times the upper reference limit. Aminotransferase enzyme concentrations are mildly increased and may precede the increase of bile acids. Prothrombin time may be increased because of vitamin K malabsorption. The condition is associated with increased risk for preterm delivery and possibly fetal death, and has an increased risk for recurrence with subsequent pregnancies.

### Fatty Liver of Pregnancy

**Fatty liver of pregnancy** occurs in approximately 1 in 10,000 pregnancies and is characterized by accumulation of microvesicular fat in the hepatocytes. Many of the cases of this maternal disorder are caused by an inherited mitochondrial fatty acid oxidation disorder in the fetus, long chain 3-hydroxyacyl-CoA dehydrogenase deficiency (LCHAD). Mothers carrying fetuses with this disorder are 50 times more likely to develop fatty liver of pregnancy. The disease typically occurs at week 37 and is manifested clinically by the rapid onset of malaise, nausea, vomiting, and abdominal pain. Mild increases in aminotransferase enzyme concentrations occur, with the AST increase typically greater than that of ALT but both typically less than six times the upper reference limit. Serum bilirubin is usually >6 mg/dL (102.6 μmol/L). Life-threatening hypoglycemia may occur. Hyperuricemia, presumably from tissue destruction and renal failure, is characteristic. Liver histology shows acute fatty infiltration with little necrosis or inflammation. If untreated, fulminant hepatic failure with hepatic encephalopathy ensues (see Chapter 37). Treatment is immediate delivery, at which time rapid recovery usually occurs. Infant and maternal mortality is approximately 50% and 20%, respectively.

## Effect of Pregnancy on Preexisting Liver Disease

Conception and full-term parturition do not usually occur in women who have cirrhosis. However, liver disease is not a reason for termination of a pregnancy. The hypervolemia associated with pregnancy may aggravate cirrhosis and predispose to bleeding from esophageal varices. Autoimmune chronic hepatitis is usually associated with amenorrhea, but pregnancy may occur after disease remission following treatment with corticosteroids.

## Neonatal Thyroid Function

During the first trimester of pregnancy, the fetus is dependent on the mother for its supply of thyroid hormone. Low maternal thyroid hormone concentrations (overt or subclinical hypothyroidism) have been associated with adverse outcomes, such as preterm delivery, fetal death, and a reduced intelligence quotient (IQ) in children. Later in pregnancy, the fetal thyroid–pituitary axis functions independently from the mother's axis in most cases. However, if the mother has preexisting Graves' disease, her IgG autoantibodies can cross the placenta and stimulate the fetal thyroid gland. Thus, the fetus can develop hyperthyroidism. Measurement of TSH-receptor antibodies is useful for assessing risk of fetal or neonatal Graves' disease.

## Hemolytic Disease of the Newborn

Hemolytic disease of the newborn (HDN) is a fetal hemolytic disorder caused by maternal antibodies directed against antigen on fetal erythrocytes. Commonly used synonyms for this disorder are *isoimmunization disease, Rh isoimmune disease, Rh disease,* or *D isoimmunization.* Any of a large number of erythrocyte surface antigens may be responsible for isoimmune hemolysis. When severe, the disorder is known as erythroblastosis fetalis and is life-threatening to fetus and newborn. Disease severity is commonly assessed using noninvasive ultrasonographic determination of middle fetal cerebral artery velocity.

### Etiology

Maternal sensitization may occur in response to blood transfusion or a pregnancy in which the mother is exposed to fetal red blood cells carrying the antigen that the mother lacks. Antibodies against RhD are the most common cause of HDN, although antibodies against other erythrocyte antigens can also cause disease. The resulting maternal antibodies are actively transported across the placenta and into the fetus, where they cause destruction of the fetal erythrocytes. The severity of the resulting hemolysis is influenced by antibody specificity, titer, and transfer rate, as well as the functional maturity of the fetal spleen in which the sensitized erythrocytes are destroyed.

Destruction of the fetal erythrocytes leads to fetal anemia that imposes an extra burden on the fetal heart to provide an adequate oxygen supply to fetal tissues. Anemia stimulates the fetal marrow and extramedullary erythropoiesis in the liver and spleen to replace the destroyed erythrocytes. Extramedullary erythropoiesis destroys hepatocytes and leads to decreased production of serum albumin and decreased oncotic pressure in the intravascular space. When severe, the outcome is congestive heart failure and generalized fetal edema, a condition referred to as hydrops fetalis, which carries a very grave prognosis. Without therapeutic intervention via red blood cell transfusion into the umbilical cord, intrauterine demise soon follows.

## Clinical Management of Rh-D Sensitized Mothers

To identify sensitized women, an alloantibody screen is performed at the first prenatal visit. If an antibody to an erythrocyte antigen is identified, the titer is determined. The critical anti-RhD titer, defined as the titer associated with risk for fetal hydrops, is usually 1:8 to 1:32. For all sensitized women, the paternal erythrocyte phenotype is determined. If the father is homozygous RhD-negative, then no follow-up studies are required. If he is D-positive, then zygosity is determined. Although this has historically been estimated from Rh antigen phenotypes (D, C/c, E/e) in conjunction with gene frequency tables based on race, DNA testing for RhD zygosity is more reliable. If the father is homozygous, then all of his offspring can be assumed to be RhD positive, negating the need for fetal RhD testing. Fetal RhD genotyping from cultured amniocytes is required if the father is heterozygous or is not available for testing. To guard against a false-negative caused by a paternal RhD gene rearrangement (occurring in about 1.5% of the White population), the father can also be genotyped. A frequent occurrence in those of African ancestry is an RhD pseudogene; the patient is RhD-negative by serology, but RhD-positive on genotype. If the fetus is RhD-genotype-positive, the mother (who is RhD-negative serologically) should be tested for RhD genotype. In the United States, as well as other parts of the world, fetal Rh genotyping using cell-free DNA that circulates in maternal blood is now available.

For sensitized mothers with an at-risk fetus, serial titers are performed on maternal serum every month until 24 weeks' gestation, and then every 2 weeks thereafter. If a critical titer anti-D is detected, ultrasound Doppler measurements are used to determine the peak velocity of blood flow in the fetal middle cerebral artery. Higher velocity is a strong indicator of fetal anemia. Historically, amniocentesis was performed every 10–14 days to assess the bilirubin concentration in amniotic fluid. Therapy for fetal anemia involves intrauterine percutaneous umbilical cord red blood cell transfusion. If fetal hydrops develops later in gestation (weeks ≥35) or multiple transfusions have been required over the course of pregnancy, delivery timing is decided to balance the risks of continued intrauterine development versus the risk for prematurity.

## Preterm Delivery

The leading cause of neonatal morbidity and mortality in the United States is **preterm delivery**, defined as delivery before 37 weeks' gestation. Rupture of the fetal membranes prior to the onset of uterine contractions is known as **premature rupture of membranes (PROM)**. When PROM occurs at <37 completed weeks' gestation, it is referred to as *preterm PROM* and is responsible for nearly one-third of preterm deliveries.

Infants born before 37 weeks' gestation are usually of low birth weight (<2500 g) and are vulnerable to numerous complications, including: (1) infection, (2) necrotizing enterocolitis, and (3) intraventricular hemorrhage, and often develop (4) **respiratory distress syndrome (RDS)**. The cause of preterm labor is unknown, but it is likely that many factors are involved.

## Premature Rupture of Membranes

Preterm PROM (PPROM) is a complication in 3% of pregnancies. Risk factors for PPROM include: (1) a history of PPROM, (2) genital tract infection, (3) antepartum bleeding, and (4) smoking. Most women who experience PPROM will deliver their infants within 1 week. Management of PPROM varies according to the gestational age of the fetus and the presence or absence of maternal/fetal infection.

The diagnosis of PROM is often difficult, and the commonly used tests to detect it lack clinical sensitivity and specificity. These include: (1) direct observation of fluid leaking from the cervix or pooling in the posterior fornix of the vagina; (2) ultrasound for the detection of oligohydramnios; (3) nitrazine (pH) and (4) fern tests; and (5) detection of placental alpha microglobulin-1 protein.

## Respiratory Distress Syndrome

Respiratory distress syndrome (RDS), also called *hyaline membrane disease*, is the most common critical problem encountered in clinical management of preterm newborns. The worldwide incidence of RDS is 1% of live births and 10%–15% of live preterm births (<37 weeks or <2500 g). The risk of RDS is affected strongly by the gestational age at the time of birth, with a likelihood of <5% at 37 weeks, 20% at 34 weeks, and 60% at 29 weeks. In 2019, RDS was the eighth leading cause of death in infants in the United States. Affected infants require supplemental oxygen and mechanical ventilation to remain properly oxygenated. The disorder is caused by a deficiency of pulmonary surfactant. In normal lungs, surfactant coats the alveolar epithelium and responds to alveolar volume changes by reducing the surface tension in the alveolar wall during expiration. When the quantity of surfactant is deficient, many of the alveoli collapse on expiration and thereby overinflate the remaining airways. The lungs become progressively noncompliant (stiff), and blood flowing through the capillary beds of collapsed alveoli fails to oxygenate. Infants at risk for developing RDS are treated with intratracheal administration of exogenous surfactant immediately at birth.

---

### POINTS TO REMEMBER

**Complications of Pregnancy**
- When a fertilized egg implants in a location other than the body of the uterus, the condition is called an *ectopic pregnancy*.
- Preeclampsia is characterized by hypertension, proteinuria, and often edema. Eclampsia is characterized by the development of seizures in conjunction with preeclampsia.
- The diagnosis of PROM is often difficult, and the commonly used tests to detect it lack clinical sensitivity and specificity.
- Respiratory distress syndrome in a neonate is most commonly caused by a deficiency of pulmonary surfactant due to prematurity, which results in collapse of the alveoli.

**Differential Diagnosis of Liver Disease**
- Acute fatty liver is suggested in a patient with nausea and vomiting in the presence of jaundice, hypoglycemia, and encephalopathy with a small or normal-sized liver.
- Preeclampsia and the HELLP syndrome are characterized by an enlarged liver, lower ALT concentrations than in liver disease, mildly increased or normal bilirubin, normal glucose, and hypertension.
- Liver biopsy may differentiate non-pregnancy-related causes of liver disease. Biopsy is not necessary to differentiate acute fatty liver from preeclampsia or HELLP syndrome because the treatment is the same for all of these conditions—delivery of the infant.

**Hemolytic Disease of the Newborn**
- HDN is a fetal hemolytic disorder caused by maternal antibodies directed against antigen on fetal erythrocytes.
- Maternal sensitization may occur in response to blood transfusion or exposure of the mother to fetal RBCs carrying antigen that the mother lacks.
- An alloantibody screen is performed to identify sensitized mothers. In positive women, a titer is determined to monitor risk for fetal hydrops.
- Fetal RhD genotyping using cultured amniocytes or circulating cell-free DNA may be required in a sensitized mother if the father is heterozygous or is not available for testing.
- Noninvasive ultrasonographic determination of middle fetal cerebral artery velocity is useful to assess disease severity.

## PRENATAL SCREENING FOR FETAL DEFECTS

Prenatal screening is the process of identifying pregnancies at sufficiently high risk of a serious birth defect such as an open NTD or **Down syndrome**. The risk for Down syndrome, calculated using screening tests, is more accurate than the use of maternal age alone, and women of all ages should be offered screening. In addition to prenatal screening tests for maternal serum analytes, detection of cell-free DNA (cfDNA) in maternal blood has been implemented as a noninvasive screen for common fetal aneuploidies. Prenatal screening of cfDNA is highly sensitive and specific for Down syndrome in both high-risk and routine pregnancies. (The reader is referred to Chapters 59 and 72 of the *Tietz Textbook of Laboratory Medicine*, 7th edition, for a more detailed discussion of this technique and its applications.) However, cfDNA testing does not assess risk of NTDs.

## Terminology and Method of Risk Calculation in Prenatal Screening
### Multiple of the Median

Understanding prenatal screening requires an understanding of the multiple of the median (MoM), the statistic used to normalize analyte values. The initial step in calculating a MoM is to develop a set of median values for each week (or day) of gestation, using the laboratory's own assay values measured on the population to be screened. Fig. 44.2 graphically illustrates typical median values for the second-trimester markers used in prenatal screening. Individual test results are then expressed as a MoM by dividing each individual test result by the median for the relevant gestational age. The MoM is universally used as a common factor for converting analyte values into an interpretative unit and serves as the starting point for calculating screening results for NTDs, Down syndrome, and trisomy 18.

## Calculating Individualized Patient-Specific Risks Using Multiple Biochemical Measurements

Measurements of each analyte are made on a serum sample, and the results in mass units are converted to MoM for the appropriate week of gestation. This MoM value is then adjusted for other variables, such as maternal weight and race. The individualized risk (patient-specific risk) for any given condition is determined by multiplying the *a priori* risk for that condition by a likelihood ratio that is calculated using the woman's MoM values, as shown in the following equation:

Patient risk = *a priori* risk × Likelihood ratio

The *a priori* risk is obtained from large epidemiological studies that ascertain the prevalence for the condition under consideration. For example, a woman's age is used to define her *a priori* risk for having a fetus with Down syndrome. The likelihood ratio is determined by calculating the ratio of the heights of the affected and unaffected overlapping population distributions for any specified MoM value. When multiple tests are used, a single likelihood ratio is calculated using the overlapping distributions for each test but with the

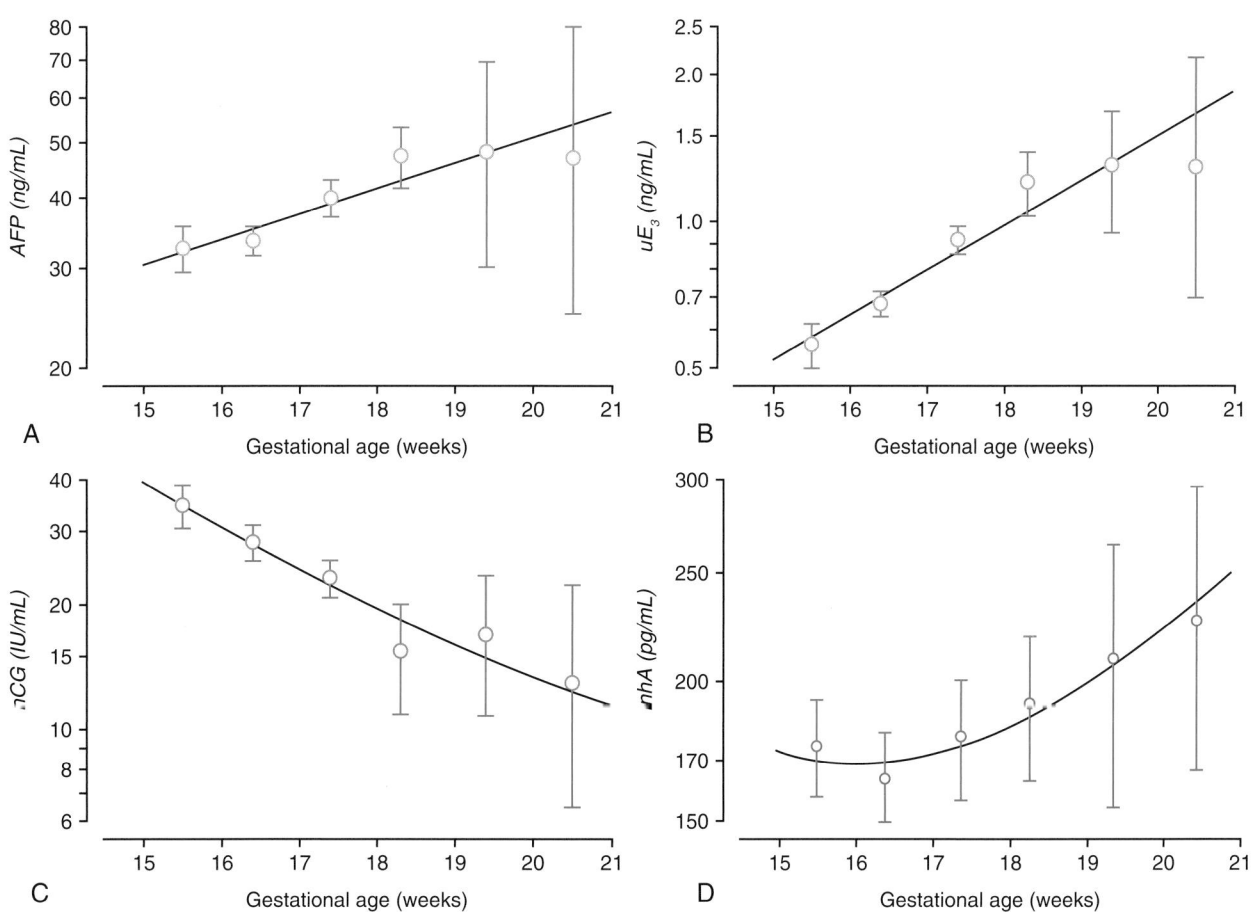

Fig. 44.2 Typical median values for maternal serum alpha-fetoprotein (*AFP*). (A) Unconjugated estriol (*uE3*); (B) human chorionic gonadotropin (*hCG*) (C); and inhibin A (inhA) (D) in the second trimester. The observed average gestational age is plotted on the horizontal axis, and the median of that week's marker measurements is plotted on the vertical axis. The thin vertical lines represent the 95% confidence interval of the medians.

correlation between tests taken into account. This final calculated risk, rather than the analyte concentrations themselves, is the screening variable upon which clinical decisions are made.

# PRENATAL SCREENING TESTS

Maternal serum screening for NTDs began in the 1970s using second trimester serum specimens. Since then, maternal serum screening has expanded to include partial detection of Down syndrome and trisomy 18, among others.

## Neural Tube Defects

NTDs are serious abnormalities that occur early in embryonic development. By 19 days after fertilization, the area that is to form the central nervous system (brain and spinal cord) has differentiated into a plate of cells. The flat plate then rolls up, and its edges fuse into a hollow neural tube that drops into the embryo to develop just underneath what will become the skin of the back. Neural tube formation is normally complete 4 weeks after fertilization. Failure of neural tube fusion leads to permanent developmental defects of the brain, spinal cord, or both. These defects include *anencephaly, meningomyelocele* (which is commonly called **spina bifida**), and *encephalocele*. Although there are many heterogeneous causes, about 90% fall into the classification of multifactorial inheritance. Folic acid deficiency is clearly associated with increased frequency of neural tube closure defects.

The birth prevalence of open NTDs varies with factors such as geographic location (higher in the Eastern United States, lower in the West), race (lower in African Americans), ethnicity (higher in Scotch-Irish), family history (higher with prior births of affected individuals), and maternal weight (higher in obese women). An average figure for the United States is 1 open NTD per 1000 pregnancies. Almost all cases of anencephaly and about 95% of meningomyeloceles are open, with no overlying skin, and therefore are in direct communication with the amniotic fluid. Thus, the concentrations of fetal serum proteins normally present in amniotic fluid are increased in pregnancies affected by open NTDs.

### Prenatal Screening

AFP concentrations are increased in amniotic fluid and serum (in the second trimester) of mothers carrying fetuses affected with an open NTD (e.g., anencephaly, open spina bifida). Maternal serum AFP testing thus provides a screening method to identify pregnancies at high risk or to estimate the numerical risk of having a fetus with an open NTD. Because concentrations in serum in affected and unaffected pregnancies overlap considerably, maternal serum AFP is useful as an initial screening test to identify women at high risk for having an affected fetus (Fig. 44.3). These women are then referred for diagnostic procedures. High resolution ultrasound is almost always diagnostic but if inconclusive, amniocentesis for measurement of AFP and acetylcholinesterase in amniotic fluid may be required to determine if the fetus has an open NTD.

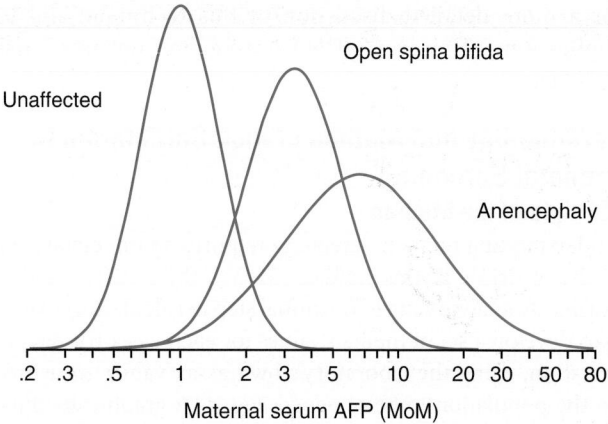

**Fig. 44.3** Distribution of maternal serum alpha-fetoprotein (*AFP*) measurements in unaffected pregnancies and in pregnancies affected with open spina bifida or anencephaly. *MoM,* Multiple of the median.

## Down Syndrome

Down syndrome is the most common serious disorder of the autosomal chromosomes in liveborn infants, occurring in 1 in 700 live births. An extra copy of chromosome 21 results in a phenotype consisting of moderate to severe intellectual and developmental disabilities, hypotonia, congenital heart defects, and flat facial profile. Most often, an affected child has three copies of chromosome 21 (i.e., trisomy 21), but 5% of cases are caused by translocations and 1% of cases are mosaics. A woman's risk increases slowly up to age 30 and then steadily increases between ages 30 and 45, to a plateau.

### Prenatal Screening

Maternal serum AFP concentrations are about 25% lower in Down syndrome than in unaffected pregnancies. The association of AFP and Down syndrome is independent of maternal age. The independence of maternal serum AFP measurements and maternal age established that it was possible to offer a screening method to younger women, in whom most cases of Down syndrome occur.

Unconjugated estriol (uE3), a product of the fetoplacental unit, is also about 25% lower in pregnancies with Down syndrome. In contrast, concentrations of hCG and inhibin A are about twice as high. A screening method that combines maternal age with measurements of these four analytes permits determination of a single Down syndrome risk estimate. This "quadruple test" provides approximately 80% detection at a 5% false-positive rate. Table 44.3 illustrates general patterns of first- and second-trimester analytes associated with various disorders.

## Trisomy 18

**Trisomy 18 (Edwards syndrome)** is caused by a nondisjunction event during meiosis that results in a fetus having an extra copy of chromosome 18. Although it occurs in only 1 in 8000 births, it is probably the most common chromosome defect at the time of conception. The dramatic change in prevalence is due to the very high fetal loss rate both before 8 weeks (>80%) and during the second and third trimesters

## TABLE 44.3  Conditions Associated with Various Maternal Serum Screening Result Patterns

| Condition | SECOND TRIMESTER | | | | FIRST TRIMESTER | | |
|---|---|---|---|---|---|---|---|
| | AFP | hCG | uE3 | inhA | PAPP-A | hCG | NT |
| Amniocentesis | Normal to high | — | — | — | — | — | — |
| Anencephaly | Very high | — | Very low | — | — | — | — |
| Congenital nephrosis, duodenal atresia, encephalocele, esophageal atresia, gastroschisis, hydrocephalus, Meckel syndrome, omphalocele, sacrococcygeal teratoma | High | — | — | — | — | — | — |
| Cystic hygroma | High | — | — | — | — | — | Increased |
| Down syndrome | Low | High | Low | High | Low | High | Increased |
| Fetal blood contamination | High to very high | Unchanged | Unchanged | Unchanged | — | — | — |
| Molar pregnancy | Very low | Very high | Very low | Normal | — | — | — |
| Molar pregnancy (partial) | Low to normal | Very high | Low to normal | Normal | — | — | — |
| Myelomeningocele (open spina bifida) | High | — | — | — | — | — | — |
| Normal pregnancy | Low, normal, or high | Low, normal, or high | Low, normal, or high | Low, normal, or high | — | — | — |
| Overestimated gestational age | Low | High | Low | Normal | — | — | — |
| Preeclampsia | Normal to high | High | — | — | — | — | — |
| Pseudocyesis (imaginary pregnancy) | Undetectable | Undetectable | Undetectable | Undetectable | — | — | — |
| Smith–Lemli–Opitz syndrome | Low | Low | Very low | — | — | — | — |
| Spontaneous or impending pregnancy loss | Variable | Low or high | Low | Low or high | — | — | — |
| Steroid sulfatase deficiency (fetal) | Unchanged | Unchanged | Very low | Unchanged | — | — | — |
| Triploidy (paternal) | Variable | High | Low | High | Variable | Very high | — |
| Triploidy (maternal) | Variable | Low | Low | Low | Variable | Very low | — |
| Trisomy 13 | Variable | Variable | Variable | Variable | Very low | Low | Increased |
| Trisomy 18 | Low | Low | Very low | Normal | Very low | Very low | Increased |
| Turner syndrome without hydrops | Low | Low | Very low | Low | Variable | Variable | Increased |
| Turner syndrome with hydrops | Low | High | Very low | High | Variable | Variable | Increased |
| Twins and other multiple gestations | High | High | High | High | High | High | — |
| Underestimated gestational age | High | Low | High | Normal | — | — | — |

*AFP*, α-Fetoprotein; *hCG*, human chorionic gonadotropin; *inhA*, inhibin A; *NT*, nuchal translucency; *PAPP-A*, pregnancy-associated plasma protein A; *uE3*, unconjugated estriol.

(≈70%). Following birth, half of the infants die within the first 5 days, and 90% die within 100 days.

## Prenatal Screening

Prenatal screening studies have found that fetal trisomy 18 has a distinctive quad screen pattern that is different from the Down syndrome pattern (see Table 44.3). In trisomy 18 pregnancies, the AFP, uE3, and hCG concentrations are low, while inhibin A is normal. A method for trisomy 18 risk calculation is available and is often included in prenatal screening programs.

## Other Aneuploidies

Although chromosome disorders other than trisomies 21 and 18 are not part of routine screening, the marker patterns exhibited in maternal serum for some aneuploidies are similar. In particular, hydropic Turner syndrome and triploidy of paternal origin have serum marker patterns resembling that of Down syndrome pregnancy and are sometimes identified as high risk using this algorithm. Similarly, Turner syndrome without hydrops and triploidy of maternal origin are sometimes identified by the trisomy 18 risk algorithm. The pattern for trisomy 13 is variable (see Table 44.3).

## Other Screening Algorithms

Following extensive use of screening tests in the second trimester, other tests have been introduced that use serum collected in the first trimester.

## First Trimester Combined Test

For patients seeking early diagnosis, screening for Down syndrome in the first trimester (10–13 weeks' gestation) is available. First trimester screening involves measurement of maternal serum **pregnancy-associated plasma protein-A (PAPP-A)** concentration, which is relatively low in Down syndrome pregnancy, and hCG (free beta subunit or total) concentration, which is relatively high in Down syndrome. A third marker used to improve first trimester screening performance is ultrasound measurement of **nuchal translucency (NT)**, the subcutaneous space between the skin and cervical spine, which is increased in fetuses with Down syndrome. A combination of NT and serum tests (the combined test) was comparable or slightly better than the second-trimester quadruple test for Down syndrome screening, detecting 85% of cases at a 5% false-positive rate.

The pattern of markers in trisomy 18 affected pregnancies consists of an increased NT measurement and reduced PAPP-A and hCG in the first trimester. Estimates for the performance of first trimester combined testing in the detection of trisomy 18 are varied, but detection rates have been suggested to be about 80% for a 0.3% false-positive rate.

## Adding First and Second Trimester Markers into a Single Integrated Screening Test

The integrated test takes advantage of first- and second-trimester markers and avoids most of the limitations of standalone first-trimester screening (Fig. 44.4). With this approach, measurements of NT and PAPP-A are made in the first trimester but are not interpreted or acted upon until testing in the second trimester is complete. In the second trimester, a quadruple test is performed on maternal serum. Results from all six tests (NT, PAPP-A, AFP, uE3, hCG, and inhibin A) are then combined into a single risk estimate. This approach detects 85% of Down syndrome cases with only a 1% false-positive rate.

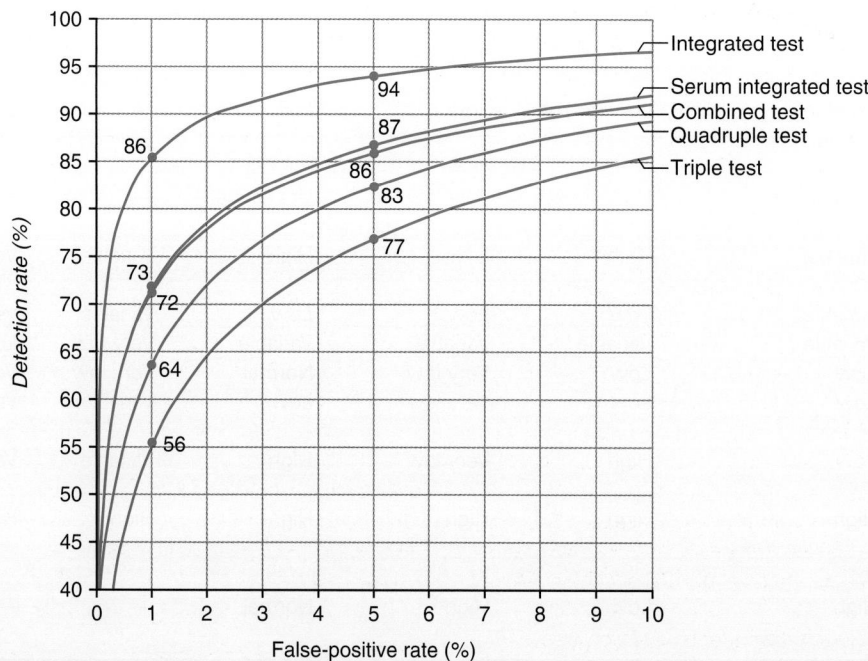

**Fig. 44.4** Receiver operating characteristic curves for tests used to screen for Down syndrome. (Reprinted with permission from Wald NJ, Rodeck C, Hackshaw AK, Rudnicka A. SURUSS in perspective. *Semin Perinatol.* 2005;29:225–235.)

The integrated screening approach can be offered effectively and at a lower cost by using a modified test based only on the serum markers (serum integrated). Maternal serum PAPP-A concentrations are measured at 10–13 weeks and combined with a second trimester quad test for a five-marker screening panel. The serum integrated test gives an 85% detection of Down syndrome cases with about a 3% false-positive rate. A summary of detection and false-positive rates for second-trimester and integrated screening tests is illustrated in Fig. 44.4.

Hybrid screening approaches that combine traditional serum screening in the first trimester with reflex to diagnostic testing or cfDNA, such as the sequential and contingent models have also been proposed.

### Adjustments for Factors That Influence Analyte Measurements

Prenatal screening for both open NTDs and Down syndrome is optimized when each woman's analyte concentration is compared with those of other women (the reference group) who are "similar" to her in many respects. In addition to gestational age, this "similarity" extends to other factors that have been shown to affect analyte concentrations, including: (1) maternal weight, (2) race, (3) insulin-dependent diabetes (IDD), and (4) multiple pregnancy. Taking these factors into account increases the accuracy of the interpretation.

### Pregnancies Achieved by Assisted Reproductive Technologies

The use of assisted reproductive technologies (ART), such as in vitro fertilization (IVF), for conception is increasing. Women who achieve pregnancy by IVF are about twice as likely to have a positive result after second-trimester Down syndrome screening as are women who achieve pregnancy spontaneously. Thus, MoM values of certain analytes are adjusted to restore an appropriate screen positive rate. In particular, concentrations of uE3 tend to be reduced, while hCG and inhibin A are increased in pregnancies achieved by IVF. Pregnancies achieved by intrauterine insemination, with or without ovulation induction, show a similar trend in marker concentrations.

---

### POINTS TO REMEMBER

**Prenatal Screening**
- Screening of maternal serum for AFP, hCG, uE3, PAPP-A, and inhibin A, together with nuchal translucency measurement is useful to identify women with increased risk for having a fetus with anomalies such as a neural tube defect, Down syndrome, or trisomy 18.
- Down syndrome is associated with increased nuchal thickness, decreased concentrations of PAPP-A, AFP, and uE3, and increased concentrations of hCG and inhibin-A in maternal serum.
- Increased risk for neural tube defects is associated with increased maternal serum AFP.
- Trisomy 18 is associated with decreased concentrations of maternal serum AFP, estriol, uE3, and hCG.

---

## ANALYTICAL METHODOLOGY

In this section of the chapter, methods for measurement of: (1) hCG, (2) AFP, (3) uE3, (4) inhibin A, (5) PAPP-A, and (6) tests for FLM are reviewed.

### Human Chorionic Gonadotropin

Measurement of hCG is used to: (1) detect pregnancy and its abnormalities (e.g., ectopic and molar pregnancies), (2) screen for Down syndrome and trisomy 18, and (3) monitor the course of a patient with a hCG-producing cancer. Because of these diverse applications, many assays are used to measure hCG, including qualitative urine and serum devices and quantitative serum assays.

### Biochemistry

hCG is a glycoprotein containing a protein core with branched carbohydrate side chains that usually terminate with sialic acid. The hormone is a heterodimer composed of two nonidentical, noncovalently bound glycoprotein subunits—alpha (α) and beta (β). When the hCG dimer is dissociated, the hormone activity is lost. However, a major part of the original activity is restored by equimolar recombination of the two subunits.

hCG is synthesized in the placenta. A single gene located on chromosome 6 encodes the α subunit of all four glycoprotein hormones (TSH, LH, FSH, and hCG). Chromosome 19 contains a family of seven genes that encode the hCGβ subunit, though only three appear to be active. Separate messenger RNAs are transcribed from the respective genes, and the α and β subunits are translated from each. The subunits spontaneously combine in the rough endoplasmic reticulum and are then continuously secreted into the maternal circulation.

In the first weeks of pregnancy, hCG stimulates the corpus luteum in the ovary to make progesterone, a steroid that prevents menses and thus facilitates pregnancy. hCG binds weakly to TSH receptors in the maternal thyroid, and extremely increased hCG concentrations have the potential to be thyrotropic.

### Methods

*Qualitative human chorionic gonadotropin tests.* Numerous tests for the qualitative detection of hCG in urine or serum are available as over-the-counter (home) or point-of-care (POC) devices, and their use for the rapid identification of pregnancy is well established. POC devices are single-use tests that utilize immunochromatography for the rapid qualitative detection of hCG when its concentration exceeds a detection threshold, frequently 10–25 IU/L. First-morning specimens are preferred for qualitative urine pregnancy tests because they are concentrated and contain abundant hCG.

*Quantitative human chorionic gonadotropin tests.* Commonly used quantitative hCG tests are high-performance immunometric assays designed to measure hCG over a wide range of concentrations. Upper limits of detection vary from 400–15,000 IU/L. Thus, specimen dilution is frequently required to obtain an absolute measurement. The lowest detectable concentration of these assays is from 1 to 2 IU/L.

The measurement of hCG is complicated by its molecular heterogeneity, and considerable variation in measured hCG concentrations is observed between the different assays. Because of variation between hCG assays, median hCG values calculated for maternal serum screening are not transferable and should be considered method-specific.

## Alpha Fetoprotein

Measurement of AFP in maternal serum and amniotic fluid is used extensively for prenatal detection of some serious fetal anomalies. Maternal serum AFP is increased in 85%–95% of cases of fetal open NTD and is decreased in about 30% of cases of fetal Down syndrome. Additionally, AFP measurements are used in non-pregnant patients for monitoring certain cancers.

### Chemistry

AFP is a glycoprotein encoded by a gene located within q11-22 on chromosome 4 that is part of a family of genes that also includes albumin and vitamin D-binding protein. The protein is composed of carbohydrate and a single polypeptide chain containing 591 amino acids. The carbohydrate composition varies depending on the organ of synthesis, the length of gestation, and source of the specimen (maternal serum vs amniotic fluid).

### Biochemistry

AFP is produced initially by the fetal yolk sac in small quantities and then by the fetal liver in larger quantities as the yolk sac degenerates. Trace amounts are also produced in the fetal gut and kidneys. Maximal concentration in the fetal serum ($\approx$3 million $\mu$g/L) is reached at about 9 weeks' gestation. The concentration then declines steadily to about 20,000 $\mu$g/L at term. The increase and decrease in concentration of AFP in the amniotic fluid roughly parallel those in the fetal serum but the concentration is two to three orders of magnitude lower ($\approx$15,000 $\mu$g/L at 16 weeks' gestation). Amniotic fluid AFP has been measured as early as 8 weeks. It rapidly decreases to a low point at 11 weeks and then increases to reach a second maximum at 13 weeks. The concentration then falls in a log-linear fashion until 25 weeks, when the decline steepens.

AFP is first detectable ($\approx$5 $\mu$g/L) in maternal serum at about the 10th week of gestation. The concentration increases about 15% per week to a peak of approximately 180 $\mu$g/L around 25 weeks. The concentration in maternal serum then subsequently declines slowly until term. After birth, the maternal serum AFP rapidly decreases to <2 $\mu$g/L. In an infant, serum AFP declines exponentially to reach adult concentrations by the 10th month of life.

### Methods

Although AFP was traditionally measured by radioimmunoassay (RIA), newer methods use immunoenzymometric assay (IEMA) or chemiluminescent immunoassay (CIA) because of their (1) lower detection limits, (2) increased precision, (3) speed, (4) avoidance of radioactivity, and (5) ease of automation.

Amniotic fluid AFP is measured using the same immunoassays as for maternal serum AFP after a suitable dilution (usually 1:50 to 1:200). AFP in amniotic fluid is less stable than in serum, and leaving samples at room temperature for prolonged periods results in degradation of amniotic fluid AFP. The presence of fetal blood in amniotic fluid samples has been known to increase AFP results, and laboratories should note the presence of blood on the report. In the event of an increased amniotic fluid AFP result (usually >2.0 or 2.5 MoM), the laboratory should test for the presence of fetal blood.

Measurement of acetylcholinesterase (AChE) is a confirmatory test for samples with increased amniotic fluid AFP. Cerebrospinal fluid contains high concentrations of the neural enzyme AChE, and in cases of fetal open NTDs, fluid leaks from the open lesion and allows AChE to enter the amniotic fluid.

## Unconjugated Estriol

Any disruption in the biosynthetic pathway will lead to very low maternal serum uE3. Conditions that cause disruption include: (1) fetal anencephaly, (2) placental sulfatase deficiency, (3) fetal death, (4) chromosome abnormalities, (5) molar pregnancy, and (6) Smith–Lemli–Opitz syndrome (SLOS). SLOS is a serious, rare birth defect that is the result of an inborn error in cholesterol metabolism, 7-dehydrosterol-7-reductase deficiency. Down syndrome leads to a modest decrease in uE3. This steroid, rather than total estriol (unconjugated plus conjugated estriol), is the most specific of the estrogens for identifying a fetus with Trisomy 21.

### Chemistry

Estriol is an estrogen with hydroxyl groups at positions 3, 16, and 17. Although present in non-pregnant patients in very low concentrations, during late pregnancy this estrogen predominates. Only a minor amount ($\approx$10%) of the hormone circulates in plasma unconjugated, and this form is strongly bound to sex hormone binding globulin (SHBG) because of its low solubility. The majority exist as conjugates of glucuronate and sulfate. Conjugation, which occurs in the maternal liver, makes the hormone more soluble and permits renal clearance.

### Biochemistry

Estriol is produced in very large amounts during the last trimester of pregnancy. The biosynthetic pathway requires three organs to be fully functioning: fetal adrenal, fetal liver, and placenta. The fetal adrenal avidly binds low-density lipoprotein to take in cholesterol, which is converted to two major steroid intermediates: pregnenolone sulfate and dehydroepiandrosterone sulfate (DHEA-S). These intermediates are secreted into the fetal circulation. The fetal liver, possessing 16$\alpha$-hydroxylase, converts DHEA-S to 16$\alpha$-hydroxy-DHEA-S, which is secreted back into the fetal circulation. Finally, the placenta synthesizes estriol from 16$\alpha$-hydroxy-DHEA-S. Approximately 90% of maternal serum estriol is derived from this fetal-placental pathway. A minor amount is made using precursors from the maternal ovary.

## Methods

The determination of uE3 is made difficult by its low concentration and values obtained with various uE3 assays vary widely. Conversion to MoM reduces the between-method differences, but uE3 is still the most variable of the screening analytes.

Of the four analytes currently used for screening, uE3 is the least stable, and consequently requirements for collection, storage, and shipment are dictated by this analyte. The uE3 concentration increases in blood at room temperature and at 4°C because the conjugated forms are able to spontaneously deconjugate to form the parent hormone. Therefore, collected blood should be allowed to clot, and serum should be removed promptly. uE3 is stable in serum for up to 7 days at 2°C–4°C. The concentration of uE3 increases when sera has been stored for longer than 4 days at room temperature.

## Inhibin A

Inhibins are members of the transforming growth factor-β (TGFβ) superfamily of proteins. Inhibin is a negative feedback regulator of FSH secretion in both males and females. The placenta produces large quantities of inhibin A that completely suppress FSH. In addition to the usefulness of inhibin A as a predictor of Down syndrome risk, inhibin A and B measurements have found additional applications as tumor markers for ovarian cancer and in the evaluation of male infertility.

### Chemistry

Inhibins are proteins consisting of dimers of dissimilar subunits (α and β) linked by disulfide bridges. The mature form of inhibin is produced by cleavage of larger precursor forms. In follicular fluid and serum, mature inhibins, precursors of inhibins, and intermediate molecules of varying molecular weight are present. Another group of related molecules, the activins, are dimers consisting of just the β-subunits. Inhibin A is the only form within the inhibin/activin family of proteins that provides sufficient discrimination to be useful for use in Down syndrome screening.

### Biochemistry

In the reproductive system, inhibin and activin subunits are expressed in the placenta, as well as in the granulosa cells of the ovary and by the Sertoli cells of the testis. Inhibin A and inhibin B have distinctive serum profiles during the human menstrual cycle. Inhibin A rises in the follicular phase and peaks at ovulation, before decreasing to basal amounts in the luteal phase. In postmenopausal women, the concentrations of both forms of inhibin are nondetectable.

Inhibin A is produced by the fetoplacental unit beginning in early pregnancy. Inhibin A concentrations exhibit a complex pattern during the course of pregnancy, rising to a peak at 8–10 weeks' gestation, declining to a minimum at 17 weeks of pregnancy, and then resuming to slowly increase at term. Unlike the other screening tests, average inhibin concentrations change relatively little from 15 to 20 weeks' gestation.

## Methods

Inhibin assays used for Down syndrome screening must measure only dimeric inhibin A and not the free α subunits and the precursors of higher molecular weight, which also circulate in blood. Highly specific assays using monoclonal antibodies are available that measure only dimeric inhibin A. Specific inhibin A assays provide better screening performance than the nonspecific total inhibin assays.

## Pregnancy-Associated Plasma Protein A

PAPP-A concentrations in the maternal serum during the first trimester of pregnancy are associated with fetal and placental health and development. Low PAPP-A concentrations early in pregnancy have been associated with: (1) Down syndrome, (2) a high rate of fetal loss, (3) poor fetal growth (intrauterine growth restriction [IUGR]), (4) premature delivery, (5) hypertension, and (6) preeclampsia.

### Biochemistry

PAPP-A is a zinc-containing metalloproteinase glycoprotein. It is expressed at low concentrations in all tissues, but high amounts of PAPP-A protein and mRNA are localized in placental tissues throughout gestation. Circulating PAPP-A is part of a larger molecular complex that includes two subunits of PAPP-A covalently bound to two subunits of pro major basic protein (pro MBP), forming a heterotetramer. PAPP-A immunoreactivity is found in syncytiotrophoblast cells.

Maternal serum PAPP-A concentrations increase as gestation proceeds to term (Fig. 44.5). Concentrations of PAPP-A are critical to normal fetal growth because of its role as an insulin-like growth factor binding protein (IGFBP) protease. PAPP-A regulates the action of insulin-like growth factor II (IGF-II) by cleaving its binding protein, primarily IGFBP-4, thereby increasing bioavailable forms.

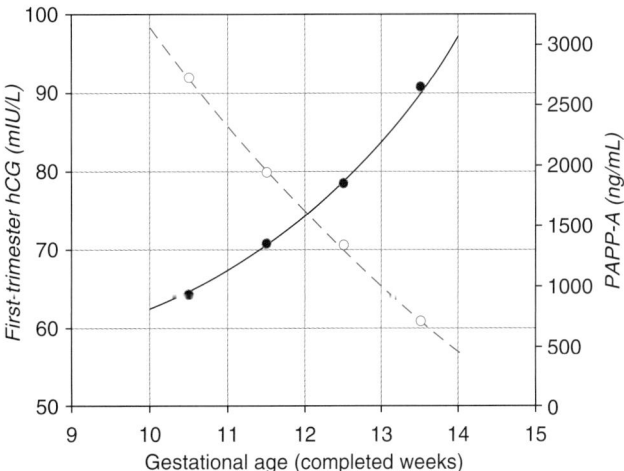

Fig. 44.5 Typical median values for maternal serum pregnancy-associated plasma protein-A (*PAPP-A*) and total human chorionic gonadotropin (*hCG*) in the first trimester. The observed average gestational age is plotted on the horizontal axis and the median of that week's PAPP-A (*black solid line*) or total hCG (*blue dashed line*) measurements on the vertical logarithmic axis.

## Methods

PAPP-A immunoassays are available on routine clinical chemistry platforms. There are significant between-method differences, and efforts to achieve standardization are currently underway. A small increase in PAPP-A concentrations has been reported for collection in plastic versus glass tubes. First-trimester serum PAPP-A concentrations are stable in serum at 4°C for 1 week or longer, depending on the assay used for testing.

## Fetal Fibronectin

Determining the risk of preterm delivery would help clinicians manage those at high risk more aggressively, thereby lowering the incidence of adverse maternal and fetal outcomes. Fetal fibronectin (fFN) concentration in cervical and vaginal secretions was proposed as a test to aid in predicting preterm delivery. Patients with a negative test result have a ≈1% chance of delivering in 1 week but this does not substantially impact clinical decision making as the number of symptomatic women who deliver within 1 week is consistently less than 5%. As a negative result does not substantially increase the negative predictive value and the positive predictive value is low, fFN is of limited utility in predicting preterm birth within 7 days of sample collection.

## Placental Alpha Microglobulin-1

Placental alpha microglobulin-1 (PAMG-1) is a placental glycoprotein. During pregnancy, PAMG-1 is secreted into the amniotic fluid, where it is present at a high concentration (2000–25,000 ng/mL) relative to that of maternal blood (5–25 ng/mL) or cervicovaginal fluid with intact membranes (0.05–2 ng/mL). A test for PAMG-1 that exploits these large differences in concentrations has been developed for clinical use as an aid for the detection of PROM and preterm delivery.

A rapid immunochromatographic method is commercially available for the rapid detection of PAMG-1 in cervicovaginal fluid. The specimen is collected using a polyester swab, and the fluid is eluted off the swab by rinsing it in a vial containing a buffer solution. A test strip is then placed into the buffer for 10 minutes. The test result is determined by visual inspection of a test and a control line on the lateral flow device. The analytical limit of detection of the test is 5 ng/mL.

This test is more sensitive and specific for the detection PROM than clinical assessment or the nitrazine or ferning tests. Contamination with large amounts of blood will cause a false-positive result. False-negative results may occur if the specimen is collected 12 or more hours after a rupture that is subsequently obstructed by the fetus or is resealed.

## Fetal Lung Maturity

FLM tests help assess the risk of a fetus developing RDS. Despite performing well, the number of FLM tests performed each year in the United States has declined, and several studies have demonstrated that FLM testing does not improve fetal morbidity or mortality.

## Fetal Lung Maturity Assessment

Interested readers are referred to previous editions of this textbook for a detailed discussion of FLM testing methodology.

## REVIEW QUESTIONS

1. The most severe form of hemolytic disease of the newborn (HDN) is referred to as:
   a. respiratory distress syndrome (RDS).
   b. ectopic pregnancy.
   c. jaundice.
   d. erythroblastosis fetalis.
2. In a developing fetus, the major blood-forming organ until 24 weeks' gestation is the:
   a. bone marrow.
   b. liver.
   c. lung.
   d. kidney.
3. Preeclampsia is diagnosed by the presence of which findings?
   a. Hypertension and proteinuria ≥300 mg of protein in 24-hour urine
   b. Hypertension and proteinuria ≥100 mg of protein in 24-hour urine
   c. Hypertension and new onset of platelet count >100,000/μL
   d. Hypertension and decreased liver transaminases
4. Which of the following accurately describes thyroid function during pregnancy?
   a. Total T4 concentrations decrease with increasing gestational age
   b. TSH concentrations increase in the first trimester
   c. Free T4 concentrations decrease with increasing gestational age
   d. Maternal thyroid-stimulating antibodies do not cross the placenta
5. Hemolytic disease of the newborn (HDN) is caused by:
   a. lack of folic acid in the maternal diet.
   b. increased formation of fetal hemoglobin (Hb F).
   c. maternal antibodies against fetal erythrocytes.
   d. blockage of placental transfer of immunoglobulin A (IgA) antibodies.
6. What is the function of the hormone hCG (human chorionic gonadotropin) in pregnancy?
   a. It signals the corpus luteum to produce progesterone to maintain pregnancy.
   b. It inhibits the production of estrogen and progesterone by the ovary.
   c. It stimulates the production of estrogen to promote uterine growth.
   d. Its concentration peaks near birth, which helps initiate the birth process.

7. Which of the following best describes changes in concentrations of placental hormones during pregnancy?
   a. Estrogen peaks in the first trimester, and then remains stable throughout gestation.
   b. Estrogen concentration increases throughout gestation.
   c. hCG concentration is stable throughout gestation.
   d. Progesterone concentration declines throughout gestation.

8. Which of the following describes the full integrated screen?
   a. PAPP-A in the first trimester and hCG, AFP, and uE3 in the second trimester
   b. AFP, hCG, uE3, and inhibin A in the second trimester
   c. PAPP-A and nuchal translucency in the first trimester and AFP, hCG, uE3, and inhibin A in the second trimester
   d. hCG and nuchal translucency in the first trimester, AFP, and PAPP-A in the second trimester

9. The majority of waste produced by a fetus is in the amniotic fluid. Which one of the following structures is responsible for removal of this waste from the amniotic fluid?
   a. Fetal kidneys
   b. Fetal liver
   c. Fetal lungs
   d. Placenta

10. When a fertilized egg implants in a location other than the body of the uterus, the condition is called:
   a. Down syndrome.
   b. spina bifida.
   c. ectopic pregnancy.
   d. hyperemesis gravidarum.

## SUGGESTED READINGS

American College of Obstetricians and Gynecologists. ACOG Practice Bulletin no. 97: fetal lung maturity. *Obstet Gynecol.* 2008;112:717–726.

American College of Obstetricians and Gynecologists. ACOG Practice Bulletin 222. Gestational hypertension and preeclampsia. *Obstet Gynecol.* 2020;135:e237–e260.

American College of Obstetricians and Gynecologists. ACOG Practice Bulletin no. 226: Screening for fetal chromosomal abnormalities. *Obstet Gynecol.* 2020;136:e48–e69.

Chiu RWK, Lo YMD. Circulating nucleic acid for prenatal diagnostics. In: Rifai N, Horvath AR, Wittwer CT, eds. *Tietz Textbook of Clinical Chemistry and Molecular Diagnostics.* 6th ed. St. Louis: Elsevier; 2017:1655–1696.

Gala R. Ectopic pregnancy. In: Schorge JSJ, Halvorson L, Hoffman B, Bradshaw K, Cunningham F, eds. *Williams Gynecology.* 1st ed. New York: McGraw-Hill; 2008.

Grenache DG. Hemolytic disease of the newborn. In: Gronowski AM, ed. *Handbook of Clinical Laboratory Testing During Pregnancy.* Totowa, NJ: Humana Press; 2004:219–243.

Haddow JE, Palomaki GE, Knight GJ, et al. Prenatal screening for Down's syndrome with use of maternal serum markers. *N Engl J Med.* 1992;327:588–593.

Lockitch GM, ed. *Handbook of Diagnostic Biochemistry and Hematology in Normal Pregnancy.* Boca Raton, FL: CRC Press; 1993.

Malone FD, Canick JA, Ball RH, et al. First-trimester or second-trimester screening, or both, for Down's syndrome. *N Engl J Med.* 2005;353:2001–2011.

McChesney R, Wilcox AJ, O'Connor JF, et al. Intact hCG, free hCG beta subunit and hCG beta core fragment: longitudinal patterns in urine during early pregnancy. *Human Reprod.* 2005;20:928–935.

Norton ME, Jacobsson B, Swamy GK, et al. Cell-free DNA analysis for noninvasive examination of trisomy. *N Engl J Med.* 2015;372:1589–1597.

Palmer OM, Grenache DG, Gronowski AM. The NACB laboratory medicine practice guidelines for point-of-care reproductive testing. *Point of Care.* 2007;6:265–272.

Wald NJ, Huttly WJ, Hackshaw AK. Antenatal screening for Down's syndrome with the quadruple test. *Lancet.* 2003;361:835–836.

Workowski KA, Berman S, Centers for Disease Control and Prevention (CDC). Sexually transmitted diseases treatment guidelines, 2010. *MMWR Recommend Rep.* 2010;59:1–110.

Yarbrough ML, Grenache DG, Gronowski AM. Fetal lung maturity testing: the end of an era. *Biomark Med.* 2014;8:509–515.

Yarbrough ML, Stout M, Gronowski AM. Pregnancy and its disorders. In: Rifai N, Horvath AR, Wittwer CT, eds. *Tietz Textbook of Clinical Chemistry and Molecular Diagnostics.* 6th ed. St. Louis: Elsevier; 2017:1655–1696.

# 45

# Newborn Screening and Inborn Errors of Metabolism

*Marzia Pasquali and Nicola Longo*

## KEY WORDS AND DEFINITIONS

**Autosomal recessive inheritance** A mendelian inheritance pattern in which (1) nonsex chromosomes (autosomes) carry a DNA sequence (gene) for the inherited trait and (2) two abnormalities (one from each parent) in the DNA sequence must be present for the trait to appear in an individual; heterozygous parents have a 25% chance of having an affected offspring.

**Disorders of amino acid metabolism** A group of disorders of amino acid metabolism caused by defective activity of an enzyme leading to increased concentration of amino acids in blood (and urine).

**Disorders of carbohydrate metabolism** A group of disorders caused by loss of an enzyme in the metabolic pathway of a carbohydrate, leading to increased accumulation of that carbohydrate within organs and tissues.

**Disorders of fatty acid oxidation** A group of disorders caused by deficiency of an enzyme in the oxidation pathway of fatty acids, leading to inability to use fat as an energy source.

**Dried blood spot (DBS)** A form of biosampling where blood samples are blotted and dried on filter paper.

**Inborn error of metabolism (IEM)** Inherited disorder due to deficiency of an enzyme or transporter impairing the transformation of body chemicals.

**Lysosomal disorder** A disorder characterized by impaired degradation of complex macromolecules in the lysosomes leading to accumulation of these substrates in organs and tissues.

**Multiplex analysis** Simultaneous assessment of multiple analytes in a single sample.

**Organic acidemia** A disorder of intermediary metabolism in which lack of an enzyme leads to buildup of an organic acid (from deamination of the amino acid) as opposed to the buildup of the parent amino acid.

**Peroxisomal disorders** A group of conditions caused by impaired function of peroxisomes resulting from either impaired peroxisomes biogenesis or impaired activity of one of the peroxisomal enzymes.

# BACKGROUND

Inborn errors of metabolism (IEM) are genetically determined disorders affecting an individual's ability to convert nutrients or to use them for energy production. They are caused by the impaired function of: (1) enzymes, (2) transporters, or (3) cofactors, and result in accumulation of abnormal metabolites (substrates) proximal to the metabolic block or by lack of necessary products (path A–D, Fig. 45.1). Abnormal byproducts can also be generated when alternative pathways are used to dispose of the excess metabolites (path A–F, see Fig. 45.1).

Typically, IEMs present in the newborn period or in infancy. Some diseases, however, such as fatty acid oxidation defects or milder variants of classic metabolic disorders, may not be detected until adulthood. Despite the long asymptomatic period, their consequences are still devastating and may result in death. Therefore, it is critical to identify and treat these diseases before irreversible damage occurs. The frequency of individual diseases is rare, varying from 1:10,000 to 1:200,000 or even rarer. Their cumulative frequency, however, is substantial and approaches a frequency of 1:2000.

# INHERITANCE PATTERN OF METABOLIC DISORDERS

Metabolic disorders are caused by pathogenic variants in genes that code for specific enzymes or transporters involved in metabolic pathways. The majority of metabolic disorders have autosomal recessive inheritance, in which affected individuals have a variant in both alleles encoding for a specific enzyme or transporter (Fig. 45.2) and girls are affected as often as boys. In the vast majority of cases, the parents of children with one of these metabolic conditions are carriers of the condition—that is, they carry one normal allele and one variant allele, and they do not show clinical signs of the condition. In each singleton pregnancy when both parents are carriers, there is:
- a 25% chance that the child is affected;
- a 50% chance that the child is a carrier like the parents; and
- a 25% chance that the child has two normal alleles (see Fig. 45.2).

## Clinical Presentation of Metabolic Disorders

The medical consequences of IEMs vary from failure to thrive to acute illness leading in some cases to brain damage, coma, and death. In many cases, the acute presentation is preceded by a symptom-free period that is variable in length depending on the specific disease. In many cases, there is a treatment available for these disorders consisting of special diets (formulas) that do not contain the specific nutrients that the patients are unable to metabolize. The treatment is effective if begun early before symptoms occur, but damage that has already occurred is usually irreversible. Thus, the ideal time for identifying patients with metabolic disorders is at birth or earlier.

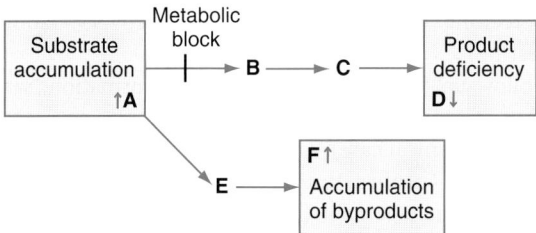

Fig. 45.1 General schematic of a metabolic pathway. The substrate A is converted by a series of reactions into product D. If one of the enzymes (arrows) is defective (metabolic block), the substrate of the reaction will accumulate (A in this case) and can enter alternative pathways of metabolism, leading to the formation of byproducts (E and F in this case). At the same time, the concentration of the product of the reaction (D) will decrease.

## POINTS TO REMEMBER

- IEMs are disorders affecting the conversion of nutrients into energy.
- IEMs usually present in the newborn period or in early infancy, although there are cases that can become symptomatic in adulthood.
- The majority of IEMs are inherited as autosomal recessive traits.
- Symptoms vary and include vomiting, lethargy, delays in development, seizures, and coma leading to death.
- For some IEMs symptoms are triggered by environmental stress, such as fasting, infections, exercise.
- The diagnosis requires analysis of specific metabolites (amino acids, carnitine, acylcarnitines, organic acids), measurement of enzyme activity, and DNA testing.
- Treatment is available for many IEMs, and it is effective if it is initiated early.
- Newborn screening can identify many of these disorders pre-symptomatically.

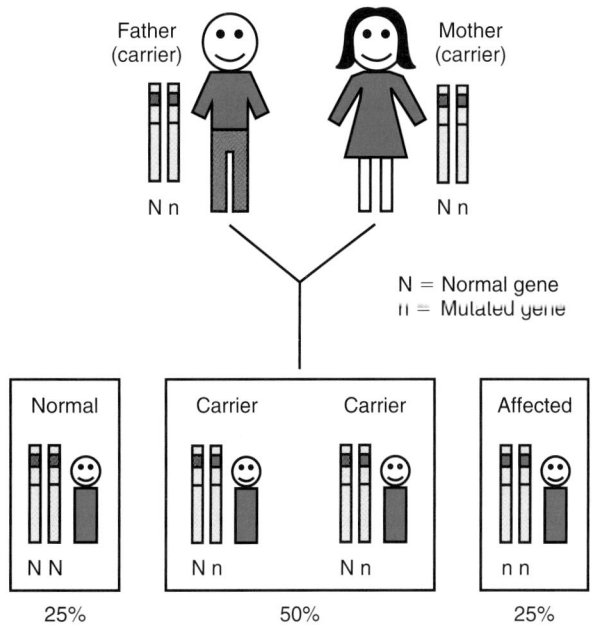

Fig. 45.2 Autosomal recessive inheritance pattern.

## Biochemical Diagnosis

The biochemical diagnosis of IEMs and treatment monitoring involve analysis of:

- metabolites;
- enzymatic activity; and/or
- DNA sequences.

Technological advances, such as *tandem mass spectrometry (MS/MS)*, allow for the simultaneous detection of multiple analytes. As such, many IEMs are now included in newborn screening programs.

# NEWBORN SCREENING

Newborn screening is a public health activity aimed at early identification of conditions for which timely intervention is expected to result in elimination or reduction of morbidity, mortality, and disabilities.

## Background

Newborn screening was originally instituted in the 1960s as a result of the pioneering efforts of Robert Guthrie and his colleagues, who developed a screening assay for measuring the phenylalanine content of a **dried blood spot (DBS)** collected from the blood of newborn babies on filter paper.

## Criteria of Newborn Screening Programs

The disease to be screened must be serious, must be fairly common, must have a natural history that is understood, and must have helpful treatment and genetic counseling (in the case of genetic disease) available. In addition, the screening test must be acceptable to the public, reliable, valid, and affordable. The newborn screening program requires the availability of expedient diagnosis and treatment of the disease and effective communication of results. Newborn screening programs must be effectual public health approaches to the diagnosis of treatable disorders early in life. Because newborn screening is a program, its efficacy depends on the integration and collaboration among its different components, involving: (1) public health, (2) screening and diagnostic laboratories, (3) physicians, and (4) families of affected children.

The recommended newborn screening panel is periodically updated by the Advisory Committee on Heritable Disorders in Newborns and Children, and it is known as the recommended uniform screening panel (RUSP). States then decide if, when, and how they will implement the recommendations of the committee. Current recommendations for the uniform screening panel of core conditions (https://www.hrsa.gov/advisory-committees/heritable-disorders/rusp/index.html/) include at least:

1. five fatty acid oxidation disorders
2. nine organic acidemias
3. six aminoacidopathies
4. two endocrinopathies (congenital hypothyroidism and congenital adrenal hyperplasia)
5. three hemoglobinopathies/thalassemias
6. three lysosomal storage disorders (Pompe disease, Hurler syndrome, and Hunter syndrome)
7. eight other disorders (Table 45.1), two of which (hearing loss and critical congenital heart disease) are not tested on dried blood spots and are tested directly at the birth facility.

In addition, many secondary conditions can be identified using MS/MS and are routinely reported by most newborn screening programs (Table 45.2).

Advances in therapeutic interventions for IEMs are continuously expanding the role of newborn screening. Of note, newborn screening does not identify all metabolic disorders, and some patients with these disorders can be missed. Therefore, a symptomatic patient at any age should be investigated despite normal newborn screening results.

Newborn screening is accomplished using MS/MS, which as a multiplex methodology allowing the measurement of multiple metabolites, which identifies the largest number of diseases, and other screening methods, such as enzyme assays, immunoassays, electrophoresis, and DNA tests.

## Steps to be Followed in a Newborn Screening Program

The different steps that need to be coordinated and tracked in a newborn screening program are:

1. Screening (sample collection and delivery, laboratory testing)
2. Follow-up (complete demographic information, satisfactory specimens, abnormal screening results, access to testing and clinical care)
3. Diagnosis (confirmatory tests, clinical consultation)
4. Clinical management (primary care physician, specialist physician, genetic counselor, dietitian)
5. Education (health care professionals, parents)
6. Quality assurance: analytical (proficiency testing, quality controls, standards), efficiency of follow-up system, efficacy of treatment, long-term outcome.

Each of these components should have specifically-written protocols that deal directly with the performance of the tasks involved. To assist laboratories in writing such protocols and procedures, the Clinical and Laboratory Standards Institute has published guidelines for newborn screening, including guidelines on:

- blood collection on filter paper (NBS01-A7);
- laboratory testing by tandem mass spectrometry (NBS04-A2);
- follow-up activities (NBS02-A2); and
- document preparation (QMS02-A6).

These documents describe the basic principles, scope, and range of activities within a newborn screening program and how to prepare the prerequisite documents. They are available at https://clsi.org/standards/products/newborn-screening/documents/.

## Second-Tier Testing

One disadvantage in newborn screening is the number of false-positive results associated with certain screening tests. To reduce the number of infants requiring additional and unnecessary confirmatory testing, second-tier tests have been developed. These second-tier tests involve further analysis of

**TABLE 45.1    Uniform Screening Panel Recommended by the Secretary of the Department of Health and Human Services for States to Screen as Part of their State Universal Newborn Screening Programs: Core Conditions[a]**

| ACMG Code | Core Condition | METABOLIC DISORDER | | | | | |
| | | Organic Acid Condition | Fatty Acid Oxidation Disorders | Amino Acid Disorders | Endocrine Disorder | Hemoglobin Disorder | Other Disorder |
|---|---|---|---|---|---|---|---|
| PROP | Propionic acidemia | X | | | | | |
| MUT | Methylmalonic acidemia (methylmalonyl-CoA mutase) | X | | | | | |
| Cbl A,B | Methylmalonic acidemia (cobalamin disorders) | X | | | | | |
| IVA | Isovaleric acidemia | X | | | | | |
| 3-MCC | 3-Methylcrotonyl-CoA carboxylase deficiency | X | | | | | |
| HMG | 3-Hydroxy-3-methylglutaric aciduria | X | | | | | |
| MCD | Holocarboxylase synthase deficiency | X | | | | | |
| βKT | β-Ketothiolase deficiency | X | | | | | |
| GA1 | Glutaric acidemia type 1 | X | | | | | |
| CUD | Carnitine uptake defect/carnitine transport defect | | X | | | | |
| MCAD | Medium-chain acyl-CoA dehydrogenase deficiency | | X | | | | |
| VLCAD | Very long-chain acyl-CoA dehydrogenase deficiency | | X | | | | |
| LCHAD | Long-chain l-3 hydroxyacyl-CoA dehydrogenase deficiency | | X | | | | |
| TFP | Trifunctional protein deficiency | | X | | | | |
| ASA | Argininosuccinic aciduria | | | X | | | |
| CIT | Citrullinemia, type 1 | | | X | | | |
| MSUD | Maple syrup urine disease | | | X | | | |
| HCY | Homocystinuria | | | X | | | |
| PKU | Classic phenylketonuria | | | X | | | |
| TYR1 | Tyrosinemia, type 1 | | | X | | | |
| CH | Primary congenital hypothyroidism | | | | X | | |
| CAH | Congenital adrenal hyperplasia | | | | X | | |
| Hb SS | S,S disease (sickle cell anemia) | | | | | X | |
| Hb S/βTh | S, Beta-thalassemia | | | | | X | |
| Hb S/C | S,C disease | | | | | X | |
| BIOT | Biotinidase deficiency | | | | | | X |
| CCHD | Critical congenital heart disease | | | | | | X |
| CF | Cystic fibrosis | | | | | | X |
| GALT | Classic galactosemia | | | | | | X |

*Continued*

TABLE 45.1   **Uniform Screening Panel Recommended by the Secretary of the Department of Health and Human Services for States to Screen as Part of their State Universal Newborn Screening Programs: Core Conditions[a]—cont'd**

| ACMG Code | Core Condition | METABOLIC DISORDER | | | | | |
|---|---|---|---|---|---|---|---|
| | | Organic Acid Condition | Fatty Acid Oxidation Disorders | Amino Acid Disorders | Endocrine Disorder | Hemoglobin Disorder | Other Disorder |
| GSD2 | Glycogen storage disease Type 2 (Pompe) | | | | | | X |
| HEAR | Hearing loss | | | | | | X |
| SCID | Severe combined immunodeficiencies | | | | | | X |
| MPS1 | Mucopolysaccharidosis type 1 | | | | | | X |
| MPS2 | Mucopolysaccharidosis type 2 | | | | | | X |
| X-ALD | X-linked adrenoleukodystrophy | | | | | | X |
| SMA | Spinal muscular atrophy SMN1 | | | | | | X |

[a]Disorders that should be included in every Newborn Screening Program. Selection of conditions based upon American College of Medical Genetics. Newborn screening: towards a uniform screening panel and system. *Genetic Med.* 2006;8(5, Suppl):S12–S252, as authored by the ACMG and commissioned by the Health Resources and Services Administration. Nomenclature for conditions based upon Sweetman L, Millington DS, Therrell BL, et al. Naming and counting disorders (conditions) included in newborn screening panels. *Pediatrics.* 2006;117(5, Suppl):S308–S314. https://www.hrsa.gov/advisorycommittees/mchbadvisory/heritabledisorders/recommendedpanel/.
*CoA,* Coenzyme.

the same blood spot with an abnormal result targeting different, more specific analytes and, often, using a methodology different from the one used in the primary screening test. They include: (1) DNA analysis for cystic fibrosis (see Chapter 48); (2) LC-MS/MS steroid profiling for congenital adrenal hyperplasia (see Chapter 41); and (3) LC-MS/MS analysis targeting specific metabolic disorders. Second-tier testing has become a crucial component of newborn screening programs to increase the sensitivity and the specificity of the screening.

## INBORN ERRORS OF METABOLISM

In this section, disorders of metabolism included in the RUSP are discussed in general, with selected individual disorders of each class reviewed in more detail as examples. An online database containing a catalog of human genetic disorders can be found at www.ncbi.nlm.nih.gov/omim/. This database is entitled "Online Mendelian Inheritance in Man" (OMIM) and is a comprehensive and authoritative compendium of human genes and genetic phenotypes. In this database, individual disorders are assigned a specific OMIM number.

### Disorders of Amino Acid Metabolism

Disorders of amino acid metabolism collectively affect approximately 1 in 8000 newborns. Almost all are transmitted as autosomal recessive traits and result from a lack of a specific enzyme in the metabolic pathway of an amino acid, leading either to the accumulation of: (1) the parent amino acid, (2) its byproducts, or (3) the catabolic products

(organic acids), depending on the location of the enzyme block. Disorders of amino acid metabolism are divided into two groups: *aminoacidopathies*, in which the parent amino acid accumulates in excess in blood and spills over into urine; and organic acidemias, in which intermediary products (organic acids) in the catabolic pathway of certain amino acids accumulate.

An example of an aminoacidopathy is *phenylketonuria (PKU)*, a disorder of phenylalanine metabolism caused in the majority of cases by deficiency of phenylalanine hydroxylase, the enzyme responsible for the conversion of phenylalanine to tyrosine. Other examples include: *maple syrup urine disease (MSUD)*, *homocystinuria*, and *tyrosinemia type 1*.

*Glutaric acidemia type 1 (GA1)*, a disorder of lysine and tryptophan metabolism, is an example of an organic acidemia. Other organic acidemias include: isovaleric acidemia, methylmalonic acidemia, and propionic acidemia (see Table 45.1). The clinical manifestations of the organic acidemias vary from no observable clinical consequences to neonatal mortality. Conditions such as developmental retardation, seizures, alterations in sensorium, failure to thrive, or behavioral disturbances, occur in more than half the disorders. Metabolic ketoacidosis, often accompanied by hyperammonemia, is a frequent finding in organic acidemias. The compound(s) accumulated depend on: (1) the site of the enzymatic block; (2) the reversibility of the reactions proximal to the lesion; and (3) the availability of alternative pathways of metabolic "runoff."

## TABLE 45.2  Uniform Screening Panel: Secondary Conditions as Recommended by the Advisory Committee on Heritable Disorders in Newborns and Children[a]

| ACMG Code | Secondary Condition | METABOLIC DISORDER | | | | |
| | | Organic Acid Condition | Fatty Acid Oxidation Disorders | Amino Acid Disorders | Hemoglobin Disorder | Other Disorder |
| --- | --- | --- | --- | --- | --- | --- |
| Cbl C,D | Methylmalonic acidemia with homocystinuria | X | | | | |
| MAL | Malonic acidemia | X | | | | |
| IBG | Isobutyrylglycinuria | X | | | | |
| 2MBG | 2-Methylbutyrylglycinuria | X | | | | |
| 3MGA | 3-Methylglutaconic aciduria | X | | | | |
| 2M3HBA | 2-Methyl-3-hydroxybutyric aciduria | X | | | | |
| SCAD | Short-chain acyl-CoA dehydrogenase deficiency | | X | | | |
| M/SCHAD | Medium/short-chain l-3-hydroxyacyl-CoA dehydrogenase deficiency | | X | | | |
| GA2 | Glutaric acidemia type 2, multiple AcylCoA dehydrogenase deficiency | | X | | | |
| MCAT | Medium-chain ketoacyl-CoA thiolase deficiency | | X | | | |
| DE RED | 2,4-Dienoyl-CoA reductase deficiency | | X | | | |
| CPT1A | Carnitine palmitoyltransferase type 1 deficiency | | X | | | |
| CPT2 | Carnitine palmitoyltransferase type II deficiency | | X | | | |
| CACT | Carnitine acylcarnitine translocase deficiency | | X | | | |
| ARG | Argininemia | | | X | | |
| CIT2 | Citrullinemia, type 2 | | | X | | |
| MET | Hypermethioninemia | | | X | | |
| H-PHE | Benign hyperphenylalaninemia | | | X | | |
| BIOPT (BS) | Biopterin defect in cofactor biosynthesis | | | X | | |
| BIOPT (REG) | Biopterin defect in cofactor regeneration | | | X | | |
| TYR2 | Tyrosinemia, type 2 | | | X | | |
| TYR3 | Tyrosinemia, type 3 | | | X | | |
| Var Hb | Various other hemoglobinopathies | | | | X | |
| GALE | Galactoepimerase deficiency | | | | | X |
| GALK | Galactokinase deficiency | | | | | X |
| | T-cell-related lymphocyte deficiencies | | | | | X |

[a]These secondary conditions are detected in the differential diagnosis of the core disorders listed in Table 45.1. Selection of conditions based upon American College of Medical Genetics. Newborn screening: towards a uniform screening panel and system. *Genetic Med.* 2006;8(5, Suppl):S12–S252 as authored by the ACMG and commissioned by the Health Resources and Services Administration. Nomenclature for Conditions based upon Sweetman L, Millington DS, Therrell BL, et al. Naming and counting disorders (conditions) included in newborn screening panels. *Pediatrics.* 2006;117(5, Suppl):S308–S314. https://www.hrsa.gov/advisorycommittees/mchbadvisory/heritabledisorders/recommendedpanel/.

## Phenylketonuria

PKU (OMIM #261600) is a disorder of phenylalanine metabolism that results from impaired phenylalanine hydroxylase activity leading to the accumulation of phenylalanine, lack of tyrosine, and production of phenylketones that are excreted in urine.

Phenylalanine is an essential amino acid, constituting 4%–6% of all dietary protein. Phenylalanine not used for protein synthesis is converted to tyrosine by the enzyme phenylalanine hydroxylase, and further degraded via a ketogenic pathway (Fig. 45.3). The frequency of hyperphenylalaninemia/PKU is 1:16,500 live births. The majority (98%) of cases of PKU are caused by pathogenic variants in the phenylalanine hydroxylase (*PAH*) gene, with the remaining 2% being caused by defects in biosynthesis or recycling of tetrahydrobiopterin ($BH_4$), the cofactor for phenylalanine hydroxylase, or by a defect in chaperone protein.

Primary or secondary (due to a deficiency of the cofactor/chaperone) impairment of phenylalanine hydroxylase causes:

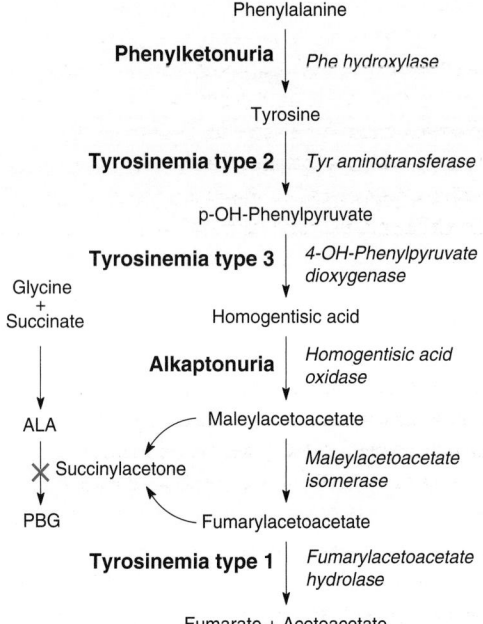

**Fig. 45.3** Inborn errors of metabolism (IEMs) resulting from deficiency of key enzymes required in the catabolism of phenylalanine. Specific disorders caused by enzyme deficiency are shown on the left side of the figure. Phenylalanine is an essential amino acid obtained from the hydrolysis of almost all the protein part of a normal diet. It is transformed to tyrosine by phenylalanine hydroxylase, the enzyme defective in phenylketonuria. The amino group of tyrosine is then removed by tyrosine aminotransferase, the enzyme defective in tyrosinemia type 2, to become *p*-hydroxyphenylpyruvate. *p*-Hydroxyphenylpyruvate dioxygenase (the enzyme defective in tyrosinemia type 3) adds oxygen to generate homogentisic acid. Homogentisic acid oxidase generates maleylacetoacetate, and a deficiency of this enzyme causes alkaptonuria, a condition in which urine turns black after standing at room temperature or with the addition of alkali. Maleylacetoacetate isomerase generates fumarylacetoacetate; a deficiency of this enzyme has been recently reported in individuals with mild elevation of succinylacetone in urine and normal clinical phenotype to date, although the definitive clinical impact of this deficiency is not yet fully known. Fumarylacetoacetate is very unstable and becomes succinylacetone, a very toxic compound capable of causing cancer and cell death. Succinylacetone also inhibits delta-aminolevulinic acid synthase, the enzyme that converts delta-aminolevulinic acid (ALA) into porphobilinogen (PBG). Accumulation of delta-aminolevulinic acid causes severe pain and neurological symptoms. Succinylacetone accumulates in tyrosinemia type 1 caused by deficiency of fumarylacetoacetate hydrolase. This enzyme normally generates fumarate and acetate that can enter the citric acid cycle for the production of energy, water, and carbonic anhydride.

(1) increased phenylalanine, (2) increased phenylketones, and (3) deficiency of tyrosine (see Fig. 45.3). The greatly increased concentration of phenylalanine impairs brain development and function, affecting other organs minimally. Patients with classic PKU are clinically asymptomatic at birth, with developmental delays and neurological manifestations typically becoming evident at several months of life when brain damage has already occurred. Untreated PKU patients develop: (1) microcephaly, (2) eczematous skin rash, (3) "mousy" odor (due to accumulation of phenylacetate), and (4) severe intellectual disability. The treatment of PKU includes a diet: (1) low in protein and phenylalanine, and (2) supplemented with tyrosine, minerals, vitamins, and other nutrients to sustain healthy growth. Some patients respond to treatment with pharmacological amounts of a synthetic form of tetrahydrobiopterin. Enzyme substitution therapy with injectable phenylalanine ammonia lyase is also available. Treatment should be continued for life.

Ideally, treatment should start before 2 weeks of age. Pregnant women with PKU should adhere to a strictly controlled diet that is low in phenylalanine and proteins, because phenylalanine is teratogenic and results in an increased risk of spontaneous abortions or of having a child with growth retardation, microcephaly, significant developmental delays, and birth defects.

The diagnosis of PKU is confirmed biochemically by demonstration of increased plasma phenylalanine (by plasma amino acids analysis) and an increased phenylalanine:tyrosine ratio. Urine specimens from affected individuals contain increased concentrations of phenylketones (hence the name *phenylketonuria*) detectable by urine organic acids analysis. Enzymatic confirmation of phenylalanine hydroxylase deficiency is not usually performed (the enzyme is expressed only in the liver), but molecular analysis of the gene is increasingly used because there is a correlation between severity of the pathogenic variant and phenylalanine tolerance, and it can exclude deficiency of the chaperone (DNAJC12 deficiency). All children with hyperphenylalaninemia should be screened for defects in $BH_4$ synthesis or recycling. This is performed by measuring the urinary pterin profile and by measuring the enzyme activity of *dihydropteridine reductase (DHPR)* in blood spotted on filter paper. Deficiency of $BH_4$ affects the synthesis of several neurotransmitters, including dopamine and serotonin because it is a cofactor of: (1) phenylalanine hydroxylase, (2) tyrosine hydroxylase, (3) tryptophan hydroxylase, and (4) nitric oxide synthase. Patients with a defect in $BH_4$ synthesis or recycling have neurological symptoms and developmental regression in the first few months of life, despite adequate control of phenylalanine intake and plasma concentrations. They can develop seizures and have a characteristic hypotonia of the trunk with hypertonia of the extremities. These patients require therapy with $BH_4$ and appropriate neurotransmitters. They may or may not require a low phenylalanine diet once $BH_4$ therapy is initiated.

## Tyrosinemia

Tyrosinemia is characterized by increased blood concentrations of tyrosine. There are three types of tyrosinemia (types 1–3); each is caused by the deficiency of a different enzyme (Fig. 45.3).

Tyrosinemia type 1 (TYR-1) is the most severe form and is caused by a deficiency of fumarylacetoacetate hydrolase. Tyrosinemia type 2 is caused by a deficiency of tyrosine aminotransferase. Tyrosinemia type 3 is caused by a deficiency of 4-hydroxyphenylpyruvate dioxygenase.

The incidence of TYR-1 is approximately 1 in 100,000 with a clustering of cases in the Lac-St. Jean region of Quebec (Canada). Patients with TYR-1 present usually before 6 months of age with severe liver involvement or with failure to thrive, liver dysfunction, and rickets due to renal Fanconi syndrome. They have extreme irritability caused by peripheral neuropathy mimicking acute intermittent porphyria. Untreated patients develop liver cirrhosis and are at very high risk for liver cancer.

Patients with TYR-1 have increased concentrations of tyrosine in the plasma, but this increase usually is not as marked as in patients with other forms of tyrosinemia. Increased tyrosine can also be seen in: (1) other types of tyrosinemia (types 2 and 3), (2) transient tyrosinemia of the newborn, (3) prematurity, (4) liver disease from any cause, (5) mitochondrial DNA depletion syndrome, and (6) diets very rich in proteins. The biochemical diagnosis of TYR-1 is based on the detection in urine of succinylacetone, derived from fumarylacetoacetic acid, the intermediate immediately upstream of the enzyme defect. TYR-1 is identified by newborn screening only when succinylacetone is used as the primary marker, because tyrosine might not be elevated in the newborn period in these patients. Therapy consists of:
1. low dietary tyrosine,
2. low dietary phenylalanine, and
3. drug therapy with 2-(2-nitro-4-trifluoro-methylbenzoyl)-1,3-cyclohexanedione (NTBC), an inhibitor of 4-hydroxyphenylpyruvate dioxygenase (see Fig. 45.3).

NTBC prevents the synthesis of succinylacetone, which is rapidly reduced within the normal range after initiation of treatment. Measurement of alpha fetoprotein is also used to monitor these patients, because liver cancer is a complication of this condition. Liver transplantation is indicated in patients who progress to liver failure and in those acquiring liver cancer.

## Homocystinuria

Homocystinuria is characterized by increased concentrations of the sulfur-containing amino acid, homocysteine, in blood and urine (Fig. 45.4). It can be caused by deficiency of cystathionine β-synthase (classic homocystinuria) or defects in homocysteine remethylation. The incidence is approximately 1:450,000 live births in the United States with a very high incidence in the country of Qatar (1:1800). Clinical manifestations are nonspecific at first and may include failure to thrive and developmental delay. Patients usually develop lens dislocation (often requiring surgery) and a body habitus like that seen in Marfan syndrome (homocysteine interferes with disulfide formation in fibrillin, the protein defective in Marfan syndrome). Patients whose blood total homocysteine concentration remains increased are at risk of blood clots, which are a life-threatening complication of the condition.

The biochemical diagnosis of homocystinuria is obtained by plasma amino acid analysis showing increased plasma concentrations of methionine (especially in children), the presence of the disulfide homocystine (not always detectable), and by elevated total plasma homocysteine. Classic homocystinuria is detected in newborn screening by increased concentrations of methionine in dried blood spots, although often the concentration of methionine is not high in the newborn screening period and this condition could be missed. Therapy for classic homocystinuria requires:
1. high doses of pyridoxine (the cofactor of cystathionine β-synthase),
2. a special diet low in methionine; and
3. administration of betaine that donates a methyl group to homocysteine to generate methionine.

## Maple Syrup Urine Disease

Maple syrup urine disease (MSUD) is an autosomal recessive disorder with an incidence of approximately 1:200,000 live births. It is caused by a deficiency of the branched-chain alpha-keto acid dehydrogenase complex (BCKDC), leading to a buildup of the branched-chain amino acids leucine, isoleucine, valine, and the pathognomonic compound alloisoleucine, and their toxic ketoacids in the blood and urine. The disease is named for the presence of sweet-smelling urine with an odor similar to that of maple syrup. Several forms of this disease may occur, depending on the gene affected and the severity of the pathogenic variants. The enzyme complex consists of four subunits designated $E_1\alpha$, $E_1\beta$, $E_2$, and $E_3$. MSUD results from pathogenic variants in any of the genes that code for the enzyme subunits.

Individuals with classic MSUD present with poor feeding and vomiting during the first week of life followed by lethargy and coma within a few days. This usually follows a normal birth and an uneventful first few days of life. Routine laboratory work is mostly unremarkable except for the presence of ketones in urine. Diagnosis is established by measuring plasma amino acids and finding increased branched chain amino acids and the presence of alloisoleucine, which is characteristic of this disease.

Cornerstones of treatment include diets that have a restricted content of branched-chain amino acids and include supplementation with: (1) high-dose thiamine and, in many patients, (2) valine and (3) isoleucine.

## Urea Cycle Disorders

**Urea cycle disorders**, or urea cycle defects, are caused by a deficiency of one of the enzymes or a transporter involved in the urea cycle, which is responsible for removing ammonia from the blood stream. The urea cycle involves a series of biochemical steps in which nitrogen derived from protein metabolism is removed from the blood and converted to urea, which is then excreted in urine. In urea cycle disorders, the nitrogen accumulates in the form of ammonia, a toxic substance, and is not removed from the body.

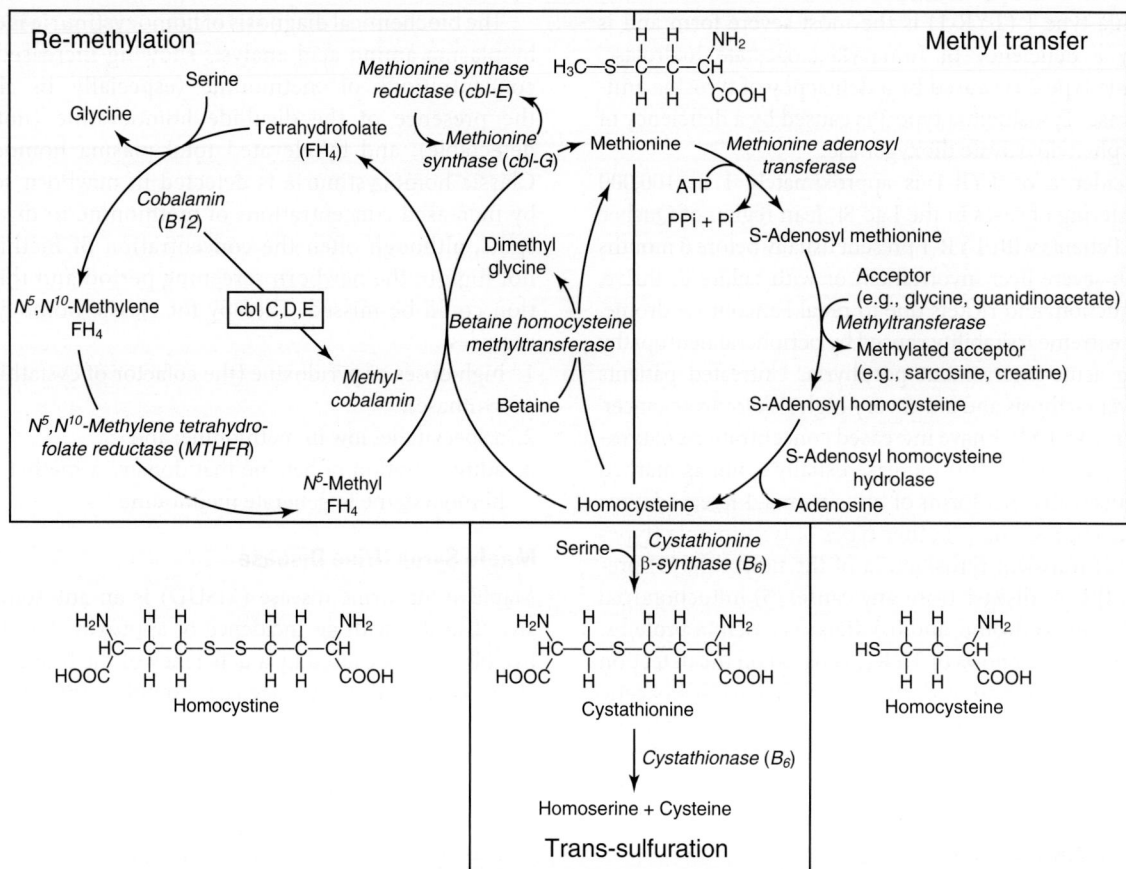

**Fig. 45.4** Sulfur amino acid metabolism. Defects in methionine metabolism (classic homocystinuria caused by cystathionine beta synthase deficiency) or defects in homocysteine remethylation (defects in vitamin $B_{12}$ or folic acid metabolism) cause homocystinuria. Methionine transfers a methyl group during its conversion to homocysteine. Defects in methyl transfer or in the subsequent metabolism of homocysteine by the pyridoxal phosphate (vitamin $B_6$)-dependent cystathionine β-synthase increase plasma methionine concentrations. Excess homocysteine is transformed back to methionine via remethylation. This reaction is catalyzed by methionine synthase and requires methylcobalamin and folic acid. Deficiencies in these enzymes or lack of vitamin $B_{12}$ (cobalamin) or folic acid or defects in their metabolism (defects in vitamin $B_{12}$ metabolism are named *cblC, cblD, cblF*; methylenetetrahydrofolate reductase [*MTHFR*] deficiency is the most common defect of folic acid metabolism) are associated with decreased or normal methionine concentrations and with elevated homocysteine. In an alternative pathway, homocysteine is remethylated by betaine:homocysteine methyltransferase.

Urea cycle disorders can result in mental and behavioral dysfunction, coma, and death. The urea cycle disposes of the nitrogen groups of amino acids before their carbon skeleton is metabolized to gluconeogenic (most amino acids) or ketogenic precursors (leucine and lysine), or both (isoleucine, phenylalanine, tyrosine, and tryptophan). This cycle requires the combined action of different enzymes and mitochondrial transporters (Fig. 45.5). Deficiency of any of these enzymes or transporters impairs the function of the urea cycle, causing hyperammonemia.

Newborn screening can effectively identify argininosuccinate synthetase (ASS) deficiency (or citrullinemia type 1), citrullinemia type 2 (mitochondrial aspartate transporter/citrin deficiency), argininosuccinate lyase (ASL) deficiency, and arginase deficiency. OTC (ornithine transcarbamoylase) deficiency, an X-linked disorder that is also the most common

of the urea cycle defects, CPS-1 (carbamoylphosphate synthase 1) and NAGS (N-acetylglutamate synthase) deficiencies are not always effectively detected by NBS. Patients with urea cycle defects may have symptoms at any age. In the neonatal period, there is usually a brief interval between birth and clinical manifestations, with the most severe cases having symptoms before the results of newborn screening are available. Hyperammonemia and the accumulation of glutamine in the brain lead to poor feeding, vomiting, lethargy, or irritability, progressing to coma and death.

Diagnosis is accomplished by measuring plasma amino acids and identifying the amino acid present in excess or in defect. Patients are treated with a diet low in proteins and administration of nitrogen scavengers, such as sodium benzoate and phenylacetate or its precursor phenylbutyrate, which bind and remove glycine and glutamine, respectively.

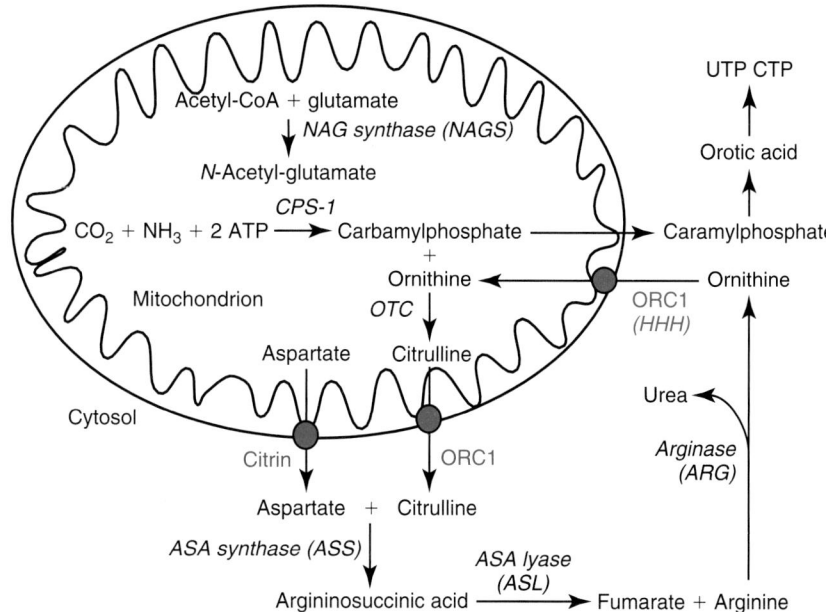

**Fig. 45.5** The urea cycle. In this cycle, urea is formed starting from ammonia ($NH_3$). It requires several enzymes (in italics) and mitochondrial transporters (*blue*), any of which can be defective and may impair the function of the urea cycle. Within the mitochondrial matrix, ammonia, derived from amino acid catabolism, is combined with carbonic anhydride and phosphorus to generate carbamoylphosphate by carbamoyl phosphate synthase 1 (*CPS-1*). This enzyme is active only in the presence of *N*-acetylglutamate, an allosteric activator synthesized by *N*-acetylglutamate synthase (*NAGS*). Carbamoylphosphate is then attached to ornithine by ornithine transcarbamoylase (*OTC*) to generate citrulline. Citrulline then exits the mitochondrial matrix using the ornithine/citrulline mitochondrial transporter (*ORC1*). This transporter is an exchanger and couples the exit of citrulline from mitochondria to the entry of ornithine. Citrulline in the cytoplasm combines with aspartate (transported from the mitochondrial matrix by the citrin transporter) to generate argininosuccinic acid by the action of argininosuccinic acid synthase (*ASS*). Argininosuccinic acid is then split to arginine and fumarate by argininosuccinic acid lyase (*ASL*). Fumarate enters the citric acid cycle, and arginine is converted to urea (excreted in urine) and ornithine by arginase (*ARG*). Ornithine can then enter the mitochondrial matrix again to restart another cycle. The two nitrogens in urea excreted in urine derive from ammonia in carbamoylphosphate and the amino group of aspartate. Carbamoylphosphate not utilized in the urea cycle (usually because of deficiency in ornithine transcarbamoylase or any of the downstream enzymes) exits to the cytoplasm to generate nucleotides (UTP and CTP). The concentration of orotic acid (an intermediate in nucleotide synthesis) can be measured in the urine of patients with OTC, ASS, ASL or ARG deficiency. *citrin*, Aspartate/glutamate exchanger; *CP*, carbamoylphosphate; *CPS-1*, carbamoyl phosphate synthase 1; *CTP*, cytidine triphosphate; *UTP*, uridine triphosphate.

## Glutaric Acidemia Type 1

Glutaric acidemia type 1 (GA1; OMIM #231670) is an autosomal recessive disorder of the metabolism of (1) lysine, (2) hydroxylysine, and (3) tryptophan; it is caused by deficiency of glutaryl-coenzyme A (CoA) dehydrogenase. In this condition, glutaric acid (GA) and 3-hydroxyglutaric acid (3-OH-GA), formed in the catabolic pathway of the abovementioned amino acids, accumulate, especially in urine. Affected patients have brain atrophy and macrocephaly (head circumference often increases dramatically following birth), and they can develop acute dystonia secondary to degeneration of the corpus striatum (a component of the motor system in the brain). In most cases, this is triggered by an infection with fever between 6 and 18 months of age.

GA1 is identified by an increased concentration of glutarylcarnitine (C5DC) on newborn screening. The diagnosis is biochemically confirmed by urine organic acid analysis that indicates the presence of excess 3-OH-GA, with elevated glutarylcarnitine in plasma that becomes the major component in urine. Therapy consists of:

1. carnitine supplementation to remove GA;
2. a diet restricted in amino acid precursors of GA; and
3. prompt administration of intravenous calories in the patient who is unable to eat for any reason such as infections, fever, and gastroenteritis.

Early diagnosis and therapy greatly reduce the risk of acute dystonia in patients with GA1.

### Treatment of Organic Acidemias and Aminoacidopathies

Therapy for aminoacidopathies, and organic acidemias consists of:
1. special diets restricting the compounds (usually amino acids) that result in the abnormal accumulation or amino acids or the formation of the abnormal organic acid,
2. supplementation with vitamins specific for each disorder,
3. carnitine supplements, and
4. avoidance of fasting.

Repeated laboratory monitoring is necessary to determine adequacy of diet and other therapies. For some of these conditions, aggressive therapy of illnesses with intravenous fluids containing glucose is essential to avoid catabolism that aggravates clinical symptoms.

## Disorders of Fatty Acid Oxidation

Fatty acids are metabolized within mitochondria to produce energy. Carnitine and the carnitine cycle are required to transfer long-chain fatty acids into mitochondria for subsequent beta-oxidation (Fig. 45.6). Within the mitochondrial matrix, long-chain fatty acids are progressively shortened by two carbon units at each cycle to generate acetyl-CoA, which is used by the Krebs cycle to produce energy (Fig. 45.7). Disorders of fatty acid oxidation, such as *medium-chain acyl-CoA dehydrogenase (MCAD) deficiency*, occur when an enzyme is missing in the metabolic pathway and fatty acids fail to undergo oxidation to supply energy. These disorders are usually silent and become evident only when the body needs energy from fat during times of increased energy demand, such as: (1) fasting, (2) infections/fever, or (3) strenuous exercise. In these cases, apparently healthy children with these disorders become acutely sick, lose consciousness, become comatose, and may die. When symptomatic, patients with fatty acid oxidation disorders develop hypoglycemia and might show increased serum transaminases indicating liver damage. Some fatty acid oxidation disorders (such as *long-chain 3-hydroxyacyl-CoA dehydrogenase [LCHAD] deficiency*) also affect: (1) skeletal muscle, (2) cardiac muscle, and (3) the mother during pregnancy. Other disorders include carnitine transporter defects and very long-chain acyl-CoA dehydrogenase deficiency (see Table 45.1).

### Medium-Chain Acyl-CoA Dehydrogenase Deficiency

MCAD (OMIM #201450) deficiency is the most common disorder of fatty acid oxidation with a frequency of about 1:18,000 in the United States. The clinical presentations of this disease are: (1) asymptomatic, (2) hypoglycemia, (3) lethargy, (4) coma, and (5) sudden death, which is usually triggered by prolonged fasting, acute illness, or both. The

majority of patients have symptoms in the first year of life, but clinical symptoms can occur at any time during life, and often the first episode is fatal. The treatment consists of:
1. avoidance of fasting;
2. consumption of a heart-healthy diet after 1 year of age;
3. carnitine supplementation; and
4. institution of an emergency plan in case of illness or other metabolic stress.

Early diagnosis through newborn screening and early initiation of treatment leads to a favorable prognosis. Patients with MCAD deficiency are identified by MS/MS newborn screening because of the characteristic acylcarnitine profile with increased concentrations of: (1) C6- (hexanoyl), (2) C8- (octanoyl), and (3) C10:1- (decenoyl) carnitine (with C8-carnitine being the highest) and increased C8/C2 and C8/C10 ratios.

The diagnosis of MCAD is confirmed biochemically by urine organic acid and acylglycine analyses showing: (1) excess hexanoylglycine and suberylglycine; (2) plasma acylcarnitine profile (confirming increased C6-, C8-, and C10:1 carnitine); and (3) DNA analysis of the *ACADM* gene. A common pathogenic variant (c.985A>G, p.Lys329Glu) is prevalent in symptomatic patients (80% of symptomatic patients are homozygous for this mutation; 98% carry at least one copy).

### Treatment of Fatty Acid Oxidation Disorders

Treatment of fatty acid oxidation disorders consists of:
1. avoidance of fasting;
2. adherence to a low-fat diet; and
3. carnitine supplementation.

For some disorders of fatty acid oxidation, therapy includes administration of medium chain triglycerides (oil) and triheptanoin (3 molecules of heptanoate bound to glycerol) that enter mitochondria independently from carnitine and bypass the metabolic block. In addition, conditions that increase catabolism such as fever, vomiting, and infections need to be aggressively treated with intravenous glucose, antipyretics, and antibiotics (if necessary).

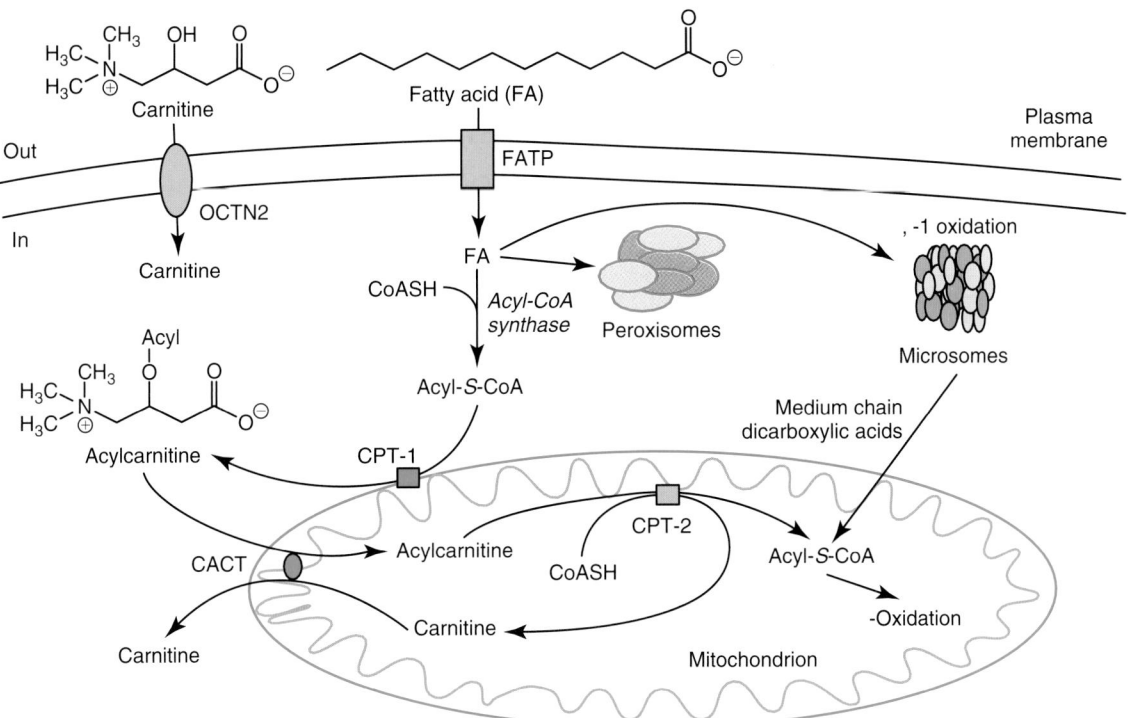

**Fig. 45.6** The carnitine cycle in fatty acid (*FA*) oxidation. The carnitine cycle is responsible for delivering long-chain fatty acids to the mitochondrial matrix for subsequent beta oxidation. FAs bound to albumin are transferred across the plasma membrane by the action of fatty acid transport proteins (*FATP*). Inside the cell, fatty acids undergo vectorial acylation, a process catalyzed by acyl-coenzyme A (CoA) synthases, that traps them in the cytoplasm as acyl-CoA thioesters (acyl-*S*-CoA). The acyl-CoA thioesters are then conveyed through different metabolic pathways in mitochondria, peroxisomes, and microsomes based on the cell energy status. Metabolism of fatty acid by peroxisomes and microsomes is usually minimal, except in disorders of fatty acid oxidation. The mitochondrial membrane is impermeable to acyl-CoAs and fatty acids must be conjugated to carnitine to enter mitochondria. Carnitine is accumulated inside the cell by the high-affinity organic cation transporter novel 2 (OCTN2) carnitine transporter. Carnitine forms a high-energy ester bond with long-chain fatty acids by the action of carnitine palmitoyl transferase 1 (*CPT-1*), located in the inner aspect of the outer mitochondrial membrane, with the formation of acylcarnitines. Acylcarnitines are then translocated across the inner mitochondrial membrane by carnitine acylcarnitine translocase (*CACT*). Once inside mitochondria, carnitine palmitoyl transferase 2 (*CPT-2*), located in the inner mitochondrial membrane, removes carnitine from acylcarnitines and re-generates acyl-CoAs. Carnitine then returns to the cytoplasm for another cycle (using CACT), while the acyl-CoAs can enter (in aerobic conditions and in the presence of low levels of ATP) β-oxidation with final production of acetyl-CoA for oxidative phosphorylation or production of ketone bodies in the liver.

## Lysosomal Disorders

Lysosomal disorders are a group of diseases caused by deficiency of one or more lysosomal enzymes responsible for the degradation of complex macromolecules, such as mucopolysaccharides. The impaired degradation of these macromolecules results in their accumulation in organs and tissues. The disease phenotype depends on the substrate accumulated and its sites of turnover—for example, muscle and heart in Pompe disease and connective tissue in mucopolysaccharidoses. In addition to symptomatic therapy to alleviate the most severe clinical symptoms, specific therapies for lysosomal storage disorders are available or in development: (1) enzyme replacement therapy; (2) substrate reduction therapy; (3) chaperone therapy; (4) bone marrow and hematopoietic stem cell transplantation; (5) gene therapy. Currently newborn screening for two lysosomal storage disorders, Pompe disease and mucopolysaccharidosis type 1 (Hurler, Hurler-Scheie, and Scheie

syndrome), is included in the RUSP. A third one (mucopolysaccharidosis type 2 or Hunter syndrome) was recommended for inclusion in 2022.

### Pompe Disease

Pompe disease is an autosomal recessive lysosomal storage disorder caused by deficiency of the enzyme, acid alpha-glucosidase (GAA), with an estimated incidence of approximately 1:17,000 births. In this condition, glycogen accumulates within the lysosomes in the skeletal muscle and heart. There are two main forms of Pompe disease: infantile and late-onset. In infantile Pompe disease, hypertrophic cardiomyopathy, muscle weakness, and hypotonia are usually evident by 2 months of age and most patients die within the first year of life. Late-onset Pompe disease is characterized by variable age of onset and presentation, with symptoms including progressive proximal muscle weakness and respiratory insufficiency. The neonatal screening for Pompe disease

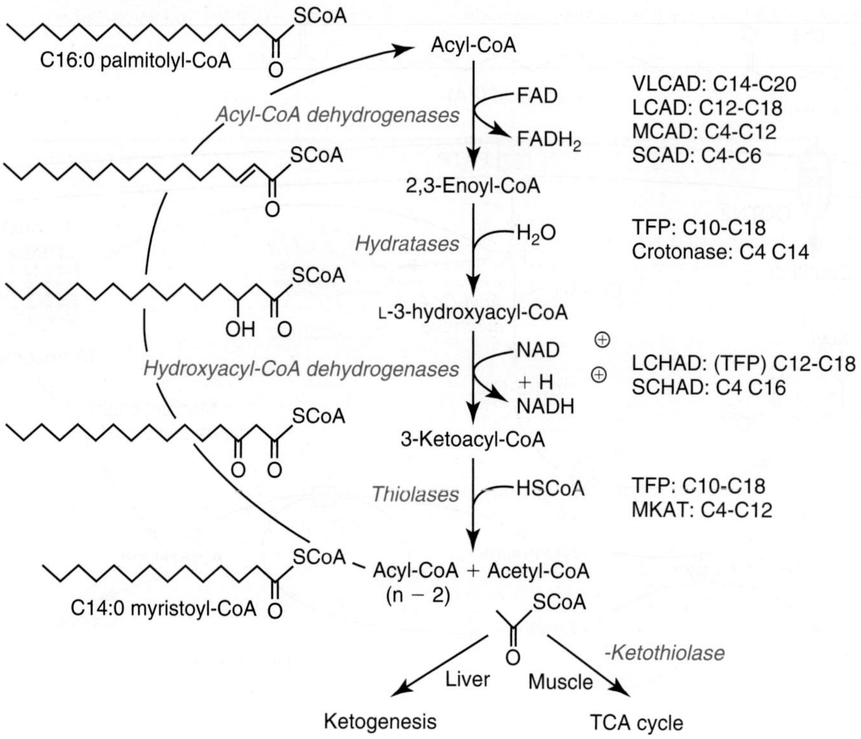

**Fig. 45.7** Beta oxidation of fatty acids. In the mitochondrial matrix, long-chain fatty acids undergo a series of steps to progressively shorten the fatty acids by two carbon units (acetyl-coenzyme A [CoA]) through a series of enzymatic reactions. Chemical structures are shown on the left, enzymes (*blue*) and reactions are in the middle, and the carbon chain lengths for various disorders are on the right. Dehydrogenases introduce a double bond between C2 and C3 and are specific for fatty acids with different chain lengths: *LCAD*, long-chain acyl CoA dehydrogenase; *MCAD*, medium-chain acyl-CoA dehydrogenase; *MKAT*, medium-chain acyl-CoA thiolase; *SCAD*, short-chain acyl-CoA dehydrogenase; *SCHAD*, short-chain 3-hydroxyacyl-CoA dehydrogenase; *VLCAD*, very long-chain acyl-CoA dehydrogenase. A trifunctional protein (TFP) adds water and cleaves two carbon atoms from the long-chain fatty acid. This is done through sequential action of a hydratase (enoyl-CoA hydratase), a l-3-hydroxyacyl-CoA dehydrogenase (*LCHAD*, long-chain 3-hydroxyacyl-CoA dehydrogenase), and a thiolase (acyl-CoA acetyltransferase). The two carbon units generated can be completely oxidized in the muscle to $CO_2$ or can generate ketone bodies in the liver that may be exported to other organs to provide energy.

is based on the measurement of enzyme activity in blood spots by: (1) LC-MS/MS, which measures the enzymatic conversion of a substrate to a product; or (2) fluorimetric methods, which detect the release of a fluorescent compound from the substrate mediated by the enzyme. In the United States, adult-onset Pompe disease is about 8 times more frequent than the infantile onset form. The diagnosis of Pompe disease is confirmed by measurement of enzyme activity in leukocytes or in fibroblasts and by DNA testing. DNA testing is important to identify patients with pseudodeficiency of enzymatic activity: a condition in which the enzyme functions normally against the natural substrate, but not against the synthetic substrate used to measure activity in the laboratory. Enzyme replacement therapy with human recombinant acid alpha-glucosidase improves the manifestations of the disease, including survival in affected children.

## Mucopolysaccharidosis Type 1

Mucopolysaccharidosis type 1 (MPS1) is an autosomal recessive lysosomal storage disorder caused by deficiency of the lysosomal hydrolase alpha-iduronidase. The incidence is

estimated at 0.7 to 4:100,000. Alpha-iduronidase is involved in the degradation of the glycosaminoglycans heparan sulfate and dermatan sulfate, and its impaired activity leads to their accumulation in organs and tissues. MPS1 is a progressive, debilitating, and often life-threatening disease. Typical features of MPS1 include coarse facial features, hepatosplenomegaly, cardiac involvement, joint stiffness, skeletal deformities, and corneal clouding. There is a wide spectrum of phenotypes, with the most severe, MPS-1H or Hurler syndrome, presenting in the first 6 months of life with a rapid disease progression involving the central nervous system (CNS) and death by 10 years of age. In patients with the attenuated presentation, Hurler-Scheie (MPS-1HS) and Scheie (MPS-1S), the disease progression is slower, does not involve the CNS, and life expectancy is close to normal in the milder affected individuals. Newborn screening methods for MPS1 are based on measurement of alpha-iduronidase activity. As for Pompe disease, there are two methods available for high throughput screening: (1) LC-MS/MS based, and (2) fluorimetric. The diagnosis is confirmed by measuring enzyme activity in freshly isolated leukocytes and by sequencing of the *IDUA* gene. As for Pompe disease, DNA can identify individuals with enzyme pseudodeficiency. Measurement of urinary glycosaminoglycan species can be used to distinguish affected from unaffected individuals and to follow response to therapies in treated individuals. Enzyme replacement therapy with human recombinant alpha-iduronidase improves organ and skeletal involvement in MPS1 patients, but is not effective in the neuropathic form (Hurler syndrome). In this case, hematopoietic stem cell transplantation early in life remains the only option to prevent CNS involvement, often in conjunction with enzyme replacement therapy to prevent peripheral complications.

## Mucopolysaccharidosis Type 2

Mucopolysaccharidosis type 2 (MPS2, Hunter syndrome) is an X-linked recessive lysosomal storage disorder caused by deficiency of the lysosomal enzyme iduronate 2-sulfatase. The incidence is estimated at 0.7 to 1.2:100,000. Iduronate 2-sulfatase is involved in the first step of the degradation of heparan sulfate and dermatan sulfate, and its deficiency leads to the accumulation of these glycosaminoglycans in organs and tissues. MPS2 is a progressive, debilitating, and often life-threatening disease. Typical features of MPS2 are very similar to those of MPS1, with the exception that corneal clouding is usually not observed in MPS2. There is a spectrum of phenotypes, with variable age of onset and rate of progression. The most severe forms affect the brain and cause progressive cognitive decline that, with narrowing of the airways and cardiac disease, usually results in death in the first or second decade of life. The slowly progressive form causes minimal to no effects on the brain, but results in severe physical disability with most individuals surviving into early adulthood.

Newborn screening methods for MPS2 are based on measurement of iduronate 2-sulfatase using either: (1) LC-MS/MS based, or (2) fluorimetric methods. The diagnosis is confirmed by measuring enzyme activity in freshly isolated leukocytes and by sequencing of the *IDS* gene. Measurement of urinary glycosaminoglycan species can be used to distinguish affected from unaffected individuals and to follow response to therapies in treated individuals. Sensitive and specific methods need to be utilized to measure glycosaminoglycans or the specific modified sugars that accumulate in them since the overall patter can be similar in MPS1 and MPS2 with commonly utilized laboratory tests. Enzyme replacement therapy with human iduronate 2-sulfatase improves organ and skeletal involvement in MPS2 patients, without affecting much brain involvement. It is still unclear whether hematopoietic stem cell transplantation early in life can prevent CNS involvement in MPS2.

## Peroxisomal Disorders

Peroxisomes are single membrane organelles containing enzymes responsible for the alpha- and beta-oxidation of very long-chain fatty acids, the synthesis of the membrane glycerophospholipids plasmalogens, and the oxidation of bile acids and cholesterol. Defects in the biogenesis of peroxisomes or defects in one or more peroxisomal function lead to severe clinical manifestations.

## X-Linked Adrenoleukodystrophy

X-linked adrenoleukodystrophy (X-ALD) is an X-linked peroxisomal disorder resulting in defective oxidation of very long-chain fatty acids. Its incidence is approximately 1:20,000. X-ALD is caused by mutations in the *ABCD1* gene located on Xq28 that encodes for the adrenoleukodystrophy protein (ALDP) in the peroxisomal membrane, which transfers very long-chain fatty acids inside the peroxisomes for degradation. X-ALD can present in males before 5 years of age with progressive cognitive and neurological deterioration leading to a vegetative state and death. A milder variant, adrenomyeloneuropathy (AMN) presents usually in the 2nd to 3rd decade of life with progressive spastic paraplegia. Adrenal dysfunction occurs in about 2/3 of males with AMN. A total of 50% to 65% of female carriers develop symptoms similar to AMN; however, the onset is usually in the 4th or 5th decade of life. X-ALD can be diagnosed by newborn screening measuring C26:0 lysophosphatidylcholine (C26:0 LPC) by LC-MS/MS. C26:0 LPC is elevated in DBS of patients with X-ALD, with peroxisomal biogenesis defects, and in approximately 80% of female carriers for X-ALD. The diagnosis is confirmed by measurement of very long-chain fatty acids (VLCFA) in plasma and by DNA sequencing of the *ABCD1* gene. VLCFAs in plasma are elevated and diagnostic in all males. However, they are elevated and informative only in 80% to 85% of heterozygous females for whom DNA testing should be considered. The only effective treatment for X-ALD is hematopoietic stem cell transplantation, to be performed before the appearance of neurological symptoms.

## Biotinidase Deficiency

Biotinidase deficiency or late-onset multiple carboxylase deficiency is an autosomal recessive disorder caused by deficiency of the enzyme biotinidase. This enzyme releases the vitamin biotin from the proteins (in most cases enzymes) to which it is attached. This enzyme allows the human body to generate free biotin from food and from the recycling of endogenous enzymes. When the enzyme is defective, there is no sufficient free biotin to incorporate into enzymes that need it, such as many carboxylases. As a result, these enzymes can become inactive resulting in clinical manifestations that can include a skin rash, loss of hair, neurological symptoms (low muscle tone, seizures, ataxia), hearing and vision loss. These signs and symptoms can be seen with profound biotinidase deficiency when enzymatic activity is totally absent. Patients with partial biotinidase deficiency retain significant residual enzymatic activity and can show symptoms at time of stress (such as that caused by infections), may have hypotonia, skin rash, and hair loss, particularly during times of stress.

Profound biotinidase deficiency affects 1:67,000 newborns, the partial form 1:25,000. The diagnosis is confirmed by measuring biotinidase activity in serum. Treatment consists in the administration of biotin 5–10 mg/day for life. Treated patients experience none of the symptoms typical of this condition.

## Disorders of Carbohydrate Metabolism

Enzyme deficiency in the metabolic pathways for carbohydrates results in accumulation of sugars within organs or tissues impairing their function, inability to obtain energy from them, or toxicity from the excess of monosaccharides or their derivatives (phosphorylated sugars). **Disorders of carbohydrate metabolism** include (1) the glycogen storage diseases; (2) glucose-6-phosphate dehydrogenase (G-6-PD) deficiency; and (3) classic galactosemia.

Glycogen storage disorders affect primarily the liver or the skeletal muscle. The accumulation of glycogen impairs organ function and, if the liver is affected, prevents release of glucose with resulting hypoglycemia. They are usually treated with avoidance of fasting and a special diet rich in protein, devoid of simple sugars and supplements with uncooked cornstarch.

G-6-PD deficiency affects red blood cells, causing them to break down (hemolysis). It can cause mild to severe jaundice in newborns and in some cases hemolytic anemia. Symptoms can be triggered by: (1) infections, (2) certain drugs (some antibiotics and medications used to treat malaria), or (3) exposure to fava beans (a reaction called *favism*). The gene for this condition is on the X chromosomes, and the condition affects mostly males. Avoidance of stressors can mitigate or avoid symptoms.

Classic galactosemia results from absence of galactose-1-phosphate uridyl transferase. Galactose is derived from the disaccharide lactose found in milk. In galactosemia, galactose is phosphorylated to galactose-1-phosphate or transformed in other metabolites such as galactitol that are not further metabolized. Increased concentrations of galactose-1-phosphate and galactitol in cells are toxic. Infants have failure to thrive, jaundice, liver failure, and predisposition to life-threatening infections with *Escherichia coli* and other Gram-negative bacteria. The treatment of galactosemia involves removal of lactose (contained in human or animal-derived milk, but not in soy milk) and avoidance of all foods containing galactose. In galactosemia, intervention early in life provides the best prognosis, although some long-term complications (speech apraxia, learning disorders, and ovarian insufficiency in females) can still occur in treated individuals.

## DIAGNOSTIC TESTS FOR INHERITED DISORDERS OF METABOLISM

A newborn screening result highly suggestive of a metabolic disorder typically leads to an immediate evaluation using confirmatory tests and a referral of the newborn to a metabolic center.

In asymptomatic patients, the confirmation of diagnosis relies on specific tests, such as (1) ion-exchange chromatography; (2) liquid chromatography-tandem mass spectrometry (LC-MS/MS) for amino acids analysis; (3) gas chromatography-mass spectrometry (GC-MS) for organic acids analysis; and (4) MS/MS without or with liquid chromatographic separation for acylcarnitines and acylglycines analyses, respectively. A combination of tests is often key in the confirmation of abnormal newborn screening results, especially for those with borderline values. DNA testing and enzyme assays are available for further diagnostic confirmation of most of these conditions.

These techniques are described in Chapters 12, 13, 14, 18, 19, and 48. MS/MS is a technique of choice in newborn screening programs.

## REVIEW QUESTIONS

1. An inherited disorder that affects the conversion of nutrients into energy is referred to as a(n):
   a. aminoacidopathy.
   b. autosomal recessive disorder.
   c. inborn error of metabolism (IEM).
   d. hemolytic disease of a newborn.

2. An inborn disorder of metabolism that is triggered by prolonged fasting and/or acute illness and that is confirmed by abnormal acylcarnitine concentrations is:
   a. galactosemia.
   b. medium-chain acyl-CoA dehydrogenase (MCAD) deficiency.
   c. phenylketonuria (PKU).
   d. homocystinuria.

3. Deficiency of an enzyme that results in excess of monosaccharides in the blood of a newborn leads to a specific disorder of metabolism. An example of this type of disorder would be:
   a. galactosemia.
   b. medium-chain acyl-CoA dehydrogenase (MCAD) deficiency.
   c. phenylketonuria (PKU).
   d. glutaric acidemia type 1 (GA1).

4. The disorder that is identified by increased blood glutaryl-carnitine on newborn screening is characterized by dysfunctional metabolism of:
   a. hydroxylysine and phenylalanine.
   b. tyrosine and tryptophan.
   c. tryptophan, hydroxylysine, and lysine.
   d. cystine and hydroxylysine.

5. In a disorder that has an autosomal recessive inheritance pattern, what is the risk of two carrier parents having an affected child with that disorder?
   a. 0%
   b. 25%
   c. 50%
   d. 100%

6. In relation to newborn screening for inborn errors of metabolism (IEMs), second-tier testing is done to:
   a. assess the parents of the newborn for possible carrier status.
   b. assess the siblings of the newborn for similar symptoms or disorders.
   c. determine the number of false negatives that might have occurred with initial screening.

d. further assess a positive screening test result by targeting more specific analytes.

7. The disorder of amino acid metabolism in which the parent amino acid accumulates in blood and spills over into urine is classified as:

a. an organic acidemia.

b. an aminoacidopathy.

c. a carbohydrate disorder.

d. a disorder of fatty acid oxidation.

8. The simultaneous analysis of multiple analytes using a single sample, such as a blood spot from a newborn, is referred to as:

a. multiplex analysis.

b. newborn screening.

c. tandem mass spectrometry (MS/MS).

d. multiple of means.

9. The enzyme that is absent in the aminoacidopathy phenylketonuria (PKU) is:

a. phenylalanine decarboxylase.

b. ornithine translocase.

c. phenylalanine hydroxylase.

d. succinyl-coenzyme A (CoA) mutase.

## SUGGESTED READINGS

Anderson DR, Viau K, Botto LD, Pasquali M, Longo N. Clinical and biochemical outcomes of patients with medium-chain acyl-CoA dehydrogenase deficiency. *Mol Genet Metab.* 2020;129(1):13–19.

Berry GT. Classic galactosemia and clinical variant galactosemia. In: Adam MP, Ardinger HH, Pagon RA, Wallace SE, eds. *GeneReviews [Internet].* Seattle: University of Washington; 1993–2017.

Burton BK. Newborn screening for Pompe disease: an update, 2011. *Am J Med Genet C Semin Med Genet.* 2012;160C:8–12.

Chace DH. Mass spectrometry in newborn and metabolic screening: Historical perspective and future directions. *J Mass Spectrom.* 2009;44:163–170.

Chien YH, Hwu WL, Lee NC. Pompe disease: Early diagnosis and early treatment make a difference. *Pediatr Neonatol.* 2013;54:219–227.

De Biase I, Gherasim C, La'ulu SL, Asamoah A, Longo N, Yuzyuk T. Laboratory evaluation of homocysteine remethylation disorders and classic homocystinuria: Long-term follow-up using a cohort of 123 patients. *Clin Chim Acta.* 2020;509:126–134.

de Ru MH, Boelens JJ, Das AM, et al. Enzyme replacement therapy and/or hematopoietic stem cell transplantation at diagnosis in patients with mucopolysaccharidosis type I: Results of a European consensus procedure. *Orphanet J Rare Dis.* 2011;6:55.

Guthrie R, Susi A. A simple phenylalanine method for detecting phenylketonuria in large populations of newborn infants. *Pediatrics.* 1963;32:338–343.

Hedlund GL, Longo N, Pasquali M. Glutaric acidemia type 1. *Am J Med Genet C Semin Med Genet.* 2006;142C:86–94.

Hobert JA, De Biase I, Yuzyuk T, Pasquali M. Quantitative analysis of urine acylglycines by ultra-performance liquid chromatography-tandem mass spectrometry (UPLC-MS/MS): Reference intervals and disease specific patterns in individuals with organic acidemias and fatty acid oxidation disorders. *Clin Chim Acta.* 2021;523:285–289.

Kubaski F, Vairo F, Baldo G, de Oliveira Poswar F, Corte AD, Giugliani R. Therapeutic options for mucopolysaccharidosis II (Hunter Disease). *Curr Pharm Des.* 2020;26(40):5100–5109.

Longo N, Frigeni M, Pasquali M. Carnitine transport and fatty acid oxidation. *Biochim Biophys Acta.* 2016;1863:2422–2435.

Manzoni F, Salvatici E, Burlina A, Andrews A, Pasquali M, Longo N. Retrospective analysis of 19 patients with 6-pyruvoyl tetrahydropterin synthase deficiency: prolactin levels inversely correlate with growth. *Mol Genet Metab.* 2020;131(4):380–389.

Matern D, Gavrilov D, Oglesbee D, Raymond K, Rinaldo P, Tortorelli S. Newborn screening for lysosomal storage disorders. *Semin Perinatol.* 2015;39:206–216.

Saleem H, Simpson B. *Biotinidase Deficiency.* Treasure Island: StatPearls; 2022. PMID: 32809442.

Schwarz E, Liu A, Randall H, et al. Use of steroid profiling by UPLC-MS/MS as a second tier test in newborn screening for congenital adrenal hyperplasia: The Utah experience. *Pediatr Res.* 2009;66:230–235.

Shigematsu Y, Hata I, Tajima G. Useful second-tier tests in expanded newborn screening of isovaleric acidemia and methylmalonic aciduria. *J Inherit Metab Dis.* 2010;33:S283–S288.

Therrell Jr BL, Lloyd-Puryear MA, Camp KM, Mann MY. Inborn errors of metabolism identified via newborn screening: ten-year incidence data and costs of nutritional interventions for research agenda planning. *Mol Genet Metab.* 2014;113:14–26.

van Spronsen FJ, Blau N, Harding C, Burlina A, Longo N, Bosch AM. Phenylketonuria. *Nat Rev Dis Primers.* 2021;7(1):36.

Viau K, Ernst SL, Vanzo RJ, Botto LD, Pasquali M, Longo N. Glutaric acidemia type 1: outcomes before and after expanded newborn screening. *Mol Genet Metab.* 2012;106:430–438.

Vogel BH, Bradley SE, Adams DJ, et al. Newborn screening for X-linked adrenoleukodystrophy in New York state: diagnostic protocol, surveillance protocol and treatment guidelines. *Mol Genet Metab.* 2015;114:599–603.

Wong D, Tortorelli S, Bishop L, et al. Outcomes of four patients with homocysteine remethylation disorders detected by newborn screening. *Genet Med.* 2016;18:162–167.

# 46

# Pharmacogenetics

*Gwendolyn A. McMillin, Mia Wadelius, and Victoria M. Pratt*

## OBJECTIVES

1. Define the following:
   a. Adverse drug reaction (ADR)
   b. Prodrug
   c. Haplotype
   d. Pharmacogenetics
   e. Pharmacokinetics
   f. Pharmacodynamics
2. Provide examples of pharmacogene-drug pairs that are associated with each of these three drug response processes: pharmacokinetics, pharmacodynamics, and immune response.
3. Explain how the CYP2D6 phenotype could predict a poor response to codeine and other prodrugs that are substrates of CYP2D6.
4. Explain how multiple pharmacogenes affect the therapeutic dose of warfarin.
5. Explain how genetic testing is used to evaluate whether or not a patient is a good candidate for ivacaftor.

## KEY WORDS AND DEFINITIONS

**Activity score** A numeric description of enzymatic activity (phenotype). A normal function allele is assigned a score of 1. Decreased function, no function and increased function alleles are assigned scores less than or greater than 1, as described for a specific pharmacogene. The composite activity score is the sum of the scores associated with each allele that is detected in a haplotype. As such, an activity score of 2 correlates with a prediction of normal enzyme activity.

**Adverse drug reaction (ADR)** Any undesirable side effect or toxic reaction that is caused by the administration of a drug.

**Allele** One of the alternative versions of a gene at a given location (locus) along a chromosome. An individual typically inherits two alleles for each gene, one from each parent. If the two alleles are the same, the individual is homozygous for that locus. If the alleles are different, the individual is heterozygous. The term now also refers to variation among noncoding DNA sequences in addition to genes.

**Cytochrome P450 (CYP)** A large family of metabolic enzymes that catalyze the oxidation of organic substrates. They are important in the metabolism of drugs, steroid hormones, fatty acids, and other substances.

**Drug metabolism** The process by which drugs are chemically modified in the body, typically by drug-metabolizing enzymes. Most but not all drugs are metabolized.

**Gene duplication** A process by which a chromosome or a portion of DNA is duplicated, resulting in an additional partial or full copy or copies of a gene. Duplication events are not always quantified and the actual number of copies cannot always be translated into clinical function. A gene duplication event may be described as a copy number greater than 2.

**Genotype** The genetic makeup of an individual. An individual's genotype codes for that individual's phenotype. The genotype for a specific gene requires knowledge of both alleles of the gene.

**Genotyping** Laboratory testing designed to detect specific genetic variants that are used to identify and classify variant alleles. The alleles are reported together as a genotype that may or may not be predictive of a phenotype.

**Haplotype** A combination of alleles on the same chromosome that are usually located close together and tend to be inherited together.

**International normalized ratio (INR)** A method of reporting prothrombin time results for patients receiving oral anticoagulant therapy such as warfarin.

**Metabolite** A chemically modified form of a compound. Drug metabolites may or may not exhibit pharmacological activity. There are often many metabolites of a single drug, some of which may be identical to independently administered drugs.

**Metabolizer classification** A classification of drug-metabolism phenotypes as they relate to an individual's metabolic efficiency for processing a specific therapeutic drug. The five best recognized types are poor metabolizers (PMs), intermediate metabolizers (IMs), normal metabolizers (NMs), rapid metabolizers (RMs), and ultrarapid metabolizers (UMs).

**Pharmacodynamics** A process in pharmacology that defines how a drug acts on its target and its mechanisms of action.

**Pharmacogene** A gene that is known to influence the pharmacokinetics and/or pharmacodynamics of a drug.

**Pharmacogenetics** Study of the variations in single genes or small groups of related genes that affect the response to a drug, including its metabolism.

**Pharmacogenomics** The study of how combinations of variations in several genes, potentially extending to the complete genome, influence the pharmacology of a drug or drugs.

**Pharmacokinetics** A process in pharmacology that describes primarily how a drug is absorbed, distributed, metabolized, and eliminated.

**Phenotype** The observable physical or biochemical characteristics of an individual as determined by his or her genetic makeup and environmental influences, including drug-drug or food-drug interactions.

**Prodrug** A drug that is administered in an inactive or poorly active form and converted to an active drug by metabolism.

**Pseudogene** A defective segment of DNA that resembles a gene but cannot be transcribed.

**Star (\*)-allele nomenclature** A nomenclature developed to standardize genetic polymorphism annotation for many pharmacogenes, such as the cytochrome P450 genes.

## PRINCIPLES OF PHARMACOGENETICS

The term **pharmacogenetics** comes from merging the terms *pharmacology* and *genetics*. Pharmacogenetics can predict and/or explain how individuals respond to drugs and is a prominent component of personalized precision medicine. Related work associating drug response with **pharmacogenes**, and ultimately the whole genome, is known as **pharmacogenomics**, although the terms are commonly used interchangeably. Pharmacogenetics and pharmacogenomics can apply to the human germline genome, tumor genomes (e.g., somatic mutations), and pathogen genomes (e.g., viral genomes). The goal of this chapter is to explain concepts and provide examples of human pharmacogenetics, with an emphasis on germline variants. Targeted variants of some pharmacogenes and specific applications to drugs are described.

### Drug Response

For simplicity, the term *drug(s)* is used throughout this chapter to reflect any foreign compound absorbed by the human body that is capable of evoking a physiologic or behavioral response. Responses to drugs depend on many variables such as drug formulation, route of administration, age, gender, clinical status (e.g., kidney function, liver function,

protein status), comedications, and genetics. Most drugs are selected and initially dosed according to drug labeling, clinical experience, and institutional protocols that stem from population-based dosage and dose frequency recommendations. However, dose optimization still largely relies on trial and error. Minimizing this process of trial and error with pharmacogenetics can improve efficacy of drugs and prevent **adverse drug reactions**.

Pharmacogenetic testing is designed to predict specific aspects of the two major processes upon which drug response is based: pharmacokinetics and pharmacodynamics. **Pharmacokinetics** describes how the body acts on a drug, often called ADME, referring to absorption, distribution, metabolism, and elimination. Pharmacogenes that encode drug-metabolizing enzymes and transport proteins are involved in pharmacokinetics. Parent drugs that are administered as inactive compounds and require metabolism to convert the compound to an active drug are called **prodrugs**. Drug **metabolites** can be pharmacologically active or inactive. Therefore, it is important to consider whether pharmacogenetic variation influences the concentrations or kinetics of pharmacologically active or inactive compounds. Fig. 46.1 illustrates the common metabolic relationship for prodrugs, active drugs, and metabolites (active

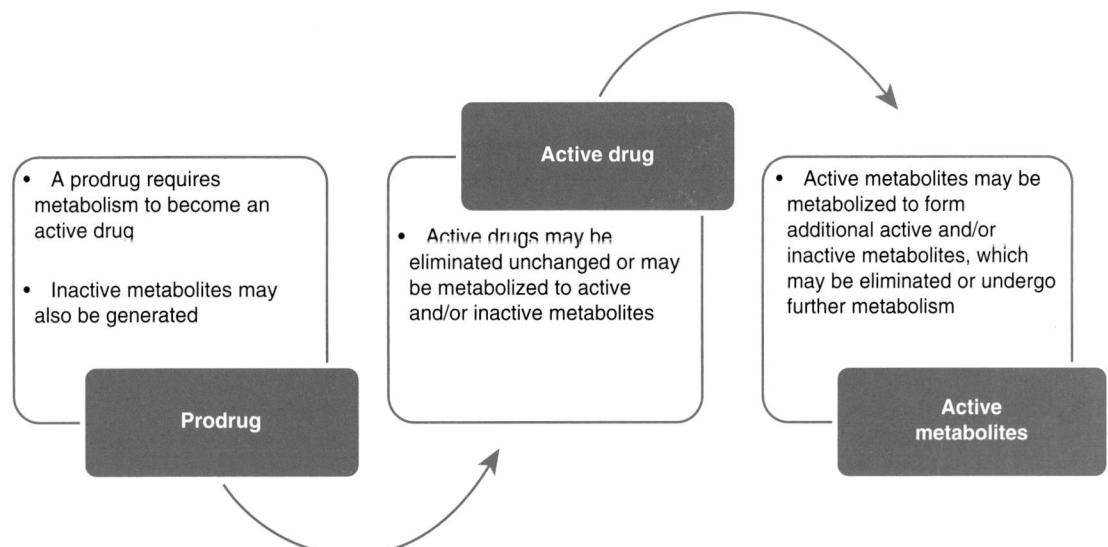

**Fig. 46.1** Schematic relationships between prodrugs, active drugs, and metabolites.

and/or inactive). **Pharmacodynamics** describes how the body responds to drugs, both desirable (e.g., therapeutic) and undesirable (e.g., therapeutic failure and/or toxicity). Pharmacogenes that encode for mechanistic proteins such as enzymes, receptors, and ion channels are involved in pharmacodynamics. Sometimes drugs cause adverse effects due to mechanisms that are unrelated to the intended use of the drug. For example, carbamazepine, a drug used to treat seizures and neuropathic pain largely by inhibiting voltage-gated sodium channels, can stimulate the immune system, leading to a severe cutaneous adverse reaction that can be life-threatening. The risk of this adverse reaction is increased in the presence of the *HLA-B\*15:02* allele, representing variation in the genes that code for the human leukocyte antigen (HLA) system, and is unrelated to the mechanisms responsible for managing seizures and pain. The adverse reaction is also unrelated to the pharmacokinetics of carbamazepine. Pretherapeutic testing to detect this allele in people being considered for carbamazepine therapy is recommended for vulnerable populations, particularly people of Asian descent.

Many different pharmacogenes can be associated with the pharmacokinetics and pharmacodynamics of a single drug. In selecting drugs and drug dosing for an individual, one should consider the clinically significant pharmacogenes in combination with relevant clinical, demographic and nongenetic factors. After drug and dose are selected, response to the drug should be monitored. If the response is desirable (therapeutic), the pharmacokinetics and pharmacodynamics are appropriate. Therapeutic failure may occur if the concentrations of active drug are insufficient (e.g., pharmacokinetic variability) or if the physiology required to elicit the response to the drug is absent or impaired (e.g., pharmacodynamic variability). If the response is not optimal or is undesirable, therapy may have to be adjusted. The dose of a drug is adjusted based on results of clinical measurements (e.g., blood pressure for antihypertensive drugs), therapeutic drug monitoring (TDM), or monitoring of biochemical markers indicating response.

The goal of TDM is to adjust the dose to achieve blood concentrations of active drug that fall within an established therapeutic range at particular times after dose administration. This practice of dose adjustment is common to immunosuppressant drugs such as tacrolimus or anticonvulsant drugs such as carbamazepine. Thus, blood specimens are collected at specific times after the drug is administered. The dose is adjusted to achieve concentrations that consistently fall within the therapeutic range selected for the patient population and clinical indication, noting that pharmacokinetic variation can contribute to differences in time to achieve stable drug concentrations, called achieving steady state. For certain drugs, pretherapeutic pharmacogenetic testing can guide drug selection, determine the initial drug dose, and predict the time required to achieve steady state.

An example of a biochemical marker of response is the **international normalized ratio (INR)**, which is calculated from the prothrombin time (PT) test (Box 46.1); it is used to guide and adjust doses of the common anticoagulant drug warfarin. As with TDM, blood samples are collected at specific times

after the administration of warfarin. The dose is adjusted until the INR consistently falls within a target range, selected for the patient population and clinical indication. The target INR range is set to 2.0 to 3.0 for most indications. Pretherapeutic pharmacogenetic testing can guide the initial dose of warfarin and predict the time required to achieve steady state.

Adverse drug reactions that are dose-dependent are managed by adjusting the dose of a drug based on clinical response or laboratory monitoring of drug concentrations and/or biomarkers. Inappropriate dosing of tacrolimus, carbamazepine, or warfarin can lead to adverse drug reactions. Adverse drug reactions that occur independent of dose require an alternate drug. The carbamazepine-induced hypersensitivity is an example. Thus, carbamazepine can produce both types of adverse reactions (dose dependent and dose independent).

---

**POINTS TO REMEMBER**

**Phenotypes** for drug metabolizing enzyme activity and/or gene expression may be classified as:
- Ultrarapid (UM) or rapid (RM) metabolizer: more than normal is expected/observed.
- Normal metabolizer (NM): normal is expected/observed.
- Intermediate metabolizer (IM): less than normal is expected/observed.
- Poor metabolizer (PM): little or no enzyme activity is expected/observed.

---

## Implementation and Logistics of Pharmacogenetics

Pharmacogenetic testing is intended to predict and/or explain discrete aspects of pharmacokinetics and pharmacodynamics to guide drug and dose selection. Once a drug is initiated, the response is monitored and dosing optimized with clinical and/or laboratory tools. It is not practical, medically indicated, or cost-effective to apply pharmacogenetics to every drug therapy situation. The pharmacogenetic tests that are the most successful are those that produce actionable results. Many resources for labeling information, gene–drug

---

**BOX 46.1    International Normalized Ratio (INR)**

INR = [(PT result for the patient)/(PT result for a normal control)]ISI
- Established by the World Health Organization and the International Committee on Thrombosis and Hemostasis.
- Standardizes reporting of the prothrombin time (PT) test, a common method of evaluating how many seconds it takes for a person's blood to clot.
- Includes an international sensitivity index (ISI) that compensates for variability in laboratory methods (usually 1.0–2.0).
- A typical therapeutic range of the INR for a patient treated with warfarin is 2.0–3.0.

associations, and clinical consensus guidelines are maintained and updated electronically. Some specific examples of gene–drug relationships for which US Food and Drug Administration (FDA) and European Medicines Agency (EMA) labeling includes pharmacogenetic information are shown in Table 46.1. Nearly all medical specialties can benefit from pharmacogenetic testing, and the number of clinically useful targets will only increase as comprehensive pharmacogenetic testing becomes more widely available with analytic techniques such as massively parallel sequencing.

## Specimens

Most pharmacogenetic testing revolves around genetic testing (as opposed to phenotype testing). DNA extracted from blood, saliva, buccal cells, or other specimens from which DNA can be obtained are used. Specimens for DNA testing do not require special timing or patient preparation in most situations. Saliva or buccal cells may be preferred due to the noninvasive nature of collection, but this may not produce a sufficient quantity or quality of DNA for all applications.

## Analytic Strategies

The analytic strategy used in pharmacogenetic testing depends on a variety of factors, such as the complexity of the gene; the extent, frequency, and type of genetic variation; and the time needed for return of the results. Most genotyping assays cannot detect all variants in a gene. If the need for a rapid time to result is clinically indicated, an assay may be designed to limit complexity, as through targeted detection of the most common and clinically relevant variants. Commercially available in vitro diagnostics (IVDs) are available for some pharmacogenetic applications and may reduce the complexity of testing and data analysis in order to reduce the time to result. However, most pharmacogenetic testing is based on laboratory-developed approaches designed to target specific gene variants, and performed at a central or reference laboratory. Clinical laboratories that offer pharmacogenetic testing in the US can be found through the voluntary National Institutes of Health Genetic Testing Registry.

Laboratory services may include a single-gene or multiple-gene panels where known variants are interrogated. Targeted genotyping will not detect any variant or alleles that are not directly interrogated, so a negative genotyping result does not rule out the possibility that an individual has another variant not detected by the assay. Multiple-gene panels may be achieved through exome or whole-genome sequencing. Exome sequencing is able to identify only those variants near to and including the coding regions of genes. This approach cannot identify intergenic differences, including structural and noncoding variants, which can be found by whole-genome sequencing. Massively parallel sequencing platforms available today have additional limitations, including the following: decreased coverage in regions with high GC content (e.g., the 5′ ends of genes), limited detection of copy number variants, limited detection of insertions/deletions, and interference from pseudogenes. These technical limitations are expected to improve if not resolve over time. However, rare and novel variants will likely be of uncertain clinical significance, causing difficulty in interpretation. Novel combinations of variants may also be identified by sequencing, which will necessitate the evolution of nomenclature and may affect phenotype predictions. Currently whole-genome sequencing is not practical for routine pharmacogenetics applications owing to the high costs and time associated with sequencing and interpretation.

## Gene Dose (Copy Number)

Human DNA is normally associated with two copies of each gene, one copy inherited from each parent for autosomal regions on each chromosome. However, many genetic

## TABLE 46.1 Gene–Drug Examples with Published Guidelines and Drug Labeling Comments

| Gene (or Allele) | Generic Drug Name | PUBLISHED GUIDELINES | | | COMMENT IN DRUG LABELING[a] | |
| | | CPIC | DPWG | EMA | Testing Required or Recommended | Actionable |
|---|---|---|---|---|---|---|
| HLA-B*57:01 | Abacavir | Yes | Yes | Yes | X | — |
| CYP2D6 CYP2C19 | Amitriptyline | Yes | Yes | No | — | X |
| HLA-B*15:02 | Carbamazepine | Yes | No | Yes | X[b] | — |
| CYP2C19 | Clopidogrel | Yes | Yes | Yes | — | X |
| CYP2D6 | Codeine | Yes | Yes | No | — | X |
| DPYD | Capecitabine/5-Fluorouracil | Yes | Yes | Yes | X | |
| CFTR | Ivacaftor | Yes | No | Yes | X | — |
| TPMT | Mercaptopurine | Yes | Yes | Yes | X | — |
| CYP2C9 | Siponimod | No | Yes | Yes | X | — |
| CYP2C9 VKORC1 | Warfarin | Yes | No | No | — | X |

[a]Comments in drug labeling are provided as examples and are subject to change.
[b]In patients with ancestry in genetically at-risk populations, mainly the Asian population.
CPIC, Clinical Pharmacogenetics Implementation Consortium; DPWG, Dutch Pharmacogenomics Working Group; EMA, European Medicines Agency.

regions display a variation in the number of copies and are termed copy number variants (CNVs). CNVs can range in size from 1 kilobase to several megabases due to deletion, insertion, duplication, or complex recombination. CNVs in some pharmacogenes play a clear role in predicting drug efficacy and toxicity. One example is the human CYP2D locus, which contains two pseudogenes, *CYP2D7* and *CYP2D8*, closely located and evolutionarily related to *CYP2D6*, and thus facilitates homologous crossovers and the formation of large gene conversions, deletions, duplications, and multiplications of CYP2D6. CNVs are not always included in analytic methods designed for genotyping.

## Haplotyping

Many of the pharmacogenes exhibit combinations of variants—for example, single-nucleotide variants (SNVs) and insertion-deletions (indels) within a gene that are inherited together on the same chromosome and are referred to as haplotypes. Many nomenclature systems have been developed to describe pharmacogenetic haplotypes. In the most commonly used nomenclature system, combinations of pharmacogenetic sequence variants are designated by star (*) alleles, where *1 is usually designated as normal (commonly referred to as wild-type or fully functional), and numbered star alleles are assigned as new variants are identified. Pragmatically the *1 allele is assigned by default when none of the targeted variant alleles are detected. Therefore, the true accuracy of a *1 allele designation depends on whether the assay detects all variants that are known.

## Reporting

The results of clinical pharmacogenetic testing should be reported using current nomenclature. Pharmacogenetic nomenclature is constantly evolving, and laboratories or users of laboratory services might not be familiar with most current nomenclature. Therefore, test results should be provided in current nomenclature, which should include clarifications of commonly used terms and should indicate the genotypes detected.

In general, which variants/alleles should be interrogated and reported for the pharmacogenes is not standardized. In addition, some assays use different combinations of variants to define or infer the haplotypes that the assay detects, which ultimately can lead to discrepancies in star allele genotypes between platforms. Laboratories are required by the Clinical Laboratory Improvement Amendment (CLIA) to include interpretation of the test results on the test report. Clinical pharmacogenetic laboratories often provide an interpreted phenotype (e.g., poor metabolizer) based on the genotype results. Laboratories that are accredited by the College of American Pathologists (CAP) are required to include a summary of methods and the variants that can be detected on the report, but overall the lack of consensus for pharmacogenetic nomenclature and variable assay designs add to the complexity of analyzing and reporting results from pharmacogenetic assays. Efforts to standardize assay content are being led by the Association for Molecular Pathology (AMP) and testing

recommendations for clinical laboratories have been published. Tier 1 recommendations define the minimum set of variant alleles to be included in clinical testing.

## Clinical Interpretation

Pharmacogenetic testing is clinically useful only when information is sufficient to support clinical interpretation of the results. This information must be derived from human studies. Many examples of this type of information can be found in the peer-reviewed literature. One limitation of the existing literature, however, is that most data are based on retrospective studies, and there is no single source in which all of this information has been collated. The Pharmacogenetics and Pharmacogenomics Knowledge Base (PharmGKB) is a publicly available electronic research tool developed at Stanford University through a nationwide collaborative research consortium. Its aim is to share information about how genetic variation among individuals contributes to differences in response to drugs. In addition, the Pharmacogene Variation (PharmVar) Consortium was introduced in September 2017 as a central electronic repository and resource for nomenclature and allele classifications.

Many ongoing clinical trials designed to study the efficacy and toxicity of new pharmaceutical products or new indications for previously developed pharmaceuticals have employed pharmacogenetic testing. In addition, drugs that were previously removed from development because of adverse drug reactions or poor therapeutic response may be reconsidered if a genetic test can be demonstrated to identify individuals who are likely to respond favorably to the drug. For each of the major pharmacogenes discussed in this chapter, Table 46.1 provides a list of some common drugs with pharmacogenetic associations that are included in drug labels in the US and European Union. Because many other drug-gene combinations are recognized, the discussion provided here is in no way comprehensive. The specific examples discussed further on can be used as a guide for translating the principles of pharmacogenetics to additional gene–drug pairs in this continually evolving field of laboratory medicine.

## SPECIFIC EXAMPLES OF PHARMACOGENE ASSOCIATIONS

### Associations with Pharmacokinetics

#### Drug-Metabolizing Enzymes

Most drugs are metabolized by at least one cytochrome P450 (CYP) enzyme. CYPs are classified into families and further into subfamilies based on amino acid homology. Using *CYP2D6* as an example, the naming convention for CYPs is shown in Fig. 46.2, illustrating that the core name of the gene and protein is shared, identifying the family, subfamily and polypeptide, also referred to as the isozyme. The variant allele designations follow the name of the protein. When referring to a gene, the name should be italicized, whereas the name of the associated protein should not be.

Genetic variants of CYPs have been associated with changes in enzyme activity, stability, and/or substrate (e.g.,

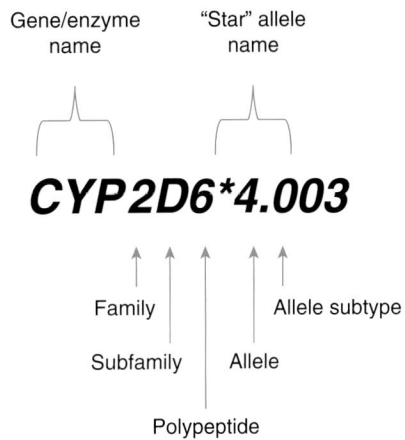

Gene/enzyme name      "Star" allele name

**CYP2D6\*4.003**

Family      Allele subtype

Subfamily      Allele

Polypeptide

Fig. 46.2 Description of the nomenclature for the *CYP2D6\*4.003* allele.

drug or drug metabolite) affinity that can lead to clinically significant phenotypes. Alleles for all CYP genes are described according to international consensus, based on the star (*) nomenclature described earlier, often followed by a number after a decimal point to describe an allele subtype. Subtypes do not usually influence the clinical phenotype but could be important for haplotype assignment or to support research studies.

*Cytochrome P450 2D6 (CYP2D6).* CYP2D6 is one of the most important drug-metabolizing enzymes, as it is responsible for metabolizing approximately 25% of all drugs and is commonly involved in drug–drug interactions. Tier 1 recommended alleles for *CYP2D6* are shown in Table 46.2 with the predicted functional consequences. Although the definition of an allele may involve detection of many variants, a common SNV is frequently chosen as the primary analytic target used to detect each allele (bolded). In many cases, however, detection of other variants is required to accurately classify an allele. For example, the *CYP2D6* c.100C>T variant is present in many alleles, some are shown in Table 46.2. Misclassification of *CYP2D6\*4* or *CYP2D6\*36* as *CYP2D6\*10* would incorrectly predict the phenotype. Allele frequencies vary among populations.

The assignment of phenotype predictions from the *CYP2D6* genotype is described in Table 46.3. An alternate approach to phenotype characterization is the assignment of activity scores. Drug-specific dosing guidelines for *CYP2D6*, and many other pharmacogenes have been published by the Clinical Pharmacogenetics Implementation Consortium (CPIC) and other organizations such as the Dutch Pharmacogenomics Working Group (DPWG).

Drug–drug or food–drug interactions often occur at the level of drug metabolism and are of particular concern under circumstances when multiple medications are prescribed and used by a single patient at one time. Drugs can be classified as inducers as well as strong, moderate, or weak inhibitors (Box 46.2). Some drugs may be both substrates and inducers or inhibitors for the same enzyme. A well-recognized food–drug interaction is the inhibition of CYP3A4 by grapefruit juice. For a person who is genetically an intermediate, normal, or rapid metabolizer, the metabolic phenotype may be modified by drug–drug interactions. For a person who is genetically a poor metabolizer, drug–drug and/or food–drug interactions are not expected to affect drug and dose selections because the lack of enzyme activity cannot be induced, or further inhibited.

**Codeine application.** Codeine is a widely used medication, prescribed for pain management and to suppress coughing. Codeine must be activated by metabolism to morphine. This occurs through a demethylation reaction mediated primarily by CYP2D6 (Fig. 46.3). Therefore, a CYP2D6 poor metabolizer would not activate codeine and should avoid this drug owing to the lack of predicted efficacy. An intermediate metabolizer may require higher doses of codeine than a normal metabolizer. The guidelines published by the CPIC suggest that alternative analgesia be sought should a CYP2D6 intermediate metabolizer fail to respond to codeine. In a typical normal metabolizer, approximately 10% of a codeine dose is converted to morphine. Administration of codeine to a person with the ultrarapid metabolizer phenotype is a significant safety concern because higher than expected concentrations of morphine can be produced, leading to the risk of unintentional overdose and opioid toxicity. For example, when nursing women with an ultrarapid metabolizer phenotype for CYP2D6 are prescribed codeine, their babies can be exposed to higher than expected morphine concentrations in the breast milk. Children who receive codeine for pain control after tonsillectomy and adenoidectomy and are ultrarapid metabolizers, are also vulnerable to potentially deadly opioid-induced respiratory depression. An ultrarapid metabolizer should therefore avoid codeine owing to the potential for toxicity. A similar pharmacogenetic vulnerability to toxicity exists for other opioids that utilize CYP2D6 for activation, such as tramadol.

*Cytochrome P450 2C family.* The CYP2C family includes four genes that code for enzymes named CYP2C8, CYP2C9, CYP2C18, and CYP2C19. CYP2C9 and CYP2C19 are commonly involved in drug metabolism. Genotype-based dosing guidelines have been proposed for some CYP2C9 and CYP2C19 substrates, sometimes in combination with other pharmacogenes. Tier 1 recommendations for *CYP2C9* testing include low activity alleles *CYP2C9\*2*, *CYP2C9\*3*, *CYP2C9\*5*, *CYP2C9\*6*,

**TABLE 46.2  Examples of Common Star (\*) Allele Definitions for *CYP2D6***

| Allele | Nucleotide Changes (RefSeqGene LRG_303 (NG_008376.4) ATG Start\*)[a] | Effect | Enzyme Function |
|---|---|---|---|
| *CYP2D6\*1* | None | — | Normal function |
| *CYP2D6xN* | More than two copies (multiple copies) | Depends on allele | Increased for functional alleles; no effect for no function alleles |
| *CYP2D6\*2* | 2851C>T, 4181G>C | p.Arg296Cys, p.Ser486Thr | Normal function |
| *CYP2D6\*3* | **2550delA** | p.Arg259fs | No function |
| *CYP2D6\*4* | **1847G>A** | Splicing defect | No function |
| *CYP2D6\*5* | Gene deletion | — | No function |
| *CYP2D6\*6* | **1708delT** | p.Trp152fs | No function |
| *CYP2D6\*9* | **2616delAAG** | p.Lys281del | Decreased function |
| *CYP2D6\*10* | **100C>T**, 4181G>C | p.Pro34Ser, p.Ser486Thr | Decreased function |
| *CYP2D6\*17* | **1022C>T**, 2851C>T, 4181G>C | p.Thr107Ile, p.Arg296Cys, p.Ser486Thr | Decreased function |
| *CYP2D6\*29* | **3184G>A**, **1660G>A**, **1662G>C**, 2851C>T, 4181G>C | p.Val338Met, p.Val136Ile, p.Arg296Cys, p.Ser486Thr | Decreased function |
| *CYP2D6\*41* | **2989G>A**, 2851C>T, 4181G>C | Splicing defect, p.Arg296Cys, p.Ser486Thr | Decreased function |

[a]When known, *bold* nucleotide variants represent the major alterations responsible for the effect.

**TABLE 46.3  Summarized Assignment of CYP2D6 Phenotype**

| Predicted Function of Star (\*) Allele | Diplotype Description | Predicted Phenotype Based on Diplotype | Predicted Activity Score Based on Diplotype |
|---|---|---|---|
| Increased function | More than two copies of normal functional alleles (e.g., \*1/\*1xN) | Ultrarapid metabolizer (~2% of people[a]) | >2.25 |
| Normal function | Two copies of functional or one functional and one decreased-function alleles (e.g., \*1/\*1, \*1/9) | Normal metabolizer (~80% of people[a]) | 1.25 ≤ x ≤ 2.25 |
| Decreased function | One decreased-function allele and one no function allele, two decreased function alleles, one normal or decreased function allele and one no function allele (e.g., \*9/\*4, \*9/\*9, \*1/\*4) | Intermediate metabolizer (~10% of people[a]) | 0 < x < 1.25 |
| No function | Two or more copies of no function alleles (e.g., \*4/\*4) | Poor metabolizer (~8% of people[a]) | 0 |

[a]Actual prevalence is population-dependent; percentages shown here represent published estimates for the general population.

*CYP2C9\*8*, and *CYP2C9\*11*. Tier 1 recommendations for *CYP2C19* testing include the low activity alleles *CYP2C19\*2* and *CYP2C19\*3*, and the increased activity allele *CYP2C19\*17*.

**Clopidogrel application.** Clopidogrel inhibits platelet aggregation and is widely used in combination with aspirin to reduce the incidence of thrombotic and ischemic events in patients with coronary artery disease or acute coronary syndrome and/or after percutaneous coronary intervention with stenting. Yet many patients do not achieve adequate platelet inhibition; rates of drug resistance are estimated at 30% and are partly due to the fact that clopidogrel is a prodrug. Intermediate and poor CYP2C19 metabolism is associated with reduced formation of the active metabolite of clopidogrel, poor clopidogrel-induced platelet inhibition, and a higher incidence of major thrombotic events. The CPIC guidelines recommend drugs that do not require bioactivation by CYP2C19, such as prasugrel or ticagrelor, for CYP2C19 intermediate and poor metabolizers. No dose adjustment for clopidogrel is recommended for patients with the CYP2C19 increased activity allele.

**Antidepressant application.** Antidepressant therapy is challenging because several weeks of consistent drug dosing are typically required to assess efficacy, and side effects are common. Optimizing drug therapy is typically an exercise of trial and error. Many antidepressant medications available today are substrates of CYP2D6 and/or CYP2C19. As such, these two genes are widely included in guidelines used to select appropriate medications to minimize trial and error. For example, both CYP2D6 and CYP2C19 are critical for metabolism of amitriptyline, a common tricyclic antidepressant (TCA). CYP2D6 is critical for paroxetine and CYP2C19 is critical for citalopram, examples of selective serotonin reuptake inhibitors (SSRI). As such, it may be prudent to avoid these drugs in patients predicted to exhibit either poor or rapid metabolizer phenotypes for the relevant CYP enzyme(s). Drug–drug interactions must also be considered when selecting antidepressant therapy because antidepressant drugs may be used in combination, which could impact the drug response phenotype and associated dose requirements. Bupropion, fluoxetine and paroxetine are examples of CYP2D6 strong inhibitors; fluoxetine is also a strong inhibitor of CYP2C19.

*Dihydropyrimidine dehydrogenase.* Dihydropyrimidine dehydrogenase (DPD) is an important enzyme in the

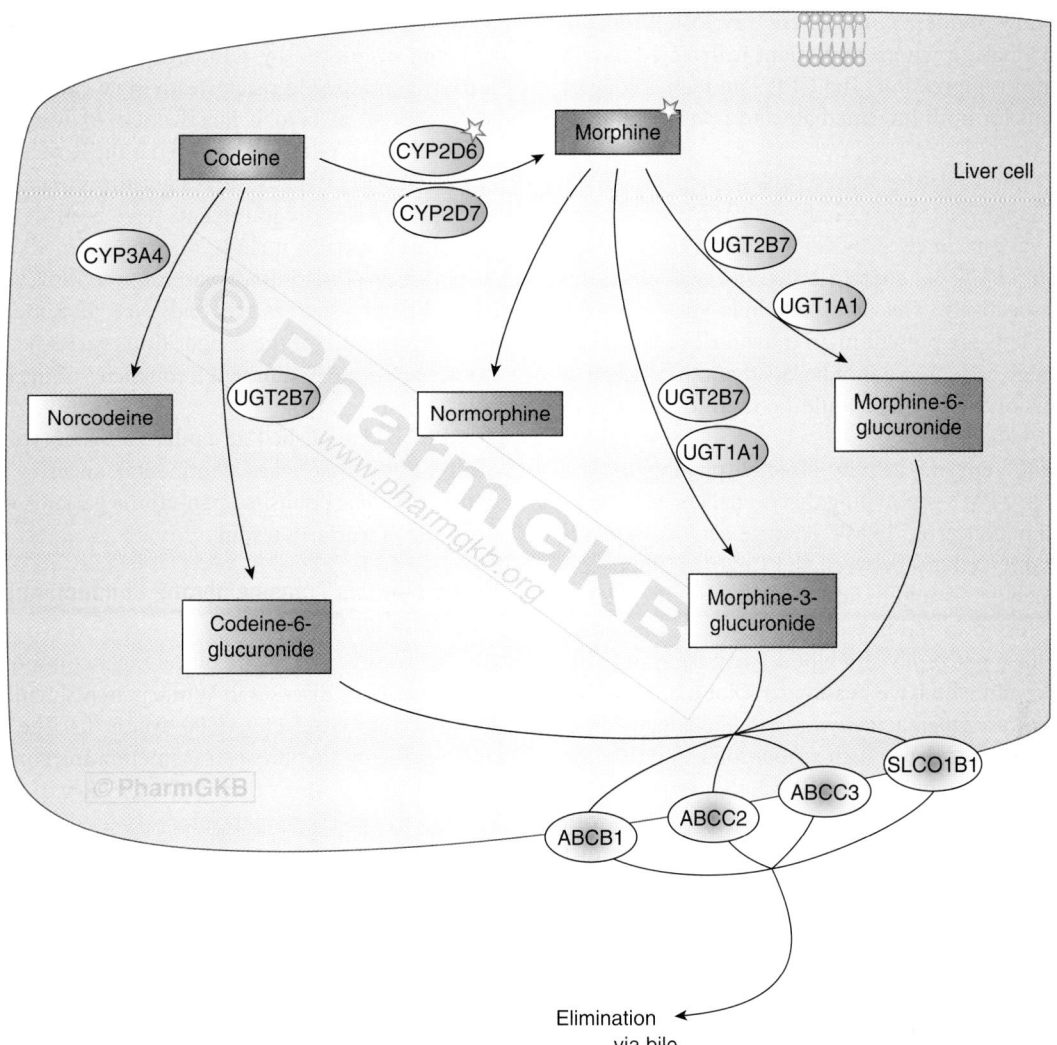

**Fig. 46.3** Schematic illustration of codeine pharmacokinetics. *Boxes* indicate the drug analytes (codeine and metabolites) and the *ovals* indicate the genes that code for drug metabolizing enzymes. Codeine is the prodrug. Morphine is the primary active metabolite, formed through a reaction mediated by CYP2D6. The *stars* indicate the importance of this metabolic activation. All other metabolites are thought to have little to no pharmacological activity. (From Thorn CF, Klein TE, Altman RB. Codeine and morphine pathway. *Pharmacogenet Genomics* 2009;19:556–558. Reproduced with permission from the copyright holder, PharmGKB and Stanford University.)

metabolic pathway of pyrimidines (e.g., thymine and uracil) and is also involved in the metabolic inactivation of fluoropyrimidine drugs. This enzyme is coded by *DPYD* and it is known that variation in the gene can lead to partial or complete enzyme deficiency. DPD deficiency contributes to dose-related toxicity when exposed to fluoropyrimidine drugs (i.e., 5-fluorouracil, capecitabine, tegafur) that are widely used to treat breast, colorectal and other types of cancer. Both capecitabine and tegafur are inactive prodrugs that are metabolized to 5-fluorouracil. There are several routes through which 5-fluorouracil is subsequently activated to exert its intended pharmacodynamic effects. However, more than 80% of 5-fluorouracil is typically inactivated by DPD. Human genome variation society (HGVS) or Single Nucleotide Polymorphism Database (dbSNP) nomenclature is used to describe *DPYD* variants. Loss of function alleles such as c.1905+1G>A (rs3918290) will lead to accumulation of active drug and

potentially fatal adverse effects. As such, clinical guidelines that recommend a 50% reduction in starting dose for patients who are heterozygous for a no function *DPYD* variant (partial DPD deficiency), along with careful patient monitoring. An alternate therapy is recommended when complete DPD deficiency is predicted (homozygous or compound heterozygous).

***Thiopurine S-methyltransferase and nudix hydrolase 15.***
Thiopurine S-methyltransferase (TPMT) and nudix hydrolase 15 (NUDT15) are metabolic enzymes that catalyze the inactivation of thiopurine drugs (i.e., azathioprine, mercaptopurine, and thioguanine) which are used for the treatment of childhood acute lymphoblastic leukemia, autoimmune diseases, inflammatory bowel diseases, lupus, and for preventing rejection after transplantation. With conventional doses of thiopurines, individuals who inherit two loss-of-function *TPMT* or *NUDT15* alleles universally experience severe myelosuppression; a high proportion of heterozygous

individuals show moderate to severe myelosuppression, whereas individuals in whom no variant is detected have a low risk of myelosuppression. The CPIC guidelines suggest dose reductions for both intermediate and poor metabolizers (Table 46.4).

The star (*) nomenclature is used to describe both *TPMT* or *NUDT15* haplotypes. For example, *TPMT*3A* contains two missense variants *in cis*, c.460G>A and c.719A>G, while *TPMT*3B* and *TPMT*3C* contain only one, c.460G>A and c.719A>G, respectively. The assumed diplotype is *1/*3A when both variants are present in an individual of European descent, although *3B/*3C cannot be ruled out. If *3B/*3C is suspected, phenotypic testing should be used to distinguish between *1/*3A and *3B/*3C.

Testing TPMT enzyme activity directly (phenotyping) is an alternative to *TPMT* genotyping that is challenged by storage and stability concerns. TPMT enzyme activity depends on stable enzyme activity between the times of blood collection and analytic testing. In addition, because the TPMT enzyme is expressed in red blood cells, testing is limited to patients who have not received a blood transfusion over the previous weeks and who have healthy red blood cells, which is often not the case when acute lymphoid leukemia is diagnosed. Coadministered drugs such as ibuprofen and thiazide diuretics may inhibit enzyme activity such that an inaccurate phenotype prediction may be assigned. Nonetheless, as with other pharmacogenetics applications designed to predict metabolic phenotype, dose optimization requires clinical and/or therapeutic drug monitoring.

## Associations with Pharmacodynamics
### Vitamin K Epoxide Reductase Complex Subunit 1 and Warfarin Application

Warfarin is an oral anticoagulant now largely replaced by the modern non-vitamin K dependent oral anticoagulants. Individual response to warfarin is highly variable and is monitored by the INR (see Box 46.1). A primary target for warfarin's actions is the vitamin K epoxide reductase complex subunit 1 (Fig 46.4). Individuals having a promoter variant allele of vitamin K epoxide reductase gene (*VKORC1*) are more sensitive to warfarin because less of the target protein

is expressed. As a consequence, such individuals are at risk of being overdosed by standard doses. Therapeutic dose of warfarin and time to reach steady state concentrations is also impacted by metabolic inactivation of warfarin, mediated primarily by CYP2C9, and by vitamin K recycling, which is impacted by CYP4F2. Several algorithms that predict individual warfarin dose requirements have been developed. These algorithms usually include the common *VKORC1* genetic variant, as well as common variants of *CYP2C9*, *CYP4F2*, and clinical factors such as age, body size, and interacting drugs. The performance of these algorithms varies between populations, partly due to different frequencies of the included variables.

CPIC has published an update on genotype-guided warfarin dosing that takes continental ancestry into account while AMP has published pan-ethnic variants that should be included in warfarin testing.

### Cystic Fibrosis Transmembrane Conductance Regulator and Ivacaftor Application

Cystic fibrosis (CF) is one of the most common lethal autosomal recessive diseases in White patients, with an estimated incidence of 1 in 2500 to 3300 live births. The gene mutated in CF is the cystic fibrosis transmembrane conductance regulator (*CFTR*). More than 1800 *CFTR* variants have been identified. HGVS nomenclature is used to describe these pathogenic variants leading to a complex multisystem disease that affects the respiratory tract, pancreas, intestine, male genital tract, hepatobiliary system, and exocrine system. There is, however, wide variability in clinical presentation, severity, and the rate of disease progression between affected individuals, which can be influenced by the underlying *CFTR* genotype as well as other genetic modifiers and environmental factors.

Traditionally, the treatment of CF has focused on ameliorating symptoms (e.g., fighting infection, thinning mucus, and reducing inflammation) rather than directly targeting the genetic cause. CF modulator therapies (e.g., ivacaftor, lumacaftor/ivacaftor, tezacaftor/ivacaftor, elexacaftor/tezacaftor/ivacaftor) are designed to correct the malfunctioning protein made by *CFTR* by improving the transport of sodium

---

**TABLE 46.4    Dosing for Mercaptopurine by TPMT Phenotype as Recommended by the Clinical Pharmacogenetics Implementation Consortium**

| Predicted TPMT Phenotype | Examples of Diplotypes | Dosing Recommendations |
|---|---|---|
| Normal metabolizer | *1/*1 | Use label-recommended dosage and administration. Adjust based on degree of myelosuppression and disease-specific guidelines. Allow 2–4 weeks to reach steady state after each dose adjustment. |
| Intermediate metabolizer | *1/*2, *1/*3A, *1/*3B, *1/*3C, *1/*4 | Reduce dose by 30%–80% and adjust based on degree of myelosuppression and disease-specific guidelines. Allow 2–4 weeks to reach steady state after each dose adjustment. |
| Poor metabolizer | *3A/*3A, *2/*3A, *3C/*3A, *3C/*4, *3C/*2, *3A/*4 | Reduce daily dose by 10-fold and dose thrice weekly instead of daily; adjust based on degree of myelosuppression and disease-specific guidelines. Allow 4–6 weeks to reach steady state after each dose adjustment. For nonmalignant conditions, consider a nonthiopurine alternative. |

through the CFTR ion channel. CFTR modulators have been approved by the US Food and Drug Administration (FDA) for individuals with the specific CF pathogenic variants, including p.F508del, one of the most common pathogenic variants in most populations. Coadministration of CYP3A inducers (e.g., rifampin, St. John's wort) that substantially decrease exposure is not recommended.

## Human Leukocyte Antigen Complex and Applications

The HLA complex is a cornerstone of the immune system because of its involvement in the identification of foreign proteins. The HLA proteins produced from the associated genes are expressed on the surface of nearly all cells, where they bind to peptides that are displayed to the circulating cells of the immune system. If the immune system recognizes the peptides

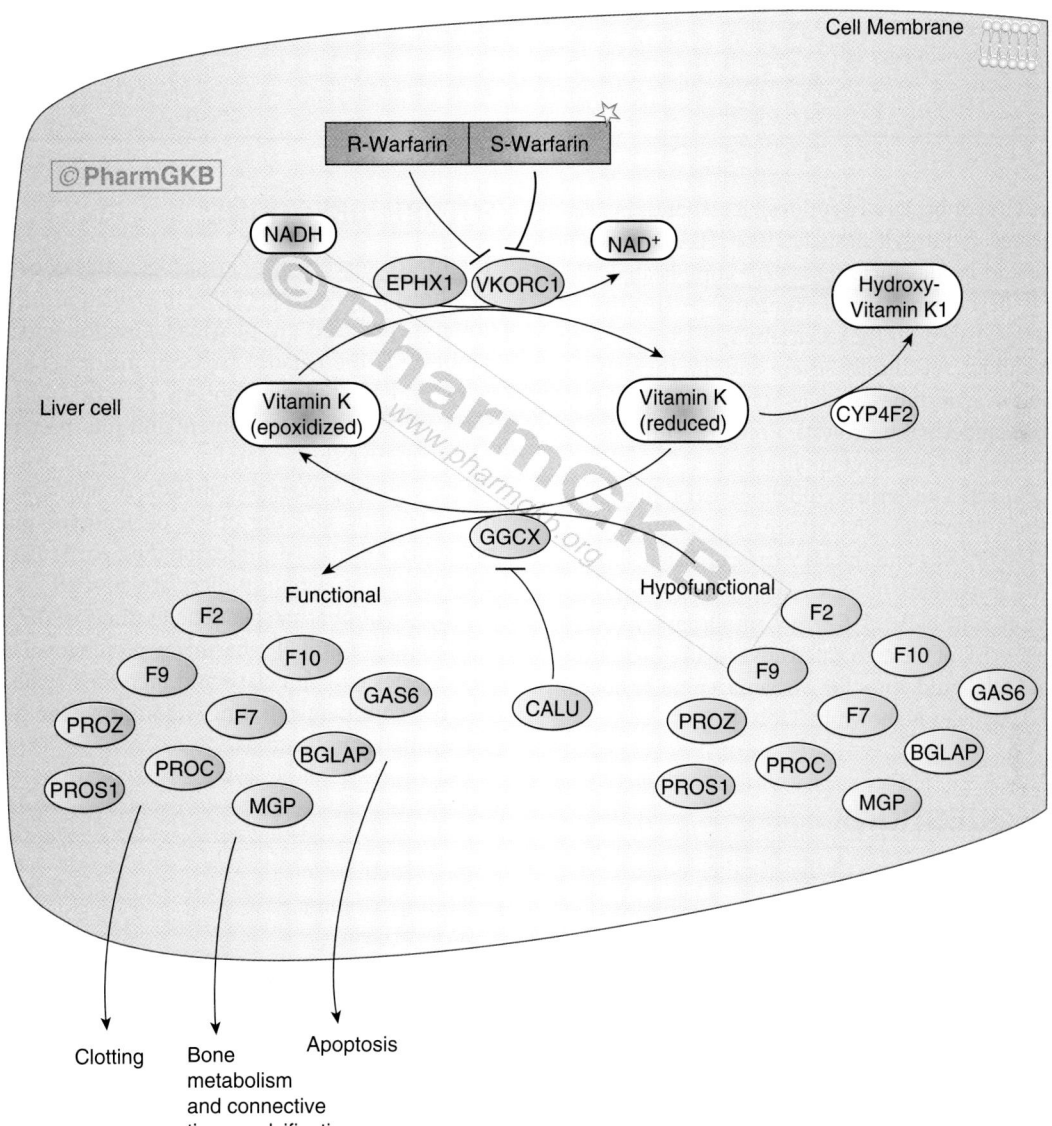

**Fig. 46.4** Schematic illustration of warfarin pharmacodynamics. *Boxes* show the two enantiomers of warfarin. *Rounded boxes* indicate cofactors important for reductive metabolism and *ovals* indicate genes that code for enzymes or coagulation factors. Warfarin is administered as a racemic mixture of R- and S-enantiomers with S-warfarin being the more potent inhibitor of vitamin K epoxide reductase (VKORC1) in the vitamin K cycle. Other enzymes involved in the vitamin K cycle are epoxide hydrolase 1 (EPHX) and gamma-glutamyl carboxylase (GGCX). The vitamin K cycle is further regulated by calumenin (CALU) that inhibits GGCX and by oxidation of reduced vitamin K by cytochrome P450 4F2. The vitamin K cycle activates the coagulation factors FII, FVII, FIX and FX, and proteins C, S and Z into their functional forms. Other vitamin K-dependent proteins activated are the apoptotic growth arrest specific 6 (GAS6); the bone gamma-carboxyglutamate (Gla) protein (BGLAP), which regulates bone remodelling; and the matrix Gla protein (MGP), which inhibits osteogenic factors. (From Whirl-Carrillo M, McDonagh EM, Hebert JM, et al. Pharmacogenomics knowledge for personalized medicine. *Clin Pharmacol Ther* 2012;92:414–417. Reproduced with permission from the copyright holder, PharmGKB, and Stanford University.)

**TABLE 46.5    Dosing for Carbamazepine and Phenytoin with *HLA-B\*15:02* and Abacavir with *HLA-B\*57:01* as Recommended by the Clinical Pharmacogenetics Implementation Consortium**

| Phenotype/Genotype | Implications for Outcome | Dosing Recommendations |
|---|---|---|
| **HLA-B\*15:02** | | |
| Absence of *15:02* alleles (may be reported as "negative" on a genotyping test) | Low or reduced risk of carbamazepine and phenytoin-associated hypersensitivity | Use label-recommended dosage and administration. |
| Presence of at least one *15:02* allele (may be reported as "positive" on a genotyping test) | Increased risk of carbamazepine or and phenytoin hypersensitivity | Select alternative drug; avoid use of carbamazepine and phenytoin. |
| **HLA-B\*57:01** | | |
| Absence of *57:01* alleles (may be reported as "negative" on a genotyping test) | Low or reduced risk abacavir hypersensitivity | Use label-recommended dosage and administration. |
| Presence of at least one *57:01* allele (may be reported as "positive" on a genotyping test) | Increased risk of abacavir hypersensitivity | Select alternate drug; avoid use of abacavir. |

as foreign (e.g., viral or bacterial peptides), it responds by triggering the infected cell to self-destruct. The HLA complex is highly variable and its classification is very complicated. The *HLA-B* gene is best characterized from the perspective of pharmacogenetics, based on the association of variants with drug hypersensitivity, specifically severe and life-threatening cutaneous reaction syndromes, such as Stevens–Johnson syndrome and toxic epidermal necrolysis. Pretherapeutic testing has been recommended for select applications.

Published clinical consensus guidelines exist for *HLA-B\*15:02* and the anticonvulsants carbamazepine and phenytoin and for *HLA-B\*57:01* and the HIV drug abacavir. Typing of *HLA-B\*15:02* in patients of East Asian origin, where this allele is common, and of *HLA-B\*57:01* in all patients, substantially reduces risk of the associated adverse drug reaction. A summary of CPIC guidelines for carbamazepine or abacavir based on HLA alleles is shown in Table 46.5.

## FUTURE DIRECTIONS

The future success of pharmacogenetics depends on understanding the following: (1) the interrelationship of the various proteins involved in pharmacokinetics and pharmacodynamics, (2) the balance between major versus minor pathways, and (3) the mechanisms of action of specific drugs. Standardization of test content and interpretation is needed. Although massively parallel sequencing will increase the complexity of pharmacogenetics, it will also improve our understanding and the utility of genotype-phenotype relationships. Additional clinical studies, particularly prospective and outcome-related studies, are needed to guide implementation of pharmacogenetic findings in the clinic. Finally, closer integration of pharmacy professionals with clinical laboratories and clinicians and increased availability of cost-effective commercial testing will improve the success of pharmacogenetic applications.

## REVIEW QUESTIONS

1. How a drug elicits responses, whether the responses are desirable or undesirable, is described by which one of the following?
   a. Pharmacodynamics
   b. Phenocopying
   c. Pharmacokinetics
   d. Pharmacogenetics
   e. Pharmacogenomics
2. A drug that is administered in an inactive form that must be metabolized to an active form is referred to as a(n):
   a. cytochrome P450 (CYP) enzyme.
   b. haplotype.
   c. prodrug.
   d. poor metabolizer.
   e. drug metabolite.
3. Which of the following is an active drug that gets inactivated by metabolism?
   a. Clopidogrel
   b. Codeine
   c. Capecitabine
   d. Warfarin
   e. Tramadol
4. What is the drug-metabolizing phenotype when an individual has two no function alleles?
   a. Normal metabolizer
   b. Intermediate metabolizer
   c. Rapid metabolizer
   d. Poor metabolizer
   e. Ultrarapid metabolizer
5. What drug has a severe dose-independent adverse drug reaction that can be predicted by genotyping?
   a. Abacavir
   b. Azathioprine
   c. Capecitabine
   d. Ivacaftor
   e. Warfarin

# SUGGESTED READINGS

Alfirevic A, Pirmohamed M. Genomics of adverse drug reactions. *Trends Pharmacol Sci.* 2017;38:100–109.

Caudle KE, Dunnenberger HM, Freimuth RR, et al. Standardizing terms for clinical pharmacogenetic test results: consensus terms from the Clinical Pharmacogenetics Implementation Consortium (CPIC). *Genet Med.* 2017;19:215–223.

Caudle KE, Keeling NJ, Klein TE, Whirl-Carrillo M, Pratt VM, Hoffman JM. Standardization can accelerate the adoption of pharmacogenomics: current status and the path forward. *Pharmacogenomics.* 2018;19:847–860.

Caudle KE, Sangkuhl K, Whirl-Carrillo M, et al. Standardizing CYP2D6 genotype to phenotype translation: consensus recommendations from the Clinical Pharmacogenetics Implementation Consortium and Dutch Pharmacogenomics Working Group. *Clin Transl Sci.* 2020;13:116–124.

Gaedigk A, Casey ST, Whirl-Carrillo M, Miller NA, Klein TE. Pharmacogene Variation Consortium: A global resource and repository for pharmacogene variation. *Clin Pharmacol Ther.* 2021;110:542–545.

Luzum JA, Pakyz RE, Elsey AR, et al. Pharmacogenomics Research Network Translational Pharmacogenetics Program. *Clin Pharmacol Ther.* 2017;102:502–510.

Maggo SD, Savage RL, Kennedy MA. Impact of new genomic technologies on understanding adverse drug reactions. *Clin Pharmacokinet.* 2016;55:419–436.

Mathias PC, Hendrix N, Wan WJ, et al. Characterizing pharmacogenomic-guided medication use with a clinical data repository. *Clin Pharmacol Ther.* 2017;102:340–348.

Pratt VM, Cavallari LH, Del Tredici AL, et al. Recommendations for clinical CYP2C9 genotype allele selection: a joint recommendation of the Association for Molecular Pathology and the College of American Pathologists. *J Mol Diagn.* 2019;21:746–755.

Pratt VM, Cavallari LH, Del Tredici AL, et al. Recommendations for clinical warfarin genotyping allele selection: a report of the Association for Molecular Pathology and the College of American Pathologists. *J Mol Diagn.* 2020;22:847–859.

Pratt VM, Cavallari LH, Del Tredici AL, et al. Recommendations for clinical CYP2D6 genotyping allele selection: a joint consensus recommendation of the Association for Molecular Pathology, College of American Pathologists, Dutch Pharmacogenomics Working Group of the Royal Dutch Pharmacists Association, and the European Society for Pharmacogenomics and Personalized Therapy. *J Mol Diagn.* 2021;23:1047–1064.

Pratt VM, Del Tredici AL, Hachad H, et al. Recommendations for clinical CYP2C19 genotyping allele selection: a report of the Association for Molecular Pathology. *J Mol Diagn.* 2018;20:269–276.

Relling MV, Klein TE, Gammal RS, Whirl-Carillo M, Hoffman JM, Caudle KE. The Clinical Pharmacogenetics Implementation Consortium: 10 years later. *Clin Pharmacol Ther.* 2020;107:171–175.

Shekhani R, Steinacher L, Swen JJ, Ingelman-Sundberg M. Evaluation of current regulation and guidelines of pharmacogenomic drug labels: opportunities for improvements. *Clin Pharmacol Ther.* 2020;107:1240–1255.

Tayeh MK, Gaedigk A, Goetz MP, et al. Clinical pharmacogenomic testing and reporting: a technical standard of the American College of Medical Genetics and Genomics (ACMG). *Genet Med.* 2022;24:759–768.

# Principles of Molecular Biology

*John Greg Howe*

## OBJECTIVES

1. Compare and contrast the structure and function of DNA and RNA.
2. Identify five different types of RNA in the cell and describe their functions.
3. Detail how the information in DNA is used to make protein through transcription and translation.
4. Describe the genetic code and why it is important.
5. Describe three reversible reactions on histones that can increase accessibility for transcription, repair, or replication.
6. Describe the spectrum of genomic variations found in cancer.

## KEY WORDS AND DEFINITIONS

**Alleles**  Different variants of a gene.

**Base pair**  Complementary base pairing of guanine and cytosine and adenine and thymine through hydrogen bonding.

**Centromere**  The region of a chromosome between the small and long arms that is used during mitosis to attach the spindle fibers.

**Chromatin**  A structure in the eukaryotic nucleus composed of DNA and histone proteins.

**Chromosome**  A nucleic acid structure bound by protein containing all or a portion of an organism's genetic information.

**Codon**  A three-base code found in messenger RNA, used in translation to specify the amino acid to be incorporated in the growing polypeptide chain.

**Deoxyribonucleic acid (DNA)**  Repository of the genetic material in an organism.

**DNA methylation**  Addition of a methyl group to a cytosine, used to regulate gene expression.

**Epigenetics**  Modifications that affect DNA packaging and accessibility without changing the DNA sequence.

**Eukaryote**  An organism that contains a nucleus and whose DNA is in chromosomes.

**Exon**  Portion of a gene that codes for protein.

**Restriction endonuclease**  An enzyme that cuts in the middle of a stretch of DNA at a specific sequence of bases.

**Gene**  DNA structure that codes for the production of a protein.

**Gene expression**  Synthesis of a gene product in the form of an RNA or protein from a gene.

**Genetic code**  Collection of three base sequences called *codons* used to translate the nucleic acid information into amino acids during protein synthesis.

**Genome**  The complete genetic content of an organism.

**Genotype**  The unique genetic information of an organism or cell.

**Histones**  Basic proteins that bind to DNA to form nucleosomes, basic units of chromatin.

**Intron**  DNA between exons that do not code for protein and are removed by RNA splicing.

**Mutation**  A disease-causing sequence variation. Historically the term has been interchangeable with *variant* to describe any change in a DNA sequence regardless of its relation to disease causation. For current clinical descriptions or reporting, the use of *mutation* is reserved for the scenario when disease causation is known. The preferred nomenclature for a disease-causing variation is now "pathogenic" or "likely pathogenic" variant. There is also an evolving tendency to describe whether a DNA variant causes disease within a specific clinical context.

**Nucleases**  Enzymes that cleave DNA to smaller fragments.

**Nucleic acid**  A polymer made of nucleotides consisting of a sugar, a phosphate group, and a nitrogenous base.

**Nucleosome**  A unit of DNA that contains 146 bases and is wound around 8 histone proteins.

**Nucleotide**  A basic unit of DNA and RNA consisting of a sugar, a phosphate group, and a nitrogenous base.

**Polymerase**  A protein that is able to connect individual molecules into a single strand.

**Promoter**  A DNA sequence usually upstream from the start of transcription of the gene that regulates its expression.

**Purine**  A double-ring structure that constitutes the foundation for adenine and guanine, two of the bases in DNA.

**905**

**Pyrimidine** A single ring structure that constitutes the foundation for thymine and cytosine, two of the bases in DNA and uracil, one of the bases of RNA.

**Recombination** The rearrangement of DNA through the breaking and rejoining of DNA strands to create a different sequence.

**Replication** The process that synthesizes a copy of an organism's DNA.

**Ribonucleic acid (RNA)** A polymer made of ribonucleotides consisting of ribose, a phosphate group, and four bases—guanine, adenine, cytosine, and uracil.

**Ribosome** A subcellular structure that functions to convert messenger RNA to protein.

**Spliceosome** A structure that functions to remove introns from a heterogeneous RNA and splice the remaining exons together to form a messenger RNA.

**Telomere** A repetitive DNA sequence at the end of a chromosome.

**Transcription** The biologic process that copies the information in DNA into RNA.

**Translation** The biologic process that uses ribosomes to convert RNA to protein.

**Variant** Any sequence variation, whether or not it results in disease.

## BACKGROUND

Molecular diagnostics and its parent field, molecular pathology, examine the origins of disease at the molecular level, primarily by studying nucleic acids. Deoxyribonucleic acid (DNA), which contains the blueprint for constructing a living organism, is the centerpiece for research and clinical analysis. Molecular pathology is an outgrowth of the enormous amount of successful research in the field of molecular biology that has discovered the basic biologic and chemical processes of how a living cell functions. Molecular biology is now used for clinical diagnosis and the development and use of therapeutics. In this chapter the fundamentals of molecular biology are reviewed.

## MOLECULAR BIOLOGY ESSENTIALS

Whether it is a bacterium, virus, or eukaryotic cell, their genetic material dictates their form and function. For the most part, the genetic material is DNA, which is composed of two strands of a sugar-phosphate backbone that are bound together by hydrogen bonds between purines and pyrimidines attached to the sugar molecule, deoxyribose, in a double helix (Figs. 47.1 and 47.2). DNA in human cells is wrapped around histone proteins and packaged into nucleosome units, which are compacted further to form chromosomes (Fig. 47.3). Each chromosome is a single length of DNA with a stretch of short repeats at the ends called telomeres and additional repeats in the centromere region. In humans, there are two sets of 23 chromosomes that are a mixture of DNA from the mother's egg and father's sperm. Each egg and sperm is therefore a single or haploid set of 23 chromosomes and the combination of the two creates a diploid set of human DNA, allowing each individual to possess two different sequences, genes, and alleles on each chromosome, one from each parent. Each child has a unique combination of alleles because of recombination between homologous chromosomes during meiosis in the development of gametes (egg and sperm cells). This creates genetic diversity within the human population. If a child has a random DNA sequence change, the child's genotype will be different from that inherited from either of the parents (de novo variant).

DNA is composed of genes that code for proteins and ribonucleic acid (RNA). For DNA to convert its store of vital information into functional RNA and protein, the DNA strands must separate so that RNA polymerase can bind to the gene. With the help of transcription factors that bind upstream to promoters, an RNA polymerase produces single strands of RNA that are further processed to remove the introns and retain the protein-encoding exons. The mature, processed RNA molecule, the messenger RNA (mRNA), migrates to the cytoplasm, where it is used in the production of protein.

To start the process of protein synthesis or translation, the mRNA is bound by various protein factors and a ribosome containing ribosomal RNA (rRNA) and additional protein. The mRNA-bound ribosome begins to produce a polypeptide chain by binding a methionine-bound transfer RNA (tRNA) to the mRNA's initiating AUG codon or triplet code. The conversion of the nucleic acid triplet code to a polypeptide is accomplished by additional specific tRNAs, which contain nucleic acid triplet codes (anticodons) and specific amino acids that are transferred to the growing polypeptide chain. After synthesis is complete, the protein migrates to its functional location and eventually is removed and degraded.

## NUCLEIC ACID STRUCTURE AND FUNCTION

DNA is a rather simple molecule with a limited number of components compared with those of proteins. DNA is composed of a deoxyribose sugar, phosphate linkages, and four nitrogen-containing bases. Deoxyribose contains five carbon atoms that are numbered from 1′ to 5′, starting with the carbon that will be attached to the base in DNA and progressing around the ring until the last carbon, which is attached to a phosphate. The bases consist of the purines, adenine and guanine and the pyrimidines, cytosine and thymine; an additional base, uracil, replaces thymine in RNA. The basic building block is the nucleotide, which consists of a deoxyribose sugar with an attached base at the 1′ carbon and a triphosphate group at the 5′ carbon. The triphosphate nucleotide is the building block for making newly

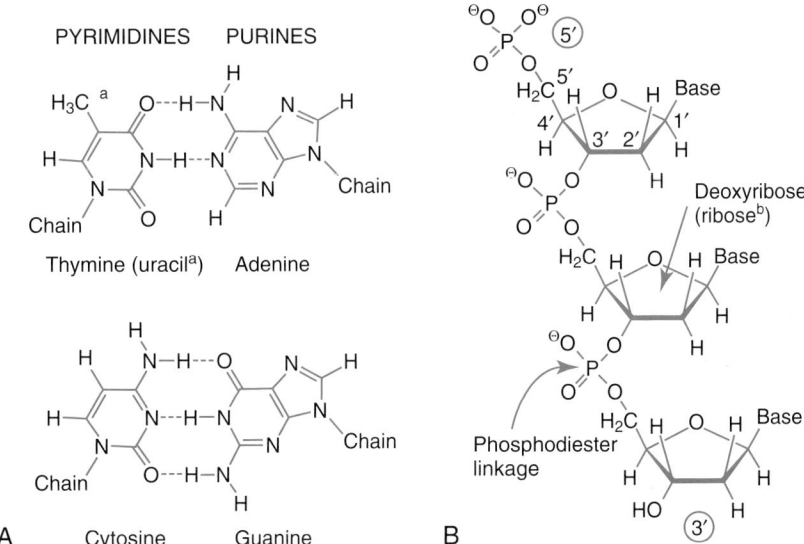

**Fig. 47.1** (A) Purine and pyrimidine bases and the formation of complementary base pairs. *Dashed lines* indicate the formation of hydrogen bonds. ([a]In RNA, thymine is replaced by uracil, which differs from thymine only in its lack of a methyl group.) (B) A single-stranded DNA chain. Repeating nucleotide units are linked by phosphodiester bonds that join the 5′ carbon of one sugar to the 3′ carbon of the next. Each nucleotide monomer consists of a sugar moiety, a phosphate residue, and a base. ([b]In RNA, the sugar is ribose, which adds a 2′-hydroxyl to deoxyribose.)

synthesized DNA, which then forms a polynucleotide chain that connects the individual nucleotides through the 5′ and 3′ carbons of each deoxyribose sugar via phosphodiester bonds.

## Structure of Deoxyribonucleic Acid

DNA is double-stranded, and the two strands bind to one another through hydrogen bonds between the bases on each strand. Hydrogen bonding is augmented by hydrophobic attraction (stacking) between bases on adjacent rungs of the DNA ladder. Both hydrogen bonds and base stacking are not covalent but are weak bonds that can be broken and reestablished. This important property is exploited by many of the methods that are used in molecular diagnostics. There are two hydrogen bonds between adenine (A) and thymine (T) and three hydrogen bonds between cytosine (C) and guanine (G); because of this difference in the number of hydrogen bonds, separating a guanine–cytosine (G–C) pair takes more energy than an adenine–thymine (A–T) pair (see Fig. 47.1).

Each of the two DNA strands is formed by a phosphate sugar backbone that starts at the 5′ phosphate and ends at a 3′ hydroxyl group, with the complementary bases binding to one another between the two phosphate sugar backbones (see Fig. 47.2). When the two strands are bound to one another, they run in opposite 5′ to 3′ directions called *an antiparallel configuration*. By convention, the DNA sequence is written in a 5′ to 3′ direction. As discussed later, both the **replication** of new DNA and the **transcription** of DNA to RNA progress in the 5′ to 3′ direction. In addition, the conversion of RNA to protein, a process called **translation**, proceeds from the 5′ end of the RNA to the 3′ end. Double-stranded DNA in living cells is generally found as a right-handed, B-DNA helix, which has specific dimensions. Each turn of the helix is 3.4 nm long and consists of 10 bases. The DNA sugar-phosphate

backbone is on the outside of the helix with the internal bases bound to their complement on the other strand by hydrogen bonds. Non-B DNA also occurs and can affect transcriptional control and genetic instability; it can also be disease-associated.

## Composition and Structure of Ribonucleic Acid

The composition of RNA is similar to that of DNA because it contains four nucleotides linked together by a phosphodiester bond, but with several important differences. RNA consists of a ribose sugar with a hydroxyl group at the 2′ carbon instead of the hydrogen atom in DNA. The bases attached to the ribose sugar are adenine, cytosine, and guanine but not thymine, because RNA uses another pyrimidine—uracil—as a substitute for thymine. Another difference between DNA and RNA is that RNA does not normally exist as two strands bound to one another, although a single strand can bind internally to itself, creating functionally important secondary structures. Although in the past several decades the complexity and number of different RNAs has greatly expanded, the most important cellular RNAs include mRNA, rRNA, and tRNA.

## Ribonucleic Acids Associated with Protein Production

mRNA is the most diverse group of the three major types of RNAs, but it constitutes only a small percentage of the total RNA. mRNAs are transcribed from DNA that codes for proteins and therefore are used as the template for the translation of proteins. mRNA is often modified by the addition of a 5′ end cap, which protects the mRNA from degradation, and a polyadenosine (polyA) sequence at the 3′ end. The production and processing of mRNA takes place in the nucleus, followed by transport to the cytoplasm, where it is translated.

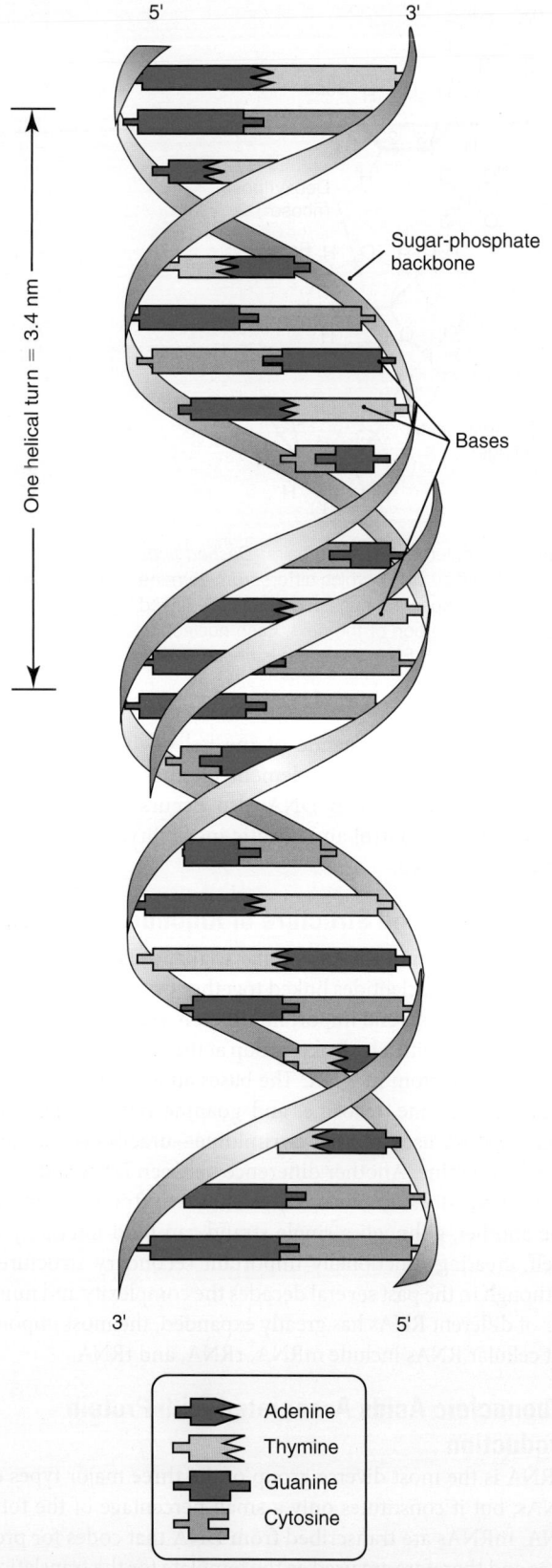

5'    3'

One helical turn = 3.4 nm

Sugar-phosphate
backbone

Bases

3'    5'

Adenine
Thymine
Guanine
Cytosine

**Fig. 47.2** The DNA double helix, with a sugar-phosphate backbone and pairing of the bases in the core-forming planar structures. (From Jorde LB, Carey JC, Bamshad MJ, eds. *Medical Genetics*, 4th ed. Philadelphia: Mosby; 2010.)

rRNA is associated with ribosomes, which are the primary structures that produce protein through the biologic process of translation. rRNA, unlike mRNA, does not code for proteins. In **eukaryotes**, the ribosome is composed of two structures, the 60S and 40S subunits, where the "S" stands for Svedberg units and is determined by the centrifugal sedimentation rate. The ribosome is a mixture of RNA and protein. rRNAs have secondary and tertiary structures that are well conserved with various loops, stem loops, and pseudoknots that contribute to their function. rRNA and protein, as the components of ribosomes, function to carry out the translation of proteins. The structure of the ribosome is now known, and the rRNA is more important than ribosomal proteins in ribosome functioning. The RNA acts as a catalytic agent called a *ribozyme*.

Another important group of RNAs are the tRNAs. These are molecules with a unique cloverleaf structure that translate the **genetic code** from nucleic acid triplets into amino acids that make up proteins. The 3′ ends of tRNAs are covalently attached to specific amino acids. In the middle of the tRNA structure is the anticodon sequence that binds to a specific codon in the mRNA. Therefore, the codon directs the binding of a specific tRNA linked to its corresponding amino acid. The genetic code specifies the appropriate amino acid in the growing polypeptide chain.

## CENTRAL DOGMA OF MOLECULAR BIOLOGY

The "central dogma" of molecular biology describes the transfer of genetic information into functional macromolecules. Genetic information moves from DNA to RNA via transcription using RNA polymerase and is further translated into protein via ribosomes. Since the initial introduction of the central dogma, a number of other postulated transfers have been described. DNA can enzymatically replicate itself by DNA polymerase, and RNA can be made into DNA using reverse transcriptase.

### Deoxyribonucleic Acid Replication

Synthesis or replication of new DNA uses one of the two original DNA strands as a template to make a new homologous strand and is termed *semiconservative replication*. Since DNA can be supercoiled into complex structures, a topoisomerase is required to first unfold the **chromatin** and nucleosomes so that the DNA is accessible. A DNA helicase then binds to the double-stranded DNA and separates the two strands, providing two single-stranded DNA templates. Replication progresses in a 5′ to 3′ direction; therefore, one strand, the leading strand, is synthesized as one continuous strand. The other strand, called the *lagging strand*, is synthesized discontinuously in small segments. The small fragments on the lagging strand are then linked by a ligase (Fig. 47.4).

DNA polymerases of various types have been identified; they function in many different roles, the most important being the replication of new DNA and the repair of existing DNA. Using the template strand as a guide, the DNA polymerase binds a nucleotide triphosphate to the primer at a

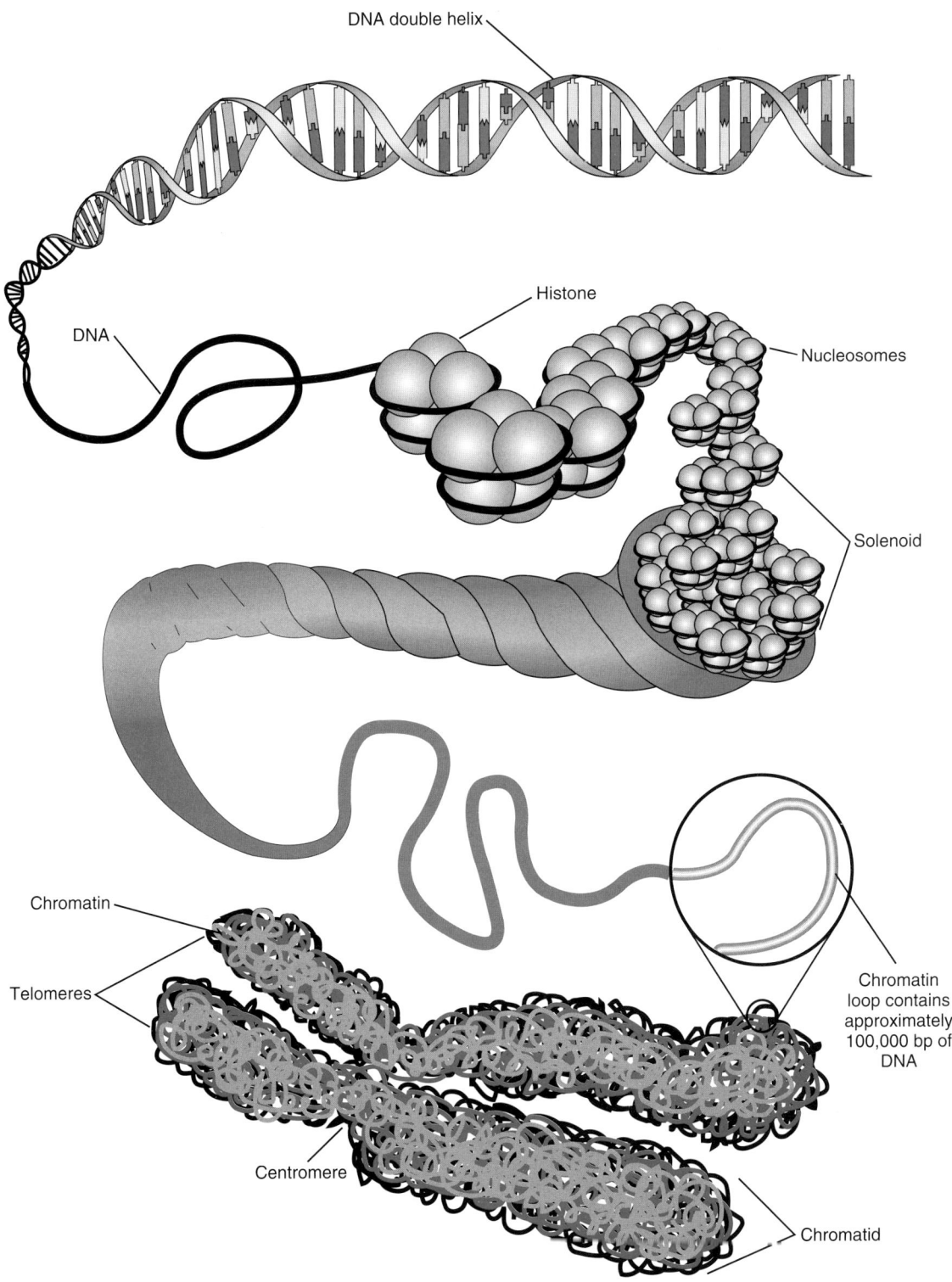

**Fig. 47.3** Structural organization of human chromosomal DNA. Double-stranded DNA is wound around the octamer core of histone proteins to form nucleosomes, which are further compacted into a helical structure called a *solenoid*. Nuclear DNA in conjunction with its associated structural proteins is known as *chromatin*. Chromatin is the most compact state of chromosomes. The primary constriction of a chromosome is the centromere, and the chromosome's ends are the telomeres. (From Jorde LB, Carey JC, Bamshad MJ, eds. *Medical Genetics*, 4th ed. Philadelphia: Mosby; 2010.)

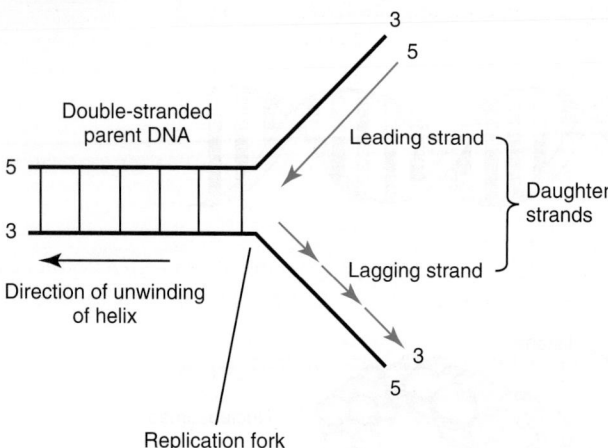

Fig. 47.4 DNA replication. Double-stranded DNA is separated at the replication fork. The leading strand is synthesized continuously, whereas the lagging strand is synthesized discontinuously but is joined later by DNA ligase.

free 3′ hydroxyl group, releasing pyrophosphate. The specific nucleotide selected depends on the base on the template strand; for example, an adenine nucleotide is used if a thymine nucleotide is in the template strand. In summary, a complementary sequence is synthesized opposite the template strand. Mistakes occur approximately every 100,000 nucleotides and a major function of some DNA polymerases is error correction or proofreading, accomplished by an intrinsic 3′ to 5′ exonuclease activity. DNA polymerases are important in molecular diagnostics because they are used in the polymerase chain reaction (PCR) and DNA sequencing.

DNA replication is part of the cell cycle and defines the synthesis (S) phase. Before the S phase is the first growth phase (G1). After the S phase is a second growth phase (G2), followed by a mitosis (M) phase. The M phase, which involves the splitting of one cell into two cells, occurs after the G2 phase and before the next G1 phase. Important control points in the cell cycle are between the G1 and S phases, just before it begins DNA replication, and between G2 and M phases, just as the cell commits to creating two cells from one. The G1/S boundary control point is disrupted in many cancers.

## Deoxyribonucleic Acid Repair

DNA can be damaged in a variety of ways that culminate in changes or mutations in the DNA sequence. DNA bases may be damaged, removed, cross-linked, or incorrectly paired with one another; single- or double-stranded breaks may also occur. When the cell senses that its DNA has become damaged, it stops the progression of its cell cycle and initiates DNA repair processes. Cells repair these lesions by employing multiple repair mechanisms that are specific for the type of DNA lesion and include base excision repair, nucleotide excision repair, mismatch repair, and homologous recombination repair.

Base excision repair removes bases that are chemically altered or damaged. Deamination of guanine, cytosine, and adenine transforms them into bases that cause incorrect base pairing, creating transition mutations, which are changes

between similar nitrogenous bases such as a purine to a purine. A transversion mutation is a change from a purine to a pyrimidine or vice versa. DNA glycosylases, such as uracil-DNA-glycosylase, cleave the damaged base, and a 5′-deoxyribose phosphate lyase removes the nucleotide upstream of the removed base. DNA polymerase and ligase then add a new nucleotide, repairing the damage.

Nucleotide excision repair removes base modifications that change the helical structure of DNA, including bulky DNA distortions and covalently bound structures that may be created by ultraviolet radiation and certain cancer drugs. After the repair is initiated, DNA is unwound and the gap is filled by DNA polymerase and finally sealed by DNA ligase.

Mismatch repair recognizes base incorporation errors and base damage. The mismatched nucleotides must be repaired on the newly synthesized strand of DNA. These mutations are corrected with DNA mismatch repair proteins that excise the surrounding sequence and then repair the excision with new sequence.

Double-stranded breaks may destabilize the genome, resulting in gross chromosomal changes such as translocations, which are frequently found in cancer. Double-stranded breaks are caused by ionizing radiation and chemotherapy drugs and are repaired by either homologous recombination or nonhomologous end joining. The homologous recombination repair pathway is initiated by recognition of a double-stranded break, followed by resection using exonucleases to create a 3′ single-stranded overhang. With the assistance of many proteins, the overhang invades the intact homologous double-stranded DNA of the sister chromatid and uses it as a template for new double-stranded DNA repair.

DNA repair mechanisms operate independently to repair simple lesions. However, the repair of more complex lesions involves multiple DNA processing steps regulated by the DNA damage-response pathway. When single- and double-stranded DNA breaks occur, a cascade of responses is initiated that culminate in either DNA repair, stopping the cell cycle, or programmed cell death.

## Deoxyribonucleic Acid Modification Enzymes

There are two groups of nucleases, the endonucleases that cut through the sugar-phosphate backbone and exonucleases that digest the ends of DNA. The commercially important restriction endonucleases, which bacteria have acquired to protect themselves from viral infections, are used to cleave DNA at a specific nucleotide sequence or restriction sites. Several thousand restriction endonucleases have been characterized and are used extensively to manipulate DNA in molecular biology and molecular diagnostics. Recent work has described new nucleases, such as the RNA-guided engineered nuclease CRISPR/Cas system, which can precisely cleave genomic DNA. The CRISPR-Cas technology has been used for human genome editing of patients with hematopoietic genetic diseases, such as sickle cell disease as well as for diagnostics such as COVID-19 testing.

DNA glycosylases are a family of enzymes associated with base excision repair; they are used in the first step of DNA repair to remove the damaged base without disrupting the sugar-phosphate backbone. An important member of that family, uracil DNA glycosylase, repairs the most common mutation found in humans, the spontaneous deamination of cytosine to uracil, by removing the uracil base.

## Gene Structure

The structure of prokaryotic genes is straightforward; almost all of the gene sequence is used to make protein; however, this is not the case with eukaryotic genes. One of the unique hallmarks of eukaryotic genes is that the protein-coding DNA is interspersed with regions that do not code for DNA. A mature mRNA retains only the protein-coding sequences, called *exons*; the sequences between the exons are non–protein-encoding sequences called *introns*, which are removed during mRNA maturation (Fig. 47.5).

## Ribonucleic Acid Transcription and Splicing

RNA transcription involves synthesizing an RNA strand using DNA as a template. This requires many different proteins, the most important being an RNA polymerase. Additional proteins function in combination to recognize and regulate the transcription of different genes. The synthesis of RNA proceeds in a 5′ to 3′ direction using DNA as a template, and a specific DNA sequence acts as a transcription start site. Transcription progresses through three phases: initiation, elongation, and termination. The initiation phase includes the binding of transcription factors to promoters upstream from the start site and includes the core promoter immediately upstream and the ancillary promoters further away. Transcription factors binding to upstream promoters act as regulators of the transcription of genes.

Important recurring sequences are found in some promoters. For example, some core promoters contain a TATAAA sequence, called a *TATA box*, located 25–40 nucleotides upstream from the transcriptional start site. Transcription factors bind to the TATA box, which in turn promotes the binding of RNA polymerase and additional proteins. A functional transcription complex forms when the double-stranded DNA in the promoter region separates and the transcription complex moves away from the core promoter region. Once started, the RNA polymerase adds nucleotides to the free 3′-hydroxyl group in a manner similar to that of DNA replication. Transcription is eventually terminated by a polyadenylation step (see Fig. 47.5).

Transcription initially produces RNA that contains both exons and introns. This pre-RNA transcript must be processed or spliced into mature mRNA for it to be properly translated into protein. RNA splicing involves the cleavage and removal of intron RNA segments and splicing of exon RNA segments. Splicing requires the effort of a number of proteins and small RNAs that come together to form a spliceosome, which directs the splicing of exons and removal of introns.

An important modification of the splicing process, alternative splicing, allows for the generation of different mRNAs from the same primary RNA transcript by the cutting and joining of the RNA strand at different locations. Among the types of alternative splicing are exon skipping, alternative 3′ and 5′ splice sites, and intron retention. Approximately 92%–95% of all human genes are alternatively spliced, resulting in additional protein complexity that may be tightly regulated and specific to different cells and tissues.

## Translation

The final phase of the transfer of information from DNA is to proteins, the structural and functional molecules that make up most of a living organism. Proteins are long single strands of various amino acids and are synthesized by a process called *translation*, which requires the functioning of many protein factors, tRNAs, and ribosomes.

Amino acids have a common structure consisting of a carbon atom bound to amino and carboxylic acid groups with a side chain. There are 20 amino acids, each with a different side chain that gives them their unique properties. The side chains can be divided into four types: nonpolar (hydrophobic), polar (hydrophilic uncharged), negatively charged, and positively charged. A protein's amino acid makeup and sequence in the polypeptide chain determine the overall structure and function of the protein. Some amino acids commonly induce structural changes, such as proline, which disrupts secondary

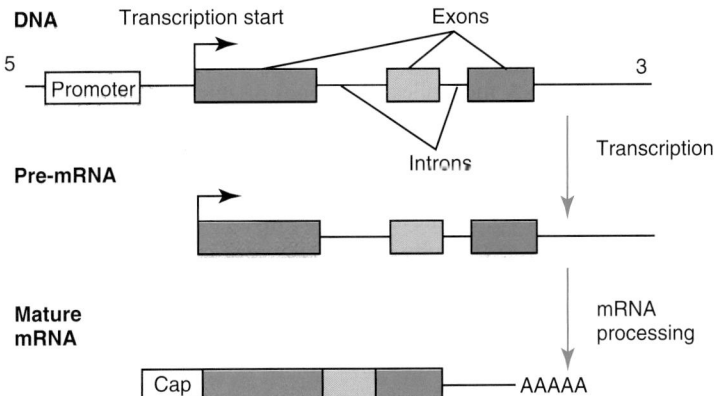

**Fig. 47.5** DNA transcription and messenger RNA (*mRNA*) processing. A gene that encodes for a protein contains a promoter region and variable numbers of introns and exons. Transcription commences at the transcription start site. Pre-mRNA is processed by capping, polyadenylation, and intron splicing to become a mature mRNA.

| First letter | Second letter: U | Second letter: C | Second letter: A | Second letter: G | Third letter |
|---|---|---|---|---|---|
| U | UUU Phenylalanine | UCU Serine | UAU Tyrosine | UGU Cysteine | U |
| U | UUC Phenylalanine | UCC Serine | UAC Tyrosine | UGC Cysteine | C |
| U | UUA Leucine | UCA Serine | UAA Stop Codon | UGA Stop Codon | A |
| U | UUG Leucine | UCG Serine | UAG Stop Codon | UGG Tryptophan | G |
| C | CUU Leucine | CCU Proline | CAU Histidine | CGU Arginine | U |
| C | CUC Leucine | CCC Proline | CAC Histidine | CGC Arginine | C |
| C | CUA Leucine | CCA Proline | CAA Glutamine | CGA Arginine | A |
| C | CUG Leucine | CCG Proline | CAG Glutamine | CGG Arginine | G |
| A | AUU Isoleucine | ACU Threonine | AAU Asparagine | AGU Serine | U |
| A | AUC Isoleucine | ACC Threonine | AAC Asparagine | AGC Serine | C |
| A | AUA Isoleucine | ACA Threonine | AAA Lysine | AGA Arginine | A |
| A | AUG Methionine | ACG Threonine | AAG Lysine | AGG Arginine | G |
| G | GUU Valine | GCU Alanine | GAU Aspartic acid | GGU Glycine | U |
| G | GUC Valine | GCC Alanine | GAC Aspartic acid | GGC Glycine | C |
| G | GUA Valine | GCA Alanine | GAA Glutamic Acid | GGA Glycine | A |
| G | GUG Valine | GCG Alanine | GAG Glutamic Acid | GGG Glycine | G |

**Fig. 47.6** Genetic code. Translation of messenger RNA to amino acids during protein synthesis.

structure, and cysteine, which can cross-link to another cysteine through disulfide bonds. For additional information on protein structure, see Chapter 18.

The genetic code, which was deciphered in the early 1960s, is required to convert a nucleic acid sequence into an amino acid sequence. Humans have four unique nucleotides, which are arranged into sets of three per codon. Theoretically, there are 64 combinations; however, rather than encoding 64 amino acids, humans have 20. A hallmark of this genetic code is that it is redundant, meaning that there are several codes for one amino acid. That is the case for most amino acids but not all; for example, methionine and tryptophan have only one code. The redundancy is usually in the third base of the code. All of the 64 three-nucleotide codon possibilities code for an amino acid except for the three that serve as stop codons (UAA, UGA, and UAG) (Fig. 47.6).

Protein synthesis or translation occurs in the cytoplasm and proceeds in three steps: initiation, elongation, and termination. The process requires tRNA and rRNA molecules as well as ribosomes and initiation, elongation, and termination factors. The first codon (AUG) always codes for methionine; therefore, to initiate translation, a methionine tRNA first binds to the ribosome. The tRNA specific for the next three-base codon—for example, lysine—binds to the ribosome, and a peptide bond is created between the amino group of one amino acid and the carboxyl group of the next amino acid. The ribosome moves forward one codon and the next tRNA specific for the next codon binds in the ribosome; this process is repeated until a termination codon is reached (Fig. 47.7). Protein synthesis occurs in the endoplasmic reticulum, where multiple ribosomes called *polyribosomes* are involved in translating an individual mRNA.

**POINTS TO REMEMBER**

- The two strands of DNA are bound together by hydrogen bonds and stacking forces that can be broken and reformed without permanent damage to the DNA.
- The conversion of DNA information into protein is facilitated by aminoacyl tRNA synthetases and their ability to create amino acid-specific tRNAs.
- The genetic code is redundant; the three-base code can have 64 different combinations, but only 20 amino acids are used in human biology.

## EPIGENETICS

Global and mRNA-specific regulation of translation often occurs by **epigenetic** changes—that is, changes that do not modify the DNA sequence. Currently, there are three major types of epigenetic modifications: (1) DNA methylation, (2) histone modifications, and (3) noncoding RNAs.

**DNA methylation** is a well-known epigenetic change. Methylation of cytosine to 5-methylcytosine occurs frequently; about 70% of CpG dinucleotides in the human genome are methylated. CpG islands are about 1000 bases in length and are often found near the 5′ end of genes. These regions consist of clusters of CG dinucleotides that are usually not methylated in normal cells. However, CpG methylation correlates with condensed chromatin structure and promoter inactivation (Fig. 47.8). Cancer is the most common human disease associated with aberrant DNA methylation.

DNA replication, repair, and transcription require free access to DNA. However, DNA is usually wound around

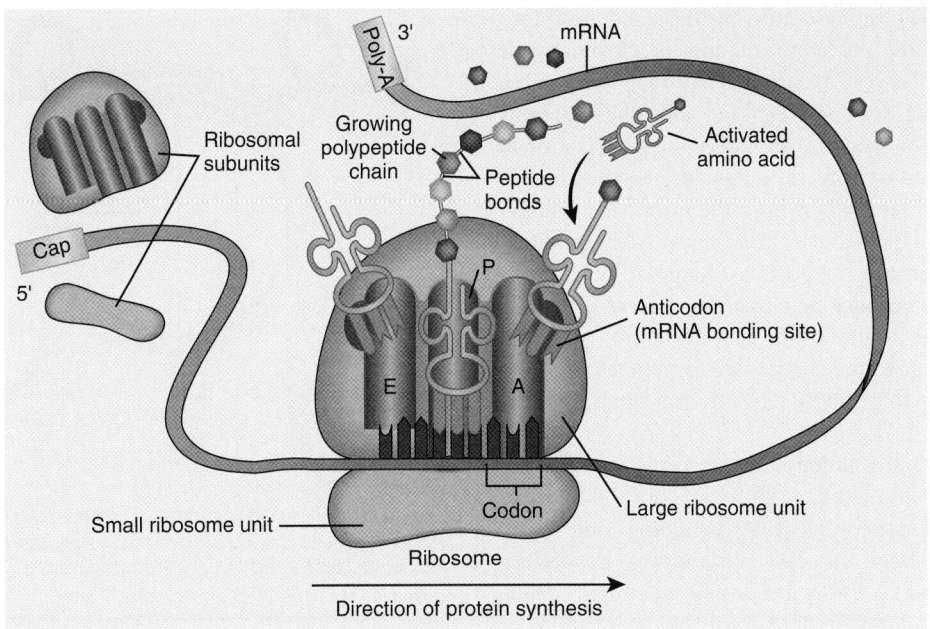

**Fig. 47.7** Translation. Shown is a ribosome bound to a messenger RNA (*mRNA*) converting the mRNA triplet code (*Codon*) via a specific amino acid-bound transfer RNA containing a complementary anticodon sequence. There are three transfer RNA positions. A new amino acid-bound transfer RNA first arrives on the ribosome at the *A* or acceptor site, at the front of the moving ribosome, and then moves to the *P* or peptidyl site, where the amino acid on the newly arrived transfer RNA combines with the growing polypeptide chain. Finally, the now empty transfer RNA moves to the *E*, or exit site, where it prepares to leave the ribosome. (Modified from Huether SE, McCance L. *Understanding Pathophysiology*, 6th ed. St. Louis: Elsevier; 2017.)

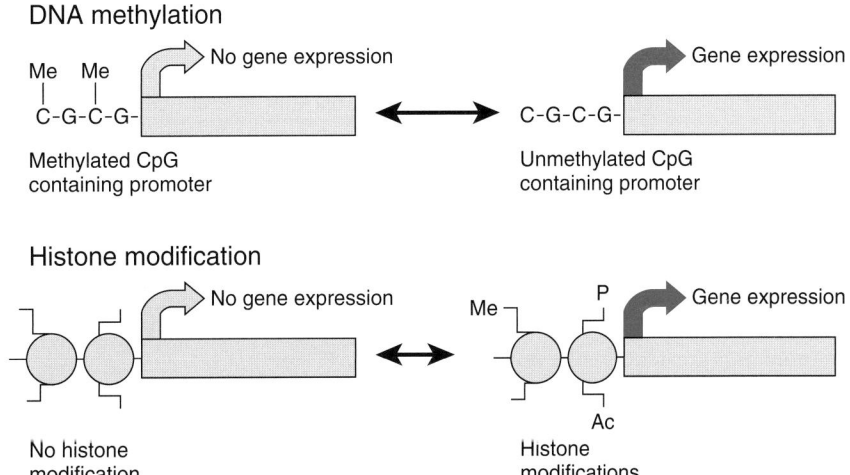

**Fig. 47.8** Epigenetics. *Top*, DNA methylation of CpG island regions indicated by *Me* in and around gene promoters is associated with loss of gene expression and silencing of the gene. When *CpG* islands are unmethylated, shown by absence of Me, gene expression is unaffected. *Bottom*, Histone modifications of the tails of histone proteins, such as methylation, acetylation, and phosphorylation, shown as *Me, Ac,* and *P*, respectively, can increase gene expression. (Modified from Zaidi SK, Young DW, Montecino M, et al. Bookmarking the genome: maintenance of epigenetic information. *J Biol Chem*. 2011;286:18355–18361.)

*histones* to form nucleosomes and is further condensed into chromatin. Therefore, the conformation of chromatin is tightly regulated and is very dynamic; at any one point in time portions of the DNA are being exposed and other portions are being covered. For example, reversible phosphorylation at serine, threonine, and tyrosine residues adds negative charges to histones that can repel them from the negatively charged DNA. Similarly, specific histones may be reversibly modified by acetylation to remove the positive charge on lysine residues and thus to lower histone attraction to DNA. Histone, lysine, and arginine residues can also be mono-, di-, and trimethylated. Although the charges are unchanged, methylation further serves to promote DNA transcription, replication, and repair.

Noncoding RNAs also function in the regulation of translation. In addition to noncoding ribosomal and tRNAs, there are many forms of noncoding RNA, including long (>200 nucleotides) and short (20–200 nucleotides) noncoding RNAs. Long noncoding RNAs are diverse and highly regulated during the development of an organism. At least 93% of the genome is transcribed, producing more than 10 times the amount of RNA than is produced from the coding segments of genes. Recently, it was determined that there are approximately 21,000 noncoding genes, which is slightly more than the 19,969 protein encoding genes.

### Human Chromosomes

Cellular DNA is bound by many proteins to form chromatin (see Fig. 47.3). The proteins in chromatin consist of histones, which are bound in precise amounts per length of DNA, and other proteins called *nonhistone proteins* that are bound more irregularly. The histone proteins consist of two copies of four proteins that bind as a unit to 147 **base pairs** (bp) of DNA to make up a nucleosome. One additional protein binds between the nucleosomes (Fig. 47.9). Access to DNA by transcription factors is controlled by proteins that remodel the histone proteins through phosphorylation, acetylation, and methylation. The nucleosomes are condensed into filaments and even more compact structures to form a chromosome (see Fig. 47.3). The

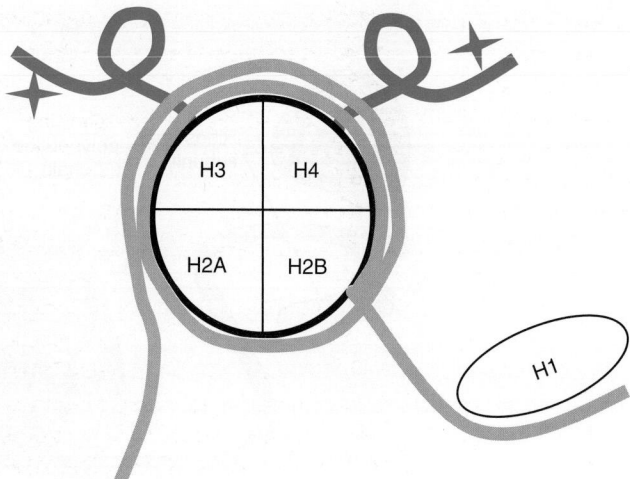

**Fig. 47.9** Schematic illustration of a nucleosome unit. A segment of DNA is wound around a nucleosome core particle consisting of an octamer containing two copies of histone proteins H2A, H2B, H3, and H4. Tails with modifications (indicated by a *blue star*) are shown to protrude from H3 and H4. Adjacent nucleosomes are separated by a segment of linker DNA and the linker histone, H1.

DNA in chromosomes is continuous for each chromosome and can be as much as several hundred million base pairs in length.

Chromosome regions can be classified by their transcriptional activity. The ends of chromosomes, called *telomeres*, contain the repeat sequence TTAGGG, which shortens with age. The centromeres, at the centers of most chromosomes, are important during mitosis and contain mostly repeated segments of DNA.

## SUMMARY

The field of molecular diagnostics is an important and exciting area that is destined to have an even greater impact on medicine in the future. As an increasing number of diseases are characterized at the molecular (e.g., nucleic acid and protein) level, new therapeutics and diagnostics specifically targeting these molecular changes will continue to emerge.

## REVIEW QUESTIONS

1. The number of human proteins is greater than the number of genes because
   **a.** alternative splicing and posttranslational modifications occur.
   **b.** of the 3′ polyadenylation of mRNA.
   **c.** only some genes are expressed.
   **d.** the ribosome adds additional noncoded amino acids to some mRNAs.

2. If there were only 12 amino acids in proteins, what would be the minimal length of nucleotides needed for a complete genetic code?
   **a.** 1
   **b.** 2
   **c.** 3

   **d.** 4

3. How would the sequence GAATATGCCAGCATATTAG translate?
   **a.** MetProAlaTyr
   **b.** GluTyrAlaSerIle
   **c.** It would not translate because the number of bases is not divisible by 3.
   **d.** It would not translate because it will not be transcribed.

4. Nucleotides that encode protein account for what percentage of the genome?
   **a.** 1%
   **b.** 10%
   **c.** 50%
   **d.** 90%

5. Hydrogen bonding between which DNA elements is required for most molecular diagnostic assays?
   a. Bonds between ribose sugars on different nucleotides of a strand of DNA
   b. Bonds between ribose and nucleotide bases
   c. Bonds between two cysteine residues
   d. Bonds between the complementary nucleotide bases

6. What nucleotide base is methylated in DNA and at what specific location?
   a. Adenine and polyadenylation
   b. Guanine and RNA transcription start site
   c. Thymine and the production of thymine dimers
   d. Cytosine and upstream CpG islands

7. Mutations can be generated by incorporating the wrong base into DNA during replication, and the mechanism to repair this error is
   a. mismatch repair.
   b. nucleotide excision repair.
   c. base excision repair.
   d. homologous recombination repair.

8. The structure of a human mRNA encoding gene generally contains promoters that are upstream from the transcriptional start site; however, there are other promoters that can be both upstream and downstream of the gene. Which of the following is one of these promoters?
   a. The TATA box
   b. The polyadenylation site
   c. The enhancer
   d. The proximal core promoter

9. An important group of DNA modification enzymes, the restriction endonucleases, are used to manipulate DNA fragments. What is their function in the organisms from which they are isolated?
   a. They digest the ends of DNA to prepare them for ligation.
   b. They are used to protect themselves from viral infections.
   c. They are used in the base excision repair found in bacteria.
   d. They are RNA-guided nucleases that can precisely cleave genomic DNA.

## SUGGESTED READINGS

Cech TR, Steitz JA. The noncoding RNA revolution-trashing old rules to forge new ones. *Cell.* 2014;157:77–94.

Crick F. Central dogma of molecular biology. *Nature.* 1970;227:561–563.

Djebali S, Davis CA, Merkel A, et al. Landscape of transcription in human cells. *Nature.* 2012;489:101–108.

Green ED, Guyer MS, National Human Genome Research Institute. Charting a course for genomic medicine from base pairs to bedside. *Nature.* 2011;470:204–213.

International Human Genome Sequencing Consortium. Finishing the euchromatic sequence of the human genome. *Nature.* 2004;431:931–945.

Jackson RJ, Hellen CU, Pestova TV. The mechanism of eukaryotic translation initiation and principles of its regulation. *Nat Rev Mol Cell Biol.* 2010;11:113–127.

Redon R, Ishikawa S, Fitch KR, et al. Global variation in copy number in the human genome. *Nature.* 2006;444:444–454.

Schubeler D. Function and information content of DNA methylation. *Nature.* 2015;517:321–326.

Venter JC, Adams MD, Myers EW, et al. The sequence of the human genome. *Science.* 2001;291:1304–1351.

Watson JD, Crick FH. Genetical implications of the structure of deoxyribonucleic acid. *Nature.* 1953;171:964–967.

# Genomes, Variants, and Massively Parallel Methods

*Jason Y. Park, Rossa W.K. Chiu, Dennis Lo, and Carl T. Wittwer*

## OBJECTIVES

1. Describe the size of the human genome and the percent that encodes proteins.
2. Compare the similarities and differences between human and non-human genomes.
3. Understand the correlation between genetic variation and human disease.
4. List the major types of genetic variation.
5. Describe the number of genes and the proportion that are clinically significant.
6. Understand the HGVS nomenclature system for describing genetic variation.
7. Describe the types of massively parallel methods used in genomics.
8. Describe common genomic techniques enabled by massively parallel methods.
9. Describe the clinical applications of cell-free nucleic acids.
10. Know the commonly used file formats used in genomic informatics.

## KEY WORDS AND DEFINITIONS

**Adapter** Oligonucleotides that are ligated to library fragments to provide consensus priming sites.

**Assembly** Reconstruction of short sequence reads on a scaffold of reference DNA.

**Contig** A linear stretch of consensus sequence assembled from smaller overlapping sequence fragments.

**Copy number variant (CNV)** A structural variant of a large region of the genome that has been deleted or duplicated.

**Coverage** The percent of target bases that were sequenced at least a given number of times.

**Deletion** A DNA sequence that is missing in one sample compared to another. Deletions may be as small as one nucleotide or as large as an entire chromosome.

**De novo assembly** Formation of a contig without using a reference sequence.

**DNA library** A collection of DNA fragments with ligated adapters that will be sequenced.

**DNA microarray** An array of microscopic DNA spots attached to a solid surface. Each DNA spot contains a specific DNA sequence known as a probe. Probe-target hybridization is usually detected and quantified by fluorescently-labeled targets to assess the relative abundance of target nucleic acid sequences.

**Fusion** A translocation, inversion, large deletion or large duplication resulting in a hybrid gene formed from originally separate genes.

**Gb** Gigabase (1,000,000,000 bases).

**Indel** Originally referred to a unique class of sequence variants that included both an insertion and a deletion, usually (but not always) resulting in an overall change in the number of base pairs. Today more commonly refers to either insertions or deletions or any combination thereof at a particular locus.

**Insert** Part of the original DNA that has been fragmented before ligation to adapters.

**Insertion** An extra DNA sequence that is present in one sample compared with a reference sequence.

**Heteroplasmy** A mixture of more than one type of mitochondrial sequence in one cell.

**Intergenic** DNA sequence between genes.

**Kb** Kilobase (1000 bases).

**Mb** Megabase (1,000,000 bases).

**Missense** A nucleotide substitution that changes a codon to the code for a different amino acid. Although these sequence changes are commonly referred to as missense "mutations," this is strictly a misnomer because missense variants may be benign and cause no disease.

**Mutation** A disease-causing sequence variation. Historically, the term has been interchangeable with variant to describe any change in DNA sequence, regardless of relation to disease causation. For current clinical descriptions or reporting, the use of mutation is reserved for the scenario when disease causation is known. Many clinical laboratories no longer use the term "mutation" and instead favor "likely pathogenic variant" or "pathogenic variant".

**Nonsense** A nucleotide substitution that results in a stop codon, prematurely terminating the protein.

**Nonsynonymous** Nucleotide substitutions that are predicted to change the coding amino acid to a different amino acid (missense) or stop codon (nonsense).

**Oligonucleotide** A short single-stranded polymer of nucleic acid.

**Paired-end sequence**  Sequence from both ends of a DNA fragment typically hundreds of bases long.

**Phred score**  Estimate of the error probability for a base called in DNA sequencing. It is represented as a Q-score; the higher the number, the higher the probability of a correct call.

**Plasmid**  An extrachromosomal ring of double-stranded, closed DNA found in bacteria.

**Polony**  A microscopic colony of clonal temples used in massively parallel sequencing. A polony may be generated by PCR, bridge amplification, or isothermal amplification.

**Pseudogene**  A genetic element that does not code for a functional gene product, usually because of accumulated sequence variations.

**Short tandem repeat (STR)**  A simple sequence repeat that is 1–13 bases long.

**Simple sequence repeat (SSR)**  A sequence from 1–500 bases that is repeated end-to-end. If the repeat unit is 1–13 bases, it is also called a *microsatellite* or *STR*. If the repeat is 14–500 bases it is a *minisatellite*.

**Single nucleotide polymorphism (SNP)**  A benign single nucleotide variant (substitution, deletion, or insertion) that occurs in a population at a frequency of at least 1%.

**Single nucleotide variation (SNV)**  A single nucleotide variant (substitution, deletion, or insertion). SNVs may be benign or may cause disease.

**Structural variation**  A region of DNA greater than 1000 bases in size that is inverted, translocated, inserted, or deleted.

**Synonymous variant**  A nucleotide change that results in no change to the amino acid sequence. Although synonymous variants are usually benign since there is no protein coding change, some are pathogenic because of changes in splicing, gene expression or mRNA stability.

**Transposon**  A mobile genetic element that can delete and insert itself variably into the genome.

**Variant call format (VCF)**  After aligning all reads onto a reference sequence, variants that are different from the reference genome at a given nucleotide position are stored in a text file in a specific format.

**Variation**  A change in DNA sequence. It may be benign or may cause disease.

## BACKGROUND

This chapter focuses on genomes, and the variations that occur within and between the genomes of different species. Genetic variation is fundamental to the diversity of life, but also plays a large role in the development of disease. This chapter also describes the technologies that enable genomic analysis—these technologies require very large (massively parallel) processes.

## HUMAN GENOME

The word *genome* signifies the collection of genes in an organism. The human genome encompasses all the information needed for growth, development, and heredity. This information is copied in every cell in the body that has a nucleus. Human genetic material is organized into 46 chromosomes. There are 22 paired chromosomes that occur regardless of biological sex (autosomes). The remaining two are sex chromosomes: 2 X chromosomes in females; 1 X and 1 Y in males.

The basic concepts of chromosomes and the naming of chromosomal variation are described by the International System for Human Cytogenetic Nomenclature (ISCN): autosomes are numbered from 1 to 22 in descending order of length. The symbols p and q designated the short (p for "petit", meaning small in French) and long q arms of the chromosomes, respectively. A chromosome band is the part of the chromosome that is clearly distinguishable from adjacent segments which are darker or lighter in appearance. G-bands are the bands resulting from Giemsa dye staining. Abnormal chromosomal rearrangements include inversions, deletions, translocations, and fusions.

The first sequencing drafts of the human genome were released in 2001 and 2004. The 2004 version contains 2.85 billion nucleotides (bases) and was considered 99% complete for euchromatic DNA. The overall size of the genome, including both euchromatic and heterochromatic sequence (tightly compact DNA found at centromeres and telomeres), was estimated to be 3.08 billion nucleotides. Thus, the total overall genome was only 92.5% sequenced when it was first declared "essentially" complete. Within the 2.85 billion nucleotides of euchromatic DNA there were 19,438 known genes and an additional 2188 predicted genes. The total number of nucleotides encoding protein was approximately 34 million (1.2%) of the genome. This portion of the genome encoding proteins is also known as the *exome*.

The 2004 genome contained 341 gaps in heterochromatic regions. These regions contain DNA that is difficult to sequence (e.g., repetitive elements, GC-rich sequence) or where no clone/template could be made. Commonly used DNA sequencing technologies require a scaffold on which sequence fragments are pieced together. The first human reference sequences were assembled by the University of California at Santa Cruz (UCSC) and were numbered starting with "hg1" in May of 2000. Reference sequences have subsequently undergone continuous improvement, currently coordinated by the international Genome Reference Consortium (GRC), producing a reference with combined designation by both UCSC and GRC: Genome Reference Consortium Human Build 37/ Human Genome 19, abbreviated GRCh37/ hg19. In the future, only one designation will be given, such as the currently released GRCh38.

Since the 2004 genome publication, there have been continuing efforts to create "Platinum Genomes" that address the missing information (gaps) and improve the quality of data. Prior gaps have been sequenced by utilizing DNA from a haploid cell line. Long-read sequencing technologies can create de novo assemblies that do not require the use of reference genomes. Hybrid sequencing methods are emerging that combine the advantages of short-read sequencing for single nucleotide base accuracy with the advantages of long-read sequencing to further decrease gaps in human genome data and reveal new mechanisms of human variation. For example, the use of long-read sequencing technology provided the first assembly of the highly repetitive centromere region of the Y-chromosome. Complete "telomere-to-telomere" genome sequencing was first accomplished on the malaria parasite, *Plasmodium falciparum*. A draft of all human chromosomes completely sequenced from telomere-to-telomere, including all repetitive centromeric and telomeric regions, was completed in 2021, revealing a 3.055 gigabase (1 gigabase = 1 billion bases) haploid female genome.

Each female human cell contains two copies of the 3.05-billion base pair genome divided into 46 chromosomes. Table 48.1 summarizes statistics for the human genome and the types of variations that are important in clinical diagnostics. Three-quarters of human DNA is intergenic or between genes. More than 60% of this intergenic sequence consists of "parasitic" DNA regions of mostly defective transposable elements 100 to 11,000 bases in length. Between 2 million and 3 million of these "retrotransposons" are present in each copy of the genome. They contribute to genetic recombination and chromosome structure and provide an evolutionary record of sequence variation and selection.

Segmental duplications constitute 6.6% of the human genome. They are over 1 kilobase (1000 bases, or Kb) in length, have a sequence identity of at least 90% and are not transposable. Segmental duplications are common in the human genome and are prone to deletion or rearrangements, often with medical consequences. Intergenic DNA also carries most of the simple sequence repeats (SSRs) present in the genome. A subset of SSRs, the short tandem repeats (STRs) have repeat units of 1 to several bases that may be repeated up to thousands of times. STRs have played a large role in genetic linkage studies and in forensic and medical identity testing. They are formed by slippage during replication and are highly polymorphic between individuals. The most common STRs are dinucleotide repeats, such as ACACAC and ATAT. On average, one STR occurs every 2000 bases.

Approximately 5% of DNA is required to maintain the structure of chromosomes and is located at chromosome centers (centromeres) and ends (telomeres) and makes up heterochromatic DNA. Centromeric DNA includes many tandem copies of nearly identical 171 base pair (bp) repeats encompassing 0.24–5.0 Mb per chromosome. Each chromosome end is capped with several Kb of the telomeric 6 base repeat TTAGGG. Although intergenic DNA does not code for protein and was originally considered "junk," much of this DNA is transcribed to RNA, producing a complex "transcriptome" network of RNA control elements, whose function and mechanics are active areas of investigation.

There are about 20,000 protein coding genes and 230,000 RNA transcripts. The excess of RNA transcripts come from both alternative splicing of protein coding genes and genes that are only transcribed. The average gene covers 27,000 bases, but only about 1300 of these bases code for amino acids. The primary RNA transcript is processed by splicing to retain exons that are interspersed throughout the gene and have a higher GC content than noncoding regions. On average, 95% of a gene is excised as introns, retaining a mean of 10.4 exons, of which on average 9.1 are translated into proteins. Exons make up only 1.9% of the total genome, with 1.2% of the genome coding for proteins. Some important genes are present in many copies, so that overall protein expression is not affected if a chance variation occurs in one copy. If extra copies of genes lose their function, they are known as pseudogenes. At least as many pseudogenes as functional genes are present in the human genome. It is important to distinguish pseudogenes from functional genes because variants in pseudogenes are seldom of clinical importance, and they often complicate DNA diagnostic assays.

> **POINTS TO REMEMBER**
>
> **Human Genome**
> - Contains approximately 3 billion base pairs per haploid genome
> - Protein coding nucleotides are about 1% (30 million base pairs)
> - Noncoding sequence has important regulatory roles

## NON-HUMAN GENOMES

Before the human genome was completed, other genomes of smaller size were sequenced, enabling advancements in technology and logistical organization to sequence the human genome. The genomes of different species vary in size and the complexity can be surprising. One of the largest known genomes is the white spruce tree (*Picea glauca*) at 26.9 billion bases. On the opposite end of the spectrum is Porcine circovirus-1, a single stranded DNA virus with a genome that is less than 2000 bases. There is overlap in the genome size of eukaryotes (animals, plants, fungi), viruses, and bacteria (Tables 48.2 and Fig. 48.1).

### Primates

Comparison of the chimpanzee genome with the human genome shows a genome-wide difference of only 1.23% with 35 million nucleotide substitutions and 5 million insertion/deletions. There are also differences at the level of proteins between humans and chimpanzees. Only 29% of proteins are identical at the amino acid level, but proteins that are different only differ by an average of two amino acids.

Two orangutan species have been sequenced. Their genome sizes are similar to humans at ≈3 billion bases. During evolutionary development, the number of structural rearrangements in orangutans has been less than humans and chimpanzees. For example, the number of genome rearrangements >100kb was 38 in the orangutan, but 85 and 54 in the chimpanzee and human, respectively.

Using long-read DNA sequencing, the genomes of two human, one chimpanzee and one orangutan were assembled

## TABLE 48.1   The Human Genome and Its Sequence Variation

**The Human Genome**

3.05 billion base pairs in 24 chromosomes
23 chromosome pairs (46–244 million base pairs per chromosome)

**75% Intergenic Sequences**

| | |
|---|---|
| Transposable elements | 42% |
| Segmental duplications | 7% |
| Simple sequence repeat | 3% |
| Structural (centromeres, telomeres) | 5% |
| Other | 18% |

**25% Genes that Code for Proteins**

| | |
|---|---|
| Introns | 23% |
| Exons | 1.9% |
|     Coding | 1.2% |
|     Untranslated | 0.7% |
| Number of protein coding genes | 19,969 |

***Composition of the Average Gene***

| | |
|---|---|
| Base pairs | 27,000 |
| Exons | 10.4 |
| Transcribed exons | 9.1 |
| Exonic bases | 1340 |
| Amino acids | 446 |

**Genomic Variation**

99.9% identity (one difference every 1250 bases between haploid genomes)
Single-Nucleotide Variants (SNVs): every 5 bases among genomes
Copy Number Variants (CNVs): involves 5%–12% of the genome

**Disease-Causing Variants**

| | |
|---|---|
| SNVs | 68% |
|     Missense (amino acid substitution) | 45% |
|     Nonsense (termination) | 11% |
|     Splicing | 10% |
|     Regulatory | 2% |
| Small insertions or deletions (or both) | 24% |
| Structural variants (copy number variations, inversions, translocations, rearrangements, repeats) | 8% |

**Epigenetic Alterations**

Variable initiation and alternative splicing
Cytosine methylation
Histone phosphorylation, methylation, acetylation

---

independently without the use of reference genomes. There were 17,789 structural variants in the apes that were predicted to disrupt 479 genes in humans. When DNA genomics were compared to RNA expression in neural progenitor cells, 41% of genes with downregulated expression in humans had an associated disrupting structural variant. This loss of expression in humans compared to apes supports the theory that human evolution involved the loss of neuronal gene expression. Comparing five primate genomes (chimpanzee, gorilla, orangutan, gibbon, and macaque) to human DNA identified more than 200,000 human-specific DNA insertions. Although most were <10 nucleotides in length, there were 5582 genes with larger insertions and 2450 of these were expressed in brain tissue. Many of the human-specific insertions were transposable elements and long terminal repeats.

## Rodents

The mouse genome is 14% smaller than the human genome, while the rat's is in between the size of the human and mouse. The number of genes is similar between all three species. About 40% of the rat, mouse, and human genomes are homologous. Another 30% of the rat and mouse genomes match each other but not the human genome.

| TABLE 48.2 *Homo sapiens* in Comparison to Other Genomes | | |
|---|---|---|
| **Organism/Name** | **Group** | **Size (Mb)** |
| Human (*Homo sapiens*) | Animals | 3050 |
| White spruce tree (*Picea glauca*) | Plants | 26,900 |
| Migratory locust (*Locusta migratoria*) | Animals | 5760 |
| Mouse (*Mus musculus*) | Animals | ≈2500 |
| Rat (*Rattus norvegicus*) | Animals | ≈2750 |
| Apple tree (*Malus domestica*) | Plants | 742 |
| Roundworm (*Caenorhabditis elegans*) | Animals | 97 |
| *Aspergillus fumigatus* | Fungi | ≈30 |
| Baker's yeast (*Saccharomyces cerevisiae*) | Fungi | 12.3 |
| *Haemophilus influenzae* | Bacteria | 1.8 |
| Human immunodeficiency virus (HIV) 1 | Viruses | 0.0092 |
| Porcine circovirus-1 | Viruses | 0.00173 |

Data from the National Center for Biotechnology Information; (http://www.ncbi.nlm.nih.gov/genome)

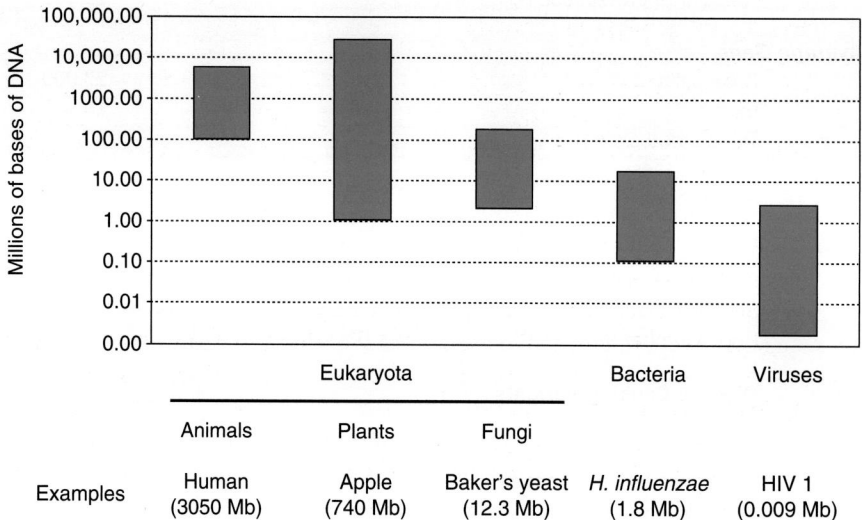

**Fig. 48.1** Range of genome sizes. Among different organisms, there is wide variation in genome size. In this plot of publicly available genomes, the *y*-axis is in megabases, and the *x*-axis lists various organisms: Eukaryota (animals, plants, fungi), bacteria, and viruses. On average, Eukaryota have larger genomes compared with bacteria and viruses; however, there are exceptions in which virus genomes are larger than bacteria or Eukaryota. The difference between the smallest and largest known genomes is more than six orders of magnitude. Several specific genome sizes are illustrated in Mb (megabases, million). (Data extracted from the National Center for Biotechnology Information; http://www.ncbi.nlm.nih.gov/genome.)

## Fungi

Fungi are eukaryotes and their genomes are less complex than the human genome. Common fungi that cause human disease have genomes of 7.5–30 million bases with 8–16 chromosomes, as well as mitochondrial genomes. Some fungi have diploid genomes, while others are haploid. Many of their genes have introns. For instance, *Aspergillus fumigatus* (a fungus that causes allergic reactions and systemic disease with a high mortality rate) has a haploid genome of about 30 million bases with more than 9900 predicted genes on eight chromosomes. Its genes are smaller than human genes, with an average length of 1400 bp and 2.8 exons per gene.

The first eukaryotic genome sequenced was *Saccharomyces cerevisiae* (baker's yeast). This fungal genome has 12 million bases arranged into 16 chromosomes. In addition to its importance in baking bread and brewing alcohol, yeast is an important model organism and pathogen. The 6000 genes of *S. cerevisiae* can be systematically altered to examine their role in yeast and their homologs in higher organisms.

## Bacteria

Bacterial genomes are considerably less complex than human or fungal genomes. Common bacteria have only one chromosome, usually a circular DNA double helix of 4–5 million base pairs, about 1000 times less than the amount of DNA in a human cell. About 90% of the DNA in bacteria codes for protein. There are no introns, but there are multiple small intergenic regions of repetitive sequences that are dispersed throughout the genome. *Escherichia coli*, a common bacterium in the human intestinal tract has about 4300 genes.

In addition to the large circular chromosome that carries essential genes, bacteria also carry accessory genes in smaller circles of double-stranded DNA (dsDNA) known as plasmids. Plasmids range in size from 1000 to more than 1 million base pairs. Plasmids are important in the molecular diagnosis of bacterial infections because they often encode pathogenic factors and antibiotic resistance.

The bacterial repertoire of DNA can be altered by: (1) gain or loss of plasmids; (2) single-base changes, small insertions and deletions as in eukaryotic genomes; and (3) large segmental rearrangements, including inversions, deletions, and duplications. Some genes, such as those for ribosomal RNA, are present in many copies, making them good targets for molecular assays to identify species of bacteria. In addition, the intergenic repetitive sequences serve as multiple targets for oligonucleotide probes, enabling the generation of unique DNA profiles or fingerprints for individual bacterial strains.

The first genome sequenced by random fragmentation and computational assembly was the pathogenic bacteria, *Haemophilus influenzae*. Its genomic DNA was fragmented into 19,687 templates and inserted into plasmids and bacteriophages. A total of 24,304 sequences were successfully generated over 3 months. The sequencing data required 30 hours of computational assembly. A total of 11 million bases of DNA were sequenced and used to generate the 1.8 million bases of the *H. influenzae* genome. In addition to being the first genome solved by shotgun sequencing, it was also the first bacterial genome sequenced. Multiple strains of *H. influenzae* have been subsequently sequenced. These additional genomes have revealed heterogeneity in the number of genes between different strains. Of the approximately 3000 genes identified, only 1461 are common to all strains. The differences in genes between different strains may be associated with differences in the infectious pathogenicity of *H. influenzae*.

## Viruses

Viral genomes are considerably less complex than bacterial genomes. Common viruses that infect humans vary in size from about 5000 to 250,000 bases, or 20–1000 times less than the amount of nucleic acid in *E. coli*. Because viruses use the host's cellular machinery, they do not need as many genes as bacteria do. Small viruses may encode only several genes, but the larger viruses can encode hundreds. The viral genome consists of either DNA or RNA, and the nucleic acid may be single stranded or double stranded, linear, or circular with one or multiple fragments or copies per viral particle. As in bacteria, there are no introns. In fact, some viruses have overlapping exons with different reading frames that code different products from the same nucleic acid sequence. Noncoding regions are usually present at the terminal ends of linear genomes. Repeat segments are often found as terminal or internal repeats and may be inverted.

Sequence alterations in viruses are common. Areas of high sequence variation may be interspersed between conserved domains. Higher frequencies of variation correlate with lower polymerase fidelity and may allow escape from antibody recognition and antiviral drugs. Common sequence variants in viruses include single base changes, insertions, and deletions.

Sequence diversity within a viral species may be so great that consensus sequences for molecular typing are difficult to find.

## DNA THAT CODES FOR RNA BUT NOT PROTEIN

Even though 99% of the human genome does not code for protein, most of it is transcribed into noncoding RNA. At least 93% of the genome is transcribed, producing more than 10 times the amount of RNA that is produced from the coding segments of genes. Both strands of DNA may be transcribed, and long noncoding transcripts may overlap coding regions, producing a complex transcriptome of functional RNA molecules that may variably regulate transcription of coding regions, RNA processing, mRNA stability, translation, protein stability, and secretion. In addition to long noncoding RNA, ribosomal RNA and transfer RNA, specific classes of noncoding RNAs include small nuclear RNAs critical for splicing, small nucleolar RNAs that modify rRNA, telomerase RNAs for maintenance of telomeres, small interfering RNAs (siRNAs), and microRNAs (miRNAs) that regulate gene expression. At least 54 different categories of RNA have been identified and some of the more important types are listed in Table 48.3.

MicroRNAs (or miRNAs) are particularly interesting as potential markers for disease. For example, concentrations of specific, circulating miRNAs correlate with many different types of cancer. MicroRNAs are noncoding but functional single-stranded RNAs that are 21–22 bases long and are expressed in a tissue-specific manner. They are initially transcribed as longer precursors that undergo two rounds of truncations as they are transported from the nucleus to the cytoplasm in the cell. The mature miRNA is then integrated into a protein complex called the *RNA-induced silencing complex*, which regulates translation of mRNA. MicroRNAs hybridize to a 6 to 8 base sequence in the 3′ untranslated region of target mRNAs and inhibit mRNA expression either by mRNA degradation if the bases are perfectly complementary, or by blocking of translation if they are imperfectly complementary. Despite the promise of miRNAs as tumor markers, the literature is often contradictory and inconsistent with few accepted conclusions.

## VARIATION IN THE HUMAN GENOME

If the DNA of any two individuals is compared, on average one difference is noted every 1250 bases (i.e., approximately 99.9% of the sequence is identical between randomly chosen copies of the genome). However, copy number variants involve a greater amount of the genome, with 0.5% of the genome differing on average between two individuals when copy number variants >50 kb are considered. Between individuals, at least five times as many bases are affected by copy number changes as by small sequence differences.

Most human genetic material is present in two copies, with the exception of the unpaired sex chromosome in males and mitochondrial DNA. The presence of only single gene copies on the X and Y chromosome in males leads to well-known sex-linked disorders. In contrast, the 16,500-bp mitochondrial genome is present in multiple copies per

| TABLE 48.3 | Some Common, Interesting, and Important Types of RNA |
|---|---|
| **Abbreviation** | **Description** |
| mRNA | Messenger RNA is translated to protein by the ribosome. |
| rRNA | Ribosomal RNA is a major component of ribosomes. |
| tRNA | Transfer RNA pairs an amino acid with its anticodon in protein synthesis. |
| ncRNA | Noncoding RNA is not translated to protein. |
| lncRNA | Long noncoding RNA is >200 bases and is not translated to protein. |
| hnRNA | Heterogeneous nuclear RNA is the initial RNA transcript that includes introns. |
| Ribozyme | RNA that has catalytic activity. |
| Riboswitch | RNA that switches between two conformations under certain conditions (ligand exposure). |
| Telomerase RNA | Structural part of telomerase that also provides a hexamer template. |
| Xist RNA | X-inactive-specific transcript RNA inactivates one X chromosome in females. |
| snRNA | Small nuclear RNA is found in the eukaryotic nucleus. |
| snoRNA | Small nucleolar RNA are intron fragments essential for pre-rRNA processing. |
| siRNA | Small interfering RNA can cleave perfectly complementary target RNA. |
| gRNA | Guide RNA pairs with an RNA target and guides proteins for cleavage, etc. |
| miRNA | MicroRNA affects target mRNA regulation or decay. |

cell, constituting about 0.3% of human DNA, depending on the tissue source. Allele fractions may vary over a wide range when all mitochondria in a cell are considered. That is, sequence variations in mitochondrial DNA are heteroplasmic, meaning that the ratio of the wild-type allele to a variant allele in a cell can vary almost continuously, sometimes resulting in a wide range of symptoms even when only one sequence variant is involved.

Large-scale human genome sequencing projects have cast a wide net across many diverse populations. These projects have provided a wealth of knowledge of the genetic diversity that exists in humans. An alternative approach to human genetic diversity is to examine more homogenous populations. Several studies have examined the genetics of a large number of individuals from Iceland. A whole-genome sequencing study of 2636 Icelanders observed 20 million single nucleotide variants (SNVs) and 1.5 million insertions/deletions. The data from this study were combined with a previous dataset of 104,220 Icelanders who had been SNV typed at 676,913 locations. By applying whole-genome sequencing data from only a small subset of individuals, the full genetics was inferred for a larger set of over 100,000 individuals who had only had SNV typing.

Another interesting result of the Icelandic whole-genome study was the identification of 6795 loss of function single nucleotide variants, insertions or deletions in 4924 genes. Loss of function changes (homozygous or compound heterozygous) were found in 7.7% of the individuals sequenced. In essence, this study identified a surprisingly high percentage of individuals with "knocked-out" or functionally silenced genes.

Any sequence change (compared to a reference sequence) is called a *sequence variant* or *variation*. Many variations do not affect human health and are benign or silent. For example: (1) copy-number variations; (2) SNVs; and (3) STRs found between genes are seldom associated with disease.

## Single Nucleotide Variants

The most common sequence variants are single nucleotide changes, known as SNVs. More than 320 million human SNVs have been described (www.pggsnv.org), and new SNVs continue to be reported. Some SNVs are common in the population, with allele frequencies of 0.1–0.5 (i.e., present in 10–50 of every 100 copies studied), but other single base changes are very rare. The vast majority of SNVs occur in noncoding regions and most of the SNVs within introns, except for splicing and regulatory variants, are not known to affect gene function. In addition, some of the SNVs within exons are silent alterations that do not code for a change in amino acid sequence because of the redundancy in the genetic code. Still other SNVs in exons code for amino acid changes that do not affect protein function. However, some silent SNVs may affect DNA splicing, and others are of interest as genetic markers.

Examination of SNVs reveals thousands of variants in each gene, many of which do not cause disease. The International 1000 Genomes Project sequenced 2504 individuals from twenty-six populations from Europe, East Asia, South Asia, West Africa, and the Americas. All participants were sequenced by both whole-genome sequencing and exome sequencing. Individuals had on average 4.1–5.0 million sites different from the human reference genome. Greater than 99% of single nucleotide variants occurred in >1% of individuals examined. Importantly for clinical genetic studies, all participants were self-declared as healthy at the time of sample collection. The genome aggregation database (gnomad.broadinstitute.org) (v3) lists over 640 million variants from over 76,000 genomes of unrelated individuals. Most variants are rare (found only once or twice) and <0.1% are disease-associated.

In the current age of genomics, the lack of understanding of disease causation based on variant identification is referred to as an "interpretive gap." Disease classification of variants (e.g., benign or pathogenic) lags far behind our ability to discover these variants. Sequence alterations that are known to cause disease are called *mutations, pathogenic variants,* or *disease-causing variants.* About 68% of known disease-causing variants involve only a single base change. Most of the remaining disease-causing variants (24%) are small insertions or deletions. The remainder (8%) includes more complex structural variations (see Table 48.1).

Most SNVs that cause disease are missense and result in amino acid substitutions; significantly fewer are nonsense variants that result in a termination codon and premature polypeptide chain termination. Approximately 10% of disease-causing variants are SNVs that affect splicing sites and result in altered concatenation of coding sequences. Finally, less than 2% of known disease-causing variants are SNVs that affect the regulatory efficiency of transcription by altering promoter or enhancer regions in introns or the stability of the RNA transcript.

Small insertion and deletion variants account for 24% of variants that cause disease. An insertion refers to the presence of extra bases, whereas deletion implies the absence of certain bases in comparison with a reference sequence. Insertions and deletions often cause a shift of the codon reading frame, resulting in altered amino acid sequence downstream of the variation—commonly followed by chain termination from a nonsense codon.

The remaining 8% of variants that relate to health and disease are mostly structural variants including: (1) duplications or deletions of entire exons or genes; (2) gene fusions, including chromosomal translocations and inversions; (3) STR expansions (e.g., an increased number of trinucleotide repeats); (4) gene rearrangements (e.g., rearrangements of immunoglobulin genes in B cells that are required for production of antibodies); (5) complex polymorphic loci related to health and disease (e.g., human leukocyte antigens); and (6) copy number variants (CNVs).

## Copy Number Variation (Gains and Losses)

Although SNVs are the most common sequence variant, CNVs cover more of the genome than SNVs. Examples of large gains or losses in genomic DNA have been known for many years in syndromic diseases. However, an examination of phenotypically normal individuals by array-based comparative genomic hybridization revealed an average of 12.4 large copy number variations per individual. Some CNVs in phenotypically normal individuals involved 2 million bases of DNA. CNVs may be duplicated in tandem or may involve complex gains or losses of homologous sequences at multiple sites in the genome. CNV regions exist in every chromosome and involve 5%–12% of the human genome.

Higher resolution comparative genomic hybridization has revealed the presence of hundreds of deletions across individuals. In total, these studies have found over 1000 unique deletions. Some deletions are in regions without known genes; however, hundreds of known or predicted genes exist at the site of the observed deletions. Interest in CNVs in relation to disease has increased recently as the extent of variation has become clear. CNVs can involve genes or contiguous sets of genes. When the normal dosage of the gene is two, but more than two functional copies of a gene are present, then the gene is "amplified." If a dosage-sensitive gene, such as HER2 (*ERBB2*) is amplified, it usually leads to overexpression of mRNA and protein, resulting in cellular abnormalities and possible progression to disease, such as cancer. When the normal gene dosage is two, and loss of one of the functional copies of the gene occurs, disorders such as mental retardation and developmental delay may result. Structural variants can be determined by cytogenetic techniques, including karyotyping, fluorescent in situ hybridization, comparative genomic hybridization, and virtual karyotyping by SNV microarrays.

## Fusions

Gene fusions arise by deletions, duplications, inversions, and translocations, and are commonly found in cancer. Often, they arise by balanced translocations, whereby a chimeric protein is created by the fusion of two coding regions. Gene fusions promote tumor proliferation by either activating an oncogenic driver or inactivating a tumor suppressor. Although translocations are rare outside of cancer, massively parallel sequencing now allows insight into the myriad of translocations that occur in both hematologic and solid tumors. By identifying gene fusions that act as primary oncogenic drivers, the hope is that targeted therapies may be available for precision treatment. Fusions across the genome can be visualized on Circos plots, where sequential chromosomes form arcs around a positional genomic circle. Intra- and interchromosomal fusions are indicated by curves connecting different genomic locations. Fig. 48.2 shows a Circos plot of a prostate cancer genome that includes many intrachromosomal fusions and several interchromosomal fusions. Additionally, concentric circles on Circos plots can indicate additional tracts of data, such as copy number information, allowing related genomic metadata to be presented in a very condensed format.

## Short Tandem Repeats

Short tandem repeats are DNA motifs that are defined by 1 to several bases that are repeated many times in tandem. STRs

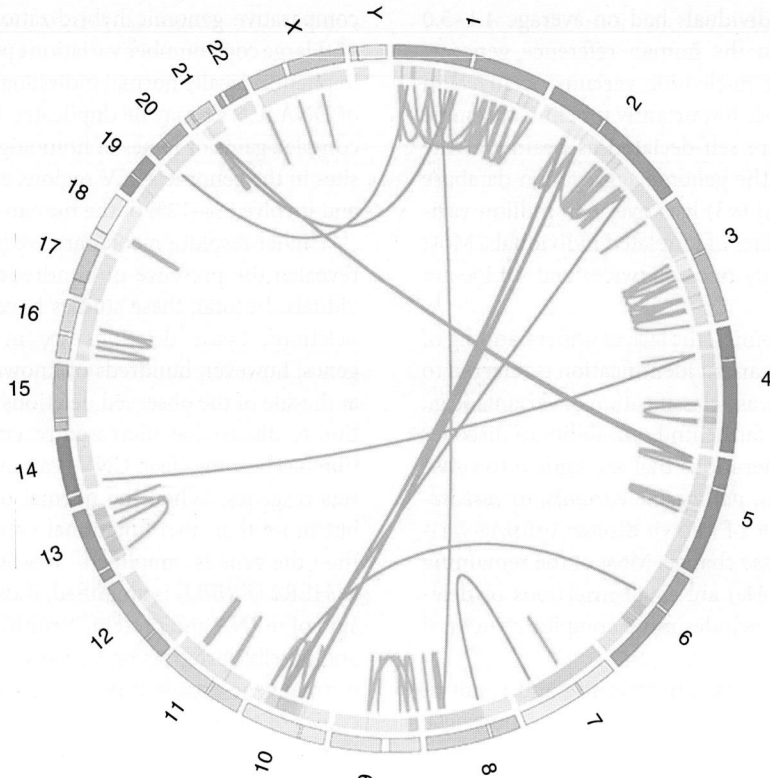

**Fig. 48.2** A Circos plot for graphical representation of genomic fusions and copy number changes. Chromosomes and their positions are indicated around the outside of the circle. Intrachromosomal fusions are indicated by short connections within chromosomes, while interchromosomal fusions cross through the interior of the circle. Copy number changes are indicated on an internal concentric circle by color and intensity. Full color version available on the Evolve Resources site. (Reprinted with permission from Berger MF, Lawrence MS, Demichelis F, et al. The genomic complexity of primary human prostate cancer. *Nature* 2011;470:214–220.)

have been implicated in >40 genetic diseases. In the case of Fragile X, there is an expansion of CGG repeats that results in disruption of protein expression of the *FMR1* gene. For Huntington's disease, an expansion of a CAG repeat results in abnormal protein expression of the *HTT* gene. Many massively parallel sequencing platforms use short reads of information that are <200 bases in length, and these short reads make the analysis of repetitive sequences difficult.

One way to catalog repetitive DNA elements is a 'thesaurus' approach that uses an extensive listing of repetitive DNA elements in the human genome. This approach detects novel variants without extensive changes to typical analysis approaches. Massively parallel sequencing technology and informatics are limited in the amount of STR data that is sequenced and analyzed. The informatics tool lobSTR (https://lobstr.teamerlich.org) can accurately genotype STRs from massively parallel sequencing datasets. When lobSTR was applied across whole-genome datasets from the 1000 Genomes Project, 700,000 STR loci were catalogued, and 350,000 STR loci were found per individual. Some STR loci were common with 300,000 having a mean allele frequency of >1% and 2237 were located within 20 bases of an exon-intron junction. The high frequency of STR loci and their proximity to coding DNA suggest a larger role for STR variants in influencing growth, development, and disease.

## Transposable Elements and their Genetic Fossils

Transposable elements include several classes of similar sequences that originally facilitated homologous recombination, creating deletions, duplications, inversions, and translocations. Most of these elements are no longer active and are categorized as retrotransposons, including long terminal repeats (LTRs), long interspersed nuclear elements (LINEs), and short interspersed nuclear elements (SINEs). In a conservative estimate not including repeat-rich regions like centromeres, these elements comprised 30%–50% of the total DNA in mammals. In comparison, the genomes of birds were <10% derived from transposable elements.

In one human study, repetitive DNA including transposable elements and their nonfunctional descendants consumed 66%–69% of the human genome. In humans, active transposable elements include a subset of L1 LINEs and *Alu* (a type of SINE). These active elements have de novo germline insertions ranging from 1 in 20 to 1 in 916 births. The insertion of these elements has multiple possible effects on the transcriptional regulation of genes including disruption of the open reading frame, creation of a novel promoter, alternative splicing, an alternative poly(A) tail, disruption of transcription factor bindings sites and changes in small RNA regulation. A study of mobile element insertions investigated their occurrence in >30,000 clinical exomes; only 14 mobile element insertions were classified as clinically significant with an overall diagnostic yield of 0.15%. Common repeat sequences in humans and other species are shown in Fig. 48.3.

## Human Epigenetic Alterations

In addition to the sequence variants considered above, epigenetic alterations, including alternative splicing and methylation, affect gene expression. Even though the number of genes may be limited to less than 20,000, variable transcription initiation and exon splicing produce about 200,000 unique mRNA transcripts and protein products.

Methylation of cytosine to 5-methylcytosine occurs frequently; about 70% of CpG dinucleotides in the human genome are methylated. Although not inherited, interest in this "fifth base" has increased as correlations with cancer have been reported. CpG islands are about 1000 bases in length and are often found near the 5′ end of genes. These regions consist of clusters of CG dinucleotides that are usually not methylated in normal cells. However, CpG methylation correlates with condensed chromatin structure and promoter inactivation; an important example occurs in tumor-suppressor

genes. Other epigenetic targets include nucleosome histone phosphorylation, acetylation, and methylation that can all affect gene expression.

## ENCODE Project

ENCODE (Encyclopedia of DNA Elements) is a project that was initiated by the National Human Genome Research Institute in 2003 to examine all functional elements in the human genome. The functional elements defined were not only the discrete genomic areas that encode a product, such as protein, but any genomic area with a reproducible biological effect on processes such as transcription or chromatin structure. These genomic areas include both exons as well as non-protein coding areas such as promoters, enhancer, and silencers. The genomic areas that do not encode protein have significant contributions to human variation. From a survey of 150 genome-wide association studies using SNVs to identify genes linked to disease, 465 unique disease-associated SNVs were identified. Of these 465 variants, 88% ($n=407$) were present in the regions between genes (intergenic) or within introns. These results suggest the importance of noncoding variants in disease.

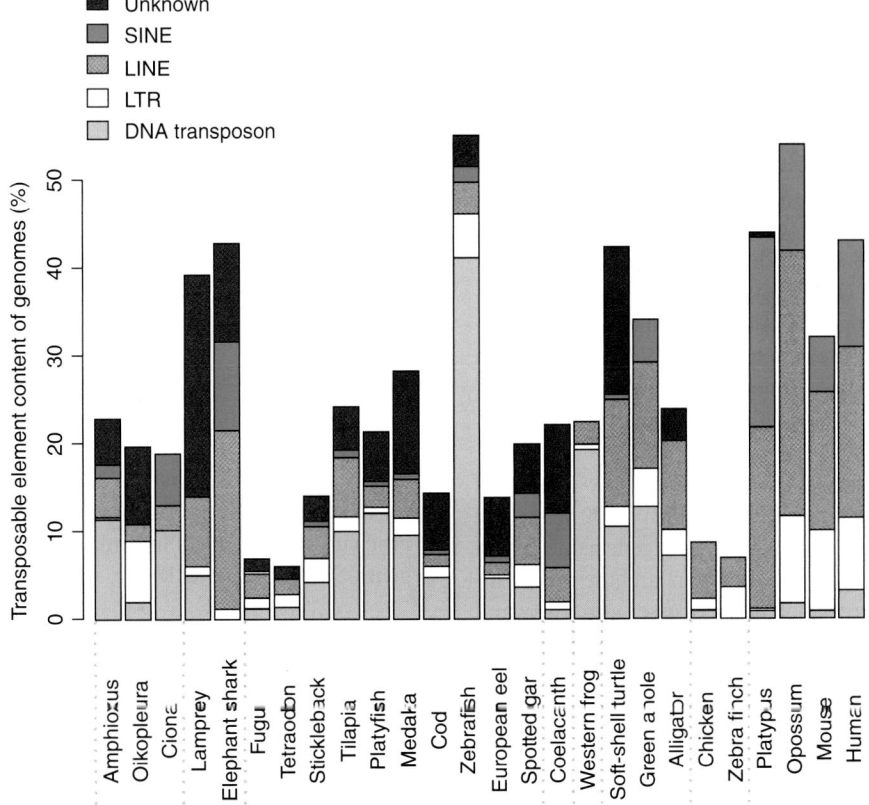

**Fig. 48.3** Transposable element diversity among species, including both retrotransposons and active transposons. The percentage of inactive retrotransposons (SINE, LINE, LTR) and active DNA transposons is shown for each organism. The organisms are grouped into invertebrates (e.g., Amphioxus), nonbony vertebrates (e.g., Lamprey), actinopterygian fish (e.g., Fugu), lobe-finned fish (e.g., Coelacanth), amphibians (e.g., Western frog), nonbird reptiles (e.g., Soft-shell turtle), birds (e.g., Chicken), and mammals (e.g., Platypus). In mammals, transposable elements contribute to >30% of the total genome. In comparison, in other organisms such as chicken and fugu, transposable elements are <10% of the genome. (Reprinted with permission from Chalopin D, Naville M, Plard F, et al. Comparative analysis of transposable elements highlights mobilome diversity and evolution in vertebrates. *Genome Biol Evol.* 2015;7:567–580.)

# NOMENCLATURE

Amino acid variations were associated with human disease long before DNA variation. Amino acid variants were found first because techniques for amino acid sequencing matured prior to DNA sequencing. Advances in DNA technology enabled the investigation of DNA variations associated with disease. For example, the characterization of amino acid variants in the globin gene products (*HBB* and *HBA*) preceded the descriptions of DNA variation in the globin genes.

## Small Variants

The Human Genome Variation Society (HGVS) provides a nomenclature system for standardized reporting of genetic variation (Box 48.1). In the HGVS system, disease alleles are described at the DNA level rather than as amino acid changes. Preferred terminology does not ascribe disease potential to the naming of a variant because only a fraction of variants cause disease. The preferred terms include: sequence variant, copy number variant, and single nucleotide variant. Hemoglobin variants were initially named by a combination of letters (Hemoglobin A, B, S, C, F) and the city of discovery. Hematologists continue to use the traditional or legacy nomenclature (Table 48.4) that does not distinguish between variants from β-globin (*HBB*) and α-globin (*HBA*). In addition to the hemoglobin genes, other genes have both a traditional/legacy nomenclature system and HGVS recommended nomenclature.

## Naming Genes

As significant as the naming of DNA variants, the naming of genes has also become standardized over the past 30 years. The basic components of gene names include the gene name, which may include information on gene function, and the gene symbol, which is a short abbreviation in upper case Latin letters and Arabic numbers that are both italicized. The currently accepted gene naming system is by the HUGO Gene Nomenclature Committee (HGNC). As with all standardization activities, there is a trade-off. The more familiar historic names are established in the literature, and used by practitioners in the specialty concerned with that gene. However, for a particular disease-associated gene, communication outside of the specialized field of knowledge may by difficult and lead to errors. Especially in the current era with genomic tests examining hundreds to tens of thousands of genes, a common gene naming system is necessary. In reporting specific genes, a hybrid approach that uses both the consensus nomenclature and the traditional

name may be useful. A current database of recommended gene names and symbols as well as traditional names can be found on the HGNC online database. As of 2022, the HGNC database currently contains information on 19,356 protein-coding genes, 9080 noncoding RNAs, and 14,339 pseudogenes.

| TABLE 48.4 | Describing Hemoglobin Variants by Different Nomenclature Systems | | | | | | |
|---|---|---|---|---|---|---|
| Traditional Name | Disease Associated | Gene | Amino Acid Change (Traditional)[a] | Amino Acid Change (HGVS) | HGVS Nucleotide Change (mRNA Transcript)[b] | Genomic Coordinate (GRCh37/hg19)[c] |
| Hemoglobin SS | Sickle cell anemia | *HBB* | Gln6Val | p.(Glu7Val) | NM_000518.4(HBB):c.20A>T | Chr11:g.5248232T>A |
| Hemoglobin CC | Hemolytic anemia | *HBB* | Glu6Lys | p.(Glu7Lys) | NM_000518.4(HBB):c.19G>A | Chr11:g.5248233C>T |
| Hemoglobin Austin | None | *HBB* | Arg40Ser | p.(Arg41Ser) | NM_000518.4(HBB):c.123G>T | Chr11:g.5247999C>A |
| Hemoglobin G Philadelphia | None | *HBA2* | Asn68Lys | p.(Asn69Lys) | NM_000517.4(HBA2):c.207C>A | Chr16:g.223235C>A |

[a]The amino acid change for hemoglobin diseases was characterized by amino acid sequencing before the advent of DNA sequencing. The first amino acid, methionine, was not included, so that the Glu to Val change in sickle cell anemia was described as the "6" position rather than the "7" position.
[b]The "c." annotation is based on a reference transcript (NM number).
[c]The HGVS nucleotide position is from 5′ to 3′ on the strand. However, the genomic coordinates are not oriented to the gene. The nucleotide position number based on mRNA transcript may increase while the genomic position number increases or decreases, depending on the orientation of the gene on the chromosome.

## Variant Databases

Databases of DNA variations may focus on specific genes or diseases (e.g., hemoglobinopathy variants cataloged in HbVar) or catalog variants throughout the entire genome. Some genomic databases target somatic variants found in cancer, including The Cancer Genome Atlas (TCGA) and the Catalog of Somatic Mutations in Cancer (COSMIC). Constitutional or germline variants that are passed from generation to generation are the focus of most genomic databases. Some of the most common are dbSNP (Database of Single Nucleotide Polymorphisms), HGMD (Human Gene Mutation Database), ClinVar (Clinical Genome Resource's variant database), gnomAD (Genome Aggregation Database), and OMIM (Online *Mendelian Inheritance in Man*).

A systematic catalog of SNVs including small insertions and deletions was created as the dbSNP in 1998 as a collaboration between the NCBI and the National Human Genome Research Institute (NHGRI). The reference identifier for variants in dbSNP begins with the prefix "rs" and as of 2022, over 1 billion variants are currently cataloged.

HGMD is a database of variants with reported disease associations. The number of new reports of germline mutations was <250 per year through 1990, but throughout the 1990s reports grew into the thousands and now >350,000 variants across over 12,000 genes are cataloged in release 2021.4 of HGMD Professional, a privatized derivative of the originally public database. As databases grow, curation and the avoidance of errors become critical; incorrect annotations do arise from database issues or problems with the primary literature. At one point in time, 80% of the HGMD disease-causing variants from the 1000 Genomes Project dataset had an allele frequency of more than 5%; however, rare diseases are expected to have allele frequencies much less than 5%.

The chief limitation of databases such as dbSNP and HGMD is that they rely on published reports. As new variants of known genes are discovered in research or clinical laboratories, they are rarely published. This recognition of the underrepresentation of clinically significant variants resulted in the ClinVar project, which allows for the contribution of annotated variants by clinical laboratories, research laboratories, and the literature into a publicly available database. The dataset combines submitter, variant, and phenotype and is given an accession number with the prefix "SCV" (Submitted Clinical Variant); when multiple records exist for a single variant then a reference accession prefix "RCF" is assigned. As of January 2022, ClinVar included over 1.8 million records with interpretations.

Instead of cataloging variants, OMIM is organized by disease state and is manually curated by a team of professionals located at Johns Hopkins University. It was started by the geneticist Victor McKusick in the 1970s as "*Mendelian Inheritance in Man*," first a series of published books and later an online resource. By design, the OMIM is not a comprehensive catalog of every variant ever described with disease but rather a catalog of genes and variants representative of a disease type. As of 2022, OMIM contained 7075 phenotype descriptions of known molecular basis involving 4574 genes.

## MASSIVELY PARALLEL METHODS

It is a daunting task to experimentally investigate the enormous complexity of biological genomes and their variants. Nevertheless, methods that interrogate entire genomes are now in common use. Perhaps the simplest genomic DNA analysis uses flow cytometry to quantify the total amount of DNA in cells. Somewhat more complex is the analysis of individual chromosomes by conventional cytogenetics. Even more detailed are nucleic acid microarrays, allowing SNV genotyping, gene expression analysis, and copy number quantification. Finally, the ultimate genomic analysis is whole-genome sequencing, enabled today by massively parallel sequencing. In this section, we focus on microarrays and massively parallel sequencing.

## Nucleic Acid Microarrays

Nucleic acid microarrays (also called *DNA arrays*, *DNA chips*, or *oligonucleotide arrays*) were introduced in the mid-1990s. They function by nucleic acid hybridization with spot sizes of about100 microns (μm) in diameter, such that one array contains thousands to millions of spots. Such small dimensions require specialized detection equipment, software, and informatics to analyze the data. Because of their high density and information content, microarrays have attracted intense interest among researchers who wish to monitor the whole genome for SNVs, gene expression, or copy number variation.

Because SNVs represent the most common genetic difference among individuals, much effort has focused on correlating SNV genotypes to phenotype and disease association. SNV microarrays have been used in many genome-wide association studies (GWAS). Microarrays that analyze human SNVs ("SNV chips") provide the technology to genotype most frequent human SNVs in one experiment. Nearby SNV alleles tend to cluster together as haplotypes, so disease association by haplotype simplifies the analysis. Although some valuable markers have been found by GWAS, the yield of useful disease markers obtained by these methods has been disappointing, and many difficulties remain, such as identifying adequate control populations. SNV arrays can also be used to genotype SNVs of known association with disease and to assess copy number variation. Cytogenomic arrays, including SNV and comparative genomic hybridization (CGH) arrays, can analyze the entire genome, providing chromosome maps of copy number changes (large insertions and deletions) across each chromosome.

Gene expression microarrays quantify the relative amounts of different messenger RNAs in test and reference samples. An example of a two-color microarray for gene expression is shown in Fig. 48.4. Probes that hybridize to mRNA are usually directly synthesized on microarrays. Modern gene expression arrays have been used to measure the mRNA transcribed from all human genes in one experiment. They have been applied to almost every conceivable human circumstance, including: (1) neoplastic, (2) inflammatory, and (3) psychiatric conditions. It is expected that application of this technology will lead to better: (1) diagnosis, (2) molecular staging,

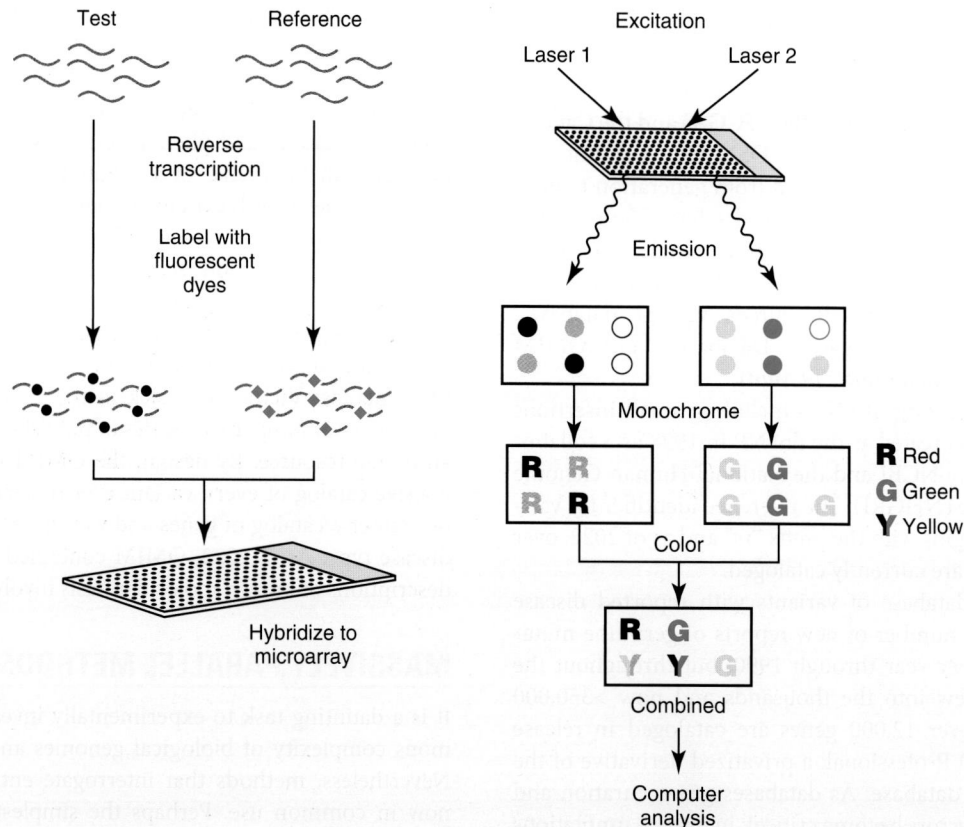

**Fig. 48.4** A two-color microarray experiment. An array of DNA oligonucleotides with sequences of messenger RNA are affixed to a glass slide. Messenger RNAs in the test and reference specimen are converted into differentially labeled cDNA by reverse transcription and incorporation of two different fluorescent dyes. The two samples are hybridized together onto the array. The array is washed, and the image is captured twice, each time with a laser of a wavelength that excites one of the dyes but not the other. The monochromatic images are then converted to two colors (green (G) for the test sample, and red (R) for the reference), and the images are combined. If the abundance of cDNA is the same in each of the two samples, then the composite spot is yellow (Y). If one is in greater abundance, then that color will be preserved. Upregulation and downregulation of gene expression are then analyzed by software.

(3) prognosis, and (4) therapy through understanding of disease pathogenesis. In oncology, gene expression microarrays have led to new diagnostic and prognostic markers in breast cancer, bladder cancer, leukemia, and sarcoma, among others. Molecular expression signatures often divide cancer into subtypes that respond differently to therapy. For example, Fig 48.5 shows a "heat map" of 165 patients with bladder cancer and the relative expression of 768 genes for each patient. Four major subtypes are apparent by clustering the expression signatures, and one of the subtypes was more responsive to anti-PD-L1 immunotherapy. Even with much progress, expression arrays are used directly in only a few clinical diagnostic and prognostic tests. Most arrays are used in marker discovery projects for selection of a smaller panel of expression targets that are then analyzed by other quantitative methods, such as real-time PCR, that provide greater precision and dynamic range.

Another important clinical application of microarrays is the genome-wide analysis of deletions and duplications, referred to as copy number variants (CNVs). CNV analysis using microarrays is replacing traditional cytogenetic chromosome analysis (karyotyping) and fluorescence in situ hybridization (FISH) analysis for detection of genome-wide copy number alterations. Similar to gene expression arrays, many of the CNV arrays use two-color comparative hybridization to determine the gene dosage in a specimen compared with a normal reference genome (array comparative genomic hybridization; aCGH). Arrays for CGH use oligonucleotide probes for very high resolution and data density. An example of CNV analysis using aCGH is shown in Fig. 48.6. SNV arrays are also used to detect copy number changes by loss of heterozygosity (this method is sometimes referred to as *virtual karyotyping*). Unlike aCGH, SNV arrays have the advantage of analyzing the specimen without the need to mix in a reference genome. SNV arrays are also able to detect copy number neutral changes caused by inversions or uniparental disomy that are not detected by aCGH methods. When a clinically significant copy number change is found, it can be verified by an orthogonal method such as FISH or high-resolution melting.

## Massively Parallel Sequencing

The need to understand the full extent of genome-wide human variation led to the human genome project. Sequencing the human genome began with the orderly "conventional" sequencing of large (150 Kb) fragments of DNA that were divided among members of the consortium and methodically sequenced. However, random "shotgun" sequencing proved to be faster and was an important tool for completing the sequence of the first human genome. Massively parallel sequencing is the current technology used for genome sequencing. Fig. 48.7 contrasts these different sequencing approaches.

Massively parallel sequencing evolved out of earlier sequencing methods. When genomic DNA is sequenced

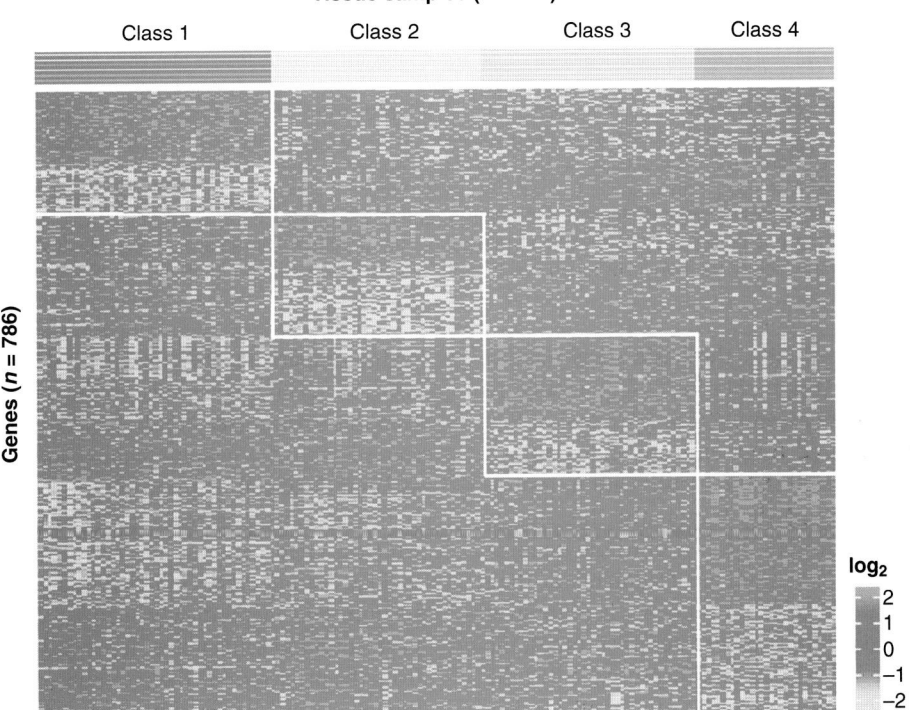

**Fig. 48.5** Heat map showing unsupervised hierarchal clustering of gene expression from 786 genes in 165 bladder cancer tissues. The molecular signature identifies four subgroups. Typically, underexpression is shown in red and overexpression is shown in green, with different intensity levels differing by log₂. Full color version available on the Evolve Resources site. (Modified with permission from Song BN, Kim SK, Mun JY, et al. Identification of an immunotherapy-responsive molecular subtype of bladder cancer. *EBioMedicine.* 2019;50:238–245.)

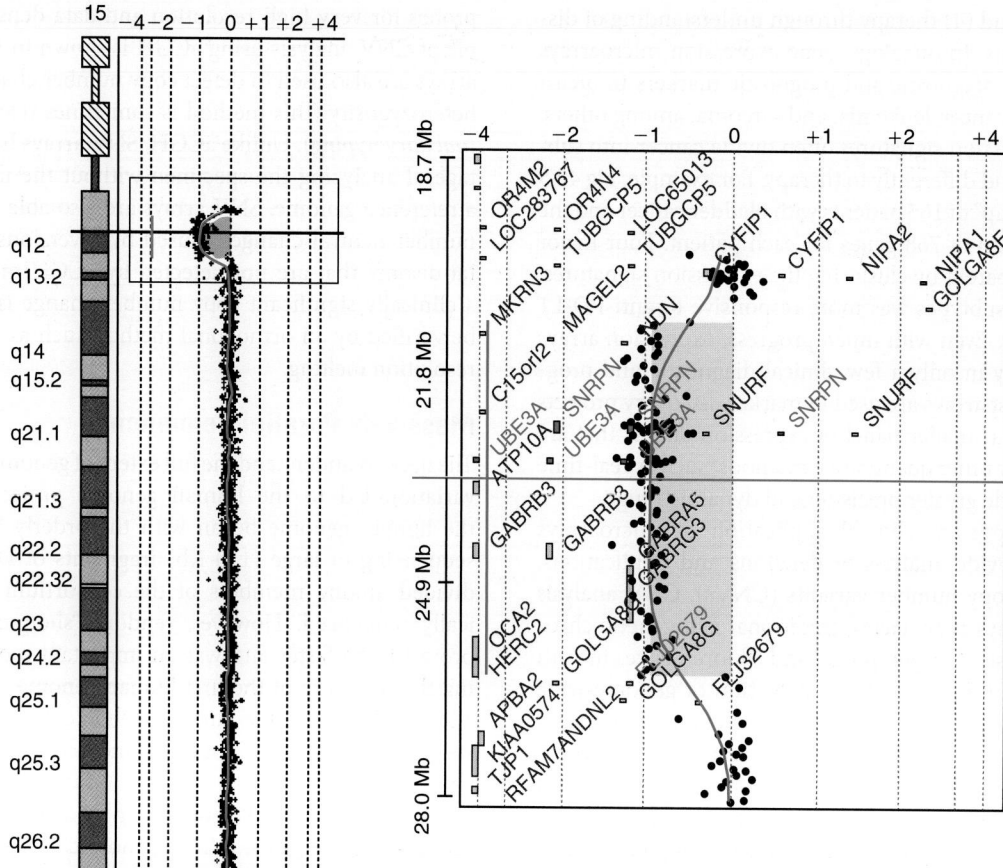

**Fig. 48.6** Copy number variation identified with a comparative genomic hybridization array made from oligonucleotides. DNA from a subject is fragmented, labeled with Cy5, and hybridized onto a microarray, together with Cy3-labeled reference DNA. On the array are 44,000 oligonucleotide probes, each about 60 bases long and tiled across the whole genome at an average spacing of 75 kb. Shown on the *left panel* are results of probes on chromosome 15 (all other chromosomes are analyzed in this assay but are not shown). Each *dot* represents a specific probe to which the subject's DNA hybridizes. Their positions (0, −1, +1, and so on) reflect the dosage of the subject's DNA relative to the reference DNA. A majority of the probes line up on "0," indicating no quantitative difference compared with the reference DNA. Probes in the 15q11 to 15q13 region, however, are on the "−1" line, indicating that the subject has a deletion of that region. A closer view of that region (*right panel*) shows that among the deleted genes are *UBE3A*, which causes Angelman syndrome, and *SNRPN*, which causes Prader–Willi syndrome. Because the method does not distinguish the methylation status of the deleted alleles, this result alone cannot determine which of the two disorders the subject has. (Courtesy Sarah South, PhD, ARUP Laboratories.)

by massively parallel sequencing, the basic steps include random DNA shearing (fragmentation), sequencing in parallel reactions, and data assembly (see *left* panel of Fig. 48.7). The randomly sheared fragments are end-modified with oligonucleotides that aid in the identification, immobilization, and sequencing of the fragments; this step is referred to as library creation. In the case of whole-genome sequencing, this "library" of modified fragments is then sequenced. However, if only a subset of genes is of interest or if only the coding nucleotides are of interest (exome), the specific targets can be hybridized and "captured" after the library step. Targeted capture of regions of interest is a key step in exome sequencing. More than 1 million sequencing reactions occur in parallel, generating more than 100 bases of data per reaction. After sequencing, the short reads of DNA are assembled based on a reference genome (e.g., GRCh38).

In comparison, the conventional sequencing of genomes was the technology used for the initiation of the Human Genome Project (see *middle panel* of Fig. 48.7). This method started with the genome cloned into large molecules such as Yeast Artificial Chromosomes (YACs) and later Bacterial Artificial Chromosomes (BACs). These larger molecules, which carried genomic inserts >150 Kb in size, were then divided among the members of the genome sequencing consortium and methodically sequenced in 700 base reactions. Each round of sequencing depended on the sequencing data from the prior round. The assembly of data is not as computationally intensive as massively parallel or shotgun sequencing.

Finally, shotgun sequencing was key to the speedy completion of the Human Genome Project (see *right panel* of Fig. 48.7). Rather than methodically sequencing targets of interest, the method relied on random shearing of DNA and subcloning the fragments into plasmids. The plasmids were then

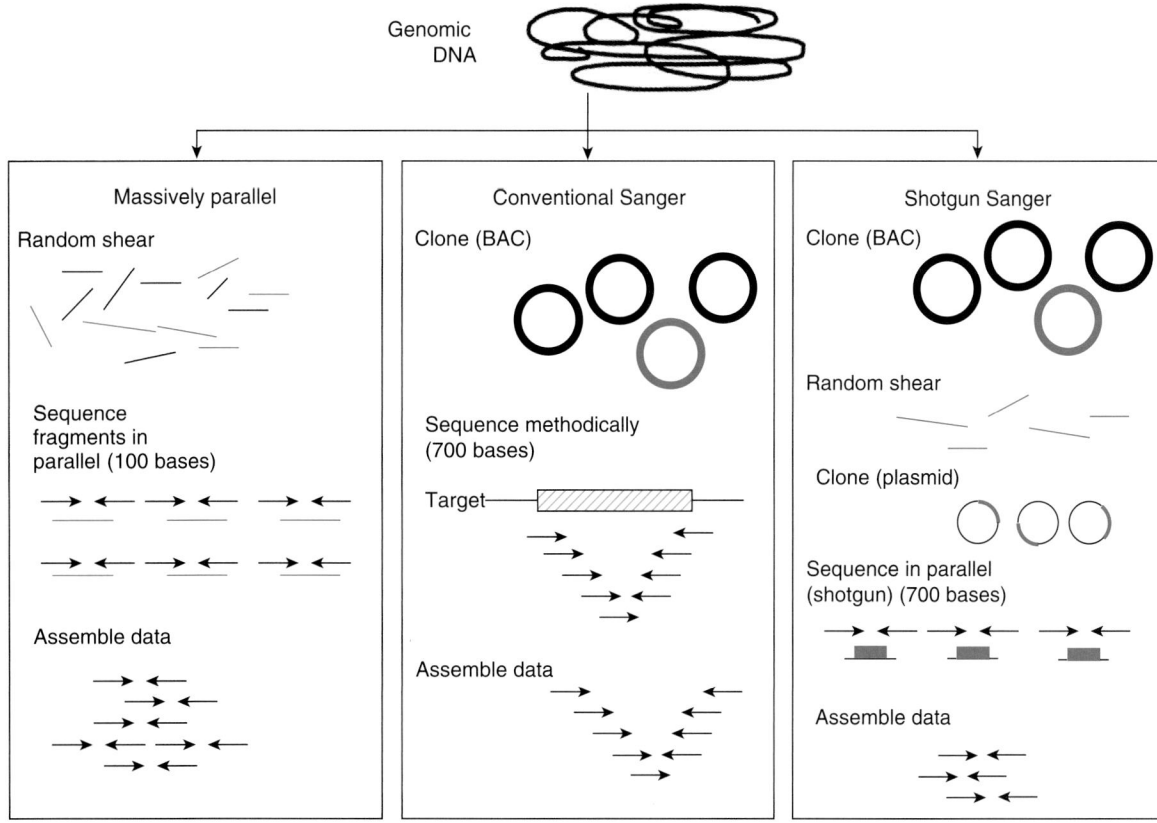

**Fig. 48.7** Genome sequencing approaches. Massively parallel sequencing (*left panel*) is the current technology used for genome sequencing, but it evolved out of earlier conventional Sanger (*middle panel*) and shotgun Sanger (*right panel*) sequencing methods. See text for details. *BAC*, bacterial artificial chromosomes.

sequenced in parallel (separate) reactions. The evolutionary roots of massively parallel sequencing technology originated in shotgun sequencing.

Compared with conventional dideoxy-termination sequencing, massively parallel sequencing generates up to 1 billion more bases of sequence data in one operation at 10,000–100,000 times lower cost per base. The method continues to improve toward even higher throughput and lower costs. Much of the progress that has been made is dependent on advances in optical data processing, bioinformatics, and overall computer power. The cost and turnaround time of these methods continue to decrease, and their convenience continues to improve, leading to increased uptake in clinical laboratories. Clinical laboratory standards for massively parallel sequencing are published, and there are practical guidelines for implementing massively parallel sequencing tests. Clonal sequencing methods replicate a single DNA strand to form a clonal template in order to generate sufficient signal for detection. In contrast, single-molecule sequencing methods must be sensitive enough to detect single molecules of DNA. Characteristics of massively parallel sequencing methods are summarized in Table 48.5, from available recent reviews.

## Sequencing From Clones

Clonal sequencing methods start with producing a random library of fragments that are typically 70–1000 bases in length, although some methods require 6- to 20-kb fragments

or greater. The starting material may be genomic DNA, a hybridization capture-based subset of genomic DNA (as in exome sequencing and some gene panels for specific diseases), or PCR products that focus on limited regions of interest. Fragmentation is usually physical or enzymatic. Common physical methods include sonication and acoustic shearing. Depending on the frequency and geometry of the sample and acoustic generator, fragments averaging from 100 to 20,000 bases can be produced. Hydrodynamic shearing can also be obtained by compressed air to atomize the liquid into a fine mist (nebulization), forcing the solution through a fine-gauge needle, or through a French pressure cell. Enzymatic fragmentation can be from restriction endonucleases, nonspecific DNAses, or a transposase enzyme that simultaneously fragments and adds adapter sequences. In each case, conditions can be modified to produce different fragment sizes.

Adapter sequences are typically added to each end of the random fragments. The primary role of these adapters is to provide common priming sites for each fragment to initiate massively parallel sequencing reactions. One primer set amplifies a massive array (beads or planer flow cell) of library inserts. Adapters also facilitate initial capture of DNA fragments onto solid surfaces and spatially restrict clonal amplification products generated from the fragments onto beads or spots on an array surface. The fragment ends typically need to be "polished" by filling in any missing bases and optionally adding a single extra A to the 3′-ends to facilitate ligation to the adapters. If multiplexing of different DNA samples is desired, a sequence "barcode" is often added as well to identify which DNA sample the clone arose from. A typical library insert with adapters and a barcode is shown in Fig. 48.8A. The libraries are then partitioned according to size to select a band optimal for the downstream sequencing technology.

Clonal amplification for massively parallel sequencing is usually performed on single DNA molecules within microreactors. The partitions may be minute aqueous droplets in a water-in-oil emulsion (*emulsion PCR*), PCR colonies (*polonies*) on a thin film of acrylamide gel, clusters on the surface of a planar flow cell generated by bridge amplification, or beads with clonally amplified template attached to their surface. When amplification is observed in these massively parallel reactions, chances are that clonal amplification has occurred from a single template molecule. Clonal amplification is usually performed by either emulsion PCR or bridge amplification.

### Emulsion Polymerase Chain Reaction

In emulsion PCR, one strand of a library element is captured on one bead and is clonally amplified inside a water-in-oil droplet, generating a bead covered with single-stranded PCR products (Fig. 48.9). The emulsion is formed by mixing beads (each covered with one primer), aqueous PCR components (including the other primer, polymerase, and dNTPs), and a mixture of oils under agitation to ideally form droplets that each contain only one bead and one library insert. The two primers are complementary to the adapters; one coats the bead surface, and one is free in solution. During emulsion PCR, all of the beads are amplified together in aqueous microdroplets dispersed in oil. The emulsion is amplified in a standard PCR thermal cycler. After PCR and denaturation, millions of copies of identical single-stranded PCR products are on each bead with each bead carrying distinct, oriented inserts flanked by the adapters. The emulsion is then broken and, after elimination of empty beads, is ready for sequencing.

### Bridge Amplification

Bridge amplification generates clusters of single-stranded PCR products tethered to the surface of a planar flow cell (Fig. 48.10). In contrast to the clonal bead generation of emulsion PCR, the amplification occurs on a flat surface. The primers, complementary to the adapters, are both attached to the surface, either randomly or in a fixed pattern. The library DNA is then denatured to form single strands that hybridize to the

---

**TABLE 48.5   Characteristics of Massively Parallel Sequencing Methods**

| Method | Principle | Detection | Clonal | Run Time | Output per Run | Read Length (bp) |
|---|---|---|---|---|---|---|
| Synthesis | Pyrophosphate release | Chemiluminescence | Emulsion PCR | 10–23 h | 40–700 Mb | 400–700 |
| Synthesis | pH Change | Electronic CMOS | Emulsion PCR | 3–4 h | 1.5–10 Gb | 125–400 |
| Synthesis | Reversible terminator | Fluorescence | Bridge amplification | 2.7–12 days | 15–1000 Gb | 200–600[a] |
| Synthesis | Reversible terminator | Florescence | Rolling circle replication | 1–4.5 days | 15–6000 Gb | 100–300[a] |
| Single molecule | Zero-mode waveguide | Fluorescence | No | 2 days | 5 Gb | 10 Kb |
| Single molecule | Conductivity | Electronic | No | "Minutes to Days" | Depends | 5 Kb |

[a]Includes both paired end reads (sequencing from both ends)

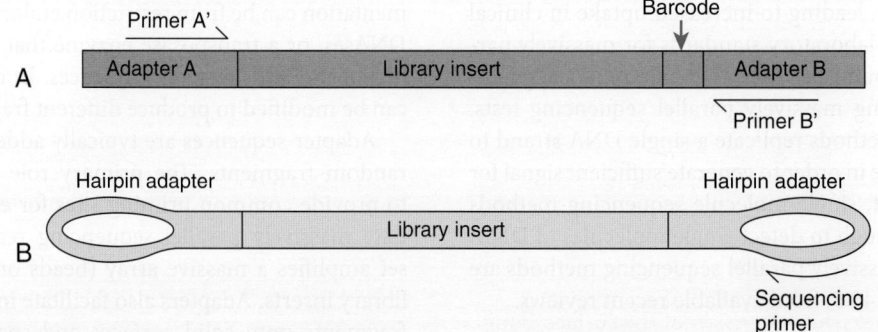

**Fig. 48.8** Diagram of different library designs used in massively parallel sequencing. In (A), two adapters that include consensus PCR priming sites are ligated onto each end of the library inserts produced by fragmentation. If multiplexing different samples is desired, a barcode is added so that each read can be assigned to a specific sample. In (B) a library insert is bounded by hairpin adapters that allow primer binding to the single-stranded loops on each end for rolling circle amplification.

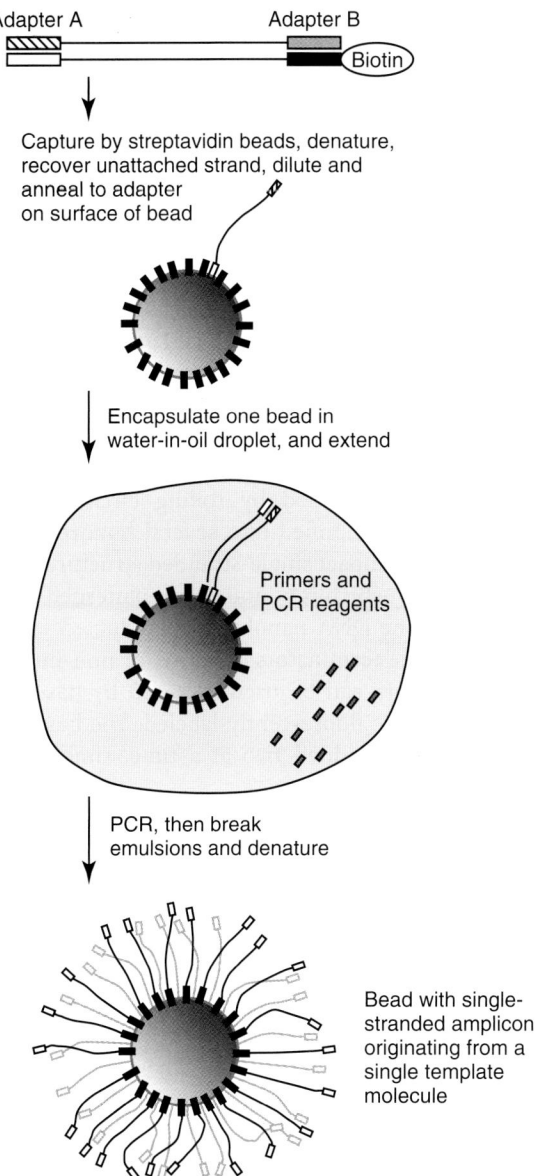

**Fig. 48.9** Emulsion polymerase chain reaction (PCR). Two adapters (*adapters A and B*) are randomly ligated to DNA fragments. Adapter B has a biotin on its 5′-end. Fragments with adapter B on one or both ends are captured by streptavidin beads, while fragments with only adapter A are washed away (not shown). Then the fragments are denatured, and the free strand with adapter A and adapter B at each end is collected (fragments with adapter B on both ends will not be released from the streptavidin bead). One molecule of the single-stranded template is then captured on a bead coated with adapter and is encapsulated inside a water-in-oil droplet that contains PCR reagents and primers. After PCR, the emulsion is disrupted, and the DNA is denatured. This generates a bead with many clonal single strands tethered to it. The bead is then deposited into one of many wells on a fiberoptic slide, or onto a glass slide for sequence analysis (not shown).

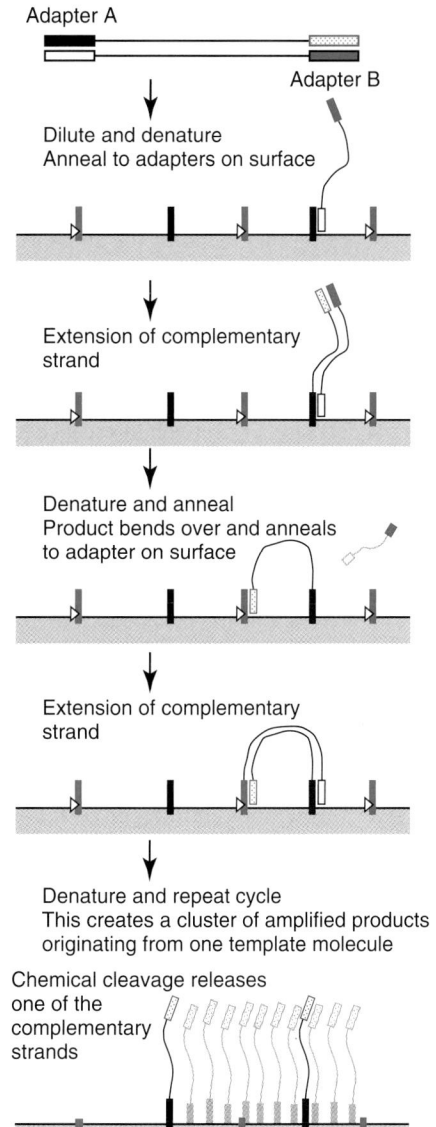

**Fig. 48.10** Bridge amplification. Two adapters (*adapters A and B*) are ligated to a DNA template. After they are diluted and denatured into single strands, the template is captured onto a flowcell surface by annealing to one of the two surface-bound primers that share sequences with adapter A or B. The polymerase reagent introduced into the flowcell extends the primer and generates the complementary strand of the template. The denaturant (usually sodium hydroxide) is introduced to the flowcell to release the original template strand. The free end of the newly synthesized strand anneals to a nearby primer by bending over, and a second round of reagent addition catalyzes the synthesis of another complementary strand. By repeating many of these cycles, a clonal cluster that consists of 1000–30,000 copies of single-stranded template tethered to the surface is generated. This cluster is still a mixture of both complementary strands. One of the strands is selectively eliminated by treatment with periodic acid that cleaves the diol linkage present in one of the surface-bound primers (*open triangle on blue primer*). The cluster now contains only one of the template strands and is ready for sequence analysis.

primers on the surface. After extension of the surface-bound primers, the original template strands are washed away under denaturing conditions. What follows is called bridge amplification, which is very similar to PCR except that both primers are bound to the surface, so that single strands bound to the

surface must bend over to find their opposite primer, resulting in a double-stranded bridge after extension. Instead of denaturing with heat as in PCR, the flow cell is kept at 60°C, and a chemical denaturant is introduced to dissociate the two bridge strands; except now both strands are attached to the planer surface. When the flow cell is flushed with a polymerase and dNTPs under favorable extension conditions, both can find new primers to form additional bridges. The process repeats until thousands of copies are formed. One of the bound primers can be designed to include a cleavable site (either chemical or enzymatic) so that one strand can be removed after denaturation. After capping the 3′-end of the single strands with ddNTPs (to prevent any undesired extension with the closely packed templates), the surface is ready for sequencing.

## Sequencing by Synthesis

Sequencing by synthesis can be detected by: (1) pyrophosphate release, (2) a pH decrease, or (3) the fluorescence of reversible terminators. The clonal amplification methods allow parallel observation of thousands to millions of strand extensions, greatly increasing the signal strength. However, the extensions must be controlled at each step because continuous strand extension would not remain synchronous between strands. This is achieved by immobilizing the clones into arrays so that reagents can be applied sequentially (no pun intended).

## Pyrosequencing

Pyrosequencing was used in the first massively parallel sequencing platform but has not remained competitive because of lower throughput and higher cost. Clonal beads were fit into picoliter reaction chambers formed in etched individual fibers of a fiberoptic cable. Solutions of dATPαS, dCTP, dGTP, or dTTP were passed over chambers one at a time under conditions that favor extension. If there was a base match, the nucleotide was incorporated, and pyrophosphate released. Pyrosequencing signal generation occurred by linked enzymatic reactions, leading to luciferase chemiluminescence. The light produced was captured by the individual light fibers and detected on a CCD. If more than one base occurred in a row (a homopolymer stretch), multiple bases of that nucleotide were incorporated, and the signal was proportionately higher. As the number of identical bases increased, it became harder to determine their exact number.

## Semiconductor Sequencing

Similar to pyrosequencing detection, clonal beads are used as template. However, the beads are arrayed on semiconductor sensors modified to detect pH changes. The chip does not detect light but a slight change in pH produced as a consequence of conversion of one of the dNTPs into pyrophosphates by the many clones on the bead. Similar to pyrosequencing, homopolymer stretches can be problematic. By leveraging semiconductor technology development, the chip has rapidly increased in performance by decreasing the size of the beads and sensor wells and increasing the size of the chip. Run times can be as short as 3–4 hours.

## Reversible Terminators

After bridge amplification on a planar flow cell, one of four nucleotides is passed through the flow cell under conditions that favor extension. Unlike pyrosequencing and semiconductor sequencing, the nucleotides are fluorescent terminators so that only one base is incorporated, avoiding the problems with homopolymer stretches. Each nucleotide has a different fluorescent label so that each can be distinguished by color. Furthermore, the fluorescent terminators are reversible, which means that the blocked 3′-end can be regenerated by simple chemical means provided by the flow cell. Each cycle involves: (1) adding polymerase and dNTPs as fluorescently labeled terminators under conditions that favor extension; (2) washing the flow cell; (3) imaging the fluorescence; (4) cleaving the fluorescent terminator; and (5) washing the flow cell. Output per run can be >1000 Gb in 1 day.

Another type of reversible terminator sequencing ligates DNA fragments from a library into circular constructs, which are then amplified by rolling circle replication. Each fragment is amplified into several hundreds of copies and forms a compact single-stranded structure termed a "DNA nanoball," which is bound onto a patterned flow cell. Sequencing of the DNA nanoballs is conducted with fluorescent reversible terminators as above, or non-fluorescent (cold) terminators can be used followed by base-specific antibodies that are fluorescently-labeled. The base-specific antibodies may be added two at a time, simplifying the required optics.

## Single Molecule Sequencing

Single-molecule sequencing methods do not require template amplification. Base reads do not require syncing with other clonal strands because there are none. Sensitive optical or electronic methods are required to detect base sequence in a single molecule. If long reads (e.g., >10,000 bases in length) and high accuracy are achieved, advantages include efficient sequence assembly, accurate analyses of repetitive sequences, de novo sequencing, mapping of chromosomal rearrangements, and fusions. In contrast, massively parallel sequencing methods usually generate short sequence reads (100–700 bases long) that have to be aligned and analyzed to derive a consensus, then stitched together, and compared with reference genome sequences. Accurate assembly of sequence data relies on sufficient coverage and/or redundancy across the sequenced region.

## Real-Time Single Molecule Sequencing with Fluorescent Nucleotides

Library preparation is unique for this method because fragmentation is tuned to provide about ≥10 kb length inserts, and the adapters are designed as hairpins. The result is a double-stranded insert bounded by identical single-stranded loops on each end (see Fig. 48.8B). Sequencing primers are annealed to the loop region and bound to a single polymerase molecule at the bottom of a zero-mode waveguide to form an active polymerase complex. The zero-mode waveguide allows single molecule detection of transient fluorescent labels that are covalently attached to the terminal phosphate of each dNTP. The four dNTPs are added to the wells with different labels that can be distinguished optically. When a fluorescent dNTP pairs with its complement near to the polymerase active site, it is in a perfect position for fluorescence detection. After being incorporated into the growing strand, the terminal fluorescent label (attached to pyrophosphate) diffuses away from the polymerase. The fluorescent signals are acquired continuously at high speed as the primer proceeds around the loop by rolling circle amplification. The process can be stopped after one loop or continued for multiple reads for error checking. Base reads of >175,000 contiguous bases have been reported.

### Nanopore Sequencing

Another single-molecule sequencing approach that does not require amplification and uses electronic, rather than optical, detection is nanopore sequencing. Single DNA strands are channeled through nanopores formed by immobilized proteins. Passage of individual DNA bases through the protein nanopore generates characteristic electrical signals that can reveal the identity of the base (or combination of bases) traversing the nanopore. In essence, this is similar to a nano-sized Coulter counter that quantifies base differences on a single strand of DNA rather than cell size. Kilobases can be sequenced in a single read. The method is nondestructive and can discriminate methylated DNA bases as well as normal bases. A number of nanopores are currently under study (α-hemolysin, *Mycobacterium smegmatis* porin A; MspA, and others), and solid-state nanopores are also being intensively investigated. Shorter and narrower nanopores that interrogate single bases would be ideal, but current material limitations allow about 4 bases within the nanopore at the same time. Ultra-long reads (>100 Kb) have enabled the assembly and phasing of the entire 4 Mb major histocompatibility complex and complete centromere sequencing.

### Applications Enabled by Massively Parallel Sequencing

Although human genome sequencing is the most obvious application of massively parallel sequencing, the impact of this technology goes far beyond the human genome. Hybridization capture of genomic subsets can reduce the sequencing burden greatly. For example, exome sequencing is a popular approach to identify disease variants that reduces the need for sequencing by almost 100-fold. Sequencing of mRNA ("RNA-Seq") is achieved by conversion of message transcripts to double-stranded DNA by priming with poly-T oligonucleotides and reverse transcriptase, a method that has quantitative advantages over microarrays, and can easily detect fusions. Variants that are traditionally hard to detect by sequencing, including copy number variants and chromosomal rearrangements, are becoming easier to identify with advances in bioinformatics. In "ChIP-seq", the readout of chromatin immunoprecipitation experiments that identify binding sites of transcription factors is greatly simplified. The genomic landscape of accessible chromatin can be determined by "ATAC-seq", a method for in vitro transposition of sequencing adaptors into native chromatin. Many of these methods can be performed on single cells, for example, "CITE-seq" (cellular indexing of transcriptomes and epitopes) combines RNA-Seq with protein identification by sequence-tagged antibodies that can simultaneously be analyzed on thousands of cells. Although it might seem like genomic sequencing only needs to be performed once on any particular individual, this is not true in cancer. Single cell sequencing of neoplastic populations may identify resistant clones that may be therapeutically important. The enormous complexity of life is being met with an equally enormous capacity for analysis.

### Non-Invasive Prenatal Screening by Massively Parallel Sequencing Analysis

Cell-free fetal DNA molecules are found in the circulation of pregnant women and provide a source of fetal genetic material that can be sampled via a maternal blood draw. During early pregnancy, cell-free fetal DNA amounts to about 10%–15% of all DNA fragments in maternal plasma with the remaining DNA being of maternal origin. Cell-free DNA molecules, both from the fetus and mother, are fragments mostly shorter than 200 bp. To non-invasively screen for fetal chromosomal aneuploidies by maternal plasma cell-free DNA analysis, approaches have been devised to detect an increase or decrease in cell-free DNA molecules originating from the potentially aneuploid chromosomes (e.g., chromosome 21 in the case of trisomy 21). In the case of a fetus with trisomy 21, the goal is to detect the elevation in fetus-derived chromosome 21 DNA among the minor fraction of highly fragmented cell-free fetal DNA molecules in maternal plasma. Currently, the major assay method is based on massively parallel sequencing.

Typically, millions of cell-free DNA molecules are sequenced per sample and the chromosomal origin of each molecule is identified bioinformatically. Some of the methods are preceded by enrichment of DNA molecules from target chromosomes, such as chromosomes 21, 18, and 13. For some methods, the proportion of molecules derived from each of the assessed chromosomes are calculated and compared with the expected range for unaffected pregnancies. A statistically significant increase or decrease in the proportion of DNA from the assessed chromosome would be interpreted as having been screened positive for aneuploidy. Other methods may additionally interrogate the SNP allele present on each of the sequenced cell-free DNA molecules. For each genomic locus showing SNP heterozygosity, an allelic ratio is calculated. The ratios among heterozygous SNPs on a test chromosome would be compared with that of other reference chromosomes. Any consistent deviation of the SNP ratios on the test chromosome would be interpreted as a positive screening result. Positive screen results need to be confirmed by conventional definitive diagnosis using fetal DNA obtained via chorionic villus sampling or amniocentesis.

Maternal plasma cell-free DNA analysis is one of the clinically accepted approaches for prenatal screening of the common fetal aneuploidies, namely trisomies 21, 18, and 13. Because millions of pregnant women annually undergo plasma cell-free DNA testing, it is likely to be the highest volume massively parallel sequencing test being conducted in routine laboratories.

## INFORMATICS

The modern era of human genome sequencing is underpinned by massively parallel sequencing. As suggested by the name, both the method as well as the amount of data is massive. Fortunately, as the scale of sequencing has increased, tools have been developed to manage and analyze the information. Many recent reviews and evaluations of existing software tools are available.

Both publicly available tools and commercial software are assembled into what is referred to as a pipeline. In the pipeline, the information is processed in a serial manner (Fig. 48.11). First, raw data (fluorescence, time, position) is analyzed by instrument-specific methods to generate serial base calls, each with an estimated uncertainty or quality of each base call. This information is saved in a text file, typically a FASTQ file. One FASTQ file typically contains data from millions of short sequencing reads, so the files are very big and not usually readable by standard text editors. Depending on the coverage required, there may be tens to thousands of sequencing reads covering a single nucleotide position.

Different sequencing reads start and stop at different genomic positions, so an alignment program is used to register each sequencing read to the reference genome. An example alignment is shown in Fig. 48.12. After alignment, each base position is "called" or assigned depending on its quality from each read, the percentage of reads that are in agreement, and the total number of reads. At any nucleotide position, there may be more than one base, which is expected in the case of heterozygous variants (1:1 ratio), mitochondrial variants (variable ratios), or somatic variants in cancer (variant bases may be rare). After the bases are called at each nucleotide position, a variant call file (VCF) is generated and a quality or Q-score assigned (Box 48.2).

Each VCF entry is then queried against existing knowledge, a process that is often both manual and automated. Because of the large number of variants that require analysis at this stage, some sort of automated database filtering is almost always performed. Consideration of population databases is a useful initial filter. A database minor allele frequency >5% is considered standalone evidence that a variant is benign. In contrast, identification of a nonsense, frameshift, or severe splice site variant is very strong, but not absolute, evidence of a pathogenic variant. Computational and predictive data for missense variants can also be automated. These predictive tools are not always accurate, but they may be helpful to prioritize the examination of a long queue of variants from a sequencing study. Finally, some manual curation is usually necessary and may include functional and segregation data from the literature, and parental testing to establish de novo variants or *cis/trans* relationships.

In 2015, standards and guidelines for the interpretation of sequence variants were recommended by the American

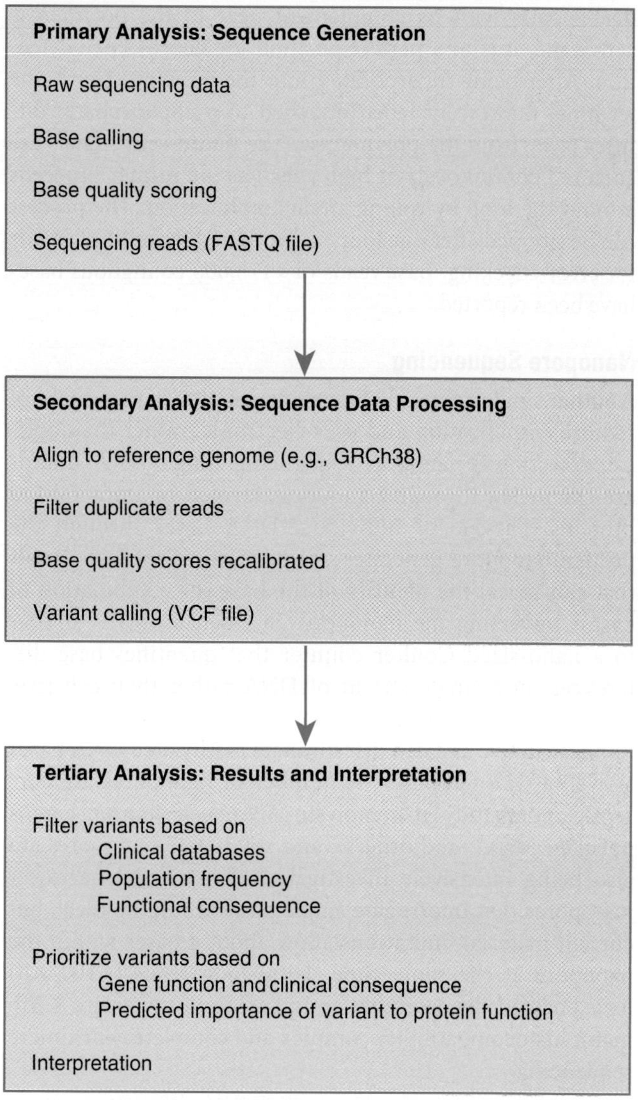

---

**Primary Analysis: Sequence Generation**

Raw sequencing data

Base calling

Base quality scoring

Sequencing reads (FASTQ file)

$\downarrow$

**Secondary Analysis: Sequence Data Processing**

Align to reference genome (e.g., GRCh38)

Filter duplicate reads

Base quality scores recalibrated

Variant calling (VCF file)

$\downarrow$

**Tertiary Analysis: Results and Interpretation**

Filter variants based on
  Clinical databases
  Population frequency
  Functional consequence

Prioritize variants based on
  Gene function and clinical consequence
  Predicted importance of variant to protein function

Interpretation

**Fig. 48.11** Bioinformatics pipeline. The analysis of data from massively parallel sequencing occurs in three phases. *Primary analysis*: The raw output (e.g., optical or electronic signals) from the sequencing instrument is transformed into data that describe the individual bases of DNA, as well as the quality and confidence of the base call at each position. These reads of DNA are assembled into a FASTQ data file. *Secondary analysis*: The data file is then assembled onto a reference sequence. For human DNA sequencing, this is typically a reference genome, such as GRCh38. If the fragments of DNA were prepared by randomly sheared fragments, then the sampling of a wide diversity of fragments improves quality and is ensured by sequencing that is from exact duplicates. When the fragments are assembled against the reference genome, the quality of each of the base calls at specific nucleotide positions can be determined. The variant at each position is then determined and reported in a single variant call file (VCF). *Tertiary analysis*: The variants are then queried against multiple databases that have information on population frequency and clinical significance. Based on these queries, the variants can be prioritized in terms of importance to the given scientific question or clinical scenario. (Modified with permission from Oliver GR, Hart SN, Klee EW. Bioinformatics for clinical next generation sequencing. *Clin Chem*. 2015;61:124–135.)

College of Medical Genetics and Genomics and the Association for Molecular Pathology. Specific standard terminology for variant pathogenicity into five categories was

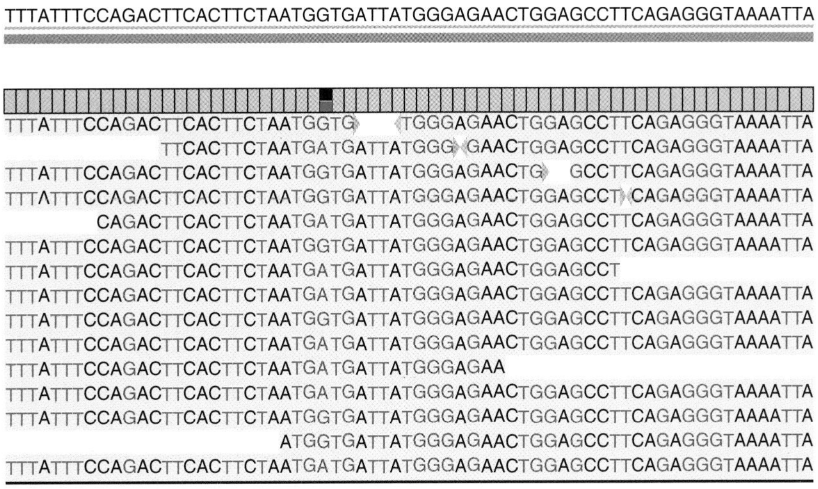
TTTATTTCCAGACTTCACTTCTAATGGTGATTATGGGAGAACTGGAGCCTTCAGAGGGTAAAATTA
TTTATTTCCAGACTTCACTTCTAATGGTG TGGGAGAACTGGAGCCTTCAGAGGGTAAAATTA
TTCACTTCTAATGATGATTATGGG GAACTGGAGCCTTCAGAGGGTAAAATTA
TTTATTTCCAGACTTCACTTCTAATGGTGATTATGGGAGAACTG GCCTTCAGAGGGTAAAATTA
TTTATTTCCAGACTTCACTTCTAATGGTGATTATGGGAGAACTGGAGCCT CAGAGGGTAAAATTA
CAGACTTCACTTCTAATGATGATTATGGGAGAACTGGAGCCTTCAGAGGGTAAAATTA
TTTATTTCCAGACTTCACTTCTAATGGTGATTATGGGAGAACTGGAGCCTTCAGAGGGTAAAATTA
TTTATTTCCAGACTTCACTTCTAATGATGATTATGGGAGAACTGGAGCCT
TTTATTTCCAGACTTCACTTCTAATGATGATTATGGGAGAACTGGAGCCTTCAGAGGGTAAAATTA
TTTATTTCCAGACTTCACTTCTAATGGTGATTATGGGAGAACTGGAGCCTTCAGAGGGTAAAATTA
TTTATTTCCAGACTTCACTTCTAATGATGATTATGGGAGAACTGGAGCCTTCAGAGGGTAAAATTA
TTTATTTCCAGACTTCACTTCTAATGATGATTATGGGAGAA
TTTATTTCCAGACTTCACTTCTAATGATGATTATGGGAGAACTGGAGCCTTCAGAGGGTAAAATTA
TTTATTTCCAGACTTCACTTCTAATGGTGATTATGGGAGAACTGGAGCCTTCAGAGGGTAAAATTA
ATGGTGATTATGGGAGAACTGGAGCCTTCAGAGGGTAAAATTA
TTTATTTCCAGACTTCACTTCTAATGATGATTATGGGAGAACTGGAGCCTTCAGAGGGTAAAATTA

**Fig. 48.12** Sequence alignment of short reads from massively parallel sequencing. Multiple sequence reads are aligned to each other and the reference sequence (top). The read starts and stops are variable, reflecting random library inserts. Most base positions are identical across reads, although at one position, two bases are present at a 50:50 ratio, suggesting a heterozygous base, which differs from the reference sequence. (Alamut Visual version 2.12 (SOPHiA GENETICS, Lausanne, Switzerland.)

### BOX 48.2 Phred Quality Score (Q-Score)

In the 1990s, Phil Green at the University of Washington developed software to automatically read the fluorescent sequence chromatograms generated from Sanger sequencing. The original software, Phred (**Ph**il's **r**ead **ed**itor), used the following basic parameters:

1. Find the predicted location of peaks.
2. Find the observed location of peaks.
3. Match predicted and observed peaks.
4. Find missing peaks.

A component of Phred was an estimator of the error probability of a base call. A quality value (Q-score) was generated from the formula:

$q = -10 \times \log_{10}(p)$

q = quality value

$p$ = estimated error for a base call

Some representative examples of quality value (Q) scores:

Q-score of 30 (Q30): The probability ($p$) is 1/1,000 of being incorrect.

Q-score of 20 (Q20): The probability ($p$) is 1/100 of being incorrect.

Q-score of 10 (Q10): The probability ($p$) is 1/10 of being incorrect.

Although massively parallel sequencing does not generate a Sanger sequencing type chromatogram, the convention of a Phred Q-score is still used to calculate the quality (and accuracy) of a sequenced base. Under ideal conditions, current massively parallel sequencing can achieve >90% of bases at Q30.

recommended for Mendelian disorders: pathogenic, likely pathogenic, uncertain significance, likely benign, and benign. Criteria for classifying pathogenic (P) variants include: very strong (PVS), strong (PS), and supporting (PP) criteria with combinatorial rules to establish pathogenic and likely pathogenic variants. Similarly, criteria for classifying benign (B) variants include: standalone (BA), strong (BS), and supporting (BP) criteria with combinatorial rules to establish benign and likely benign variants. When the criteria and rules are insufficient to establish any of these four categories, the variant is classified as that of uncertain significance. The intent for the likely pathogenic and likely benign categories is to have a >90% probability of being pathogenic or benign, respectively. These guidelines have been adopted internationally, adapted to copy number variants, and refined for compatibility with Bayesian statistical reasoning.

In 2017, standards and guidelines for the interpretation and reporting of sequence variants in cancer were jointly recommended by the Association for Molecular Pathology, the American Society of Clinical Oncology, and the College of American Pathologists. Somatic sequence variants were categorized into tiers based on their clinical significance: variants with strong clinical significance, variants with potential clinical significance, variants of unknown clinical significance, and variants deemed benign or likely benign. Evidence for clinical significance is collected along 10 evidential lines, including FDA approval, professional guidelines, investigational studies, mutation type, variant frequency, presence in databases, predictive software, pathway involvement, and publications. The process has been semi-automated in software to standardize the interpretation.

Massively parallel methods require informatics to process the enormous amount of data generated. Large laboratories often assign the different stages of the analysis pipeline to different specialists, including sequence analysts to extract the best sequence information, variant scientists to interpret the pathogenicity of variants, genetic counselors to draft reports and follow-up with clients, and medical directors to coordinate and take medical responsibility for the results.

## REVIEW QUESTIONS

1. What percent genomic similarity exists between humans and non-human primates?
   a. 1%
   b. 10%
   c. 50%
   d. 90%
   e. 98%

2. Nucleotides that encode protein account for what percentage of the genome?
   a. 1%
   b. 10%
   c. 50%
   d. 90%
   e. 98%

3. What approximate percentage of the human genome is comprised of transposable elements?
   a. 1%
   b. 10%
   c. 20%
   d. 30%
   e. 40%

4. With a Phred Quality Score of Q20, the probability of being incorrect is which of the following?
   a. 1 in 10
   b. 1 in 100
   c. 1 in 1000
   d. 1 in 10,000
   e. 1 in 100,000

5. What is the correct nomenclature for the variant in the following sequence if the base in blue underlined text is converted to a C? Hint: The sequence includes the initiation codon of a gene.
   ACAGCATAGCATATGACGCATCAGCACATT
   a. GRCh37/hg19 g.32335623
   b. p.W4A
   c. c.12G>C
   d. c.-7G>C
   e. p.T12P

6. Which massively parallel sequencing method uses nucleotides labeled on the terminal phosphate?
   a. Sequencing by synthesis
   b. Sequencing by ligation
   c. Semiconductor sequencing
   d. Nanopore sequencing
   e. Single molecule sequencing with zero-mode waveguide

7. Which massively parallel sequencing method detects a change in pH?
   a. Semiconductor sequencing
   b. Sequencing by ligation
   c. Sequencing by synthesis with fluorescent reversible terminators
   d. Single molecule sequencing
   e. Nanopore sequencing

8. How much of the human genome is transcribed?
   a. 1%
   b. 2%
   c. 20%
   d. 50%
   e. >90%

9. The average gene has about how many exons?
   a. 1
   b. 5
   c. 10
   d. 20
   e. 100

10. In each resting (non-replicating) human cell, there are about how many incorporated bases in DNA?
    a. 3 billion
    b. 6 billion
    c. 12 billion
    d. Varies according to cellular metabolism
    e. 24 billion

## SUGGESTED READINGS

Brandt T, Sack LM, Arjona D, et al. Adapting ACMG/AMP sequence variant classification guidelines for single-gene copy number variants. *Genet Med.* 2020;22:336–344.

ENCODE Project Consortium. A user's guide to the encyclopedia of DNA elements (ENCODE). *PLoS Biol.* 2011;9:e1001046.

Fotsing SF, Margoliash J, Wang C, et al. The impact of short tandem repeat variation on gene expression. *Nat Genet.* 2019;51:1652–1659.

Gao G, Smith D. Clinical massively parallel sequencing. *Clin Chem.* 2020;66:77–88.

Gargis AS, Kalman L, Berry MW, et al. Assuring the quality of next-generation sequencing in clinical laboratory practice. *Nat Biotechnol.* 2012;30:1033–1036.

Jain M, Koren S, Miga KH, et al. Nanopore sequencing and assembly of a human genome with ultra-long reads. *Nat Biotechnol.* 2018;36:338–345.

Kerzendorfer C, Konopka T, Nijman SM. A thesaurus of genetic variation for interrogation of repetitive genomic regions. *Nucleic Acids Res.* 2015;43:e68.

Kronenberg ZN, Fiddes IT, Gordon D, et al. High-resolution comparative analysis of great ape genomes. *Science.* 2018;360:eaar6343.

Landrum MJ, Lee JM, Benson M, et al. ClinVar: improving access to variant interpretations and supporting evidence. *Nucleic Acids Res.* 2018;46:D1062–1067.

Li MM, Datto M, Duncavage EJ, et al. Standards and guidelines for the interpretation and reporting of sequence variants in cancer: A joint consensus recommendation of the Association for Molecular Pathology, American Society of Clinical Oncology, and College of American Pathologists. *J Mol Diagn*. 2017;19:4–23.

Miga KH, Koren S, Rhie A, et al. Telomere-to-telomere assembly of a complete human X chromosome. *Nature*. 2020;585:79–84.

Mikhail FM, Biegel JA, Cooley LD, et al. Technical laboratory standards for interpretation and reporting of acquired copy-number abnormalities and copy-neutral loss of heterozygosity in neoplastic disorders: a joint consensus recommendation from the American College of Medical Genetics and Genomics (ACMG) and the Cancer Genomics Consortium (CGC). *Genet Med*. 2019;21:1903–1916.

Rehm HL, Bale SJ, Bayrak-Toydemir P, et al. ACMG clinical laboratory standards for next-generation sequencing. *Genet Med*. 2013;15:733–747.

Richards S, Aziz N, Bale S, et al. Standards and guidelines for the interpretation of sequence variants: a joint consensus recommendation of the American College of Medical Genetics and Genomics and the Association for Molecular Pathology. *Genet Med*. 2015;17:405–424.

Santani A, Simen BB, Briggs M, et al. Designing and implementing NGS tests for inherited disorders: A practical framework with step-by-step guidance for clinical laboratories. *J Mol Diagn*. 2019;21:369–374.

Torene RI, Galens K, Liu S, et al. Mobile element insertion detection in 89,874 clinical exomes. *Genet Med*. 2020;22:974–978.

Venter JC, Adams MD, Myers EW, et al. The sequence of the human genome. *Science*. 2001;291:1304–1351.

# 49

# Molecular Microbiology

*Heba H. Mostafa, Stefan Zimmerman, and Melissa B. Miller*

## OBJECTIVES

1. Explain the role of molecular-based methods in the diagnostic microbiology laboratory.
2. Detail the different types of molecular technologies used for the diagnosis of infectious diseases.
3. Understand approaches for target and signal amplification.
4. Discuss the role of molecular diagnostics in combating health care-associated infections.
5. Explain molecular based syndromic panels for the diagnosis of infectious diseases.
6. Review the available point-of-care molecular testing approaches and describe their clinical utility.
7. Discuss emerging technologies with significant promise for the microbiology laboratory.

## KEY WORDS AND DEFINITIONS

**Metagenomics** The study of genomic materials of microbial communities recovered from the environment.

**Multiplex PCR** The process of amplifying multiple nucleic acid sequence targets simultaneously.

**Nucleic acid (NA) sequencing** A process by which the order of nucleotides or stretches of DNA or RNA is determined.

**Nucleic acid (NA) amplification test (NAAT)** Amplification of a specific nucleic acid sequence target (DNA or RNA).

**Massively parallel sequencing** A high throughput sequencing approach.

**Polymerase chain reaction (PCR)** The process of amplifying a target nucleic acid sequence using a heat-stable polymerase and temperature cycling.

**Point-of-care** Diagnostic testing that is run near to the patient.

**Probe** A single stranded DNA or RNA sequence that hybridizes to a complementary target sequence.

**Syndromic panel** The process of using one assay that simultaneously detects multiple pathogens that can cause overlapping clinical presentations.

## BACKGROUND

Nucleic acid (NA) amplification techniques are routinely used to diagnose and manage patients with infectious diseases. Technological advances in NA amplification techniques, automation, NA sequencing, and **multiplex** analysis have reinvigorated the field and created new opportunities for growth. Simple, sample-in, answer-out molecular test systems are now widely available that can be deployed in a variety of laboratory and clinical settings, including at the **point-of-care**. Molecular microbiology remains a leading area in molecular pathology in terms of both the numbers of tests performed and clinical relevance. NA-based tests have reduced the dependency of the clinical microbiology laboratory on more traditional antigen detection and culture methods and created new opportunities for the laboratory to impact patient care.

This chapter reviews the molecular technology currently available in clinical laboratories to diagnose infectious diseases and emerging technology that may impact the field. The application of these technologies to diagnose health care-associated infections, syndromic infectious diseases, and infectious diseases at the point-of-care are reviewed. In addition, this chapter highlights the unique challenges and opportunities that these tests present for clinical laboratories.

## OVERVIEW OF METHODOLOGIES FOR THE DIAGNOSIS OF INFECTIOUS DISEASES

The diagnosis of infectious diseases has witnessed multiple phases over the years, which largely started with Gram stain and growth of organisms in culture in the late 1800s, and expanded to antigen detection methods, serology, and **polymerase chain reaction (PCR)**. Different approaches for molecular detection in clinical microbiology laboratories have become available that extend from non-amplification techniques to PCR and real-time PCR. Real-time PCR facilitated a transformation in the clinical microbiology laboratory and enabled the introduction of quantitative assays that particularly revolutionized the virology laboratory. Multiple commercially available molecular platforms, technologies, and assays now exist; some of them are also used as point-of-care or near-patient tests. Methods for single target detection, small panels, and large syndromic molecular panels are also available. Broader non-targeted strategies are also expanding, such as **metagenomics** and the characterization of the host response to infectious diseases.

## Probe Hybridization

Identification of microorganisms by specifically targeting certain regions in their genome by DNA or RNA probes is a common method of microbial identification and can generate either qualitative or quantitative results. Probe hybridization methods are formed of four main components: the target, the probe, the reporter or detection method, and the hybridization method. Common hybridization methods include: (1) liquid phase, (2) solid phase, and (3) in situ hybridization. Compared to amplification-based approaches, probe hybridization methods have lower sensitivity and require high loads of microorganisms. To increase sensitivity, many hybridization-based assays include an amplification step either prior to or after hybridization.

### Liquid-Phase Hybridization

In liquid-phase hybridization, the reaction is carried out in solution, which enhances the chance of the probe binding to the target. A successful reaction is dependent on the ability of the probe and target to exist in a single stranded form. A common method for hybridization detection in solution is using an acridinium ester moiety attached to the probe, and then treating the mixture with an alkali reagent after hybridization, which hydrolyzes the acridinium ester of unhybridized probes. Emission of light occurs from the probe-target hybridized product only (hybridization protection assay [HPA]). The Hologic (San Diego, CA) assays are the most encountered liquid phase hybridization methods in the clinical microbiology laboratory. An example is the Hologic Aptima assays for sexually transmitted infections (STI).

### Solid-Phase Hybridization

In solid-phase hybridization, the target is fixed to a solid surface such as a membrane (nylon or nitrocellulose). The membrane is exposed to the probe in solution, and specific binding is detected by different methods; the most common detection methods include colorimetric, fluorescence and chemiluminescence. Examples include the line probe assays (e.g., Innogenetics/Fujirebio, Ghent, Belgium) that are used for genotyping (e.g., hepatitis C virus [HCV]), and drug resistance mutations detection (e.g., human immunodeficiency virus [HIV] and *Mycobacterium*).

### In Situ Hybridization

In situ hybridization is solid-phase hybridization where nucleic acids are targeted within fixed cells or tissues. Because the target can be visualized within intact tissues or cells, additional information can be collected that might include a change in the tissue morphology. A widely used approach for identifying microorganisms using this method is fluorescence in situ hybridization (FISH). FISH allows for identification of microbial targets and by using specific probes, species level identifications can be made. Peptide-nucleic-acid (PNA) probes are a substitute for traditional nucleic acid probes that have enhanced detection because the PNA probes have a neutrally charged glycine backbone that allows the probes

to more readily penetrate through the cell membrane (Table 49.1). Examples include OpGen (AdvanDx, Wolburn, MA) *Candida* PNA FISH for the direct and rapid detection of *Candida* spp.

### Hybridization Arrays

DNA hybridization arrays, also called *microarrays*, *macroarrays*, or *high-density oligonucleotide arrays*, offer high throughput ways to look at multiple targets simultaneously. These methods rely on immobilizing an array of target-specific probes on a surface (membrane, a slide, or a chip); these sequences are then hybridized with nucleic acids (amplified and/or labeled) from clinical specimens. Different array methods were developed that differ in the number of detectable targets, which varies from a few to thousands (low/moderate density vs high density microarrays) and the method of detection. The routine use of arrays in clinical microbiology laboratories is currently limited to low and moderate density microarrays. Clinical applications include microbial identification, antimicrobial resistance detection, and strain typing. Syndromic infectious disease testing is among the most commonly used arrays in diagnostic laboratories. An example is eSensor technology (Roche Diagnostics, Indianapolis, IN) which uses an electrochemical detection system with a gold-plated microarray of electrodes. The targets are initially amplified and converted by exonuclease to single strands which hybridize to ferrocene-labeled probes. This oligonucleotide "sandwich" brings ferrocene closer to the surface of the electrode and results in specific electric currents that can identify each target.

High-density microarrays that use hundreds to thousands of hybridization probes offer a large multiplexing capacity that permits applications including microbial identification, antimicrobial resistance detection, epidemiologic surveillance, and viral discovery, among others. Due to the high cost associated with most of the high-density microarray methods, routine clinical laboratory applications and commercially available assays are not yet available.

---

**POINTS TO REMEMBER**

- Hybridization methods include liquid, solid, and in situ hybridization.
- Hybridization sensitivity can be increased with target or signal amplification.
- Hybridization arrays offer multiplexing panels that detect targets that range from a few to thousands.

---

## TARGET NUCLEIC ACID AMPLIFICATION STRATEGIES

Nucleic acid (NA) amplification via PCR has markedly advanced molecular diagnostics and significantly improved their analytical sensitivity. Different groups have developed novel strategies for NA amplification; however, they all share the requirement for a polymerase. In addition, all

## TABLE 49.1    Examples of Probes and Dyes for Real-Time PCR

|  | Mechanism | Advantage/Disadvantage |
|---|---|---|
| **Nonspecific detection of dsDNA products** | | |
| SYBR® Green | Binds to the minor grooves of dsDNA with subsequent fluorescence | • Less cost<br>• Melting curve analysis is required to confirm the PCR specificity |
| **Primer-probe** | | |
| Scorpions | Fluorescence emission starts after the second denaturation step due to binding of complementary sequences of the probe to the newly synthesized DNA | • Combining the primer and probe reduces the cost<br>• Less background fluorescence |
| **Hydrolysis probes** | | |
| TaqMan | Due to the close proximity of the fluorophores (of which one serves as the reporter and the other serves as the quencher), the signal is quenched. During PCR extension, the 5'-3' exonuclease activity of the DNA polymerase is associated with the emission of fluorescence due to the release of the reporter | • Probes are easy to design<br>• Primer-dimers can form if not appropriately designed |

Low fluorescence

Emission of fluorescence

**Scorpions primer-probe**

(Reprinted from Navarro E, Serrano-Heras G, Castano MJ, Solera J. *Real-time PCR Detection Chemistry*, with permission from Elsevier.)

**TaqMan probe**

(Reprinted from Navarro E, Serrano-Heras G, Castano MJ, Solera J. *Real-time PCR Detection Chemistry*, with permission from Elsevier.)

*Continued*

## TABLE 49.1  Examples of Probes and Dyes for Real-Time PCR—cont'd

| | Mechanism | Advantage/Disadvantage |
|---|---|---|
| **Hybridization probes** | | |
| FRET | Annealing of the probes to complementary target sequences is designed to bring the quencher and reporter closer with an associated emission of fluorescence secondary to energy transfer by FRET | • Probes are easy to design<br>• Melting curve analysis could be performed |
| | <br>Reporter<br>5' Oligo probe 1 3'<br>Quencher Phosphate group<br>5' Oligo probe 2 3'<br>Amplified target DNA<br>**Hybprobes or FRET probes**<br>(Reprinted from Navarro E, Serrano-Heras G, Castano MJ, Solera J. *Real-time PCR Detection Chemistry*, with permission from Elsevier.) | |
| Molecular Beacons | Upon annealing, fluorescence is released when the probe binds to the target sequence | • Melting curve analysis could be performed<br>• Single nucleotide mismatch could be discriminated |
| | <br>Loop sequence<br>Stem sequence<br>5' 3'<br>Reporter Quencher<br>Reporter Loop sequence Quencher<br>5' 3'<br>Amplified target DNA<br>**Molecular beacon probe**<br>(Reprinted from Navarro E, Serrano-Heras G, Castano MJ, Solera J. *Real-time PCR Detection Chemistry*, with permission from Elsevier.) | |
| Molecular Torches | Hybridization separates the quencher from the reporter and is associated with the emission of fluorescence | • The linker facilitates the closed conformation in the absence of the target<br>• The linker enables the use of smaller target binding region which increases the sensitivity |
| | <br>Non-nucleotide linker<br>Nucleic acid target<br>Fluorescence<br>**Molecular torch**<br>(This figure courtesy HOLOGIC®, Inc. and affiliates.) | |

| | **Mechanism** | **Advantage/Disadvantage** |
|---|---|---|
| Partially Double Stranded | Fluorescence is generated when the hybridization probe (blocked at the 3' to prevent extension) with the fluorescent marker attached binds to target DNA | • Mismatch discrimination capability can be controlled<br>• High tolerance to mismatches allows the detection of genetically diverse targets |
| **Nucleic acid analogues**<br>PNAs | Mechanism is dependent on the probe design (e.g., primer-probe) and is similar to oligonucleotide probes | • Resistant to proteases and nucleases<br>• DNA binding is possible at lower salt concentrations<br>• Due to their neutral charge, binding to DNA or RNA is of superior affinity than regular oligonucleotides |

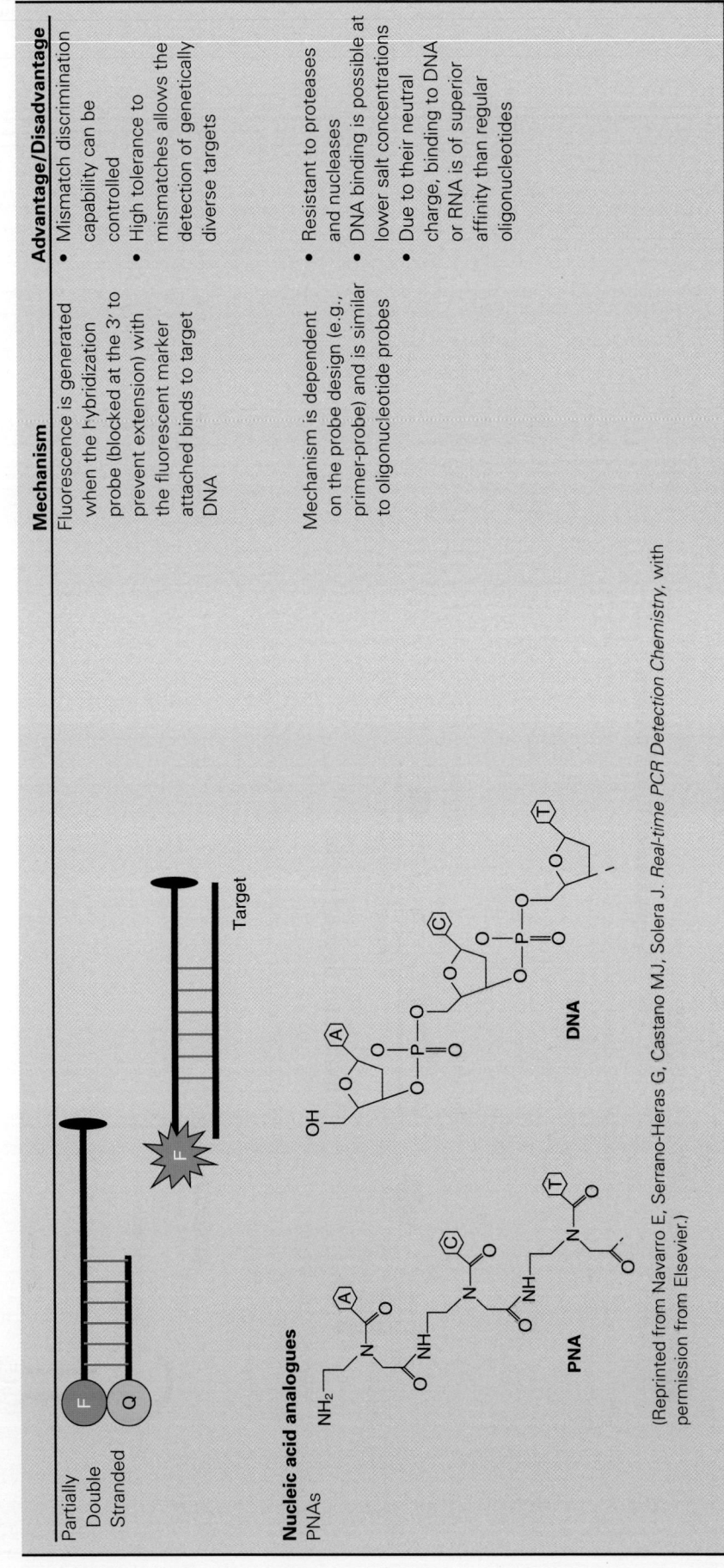

(Reprinted from Navarro E, Serrano-Heras G, Castano MJ, Solera J. *Real-time PCR Detection Chemistry*, with permission from Elsevier.)

target-specific amplification-based assays require specific primers. Primer binding sites flank the region to be amplified by the polymerase in a reaction that results in the production of up to billions of copies of the target. The basic PCR reaction requires a buffer that, in addition to the primers and a thermostable polymerase, contains deoxyribonucleotides triphosphate (dNTPs) and magnesium. Cycles of time periods at specific temperatures (thermocycling) are required for double-stranded DNA denaturation, primer binding (annealing) and primer extension (polymerization). With each PCR cycle, the number of target NA amplicons ideally doubles. This means that for a PCR reaction with 30 cycles, there is a theoretical $10^9$-fold amplification. This exponential

amplification is limited by the efficiency of the reaction and may plateau with the depletion of the reaction components (Fig. 49.1). Because this reaction starts with a DNA target, a reverse transcription reaction step is required before the PCR amplification of RNA targets (RT-PCR), which requires a reverse transcriptase enzyme. Reverse transcriptase requires primers for synthesizing the complementary DNA strand (cDNA); those primers can be either random, target-specific, or oligonucleotides that bind to the poly A tail if mRNAs are targeted for amplification (Oligo (dT) primers).

Traditionally, the detection of amplicons was based on visualizing the PCR products after agarose or polyacrylamide gel electrophoresis. DNA staining was required for

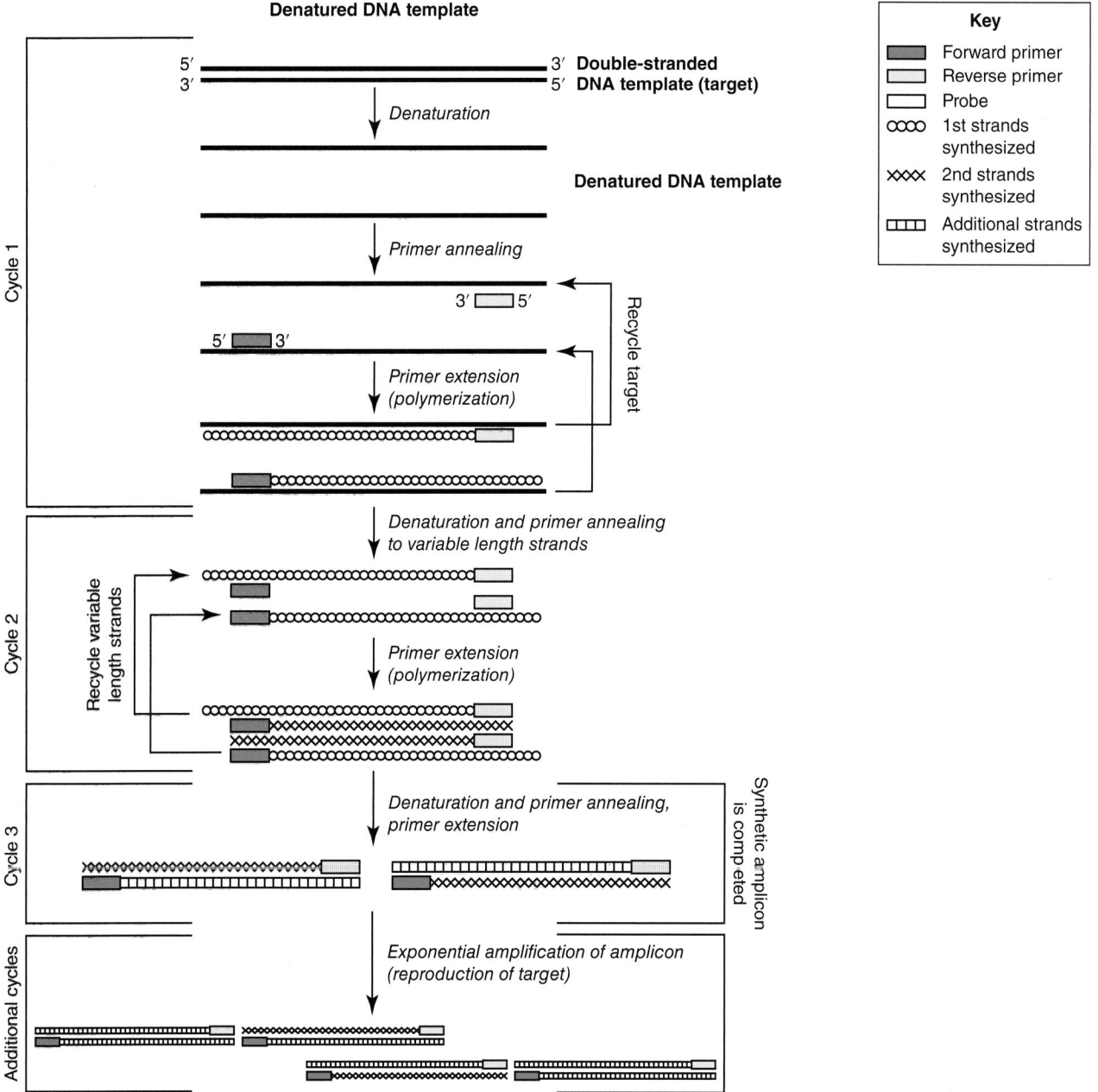

**Fig. 49.1** Polymerase chain reaction (PCR) amplification. Cycles of DNA denaturation, primer annealing, and extension lead to exponential amplification of targets. (Reprinted from Wolk D, Mitchell S, Patel R. *Principles of Molecular Microbiology Testing Methods*, with permission from Elsevier.)

visualizing the PCR products and different DNA binding stains, the most widely used of which is ethidium bromide, were used. The correct product was identified based on the amplicon size. This methodology is still widely used for research purposes but is not practical for the clinical microbiology laboratory. Several methods were developed to provide PCR assays that fulfill the criteria needed for diagnostic assays, which include detection with minimal manipulation of amplicons to reduce the risk of cross-contamination and reduce the hands-on time.

## Real-Time PCR

Real-time PCR has transformed the diagnostic capabilities of clinical microbiology laboratories. Real-time PCR offers simultaneous target amplification and product detection in real-time. In addition, real-time PCR assays add the great advantage of not only target detection, but also highly accurate and sensitive quantification. In general, the detection relies on fluorescence that is measured with every PCR cycle and normalized to the baseline. Fluorescence emission is associated with the use of fluorescent dyes that bind to double-stranded DNA products with every cycle (e.g., SYBR green) or fluorescently-labeled oligonucleotides designed to specifically bind to the target of interest with different mechanisms such that fluorescence is altered (i.e., quenched or emitted) with target amplification (Table 49.1 shows examples of probes and dyes used for real-time PCR).

Because amplification and detection overlap, the thermocyclers used for performing real-time PCR require special optical detectors and software for fluorescence analysis and generation of the real-time PCR amplification plots. Typically, the amplification plot shows the cycle numbers on the X-axis and the intensity of fluorescence on the Y-axis (normalized). The initial cycles will not show a change in fluorescence signal; this defines the baseline. A positive real-time PCR is defined by a reaction in which the fluorescence signal increases above the background threshold of the assay. The cycle threshold ($C_T$) value is the fractional cycle number at which the fluorescence crosses the plot's fixed threshold (Fig. 49.2). Calibrator samples, which contain a specified amount of the target, can be used to convert the $C_T$ to a target quantified value (e.g., copies or units). Several companies currently offer real-time PCR platforms including Applied Biosystems (Foster City, CA), Bio-Rad (Hercules, California), and Roche Diagnostics (Indianapolis, IN). In addition, continuous systems and high-throughput closed platforms that offer qualitative and quantitative real-time PCR assays for different targets are commercially available (e.g., GeneXpert from Cepheid, Roche *Cobas* systems, and Abbott molecular platforms (Lake Forest, Illinois)).

dsDNA dyes bind non-specifically to the minor grove of dsDNA, with a progressive increase in fluorescence during DNA amplification. The use of these dyes is associated with non-specific fluorescence due to amplification of non-specific products, and hence a melting curve analysis is highly recommended to confirm the specificity of the fluorescent signal. Different PCR products have different melting (denaturation) temperatures and should give distinct peaks of loss of fluorescence (due to the dissociation of dye) when exposed to a certain range of temperature. In contrast, fluorophore-labeled oligonucleotides bind with high specificity to the PCR target of interest. The fluorophore-labeled oligonucleotides available for real-time PCR belong to three main groups based on their structure and mechanism of signal quenching and production: primer-probe (e.g., Scorpions), probes (hydrolysis, e.g., TaqMan probes; hybridization, e.g., FRET and molecular beacons), and nucleic acid analogues (e.g., PNA) (Table 49.1).

## Digital PCR

Digital PCR offers a different nucleic acid quantification approach without the need for standards, an advantage that adds precision to quantification of reference materials and controls for clinical microbiology quantitative assays. Other applications include absolute quantification of viral load and detection of mutations that confer drug resistance. As in real-time PCR, fluorescent dyes or probes are added to the PCR reaction; however, in digital PCR, the reaction is divided into thousands of partitions so that each partition likely ends up with either no copies or one copy. Quantification is achieved

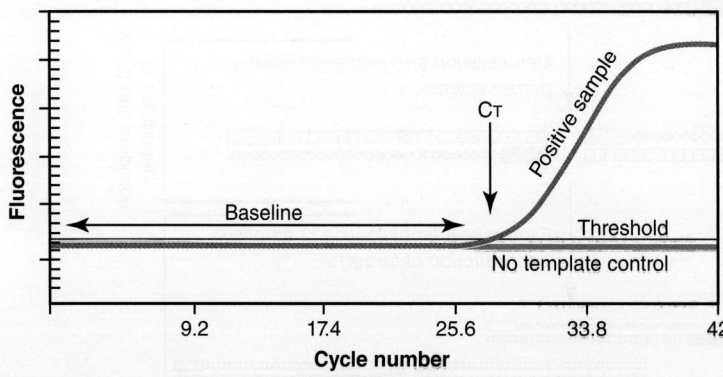

**Fig. 49.2** Real-time PCR amplification plot. The plot shows the cycle numbers on the x-axis and the intensity of fluorescence on the y-axis (normalized). The initial cycles will not show a change in fluorescence signal, which defines the baseline. The cycle threshold (CT) value is the cycle number at which the fluorescence crosses the plot fixed threshold.

by counting the number of positive and negative partitions and applying the Poisson distribution to accurately calculate the concentration in the original sample. Partitioning can be attained by using chips, arrays, capillaries, or oil droplets (droplet digital PCR).

---

### POINTS TO REMEMBER

- PCR is a reaction that requires thermocycling conditions, primers, and a polymerase.
- Real-time PCR permits real-time detection of amplification as well as quantification.
- RT-PCR is a reaction that adds a step of reverse transcription prior to PCR for amplification of RNA targets.
- The sensitivity of microbial detection by PCR is high. The amplification is robust, which increases the risk of workspace contamination.
- Digital PCR is an absolute quantitative approach that does not require calibrators.

---

## NON-PCR TARGET AND SIGNAL AMPLIFICATION APPROACHES

Several amplification methods that are not PCR-based have been developed, including non-PCR target amplification and signal amplification. These approaches were developed to reduce the need for thermocycling, which is associated with a reduction in cost, or to reduce the risk of amplicon contamination. Signal amplification techniques amplify the detection of signal rather than the target and include technologies such as hybrid capture and Invader assays. The non-PCR target amplification methods are largely isothermal and result in an efficient target amplification. These methods include isothermal transcription-mediated amplification (TMA), loop-mediated amplification (LAMP), and helicase-dependent amplification.

### Signal Amplification Techniques
#### Hybrid Capture
The hybrid capture methodology uses RNA probes for the detection of specific DNA target sequences, followed by the detection of RNA/DNA hybrids by specific antibodies. The methodology has progressed to offer the ability to detect RNA targets using DNA probes or the reverse with the introduction of Hybrid Capture 2 (HC2). The use of enzyme-conjugated antibodies (e.g., alkaline phosphatase) allows for signal amplification after adding a chemiluminescent substrate. HC2 assays were developed for the detection of *Chlamydia trachomatis*, *Neisseria gonorrhoeae*, hepatitis B virus (HBV), cytomegalovirus (CMV), and herpes simplex viruses (HSV) 1 and 2 (Fig. 49.3).

#### Invader Technology
The Invader technology is an isothermal assay that uses highly specific DNA probes, an upstream invader oligonucleotide and a downstream probe. Both probes hybridize to the target DNA to form a structure that has a single nucleotide

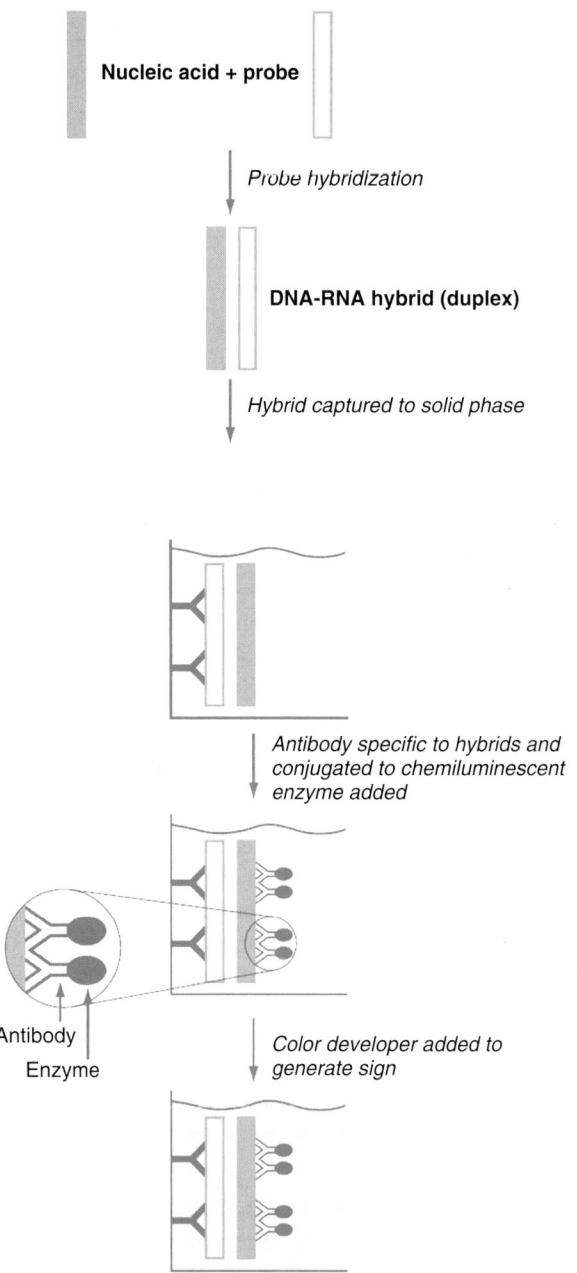

**Fig. 49.3** Hybrid capture assay. DNA-RNA hybrid is captured by specific antibodies. Chemiluminescent enzyme tagged specific antibodies bind to the hybrids, and the signal is amplified by adding the appropriate substrate. (Reprinted from Wolk D, Mitchell S, Patel R. *Principles of Molecular Microbiology Testing Methods*, with permission from Elsevier.)

overlap at the cleavage site. The 3′ end of the probe has a specific complementarity to the target DNA; however, the 5′ end makes a flap. When the invader oligo binds, the structure will be a substrate for the cleavase enzyme, and the probe will be cleaved to release the flap. Signal amplification is feasible due to the ability of the reaction to continuously proceed due to the temporary binding of the probes, as the temperature of the reaction is set very close to the melting temperature of the probe. As the oligos are present in the reaction in molar excess, cycles of binding of the signal and invader probes, formation of the cleavage substrate, and cleavage continue with the production of cleavage products (cleaved flaps). The signal stems from the binding of the flaps to FRET cassettes, which also upon binding form a cleavage substrate-specific structure. Cleavage of the FRET probe is associated with fluorescence. A robust linear signal amplification reaction can develop with this approach with each flap being able to cleave $10^3$–$10^4$ FRET probes per hour. Invader technology has been used for qualitative and quantitative detection and identification of single base polymorphisms.

## Non-PCR Target Amplification
### Transcription-Based Amplification

Isothermal transcription-based amplification is achieved by three enzymatic reactions: a primer-based reverse transcription step mediated by a reverse transcriptase to convert the RNA targets to cDNA, degradation of the RNA strand bound to the cDNA by RNAse H, and a second primer-based amplification of cDNA using the DNA- dependent DNA polymerase activity of the reverse transcriptase. In the first step, the primer has T7 polymerase promotor sequence incorporated which allows the subsequent transcription of the DNA synthesized copies by the bacteriophage T7 RNA polymerase to new RNA copies at a fixed temperature. This method can achieve $10^9$-fold amplification of target in less than 2 hours. RNA-based methods detect pathogens at low abundance due to the richness of rRNA in relation to a single copy of DNA per pathogen. Another advantage is the detection of the transcriptional activities of organisms, which rules out dead pathogens or latent viral infections. Transcription-mediated amplification (TMA) is a transcription-based amplification technology used by Hologic for the detection of many pathogens including SARS-CoV-2, *Chlamydia trachomatis*, *Neisseria gonorrhoeae*, *Trichomonas vaginalis*, and *Mycoplasma genitalium*. Real-time TMA assays are also available from Hologic, both quantitative (HIV, HCV, and HBV) and qualitative (HSV-1 and 2).

### Loop-Mediated Isothermal Amplification (LAMP)

LAMP is an isothermal non-PCR amplification method that requires the use of special DNA polymerases with high strand displacement capability (e.g., *BstI* polymerase). The amplification reaction requires multiple sets of primers (4–6). The inner primers have a 5′ region that is complementary to the immediate downstream sequence of the primer binding site. This design results in the formation of a loop structure when an upstream primer anneals and the polymerase starts displacing the annealed strand. As amplification continues, multiple loop structures are formed, and positivity can be detected as turbidity due to the precipitation of magnesium pyrophosphate. Other methods for detection include bioluminescence or the use of fluorescent probes. Detection of RNA targets using LAMP was developed by adding a reverse transcription step in the same reaction.

### Helicase-Dependent Amplification (HDA)

In HDA, a helicase enzyme is used for separating dsDNA instead of the conventional PCR denaturation step that requires heat. The specificity of the reaction is enhanced by using a thermophilic helicase that allows greater specificity of primer binding to target DNA. Clinical assays that use HDA are available from Quidel (San Diego, CA) which include Solana for detection of HSV-1 and 2, varicella zoster virus from cutaneous and mucocutaneous lesions and *Clostridioides difficile*, among others (Fig. 49.4).

### Strand Displacement Amplification (SDA)

SDA is an isothermal amplification approach that relies on strand displacing exonuclease-deficient polymerases for amplification. Replication initiates at nicks made by restriction enzyme sites introduced by a 5′ extension of target-specific primers. An outside primer (bump primer) binds upstream, and extension of the primer results in products containing

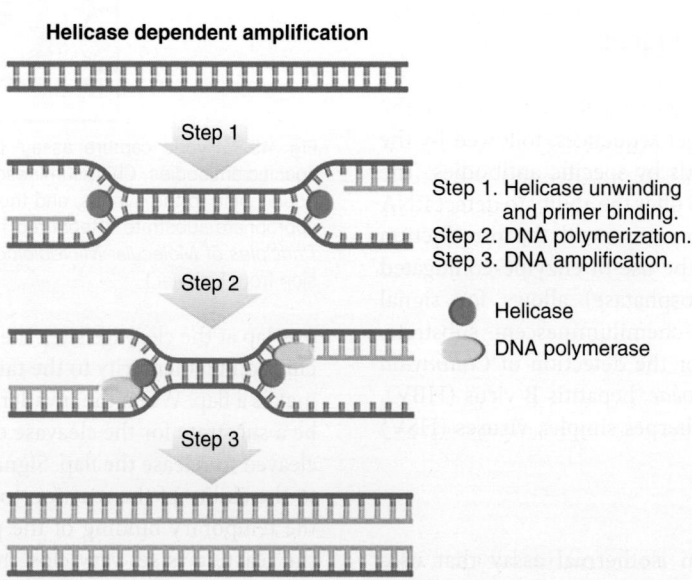

**Helicase dependent amplification**

Step 1
Step 2
Step 3

Step 1. Helicase unwinding and primer binding.
Step 2. DNA polymerization.
Step 3. DNA amplification.

⬤ Helicase
⬭ DNA polymerase

**Fig. 49.4** Helicase dependent amplification (HDA). Isothermal amplification using helicase to unwind DNA to enable primer annealing and strand-displacing DNA polymerase mediated extension. (Reprinted from www.neb.com (2023) with permission from New England Biolabs, Inc..)

restriction enzyme sites. During DNA amplification, a substitution of a dNTP with a 5′-alpha-thio-triphosphate modified form (e.g., dATPαS) results in incorporation of a linkage that allows the endonuclease to only nick a single strand.

---

**POINTS TO REMEMBER**

- Signal amplification methods were developed to avoid target amplification, which reduces the risk of contamination.
- Signal amplification methods include hybrid capture and invader technologies.
- Non-PCR amplification methods are isothermal methods that do not require thermocycling conditions. They still require a polymerase and target-specific primers.
- Non-PCR amplification methods include TMA, LAMP, and HDA.
- TMA targets RNA.
- LAMP is unique in that it uses more than two sets of primers.
- HDA uses a helicase for unwinding the DNA.

---

# SEQUENCING

## Sanger Sequencing

Nucleic acid (NA) sequencing allows microorganism identification, species characterization, and identifying variants associated with antimicrobial resistance. Multiple applications for targeted sequencing using Sanger dideoxynucleotide chain termination in the clinical microbiology laboratory are available. The method relies on chain termination, where the DNA polymerase makes variable length chains of PCR products due to the incorporation of dideoxynucleotide triphosphates (ddNTPs). The sequencing reaction includes a single stranded DNA and a specific primer. The four standard dNTPs are added to the reaction in excess in relation to the ddNTPs. Random insertion of ddNTPs terminates the reaction as they lack a 3′ hydroxyl group required for the formation of a phosphodiester bond with a newly added nucleotide for chain elongation. The products are separated by size using capillary electrophoresis, which is sensitive enough to separate the fragments that differ in size by only one base. As each of the four ddNTPs is fluorescently labeled with a different fluorophore, the sequence is converted to a chromatogram that is interpreted as a sequence. This method can identify sequences up to 800 bases in length with high accuracy. Integrated and well-curated databases are essential for the routine use of this method in the diagnostic laboratory. Sanger sequencing applications in the clinical microbiology laboratory include ribosomal RNA (rRNA) gene amplification followed by sequencing for bacterial and fungal identification, and Sanger sequencing for viral genotyping and antiviral resistance.

## Pyrosequencing

Pyrosequencing is an example of sequencing by the DNA synthesis method that relies on the detection of pyrophosphate released upon nucleotide incorporation. This method is high throughput and fast, as sequencing signals are generated immediately downstream of primers. The method offers a robust strategy for sequencing short genomic regions. Pyrosequencing has been used for bacterial identification, antimicrobial resistance characterization, fungal identification, detection of antifungal resistance mutations, and viral typing.

## Massively Parallel Sequencing (see also Chapter 48)

Sequencing has witnessed a robust advancement with new methodologies that offer the capacity for both parallel and deep sequencing. These advancements were initially named next generation sequencing (NGS), although massively parallel sequencing (MPS) is more descriptive and recognizes the potential of future sequencing technologies. MPS applications have been developed for the clinical microbiology laboratory and typically generate clonal clusters via bridge amplification or emulsion PCR. A single DNA molecule with attached adaptors is bound to either a planar surface (bridge PCR) or a bead (emulsion PCR). Illumina systems use bridge PCR and reversible dye-terminators. Cycles of sequencing occur, and the data are collected by imaging of the full array. The Ion Torrent sequencing systems (e.g., ThermoFisher Scientific, Waltham, MA) use a different data collection system based on voltage detection associated with release of protons with every incorporated nucleotide.

MPS in the clinical microbiology laboratory offers applications for both whole genome sequencing (WGS), as well as both targeted and non-targeted deep sequencing. WGS has been used successfully by microbiology and public health laboratories in outbreak investigations and epidemiologic surveillance. The development of advanced and easy to use bioinformatic pipelines for data analysis with the continuous expansion of curated databases has enabled the implementation of WGS in the public health laboratory and for resistance detection of mycobacteria. Targeted MPS on the other hand has multiple potential clinical applications including viral resistance detection and microbiome analyses. The detection of viral variants that constitute minor populations missed by conventional sequencing methods is important because these variants may be correlated with the emergence of antiviral resistance.

## Single Molecule Sequencing

Single molecule sequencing was introduced by Oxford Nanopore Technologies' products (Oxford, UK). This technology sequences long stretches of nucleic acid (10,000 bases) in contrast to MPS, which requires shearing of the DNA to small fragments (100s of bases). Single strands of DNA or RNA are directed to protein nanopores, and the sequence is called by characteristic electric current changes that distinguishes different nucleotide bases. Nanopore technology offers the benefits of obtaining much longer reads, faster runs, real-time analysis, ability to directly sequence RNA, and much smaller sizes of the platforms (MinION, GridION, and PromethION). The development of analysis software modules that offer real-time identification of microorganisms and antimicrobial resistance markers (e.g., EPI2ME) has provided customization of nanopore-based sequencing for infectious diseases. Clinical applications include bacterial and fungal identification, antimicrobial resistance prediction, complete plasmid sequencing, and viral identification.

## MASS SPECTROMETRY

Matrix-assisted laser desorption/ionization – time of flight (MALDI-TOF) mass spectrometry (MS) has become a cornerstone for bacterial identification in clinical microbiology laboratories (see Chapter 13). The use of MS has improved laboratory workflow, decreased identification turn-around time and improved reproducibility and accuracy. The use of MALDI-TOF MS has been applied to the identification of bacteria, mycobacteria, yeast, and molds. Additional MS applications include liquid chromatography with tandem mass spectrometry (LC-MS/MS) that allows identification of bacteria at the level of protein sequence and targeted LC-MS/MS that could allow both identification and target quantification. MS technologies rely on measuring the analyte's mass and charge. The two most commonly used ion sources are MALDI and electrospray ionization (ESI). MALDI ionizes condensed samples, while ESI ionizes liquid samples, which allows its combined use with liquid phase chromatography for separating ions. Both can be used with different MS analyzers.

Whole cell MALDI-TOF MS has become a very popular method for identification of bacteria. Although growth of bacteria is required, once a bacterial colony develops, identification takes ≈10 minutes. Bacterial colonies are streaked onto a target slide premixed or covered with a matrix. The matrix assists with ionization where the analytes are transformed into a gas phase, then ions are separated based on their mass to charge ratio defined by their time of flight (TOF). As detection of the ions takes place, a distinct mass spectrum is generated. The spectrum of the unknown organism is compared to pre-defined spectra in databases, and an identification is reported with a confidence score. Bacterial identification directly from positive blood culture bottles has been reported with promising results.

The MassARRAY system from Agena Biosciences (San Diego, CA) is based on nucleic acid fingerprinting using electrospray ionization MS (PCR-electrospray ionization mass spectrometry (PCR-ESI/MS)). This technology can achieve a sensitive quantification of gene expression by an innovative approach that defines the signatures of transcribed PCR-amplified sequences. The resultant RNA fragments provide a unique identification of the microorganisms. These methods allow direct analysis of patients' specimens and offer multiplexing potential and fast turnaround.

## HEALTH CARE-ASSOCIATED INFECTIONS

Health care-associated infections (HAI) are one of the most severe threats in modern medicine. In most cases, the bacteria inducing HAI are already present in or on the patient at the time of hospital admission and, when relocated, can cause life-threatening infections. Modern health care employs many types of invasive devices and procedures to treat patients and to help them recover. Infections can be associated with the devices used in medical procedures, such as catheters or ventilators. To reduce the incidence of device or procedure-associated infections, hospitals monitor Central Line-associated Bloodstream Infections (CLABSI), Catheter-associated Urinary Tract Infections (CAUTI), Surgical Site Infection (SSI), and Ventilator-associated Pneumonia (VAP).

Antimicrobial resistance and the emergence of new pathogens challenge controlling HAI and complicate patients' management. The COVID-19 pandemic highlighted this challenge and emphasized the importance of adapting measures to reduce health care workers' exposure risk. Hence, infection control plans are essential for preventing HAI and are primarily based on early detection, screening, and outbreak investigations. The clinical microbiology laboratory is central to this and has been adapting and implementing sensitive techniques for screening, early diagnosis, and characterizing antimicrobial resistance. Of the most commonly encountered diseases and organisms in the health care settings, this section focuses on methicillin-resistant *Staphylococcus aureus* (MRSA), vancomycin-resistant enterococci (VRE), β-lactam resistant Gram-negative bacilli, and *C. difficile*.

### Methicillin-Resistant *S. aureus*

Because *S. aureus* is among the most common causes of bacterial infection in the industrialized world, attention has been focused on assays to rapidly detect *S. aureus* and differentiate MRSA from methicillin-susceptible *S. aureus* (MSSA). Molecular assays that recognize MRSA based on detection of a single target detect the junction between the staphylococcal cassette chromosome *mec* element (SCC*mec*), which carries the *mecA* resistance and other genes, and the flanking *orfX* gene. This assay design has several limitations, including false-negative results caused by SCC*mec* variants and false-positive results caused by MSSA strains that carry SCC*mec* remnants lacking the *mecA* gene, sometimes referred to as "empty cassettes," or that carry SCC*mec* with a nonfunctional *mecA* gene. An alternative approach to molecular detection of MRSA combines a *mecA* target and a second gene target specific for *S. aureus* such as *sa442*, *nuc*, *femA-femB*, *spa*, or *Idh1*. An SCC*mec* cassette with a *mecC* gene (originally from *S. sciuri*) can also confer methicillin resistance in *S. aureus*, as well as *mecB*. While infections with *mecC*-positive strains are regularly reported, the number of clinical infections with *mecB*-harboring MRSA isolates is very rare. Therefore, it is not surprising that *mecC* detection has already been included in commercially available assays. While most of the *mecA*-based resistance can be detected phenotypically, *mecC* sometimes is not detectable *in vitro*. Therefore, molecular analysis is superior. These assays are intended for use in surveillance testing or to assist in the diagnosis of infections. Studies indicate that use of molecular methods for rapid identification of patients who are colonized with MRSA may be a cost-effective infection control strategy. All current MRSA nucleic acid amplification tests (NAATs) lack the ability to differentiate between DNA from dead or live bacteria, although only the latter can spread in the hospital and cause HAI. Therefore, a risk of overtreatment for patients and unjustified barrier isolation still exists.

## Vancomycin-Resistant Enterococci

Enterococci are commensal residents of the GI tract and female genital tract that account for about 10% of HAI. The vast majority of enterococcal infections are caused by *Enterococcus faecalis* and *E. faecium* and occur primarily in patients requiring long-term care. The emergence of VRE in hospitals is concerning because vancomycin is often used empirically to treat a wide variety of infections. Infection with VRE is associated with increased morbidity and mortality because of the propensity of VRE to infect patients already at high risk for comorbidity.

In the United States, about 30% of enterococci are resistant to vancomycin. High-level vancomycin resistance in enterococci occurs via acquisition of mobile transposable elements carrying the *vanA* or *vanB* genes. *E. faecium* is more frequently resistant to vancomycin than *E. faecalis*, and *vanA* is more commonly found than *vanB* in resistant strains. As with MRSA, the rapid detection of VRE colonization to prevent HAI is widely recommended and molecular assays are marketed for rapid detection of *vanA* and/or *vanB* from perianal and rectal swabs. Aside from rare reports of *vanA* in *S. aureus* and *Streptococcus* spp., detection of *vanA* is highly specific for VRE. However, *vanB* can be found in a wide variety of commensal nonenterococcal bacteria, e.g., *Eggerthella* spp. or with a lower homology also in *Clostridium innocuum*. Therefore, detection of *vanB* requires confirmation of VRE by culture to limit false-positive results.

## Beta-Lactam Resistant Gram-Negative Bacilli

One of the greatest threats to our antimicrobial formulary is the emergence of β-lactamases in Gram-negative bacteria with the capabilities of hydrolyzing broad-spectrum penicillins, cephalosporins, and carbapenems. These enzymes include extended-spectrum β-lactamases (ESBLs), AmpCs, and carbapenemases. Detection of organisms harboring these broad-spectrum β-lactamases by phenotypic methods is imperfect. A rapid, inexpensive, multiplex molecular assay to detect the genes encoding these enzymes would be clinically useful but presently is an unmet need. One of the biggest challenges to molecular detection is the great diversity

of β-lactamases, with more than 200 described ESBLs and numerous classes of carbapenemases. Overlooking these carbapenemases may result in clinical treatment failures, therefore, molecular assays for confirmation are recommended. An additional challenge is that the detection of the gene(s) does not provide information about copy number and expression, which are important to phenotypic expression of resistance to β-lactam and carbapenem antibiotics.

Many kits have been developed for molecular detection of a variety of broad-spectrum β-lactamase genes. All these assays sufficiently detect threatening carbapenemases, but do not necessarily reveal the species harboring the specific resistance gene (e.g., in rectal swabs). In the future, the rapidly rising number of clinically relevant carbapenemases will limit the possibility of PCR platforms to detect this broad spectrum, even if multiplex technologies are combined with melting curve analysis. New analyzers will become necessary; one possibility is the combination of qPCR and microarray approaches.

## *Clostridioides difficile*

*Clostridioides difficile* (*C. difficile*) is a Gram-positive spore-forming anaerobic bacillus that is frequently found in the stool microbiota of healthy infants but is rarely found in the stool microbiota of healthy adults and children older than 12 months. The organism is acquired by ingesting spores, which survive the gastric acid barrier and germinate in the colon. Alteration of the intestinal flora with the use of antibiotics facilitates colonization of the intestinal tract, causing diarrhea or colitis. Most strains of *C. difficile* make two toxins: toxin A and toxin B; the regulatory proteins TcdR and TcdC control expression of the toxin A (*tcdA*) and B (*tcdB*) genes. These toxins are responsible for symptomatic disease; strains that lack these toxin genes do not cause diarrhea or colitis. Toxin B may be more important for the production of disease than toxin A. Detection of these toxins or their activity is essential in diagnostic tests for *C. difficile*-associated disease. An additional toxin, the binary toxin, has been described in some strains of *C. difficile*, and recent reports have suggested that strains encoding the binary toxin (CDT) have a deletion in the *tcdC* gene, leading to overexpression of toxins A and B (ribotype 027) and are causing outbreaks of more severe disease.

The risk of infection with *C. difficile* increases with the length of hospital stay and use of antimicrobial therapy. *C. difficile* causes a spectrum of diseases ranging from asymptomatic carrier state to fulminant, relapsing and fatal colitis. Diarrhea may be mild to severe. Pseudomembranous colitis is a classic presentation of *C. difficile* disease, and toxic megacolon may also be seen. Although clindamycin, penicillins, and cephalosporins have commonly been associated with disease, almost all antibiotics can cause similar disease. Due to its high ability to survive in the hospital environment, *C. difficile* is the most important cause of hospital-acquired diarrhea. To implement timely infection control measures and appropriate treatment, rapid identification of toxigenic *C. difficile* is necessary.

The *tcdB* gene is most commonly used as the target gene for the molecular detection of *C. difficile*, but some assays also detect toxin A and/or the binary toxin gene. There is an ongoing and intensive discussion if NAATs alone or algorithms including NAATs are the best practice for the diagnosis of *C. difficile* infections in adults. Critics of NAATs cite an overtreatment of patients, who may be positive by molecular assays, but do not produce sufficient amounts of toxin to cause harm. However, semi-quantitative molecular analysis and consideration of threshold cycles can predict free toxin levels and reduce the risk of unnecessary antibiotic use.

### POINTS TO REMEMBER

- Multiple assays are commercially available for rapid detection of MRSA for both infection control and diagnostic purposes.
- Precise VRE detection is still a problem with direct molecular assays, as *vanB* is not specific for *Enterococcus*.
- Multi-drug resistant Gram-negative bacilli are a major threat in health care-associated infections. An increasing number of assays are commercially available, but none covers the broad range of relevant carbapenemases.
- *C. difficile* outbreaks have declined, mainly due to hygiene control measures. The optimal diagnostic approach for toxigenic *C. difficile* detection remains an area of controversy.

## SYNDROMIC PANELS

Clinical microbiology laboratories have performed syndromic-based testing for decades using a combination of microscopy, culture, and serologic methods. However, when NA-based methods were initially employed in clinical microbiology laboratories, most tests assayed for a single analyte requiring health care providers to order each molecular test separately. Although the increased sensitivity of molecular infectious disease testing was embraced, it was challenging to go from a "culture all" mentality to specifying potential pathogens to be tested. Molecular syndromic panels combine the advantages of the broad diagnostic approach of culture/microscopy with the improved sensitivity of molecular-based detection. Commercial molecular syndromic panels are available for positive blood culture identification, sepsis, upper respiratory tract infections, pneumonia, gastroenteritis, and meningitis/encephalitis. How best to use these tests to have the greatest impact on patient care remains a subject of debate.

### Positive Blood Culture Identification

One of the most important functions of clinical microbiology laboratories is the detection of bloodstream infections. Automated culture-based systems require 12–72 hours of incubation for most pathogens, followed by an additional 24–48 hours to isolate, identify, and determine

the antimicrobial susceptibility profile of the organism(s). A variety of NA-based tests have been developed to expedite identification of organisms in positive blood cultures. Commercially available tests include PNA-FISH probes, FISH-based identification coupled with susceptibility results, real-time PCR assays for detection of single or limited numbers of pathogens, and high-order multiplex blood culture identification panels. The key features of these methods are listed in Table 49.2. Four high-order multiplex assays are commercially available for identification of microorganisms from positive blood culture bottles—Verigene Gram-Positive (GP) and Gram-Negative (GN) Blood Culture tests (Luminex Molecular Diagnostics); FilmArray Blood Culture Identification (BCID) panel (BioFire Diagnostics); ePlex BCID-GP, BCID-GN and BCID-FP (Fungal Pathogen) panels (Roche); and iCubate iC-GPC and iC-GN assays. All but the Verigene tests rely on NA amplification; the Verigene tests employ microarray hybridization followed by signal amplification. MALDI-TOF MS has also been applied to the direct identification of microorganisms from positive blood culture bottles.

These multiplex panels provide comprehensive approaches to rapid identification of the vast majority of blood pathogens and important information about resistance of these pathogens to antibiotics. When coupled with active antimicrobial stewardship program interventions, the results of these tests will likely have a positive impact on the clinical outcomes of patients with sepsis. Challenges to implementing these tests include cost, throughput, and false-positive results.

## DIRECT PATHOGEN DETECTION

The methods discussed in the preceding section provide opportunities to expedite the identification of microorganisms when a blood culture signals positive. However, blood cultures require up to 5 days of incubation, and this timeline is inconsistent with the need to obtain rapid answers to inform treatment decisions in patients with sepsis. Direct detection of pathogens in blood without the need for culture would be ideal but presents a number of challenges. Specimen preparation, enrichment for pathogen DNA, and integration of the front-end specimen preparation with a back-end molecular analysis that identifies virtually all pathogens are major obstacles. Furthermore, many current molecular methods are not sensitive enough to detect low-level bacteremia from whole blood (i.e., 1–10 colony forming units/mL) and, therefore, require a high input volume of specimen. In contrast, highly sensitive molecular methods for direct detection of microbial DNA in blood present significant challenges for assay verification given the known limitations of the sensitivity of culture, the current gold standard.

The Roche SeptiFast system has been available longer than any other method for direct detection of microorganisms in the blood. It uses real-time PCR performed on a LightCycler instrument that targets the ribosomal internal transcribed spacer region. The target DNA is amplified in three parallel, multiplex, real-time PCR assays for detection of 10

## TABLE 49.2    Key Features of Rapid Blood Culture Identification Methods

| Technology (Manufacturer) | Test Name | Number of Organism Targets | Number of Resistance Targets | Time to Result |
|---|---|---|---|---|
| Gold nanoparticle microarray (Luminex Corp.) | Verigene BC-GP | 12 | 3 | 2.5 h |
|  | Verigene BC-GN | 9 | 6 |  |
| PCR (GenMark Dx) | ePLex BCID-GP | 20 | 4 | 1.5 h |
|  | ePlex BCID-GN | 21 | 6 |  |
|  | ePlex BCID-FP | 15 | 0 |  |
| Nested PCR (BioFire Diagnostics) | FilmArray BCID | 24 | 3 | 1 h |
| Rescue PCR (iCubate) | iC-GPC | 5 | 3 | 3–4.5 h |
|  | iC-GN | 8 | 3 |  |
| PNA-FISH (AdvanDX/Opgen) | *S. aureus*/CNS | 2 | 0 | 20–90 min |
|  | *E. faecalis*/OE | 2 | 0 |  |
|  | Gram-negative | 3 | 0 |  |
|  | *Candida* | 5 | 0 |  |
| Automated PNA-FISH (Accelerate Dx) | PhenoTest BC | 16 | 20 (MIC) | ID: 2 h MIC: 4–5 h after ID |

*PCR*, Polymerase chain reaction; *PNA FISH*, peptide nucleic acid fluorescent in situ hybridization; ID, identification; MIC, minimum inhibitory concentration

Gram-positive, 10 Gram-negative and 5 fungal pathogens. Melting curve analysis is used to differentiate the pathogens. The assay is technically complex, requires large amounts of hands-on time and has an analysis time of about 6 hours. Several evaluations have reported lower sensitivities and specificities compared with blood cultures.

A novel technology that shows promise for direct detection of pathogens in blood is T2 magnetic resonance (T2MR)-based biosensing. T2 Biosystems has developed an assay to directly identify *Candida* spp. (*C. albicans, C. tropicalis, C. krusei, C. glabrata, C. parapsilosis*) in the blood of patients with suspected candidemia and another to detect the five most common bacteria in bloodstream infections (*E. faecium, S. aureus, K. pneumoniae, P. aeruginosa, E. coli*). The T2 system lyses microbial cells and amplifies their DNA by PCR, then the amplified product is detected directly in the whole-blood matrix by amplicon-induced agglomeration of superparamagnetic nanoparticles. Nanoparticle clustering yields changes in the T2 (spin-spin) relaxation time, making it detectable by magnetic resonance. A small portable T2MR instrument for rapid and precise T2 relaxation measurements has been designed for standard PCR tubes. The T2Dx instrument automates the steps in the assay with approximately 5 minutes of hands-on time, and results are available within 3–5 hours.

While more data are needed regarding the routine performance of the T2 assays and its potential role in antimicrobial stewardship, the decrease in time to result it offers over traditional blood cultures indicates it may have a significant impact in certain patient populations. Obstacles to implementation include cost, laboratory throughput and defining clinically appropriate patient populations for testing. T2 Biosystems also has a panel in development for antimicrobial resistance detection.

## UPPER RESPIRATORY TRACT INFECTIONS

The viruses that infect the respiratory tract consist of large and diverse groups that cause disease in humans, and new ones continue to be discovered. The more common viruses that infect humans include: influenza A and B, parainfluenza virus (PIV) types 1 to 4, respiratory syncytial virus (RSV), metapneumovirus, adenoviruses (>50 different types), rhinoviruses (>100 different types), and coronaviruses (5 types). The disease spectrum ranges from the common cold to severe life-threatening pneumonia. It can be difficult to differentiate the viral origin based on signs and symptoms alone, and treatment options vary depending on the viral etiology. Viral respiratory tract infections have demonstrated the potential for global public health threats of epidemic and pandemic proportions. Detection of emerging respiratory viruses will require multiple modalities, but molecular methods have been crucial to their discovery and characterization and in the development of diagnostic tools.

Acute respiratory viral infection: (1) is a leading cause of hospitalization and death in infants and young children; (2) contributes to problems of asthma exacerbation, otitis media, and lower respiratory tract infection; and (3) contributes to acute disease in immunocompromised and elderly patients. Rapid diagnosis aids in effective treatment (e.g., with antiviral medications such as oseltamivir for influenza A virus infection) and management (e.g., reduction in inappropriately prescribed antibiotics for viral infection and infection control).

Nonmolecular methods such as rapid antigen-based EIAs, direct fluorescent antibody and culture-based methods are available for the detection of respiratory viruses, but they suffer from decreased sensitivity and/or long turnaround times. The analytical sensitivity of molecular assays, primarily using PCR or real-time PCR, is consistently better than that of traditional methods. Results from molecular testing are more accurate, and thus the patient benefits from the most appropriate treatment decision; also, infection control practitioners can more effectively implement strategies to prevent or reduce health care-associated transmission. Molecular assays can be designed to detect a wide range of respiratory pathogens, including organisms that are difficult to culture.

Despite the advantages of NAATs for respiratory virus detection, their adoption by clinical laboratories was initially slow because of the limited capacity for multiplexing. There are numerous commercially available molecular tests capable of detecting one to four respiratory viruses in single reactions, but to provide comprehensive coverage for respiratory viruses, a panel of such assays needed to be deployed, an approach not practical for most laboratories. In 2008, the first molecular multiplex panel was FDA-cleared (Table 49.3). Now there are several commercially available multiplexed panels capable of detecting up to 20 different viral and bacterial respiratory pathogens. Although multiplex panels offer the advantages of improved diagnostic yield and laboratory workflow, decreased turnaround time, and increased sensitivity, the need for molecular tests designed to detect a limited number of viruses of particular importance (e.g., SARS-CoV-2, influenza A and B, and RSV) will likely continue. In addition, there are now simple, "sample in, answer out" molecular systems that can be used at the point-of-care (see Chapter 17).

Some disadvantages of syndromic multiplexed panels for respiratory pathogens include cost, throughput for some platforms, false-positive results, and lack of reimbursement. Outcome studies have demonstrated multiplex respiratory pathogen tests have a positive impact in the pediatric population (i.e., decreased antibiotic use and length of stay), but outcome data are inconclusive or still lacking in adult populations.

## PNEUMONIA PANELS

Lower respiratory tract infections (LRTIs) can vary in severity, symptoms, and causative agents. Although bacteria and viruses are the most common causes of LRTIs, fungi and parasites can also cause LRTIs in certain patient populations. Further, the typical causative agents can vary depending on whether the patient has community-acquired, hospital-acquired, ventilator-associated, or health care-associated pneumonia. Therefore, a wide range of diagnostic methods is needed, which usually includes antigen detection, microscopy, cultures, and molecular methods.

The respiratory panels discussed in the section above are only indicated for the testing of nasopharyngeal swabs (NPS). While many pathogens on the upper respiratory pathogen panels cause both upper and lower respiratory tract infections, a patient with pneumonia may not always have a positive NPS, so it is essential to sample and test specimens from the lower airways (e.g., sputa, tracheal aspirates, bronchoscopically-obtained washes/lavages), to obtain an accurate laboratory diagnosis. Recently, two molecular multiplex tests were FDA-cleared for the diagnosis of pneumonia—Curetis Unyvero LRT panel (endotracheal aspirates and

bronchoalveolar lavages [BALs]), and BioFire Pneumonia (PN) panel (BAL, mini-BAL, sputa, endotracheal aspirates).

The Unyvero LRT panel includes 19 bacteria, 10 antimicrobial resistance genes, and 1 fungus (*Pneumocystic jiroveci*, BAL only). The BioFire Pneumonia panel detects 18 bacteria, 7 resistance genes, and 8 (PN panel) or 9 (PN*plus*) viruses or virus groups. The BioFire PN*plus* includes MERS-CoV (Table 49.4). Since many potential bacterial pathogens can also be colonizers, it is important to determine the relative quantitative load of these organisms. Traditional bacterial culture performed on LRT specimens include quantitative or semi-quantitative results to ascertain likely colonization vs infection. Both the Curetis and BioFire platforms address this in their molecular panels. The limit of detection for reporting a positive result by Unyvero LRT is $10^4$ cfu/mL, which is generally accepted as an appropriate clinical cutoff; the BioFire panel reports everything below $10^{3.5}$ copies/mL as not detected. In addition, the BioFire test reports a semi-quantitative abundance (10-fold from $10^4$ to $\geq 10^7$ copies/mL) for 15 common colonizers.

The primary benefit of the LRT and PN panels appears to be decreased time to result for detecting potential pathogens and associated resistance markers. Since the panels do not encompass all potential pneumonia etiologies, they are not a replacement for traditional methods. Adding these panels to a laboratory test menu will increase costs, so it is imperative that clinical outcome data is collected, and testing algorithms are developed, so that the appropriate patient populations are tested.

## Gastrointestinal Pathogen Panels

Infectious gastroenteritis (IGE) is a leading cause of global morbidity and mortality. Diarrheal disease disproportionally affects developing nations, but IGE remains a significant problem in industrialized countries as well. IGE is associated with a diverse array of etiologic agents, including bacteria, viruses, and parasites. Clinical presentation does little to aid with a specific etiologic diagnosis because diarrhea is the predominant symptom regardless of the etiology. Accurate identification of the etiology of IGE provides important information that impacts individual patient management, infection control, and public health interventions.

Before multiplexed molecular approaches became available for the diagnosis of IGE, providers chose among a variety of tests, including antigen detection tests, culture, ova and parasite microscopic examination, and single-target NAATs, for detection of the responsible organism or toxin. The selection of tests may be informed by patient's age, severity of disease, immunocompromised state, duration and type of diarrhea, travel history, and time of year. Often the clinician is unsure of what pathogens are included in each test and consequently may miss testing for specific pathogens of interest. In the laboratory, the battery of tests required to detect all possible pathogens is laborious and expensive to maintain, can require special expertise, and may have an unacceptably long TAT. In addition, the conventional microbiologic tests have limited sensitivity for many of the major pathogens.

## TABLE 49.3  Parameters of Currently Marketed FDA-Cleared Respiratory Panels

| Parameter | Applied BioCode RPP | BioFire FilmArray RP EZ | BioFire FilmArray RP/RP2[b] | GenMark eSensor RVP | GenMark ePlex RPP | Luminex Verigene RP-Flex | Luminex NxTAG RPP | QIAGEN QIAstat-Dx RP |
|---|---|---|---|---|---|---|---|---|
| Amplicon detection method | Barcoded magnetic beads | Melting curve analysis | Melting curve analysis | Voltammetry | Voltammetry | Gold nanoparticle microarray hybridization | Fluorescence-labeled bead array | Real-time PCR probes |
| On-board sample processing | No | Yes | Yes | No | Yes | Yes | No | Yes |
| Post-PCR manipulation | Yes (automated) | No | No | Yes | No | Yes | Yes | No |
| Throughput | High | Low | Low (scaleable) | Moderate | Low (scaleable) | Low (scaleable) | High | Low |
| Total time to results (h)[a] | 8 | 1.1 | 0.75[b]–1.1 | 8 | 1.5 | 2 | 5 | 1 |
| CLIA Complexity | High | Waived | Moderate | High | Moderate | Moderate | High | Moderate |
| Pathogens detected: | ADV<br>INF A (H1, H3, 09H1)<br>INF B<br>MPV (A, B)<br>RSV (A, B)<br>RV/EV<br>PIV (1, 2, 3, 4)<br>COV (HKU1, NL63, 229E, OC43)<br>Bordetella pertussis<br>Chlamydia pneumoniae<br>Mycoplasma pneumoniae | ADV<br>INF A (H1, H3, 09H1)<br>INF B<br>MPV<br>RSV<br>RV/EV<br>PIV<br>COV<br>Bordetella pertussis<br>Chlamydia pneumoniae<br>Mycoplasma pneumoniae | ADV<br>INF A (H1, H3, 09H1)<br>INF B<br>MPV<br>RSV<br>RV/EV<br>PIV (1, 2, 3, 4)<br>COV (HKU1, NL63, 229E, OC43)<br>Bordetella pertussis[b]<br>Bordetella parapertussus<br>Chlamydia pneumoniae<br>Mycoplasma pneumoniae | ADV (B/E, C)<br>INF A (H1, H3, 09H1)<br>INF B<br>MPV<br>RSV (A, B)<br>RV<br>PIV (1, 2, 3) | ADV<br>INF A (H1, H3, 09H1)<br>INF B<br>MPV<br>RSV (A, B)<br>RV/EV<br>PIV (1, 2, 3, 4)<br>COV (HKU1, NL63, 229E, OC43)<br>Chlamydia pneumoniae<br>Mycoplasma pneumoniae | ADV<br>INF A (H1, H3)<br>INF B<br>MPV<br>RSV (A, B)<br>RV<br>PIV (1, 2, 3, 4)<br>Bordetella pertussis<br>Bordetella parapertussis<br>Bordetella holmesii | ADV<br>INF A (H1, H3, 09H1)<br>INF B<br>MPV<br>RSV (A, B)<br>RV/EV<br>PIV (1, 2, 3, 4)<br>COV (HKU1, NL63, 229E, OC43)<br>Bocavirus<br>Chlamydia pneumoniae<br>Mycoplasma pneumoniae<br>Legionella pneumophila | ADV<br>INF A (H1, H3, 09H1)<br>INF B<br>MPV (A, B)<br>RSV (A, B)<br>RV/EV<br>PIV (1, 2, 3, 4)<br>COV (HKU1, NL63, 229E, OC43)<br>Bordetella pertussis<br>Chlamydia pneumoniae<br>Mycoplasma pneumoniae |

[a]Includes the time required for nucleic acid extraction.
[b]Details specific to RP2 version.

ADV, Adenovirus; COV, coronavirus; EV, enterovirus; INF A, influenza A virus; INF B, influenza B virus; MPV, metapneumovirus; PCR, polymerase chain reaction; PIV, parainfluenza virus; RSV, respiratory syncytial virus; RV, rhinovirus.

## TABLE 49.4    Targets included in FDA-cleared pneumonia panels

| BioFire FilmArray Pneumonia Panel | Curetis Unyvero LRT Panel |
|---|---|
| **Bacteria** | **Bacteria** |
| ***Semi-quantitative*** | Acinetobacter spp. |
| Acinetobacter calcoaceticus-baumannii complex | Chlamydia pneumoniae |
| Enterobacter cloacae complex | Citrobacter freundii |
| Escherichia coli | Enterobacter cloacae complex |
| Haemophilus influenzae | Escherichia coli |
| Klebsiella aerogenes | Haemophilus influenzae |
| Klebsiella oxytoca | Klebsiella oxytoca |
| Klebsiella pneumoniae group | Klebsiella pneumoniae |
| Moraxella catarrhalis | Klebsiella variicola |
| Proteus spp. | Legionella pneumophila |
| Pseudomonas aeruginosa | Moraxella catarrhalis |
| Serratia marcescens | Morganella morganii |
| Staphylococcus aureus | Mycoplasma pneumoniae |
| Streptococcus agalactiae | Proteus spp. |
| Streptococcus pneumoniae | Pseudomonas aeruginosa |
| Streptococcus pyogenes | Serratia marcescens |
| ***Qualitative*** | Staphylococcus aureus |
| Chlamydia pneumoniae | Stenotrophomonas maltophilia |
| Legionella pneumophila | Streptococcus pneumoniae |
| Mycoplasma pneumoniae | |
| **Antimicrobial resistance genes** | **Antimicrobial resistance genes** |
| ***Methicillin resistance*** | ***Methicillin resistance*** |
| • mecA/C and MREJ | • mecA |
| **Carbapenemases** | ***Penicillin resistance*** |
| • KPC | • tem |
| • NDM | ***Carbapenemases*** |
| • Oxa-48-like | • KPC |
| • VIM | • NDM |
| • IMP | • Oxa-23 |
| ***ESBL*** | • Oxa-24 |
| • CTX-M | • Oxa-48 |
| | • Oxa-58 |
| | • VIM |
| | ***ESBL*** |
| | • CTX-M |
| **Viruses** | **Fungi** |
| Adenovirus | Pneumocystis jiroveci (BAL only) |
| Coronavirus | |
| Metapneumovirus | |
| Rhinovirus/enterovirus | |
| Influenza A | |
| Influenza B | |
| Parainfluenza virus | |
| Respiratory syncytial virus | |

Enteric pathogen panels are currently available (Table 49.5) and laboratories can choose from a variety of test platforms based on whether a more focused or broader approach to IGE pathogen detection is desired. Also, the technical complexity and required throughput are important variables that may influence the approach chosen for this application. The use of comprehensive pathogen panels dramatically increases diagnostic yield, but with this comes the unique challenge of interpreting the results from patients with multiple pathogens detected. Asymptomatic infections with *C. difficile*, *Cryptosporidium* spp., and *G. lamblia* are not uncommon, and some of the other IGE pathogens such as *Salmonella* spp. and norovirus can be shed for weeks after resolution of symptoms. Comprehensive panels consolidate testing platforms for agents of IGE and substantially reduce, but do not completely eliminate, the need for culture because isolates are needed for epidemiologic surveillance and occasionally for antimicrobial susceptibility testing.

## Meningitis/Encephalitis

Routine laboratory tests on cerebrospinal fluid (CSF) for the diagnosis of meningitis/encephalitis (ME) include chemistry analyses (e.g., white cell count, glucose, protein), bacterial cultures and stains, specific viral PCRs (e.g., HSV PCR, enterovirus RT-PCR), antibody tests for arboviruses, and antigen tests for *Cryptococcus*.

The scope of diagnostic tests ordered often depends on epidemiology and the patient's age, immune status, clinical presentation/radiology results, and CSF chemistry parameters. Given the complexity of the panel of tests needed to cover all potential etiologies and the extended time that may be required to achieve a diagnosis, a molecular syndromic approach is an attractive solution. Current nonmolecular methods suffer from lack of sensitivity and may be compromised by the timing of antimicrobial therapy. Further, easy to use molecular devices make testing feasible for laboratories that otherwise may not offer molecular testing for agents causing ME. However, the ME molecular syndromic panel is perhaps the most controversial of the syndromic panels in terms of analytical performance and potential impact. Currently, there is only one commercially available molecular multiplex for meningitis/encephalitis—the BioFire ME panel that detects 14 pathogens in ≈1 hour (Box 49.1).

Studies published after the regulatory clearance of the ME panel demonstrated some limitations of the panel. HSV-1, HSV-2, EV, and *Cryptococcus* were targets that showed a high false-negative rate. In addition, the potential impact of a false-positive result should be carefully considered, as it might delay efforts in obtaining the true diagnosis. Close to 25% of positive results were reported to be clinically insignificant and the short time to results led to over-utilization of the test. In addition to conflicting data on the ME panel's performance and clinical utility, other obstacles to implementation include cost and the ability to perform an adequate laboratory test verification.

Undiagnosed and improperly treated ME leads to a high mortality rate. Therefore, it is critical to accurately and quickly identify the etiology of infectious ME. It is estimated that 15%–70% of ME patients never receive a specific microbiologic diagnosis. The use of an ME panel in a diagnostic algorithm (e.g., not discontinuing traditional methods) and in appropriate patient populations could greatly improve our ability to diagnose and treat patients with ME and, therefore, reduce the mortality rate. Improvements in the sensitivity and specificity of ME panels, along with additional outcome studies, will be important.

---

### BOX 49.1 Targets included in the BioFire Meningitis/Encephalitis Panel

**Bacteria**
- *Escherichia coli* K1
- *Haemophilus influenzae*
- *Listeria monocytogenes*
- *Neisseria meningitidis*
- *Streptococcus agalactiae*
- *Streptococcus pneumoniae*

**Viruses**
- Cytomegalovirus
- Enterovirus
- Herpes simplex virus 1
- Herpes simplex virus 2
- Human herpes virus 6
- Human parechovirus
- Varicella zoster virus

**Yeast**
- *Cryptococcus neoformans/gattii*

---

### POINTS TO REMEMBER

- Syndromic molecular tests are available using a variety of platforms to diagnose blood, respiratory, gastrointestinal, and central nervous system infections.
- Advantages of syndromic testing include improved time to result, expanded access to diagnostic tests, and improved sensitivity for many pathogens.
- Disadvantages of syndromic testing included cost, required laboratory expertise for some platforms, and lack of clinical utility data for some indications.

## POINT-OF-CARE TESTING

Although point-of-care tests (POCTs) for infectious diseases have been around for decades, the development of molecular-based POCTs is relatively recent. The majority of POCTs in microbiology are lateral flow immunoassays (LFIAs) detecting one or more antigens of or antibodies produced to potential pathogens (e.g., SARS-CoV-2, Group A *Streptococcus*, *Helicobacter pylori*, bacterial vaginosis, influenza A/B, respiratory syncytial virus, hepatitis C virus, HIV 1/2, adenovirus, *Trichomonas vaginalis*). The sensitivity of LFIAs is dependent on the concentration of the antigen or antibody in the specimen. With routine implementation of NA amplification tests in microbiology, the analytic limitations of LFIAs became apparent.

A meta-analysis estimated 84% sensitivity and 96% specificity for rapid antigen detection tests (RADTs) for Group A *Streptococcus* (GAS) when compared to throat culture. Due to the lower sensitivity of RADTs, culture is still recommended after a negative test in pediatric patients. However, the GAS PCR is more sensitive than RADTs (93% vs 55% in one study) and culture. Improved analytical performance offered by molecular detection of GAS may allow a single test to be performed. However, even when laboratory workflow is optimized, the time to result for PCR tests performed by a central lab is not optimal for patient care. Accurate, rapid and inexpensive molecular tests at the point-of-care is critical. The Alere i Strep A test (now, Abbott ID NOW Strep A 2) uses an isothermal nicking enzyme amplification reaction (NEAR) and molecular beacon probes for amplicon detection with a sensitivity of 98.7% and a specificity of 98.5%. Results are available in 6–8 minutes. The Roche Liat molecular POCT test uses PCR for GAS detection with 97.7%–100% sensitivity when compared to throat culture and results are available in 15 minutes.

Another successful application of molecular POCTs in infectious diseases is the detection of respiratory viruses. RADTs for influenza have been criticized for their low sensitivity (50%–70% in most seasons and as low as 18% in the 2009 H1N1 influenza A pandemic). Due to the diagnostic limitations of influenza RADTs, the US CDC has provided guidelines for the interpretation of RADTs and the need for additional testing. The COVID-19 pandemic highlighted the need for POCT for SARS-CoV-2 and the significant utility of detecting both influenza and SARS-CoV-2 by the same test. Similar to RADTs for influenza, SARS-CoV-2 RADTs were also less sensitive than molecular approaches (60%–70%). Molecular tests with greater accuracy for the diagnosis of SARS-CoV-2, influenza, RSV, and other respiratory viruses have improved diagnostic yield. Subsequently, several CLIA-waived molecular tests became commercially available (Table 49.6).

## TABLE 49.5    Comparison of FDA-Cleared Enteric Pathogen Panel Platforms

| Feature | Applied Biocode GPP | Enteric Bacterial Panel (EBP) | Extended EBP | Enteric Parasite Panel | Enteric Viral Panel |
|---|---|---|---|---|---|
| | | | **BD MAX** | | |
| Technology | PCR and barcoded magnetic beads | Real-time PCR | | | |
| Automation | Separate extraction, manual PCR setup followed by automated amplification, hybridization, and detection | Sample to result | | | |
| Relative throughput | High | Moderate | | | |
| Total time to results (h)[a] | 8 | 3 | 3.5 | 4.5 | 3 |
| Bacterial targets | *Campylobacter* *Clostridioides difficile* toxins A and B *E. coli* O157 Enterotoxigenic *E. coli* LT/ST (ETEC) *Salmonella* Shiga-like toxin producing *E. coli* stx1/stx2 (STEC) *Shigella*/ Enteroinvasive *E. coli* (EIEC) *Vibrio*/*Vibrio parahemolyticus* *Yersinia enterocolitica* | *Campylobacter* spp. *(jejuni, coli)* *Salmonella* spp. Shiga-toxin producing organisms (STEC, *Shigella*) *Shigella* spp./EIEC | ETEC *Plesiomonas shigelloides* *Vibrio* (*cholerae*/ *parahemolyticus*/ *vulnificus*) *Yersinia enterocolitica* | | |
| Viral targets | Adenovirus 40/41 Norovirus GI/GII Rotavirus A | | | | Norovirus GI/GII Rotavirus A Adenovirus 40/41 Sapovirus (I, II, IV, V) Astrovirus |
| Parasitic targets | *Cryptosporidium* *Entamoeba histolytica* *Giardia lamblia* | | | *Giardia lamblia* *Cryptosporidium* spp. (*parvum* and *hominis*) *Entamoeba histolytica* | |

[a]Includes the time required for nucleic acid extraction.
*PCR*, Polymerase chain reaction; *GPP*, gastrointestinal pathogen panel; *GI*, gastrointestinal

Challenges to the implementation of molecular tests at the point-of-care include throughput, cost, and quality assurance monitors. Most of the currently available platforms only test one specimen at a time, limiting throughput unless multiple analyzers are purchased. Molecular tests are more expensive than RADTs, but consideration should be given to the cost of additional follow-up testing and the cost of a missed diagnosis associated with RADTs. Contamination from amplified material, specimens or the clinic environment can contribute to false-positive results if appropriate quality monitors are not in place. In 2019, the College of American Pathologists updated accreditation checklists to include CLIA-waived molecular microbiology tests. New checklist items include requirements for quality monitoring statistics to monitor false-positive results, written

| BioFire Film Array GI | Serosep EntericBio Dx Molecular GI Panel | Great Basin Stool Bacterial Pathogens | Hologic ProGastro SSCS | Luminex Verigene Enteric Pathogens | Luminex xTAG GPP |
|---|---|---|---|---|---|
| Nested PCR and melting curve analysis | Real-time PCR | Real-time PCR with chip-based detection | Real-time PCR | PCR and gold nanoparticle microarray | PCR and fluorescence-labeled bead array |
| Sample to result | Separate extraction, automated pipetting system, amplification on ABI 7500 FAST Dx | Sample to result | Separate extraction, manual PCR setup | Sample to result | Separate extraction, manual PCR setup, post-PCR amplicon transfer |
| Low (scaleable) | Moderate | Low | Moderate | Low (scaleable) | High |
| 1 | 4-5 | 2 | 3 | 2 | 5 |
| *Campylobacter* (*jejuni, coli* and *upsaliensis*) | *Campylobacter* (*jejuni, coli, lari*) | *Campylobacter* spp. (*jejuni, coli*) | *Campylobacter* spp. (*jejuni, coli*) | *Campylobacter* spp. | *Campylobacter* |
| *Clostridioides difficile* (toxin A/B) | *Salmonella* | *Salmonella* spp. | *Salmonella* spp. | *Salmonella* spp. | *Clostridioides difficile* toxins A and B |
| Enteroaggregative *E. coli* | *Shigella* spp./ EIEC STEC | Shiga toxin 1 (stx1) | Shiga toxin 1 (stx1) | Shiga toxin 1 (stx1) | *E. coli* |
| Enteropathogenic *E. coli* | *Vibrio* (*cholerae, parahaemolyticus*) | Shiga toxin 2 (stx2) | Shiga toxin 2 (stx2) | Shiga toxin 2 (stx2) | O157 ETEC |
| ETEC | | *E. coli* O157 | *Shigella* | *Shigella* spp. | *Salmonella* |
| STEC | | *Shigella* | | *Vibrio* spp. | *Shigella* |
| *E. coli* O157 | | | | *Yersinia enterocolitica* | STEC |
| *Shigella*/EIEC | | | | | *Vibrio cholerae* |
| *Plesiomonas shigelloides* | | | | | *Yersinia enterocolitica* |
| *Salmonella* | | | | | |
| *Yersinia enterocolitica* | | | | | |
| *Vibrio* (*parahaemolyticus, vulnificus, cholerae*) | | | | | |
| Adenovirus 40/41 | | | | Norovirus | Adenovirus 40/41 |
| Astrovirus | | | | Rotavirus | Norovirus GI/GII |
| Norovirus GI/GII | | | | | Rotavirus A |
| Rotavirus A | | | | | |
| Sapovirus (I, II, IV, V) | | | | | |
| *Cryptosporidium* | *Giardia lamblia* | | | | *Cryptosporidium* |
| *Cyclospora cayetanensis* | *Entamoeba histolytica* | | | | *Entamoeba histolytica* |
| *Entamoeba histolytica* | | | | | *Giardia* |
| *Giardia lamblia* | | | | | |

procedures for specimen handling, policies for processing specimens from patients suspected of having a highly communicable infectious disease (e.g., avian influenza, SARS, Ebola) and reporting verbiage to include test method and information about clinical interpretation when appropriate. The American Academy of Microbiology also published recommendations for the implementation, oversight, and evaluation of molecular

POCTs, which are summarized in Box 49.2. With appropriate oversight, accurate molecular diagnostics performed at the point-of-care have the potential to improve patient care, clinical decision-making and patient satisfaction. For widespread adoption in clinics, manufacturers will need to make pricing competitive with RADTs and improve the throughput to handle epidemiologic peaks and clinic demands.

TABLE 49.6    **Parameters of CLIA-Waived Molecular Infectious Disease Tests for Respiratory Viruses**

| Manufacturer | Product | Platform/ Instrument | Molecular Technology | Organisms Detected | Approved Specimens | Test Time |
|---|---|---|---|---|---|---|
| Abbott (previously Alere) | ID NOW™ Influenza A and B 2 | ID NOW™ Platform | Isothermal NEAR amplification | Influenza A and B | NPS and NS direct, or NPS and NS in VTM | 15 min |
| | ID NOW RSV | | | RSV | | |
| | ID NOW COVID-19 | | | SARS-CoV-2 | NPS, NS, throat direct | 13 min |
| BioFire, Inc. | FilmArray® Respiratory Panel EZ | FilmArray 2.0 EZ | Nested multiplex PCR and post-PCR melt curve analysis | Influenza A (H1, H1pdm09, H3) and B, adenovirus, coronavirus, metapneumovirus, rhinovirus/enterovirus, parainfluenza virus, respiratory syncytial virus, *Mycoplasma pneumoniae*, *Chlamydia pneumoniae*, *Bordetella pertussis* | NPS in VTM | 1 h |
| | BioFire® Respiratory Panel 2.1-EZ (RP2.1-EZ) | FilmArray 2.0 EZ | Nested multiplex PCR and post-PCR melt curve analysis | Adenovirus, coronavirus 229E, coronavirus HKU1, coronavirus NL63, coronavirus OC43, coronavirus SARS-CoV-2, Human metapneumovirus, Human rhinovirus/enterovirus, Influenza A including subtypes H1, H3, and H1-2009, Influenza B, parainfluenza virus, respiratory syncytial virus, *Bordetella parapertussis*, *Bordetella pertussis*, *Chlamydia pneumoniae*, *Mycoplasma pneumoniae* | NPS in UTM | 45 min |
| Cepheid | Xpert Xpress Flu | GeneXpert Xpress | Real-time RT-PCR | Influenza A and B | NPS and NS in VTM | 20–30 min |
| | Xpert Xpress Flu/ RSV | | | Influenza A and B, RSV | | |
| | Xpert Xpress SARS-CoV-2 test | | | SARS-CoV-2 | | |
| | Xpert Xpress SARS-CoV-2/Flu/RSV | | | SARS-CoV-2, Influenza A and B, RSV | | |
| Mesa Biotech. Inc | Accula Flu A/Flu B | Accula Dock | RT-PCR followed by hybridization and colorimetric visualization on a test strip | Influenza A and B | NS direct | <30 min |
| | Accula SARS-CoV-2 Test | | | SARS-CoV-2 | NS and NMT in SARS-CoV-2 buffer | |
| Roche Molecular Diagnostics | Cobas® Influenza A/B Assay | Cobas® Liat® Analyzer | Real-time RT-PCR | Influenza A and B | NPS in VTM | 20 min |
| | Cobas® Influenza A/B & RSV Assay | | | Influenza A and B, RSV | | |
| | Cobas SARS-CoV-2 | | | SARS-CoV-2 | NPS, NMT, and NS in UTM | |
| | Cobas SARS-CoV-2, Influenza A/B | | | SARS-CoV-2, Influenza A and B | | |
| Sekisui Diagnostics | Silaris Influenza A/B | Silaris Dock | PCR using proprietary OscAR technology | Influenza A and B | NS direct | <30 min |

*NPS*, Nasopharyngeal swab; *NS*, nasal swab; *NMT*, nasal mid-turbinate; *OPS*, oropharyngeal swab; *VTM*, viral transport media; *UTM*, universal transport media

## BOX 49.2  Recommendations from the American Academy of Microbiology for Advanced POCTs

**Implementation**

- Redesign clinic workflows to incorporate near-patient and point-of-care testing.
- Promote proper interpretation of tests to avoid adverse outcomes.
- Provide resources, such as training videos, to support appropriate self-collection of patient specimens.
- Ensure that public health surveillance of infectious diseases is maintained with point-of-care testing.
- Link near-patient and POCT results to the patient's electronic medical record.

**Oversight**

- Maintain clinical microbiology laboratory expertise and oversight of infectious disease tests.
- Utilize competent personnel to oversee ordering, testing, and interpretation.
- Educate providers and patients on different types of tests.

**Evaluation**

- Conduct clinical outcomes and cost-effectiveness studies for near-patient and POCTs.
- Evaluate near-patient and POCTs periodically and undertake regulatory action or reclassification for tests that do not meet performance standards.

## POINTS TO REMEMBER

- Molecular POCTs have improved sensitivity compared to traditional POCTs (based on antigen detection) for infectious diseases.
- Using amplified molecular methods at the point-of-care requires careful oversight to mitigate contamination risk.
- Clinical outcome studies are needed to determine how best to utilize molecular testing at the point-of-care.

## EMERGING TECHNOLOGIES

### Contrast to Targeted Approaches

Traditional molecular diagnostic methods in clinical microbiology laboratories focus on detection of specific targets based on the clinical scenario and clinical suspicion. In many cases, this approach is successful in identifying the pathogen, and if large syndromic panels are used, additional targets and co-infections might be identified. In certain situations, traditional targeted diagnosis might not generate an answer and physicians are left to wonder about the possibility of noninfectious versus infectious causes of the patient's symptoms. To address that, multiple approaches have rapidly progressed during the past few years aimed at nontargeted diagnosis. These approaches include metagenomics or nontargeted massively parallel sequencing of clinical specimens and class specific immune response signature characterization.

### Metagenomics

Metagenomics MPS (mMPS), also called *shotgun metagenomic sequencing*, reflects non-targeted analysis of all the microbial genomes in clinical specimens (DNA and RNA; microbiome). This approach has only recently become feasible facilitated by advances in MPS technologies combined with lower cost and improvement in bioinformatic approaches for analysis. A plethora of information can be obtained using mMPS, including the detection of mixed infections and infections with fastidious organisms or esoteric viruses. Additional breakthrough applications of mMPS in antimicrobial resistance detection include developing bioinformatics pipelines that correlate the genomic data to phenotypic drug resistance. mMPS has also been extended to analyze the host response associated with an infection.

mMPS is faced with many challenges. A major challenge is the abundance of human nucleic acids in relation to microbial sequences. Since microbial genomic reads are much fewer than the human reads (could reach <0.01% of the total reads in some cases), increased sequencing depth is required to provide acceptable coverage of microbial sequences. In principle, the more sequencing reads, the better the sensitivity, and the greater the ability to cover less abundant microorganisms. Another major challenge is the liability of the assay for contamination due to the ubiquitous nature of microorganisms. Contamination might stem from skin flora during specimen collection, reagents or other environmental sources, which complicates the interpretation of the results.

In general, the process starts with a nucleic acid extraction step, followed by random amplification. Due to the abundance of human reads, different groups have attempted host depletion steps before nucleic acid extraction, including lysis of human cells or chemically targeting human DNA. For RNA sequencing libraries that enable sequencing of RNA targets (e.g., RNA viruses), host RNA depletion steps were also attempted to reduce the abundance of human RNA, especially mitochondrial and rRNA. Different sequencing platforms and library prep kits are available and should be carefully selected based on the required total number of reads and lengths of sequenced fragments. Data analysis usually starts with filtering of the good quality reads based on predefined quality matrices and removing the adaptor sequences, followed by human read depletion by computational methods that involve aligning the data to the human genome. The remaining reads are then aligned to pathogen databases for classification. Multiple pipelines for microbial MPS data analysis are currently available either as open-source or private software which include Kraken, Taxonomer, CosmosID, and different in-house developed pipelines. Some analysis pipelines integrate algorithms for result interpretation by using predefined QC criteria and generate a user-friendly report (e.g., Explify Illumina, San Diego). Curated, comprehensive, and updated databases are the cornerstone for a successful and meaningful analysis.

Nontargeted mMPS as a clinical assay has recently become available for infectious disease diagnosis using specimens that include plasma (cell free DNA, cfDNA, discussed below), cerebrospinal fluid for diagnosis of cases of meningitis and encephalitis, and respiratory specimens for undiagnosed pneumonia. Some studies have also used mMPS for stool analysis and diagnosing ocular infections. In all cases, mMPS is beneficial when patients are on antimicrobial therapy.

Challenges of implementing MPS in the clinical microbiology laboratory include the complexity of the assay, cost, and the complicated data analysis with the lack of sufficient clinical outcome studies that justify the validity of the assay for clinical implementation. In addition, the workflow for preparing the libraries, sequencing, and data analysis has not been standardized between laboratories, which could introduce variability in the results. Additional challenges include developing clinical thresholds that correlate with an infection, determining appropriate specimen types and the time requirement of the assay. Cost, reimbursement, and quality assurance are ongoing concerns.

## Cell-Free Nucleic Acid for Microbial Identification

Cell-free DNA (cfDNA) for diagnosis of microbial infection is a method for the detection of short fragments of DNA that result from degradation of microbes by apoptosis or necrosis, which facilitate their accessibility for analysis by WGS. Because of the random fragmentation of the DNA, these specimens are of poor quality for assays that require intact primer or probe binding sites like PCR, Sanger sequencing or microarrays. Additionally, using nontargeted MPS is more suitable for identifying novel microorganisms. This approach differs from conventional sequencing-based diagnostics in that it does not require collection of samples from presumptively infected tissues and mainly relies on pathogen detection from peripheral blood (liquid biopsy, noninvasive). Other fluids have also been investigated as liquid biopsies for detection of microbial cfDNA including urine. cfDNA from infectious agents was successfully detected in the blood, and several studies during the past few years showed the diagnostic potential of cfDNA detection in microbe identification in pneumonia, sepsis, and invasive fungal infections, among others. The Karius test (Karius Inc., Redwood City, CA) was recently introduced to the market and is an MPS blood test for detection of microbial cfDNA. The assay is currently used for diagnosing pneumonia, endocarditis, and various infections in immunocompromised patients. Challenges that face mMPS for diagnosis, including contamination, abundance of human reads, and data analysis, also apply to cfDNA-based sequencing.

## Host Response

This approach is based on detecting the host immune response or signature change in biomarkers that characterizes infection with specific pathogen groups, largely dependent on the concept that the immune response to a particular pathogen class (bacterial, viral, or fungal) is generally consistent. Differentiating bacterial versus viral or fungal infection and diagnosis of sepsis are a few applications of such technology. Advantages of this approach include providing evidence of infection when direct detection of pathogens might not differentiate colonization, contamination, and infection. In addition, characterizing the host response could diagnose an infectious process when methods of direct molecular identification fail to recognize a causative pathogen (novel strain or emerging pathogen). In fact, this approach is not entirely novel for infectious disease diagnosis. The erythrocyte sedimentation rate (ESR) and C-reactive protein (CRP) as markers of inflammation were discovered early during the past century and have been used to suggest a bacterial infection. The newest direction for using the host response for diagnosing infectious diseases is indeed more complex and could be

thought about as a multi-analyte panel approach. The applications of this approach would be most rewarding if used as a point-of-care test. A rapid result could decrease antibiotic utilization (if viral infection can be ruled in or bacterial infection can be ruled out). Different strategies have been developed to diagnose infections by dissecting the host response that include gene expression profiles, protein and metabolite panels, and cytokine panels.

## Gene Expression Analysis (Transcriptomics)

Transcript signatures associated with infections can be defined and measured by various methods of RNA quantification. This includes real-time PCR, RNA-sequencing (RNA-seq) and microarrays. Recent studies have shown that this approach is robust in differentiating class level infections (e.g., bacterial versus viral), and several studies have shown promising applications including the diagnosis of tuberculosis and early detection of leprosy. However, these approaches are still largely research based. SeptiCyte is currently the only FDA cleared gene expression host response assay for early diagnosis of sepsis available from Immunexpress (Seattle, WA). The assay measures RNA transcripts from four genes: *CEACAM4*, *LAMP1*, *PLA2G7*, and *PLAC8*.

## Host Protein Signature (Proteomics)

Host proteins used for differentiating bacterial and viral infections include tumor necrosis factor-related apoptosis-inducing ligand (TRAIL), interferon gamma-induced protein-10 (IP-10), and C-reactive protein (CRP). A few assays have shown good performance in differentiating viral from bacterial infections in a format that permits use as a point-of-care test, including the ImmunoXpert (MeMed diagnostics, Haifa, Israel) and FebriDx (RPS Diagnostics, Sarsota, FL) that combines CRP (as a marker of bacterial infection) and myxovirus resistance protein A (as a marker of viral infection), available in Europe and Canada.

A major disadvantage of host response for diagnosis of infectious diseases is the diagnostic performance in immunocompromised patients. This population of patients can develop very severe and diverse infections with a blunt immune response. Additional studies are required to define the immune signatures in immunocompromised populations, patients with chronic inflammatory disease, or chronic infections, old age, and patients with comorbidities, to add to our understanding about the spectrum of the clinical utility of this approach.

---

### POINTS TO REMEMBER

- mMPS is an approach for detection of microbial genomes in clinical samples by nontargeted MPS.
- Challenges of mMPS include complexity, cost, and lack of standardization.
- cfDNA is an MPS approach that specifically targets the free, fragmented DNA of pathogens in the blood or other accessible specimens, minimizing the need for invasive specimen collection.
- The detection of host response is an indirect way to diagnose an infection.

## CRISPR-CAS APPLICATIONS

Clustered regularly interspaced short palindromic repeats (CRISPR) were first described in the genome of *E. coli* in 1987. Five repeats of 29 nucleotides that are highly homologous, separated by spacers of 32 nucleotides were defined. Interestingly, the spacers were later identified to constitute a part of an adaptive and heritable immune response to phages and foreign genetic material. Cas (CRISPR-associated proteins) are nucleases that are directed to silence invading genetic elements. This immune response is sequence specific, based on CRISPR-Cas stored information of past infections. Cas proteins are encoded by genes that are adjacent to the CRISPR array and they drive the immune response that develops through three steps: adaptation, CRISPR RNA (crRNA) synthesis, and interference. During the adaptation phase, the invader DNA is integrated into the CRISPR region. When the CRISPR array is transcribed, the invader RNA is incorporated into a long precursor crRNA, which is modified by Cas proteases to generate mature crRNA. Re-exposure to the same genetic sequences triggers an interference response that directs crRNA to cleave complementary nucleic acid.

The CRISPR-Cas system introduced a marked advance as a genome editing tool with applications that extended to infectious disease diagnosis and treatment. For example, multiple groups attempted using this technology to develop approaches for characterizing antimicrobial resistance genes. An assay that combines CRISPR-Cas9 with MPS was developed (FLASH, finding low abundance sequencing by hybridization) where antimicrobial resistance genes are targeted by a set of RNA molecules that direct Cas9 to DNA fragmentation. Fragmented DNA then gets amplified and sequenced. In addition, CRISPR-Cas9 was combined with DNA mapping or FISH for the detection of ESBLs, carbapenemases and MRSA. CRISPR-Cas for diagnosis of viral infections is also a quickly developing field. A group at Harvard and MIT developed a technology based on CRISPR-Cas13, which they called CARVER (Cas13-assisted restriction of viral expression and readout), which could not only identify an infection, but can also direct RNA viral destruction. In addition, DETECTR (DNA endonuclease-targeted CRISPR *trans* reporter) is a CRISPR-Cas12 based assay that was used to detect HPV16 and 18 in clinical specimens with great success. CRISPR was also combined with target nucleic acid pre-amplification in a platform that was named SHERLOCK (specific high sensitivity enzymatic reporter unlocking). A SARS-CoV-2 SHERLOCK-based assay was the first CRISPR-based diagnostic assay to receive FDA Emergency Use Authorization.

## REVIEW QUESTIONS

1. Which of the following describes Loop-Mediated Isothermal Amplification (LAMP):
   a. A thermocycler is required for amplification.
   b. More than four primers are required.
   c. A helicase unwinds the DNA.
   d. Amplification starts at a nick introduced by a restriction enzyme.
   e. Signal is released when a cleavase enzyme cleaves a FRET probe separating the quencher from the reporter.

2. The following allows target visualization within fixed cells:
   a. Digital PCR.
   b. 16S rRNA sequencing.
   c. Fluorescence in situ hybridization (FISH).
   d. Transcription-mediated amplification.
   e. Real-time PCR.

3. Detection of a minor population of HIV variants can be best achieved by the following method:
   a. MALDI-TOF.
   b. Real-time PCR.
   c. Massively parallel sequencing.
   d. 16S rRNA Sanger sequencing.
   e. Digital PCR.

4. Which of the following methods permits target quantification without a need for calibrators?
   a. Transcription-mediated amplification
   b. MALDI-TOF
   c. Real-time PCR
   d. Strand displacement amplification
   e. Digital PCR

5. Which is true for molecular assays that detect MRSA?
   a. They detect mecA, mecB, and mecC.
   b. Only tests for infection control surveillance exist.
   c. They are less sensitive than culture-based methods.
   d. Differentiating from MR-*S. epidermidis* is not possible.
   e. False-positives may occur due to empty cassettes or non-functional *mec* genes.

6. What is correct for glycopeptide resistance in enterococci?
   a. *Van* genes are only found in the genus *Enterococcus*.
   b. All *van* genes play a role in health care-associated infections.
   c. *VanA and vanB* confer resistance to all common glycopeptides.
   d. *VanB* can be found in other genera and confers resistance only to vancomycin.
   e. *VanA* has been detected in *Streptococcus pneumoniae*.

7. Which of the following statements best describes current knowledge about carbapenemases?
   a. Detection of carbapenemases in Enterobacterales is not important for treatment decisions.
   b. KPC, NDM, VIM, IMP, and OXA are the most common genes detected by rapid molecular diagnostic tests.
   c. New cephalosporin/beta-lactamase inhibitor combinations are effective against all types of carbapenemases.
   d. Multiplex PCR assays can easily cover the current spectrum of known carbapenemases.
   e. Carbapenemases occur only in Enterobacterales.

8. Molecular syndromic tests have the following disadvantage:
   a. They are overall less sensitive than traditional methods.
   b. Limited numbers of pathogens are detected.
   c. The time to result is longer than a combination of traditional methods.
   d. An organism is not recovered limiting additional testing like antimicrobial susceptibility testing or strain typing.
   e. There are no commercially available platforms.

9. Which of the following is true of multiplex tests for the detection of respiratory pathogens?
   a. The only acceptable specimen type is a nasopharyngeal swab.
   b. None includes bacterial agents that cause acute respiratory tract illness.
   c. Both upper respiratory tract infection and pneumonia tests are available.
   d. They are not available for testing at the point-of-care.
   e. All platforms have low throughput.

10. Molecular point-of-care tests for infectious diseases are:
    a. easy to use.
    b. inexpensive.
    c. less sensitive than antigen-based tests.
    d. high-throughput.
    e. difficult to interpret.

## SUGGESTED READINGS

Becker K, van Alen S, Idelevich EA, et al. Plasmid-encoded transferable mecB-mediated methicillin resistance in *Staphylococcus aureus. Emerg Infect Dis.* 2018;24:242–248.

Dalpke AH, Hofko M, Zorn M, Zimmermann S. Evaluation of the fully automated BD MAX Cdiff and Xpert *C. difficile* assays for direct detection of *Clostridium difficile* in stool specimens. *J Clin Microbiol.* 2013;51:1906–1908.

Dolen V, Bahk K, Carroll KC, Klugman K, Ledeboer NA, Miller MB. Changing diagnostic paradigms for microbiology: report on an American Academy of Microbiology colloquium held in Washington, DC, from 17 to 18 October 2016. Washington, DC: American Society for Microbiology; 2017.

Espy MJ, Uhl JR, Sloan LM, et al. Real-time PCR in clinical microbiology: applications for routine laboratory testing. *Clin Microbiol Rev.* 2006;19:165–256.

Evans SR, Tran TTT, Hujer AM, et al. Rapid molecular diagnostics to inform empiric use of ceftazidime/avibactam and ceftolozane/tazobactam against *Pseudomonas aeruginosa*: PRIMERS IV. *Clin Infect Dis.* 2019;68:1823–1830.

Girlich D, Oueslati S, Bernabeu S, et al. Evaluation of the BD MAX Check-Points CPO Assay for the detection of carbapenemase producers directly from rectal swabs. *J Mol Diagn.* 2020;22:294–300.

Gu W, Miller S, Chiu CY. Clinical metagenomic next-generation sequencing for pathogen detection. *Annu Rev Pathol.* 2019;14:319–338.

Kozel TR, Burnham-Marusich AR. Point-of-care testing for infectious diseases: past, present, and future. *J Clin Microbiol.* 2017;55:2313–2320.

Kraft CS, Parrott JS, Cornish NE, et al. A laboratory medicine best practices systematic review and meta-analysis of nucleic acid amplification tests (NAATs) and algorithms including NAATs for the diagnosis of *Clostridioides (Clostridium) difficile* in adults. *Clin Microbiol Rev.* 2019;32.

Miller JM, Binnicker MJ, Campbell S, et al. A guide to utilization of the microbiology laboratory for diagnosis of infectious diseases: 2018 update by the Infectious Diseases Society of America and the American Society for Microbiology. *Clin Infect Dis.* 2018;67:813–816.

Miller MB, Tang YW. Basic concepts of microarrays and potential applications in clinical microbiology. *Clin Microbiol Rev.* 2009;22:611–633.

Navarro E, Serrano-Heras G, Castano MJ, Solera J. Real-time PCR detection chemistry. *Clin Chim Acta.* 2015;439:231–250.

Nolte FS. Molecular microbiology. In: Carroll KC, Pfaller MA, Landry ML, et al., eds. *Manual of Clinical Microbiology.* Washington, DC: American Society for Microbiology; 2019.

Ramanan P, Bryson AL, Binnicker MJ, Pritt BS, Patel R. Syndromic panel-based testing in clinical microbiology. *Clin Microbiol Rev.* 2018;31.

Schlaberg R. Microbiome diagnostics. *Clin Chem.* 2020;66:68–76.

Schreckenberger PC, McAdam AJ. Point-counterpoint: large multiplex PCR panels should be first-line tests for detection of respiratory and intestinal pathogens. *J Clin Microbiol.* 2015;53:3110–3115.

Senchyna F, Gaur RL, Gombar S, Truong CY, Schroeder LF, Banaei N. *Clostridium difficile* PCR cycle threshold predicts free toxin. *J Clin Microbiol.* 2017;55:2651–2660.

She RC, Schutzbank TE, Marlowe EM. Non-PCR amplification techniques. In: Tang Y-W, Stratton CW, eds. *Advanced Techniques in Diagnostic Microbiology.* Cham: Springer; 2018.

Tsalik EL, Petzold E, Kreiswirth BN, et al. Advancing diagnostics to address antibacterial resistance: The Diagnostics and Devices Committee of the Antibacterial Resistance Leadership Group. *Clin Infect Dis.* 2017;64:S41–S47.

Wolk D, Mitchell S, Patel R. Principles of molecular microbiology testing methods. *Infect Dis Clin North Am.* 2001;15:1157–1204.

# Reference Information for the Clinical Laboratory

*Khosrow Adeli, Victoria Higgins, and Mary Kathryn Bohn*

## OVERVIEW

Laboratory tests are ubiquitously used in clinical practice to screen, diagnose, and monitor patients for several medical conditions. To correctly interpret laboratory test results, physicians often use reference intervals (i.e., normal ranges) as a health-associated benchmark by which to compare patient test results. If a laboratory test result falls within the reference interval, the patient is considered to be within a healthy range for that particular test. On the other hand, if a laboratory test result falls outside the reference interval, the patient may require follow-up testing to confirm the presence of a particular medical condition. Therefore, population-based reference intervals are a fundamental tool in laboratory medicine to assess health status.

Although the concept and utility of reference intervals appear straightforward, their establishment can be challenging and complex, particularly for the pediatric population. Determining robust reference intervals requires a sufficiently large reference population (120 individuals per partition according to CLSI EP28-A3c) comprised of representative, healthy individuals. Recruiting a healthy pediatric population can pose additional challenges due to parental consent, small blood sample volume, and the large number of healthy subjects required. Due to the profound stages of growth and development throughout childhood and adolescence, these populations often additionally require several age and sex partitions.

Given the complexity of reference interval establishment, it is difficult for most laboratories to undertake this task, and instead, they often use reference intervals established from other laboratories, textbooks, or manufacturer product inserts. Unfortunately, several of these sources often do not use appropriate sampling methods (e.g., sample from patient populations) and/or statistical procedures to establish reference intervals, leading to inaccurate test result interpretation. In addition to the lack of evidence-based reference intervals in clinical use, many laboratories use reference intervals that were established using a different analytical instrument or population. Prior to adopting a reference interval, each clinical laboratory must ensure that the analytical method used to establish the reference interval is comparable with the method used for patient testing. Moreover, it is not yet clear to what extent ethnicity and/or local environmental factors influence reference intervals for specific analytes, and therefore reference intervals developed based on one reference population may not be applicable to a laboratory serving a different population.

It is important to note that despite the application of exclusion criteria to reference populations (i.e., populations used to establish reference intervals), they may still include individuals with subclinical conditions. Therefore, although reference intervals are a useful tool for clinicians, they should not be used as definitive limits of health and disease.

The reference intervals presented in the following tables are for general informational purposes only. Each individual laboratory should generate its own set of reference intervals or validate published reference intervals based on the *CLSI EP28-A3c Guidelines* (Wayne PA. Clinical and Laboratory Standards Institute (CLSI) document *EP28-A3c*. 2010:30–34).

## REFERENCE INTERVAL AND CRITICAL VALUE TABLES

- Table A.1: Pediatric and Adult Reference Intervals for Biochemical Markers (Serum, Plasma, Urine, and Whole Blood)
- Table A.2: Pediatric and Adult Critical Values (Risk Thresholds) for Biochemical Markers

## APPENDIX OUTLINE

Tables A.1 and A.2 include up-to-date reference intervals and critical values obtained from recent studies of pediatric and adult reference values for several biochemical markers. Wherever possible, data from recent, large *a priori* reference interval studies based on healthy populations have been used to update each table with robust reference information. Where no new data were available, reference intervals from the *Tietz Textbook of Clinical Chemistry and Molecular Diagnostics*, 8th edition tables are presented.

Table A.1 provides pediatric and adult reference intervals for several biochemical markers. The majority of pediatric reference intervals presented in Table A.1 are based on recent data published by the Canadian Laboratory Initiative on Pediatric Reference Intervals (CALIPER), a national research project that has established age- and sex-specific pediatric reference intervals based on thousands of healthy community children and adolescents. As noted in the table, the majority of CALIPER reference intervals were determined on Abbott Architect assays. For specific biochemical and endocrine markers, both pediatric and adult reference values were obtained through the recent Canadian Health Measures Survey (CHMS), a study of approximately 12,000 children, adults, and the elderly. CHMS reference intervals were determined based on numerous platforms, including Ortho Clinical Diagnostics and Siemens, as noted in the table. Other reference intervals were adopted primarily from reference tables in *Tietz*

*Textbook of Clinical Chemistry and Molecular Diagnostics,* 8th edition.

Table A.2 provides a table of pediatric and adult critical risk values. Notifying clinical staff of critical results is an important post-analytical process in all acute care clinical laboratories. Data from numerous sources (including Wayne PA. *CLSI Guideline GP47*. Clinical and Laboratory Standards Institute (CLSI). 2015:100) are included in this table of critical risk values to assist laboratories in establishing and updating their critical risk result management policy.

## TABLE A.1   Pediatric and Adult Reference Intervals for Biochemical Markers

| Analyte | Specimen | Condition | Conventional Units | Conversion Factor | SI Units |
|---|---|---|---|---|---|
| α1-Acid glycoprotein | S | | mg/dL | 0.01 | g/L |
| Pediatric values (0–19 | | 0–<6 months | 21–85 | | 0.2–0.9 |
| years) based on Abbott | | 6 months–<5 years | 48–201 | | 0.5–2.0 |
| Architect method | | 5–<19 years | 48–114 | | 0.5–1.1 |
| | | Adult (20–60 years) | 50–120 | | 0.5–1.2 |
| Adrenocorticotropic hormone | P, EDTA | | pg/mL | 0.22 | pmol/L |
| ACTH reference intervals | | Cord | 50–570 | | 11–125 |
| may vary depending on | | Newborn | 10–185 | | 2.2_41 |
| immunoassay methods | | Adult (0800–0900) | <120 | | <26 |
| | | Adult (24 h, supine) | <85 | | <19 |
| Alanine | P | | mg/dL | 112.2 | µmol/L |
| | | Premature, 1 day | 2.44–4.24 | | 274–476 |
| | | Newborn, 1 day | 2.10–3.65 | | 236–410 |
| | | 1–3 months | 1.19–3.71 | | 134–416 |
| | | 2–6 months | 1.58–3.68 | | 177–413 |
| | | 9 months–2 years | 0.88–2.79 | | 99–313 |
| | | 3–10 years | 1.22–2.71 | | 137–305 |
| | | 6–18 years | 1.72–4.85 | | 193–545 |
| | | Adult | 1.87–5.88 | | 210–661 |
| | S | 0–<1 week | 1.56–3.81 | | 175–427 |
| | | 1 week–<19 years | 1.85–5.24 | | 208–588 |
| | U, 24 h | | mg/day | 11.2 | µmol/day |
| | | 10 days–7 weeks | 4.1–9.3 | | 46–104 |
| | | 3–12 years | 9.1–39.2 | | 102–439 |
| | | Adult | 7.9–48.3 | | 88–541 |
| | | | µmol/g creatinine | 0.113 | µmol/mol creatinine |
| | | 0–1 month | 554–2957 | | 62.6–334.1 |
| | | 1–6 months | 613–2874 | | 59.3–324.8 |
| | | 6 months–1 year | 428–2064 | | 48.4–233.2 |
| | | 1–2 years | 389–1497 | | 44.0–169.2 |
| | | 2–3 years | 255–1726 | | 28.8–195.0 |
| Alanine aminotransferase | S | | U/L | 0.017 | µkat/L |
| With pyridoxal phosphate | | 0–<1 year | 5–51 | | 0.08–0.85 |
| Values (0–<3 years) based on Abbott Architect method | | 1–<3 years | 11–30 | | 0.18–0.50 |

## TABLE A.1   Pediatric and Adult Reference Intervals for Biochemical Markers—cont'd

| Analyte | Specimen | Condition | REFERENCE INTERVALS | | |
| --- | --- | --- | --- | --- | --- |
| | | | Conventional Units | Conversion Factor | SI Units |
| Values (3–79 years) based | | 3–5 years | 15–33 | | 0.26–0.56 |
| on Ortho Clinical Diag- | | 6–8 years | 16–37 | | 0.27–0.63 |
| nostics (OCD) VITROS | | 9–11 years | 18–39 | | 0.31–0.66 |
| method | | 12–17 years M | 17–50 | | 0.29–0.85 |
| | | 12–49 years F | 14–41 | | 0.24–0.70 |
| | | 18–49 years M | 18–78 | | 0.31–1.33 |
| | | 50–79 years M | 20–62 | | 0.34–1.05 |
| | | 50–79 years F | 16–44 | | 0.27–0.75 |
| Without pyridoxal phosphate | S | 0–<1 year | 5–33 | | 0.08–0.56 |
| | | 1–<13 years | 9–25 | | 0.15–0.43 |
| | | 13–19 years M | 9–24 | | 0.15–0.41 |
| | | 13–19 years F | 8–22 | | 0.14–0.37 |
| Albumin (BCG) | S | | g/dL | 10 | g/L |
| Values (3–79 years) based | | 0–<15 days | 3.3–4.5 | | 33–45 |
| on OCD VITROS method | | 15 days–<1 year | 2.8–4.7 | | 28–47 |
| | | 1–<3 years | 3.8–4.7 | | 38–47 |
| | | 3–5 years | 3.9–5.0 | | 39–50 |
| | | 6–15 years | 4.1–5.1 | | 41–51 |
| | | 16–29 years M | 4.6–5.3 | | 46–53 |
| | | 16–54 years F | 3.9–5.0 | | 39–50 |
| | | 30–54 years M | 4.4–5.1 | | 44–51 |
| | | 55–79 years | 4.2–5.0 | | 42–50 |
| | U | | mg/L | 1 | mg/L |
| | | 3–5 years | 1.5–21.5 | | 1.5–21.5 |
| | | 6–8 years | 1.5–37.8 | | 1.5–37.8 |
| | | 9–19 years | 1.5–169.6 | | 1.5–169.6 |
| | | 20–29 years | 1.5–74.6 | | 1.5–74.6 |
| | | 30–39 years | 1.5–36.8 | | 1.5–36.8 |
| | | 40–79 years | 1.5–47.2 | | 1.5–47.2 |
| Albumin-creatinine ratio | | | mg/mmol | | mg/g creatinine |
| (NKDEP guidelines) | M | | <2.5 | | <22 |
| | F | | <3.5 | | <30 |
| Aldosterone | S | | ng/dL | 0.0277 | nmol/L |
| | | Cord blood | 40–200 | | 1.11–5.54 |
| | | Premature infants | 19–141 | | 0.53–3.91 |
| Full-term infants | | | | | |
| | | 3 days | 7–184 | | 0.19–5.10 |
| | | 1 week | 5–175 | | 0.03–4.85 |
| | | 1–12 months | 5–90 | | 0.14–2.49 |
| | | 1–2 years | 7–54 | | 0.19–1.50 |
| | | 2–10 years (supine) | 3–35 | | 0.08–0.97 |
| | | 2–10 years (upright) | 5–80 | | 0.14–2.22 |
| | | 10–15 years (supine) | 2–22 | | 0.06–0.61 |
| | | 10–15 years (upright) | 4–48 | | 0.11–1.33 |
| Adults | | | | | |
| | | (supine) | 3–16 | | 0.08–0.44 |
| | | (upright) | 7–30 | | 0.19–0.83 |
| | U, 24 h | | µg/day | | µg/g creatinine |
| | | Newborns (1–3 days) | 0.5–5 | 2.77 | 1–14 |
| | | Prepubertal children | | | |
| | | 4–10 years | 1–8 | | 3–22 |
| | | Adults | 3–19 | | 8–51 |

*Continued*

## TABLE A.1  Pediatric and Adult Reference Intervals for Biochemical Markers—cont'd

| Analyte | Specimen | Condition | REFERENCE INTERVALS Conventional Units | Conversion Factor | SI Units |
|---|---|---|---|---|---|
| Aluminum | S, P | | µg/L | 0.0371 | µmol/L |
| | | | <5.51 | | <0.2 |
| | | Patients on hemodialysis | 20–550 | | 0.74–20.4 |
| | | All medication | <30 | | <1.11 |
| | U | | 5–30 | | 0.19–1.11 |
| Amylase | S | | U/L | 0.017 | µkat/L |
| Values (0≤19 years) based | | 0–14 days | 3–10 | | 0.05–0.17 |
| on Abbott Architect | | 15 days–<13 weeks | 2–22 | | 0.03–0.37 |
| method | | 13 weeks–<1 year | 3–50 | | 0.05–0.83 |
| | | 1–<19 years | 25–101 | | 0.42–1.68 |
| IFCC, 37°C | | Adult | 31–107 | | 0.52–1.78 |
| Androgen index, free (FAI) | | | | | % |
| | | 0–<1 year F | | | 0.04–1.32 |
| | | 1–<9 years F | | | 0.04–1.32 |
| | | 9–<14 years F | | | 0.12–2.63 |
| | | 14–19 years F | | | 0.59–6.50 |
| | | 0–<1 year M | | | 0.02–32.72 |
| | | 1–<9 years M | | | 0.03–0.60 |
| | | 9–<14 years M | | | 0.15–34.68 |
| | | 14–<19 years M | | | 3.58–83.30 |
| | | NOTE: FAI should not be used in men where testosterone levels exceed sex hormone binding globulin (SHBG) binding capacity | | | |
| Androstenedione (LC-MS/MS) | S | | ng/L | | |
| | | 6–24 months M | 25–150 | | |
| | | 2–3 years M | <110 | | |
| | | 4–5 years M | 23–170 | | |
| | | 6–7 years M | 10–290 | | |
| | | 7–9 years M | 30–300 | | |
| | | 10–11 years M | 70–390 | | |
| | | 12–13 years M | 100–640 | | |
| | | 14–15 years M | 180–940 | | |
| | | 16–17 years M | 300–1130 | | |
| | | 18–40 years M | 330–1340 | | |
| | | 40–67 years M | 230–890 | | |
| | | 6–24 months F | <150 | | |
| | | 2–3 years F | <160 | | |
| | | 4–5 years F | 20–210 | | |
| | | 6–7 years F | 20–280 | | |
| | | 7–9 years F | 40–420 | | |
| | | 10–11 years F | 90–1230 | | |
| | | 12–13 years F | 240–1730 | | |
| | | 14–15 years F | 390–2000 | | |
| | | 16–17 years F | 350–2120 | | |
| | | Menstrual Status | | | |
| | | Before menarche | 48–1080 | | |
| | | After menarche, ≤18 years | 330–2130 | | |
| | | Premenopausal, >18 years | 260–2140 | | |
| | | Postmenopausal | 130–820 | | |
| Vasopressin (antidiuretic hormone ADH) | P, EDTA | mOsm/kg | ng/L | 0.926 | pmol/L |
| | | 270–280 | <1.5 | | <1.4 |

## TABLE A.1   Pediatric and Adult Reference Intervals for Biochemical Markers—cont'd

| Analyte | Specimen | Condition | REFERENCE INTERVALS Conventional Units | Conversion Factor | SI Units |
|---|---|---|---|---|---|
| | | 280–285 | <2.5 | | <2.3 |
| | | 285–290 | 1–5 | | 0.9–4.6 |
| | | 290–294 | 2–7 | | 1.9–6.5 |
| | | 295–300 | 4–12 | | 3.7–11.1 |
| Antistreptolysin-O (ASO) | S | | IU/mL | 1 | kIU/L |
| Values (0–<19 years) | | 0–<6 months | 0–0 | | 0–0 |
| based on Abbott | | 6 months–<1 year | 0–30 | | 0–30 |
| Architect method | | 1–<6 years | 0–104 | | 0–104 |
| | | 6–<19 years | 0–331 | | 0–331 |
| | | Adult | <20–364 | | <20–364 |
| Antithyroglobulin (Anti-Tg) | S | | IU/mL | 1 | kIU/L |
| Values based on Abbott | | 0–<19 years | 0.4–17.7 | | 0.4–17.7 |
| Architect method | | | | | |
| α1-Antitrypsin | S | | mg/dL | 0.01 | g/L |
| Values (0–<19 years) based | | 0–<19 years | 110–181 | | 1.1–1.8 |
| on Abbott Architect | | Adult (20–60 years) | 90–200 | | 0.9–2.0 |
| method | | | | | |
| Apolipoprotein AI | S | | mg/dL | 0.01 | g/L |
| Values (0–<6 years) | | 0–14 days F | 71–97 | | 0.7–1.0 |
| based on Abbott | | 0–14 days M | 62–91 | | 0.6–0.9 |
| Architect method | | 15 days–<1 year | 53–175 | | 0.5–1.8 |
| | | 1–<6 years | 80–164 | | 0.8–1.6 |
| Values (6–79 years) based | | 6–15 years | 100–180 | | 1.0–1.8 |
| on OCD VITROS method | | 16–39 years M | 80–170 | | 0.8–1.7 |
| | | 16–39 years F | 100–200 | | 1.0–2.0 |
| | | 40–79 years M | 120–200 | | 1.2–2.0 |
| | | 40–79 years F | 110–230 | | 1.1–2.3 |
| Apolipoprotein B-100 | S | | mg/dL | 0.01 | g/L |
| Values (0–<6 years) based | | 0–14 days | 9–67 | | 0.1–0.7 |
| on Abbott Architect | | 15 days–<1 year | 19–123 | | 0.2–1.2 |
| method | | 1–<6 years | 41–93 | | 0.4–0.9 |
| Values (6–79 years) based | | 6–13 years | 50–100 | | 0.5–1.0 |
| on OCD VITROS method | | 14–29 years | 40–110 | | 0.4–1.1 |
| | | 30–79 years | 60–140 | | 0.6–1.4 |
| Arginine | P | | mg/dL | 57.4 | µmol/L |
| | | Premature, 1 day | 0.17–1.57 | | 10–90 |
| | | Newborn, 1 day | 0.38–1.53 | | 22–88 |
| | | 1–3 months | 0.38–1.30 | | 22–74 |
| | | 2–6 months | 0.98–2.47 | | 56–142 |
| | | 9 months–2 years | 0.19–1.13 | | 11–65 |
| | | 3–10 years | 0.40–1.50 | | 23–86 |
| | | 6–18 years | 0.77–2.26 | | 44–130 |
| | | Adult | 0.37–2.40 | | 21–138 |
| | U, 24 h | | mg/day | 5.74 | µmol/day |
| | | 10 days–7 weeks | <1.2 | | <7 |
| | | 3–12 years | <5.1 | | <29 |
| | | Adult | <50.2 | | <288 |
| | | | mg/g creatinine | 0.65 | mmol/mol creatinine |
| | | Adult | 0–4 | | 0–2.7 |
| Arsenic | WB (Hep) | | µg/L | 0.0113 | µmol/L |
| | | Not exposed | 2–23 | | 0.03–0.31 |
| | | Chronic poisoning | 100–500 | | 1.33–6.65 |
| | | Acute poisoning | 600–9300 | | 7.98–124 |

*Continued*

## TABLE A.1   Pediatric and Adult Reference Intervals for Biochemical Markers—cont'd

| Analyte | Specimen | Condition | Conventional Units | Conversion Factor | SI Units |
|---|---|---|---|---|---|
| Ascorbic acid (see vitamin C) | | | | | |
| Asparagine | P | | mg/dL | 75.7 | µmol/L |
| | | 1–3 months | 0.08–0.44 | | 6–33 |
| | | 3 months–6 years | 0.95–1.90 | | 72–144 |
| | | 6–18 years | 0.42–0.82 | | 32–62 |
| | | Adult | 0.40–0.91 | | 30–69 |
| | S | 0–<19 years | 0.50–1.20 | | 38–91 |
| | U, 24 h | | mg/day | 7.57 | µmol/day |
| | | Adult | 4.5–13.2 | | 34–100 |
| | | | mg/g creatinine | 0.86 | mmol/mol creatinine |
| | | Adult | 2–10 | | 1.8–8.6 |
| Aspartate aminotransferase | S | | U/L | 0.017 | µkat/L |
| with pyridoxal phosphate | | 0–14 days | 23–186 | | 0.38–3.10 |
| Values (0–<3 years) based | | 15 days–<1 year | 23–83 | | 0.38–1.38 |
| on Abbott Architect method | | 1–<3 years | 26–55 | | 0.43–0.92 |
| Values (3–79 years) based | | 3–5 years | 28–52 | | 0.48–0.88 |
| on OCD VITROS method | | 6–11 years M | 25–47 | | 0.43–0.80 |
| | | 6–11 years F | 23–44 | | 0.39–0.75 |
| | | 12–17 years M | 18–36 | | 0.31–0.61 |
| | | 12–19 years F | 15–34 | | 0.26–0.58 |
| | | 18–54 years M | 18–54 | | 0.31–0.92 |
| | | 20–54 years F | 18–34 | | 0.31–0.58 |
| | | 55–79 years | 18–39 | | 0.31–0.66 |
| Without pyridoxal phosphate | S | 0–14 days | 32–162 | | 0.54–2.75 |
| Values (0–<19 years) | | 15 days–<1 year | 20–67 | | 0.34–1.14 |
| based on Abbott | | 1–<7 years | 21–44 | | 0.36–0.75 |
| Architect method | | 7–<12 years | 18–36 | | 0.31–0.61 |
| | | 12–19 years M | 14–35 | | 0.24–0.60 |
| | | 12–19 years F | 13–26 | | 0.22–0.44 |
| Aspartic acid | P | | mg/dL | 75.1 | µmol/L |
| | | Premature, 1 day | 0–0.39 | | 0–30 |
| | | Newborn, 1 day | <0.21 | | <16 |
| | | 1–3 months | 0–0.15 | | 0–8 |
| | | 9 months–2 years | <0.12 | | <9 |
| | | 19 months–10 years | <0.27 | | <20 |
| | | 6–18 years | <0.19 | | <14 |
| | | Adult | <0.32 | | <24 |
| | S | 0–< 2 week | 0.25–1.61 | | 19–121 |
| | | 2 week–<19 years | 0.27–0.56 | | 20–42 |
| | U, 24 h | | mg/day | 7.51 | µmol/day |
| | | 3–12 years | <5.1 | | <38 |
| | | Adult | <26.2 | | <197 |
| | | | mg/g creatinine | 0.85 | mmol/mol creatinine |
| | | Adult | 0–4 | | 0.1–3.7 |
| Bilirubin, direct (conjugated) | S | | mg/dL | 17.1 | µmol/L |
| Values (0–<19 years) | | 0–14 days | 0.33–0.71 | | 5.7–12.1 |
| based on Abbott | | 15 days–<1 year | 0.05–0.30 | | 0.8–5.2 |
| Architect method | | 1–<9 years | 0.05–0.20 | | 0.8–3.4 |
| | | 9–<13 years | 0.05–0.29 | | 0.8–5.0 |
| | | 13–<19 years M | 0.11–0.42 | | 1.9–7.1 |
| | | 13–<19 years F | 0.10–0.39 | | 1.7–6.7 |
| | | Adult | 0.0–0.2 | | 0.0–3.4 |

## TABLE A.1   Pediatric and Adult Reference Intervals for Biochemical Markers—cont'd

| Analyte | Specimen | Condition | REFERENCE INTERVALS Conventional Units | Conversion Factor | SI Units |
|---|---|---|---|---|---|
| Bilirubin, total | S | | mg/dL | 17.1 | µmol/L |
| Values (0–<3 years) | | 0–14 days | 0.19–16.6 | | 3.3–283.8 |
| based on Abbott | | 15 days–<1 year | 0.05–0.68 | | 0.8–11.7 |
| Architect method | | 1–<3 years | 0.05–0.40 | | 0.8–6.8 |
| Values (3–79 years) based | | 3–5 years | 0.1–0.5 | | 1.0–8.8 |
| on OCD VITROS method | | | | | |
| | | 6–15 years | 0.1–0.9 | | 1.0–15.6 |
| | | 16–48 years M | 0.2–1.1 | | 3.0–18 |
| | | 16–48 years F | 0.1–0.9 | | 1.0–16 |
| | | 49–79 years M | 0.1–1.2 | | 2.0–19.9 |
| | | 49–79 years F | 0.1–1.0 | | 1.0–16.6 |
| | U | | Negative | | Negative |
| Biotin | WB | | | | nmol/L |
| | | Healthy | | | 0.5–2.20 |
| | | Deficiency | | | <0.5 |
| Cadmium | WB (Hep) | | µg/L | 8.897 | nmol/L |
| | | Nonsmokers | 0.3–1.2 | | 2.7–10.7 |
| | | Smokers | 0.6–3.9 | | 5.3–34.7 |
| | U, 24 h | | µg/L | | µmol/L |
| | | Toxic range | 100–3000 | | 0.9–26.7 |
| Calcitonin | S, P | | pg/mL | 1 | ng/L |
| | | M | <8.8 | | <8.8 |
| | | F | <5.8 | | <5.8 |
| | | Athyroidal | <0.5 | | <0.5 |
| Calcium, ionized (free) | S, P (Hep) | | mg/dL | 0.25 | mmol/L |
| | | Adults | 4.6–5.3 | | 1.15–1.33 |
| Values based on Radio-meter ABL90 Plus | WB, venous | 0–<19 years | 1.19–1.33 | | 1.19–1.33 |
| Calcium, total | S, P (Hep) | | mg/dL | 0.25 | mmol/L |
| Values (0–<3 years) based | | 0–<1 year | 8.5–11.0 | | 2.13–2.74 |
| on Abbott Architect | | 1–<3 years | 9.2–10.5 | | 2.29–2.63 |
| method | | | | | |
| Values (3–79 years) based | | 3–5 years | 9.4–10.6 | | 2.35–2.64 |
| on OCD VITROS method | | 6–15 years | 9.3–10.5 | | 2.33–2.62 |
| | | 16–19 | 9.2–10.4 | | 2.3–2.60 |
| | | 20–39 years M | 9.1–10.4 | | 2.28–2.60 |
| | | 20–39 years F | 9.0–10.1 | | 2.24–2.53 |
| | | 40–79 years | 9.0–10.2 | | 2.24–2.56 |
| β-Carotene HPLC | S | | µg/dL | 0.0186 | µmol/L |
| | | | 10–85 | | 0.19–1.58 |
| Cancer antigen 15–3 | S | | U/mL | 1 | kU/L |
| Values (0–<19 years) | | 0–<1 week | 3.4–24 | | 3.4–24 |
| based on Abbott | | 1 week–<1 year | 4.9–33 | | 4.9–33 |
| Architect method | | 1–<19 years | 3.9–21 | | 3.9–21 |
| | | Adult | <30 | | <30 |
| Cancer antigen 19–9 | S | | U/mL | 1 | kU/L |
| Values (0–<19 years) | | 0–<1 year | <2.0–64 | | <2.0–64 |
| based on Abbott | | 1–<19 years | <2.0–41 | | <2.0–41 |
| Architect method | | Adult | <37 | | <37 |
| Cancer antigen 125 | S | | U/mL | 1 | kU/L |
| Values (0–<19 years) | | 0–<4 months | 2.4–22 | | 2.4–22 |
| based on Abbott | | 4 months–<5 years | 7.7–33 | | 7.7–33 |
| Architect method | | 5–<11 years | 4.7–30 | | 4.7–30 |
| | | 11–<19 years | 5.4–28 | | 5.4–28 |
| | | Adult | <35 | | <35 |

*Continued*

## TABLE A.1    Pediatric and Adult Reference Intervals for Biochemical Markers—cont'd

| Analyte | Specimen | Condition | REFERENCE INTERVALS | | |
|---|---|---|---|---|---|
| | | | Conventional Units | Conversion Factor | SI Units |
| Carbon dioxide, partial pressure $PCO_2$ | WB, arterial (Hep) | | mm Hg | 0.133 | kPa |
| | | Newborn | 27–40 | | 3.59–5.32 |
| | | Infant | 27–41 | | 3.59–5.45 |
| | | Adult M | 35–48 | | 4.66–6.38 |
| | | Adult F | 32–45 | | 4.26–5.99 |
| Carbon dioxide, total ($tCO_2$) | | | mEq/L | 1 | mmol/L |
| Values (0–<6 years) based on Abbott Architect method | | 0–14 days | 5–20 | | 5–20 |
| | | 15 days–<1 year | 10–24 | | 10–24 |
| | | 1–<5 years | 14–24 | | 14–24 |
| | | 5–<6 years | 17–26 | | 17–26 |
| Values (6–79 years) based on OCD VITROS method | 6–79 years | | 19–26 | | 19–26 |
| | WB | | | | |
| | Arterial | | 19–24 | | 19–24 |
| | Venous | | 22–26 | | 22–26 |
| Carcinoembryonic antigen (CEA) | S | | ng/mL | 1 | µg/L |
| Pediatric values based on Abbott Architect values | | 0–<1 week | 8.1–62 | | 8.1–62 |
| | | 1 week–<2 years | <0.5–4.7 | | <0.5–4.7 |
| | | 2–<19 years | <0.5–2.6 | | <0.5–2.6 |
| | | Adult, nonsmokers | <3 | | <3 |
| | | Adult, smokers | <5 | | <5 |
| Catecholamines | | | | | |
| Epinephrine | P | Adults | pg/mL | 5.46 | pmol/L |
| | | Supine (30 min) | <50 | | <273 |
| | | Sitting (15 min) | <60 | | <328 |
| | | Standing (30 min) | <90 | | <491 |
| Norepinephrine | P | Adults | pg/mL | 5.91 | pmol/L |
| | | Supine (30 min) | 110–410 | | 650–2423 |
| | | Sitting (15 min) | 120–680 | | 709–4019 |
| | | Standing (30 min) | 125–700 | | 739–4137 |
| Dopamine | P | Adults | pg/mL | 6.53 | pmol/L |
| | | Supine (30 min) | <87 | | <475 |
| | | Sitting (15 min) | <87 | | <475 |
| | | Standing (30 min) | <87 | | <475 |
| Ceruloplasmin | P | | mg/L | 0.001 | g/L |
| | | Cord (term) | 50–330 | | 0.05–0.33 |
| Pediatric values (0–<19 years) based on Abbott Architect method | | 0–<2 months | 74–237 | | 0.07–0.24 |
| | | 2–<6 months | 135–329 | | 0.13–0.33 |
| | | 6 months–<1 year | 137–389 | | 0.14–0.39 |
| | | 1–<8 years | 217–433 | | 0.22–0.43 |
| | | 8–<14 years | 205–402 | | 0.21–0.40 |
| | | 14–<19 years M | 170–348 | | 0.17–0.35 |
| | | 14–<19 years F | 208–432 | | 0.21–0.43 |
| | | Adult M | 220–400 | | 0.22–0.40 |
| | | Adult F (no contraceptive) | 250–600 | | 0.25–0.60 |
| | | Adult F (contraceptives [estrogen]) | 270–660 | | 0.27–0.66 |
| | | Adult F (pregnant) | 300–1200 | | 0.3–1.20 |
| | | | mg/dL | 0.01 | g/L |
| | | Adult (20–60 years) | 20–60 | | 0.2–0.6 |
| Chloride (Cl) | S, P | | mEq/L | 1 | mmol/L |
| Values (0–2 years) based on Siemens EXL method | | 0–2 years | 102–111 | | 102–111 |

## TABLE A.1    Pediatric and Adult Reference Intervals for Biochemical Markers—cont'd

| Analyte | Specimen | Condition | REFERENCE INTERVALS Conventional Units | Conversion Factor | SI Units |
|---|---|---|---|---|---|
| Values (3–79 years) based on OCD VITROS method | | 3–5 years | 100–107 | | 100–107 |
| | | 6–11 years | 101–107 | | 101–107 |
| | | 12–29 years M | 101–106 | | 101–106 |
| | | 12–29 years F | 100–107 | | 100–107 |
| | | 30–79 years | 102–108 | | 102–108 |
| | U, 24 h | | mEq/day | 1 | mmol/day |
| | | Infant | 2–10 | | 2–10 |
| | | Child <6 years | 15–40 | | 15–40 |
| | | 6–10 years M | 36–110 | | 36–110 |
| | | 6–10 years F | 18–74 | | 18–74 |
| | | 10–14 years M | 64–176 | | 64–176 |
| | | 10–14 years F | 36–173 | | 36–173 |
| | | Adult | 110–250 | | 110–250 |
| | | >60 years | 95–195 | | 95–195 |
| Values based on Radiometer ABL90 Plus | WB | 0–<1 year | 96–108 | | 96–108 |
| | | 1–<5 years | 101–111 | | 101–111 |
| | | 5–<19 years | 101–107 | | 101–107 |
| Cholesterol *Reference Limits* | S | | mg/dL | 0.0259 | mmol/L |
| Values (0–<3 years) based on Abbott Architect method | | 0–14 days M | 42–109 | | 1.09–2.82 |
| | | 0–14 days F | 46–125 | | 1.19–3.24 |
| | | 15 days–<1 year | 64–237 | | 1.66–6.14 |
| | | 1–<3 years | 112–208 | | 2.90–5.39 |
| Values (3–79 years) based on OCD VITROS method | | 3–5 years | 120–216 | | 3.11–5.59 |
| | | 6–15 years | 116–205 | | 3.00–5.31 |
| | | 16–19 years | 100–182 | | 2.59–4.71 |
| | | 20–29 years | 116–228 | | 3.00–5.91 |
| | | 30–39 years | 147–266 | | 3.81–6.89 |
| | | 40–79 years | 139–274 | | 3.60–7.10 |

NOTE: See more recent guidelines for recommendations on reducing the risk of atherosclerotic disease through cholesterol management (2018 AHA/ACC/AACVPR/AAPA/ABC/ACPM/ADA/AGS/APhA/ASPC/NLA/PCNA Guideline on the Management of Blood Cholesterol).

| *Clinical Decision Limits* | | Coronary heart disease risk, child | | | |
|---|---|---|---|---|---|
| | | Desirable | <170 | | <4.40 |
| | | Borderline high | 170–199 | | 4.40–5.15 |
| | | High | >200 | | >5.15 |
| | | Coronary heart disease risk, adult | | | |
| | | Desirable | <200 | | <5.18 |
| | | Borderline high | 200–239 | | 5.18–6.19 |
| | | High | >239 | | >6.19 |

NOTE: Cholesterol should not be used on its own for risk prediction.

| Cholinesterase (37°C) | S | | U/L | 0.017 | μkat/L |
|---|---|---|---|---|---|
| Pediatric values (0–<19 years) based on Abbott Architect method | | 0–14 days | 4421–9722 | | 75–165 |
| | | 15 days–<1 year | 5182–16,027 | | 88–272 |
| | | 1–<17 years | 7769–15,206 | | 132–259 |
| | | 17–<19 years, F | 7511–10,904 | | 128–185 |
| | | 17–<19 years, M | 8186–12,639 | | 139–215 |
| | | M | 40–78 | | 0.68–1.33 |
| | | F | 33–76 | | 0.56–1.29 |
| Cholinesterase activity with dibucaine inhibitor (ChEDi) | S | | U/L | 0.017 | μkat/L |
| | | 0–<1 month | 797–2,478 | | 13–41 |

*Continued*

## TABLE A.1    Pediatric and Adult Reference Intervals for Biochemical Markers—cont'd

| Analyte | Specimen | Condition | REFERENCE INTERVALS Conventional Units | Conversion Factor | SI Units |
|---|---|---|---|---|---|
| Pediatric values (0–<19 years) based on Abbott Architect method | | 1 month–<19 years | 1523–3280 | | 25–55 |
| Chorionic gonadotropin intact molecule | S | | mIU/mL | 1 | IU/L |
| | | Male and non-pregnant female | <5.0 | | <5.0 |
| | | Female, pregnancy (weeks of gestation) | | | |
| | | 4 weeks | 5–100 | | 5–100 |
| | | 5 weeks | 200–3000 | | 200–3000 |
| | | 6 weeks | 10,000–80,000 | | 10,000–80,000 |
| | | 7–14 weeks | 90,000–500,000 | | 90,000–500,000 |
| | | 15–26 weeks | 5000–80,000 | | 5000–80,000 |
| | | 27–40 weeks | 3000–15,000 | | 3000–15,000 |
| | | | NOTE: Values based on the Second International Standard for hCG | | |
| | | Trophoblastic disease | >100,000 | | >100,000 |
| | U | | Negative | | Negative |
| | | | One half of pregnancies are detected on the first day of the missed menstrual period | | One half of pregnancies are detected on the first day of the missed menstrual period |
| Chromium | | | µg/L | 19.23 | nmol/L |
| | WB (Hep) | | 0.7–28.0 | | 14–538 |
| | S | | 0.1–0.2 | | 2–3 |
| | | | µg/day | 19.23 | nmol/day |
| | U, 24 h | | 0.1–2.0 | | 1.9–38.4 |
| | | | µg/L | 19.23 | nmol/L |
| | RBC | | 20–36 | | 384–692 |
| Citric acid | U | | | | mmol/mol creatinine |
| | | 0–1 month | | | <1,046 |
| | | 1–6 months | | | 104–268 |
| | | 6 months–5 years | | | 0–656 |
| | | >5 years | | | 87–639 |
| Cobalt | | | µg/L | 16.97 | nmol/L |
| | S | | 0.11–0.45 | | 1.9–7.6 |
| | U | | 1–2 | | 17.0–34.0 |
| | | | µg/kg | | nmol/kg |
| | RBC | | 16–46 | | 272–781 |
| Complement C3 | S | | mg/dL | 0.01 | g/L |
| Values (0–<19 years) | | 0–14 days | 50–121 | | 0.5–1.2 |
| based on Abbott | | 15 days–<1 year | 51–160 | | 0.5–1.6 |
| Architect method | | 1–<19 years | 83–152 | | 0.8–1.5 |
| | | Adult (20–60 years) | 90–180 | | 0.9–1.8 |
| Complement C4 | S | | mg/dL | 0.01 | g/L |
| Values (0–<19 years) | | 0–<1 year | 7–30 | | 0.1–0.3 |
| based on Abbott | | 1–<19 years | 13–37 | | 0.1–0.4 |
| Architect method | | Adult (20–60 years) | 10–40 | | 0.1–0.4 |
| Copper | S | | µg/dL | 0.157 | µmol/L |

## TABLE A.1   Pediatric and Adult Reference Intervals for Biochemical Markers—cont'd

| Analyte | Specimen | Condition | REFERENCE INTERVALS Conventional Units | Conversion Factor | SI Units |
|---|---|---|---|---|---|
| | | Birth–6 months | 20–70 | | 3.1–11.0 |
| | | Deficiency | <30 | | <5 |
| | | 6 years | 90–190 | | 14.1–29.8 |
| | | 12 years | 80–160 | | 12.6–25.1 |
| | | Adult M | 70–140 | | 11.0–22.0 |
| | | Adult F | 80–155 | | 12.6–24.3 |
| | | Deficiency | 50 | | 8 |
| | | Pregnancy, at term | 118–302 | | 18.5–47.4 |
| | | Black population | Black pop. 8–12% higher | | Black pop. 8–12% higher |
| | U, 24 h | | µg/24 h | 0.0157 | µmol/24 h |
| | | Adults | <60 | | <1.0 |
| | | Wilson's disease | >200 | | >3 |
| Corticosterone | S | | µg/dL | 28.84 | nmol/L |
| Pediatric values based on LC-MS/MS | | 0–<1 month | 0.00–0.69 | | 0.14–20.0 |
| | | 1 month–<1 year | 0.01–0.53 | | 0.28–15.4 |
| | | 1–<4 years | 0.02–0.13 | | 0.62–3.72 |
| | | 4–<6 years | 0.03–0.14 | | 0.95–4.11 |
| | | 6–<15 years | 0.02–0.32 | | 0.44–9.19 |
| | | 15–<19 years | 0.03–0.53 | | 0.85–15.24 |
| Cortisol, free | S | | µg/dL | 27.6 | nmol/L |
| | | 0800 h | 0.6–1.6 | | 17–44 |
| | | 1600 h | 0.2–0.9 | | 6–25 |
| | U, 24 h | | µg/day | 2.76 | nmol/day |
| | | 1–10 years | 2–27 | | 6–74 |
| | | 2–11 years | 1–21 | | 3–58 |
| | | 11–20 years | 5–55 | | 14–152 |
| | | 12–16 years | 2–38 | | 6–105 |
| | | Adult | µg/day | 2.76 | nmol/day |
| | | Extracted | 20–90 | | 55–248 |
| | | Unextracted (HPLC) | 75–270 | | 207–745 |
| Cortisol, total | S | | µg/dL | 27.6 | nmol/L |
| | | Cord blood | 5–17 | | 138–469 |
| Pediatric values (2 days–<19 years) based on Abbott Architect method | | 2–<15 days | 1–12 | | 13–340 |
| | | 15 days–<1 year | 1–17 | | 14–458 |
| | | 1–<9 years | 2–11 | | 48–297 |
| | | 9–<14 years | 2–13 | | 60–349 |
| | | 14–<17 years | 3–16 | | 77–453 |
| | | 17–<19 years | 4–18 | | 97–506 |
| | | | µg/dL | 27.6 | nmol/L |
| | | Child (1–16 years), 08:00 h | 3–21 | | 83–580 |
| | | Adult | | | |
| | | 08:00 h | 5–23 | | 138–635 |
| | | 16:00 h | 3–16 | | 83–441 |
| | | 20:00 h | <50% of 08:00 h values | | <50% of 08:00 h values |
| *For LC-MSMS pediatric reference intervals, see: Clin Biochem 2013;46:642–651* | | | | | |
| C-reactive protein (CRP) high sensitivity | S | | mg/L | 1 | mg/L |
| Values (0–<3 years) based on Abbott Architect method | | 0–14 days | 0.3–6.1 | | 0.3–6.1 |
| | | 15 days–<3 years | 0.1–1.0 | | 0.1–1.0 |

*Continued*

## TABLE A.1    Pediatric and Adult Reference Intervals for Biochemical Markers—cont'd

| Analyte | Specimen | Condition | Conventional Units | Conversion Factor | SI Units |
|---|---|---|---|---|---|
| Values (3–79 years) based | | 3–5 years | 0.1–2.4 | | 0.1–2.4 |
| on OCD VITROS method | | 6–11 years | 0.1–5.9 | | 0.1–5.9 |
| | | 12–13 years | 0.1–1.9 | | 0.1–1.9 |
| | | 14–16 years | 0.1–2.9 | | 0.1–2.9 |
| | | 17–39 years M | 0.1–6.0 | | 0.1–6.0 |
| | | 17–39 years F | 0.1–12.1 | | 0.1–12.1 |
| | | 40–79 years | 0.1–8.8 | | 0.1–8.8 |
| | | American M | 0.3–8.6 | | 0.3–8.6 |
| | | White American M | 0.2–12.3 | | 0.2–12.3 |
| | | African American M | 0.1–8.2 | | 0.1–8.2 |
| | | Mexican American M | 0.2–6.3 | | 0.2–6.3 |
| | | European M | 0.3–8.6 | | 0.3–8.6 |
| | | Japanese M | <7.8 | | <7.8 |
| | | American F | 0.2–9.1 | | 0.2–9.1 |
| | | European F | 0.3–8.8 | | 0.3–8.8 |
| Creatine kinase (CK) | S | | U/L | 0.017 | μkat/L |
| Pediatric reference values | | 0–<13 years | 68–293 | | 1.16–4.98 |
| (0–<19 years) based on | | 13–<19 years, F | 48–200 | | 0.82–3.40 |
| Siemens ADVIA method | | 13–<19 years, M | 80–354 | | 1.36–6.02 |
| IFCC, 37°C | | M | 46–171 | | 0.78–2.90 |
| | | F | 34–145 | | 0.58–2.47 |
| CK isoenzymes | S | Fraction 2 (MB) | <5.0 μg/L | 1 | <5.0 μg/L |
| | | Relative index MB/total | <3.9% | 0.01 | <0.039 Fractional activity |
| Creatinine | | | mg/dL | 88.4 | μmol/L |
| Enzymatic | S | 0–14 days | 0.32–0.92 | | 28–81 |
| Values (0–<3 years) based | | 15 days–<2 years | 0.10–0.36 | | 9–32 |
| on Abbott Architect method | | 2–<3 years | 0.20–0.43 | | 18–38 |
| Values (3–79 years) based | | 3–5 years | 0.31–0.51 | | 28–45 |
| on OCD VITROS method | | 6–7 years | 0.36–0.56 | | 32–49 |
| | | 8–9 years | 0.37–0.63 | | 32–56 |
| | | 10–11 years | 0.43–0.68 | | 38–60 |
| | | 12–15 years M | 0.47–0.91 | | 42–81 |
| | | 12–16 years F | 0.48–0.84 | | 42–74 |
| | | 16–79 years M | 0.71–1.16 | | 63–102 |
| | | 17–79 years F | 0.56–0.96 | | 49–85 |
| | U | | mg/dL | 0.0884 | mmol/L |
| Values (3–79 years) based | | 3–5 years | 14.71–151.58 | | 1–13 |
| on OCD VITROS method | | 6–11 years | 13.57–195.70 | | 1–17 |
| | | 12–13 years | 21.49–214.93 | | 2–19 |
| | | 14–29 years | 19.23–305.43 | | 2–27 |
| | | 30–79 years M | 14.71–294.12 | | 1–26 |
| | | 30–79 years F | 12.44–229.64 | | 1–20 |
| Jaffe | | | mg/dL | 88.4 | μmol/L |
| | S | Cord | 0.60–1.20 | | 53–106 |
| | | 0–14 days | 0.42–1.05 | | 37–93 |
| | | 15 days–<1 year | 0.31–0.53 | | 28–47 |
| | | 1–<4 years | 0.39–0.55 | | 34–48 |
| | | 4–<7 years | 0.44–0.65 | | 39–57 |
| | | 7–<12 years | 0.52–0.69 | | 46–61 |
| | | 12–<15 years | 0.57–0.80 | | 50–71 |
| | | 15–<17 years M | 0.65–1.04 | | 58–92 |
| | | 15–<17 years F | 0.59–0.86 | | 52–76 |
| | | 17–<19 years M | 0.69–1.10 | | 61–97 |
| | | 17–<19 years F | 0.60–0.88 | | 53–78 |
| | | 18–60 years M | 0.90–1.30 | | 80–115 |

## TABLE A.1  Pediatric and Adult Reference Intervals for Biochemical Markers—cont'd

| Analyte | Specimen | Condition | REFERENCE INTERVALS Conventional Units | Conversion Factor | SI Units |
|---|---|---|---|---|---|
| | | 18–60 years F | 0.60–1.10 | | 53–97 |
| | | 60–90 years M | 0.80–1.30 | | 71–115 |
| | | 60–90 years F | 0.60–1.20 | | 53–106 |
| | | >90 years M | 1.00–1.70 | | 88–150 |
| | | >90 years F | 0.60–1.30 | | 53–115 |
| Jaffe, manual | U, 24 h | | mg/kg per day | 8.84 | µmol/kg per day |
| | | Infant | 8–20 | | 71–177 |
| | | Child | 8–22 | | 71–194 |
| | | Adolescent | 8–30 | | 71–265 |
| | | Adult M | 14–26 | | 124–230 |
| | | Adult F | 11–20 | | 97–177 |
| Creatinine clearance (see Glomerular filtration rate) | | | | | |
| C-Telopeptide | S | | ng/L | 1 | ng/L |
| Values (0–<19 years) based on Abbott Architect method | 0–<1 year | 210–4390 | | 210–4390 | |
| | 1–<6 years | 350–4480 | | 350–4480 | |
| | 6–<19 years | 780–6790 | | 780–6790 | |
| | | M | <1009 | | <1009 |
| | | Premenopausal female | <574 | | <574 |
| | U | | mg/mol creatinine | 1 | mg/mol creatinine |
| | | M | 0–505 | | 0–505 |
| | | Premenopausal female | 0–476 | | 0–476 |
| Cyanide | WB (Ox) | | mg/L | 38.5 | µmol/L |
| | | Nonsmokers | <0.2 | | <7.7 |
| | | Smokers | <0.4 | | <15.4 |
| | | Nitroprusside therapy | Up to 100 without toxicity | | Up to 3850 |
| | | Toxic | >1 | | >38.5 |
| Cystatin C | S | | mg/L | 1 | mg/L |
| Pediatric values (0–<19 years) based on Abbott Architect method | | 0–<1 month | 1.49–2.85 | | 1.49–2.85 |
| | | 1–<5 months | 1.01–1.92 | | 1.01–1.92 |
| | | 5 months–<1 year | 0.75–1.53 | | 0.75–1.53 |
| | | 1–<2 years M | 0.77–1.85 | | 0.77–1.85 |
| | | 1–<2 years F | 0.60–1.20 | | 0.60–1.20 |
| | | 2–<19 years | 0.62–1.11 | | 0.62–1.11 |
| | | Adult F | 0.61–1.05 | | 0.61–1.05 |
| | | Adult M | 0.71–1.21 | | 0.71–1.21 |
| Cystine | S | | mg/dL | 83.3 | µmol/L |
| | | Premature, 1 day | 0.54–1.02 | | 45–85 |
| | | Newborn, 1 day | 0.43–1.01 | | 36–84 |
| | | 0–<6 days, F | 0.19–0.61 | | 16–51 |
| | | 0–<6 days, M | 0.19–0.64 | | 16–53 |
| | | 6 days–<2 week | 0.08–0.68 | | 6.7–57 |
| | | 2 week–<8 years | 0.04–0.24 | | 3.3–20 |
| | | 8–<19 years | 0.05–0.34 | | 4.2–28 |
| | | Adult | 0.40–1.40 | | 33–117 |
| | U, 24 h | | mg/day | 8.33 | µmol/day |
| | | 10 days–7 weeks | 2.16–3.37 | | 18–28 |
| | | 3–12 years | 4.9–30.9 | | 41–257 |
| | | Adult | <38.1 | | <317 |
| | | | mg/g creatinine | 0.94 | mmol/mol creatinine |
| | | Adult | 2–14 | | 1.9–13.1 |
| Dehydroepiandrosterone, unconjugated | S | | ng/dL | 0.0347 | nmol/L |
| | | Children | | | |

Continued

## TABLE A.1    Pediatric and Adult Reference Intervals for Biochemical Markers—cont'd

| Analyte | Specimen | Condition | REFERENCE INTERVALS Conventional Units | REFERENCE INTERVALS Conversion Factor | REFERENCE INTERVALS SI Units |
|---|---|---|---|---|---|
| | | 6–9 years M | 13–187 | | 0.45–6.49 |
| | | 6–9 years F | 18–189 | | 0.62–6.55 |
| | | 10–11 years M | 31–205 | | 1.07–7.11 |
| | | 10–11 years F | 112–224 | | 3.88–7.77 |
| | | 12–14 years M | 83–258 | | 2.88–8.95 |
| | | 12–14 years F | 98–360 | | 3.40–12.5 |
| | | Adult M | 180–1250 | | 6.25–43.4 |
| | | Adult F | 130–980 | | 4.51–34.0 |
| Dehydroepiandrosterone sulfate | S | | µg/dL | 0.027 | µmol/L |
| Pediatric values (0–<19 years) based on Abbott Architect method | | 0–<2 months | 1,070–>1,507 | | 28.9–>40.7 |
| | | 2–<6 months | 26–578 | | 0.7–15.6 |
| | | 6 months–<1 year | 7–178 | | 0.2–4.8 |
| | | 1–<6 years | 4–111 | | 0.1–3.0 |
| | | 6–<9 years | 4–152 | | 0.1–4.1 |
| | | 9–<13 years | 33–270 | | 0.9–7.3 |
| | | 13–<16 years | 56–463 | | 1.5–12.5 |
| | | 16–<19 years M | 126–674 | | 3.4–18.2 |
| | | 16–<19 years F | 148–574 | | 4.0–15.5 |
| | | Pubertal levels, Tanner Stage | | | |
| | | 1, M | 5–265 | | 0.1–7.2 |
| | | 1, F | 5–125 | | 0.1–3.4 |
| | | 2, M | 15–380 | | 0.4–10.3 |
| | | 2, F | 15–150 | | 0.4–4.0 |
| | | 3, M | 60–505 | | 1.6–13.6 |
| | | 3, F | 20–535 | | 0.5–14.4 |
| | | 4, M | 65–560 | | 1.8–15.1 |
| | | 4, F | 35–485 | | 0.9–13.1 |
| | | 5, M | 165–500 | | 4.4–13.5 |
| | | 5, F | 75–530 | | 2.0–14.3 |
| | | Adults | | | |
| | | 18–30 years M | 125–619 | | 3.4–16.7 |
| | | 18–30 years F | 45–380 | | 1.2–10.3 |
| | | 31–50 years M | 5–532 | | 1.6–12.2 |
| | | 31–50 years F | 12–379 | | 0.8–10.2 |
| | | 51–60 years M | 20–413 | | 0.5–11.1 |
| | | 61–83 years M | 10–285 | | 0.3–7.7 |
| | | Postmenopausal F | 30–260 | | 0.8–7.0 |
| 11-Deoxycortisol | S | | ng/dL | 0.0289 | nmol/L |
| | | Cord blood | 295–554 | | 9–16 |
| | | Child and adult | 20–158 | | 0.6–4.6 |
| Pediatric values based on LCMS/MS | | 0–<1 year | 0.00–183 | | 0.00–5.30 |
| | | 1–<2 years | 3.46–30.4 | | 0.10–0.88 |
| | | 2–<7 years | 2.42–37.0 | | 0.07–1.07 |
| | | 7–<12 years | 3.11–78.5 | | 0.09–2.27 |
| | | 12–<19 years | 0.00–78.9 | | 0.00–2.28 |
| Dihydrotestosterone | S | | ng/dL | 0.0334 | nmol/L |
| | | Child, prepubertal | <3 | | <0.10 |
| | | Adult M | 30–85 | | 1.03–2.92 |
| | | Adult F | 4–22 | | 0.14–0.76 |
| Dopamines | P, S | | pg/mL | | nmol/L |
| L-Dopa (1-dodecenoylcarnitine) | | Normotensive adults | 1042–2366 | 0.0051 | 5.3–12.0 |
| DOPAC (3,4-dihydroxyphenylacetic acid) | | | 674–2636 | 0.0059 | 4.0–15.7 |

## TABLE A.1   Pediatric and Adult Reference Intervals for Biochemical Markers—cont'd

| Analyte | Specimen | Condition | REFERENCE INTERVALS | | |
| --- | --- | --- | --- | --- | --- |
| | | | Conventional Units | Conversion Factor | SI Units |
| DHPG | | | 797–1208 | 0.0059 | 4.7–7.1 |
| (3,4-dihydroxyphenylglycol) | | | | | |
| DU-PAN-2 (Duke pancre- | | | U/mL | 1 | kU/L |
| atic cancer associated | | | <401 | 3.69 | <401 |
| antigen) | | | | | |
| Estradiol | S | | pg/mL | 3.69 | pmol/L |
| Values (15 days–<19 years) | | 15 days–<1 year | <25 | | <92 |
| based on Abbott | | 1–<9 years F | <10 | | <37 |
| Architect method | | 9–<11 years F | <48 | | <176 |
| | | 11–<12 years F | <94 | | <345 |
| | | 12–<14 years F | 11–172 | | 39–631 |
| | | 14–19 years F | <255 | | <936 |
| | | 1–<11 years M | <13 | | <46 |
| | | 11–<13 years M | <26 | | <95 |
| | | 13–<15 years M | <28 | | <102 |
| | | 15–<19 years M | <38 | | <141 |
| | | Adult M | 10–50 | | 37–184 |
| | | Adult F | | | |
| | | Early follicular phase | 20–150 | | 73–550 |
| | | Late follicular phase | 40–350 | | 147–1285 |
| | | Midcycle | 150–750 | | 550–2753 |
| | | Luteal phase | 30–450 | | 110–1652 |
| | | Postmenopausal | <21 | | <74 |
| | | Pubertal levels, Tanner Stage | | | |
| Tanner (values based on | | 1, M | <19 | | <68 |
| Abbott Architect method) | | 1, F | <20 | | <74 |
| | | 2, M | <18 | | <67 |
| | | 2, F | <26 | | <96 |
| | | 3, M | <21 | | <76 |
| | | 3, F | <86 | | <317 |
| | | 4, M | <35 | | <128 |
| | | 4, F | 13–141 | | 49–517 |
| | | 5, M | 17–34 | | 64–126 |
| | | 5, F | 19–208 | | 69–762 |
| Estriol, free (unconjugated, uE3) | S | | ng/mL | 3.47 | nmol/L |
| | | Males and non-pregnant females | <2.0 | | <6.9 |
| | | Pregnancy, week of gestation | | | |
| | | 16 | 0.30–1.05 | | 1.04–3.64 |
| | | 18 | 0.63–2.30 | | 2.19–7.98 |
| | | 34 | 5.3–18.3 | | 18.4–63.5 |
| | | 35 | 5.2–26.4 | | 18.0–91.6 |
| | | 36 | 8.2–28.1 | | 28.4–97.5 |
| | | 37 | 8.0–30.1 | | 27.8–104.0 |
| | | 38 | 8.6–38.0 | | 29.8–131.9 |
| | | 39 | 7.2–34.3 | | 25.0–119.0 |
| | | 40 | 9.6–28.9 | | 33.3–100.3 |
| *For LC-MSMS reference intervals see: Clin Biochem 2013;46:642–651* | | | | | |
| Estriol, total (E3) | S | | ng/mL | 3.47 | nmol/L |

*Continued*

## TABLE A.1 Pediatric and Adult Reference Intervals for Biochemical Markers—cont'd

| Analyte | Specimen | Condition | REFERENCE INTERVALS | | |
|---|---|---|---|---|---|
| | | | Conventional Units | Conversion Factor | SI Units |
| | | Pregnancy, week of gestation | | | |
| | | 34 | 38–140 | | 132–486 |
| | | 35 | 31–140 | | 108–486 |
| | | 36 | 35–330 | | 121–1145 |
| | | 37 | 45–260 | | 156–902 |
| | | 38 | 48–350 | | 167–1215 |
| | | 39 | 59–570 | | 205–1978 |
| | | 40 | 95–460 | | 330–1596 |
| | U, 24 h | | µg/day | 3.47 | nmol/day |
| | | M | 1.0–11.0 | | 3.5–38.2 |
| | | F | | | |
| | | Follicular phase | 0–15.0 | | 0–52.0 |
| | | Ovulatory phase | 13.0–54.0 | | 45.1–187.4 |
| | | Luteal phase | 8.0–60.0 | | 27.8–208.2 |
| | | Postmenopausal | 0–11.0 | | 0–38.2 |
| | | Pregnancy | | | |
| | | First trimester | 0–800 | | 0–2776 |
| | | Second trimester | 800–12,000 | | 2776–41,640 |
| | | Third trimester | 5000–50,000 | | 17,350–173,500 |
| Estrone | S | | pg/mL | 3.69 | pmol/L |
| | | M | 15–65 | | 55–240 |
| | | F | | | |
| | | Early follicular phase | 15–150 | | 55–555 |
| | | Late follicular phase | 100–250 | | 370–925 |
| | | Luteal phase | 15–200 | | 55–740 |
| | | Postmenopausal | 15–55 | | 55–204 |
| Ethanol | WB (Ox) | | mg/dL | 0.217 | mmol/L |
| | | Impairment | 50–100 | | 11–22 |
| | | Depression of CNS | >100 | | >21.7 |
| | | Fatalities reported | >400 | | >86.8 |
| Ferritin | S | | ng/mL | 1 | µg/L |
| Values (4 days–<3 years) based on Abbott Architect method | | 4–<15 days | 99.6–717.0 | | 99.6–717.0 |
| | | 15 days–<6 months | 14.0–647.2 | | 14.0–647.2 |
| | | 6 months–<1 year | 8.4–181.9 | | 8.4–181.9 |
| | | 1–<3 years | 5.3–99.9 | | 5.3–99.9 |
| Values (3–79 years) based on the Siemens IMMULITE method | | 3–5 years | 10.7–85.2 | | 10.7–85.2 |
| | | 6–16 years M | 16.2–106.7 | | 16.2–106.7 |
| | | 6–24 years F | 9.6–81.9 | | 9.6–81.9 |
| | | 17–37 years M | 39.3–439.4 | | 39.3–439.4 |
| | | 25–49 years F | 6.5–147.1 | | 6.5–147.1 |
| | | 38–79 years M | 45.8–714.8 | | 45.8–714.8 |
| | | 50–79 years F | 6.0–362.6 | | 6.0–362.6 |
| α-fetoprotein | S | | mg/dL | 0.01 | g/L |
| | | Fetal, first trimester | 200–400 | | 2.0–4.0 |
| | | Cord blood | <5 | | <0.05 |
| Pediatric values based on Abbott Architect method | | | ng/mL | 1 | µg/L |
| | | 0–<1 month | >2,000 | | >2,000 |
| | | 1–<3 months | 9.80–1,359.0 | | 9.80–1,359.0 |
| | | 3–<6 months | 4.15–274.70 | | 4.15–274.70 |
| | | 6 months–<1 year | 2.66–148.21 | | 2.66–148.21 |
| | | 1–<3 years | 2.88–20.94 | | 2.88–20.94 |
| | | 3–<19 years | 0.89–4.48 | | 0.89–4.48 |
| | | Adult (85% of population) | <8.5 | | <8.5 |
| | | Adult (100% of population) | <15 | | <15 |

## TABLE A.1   Pediatric and Adult Reference Intervals for Biochemical Markers—cont'd

| Analyte | Specimen | Condition | REFERENCE INTERVALS | | |
|---|---|---|---|---|---|
| | | | Conventional Units | Conversion Factor | SI Units |
| | Maternal serum | | ng/mL (median) | 1 | µg/L (median) |
| | | Weeks of gestation | | | |
| | | 14 | 25.6 | | 25.6 |
| | | 15 | 29.9 | | 29.9 |
| | | 16 | 34.8 | | 34.8 |
| | | 17 | 40.6 | | 40.6 |
| | | 18 | 47.3 | | 47.3 |
| | | 19 | 55.1 | | 55.1 |
| | | 20 | 64.3 | | 64.3 |
| | | 21 | 74.9 | | 74.9 |
| | S | Tumor marker | ng/mL | 1 | µg/L |
| | | Early marker | 10–20 | | 10–20 |
| | | Cancer | >1000 | | >1000 |
| Fluoride | S | | mg/L | 52.6 | µmol/L |
| | | | 0.2–3.2 | | 10.5–168 |
| Folate | | | ng/mL | 2.265 | nmol/L |
| Values (5 days–<6 years) based on Abbott Architect method | S | 5 days–<1 year | >10.6 | | >23.9 |
| | | 1–<3 years | >3.9 | | >8.7 |
| | | 3–<6 years | >11.9 | | >27.0 |
| Values (6–79 years) based on Siemens IMMULITE method | | 6–18 years | 8.2–30.6 | | 18.6–69.3 |
| | | 19–79 years | 9.5–39.0 | | 21.5–88.4 |
| | Erythrocyte | 3–5 years | 294.7–883.4 | | 703.1–2012.9 |
| | | 6–79 years | 228.2–998.7 | | 541.4–2110.6 |
| | | NOTE: Reference limits for erythrocytes depend on the level of supplementation in the country | | | |
| | S deficiency | | <1.4 | | <3.2 |
| | Erythrocyte deficiency | | <110 | | <252 |
| Follicle stimulating hormone | S | | mIU/mL | 1 | IU/L |
| Values (30 days–<19 years) based on Abbott Architect method | | 30 days–<1 year F | 0.4–10.4 | | 0.4–10.4 |
| | | 1–<9 years F | 0.4–5.5 | | 0.4–5.5 |
| | | 9–<11 years F | 0.4–4.2 | | 0.4–4.2 |
| | | 11–19 years F | 0.3–7.8 | | 0.3–7.8 |
| | | 30 days–<1 year M | 0.1–2.4 | | 0.1–2.4 |
| | | 1–<5 years M | <0.9 | | <0.9 |
| | | 5–<10 years M | <1.6 | | <1.6 |
| | | 10–<13 years M | 0.4–3.9 | | 0.4–3.9 |
| | | 13–<19 years M | 0.8–5.1 | | 0.8–5.1 |
| | | Pubertal levels, Tanner Stage | | | |
| | | 1, M | <1.5 | | <1.5 |
| | | 1, F | 0.6–4.1 | | 0.6–4.1 |
| | | 2, M | <3.0 | | <3.0 |
| | | 2, F | 0.3–5.8 | | 0.3–5.8 |
| | | 3, M | 0.4–6.2 | | 0.4–6.2 |
| | | 3, F | 0.1–7.2 | | 0.1–7.2 |
| | | 4, M | 0.6–5.1 | | 0.6–5.1 |
| | | 4, F | 0.3–7.0 | | 0.3–7.0 |
| | | 5, M | 0.8–7.2 | | 0.8–7.2 |
| | | 5, F | 0.4–8.6 | | 0.4–8.6 |
| | | Adult (23–70 years) M | 1.4–15.4 | | 1.4–15.4 |
| | | Adult (23–70 years) F | | | |
| | | Follicular phase | 1.4–9.9 | | 1.4–9.9 |

*Continued*

## TABLE A.1   Pediatric and Adult Reference Intervals for Biochemical Markers—cont'd

| Analyte | Specimen | Condition | REFERENCE INTERVALS | | |
|---|---|---|---|---|---|
| | | | Conventional Units | Conversion Factor | SI Units |
| | | Midcycle peak | 0.2–17.2 | | 0.2–17.2 |
| | | Luteal phase | 1.1–9.2 | | 1.1–9.2 |
| | | Postmenopausal | 19.3–100.6 | | 19.3–100.6 |
| Fructosamine | S | Child | 5% below adult levels | | |
| | | Adult | 205–285 µmol/L | | 205–285 µmol/L |
| Glomerular filtration rate (endogenous) | Categories | | mL/min per 1.73 m$^2$ | 0.00963 | mL/s per m$^2$ |
| —based on KDIGO | G1 | Normal or high | ≥90 | | ≥0.87 |
| | G2 | Mildly decreased | 60–89 | | 0.58–0.86 |
| | G3a | Mildly to moderately decreased | 45–59 | | 0.43–0.57 |
| | G3b | Moderately to severely decreased | 30–44 | | 0.29–0.42 |
| | G4 | Severely decreased | 15–29 | | 0.14–0.28 |
| | G5 | Kidney failure | <15 | | <0.14 |
| Glucagon | P (Hep or EDTA) | Adult | ng/L | | ng/L |
| | | | 70–180 | | 70–180 |
| Glucose | S, fasting | | mg/dL | 0.0555 | mmol/L |
| | | Cord | 45–96 | | 2.5–5.3 |
| | | Premature | 20–60 | | 1.1–3.3 |
| | | Neonate | 30–60 | | 1.7–3.3 |
| | | Newborn | | | |
| | | 1 day | 40–60 | | 2.2–3.3 |
| | | >1 day | 50–80 | | 2.8–4.5 |
| | | Child | 60–100 | | 3.3–5.6 |
| | | Adult | 74–100 | | 4.1–5.6 |
| | | >60 years | 82–115 | | 4.6–6.4 |
| | | >90 years | 75–121 | | 4.2–6.7 |
| *Clinical Decision Limits* | S | Normal glucose metabolism | ≤100 | | ≤5.55 |
| | | Diabetes | ≥126 | | ≥7.00 |
| Values based on Radiometer ABL90 Plus | WB, venous (random) | 0–<6 months | 52.2–100.9 | | 2.9–5.6 |
| | | 1–<6 months | 64.9–106.3 | | 3.6–5.9 |
| | | 6 months–<19 years | 72.0–111.7 | | 4.0–6.2 |
| Values based on Nova Biomedical StatStrip | WB, venous (random) | 0–<6 months | 55.8–95.5 | | 3.1–5.3 |
| | | 1–<6 months | 64.9–106.3 | | 3.6–5.9 |
| | | 6 months–<19 years | 66.7–111.7 | | 3.7–6.2 |
| *Clinical Decision Limits* | U | | 1–15 | | 0.1–0.8 |
| | | | g/day | 5.55 | mmol/day |
| | U, 24 h | | <0.5 | | <2.8 |
| Glutamic acid | P | | mg/dL | 68 | µmol/L |
| | | Premature, 1 day | 0–1.98 | | 0–135 |
| | | Newborn, 1 day | 0.29–1.57 | | 20–107 |
| | | 6 months–3 years | 0.28–1.47 | | 19–100 |
| | | 3–10 years | 0.34–3.68 | | 23–250 |
| | | 6–18 years | 0.10–0.96 | | 7–65 |
| | | Adult | 0.21–2.82 | | 14–192 |
| | S | 0–<2 week | 1.34–5.90 | | 91–401 |
| | | 2 week–<1 year | 1.09–3.91 | | 74–266 |
| | | 1<19 years | 0.76–2.01 | | 52–137 |
| | U 24 h | | mg/day | 6.8 | µmol/day |
| | | 10 days–7 weeks | 0.3–1.5 | | 2–10 |
| | | Adult | <33.8 | | <230 |
| | | | mg/g creatinine | 0.77 | mmol/mol creatinine |

## TABLE A.1   Pediatric and Adult Reference Intervals for Biochemical Markers—cont'd

| Analyte | Specimen | Condition | Conventional Units | Conversion Factor | SI Units |
|---------|----------|-----------|--------------------|--------------------|----------|
| | | Adult | 2–6 | | 1.5–4.7 |
| Glutamine | P | | mg/dL | 68.5 | µmol/L |
| | | 3 months–6 years | 6.93–10.89 | | 475–746 |
| | | 6–18 years | 5.26–10.80 | | 360–740 |
| | | Adult | 5.78–10.38 | | 396–711 |
| | S | 0–<1 week | 6.58–16.2 | | 451–1113 |
| | | 1 week–<1 year | 4.85–11.5 | | 332–789 |
| | | 1–<9 years | 6.09–9.90 | | 417–678 |
| | | 9–<19 years | 6.82–11.0 | | 467–755 |
| | U, 24 h | | mg/day | 6.85 | µmol/day |
| | | 10 days–7 weeks | 12.4–25.8 | | 85–177 |
| | | 3–12 years | 20.4–113.7 | | 140–779 |
| | | Adult | 43.8–151.8 | | 300–1040 |
| | | | mg/g creatinine | 0.77 | mmol/mol creatinine |
| | | Adult | 2–78 | | 2–60 |
| γ-Glutamyltransferase | S | | U/L | 0.017 | µkat/L |
| Values (0–<3 years) based | | 0–<14 days | 23–219 | | 0.38–3.65 |
| on Abbott Architect | | 15 days–<1 year | 8–127 | | 0.13–2.12 |
| method | | 1–<3 years | 6–16 | | 0.10–0.27 |
| Values (3–79 years) based | | 3–5 years | 11–20 | | 0.19–0.34 |
| on OCD VITROS method | | 6–14 years M | 10–26 | | 0.17–0.44 |
| | | 6–17 years F | 9–24 | | 0.15–0.41 |
| | | 15–19 years M | 10–33 | | 0.17–0.56 |
| | | 18–35 years F | 12–38 | | 0.20–0.65 |
| | | 20–35 years M | 12–62 | | 0.20–1.05 |
| | | 36–79 years M | 13–109 | | 0.22–1.85 |
| | | 36–79 years F | 10–54 | | 0.17–0.92 |
| Glycated hemoglobin | WB (EDTA, | | % | | mmol/mol (IFCC) |
| (HbA$_{1c}$) | Hep or Ox) | | | | |
| Values (6–79 years) based | | 6–39 years | 4.9–6.1 | | 30–43 |
| on OCD VITROS method | | 40–79 years | 5.0–6.3 | | 31–45 |
| | | Cut off for diagnosis | ≥6.5 (NGSP) | | ≥48 |
| Glycine | P | | mg/dL | 133.3 | µmol/L |
| | | Premature 1 day | 0–7.57 | | 0–1010 |
| | | Newborn 1 day | 1.68–3.86 | | 224–514 |
| | | 1–3 months | 0.79–1.67 | | 106–222 |
| | | 2–6 months | 1.31–2.22 | | 175–296 |
| | | 9 months–2 years | 0.42–2.31 | | 56–308 |
| | | 3–10 years | 0.88–1.67 | | 117–223 |
| | | 6–18 years | 1.18–2.27 | | 158–302 |
| | | Adult | 0.90–4.16 | | 120–554 |
| | S | 0–<2 week | 2.24–5.87 | | 299–782 |
| | | 2 week–<13 years | 1.47–2.99 | | 196–398 |
| | | 13–<19 years | 1.64–3.05 | | 218–407 |
| | U, 24 h | | mg/day | 13.3 | µmol/day |
| | | 10 days–7 weeks | 14.6–59.2 | | 194–787 |
| | | 3–12 years | 12.4–106.8 | | 165–1,420 |
| | | Adult | 59.0–294.6 | | 785–3,918 |
| | | | mg/g creatinine | 1.51 | mmol/mol creatinine |
| | | Adult | 12–108 | | 18.2–163 |
| Growth hormone | S | | ng/mL | 1 | µg/L |
| | | Basal | 2–5 | | 2–5 |
| | | Insulin tolerance test | >10 | | >10 |
| | | Arginine | >7.5 | | >7.5 |
| | | L-Dopa | >7.5 | | >7.5 |

*Continued*

## TABLE A.1   Pediatric and Adult Reference Intervals for Biochemical Markers—cont'd

| | | | REFERENCE INTERVALS | | |
|---|---|---|---|---|---|
| Analyte | Specimen | Condition | Conventional Units | Conversion Factor | SI Units |
| Pediatric values (0–<19 years) based on Beckman DxI method | S | 0–<3 months | 0.80–33.5 | | 0.80–33.5 |
| | | 3 month–<2 years | 0.14–6.27 | | 0.14–6.27 |
| | | 2–<7 years | 0.05–5.11 | | 0.05–5.11 |
| | | 7–<12 years | 0.02–4.76 | | 0.02–4.76 |
| | | 12–<14 years | 0.01–6.20 | | 0.01–6.20 |
| | | 14–<19 years, F | 0.03–5.22 | | 0.03–5.22 |
| | | 14–<19 years, M | 0.02–3.81 | | 0.02–3.81 |
| Haptoglobin | S | | mg/dL | 0.01 | g/L |
| Values (0–<19 years) based on Abbott Architect method | | 0–14 days | 0–10 | | 0–0.1 |
| | | 15 days–<1 year | 7–221 | | 0.1–2.2 |
| | | 1–<12 years | 7–163 | | 0.1–1.6 |
| | | 12–<19 years | 7–179 | | 0.1–1.8 |
| | | Adult (20–60 years) | 30–200 | | 0.3–2.0 |
| High-density lipoprotein cholesterol (HDL-C) | S | | mg/dL | 0.0259 | mmol/L |
| *Reference Intervals* | | | | | |
| Values (0–<3 years) based on Abbott Architect method | | 0–14 days | 15–42 | | 0.4–1.1 |
| | | 15 days–<1 year | 12–71 | | 0.3–1.9 |
| | | 1–<3 years | 32–63 | | 0.8–1.6 |
| Values (3–79 years) based on OCD VITROS method | | 3–5 years | 31–73 | | 0.8–1.9 |
| | | 6–14 years | 35–81 | | 0.9–2.1 |
| | | 15–79 years M | 31–70 | | 0.8–1.8 |
| | | 15–79 years F | 35–89 | | 0.9–2.3 |
| *Clinical Decision Limits* | | Pediatric | mg/dL | 0.0259 | mmol/L |
| | | Acceptable | >45 | | >1.2 |
| | | Borderline | 40–45 | | 1.0–1.2 |
| | | Low | <40 | | <1.0 |
| | ATP III Classification | | | | |
| | S | Low | <40 | | <1.0 |
| | | High | >59 | | >1.5 |
| Non-HDL cholesterol (calculated) | S | | mg/dL | 0.0259 | mmol/L |
| Calculated pediatric values based on Abbott Architect method | | 0–<1 year | 27.8–202 | | 0.72–5.22 |
| | | 1–<10 years, F | 79.9–165 | | 2.07–4.28 |
| | | 1–<10 years, M | 69.1–142 | | 1.79–3.68 |
| | | 10–<19 years | 64.9–156 | | 1.68–4.04 |
| Histidine | P | | mg/dL | 64.5 | µmol/L |
| | | Premature, 1 day | 0.16–1.40 | | 10–90 |
| | | Newborn, 1 day | 0.76–1.77 | | 49–114 |
| | | 1–3 months | 0.66–1.30 | | 43–83 |
| | | 2–6 months | 1.49–2.12 | | 96–137 |
| | | 9 months–2 years | 0.37–1.74 | | 24–112 |
| | | 3–10 years | 0.37–1.32 | | 24–85 |
| | | 6–18 years | 0.99–1.64 | | 64–106 |
| | | Adult | 0.50–1.66 | | 32–107 |
| | S | 0–<2 week | 0.70–2.60 | | 45–168 |
| | | 2 week–<19 years | 1.01–1.75 | | 65–113 |
| | U, 24 h | | mg/day | 6.45 | µmol/day |
| | | 10 days–7 weeks | 16.0–38.6 | | 103–249 |
| | | 3–12 years | 47.4–199.2 | | 306–1285 |
| | | Adult | 72.9–440.8 | | 470–2843 |
| | | | mg/g creatinine | 0.73 | mmol/mol creatinine |
| | | Adult | 1–141 | | 1–103 |
| Homocysteine, total | S, P | | µg/mL | 7.397 | µmol/L |
| | | Folate supplemented diet | | | |
| | | <15 years | <1.08 | | <8 |

## TABLE A.1 Pediatric and Adult Reference Intervals for Biochemical Markers—cont'd

| Analyte | Specimen | Condition | REFERENCE INTERVALS | | |
| --- | --- | --- | --- | --- | --- |
| | | | Conventional Units | Conversion Factor | SI Units |
| | | 15–65 years | <1.62 | | <12 |
| | | >65 years | <2.16 | | <16 |
| | | No folate supplementation | | | |
| | | <15 years | <1.35 | | <10 |
| | | 15–65 years | <2.03 | | <15 |
| | | >65 years | <2.70 | | <20 |
| Values (5 days–<6 years) based on Abbott Architect method | | 5 days–<1 year | 0.39–1.35 | | 2.9–10.0 |
| | | 1–<6 years | 0.37–1.03 | | 2.8–7.6 |
| Values (6–79 years) based on OCD VITROS method | | 6–12 years | 0.23–0.93 | | 1.7–6.9 |
| | | 13–25 years M | 0.49–1.43 | | 3.6–10.6 |
| | | 13–39 years F | 0.39–1.28 | | 2.9–9.5 |
| | | 26–79 years M | 0.70–1.91 | | 5.2–14.1 |
| | | 40–79 years F | 0.50–1.47 | | 3.7–10.9 |
| Homovanillic acid | U, 24 h | | mg/day | 5.49 | µmol/day |
| | | 3–6 years | 1.4–4.3 | | 8–24 |
| | | 6–10 years | 2.1–4.7 | | 12–26 |
| | | 10–16 years | 2.4–8.7 | | 13–48 |
| | | 16–83 years | 1.4–8.8 | | 8–48 |
| 17–Hydroxyprogesterone | | | ng/dL | 0.03 | nmol/L |
| | | Cord blood | 900–5000 | | 27.3–151.5 |
| | | Premature | 26–568 | | 0.8–17.0 |
| Values (4 days–<19 years) based on Abbott Architect method | | 4 days–<1 year F | <132 | | <4.0 |
| | | 30 days–<1 year M | <66 | | <2.0 |
| | | 1–<10 years | <35 | | <1.1 |
| | | 10–<15 years | 13–85 | | 0.4–2.7 |
| | | 15–<19 years F | 20–1,026 | | 0.6–32.6 |
| | | 15–<19 years M | 16–57 | | 0.5–1.8 |
| | | Puberty–Tanner Stage | | | |
| Tanner values based on Abbott Architect method | | 1, M | <44 | | <1.4 |
| | | 1, F | <28 | | <0.9 |
| | | 2, M | <44 | | <1.4 |
| | | 2, F | 13–41 | | 0.4–1.3 |
| | | 3, M | <50 | | <1.6 |
| | | 3, F | 16–47 | | 0.5–1.5 |
| | | 4, M | <41 | | <1.3 |
| | | 4, F | 19–72 | | 0.6–2.3 |
| | | 5, M | 13–50 | | 0.4–1.6 |
| | | 5, F | <1,082 | | <34.4 |
| | | Adult M | 27–199 | | 0.8–6.0 |
| | | Adult F | | | |
| | | Follicular phase | 15–70 | | 0.4–2.1 |
| | | Luteal phase | 35–290 | | 1.0–8.7 |
| | | Pregnancy | 200–1,200 | | 6.0–36.0 |
| | | Post-ACTH | <320 | | <9.6 |
| *For LC-MSMS reference intervals, see: Clin Chem 2006;52:1559–1567; Clin Biochem 2013;46:642–651* | | Postmenopausal | <70 | | <2.1 |
| 21-Hydroxyprogesterone | S | | nmol/L | 1 | nmol/L |
| Pediatric values based on LC-MS/MS method | | 0–<1 year | 0.07–0.76 | | 0.07–0.76 |
| | | 1–<2 years | 0.03–0.25 | | 0.03–0.25 |
| | | 2–<12 years | 0.00–0.15 | | 0.00–0.15 |
| | | 12–<19 years | 0.00–0.24 | | 0.00–0.24 |

*Continued*

## TABLE A.1   Pediatric and Adult Reference Intervals for Biochemical Markers—cont'd

| Analyte | Specimen | Condition | REFERENCE INTERVALS | | |
|---|---|---|---|---|---|
| | | | Conventional Units | Conversion Factor | SI Units |
| Immunoglobulin A | S, P | | mg/dL | 0.01 | g/L |
| Values (0–<19 years) | | 0–<1 year | 1–29 | | 0.0–0.3 |
| based on Abbott | | 1–<3 years | 4–90 | | 0.0–0.9 |
| Architect method | | 3–<6 years | 26–147 | | 0.3–1.5 |
| | | 6–<14 years | 47–221 | | 0.5–2.2 |
| | | 14–<19 years | 53–287 | | 0.5–2.9 |
| | | Adult (20–60 years) | 70–400 | | 0.7–4.0 |
| | | Adult (>60 years) | 90–410 | | 0.9–4.1 |
| Immunoglobulin D | S | | IU/mL | 1 | kIU/L |
| | | Adult (20–60 years) | 0–160 | | 0–160 |
| | | | ng/mL | 1 | µg/L |
| | | | 0–384 | | 0–384 |
| Immunoglobulin E | S | | kIU/L | 2.4 | µg/L |
| Values (0–<19 years) | | 0–<7 years | <25–440 | | <60–1057 |
| based on Abbott | | 7–<19 years | <25–450 | | <60–1079 |
| Architect method | | Adult (20–60 years) | 0–160 | | 0–380 |
| Immunoglobulin G | S | | mg/dL | 0.01 | g/L |
| Values (0–<19 years) | | 0–14 days | 320–1407 | | 3.2–14.1 |
| based on Abbott | | 15 days–<1 year | 108–702 | | 1.1–7.0 |
| Architect method | | 1–<4 years | 316–1148 | | 3.2–11.5 |
| | | 4–<10 years | 542–1358 | | 5.4–13.6 |
| | | 10–<19 years | 658–1534 | | 6.6–15.3 |
| | | Adult (20–60 years) | 700–1600 | | 7.0–16.0 |
| | | Adult (>60 years) | 600–1560 | | 6.0–15.6 |
| Immunoglobulin M | S | | mg/dL | 0.01 | g/L |
| Values (0–<19 years) | | 0–14 days | 5–35 | | 0.1–0.4 |
| based on Abbott | | 15 days–13 weeks | 12–71 | | 0.1–0.7 |
| Architect method | | 13 weeks–<1 year | 16–86 | | 0.2–0.9 |
| | | 1–<19 years M | 39–151 | | 0.4–1.5 |
| | | 1–<19 years F | 48–186 | | 0.5–1.9 |
| | | Adult (20–60 years) | 40–230 | | 0.4–2.3 |
| | | Adult (>60 years) | 30–360 | | 0.3–3.6 |
| Inhibin A | S | | pg/mL | 1 | ng/L |
| | | M | 1.0–3.6 | | 1.0–3.6 |
| | | F (Cycling; days of cycle) | | | |
| | | Early follicular phase (−14 to −10 days) | 5.5–28.2 | | 5.5–28.2 |
| | | Midfollicular phase (−9 to −4 days) | 7.9–34.5 | | 7.9–34.5 |
| | | Late follicular phase (−3 to −1 day) | 19.5–102 .3 | | 19.5–102 .3 |
| | | Midcycle (day 0) | 49.9–155.5 | | 49.9–155.5 |
| | | Early luteal (1–3 days) | 35.9–132.7 | | 35.9–132.7 |
| | | Midluteal (4–11 days) | 13.2–159.6 | | 13.2–159.6 |
| | | Late luteal (12–14 days) | 7.3–89.9 | | 7.3–89.9 |
| | | IVF, peak levels | 354–1690 | | 354–1690 |
| | | PCOS, ovulatory | 5.7–16.0 | | 5.7–16.0 |
| | | Postmenopausal | 1.0–3.9 | | 1.0–3.9 |
| Insulin | S | | µIU/mL | 7 | pmol/L |
| Values (0–<6 years) based | | 0–<1 year | 1.0–23.4 | | 7–164 |
| on Abbott Architect method | | 1–<6 years | 1.3–40.2 | | 9–281 |
| Values (6–79 years) based | | 6–10 years | 0.4–13.0 | | 3–91 |
| on Siemens IMMULITE | | 11–19 years | 2.1–19.5 | | 15–137 |
| and ADVIA Centaur methods | | 20–79 years | 2.4–21.8 | | 17–153 |

## TABLE A.1  Pediatric and Adult Reference Intervals for Biochemical Markers—cont'd

| Analyte | Specimen | Condition | REFERENCE INTERVALS | | |
|---|---|---|---|---|---|
| | | | Conventional Units | Conversion Factor | SI Units |
| Insulin-like growth factor-1 | S | | ng/mL | 1 | µg/L |
| | | 1–2 years M | 31–160 | | 31–160 |
| | | 1–2 years F | 11–206 | | 11–206 |
| | | 3–6 years M | 16–288 | | 16–288 |
| | | 3–6 years F | 70–316 | | 70–316 |
| | | 7–10 years M | 136–385 | | 136–385 |
| | | 7–10 years F | 123–396 | | 123–396 |
| | | 11–12 years M | 136–440 | | 136–440 |
| | | 11–12 years F | 191–462 | | 191–462 |
| | | 13–14 years M | 165–616 | | 165–616 |
| | | 13–14 years F | 286–660 | | 286–660 |
| | | 15–18 years M | 134–836 | | 134–836 |
| | | 15–18 years F | 152–660 | | 152–660 |
| | | 19–25 years M | 202–433 | | 202–433 |
| | | 19–25 years F | 231–550 | | 231–550 |
| | | Adult (25–85 years) M | 135–449 | | 135–449 |
| | | Adult (25–85 years) F | 135–449 | | 135–449 |
| Insulin-like growth factor-II | S | | ng/mL | 1 | µg/L |
| | | Child | | | |
| | | Prepubertal | 334–642 | | 334–642 |
| | | Pubertal | 245–737 | | 245–737 |
| | | Adult | 288–736 | | 288–736 |
| | | GH deficiency | 51–299 | | 51–299 |
| Iodine | U | | µg/dL | 0.079 | µmol/L |
| Values based on manual | | 3–5 years | 5–83 | | 0.39–6.58 |
| microplate analysis | | 6–79 years | 1–49 | | 0.09–3.88 |
| Iron | | | µg/dL | 0.179 | µmol/L |
| Values based on Abbott | | 0–<14 years | 16–128 | | 2.8–22.9 |
| Architect method | | 14–<19 years M | 31–168 | | 5.5–30.0 |
| | | 14–<19 years F | 20–162 | | 3.5–29.0 |
| Iron Binding Capacity, total | S | | µg/dL | 0.179 | µmol/L |
| Values based on Siemens | | 0–<19 years | 300–439 | | 53.7–78.6 |
| ADVIA method | | | | | |
| Isoleucine | P | | mg/dL | 76.3 | µmol/L |
| | | Premature, 1 day | 0.26–0.78 | | 20–60 |
| | | Newborn, 1 day | 0.35–0.69 | | 27–53 |
| | | 1–3 months | 0.59–0.95 | | 45–73 |
| | | 2–6 months | 0.50–1.61 | | 38–123 |
| | | 9 months–2 years | 0.34–1.23 | | 26–94 |
| | | 3–10 years | 0.37–1.10 | | 28–84 |
| | | 6–18 years | 0.50–1.24 | | 38–95 |
| | | Adult | 0.48–1.28 | | 37–98 |
| | S | 0–<2 week | 0.33–1.69 | | 25–129 |
| | | 2 week–<1 year | 0.39–1.48 | | 30–113 |
| | | 1<12 years | 0.56–1.69 | | 43–129 |
| | | 12–<19 years, F | 0.42–0.89 | | 32–68 |
| | | 12–<19 years, M | 0.69–1.66 | | 53–127 |
| | U | | mg/day | 7.62 | µmol/day |
| | | 10 days–7 weeks | Trace–0.4 | | Trace–3 |
| | | 3–12 years | 2–7 | | 15–53 |
| | | Adult | 5–24 | | 38–183 |
| | | | mg/g creatinine | 0.86 | mmol/mol creatinine |
| | | Adult | 1–5 | | 0.8–4.4 |
| Lactate | | | mg/dL | 0.111 | mmol/L |
| Values based on Radio-meter ABL90 Plus | WB, venous | 0–<19 years | 5.4–18.9 | | 0.6–2.1 |

*Continued*

# 

## TABLE A.1 Pediatric and Adult Reference Intervals for Biochemical Markers—cont'd

| Analyte | Specimen | Condition | Conventional Units | Conversion Factor | SI Units |
|---|---|---|---|---|---|
| L-Lactate | WB (Hep) | | mg/dL | 0.111 | mmol/L |
| | | At bed rest | 5–12 | | 0.56–1.39 |
| | | Venous | 3–7 | | 0.36–0.75 |
| | | Arterial | 16–17 | | 1.78–1.88 |
| | U, 24 h | Adult | | | |
| | | | | | mmol/mol creatinine |
| | | 0–1 month | | | 46–348 |
| | | 1–6 months | | | 57–346 |
| | | 6 months–5 years | | | 21–38 |
| | | >5 years | | | 20–101 |
| Lactate dehydrogenase (LD) | S | | U/L | 0.017 | µkat/L |
| Pediatric values based on Abbott Architect method | | 0–<15 days | 309–1222 | | 5.25–20.8 |
| | | 15 days–<1 year | 163–452 | | 2.77–7.68 |
| | | 1–<10 years | 192–321 | | 3.26–5.46 |
| | | 10–<15 years, F | 157–272 | | 2.67–4.62 |
| | | 10–<15 years, M | 170–283 | | 2.89–4.81 |
| | | 15–<19 years | 130–250 | | 2.21–4.25 |
| | | Adult | 125–220 | | 2.1–3.7 |
| Lead | WB (Hep) | | µg/dL | 0.0483 | µmol/L |
| | | Child | <25 | | <1.21 |
| | | Adult | <25 | | <1.21 |
| | | Toxic | >99 | | >4.78 |
| | U, 24 h | | µg/L | | µmol/L |
| | | | <80 | | <0.39 |
| Leucine | P | | mg/dL | 76.3 | µmol/L |
| | | Premature, 1 day | 0.26–1.58 | | 20–120 |
| | | Newborn, 1 day | 0.62–1.43 | | 47–109 |
| | | 1–3 months | 10.58–2.14 | | 44–164 |
| | | 9 months–2 years | 0.59–2.03 | | 45–155 |
| | | 3–10 years | 0.73–2.33 | | 56–178 |
| | | 6–18 years | 1.03–2.28 | | 79–174 |
| | | Adult | 0.98–2.29 | | 75–175 |
| | S | 0–<1 week | 0.60–2.16 | | 46–165 |
| | | 1 week–<1 year | 0.72–2.46 | | 55–188 |
| | | 1–<11 years | 1.11–2.96 | | 85–226 |
| | | 11–<19 years, F | 1.10–1.99 | | 84–152 |
| | | 11–<19 years, M | 1.35–2.98 | | 103–227 |
| | U, 24 h | | mg/day | 7.624 | µmol/day |
| | | 10 days–7 weeks | 0.9–2.0 | | 7–15 |
| | | 3–12 years | 3–11 | | 23–84 |
| | | Adult | 2.6–8.1 | | 20–62 |
| | | | mg/g creatinine | 0.86 | mmol/mol creatinine |
| | | Adult | 0–8 | | 0–6.8 |
| Lipase, | S | | U/L | 0.017 | µkat/L |
| Values (0–<19 years) based on Abbott Architect method | | 0–<19 years | 4–39 | | 0.07–0.65 |
| 37°C | | Adult | <38 | | <0.65 |
| Low-density lipoprotein cholesterol (LDL-C) (Measured) | S | | mg/dL | 0.0259 | mmol/L |
| *Reference Intervals* | | | | | |
| Calculated pediatric values based on Abbott Architect Method | | 0–<1 year | 13.1–173 | | 0.34–4.48 |
| | | 1–<10 years, F | 58.7–128 | | 1.52–3.32 |
| | | 1–<10 years, M | 47.1–121 | | 1.22–3.14 |
| | | 10–<19 years | 45.6–131 | | 1.18–3.40 |

## TABLE A.1    Pediatric and Adult Reference Intervals for Biochemical Markers—cont'd

| Analyte | Specimen | Condition | Conventional Units | Conversion Factor | SI Units |
|---|---|---|---|---|---|
| Values (6–79 years) based | | 6–24 years, F | 46–143 | | 1.2–3.7 |
| on OCD VITROS method | | 25–49 years M | 62–189 | | 1.6–4.9 |
| | | 23–49 years F | 50–178 | | 1.3–4.6 |
| | | 50–79 years | 73–189 | | 1.9–4.9 |
| | | NOTE: See more recent guidelines for recommended LDL-C cutoffs for treatment initiation and LDL-C treatment targets to reduce risk of atherosclerotic cardiovascular disease through cholesterol management. (2018 AHA/ACC/AACVPR/AAPA/ABC/ACPM/ADA/AGS/APhA/ASPC/NLA/PCNA Guideline on the Management of Blood Cholesterol). | | | |
| *Clinical Decision Limits* | | | mg/dL | 0.0259 | mmol/L |
| | | Risk of coronary heart disease, Child | | | |
| | | Acceptable | <110 | | <2.8 |
| | | Borderline | 110–129 | | <3.3 |
| | | High | ≥130 | | ≥3.4 |
| | | Risk coronary heart disease, Adults | | | |
| | | Optimal | <100 | | <2.59 |
| | | Near/above optimal | 100–129 | | 2.59–3.34 |
| | | Borderline high | 130–159 | | 3.37–4.12 |
| | | High | 160–189 | | 4.15–4.90 |
| | | Very high | >189 | | >4.90 |
| Luteinizing hormone (LH) | | | mIU/mL | 1 | IU/L |
| Values (4 days–<19 years) | | 4 days–<3 months F | <2.4 | | <2.4 |
| based on Abbott | | 4 days–<3 months M | 0.2–3.8 | | 0.2–3.8 |
| Architect method | | 3 months–<1 year F | <1.2 | | <1.2 |
| | | 3 months–<1 year M | <2.9 | | <2.9 |
| | | 1–<10 years | <0.3 | | <0.3 |
| | | 10–<13 years | <4.3 | | <4.3 |
| | | 13–<15 years F | 0.4–6.5 | | 0.4–6.5 |
| | | 13–<15 years M | <4.1 | | <4.1 |
| | | 15–<17 years F | <13.1 | | <13.1 |
| | | 15–<17 years M | 0.8–4.8 | | 0.8–4.8 |
| | | 17–<19 years F | <8.4 | | <8.4 |
| | | 17–<19 years M | 0.9–7.1 | | 0.9–7.1 |
| | | Pubertal levels, Tanner Stage | | | |
| Tanner values based on | | 1, M | <1.2 | | <1.2 |
| Abbott Architect method | | 1, F | <0.1 | | <0.1 |
| | | 2, M | <1.2 | | <1.2 |
| | | 2, F | <2.3 | | <2.3 |
| | | 3, M | <2.3 | | <2.3 |
| | | 3, F | <7.4 | | <7.4 |
| | | 4, M | <4.9 | | <4.9 |
| | | 4, F | 0.3–6.7 | | 0.3–6.7 |
| | | 5, M | 0.6–5.9 | | 0.6–5.9 |
| | | 5, F | 0.4–21.2 | | 0.4–21.2 |
| | | Adult (23–70 years) M | 1.2–7.8 | | 1.2–7.8 |
| | | Adult (23–70 years) F | | | |
| | | Follicular phase | 1.7–15.0 | | 1.7–15.0 |
| | | Midcycle peak | 21.9–56.6 | | 21.9–56.6 |
| | | Luteal phase | 0.6–16.3 | | 0.6–16.3 |
| | | Postmenopausal | 14.2–52.3 | | 14.2–52.3 |
| Lysine | P | | mg/dL | 68.5 | µmol/L |
| | | Premature,1 day | 1.01–4.53 | | 70–310 |

## TABLE A.1  Pediatric and Adult Reference Intervals for Biochemical Markers—cont'd

| Analyte | Specimen | Condition | Conventional Units | Conversion Factor | SI Units |
|---------|----------|-----------|--------------------|--------------------|----------|
| | | Newborn, 1 day | 1.66–3.93 | | 114–269 |
| | | 1–3 months | 0.54–2.46 | | 37–169 |
| | | 9 months–2 years | 0.66–2.10 | | 45–144 |
| | | 3–10 years | 1.04–2.20 | | 71–151 |
| | | 6–18 years | 1.58–3.40 | | 108–233 |
| | | Adult | 1.21–3.47 | | 83–238 |
| | S | 0–<2 week | 1.31–4.66 | | 90–319 |
| | | 2 week–<19 years | 1.49–3.78 | | 102–259 |
| | U, 24 h | | mg/day | 6.85 | μmol/day |
| | | 10 days–7 weeks | 5.7–10.9 | | 39–75 |
| | | 3–12 years | 9.3–93.7 | | 64–642 |
| | | Adult | 3.1–153.0 | | 21–1,048 |
| | | | mg/g creatinine | 0.77 | mmol/mol creatinine |
| | | Adult | 4–12 | | 3.2–9.2 |
| α2-Macroglobulin | S | | mg/dL | 0.01 | g/L |
| | | Adult (20–60 years) | 130–300 | | 1.3–3.0 |
| Magnesium, free | S | | mmol/L | 1.0 | mmol/L |
| | | | 0.45–0.60 | | 0.45–0.60 |
| Magnesium, total (enzymatic) | S | | mg/dL | 0.4114 | mmol/L |
| | | 0–14 days | 1.99–3.94 | | 0.82–1.62 |
| | | 15 days–<1 year | 1.97–3.09 | | 0.81–1.27 |
| | | 1–<19 years | 2.09–2.84 | | 0.86–1.17 |
| Manganese | | | μg/L | 18.0 | nmol/L |
| | WB (Hep) | | 5–15 | | 90–270 |
| | S | | 0.5–1.3 | | 9–24 |
| | U, collect in metal-free container | | 0.5–9.8 | | 9.1–178 |
| | | Toxic conc. | >19 | | >342 |
| Mercury | | | μg/L | 4.99 | nmol/L |
| | WB (EDTA) | | 0.6–59 | | 3.0–294.4 |
| | U, 24 h | | <20 | | <99.8 |
| | | Toxic conc. | >150 | | >748.5 |
| | | Lethal conc. | >800 | | >3992 |
| Methemoglobin (MetHb) | WB (EDTA, Hep or ACD) | | g/dL | 155 | μmol/L |
| | | | 0.06–0.24 | | 9.3–37.2 |
| | | | % of total Hb | 0.01 | Mass fraction of total Hb |
| | | | 0.04–1.52 | | 0.0004–0.0152 |
| Methionine | | | mg/dL | 67.7 | μmol/L |
| | P | Premature, 1 day | 0.38–0.66 | | 25–45 |
| | | Newborn, 1 day | 0.13–0.61 | | 9–41 |
| | | 1–3 months | 0.05–0.57 | | 3–39 |
| | | 2–6 months | 0.24–0.73 | | 16–49 |
| | | 9 months–2 years | 0.04–0.43 | | 3–29 |
| | | 3–10 years | 0.16–0.24 | | 11–16 |
| | | 6–18 years | 0.24–0.55 | | 16–37 |
| | | Adult | 0.09–0.60 | | 6–40 |
| | S | 0–<19 years | 0.19–0.65 | | 13–44 |
| | U | | mg/day | 6.7 | μmol/day |
| | | 10 days–7 weeks | 0.1–1.9 | | 0.7–13 |
| | | 3–12 years | 3–14 | | 20–95 |
| | | Adult | <9.1 | | <63 |
| | | | mg/g creatinine | 0.76 | mmol/mol creatinine |

## TABLE A.1   Pediatric and Adult Reference Intervals for Biochemical Markers—cont'd

| Analyte | Specimen | Condition | REFERENCE INTERVALS Conventional Units | Conversion Factor | SI Units |
|---|---|---|---|---|---|
| | | Adult | 0–9.5 | | 0–7.2 |
| β2-Microglobulin | S | | mg/dL | 10 | mg/L |
| Values (0–<19 years) | | 0–<3 months M | 0.19–0.47 | | 1.9–4.7 |
| based on Abbott | | 0–<3 months F | 0.19–0.58 | | 1.9–5.8 |
| Architect method | | 3 months–<2 years | 0.13–0.45 | | 1.3–4.5 |
| | | 2–<19 years | 0.12–0.23 | | 1.2–2.3 |
| | | | mg/dL (mean) | 10 | mg/L (mean) |
| | | 0–59 years | 0.19 | | 1.9 |
| | | 60–69 years | 0.21 | | 2.1 |
| | | >70 years | 0.24 | | 2.4 |
| Molybdenum | | | µg/L | 10.42 | nmol/L |
| | S | | 0.1–3.0 | | 1.0–31.3 |
| | | | µg/day | 10.42 | nmol/day |
| | U, 24 h | | 40–60 | | 416–625 |
| Myoglobin | S | | ng/mL | 1.0 | µg/L |
| Values based on OCD | | 0–<2 week | 13.9–234 | | 13.9–234 |
| Vitros method | | 2 week–<1 year | 7.29–60.9 | | 7.29–60.9 |
| | | 1–<13 years | 15.1–50.3 | | 15.1–50.3 |
| | | 13–<19 years, F | 11.7–47.3 | | 11.7–47.3 |
| | | 13–<19 years, M | 16.7–206 | | 16.7–206 |
| Niacin | U, 24 h | | mg/day | 7.3 | µmol/day |
| | | | 2.4–6.4 | | 17.5–46.7 |
| Nickel | | | µg/L | 17 | nmol/L |
| | S or P (Hep) | | 0.14–1.0 | | 2.4–17.0 |
| | WB | | 1.0–28.0 | | 17–476 |
| | | | µg/day | 17 | nmol/day |
| | U, 24 h | | 0.1–10 | | 2–170 |
| N-telopeptide (BCE = bone collagen equivalents) | S | | nmol BCE/L | 1.0 | nmol BCE/L |
| | | M | 5.4–24.2 | | 5.4–24.2 |
| | | Premenopausal female | 6.2–19.0 | | 6.2–19.0 |
| | | | nmol BCE/mmol creatinine | 1.0 | nmol BCE/mmol creatinine |
| | U | M | 3–63 | | 3–63 |
| | | Premenopausal female | 5–65 | | 5–65 |
| Orotic acid | | | | | mmol/mol creatinine |
| | U | 0–1 month | | | 1.4–5.3 |
| | | 1–6 months | | | 1.0–3.2 |
| | | 6 months–5 years | | | 0.5–3.3 |
| | | >5 years | | | 0.4–1.2 |
| Osteocalcin | S | | ng/mL | 1.0 | µg/L |
| | | Adult M | 3.0–13.0 | | 3.0–13.0 |
| | | Adult F | | | |
| | | Premenopausal | 0.4–8.2 | | 0.4–8.2 |
| | | Postmenopausal | 1.5–11.0 | | 1.5–11.0 |
| Oxalic acid | | | | | mmol/mol creatinine |
| | U | 0–1 month | | | 51–931 |
| | | 1–6 months | | | 7–567 |
| | | 6 months–5 years | | | 7–352 |
| | | >5 years | | | <188 |
| Oxygen, partial pressure ($PO_2$) | Cord blood | | mm Hg | 0.133 | kPa |
| | Arterial | | 5.7–30.5 | | 0.8–4.0 |
| | Venous | | 17.4–41.0 | | 2.3–5.5 |
| | WB, arterial | Birth | 8–24 | | 1.06–3.19 |

Continued

## TABLE A.1    Pediatric and Adult Reference Intervals for Biochemical Markers—cont'd

| Analyte | Specimen | Condition | REFERENCE INTERVALS | | |
| --- | --- | --- | --- | --- | --- |
| | | | Conventional Units | Conversion Factor | SI Units |
| | | 5–10 min | 33–75 | | 4.39–9.96 |
| | | 30 min | 31–85 | | 4.12–11.31 |
| | | 1 h | 55–80 | | 7.32–10.64 |
| | | 1 day | 54–95 | | 7.18–12.64 |
| | | 2 days–60 years | 83–108 | | 11.04–14.36 |
| | | >60 years | >80 | | > 10.64 |
| | | >70 years | >70 | | >9.31 |
| | | >80 years | >60 | | >7.98 |
| | | >90 years | >50 | | >6.65 |
| Oxygen, saturation (sO₂) | WB, arterial | | Percent saturation | 0.01 | Fraction saturation |
| | | Newborn | 40–90 | | 0.40–0.90 |
| | | Thereafter | 94–98 | | 0.94–0.98 |
| Oxytocin | P, EDTA | | μU/mL | 1.0 | mU/L |
| | | M | 1.1–1.9 | | 1.1–1.9 |
| | | F | | | |
| | | Non-pregnant | 1.0–1.8 | | 1.0–1.8 |
| | | Second stage of labor | 3.2–5.3 | | 3.2–5.3 |
| Parathyroid hormone, intact Values (6 days–<3 years) based on Abbott Architect method | S | | pg/mL | 0.106 | pmol/L |
| | | 6 days–<1 year | 6–89 | | 0.7–9.4 |
| | | 1–<3 years | 16–63 | | 1.7–6.7 |
| Values (3–79 years) based on DiaSorin LIAISON method | | 3–5 years | 7–29 | | 0.7–3.1 |
| | | 6–11 years | 7–30 | | 0.7–3.2 |
| | | 12–15 years | 8–36 | | 0.8–3.8 |
| | | 16–29 years | 8–32 | | 0.8–3.4 |
| | | 30–79 years | 9–42 | | 1.0–4.4 |
| Parathyroid hormone, (1–84) | S | | pg/mL | 1.0 | ng/L |
| | | | 6–40 | | 6–40 |
| pH (37°C) | WB | | pH | 1.0 | pH |
| | | Cord blood | | | |
| | | Arterial | 7.18–7.38 | | 7.18–7.38 |
| | | Venous | 7.25–7.45 | | 7.25–7.45 |
| | | Newborn | | | |
| | | Premature, 48 h | 7.35–7.50 | | 7.35–7.50 |
| | | Full-term | | | |
| | | Birth | 7.11–7.36 | | 7.11–7.36 |
| | | 5–10 min | 7.09–7.30 | | 7.09–7.30 |
| | | 30 min | 7.21–7.38 | | 7.21–7.38 |
| | | 1 h | 7.26–7.49 | | 7.26–7.49 |
| | | 1 day | 7.29–7.45 | | 7.29–7.45 |
| | | Children, adults | | | |
| | | Arterial | 7.35–7.45 | | 7.35–7.45 |
| Pediatric values for venous pH were established by CALIPER on Radiometer ABL90 Plus (POCT system) | | Venous, children | 7.31–7.41 | | 7.31–7.41 |
| | | Venous, adults | 7.32–7.43 | | 7.32–7.43 |
| | | Adults | | | |
| | | 60–90 years | 7.31–7.42 | | 7.31–7.42 |
| | | >90 years | 7.26–7.43 | | 7.26–7.43 |
| Phenylalanine | | | mg/dL | 60.5 | μmol/L |
| | Dry blood spot | | <2.1 | | <122 |
| | P | Premature | 2.0–7.5 | | 121–454 |

## TABLE A.1   Pediatric and Adult Reference Intervals for Biochemical Markers—cont'd

| Analyte | Specimen | Condition | REFERENCE INTERVALS | | |
|---|---|---|---|---|---|
| | | | Conventional Units | Conversion Factor | SI Units |
| | | Newborn | 1.2–3.4 | | 73–205 |
| | | Phenylketonuric 2–3 days | >4.5 | | >272 |
| | | Phenylketonuric untreated | 15–30 | | 907–1815 |
| | | Adult | 0.8–1.8 | | 48–109 |
| | S | 0–<2 week | 0.81–1.77 | | 49–107 |
| | | 2 week–<1 year | 0.86–1.92 | | 52–116 |
| | | 1–<19 years | 0.91–1.67 | | 55–101 |
| | | | mg/day | 6.05 | µmol/day |
| | U, 24 h | 10 days–7 weeks | 1.2–1.7 | | 7–10 |
| | | 3–13 years | 4.0–17.5 | | 24–106 |
| | | Adult | <16.5 | | <100 |
| | | | mg/g creatinine | 0.68 | mmol/mol creatinine |
| | | Adult | 2–10 | | 1.3–6.9 |
| Phosphate | S | | mg/dL | 0.323 | mmol/L |
| Values (0–<3 years) based on Abbott Architect method | | 0–14 days | 5.6–10.5 | | 1.80–3.40 |
| | | 15 days–<1 year | 4.8–8.4 | | 1.54–2.72 |
| | | 1–<3 years | 4.3–6.8 | | 1.38–2.19 |
| Values (3–79 years) based on OCD VITROS method | | 3–5 years | 4.4–6.0 | | 1.41–1.94 |
| | | 6–10 years | 4.4–5.7 | | 1.41–1.85 |
| | | 11–15 years M | 3.8–5.9 | | 1.24–1.91 |
| | | 11–15 years F | 3.6–5.6 | | 1.16–1.81 |
| | | 16–47 years | 2.9–4.7 | | 0.95–1.52 |
| | | 48–79 years M | 2.8–4.7 | | 0.89–1.52 |
| | | 48–79 years F | 3.1–4.8 | | 0.99–1.54 |
| | U, 24 h | | g/day | 32.3 | mmol/day |
| | | Adults | 0.4–1.3 | | 12.9–42.0 |
| Phosphatase, acid tartrate resistant 37°C | S | | U/L | 0.017 | µkat/L |
| | | Children | 3.4–9.0 | | 0.05–0.15 |
| | | Adult | 1.5–4.5 | | 0.03–0.08 |
| Phosphatase, alkaline IFCC, 37°C | S | | U/L | 0.017 | µkat/L |
| Values (0–<3 years) based on Abbott Architect method | | 0–14 days | 90–273 | | 1.50–4.55 |
| | | 15 days–<1 year | 134–518 | | 2.23–8.63 |
| | | 1–<3 years | 156–369 | | 2.60–6.15 |
| Values (3–79 years) based on OCD VITROS method | | 3–5 years | 144–327 | | 2.45–5.56 |
| | | 6–10 years | 153–367 | | 2.60–6.24 |
| | | 11–15 years M | 113–438 | | 1.92–7.45 |
| | | 11–15 years F | 64–359 | | 1.09–6.10 |
| | | 16–21 years M | 56–167 | | 0.95–2.84 |
| | | 16–29 years F | 44–107 | | 0.75–1.82 |
| | | 22–79 years M | 50–116 | | 0.85–1.97 |
| | | 30–79 years F | 46–122 | | 0.78–2.07 |
| Phosphatase, alkaline (bone specific, by immunoabsorption) | S | | U/L | 1.0 | U/L |
| | | M | 15.0–41.3 | | 15.0–41.3 |
| | | Premenopausal female | 11.6–29.6 | | 11.6–29.6 |

| Phosphatase, alkaline isoenzymes | | | | | |
|---|---|---|---|---|---|
| Percentage of Total Activity | <1 year | 1–15 years | Adult | Pregnant female | Postmenopausal female |
| Biliary | 3–6 | 2–5 | 1–3 | 1–3 | 0–12 |

*Continued*

## TABLE A.1　Pediatric and Adult Reference Intervals for Biochemical Markers—cont'd

| Analyte | Specimen | Condition | REFERENCE INTERVALS | | |
|---|---|---|---|---|---|
| | | | Conventional Units | Conversion Factor | SI Units |
| Liver | 20–34 | 22–34 | 17–35 | 5–17 | 17–48 |
| Bone | 20–30 | 21–30 | 13–19 | 8–14 | 8–21 |
| Placental | 8–19 | 5–17 | 13–21 | 53–69 | 7–15 |
| Renal | 1–3 | 0–1 | 0–2 | 3–6 | 0–2 |
| Intestinal | 0–2 | 0–1 | 0–1 | 0–1 | 0–1 |
| *Fraction Activity* | <1 year | 1–15 years | Adult | Pregnant female | Postmenopausal female |
| Biliary | 0.03–0.06 | 0.02–0.05 | 0.01–0.03 | 0.01–0.03 | 0.0–0.12 |
| Liver | 0.20–0.34 | 0.22–0.34 | 0.17–0.35 | 0.05–0.17 | 0.17–0.48 |
| Bone | 0.20–0.30 | 0.21–0.30 | 0.13–0.19 | 0.08–0.14 | 0.08–0.21 |
| Placental | 0.08–0.19 | 0.05–0.17 | 0.13–0.21 | 0.53–0.69 | 0.07–0.15 |
| Renal | 0.01–0.03 | 0.0–0.01 | 0.0–0.02 | 0.03–0.06 | 0.0–0.02 |
| Intestinal | 0.0–0.02 | 0.0–0.01 | 0.0–0.01 | 0.0–0.01 | 0.0–0.01 |
| Porphobilinogen | U, 24 h | | mg/L<br><2.26 | 4.42 | μmol/L<br><10 |
| Porphyrins, total | U, 24 h | | | | nmol/L<br>20–320 |
| | Feces | | | | nmol/L g dry wt<br>10–200 |
| | Erythro-cytes | | | | μmol/L erythrocytes<br>0.4–1.7 |
| Potassium (K) | S | | mEq/L | 1.0 | mmol/L |
| | | Premature cord | 5.0–10.2 | | 5.0–10.2 |
| | | Premature, 48 h | 3.0–6.0 | | 3.0–6.0 |
| | | Newborn cord | 5.6–12.0 | | 5.6–12.0 |
| | | Newborn | 3.7–5.9 | | 3.7–5.9 |
| | | Infant | 4.1–5.3 | | 4.1–5.3 |
| Values (0–2 years) based on Siemens ADVIA method | | 0–<1 year, F | 4.2–6.2 | | 4.2–6.2 |
| | | 0–<1 year, M | 4.3–6.7 | | 4.3–6.7 |
| | | 1–2 years | 4.0–5.3 | | 4.0–5.3 |
| Values (3–79 years) based on OCD VITROS method | | 3–5 years | 3.9–4.6 | | 3.9–4.6 |
| | | 6–79 years | 3.8–4.9 | | 3.8–4.9 |
| | U, 24 h | | mEq/day | 1.0 | mmol/day |
| | | 6–10 years M | 17–54 | | 17–54 |
| | | 6–10 years F | 8–37 | | 8–37 |
| | | 10–14 years M | 22–57 | | 22–57 |
| | | 10–14 years F | 18–58 | | 18–58 |
| | | Adult | 25–125 | | 25–125 |
| Values based on Radiometer ABL90 Plus | WB, venous | 0–<19 years | 3.5–4.7 | | 3.5–4.7 |
| Progastrin-Releasing Peptide (ProGRP) | S | | pg/mL | 1.0 | ng/L |
| Values based on Abbott Architect method | | 0–<1 week | 535–1889 | | 535–1889 |
| | | 1 week–<6 m | 57–817 | | 57–817 |
| | | 6 m–<1 year | 25–198 | | 25–198 |
| | | 1–<12 years | 22–129 | | 22–129 |
| | | 12–<19 years | 17–83 | | 17–83 |
| Proinsulin | S | | pmol/L<br>1.1–6.9 | 1.0 | pmol/L<br>1.1–6.9 |
| Prolactin | S | | ng/mL | 21.0 | mIU/L |
| | | Cord blood | 45–539 | | 945–11,319 |
| Values (4 days–<19 years) based on Abbott Architect method | | 4–<30 days | 13–213 | | 273–4473 |
| | | 30 days–<1 year | 6–114 | | 126–2394 |
| | | 1–<19 years | 4–23 | | 84–483 |
| | | Puberty, Tanner Stage 1, M | 3–20 | | 63–420 |

## TABLE A.1   Pediatric and Adult Reference Intervals for Biochemical Markers—cont'd

| Analyte | Specimen | Condition | REFERENCE INTERVALS Conventional Units | Conversion Factor | SI Units |
|---|---|---|---|---|---|
| | | 1, F | 2–20 | | 42–420 |
| | | 2, M | 4–19 | | 84–399 |
| | | 2, F | 4–23 | | 84–483 |
| | | 3, M | 4–23 | | 84–483 |
| | | 3, F | 4–23 | | 84–483 |
| | | 4, M | 6–20 | | 126–420 |
| | | 4, F | 6–23 | | 126–483 |
| | | 5, M | 7–32 | | 147–672 |
| | | 5, F | 5–23 | | 105–483 |
| | | Adult M | 3.0–14.7 | | 63.0–308.7 |
| | | Adult F | 3.8–23.0 | | 79.8–483.0 |
| | | Pregnancy, third trimester | 95–473 | | 1995–9933 |
| Proline | P | | mg/dL | 86.9 | µmol/L |
| | | Premature, 1 day | 0.92–4.36 | | 80–380 |
| | | Newborn, 1 day | 1.23–3.18 | | 107–277 |
| | | 1–3 months | 0.89–3.73 | | 77–325 |
| | | 9 months–2 years | 0.59–2.13 | | 51–185 |
| | | 3–10 years | 0.78–1.70 | | 68–148 |
| | | 6–18 years | 0.67–3.72 | | 58–324 |
| | S | 0–<1 year | 1.46–3.36 | | 127–292 |
| | | 1–<13 years | 1.36–4.28 | | 118–372 |
| | | 13–<19 years | 1.33–4.14 | | 116–360 |
| | | Adult | 1.17–3.86 | | 102–336 |
| | U, 24 h | | mg/day | 8.69 | µmol/day |
| | | 10 days–7 weeks | 3.2–11.0 | | 28–96 |
| | | 3–12 years | Trace | | Trace |
| | | Adult | Trace | | Trace |
| | | | µmol/g creatinine | 0.113 | µmol/mol creatinine |
| | | 0–1 month | 70–2300 | | 7.91–259.9 |
| | | 1–6 months | <600 | | <67.8 |
| | | 6 months–1 year | <300 | | <33.9 |
| | | 1–2 years | <270 | | <30.5 |
| | | 2–3 years | <220 | | <24.9 |
| Prostate-specific antigen (PSA) | S | | ng/mL | 1.0 | µg/L |
| Pediatric values based on Abbott Architect | | Free PSA | | | |
| | | 0–<12 years M | <0.008 | | <0.008 |
| | | 12–<19 years M | <0.008–0.279 | | <0.008–0.279 |
| | | 0–<19 years F | <0.008–0.097 | | <0.008–0.097 |
| | | Total PSA | | | |
| | | 1 week–<6 months M | <0.008–0.038 | | <0.008–0.038 |
| | | 6 months–<12 years M | <0.008–0.353 | | <0.008–0.353 |
| | | 12–<19 years M | <0.008–0.566 | | <0.008–0.566 |
| | | 0–<1 week F | <0.008–0.039 | | <0.008–0.039 |
| | | 1 week–<1 year F | <0.008–0.010 | | <0.008–0.010 |
| | | 1–<19 years F | <0.008–0.015 | | <0.008–0.015 |
| | | Adult M | | | |
| | | 40–49 years | 0–2.5 | | 0–2.5 |
| | | 50–59 years | 0–3.5 | | 0–3.5 |
| | | 60–69 years | 0–4.5 | | 0–4.5 |
| | | 70–79 years | 0–6.5 | | 0–6.5 |
| Protein, total | | | g/dL | 10 | g/L |
| | | Cord | 4.8–8.0 | | 48–80 |

*Continued*

## TABLE A.1    Pediatric and Adult Reference Intervals for Biochemical Markers—cont'd

| Analyte | Specimen | Condition | Conventional Units | Conversion Factor | SI Units |
|---|---|---|---|---|---|
| | S | Premature | 3.6–6.0 | | 36–60 |
| Values (0–<3 years) based on Abbott Architect method | | 0–14 days | 5.3–8.3 | | 53–83 |
| | | 15 days–<1 year | 4.4–7.1 | | 44–71 |
| | | 1–<3 years | 6.1–7.5 | | 61–75 |
| Values (3–79 years) based on OCD VITROS method | | 3–5 years | 6.3–8.1 | | 63–81 |
| | | 6–19 years | 6.8–8.2 | | 68–82 |
| | | 20–29 years | 6.5–8.3 | | 65–83 |
| | | 30–79 years | 6.5–7.8 | | 65–78 |
| | U, 24 h | | mg/dL | 10 | mg/L |
| | | Adult | 1–14 | | 10–140 |
| | Excretion | | mg/day | 0.001 | g/day |
| | | Adult | <100 | | <0.1 |
| | | Pregnancy | <150 | | <0.15 |
| Pyruvic acid | | | mg/dL | 0.114 | µmol/L |
| | WB, arterial | Adult | 0.2–0.7 | | 0.02–0.08 |
| | WB, venous | Adult | 0.3–0.9 | | 0.03–0.10 |
| | | | | | mmol/day |
| | U, 24 h | Adult | | | <1.1 |
| | | | | | mmol/mol creatinine |
| | U | 0–1 month | | | 24–123 |
| | | 1–6 months | | | 8–90 |
| | | 6 months–5 years | | | 3–19 |
| | | >5 years | | | 6–9 |
| Remnant cholesterol (calculated) | S | | mg/dL | 0.0259 | mmol/L |
| Calculated pediatric values based on Abbott Architect method | 0–<14 days | | 16.2–50.6 | | 0.42–1.31 |
| | 14 days–<1 year | | 10.4–51.7 | | 0.27–1.34 |
| | 1–<19 years | | 8.88–39.0 | | 0.23–1.01 |
| Retinol-binding protein (RBP) | S | | mg/dL | 10 | mg/L |
| | | Birth | 1.1–3.4 | | 11–34 |
| | | 6 months | 1.8–5.0 | | 18–50 |
| | | Adult | 3.0–6.0 | | 30–60 |
| Rheumatoid factor (RF) | S | | IU/mL | 1 | kIU/L |
| Values (0–<19 years) based on Abbott Architect method | | 0–14 days | 9.0–17.1 | | 9.0–17.1 |
| | | 15 days–<19 years | 9.0–9.0 | | 9.0–9.0 |
| | | Adult | <7.5–14 | | <7.5–14 |
| Riboflavin (vitamin B2) | | | µg/dL | 26.6 | nmol/L |
| | S | | 4–24 | | 106–638 |
| | Erythrocytes | | 10–50 | | 266–1330 |
| | | | µg/g creatinine | 0.3 | µmol/mol creatinine |
| | U | | >80 | | >24 |
| | | | µg/day | 2 .66 | nmol/day |
| | U, 24 h | | >100 | | >266 |
| Selenium | S | | µg/L | 0.0127 | µmol/L |
| | | Neonates | <8.0 (deficiency) | | <0.10 (deficiency) |
| | | <2 years | 16–71 | | 0.2–0.9 |
| | | 2–4 years | 40–103 | | 0.5–1.3 |
| | | 4–16 years | 55–134 | | 0.7–1.7 |
| | | Adults | 63–160 | | 0.8–2.0 |
| | WB (Hep) | | 58–234 | | 0.74–2.97 |
| | U, 24 h | | 7–160 | | 0.09–2.03 |
| | | Toxic conc. | >400 | | >5.08 |
| Sex hormone-binding globulin (SHBG) | S | | nmol/L | 1 | nmol/L |

## TABLE A.1   Pediatric and Adult Reference Intervals for Biochemical Markers—cont'd

| Analyte | Specimen | Condition | REFERENCE INTERVALS Conventional Units | Conversion Factor | SI Units |
|---|---|---|---|---|---|
| Values (4 days–<19 years) based on Abbott Architect method | | 4 days–<1 month | 14.4–120.2 | | 14.4–120.2 |
| | | 1 month–<1 year | 36.2–229.0 | | 36.2–229.0 |
| | | 1–<8 years | 41.8–188.7 | | 41.8–188.7 |
| | | 8–<11 years | 26.4–162.4 | | 26.4–162.4 |
| | | 11–<13 years | 14.9–107.8 | | 14.9–107.8 |
| | | 13–<15 years | 11.2–98.2 | | 11.2–98.2 |
| | | 15–<19 years M | 9.7–49.6 | | 9.7–49.6 |
| | | 15–<17 years F | 9.8–84.1 | | 9.8–84.1 |
| | | 17–<19 years F | 10.8–154.6 | | 10.8–154.6 |
| | | Puberty, Tanner Stage | | | |
| Tanner values based on Abbott Architect method | | 1 M | 23.4–156.8 | | 23.4–156.8 |
| | | 1, F | 21.1–210.1 | | 21.1–210.1 |
| | | 2, M | 27.5–133.4 | | 27.5–133.4 |
| | | 2, F | 29.6–140.7 | | 29.6–140.7 |
| | | 3, M | 17.4–160.1 | | 17.4–160.1 |
| | | 3, F | 23.7–101.7 | | 23.7–101.7 |
| | | 4, M | 12.2–79.4 | | 12.2–79.4 |
| | | 4, F | 12.1–125.6 | | 12.1–125.6 |
| | | 5, M | 7.7–49.4 | | 7.7–49.4 |
| | | 5, F | 15.3–92.5 | | 15.3–92.5 |
| | | Adult | | | |
| | | 20 years | 13.1–53.2 | | 13.1–53.2 |
| | | 30 years | 13.5–57.4 | | 13.5–57.4 |
| | | 40 years | 15.3–65.3 | | 15.3–65.3 |
| | | 50 years | 18.4–75.6 | | 18.4–75.6 |
| | | 60 years | 22.6–87.6 | | 22.6–87.6 |
| | | 70 years | 27.8–101.0 | | 27.8–101.0 |
| | | 80 years | 33.8–115.4 | | 33.8–115.4 |
| Sodium (Na) | | | mEq/L | 1.0 | mmol/L |
| | | Premature cord | 116–140 | | 116–140 |
| | | Premature, 48 h | 128–148 | | 128–148 |
| | | Newborn cord | 126–166 | | 126–166 |
| | | Newborn | 133–146 | | 133–146 |
| | | Infant | 139–146 | | 139–146 |
| Values (0–3 years) based on Siemens ADVIA method | | 0–3 years | 139–146 | | 139–146 |
| Values (3–79 years) based on OCD VITROS method | | 3–5 years | 135–142 | | 135–142 |
| | | 6–15 years | 136–143 | | 136–143 |
| | | 16–49 years M | 137–143 | | 137–143 |
| | | 16–49 years F | 137–142 | | 137–142 |
| | | 50–79 years | 136–143 | | 136–143 |
| | U, 24 h | | mEq/day | 1.0 | mmol/day |
| | | 6–10 years M | 41–115 | | 41–115 |
| | | 6–10 years F | 20–69 | | 20–69 |
| | | 10–14 years M | 63–177 | | 63–177 |
| | | 10–14 years F | 48–168 | | 48–168 |
| | | Adult M | 40–220 | | 40–220 |
| | | Adult F | 27–287 | | 27–287 |
| Values based on Radiometer ABL90 Plus | WB, venous | 0–<5 years | 135–143 | | 135–143 |
| | | 5–<19 years | 138–143 | | 138–143 |
| Testosterone, bioavailable (Vermeulen Equation) | S | | ng/dL | 0.0347 | nmol/L |

*Continued*

## TABLE A.1   Pediatric and Adult Reference Intervals for Biochemical Markers—cont'd

| Analyte | Specimen | Condition | REFERENCE INTERVALS | | |
|---|---|---|---|---|---|
| | | | Conventional Units | Conversion Factor | SI Units |
| Values (0–<19 years) | | 0–<1 year M | 0–121.9 | | 0.01–4.23 |
| based on Abbott | | 1–<9 years M | 0.29–2.88 | | 0.01–0.10 |
| Architect method | | 9–<14 years M | 0.58–161.69 | | 0.02–5.62 |
| | | 14–<19 years M | 12.1–346.69 | | 0.42–12.03 |
| | | 0–<1 year F | 0.29–6.05 | | 0.01–0.21 |
| | | 1–<9 years F | 0.29–6.05 | | 0.01–0.21 |
| | | 9–<14 years F | 0.58–10.95 | | 0.02–0.38 |
| | | 14–<19 years F | 3.75–23.05 | | 0.13–0.80 |
| | | Adult M | 66–417 | | 2.29–14.5 |
| | | Adult F | 0.6–5.0 | | 0.02–0.17 |
| Testosterone, free (Vermeulen Equation) | S | | pg/mL | 3.47 | pmol/L |
| | | Cord M | 5–22 | | 17.4–76.3 |
| | | Cord F | 4–19 | | 13.9–55.5 |
| Values (0–<19 years) | | 0–<1 year M | 0.03–57.2 | | 0.1–198.4 |
| based on Abbott | | 1–<9 years M | 0.1–1.2 | | 0.3–4.0 |
| Architect method | | 9–<14 years M | 0.4–72.2 | | 1.5–250.6 |
| | | 14–<19 years M | 5.0–142.4 | | 17.4–494.0 |
| | | 0–<1 year F | 0.1–2.6 | | 0.3–9.1 |
| | | 1–<9 years F | 0.1–2.6 | | 0.3–9.1 |
| | | 9–<14 years F | 0.3–4.7 | | 1.0–16.4 |
| | | 14–<19 years F | 1.4–9.9 | | 4.9–34.3 |
| | | Adult M | 50–210 | | 174–729 |
| | | Adult F | 1.0–8.5 | | 3.5–29.5 |
| Testosterone, total | S | | ng/dL | 0.0347 | nmol/L |
| | | Cord M | 13–55 | | 0.45–1.91 |
| | | Cord F | 5–45 | | 0.17–1.56 |
| | | Premature M | 37–198 | | 1.28–6.87 |
| | | Premature F | 5–22 | | 0.17–0.76 |
| Values (4 days–<19 years) | | 4 days–<6 months M | 9–299 | | 0.3–10.37 |
| based on Abbott | | 6 months–<9 years M | <36 | | <1.24 |
| Architect method | | 9–<11 years M | <23 | | <0.81 |
| | | 11–<14 years M | <444 | | <15.42 |
| | | 14–<16 years M | 36–632 | | 1.25–21.94 |
| | | 16–<19 years M | 148–794 | | 5.13–27.55 |
| | | 4 days–<9 years F | 1–62 | | 0.0–2.15 |
| | | 9–<13 years F | <28 | | <0.98 |
| | | 13–<15 years F | 10–44 | | 0.36–1.54 |
| | | 15–<19 years F | 14–49 | | 0.49–1.70 |
| Tanner values based on | | 1, M | <18 | | <0.62 |
| Abbott Architect method | | 1, F | <19 | | <0.67 |
| | | 2, M | <25 | | <0.85 |
| | | 2, F | <20 | | <0.69 |
| | | 3, M | <543 | | <18.85 |
| | | 3, F | <42 | | <1.45 |
| | | 4, M | 9–636 | | 0.30–22.08 |
| | | 4, F | 9–42 | | 0.31–1.44 |
| | | 5, M | 100–760 | | 3.46–26.36 |
| | | 5, F | 4–50 | | 0.13–1.72 |
| | | Adult M | 260–1000 | | 9–34.72 |
| | | Adult F | 15–70 | | 0.52–2.43 |
| *For LC-MSMS pediatric reference intervals, see: Clin Biochem 2013;46:642–651* | | | | | |
| Thallium | | | µg/L | 4.89 | nmol/L |

## TABLE A.1   Pediatric and Adult Reference Intervals for Biochemical Markers—cont'd

| Analyte | Specimen | Condition | Conventional Units | Conversion Factor | SI Units |
|---|---|---|---|---|---|
| | WB (Hep) | | <5 | | <24 .5 |
| | | | mg/L | | µmol/L |
| | | Toxic | 0.1–8.0 | | 0.5–390 |
| | | | µg/L | 4.89 | nmol/L |
| | U, 24 h | | <2.0 | | <9.8 |
| | | | mg/L | | µmol/L |
| | | Toxic | 1.0–20.0 | | 4.9–97.8 |
| Threonine | P | | mg/dL | 84 | µmol/L |
| | | Premature, 1 day | 1.14–3.98 | | 95–335 |
| | | Newborn, 1 day | 1.36–3.99 | | 114–335 |
| | | 1–3 months | 0.75–2.67 | | 64–224 |
| | | 2–6 months | 2.27–4.33 | | 191–364 |
| | | 3–10 years | 0.50–1.13 | | 42–95 |
| | | 6–18 years | 0.88–2.40 | | 74–202 |
| | | Adult | 0.94–2.30 | | 79–193 |
| | S | 0–<1 year | 0.96–3.73 | | 81–313 |
| | | 1–<19 years | 0.86–2.20 | | 72–185 |
| | U, 24 h | | mg/day | 8.40 | µmol/day |
| | | 10 days–7 weeks | 1.5–11.9 | | 13–100 |
| | | 3–12 years | 10.1–29.6 | | 85–249 |
| | | Adult | 14.3–46.7 | | 120–392 |
| | | | mg/g creatinine | 0.95 | mmol/mol creatinine |
| | | Adult | 0–28 | | 0–27 |
| Thyroglobulin (TG) | S | | ng/mL | 1.0 | µg/L |
| | | 0–<2 years, F | 7.82–79.5 | | 7.82–79.5 |
| | | 0–<2 years, M | 2.99–56.0 | | 2.99–56.0 |
| | | 2–<6 years | 6.74–34.2 | | 6.74–34.2 |
| | | 6–<9 years | 5.01–28.5 | | 5.01–28.5 |
| | | 9–<19 years | 2.50–25.8 | | 2.50–25.8 |
| | | Adult euthyroid | 3–42 | | 3–42 |
| | | Athyroidic patient | <5 | | <5 |
| Thyroid uptake | S | | % | 1.0 | % |
| Pediatric values based on Beckman DxI method | | 0–<12 years | 38.1–49.5 | | 38.1–49.5 |
| | | 12–<19 years, F | 38.1–48.5 | | 38.1–48.5 |
| | | 12–<19 years, M | 39.6–48.8 | | 39.6–48.8 |
| Thyrotropin (thyroid-stimulating hormone) (TSH) | | | µIU/mL | 1.0 | mIU/L |
| | S | Premature, 28–36 weeks | 0.7–27.0 | | 0.7–27.0 |
| | | Cord blood (>37 weeks) | 2.3–13.2 | | 2.3–13.2 |
| Values (4 days–<19 years) based on Abbott Architect method | | 4 days–<6 months | 0.7–4.8 | | 0.7–4.8 |
| | | 6 months–<14 years | 0.7–4.2 | | 0.7–4.2 |
| | | 14–<19 years | 0.5–3.4 | | 0.5–3.4 |
| | | Adults | | | |
| | | 21–54 years | 0.4–4.2 | | 0.4–4.2 |
| | | 55–87 years | 0.5–8.9 | | 0.5–8.9 |
| | | Pregnancy | µU/mL | 1.0 | mU/L |
| | | First trimester | 0.1–2.5 | | 0.1–2.5 |
| | | Second trimester | 0.2–3.0 | | 0.2–3.0 |
| | | Third trimester | 0.3–3.0 | | 0.3–3.0 |
| | WB (heel puncture) | Newborn screen | <20 | | <20 |
| Thyroxine-binding globulin | | | mg/dL | 10 | mg/L |
| | S | Cord | 3.6–9.6 | | 36–96 |
| | | Children | | | |
| | | 4 months–1 year | 3.1–5.6 | | 31–56 |
| | | 1–5 years | 2.9–5.4 | | 29–54 |

*Continued*

## TABLE A.1  Pediatric and Adult Reference Intervals for Biochemical Markers—cont'd

| Analyte | Specimen | Condition | REFERENCE INTERVALS Conventional Units | Conversion Factor | SI Units |
|---|---|---|---|---|---|
| | | 5–10 years | 2.5–5.0 | | 25–50 |
| | | 10–15 years | 2.1–4.6 | | 21–46 |
| | | Adult M | 1.2–2.5 | | 12–25 |
| | | Adult F | 1.4–3.0 | | 14–30 |
| | | Adult F (oral contraceptive) | 1.5–5.5 | | 15–55 |
| Thyroxine (T4), total | | | µg/dL | 12.9 | nmol/L |
| Values (7 days–<19 years) | S | 7 days–<1 year | 5.9–13.7 | | 76–176 |
| based on Abbott | | 1–<9 years | 6.2–10.3 | | 79–133 |
| Architect method | | 9–<12 years | 5.5–9.3 | | 71–120 |
| | | 12–<14 years M | 5.0–8.3 | | 65–107 |
| | | 12–<14 years F | 5.1–8.3 | | 65–107 |
| | | 14–<19 years M | 4.7–8.6 | | 61–111 |
| | | 14–<19 years F | 5.5–13.0 | | 70–167 |
| | | Adult (15–60 years) F | 4.6–10.5 | | 59–135 |
| | | Adult (15–60 years) F | 5.5–11.0 | | 65–138 |
| | | >60 years | 5.0–10.7 | | 65–138 |
| | | Newborn screen | | | |
| | | 1–5 days | >7.5 | | >97 |
| | | 6 days | >6.5 | | >84 |
| Thyroxine, free (FT4) | S | | ng/dL | 12.9 | pmol/L |
| | | Newborns (1–4 days) | 2.2–5.3 | | 28.4–68.4 |
| Values (5 days–<19 years) | | 5–15 days | 1.1–3.2 | | 13.5–41.3 |
| based on Abbott | | 15–<30 days | 0.7–2.5 | | 8.7–32.5 |
| Architect method | | 30 days–<1 year | 0.9–1.7 | | 11.4–21.9 |
| | | 1–<19 years | 0.9–1.4 | | 11.4–17.6 |
| | | Adults (21–87 years) | 0.8–2.7 | | 10.3–34.7 |
| | | Pregnancy | | | |
| | | First trimester | 0.7–2.0 | | 9.0–25.7 |
| | | Second and third trimesters | 0.5–1.6 | | 6.4–20.6 |
| Transferrin | S | | mg/dL | 0.01 | g/L |
| Values (0–<19 years) | | 0–<9 weeks | 104–224 | | 1.0–2.2 |
| based on Abbott | | 9 weeks–<1 year | 107–324 | | 1.1–3.2 |
| Architect method | | 1–<19 years | 220–337 | | 2.2–3.4 |
| | | 20–60 years | 200–360 | | 2.0–3.6 |
| | | >60 years | 160–340 | | 1.6–3.4 |
| Soluble Transferrin Receptor (STfR) | S | | mg/L | | mg/L |
| Values based on Beckman | | 0–<1 year | 0.98–1.99 | | 0.98–1.99 |
| DxI method | | 1–<2.5 years | 1.37–2.64 | | 1.37–2.64 |
| | | 2.5–<14 years | 1.03–2.09 | | 1.03–2.09 |
| | | 14–<19 years | 0.79–1.68 | | 0.79–1.68 |
| Transthyretin (prealbumin) | S | | mg/dL | 10 | mg/L |
| Values (0–<19 years) | | 0–14 days | 2–12 | | 20–120 |
| based on Abbott | | 15 days–<1 year | 5–24 | | 50–240 |
| Architect method | | 1–<5 years | 12–23 | | 120–230 |
| | | 5–<13 years | 14–26 | | 140–260 |
| | | 13–<16 years | 18–31 | | 180–310 |
| | | 16–<19 years M | 20–35 | | 200–350 |
| | | 16–<19 years F | 17–33 | | 170–330 |
| | | Adult (20–60 years) | 20–40 | | 200–400 |
| Triglycerides | S | | mg/dL | 0.0113 | mmol/L |
| *Reference Intervals* | | | | | |
| Values (0–<6 years) based | | 0–14 days | 82–259 | | 0.9–2.9 |
| on Abbott Architect | | 15 days–<1 year | 53–258 | | 0.6–2.9 |
| method | | 1–<6 years | 44–197 | | 0.5–2.2 |

## TABLE A.1   Pediatric and Adult Reference Intervals for Biochemical Markers—cont'd

| Analyte | Specimen | Condition | REFERENCE INTERVALS Conventional Units | Conversion Factor | SI Units |
|---|---|---|---|---|---|
| Values (6–79 years) based on OCD VITROS method | | 6–29 years | 35–186 | | 0.4–2.1 |
| | | 30–79 years M | 44–301 | | 0.5–3.4 |
| | | 30–79 years F | 35–212 | | 0.4–2.4 |
| *Clinical Decision Limits* | | Recommended cut-off points, Child 0–9 years | mg/dL | 0.0113 | mmol/L |
| | | Acceptable | <75 | | <0.9 |
| | | Borderline | 75–99 | | 0.9–1.1 |
| | | High | ≥100 | | ≥1.1 |
| | | 10–19 years | | | |
| | | Acceptable | <90 | | <1.0 |
| | | Borderline | 90–129 | | 1.0–1.5 |
| | | High | ≥130 | | ≥1.5 |
| | | Recommended cut-off points, Adult | mg/dL | 0.0113 | mmol/L |
| | | Normal | <150 | | <1.70 |
| | | High | 150–199 | | 1.70–2.25 |
| | | Hypertriglyceridemic | 200–499 | | 2.26–5.64 |
| | | Very high | >499 | | >5.64 |
| Triiodothyronine (T3), free | | | pg/dL | 0.0154 | pmol/L |
| | S | Cord | 15–391 | | 0.2–6.0 |
| Values (4 days–<19 years) based on Abbott Architect method | | 4 days–<1 year | 232–487 | | 3.6–7.5 |
| | | 1–<12 years | 279–442 | | 4.3–6.8 |
| | | 12–<15 years M | 289–433 | | 4.4–6.7 |
| | | 12–<15 years F | 247–395 | | 3.8–6.1 |
| | | 15–<19 years M | 225–385 | | 3.5–5.9 |
| | | 15–<19 years F | 231–371 | | 3.6–5.7 |
| | | Adult | 210–440 | | 3.2–6.8 |
| | | Pregnancy | 200–380 | | 3.1–5.9 |
| Triiodothyronine (T3), total | S | | ng/dL | 0.0154 | nmol/L |
| | | Cord (>37 weeks) | 5–141 | | 0.08–2.17 |
| Values (4 days–<19 years) based on Abbott Architect method | | 4 days–<1 year | 85–234 | | 1.33–3.60 |
| | | 1–<12 years | 113–189 | | 1.74–2.91 |
| | | 12–<15 years | 98–176 | | 1.50–2.71 |
| | | 15–<17 years M | 94–156 | | 1.44–2.40 |
| | | 15–<17 years F | 92–142 | | 1.42–2.18 |
| | | 17–<19 years | 90–168 | | 1.38–2.58 |
| | | Adults | | | |
| | | 20–50 years | 70–204 | | 1.08–3.14 |
| | | 50–90 years | 40–181 | | 0.62–2.79 |
| | | Pregnancy | | | |
| | | First trimester | 81–190 | | 1.25–2.93 |
| | | Second and third trimesters | 100–260 | | 1.54–4.00 |
| Troponin I, high sensitivity | S | | ng/L | 1 | ng/L |
| Values based on Abbott Architect method, 99th percentile | | 0–<19 years | <33.6 | | <33.6 |
| Troponin T, high sensitivity | S | | ng/L | 1 | ng/L |
| Values based on Roche Cobas method, 99th percentile | | 0–<6 m | <93 | | <93 |
| | | 6 m–<1 year | <21 | | <21 |
| | | 1–<19 years, F | <11 | | <11 |
| | | 1–<19 years, M | <14 | | <14 |
| | | NOTE: Refer to manufacturer 99th percentiles for interpretation in adult males and females | | | |
| Tryptophan | | | mg/dL | 49 | µmol/L |
| | P | Premature, 1 day | 0–1.23 | | 0–60 |
| | | Newborn, 1 day | <1.37 | | <67 |

*Continued*

## TABLE A.1   Pediatric and Adult Reference Intervals for Biochemical Markers—cont'd

| Analyte | Specimen | Condition | Conventional Units | Conversion Factor | SI Units |
|---|---|---|---|---|---|
| | | 1–16 years | 0.49–1.61 | | 24–79 |
| | | >16 years | 0.41–1.94 | | 20–95 |
| | | | mg/day | 4.9 | µmol/day |
| | U, 24 h | Adult | 5–39 | | 25–191 |
| | | | mg/g creatinine | 0.55 | mmol/mol creatinine |
| | | Adult | <30 | | <16.5 |
| Tyrosine | P | | mg/dL | 55.2 | mmol/L |
| | | Premature, 1 day | 0–5.79 | | 0–320 |
| | | Newborn, 1 day | 0.76–1.79 | | 42–99 |
| | | 1–3 months | 0.54–2.42 | | 30–134 |
| | | 2–6 months | 1.30–3.91 | | 72–216 |
| | | 9 months–2 years | 0.20–2.21 | | 11–122 |
| | | 3–10 years | 0.56–1.29 | | 31–71 |
| | | 6–18 years | 0.78–1.59 | | 43–88 |
| | | Adult | 0.40–1.58 | | 22–87 |
| | S | 0–<2 week | 0.49–3.39 | | 27–187 |
| | | 2 week–<1 year | 0.62–2.74 | | 34–151 |
| | | 1–<13 years | 0.82–2.28 | | 45–126 |
| | | 13–<19 years | 0.62–1.59 | | 34–88 |
| | U, 24 h | | mg/day | 5.52 | µmol/day |
| | | 10 days–7 weeks | 4.0–7.2 | | 22–40 |
| | | 3–12 years | 7.2–30.4 | | 40–168 |
| | | Adult | 12.0–55.1 | | 66–304 |
| | | | mg/g creatinine | 0.62 | mmol/mol creatinine |
| | | Adult | 0–23 | | 0–14.2 |
| Urea | S | | mg/dL | 0.357 | mmol/L |
| Values (0–<3 years) based | | 0–<14 days | 3–23 | | 1.0–8.2 |
| on Abbott Architect | | 15 days–<1 year | 3–17 | | 1.2–6.0 |
| method | | 1–<3 years | 9–22 | | 3.2–7.9 |
| Values (3–79) based on | | 3–5 years | 9–19 | | 3.1–6.9 |
| OCD VITROS method | | 6–7 years | 8–21 | | 2.8–7.5 |
| | | 8–19 years M | 8–20 | | 2.9–7.0 |
| | | 20–39 years M | 9–22 | | 3.3–7.9 |
| | | 40–59 years M | 10–24 | | 3.5–8.6 |
| | | 8–59 years F | 8–19 | | 2.7–6.7 |
| | | 60–79 years | 10–26 | | 3.6–9.2 |
| | U, 24 h | | g/day | 0.0357 | mol/day |
| | | | 10–20 | | 0.43–0.71 |
| Urea Creatinine Ratio | S | | mg/dL/mg/dL | 4.04 | µmol/L/ µmol/L |
| (UCR) | | | | | |
| Values based on Abbott | | 0–<15 days | 5–40 | | 21–162 |
| Architect method, | | 15 days–<1 year | 12–108 | | 49–438 |
| Enzymatic | | 1–<3 years | 31–104 | | 127–419 |
| | | 3–<5 years | 32–74 | | 130–299 |
| | | 5–<8 years | 22–61 | | 87–246 |
| | | 8–<10 years, F | 17–44 | | 69–177 |
| | | 8–<10 years, M | 21–47 | | 83–189 |
| | | 10–<15 years | 12–36 | | 50–146 |
| Uric acid | | 15–<19 years | 11–26 | | 44–107 |
| Values (0–<3 years) based | | 0–14 days | 2.8–12.7 | | 167–755 |
| on Abbott Architect | | 15 days–<1 year | 1.6–6.3 | | 95–375 |
| method | | 1–<3 years | 1.8–4.9 | | 107–291 |
| Values (3–79 years) based | | 3–<5 years | 2.0–4.9 | | 117–291 |
| on OCD VITROS method | | 6–8 years | 1.9–5.0 | | 116–295 |
| | | 9–10 years | 2.4–5.5 | | 142–326 |
| | | 11–12 years | 2.6–5.8 | | 156–345 |
| | | 13–79 years M | 3.7–7.7 | | 218–459 |
| | | 13–79 years F | 2.5–6.2 | | 147–366 |

## TABLE A.1    Pediatric and Adult Reference Intervals for Biochemical Markers—cont'd

| Analyte | Specimen | Condition | REFERENCE INTERVALS | | |
| --- | --- | --- | --- | --- | --- |
| | | | Conventional Units | Conversion Factor | SI Units |
| Valine | P | | mg/dL | 85.5 | µmol/L |
| | | Premature, 1 day | 0.34–2.70 | | 30–230 |
| | | Newborn, 1 day | 0.94–2.88 | | 80–246 |
| | | 1–3 months | 1.13–3.4 1 | | 96–292 |
| | | 9 months–2 years | 0.67–3.07 | | 57–262 |
| | | 3–10 years | 1.50–3.31 | | 128–283 |
| | | 6–18 years | 1.83–3.37 | | 156–288 |
| | | Adult | 1.65–3.71 | | 141–317 |
| | S | 0–<2 week | 1.02–3.81 | | 87–326 |
| | | 2 week–<13 years | 1.50–4.22 | | 128–361 |
| | | 13–<19 years, F | 1.81–3.03 | | 155–259 |
| | | 13–<19 years, M | 1.94–3.52 | | 166–301 |
| | U | | mg/day | 8.55 | µmol/day |
| | | 10 days–7 weeks | 1.4–3.2 | | 12–27 |
| | | 3–12 years | 1.8–6.0 | | 15–51 |
| | | Adult | 2.5–11.9 | | 21–102 |
| | | | mg/g creatinine | 0.97 | mmol/mol creatinine |
| | | Adult | 2–6 | | 1.9–5.9 |
| Vanillylmandelic acid (VMA) | U, 24 h | | mg/day | 5.05 | µmol/day |
| | | 3–6 years | 1.0–2.6 | | 5–13 |
| | | 6–10 years | 2.0–3.2 | | 10–16 |
| | | 10–16 years | 2.3–5.2 | | 12–26 |
| | | 16–83 years | 1.4–6.5 | | 7–33 |
| | | | mg/g creatinine | 0.571 | mmol/mol creatinine |
| | U | 0–1 month | <27 | | <16 |
| | | 1–6 months | <19 | | <11 |
| | | 6 months–5 years | <13 | | <8 |
| | | 3–6 years | 4.0–10.8 | | 2.3–6.2 |
| | | 6–10 years | 4.0–7.5 | | 2.3–4.3 |
| | | 10–16 years | 3.0–8.8 | | 1.7–5.0 |
| Vitamin A | S | | µg/dL | 0.0349 | µmol/L |
| Values (0–<19 years) | | 0–<1 year | 8–54 | | 0.3–1.9 |
| based on Abbott | | 1–<11 year | 28–44 | | 1.0–1.6 |
| Architect method | | 11–<16 years | 25–55 | | 0.9–1.9 |
| | | 16–<19 years | 29–75 | | 1.0–2.6 |
| | | Adult | 30–80 | | 1.05–2.8 |
| Vitamin B1 (thiamine diphosphate) | | | nmol/L | 1 | nmol/L |
| | WB | | 90–140 | | 90–140 |
| | | | ng/g Hb | 0.146 | µmol/mol Hb |
| | Erythro-cytes | | 280–590 | | 40.3–85.0 |
| Vitamin B2 (see riboflavin) | | | | | |
| Vitamin B6 | P (EDTA) | | ng/mL | 4.046 | nmol/L |
| | | | 5–30 | | 20–121 |
| | | Deficiency | <5 | | <20 |
| Vitamin B12 | S | | ng/L | 0.733 | pmol/L |
| *Reference Intervals* | | | | | |
| Values (5 days–< 3 years) | | 5 days–<1 year | 259–1576 | | 191–1163 |
| based on Abbott | | 1–<3 years | 283–1613 | | 209–1190 |
| Architect method | | | | | |
| Values (3–79 years) based | | 3–5 years | 310–988 | | 229–729 |
| on Siemens IMMULITE | | | | | |
| method | | | | | |
| | | 6–8 years | 321–985 | | 237–727 |
| | | 9–11 year | 276–969 | | 204–715 |
| | | 12–79 years | 188–908 | | 139–670 |

*Continued*

## TABLE A.1 Pediatric and Adult Reference Intervals for Biochemical Markers—cont'd

| Analyte | Specimen | Condition | Conventional Units | Conversion Factor | SI Units |
|---|---|---|---|---|---|
| | | | **REFERENCE INTERVALS** | | |
| *Clinical Decision Limits* | | | | | |
| | | Acceptable (WHO) | >201 | | >147 |
| | | Deficiency (WHO) | <150 | | <110 |
| Vitamin C (ascorbic acid) | S | | mg/dL | 56.78 | µmol/L |
| | | | 0.4–1.5 | | 23–85 |
| | | Deficiency | <0.2 | | <11 |
| | | | µg/$10^8$ leukocytes | 0.057 | fmol/$10^8$ leukocytes |
| | Leukocyte | | 20–53 | | 1.14–3.01 |
| | | | µg/$10^8$ leukocytes | 0.057 | fmol/$10^8$ leukocytes |
| | | Deficiency | <10 | | <0.57 |
| Vitamin D 25(OH)D | S | | ng/mL | 2.5 | nmol/L |
| Values (5 days–<3 years) | | 5–<15 days | 2–34 | | 4–85 |
| based on Abbott | | 15 days–<3 months | 6–41 | | 15–101 |
| Architect method | | 3 months–<1 year | 7–47 | | 17–118 |
| | | 1–<3 years | 13–55 | | 33–137 |
| Values (3–79 years) based on | P | 3–5 years | 13–42 | | 33–104 |
| DiaSorin LIAISON method | | 6–79 years | 8–46 | | 21–116 |
| | | Deficiency | <20 | | <50 |
| Vitamin D (1,25(OH)$_2$) | | | pg/mL | 2.4 | pmol/L |
| Pediatric values based | | 0–<1 year | 32.1–196 | | 77–471 |
| on DiaSorin LIAISON | | 1–<3 years | 47.1–151 | | 113–363 |
| method | | 3–<19 years | 45.0–102 | | 108–246 |
| | | | 15–60 | | 36–144 |
| Vitamin E | S | | mg/dL | 23.2 | µmol/L |
| | | Premature neonates | 0.1–0.5 | | 2.3–11.6 |
| Values (0–<19 years) | | 0–<1 year | 0.2–2.1 | | 4.9–49.6 |
| based on Abbott | | 1–<19 years | 0.6–1.4 | | 14.5–33.0 |
| Architect method | | Adults | 0.5–1.8 | | 12–42 |
| Vitamin E: Total cholesterol ratio | | 1–19 years | | | 3.7–6.7 |
| Vitamin E: Triglyceride ratio | | 1–19 years | | | 8.5–44.5 |
| Vitamin K | S | | ng/mL | 2.22 | nmol/L |
| | | | 0.13–1.19 | | 0.29–2.64 |
| Zinc | S | | µg/dL | 0.153 | µmol/L |
| | | | 80–120 | | 12–18 |
| | | Deficiency | <30 | | <5 |
| | | | mg/24 h | 15.3 | µmol/24 h |
| | U, 24 h | | 0.2–1.3 | | 3–21 |

KDIGO Clinical practice guideline for the evaluation and management of chronic kidney disease. *Kidney Int Suppl*. 2013;3. Available http://www.kdigo.org/clinical_practice_guidelines/pdf/CKD/KDIGO_2012_CKD_GL.pdf.

Raizman JE, Cohen AH, Teodoro-Morrison T, et al. Pediatric reference value distributions for vitamins A and E in the CALIPER cohort and establishment of age-stratified reference intervals. *Clin Biochem*. 2014;47:812–815.

Raizman JE, Quinn F, Armbruster DA, Adeli K. Pediatric reference intervals for calculated free testosterone, bioavailable testosterone and free androgen index in the CALIPER cohort. *Clin Chem Lab Med*. 2015;53:e239–e243.

Stagnaro-Green A, Abalovich M, Alexander E, et al. Guidelines of the American Thyroid Association for the diagnosis and management of thyroid disease during pregnancy and postpartum. *Thyroid*. 2011;21:1081–1125.

Thomas L. Critical limits of laboratory results for urgent clinician notification. *eJIFCC*. 2003;14. Available http://www.ifcc.org/ifccfiles/docs/140103200303.pdf.

World Health Organization. Use of glycated hemoglobin A$_{1c}$ in the diagnosis of diabetes mellitus. World Health Organization. 2011;1–25.

For additional information regarding the sources of specific presented data, refer to *Tietz Textbook of Clinical Chemistry and Molecular Diagnostics*, 8th ed., 2020.

## TABLE A.2   Pediatric and Adult Critical Risk Values

| Parameter | CONVENTIONAL UNITS | | SI UNITS | |
| --- | --- | --- | --- | --- |
| | Lower Limit | Upper Limit | Lower Limit | Upper Limit |
| Albumin (children) | g/dL | | g/L | |
| | 1.7 | 6.8 | 17 | 68 |
| Aminotransferases | U/L | | μkat/L | |
| | — | 1,000 | — | 16.7 |
| Ammonia | μg/dL | | μmol/L | |
| | — | 187 | — | 110 |
| Anion gap | | | mmol/L | |
| | | | — | 20 |
| Bilirubin (newborn) | mg/dL | | mmol/L | |
| | — | 15 | — | 257 |
| Calcium (total) | mg/dL | | mmol/L | |
| | 6.6 | 14 | 1.65 | 3.5 |
| Calcium (children) | mg/dL | | mmol/L | |
| | 6.5 | 12.7 | 1.63 | 3.18 |
| Calcium (free) | mg/dL | | mmol/L | |
| | 3.1 | 6.3 | 0.75 | 1.6 |
| Carbon dioxide, total | | | mmol/L | |
| | | | 10 | 40 |
| Chloride (adult) | | | mmol/L | |
| | | | 80 | 120 |
| Creatinine (adult) | mg/dL | | mmol/L | |
| | — | 5 | — | 442 |
| Creatinine (children) | mg/dL | | μmol/L | |
| | — | 3.8 | — | 336 |
| Creatine kinase | U/L | | μkat/L | |
| | — | 1,000 | — | 16.7 |
| Glucose | mg/dL | | mmol/L | |
| | 40 | 500 | 2.22 | 27.8 |
| Glucose (children) | mg/dL | | mmol/L | |
| | 46 | 445 | 2.56 | 24.72 |
| Glucose (newborn) | mg/dL | | mmol/L | |
| | 30 | 325 | 1.67 | 18.06 |
| Glucose, CSF (adult) | mg/dL | | mmol/L | |
| | 40 | 200 | 2.22 | 11.11 |
| Glucose, CSF (children) | mg/dL | | mmol/L | |
| | 31 | — | 1.72 | — |
| Lactate plasma | mg/dL | | mmol/L | |
| | — | 45 | — | 5 |
| Lactate plasma (children) | mg/dL | | mmol/L | |
| | — | 36.9 | — | 4.1 |
| Lactate dehydrogenase | U/L | | μkat/L | |
| | — | 1,000 | — | 16.7 |
| Lipase | U/L | | μkat/L | |
| | — | 700 | — | 11.7 |
| Magnesium | mg/dL | | mmol/L | |
| | 1 | 4.9 | 0.41 | 2 |
| Osmolality | | | mOsm/kg | |
| | | | 240 | 330 |
| Osmolar gap | | | mOsm/kg | |
| | | | — | 10 |
| Phosphate | mg/dL | | mmol/L | |
| | 1 | 9 | 0.32 | 2.9 |
| Potassium | | | mmol/L | |
| | | | 2.8 | 6.2 |
| Potassium (newborn) | | | mmol/L | |
| | | | 2.8 | 7.8 |
| Protein (children) | g/dL | | g/L | |

*Continued*

## TABLE A.2 Pediatric and Adult Critical Risk Values—cont'd

| Parameter | CONVENTIONAL UNITS Lower Limit | Upper Limit | SI UNITS Lower Limit | Upper Limit |
|---|---|---|---|---|
| Protein, CSF (children) | 3.4 mg/dL | 9.5 | 34 mg/L | 95 |
| Sodium | — | 188 mmol/L | — | 1,880 |
| T4 (free) | 120 ng/dL | 160 | pmol/L | |
| Urea nitrogen | — mg/dL | 3.5 | — mmol/L | 45 |
| Urea | — mg/dL | 100 | — mmol/L | 35.6 |
| Urea nitrogen (children) | — mg/dL | 214 | — mmol/L | 35.6 |
| Uric acid | — mg/dL | 55 | — mmol/L | 19.6 |
| Uric acid (children) | — mg/dL | 13 | — | 0.767 |
| pH | — | 12 | — | 0.708 |
| $PCO_2$ | 7.2 mm Hg | 7.6 | 7.2 kPa | 7.6 |
| $PO_2$ | 20 mm Hg | 70 | 2.7 kPa | 9.45 |
| $PO_2$ children | 40 mm Hg | — | 5.3 kPa | — |
| $PO_2$ newborn | 45 mm Hg | 125 | 6.0 kPa | 16.7 |
| | 35 | 90 | 4.7 | 12.0 |

For additional information regarding the sources of specific presented data refer to *Tietz Textbook of Clinical Chemistry and Molecular Diagnostics*, 8th ed, 2020.

## ABBREVIATIONS

| | |
|---|---|
| **ATP III** | Adult Treatment Panel III |
| **Amf** | Amniotic fluid |
| **CSF** | Cerebrospinal fluid |
| **EDTA** | Ethylenediaminetetraacetic acid |
| **KDIGO** | Kidney disease improving global outcomes |
| **F** | Fluoride ion |
| **Hep** | Heparin |
| **ICSH** | International Council for Standardization in Haematology |
| **NGSP** | National Glycohemoglobin Standardization Program |
| **Ox** | Oxalate |
| **P** | Plasma |
| **PCOS** | Polycystic ovary syndrome |
| **RBC** | Red blood cells |
| **S** | Serum |
| **U** | Urine |
| **WB** | Whole blood |
| **WHO** | World Health Organization |

## SUGGESTED READINGS

Adeli K, Higgins V, Bohn MK. Reference information for the clinical laboratory. In: N. Rifai AR, Horvath CT, Wittwer, eds. *Tietz Textbook of Clinical Chemistry and Molecular Diagnostics*. 8th ed. St. Louis: Elsevier; 2020.

Adeli K, Higgins V, Nieuwesteeg M, Raizman JE, Chen Y, Wong SL. Biochemical marker reference values for pediatric, adult and geriatric age groups: establishment of robust pediatric and adult reference intervals based on the Canadian Health Measures Survey. *Clin Chem*. 2015;61:1049–1062.

Adeli K, Higgins V, Nieuwesteeg M, Raizman JE, Chen Y, Wong SL. Complex reference value distributions for endocrine and special chemistry biomarkers across pediatric, adult and geriatric age: establishment of robust pediatric and adult reference intervals based on the Canadian Health Measures Survey. *Clin Chem*. 2015;61:1063–1074.

Adeli K, Higgins V, Trajcevski K, White-Al Habeeb N. The Canadian laboratory initiative on pediatric reference intervals: a CALIPER white paper. *Crit Rev Clin Lab Sci*. 2017;54:358–413.

Bailey D, Colantonio D, Kyriakopoulou L, Cohen AH, Chan MK, Armbruster D. Marked biological variance in endocrine and biochemical markers in childhood: establishment of pediatric reference intervals using healthy community children from the CALIPER cohort. *Clin Chem.* 2013;59:1393–1405.

Bevilacqua V, Chan MK, Chen Y, Armbruster D, Schodin B, Adeli K. Pediatric population reference value distributions for cancer biomarkers and covariate-stratified reference intervals in the CALIPER cohort. *Clin Chem.* 2014;60:1532–1542.

Bjerner J, Biernat D, Fosså SD, Bjøro T. Reference intervals for serum testosterone, SHBG, LH and FSH in males from the NORIP project. *Scand J Clin Lab Invest.* 2009;69:873–879.

Colantonio DA, Kyriakopoulou L, Chan MK, et al. Closing the gaps in pediatric laboratory reference intervals: a CALIPER database of 40 biochemical markers in a healthy and multiethnic population of children. *Clin Chem.* 2012;58:854–868.

Fuentes-Arderiu X, Ferré-Masferrer M, Gonzàlez-Alba JM, et al. Multicentric reference values for some quantities measured with Tina-Quant reagents systems and RD/Hitachi analysers. *Scand J Clin Lab Invest.* 2001;61:273–276.

Hashim IA, Cuthbert JA. Critical values working group. establishing, harmonizing and analyzing critical values in a large academic health center. *Clin Chem Lab Med.* 2014;52:1129–1135.

Ichihara K, Ceriotti F, Kazuo M, et al. The Asian project for collaborative derivation of reference intervals: (2) results of non-standardized analytes and transference of reference intervals to the participating laboratories on the basis of cross-comparison of test results. *Clin Chem Lab Med.* 2013;51:1443–1457.

Jones GR, Haeckel R, Loh TP, et al. Indirect methods for reference interval determination–review and recommendations. *Clin Chem Lab Med.* 2019;57:20–29.

Kelly J, Raizman JE, Bevilacqua V, et al. Complex reference value distribution and partitioned reference intervals across the pediatric age for 14 special chemistry and endocrine markers in the CALIPER cohort of healthy community children and adolescents. *Clin Chim Acta.* 2015;450:196–202.

Konforte D, Shea JL, Kyriakopoulou L, et al. Complex biological pattern of fertility hormones in children and adolescents: a study of healthy children from the CALIPER cohort and establishment of pediatric reference intervals. *Clin Chem.* 2013;59:1215–1227.

Kushnir MM, Blamires T, Rockwood AL, et al. Liquid chromatography – tandem mass spectrometry assay for androstenedione, dehydroepiandrosterone, and testosterone with pediatric and adult reference intervals. *Clin Biochem.* 2010;56:1138–1147.

NIH National Heart, Lung and Blood Institute. *Integrated Guidelines for Cardiovascular Health and Risk Reduction in Children and Adolescents.* 2013. Available https://www.nhlbi.nih.gov/health-topics/integrated-guidelines-for-cardiovascular-health-and-risk-reduction-in-children-and-adolescents.

Ozarda Y, Sikaris K, Streichert T, Macri J. IFCC Committee on Reference Intervals and Decision Limits (C-RIDL). Distinguishing reference intervals and clinical decision limits. A review by the IFCC Committee on Reference Intervals and Decision Limits. *Crit Rev Clin Lab Sci.* 2018;55:420–431.

Rustad P, Felding P, Franzson L, et al. The Nordic Reference Interval Project 2000: recommended reference intervals for 25 common biochemical properties. *Scand J Clin Lab Invest.* 2004;64:271–284.

Tate JR, Sikaris KA, Jones GR, et al. Harmonising adult and paediatric reference intervals in Australia and New Zealand: an evidence-based approach for establishing a first panel of chemistry analytes. *Clin Biochem Rev.* 2014;35:213–235.

# ANSWERS

## CHAPTER 1

1. c. Molecular diagnostics
2. d. Conflict of interest
3. b. Nucleic acids
4. c. Discussion of one's salary
5. b. Publicly disclose without obtaining the patient's consent
6. d. Establishing the subscription price
7. d. Studies the quantity or sequence of nucleic acids
8. c. Contact the author if they have a question
9. c. Decide the pricing of the test and market laboratory services

## CHAPTER 2

1. d. The *t* distribution is useful for estimation of the 95% CI for the mean value.
2. a. the ability of an assay procedure to determine the concentration of a target analyte in the presence of interfering substances in the sample matrix.
3. d. In case of constant CV%s, the Bland-Altman difference plot shows an increasing scatter of the measured differences at increasing measurement values.
4. c. systematic difference.
5. d. Uncertainty.
6. c. Harmonization of laboratory measurements do not presuppose traceability to a reference measurement procedure.
7. b. The ROC area provides a measure of the diagnostic accuracy, which is not dependent on a selected cut-off value.
8. b. odds ratio.
9. a. false-positive rate.
10. d. The difference between the ROC curve area after addition of the new test and the area of the ROC curve of the original diagnostic procedure expresses the added value of the new test.

## CHAPTER 3

1. c. By selecting a more specific method
2. e. 415, 540, and 570 nm
3. a. Plasma
4. b. Testing should always be done on the native sample before delipidation.
5. e. In vivo hemolysis
6. a. dipotassium EDTA.

## CHAPTER 4

1. d. Random variations
2. b. Fractions of biological variation component estimates
3. e. Between-subject biological variation

4. c. The analytical imprecision obtained in your laboratory during the same time period as the time interval between the samples examined
5. b. The index of individuality is low

## CHAPTER 5

1. c. based on several samples collected over time in a single individual.
2. d. selection criteria.
3. c. The indirect method is more expensive than the direct methods.
4. a. partitioning.
5. b. parametric method.

## CHAPTER 6

1. d. Check the room and bed number of the patient to be collected and proceed with collection.
2. a. A sodium fluoride tube helps to prevent glycolysis and is used for glucose measurement.
3. c. metabolic activity of the blood and muscles will affect analytes such as potassium and calcium through effects on pH.
4. b. Proper collection technique on an infant utilizes "bagging" with a small plastic collection bag.
5. c. sufficient sample volume left on a sample of the correct type for the add-on assay.

## CHAPTER 7

1. c. To have a high probability that correct patient results are released
2. c. When my result is close to the target value for the peers in my measurement procedure group, I can be confident my laboratory is performing as well as my peers.
3. d. Their results provide information on the accuracy for patient samples if the target value is set by a reference measurement procedure; e. Their results can be compared among different measurement procedures to assess harmonization
4. c. To assess the performance of your measurement procedure compared with other measurement procedures
5. b. From the long-term SD that includes most types of variability expected to influence the measurement procedure

## CHAPTER 8

1. c. Gloves, eye protection, and a lab coat
2. c. Balances must be calibrated each day of use for accurate analytical work.
3. b. CLSI
4. d. dilution.

**5.** b. number of moles of solute/number of liters of solution

**6.** d. Primary Reference Material

**7.** c. Only one purification process is necessary for obtaining CLRW.

**8.** d. ultrapure and analytical reagent grades.

**9.** a. Gravities (*g*)

**10.** b. Exposure control plan

## CHAPTER 9

**1.** a. "*a*" is the absorptivity constant which is fixed for a given compound at a given wavelength under specific conditions.

**2.** c. Laser (light amplification by stimulated emission of radiation) is a device that provides coherent light of narrow wavelength.

**3.** e. Charge-coupled detectors are solid-state devices with a superior high signal to noise ratio compared to photomultiplier tubes.

**4.** b. The intensity of light scattering is inversely proportional to the distance between the light scattering particles and the detector.

**5.** b. Laser diodes provide coherent light, whereas LEDs provide incoherent light.

**6.** b. 16 μM

**7.** c. Electrochemiluminescence results from a chemical reaction generated at the surface of an electrode.

**8.** d. A solution appears blue when it transmits light between 450 and 495 nm.

**9.** b. Turbidimetry is the measurement of light intensity at 180 degrees to the path of incident light.

**10.** c. Store fluorophores in protected (dark) containers to decrease exposure to ambient light.

## CHAPTER 10

**1.** b. potentiometry.

**2.** d. reference electrode.

**3.** d. Electrolytic electrochemical cells

**4.** a. antibody.

**5.** c. direct-reading potentiometer.

**6.** b. Abnormal protein levels

**7.** b. electromotive force.

**8.** a. Amperometry

**9.** a. Nernst equation

**10.** c. Interstitial fluid

## CHAPTER 11

**1.** c. pH at which a molecule has no net charge.

**2.** c. that a protein has both positive and negative charges because of its side chains.

**3.** a. dirty electrodes causing uneven application of the electrical field.

**4.** b. the faster it will migrate.

**5.** d. Separation

**6.** b. capillary electrophoresis.

**7.** c. Densitometry

**8.** d. DNA

**9.** a. 500 bp (0.5 kbp) to 20 kbp

**10.** b. support medium

## CHAPTER 12

**1.** b. Mobile phase

**2.** c. Increase the amount of sample that is applied

**3.** b. retention factor.

**4.** a. be volatile or be converted into a volatile form.

**5.** b. Gas-solid chromatography

**6.** c. Mass spectrometer

**7.** b. Normal-phase chromatography uses a nonpolar stationary phase and is one of the most popular types of LC.

**8.** d. Affinity chromatography

**9.** a. The strength of the mobile phase is varied during solvent programming.

**10.** c. This method is mainly used for quantitative analysis.

## CHAPTER 13

**1.** b. Beam type

**2.** d. total ion chromatogram.

**3.** a. Electron ionization

**4.** a. determination of trace elements.

**5.** d. electron ionization.

**6.** a. quadrupole mass spectrometer.

## CHAPTER 14

**1.** b. transferase.

**2.** c. tertiary structure.

**3.** a. small compared to the entire enzyme.

**4.** e. All of the above

**5.** b. a property of an enzyme and substrate under certain conditions.

**6.** c. Coenzymes may be derivatives of vitamins.

**7.** a. fixed-time assay.

**8.** c. substrate.

**9.** a. one micromole of substrate per minute.

**10.** a. Competitive

**11.** d. self-indicating reaction.

## CHAPTER 15

**1.** d. Enzyme inhibitor present in the sample

**2.** d. Effective competition between the conjugate and the TSH for capture antibody

**3.** b. specificity.

**4.** c. Cloned enzyme donor immunoassay (CEDIA)

**5.** a. a decrease

**6.** b. enzyme-linked immunosorbent assay.

**7.** c. binding to the mouse monoclonal capture antibody reagents.

**8.** d. Particle-enhanced turbidimetric inhibition immunoassay (PETINIA)

9. c. IgM.
10. a. Dyed-latex microparticles are effective labels in simplified immunoassays because they are visible to the naked eye.

## CHAPTER 16

1. c. Labels containing barcodes that are unique identifiers
2. b. Hemolysis
3. e. All of the above
4. b. Carryover
5. a. Laboratory automation system (LAS)
6. b. Reproducibility of process

## CHAPTER 17

1. c. Testing that enables the clinician or caregiver to make a decision at the point-of-care
2. b. performing a study of clinical and cost effectiveness.
3. a. comparing the results obtained by the person(s) who will be operating the device in the intended setting.
4. a. analysis of a designated QC specimen on at least one occasion in each shift.
5. c. the unmet clinical need.

## CHAPTER 18

1. c. Histidine
2. c. Isoleucine
3. a. isoelectric point.
4. d. monoclonal immunoglobulin.
5. b. Leucine
6. c. Ferritin
7. b. catabolism/destruction.
8. d. albumin.
9. d. Serine proteases
10. c. IgG.

## CHAPTER 19

1. a. alkaline phosphatase (ALP).
2. a. LDH-1
3. b. lipase (LIP).
4. c. Alanine aminotransferase (ALT)
5. b. 4-nitrophenyl phosphate.
6. d. CHE
7. a. ALP leaks from osteoblasts during physiological bone growth.
8. c. P-AMY.
9. d. CK
10. a. LDH.

## CHAPTER 20

1. c. Monitoring treatment effectiveness and the course of disease.
2. e. Choriocarcinoma
3. a. Estrogen receptors

4. b. AFP in neonates and infants under 12 months old
5. d. To assist in triaging women with pelvic masses
6. e. They provide a benchmark against which the accuracy of calibration can be assessed

## CHAPTER 21

1. c. The glomerular filtration rate
2. b. Precipitation of excessive uric acid in joints and the urinary tract
3. d. Urea
4. c. Hypouricemia
5. a. Liver
6. b. Subtract a fixed value from each result to compensate for noncreatinine interference
7. a. 2.99
8. a. Jaffe reaction and uricase methods
9. b. Ascorbic acid and bilirubin
10. d. The major product of purine catabolism

## CHAPTER 22

1. a. Gluconeogenesis
2. d. Insulin
3. c. Combined citrate-fluoride-EDTA
4. c. Lactose
5. a. Glycogenesis
6. d. The brain functions normally with a low concentration of plasma glucose (<20 to 30 mg/dL).
7. a. Hexokinase method
8. c. Absence of an enzyme involved in carbohydrate metabolism
9. c. 70 mg/dL
10. a. Glycogen storage disease

## CHAPTER 23

1. e. All the above
2. b. apolipoprotein
3. d. lipoprotein(a)
4. a. LDL
5. c. lipoprotein lipase
6. d. HMG-CoA reductase
7. d. Reverse cholesterol transport pathway
8. b. Total cholesterol, triglycerides, HDL-C, non-HDL-C, and LDL-C
9. c. fatty acid
10. c. hydrolysis of triglyceride to form free glycerol

## CHAPTER 24

1. d. ion-selective electrode.
2. a. Hyperthermia
3. a. 30 minutes at ambient temperature
4. c. It contains a thermistor, a galvanometer, and a measuring potentiometer.
5. d. decreased freezing point.

6. d. postcollection evaporation.
7. c. An insignificant increase in plasma K+ of ~0.2 mmol/L
8. d. Potassium; it is localized mainly within cells, particularly RBCs
9. c. pH = p$K'$+ log [$c$HCO$_3$]/[$c$H$_2$CO$_3$]
10. d. Electrolyte exclusion effect

## CHAPTER 25

1. b. Gene expression changes
2. a. Phosphorylation of intracellular enzymes
3. b. Thyroid hormone
4. c. Adrenocorticotropic hormone
5. a. Receptor-based assay
6. d. Homeostatic control of metabolism
7. d. Long half-life in the circulation

## CHAPTER 26

1. d. vanillylmandelic acid (VMA).
2. c. an individual has recently eaten fruit, such as bananas, kiwis, and plums.
3. a. HVA and VMA.
4. b. Serotonin
5. c. liquid chromatography.
6. d. collection in heparin or EDTA anticoagulant from a fasting supine individual.
7. b. pheochromocytoma.
8. a. True
9. c. Adrenal gland; epinephrine
10. b. adrenaline.

## CHAPTER 27

1. c. Transketolase
2. a. SIR causes a decrease in the vitamins A, E, B2, B6, C, D, and carotenoids.
3. c. It may result due to decreased retinol binding protein (RBP) concentration in circulating blood.
4. c. Renal insufficiency
5. c. Wernicke-Korsakoff syndrome—vitamin B2
6. c. Glutathione reductase
7. c. Urine copper post penicillamine challenge
8. c. Keshan disease
9. d. whole blood and plasma content of the named traced elements.

## CHAPTER 28

1. a. chelate of iron with the four pyrrole groups of a porphyrin.
2. c. reversibly bind oxygen.
3. b. Decreased hemoglobin concentration, MCV, and MCHC with the peripheral blood smear indicating microcytosis, target cells, and polychromasia
4. b. Iron-deficiency anemia

5. a. Ferritin
6. d. [Serum iron: TIBC] × 100
7. c. in a hemoglobinopathy the globin chains of hemoglobin are structurally altered.
8. d. low TSAT and elevated or normal ferritin.
9. a. elevated TSAT and elevated ferritin.

## CHAPTER 29

1. c. succinyl CoA and glycine.
2. b. urine porphobilinogen (PBG).
3. a. heme.
4. d. excess presence of porphyrins in skin that generate oxygen radicals.
5. b. Zinc
6. c. porphyria cutanea tarda.
7. a. mitochondrion.
8. c. a fresh early morning urine specimen collected without preservative and protected from light.
9. b. Acute photosensitivity caused by protoporphyrin-IX accumulation in skin
10. d. porphyrinogen.

## CHAPTER 30

1. e. Lithium toxicity is related to serum concentration.
2. b. S-methylation via thiopurine S-methyltransferase (TPMT) deficiency
3. a. Tacrolimus is typically measured in whole blood.
4. b. typically combined with leucovorin treatment when used in high doses.
5. d. Valproic acid is highly protein bound and its serum concentrations are affected in uremia, cirrhosis, and other drug therapy.

## CHAPTER 31

1. b. meconium.
2. d. N-acetylcysteine.
3. a. HPLC does not require a derivatization step.
4. b. Clonazepam
5. d. 6-Acetylmorphine
6. b. GC-MS.

## CHAPTER 32

1. a. Arsenic
2. d. aminolevulinic acid dehydratase
3. c. Signs and symptoms in elemental toxicity mirror numerous disease states.
4. b. Unexplained, bilateral neuropathy
5. d. Antidotal treatment
6. b. Kidney
7. a. Cr
8. d. Hg
9. c. soluble, less soluble

10. d. The effectiveness of environmental control strategies used in the workplace

## CHAPTER 33

1. b. 8 to 12 weeks
2. b. Fasting glucose = 138 mg/dL (7.7 mmol/L)
3. a. is associated with resistance to the action of insulin.
4. c. urine glucose >250 mg/dL. (13.9 mmol/L).
5. b. glycogenolysis.
6. d. All of the above hormones produce hyperglycemia.
7. b. 11% lower
8. a. increased lipolysis of fatty acids from adipose stores and decreased re-esterification of these fatty acids to triglycerides.
9. d. Insulin
10. c. assess the possibility of overt diabetic nephropathy.

## CHAPTER 34

1. d. All of the above
2. b. Type 2 MI
3. c. 99th percentile URL
4. c. *H. pylori* infection
5. a. cTn
6. a. TnC
7. d. Have ability to have a measurable concentration above the LoD in >50% of both male and female normal subjects independently
8. c. ANP
9. d. Baseline concentration <99th perentile in low-risk patient
10. a. proBNP

## CHAPTER 35

1. c. Serum creatinine
2. a. Urine osmolality
3. b. The glomeruli, tubules, and associated blood vessels
4. d. inflammation of both the lining of the renal pelvis and the parenchyma of the kidney especially due to bacterial infection.
5. c. Renin
6. b. elevated nitrogenous compounds in blood.
7. a. IgA nephropathy.
8. c. diabetes insipidus.
9. d. Antidiuretic hormone
10. b. diuretic.

## CHAPTER 36

1. b. Intracellular fluid (ICF)
2. b. $Na^+ - (Cl^- + HCO_3^-)$
3. a. decreased production of antidiuretic hormone
4. d. Respiratory alkalosis
5. c. Potassium; hyperkalemia

6. c. Chronic obstructive pulmonary disease (COPD)
7. a. 55 mm Hg, hypoxia
8. c. 20:1
9. b. Renal tubular acidosis type II

## CHAPTER 37

1. d. glucuronide.
2. b. immunoglobulins.
3. b. canaliculi.
4. c. a chronic hepatitis B infection.
5. b. Hepatitis B
6. d. bilirubin, liver enzymes, prothrombin time (PT), and albumin.
7. c. cholestasis.
8. a. Wilson disease.
9. c. cholestasis due to gallstones.
10. d. cirrhosis.

## CHAPTER 38

1. c. stimulates gastric acid secretion.
2. a. intestinal bacterial overgrowth.
3. c. vasoactive intestinal polypeptide (VIP).
4. d. when weakly acidic digestive products of proteins and lipids enter the duodenum.
5. b. microbiologic culture of a gastric biopsy sample.
6. c. Celiac disease
7. d. alcohol consumption.
8. c. Secretin
9. a. the Zollinger-Ellison syndrome.

## CHAPTER 39

1. b. Osteoblast
2. e. Thick ascending limb of the Loop of Henle
3. c. In patients with hypercalcemia thought to be caused by a tumor but with no obvious clear diagnosis of malignancy
4. a. Monitoring a metabolic bone disease treatment response
5. c. Alkaline phosphatase
6. e. High concentration of 24,25-dihydroxyvitamin D in the sample

## CHAPTER 40

1. b. Prolactin
2. e. Thyroid hormone
3. c. IGF-1 and IGF-2 circulate together bound to IGFBP-3 and the acid-labile subunit (ALS).
4. a. Physiologically, GH secretion is episodic and pulsatile.
5. b. GH raises blood glucose by stimulating gluconeogenesis and reducing insulin sensitivity.
6. c. Anterior pituitary GH-secreting tumors (somatotropinomas)
7. a. This is often caused by a complex between prolactin and immunoglobulin.

8. e. LH and FSH are secreted episodically.

9. d. Increased ACTH increases cortisol secretion.

10. c. Urine osmolality less than 300 mOsm/kg (mmol/kg) plus serum osmolality greater than 300 mOsm/kg

## CHAPTER 41

1. b. Cortisol hypersecretion
2. a. increase
3. d. Aldosterone
4. a. Liver
5. c. Cosyntropin test
6. b. Addison disease
7. d. Congenital adrenal hyperplasia (CAH)
8. a. Corticotropin
9. c. Sodium retention.
10. a. Cushing syndrome

## CHAPTER 42

1. b. Immunoassay
2. a. Thyroid-stimulating hormone (TSH)
3. a. The absence or dysfunction of the thyroid gland
4. c. Thyrotoxicosis
5. d. Regulate carbohydrate, lipid, and protein metabolism within cells
6. c. Decreased FT4, and increased TSH
7. a. TSH
8. b. Tyrosine
9. d. Thyroglobulin
10. b. Calcitonin

## CHAPTER 43

1. a. FSH
2. c. Mass spectrometry-based methods are usually more sensitive and specific than immunoassays.
3. d. Progesterone on cycle day 21
4. b. Free testosterone provides an accurate reflection of androgen status in patients with altered SHBG concentrations.
5. c. Pituitary failure
6. e. Pregnancy
7. a. Females with PCOS have otherwise unexplained hyperandrogenism and anovulation.

## CHAPTER 44

1. d. erythroblastosis fetalis.
2. b. liver.
3. a. Hypertension and proteinuria ≥300 mg of protein in 24-hour urine
4. c. Free T4 concentrations decrease with increasing gestational age
5. c. maternal antibodies against fetal erythrocytes.

6. a. It signals the corpus luteum to produce progesterone to maintain pregnancy.
7. b. Estrogen concentration increases throughout gestation.
8. c. PAPP-A and nuchal translucency in the first trimester and AFP, hCG, uE3, and inhibin A in the second trimester
9. d. Placenta
10. c. ectopic pregnancy.

## CHAPTER 45

1. c. inborn error of metabolism (IEM).
2. b. medium-chain acyl-CoA dehydrogenase (MCAD) deficiency.
3. a. galactosemia.
4. c. tryptophan, hydroxylysine, and lysine.
5. b. 25%
6. d. further assess a positive screening test result by targeting more specific analytes.
7. b. an aminoacidopathy.
8. a. multiplex analysis.
9. c. phenylalanine hydroxylase.

## CHAPTER 46

1. a. Pharmacodynamics
2. c. prodrug.
3. d. Warfarin
4. d. Poor metabolizer
5. a. Abacavir

## CHAPTER 47

1. a. alternative splicing and posttranslational modifications occur.
2. b. 2
3. a. MetProAlaTyr
4. a. 1%
5. d. Bonds between the complementary nucleotide bases
6. d. Cytosine and upstream CpG islands
7. a. mismatch repair.
8. c. The enhancer
9. b. They are used to protect themselves from viral infections.

## CHAPTER 48

1. e. 98%
2. a. 1%
3. e. 40%
4. b. 1 in 100
5. c. c.12G>C
6. e. Single molecule sequencing with zero-mode waveguide

**7.** a. Semiconductor sequencing
**8.** e. >90%
**9.** c. 10
**10.** c. 12 billion

## CHAPTER 49

**1.** b. More than four primers are required.
**2.** c. Fluorescence in situ hybridization (FISH).
**3.** c. Massively parallel sequencing.
**4.** e. Digital PCR

**5.** e. False-positives may occur due to empty cassettes or non-functional *mec* genes.
**6.** d. *VanB* can be found in other genera and confers resistance only to vancomycin.
**7.** b. KPC, NDM, VIM, IMP, and OXA are the most common genes detected by rapid molecular diagnostic tests.
**8.** d. An organism is not recovered limiting additional testing like antimicrobial susceptibility testing or strain typing.
**9.** c. Both upper respiratory tract infection and pneumonia tests are available.
**10.** a. easy to use.

# INDEX

*Note*: Page numbers followed by "f" indicate figures, "t" indicate tables, and "b" indicate boxes.

## A

Autosomal dominant acute porphyrias, predictive testing of, 533
Autosomal dominant polycystic kidney disease (ADPKD), 665
Autosomal recessive disorder, 883
Autosomal recessive inheritance, 876–877, 877f
Autosomes, 917
Autoverification, 279
Avidity, 248, 250
Avogadro's hypothesis, 432t
AVP. *See* Arginine vasopressin
AZA. *See* Azathioprine
Azathioprine (AZA), for inflammatory bowel disease, 733
Azotemia, 649, 660

**B**
Bacteria, 920–921
Bacterial overgrowth, 731
Band-broadening, in chromatography, 194
Bandpass, 136, 140
Bar code identification systems, 288
Bar coding
  reading stations, 269
  specimen identification using, 266
Barbiturates, 561, 574
  analytical methods for, 574
  half-life of, 574t
Bartter syndrome, 649, 666
Basal body temperature, 849
Base pair, 905, 914
Base peak, 211–212
Bases, 684
Basic lipid panel, 416t, 416b
Basic techniques, in laboratory, 118–124
Batch analysis, 264
Beam-type mass spectrometers, 217–219
Beer's law, 136, 138–139, 138f
Bence-Jones proteins, 319, 353t–354t, 649
  as tumor marker, 348
Benzethonium chloride, 373
Benzodiazepines, 574–575, 580
  analytical methods for, 575
  half-life of, 575t
Benzylpiperazines, designer drugs related to, 573t
Beriberi, 469, 480
Beta-blockers, 539–540
Beta-lactam resistant gram-negative bacilli, 951
Beta-thalassemias, 505–506
  intermedia, 506
  major, 502, 505–506
  minor, 502, 506
Between-subject variation (CV$_G$), 52–53, 53f
Bias, 16t
  calibration, 18–19
  definition of, 9, 14–15
  random, 18–19

Bicarbonate, 428, 684
  buffer system, 685
  filtered, reclamation of, 687
  reabsorption of, 653
Big GH, 771
Bilateral inferior petrosal venous sinus sampling (BIPSS), for adrenal hyperactivity, 800
Bile acids, 695
  cholesterol, converted to, 405
  malabsorption, 731–732, 732b
  metabolism, by liver, 699
  for micelle formation, 404
Biliary drainage, in liver, 696–697
Bilirubin, 698–699
  analytical methods for, 718–719
    diazo methods, 718, 718f
    total Bilirubin, 719
  critical risk values, 1005t–1006t
  direct, reference intervals for, 966t–1004t
  metabolism, 701–702, 702f
  total, 719
    reference intervals for, 966t–1004t
Bioavailability, 539, 541
Bio-barcode immunoassay, 259–261, 260f
Biocatalytic reaction, 167
Biochemistry, 637
BioFire Pneumonia panel, 954
BioFire PN*plus*, 954
Bioinformatics, pipeline, 936f
Biological hazards, 128–129, 129f
Biological variation, 52–65, 64b
  definition of, 52
  generation of data on components of, 53–56
    data analysis, 56, 57f
    design of studies, 53–54
    methods for analysis, 54–56
  in health and disease, 58
  nature of, 52–53
  random, 52–53
Bioluminescence, 151
Biomarkers. *See* Cardiac biomarkers
Biopsies, for *Helicobacter pylori*, 726
Biosensors, 155, 167–175, 167b, 290
  enzyme-based, 167
    with amperometric detection, 167–170, 168f–169f
    with potentiometric and conductometric detection, 170–171, 170f
Biotin, 256, 489–490, 489f, 966t–1004t
  absorption of, 489
  deficiency in, 489–490
  excretion of, 489
  functions of, 489
  laboratory assessment for, 490
  metabolism of, 489
  toxicity of, 490
  transport of, 489
Biotinidase deficiency, 889
Biotin-responsive basal ganglia disease, 490
Biotransformation, 539, 541, 543

BIPSS. *See* Bilateral inferior petrosal venous sinus sampling
Bitot spots, 476
Biuret method, for total protein, 319
Biuret reaction, 319
Bladder cancer, tumor markers in, 357
  relevant to, 357
Bladder tumor associated antigens (BTA), 357
Bland-Altman plot, 20, 20f
Blank reagent, 136, 139
Blastocyst, 856–857
Blood. *See also* Plasma; Serum.
  androgen transport in, 830
  estrogen transport in, 835
  ethanol, 568
  fetal development of, 862
  oxygen in, 433–434
  pregnancy-related changes in, 860
  testosterone transport in, 830
  venipuncture for collection of. *See* Venipuncture
Blood collection tubes, 83
Blood gases, 422–441
  aqueous fluid control materials for, 439
  behavior of, 431–433, 431b
  blood-based and fluorocarbon-based control materials for, 439
  conversion of, 431b
  definition of, 422
  descriptors used in, 431b
  instrumentation for, 437–438, 438f, 439b
  measurements
    analytical error in, 439
    Henderson-Hasselbalch equation, 423, 433
    physical principles in, 432t
    prefixes for, 431b
    reference intervals for, 437t
  pH and, 430–431
  quality assurance and quality control in, 438–439
  specimen of, 435–437
  symbols in, 431b
Blood glucose
  concentration, regulation of, 393
  glycated hemoglobin and, 616
  hormones regulating, 600–603, 601f
  self-monitoring of, 612–614
Blood lead level, of concern, 591
Blood porphyrins, analysis of, 535, 537f
Blood sampling, patient preparation for, 41
Blood specimen, 80–85
  anticoagulants and preservatives added to, 84–85
    acid citrate dextrose, 85
    EDTA, 84–85
    iodoacetate, 85
    oxalates, 85
    sodium citrate, 85
    sodium fluoride, 85
  centrifugation of, 88